1986

CONN'S CURRENT THERAPY

Edited by ROBERT E. RAKEL, M.D.

Chairman, Department of Family Medicine
Associate Dean for Academic and Clinical Affairs
Baylor College of Medicine, Houston, Texas

LATEST APPROVED METHODS OF TREATMENT FOR THE PRACTICING PHYSICIAN

W.B. SAUNDERS COMPANY
Philadelphia London Toronto Mexico City Rio de Janeiro Sydney Tokyo Hong Kong

W. B. Saunders Company: West Washington Square
Philadelphia, PA 19105

Library of Congress Cataloging in Publication Data

Current therapy; latest approved methods of treatment for the practicing physician. 1949–

v. 28 cm. annual.

Editors: 1949– H. F. Conn and others.

1. Therapeutics. 2. Therapeutics, Surgical. 3. Medicine—Practice. I. Conn, Howard Franklin, 1908–1982 ed.

RM101.C87 616.058 49–8328 rev*

Editor: Carroll Cann
Editorial Coordinator: Carolyn Naylor
Developmental Editor: Ken McNally
Designer: Bill Donnelly
Production Manager: Bob Butler
Manuscript Editor: Wynette Kommer
Indexer: Dennis Dolan

Conn's Current Therapy 1986 ISBN 0–7216–1769–7

Last digit is the print number: 9 8 7 6 5 4 3 2 1

Contributors

ABDULLA M. ABDULLA, M.D.
Professor of Medicine and Cardiology and Director, Hemodynamics Laboratory, Medical College of Georgia, Augusta, Georgia
Congestive Heart Failure

JOEL N. ABRAMOVITZ, M.D.
Assistant Professor of Neurosurgery, Tufts University School of Medicine; Chief of Neurosurgery, Boston Veterans Administration Medical Center, New England Medical Center, and St. Elizabeth's Hospital, Boston, Massachusetts
Brain Abscess

RAYMOND H. ALEXANDER, M.D.
Associate Professor, University of Florida College of Medicine; Associate Professor and Chairman, Department of Surgery, University Hospital of Jacksonville, Jacksonville, Florida
Thrombophlebitis

MARTIN A. ALPERT, M.D.
Associate Professor, University of Missouri School of Medicine, Department of Internal Medicine; Staff Physician, University of Missouri Hospital and Clinics; Chief, Cardiology Section, Harry S Truman Memorial Veterans Hospital, Columbia, Missouri
Premature Beats

FRANCISCO AMPUERO, M.D.
Attending, St. Joseph Hospital, Albuquerque, New Mexico
Cancer of the Uterine Corpus

RICHARD D. ANDERSEN, M.D.
Assistant Professor, Department of Pediatrics, University of Iowa Hospitals and Clinics, Iowa City, Iowa
Herpes Simplex and Herpes Zoster

JOHN A. ANDERSON, M.D.
Clinical Associate Professor, University of Michigan, Ann Arbor; Chairman, Department of Pediatrics, and Head, Division of Allergy and Clinical Immunology, Henry Ford Hospital, Detroit, Michigan
Allergic Reactions to Drugs

THOMAS F. ANDERSON, M.D.
Associate Professor, Department of Dermatology, University of Michigan; Attending Physician, Department of Dermatology, University of Michigan, and Veterans Administration Medical Center, Ann Arbor, Michigan
Papulosquamous Eruptions

JEFFREY L. ANGEL, M.D.
Fellow/Assistant Professor, Division of Maternal-Fetal Medicine, University of South Florida College of Medicine; Attending, Tampa General Hospital; Medical Staff, Humana Women's Hospital, Tampa, Florida
Vaginal Bleeding Late in Pregnancy

I. KAUFMAN ARENBERG, M.D., FACS
Associate Clincal Professor of Otolaryngology—Head and Neck Surgery (Otology and Neurotology), University of Colorado Health Sciences Center; Director, International Merniere's Disease Research Institute of the Colorado Otologic Research Center at Porter Memorial Hospital—Swedish Medical Center, Denver, Colorado
Meniere's Disease

JAMES L. AUSTIN, M.D.
Assistant Professor of Surgery, University of Missouri School of Medicine; Staff Surgeon, Harry S Truman Memorial Veterans Hospital, Columbia, Missouri
Chronic Pancreatitis

C. KIRK AVENT, M.D.
Professor of Medicine, University of Alabama School of Medicine; Active Staff, University Hospital and Birmingham Veterans Administration Hospital, Birmingham, Alabama
Tetanus

LAURA K. BACHRACH, M.D.
Assistant Clinical Professor, Stanford University Hospital, Stanford, California
Nontoxic Goiter

R. ROBINSON BAKER, M.D.
Professor of Surgery and Oncology, Johns Hopkins University School of Medicine; Surgeon-in-Charge, Thoracic Surgical Service, and Director, Breast Clinic, Johns Hopkins Hospital, Baltimore, Maryland
Diseases of the Breast

JAMES C. BALLENGER, M.D.
Chairman and Professor, Department of Psychiatry and Behavioral Sciences, Medical University of South Carolina and Medical University Hospital; Consultant, Veterans Administration Hospital; Clinical Staff, Charleston Memorial Hospital, Charleston, South Carolina.
Panic Disorder and Agoraphobia

G. WILLIAM BATES, M.D.
Professor of Obstretrics and Gynecology; Director, Division of Reproductive Endocrinology, University of Missouri Medical Center, Jackson, Mississippi
Dysfunctional Uterine Bleeding

STUART B. BAUER, M.D.
Assistant Professor of Urology, Harvard Medical School; Associate in Urology, The Children's Hospital, Boston, Massachusetts
Bacterial Infections of the Urinary Tract—Female Children

DOROTHY J. BECKER, M.B., B.Ch., FCP(Paed)
Associate Professor of Pediatrics, University of Pittsburgh School of Medicine; Director, Diabetes Laboratory, and As-

sociate Director, Clinical Research Center, Children's Hospital of Pittsburgh, Pittsburgh, Pennsylvania
Diabetes Mellitus in Children and Adults

MICHAEL A. BECKER, M.D.
Professor of Medicine, The University of Chicago Pritzker School of Medicine; Attending Physician and Head of Rheumatology, University of Chicago Medical Center, Chicago, Illinois
Hyperuricemia and Gout

CHARLES R. B. BECKMANN, M.D., M.H.P.E.
Assistant Professor of Obstetrics-Gynecology; Director, Undergraduate Medical Education, University of Illinois; University of Illinois Hospital, Chicago, Illinois
Pelvic Inflammatory Disease

WILLIAM BELL, M.D.
Professor, Departments of Pediatrics and Neurology, University of Iowa College of Medicine, Iowa City, Iowa
Viral Meningitis/Encephalitis

WILLIAM R. BELL, M.D.
Professor of Medicine and Radiology, Department of Medicine, Johns Hopkins University; Physician, Department of Medicine, Johns Hopkins University Hospital, Baltimore, Maryland
Thrombophlebitis in Obstetrics and Gynecology

COSTANTINO BENEDETTI, M.D.
Associate Professor, University of Washington School of Medicine; Staff Anesthesiologist, Department of Anesthesiology, University of Washington, Medical Center and Affiliated Hospitals; Chief, Pain Service, Veterans Administration Hospital, Seattle, Washington
Pain

RICHARD G. BENNETT, M.D.
Adjunct Assistant Professor, University of California, Los Angeles; Staff Physician, UCLA Medical Center; Consultant, Veterans Administration Wadsworth Medical Center, Los Angeles, Veterans Administration Hospital, Sepulveda, and USC County Medical Center, Los Angeles, California
Skin Cancer

JOSEPH R. BENOTTI, M.D.
Associate Professor of Medicine, University of Massachusetts Medical School; Associate Director, Cardiac Catheterization Laboratories, University of Massachusetts Medical Center, Worcester, Massachusetts
Acute Myocardial Infarction

PHILLIP M. BERMAN, M.D.
Clinical Associate Professor of Medicine, University of Illinois School of Medicine, Chicago; Attending, Louis A. Weiss Memorial Hospital, Chicago; Associate Staff, St. Francis Hospital, Evanston, Illinois
Peptic Ulcer

DAVID I. BERNSTEIN, M.D.
Assistant Professor of Clinical Medicine, University of Cincinnati Medical Center, Cincinnati, Ohio
Allergic Rhinitis Caused by Inhalant Factors

I. LEONARD BERNSTEIN, M.D.
Clinical Professor of Medicine and Environmental Health Sciences, Co-Director of the Allergy Research Laboratory and the Allergy Training Program, University of Cincinnati Medical Center, Cincinnati, Ohio
Allergic Rhinitis Caused by Inhalant Factors

ERNEST BEUTLER, M.D.
Scripps Clinic and Research Foundation, La Jolla, California
Acute Leukemia in Adults

NASREEN A. BHUMBRA, M.D.
Assistant Professor, Infectious Diseases Division, Department of Pediatrics, Medical College of Ohio; Attending, Medical College Hospital, Toledo, Ohio
Measles (Rubeola)

DAVID R. BICKERS, M.D.
Professor and Chairman, Department of Dermatology, Case Western Reserve University School of Medicine; Director of Dermatology, University Hospitals of Cleveland and Veterans Administration Medical Center, Cleveland, Ohio
Sunburn and Photosensitivity

DANIEL D. BIKLE, M.D., PH.D.
Assistant Professor of Medicine, University of California, San Francisco; Attending Physician, University of California, San Francisco; Codirector, Special Diagnostic and Treatment Unit, Veterans Administration Medical Center, San Francisco, California
Hyper- and Hypoparathyroidism

H. STEPHEN BJORNSON, M.D., Ph.D.
Associate Professor of Surgery, Division of Surgical Infectious Diseases, University of Cincinnati College of Medicine; Active Medical Staff, University of Cincinnati Hospitals, Cincinnati, Ohio
Necrotizing Infections of the Soft Tissues, Including Gas Gangrene

MARTIN J. BLASER, M.D.
Associate Professor of Medicine, Division of Infectious Diseases, University of Colorado School of Medicine; Chief, Infectious Disease Section, Veterans Administration Medical Center, Denver, Colorado
Acute Infectious Diarrhea

MELVIN A. BLOCK, M.D., Ph.D.
Clinical Professor of Surgery, Department of Surgery, University of California, San Diego; Chairman, Department of Surgery, Scripps Clinic and Research Foundation, Green Hospital of Scripps Clinic, La Jolla, California
Thyroid Cancer

CHARLES D. BLUESTONE, M.D.
Professor of Otolaryngology, University of Pittsburgh School of Medicine; Director, Department of Otolaryngology, Children's Hospital of Pittsburgh, Pittsburgh, Pennsylvania
Otitis Media

FRANK G. BOINEAU, M.D.
Associate Professor of Pediatrics, Tulane University School Medicine; Attending Staff, Tulane University Hospital, Children's Hospital of New Orleans, and Charity Hospital of Louisiana in New Orleans, New Orleans, Louisiana
Parenteral Fluid Therapy for Infants and Children

ROBERT W. BRADSHER, Jr., M.D.
Associate Professor of Medicine, University of Arkansas for Medical Sciences, Little Rock, Arkansas
Blastomycosis

THOMAS BRANDT, M.D.
Professor and Chairman of Neurology, University of Munich; Director, Department of Neurology, Klinikum Grosshadern, Ludwig Maximilian University, Munich, Federal Republic of Germany
Episodic Vertigo

EMMANUEL L. BRAVO, M.D.
Assistant Clinical Professor of Medicine, Department of Medicine, Case Western Reserve University School of Medicine; Staff, Cleveland Clinic Foundation; Assistant Clinical Professor of Medicine, Cleveland Metropolitan General Hospital, Cleveland, Ohio
Adrenocortical Insufficiency

DALE BROWN, Jr., M.D.
Associate Clinical Professor, Baylor College of Medicine; Associate Chief of Obstetrics-Gynecology, St. Luke's Episcopal Hospital; Attending Physician, Methodist and Ben Taub Hospitals; Courtesy Staff, Women's Hospital and Texas Children's Hospital, Houston, Texas
Vulvovaginitis

LOUIS A. BROWN, Jr., M.D.
Consultant Dermatologist, Philadelphia Public Health Department; Attending Dermatologist, Lawndale Community Hospital, Philadelphia, Pennsylvania
Keloids

ROBERT S. BROWN, Jr., M.D.
Senior Resident in Internal Medicine and Psychiatry and Forensic Psychiatry Fellow, University of Virginia Medical Center, Charlottesville, Virginia
Panic Disorder and Agoraphobia

JOHN R. BURNS, M.D.
Associate Professor, Department of Surgery, Division of Urology, University of Alabama at Birmingham; Attending, University of Alabama at Birmingham and Veterans Administration Hospital, Birmingham, Alabama
Renal Calculi

GERARD N. BURROW, M.D.
Sir John and Lady Eaton Professor and Chairman, Department of Medicine, University of Toronto; Physician-in-Chief, Toronto General Hospital, Toronto, Ontario, Canada
Nontoxic Goiter

CHARLES A. BUSH, M.D.
Professor of Medicine, Department of Medicine, Division of Cardiology, Ohio State University College of Medicine; Director, Cardiac Catheterization Laboratories, Ohio State University Hospital Medical Center, Columbus, Ohio
Pericarditis

STEPHEN H. BUTLER, M.D.
Associate Professor, Department of Anesthesiology, University of Washington; Staff Anesthesiologist, Pain Clinic, University Hospital; Staff Anesthesiologist, Department of Anesthesiology, Harborview Medical Center, Seattle, Washington
Pain

JOHN L. CAMERON, M.D., FACS
Professor and Chairman, Department of Surgery, The Johns Hopkins University; Chief of Surgery, The Johns Hopkins Hospital, Baltimore, Maryland
Acute Pancreatitis

CARLOS C. CAMPBELL, M.D., M.P.H.
Chief, Malaria Branch, Division of Parasitic Diseases, Center for Infectious Diseases, Centers for Disease Control, Atlanta, Georgia
Malaria

GEORGE P. CANELLOS, M.D.
Professor of Medicine, Harvard Medical School; Chief of Medical Oncology, Dana-Farber Cancer Institute; Physician, Brigham and Women's Hospital, Boston, Massachusetts
The Chronic Leukemias

ROBERT E. CANFIELD, M.D.
Professor of Medicine and Director of Center for Clinical Research, Columbia University College of Physicians and Surgeons; Attending Physician, Professor of Medicine, and Director of Center for Clinical Research, Presbyterian Hospital, New York, New York
Paget's Disease of Bone

JOHN E. CANHAM, M.D.
Director of Medical Affairs, KabiVitrum, Inc., Alameda, California
Pellagra

STEPHEN A. CANNISTRA, M.D.
Instructor in Medicine, Harvard Medical School; Clinical Associate, Dana-Farber Cancer Institute; Associate Physician, Brigham and Women's Hospital, Boston, Massachusetts
The Chronic Leukemias

LOUIS R. CAPLAN, M.D.
Chairman and Professor of Neurology, Tufts University School of Medicine; Neurologist in Chief, New England Medical Center Hospital, Boston, Massachusetts
Intracerebral Hemorrhage (Nontraumatic)

THOMAS R. CARACCIO, R.P.H., Pharm.D.
Preceptor, St. John's University College of Pharmacy, Jamaica; Field Supervisor, Hofstra University Community Health Administration Department, Hempstead; Clinical Coordinator, Long Island Regional Poison Control Center and Clinical Pharmacist, Departments of Pediatrics and Pharmacology, Nassau County Medical Center, East Meadow, New York
Acute Poisonings

ROBERT G. CARNEY, Jr., M.D.
Decatur, Illinois
The Erythemas

BARRY L. CARTER, Pharm.D.
Assistant Professor, College of Pharmacy, University of Iowa, Iowa City, Iowa
Insomnia

ALEXANDER S. CASS, M.B.B.S.
Associate Professor, University of Minnesota Medical School, Minneapolis; Chief, Department of Urology, St. Paul-Ramsey Medical Center, and Chief, Urology Service, Gillette Chldren's Hospital, St. Paul; Chief, Urology Service, Hennepin County Medical Center, Minneapolis, Minnesota
Trauma to the Genitourinary Tract

THOMAS R. CATE, M.D.
Professor of Medicine and Microbiology-Immunology, Baylor College of Medicine; Attending, Ben Taub General Hospital and The Methodist Hospital, Houston, Texas
Influenza

JAMES J. CERDA, M.D.
Professor and Associate Chairman, Department of Medicine, University of Florida College of Medicine, Gainesville; Staff Physician, Shands Hospital, University of Florida; Consultant, Veterans Administration Hospital, Gainesville; Consultant, US Naval Hospital, Jacksonville, Florida
Amebiasis

MELVIN D. CHEITLIN, M.D.
Professor of Medicine, University of California, San Francisco, School of Medicine; Associate Chief, Cardiology Division, Department of Medicine, San Francisco General Hospital, San Francisco, California
Infective Endocarditis

P. JOAN CHESNEY, M.D.
Associate Professor of Pediatriacs, Division of Pediatric Infectious Diseases, University of Wisconsin–Madison and University Hospital and Clinics, Madison, Wisconsin
Toxic Shock Syndrome

GEORGE P. CHROUSOS, M.D.
Senior Investigator, Developmental Endocrinology Branch, National Institute of Child Health and Human Development, National Institutes of Health, Bethesda, Maryland; Clincal Associate Professor, Georgetown University Medical Center, Washington, D.C.
Cushing's Syndrome

DOUGLAS B. CINES, M.D.
Assistant Professor of Medicine, University of Pennsylvania School of Medicine; Attending Physician, Hematology-Oncology Section, Department of Medicine, Hospital of the University of Pennsylvania, Philadelphia, Pennsylvania
Autoimmune Hemolytic Anemia

RICHARD B. CLARK, M.D.
Professor of Anesthesiology and Obstetrics/Gynecology, University of Arkansas for Medical Sciences; Attending Physician, University Hospital, Little Rock, Arkansas
Obstetric Anesthesia

H. CECIL COGHLAN, M.D., FACP
Professor of Medicine, University of Alabama in Birmingham; Professor of Medicine, Division of Cardiology, and Director, Autonomic Laboratory, University of Alabama Hospital, Birmingham, Alabama
Mitral Valve Prolapse

ALAN COHEN, M.D.
Associate Professor of Pediatrics, University of Pennsylvania School of Medicine; Associate Hematologist, Children's Hospital of Philadelphia, Philadelphia, Pennsylvania
Scurvy

MIRIAM R. COHEN, M.D.
Fellow, Combined Rheumatology Program, University of Chicago, Michael Reese Hospital, and LaRabida Children's Hospital, Chicago, Illinois
Bursitis and Calcific Tendinitis

MICHAEL COLEMAN, M.D.
Assistant Professor of Pediatrics, University of Minnesota; Associate Director, Neonatal Medicine, St. Paul Children's Hospital, St. Paul, Minnesota
Neonatal Resuscitation

BLAISE L. CONGENI, M.D.
Associate Professor of Pediatrics and Associate Professor of Medical Microbiology, Northeastern Ohio Universities College of Medicine, Rootstown; Head, Infections Disease Division, Children's Hospital Medical Center of Akron, Akron, Ohio
Mumps (Epidemic Parotitis)

REX B. CONN, M.D.
Professor of Pathology and Laboratory Medicine, Emory University School of Medicine; Director, Clinical Pathology Laboratories, Emory University Hospital, Atlanta, Georgia
Laboratory Values of Clinical Importance

JOSEPH S. COSELLI, M.D.
Assistant Professor of Surgery, Baylor College of Medicine; Attending Surgeon, The Methodist Hospital, Houston, Texas
Acquired Diseases of the Aorta

DANIEL B. CRAIG, M.D.
Associate Clinical Professor, Medical College of Georgia, Augusta; Chief, Infectious Disease Section, Dwight David Eisenhower Army Medical Center, Ft. Gordon, Georgia
Pyelonephritis

ALBERT E. CRAM, M.D.
Associate Professor of Surgery, University of Iowa College of Medicine and University of Iowa Hospitals; Consultant, Veterans Administration Hospital, Iowa City, Iowa
Burns

E. STANLEY CRAWFORD, M.D.
Professor of Surgery, Baylor College of Medicine; Senior Attending Surgeon, The Methodist Hospital, Houston, Texas
Acquired Diseases of the Aorta

CHARLES H. CROFT, M.D., FACC
Assistant Professor of Medicine, University of Texas Health Science Center at Dallas, and Southwestern Medical School; Cardiologist, Division of Cardiology, Department of Medicine, Veterans Administration Medical Center, Dallas, Texas
Angina Pectoris

MICHAEL H. CYNAMON, M.D.
Assistant Professor of Medicine, SUNY Upstate Medical Center; Chief of Infectious Diseases, Veterans Administration Medical Center, Syracuse, New York
Tuberculosis and Other Mycobacterial Diseases

ALBERT J. CZAJA, M.D.
Associate Professor of Medicine, Mayo Medical School; Consultant in Gastroenterology, Mayo Clinic, Rochester Methodist Hospital, and St. Mary's Hospital, Rochester, Minnesota
Bleeding Esophageal Varices

CHI V. DANG, M.D., Ph.D
Fellow in Medicine, Cancer Research Institute, University of California, San Francisco, San Francisco, California
Thrombophlebitis in Obstetrics and Gynecology

JAMES H. DAUBER, M.D.
Associate Professor of Medicine, University of Pittsburgh; Chief, Pulmonary Service, Veterans Administration Hospital; Attending Physician, Presbyterian-University Hospital, Pittsburgh, Pennsylvania
Silicosis

JOHN M. DAVIS, M.D.
Gilman Professor of Psychiatry, University of Illinois School of Medicine at Chicago; Director of Research, Illinois State Psychiatric Institute, Chicago, Illinois
Schizophrenia

M. YUSOFF DAWOOD, M.D., Ch.B., M. Med., FRCOG
Professor of Obstetrics and Gynecology, University of Illinois College of Medicine at Chicago; Attending Obstetrician and Gynecologist and Director, Division of Reproductive Endocrinology, University of Illinois Hospital, Chicago, Illinois
Amenorrhea

R. BEN DAWSON, M.D.
Professor of Pathology, Associate Professor of Medicine, and Director of Blood Research Laboratory, School of Medicine, University of Maryland; Senior Consultant in Hematology, University of Maryland Hospital; Attending Internist, Loch Raven Veterans Administration Hospital, Baltimore, Maryland
Adverse Reactions to Blood Transfusion

JOHN B. De HOFF, M.D., M.P.H.
Associate in Preventive Medicine, University of Maryland School of Medicine; Consultant in Preventive Medicine, Church Hospital; Courtesy Staff (Emeritus) in Medicine, Greater Baltimore Medical Center, Baltimore, Maryland
Disturbances Due to Heat

ALBERT A. DEL NEGRO, M.D., FACC
Assistant Professor of Medicine, Georgetown University Medical Center; Director, Clinical Electrophysiology, and Director, Cardiology Fellowship Program, Georgetown University Medical Center, Washington, D.C.
Heart Block

L. DANA DeWITT, M.D.
Assistant Professor of Neurology, Tufts University Medical School; Medical Staff, New England Medical Center, Boston, Massachusetts
Intracerebral Hemorrhage (Nontraumatic)

CHARLES DIAMOND, M.B., Ch.B., D.Obst. R.C.O.G., FRCS(GLAS)
Honorary Clinical Lecturer, Department of ENT Studies, University of Newcastle upon Tyne; Consultant ENT Surgeon, Newcastle General Hospital, Newcastle upon Tyne, England
Acute Peripheral Facial Paralysis (Bell's Palsy)

GORDON M. DICKINSON, M.D.
Associate Professor of Medicine, University of Miami School of Medicine; Attending, Jackson Memorial Hospital and Miami Veterans Administration Hospital, Miami, Florida
Acquired Immunodeficiency Syndrome (AIDS)

WILLIAM H. DOOLITTLE, M.D.
Chief of Staff, Fairbanks Memorial Hospital, Fairbanks, Alaska
Disturbances Due to Cold

DEBORAH J. DOTTERS, M.D.
Clinical Instructor, University of North Carolina School of Medicine; Physician, North Carolina Memorial Hospital, Chapel Hill, North Carolina
Leiomyomas of the Uterus

F. E. DREIFUSS, M.B., FRCP
Professor of Neurology, School of Medicine, University of Virginia; Neurologist, and Director, Comprehensive Epilepsy Program, University of Virginia Hospital, Charlottesville, Virginia
Epilepsy in Infants and Children

BERNARD J. DREILING, M.D.
Associate Professor of Medicine, University of Mississippi School of Medicine; Staff Hematologist, Veterans Administration Medical Center, Jackson, Mississippi
Nonimmune Hemolytic Anemia

CHARLES E. DRISCOLL, M.D.
Associate Professor and Acting Head, Department of Family Practice, University of Iowa College of Medicine; Physician, University of Iowa Hospitals and Clinics and Mercy Hospital of Iowa City, Iowa City, Iowa
Insomnia

WILLIAM DROEGEMUELLER, M.D.
Professor and Chairman, University of North Carolina School of Medicine, Department of Obstetrics and Gynecology; and North Carolina Memorial Hospital, Chapel Hill, North Carolina
Leiomyomas of the Uterus

GEOFFREY M. DUSHEIKO, M.D.
Senior Physician, University of the Witwatersrand Medical School; Senior Physician, Liver Unit, Hillbrow and Johannesburg Hospitals, Johannesburg, South Africa
Acute and Chronic Viral Hepatitis

JAMES EASTON, M.D.
Clinical Professor of Pediatrics, University of California, Los Angeles, School of Medicine; Chief, Department of Allergy and Clinical Immunology, Kaiser-Permanente Medical Center, Los Angeles, California
Anaphylaxis and Serum Sickness

PAUL H. EDELSTEIN, M.D.
Associate Professor of Medicine, University of California, Los Angeles, School of Medicine; Staff Physician, Veterans Administration Wadsworth Medical Center, Los Angeles, California
Legionellosis (Legionnaires' Disease and Pontiac Fever)

JOHN EDMEADS, M.D., FRCP(C), FACP
Professor of Medicine (Neurology), University of Toronto; Neurologist-in-Chief, Sunnybrook Medical Center, University of Toronto, Toronto, Ontario, Canada
Headache

HENRY W. EISENBERG, M.D.
Assistant Clinical Professor, Department of Surgery, Case Western Reserve University School of Medicine; Visiting Surgeon, Mt. Sinai Medical Center and St. Luke's Hospital, Cleveland, Ohio
Hemorrhoids, Anal Fissure, and Anorectal Abscess and Fistula.

HOWARD M. EISENBERG, M.D.

Professor of Surgery/Neurosurgery and Pediatrics; Chief of Neurosurgery, University of Texas Medical Branch, Galveston, Texas
Head Injuries in Children

E. GEORGE ELIAS, M.D., Ph.D

Professor of Surgery and Oncology, University of Maryland School of Medicine; Director of Surgical Oncology Program, University of Maryland Hospital, Baltimore, Maryland
Tumors of the Stomach

MICHAEL H. ELLMAN, M.D.

Associate Professor of Clinical Medicine, Pritzker School of Medicine, University of Chicago; Director, Division of Rheumatology, Attending Physician, Michael Reese Hospital and Medical Center, Chicago; Consultant Physician, St. Mary's Hospital, Kankakee, and Oak Forest Hospital, Oak Forest, Illinois
Bursitis and Calcific Tendinitis

WILLIAM L. EPSTEIN, M.D.

Professor and Chairman, Department of Dermatology, University of California, San Francisco, School of Medicine, San Francisco, California
Contact Dermatitis

GEORGE A. FARBER, M.D.

Clinical Associate Professor, Department of Dermatology, Tulane University Medical School; Visiting Physician, Charity Hospital of New Orleans and Tulane Medical Referral Center Hospital, New Orleans, Louisiana
Premalignant Lesions

BARRY FARR, M.D., M.Sc.

Assistant Professor of Medicine, University of Virginia; and University of Virginia Hospital, Charlottesville, Virginia
Viral Respiratory Infections

RICHARD W. FINCHAM, M.D.

Professor of Neurology, College of Medicine, University of Iowa; Physician, University Hospitals, Iowa City, Iowa
Epilepsy in Adolescents and Adults

MARGARET A. FISCHL, M.D.

Associate Professor of Medicine, University of Miami School of Medicine; Director, AIDS Clinical Research Unit; Director, Special Immunology Clinic; Attending, Jackson Memorial Hospital, Miami, Florida
Acquired Immunodeficiency Syndrome (AIDS)

JOHN P. FITZGIBBONS, M.D.

Assistant Professor of Medicine, Tufts University School of Medicine, Boston; Chief, Renal Service, Baystate Medical Center, Springfield, Massachusetts
Diabetes Insipidus

BERTRAM FLESHLER, M.D., FACP

Clinical Associate Professor of Medicine, Case Western Reserve University; Chairman, Department of Gastroenterology, Cleveland Clinic Foundation, Cleveland, Ohio
Ulcerative Colitis

MARTIN J. FRANK, M.D.

Professor of Medicine and Cardiology, Professor of Radiology, and Chief, Section of Cardiology and Nuclear Medicine, Medical College of Georgia, Augusta, Georgia
Congestive Heart Failure

CLAUDE A. FRAZIER, M.D.

Staff Member, Memorial Mission and St. Joseph's Hospitals, Asheville, North Carolina
Spider Bites and Scorpion Stings

IVOR FREW, M.B., B.S., FRCS(Eng)

Emeritus Honorary Lecturer, Department of ENT Studies, University of Newcastle upon Tyne; Honorary Consultant ENT Surgeon, Newcastle General Hospital, Newcastle upon Tyne, England
Acute Peripheral Facial Paralysis (Bell's Palsy)

WALTER G. FREY, M.D.

Professor of Clinical Medicine, Dartmouth Medical School, Hanover, New Hampshire; Assistant Chief of Medicine, White River Junction Veterans Administration Hospital, White River Junction, Vermont; Consultant in Medicine, Mary Hitchock Memorial Hospital, Hanover, New Hamphire
Hemochromatosis

ANDREW J. FRIEDMAN, M.D.

Instructor, Obstetrics and Gynecology, Harvard Medical School; Associate Obstetrician and Gynecologist, Brigham and Women's Hospital, Boston, Massachusetts
Dysmenorrhea

ANTHONY J. FURLAN, M.D.

Director, Cerebrovascular Program, Department of Neurology, Cleveland Clinic Foundation, Cleveland, Ohio
Focal Ischemic Cerebrovascular Disease

THOMAS R. GADACZ, M.D.

Associate Professor of Surgery, Johns Hopkins University; Chief, Surgical Service, Baltimore Veterans Administration Medical Center, Baltimore, Maryland
Cholelithiasis and Cholecystitis

GEORGE R. GAY, M.D.

Associate Professor of Anesthesiology, University of Missouri Hospital and Clinics, Columbia, Missouri
Narcotic Poisoning

LAYNE O. GENTRY, M.D.

Associate Professor of Medicine, Microbiology, and Immunology, Baylor College of Medicine; Chief, Infectious Disease Section, St. Luke's Episcopal Hospital, Houston, Texas
Bacteremia

RAY W. GIFFORD, Jr., M.D.

Chairman, Department of Hypertension and Nephrology, The Cleveland Clinic Foundation, Cleveland, Ohio
Hypertension

GERALD S. GILCHRIST, M.D.

Professor and Chairman, Department of Pediatrics, Mayo Medical School; Consultant in Pediatric Hematology and Oncology, Mayo Clinic and Foundation, Rochester, Minnesota
Acute Leukemia in Childhood

ALAN R. GILES, M.D.

Associate Professor, Departments of Pathology and Medicine, Queen's University at Kingston Medical School; Director of Blood Bank and Apheresis Program and Attending Staff, Kingston General Hospital; Director of Kingston and Region Hemophilia Program, Kingston, Ontario, Canada
Disseminated Intravascular Coagulation; Thrombotic Thrombocytopenic Purpura

ROBERT L. GIUNTOLI, M.D.

Associate Professor of Gynecologic Oncology, University of Pennsylvania School of Medicine and Hospital of the University of Pennsylvania; Consultant, American Oncologic Hospital, Philadelphia, Pennsylvania
Cancer of the Uterine Cervix

JOHN P. GOFTON, M.D., C.M., FACP, FRCP(C)

Clinical Professor of Medicine, University of British Columbia; Senior Consultant, Vancouver General Hospital, Vancouver, British Columbia, Canada
Ankylosing Spondylitis

SIR ABRAHAM GOLDBERG, M.D.

Regius Professor of the Practice of Medicine, University of Glasgow; Consultant Physician, Western Infirmary, Glasgow, Scotland, United Kingdom
The Porphyrias

ROBERT A. GOODWIN, Jr., M.D.

Emeritus Professor of Medicine, Vanderbilt University, Nashville, Tennessee
Histoplasmosis

JAMES G. GOW, M.D., Ch.M., FRCS

University of Liverpool (Ret.), Liverpool, England
Genitourinary Tuberculosis

WILLIAM L. GREEN, M.D.

Professor of Medicine, State University of New York, Downstate Medical Center; Associate Chief of Staff for Research and Development, Veterans Administration Medical Center, Brooklyn, New York
Hypothyroidism

ROBERT B. GREENBLATT, M.D., C.M.

Professor Emeritus, Endocrinology, Medical College of Georgia, Augusta, Georgia
The Menopause

WILLIAM B. GREENOUGH, M.D., FACP

Professor of Medicine, The Johns Hopkins University, on Deputation as Director, International Centre for Diarrhoeal Disease Research, Dhaka, Bangladesh
Cholera

JOSEPH GREENSHER, M.D., FAAP

Associate Professor of Clinical Pediatrics, State University of New York at Stony Brook; Chairman, Department of Pediatrics, Nassau Hospital, Mineola; Associate Director, Long Island Regional Poison Control Center, Nassau County Medical Center, East Meadow, New York
Acute Poisonings

DAVID GROB, M.D.

Professor of Medicine and Clinical Associate Dean, State University of New York, Downstate Medical Center College of Medicine; Director, Departments of Medicine and Medical Education, Maimonides Medical Center, Brooklyn, New York
Myasthenia Gravis

CHARLES GROSE, M.D.

Associate Professor and Head, Division of Infectious Diseases, Department of Pediatrics, University of Iowa and University of Iowa Hospitals, Iowa City, Iowa
Varicella (Chickenpox)

MOSES GROSSMAN, M.D.

Professor of Pediatrics, University of California, San Francisco; Chief of Pediatrics, San Francisco General Hospital, San Francisco, California
Whooping Cough (Pertussis)

SCOTT M. GRUNDY, M.D., Ph.D.

Professor of Internal Medicine and Biochemistry, University of Texas Health Science Center at Dallas; Physician, Veterans Administration Medical Center–Dallas and Parkland Memorial Hospital, Dallas, Texas
Hyperlipoproteinemia

ROBERT A. GUTMAN, M.D.

Clinical Professor of Medicine, Duke University; Staff Physician and Chief of Nephrology, Durham County General Hospital, Durham, North Carolina
Acute Renal Failure

JEAN K. HADDAD, M.D.

Associate Clinical Professor of Medicine, University of California, San Francisco; Active Staff, St. Francis Memorial Hospital; Courtesy Staff, University of California Medical Center, St. Mary's Hospital, and Chinese Hospital, San Francisco, California
Dysphagia and Esophageal Obstruction

WILLIAM J. HALL, M.D.

Professor of Medicine and Pediatrics, University of Rochester School of Medicine; Chairman, Department of Medicine, Rochester General Hospital, Rochester, New York
Acute Respiratory Failure

BRUCE H. HAMORY, M.D.

Associate Professor of Medicine, University of Missouri–Columbia School of Medicine; Attending Physician and Hospital Epidemiologist, University of Missouri–Columbia Hospital and Clinics, Columbia, Missouri
Viral and Mycoplasmal Pneumonias

DAVID HARMON, M.D.

Assistant Professor of Medicine, Harvard Medical School; Assistant Physician, Massachusetts General Hospital, Boston, Massachusetts
Neutropenia

HARRY W. HERR, M.D.

Associate Professor of Surgery, Cornell University Medical College; Associate Member, Sloan-Kettering Institute for Cancer Research; Attending, Memorial Sloan-Kettering Cancer Center and The New York Hospital, New York, New York
Malignant Tumors of the Urogenital Tract

FRANK HINMAN, Jr., M.D.

Clinical Professor of Urology, University of California, San Francisco; Chief of Urology, Children's Hospital, San Francisco, California
Benign Prostatic Hypertrophy

LOREN F. HIRATZKA, M.D.

Associate Professor of Surgery, Division of Thoracic-Cardiovascular Surgery, Department of Surgery, The University of Iowa Hospitals and Clinics, Iowa City, Iowa
Atelectasis

MARGARET M. MAIER HOEHN, M.D., FRCP(C)
Clinical Professor of Neurology and Director of Parkinson's Disease and Movement Disorder Program, University of Colorado School of Medicine; University Hospitals, Swedish-Porter Hospital, St. Joseph Hospital, and St. Luke's-Presbyterian Hospital, Denver, Colorado
Parkinsonism

KRISTEN L. ENGDAHL HOFFMAN, M.D.
Assistant Professor, University of Nebraska Medical Center, Department of Obstetrics and Gynecology; Active Staff, University of Nebraska Medical Center; Courtesy Staff, Immanuel Medical Center and Bishop Clarkson Memorial Hospital, Omaha, Nebraska
Contraception

THOMAS H. HOLMES, M.D.
Professor Emeritus, Department of Psychiatry and Behavioral Sciences, University of Washington, Seattle, Washington
Psychoneurosis

HOWARD D. HOMESLEY, M.D.
Professor and Head, Section on Gynecologic Oncology, Bowman Gray School of Medicine of Wake Forest University; Physician, North Carolina Baptist Hospital, Winston-Salem, North Carolina
Carcinoma of the Vulva

RICHARD T. HOPPE, M.D.
Associate Professor of Radiology, Division of Radiation Therapy, Stanford University, Stanford, California
Hodgkin's Disease: Radiation Therapy

DAVID O. HOUGH, M.D.
Associate Professor of Family Practice and Director of Sports Medicine, Michigan State University, East Lansing; St. Lawrence Hospital, E. W. Sparrow Hospital, Ingham Medical Center, and Lansing General Hospital, Lansing, Michigan
Common Sports Injuries

JEFFREY L. HOUPT, M.D.
Professor and Chairman, Department of Psychiatry, Emory University School of Medicine; Member, Medical Staff of Emory University Hospital, Grady Memorial Hospital, and Georgia Mental Health Institute, Atlanta, Georgia
Delirium

ROBERT P. HUMMEL, M.D.
Professor of Surgery, University of Cincinnati College of Medicine; Active Staff, University of Cincinnati Hospital, The Children's Hospital, and Our Lady of Mercy Hospitals; Courtesy Staff, Bethesda Hospital and The Christ Hospital, Cincinnati, Ohio
Necrotizing Infections of The Soft Tissues, Including Gas Gangrene

ABDOLLAH IRAVANI, M.D.
Associate Professor, University of Florida College of Medicine; Attending Physician, Shands Teaching Hospital, Gainesville, Florida
Bacterial Infections of the Urinary Tract—Female

KEVIN J. IVEY, M.D., FACP
Professor of Medicine, University of California, Irvine; Staff Physician, Long Beach Veterans Administration Medical Center, Long Beach, California
Gastritis

JERRY C. JACOBS, M.D.
Professor of Clinical Pediatrics and Director, Section of Pediatric Rheumatology, Columbia University College of Physicians and Surgeons; Attending Pediatrician, Babies Hospital, Columbia-Presbyterian Medical Center, New York, New York
Juvenile Rheumatoid Arthritis

ROBERT J. JACOBSON, M.B., B.Ch.
Associate Professor of Medicine and Pathology, Georgetown University School of Medicine; Chief, Division of Hematology, and Director, Hematology Laboratory, Georgetown University Hospital, Washington, D.C.
Pernicious Anemia and Other Megaloblastic Anemias

ROBERT R. JACOBSON, M.D., Ph.D.
Instructor in Medicine, Louisiana State University School of Medicine, New Orleans; Chief of the Clinical Branch and Department of Medicine, National Hansen's Disease Center, Carville, Louisiana
Leprosy (Hansen's Disease)

D. GERAINT JAMES, M.A., M.D., FRCP
Dean and Consultant Physician, Royal Northern Hospital, London, England
Sarcoidosis

DAVID S. JANOWSKY, M.D.
Professor of Psychiatry, University of California, San Diego La Jolla; San Diego Veterans Administration Medical Center, University of California Medical Center, San Diego, California
Affective Disorders

CHRISTINE A. JOHNSON, M.D.
Associate Professor of Pediatrics and Director, Comprehensive Sickle Cell Program, Bowman Gray School of Medicine; Attending, North Carolina Baptist Hospital, Winston-Salem, North Carolina
Sickle Cell Disease

KENNETH P. JOHNSON, M.D.
Professor and Chairman, Department of Neurology, University of Maryland School of Medicine; Chief of Neurology, University of Maryland Hospital, Baltimore, Maryland
Multiple Sclerosis

GERALD H. JORDAN, M.D.
Assistant Professor, Eastern Virginia Medical School Department of Urology, Norfolk; Staff Urologist, United States Naval Hospital, Portsmouth, Virginia
Epididymitis

ROBERT E. JORDON, M.D.
Chairman and Professor of Dermatology, The University of Texas Health Science Center Medical School at Houston; Physician, Hermann Hospital and M. D. Anderson Cancer and Tumor Institute, Houston, Texas
Bullous Diseases

JOSEPH L. JORIZZO, M.D.
Associate Professor, Department of Dermatology, University of Texas Medical Branch, Galveston, Texas
Cutaneous Vasculitis

ROBERT J. JOYNT, M.D., Ph.D.
Dean and Professor of Neurology, University of Rochester; Neurologst, Strong Memorial Hospital, Rochester, New York
Alzheimer's Disease

M. BASHAR KAHALEH, M.D.
Associate Professor of Medicine, Medical University of South Carolina; Attending Physician, Medical University of South Carolina Hospital, Charleston, South Carolina
Polymyalgia Rheumatica and Temporal Arteritis

GEORGE W. KAPLAN, M.D., M.S,, FAAP, FACS
Clinical Professor of Surgery/Urology and Pediatrics, University of California, San Diego, School of Medicine; Chief of Pediatric Urology, Children's Hospital, San Diego, California
Childhood Enuresis

RAYMOND H. KAUFMAN, M.D.
Ernst W. Bertner Chairman and Professor, Department of Obstetrics-Gynecology, Baylor College of Medicine; Chief of Obstetrics-Gynecology Service, Harris County Hospital District, St. Luke's Episcopal Hospital, and The Methodist Hospital; Houston, Texas
Vulvovaginitis

RUSSEL E. KAUFMAN, M.D.
Assistant Professor of Medicine and Assistant Professor of Biochemistry, Duke University Medical Center and School of Medicine; Physician, Duke University Hospital and Durham Veterans Administration Hospital, Durham, North Carolina
Thalassemia

ROBERT C. KAUFMANN, M.D.
Assistant Professor, Maternal/Fetal Medicine, Southern Illinois University School of Medicine, Department of Obstetrics/Gynecology; Staff, Memorial Medical Center and St. John's Hospital, Springifield, Illinois
Ectopic Pregnancy

THOMAS KAYE, M.D.
Neurosurgery Resident, Montefiore Hospital Medical Center, Albert Einstein College of Medicine, New York, New York
Acute Head Injuries in Adults

JOHN G. KELTON, M.D.
Associate Professor of Medicine and Pathology, McMaster University; Director of the McMaster Medical Centre Blood Bank, Hamilton, Ontario, Canada
Platelet-Mediated Bleeding Disorders

CLARK M. KERR, M.D.
Director, Infectious Disease Section, Department of Medicine, St. Joseph's Hospital; President, Associate Staff, St. Luke's Hospital; Associate Staff, Mercy and Humana Aurora Hospitals, Denver, Colorado
Psittacosis (Ornithosis)

HAROLD A. KESSLER, M.D.
Assistant Professor of Medicine and Immunology/Microbiology, Rush Medical College; Senior Attending Physician, Department of Medicine, Rush-Presbyterian-St. Luke's Medical Center, Chicago, Illinois
Infectious Mononucleosis

C. THOMAS KISKER, M.D.
Director of Pediatrics, University of Iowa College of Medicine; Director, Division of Pediatric Hematology/Oncology and Director, Regional Hemophilia Center, University of Iowa Hospitals and Clinics, Iowa City, Iowa
Vitamin K Deficiency

ROBERT A. KNUPPEL, M.D., M.P.H.
Professor of Obstetrics and Gynecology and Director, Division of Maternal-Fetal Medicine, University of South Florida College of Medicine, Tampa; Attending, Tampa General Hospital and Humana Women's Hospital; Director, Maternal-Fetal Medicine, Bayfront Medical Center, St. Petersburg, Florida
Vaginal Bleeding Late in Pregnancy

FREDERICK T. KOSTER, M.D.
Associate Professor, Department of Medicine, University of New Mexico School of Medicine; Staff Physician, University of New Mexico Hospital, Albuquerque, New Mexico
Q Fever

BENJAMIN KOZINER, M.D.
Associate Attending Physician, Hematology/Lymphoma Service, Department of Medicine, Memorial Hospital for Cancer and Allied Disease, New York, New York
Non-Hodgkin's Lymphomas

KENNETH KREINES, M.D.
Clinical Professor of Medicine, University of Cincinnati Medical Center, Metabolism Division; Senior Attending Physician, Bethesda Hospital and Jewish Hospital; Consultant, Children's Hospital Medical Center, Cincinnati, Ohio
Diabetes Mellitus in Adults

CHARLES L. KRONE, M.D., FACP
Clinical Associate, Internal Medicine, University of Arizona College of Medicine; Medical Director, School of Enterostomal Therapy, Tucson Medical Center, St. Joseph's Hospital, and El Dorado Hospital, Tucson, Arizona
Gaseousness and Indigestion

GREGORY J. KUNDRAT, M.D.
Precepting Physician, Middlesex Memorial Hospital Family Practice Residency, Middletown; Chief of Department of Family Practice, Attending Staff, Lawrence and Memorial Hospital, New London, Connecticut
Lyme Disease

ROBERT A. KYLE, M.D.
William H. Donner Professor of Medicine and Laboratory Medicine, Mayo Medical School; Consultant, Division of Hematology and Internal Medicine and Department of Laboratory Medicine, Mayo Clinic and Mayo Foundation, Rochester, Minnesota
Multiple Myeloma

STANFORD I. LAMBERG, M.D.
Associate Professor of Dermatology, The Johns Hopkins University School of Medicine and The Johns Hopkins Hospital; Chief, Department of Dermatology, Francis Scott Key Medical Center, Baltimore, Maryland
Cutaneous T Cell Lymphomas (CTCL): Mycosis Fungoides and the Sézary Syndrome

STEPHEN A. LANDAW, M.D., Ph.D.
Professor of Medicine and Associate Professor of Radiology, State University of New York Upstate Medical Center; Associate Chief of Staff, Research and Development and Attending in Internal Medicine/Hematology, Veterans Administration Medical Center; Attending in Medicine/Hematology, University Hospital and Crouse-Irving Memorial Hospital, Syracuse, New York
Polycythemia Vera and Other Polycythemic Conditions

LEWIS LANDSBERG, M.D.
Associate Professor of Medicine, Harvard Medical School; Chief, Division of Endocrinology and Metabolism, Beth Israel Hospital, Boston, Massachusetts
Pheochromocytoma

TIMOTHY W. LANE, M.D.
Associate Professor of Medicine, University of North Carolina, Chapel Hill; Chief, Internal Medicine Training Program, Moses Cone Hospital, Greensboro, North Carolina
Rocky Mountain Spotted Fever

JOHN LASZLO, M.D.
Professor of Medicine, Duke University School of Medicine and Medical Center; Physician, Durham County General Hospital, Durham, North Carolina
Nausea and Vomiting

LAURA LAYDEN, M.D.
Surgical Resident, Harbor-UCLA Department of Surgery, Torrance, California
Bacterial Diseases of the Skin

JOSIANE S. LEDERMAN, M.D.
Clinical and Research Fellow, Massachusetts General Hospital, Harvard Medical School, Boston, Massachusetts
Pigmentary Disorders

BURTON J. LEE, M.D.
Clinical Associate Professor of Medicine, Cornell University Medical College; Attending Physician, Hematology/Lymphoma Service, Department of Medicine, Memorial Hospital, New York, New York
Non-Hodgkin's Lymphomas

ROBERT B. LEMAN, M.D.
Assistant Professor of Medicine, Medical University of South Carolina, Charleston, South Carolina
Atrial Fibrillation

MICHAEL L. LEVIN, M.D.
Assistant Professor of Medicine, Johns Hopkins University; Founder and Former Head, Division of Infectious Diseases, Sinai Hospital of Baltimore, Inc., Baltimore, Maryland
Trichinellosis

STUART LEVIN, M.D.
Professor of Medicine, Rush Medical College; Associate Chairman of Medicine, Director of Infectious Disease, and Senior Attending—Medicine, Rush-Presbyterian-St. Luke's Medical Center, Chicago, Illinois
Infectious Mononucleosis

GARY M. LEVINE, M.D.
Professor of Medicine, Temple University School of Medicine; Head, Division of Gastroenterology and Nutrition, Albert Einstein Medical Center, Philadelphia, Pennsylvania
The Malabsorption Syndromes

CARL J. LEVINSON, M.D.
Clinical Professor of Obstetrics and Gynecology, University of California, San Francisco; Chairman, Department of Obstetrics and Gynecology, Children's Hospital of San Francisco, San Francisco, California
Endometriosis

JOHN E. LEWY, M.D.
Professor and Chairman, Department of Pediatrics, Tulane University School of Medicine; Pediatrician in Chief, Tulane Medical Center and Tulane Service, Charity Hospital, New Orleans, Louisiana
Parenteral Fluid Therapy for Infants and Children

FRANK W. LING, M.D.
Associate Professor, Department of Obstetrics and Gynecology, University of Tennessee College of Medicine; Physician, E. H. Crump Women's Hospital and Perinatal Center, Memphis, Tennessee
Postpartum Care

BARRY I. LISKOW, M.D.
Associate Professor of Psychiatry, University of Kansas Medical Center, Kansas City, Kansas; Chief, Alcohol Dependence Treatment Unit, Kansas City Veterans Administration Medical Center, Kansas City, Missouri
Alcoholism

JOHN R. LITTLE, M.D.
Head, Section of Cerebrovascular Surgery, Department of Neurosurgery, Cleveland Clinic Foundation, Cleveland, Ohio
Focal Ischemic Cerebrovascular Disease

WILLIAM E. LOCKHART, Jr., M.D., FAAFP
Physician, Big Bend Memorial Hospital, Alpine, Texas
Snakebite

D. LYNN LORIAUX, M.D., Ph.D.
Chief, Developmental Endocrinology Branch, and Clinical Director, National Institute of Child Health and Human Development, National Institutes of Health, Bethesda, Maryland
Cushing's Syndrome

PHILLIP A. LOW, M.D., FRACP
Professor of Neurology, Mayo Medical School; Attending, Mayo Clinic and affiliated hospitals, Rochester, Minnesota
Peripheral Neuropathies

STEVEN W. LUGER, M.D.
Precepting Physician, Family Practice Residency, Middletown; Attending Physician, Lawrence and Memorial Hospital, New London, Connecticut
Lyme Disease

MICHAEL P. MADAIO, M.D.
Assistant Professor of Medicine, Tufts University School of Medicine; Assistant Physician, New England Medical Center, Boston, Massachusetts
Glomerular Disorders

LARRY T. MAHONEY, M.D.
Assistant Professor, Department of Pediatrics, University of Iowa School of Medicine; Division of Pediatric Cardiology, University of Iowa Hospitals and Clinics, Iowa City, Iowa
Congenital Heart Disease

MARK C. MAMMEL, M.D.
Assistant Professor of Pediatrics, University of Minnesota School of Medicine; Associate Director, Neonatal Medicine, St. Paul Children's Hospital, St. Paul, Minnesota
Neonatal Resuscitation

JOSEPH C. MAROON, M.D.
Clinical Professor of Neurosurgery, University of Pittsburgh School of Medicine; Director, Department of Neurosurgery, Allegheny General Hospital, Pittsburgh, Pennsylvania
Trigeminal Neuralgia

PHILIP D. MARSDEN, M.D. (London), FRCP, FRCPE

Titled Professor of Medicine, University of Brasilia; Consultant Physician, Hospital Presidente Medici, Brasilia, Brazil
Leishmaniasis

HAROLD M. MAURER, M.D.

Professor and Chairman, Department of Pediatrics, Children's Medical Center, Medical College of Virgina, Virgina Commonwealth University, Richmond, Virginia
Hemolytic Disease of the Newborn (Erythroblastosis Fetalis)

MICHAEL D. MAVES, M.D., FACS

Assistant Professor, Otolaryngology—Head and Neck Surgery, and Director, Division of Head and Neck Surgical Oncology, University of Iowa College of Medicine and University of Iowa Hospitals and Clinics; Iowa City Veterans Administration Hospital; Iowa City, Iowa
Hoarseness and Laryngitis

C. KENNETH McALLISTER, M.D.

Clinical Associate Professor of Medicine, University of Texas Health Science Center at San Antonio; Chief, Infectious Disease Service, Brooke Army Medical Center, San Antonio, Texas
Rabies

BRIAN F. McCABE, M.D.

Professor and Head, Department of Otolaryngology—Head and Neck Surgery, University of Iowa College of Medicine and University of Iowa Hospitals and Clinics, Iowa City, Iowa
Tinnitus

RICHARD V. McCLOSKEY, M.S., M.D.

Professor of Medicine, Jefferson Medical College; Physician, Albert Einstein Medical Center, Mt. Sinai/Daroff Division, Philadelphia, Pennsylvania
Diphtheria

KENNETH E. L. McCOLL, M.D.

Senior Lecturer in Medicine, University of Glasgow; Consultant Physician and Gastroenterologist, Western Infirmary, Glasgow, Scotland, United Kingdom
The Porphyrias

EDWARD J. McGUIRE, M.D.

Professor and Head, Section of Urology, University of Michigan and University Hospitals, Ann Abor, Michigan
Urinary Incontinence

KEVIN M. McINTYRE, M.D.

Assistant Professor of Medicine, Havard Medical School; Veterans Administration and Brigham and Women's Hospital, Departments of Medicine, Boston, Massachusetts
Pulmonary Embolism

PHILIP G. McMANIS, M.B.B.S., FRACP

Special Clinical Fellow, Mayo Graduate School; Mayo Clinic and affiliated hospitals, Rochester, Minnesota
Peripheral Neuropathies

W. JAMES METZGER, M.D.

Associate Professor of Medicine and Head, Section of Allergy/Immunology, East Carolina University School of Medicine, Greenville, North Carolina
Asthma in the Adolescent and Adult

RODNEY A. MICHAEL, M.D.

Senior Fellow, Infectious Diseases, Brooke Army Medical Center, San Antonio, Texas
Rabies

KIRK D. MILLER, M.D.

EIS Officer, Malaria Branch, Division of Parasitic Diseases, Center for Infectious Disease, Centers for Disease Control, Atlanta, Georgia
Malaria

LARRY E. MILLIKAN, M.D.

Professor and Chairman, Department of Dermatology, Tulane University School of Medicine; Attending, Tulane University Hospital and Clinics; Senior Visiting Physician, Charity Hospital of New Orleans; Consultant, Veterans Administration Hospitals, New Orleans and Pineville; Staff Dermatologist, Veterans Administration Hospital, Biloxi, Mississippi; Courtesy Staff, Huey P. Long Charity Hospital, New Orleans, Louisiana
Urticaria and Angioedema

DONALD L. MITTS, M.D.

Assistant Clinical Professor of Surgery, Division of Thoracic and Cardiovascular Surgery, University of Cincinnati College of Medicine; Staff, Department of Cardiac Surgery, The Christ Hospital; Staff, The Jewish Hospital of Cincinnati, Division of Cardiac Surgery, Cincinnati, Ohio
Pleural Effusions and Empyema Thoracis

HOWARD C. MOFENSON, M.D., FAAP, FAACT

Professor of Clinical Pediatrics, Medical School of State University of New York at Stony Brook; Acting Dean, Nassau County Medical Center; Director, Long Island Regional Poison Control Center, East Meadow, New York
Acute Poisonings

MICHAEL R. MOORE, Ph.D.

Senior Lecturer in Medicine, University of Glasgow, Glasgow, Scotland, United Kingdom
The Porphyrias

REMO L. MORELLI, M.D.

Assistant Professor of Medicine, University of California, San Francisco, and Division of Cardiology, San Francisco General Hospital, San Francisco, California
Infective Endocarditis

DAWN G. MUELLER, M.D.

Associate Professor of Pediatrics, Medical College of Virginia, Virginia Commonwealth University; Assistant Director, Newborn Intensive Care Unit, Children's Medical Center, Medical College of Virginia Hospital, Richmond, Virginia
Hemolytic Disease of The Newborn (Erythroblastosis Fetalis)

TIMOTHY F. MURPHY, M.D.

Assistant Professor of Medicine, School of Medicine, State University of New York at Buffalo; Internist, Division of Infectious Diseases, Erie County Medical Center, Buffalo, New York
Tularemia

HENRY W. MURRAY, M.D.

Associate Professor of Medicine, Cornell University Medical College; Chief, Division of Infectious Diseases, The New York Hospital, New York, New York
Toxoplasmosis

GEORGE A. NANKERVIS, Ph.D., M.D.
Professor and Chairman, Department of Pediatrics, Medical College of Ohio and Medical College Hospital, Toledo, Ohio
Measles (Rubeola)

KENRAD E. NELSON, M.D.
Professor, Internal Medicine and Preventive Medicine, University of Illinois College of Medicine; Attending Physician, Department of Medicine, University of Illinois Hospital, Chicago, Illinois
Brucellosis

LEE S. NEWMAN, M.D.
Fellow in Pulmonary Medicine, University of Colorado Health Sciences Center; Denver General Hospital, Denver, Colorado
Chronic Obstructive Pulmonary Disease and Bronchiectasis

CARTER NEWTON, M.D.
Assistant Clinical Professor of Medicine, University of California, Los Angeles, School of Medicine, Los Angeles; Director, Cardiac Rehabilitation, St. Johns Hospital and Health Center, Santa Monica, California
Care and Rehabilitation After Myocardial Infarction

THOMAS F. NIKOLAI, M.D., FACP
Associate Clinical Professor of Medicine, University of Wisconsin; Section of Endocrinology, Marshfield Clinic, Marshfield, Wisconsin
Thyroiditis

HOOSHANG M. NIKOO, M.D.
Director of Medical Education, Department of Obstetrics/Gynecology, Episcopal Hospital; Attending Physician, Obstetrics/Gynecology Department, Nazareth Hospital and Jeanes Hospital, Philadelphia, Pennsylvania
Abortion

STEVEN M. OPAL, M.D.
Visiting Assistant Professor of Medicine, University of Colorado School of Medicine, Denver; Chief of Infectious Diseases, Fitzsimons Army Medical Center, Aurora, Colorado
Bacterial Meningitis

DAVID S. ORENTREICH, M.D.
Clinical Instructor, Department of Dermatology, Mount Sinai School of Medicine; Clinical Assistant, Department of Dermatology, Mount Sinai Medical Center, New York, New York
Diseases of the Hair

NORMAN ORENTREICH, M.D.
Clinical Professor of Dermatology, New York University School of Medicine; Associate Attending, Department of Dermatology, University Hospital, New York University Medical Center; Associate Attending, Department of Dermatology, Bellevue Hospital Center, New York, New York
Diseases of the Hair

LAWRENCE CHARLES PARISH, M.D.
Clinical Professor of Dermatology, Jefferson Medical College of Thomas Jefferson University, and Adjunct Associate Professor of Dermatology, University of Pennsylvania School of Veterinary Medicine; Chief of Dermatology, St. Agnes Medical Center, Frankford Hospital, Albert Einstein Medical Center—Mt. Sinai–Daroff Division, Philadelphia, Pennsylvania
Parasitic Diseases

J. R. PARMAR, M.D.
Fellow in Gastroenterology, University of Illinois, College of Medicine, Chicago, Illinois
Constipation

PERRY G. PATE, M.D.
Assistant Professor, Department of Medicine, Tulane University School of Medicine; Visiting Physician, Charity Hospital of Louisiana in New Orleans; Staff Physician, Tulane University Hospital, New Orleans, Louisiana
Rat-Bite Fever

JOHN A. PENNER, M.D.
Professor of Medicine, Michigan State University School of Medicine; Chief, Hematology/Oncology Division, Michigan State University Associated Hospitals, East Lansing, Michigan
Hemophilia and Related Conditions

PETER L. PERINE, M.D., M.P.H.
Professor and Director, Division of Tropical Public Health, Department Preventive Medicine and Biometrics; Adjunct Professor of Medicine, Uniformed Services University of the Health Sciences; Attending Physician, Naval Hospital, Bethesda, Maryland
Typhus Fevers

STANLEY PERLMAN, M.D., Ph.D.
Assistant Professor of Pediatrics, University of Iowa College of Medicine and University of Iowa Hospitals and Clinics, Iowa City, Iowa
Viral Meningitis/Encephalitis

JEFFREY P. PHELAN, M.D.
Associate Professor, Department of Obstetrics and Gynecology, University of Southern California School of Medicine; Los Angeles County–University of Southern California Medical Center, Los Angeles, California
Antepartum Care

DANIEL A. PIETRO, M.D.
Assistant Professor of Medicine, Harvard Medical School, Boston; Associate Chief of Cardiology, Brockton/West Roxbury Veterans Administration Medical Center, Brockton, Massachusetts
Pulmonary Embolism

WARREN W. PIETTE, M.D.
Assistant Professor of Dermatology, University of Iowa Hospital and Clinics, Iowa City, Iowa
Herpes Simplex and Herpes Zoster

MICHAEL A. POLIS, M.D.
Fellow, Division of Infectious Diseases, George Washington University School of Medicine, Washington, D.C.
Food Poisoning

STUART M. POLLY, M.D.
Associate Professor, Department of Internal Medicine, Texas Tech University School of Medicine; Chief, Medical Service, R. E. Thomason General Hospital, El Paso, Texas
Relapsing Fever

HERBERT H. POMERANCE, M.D.
Emeritus Professor of Pediatrics, West Virginia University, Charleston, West Virginia; Visiting Professor of Pediatrics, University of South Florida, Tampa, Florida
Normal Infant Feeding

FRANK C. POWELL, M.B., MRCPI
Consultant Dermatologist, Mater Hospital, Dublin, Ireland
Dermatomyositis

THOMAS H. PRICE, M.D.
Associate Professor of Medicine, University of Washington; Director of Pheresis, Puget Sound Blood Center, Seattle, Washington
Therapeutic Use of Blood Components

ERIC N. PRYSTOWSKY, M.D.
Associate Professor of Medicine and Director, Clinical Electrophysiology Laboratory, Indiana University School of Medicine; Research Associate, Krannert Institute of Cardiology; Attending Physician, Indiana University Hospital, Wishard Memorial Hospital and Roudebush Veterans Administration Medical Center, Indianapolis, Indiana
Tachycardia

EDWARD J. QUEBBEMAN, M.D., Ph.D.
Assistant Professor of Surgery and Assistant Professor of Physiology, Medical College of Wisconsin; Director, Surgical Intensive Care Unit, Milwaukee County Medical Complex and Froedtert Memorial Lutheran Hospital; Director, Nutritional Support Service, Veterans Administration Medical Center, Wood, and Milwaukee County Medical Complex; Associate Attending Staff Physician, Froedtert Memorial Lutheran Hospital; Staff Surgeon, Milwaukee County Medical Complex, Milwaukee, Wisconsin
Parenteral Nutrition in Adults

RAYMOND V. RANDALL, M.D.
Professor of Medicine, Mayo Medical School; Senior Consultant, Mayo Clinic; Consultant, St. Mary's Hospital and Rochester Methodist Hospital, Rochester, Minnesota
Hypopituitarism; Hyperprolactinemia

HENRY W. RANDLE, M.D., Ph.D.
Associate Professor of Medicine (Dermatology), Texas A & M University College of Medicine; Scott & White Hospital, Temple, Texas
Diseases of the Mouth

GEORGE B. RANKIN, M.D., FACP
Staff Physician, Department of Gastroenterology, Cleveland Clinic, Cleveland, Ohio
Crohns' Disease

RONALD P. RAPINI, M.D.
Assistant Professor of Dermatology and Pathology, University of Texas Medical School at Houston; Physician, Hermann Hospital and M. D. Anderson Hospital, Houston, Texas
Bullous Diseases

JAMES E. RASMUSSEN, M.D.
Professor of Dermatology and Pediatrics, University of Michigan Medical School and University of Michigan Hospitals, Ann Arbor, Michigan
Pruritus Ani and Vulvae

HOWARD A. REBER, M.D.
Professor of Surgery and Medicine, University of Missouri School of Medicine; Chief, Surgical Service, Harry S Truman Memorial Veterans Hospital, Columbia, Missouri
Chronic Pancreatitis

K. RAJENDER REDDY, M.D., FACP
Assistant Professor of Medicine, Division of Hepatology, Department of Medicine, University of Miami School of Medicine; Staff Physician, Veterans Administration Hospital, Jackson Memorial Hospital, and University of Miami Hospital, Miami, Florida
Cirrhosis

VINODINI REDDY, M.D., D.C.H.
Deputy Director, National Institute of Nutrition, Hyderabad, India
Hypo- and Hypervitaminosis A

JOHN F. REDMAN, M.D.
Professor and Chairman, Department of Urology, University of Arkansas College of Medicine; Chief, Urology Service, University Hospital and Arkansas Children's Hospital, Little Rock, Arkansas
Urethral Stricture

FAY O. REDWINE, M.S., M.D.
Associate Professor of Obstetrics-Gynecology and Human Genetics, Medical College of Virginia, Medical College of Virginia Hospital, Richmond, Virginia
Hemolytic Disease of the Newborn (Erythroblastosis Fetalis)

MICHAEL F. REIN, M.D.
Associate Professor of Medicine, University of Virginia; Attending Physician, University of Virginia Hospital, Charlottesville, Virginia
Syphilis

HAL B. RICHERSON, M.D.
Professor of Internal Medicine and Director, Allergy-Immunology Division, University of Iowa College of Medicine; Attending Physician, University Hospitals, and Consultant, Veterans Administration Hospital, Iowa City, Iowa
Hypersensitivity Pneumonitis

NICHOLAS J. ROBERT, M.D.
Assistant Professor in Medicine, Pathology and Radiation Medicine, Tufts Medical School; Clinical Director, Medical Oncology, Division of Hematology/Oncology, New England Medical Center, Boston, Massachusetts
Hodgkins' Disease: Chemotherapy

JUNE K. ROBINSON, M.D.
Assistant Professor of Dermatology and Surgery, Northwestern University Medical School; Attending Staff, Northwestern Memorial Hospital, Chicago, Illinois
Nevi and Malignant Melanomas

HENRY H. ROENIGK, Jr., M.D.
Professor and Chairman, Department of Dermatology, Northwestern University Medical School; Attending Staff, Northwestern Memorial Hospital, Chicago, Illinois
Stasis and Other Skin Ulcers

EDWARD H. ROMOND, M.D.
Assistant Professor of Medicine, University of Kentucky; Director, Adult Hemophilia Program, Albert B. Chandler Medical Center, University of Kentucky, Lexington, Kentucky
Hemophilia and Related Conditions

TED ROSEN, M.D.
Associate Professor of Dermatology, Baylor College of Medicine; Chief, Dermatology Service, Veterans Administration Medical Center, Houston, Texas
Chancroid

AMNON ROSENTHAL, M.D.
Director of Pediatric Cardiology and Professor of Pediatrics and Communicable Diseases, University of Michigan; Attending, C. S. Mott Children's Hospital and University of Michigan Medical Center, Ann Arbor, Michigan
Rheumatic Fever

JAMES L. A. ROTH, M.D., Ph.D.
Professor of Clinical Medicine, School of Medicine, University of Pennsylvania; Director of Institute of Gastroenterology and Chief of Gastroenterology Service, Presbyterian University of Pennsylvania Medical Center; Consultant in Gastroenterology, Lankenau Hospital, Philadelphia, Pennsylvania
Diverticula of the Alimentary Tract

VIRGINIA S. ROWLAND, M.D.
Attending, Desert Samaritan Hospital, Mesa and Valley Lutheran Hospitals, Mesa, Arizona
Coccidioidomycosis

EBEN M. RUBIN, M.D.
Assistant Professor, Pulmonary Division, University of Miami School of Medicine; Associate Director, Medical Intensive Care Unit, and Attending Physician, Pulmonary Division, Jackson Memorial Hospital, Miami, Florida
Primary Lung Abscess

RICHARD A. RUDDERS, M.D.
Associate Professor of Medicine, Tufts University School of Medicine; Physician, Head, Lymphoma Service, New England Medical Center, Boston, Massachusetts
Hodgkin's Disease: Chemotherapy

HAZIM J. SAFI, M.D.
Assistant Professor of Surgery, Baylor College of Medicine; Attending Surgeon, The Methodist Hospital, Houston, Texas
Acquired Diseases of the Aorta

SIMONE SALTZMAN, M.D.
Assistant Professor of Medicine, Albert Einstein College of Medicine; Attending Physician, Bronx Municipal Hospital Center, Hospital of the Albert Einstein College of Medicine; Chairman, Infection Control Committee, Bronx Municipal Hospital Center, Bronx, New York
Bacterial Pneumoma

ARTHUR A. SASAHARA, M.D.
Professor of Medicine, Harvard Medical School Boston; Chief, Medical Service, Brockton/West Roxbury Veterans Administration Medical Center, West Roxbury, Massachusetts
Pulmonary Embolism

EUGENE R. SCHIFF, M.D., FACP
Professor of Medicine and Chief, Division of Hepatology, Department of Medicine, University of Miami School of Medicine; Chief, Hepatology Section, Veterans Administration Hospital; Staff Physician, Veterans Administration Hospital, Jackson Memorial Hospital, and University of Miami Hospital, Miami, Florida
Cirrhosis

ISAAC SCHIFF, M.D.
Associate Professor, Obstetrics and Gynecology, Harvard Medical School; Associate Obstetrician and Gynecologist, Brigham and Women's Hospital, Boston, Massachusetts
Dysmenorrhea

DAVID J. SCHOETZ, Jr., M.D.
Staff, Section of Colon and Rectal Surgery, Lahey Clinic Medical Center, Burlington, Massachusetts
Tumors of the Colon and Rectum

NEVIN S. SCRIMSHAW, Ph.D., M.D.
Institute Professor and Director, International Food and Nutrition Program, Massachusetts Institute of Technology, Cambridge, Massachusetts
Beriberi (Thiamine [Vitamin B_1] Deficiency)

FRANCISCO SERAFIN, M.D.
Associate Professor of Pediatrics and Associate Professor of Infectious Diseases and Clinical Microbiology, National Autonomous University of Mexico; Associate Director, Hospital de Pediatria—IMSS, Mexico D.F., Mexico
Typhoid Fever

JOHN L. SEVER, M.D., Ph.D.
Professor of Pediatrics, Georgetown University Medical School, and Professor and Lecturer, Pediatrics and Obstetrics and Gynecology, George Washington University Medical School, Washington, D.C.; National Institutes of Health, Bethesda, Maryland
Rubella and Congenital Rubella

H. GUNTER SEYDEL, M.D.
Clinical Professor of Radiation Oncology, Wayne State University; Chief, Department of Therapeutic Radiology, Henry Ford Hospital, Detroit, Michigan
Primary Lung Cancer

ALAN R. SHALITA, M.D.
Professor and Chairman, Department of Dermatology, State University of New York Downstate Medical Center; Director of Dermatology Services, State University Hospital, Kings County Hospital Center, and Brookdale Hospital Medical Center; Consultant in Dermatology, Brooklyn Veterans Administration Medical Center, Brooklyn, New York
Acne Vulgaris and Rosacea

G.V.R.K. SHARMA, M.D.
Assistant Professor of Medicine, Harvard Medical School, Boston; Associate Chief of Cardiology, Brockton/West Roxbury Veterans Administration Medical Center, West Roxbury, Massachusetts
Pulmonary Embolism

JOHN T. SHARP, M.D.
Professor of Medicine, University of Colorado School of Medicine; Director, Joe and Betty Alpert Arthritis Center, Rose Medical Center, Denver, Colorado
Rheumatoid Arthritis

LINDA M. DAIRIKI SHORTLIFFE, M.D.
Assistant Professor of Surgery, Stanford University School of Medicine, Stanford; Chief, Urology Section, Palo Alto Veterans Administration Medical Center, Palo Alto, California
Prostatitis

STANFORD T. SHULMAN, M.D.
Professor of Pediatrics, Northwestern University Medical School; Chief, Infectious Diseases, Children's Memorial Hospital, Chicago, Illinois
Streptococcal Pharyngitis

ROBERT C. SIEGEL, M.D.
Associate Clinical Professor of Medicine and Orthopedics, University of California, San Francisco; Attending Physician, Department of Medicine, Mills Memorial Hospital; Director, Rheumatology Clinic, H. D. Chope Community Hospital, San Mateo, California
Scleroderma (Systemic Sclerosis)

LESLIE E. SILBERSTEIN, M.D.
Assistant Professor of Pathology and Laboratory Medicine in Department of Pathology and Department of Medicine, School of Medicine, University of Pennsylvania; Director, Blood Bank and Apheresis and Outpatient Transfusion Unit, Hospital of the University of Pennsylvania, Philadelphia, Pennsylvania
Autoimmune Hemolytic Anemia

GARY L. SIMON, M.D., PH.D.
Associate Professor of Medicine, Division of Infectious Diseases; Associate Chairman, Department of Medicine, The George Washington University School of Medicine; Attending Physician, The George Washington University Hospital, Washington, D.C.
Food Poisoning

MARGARET L. SIMPSON, M.D.
Assistant Professor of Medicine, Division of Infectious Disease, University of Minnesota; Physician, Hennepin County Medical Center, Division of Infectious Diseases, Minneapolis, Minnesota
Gonorrhea

ETHEL S. SIRIS, M.D.
Associate Professor of Clinical Medicine, Columbia University, College of Physicians and Surgeons; Associate Attending Physician, Presbyterian Hospital, New York, New York
Paget's Disease of Bone

ARNOLD SLADEN, M.D.
Professor of Anesthesiology and Critical Care Medicine and Associate Professor of Surgery, University of Pittsburgh School of Medicine; Director, Surgical Intensive Care Unit, Montefiore Hospital, Pittsburgh, Pennsylvania
Cardiac Arrest

CARL V. SMITH, M.D.
Clinical Research Fellow, Department of Obstetrics and Gynecology, University of Southern California School of Medicine; Attending, Los Angeles County–University of Southern California Medical Center, Los Angeles, California
Antepartum Care

EDGAR B. SMITH, M.D.
Professor and Chairman, Department of Dermatology, University of Texas Medical Branch and University of Texas Medical Branch Hospitals, Galveston, Texas
Fungal Diseases

THOMAS F. SMITH, M.D.
Assistant Professor of Pediatrics and Medicine and Instructor of Microbiology and Immunology, and Chief, Pediatric Allergy/Immunology, Emory University School of Medicine; Chief, Pediatric Allergy, Immunology, and Pulmonary Disease, Henrietta Egleston Hospital for Children, Atlanta, Georgia
Asthma in Childhood

WILLIAM A. SMITHSON, M.D.
Assistant Professor of Pediatrics, Mayo Medical School; Consultant in Pediatric Hematology and Oncology, Mayo Cinic, Rochester, Minnesota
Acute Leukemia in Childhood

PETER J. SYNDER, M.D.
Associate Professor of Medicine, University of Pennsylvania School of Medicine; Hospital of the University of Pennsylvania, Philadelphia, Pennsylvania
Acromegaly

ARTHUR J. SOBER, M.D.
Associate Professor of Dermatology, Massachusetts General Hospital, Harvard Medical School, Boston, Massachusetts
Pigmentary Disorders

BRUNO SPECK, M.D.
Professor of Medicine and Head, Division of Hematology, Kantonsspital, University of Basel, Basel, Switzerland
Aplastic Anemia

JOHN A. SPITTELL, Jr., M.D., FACP, FACC
Mary Lowell Leary Professor of Medicine, Mayo Medical School; Consultant, Division of Cardiovascular Diseases and Internal Medicine, Mayo Clinic and Mayo Foundation, Rochester, Minnesota
Peripheral Arterial Disease

ROBERT B. STANLEY, Jr., M.D., D.D.S.
Assistant Professor, Department of Otolaryngology—Head and Neck Surgery, University of Southern California School of Medicine; Active Staff, Los Angeles County–University of Southern California Medical Center, Hollywood Presbyterian Medical Center, and Hospital of the Good Samaritan, Los Angeles, California
Sinusitis

MARTIN H. STEINBERG, M.D.
Professor of Medicine, University of Mississippi School of Medicine; Associate Chief of Staff for Research, Jackson Veterans Administration Medical Center, Jackson, Mississippi
Nonimmune Hemolytic Anemia

JAMES A. STOCKMAN, III, M.D.
Professor and Chairman, Department of Pediatrics, Northwestern University Medical School; Chairman of Medicine and Physician in Chief, Children's Memorial Hospital, Chicago, Illinois
Iron Deficiency

ORVILLE J. STONE, M.D.
Clinical Professor of Dermatology, School of Medicine, University of California, at Irvine; Attending Staff, Pacifica Hospital, Huntington Beach, California
Nail Diseases

THOMAS STOSSEL, M.D.
Professor of Medicine, Harvard Medical School; Chief, Hematology-Oncology Unit, Massachusetts General Hospital, Boston, Massachusetts
Neutropenia

ALBERT J. STUNKARD, M.D.
Professor of Psychiatry, University of Pennsylvania School of Medicine, Philadelphia, Pennsylvania
Obesity

W. P. DANIEL SU, M.D.
Associate Professor in Dermatology, Mayo Medical School; Consultant (Staff), Department of Dermatology, Mayo Clinic, Rochester, Minnesota
Dermatomyositis

KAMRAN TABADDOR, M.D.
Associate Professor of Neurosurgery, Albert Einstein College of Medicine; Director of Neurosurgery, Bronx Municipal Hospital Center; Attending, Montefiore Hospital Medical Center, Bronx, New York
Acute Head Injuries in Adults

HERBERT B. TANOWITZ, M.D.

Associate Professor of Medicine and Pathology, Albert Einstein College of Medicine; Attending Physician, Bronx Municipal Hospital Center, Hospital of the Albert Einstein College of Medicine, Bronx, New York
Echinococcosis (Hydatid Disease)

ROBERT M. TATE, M.D.

Assistant Professor of Medicine, Division of Pulmonary Sciences, University of Colorado Health Sciences Center; Denver General Hospital, Denver, Colorado
Chronic Obstructive Pulmonary Disease and Bronchiectasis

JAMES S. TAYLOR, M.D.

Head, Section of Industrial Dermatology, Cleveland Clinic Foundation, Cleveland, Ohio
Occupational Dermatoses

MAX R. TAYLOR, M.D.

Clinical Assistant Professor of Medicine, University of Mississippi Medical Center, Jackson; Attending, North Mississippi Medical Center, Tupelo, Mississippi
Granuloma Inguinale; Lymphogramuloma Venereum

BRUCE TEMPEST, M.D.

Associate Professor, Department of Medicine, University of New Mexico, Albuquerque; Chief, Internal Medicine, Gallup Indian Medical Center, Gallup, New Mexico
Plague

JOEL A. THOMPSON, M.D.

Associate Professor of Pediatrics and Neurology, University of Utah Medical Center and Primary Childrens Medical Center, Salt Lake City, Utah
Reye's Syndrome

JEROME S. TOBIS, M.D.

Professor of Physical Medicine and Rehabilitation and Director, Program of Geriatric Medicine and Gerontology, University of California, Irvine, College of Medicine; Attending, University of California, Irvine, Medical Center, Irvine, California
Rehabilitation of the Patient with Hemiplegia

JOHN W. P. TOOLE, B.Sc., M.D., FRCP(C)

Assistant Professor, Department of Pediatrics, and Assistant Professor, Department of Medicine, Faculty of Medicine, University of Manitoba; Head, Section of Dermatology, Health Science Center, Winnipeg, Manitoba, Canada
Atopic Dermatitis

PIERRE TRIOZZI, M.D.

Research Fellow, Duke University Medical Center, Durham, North Carolina
Nausea and Vomiting

DENNY L. TUFFANELLI, M.D.

Clinical Professor of Dermatology, University of California, San Francisco; Active Staff, Presbyterian Hospital and St. Francis Hospital, San Francisco, California
Lupus Erythematosus

MARWAN UWAYDAH, M.D.

Clinical Professor of Medicine and Microbiology, American University of Beirut Medical School; Head, Division of Infectious diseases, American University of Beirut Medical Center, Beirut, Lebanon
Salmonellosis (Other Than Typhoid Fever)

MARTIN D. VALENTINE, M.D.

Associate Professor of Medicine, Johns Hopkins University School of Medicine; Active Staff, Johns Hopkins Hospital and Good Sarmaritan Hospital, Baltimore, Maryland
Insect Sting Allergy

KEITH N. VAN ARSDALEN, M.D.

Assistant Professor of Surgery (Urology), University of Pennsylvania School of Medicine; Attending in Urology, Hospital of the University of Pennsylvania; Assistant Surgeon of the Hospital (Urology), Pennsylvania Hospital; Physician, Philadelphia Veterans Administration Medical Center, Philadelphia, Pennsylvania
Bacterial Infections of The Urinary Tract—Male

PAUL R. VANDERSTEEN, M.D.

Clinical Professor of Medicine and Chief, Division of Dermatology, University of North Dakota School of Medicine; Active Staff, St. Luke's Hospitals; Courtesy Staff, Dakota Hospital and St. John's Hospital; Courtesy Staff, St. Ansgar Hospital, Moorhead; Consulting Staff, Veteran's Administration Hospital and T.N.I. Hospital, Fargo, North Dakota
Pruritus

M.A. VELLA, M.Phil., MRCP

Registrar in Internal Medicine, Royal Northern Hospital, London, England
Sarcoidosis

NICHOLAS A. VICK, M.D.

Professor of Neurology, Northwestern University Medical School, Chicago; Head, Division of Neurology, the Evanston Hospital, Evanston, Illinois
Brain Tumors

JOHN J. VOORHEES, M.D.

Professor and Chairman, Department of Dermatology, University of Michigan Medical School; Chief of Service, University of Michigan Hospitals; Consultant Physician, Ann Arbor Veterans Administration Hospital and St. Joseph Mercy Hospital, Ann Arbor; Consultant Physician, Chelsea Community Hospital, Chelsea, Michigan
Papulosquamous Eruptions

THOMAS A. WADDEN, Ph.D.

Assistant Professor of Psychology in Psychiatry, University of Pennsylvania School of Medicine, Philadelphia, Pennsylvania
Obesity

GARY W. WAHL, M.D.

Assistant Professor of Medicine, University of Rochester School of Medicine; Director, Surgical Intensive Care Unit, Rochester General Hospital, Rochester, New York
Acute Respiratory Failure

LEONARD WARTOFSKY, M.D., COL, MC, USA

Professor of Medicine, Uniformed Services University of the Health Sciences, Bethesda, Maryland, and Clinical Professor of Medicine, Georgetown University, Washington, D.C.; Chief, Endocrinology Services, Walter Reed Army Medical Center, Washington, D.C.
Hyperthyroidism

ARTHUR L. WEAVER, M.D.

Clinical Associate Professor of Internal Medicine, University of Nebraska Medical School; Chief of Staff-Elect and Chair-

man, Department of Rheumatology, Bryan Memorial Hospital, Lincoln, Nebraska
Osteoarthritis

RICHARD L. WEINER, M.D.

Assistant Professor of Surgery, University of Texas Medical Branch, Galveston; Attending Neurosurgeon, John Sealy Hospital of the University of Texas Medical Branch; Consultant, St. Mary's Hospital, Galveston, and The Institute for Rehabilitation and Research, Houston, Texas
Head Injuries in Children

JOEL M. WEINSTEIN, M.D.

Assistant Professor of Ophthalmology, Neurology, and Neurosurgery, University of Wisconsin; Director, Neuro-Ophthalmology Service, University of Wisconsin Hospital and Clinics, Madison, Wisconsin
Optic Neuritis

ROBERT S. WEINSTEIN, M.D.

Associate Professor of Medicine, Medical College of Georgia; Director, Metabolic Bone Disease Laboratory, Medical College of Georgia Hospital and Clinics, Augusta, Georgia
Osteoporosis

DUANE C. WHITAKER, M.D.

Assistant Professor, Department of Dermatology, University of Iowa College of Medicine; Director, Dermatologic Surgery, University of Iowa Hospitals and Clinics, Iowa City, Iowa
Verruca Vulgaris (Warts)

MICHAEL P. WHYTE, M.D.

Assistant Professor of Medicine and Pediatrics, Washington University School of Medicine; Director, Metabolic Research Unit, Shriners Hospital for Crippled Children; Attending Physician, The Jewish Hospital of St. Louis, Barnes Hospital, and St. Louis Children's Hospital, St. Louis, Missouri
Rickets and Osteomalacia

JACK WILBERGER, M.D.

Clinical Assistant Professor of Neurosurgery, University of Pittsburgh School of Medicine; Staff, Department of Neurosurgery, Allegheny General Hospital, Pittsburgh, Pennsylvania
Trigeminal Neuralgia

FRANK C. WILSON, M.D.

Professor and Chairman, Division of Orthopaedics, University of North Carolina School of Medicine; Chief of Orthopaedics, North Carolina Memorial Hospital, Chapel Hill, North Carolina
Osteomyelitis

SAMUEL E. WILSON, M.D.

Professor of Surgery, University of California, Los Angeles, School of Medicine; Chairman, Department of Surgery, Harbor-UCLA Medical Center, Torrance, California
Bacterial Diseases of the Skin

JAMES F. WINCHESTER, M.D., FRCP

Associate Professor of Medicine, Georgetown University Medical Center; Director of Dialysis, Co-director of Transplantation and Clinical Neurology, Georgetown University Hospital, Washington, D.C.
Chronic Renal Failure

JOSEPH A. WITKOWSKI, M.D.

Clinical Professor of Dermatology, University of Pennsylvania School of Medicine; Professor of Medicine (Dermatology), Pennsylvania College of Podiatric Medicine
Parasitic Diseases

MARTIN S. WOLFE, M.D.

Clinical Professor of Medicine, George Washington University Medical School; Clinical Associate Professor of Medicine, Georgetown University Medical School; Attending Physician, George Washington University Hospital and Georgetown University Hospital; Tropical Medicine Specialist, Office of Medical Services, Department of State, Washington, D.C.
Intestinal Parasites

RICHARD J. WORLEY, M.D.

Associate Professor of Obstetrics-Gynecology; Chairman, Department of Obstetrics-Gynecology, University of Utah Health Sciences Center, Salt Lake City, Utah
Hypertensive Disorders of Pregnancy

CREIGHTON B. WRIGHT, M.D.

Professor of Clinical Surgery, University of Cincinnati College of Medicine; Clinical Professor of Surgery, Uniformed Services University of the Health Sciences, Bethesda, Maryland; Director, Vascular Surgery, The Jewish Hospital of Cincinnati; Staff, The Christ Hospital, Cincinnati, Ohio
Pleural Effusions and Empyema Thoracis

RALPH J. WYNN, M.D.

Associate Professor of Pediatrics, State University of New York at Buffalo; Attending Neonatologist, Children's Hospital of Buffalo, Buffalo, New York
Care of the High Risk Neonate

KIM B. YANCEY, M.D.

Assistant Professor, Department of Dermatology, Uniformed Services University of the Health Sciences; Consultant, Dermatology Branch, National Cancer Institute, National Institutes of Health; Consultant, Department of Dermatology, Naval Hospital, Bethesda, Maryland; Consultant, Department of Dermatology, Walter Reed Army Medical Center, Washington, D.C.
Skin Diseases of Pregnancy

EDWIN J. ZARLING, M.D., FACP

University of Illinois School of Medicine; Attending, University of Illinois at Chicago Health Sciences Center and Veterans Administration Hospital (Westside), Chicago, Illinois
Constipation

BARRY J. ZELUFF, M.D.

Clinical Assistant Professor, Baylor College of Medicine; Courtesy Staff, St. Luke's Episcopal Hospital, Houston, Texas
Bacteremia

DOUGLAS P. ZIPES, M.D.

Professor of Medicine, Indiana University School of Medicine; Senior Research Associate, Krannert Institute of Cardiology, Indiana University, Indianapolis, Indiana
Tachycardia

NOTICE

Extraordinary efforts have been made by the authors, the editors, and the publisher of this book to insure that dosage recommendations are precise and in agreement with standards officially accepted at the time of publication.

It does happen, however, that dosage schedules are changed from time to time in the light of accumulating clinical experience and continuing laboratory studies. This is most likely to occur in the case of recently introduced products.

It is urged, therefore, that you check the manufacturer's recommendations for dosage, *especially if the drug to be administered or prescribed is one that you use only infrequently or have not used for some time.*

THE PUBLISHER

Preface

This edition of Current Therapy is the 38th of an annual series first published by Howard Conn in 1949. Our objective remains the same—to provide the practicing physician with precise and useful information regarding the management of conditions most often encountered in practice. The features essential for an accurate diagnosis may be included, but emphasis is on a concise, yet detailed, discussion of therapy, focusing on specific drugs and treatment techniques.

In keeping with our long-established policy, this is a new edition rather than a revision of the old. Different contributors are selected yearly to keep the material fresh and current, thus avoiding the temptation to merely change a few words and call it new. The writers are leading investigators who have been carefully chosen to present their methods of managing the illness, devoid of extraneous material. All information has been reviewed by the contributors just before publication to ensure accuracy. Ninety per cent of the articles in this edition are by new contributors, and those carried over from the previous edition have been reviewed and brought up-to-date.

Added this year is the section on Symptomatic Care Pending Diagnosis, which includes the management of pain, nausea and vomiting, acute diarrhea, and insomnia, among others. Another new feature is the table inside the back cover listing the most commonly used laboratory studies, intended as a quick reference for the busy practitioner. The complete list of laboratory values prepared by Rex Conn, M.D., editor of *Current Diagnosis,* is presented as usual in Section 18 preceding the index.

This year there are discussions of Lyme Disease by two physicians in Lyme, Connecticut; Common Sports Injuries by the team physician at Michigan State University; Panic Disorder and Agoraphobia coauthored by the chairman of the department of psychiatry and behavioral sciences at the Medical University of South Carolina; plus snakebite and osteomyelitis. Although the majority of contributors are from the United States, as always a significant number are from other countries. I am deeply grateful to these many respected physicians for helping us maintain the high standards of this book.

I wish to thank my wife Peggy for her valuable assistance in preparing this edition and Mr. C. F. Robinson and the staff of the W. B. Saunders Company for their help and guidance. My appreciation goes also to John Strauss, M.D., for his review and wise counsel regarding the dermatology section, and to the young practicing family physicians who reviewed the book for appropriateness of content. We are determined to ensure the continuing relevance and value of this reference to practicing primary care physicians.

Robert E. Rakel, M.D.

Table of Contents

Section 1. Symptomatic Care Pending Diagnosis

Section 2. The Infectious Diseases

Section 3. The Respiratory System

Section 4. The Cardiovascular System

Section 5. The Blood and Spleen

Section 6. The Digestive System

Section 7. Metabolic Disorders

Section 8. The Endocrine System

Section 9. The Urogenital Tract

Section 10. Sexually Transmitted Diseases

Section 11. Diseases of Allergy

Section 12. Diseases of the Skin

Section 13. The Nervous System

Section 14. The Locomotor System

Section 15. Obstetrics and Gynecology

Section 16. Psychiatric Disorders

Section 17. Physical and Chemical Injuries

Section 18. Appendices and Index

Section 1

Symptomatic Care Pending Diagnosis

PAIN

method of
STEPHEN H. BUTLER, M.D.,
and COSTANTINO BENEDETTI, M.D.,
University of Washington
Seattle, Washington

Although knowledge of the physiology and psychology of pain and the pharmacokinetics of analgesics is becoming more sophisticated, treatment is often inadequate. In addition, drugs used for pain relief are a common source of conscious and unconscious abuse by patients and prescribing physicians. The source of pain and its severity should be analyzed both from nociceptive and psychologic/behavioral viewpoints. The most appropriate medication in an optimal dosage should be selected for each patient. Optimal dosage is the minimum amount, repeated at the appropriate time interval, that gives the desired therapeutic effect with a minimum of side effects.

It is important to distinguish among acute pain, pain associated with cancer, and chronic pain. The approaches to treatment for acute pain and cancer pain are similar, whereas they are significantly different for chronic pain. Narcotic analgesics in adequate doses at appropriate intervals are the primary approach to acute pain and often to cancer pain though generally contraindicated for chronic pain. Treatment must be individualized since requirements are variable. In one study of postoperative pain, a sevenfold difference in requirement was seen for the same surgery by the same surgeon.

Acute Pain

Acute pain is produced by injury, accidental or surgical, or disease states such as infection or myocardial infarction and is associated with tissue damage. The acute phase lasts days to a few weeks and therefore treatment is relatively easy to organize.

Treatment (Tables 1 and 2)

1. Strong narcotic analgesics for severe pain (morphine, meperidine [Demerol]) and weaker narcotic analgesics (codeine, propoxyphene [Darvon]) or nonsteroidal anti-inflammatory drugs (NSAIDs) (aspirin, acetaminophen, ibuprofen) for mild pain.
2. Give sufficient drug often enough according to each drug's pharmacokinetics.
3. Since anxiety is often a part of acute suffering, anxiolytics (hydroxyzine [Vistaril], promethazine [Phenergan]), which often potentiate narcotic analgesia, are useful adjuncts.
4. Tolerance (physical dependence) or addiction (psychologic dependence) is not a concern.

Newer techniques for management of acute pain may offer better control than standard oral or parenteral therapies. Intravenous demand analgesia controlled by the patient is one approach that has excellent results. Intrathecal narcotics (epidural or subarachnoid) are another promising method of pain control. Both of these, it is hoped, will aid in improving postoperative and posttraumatic pain control as familiarity leads to dissemination from the few centers that now strongly advocate them.

Pain Associated with Cancer

Approximately 65 per cent of individuals with cancer will have some pain during the course of their illness and 55 per cent of these will have severe pain at some time. Pain problems are due primarily to neural compression or invasion by tumor or to primary or metastatic tumor in bone. Pain can increase during chemotherapy, and medications may have to be increased temporarily. Significant decrease in pain may follow chemotherapy and radiation therapy. In these cases, pain medication should be reduced to avoid central depression and to decrease tolerance that

TABLE 1. **Acute Pain—Mild to Moderate**

Drug	*Route*	*Effective Duration*	*Dosage*	*Major Side Effects*
Acetaminophen (Tylenol)	oral	3–4 hrs	650 mg q 4 hr	Liver damage with high sustained doses
NSAIDs				As a group, bleeding diatheses
ASA	oral	3–4 hr	500–1000 mg q 4 hr	Allergy, GI bleeding
Indomethacin	oral	6–8 hr	25–75 mg q 6 hr initially; 25–75 mg q 8 hr maintenance	GI irritation
Ibuprofen (Motrin)	oral	3–4 hr	25–50 mg q 3–4 hr	GI irritation
Naproxen (Naprosyn)	oral	12 hr	500 mg initially; 250–750 mg bid	GI irritation
Phenylbutazone (Butazolidin)	oral	4–6 hr	100–400 mg q 4–6 hr†	Bone marrow depression, GI irrigation
Weak Narcotics				
Codeine*	oral	4–6 hr	30–120 mg q 4 hr	Constipation

DOSES OF ALL MEDICATIONS MUST BE INDIVIDUALIZED TO PATIENT WEIGHT, PATIENT RESPONSE, AND PAIN SOURCE.

*Codeine may be combined with any of the preceding for combined central and peripheral effects.

†400 mg every 4 hours exceeds the manufacturer's recommended dosage.

may interfere with the treatment of subsequent pain increases. Patients often tailor medications spontaneously if forewarned.

Treatment (Table 3)

1. Longer-acting narcotics, preferably by the oral route (morphine, sustained-release morphine, methadone) are the mainstay for severe pain. These are easily prepared in liquid form, often in combination with acetaminophen or an NSAID and a sedative/antihistaminic, hydroxyzine (Vistaril) or diphenhydramine (Dramamine) for potentiation. Careful monitoring and individual dosage adjustment are necessary for optimal treatment.

2. Mild to moderate pain will often respond to nonsteroidal anti-inflammatory medications (aspirin, ibuprofen) or less potent narcotics (codeine).

3. The drug of choice for control of pain due to bone involvement is indomethacin (Indocin). Other nonsteroidal anti-inflammatory drugs may subsequently control this pain or be more appropriate if bone pain is not severe (aspirin, ibuprofen).

4. Depression or sleep disturbance that often accompanies this problem can be treated with tricyclic antidepressants, doxepin (Sinequan, Adapin), amitriptyline (Elavil, Endep).

5. Somnolence associated with high dose narcotics can be treated with daytime doses of amphetamines (dextroamphetamine).

6. Steroids may be helpful, if there is neural

TABLE 2. **Acute Pain—Moderate to Severe**

Drug	*Route*	*Effective Duration*	*Dosage*	*Major Side Effects*
NSAIDs—See Table 1. These drugs often are useful adjuncts to the strong narcotics in more severe pain.				
Strong Narcotics				Somnolence, respiratory depression, constipation, urinary retention, pruritus, and nausea occur with all narcotics
Morphine	IM	4–5 hr	7.5–20 mg q 4 hr	
Meperidine (Demerol)	IM	3–4 hr	50–200 mg q 3–4 hr	
Hydromorphone (Dilaudid)	IM	3–4 hr	1.5–3 mg q 3 hr	
Pentazocine (Talwin)	IM	3–4 hr	30–60 mg q 3 hr	May have strong dysphoric effects. Also an agonist/antagonist and should not be used with or after other narcotics
Antihistaminics/Phenothiazines*				
Promethazine (Phenergan)	IM	4–6 hr	25–50 mg q 3–6 hr	Sedation, dry mouth, urinary retention, extrapyramidal reactions
Hydroxyzine (Vistaril)	IM	4–6 hr	25–75 mg q 3–6 hr	As above

*Given as sedatives, antiemetics, anxiolytics, and possible potentiators of narcotics.

TABLE 3. **Cancer Pain—Moderate to Severe***

Drug	*Route*	*Effective Duration*	*Dosage*	*Major Side Effects*
NSAIDs—See Table 1. These drugs are particularly important when metastatic disease in bone is present.				
Narcotics†				
Morphine	PO	3–4 hr (12 hr with sustained release form)	30–100 mg initially q 3–4 hr; increases to 300 mg prn can be well tolerated (60 mg morphine sulfate orally = 10 mg morphine sulfate IM)	Refer to Table 2 Tolerance over time is frequent. Dosage adjustment (both increases and decreases) is necessary with disease progression or regression
	IM	3–4 hr	10–30 mg usually used for acute pain stabilization	
	IV	Usually used as a constant infusion premorbidly where dose is adjusted to the patient's need		
	Suppository (when oral route is impractical)	3–4 hr	20–60 mg q 3–4 hr	
Methadone (Dolophine)	PO	Initially 4–6 hr; after 24 + hr, 6–18 hr	2.5–40 mg q 6 hr (higher doses may be necessary)	
Buprenorphine‡	Sublingual	8–12 hr	0.4–0.8 mg q 4–8 hr	
Antihistaminics—These are usually combined in oral form with morphine or methadone. See Table 2.				
Hydroxyzine (Vistaril)	PO	4–6 hr	12.5–75 mg	
Diphenydramine (Benadryl)	PO	4–6 hr	12.5–75 mg	
Amphetamines—Helpful to counteract lethargy with high dosages				
Dextroamphetamines (Dexedrine)	PO	2–4 hr	5–10 mg q AM and at noon	Agitation, excitability, palpitations, hypertension
Tricyclic Antidepressants—Helpful for bedtime sedation as well as for depression				
Amitriptyline	PO	4–12 hr (sedation)	25–200 mg q HS	Sedation, dry mouth, confusion, cardiac arrythmias, hypotension
Doxepin (Sinequan)	PO	4–12 hr (sedation)	25–200 mg q HS	As above, but less, especially cardiac

An oral preparation of constant volume (10 ml) in a masking vehicle (cherry syrup) is useful. Combining a narcotic (morphine or methadone), a sedative antihistaminic, and acetaminophen is a common preparation. This should be given in a unit dose on a time contingent basis (*not* prn but every 4–6 hr). This preparation is simpler than multiple pills at varying times and is well accepted by patients and families.

*For mild to moderate cancer pain, the information in Table 1 applies.

†For terminal care, epidermal or subarachnoid administration of narcotics by chronic catheter placement is gaining popularity and should be considered.

‡This drug is just becoming available in this country. European experience is promising, especially in those patients with swallowing difficulties.

involvement with tumor, where swelling compresses nerves centrally or peripherally.

The use of peridural or subarachnoid narcotics is gaining popularity for treatment of severe pain associated with cancer. Terminal pain may also be treated with continuous intravenous narcotic administration; however, this is rarely necessary if the aforementioned therapies are used judiciously.

Chronic Pain

Chronic pain persists past the healing time of acute injury or other disease in which there is no longer ongoing tissue damage. It is an indication of abnormal neurologic function rather than a warning from the periphery that something is wrong and needs urgent intervention. It may represent input from myofascial structures that played a part in protecting an injured area during the acute disease phase. Continuous muscle contraction, now an established reflex but no longer serving an important physiologic function, can give continuing pain.

Chronic pain is frequently augmented by psychosocial factors that are often not appreciated or attended to by the treating physician. These psychosocial factors are not usually appreciated or are emphatically denied by the patient and his or her family. This, plus unusual activation of pain pathways, makes treatment difficult. Narcotic analgesics on demand are rarely successful

TABLE 4. **Chronic Denervation Pain**

Drug	*Route*	*Effective Duration*	*Dosage*	*Major Side Effects*
Tricyclic Antidepressants*		Effect accumulates over time		
Amitriptyline (Elavil)	PO	Not related to drug half-life	25–150 mg q HS	Drowsiness, dry mouth, confusion, arrhythmias, urinary retention
Doxepin (Sinequan)	PO	Not applicable	25–150 mg q HS	Less than with amitriptyline
Imipramine (Tofranil)	PO	Not applicable	25–150 mg q AM or q HS	
Phenothiazines†				
Fluphenazine (Prolixin)	PO	Not applicable	1 mg bid initially to 2 mg tid	Tardive dyskinesia, extrapyramidal symptoms
Perphenazine (Trilafon)	PO	Not applicable	2 mg bid initially to 4 mg tid	As above
Antiseizure Agents‡				
Carbamazepine (Tegretol)	PO	12–17 hr	100 mg bid to 1600 mg/day by increments of 200 mg/day	Dizziness, GI upset, blurred vision, hepatic dysfunction, bone marrow depression
Phenytoin (Dilantin)	PO	7–42 hr	100 to 200 mg bid	Ataxia, confusion, dyskinesia, GI upset, rash, bone marrow depression

*Doses should be increased from 25 mg slowly, as the therapeutic dose for denervation is often much below 150 mg, the minimal antidepressant dose.

†These two classes of medications are often given together. Trials of medications should be over a minimun of 4 weeks as the effects are not seen except with prolonged administration.

‡These medications need to be tried over several days, as slow accumulation in body tissue occurs. Generally a 2 to 3 week trial will suffice.

and are relatively contraindicated. Pharmacologic interventions can help relieve the problem or can be directed at the side effects.

Treatment

1. Narcotics are generally contraindicated in chronic pain syndromes.
2. Narcotic tolerance or addiction is a significant risk. (In some cases, a low dose time-contingent narcotic may control the symptoms, as in arthritis osteoporosis. These patients are somewhat difficult to identify.)
3. Where nerve damage is present, as in posttraumatic denervation, postherpetic neuralgia, or peripheral neuropathy, a wide variety of nonanalgesic medications has been useful. These include the antiseizure medications (carbamazepine [Tegretol], phenytoin [Dilantin]), the tricyclic antidepressants (amitriptyline [Elavil], doxepin [Sinequan], imipramine [Tofranil]), the phenothiazines (fluphenazine [Prolixin], perphenazine [Trilafon]), and others. Often medications from two categories are used in combination. See Table 4.
4. Treatment of depression frequently associated with chronic pain is imperative and can be done using the tricyclic antidepressants amitriptyline (Elavil), doxepin (Sinequan), imipramine (Tofranil), or the new agents trazadone (Desyrel), maprotiline (Ludiomil). If standard treatment regimens fail to decrease pain significantly within 6 months, patients should be referred to experienced professionals in pain clinics.

Nonpharmacologic Treatments

Physical reactivation is perhaps the most important treatment modality available for the majority of chronic pain problems. Individuals suffering chronic pain tend to be deactivated and significantly deconditioned. Active physiotherapy that involves both stretching and strengthening exercises plus aerobic training is the most effective combination for treating refractory chronic pain problems. Initially this form of therapy may be aided by passive physiotherapy (heat, ultrasound), by use of transcutaneous electrical stimulation, and occasionally by nerve block therapies.

Various forms of behavioral therapy are extremely important for the patient and family to change living patterns that encourage ill health. These range from counseling by a family physician to inpatient programs run by a team of physicians and psychologists.

Electromyographic or temperature biofeedback modalities can aid in treatment of many chronic pain syndromes.

NAUSEA AND VOMITING

method of
PIERRE TRIOZZI, M.D.,
and JOHN LASZLO, M.D.
Duke University
Durham, North Carolina

Teleologically we can think of vomiting as a protective mechanism to rid the body of accidentally ingested poisons or excessive food. More frequently, however, vomiting occurs as a symptom of disease—not only disease of the gastrointestinal tract but also of other organ systems. With the development of new methods of travel, including space travel, and of new methods of therapy, cancer chemotherapy in particular, vomiting also occurs commonly as a side effect.

The generic problem referred to as "vomiting" can be considered in three parts: nausea, retching, and emesis. We tend to think of these as stages of the same process when, in fact, this is not an accurate representation. Nausea, retching, and emesis can occur independently or in a number of combinations. A good deal is known about the physiology of vomiting and retching, but very little is known about the physiology of nausea. From animal studies we are aware of two distinct centers in the medulla that are responsible for coordinating the complicated vomiting process—the vomiting center (VC) and the chemoreceptor trigger zone (CTZ). The VC controls the actual act of emesis through somatic and visceral efferents. The CTZ is incapable of mediating the act of vomiting without an intact VC and is stimulated by drugs and toxins circulating in the blood or spinal fluid.

Prolonged vomiting can lead to dehydration and loss of gastric secretion, which in turn causes hypokalemia and metabolic alkalosis. Esophageal tears (Mallory-Weiss syndrome), esophageal rupture (Boerhaave's syndrome), pathologic fractures, and wound dehiscence can occur with severe retching and emesis. Aspiration pneumonia is a particularly worrisome complication when central nervous system depression is present, as in diabetic coma or drug overdose. In patients receiving cancer chemotherapy, vomiting can lead to suspension of potentially curative therapy. For example, young men with potentially curable metastatic testicular cancer sometimes discontinue their treatment program if the nausea and vomiting problems are not adequately managed.

Treatment

General medical management of most patients with vomiting consists of treating dehydration and electrolyte imbalance and preventing complications. Intravenous fluid therapy is often necessary. Normal saline alone is usually sufficient, but potassium chloride should be added when hypokalemia is present. When the vomiting abates, small feedings with dry bland foods are often best tolerated. Hot beverages like tea and broths and cold beverages, particularly carbonated beverages, are often well tolerated. Bedridden vomiting patients should be turned on their sides and placed with their heads at the edge of a pillow to prevent aspiration and to facilitate drainage from the mouth. The patient may need to be suctioned to prevent aspirating vomitus. Splinting an abdominal wound with a pillow can help relieve the strain on a wound in the postoperative patient.

Whenever possible, the specific underlying medical condition should be treated. For example, tube decompression and surgical intervention may be required for patients with gastric outlet obstruction; protein restriction and dialysis should be considered in patients with uremia; and corticosteroids should be administered to patients with adrenal crisis and those with increased intracranial pressure. Drug-induced vomiting requires a reduction in dosage of the medication or a change to lesser offenders. Vomiting on occasion may have a psychogenic basis, as anorexia nervosa or bulimia, and definitive psychotherapy may be necessary.

When the cause of vomiting cannot be ascertained, when specific therapy for the cause is not available (e.g., gastroenteritis), or when vomiting is a predictable consequence of necessary therapy (e.g., cancer chemotherapy), it is often necessary to administer an antiemetic drug or a combination of antiemetics to interrupt the process, relieve symptoms, and prevent complications (Table 1). The mechanism of action of antiemetic drugs is not entirely clear, and a given antiemetic drug may have more than one effect on the vomiting process. Some drugs apparently depress sensitivity of the CTZ (phenothiazines, butyrophenones, trimethobenzamide [Tigan], and metoclopramide [Reglan]) or of the VC (antihistamines, scopolamine [Transderm-Scōp] and phenothazines). Some can block stimuli to the VC and CTZ from the cerebral cortex (cannabinoids, sedatives, and antihistamines), vestibular apparatus (antihistamines), and the gastrointestinal tract (metoclopramide [Reglan]). The selection of a particular antiemetic depends upon the etiology and mechanism of the vomiting, the potential toxicity of the antiemetic, the familiarity of the physician with the antiemetic, and whether antiemetic therapy is to take place in the hospital or in an outpatient setting. No one antiemetic is effective or safe in all situations.

Because the VC is influenced by higher brain centers, there are important psychologic considerations in the management of vomiting. Care must be taken to minimize those psychologic factors that may make nausea and vomiting more prominent. Conversely, sufficient mental distraction, for example, may inhibit motion sickness. Behavioral therapy has been useful in the treat-

TABLE 1. **Antiemetic Drugs**

Drug Name (Commercial Name[s])	*Dosage Regimen*
Phenothiazines	
Chlorpromazine (Thorazine)	10 to 25 mg orally every 4 to 6 hours, *or* 25 mg intramuscularly every 4 to 6 hours, *or* 100 mg rectally every 6 to 8 hours
Prochlorperazine (Compazine)	5 to 10 mg orally or intramuscularly, 3 to 4 times daily (limit 40 mg a day), *or* 25 mg rectally twice daily
Thiethylperazine (Torecan)	10 mg orally, 1 to 3 times daily; *or* intramuscularly, 2 ml, up to 3 times a day; *or* 10 mg rectally 1 to 3 times daily
Promethazine (Phenergan)	25 mg orally, rectally, or intramuscularly every 4 to 6 hours
Perphenazine (Trilafon)	8 to 16 mg orally daily in divided doses or 5 mg intramuscularly
Antihistamines	
Dimenhydrinate (Dramamine)	50 mg orally, intramuscularly, or intravenously every 4 to 6 hours
Buclizine (Bucladin-S Softab)	50 mg orally every 4 to 6 hours
Meclizine (Antivert, Bonine)	25 to 50 mg orally every 4 to 6 hours
Cyclizine (Marezine)	50 mg orally or intramuscularly every 4 to 6 hours
Hydroxyzine (Atarax, Vistaril)	25 to 100 mg orally or intramuscularly 3 to 4 times daily
Butyrophenones	
Haloperidol (Haldol)	1 to 2 mg orally or intramuscularly 3 times daily
Droperidol (Inapsine)	0.5 to 1.5 mg intravenously every 4 hours
Miscellaneous	
Trimethobenzamide (Tigan)	250 mg orally or 200 mg intramuscularly 4 times a day *or* 200 mg rectally every 6 hours
Benzquinamide (Emete-con)	50 mg intramuscularly (may be repeated in 1 hour), then every 3 to 4 hours; *or* 25 mg intravenously (1 ml per minute) initially with subsequent doses intramuscularly
Diphenidol (Vontrol)	25 to 50 mg orally every 4 hours
Scopolamine (Transderm-Scōp)	1 pad postauricularly every 3 days
Metoclopramide (Reglan)	10 mg orally 3 to 4 times daily; "high dose" for emetogenic chemotherapy—1 to 2 mg per kg intravenously, 30 minutes before and 1.5 and 3.5 hours after chemotherapy
Phosphorated carbohydrates (Emetrol)	1 to 2 tablespoons every 3 hours
Investigational Agents	
Tetrahydrocannabinol (THC)	5 to 7.5 mg per M^2 every 4 to 6 hours starting 8 to 12 hours before chemotherapy
High dose methylprednisolone (Solu-Medrol)	250 mg intravenously every 6 hours starting 2 hours before chemotherapy for 4 doses

ment of chemotherapy-induced vomiting, especially anticipatory vomiting.

Motion Sickness

Motion sickness results from stimulation of the vestibular apparatus of the ear. The stimulus is transmitted through the CTZ to the VC with relays to the cerebral cortex. Antihistamines are especially useful in vomiting related to motion sickness as well as to other vestibular disturbances. Their effectiveness is thought to be due to their anticholinergic properties. Although phenothiazines have some anticholinergic effects, they generally are ineffective in the treatment of motion sickness. Antiemetic therapy with antihistamines such as dimenhydrinate (Dramamine), meclizine (Antivert, Bonine), buclizine (Bucladin-S Softab), and cyclizine (Marezine) should be started 30 to 60 minutes prior to the activity that is likely to produce motion sickness, because therapy given after vomiting has begun will not abort the attack nor alleviate further episodes. (Indeed, oral medications are difficult to keep down after any kind of vomiting.)

Individuals may vary in their responsiveness to various antihistamines, and a change in dosage or a change to another antihistamine can be tried if one is ineffective. The anticholinergic agent scopolamine (Transderm-Scōp), applied transdermally at least 4 hours prior to exposure, is useful for patients who fail to respond to antihistamines. The efficacy of scopolamine is highly variable; it seems particularly effective in space travel. Subsequent use may not always be effective, and undesirable anticholinergic effects also may occur.

Certain other measures also reduce the risk of vomiting in susceptible individuals. The dietary intake prior to and during exposure should be prudent, and reassurance and diversions may be helpful. The severity of motion sickness may be diminished by lying down or tilting the head back and supporting it in a stationary position to reduce the vestibular stimulation. Looking at the sky or at the wall of the vehicle will lessen rhythmic visual stimulation from a moving horizon.

Patients usually develop tolerance to motion after prolonged exposure and therefore only short-term treatment is usually needed. If the patient continues to suffer, further evaluation for other causes should be instituted.

Chemotherapy-Induced Vomiting

Vomiting is a serious and occasionally dose-limiting toxicity of cancer chemotherapy. Management involves not only various pharmacologic agents but also emotional support and, in some instances, behavioral therapy. Maintenance of hydration is important since dehydration can compound the nephrotoxic effects of many chemotherapeutic agents. When managing chemotherapy-induced vomiting, one should not assume that the vomiting is due entirely to the chemotherapy. Excessive vomiting following the course of chemotherapy suggests the possibility of alternative medical or psychologic causes.

Different chemotherapeutic drugs act by different mechanisms in producing vomiting. Some clearly act on the CTZ; some on the VC; and others directly by interfering with intestinal motility with or without additional central nervous system effects. Chemotherapeutic drugs vary in emetic potential, and this is an important consideration when selecting an antiemetic (Table 2). Dosage of the chemotherapeutic drug is also important. For example, vomiting produced by low doses of cisplatin may be prevented with moderately potent antiemetics, whereas the control of vomiting secondary to high doses of cisplatin is much more difficult. In addition, a chemotherapeutic agent alone may be only mildly emetogenic but may become strongly emetogenic in combination with other agents. Combinations of highly emetogenic agents, including cisplatin, doxorubicin, cyclophosphamide, or dacarbazine, are commonly employed in various anticancer programs.

Phenothiazines have been the mainstay of antiemetic therapy and have the advantage of being available in oral, parenteral, and rectal forms. They are effective against mildly to moderately emetogenic chemotherapeutic programs but are of limited efficacy when used with strongly emetogenic drugs. All phenothiazines tested in controlled trials appear to have similar efficacy, and the choice, therefore, for initial antiemetic therapy is determined by the relative potential for side effects and by the familiarity of the physician. Side effects of significant consequence include sedation, hypotension, and extrapyramidal effects. (Sedation is common to most antiemetics and is not necessarily undesirable unless the patient wishes to operate a motor vehicle.) Jaundice, blood dyscrasia, and photosensitivity are infrequent and are seen primarily with chronic administration. However, aplastic anemia, though rare, may be an irreversible complication. Chlorpromazine (Thorazine) causes the highest incidence of sedation and hypotension, although tolerance appears to develop to these side effects. Promethazine (Phenergan) also commonly causes sedation and hypotension. Extrapyramidal effects occur most often with perphenazine (Trilafon) and frequently with triethylperazine (Torecan) and prochloperazine (Compazine). These agents, however, cause less sedation and hypotension.

Antiemetic therapy with phenothiazines for mildly to moderately emetogenic chemotherapy programs should begin 8 to 12 hours before chemotherapy is administered. This is continued as long as the patient has nausea and vomiting. If the phenothiazine is effective initially, it usually continues to be effective for subsequent courses, although dosages may have to be adjusted to maintain control. Alternative initial therapy for mildly to moderately emetogenic programs includes trimethobenzamide (Tigan), which may be more effective as an antinauseant than as an antiemetic, and benzquinamide (Emete-Con), which can only be administered parenterally. These agents lack the sedative, hypotensive, and extrapyramidal effects of phenothiazines.

Strongly emetogenic chemotherapy programs containing cisplatin are best controlled with high doses of metoclopramide (Reglan) infused intravenously prior to and after cisplatin is administered; it can be given orally for 24 hours afterward. Extrapyramidal side effects may be encountered, particularly in young patients, which should be anticipated by simultaneous use of diphenhydramine (Benadryl). The occurrence of side effects does not affect the use of metoclopramide, since lower doses or administration with prophylactic diphenhydramine can eliminate this problem. Care should be taken to avoid the combined used of phenothiazines, butyrophenones,

TABLE 2. **Emetic Potential of Chemotherapeutic Drugs***

Worst	Moderate	Least
Cisplatin	Nitrosoureas	Vincristine
Dacarbazine	Procarbazine	Vinblastine
Mechlorethamine	Mitomycin–C	Bleomycin
Doxorubicin		6-Mercaptopurine
Cyclophosphamide		Cytarabine

*Potency based on usual doses.

and metoclopramide, as the risk of extrapyramidal reactions is increased. This caution does not pertain to combined usage with steroids.

Butyrophenones, cannabinoids, and high doses of corticosteroids are therapeutic options for the patient receiving strongly emetogenic, noncisplatin-containing chemotherapy or for the patient refractory to phenothiazines. Butyrophenones such as haloperidol (Haldol) and droperidol (Inapsine) are thought to be more effective than phenothiazines in many instances of chemotherapy-induced vomiting. The frequency of extrapyramidal reactions and hypotension may be less with butyrophenones than with many phenothiazines, but sedation, agitation, and motor restlessness do occur. Cannabinoids such as tetrahydrocannabinol (THC) are very good antiemetic agents for chemotherapeutics other than cisplatin. Side effects include a "high" and sedation but also include dysphoric reactions and hypotension. Presently tetrahydrocannabinol (THC) is available at special hospital-approved pharmacies only. Since cannabinoids are not yet commercially available in the United States (FDA approval is expected for tetrahydrocannabinol and the synthetic cannabinoid nabilone), they should be used only in an experimental setting for younger patients who do not have cardiovascular or psychiatric disorders and who are refractory to other emetics.

High doses of corticosteroids, such as methylprednisolone (Solu-Medrol), have been shown to have antiemetic properties. The mechanism of this antiemetic effect is unknown; it may involve inhibiting the release of prostaglandins, which are stimulated by the direct gastrointestinal toxicity of chemotherapy. Potential complications of high dose corticosteroids include their metabolic and immunosuppressive effects, interactions with chemotherapeutic agents, and the possible enhancement of tumor growth. Other than for the patient with unstable diabetes, these are more theoretic than real when only short courses are given. Combining high doses of corticosteroids with other antiemetic medications such as metoclopramide (Reglan) appears to add antiemetic effectiveness. The use of high doses of corticosteroids in antiemetic therapy is currently investigational.

Benzquinamide (Emete-con) and diphenidol (Vontrol) are antiemetics that can be used as second line agents for patients receiving strongly emetogenic chemotherapy programs and in patients refractory to other antiemetics. High doses of metoclopramide (Reglan) may also be effective in these situations for noncisplatin-containing regimens. Sedation with benzodiazepines or with short-acting barbiturates is often beneficial, and patients appreciate their anxiolytic effects. Care must be taken to prevent aspiration. (If, however, patients are able to fall asleep they will not vomit because vomiting requires a wakeful state.) Antihistamines as a class are not useful in chemotherapy-induced vomiting except for their sedative properties. There is some rationale for combining antiemetics that work in different sites and have different mechanisms of action when treating refractory patients or patients receiving strongly emetogenic chemotherapy. Behavioral therapies such as systematic desensitization, the use of relaxation tapes, biofeedback, and hypnosis appear to be effective in some cases, nor are they mutually exclusive with pharmacologic agents.

Many patients experience anticipatory vomiting upon receiving repeated courses of chemotherapy, a phenomenon that is probably a classically conditioned reflex. There is no pharmacologic treatment for anticipatory vomiting at present, and all efforts should be directed toward prevention. Adequate control of vomiting with the initial exposure to chemotherapy is important. Pleasant surroundings, free of odors, with some distractions like television are desirable when administering chemotherapy. Hard candy can temper the taste of a chemotherapeutic agent like cyclophosphamide. Behavioral therapies may be of help in treating anticipatory vomiting.

Vomiting of Early Pregnancy

The cause of vomiting of early pregnancy, or morning sickness, is not known. Increased estrogen levels may initiate vomiting via stimulation of the CTZ, and decreased gastric tone and decreased hydrochloric acid release may contribute. Neurologic and psychologic factors also have been implicated in the etiology. Morning sickness is usually benign and self-limiting, though it may be quite distressing, and psychologic support is the most important aspect of therapy. Avoidance of certain unpalatable foods or unpleasant odors may be sufficient therapy, as may a change to repeated small meals rich in carbohydrates with adequate fluid intake. Antiemetic therapy is desirable if vomiting is severe and incapacitating, or if the patient is losing weight and progressing to malnutrition. At this point the potential benefits of antiemetic therapy outweigh the risk to both the fetus and the mother.

Indeed, antiemetics used to be prescribed regularly, but there is now great reluctance to do so because of the widely held belief that any drug prescribed during the first trimester of pregnancy is potentially teratogenic. Although antihistamines and trimethobenzamide (Tigan) have been used extensively and have not been shown conclusively to be teratogenic, currently no antiemetic is available that is approved by the Food and Drug Administration for use during pregnancy. It is important that the patient be informed of the possibility of congenital malformation, even if the risk is very low. The safest agents are probably dimenhydrinate (Dramamine) and trimethobenzamide (Tigan). Pyridoxine has been proposed to be a safe and effective agent, although there is no good clinical or laboratory evidence to support its use. Women with severe nausea and vomiting who do not respond to antihistamines should receive one of the phenothiazines; because of jaundice, chlorpromazine (Thorazine) is probably less desirable than others. Teratogenicity does not appear to be a major problem with phenothiazines, possibly because they are seldom used in the first trimester.

Hospitalization should be considered in refractory cases; removal from the home environment may be therapeutic, and fluid and electrolyte abnormalities are often present. Vomiting in early pregnancy must be distinguished from the intractable vomiting of hyperemesis gravidarum, which requires aggressive medical therapy. Aggravating conditions such as gastroenteritis, cholecystitis, ulcerative colitis, urinary tract infection, and bowel obstruction may be present and require specific therapy.

Postoperative Vomiting

The nature and duration of the surgery, use of preoperative medication, and the choice of anesthetic all influence the mechanism as well as the incidence and severity of postoperative nausea and vomiting. Because the incidence is minimal and because of the risk of adverse effects, routine prophylactic treatment is not indicated and should be reserved for selected patients.

When vomiting is likely to occur postoperatively because of the nature of the surgery, a nasogastric tube is inserted beforehand and remains in place throughout the postoperative period. When vomiting does occur in the postoperative period and antiemetics are not contraindicated, antihistamines such as cyclizine (Marezine) or phenothiazines such as triethylperazine (Torecan), prochlorperazine (Compazine), or chlorpromazine (Thorazine) can be used. Phenothiazines may cause central nervous system and respiratory depression when they are used alone or in combination with other medications, particularly narcotics, which are often used in the postoperative period. The same can be said of butyrophenones, which have also been shown to be effective in the reduction of postoperative vomiting. Benzquinamide (Emete-con) may be preferred in some instances because it does not cause the central nervous system or respiratory depression that phenothiazines or butyrophenones do, nor does it cause extrapyramidal effects or hypotension. Metoclopramide (Reglan) has also been shown to have efficacy with postoperative vomiting, although results of clinical trials vary. Mild sedation with benzodiazepines or barbiturates may also be useful if not contraindicated.

Gastroenteritis

Vomiting associated with viral gatroenteritis can usually be treated with dietary manipulations. Phosphorated carbohydrate (Emetrol) may be of benefit and supposedly relieves nausea and vomiting by direct, local reduction in smooth muscle contraction of the wall of the gastrointestinal tract. Antihistamines such as dimenhydrinate (Dramamine), meclizine (Antivert, Bonine) or cyclizine (Marezine) may be required. Phenothiazines, such as triethylperazine (Torecan) or prochlorperazine (Compazine), and benzquinamide (Emete-con) should be considered if the vomiting is severe. Bismuth subsalicylate (Pepto-Bismol) therapy may help nausea but has not been found to be effective in reducing vomiting.

Narcotic-Induced Vomiting

Morphine and its analogues induce nausea and vomiting by stimulating the CTZ but also can inhibit vomiting by suppressing the VC. Curiously, morphine, which frequently causes vomiting, has shown the greatest promise of inhibiting all forms of vomiting. The severity of nausea and vomiting is directly related to dose, but once therapeutic levels are reached suppression of the VC can predominate, and nausea and vomiting can be inhibited. For this reason, narcotics rarely continue to produce nausea and vomiting after the first 3 or 4 days of regular use, but they can continue to produce nausea and vomiting if taken sporadically. In addition to stimulating the CTZ, narcotics also can increase the sensitivity of the VC to vestibular stimulation. Vomiting is thus more common in patients taking narcotics who are ambulatory than in those who are recumbent. Narcotics also affect the vomiting process by decreasing gastric motility and prolonging emptying time.

Because of the manner in which narcotics affect the vomiting process, it is desirable to restrict doses to the minimum necessary and to administer them on a regular schedule. Since vomiting may be related to the particular narcotic, it is often beneficial to try another if the patient experiences vomiting. Antihistamines such as meclizine (Antivert, Bonine) or cyclizine (Marezine) may be tried along with bed rest since there may be a vestibular component. Benzquinamide (Emete-con) and phenothiazines are effective and can be administered if other measures fail. Phenothiazines can potentiate narcotic-induced central nervous system and respiratory depression, and benzquinamide, therefore, may be preferable.

GASEOUSNESS AND INDIGESTION

method of
CHARLES L. KRONE, M.D.
University of Arizona
Tucson, Arizona

Conditioned by television commericals and folk medicine, patients will use such terms as "gas" and "indigestion" in an imprecise and often misleading manner. It is critical for the physician to delineate what the patient is actually experiencing, for many organic diseases can cause gaseousness and indigestion. It is assumed that these have been ruled out and only conditions caused by disturbances in function are discussed here. Successful management requires establishment of patient rapport and confidence, maximizing the placebo effect nurtured by the physician's supportive role, and treatment that restores normal gastrointestinal function. Many patients will manifest significant depression, anxiety, or other emotional disorder, but it should not be assumed that gaseousness and indigestion are primarily psychoneurotic in origin.

Indigestion

Indigestion is commonly used interchangeably with dyspepsia, but it is obvious that these terms have no uniform meaning. Patients often describe epigastric fullness or discomfort that usually occurs after meals. Textbook definitions suggest that indigestion represents an abnormal awareness of digestive-alimentary function, but such definitions are relatively meaningless. Further confusion is added by the recently popularized category of endoscopic-negative dyspepsia which suggests that patients with no mucosal abnormality found at direct inspection comprise some distinct group. A substantial number of patients with dyspepsia will have evidence of acid-peptic disease, for example reflux esophagitis, ulcer, or gastritis at endoscopy. However, others with unremarkable-appearing mucosa will respond to antacid or H_2 histamine receptor blocker therapy. Perhaps a more subtle manifestation of acid-peptic disease accounts for the success of over-the-counter antacids.

There remains a large group of patients unresponsive to antacid therapy. Their underlying problem is slow stomach motility, particularly in the antropyloric region, with increased contractions and delayed passage of food into the duodenum. There may be diminished gastric distensibility, duodenal spasm, and bile regurgitation. There often is an overlapping of symptoms, with some patients having a more typical irritable colon syndrome. Forceful gastrocolic reflex can mimic indigestion, although this is usually associated with disordered bowel action. In all likelihood the upper and lower gastrointestinal disturbances are simply variations of a common motility disorder.

Treatment

The foremost aspect of treatment is explanation and reassurance that there is no serious organic disease. Encouraging more relaxed and slower meals, avoiding rich, fatty foods and excessive alcohol, and eliminating irritating drugs may be helpful. Anticholinergics have long been used to treat indigestion, but there is little convincing evidence of their effectiveness. The delayed gastric emptying produced by anticholinergics could aggravate patients' distress. The effectiveness observed might be due to placebo response.

Recently, results of controlled studies have indicated effectiveness of the dopamine receptor antagonists metoclopramine (Reglan) and domperidone (Motilium). (The latter is not yet approved for use in the United States.) Metoclopramide blocks central dopaminergic receptors, enhances peripheral cholinergic activity, and modifies the motor activity of the digestive tract, accentuating the phasic activity of the antrum, relaxing the pyloric sphincter and duodenum. Gastric emptying is enhanced by improving the transit of food into the duodenum and diminishing bile regurgitation. Domperidone primarily inhibits peripheral dopaminergic receptors and avoids the risk of dystonic reactions which occur in 2 to 5 per cent of patients taking metoclopramide. The starting dosage for both is 10 mg before meals. Anticholinergic drugs antagonize the effect of metoclopramide, so the two should not be used simultaneously.

There is no evidence for the effectiveness of simethicone or pancreatic and bile acid combination tablets though they are often used as placebos. Tranquilizers should not be routinely prescribed, as there is no evidence of their effectiveness in improving motility. However, significant anxiety and depression should be managed appropriately.

Gaseousness

Symptoms of indigestion and gaseousness overlap. However, there are three more or less distinguishable gaseous conditions: excessive belching, abdominal bloat, and excessive passage of flatus, which it is useful to consider separately. Patients may manifest more than one of these symptoms, but it is helpful to consider therapy according to their separate origins.

Excessive Belching

Repetitive belching is caused by air swallowed or aspirated into the esophagus then explosively expelled before reaching the stomach. Some residual air may enter the stomach; with repetitive belching this slowly builds up, causing gastric distention and stimulating more belching. The primary cause is often emotional, and correction is through education, behavior modification, and relief of anxiety. It is imperative to rule out the multiple organic diseases that can trigger excessive belching. Less dramatic postprandial belching caused by simple aerophagia or excessive carbon dioxide production during fat digestion is managed by encouraging slower, more relaxed eating habits and eliminating carbonated beverages, chewing gum, use of straws, smoking, and rich, fatty foods.

Bloating

Patients will complain of having too much gas, abdominal distention, and borborygmi. However, when studies are made, no evidence of more than the normal 150 to 200 ml of intestinal gas can be identified in these patients. Indeed, the problem is not that of too much gas but increased smooth muscle tone. Patients are usually sensitive to insufflation of air into the gut and experience discomfort even when gas volume is normal. This condition is essentially a variation of the irritable bowel syndrome and is treated similarly with reassurance, relief of anxiety, and treatment of depression.

Anticholinergic drugs have variable results. Some patients respond adequately, but constipation and other side effects often compromise therapy. Bulking agents, such as psyllium hydrophilic mucilloids, polycarbophil, and unprocessed bran, are helpful. However, patients initially may complain of increased bloat until gut transit is substantially improved. Correction of constipation, avoidance of excessive gas-producing foods, (discussed next), and general measures such as exercise, use of a heating pad, warm bath, peppermint carminatives, drinking hot water, or tap water enema, may be helpful in some patients. Simethicone, pancreatic enzyme-bile preparations, and charcoal are of no value. Recently, metoclopramide has had demonstrated success but I believe it is more useful in treating gastroduodenal dysmotility then abdominal bloating of lower gut origin.

Excessive Passage of Flatus

Most of the gas passed from the anus is carbon dioxide and hydrogen produced by bacterial metabolism of unabsorbed carbohydrates in the colon. Patients who pass excessive flatus have increased amounts of fermentable substance in the colon as a result of incomplete absorption of ingested foods. Constipation may aggravate the problem by allowing more prolonged contact with bacteria in the colonic lumen. The ingestion of legumes, particularly beans, containing undigestible disaccharides, produces universal flatulence. Ingestion of milk products by lactase-deficient individuals produces the same effect. Less commonly appreciated is the fact that partial malabsorption of the flour of wheat, oats, corn, and potato is prevalent in the otherwise normal population. Reduction of dietary intake of foods containing flour will significantly decrease flatus. Rice flour is an exception, being universally tolerated as a nongas producer. Other foods—cabbage, Brussels sprouts, peas, raw onions, and certain fruits containing pectin, such as apples, pears, peaches, and melons—are high gas producers. Unprocessed miller's bran does not contribute significantly to gas production, but finely processed bran is highly fermentable. Other low gas-producing foods that are well tolerated are bananas, citrus fruits, grapes, hard cheese, meats, eggs, and peanut butter.

Many patients will benefit from trial and error elimination of high gas producers from the diet. The use of antibiotics to alter colonic bacterial flora is ineffective and may cause serious bacterial overgrowth. Activated charcoal has been advocated but I have not found it useful. Control of constipation with bulking agents is important. Although early treatment may increase gaseousness, once improved colonic transit is achieved gas production will diminish.

The management of gaseousness and indigestion is a major challenge to the clinician. Symptoms are difficult to interpret; serious organic disease will appear disguised as more benign, but persistent, functional disorders. These must be excluded, but lingering doubts bedevil the earnest physician. Psychiatric overlay is often severe and must be alleviated before gastrointestinal symptoms can be corrected. Lastly, it is difficult if not impossible with our present limitations in knowledge to separate the effect of placebo from the physiologic action of our therapy. Adequately controlled studies are very difficult to perform and self-deception is pervasive. It is important to steer our patients away from unnecessarily expensive or hazardous medications or needless limitations in behavior and life style if there is no demonstrable physiologic benefit from such therapy.

ACUTE INFECTIOUS DIARRHEA

method of
MARTIN J. BLASER, M.D.
University of Colorado
Denver, Colorado

Acute infectious diarrhea is a common problem in all parts of the world. A wide variety of viral, bacterial, and parasitic agents is responsible for the frequency of the complaint of acute diarrhea. Although these infections often are self-limiting, they are second only to acute respiratory infections as the leading infectious causes for patients' seeking medical attention. For the physician, making the proper diagnosis is often the key to correct management of acute infectious diarrhea.

Acute food poisoning refers to those illnesses that occur within 24 hours of ingesting contaminated food. The disease usually occurs several hours after ingestion of a noxious chemical or preformed bacterial toxin; ingestion of live microorganisms is not necessary. The most common pathogens are toxin-producing strains of *Staphylococcus aureus, Clostridium perfringens,* and *Bacillus cereus.* Either vomiting or diarrhea may predominate, and acute prostration, headache, and myalgias are common. Since symptoms usually last less than 24 hours, no specific diagnosis is needed and therapy is supportive.

Acute diarrheal illness usually implies watery diarrhea lasting more than 24 hours. Such illnesses commonly are caused by viable microorganisms that secrete toxins or invade host tissues. Strains of *Escherichia coli* that elaborate enterotoxins are the most common causes of traveler's diarrhea. The toxin of *Vibrio cholerae* causes cholera, in which affected persons may deplete their entire fluid volume within 24 hours. Viral infections may be endemic, such as those caused by the rotaviruses, affecting young children primarily, or may be epidemic and waterborne, such as those caused by the Norwalk virus and related agents or adenoviruses. *Cryptosporidium,* a protozoan, may cause symptoms resembling viral gastroenteritis. *Giardia lamblia,* a ubiquitous protozoan, causes an acute or subacute syndrome of watery diarrhea often associated with abdominal cramps, nausea, weight loss, and flatulence, but constitutional symptoms are usually minimal or absent.

The acute onset of *bloody diarrhea* with or without fever is called dysentery, most commonly caused by *Campylobacter jejuni, Shigella, Salmonella, Yersinia enterocolitica,* and *Clostridium difficile.* Less frequent causes include enteroinvasive or enteropathogenic strains of *E. coli, Aeromonas, Plesiomonas,* non-01 strains of *V. cholerae,* and *V. parahaemolyticus.* Constitutional symptoms are usually prominent. High fever in a septic-appearing patient represents the most severe end of the clinical spectrum. These infections cannot be distinguished from one another on the basis of clinical features; diagnosis must be based on the identification of the causative agent. It is important to remember that these same agents also may cause watery diarrhea in less severe infections.

Based on these diagnostic considerations, appropriate laboratory procedures to isolate or identify causative agents can be done. In most cases, however, the cost of the necessary laboratory tests outweighs the benefits of obtaining a specific diagnosis. Exceptions to that policy include patients with febrile, bloody, or prolonged diarrhea or those in whom leukocytes are found to be present on direct fecal smear. In such patients, fecal culture and examination of stools for pathogenic protozoa, *C. difficile* toxin, and vibrio forms on Gram stain are indicated.

Supportive Measures

The major cause of death from the diarrheal illness is dehydration leading to hypovolemic shock; therefore, the foremost treatment principle is fluid and electrolyte replacement. Regardless of suspected etiology, the volume status of the patient should be monitored closely. Obtaining standing and supine blood pressure and pulse determinations is a sensitive way to detect hypovolemia. For the critically ill or those vomiting, parenteral fluids such as 5 per cent dextrose with normal or half-normal saline with 20 to 30 mEq of potassium added are most useful. At the time of presentation, patients with severe diarrheal illnesses such as cholera may be depleted by up to 20 per cent of their body weight and may require liters of fluid to replace their stood volume. Diarrheal illness of that severity is rare in the United States.

For persons with milder volume depletion (5 to 10 per cent), oral rehydration solutions containing glucose and electrolytes are effective. Glucose facilitates intestinal reabsorption of electrolytes and water. Oral rehydration usually is preferred over parenteral treatment since patients need not be hospitalized, none of the complications of intravenous lines in place need occur, and it is inexpensive. Several oral rehydration solutions containing similar electrolyte concentrations (Hydra-Lyte, Lytren, and Pedialyte) are now commercially available in the United States, and beverages such as Gatorade are available in food stores. An oral rehydration solution using home ingredients may be made as follows: to 1 liter of boiled water add ½ teaspoon of table salt, 4 teaspoons of sugar, ½ teaspoon of sodium bicarbonate (baking soda) and ¼ teaspoon of potassium chloride (salt substitute). Some patients with acute diarrheal illnesses appear to have minimal or no volume depletion. Nevertheless it is necessary for the physician to monitor volume losses carefully. Appropriate monitoring by patients who return home after seeking medical care may include noting the consistency and number of stools they continue to have. A further 10 to 20 watery stools may require re-examination. For patients who cannot comply with such a regimen, a brief admission to the hospital for rehydration is a reasonable alternative.

The widely prescribed antimotility agents such as opiates and derivatives (camphorated tincture of opium [paregoric], Lomotil, and Imodium) are useful for diminishing cramps in patients with mild, nonfebrile diarrheas. Lomotil (diphenoxylate dihydrochloride with atropine) taken as needed up to 8 tablets in 24 hours is often effective. Paregoric may be taken as 2 teaspoons every 4 hours; for children, 0.5 ml per kg per day in four divided doses is recommended. Antimotility agents should be stopped if symptoms worsen or do not improve within 48 hours. In patients with inflammatory diarrheas, manifesting with fever or with red or white blood cells in stools, antimotility agents are contraindicated. Their use may prolong the duration of diarrhea and fever or could lead to intestinal perforation during shigellosis or amebiasis. Kaolin and pectin (Kaopectate) and polycarbophil are adsorbents that solidify stools. They are effective in diminishing mild diarrhea and in contrast to the antimotility agents are very safe. Bismuth subsalicylate (Pepto-Bismol) is equally effective but must be taken often (30 ml every 30 minutes for 8 doses), may lead to salicylate intoxication, and turns stools black.

Antimicrobial Therapy

After an appropriate supportive program has been initiated, other aspects of therapy should now be considered. Acute diarrheal illnesses are often self-limited, thus specific antimicrobial treatment usually is not needed. Furthermore it is not possible empirically to cover the patient for all eventualities with "shot-gun therapy." However, specific treatment is desirable once an etiologic diagnosis has been made if the patient remains febrile or has bloody or persistent diarrhea, or to prevent further transmission of infection. Even within the group of agents causing dysentery or febrile diarrhea, no single agent is effective against all the common pathogens; laboratory diagnosis is needed. Table 1 lists the treatments of choice and the best alternative treatments for these agents.

All symptomatic persons with shigellosis should be treated. Because of increasing resistance to ampicillin, trimethoprim-sulfamethoxazole (TMP-SMX) (Bactrim, Septra), to which more than 95 per cent of the isolates in the United States are susceptible, is now the treatment of choice. For children, TMP, 10 mg per kg per day, and SMX, 50 mg per kg per day, in divided doses every 12 hours for 5 days is recommended. If the *Shigella* is susceptible, ampicillin or tetracycline is an alternative treatment. Pregnant women or children under 7 years of age should not receive tetracycline because of the risk of accumulation on developing bones and teeth. Children should receive 50 to 100 mg of ampicillin per kg per day in four divided doses.

The treatment of enteropathogenic strains of *E. coli* is the same as that for *Shigella*.

Patients with severe or prolonged infections caused by *Campylobacter jejuni* or related organisms should be treated with a 5 to 7 day course of erythromycin. For children, 30 mg per kg per day in divided doses should be given. In patients in the United States, resistance to erythromycin

TABLE 1. **Antimicrobial Therapy of Agents Causing Acute Diarrheal Illnesses**

Pathogen	*Treatment(s) of Choice*	*Alternative Treatment(s)*
Shigella species	Trimethoprim (TMP; 160 mg) + sulfamethoxazole (SMX; 800 mg), q 12 hr for 5 days	Ampicillin, 500 mg q 6 hr for 5 days; tetracycline, 2.5 gm PO once
Campylobacter species	Erythromycin, 250 mg, q 6 hr for 5 days	Tetracycline, 250 mg q 6 hr for 5 days; clindamycin (Cleocin) 300 mg q 6 hr for 5 days
Salmonella species		
Bacteremia	Chloramphenicol, 500 mg IV q 6 hr for 10 days; ampicillin, 1 gm IV q 4 hr for 10 days; TMP (160 mg) + SMX (800 mg), q 12 hr for 10 days	—
Gastroenteritis	None	—
Clostridium difficile	Discontinue antibiotic or antineoplastic agent if possible, and begin vancomycin (Vancocin), 125 mg q 6 hr for 10 days	Metronidazole (Flagyl), 500 mg q 6 hr for 10 days
Yersinia enterocolitica	Tetracycline, 250 mg q 6 hr for 7 days	TMP (80 mg) + SMX (400 mg), q 6 hr for 7 days
Aeromonas species	Tetracycline, 500 mg q 6 hr for 7 days	—
Giardia lamblia	Metronidazole (Flagyl), 250 mg tid for 7 days	Quinacrine (Atabrine), 100 mg for 7 days

is uncommon. Patients with milder symptoms or in whom the illness is improving need not be treated with antibiotics.

Patients with acute nontyphoidal *Salmonella* gastroenteritis have not been shown to benefit from antimicrobial treatment; paradoxically, antibiotic treatment may prolong the duration of the carrier state. However, patients who are septic-appearing or are bacteremic should be treated. If the isolate is susceptible, ampicillin or TMP-SMX is the agent of choice; if susceptibility is unknown, treat with chloramphenicol (Chloromycetin). For children, chloramphenicol, 50 to 75 mg per kg per day in four divided doses, is recommended. If meningitis is suspected, chloramphenicol is the agent of choice.

In patients who have antibiotic-associated diarrhea or pseudomembranous colitis, the etiologic agent is usually *Clostridium difficile,* which secretes cytotoxins. Mild illnesses respond to stopping of antibiotics or antineoplastic agents, but more severe infections should be treated with metronidazole (Flagyl) or oral vancomycin.

Yersiniosis can be treated with the tetracyclines or with TMP-SMX.

Infections due to *Aeromonas* species or *Vibrio parahaemolyticus* may be treated with tetracycline for 5 days.

Giardiasis may be treated with either metronidazole or Atabrine; relapses may occur after either, and a second course of the same agent is then necessary. Patients should not drink alcohol within 24 hours after taking metronidazole as there is significant risk of an "antabuse-like" reaction. Because of the possibility of teratogenicity with metronidazole, it is contraindicated in pregnant women.

CONSTIPATION

method of
J. R. PARMAR, M.D.,
and EDWIN J. ZARLING, M.D., FACP
University of Illinois at Chicago
Chicago, Illinois

Approximately 10 to 20 per cent of the general population intermittently experiences constipation. Constipation has different meanings to various people. It may be claimed when patients pass infrequent stools, small stools, or hard stools. The normal frequency of defecation ranges from three times per day to three times per week. The frequency of stool passage is diet dependent; increased amounts of dietary fiber are associated with more frequent stooling. Increased dietary fiber also causes increases in stool weight. In general, normal subjects consuming a Western diet pass stools that weigh between 35 and 225 grams per day. For high fiber–consuming populations, such as rural African villagers, daily stool weights range from 170 to 900 grams per day. This increase in stool bulk is caused by the profound "water-holding" capacity of fiber. Depending on the fiber source, fecal fiber holds two to six times its weight of water. This water-holding capacity of fiber is a function of the noncelluloid polysaccharide fraction of the fiber. Daily stool weight also varies widely in an individual patient over time. In normal subjects eating a defined diet, we have found as much as a fivefold day-to-day variation in stool weight.

Diagnosis

Constipation can be caused by a wide variety of conditions (Table 1). Perhaps the most common cause is the irritable bowel syndrome. Teenagers and young adults are most commonly affected. In this condition, constipation can occur intermittently, with alternate periods of either normal or diarrheal stools. Cramping pain is usually present in the left lower quadrant of the abdomen and is relieved by defecation. No radiologic or laboratory abnormalities can be identified in this syndrome; the cause is unknown.

Diverticulitis of the colon may produce constipation by intestinal muscle spasm or stricture formation. This

TABLE 1. **Conditions Associated with Constipation**

Idiopathic
Irritable bowel syndrome*
Idiopathic intestinal pseudo-obstruction
Colon
Anorectal disease (hemorrhoids, fissures, anal spasm)*
Diverticular disease*
Mechanical obstruction (tumor, stricture)
Rectal prolapse
Rectocele
Drugs
Opiates*
Aluminum- or calcium-containing antacids*
Antidepressants*
Anticholinergics
Heavy metal intoxication (lead, mercury, arsenic)
Systemic disease
Amyloidosis
Diabetes mellitus
Hypokalemia
Hypothyroidism
Pregnancy*
Systemic sclerosis
Uremia
Neurogenic
Cauda equina tumors
Cerebral palsy
Chagas' disease
Hirschsprung's disease (aganglionosis)
Parkinson's disease
Stroke
Tabes dorsalis
Diet
Insufficient fiber intake*
Insufficient fluid intake

*Common cause of constipation.

form of constipation is usually seen in adults over the age of 50 years. This condition tends to occur more frequently in patients who have had the irritable bowel syndrome. The incidence of diverticulosis is significantly less in populations with high fiber intake.

Anorectal disease is another common cause of constipation. This can occur in any age group, especially young children. Patients with painful hemorrhoids, anal fissures, or anal strictures may reduce their frequency of defecation voluntarily in an effort to avoid pain. In addition, anal spasm may be associated with these conditions and can make the passage of stool difficult and uncomfortable.

Medications with a high propensity to cause constipation include opiates, aluminum- or calcium-containing antacids, antidepressants, and anticholinergic preparations. Drug-induced constipation is usually easily diagnosed from the patient's history. Stool is frequently detected in the rectum upon digital examination.

Pregnant females tend to become constipated in the second or third trimester. This has been attributed to the mass effect of the enlarged uterus causing compression of the sigmoid colon and rectum. Recent evidence also suggests that hormones may cause a slowing of bowel transit.

Elderly patients, particularly those who need the services of nursing homes, frequently become constipated. This may be due to insufficient water intake causing a concretion of stool in the lower bowel (fecaloma). Also, insufficient dietary fiber leads to small stools and decreased frequency of defecation. The formation of a fecaloma may lead to development of stercoral ulcers in the colon, which may rarely perforate and cause peritonitis.

Evaluation

As in most diseases, the history is very important in determining the cause of constipation. Patients with congenital lesions will have had bowel dysfunction beginning in the first decade of life. Constipation which began in adolescence and is intermittent is most likely due to the irritable bowel syndrome. Particularly with adult onset constipation, the patient must be questioned about drug ingestion as well as other causes listed in Table 1. The dietary history is investigated, paying particular attention to the adequacy of fiber and fluid intake.

The physical examination should include careful evaluation of the anus, looking for spasm or mucosal damage. Sensory examination of the anal region must be performed as part of the evaluation for neurologic disorders. Digital rectal examination is helpful for detecting a fecaloma and rectocele. Patients with Hirschsprung's disease will have a profuse fecal discharge after digital examination. Proctoscopy is useful for detecting tumors of the rectum and also melanosis coli, which is brownish mucosal discoloration indicative of chronic laxative abuse.

We obtain a barium enema radiograph in all new patients with constipation. This is done to diagnose the colonic causes of constipation. Colonoscopy is rarely needed. It is extremely important to rule out organic causes of obstruction in the colon, such as tumors or strictures. Dietary manipulation in such patients may precipitate complete obstruction or even perforation. Anal manometry is increasingly performed. It is particularly useful in diagnosing ultrashort segment Hirschsprung's disease for which the barium enema may be normal. Classically, the manometry will show no relaxation of the internal anal sphincter on rectal distention.

Therapy

Whenever possible, therapy is directed at the underlying disorder. For example, patients with drug-induced constipation must discontinue the offending medication. Partial bowel obstruction due to strictures or tumors must be surgically treated. Patients with Hirschsprung's disease can be temporarily treated with a daily digital examination, which will provide bowel evacuation until definitive surgical therapy can be arranged. However, in the great majority of patients with constipation, we attempt to increase fiber intake by dietary manipulation coupled with commercially prepared fiber medications (Metamucil, Konsyl, Hydrocil). Fiber speeds up intestinal transit time and also increases stool weight. The daily ingestion of 20 grams of fiber increases stool weight by approximately 127 per cent. This probably occurs because fiber tends to "hold water." Studies using the technique of colonic manometry have shown that increasing stool weight and shortening transit time lowers the high intracolonic pressure found in constipated patients. This diminishes the frequency of abdominal cramps and pain. Twenty grams of fiber per day is the amount necessary to effect a change in the bowel habits of the majority of patients.

Dietary manipulation aims to increase the ingested fiber. Table 2 lists the fiber content of several common foods, as well as the effect of these foods on intestinal transit time. Although we encourage the consumption of all high fiber foods, it becomes impractical to consume sufficient quantities of these foods to equal 20 grams of fiber. Bran consumed in cereal form is the

TABLE 2. **Effect of Food Fiber on Intestinal Transit Time**

Food	Grams of Dietary Fiber*	% Change in Transit Time†
Bran	26.7	−41%
Carrots	3.70	−17%
Apples	1.42	−14%
Lettuce (raw)	1.53	N/A
Whole wheat bread	8.50	N/A

*As gm/100 gm serving.
†As produced by 20 gm of specific fiber.
N/A, not available.
Data abstracted from Cummings JW, et al: Lancet *1*:5–8, 1978; and Kay RM, et al: Clin Invest Med *1*:9–24, 1978.

easiest way to increase dietary fiber intake. Consumption of fruits is also encouraged for patients with constipation. This is done not only to supplement fiber intake but also for the effects of other components of the fruits. Prunes have a high magnesium content, and apples contain sorbitol. Both these compounds exert a laxative effect. We encourage our patients to consume at least 6 glasses of fluid per day. This is particularly important in patients confined to nursing homes, since they often are unable to obtain fluids on their own.

Of the various commercially prepared remedies for constipation, we prefer to use psyllium hydrophilic mucilloid (Metamucil). This is a fiber supplement that we prescribe in addition to dietary fiber. Patients are usually started with 2 tablespoonfuls per day, mixed in juice or water. If no improvement is noted in 1 week, we increase the dosage up to 6 tablespoonfuls per day. Lactulose is an alternative laxative that appears to be safe for chronic use. This compound is a synthetic sugar that cannot be absorbed by the small intestine. Although its mechanism of action is not fully understood, it probably works by osmotically increasing the fluid load delivered to the colon and by inducing bowel movements due to colonic bacterial degradation of this sugar. The usual dosage of lactulose is 30 ml at bedtime. Excessive use of this medication can produce an explosive diarrhea. We use it as the primary therapy in patients who are susceptible to hepatic encephalopathy and as a secondary therapy in patients who are intolerant of fiber therapy.

Mineral oil, in doses of 15 ml per day, also is an effective laxative. This medication is not recommended for use in young children or elderly patients with swallowing disorders, since aspiration of this compound can easily occur and lead to lipoid pneumonia.

Mild cathartics can be added to the regimen in the early phases of constipation therapy. Examples of such compounds are milk of magnesia, bisacodyl sodium, senna extract, and cascara extract. However, chronic use of these compounds should be avoided because of the possibility of inducing chronic colonic damage. This may be in the form of a dilated hypotonic colon ("laxative colon") or the less serious condition of melanosis coli.

Recently, biofeedback has been used successfully to treat constipation in patients with neurologic damage. In this therapy, a balloon is inserted into the rectum and inflated to various sizes. The patient is taught to recognize the sensation of rectal distention in an effort to become more aware of the presence of stool in the rectum.

HOARSENESS AND LARYNGITIS

method of
MICHAEL D. MAVES, M.D., FACS
University of Iowa
Iowa City, Iowa

Hoarseness is a symptom rather than a diagnosis and, in general, is due to an identifiable cause. For adequate evaluation, the physician needs to examine the larynx during inspiration and phonation and formulate a diagnosis based upon that observation. Most patients with hoarseness are concerned about cancer as the cause of their laryngitis and need reassurance that the physician is investigating this possibility. Treatment with antibiotics or decongestants without a thorough evaluation is inappropriate and may delay the diagnosis.

History. How long has the hoarseness been present? Hoarseness resulting from acute laryngitis is usually of short duration and follows a prodrome of an upper respiratory tract infection, whereas long-standing hoarseness may be the result of systemic disease, chronic irritation, or cancer.

How does the patient's current voice differ in quality from normal? In many instances, the alteration in vocal quality is marked and obvious; however, even a subtle disturbance in the tone of the voice of a professional singer will cause concern to that patient. A family member may be helpful in describing changes that have occurred.

Is speaking painful or has there been an associated disturbance in swallowing? Chronic laryngitis is usually painless; however, contact ulcers are quite painful and also affect deglutition.

Does the patient smoke or drink? Although cigarette smoke is the most common laryngeal irritant, noxious industrial fumes or marijuana smoke may be just as harsh. Ethanol has no direct effect upon the larynx, but it is well known that intoxicated individuals tend to abuse their voices.

What type of work is the patient engaged in? How is the voice used or abused? At this point in the history, the patient's vocal habits need to be precisely defined. Family, friends, or associates may give more accurate information than the patient, who may minimize his or her contribution to the problem. It is important to determine whether the patient has experienced prolonged exposure to a noisy environment, which could result in noise-induced hearing loss or hoarseness from the need to shout to be heard.

Has there been a history of laryngeal instrumentation or intubation, or cervical or laryngeal trauma? Is there a significant systemic disease, such as hypothyroidism or rheumatoid arthritis, that can directly affect laryngeal function?

Vocal Quality. A considerable amount of information may be obtained by listening to the quality of the patient's voice. A whispered voice suggests laryngitis. Vocal nodules, because they interfere with complete closure and apposition of the vocal cords, produce a breathy voice. Vocal cord paralysis also results in a breathy voice. A harsh, rough voice may be the hallmark of chronic laryngitis or neoplasm. Patients with aphonia need to be carefully evaluated for a functional disorder. A spastic, grimacing voice may result from a functional disorder or from spastic dysphonia.

Acute Laryngitis

This is the most common source of hoarseness. Typically, the patient complains of loss of voice and pain in the throat. Usually there is a history of upper respiratory tract infection. The laryngitis may be viral or bacterial in nature. Other less common causes include inhalation of fumes and gases, aspiration of caustics, and allergic reactions.

Examination of the vocal cords reveals intense hyperemia of the surfaces of the true cords and perhaps the false cords and supraglottis as well. If the laryngitis is bacterial in nature, an exudate or membrane over the surface of the larynx may be visible. In children the most common bacterial organism is *Haemophilus influenzae,* whereas in adults the *Streptococcus* organism is predominant. Diphtheria, formerly a common cause of severe and often fatal laryngitis, is now rare because of widespread immunization; however, it should always be considered. Probably most cases are viral infections.

Treatment

Most patients with acute viral laryngitis improve spontaneously as the infection resolves. Supportive care in the form of throat lozenges, sprays, and antitussive medications provides comfort but does nothing to shorten the course of the illness. The patient should abstain from smoking. When symptoms of fever, dyspnea, or cervical lymphadenopathy are present, administration of antibiotics for the most common infectious organisms is advisable. In general, if the voice does not improve in 2 weeks, repeat indirect laryngoscopy, and perhaps direct laryngoscopy with biopsy is indicated.

Chronic Laryngitis

Unlike acute laryngitis, the chronic form of the disease involves a long-standing condition in which inflammatory changes occur in the laryngeal mucosa. A distinguishing difference is that hoarseness in chronic laryngitis is usually painless. Also, the throat may ache or feel tired, and the patient may find it impossible to speak for extended periods of time. Frequent coughing and clearing the throat may occur, but unless a tracheitis or bronchitis is present, little or no sputum is produced. The condition occurs more frequently in women than in men.

The most common cause of chronic laryngitis is repeated episodes of acute laryngitis. Smoking can also cause the condition or be a contributing factor. Constant use (or misuse) of the voice, most frequent in professional singers, public speakers, and politicians, aggravates the condition or may cause it in a patient with a normal larynx. Ethanol abuse with subsequent loss of inhibitions and misuse of the voice can exacerbate an already traumatized glottis. In some individuals, postnasal discharge of mucopurulent secretions irritates the laryngeal mucosa, causing chronic laryngitis. Similarly, gastroesophageal reflux and the pooling of refluxed stomach contents near the arytenoid cartilages in the supine position may cause irritation and laryngitis.

The larynx may be observed in a variety of conditions. The cords may simply be red and swollen, rather than sharp-edged and white, not unlike the usual situation in acute laryngitis. Thickening of the true cords with edema or polypoid changes to the phonatory surfaces of the cords are also common. Strands of mucus bridging the cords may be visible; pearls of mucus over the surface of the cords may be mistaken for vocal nodules. The false cords and supraglottis may also be mucus-covered, but vocal cord motion is unaffected.

Treatment

The most important factor in the successful treatment of patients with chronic laryngitis is the identification and removal of the cause. Smoking, in particular, must be eliminated, although patient compliance may be a difficult problem. For laryngitis due to vocal abuse, total voice rest is the only effective treatment. However, communication limited to writing is difficult, and in general patients will not comply with "limited" voice use. Topical medications are generally of less value than humidification, which is especially important in the overall treatment of patients with chronic laryngitis. A room vaporizer started 1 hour before retiring and continued throughout the night may prove invaluable to the patient who cannot avoid contact with noxious fumes or cigarette smoke. "Stripping" the hyperplastic polypoid mucosa from the vocal cords in these patients frequently yields a poor result. In general, the treatment of chronic laryngitis may be problematic because the cause is difficult to ascertain and patient compliance is difficult.

Traumatic Laryngitis

This category of diagnoses includes laryngitis related to external, self-inflicted, or iatrogenic trauma. The most common type is laryngitis following an acute episode of vocal abuse, such as vigorous cheering at a sporting event. Inspection of the larynx usually reveals hemorrhage or bleb formation at the margin of the vocal cord in the potential lymphatic space of Reinke. This edema and hemorrhage usually resolve within 48 hours if the voice is rested but may continue longer and develop into chronic laryngitis if vocal abuse is continued. If necessary, resolution may be hastened by the administration of corticosteroids: prednisone, 10 mg orally, or Medrol Dosepak.

Vocal nodules are a related condition. These often occur in children who abuse their voices but are also observed in singers, politicians, ministers, and teachers. When first noted they may appear round and pink, but with continued abuse they become keratinized, thicker, and white. Nodules typically occur at the junction of the anterior one third and posterior two thirds of the free margin of the true cords. They are customarily bilateral but may appear as unilateral cysts or granulomas.

Treatment

The treatment of vocal nodules depends upon the age of the patient, the age and development of the nodules, and the cause. In preadolescent children and all patients with early vocal nodules, speech therapy and conservative handling are indicated. Excision of the nodules in children usually is not successful because the patients will rarely change their vocal habits sufficiently to prevent prompt recurrence. In adults or older adolescents, excision of the nodules via laser laryngoscopy may result in restoration of the normal voice, but, again, voice rest and work with a speech pathologist to correct the long-standing problems due to voice abuse are necessary for prolonged cure.

Contact ulcers occur on the medial surface of the vocal cords in the posterior one third of the cord, usually resulting from instrumentation of the larynx, such as peroral endoscopy or endotracheal intubation. They are believed to occur following trauma from the endotracheal tube lying in the posterior glottic chink. Occasionally they result from prolonged vocal abuse and habitual throat clearing. Usually this condition can be easily differentiated from other causes of hoarseness if the history includes intubation, pain with phonation and deglutition, and ulceration of the posterior third of both vocal cords. Referred otalgia may be the only symptom, however. Exposure of the cartilage of the vocal process may lead to chronic chondritis that is indolent and refractory. Therapy is supportive, consisting of complete voice rest, antibiotics, and steroids. Occasionally these lesions progress and form granulomas, which can be removed with microlaryngoscopy. Resolution of granulomas may require months to years, however. The best course is prevention by carefully avoiding excessively large endotracheal tubes.

Vocal Cord Paralysis

Laryngeal paralysis may give rise to hoarseness. Paralysis may be caused by trauma (including iatrogenic trauma during thyroid surgery) or have organic causes, including paralysis from laryngeal cancer, or idiopathic causes, usually presumed to be viral. The paralysis may be unilateral or bilateral and involve the recurrent laryngeal nerve, the superior laryngeal nerve, or both. A breathy, air-spilling hoarseness and weakness in the voice are the usual presenting complaints. Aspiration of secretions or liquids may occur if the paralysis has resulted in an incompetent laryngeal sphincter. The diagnosis is made on indirect laryngoscopy. If the paralyzed cord lies in a paramedian position, it is probably associated with an isolated recurrent laryngeal nerve paralysis. If the cord is in a more lateral, intermediate position, combined paralysis of the recurrent and superior laryngeal nerves is present. Isolated superior laryngeal nerve paralysis is more difficult to diagnose but is characterized by rotation of the larynx to the paralyzed side on phonation.

Treatment

Treatment depends upon the lesion and prognosis. Unilateral paralysis of either superior or recurrent nerve may not require immediate treatment, and with time, the affected cord may assume a more optimal, medial position. If necessary, Teflon may be injected into the paralyzed cord to displace it into a medial position. In bilateral recurrent nerve paralysis, both cords cover the glottis like a curtain, and immediate tracheotomy with an eventual cord lateralization procedure may be necessary.

Metabolic Diseases

Hypothyroidism yields the same myxedematous changes in the laryngeal mucosa as occur on other surfaces. The patient experiences a deepening of the voice and fatigue with speaking. Examination of the cords demonstrates a thickened, edematous "floppy" appearance to both cords, without evidence of inflammation. Confirmation with thyroid function tests and treatment with thyroid replacement result in return of the voice to normal.

Rheumatoid arthritis may affect the cricoarytenoid joint as it does other synovial joints. Pain is a prominent aspect of this hoarseness and may be exacerbated by palpation and movement of the larynx. With impairment of the cricoarytenoid joint, limitation of vocal cord motion may occur and dyspnea develop. Inspection of the larynx reveals a cherry-red arytenoid cartilage and perhaps limited motion of the cord. Treatment with systemic corticosteroids and control of the arthritis will improve the voice and dyspnea. More marked or resistant cases may need direct injection of steroids into the area of the affected cricoarytenoid joint.

Neoplastic Diseases

The most important cause of hoarseness to investigate in any patient is cancer of the larynx. Only too often, treatment of early cancer is not undertaken because of failure to examine the larynx and observe neoplastic changes in the cords. Careful examination of the larynx is especially important in patients with a history of heavy smoking, since cigarette smoke is the primary carcinogen involved in cancer of the larynx. Early cancers may be treated with either surgery or radiation therapy with high cure rates and preservation of laryngeal function.

White lesions, or leukoplakia, occur most commonly over the true vocal cords. This condition results from chronic irritation. Removal of the offending agent and treatment for chronic laryngitis with broad-spectrum antibiotics should be instituted. If the condition fails to improve, a biopsy should be done, since it is difficult to distinguish between leukoplakia and carcinoma.

Both the surgeon and the patient should realize that, when an early diagnosis is made, in many instances treatment less radical than a total laryngectomy is required for cure. When laryngectomy is required, many means of vocal rehabilitation are available, including the new tracheoesophageal fistula techniques.

Functional Dysphonia and Spastic Dysphonia

Functional dysphonia is a volitional inability to speak, usually assumed to be emotional or psychogenic in origin. On examination, the vocal cords appear normal but with attempted phonation the cords appear to meet, and then separate just prior to voice initiation. The patient is able to adduct the cords, however, when asked to cough, which serves to confirm the diagnosis and differentiate the condition from hoarseness or paralysis of an organic nature. Treatment is supportive, with careful explanation of the vocal problem and, occasionally, formal psychiatric consultation.

Spastic dysphonia, on the other hand, was thought for many years to be psychologic in nature but is a vocal disorder characterized by tight, forced, low-pitched phonation requiring great physical effort on the patient's part and usually interrupted by frequent breaks in the flow of speech. This strained voice production is accompanied by facial grimacing and cervical muscular contractions. Careful evaluation by both a physician and a speech scientist is necessary to differentiate spastic dysphonia from other vocal disorders, such as essential voice tremor. Current treatment involves sectioning of the recurrent laryngeal nerve (usually the left), which eliminates the spasticity in about 90 per cent of patients. This may be tested preoperatively by unilateral temporary paralysis of the recurrent laryngeal nerve with 1 per cent lidocaine (Xylocaine) injected into the tracheoesophageal groove.

INSOMNIA

method of
CHARLES E. DRISCOLL, M.D.,
and BARRY L. CARTER, Pharm.D.
University of Iowa
Iowa City, Iowa

Problems with disturbed sleep are commonly discovered during routine history taking. Broader public awareness of newer technologies for investigation of sleep disorders prompts some patients to offer insomnia as a chief complaint. Estimates of the prevalence of insomnia range from 12 per cent to more than 35 per cent of the population. A recent consensus development conference on the treatment of insomia reported that one third of the United States population suffers some degree of insomnia, and half this group (17 per cent of the population) considers their problem serious. The physician is often confronted with the decision of whether or not to prescribe a sleep-promoting medication.

Understanding the Cause of the Sleep Complaint

Managing a patient with disordered sleep is more complex than simply prescribing a sleeping pill. The selection of an appropriate course of therapy for sleep disturbance should be based on an appreciation of the underlying cause and a pharmacologic intervention that relates to it. For purposes of general clinical practice, sleep complaints can be described as mild or severe and classified according to the following categories: transient insomnia, short-term insomnia, and long-term or chronic insomnia. The problem may be further classified according to the part of the sleep cycle affected: falling asleep, maintaining sleep, early awakening, and primary sleep disorder (e.g., sleep apnea, nocturnal myoclonus, or restless legs syndrome).

Before prescribing any therapy for a sleep complaint, it is important to assess the patient for the presence of a primary medical or psychiatric disorder. Any illness accompanied by pain, dyspnea, pruritus, or nocturia, for example, may awaken the patient at night. The sleep disturbance will resolve with appropriate therapy aimed at the medical disorder. Similarly, psychiatric conditions such as anxiety, depression, mania, and schizophrenia may cause insomnia which is not appropriately controlled by hypnotics. The patient's insomnia can also be due to excessive alcohol or hypnotic agent abuse with rebound insomnia; in such cases withdrawal of the drug must be managed.

Treatment of Primary Sleep Disorders

In a primary sleep disorder, some physiologic, anatomic, or biochemical mechanism is presumed to be dysfunctional.

Sleep Apnea. This group of disorders may have an anatomic etiology within the upper airway or involve a central mechanism, causing absent diaphragmatic movements. As the patient enters REM sleep, breathing may cease for periods that range from 10 seconds to 2 or more minutes. When respirations stop, sleep lightens and either the patient will take a breath or awaken. Patients exhibit daytime sleepiness, and their sleep partners may observe excessive loud snoring or absent respirations. Marked obesity (the pickwickian syndrome) may be associated. Obstructive apnea is most successfully treated with tracheostomy; however, some reduction in the number of apneic events can be accomplished nonsurgically with use of a tongue-retaining device designed to hold the tongue slightly forward. Medical therapy usually has been reported as unsuccessful. Tricyclic antidepressants (serotonergic) have helped a few patients, but adaptation quickly develops. Nocturnal oxygen or hypnotic agent administration, in fact, may be detrimental by effecting longer episodes of apnea.

Nocturnal Myoclonus. Characterized by regular (every 20 seconds) leg jerks in one or both legs, this syndrome may be unrecognized by the patient. A complaint of fatigue on awakening and daytime drowsiness is offered, which is due to miniarousals and sleep pattern disruption. The best evidence for this diagnosis is obtained by interviewing the patient's sleeping partner. Small bedtime doses (0.5 to 2.0 mg) of clonazepam (Clonopin), a benzodiazepine anticonvulsant, are usually effective though loss of antimyoclonic activity may occur within 3 months of starting the drug.

Restless Legs Syndrome. When the patient has complaints of severe, ill-at-ease feelings in the legs so that the only relief comes with getting up and moving around, restless legs syndrome is a likely cause of the insomnia. Some of the patients in this group will be afflicted with nocturnal myoclonus and may respond to clonazepam. Carbamazepine (Tegretol), 100 to 200 mg, has been reported to be more effective than placebo in treating this syndrome; however, serious side effects, including blood dyscrasias, may accompany use of the drug. Diphenhydramine (Benadryl), quinine, and vitamin E have been tried with some success. However, medical therapies have not been found to be very effective.

TABLE 1. **Patient's Guide for Behavioral Changes to Improve Sleep**

Decrease tobacco, caffeine, and stimulant intake
Avoid alcohol consumption
Solve relationship problems before bedtime
Curtail daytime naps
Attempt to get regular daily exercise
Have a bedtime snack or warm milk before retiring (caloric and L-tryptophan intake may be at work here)
Do not use the bed for anything except sexual activity or sleep (no eating, reading, TV watching, worrying)
Don't lie down in bed until sleepy
Avoid "trying" to go to sleep, don't go to bed too early
Practice relaxation training (deep muscle relaxation and relaxation breathing with longer expirations than inspirations)
If you can't sleep, get up and try some other activity, stay up until you feel sleepy, then return to bed; repeat as necessary
Sleep loss will do no physical harm—worry over sleep loss will induce further problems with insomnia
Establish a regular daily schedule for arising regardless of length of sleep

When to Prescribe Hypnotics

The best conditions for a favorable outcome after prescribing a hypnotic are when the patient is experiencing a transient or short-term insomnia. For milder conditions involving prolonged sleep latency, behavioral interventions should be tried first. Education and reassurance may be more important to the patient than a medication. Table 1 gives recommendations for guiding sleep behavioral changes.

Transient insomnia affects normal sleepers and may be expected to last only 3 to 5 days. Examples include acute short-term stress, anticipated surgery, or time change by travel. Short-term insomnia may be less acute than transient insomnia and may be recurrent. This type of insomnia usually lasts longer (1 to 3 weeks) and occurs with anxiety or stress related to family turmoil, job loss, financial worries, grief, or medical illness. For these conditions a hypnotic sedative is a plausible therapeutic option. Recommend an over-the-counter hypnotic, usually an antihistamine, if one has not already been tried by the patient.

As a class, barbiturates are more likely to induce unwanted induction of hepatic enzymes, cause drug-drug interactions, cause more adverse

TABLE 2. **Hypnotic Drugs for Insomnia**

Generic Name	Brand Name	Dose Form*	Usual Oral Dose Range	Half-Life	Active Metabolites	Advantages	Disadvantages
Benzodiazepines							
Triazolam	Halcion	O	0.25–0.5 mg	3–4 hr	No	Minimal daytime sedative effects	Increase in anxiety on awakening, prominent rebound insomnia, early morning awakening
Temazepam	Restoril	O	15–30 mg	8–12 hr	No	Mild carryover	Slow absorption resulting in long sleep latency
Flurazepam	Dalmane	O	15–30 mg	75–150 hr	Yes	Carryover hypnotic effect to next 2 nights—rebound insomnia mild	Daytime sedation, takes 3–4 days treatment for maximum effects
Barbiturates							
Secobarbital	Seconal and others	O, E, I, S	100–200 mg	20–35 hr	Yes	Preop sedation	Sedation, hangover, potential lethality, REM rebound
Pentobarbital	Nembutal and others	O, E, I, S	100–200 mg	20–40 hr	No	Preop sedation	Sedation, hangover, potential lethality, REM rebound
Chlorals							
Chloral hydrate	Noctec and others	O, E, S	500–1500 mg	8 hr	Yes	Useful for occasional need, no REM rebound	Loses efficacy with long-term use
Piperidinediones							
Methyprylon	Noludar	O	200–400 mg	4 hr	No	None	REM rebound, potential lethality
Glutethimide	Doriden	O	250–500 mg	5–20 hr	No	None	REM rebound, strong anti-cholinergic effects, potential lethality—avoid using
Antihistamines							
Diphenhydramine	Benadryl and others	O, E, I	25–50 mg	3.5 hr	No	Safety	
Pyrilamine	Somnicaps	O	25–50 mg	?	No	Safety	
Doxylamine	Unisom	O	25–50 mg	?	No	Safety	
Other							
L-Tryptophan†	Trofan and others	O	600–2000 mg	?	?		

*E, elixir; I, injectable; O, oral—capsule or tablet; S, suppository.
†This use of L-tryptophan is not listed by the manufacturer.

reactions in the elderly, and more easily induce lethality. For these reasons benzodiazepines have become the drugs of choice, largely replacing the barbiturates and piperidinediones. Unless combined with alcohol they have a wider margin of safety. Though probably still useful in occasional and brief use, chlorals have also been largely replaced. Table 2 compares these drugs available for use in treating insomnia.

Administration of Benzodiazepine Hypnotics

All benzodiazepines have sedative/hypnotic properties in sufficient dosage; however, only three are promoted strictly for their hypnotic effect.

No drug available produces "normal sleep." At best, the drugs will decrease sleep latency by 10 to 20 minutes and will increase sleep length by 20 to 40 minutes. All have the potential for habituation, dependence, tolerance, withdrawal, and hangover effects. Tolerance begins to appear within 2 weeks of continued use, and the patient may express less satisfaction from the medication. At this time it would be a mistake to increase the dose of the drug since tolerance will eventually develop to the higher dose as well.

All benzodiazepines have the potential to lower cognitive performance, induce memory deficits, and interfere with psychomotor skills. These will return to normal after discontinuation.

Agents with a long duration of activity, such as flurazepam, may have a carryover effect and influence daytime performance. Short-acting benzodiazepines are less likely to cause hangover and may be useful when minimal daytime sedation is important. In some cases, this effect of the long-acting agents can be used to the clinician's advantage. If the patient complains of early morning awakenings accompanied by significant daytime agitation or anxiety, a longer-acting hypnotic will be beneficial and may alleviate the need for daytime anxiolytics. Rule out depression as a cause of the early morning awakening or give a trial on a sedating antidepressant. In this situation a short-acting agent may be detrimental since it will not interrupt the early awakening. Flurazepam has a long half-life, therefore it takes a number of days for the drug to accumulate and produce maximal effects. However, it may not be necessary to give flurazepam nightly since a significant carryover hypnotic effect may be present the next night.

When the sleep complaint involves difficulty in falling asleep (prolonged sleep latency), particularly when occurring as transient insomnia, a rapidly absorbed hypnotic is appropriate. Temazepam is marketed in the U.S. as a hard gelatin capsule that is slowly absorbed, and the onset of action is delayed 2 to 3 hours. This limits the usefulness of temazepam in patients with prolonged sleep latency. More rapid onset of action is achieved with flurazepam (0.5 to 2 hours) and triazolam (1 to 3 hours).

Hypnotics should generally be used for short periods and then be withdrawn. Drug withdrawal is accompanied by a rebound insomnia which results in fewer hours of sleep than before the hypnotic was started (Fig. 1). This is followed by a gradual increase in hours of sleep, eventually returning to the patient's prehypnotic baseline. Rebound insomnia may be more prominent with short-acting benzodiazepines that are rapidly cleared from the serum. Since long-acting benzodiazepines are slowly eliminated after discontinuation, rebound insomnia, though still present, is not as intense.

For these reasons, flurazepam has the most desirable characteristics of the benzodiazepines for initial hypnotic choice. If excessive daytime hangover occurs, a trial of triazolam may be appropriate.

PRURITUS

method of
PAUL R. VANDERSTEEN, M.D.
University of North Dakota
Fargo, North Dakota

Pruritus, a synonym for itching, is the most common presenting symptom in dermatology. A modified form of pain, it promotes an oftentimes insatiable desire to scratch or rub the skin. Thermal, mechanical, and chemical stimuli may provoke this sensation as can touch, temperature change, and emotional stress. Itching may be localized or generalized, persistent or episodic. Frequently it is most severe at bedtime.

As one of the cardinal symptoms in dermatology, establishing the cause of the pruritus is of utmost importance. Itching is an attendant symptom of many eruptions, especially drug reactions, atopic dermatitis,

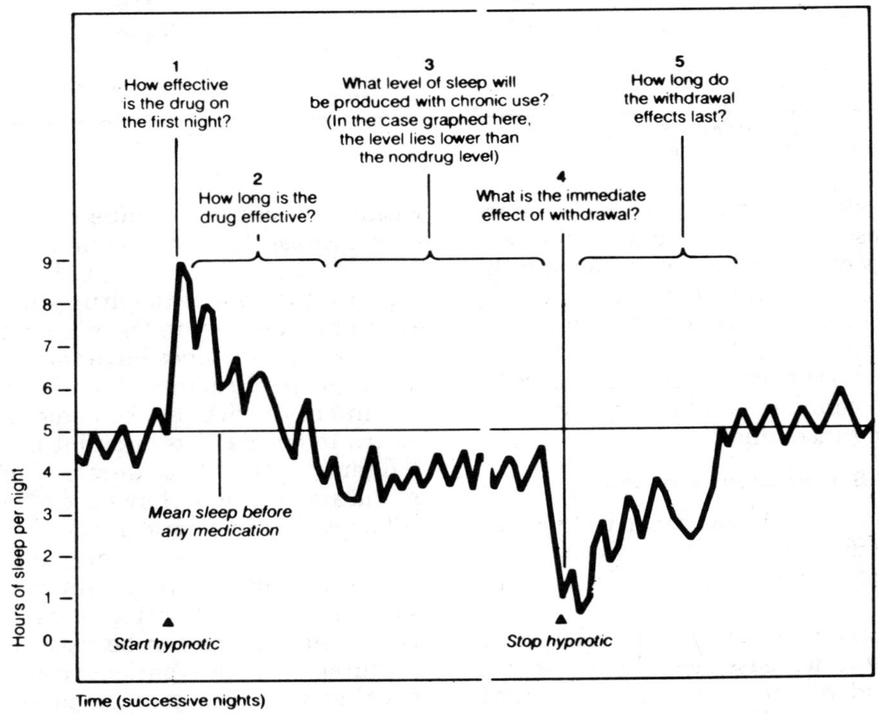

Figure 1. The five efficacy questions for hypnotic agents. (From Haurie P: The sleep disorders, *in* Current Concepts. Kalamazoo, MI, The Upjohn Company, 1977, p 31.)

dermatitis herpetiformis, lichen planus, arthropod bites, scabies, and urticaria.

Generalized pruritus occurring in the absence of a primary eruption may be of systemic genesis. Among the most frequent causes are pregnancy, obstructive biliary disease, chronic renal failure, malignancies (especially lymphoma), parasitic infestations, and hyper- and hypothyroidism. Less frequently it has been observed in diabetes mellitus and iron deficiency anemia.

A battery of tests will exclude most of the systemic causes of itching: an assessment of liver, renal, and thyroid function; a complete blood count; urinalysis; stool examination for occult blood, ova, and parasites; and a chest radiograph.

Diffuse pruritus without perceptible skin disease is usually due to pruritus hiemalis (winter itch), senile skin, or unknown causation. In individuals with this condition, as well as those being evaluated for systemic causes, treatment progresses from local to systemic therapy.

Preventive Measures

Alleviating cutaneous irritation is most significant. Patients should trim their fingernails and wear comfortable, loose-fitting clothing. As dry skin is more susceptible to itching, the control of environmental factors is consequential. Excessive exposure to solvents, soap, and hot water is eschewed. Bathing in warm, not hot, water should be confined to three times a week. Bath oils (Alpha Keri, Domol, Oilated Aveeno) must be used cautiously as they make the tub very slippery. The use of a bland soap such as Dove is best confined to uninvolved skin and intertriginous areas.

Local Therapy

For severe pruritus, especially that associated with an exudative eruption, a comfortably cool wet dressing (Prophyllin, 1 packet in 1 to 2 pints of water) is salutary. Immediately thereafter the application of a soothing moisturizing lotion (Moisturel, Complex 15) or cream (Eucerin, Aquaphor) is beneficial. Medicaments such as 0.5 per cent menthol, 1 per cent camphor, or 2 per cent chloral hydrate are useful additives for their antipruritic effect. Humectants, such as lactic acid (LactiCare lotion) and urea (Aquacare Dry Skin lotion), enhance the hydration of the skin. The topical use of local anesthetics and antihistamines is best avoided because of the risk of allergic sensitization.

In the absence of a primary dermatosis, topical corticosteroids should be used sparingly, if at all. They are beneficial in rapidly resolving symptomatic asteatotic dermatitis. Under such circumstances it is better to select a nonfluorinated preparation such as 1 per cent hydrocortisone (Hytone cream or lotion). The more potent fluorinated preparations are best reserved for inflammatory skin disorders. Chronic use of such preparations may lead to dermal atrophy, telangiectasia, and striae.

Systemic Therapy

Most medications used to treat pruritus are H_1 antihistamines. Of these, hydroxyzine (Atarax or Durax), 10 to 25 mg two to four times daily, is particularly helpful in recalcitrant cases. Since many patients note a nocturnal exacerbation of their pruritus, proportionately larger doses (50 mg) are useful before bedtime.

When one antihistamine fails, another agent should be selected from a separate pharmacologic group. Such alternatives, all given four times a day, are diphenhydramine (Benadryl), 50 mg; tripelennamine (PBZ), 50 mg; chlorpheniramine (Chlor-Trimeton), 4 mg; trimeprazine (Temaril), 2.5 mg; and cyproheptadine (Periactin), 4 mg.

Cimetidine (Tagamet), an H_2 antihistamine, given 300 mg four times daily is a useful addition in some cases. The tricyclic antidepressant doxepin (Sinequan) is a potent H_1 inhibitor and may also exert H_2 antihistaminic properties. Some patients respond to as little as 25 to 50 mg a day. Systemic corticosteroids are best avoided in the management of chronic pruritus. They are helpful if used judiciously for a limited time in the presence of severe acute pruritus. An example would be prednisone (Deltasone or Orasone), 5 mg four times a day initially. It should then be tapered and discontinued after 7 to 10 days.

Special Situations

Oral cholestyramine (Questran) produces a reduction in serum bile acids and provides relief in patients with biliary cirrhosis and renal disease. Given in dosages of 4 grams two to three times a day, it is helpful in treating more severe forms of pruritus gravidarum.

Ultraviolet B therapy is effective in uremic pruritus. It is administered in whole body exposures just under the minimal erythema dose. Treatment three times weekly for 4 weeks often results in prolonged remissions. Activated charcoal, 6 grams daily, has also given relief in many patients. Lidocaine (Xylocaine) given during hemodialysis is also of value; 200 mg is given as an infusion through the arterial line over a 20 minute period. The patients must be carefully monitored because of potential systemic toxicity.

The paroxysmal itching in multiple sclerosis has been found to respond to carbamazepine (Tegretol), 400 to 1200 mg daily. Blood counts need to be carefully followed because of potentially severe hematopoietic side effects.

Iron deficiency has been associated with pruritus even in the absence of anemia. Ferrous sulfate, 300 mg three times a day, has ameliorated the pruritus in some.

TINNITUS

method of
BRIAN F. McCABE, M.D.
University of Iowa
Iowa City, Iowa

Tinnitus is one of the oldest symptoms of humankind; descriptions go back to the early medical literature. It is simply defined as an abnormal noise in the ear. Tinnitus is an important symptom because it can be of an intensity and tenacity to preoccupy the mind of the patient and significantly diminish his or her quality of life. The attention span of some patients is so diminished as to reduce or eliminate their productivity.

The symptom can be divided into objective and subjective forms. Objective is that which can be heard by the examiner with a stethoscope; subjective is that which can be heard only by the patient. The subjective form can be further subdivided into central (central nervous system) and peripheral (end organ).

Objective tinnitus is almost always vascular and of a pulsatile or machinery-like crescendo-decrescendo nature. The best example is the noise accompanying a carotid-cavernous fistula, best heard with a bell-type stethoscope over the closed upper lid. Vascular tumors and vascular malformations of the upper neck, in and about the temporal bone, generally produce objective tinnitus. The most common example is the glomus tumor, either a glomus tympanicum or glomus jugulare. Objective tinnitus disappears when the tumor or other cause is eliminated.

Subjective tinnitus of the central variety, and of the peripheral variety for that matter, is very poorly understood. We have no animal models, and so research has been entirely through clinical observations. An example of the central variety is the ringing that is still present after removal of an acoustic neuroma when the entire eighth nerve is sacrificed. Another example is that which is still present after a surgical labyrinthectomy. In these situations tinnitus cannot be coming from the ear and must be originating in the brain.

Peripheral tinnitus is almost always accompanied by hearing loss in that ear, of either the conductive or sensorineural type. The noise is always at or quite near the frequencies of the hearing loss. It is as though the ear or brain fills up the hearing void with a noise of its own. To the degree the hearing loss can be reversed, the noise disappears. Indeed, patients commonly state it is the noise that is blocking their hearing. The character of the tinnitus can give some clue as to its cause. In conductive deafness it is of a pan-frequency nature that the patient likens to the noise of a seashell or a waterfall. Tinnitus due to sensorineural deafness is generally high frequency in type, and the patient likens it to a "singing telephone wire." Cricket-like tinnitus is also common and is probably due to a bifrequency hearing loss.

Treatment

The best treatment is to remove the cause; resect the tumor or correct the hearing loss. Correction of the hearing loss is infrequently possible because only 15 per cent of deafness is conductive in nature. For tinnitus accompanying sensorineural deafness, a number of treatments are available but each has had limited success. The most common is the use of a masking device that delivers a signal to the ear at or just off the frequency at which the ear rings. In a relatively small number of fortunate patients the masking effect persists for hours after the device is removed from the ear (poststimulation inhibition). Hypnotherapy has been used with some success, evoking posthypnotic suggestion. The oral form of lidocaine, Tocainide, has been tried in double-blind studies with significant improvement in less than the majority of patients. Studies are at present underway using a low voltage, low current stimulation of the temporal bones for several hours a day. Mild sedation may be helpful since some patients tend to listen intently to the tinnitus and develop a fixation upon it.

Section 2

The Infectious Diseases

ACQUIRED IMMUNODEFICIENCY SYNDROME (AIDS)

method of
MARGARET A. FISCHL, M.D.
and GORDON M. DICKINSON, M.D.
University of Miami
Miami, Florida

The acquired immunodeficiency syndrome (AIDS) is a newly recognized disease that has reached rather startling epidemic proportions in a short time. More than 9000 cases have been reported to the Centers for Disease Control (CDC) in Atlanta, and an additional 2000 cases are expected before the end of 1985. AIDS has been seen predominately among homosexual men and intravenous drug users as well as among persons with hemophilia A, recent Haitian immigrants, and those receiving blood products. AIDS has also been described among infants whose mothers have persistent immunologic abnormalities, AIDS, or an AIDS-related illness. AIDS is caused by a newly recognized retrovirus, human T-lymphotrophic virus type III/lymphadenopathy-associated virus (HTLV-III/LAV). HTLV-III/LAV has been isolated from the blood, semen, and saliva of infected persons. Epidemiologic data suggest that the virus is transmitted through intimate sexual contact; sharing of contaminated needles; transfusion of infected whole blood, blood components, plasma or clotted factor concentrates; or transmission from an infected mother to child during pregnancy or the perinatal period. No other blood products (immunoglobulin, albumin, hepatitis B vaccine) have been associated with infection, nor have cases been implicated on the basis of casual contact. Tests to detect antibody to HTLV-III/LAV via a modified enzyme-linked immunosorbent assay (ELISA) are now available.

Opportunistic Infections

The patient with AIDS is at risk for a number of life-threatening infections that are unique to patients with cellular immunodeficiency. Many of these causative pathogens infect healthy individuals but cause mild or no disease. In patients with AIDS, however, these pathogens often cause fulminant infections, and more than one pathogen may be present at any time. As shown in Table 1, infections tend to present as a pneumonia, gastroenteritis, central system dysfunction, or occult febrile illness.

General considerations related to opportunistic infections in AIDS include the following:

1. More than one infection may be present at any one time.
2. Infections may initially present subacutely but progress rapidly to a more fulminant process, e.g., *P. carinii* pneumonia, cryptococcal infection.
3. Several infections more typically cause a slowly progressive and debilitating illness, e.g., disseminated cytomegalovirus and *M. avium-intracellulare* infection.
4. Infections in general are less responsive to therapy, and high dose prolonged treatment is often needed.
5. Relapses are common and suppressive therapy may be needed, when available.
6. Adequate therapy is not available for all infections, e.g., cytomegalovirus, *M. avium-intracellulare* infection.
7. Numerous therapeutic and chemoprophylactic trials are under investigation, and recommendations may therefore change.
8. An unusually high incidence of allergic reactions to antimicrobials has been noted.
9. Secondary complications of infections, such as volume depletion, electrolyte imbalance, anemias, and malnutrition, are common.

TABLE 1. **Opportunistic Pathogens Associated with AIDS**

Pneumonias, Encephalitis, Meningitis	**Esophagitis**
Pneumocystis carinii	*Candida albicans*
Cytomegalovirus	Herpes simplex virus
Cryptococcus neoformans	Cytomegalovirus
Toxoplasma gondii	
Herpes simplex virus	**Enterocolitis**
Aspergillus fumigatus	Cytomegalovirus
Pseudomonas aeruginosa	*Candida albicans*
Mycobacterium tuberculosis	*Isospora belli*
	Cryptosporidium species
Cutaneous	
Herpes simplex virus	**Miscellaneous**
Herpes zoster virus	*Salmonella* species
	Mycobacterium avium complex
	Histoplasma capsulatum
	Coccidioides immitis

Antimicrobial treatment of AIDS-related opportunistic infection is given in Table 2.

Protozoa

Pneumocystis *Carinii* Pneumonia. *P. carinii* pneumonia represents one of the more commonly encountered infections among patients with AIDS and typically presents as a slowly progressive respiratory illness, although fulminant disease can occur. A dry cough, shortness of breath, fever, and hypoxemia are frequently noted. Although chest films classically show bilateral alveolar-interstitial infiltrates, normal chest films may be seen. In the face of normal studies, gallium scanning has shown diffuse pulmonary uptake, and pulmonary function testing has shown a decreased diffusing capacity. Either test may, therefore, be helpful in the patient suspected to harbor *Pneumocystis*.

The diagnosis of *Pneumocystis* infection is established by the identification of the cysts or trophozoites of *Pneumocystis* in tissue obtained from a lung biopsy stained with Giemsa or Gomori methenamine silver. Impression smears of biopsy material should be done, as they are frequently positive and are available within 2 hours. In patients with a bleeding diathesis or in those at a high risk for pneumothorax, bronchial lavage should be performed and concentrated lavage fluid carefully examined before an open lung biopsy is undertaken.

The treatment of *P. carinii* infection requires high dose trimethoprim-sulfamethoxazole (Bactrim, Septra). A dose of 20 mg per kg per day of trimethoprim and 100 mg per kg per day of sulfamethoxazole should be given in four equally divided doses. An intravenous route of administration is recommended. Each 5 ml of the preparation should be diluted in 125 ml of 5 per cent dextrose-in-water and used within 6 hours. If fluid restriction is needed, 5 ml of the drug should be diluted in 75 ml of 5 per cent dextrose-in-water and used within 2 hours. Drug shoud be administered slowly over 60 to 90 minutes. Rapid infusion or bolus injection should be avoided. High dose therapy should be continued for a total of 21 days, as shorter courses have proved ineffective in some patients. In patients who respond rapidly to intravenous treatment, a full 21-day course of antibiotic therapy can be completed with an oral preparation, if tolerated.

Treatment of the first episode of *Pneumocystis*

TABLE 2. **Antimicrobial Treatment of Opportunistic Infections Associated with AIDS**

Infection	Drug	Dose	Route/ Frequency	Duration
Pneumocystis carinii pneumonia	Trimethoprim-sulfamethoxazole	5/25 mg/kg	IV every 6 hours	21 days
	or			
	Pentamidine isethionate	4 mg/kg	IM once/day[1]	21 days
Toxoplasma encephalitis	Pyrimethamine and	100 mg (loading dose)	Orally, day 1	
		25 mg	Orally, once/day	12 weeks
	sulfadiazine	4 grams (loading dose)	Orally, day 1	
		1 gm	Orally, every 6 hours	
Cryptosporidiosis	None			
	Spiramycin (experimental)	1 gm	Orally, every 6 hours	21 days
Isosporiasis	Trimethoprim-sulfamethoxazole	5/25 mg/kg	Orally, tid	
	or			
	Pyrimethamine and	25 mg	Orally, once/day	21 days
	sulfadiazine	1 gm	Orally, every 6 hours	
Cryptococcal meningitis	Amphotericin B and	0.3 mg/kg	IV once/day	6 weeks[2]
	flucytosine	150 mg/kg	Orally, every 6 hours	6 weeks
	or			
	Amphotericin B	0.5 mg/kg	IV once/day	6 weeks[3]
Oral candidiasis	Mycostatin suspension	500,000 units (5 ml)	Swish/swallow qid	10–14 days
	or			
	Clotrimazole troches	Single troche	Dissolved slowly five times/day	10–14 days
	or			
	Ketoconazole	200–400 mg	Orally, bid	10–14 days
Candida esophagitis	Ketoconazole	200–400 mg	Orally, bid	10–14 days
Herpes virus (cutaneous disease)	Acyclovir	200 mg	Orally, six[5] times/day	10–14 days
(disseminated infection)	Acyclovir	5 mg/kg	IV every 8 hours	14 days
Mycobacerium avium complex	Isoniazid	300 mg	Orally, daily	1–2 years
	Ethambutol hydrochloride	25 mg/kg	Orally, daily	
	Ansamycin (experimental)[4]	150–300 mg	Orally, daily	
	Clofazamine (experimental)[4]	100 mg	Orally, daily	

[1]May be given safely as a 1 to 2 hour intravenous infusion.
[2]Total dose of 2–2.5 grams should be achieved; after 6 weeks of daily therapy, drug can then be given three times a day.
[3]If flucytosine is not tolerated, a higher dose of amphotericin B must be used.
[4]No defined regimen has been established; listed regimen is currently under evaluation.
[5]If oral drug not tolerated, should be given intravenously.

pneumonia is effective in 70 to 75 per cent of the cases, similar to the rate seen in other immunocompromised hosts. However, 60 to 80 per cent of patients with AIDS develop adverse reactions to treatment, including nausea, vomiting, rash, high fever, and joint and muscle pain. Nausea and vomiting can usually be controlled with antiemetics and/or metoclopramide hydrochloride (Reglan) prior to each infusion. More severe reactions leading to a Stevens-Johnson syndrome with an exfoliating dermatitis and vasculitis have also been described. If rash develops, treatment can be continued with close observation. However, if involvement of mucous membranes is noted or if a progressive rash is seen, the drug should be stopped. Other adverse reactions include hepatotoxicity and bone marrow suppression with leukopenia, thrombocytopenia, and/or a megaloblastic anemia. Simultaneous administration of folinic acid may decrease the incidence of profound leukopenia, but its efficacy has not been established. Trimethoprim-sulfamethoxazole is contraindicated in patients with known hypersensitivity, documented megaloblastic anemia, or pregnancy at term as well as in mothers who are breast feeding. Sulfonamides cross the placental barrier and are excreted in human milk and may cause kernicterus.

Pentamidine isethionate (Lomidine) is an alternative drug for the treatment of *P. carinii* infection in patients who develop reactions to trimethoprim-sulfamethoxazole or those with known sulfonamide drug allergies. Pentamidine has been approved by the Food and Drug Administration and is now commercially available. It should be given in a dose of 4 mg per kg per day for a total of 21 days (the manufacturer states that the benefits and risks of therapy for more than 14 days are not well defined). It is traditionally given intramuscularly in a single injection. However, careful intravenous infusions, given over 1 to 2 hours, can be safely administered. Adverse reactions include profound hypotension, tachycardia, and nausea and vomiting. Other reported reactions include thrombocytopenia, elevation of liver transaminases, hypoglycemia, hyperglycemia, and skin rash. Hypoglycemia may be severe and result in either seizures or coma. Mild renal dysfunction is not uncommon. Careful attention to the patient's fluid status can avoid problems with significant renal failure. Severe local myositis and sterile abscesses can occur with intramuscular administration.

In patients not responding to trimethoprim-sulfamethoxazole after 5 days or in those with progressive respiratory failure, pentamidine can be added to or substituted for trimethoprim-sulfamethoxazole. Patients who fail to respond to trimethoprim-sulfamethoxazole, however, usually do not respond to pentamidine alone or in combination with trimethoprim-sulfamethoxazole.

Recurrence of *P. carinii* pneumonia is common among patients with AIDS, and retreatment is frequently associated with severe adverse reactions. Trimethoprim-sulfamethoxazole administered at a lesser dose of 5 mg per kg of trimethoprim and 25 mg per kg of sulfamethoxazole in two equally divided doses can be used prophylactically in high-risk patients. Adverse reactions may still occur, and patients should be carefully monitored. Other drugs under current evaluation for chemoprophylaxis include the combination of pyrimethamine and sulfadoxine (Fansidar) and diaminodiphenylsulfone (dapsone).

***Toxoplasma* Infection.** Infection with *Toxoplasma gondii* frequently presents with neurologic disease, although pneumonitis, myopericarditis, and disseminated infection have been noted. Central nervous system infection typically presents as an encephalitis, as a meningoencephalitis, or as a cerebral mass lesion. Memory impairment and neurologic dysfunction, which can include seizures and coma secondary to mass effect, are common. Computed tomographic (CT) scan of the brain frequently demonstrates multiple bilateral enhancing lesions, although nonenhancing and single lesions may be seen. Cerebral spinal fluid analysis often shows a mild lymphocytic pleocytosis and an elevation of protein levels; glucose levels are typically normal. Diagnosis cannot be readily established by serology, as titers may be low in patients with disease and are often elevated in patients without disease. Diagnosis is established by demonstrating the trophozoites in tissue obtained from a brain biopsy or aspiration. False-negative biopsies can occur, especially with material containing predominantly necrotic tissue.

Combined administration of pyrimethamine (Daraprim) and sulfadiazine is the treatment of choice. Sulfadiazine is given as a 4 gram oral loading dose followed by 1 gram every 6 hours, and pyrimethamine as a 100 mg oral loading dose followed by 25 mg per day. Sulfonamides other than sulfadiazine or trisulfapyrimidines are less active against *T. gondii* infection and should be avoided. The duration of treatment is unknown. Based on preliminary experience, most patients will have complete resolution of clinical and radiographic abnormalities after 12 weeks of therapy. As these antibiotics are effective only against the actively proliferating trophozoite and not the dormant cyst forms, relapses are common in the immunocompromised host after therapy is stopped. Therefore, indefinite treatment or chronic suppressive therapy with low-dose sulfadiazine (1 gram) and pyrimethamine (25 mg) every other day or Fansidar given once per week is currently under evaluation.

The most common toxic effect of pyrimethamine and sulfadiazine is bone marrow suppression secondary to folate deficiency. Administration of 5 to 10 mg of folinic acid (Leucovorin) daily or three times per week is recommended. Other adverse reactions include anorexia, nausea, vomiting, rash, fever, and an atrophic glossitis. Vomiting may be minimized by administering the drug with meals. Reports of a Stevens-Johnson reaction to both pyrimethamine and sulfadiazine have been noted.

Alternative therapy is not available. Pyrimethamine alone is not effective. Patients with allergies to sulfonamides have been treated with pryimethamine and clindamycin, but clinical efficacy of this regimem has not been established. Spiramycin does not cross the blood-brain barrier and is therefore not useful in central nervous system disease. Trimethoprim, another antifolate drug, is also not effective.

Cryptosporidiosis. Chronic or intermittent diarrhea, often associated with malabsorption and debilitation, is a serious complication of AIDS. Pathogens that cause diarrhea in normal hosts may also infect patients with AIDS, but cryptosporidiosis is now recognized as a major cause of diarrhea and malabsorption in these patients. The organism is not identified by routine stool examination. A modified acid-fast stain of a concentrated stool specimen will readily demonstrate this parasite. Small bowel biopsy is not necessarily helpful, as involvement of the bowel can be sporadic.

There is no definitive treatment. Numerous regimens, including diodoquin, furazolidone, metronidazole, pentamidine, quinacrine, tetracycline, and trimethoprim-sulfamethoxazole, have been tried without much success. Alternative therapies under current evaluation include high-dose spiramycin (1 gram given orally four times per day) for a total of 3 weeks. Spiramycin is not available in the United States and must be obtained via the FDA from Rhone-Poulenc Pharma, Inc., Montreal, Quebec, Canada.

Isospora Belli. Another coccidial parasite seen with increasing frequency among patients with AIDS is *Isospora belli*. Presentation usually consists of watery diarrhea (typicaly less than what is seen with cryptosporidiosis), mild malabsorption, and fever. The organism can be found on routine stool examination. An Enterotest (string test) or duodenal aspirate can aid in the diagnosis. Treatment includes trimethoprim 10 mg per kg per day and sulfamethoxazole 50 mg per kg per day given orally in three equally divided doses for 3 weeks. Relapses are common. Suppressive therapy with trimethoprim 5 mg per kg and 25 mg of sulfamethoxazole given orally in two equally divided doses may be helpful. Alternative therapy includes pyrimethamine given as a 100 mg oral dose followed by 25 mg per day and sulfadiazine given as a 4 gram oral loading dose followed by 1 gram four times per day for 3 weeks.

Patients with coccidial parasite infections frequently present with dehydration, volume depletion, electrolyte abnormalities, and renal failure. Particular attention to fluid and electrolyte replacement is essential. Severe malnutrition can be seen, but parenteral hyperalimentaton is not always helpful unless infection can be eradicated and diarrhea controlled.

Fungi

Cryptococcal Infection. Infection with *Cryptococcus neoformans* typically presents as a meningitis or as a disseminated disease. Fungemia is common, and a subacute illness may abruptly end in cardiovascular collapse that is suggestive of septic shock.

The diagnosis of cryptococcal infection is established by culturing *C. neoformans* from spinal fluid, blood, or tissue such as lung, lymph node, or bone marrow. Cryptococcal antigen can be identified in the cerebral spinal fluid of most patients with meningitis and is often present in their serum. Microscopic examination of cerebral spinal fluid sediment stained with India ink often demonstrates the characteristic encapsulated yeast forms. It is noteworthy that nonencapsulated cryptococcal strains may cause infection among patients with AIDS. Diagnosis is frequently made with culture, as the India ink smear and test for antigen are negative owing to the lack of a capsule.

The treatment of choice for cryptococcal disease is a prolonged course of amphotericin B (Fungizone) and flucytosine (Ancobon). Therapy should be initiated with both amphotericin B, 0.3 mg per kg per day intravenously, and flucytosine, 150 mg per kg per day in four equally divided oral doses. Daily treatment should be continued for at least 6 weeks. In patients with severe or persistent central nervous system infection, intrathecal therapy via an Omaya reservoir may be helpful. Although a prolonged course of combination therapy may be effective in controlling the clinical manifestations, relapse has been noted in many patients within weeks or months after cessation of therapy. Therefore, careful follow-up of patients is necessary. Continuing treatment beyond a 6-week course, with infusions three times a week to achieve a total dose of 2.0 to 2.5 grams of amphotericin B, should be considered. Therapy three times a week can be given in an outpatient setting, if available. Placement of a Hickman catheter or Porto-cath is helpful with long-term amphotericin B administration.

Both amphotericin B and flucytosine are toxic drugs. Initial amphotericin B administration may cause fever, rigors, nausea, and hypotension. A test dose of 1 mg should be administered, followed by a stepwise increase of dosage. The traditional infusion time of 4 to 6 hours is not necessary, and infusions may be safely given over 1 hour. Adverse reactions resulting from intravenous therapy may be partially alleviated by giving aspirin, antihistamines, and low-dose corticosteroids just prior to each infusion. Thrombophlebitis is also not uncommon, and adding small amounts of heparin to the infusion may be helpful.

Other adverse reactions include both a distal renal tubular acidosis and a decrease in the glomerular filtration rate. Hypokalemia secondary to renal tubular acidosis typically occurs during the first few weeks of treatment and may be potentiated with concomitant corticosteroid administration. The decrease in glomerular filtration rate is dose-related and therefore tends to occur late in the course of therapy. Renal function should be determined at least weekly. If the blood urea nitrogen (BUN) increases above 40 mg per dl or the serum creatinine rises above 3.0 mg per dl, the drug should be temporarily discontinued. Treatment is resumed when the creatinine falls below 3.0 mg per dl. Other nephrotoxic drugs should be avoided. Liver function tests should be obtained weekly.

Flucytosine may cause nausea and vomiting and severe myelosuppression. Nausea and vomiting can be reduced or eliminated by administering the capsules a few at a time over 15 minutes. Myelosuppression is common, especially among patients with AIDS. It may therefore be necessary to lower the dose or stop the drug to avoid severe myelosuppression. Complete blood counts should be obtained biweekly. Because renal impairment caused by amphotericin B will raise serum levels of flucytosine, the dose should be decreased in the face of impaired renal function. If flucytosine is not tolerated and must be stopped, the dose of amphotericin B should be increased to 0.5 mg per kg per day, but not to exceed a maximum dose of 50 mg per day for the duration of therapy.

Candidiasis. The most common gastrointestinal infection seen among patients with AIDS is oral and esophageal candidiasis. Persistent or recurrent oral thrush among persons at risk for AIDS is an important and often early clue to immunodeficiency. In some patients, oral thrush may be a minor problem with subtle findings. In others, it may interfere with taste and further decrease eating. Esophageal candidiasis is also common among patients with AIDS. Patients typically complain of retrosternal chest pain or dysphagia. Barium studies are frequently positive and demonstrate characteristic findings of an esophagitis. Endoscopy may be needed in isolated cases to exclude cytomegalovirus, herpes simplex, or tumors as a cause of esophagitis.

The major treatment for oral candidiasis is nystatin or clotrimazole. Nystatin (Mycostatin) can be given as a suspension, 100,000 units per ml, 5 ml gargled and swallowed three to four times per day. Mycostatin suppositories dissolved in the mouth three to four times a day are also effective but have a chalky, often bitter, taste that may hamper therapy. Clotrimazole (Mycelex) troches are available and are often more palatable to patients. Troches should be dissolved in the mouth four to five times per day. Therapy should be continued for 10 to 14 days. In patients with more severe infection or in those in whom the foregoing therapy is not effective, ketoconazole (Nizoral), 200 to 400 mg oral dose twice per day for 10 to 14 days, can be used. Recurrent infection is common, and suppressive therapy with either ketoconazole 200 mg once per day or any of the topical preparations once to twice per day can be used.

Esophageal candidiasis can be best managed with ketoconazole, 200 to 400 mg orally twice a day for 10 to 14 days. After resolution of symptoms, dosage can be reduced to 200 mg per day to prevent recurrence. In patients with severe oral candidiasis or esophagitis, low-dose amphotericin B, 0.3 mg per kg per day for 5 to 10 days (a total dose of 100 to 300 mg), can be given and followed by ketoconazole and/or topical therapy for long-term prevention.

The major side effects of topical therapy include nausea and vomiting. No other serious adverse reactions have been noted. Ketoconazole in high doses has been associated with a fulminant hepatitis. Other adverse reactions include nausea, vomiting, abdominal pain, and pruritus.

***Histoplasma Capsulatum* and *Coccidioides Immitis*.** Disseminated infection secondary to both *H. capsulatum* and *C. immitis* has been documented among patients with AIDS. Diagnosis can be made by fungal stain and culture of biopsy specimens. Tissues most frequently positive are bone marrow, liver, blood, and lung. Treatment with amphotericin B has been effective in a few patients. Relapses are common.

Bacteria

***Mycobacterium Avium* Complex.** This is an atypical mycobacterium that is ubiquitous in the environment and found as a contaminant in dust, domesticated animals, and dairy products. Infection is uncommon, even in the immunocompromised host, but is seen with an unusual frequency among patients with AIDS. The clinical implication of *M. avium* complex in patients with AIDS is unclear. Infection is typically associated with the vague onset of nonspecific symptoms of fever, malaise, and weight loss. *M. avium* complex is readily isolated from the bone marrow and blood and less frequently identified in biopsy specimens of the liver, lymph nodes, lung, and small and large bowel. Intestinal infection with severe diarrhea, mimicking Whipple's disease, has been described. Although urine and sputum specimens may be positive, it is difficult to know whether this represents colonization or deep-seated infection. Blood cultures using a lysis centrifugation technique or a radiometric method are useful in assessing patients. How sensitive blood culture is compared with documentation in other tissues is unknown. Histiocytes and granulomas are frequently not present in biopsy specimens despite a large number of organisms identified with acid-fast stain.

There is currently no known treatment regimen that has proven clinical and microbiologic efficacy. The only drugs with *in vitro* activity against most isolates are ansamycin (an experimental rifampin derivative, available from the CDC, Atlanta, Georgia), clofazimine (an experimental antileprosy drug, which can be obtained from the Leprosy Service in Carville, Louisiana), and amikacin (Amikin). If disseminated disease is documented, treatment with four or five drugs, including isoniazid, ethambutol hydrochloride, ansamycin, and clofazimine with or without amikacin is recommended. Since rifampin is an analog of ansamycin, it should not be used in combination with ansamycin. Unfortunately, data supporting the efficacy and safety of any particular regimen does not yet exist. If disseminated disease is not identified, observation without therapy is advisable.

Mycobacterium Tuberculosis. *M. tuberculosis* infection is not uncommon in patients with AIDS, especially among risk groups with a high prevalence of tuberculous infection. It is frequently the first opportunistic infection noted and precedes other infection by several months. Disease often presents as a disseminated lymphatic or hematogenous infection or localized extrapulmonary infection. The most common sources of positive culture include lymph nodes, lung, bone marrow, liver, and pericardium. Histologic examination frequently does not reveal granuloma, and the number of acid-fast bacili may be few. Despite the pattern of disseminated or extrapulmonary manifestation, infection responds well to antituberculosis therapy. Antituberculosis regimens currently recommended for the treatment of tuberculosis in the nonimmunocompromised host appear appropriate for these patients. How long treatment should be continued is not known.

Viruses

Herpes Simplex Virus. Infections with herpes virus may be disseminated, but the most common presentation is one of chronic progressive cutaneous ulcerations. Lesions may be located in the perianal, genital, or oral areas. With perianal disease, severe rectal pain, bleeding, tenesmus, or rectal discharge may be noted by the patient.

The diagnosis of herpes simplex virus disease is based on histopathology and/or culture. Virus has been documented in the esophagus, lungs, lymph nodes, and brain. The presence of multinucleated giant cells with intranuclear inclusion bodies on a scraping or biopsy specimen confirms the diagnosis. Serology is not helpful.

Active herpes simplex infection should be treated with acyclovir (Zovirax), which is now available in topical, oral, and injectable forms. Small ulcers may respond to acyclovir creams appled topically every 2 to 3 hours. Most patients with cutaneous disease, however, will require the oral or parenteral form to control infection. Acyclovir should be given as a 200 mg oral dose five times a day for 10 to 14 days. In patients who are unable to tolerate an oral medication, acyclovir can be administered intravenously at a dose of 5 mg per kg every 8 hours for 10 to 14 days. In patients with isolated extracutaneous or disseminated disease, acyclovir should be given parenterally for 14 days. A longer course of treatment may be needed. In patients with severe recurrent infection, suppressive therapy with acyclovir, 200 mg oral dose twice per day, may reduce further outbreaks.

Adverse reactions are uncommon and include rash, fever, nausea, vomiting, and elevation in liver transaminases.

Cytomegalovirus. Most patients with AIDS will have serologic evidence of prior infection with cytomegalovirus, and viral shedding in the urine is common, especially among homosexual men. Disease caused by cytomegalovirus may involve virtually every organ. Localized infection of the brain, eyes, esophagus, large intestine, and lungs has been noted most frequently among patients with AIDS. Disseminated infections can also occur, especially in the terminally ill patient. In addition to localizing symptoms, patients may present with fever, malaise, weight loss, and fatigue.

The diagnosis of cytomegalovirus infection is based on histopathologic findings of typical intranuclear and cytoplasmic inclusion bodies. Positive culture of a biopsy specimen is also useful, but isolation from the urine is common among asymptomatic patients with AIDS and may not reflect disease. For the same reason, serology is not helpful.

No therapy exists at this time. Acyclovir, adenine arabinoside, and other antiviral drugs have been ineffective. Preliminary studies have shown that dihydroxy-propoxymethyl guanine (DHPG) effectively suppresses cytomegalovirus excretion and appears to provide some clinical benefit to patients with cytomegalovirus chorioretinitis. Its use, however, does not eradicate virus. Leukocyte alpha interferon has been shown to be effective prophylactically in renal transplant recipients but has no proven efficacy in the treatment of active disease associated with AIDS.

Varicella. Herpes zoster occurs in patients with AIDS, and dissemination beyond a single dermatome is typical. The presentation is similar to that in the nonimmunocompromised host. Diagnosis can be made on clinical grounds alone. A Tzanck preparation of a scraping of an ulcer will typically show multinucleated giant cells and confirm the presence of a herpes virus infection.

Varicella zoster will respond to acyclovir given as an oral dose four to five times per day for 7 days.

Kaposi's Sarcoma

Kaposi's sarcoma, previously a rare dermal malignancy in the United States, is now occurring in epidemic form in association with AIDS. Unlike the indolent cutaneous form described among elderly men of Jewish or Italian background, Kaposi's sarcoma in association with AIDS often presents with disseminated disease and follows an aggressive course. Over 95 per cent of patients present with skin lesions. Lesions are quite characteristic and can be flat, slightly raised, or nodular. Lesions are typically pigmented, ranging in color from a faint pink to a deep purple. Involvement of lymph nodes and the gastrointestinal tract is not common. Other visceral disease, especially lung involvement, carries a poorer prognosis.

The diagnosis of Kaposi's sarcoma can be readily made from a biospy specimen. Skin lesions are easily accessible, and a simple dermal punch biopsy obtains adequate tissue for diagnosis.

The treatment of Kaposi's sarcoma in association with AIDS is variable. Patients do respond to cytotoxic chemotherapy. Single agents, such as vinblastine, bleomycin, and etoposide (VP-16), achieve antitumor response rates of 20 to 60 per cent with short remission durations of about 1 month. Combination therapy is quite effective but is associated with a high incidence of complicating opportunistic infections and mortality. Alpha interferons have been used successfully alone or in combination with single agent cytotoxic chemotherapy. Average antitumor response rates vary from 40 to 50 per cent with remission durations up to 6 months. Local radiation therapy may be helpful in isolated cases.

Human T-Lymphotrophic Virus, Type III (HTLV-III) Infection

The natural history of HTLV-III/LAV infection is unknown. Infection may be asymptomatic, or it may be associated with a spectrum of disease that ranges from chronic lymphadenopathy to a severe progressive illness characterized by recurrent opportunistic infections or the development of malignancies. Not all patients with HTLV-III/LAV infection will develop symptoms of AIDS. Preliminary studies suggest that most persons (50 to 60 per cent) do not develop progressive symptoms—at least over a 1 to 2 year period of observation. Persons with isolated lymphadenopathy associated with mild immunodeficiency also do well, and few progress to more serious disease. Persons, however, who have symptoms including oral candidiasis, herpes zoster infection, chronic fevers, or weight loss are at a greater risk for developing AIDS and should be closely followed. Prodromal symptoms of AIDS are well recognized and are outlined in Table 3. Patients presenting with these symptoms should be evaluated carefully for opportunistic infections and tumors.

Tests to detect antibody to HTLV-III/LAV are now licensed and commercially available in the United States. The antibody tests are modifications of the enzyme-linked immunosorbent assay (ELISA), which uses antigen derived from whole disrupted HTLV-III virus. In different studies, HTLV-III antibody was found to range from 68 to 100 per cent in patients with AIDS and from 84 to 90 per cent in patients with AIDS-related illnesses. In addition, a high seroprevalence rate among persons at risk for AIDS has been found. Twenty-two to 65 per cent of homosexual men, 87 per cent of intravenous drug users in New York City, and 56 to 72 per cent of persons with hemophilia A have been noted to have positive antibody to HTLV-III. In contrast, HTLV-III antibody has been detected in less than 1 per cent of the general population. Antibody testing should be used cautiously, especially in the asymptomatic person at risk for AIDS. Individuals noted to have positive antibody should be coun-

TABLE 3. **Prodromal Symptoms Associated with AIDS***

Symptom	Incidence (%)
Fatigue	90
Anorexia	85
Weight loss	85
Fever	80
Diarrhea	50
Lymphadenopathy	50
Oral thrush	45
Paresthesias	15

*Typically present for more than 3 weeks without a definable etiology.

seled. Recommendations that have been put forth by the CDC include the following:

1. Although asymptomatic, individuals with antibody to HTLV-III may be infectious and transmit virus to others. These individuals should therefore refrain from donating blood, plasma, body organs, or other tissues or sperm.
2. There is a risk of infecting partners through sexual intercourse, through sharing of needles, and possibly through exposure with saliva through oral-genital contact or intimate kissing.
3. The efficacy of condoms in preventing infection with HTLV-III is unproved, but their use may reduce transmission.
4. Toothbrushes, razors, or other implements that could become contaminated with blood should not be shared.
5. Seropositive women, or women whose sexual partners are seropositive, are at risk for developing AIDS. If they become pregnant, their offspring is at an increased risk of acquiring AIDS.
6. After accidents resulting in bleeding, contaminated areas should be cleaned with household bleach diluted 1:10 with water.

Prevention

Since AIDS is recognized to be transmitted via contact with infected blood or blood products, a potential hazard to health care professionals exists. The present recommendations for health care workers and laboratory personnel are similar to those for hepatitis B infection. Gloves should be worn when one handles blood or blood-soiled items or when possible blood contamination may occur (for example, when an intravenous catheter is flushed). Personnel who may be exposed to bloody aerosolized secretions should also wear a face mask and eye protection. Except when caring for patients with a productive cough, face masks are generaly not needed. Private rooms are recommended for ill patients who cannot attend to their own personal needs. Blood samples, tissues, and other body secretions sent to the laboratory should be appropriately labeled.

AMEBIASIS

method of
JAMES J. CERDA, M.D.
University of Florida
Gainesville, Florida

The aim of chemotherapy in amebiasis is to eradicate infection, whether it be luminal, in the intestinal wall, or in other body organs. More than one amebicide is necessary because of important variations in both the pharmacology of the drugs and their site of action. In addition, the pathogenicity of *Entamoeba histolytica* depends on its grouping (zymodemes—18 in all). It may be that most amebic infections are of zymodeme types II, VI, VII, and XI.

Commonly available tissue amebicides include metronidazole (Flagyl) and tetracycline. It is, however, extremely difficult to obtain luminal agents that include diiodohydroxyquin (Yodoxin), emetine hydrochloride, and paromomycin (Humatin). Dehydroemetine and diloxanide furoate (Furamide) are both investigational. They can be obtained from the Parasitic Disease Drug Service, Centers for Disease Control, Atlanta, Georgia 30333. One can telephone during business hours to 404/329-3670, at other times, 404/329-2888.

Lastly, the success of the treatment must be shared with the newer diagnostic methods, including isotope hepatoscanning ultrasonography, computed axial tomography (CAT scans), and serologic titers.

Treatment

Acute Amebic Dysentery. The term *acute amebic dysentery* implies tissue invasion by the parasite. For this reason, the tissue-active drug metronidazole, 750 mg three times daily for 10 days, is recommended for adults. If amebic dysentery should become severe enough to require hospital admission, intravenous metronidazole can be administered. It can be given as a loading dose of 15 mg per kg infused over 1 hour, followed by 7.5 mg per kg every 6 hours. Supportive measures—intravenous fluids, hyperalimentation—and frequent observation for toxic megacolon, peritonitis, and ileus are indicated. In many parts of the world, emetine hydrochloride is still used. Dehydroemetine has fewer side effects and is obtainable from the Centers for Disease Control, Atlanta, Georgia. Emetine can be given in a dosage of 1 mg per kg per day intramuscularly or subcutaneously for 10 days. Dehydroemetine is given in dosages of 1 to 1.5 mg per kg per day intramuscularly or subcutaneously for 10 days. Side effects of the emetines include diarrhea, nausea, vomiting, weakness, and spontaneous pain and rigidity of skeletal muscles. Electrocardiographic findings may demonstrate T wave depression, ST segment deviation, tachycardia, and arrhythmias. Supervision of dosage administration is mandatory. Since none of the tissue amebicides will totally eradicate luminal amebae, luminal amebicides should always follow. Either diiodohydroxyquinoline (Yodoxin), 650 mg three times daily for 20 days, or diloxanide furoate (Furamide), 500 mg three times daily for 10 days is recommended.

Fulminant Amebic Colitis. Fulminant amebic colitis is characterized by rapidly progressive symptoms of urgent, bloody diarrhea; abdominal pain preceding evacuation; and tenesmus resembling that seen in acute *Shigella* dysentery. Fever ranges from 38 to 39 C. There is rapid weight loss, dehydration, and abdominal distention. Examination demonstrates a distended abdomen and tympanitic and patchy peristaltic sounds. A survey film of the abdomen may demonstrate megacolon. Perforation and peritonitis may follow. Specific antiamebic treatment may be ineffective, and surgery may be required. Resection, drainage, or, rarely, colectomy followed by medical therapy is the usual sequence of events. Concomitant hyperalimentation is recommended.

Mild to Moderate Intestinal Amebiasis. Metronidazole, 500 mg three times daily for 10 days, followed by diiodohydroxyquin or diloxanide furoate, is extremely effective. Over 95 per cent of all cases will be cured with this method. Alternatively, paromomycin followed by diiodohydroxyquin can be used. Tetracycline, 250 mg four times daily for 10 days, followed by one of the aforementioned luminal amebicides, is still used by some but can be recommended only as alternative therapy.

Side effects of metronidazole include nausea, diarrhea, a metallic taste in the mouth, dizziness, and occasional discoloration of the urine. Modest leukopenia has been noted, but white blood cell counts generally return to normal after completion of treatment. Metronidazole is contraindicated for patients with blood dyscrasias, warfarin therapy, or active disease of the central nervous system. Approximately 25 per cent of patients will develop severe abdominal pain resembling a disulfiram-like reaction. All patients should be cautioned against that possibility.

Asymptomatic Infection. The key question here is "to treat or not to treat," since carriers comprise the largest group of persons (perhaps 500 million!) who shed amebae in their stools. Asymptomatic infections are usually diagnosed in a hospital that has a clinical laboratory. If one is dealing with asymptomatic carriers in an endemic area, treatment is generally not necessary since the probability of reinfection in endemic areas is highly likely. This should be tempered by the possibility that one is dealing with a highly pathogenic strain in a particular area, or that the carrier is a food handler by profession. If asymptomatic infections are found in nonendemic areas, they probably should be treated. Diiodohydroxyquin (Yodoxin), 600 mg three times daily for 20 days, is recommended. Although side effects are uncommon, they include a reaction to iodine, an occasional case of optic atrophy (in children), and peripheral neuropathy, if used for long periods. If available, diloxanide furoate (Furamide) is very effective, with a cure rate of greater than 90 per cent. Its major side effects are excessive flatulence and occasional nausea and diarrhea. Metronidazole has been disappointing when used in tissue doses as a luminal amebicide. Some have advocated its use as a single dose for 2 days in the higher dosage of 2 grams; however, reports of its efficacy at this high dosage have been sporadic.

Amebic Liver Abscess. The liver is the most common site of extraintestinal infection with *E. histolytica*. The lack of intestinal disease in these patients is common. Amebic abscess requires hospitalization. Since most, if not all, of the patients probably exhibit some form of protein-caloric malnutrition, aggressive enteral or parenteral hyperalimentation is often indicated. The clinical features of liver abscess may include an abrupt onset, pain and tenderness in the region of the liver, wasting, and fever associated with chills and profuse night sweats. Because of its generalized nature, not only careful examination but also hepatic ultrasonography, isotope hepatoscans, and CAT scans are extremely useful in the diagnosis of amebic abscess. The exact role of CAT scans or nuclear magnetic resonance imaging remains to be resolved.

If the patient can take oral medication, metronidazole, 750 mg three times daily for 5 to 7 days should suffice. If relapse occurs, metronidazole, 750 mg three times daily should be administered for 3 weeks. Intravenous metronidazole (previously described) is indicated for patients who cannot take oral medications. Parenteral emetine or dehydroemetine is also effective against amebic abscess. These agents can be given in a dosage of 1 mg per kg per day intramuscularly or by deep subcutaneous injection for 6 to 8 days. Closed drainage of a liver abscess may be necessary if the abscess is large and there is no substantial improvement within 48 hours after starting chemotherapy. Closed aspiration is facilitated by ultrasonography or CAT scan, since the area of the abscess cavity can be mapped. The cavity should be entered at the point of maximum tenderness.

OPEN SURGICAL DRAINAGE OF AMEBIC ABSCESS. Surgical intervention should be limited to cases in which there is imminent or actual rupture of the abscess into the pleura, peritoneum, or pericardium and to the rare case of amebic abscess that does not respond to chemotherapy or closed aspiration.

Ameboma. Amebomas are granulomatous lesions that occur predominantly in the vertical regions of the colon, the cecum, and the rectum. They are associated with vague abdominal symptoms, occasional bloody diarrhea, and a probable mass. Rarely, more than one ameboma may be present. Colonoscopy with biopsy is extremely helpful in establishing the diagnosis. Amebomas should be treated with 750 mg of metronidazole three times daily for 10 days, followed by diiodohydroxyquin or diloxanide furoate.

Amebic granulomas may perforate with all the signs of an acute abdomen. More commonly, the perforations seal off and the patient is explored because of a suspicion of malignancy.

Other Forms. Cutaneous, pulmonary, genitoperineal, or brain involvement with amebiasis should be treated with metronidazole followed by a luminal agent, as described previously. These forms are extremely uncommon in the United States.

BACTEREMIA

method of
LAYNE O. GENTRY, M.D.,
and BARRY J. ZELUFF, M.D.
Baylor College of Medicine
Houston, Texas

Bacteremia—the presence of bacteria in the blood stream—is always a serious condition. Newer culture techniques are now available that make possible the detection of bacteremia within hours. Although it can be a benign occurrence, such as the transient bacteremia commonly seen after the brushing of teeth, it is the initial event in patients who develop septic shock. Because there is increased mortality in all patients with infection who have concomitant bacteremia, prompt recognition and correct management are essential. Bacteremia may be transient, intermittent, or sustained, depending on the source, underlying conditions, and timing of blood cultures. Because bacteremia associated with an identifiable focus of infection often persists until the focus is resolved, it is important to quickly search for such a site.

The most common presenting symptoms of clinically significant bacteremia are fever and chills. However, localizing signs and symptoms may be related to the specific focus if infection is the source of the bacteremia. Thus, a patient with urinary tract sepsis may be seen with urgency, frequency, or dysuria whereas a person with bacteremia resulting from pneumonia may have a productive cough, shortness of breath, or chest pain. Shock is usually a late finding and is associated with a worse prognosis. Not all patient groups have the same clinical presentation: The elderly often present hypothermia or a change in the level of consciousness, whereas neonates will show increased irritability

TABLE 1. **Site of Initial Infection and Pathogens Likely to Cause Bacteremia**

Respiratory	Cardiovascular	Urinary	Gastrointestinal	Musculoskeletal
Pharyngitis *Streptococcus pyogenes (group A)* *Neisseria meningitidis*	Subacute bacterial endocarditis *Streptococcus viridans* *Streptococcus faecalis*	Pyelonephritis *Escherichia coli* *Proteus* spp. *Klebsiella pneumoniae* *Streptococcus faecalis*	Gastroenteritis *Salmonella typhi* *Campylobacter jejuni*	Septic arthritis *Neisseria gonorrhoeae* *Staphylococcus aureus* *Streptococcus pyogenes* Gram-negative rods
Otitis *Streptococcus pneumoniae* *Streptococcus pyogenes (group A)*	Acute bacterial endocarditis *Staphylococcus aureus* *Streptococcus pneumoniae*		Peritonitis (appendicitis, diverticulitis) *Escherichia coli* *Streptococcus faecalis* *Bacteroides fragilis* Other gram-negative aerobic rods	Myositis *Staphylococcus aureus* *Streptococcus pyogenes (Group A)* *Clostridium* spp. Anaerobes
Sinusitis *Streptococcus pneumoniae* *Streptococcus pyogenes (group A)* *Staphylococcus aureus*	Prosthetic valve endocarditis *Staphylococcus epidermidis* *Staphylococcus aureus* *Streptococcus viridans* Gram-negative bacilli *Candida* spp.		Perirectal abscess *Escherichia coli* *Streptococcus faecalis* *Bacteroides fragilis* Other gram-negative aerobic rods	Osteomyelitis *Staphylococcus aureus*
Pneumonia *Streptococcus pneumoniae* *Haemophilus influenzae* *Staphylococcus aureus* *Klebsiella pneumoniae* *Branhamella catarrhalis* *Bacteroides* spp.	Associated IV catheter and drug abuse *Staphylococcus aureus* *Escherichia coli* *Klebsiella pneumoniae* *Pseudomonas aeruginosa*			
Bronchitis *Streptococcus pneumoniae* *Haemophilus influenzae*				

TABLE 2. **First and Second Choice Antibiotic Regimens to Treat Bacteremia Caused by Common Pathogens**

Organism	First Choice Regimen	Second Choice Regimen
Bacteroides fragilis (colon flora)	clindamycin chloramphenicol or metronidazole	cephalosporin (H) carbenicillin ticarcillin mezlocillin or piperacillin
Bacteroides spp. (oropharyngeal flora)	penicillin G	ampicillin clindamycin or cephalosporin (H)
Branhamella catarrhalis	trimethoprim-sulfamethoxazole	erythromycin or cephalosporin (J)
Clostridium spp. (not *C. difficile*)	penicillin G	cephalosporins (E, D, H, or J)
Campylobacter jejuni	erythromycin	
Enterobacter spp.		
community strains	cephalosporins (F, G, or I) aminoglycosides (A, W, or N)	carbenicillin ticarcillin or piperacillin
hospital strains	aminoglycosides (A, W, or N) cephalosporins (F, G, or I)	carbenicillin trimethoprim-sulfamethoxazole
Escherichia coli		
community strains	cephalosporins (D, E, J, or H)	aminoglycosides (A, W, or N) carbenicillin ticarcillin mezlocillin piperacillin
hospital strains	aminoglycosides (A, W, or N) cephalosporins (F, G, or I)	trimethoprim-sulfamethoxazole
Haemophilus influenzae	(initially) ampicillin plus chloramphenicol	
beta-lactamase (−)	ampicillin	cephalosporins (J, G, or I) trimethoprim-sulfamethoxazole
beta-lactamase (+)	chloramphenicol or cephalosporins (J, G, or E)	cephalosporins (J, G, or I) trimethoprim-sulfamethoxazole
Klebsiella pneumoniae		
community strains	cephalosporins (J, F. G, or I)	mezlocillin piperacillin aminoglycosides (W, N, or A) trimethoprim-sulfamethoxazole
hospital strains	aminoglycosides (W, N, or A)	cephalosporins (J, F, G, or I)
Proteus mirabilis	ampicillin	cephalosporins (all) aminoglycosides (all) trimethoprim-sulfamethoxazole
Proteus spp. [indole (+)]	aminoglycosides (W, N, or A)	cephalosporins (G or I) carbenicillin ticarcillin mezlocillin piperacillin trimethoprim-sulfamethoxazole
Providencia stuartii	aminoglycosides (A, W, or N)	cephalosporins (G or I) carbenicillin ticarcillin mezlocillin piperacillin trimethoprim-sulfamethoxazole

Table continued on following page

TABLE 2. **First and Second Choice Antibiotic Regimens to Treat Bacteremia Caused by Common Pathogens** *Continued*

Organism	First Choice Regimen	Second Choice Regimen
Pseudomonas aeruginosa		
community strains	aminoglycosides (W, N, or A) plus either carbenicillin, ticarcillin, mezlocillin or piperacillin	aminoglycosides (W, N, or A) plus cephalosporin (F)
hospital strains	aminoglycosides (W, N, or A) plus either carbenicillin, ticarcillin, mezlocillin or piperacillin	aminoglycosides (W, N, or A) plus cephalosporin (F)
Salmonella typhi	chloramphenicol	ampicillin trimethoprim-sulfamethoxazole
Serratia marcescens	aminoglycosides (N, A, or W) plus carbenicillin, ticarcillin or mezlocillin, piperacillin	aminoglycosides (N, A, or W) plus cephalosporins (G or I) or trimethoprim-sulfamethoxazole
Staphylococcus		
beta-lactamase (−)	penicillin G	cephalosporins (E, D, or J) vancomycin
beta-lactamase (+)	nafcillin methicillin or oxacillin	vancomycin clindamycin or cephalosporin (E, D, or J)
methicillin-resistant	vancomycin	trimethoprim-sulfamethoxazole
Streptococcus (group B)	penicillin G ampicillin	cephalosporin (E, D, or J) vancomycin
Streptococcus, anaerobic	penicillin G	clindamycin cephalosporins (E, D, or J)
Streptococcus faecalis (Streptococcus faecium, Group D *Enterococcus*	ampicillin plus aminoglycosides (N or W)	vancomycin plus aminoglycosides (N or W)
Streptococcus pneumoniae	penicillin G	erythromycin cephalosporins (E, D, or J) vancomycin
Beta-hemolytic streptococcus (groups A, C, and G)	penicillin G	cephalosporin (E, D, or J) vancomycin

*SEE TABLE 3 FOR KEY LETTERS AND DOSAGES.

or a change in eating habits. Diabetic patients, chronic renal failure patients, leukemic patients, or immunosuppressed patients with bacteremia may also have atypical signs and symptoms.

Treatment

In most patients, clues about the source of the bacteremia can be obtained from a careful history and physical examination (Table 1). Based on the most likely source for the bacteremia, a logical prediction of the responsible organism and the selection of appropriate empiric therapy can be made (Tables 2 and 3). A Gram stain of body fluids from suspected sites of infection may provide early clues; however, culture confirmation yields the final documentation of the bacterial etiology. Bacteremia associated with pneumonia may be diagnosed by looking at the Gram stain of the sputum; urinary tract sepsis, by Gram stain of the urine; and sepsis associated with a wound infection, Gram stain of the wound exudate.

Often there is no material for Gram stain, and empiric therapy must be based on knowledge of the bacterial flora common to the site of infection. Thus, patients with intra-abdominal sepsis usually have mixed infections with aerobic gram-negative rods and anaerobes, and empiric therapy must include antibiotics effective against these organisms.

Bacteremia associated with endocarditis is usually sustained; however different bacterial patterns are associated with different patient populations. Patients with endocarditis, therefore, must be divided into addicts versus nonaddicts or

TABLE 3. **Recommended Doses of Antimicrobial Agents for Patients with Bacteremia and Normal Renal Function**

Agent	Dose	Frequency
amikacin	7.5 mg/kg IV	q 12 hr
	5.0 mg/kg IV	q 8 hr
ampicillin	2.0 gm IV	q 4 hr
carbenicillin	5.0 gm IV	q 4 hr
cefamandole	2.0 gm IV	q 4–6 hr
cefazolin	2.0 gm IV	q 8 hr
cefoperazone	2.0 gm IV	q 8 hr
cefotaxime	2.0 gm IV	q 4–6 hr
cefoxitin	2.0 gm IV	q 6 hr
ceftizoxime	2.0 gm IV	q 6 hr
cefuroxime	1.5 gm IV	q 8 hr
chloramphenicol	0.5 gm IV	q 6 hr
clindamycin	600 mg IV	q 6 hr
erythromycin lactobionate	0.5 gm IV	q 6 hr
gentamicin	1.5 mg/kg IV as loading dose, then	
	1.0 mg/kg IV	q 8 hr
methicillin	2.0 gm IV	q 4 hr
metronidazole	15.0 mg/kg as loading dose, then	
	7.5 mg/kg IV	q 6 hr
mezlocillin	3.0 gm IV	q 4 hr
nafcillin	2.0 gm IV	q 4 hr
oxacillin	2.0 gm IV	q 4 hr
penicillin (aqueous)	2–5 million units IV	q 3 hr
piperacillin	3.0 gm IV	q 4 hr
ticarcillin	3.0 gm IV	q 4 hr
tobramycin	1.5 mg/kg IV as loading dose, then	
	1.0 mg/kg IV	q 8 hr
trimethoprim-sulfamethoxazole	15–20 mg/kg/day of trimethoprim divided into 3 or 4 doses given either q 8 or q 6 hr	
vancomycin	500 mg IV	q 6 hr

those with prosthetic valve endocarditis. Endocarditis in nonaddicts is usually due to *Streptococcus viridans;* thus penicillin is the drug of choice. Endocarditis in intravenous drug abusers is usually *Staphylococcus aureus,* and most strains are resistant to penicillin. Thus either a penicillinase-resistant penicillin, such as nafcillin, or vancomycin is the drug of choice. Gram-negative bacteria such as *Pseudomonas aeruginosa* and *Serratia marcescens* are also encountered in addicts with endocarditis. In prosthetic valve endocarditis, early infection (occurring less than 2 months after surgery) and late infection (occurring more than 2 months after surgery) differ. Early prosthetic valve endocarditis is usually due to *Staphylococcus epidermidis* or *S. aureus*. However, gram-negative rods and fungi are also encountered in early prosthetic valve endocarditis. Late prosthetic valve endocarditis is most commonly caused by *S. epidermidis* or *S. aureus,* but *S. viridans* and group D enterococci infection may also occur.

Bacteremia in the immunocompromised host, especially if neutropenic, is usually due to gram-negative rods like *E. coli, Klebsiella pneumoniae, Pseudomonas aeruginosa,* or *Serratia marcescens.* Because patients are seriously ill with such infections, combination therapy with an antipseudomonal penicillin or a third generation cephalosporin plus aminoglycoside is now considered standard empiric therapy. Catheter-related sepsis is usually due to gram-positive cocci like *S. aureus* or *S. epidermidis.* Because of the usually high level of methicillin-resistant *S. epidermidis* in most hospitals, vancomycin is the initial drug of choice for catheter sepsis. Gram-negative rods may also be responsible for 15 to 20 per cent of catheter-related sepsis, especially in patients with tracheostomy whose tracheal secretions are colonized with these organisms.

Adjunct therapy is often as important as antibiotic therapy in the management of bacteremia. Simple procedures, such as removing an intravascular catheter or draining an abscess that may be the source of the bacteremia, may prevent serious sequelae, including septic shock.

Shock is the most life-threatening complication associated with bacteremia. Support of the blood pressure with intravascular volume or vasopressor agents like dopamine or dobutamine is necessary to maintain renal, cardiac, and cerebral blood flow. Steroids are often used in the management of septic shock, though their efficacy has not been conclusively proved. If steroids are to be used, early treatment with methylprednisolone, 30 mg per kg, or dexamethasone, 2 mg per kg, has been suggested. The experimental use of naloxone, 0.4 to 1.2 mg, has been shown to increase transiently the blood pressure of patients with septic shock.

In patients with a known source for bacteremia, 10 to 14 days of parenteral therapy are adequate. Bacteremia associated with an abscess or empyema may not respond to such a short course, and often a total of 3 to 4 weeks of therapy is necessary. Bacterial endocarditis also requires prolonged therapy, and 4 to 6 weeks of parenteral antibiotic are considered appropriate. Antibiotic therapy in patients with bacteremia who have granulocytopenia may need to be continued until the granulocyte count is greater than 1000.

BRUCELLOSIS

method of
KENRAD E. NELSON, M.D.
University of Illinois
Chicago, Illinois

In the United States, brucellosis is relatively rare; only about 200 to 300 cases are reported each year. Human disease may be acute, with sudden onset of fever, chills, and weight loss, or it may be chronic, in which case onset is insidious. In the chronic form, organ localization of granulomatous infection is not unusual, as in bones and joints, spleen, hepatobiliary system, genitourinary tract, lymph nodes, lungs, and heart valves. Relapse of acute brucellosis after apparently successful therapy is a troublesome and not infrequent problem. Also, many patients may develop a syndrome of malaise, fatigue, and depression after treatment. Whether nonspecific symptoms such as these represent "chronic brucellosis" may at times be a diagnostic challenge for the clinician. However, this syndrome probably does not represent active brucellosis requiring retreatment, unless other objective evidence of infection is present, such as fever, elevated erythrocyte sedimentation rate, positive cultures of blood or tissues for *Brucella,* or persistently elevated or rising agglutinin antibodies to *Brucella,* especially of the IgG class.

In Vitro Antimicrobial Sensitivity of Brucella

Many drugs show evidence of in vitro activity against *Brucella,* including tetracycline, aminoglycosides, trimethoprim-sulfamethoxazole (co-trimoxazole), rifampin, erythromycin, and ampicillin. Despite evidence of activity in vitro in some studies, ampicillin has been shown to be ineffective, as are the cephalosporins, cefamycins, erythromycin, and chloramphenicol. These drugs should not be used even if they exhibit in vitro sensitivity to the strain of *Brucella* responsible for a human infection.

Discrepancies between in vitro and in vivo activity may relate in part to the fact that in brucellosis the organisms are located intracellularly in a granulomatous infection and may not be highly active metabolically. Therefore, penetration of the antibiotic into the site of infection and antibacterial activity of some drugs may be compromised in vivo.

Antimicrobial Regimens

The regimen that has been studied for many years and seems to have the greatest efficacy and lowest relapse rate for uncomplicated brucellosis is a combination of tetracycline, 500 mg every 6 hours for 3 to 6 weeks, with streptomycin, 1 gram intramuscularly daily (or 500 mg every 12 hours) for 2 to 4 weeks. Some authorities feel that aminoglycosides are not always needed for treatment of all patients with acute brucellosis and recommend tetracycline alone, 500 mg every 6 hours for 3 to 6 weeks, for uncomplicated cases. However, studies of *B. suis* infections, which are the most common species involved in human brucellosis in the United States, show significantly lower relapse rates when streptomycin is added to tetracycline therapy.

Also, in vitro studies have demonstrated synergy between aminoglycosides and tetracycline in brucellosis. In recent years, several investigators have reported the successful treatment of brucellosis with trimethoprim-sulfamethoxazole (Bactrim, Septra), 2 tablets three times daily for 4 weeks (total daily dose, trimethoprim, 480 mg; sulfamethoxazole, 2400 mg). The most recently studied regimen for brucellosis is rifampin, 1200 mg daily for 1 week followed by 900 mg daily for 3 additional weeks. Most authorities advocate the addition of either tetracycline, streptomycin, or both to the rifampin to avoid the development of rifampin-resistant strains, a definite hazard when this drug is used alone.

Acute Brucellosis

Acute brucellosis is the form of the disease most commonly encountered clinically in the United States. Patients should be treated for 3 to 4 weeks with the combination of tetracycline and streptomycin. Prompt antibiotic therapy with these drugs results in a good clinical response in most. Relapse rates and localized infections are also lower with combination therapy. Alternative antibiotic regimens include trimethoprim-sulfamethoxazole (co-trimoxazole) and the combination of rifampin and tetracycline with or without streptomycin, as described earlier.

Occasionally very ill patients will develop Herxheimer reactions when treated with antibiotics, characterized by increased fever and toxicity and sometimes hypotension. They should receive prednisone, 15 mg orally every 6 hours for 2 to 3 days, in addition to antibiotics.

Relapsing Brucellosis

Relapse of patients after apparently effective therapy is not uncommon. Often the diagnosis is not difficult, since the patient will develop another episode of fever, sweats, chills, arthralgias, and myalgia; the *Brucella* agglutinin titer will rise; and cultures of blood or bone marrow will again become positive. The relapse rate is related to the type and duration of the initial antibiotic therapy, the chronicity of symptoms before therapy, and the species of infecting organism. Relapses may affect 5 to 30 per cent of all patients with brucellosis. They usually occur within 3 to 6 months, but relapse as long as 2 years after initial infection has been described. Antibiotic sensitivity tests should always be performed on the isolate in a relapsed case; however, strains involved in a relapse are generally still sensitive to the original drugs. Retreatment with tetracycline and streptomycin for at least 21 days is usually successful.

Subacute, Chronic, or Localized Brucellosis

Brucellosis may be associated with a very insidious onset of symptoms or with infections localized to one or more organ systems. Nearly any organ or organ system may be involved; however, brucellosis involving the spleen, musculoskeletal system, genitourinary system, nervous system, and heart are well known and may present special therapeutic problems.

SPLENIC INVOLVEMENT. Although the spleen is commonly enlarged in acute brucellosis and occasionally evidence of hypersplenism is present, this condition usually responds to antibiotic therapy. Some patients with chronic brucellosis have splenomegaly and splenic calcification. Splenectomy in addition to antibiotic therapy may be necessary for cure. At operation the surgeon should also look for other suppurative foci in the abdomen, as these may be responsible for late relapses if not surgically drained or removed.

MUSCULOSKELETAL BRUCELLOSIS. Localized brucellosis commonly involves the bones and joints, usually the lumbosacral area. Disk space infection, or spondylitis, usually does not require surgical therapy and can be treated with tetracycline for 6 weeks and streptomycin for 3 to 4 weeks. Although needle biopsy or exploration may be necessary for diagnosis of *Brucella* spondylitis, surgical therapy is reserved for cases with instability of the spine, associated paravertebral abscesses, or failures of medical management. Established osteomyelitis may require debridement, especially if advanced. *Brucella* arthritis of weight-bearing joints may require synovectomy in addition to medical management.

GENITOURINARY BRUCELLOSIS. The testicle, epididymis, prostate, or kidney may be involved. In addition, proteinuria is common in acute brucellosis, and focal or diffuse embolic glomerulonephritis commonly accompanies *Brucella* endocarditis. Drainage of localized lesions in the genitourinary system or nephrectomy for chronic calcified *Brucella* granulomas may be required in selected cases.

NERVOUS SYSTEM. Brucellosis of the nervous system can manifest as clinical syndromes of meningitis, encephalitis, myelitis, radiculitis, or neuritis. The most frequent lesion is meningoencephalitis. Some patients will have evidence of basal arachnoiditis with increased cerebrospinal fluid (CSF) pressure. Such patients should be treated with anti-inflammatory doses of steroids. Shunt to reduce CSF pressure and hydrocephalus occasionally may be needed. Patients with meningoencephalitis should be given rifampin in addition to tetracycline and streptomycin, since rifampin has better CSF penetration. Therapy should be continued for 4 to 6 weeks.

BRUCELLA ENDOCARDITIS. Endocarditis is a well known but relatively rare manifestation of brucellosis. It occurs in only 1 to 3 per cent of hospitalized cases. Involvement of the aortic valve is most common but sometimes the mitral valve is involved. Large vegetations are frequent. This lesion is associated with considerable mortality and accounts for approximately 80 per cent of the deaths from brucellosis. Although very rare instances of successful medical therapy have been reported, *Brucella* endocarditis should nearly always be treated with valve replacement in addition to antibiotic therapy. Medical therapy should be based on in vitro study of the best bactericidal combination of antibiotics for the strain of *Brucella* involved. Generally combinations of tetracycline and rifampin for 2 to 3 months and streptomycin for 4 to 6 weeks will be needed, in addition to valve replacement.

Accidental Inoculation of Brucella *Vaccine*

Veterinarians who use live *Brucella* vaccine (e.g., *B. abortus,* strain 19) may accidentally inject themselves with the vaccine when they are attempting to vaccinate an animal. Some who have been hypersensitized by a previous clinical or subclinical infection may develop moderate to severe local hypersensitivity at the site of the inoculation. This may progress to moderate to severe swelling, pain, erythema, and even gangrene within 48 to 72 hours. Treatment is prednisone, 60 mg per day orally, and tetracycline, 2 grams per day for 2 to 3 weeks.

In a patient with no previous history of brucellosis or sensitization to brucella, typical acute brucellosis may occur with an incubation period of 10 days to 6 weeks. Treat as for acute brucellosis with tetracycline and streptomycin.

General Measures

Bed rest is an important component of the therapy for symptomatic brucellosis and should be recommended for the first 2 to 3 weeks of treatment. Many patients have profound weakness, anorexia, weight loss, lassitude, and mental depression. The patient should be assured that such reactions are common and that the therapy is eventually curative in most cases. Isolation of the hospitalized patient is usually not necessary. Draining lesions should be covered with a dressing, which should be disposed of aseptically. All patients in whom the source and means of acquisition are unclear should undergo epidemiologic investigation.

Follow-Up

Response to therapy should be monitored clinically and with periodic (e.g., twice yearly) blood cultures and brucella serology utilizing the 2-mercaptoethanol (2-ME) reduction test. IgG antibodies that are resistant to 2-ME should not persist at a level of 1:160 of higher beyond 6 to 12 months after antibiotic treatment. If *Brucella* agglutinating antibodies persist at a significant level (≥1:160) longer than 6 to 12 months, a continuing localized focus of infection should be sought.

Vaccines and Prevention

No vaccine is presently available for humans in the United States, although vaccines have been studied in France and Russia. Persons whose work may entail a risk of exposure of *Brucella,* such as slaughterhouse workers, meat inspectors, or veterinarians, should reduce the risk of infection by wearing protective gloves and goggles and avoiding cuts on the arms that might provide a route of entry for *Brucella* organisms.

Steroids

Steroids are used only rarely. They may be needed in Herxheimer reactions, accidental inoculations in hypersensitized individuals, and in some instances of central nervous system infection.

VARICELLA

(Chickenpox)

method of
CHARLES GROSE, M.D.
The University of Iowa
Iowa City, Iowa

Varicella, or chickenpox, is caused by primary infection with varicella-zoster virus, one of the five human herpesviruses. Chickenpox is a very common childhood exanthem, affecting about 70 per cent of all school-age children. The disease is usually easy to diagnose because of the common vesicular rash, which begins around the face, often at the hairline, then spreads over the head to the neck and trunk and finally to the extemities over the next 3 to 6 days. Each vesicle appears after a rapid progression from macule to papule and attains a final diameter of 2 to 3 mm. After 4 to 5 days a crust forms and completes the transition from macule to papule to vesicle to crusted lesion. The scab persists for 1 to 3 weeks before falling off. At sites of skin abrasion or trauma, such as the diaper area in a young child, the rash may be more confluent, presumably because of increased virus egress secondary to local inflammation.

Chickenpox in the Normal Child

The average course of chickenpox in otherwise healthy children includes about 1 week of signs and symptoms. The prodrome is mild and, if noticeable at all, consists of malaise, anorexia, pharyngitis, and rhinitis. After the appearance of rash, the child develops low grade fever, usually less than 39°C (102°F), which lasts for 4 to 6 days. The number of vesicular lesions is extremely variable but often totals between 200 and 300 pocks. Constitutional symptoms that may occur after the appearance of the rash include pruritus, sleeplessness, irritability, listlessness, anorexia, and abdominal pain. These abate with the cessation of new vesicle formation by the end of the first week of illness.

The mildly symptomatic child requires few medications. Calamine lotion is often recommended to relieve pruritus as the vesicular lesions begin to crust. For amelioration of fever, the child should be given acetaminophen at appropriate dosage for age and weight. *Aspirin should not be administered to a child with chickenpox because of the strong association between aspirin ingestion and subsequent development of Reye's syndrome in this clinical setting.*

Although chickenpox is a systemic disease with a viremic phase, untoward effects of the virus infection are rare in children. These complications include purpura, appendicitis, pneumonitis, hepatitis, pericarditis, glomerulonephritis, and orchitis, as well as involvement of the nervous system. The secondary bacterial infections are usually a greater cause of concern. The most common site of bacterial disease is the skin around a pock lesion. Superinfections arise very rapidly after the onset of chickenpox, sometimes within 24 to 48 hours. If untreated, they may progress to cellulitis, cutaneous abscesses, impetigo, and suppurative lymphadenitis. Specimens from these lesions should be submitted for bacterial culture. The most common etiologic agent is group A beta-hemolytic streptococcus; staphylococcal infections also occur. The initial antibiotic regimen, therefore, should include an agent effective against both streptococcus and staphylococcus—for example, oral semisynthetic penicillin such as dicloxacillin. When the bacterial culture results are available, the most appropriate antibiotic can be selected for the remainder of a 10 to 14 treatment course.

Chickenpox in the Immunocompromised Child

With the exception of the complications mentioned, chickenpox in otherwise healthy children is a relatively mild disease. However, chickenpox is a much more serious infection in children with immunodeficiency syndromes or children who are immunosuppressed because of corticosteroid or anticancer chemotherapy and irradiation. These children often have a more prolonged illness, called progressive varicella because it frequently involves the lungs, liver, pancreas, and central nervous system. Pneumonitis is an especially ominous complication, because it is associated with the highest mortality. Progressive chickenpox in the immunosuppressed child can be avoided by the prompt intramuscular administration of varicella-zoster immune globulin (V-ZIG) within 3 to 4 days after the child is exposed to the disease. V-ZIG is distributed at cost by the

American Red Cross through their regional centers. The dose of V-ZIG is one vial per 10 kg of body weight. (The cost to the patient is approximately $100 per vial.) The main problem with this therapeutic approach is that many children do not know when they are exposed to chickenpox, since the event occurs in a public place such as a school room, or even in a large clinic. The hyperimmune globulin must be administered within the first 3 to 4 days of the incubation period (after exposure) to be effective; V-ZIG is not efficacious after clinical disease is apparent. If an immunosuppressed child develops chickenpox, whether or not V-ZIG was administered, the child should be treated with the antiviral agent acyclovir (Zovirax). The dosage regimen of intravenous acyclovir for children is 500 mg per M^2 per dose given every 8 hours. Generally the child is treated for a total of 7 days. No regimen for treatment of progressive chickenpox with the oral tablet form of acyclovir has been published as of January, 1985, although recommendations may be forthcoming within the next 1 to 2 years.

Chickenpox in the Adult

As with many childhood diseases, chickenpox is frequently a more severe disease in adults than in children. Whereas the child usually has only a brief and mild prodromal illness, the adult often experiences considerable malaise accompanied by low grade fever for 1 to 3 days prior to the appearance of the vesicular exanthem. Viral pneumonitis, which is rare in all children except the immunocompromised, is seen in about 14 per cent of otherwise healthy individuals 20 years of age and older who contract chickenpox. The most common symptoms of varicella pneumonitis are cough, dyspnea, tachypnea, and chest pain. These symptoms usually begin 3 to 5 days after the onset of the rash. The roentgenographic findings include peribronchial nodular infiltrates in both lungs, especially near the hilum. Based on the number of published clinical reports, varicella pneumonitis appears to be more common and more severe in pregnant women who contract chickenpox. The onset of clinical symptomatic varicella pneumonitis in an adult is a medical emergency. The patient should be admitted to a hospital with specialized respiratory care facilities for continuous observation and assisted ventilation, if necessary.

The pneumonitis should be treated with intravenously administered acyclovir at a dosage of 10 mg per kg every 8 hours. Total duration of antiviral chemotherapy is generally 7 days. Patients should always be given liberal amounts of fluids to avoid even minimal dehydration. Although few adverse effects of intravenously administered acyclovir have been observed in children, adults may develop abnormal renal function within 2 to 3 days after onset of therapy. Serum creatinine levels commonly rise to twofold higher than baseline and may diminish while therapy is continued or within 1 week after completion of a normal course of acyclovir. When the serum creatinine levels rise threefold or higher above baseline, the patient may develop symptoms of nausea, vomiting, and abdominal pain. At this point, acyclovir should be reduced in dosage or discontinued altogether. In addition to monitoring renal function of patients receiving acyclovir for varicella pneumonitis, repeat roentgenograms, blood cultures, and hematologic profiles should be obtained to evaluate for possible bacterial superinfection of the lung.

CHOLERA

method of
WILLIAM B. GREENOUGH, M.D., FACP
International Centre for Diarrhoeal Disease Research
Dhaka, Bangladesh

Cholera is an acute diarrheal illness caused by *Vibrio cholerae,* a bacteria that can colonize the small intestinal lumen and mucosal lining. When this occurs a toxin is released which attaches very tightly to a specific receptor (GM_1 ganglioside) present in mucosal lining cells. The toxin produces rapid transfer of body fluids into the gut by stimulating a cyclic nucleotide system that regulates secretion. If lost fluid is not replaced, vascular collapse ensues and the patient dies. Cholera occurs both sporadically and in large, abrupt epidemics that can overwhelm and disorganize traditional treatment efforts. When not treated, about half of all cholera patients die. When properly managed, even in large epidemics mortality is less than one half of 1 per cent. Recent simplifications of therapy involving early and intensive use of oral rehydration therapy (ORT) have greatly facilitated successful management of individual patients and large epidemics.

Treatment

Before 1967 fluid losses in cholera could be replaced only by intravenous therapy. Research that applied the principles of "carrier-mediated" transport to the design of an effective oral rehydration solution (ORS) has changed this. Sodium ion and with it anions and water are absorbed even during severe cholera if the right amount of glucose (the "carrier") is present. The agreed-upon formula for treating cholera and all other diarrheal diseases by ORS is shown in Table 1.

The keys to success for oral rehydration therapy (ORT) with ORS are (1) to start promptly at

TABLE 1. **Composition of Oral Glucose–Electrolyte Solution Used for Therapy of Acute Diarrheal Diseases**

	mEq/Liter*
Sodium	90
Potassium	20
Chloride	80
Bicarbonate	30
Glucose	111

*Each liter contains:

sodium chloride	3.5 grams
sodium bicarbonate	2.5 grams
potassium chloride	1.5 grams
glucose	20.0 grams (or sucrose, 40.0 grams)

the first sign of diarrhea, (2) to drink an amount equal to the losses that occur, and (3) to continue until diarrhea stops. If this is done, then only the most severely affected patients will require medical attention and intravenous fluid replacement therapy and they will not die while getting to the doctor. When cholera is demonstrated in any community, intensive efforts must begin promptly to inform everyone about how to prepare ORS and use it for ORT.

When the complete packaged ORS formulation is not available, an effective approximation using table salt, sugar, and water can be used.

This home solution can be made by taking 1 three-finger pinch of salt (5 grams per liter) and one full hand scoop of sugar (40 grams per liter) in one half liter or one pint of drinking water. Thus in almost any situation effective if not optimal ORS can be prepared and used immediately.

Administration of ORS may be governed by thirst but patients with active cholera may not take the initiative to drink adequate amounts. An attendant, who can be an untrained family member or volunteer, should offer small amounts to the patient every 2 to 3 minutes. This reduces the risk of vomiting and can result in adequate volumes taken. If only 50 ml is given every 3 minutes, 1 liter per hour replacement is achieved, which is adequate in almost all adult cholera patients. In a 10 kg child, administration of 10 ml every 3 minutes will replace 2 per cent of the total body weight every hour. When vomiting occurs, ORT should be continued. The only limitations are if coma or convulsions are present or if a question of intestinal ileus arises. Attentive persistence is the key to success. Forcing is not needed. Periodic observation by a physician or trained health worker can avoid risks of under- or overhydration.

If a patient does not receive oral hydration and arrives for treatment in shock, then intravenous fluid is required.

Intravenous Fluid Therapy

Prompt and adequate replacement of fluid losses will restore the circulation, prevent most complications, and save the patient's life. The fluid used should approximate the stool losses in its composition (Table 2). Cutdowns and indwelling lines add risks, are rarely needed, and may waste critical moments in severely collapsed patients. In such patients fluid should be given rapidly (50 to 100 ml per minute in adults) so that the original deficit plus any new losses is corrected within the first hour of treatment. At this point, with the patient well-hydrated, intravenous fluid can be stopped and hydration maintained by ORT. This avoids risks of overhydration and infection. It is important that patients receiving either oral or intravenous treatment are carefully watched to insure that fluid deficits do not occur. Patients purging at a rate of 300 to 500 or more ml of stool per kg of body weight in 24 hours are more likely to require intravenous supplement to ORT. Fortunately, such patients are the exception.

Intravenous therapy prescribed at fixed rates without frequent assessment of the state of hydration risks both over- and underhydration. Frequent observations of losses or clinical parameters of state of hydration will avoid serious excesses or deficits. The best way to avoid risks of overhydration is to rely principally on ORT. Lack of thirst will usually prevent excessive intake.

Antimicrobial Therapy

When *Vibrio cholerae* is promptly killed in the intestinal lumen, no more cholera toxin is produced and only the residual effects of toxin already bound to the gut mucosa remain. These residual effects may cause serious fluid loss for up to 36 hours. Early antibiotic therapy is useful in shortening the total duration of diarrhea but does not reduce the immediate needs for hydration since *Vibrio cholerae* does not penetrate or invade, so the only possible effect is shortening diarrhea and lessening fluid losses. Microbial

TABLE 2. **Composition of Stool and Commonly Used Intravenous Solutions in Cholera**

Concentration *(Mmol per Liter)*	Cholera Stool	DTS	5:4:1	Ringer's Lactate
Na^+	135	118	134	131
K^+	15	13	13	4
Cl^-	100	83	99	111
HCO_3^-*	45	48	48	26
Glucose	—	22	—	—

*Acetate can be used in place of bicarbonate in cholera replacement solutions.

resistance to antibiotics occurs and is plasmid mediated. Sensitivity testing is essential in any cholera outbreak to select an effective agent. At present the least costly effective drug against which resistance has not yet been reported is furazolidone (Furoxone). A dosage of 6 mg per kg per day in children and 400 mg per day in adults, either in a single or divided dose for 2 days, is sufficient. Tetracyclines in adults are effective even when given as a single dosage of 2 grams although divided dosage of 250 mg every 6 hours over 48 hours is preferred.

Drugs That Reduce Fluid Loss

Although no drugs can yet be recommended for routine use, it has been shown that chlorpromazine, nicotinic acid, and berberine may promptly reduce fluid losses during cholera. Charcoal GM_1 ganglioside, an adsorbent for the cholera toxin, also has reduced fluid losses to a small extent early in the disease. However, none of these agents are recommended at this time. Antimotility drugs are contraindicated in cholera and should never be used.

Nutrition and a New ORS

Feeding as soon as the patient is able to eat is useful. During cholera, large quantities of active enzymes that can digest foods are produced. In ORS, glucose or sugar can be replaced by rice which, if powdered and cooked into a somewhat thick soup with the appropriate salts added, is highly effective in replacing fluid losses. It also reduces those losses, minimizes vomiting, and may shorten the duration of illness. In addition, nutrition is well sustained even during acute illness. To prepare this form of ORS, 50 grams of rice powder is cooked to a soupy consistency (5 to 6 minutes) in 1 liter of water. To this is added 3.5 grams of sodium chloride, 2.5 grams of sodium bicarbonate, and 1.5 grams of potassium chloride. It may then be flavored as wished and given in an amount to replace all losses and maintain hydration. When diarrhea ceases, the amount of rice powder can be increased to prepare a soft food. Other nutrients that contain protein and fat can be added according to the practices of the particular country or household, for effective and immediate postdiarrhea feeding. Although cholera is not as strongly associated with malnutrition as invasive diarrheal illnesses, malnutrition is often present in populations where cholera occurs, and early attention to improved nutrition may avert a vicious diarrhea-malnutrition cycle that results in many late deaths.

The full place of new cereal-based ORS is not yet known, but rice-based ORS can be safely recommended as a very useful alternate form to the glucose- or sucrose-based ORS. An approximation of the complete ORS is 0.5 liter of powdered rice cooked into a thick soup with one 3-finger pinch of salt.

Complications

Attention to adequate fluid replacement averts almost all complications of cholera and always must be the prime focus of treatment. Risks of pyrogens, excessive hydration, and overly rapid correction of hyper- or hyponatremia are minimized by use of ORT as the prime modality. The main limiting factors of ORT are altered states of consciousness, which in children may signal low blood glucose or electrolyte imbalances. Intravenous glucose sufficient to raise blood glucose to normal should be given promptly to any child with convulsions or coma. When possible, blood electrolytes will identify hyper- or hyponatremic scales. Potassium depletion can be an important complication in children and is best supplemented by foods rich in this element such as fruits and green coconut water. Feeding early is important. Breast feeding always should be maintained, even during acute illness.

Pneumonia is a common problem. It may be due to aspiration from vomiting or it may have been precipitated by altered defenses secondary to shock and acidosis. Diagnosis by sputum examination and culture should be done and an appropriate antibiotic given if the cause is bacterial.

Prevention

The only truly effective current means for preventing cholera is to insure that *Vibrio cholerae* is not eaten in food or drunk in water. Handwashing with soap by food and water handlers and water purification by boiling, filtration, or chlorination (iodination) are helpful in epidemic cholera.

The injected whole killed bacterial vaccine against cholera is not very effective, has side effects, and in my view is medically contraindicated. New oral vaccines are now being field-tested and may prove valuable when the results are in.

DIPHTHERIA

method of
RICHARD V. McCLOSKEY, M.D.
Thomas Jefferson University
Philadelphia, Pennsylvania

Diphtheria is an acute, communicable disease of the respiratory tract or skin. The sole etiologic agent is *Corynebacterium diphtheriae,* a pleomorphic, gram-positive rod. Transmission of the organism may be from the respiratory tract or skin of symptomatic patients or asymptomatic carriers. The incubation period is usually less than 1 week. The most serious pathology is caused by the elaboration of a unique and potent exotoxin which can produce myocarditis, neuropathy, mucosal necrosis, and shock. Death is most often due to respiratory obstruction, acute toxemia with cardiac dysrhythmia, or circulatory collapse. Neurotoxic injury may cause long-term morbidity as a result of peripheral or cranial nerve palsies. The clinical course depends on the location and extent of diphtheritic membrane, the amount of toxin absorbed, patients' premorbid antitoxic immunity, and the timing of treatment. From 1976 through 1981, about 56 cases annually have been reported in the United States. The actual incidence of disease is higher. Many American adults are not adequately immunized. Mortality rates from respiratory diphtheria are less than 10 per cent but may be higher at the extremes of age.

Prevention

Diphtheria is a preventable disease. Everyone must be immunized. The immunization schedule against diphtheria (as well as tetanus and pertussis) in Table 1 is that recommended by the Immunization Practices Advisory Committee to the Centers for Disease Control.

Tetanus and diphtheria toxoids adsorbed (Td) is used for persons older than 7 years of age. Td should be given as a booster at age 16 and every 10 years thereafter to maintain protective antitoxic immunity. Schick testing (for sensitivity and antitoxic immunity) is not needed for adult populations.

General Management

Hospitalization is advised for all patients with diphtheria, since the extent of toxin-mediated complications is not predictable early in the course of disease and is not always correlated with the apparent extent of tissue involvement. All patients should be isolated until respiratory secretions have become noninfectious. Antibiotic therapy will usually accomplish this within 3 to 5 days. Staff should wear gowns and masks. Thorough handwashing is imperative after attending patients isolated for diphtheria. Since diphtheria usually appears epidemically, a hospital may have to group patients together for initial treatment. Untreated patients and patients treated for 4 days or more should be separated to prevent development of a carrier state or even a second attack of diphtheria. Cultures of the pharynx and nose taken at least 48 hours after antibiotic treatment has been stopped should be negative on 2 or 3 consecutive days to discontinue isolation. Symptomatic treatment with isotonic gargles and mild analgesia (codeine, 3 mg per kg per day in four to six divided doses) may be helpful in removing pharyngeal debris and moderating sore throat. Parenteral fluid supplementation may be needed for patients with dysphagia, palatal paralysis, or airway obstruction.

TABLE 1. **Routine Diphtheria, Tetanus, and Pertussis Immunization Schedule for Children Under 7 Years of Age, 1981**

Dose	Age/Interval	Product
Primary 1	6 weeks of age or older	DTP*
Primary 2†	4–8 weeks after 1st dose	DTP
Primary 3†	4–8 weeks after 2nd dose	DTP
Primary 4†	Approximately 1 year after 3rd dose	DTP
Booster	4–6 years of age, prior to entering kindergarten or elementary school (not necessary if 4th primary immunizing dose administered after 4th birthday)	DTP
Additional boosters	Every 10 years after last dose	Td‡

*DTP, Diphtheria and tetanus toxoids and pertussis vaccine adsorbed. DT, if pertussis vaccine is contraindicated.

†Prolonging the interval does not require restarting series.

‡Td, Tetanus and diphtheria toxoids adsorbed (for adult use).

Antitoxic Therapy

The longer the interval between onset of disease and administration of antitoxin, the less effective antitoxin becomes. Antitoxin is horse serum, therefore measures to prevent immediate hypersensitivity should be taken. Epinephrine chloride (1:1000) should be available in a syringe when antitoxin is injected. The dose of epinephrine is 0.01 ml per kg; maximum dose is 0.5 ml.

Preliminary sensitivity testing of the patient to horse serum should always be done before antitoxin is administered. Both a skin test and an eye test should be done. For the skin test, 0.1 ml of a 1:1000 dilution in isotonic saline should be injected intradermally. A positive skin test consists of the appearance of a significant wheal and flare occurring at the injection site after a period of 15 to 20 minutes. For the eye test, 1 drop of a 1:10 dilution in isotonic saline of antitoxin is instilled into the conjunctival sac. A positive reaction consists of conjunctivitis occurring 15 to 20 minutes after instillation. If either of these tests is positive, the patient is considered sensitive to horse serum, and desensitization should be accomplished. Before desensitization, the patient should be given diphenhydramine hydrochloride (Benadryl) as follows: 2 to 5 years, 25 mg intramuscularly; 6 to 14 years, 50 mg intramuscularly; adults, 50 to 100 mg intramuscularly. Serial injections of diluted antitoxin as indicated may be made at intervals of 15 minutes, provided no reaction occurs. If a reaction occurs after an injection, wait an hour and then repeat the last dose that failed to cause a reaction:

1. Subcutaneously, 0.05 ml of 1:30 dilution of antitoxin.
2. Subcutaneously, 0.05 ml of 1:10 dilution of antitoxin.
3. Subcutaneously, 0.1 ml of undiluted antitoxin.
4. Subcutaneously, 0.2 ml of undiluted antitoxin.
5. Intramuscularly, 0.5 ml of undiluted antitoxin.
6. Intravenously, 0.1 ml of undiluted antitoxin.
7. A therapeutic dose is then administered slowly intravenously. The intravenous route is preferable in all cases. A single dose should suffice; retreatment should never be considered because of the serious risk of increasing sensitization to horse serum. Diphtheria antitoxin is administered on the basis of the following schedule: mild pharyngeal diphtheria or when careful examination indicates that the membrane is small or confined to the anterior nares or tonsils, 40,000 units; moderate pharyngeal diphtheria, 80,000 units; severe pharyngeal or laryngeal diphtheria, combined types, or late cases, 120,000 units. Diphtheria antitoxin is infused in 200 ml of isotonic saline over a 30 minute period.

Immediate allergic reactions to antitoxin occur in approximately 16 per cent of cases. Such early reactions bear no relation to the subsequent development of serum sickness. In children over 10 years of age and adults, the incidence of serum sickness has been 20 to 30 per cent. Clinical manifestations have occurred between the 7th and 16th days after antitoxin administration and have lasted from 2 to 6 days. All such patients have rash, most have fever, and about one third have arthralgia and one third, dermal edema. The prophylactic use of antagonists of vasoactive amines may be worthwhile for the prevention of serum sickness when orally administered during the period of significant risk after the infusion of horse serum products. Either one of two drugs, cyproheptadine (Periactin) or hydroxyzine hydrochloride (Atarax) has been found efficacious. Cyproheptadine is taken according to the following daily dose schedule: The minimal daily dose is 12 mg. For patients of 20 to 39 kg of body weight, the dose is 0.7 mg per kg; 40 to 59 kg of body weight, 0.6 mg per kg; over 60 kg of body weight, 0.5 mg per kg. For hydroxyzine, the daily dosage regimen is for 21 to 29 kg of body weight, 4 mg per kg; 30 to 39 kg of body weight, 5 mg per kg; 40 to 49 kg of body weight, 6 mg per kg; over 50 kg of body weight, 7 mg per kg. The maximum dose is 450 mg. (These doses are higher than those usually recommended.) Equal portions of the daily dose of either drug are given every 4 to 6 hours around the clock to ensure continuous effective blood levels. The drug is started on day 4 of hospitalization and is continued through day 16. If the patient is discharged prior to day 16, the course of the drug is completed outside the hospital.

Antibiotic Treatment

Antibiotic treatment eliminates *C. diphtheriae* from the respiratory tract, stops exotoxin production, and terminates the carrier state. Antibiotics will also treat secondary beta-hemolytic streptococcal infections, which may be encountered in 25 per cent of patients with diphtheria.

The preferred drug is penicillin as 250 mg of penicillin V potassium (Pen-Vee K) three times daily. Intramuscular procaine penicillin, or intravenous aqueous penicillin at 600,000 units twice daily is used for patients who cannot swallow. Erythromycin orally, 25 to 50 mg per kg per day, can be given to patients with penicillin hypersensitivity. Since erythromycin by the intravenous route may produce nausea and thrombophlebitis, clindamycin (Cleocin), 25 to 40 mg per kg per day every 6 hours, can be used until oral medication can be given using either erythromycin or clindamycin, 150 mg four times daily. The duration of treatment is 10 days.

Management of the Carrier State

Asymptomatic individuals who are household or conjugal contacts should have nose and throat cultures. If possible, household members should be confined until 3 to 5 days of antibiotic treatment are completed, but this is difficult to enforce in an open urban society. Previously unimmunized persons should begin a program of primary immunization using DTP or Td according to age. Previously immunized household members should receive DTP or Td if they have not received a booster within 4 years. The administration of antitoxin to exposed unimmunized persons is not recommended since it may unnecessarily sensitize those who may require antitoxin treatment later.

Carriers should be treated with either oral erythromycin, 20 to 50 mg per day in four doses, or oral clindamycin (Cleocin), 20 mg per kg per day in four doses for 10 days. The carrier state will not reliably be eradicated unless the full course of treatment is given. Benzathine penicillin G (Bicillin) intramuscularly is also effective and has the advantage of assuring compliance. For children less than 5 years of age, give 600,000 units; all others receive 1.2 million units. Two consecutive daily cultures of the nose and throat should be obtained on days 11 and 12 after treatment to certify that the carrier state has been eliminated. Retreatment is sometimes required.

Management of Complications

Myocarditis. From 40 to 65 per cent of patients will show minor ST and T wave changes in the electrocardiogram. Generally they are kept in the hospital routinely for 2 weeks. It is advisable, at least in children, to restrict strenuous exercise at home for the 4 weeks after discharge. More serious diphtheritic myocarditis is characterized by a rapid, thready pulse, indistinct and poor heart sounds, cardiac arrhythmias, cardiac failure, hepatomegaly, and fluid retention. Myocarditis can occur from 2 to 27 days after the onset of pharyngitis. Cardiac failure most commonly occurs during the 2nd week. ECG changes are characteristic of myocarditis. Left hemianterior block is frequent. Complete heart block signifies a poor prognosis. Strict bed rest must be enforced in an attempt to prevent sudden death from slight physical activity. The patient is nursed supine in bed with an attendant at the bedside to do everything for him or her. Digitalis is not well tolerated and should be reserved for therapy of congestive heart failure and arrhythmias with a rapid ventricular response. The value of adrenocorticosteroid therapy is difficult to assess. However, prednisone, 0.5 to 1 mg per kg per day for approximately 2 weeks, is advised to lessen the severity of myocarditis. Bed rest is continued for at least 1 month, with graduated activity allowed if there is no recurrence of myocarditis or development of peripheral neuritis.

Shock. Rarely, in the absence of either myocarditis or peripheral neuritis, severe shock may occur suddenly during the course of diphtheria. This is usually associated with overwhelming toxemia. Under these circumstances, it is best to insert a central venous catheter. The use of fluids, including blood, plasma, and plasma expanders such as dextran, in a quantity sufficient to restore central venous pressure to normal levels may be sufficient to eliminate the shock state. In patients who fail to respond to this therapy, use of sympathetic blocking agents such as phenoxybenzamine hydrochloride (Dibenzyline) may be efficacious. It may be necessary to give large doses of corticosteroids to maintain normal tissue perfusion. If heart failure occurs, the intravenous administration of a rapidly acting digitalis preparation is recommended with constant ECG monitoring.

Laryngotracheal Obstruction. Bronchoscopy may be used to remove dislodged membrane from larger bronchi, where it may cause death by asphyxia. Tracheostomy may be required early in the course of severely ill patients. Secondary bronchopneumonia caused by hospital-acquired gram-negative bacilli may complicate treatment. Corticosteroids may be of use in acute laryngeal diphtheria. Hydrocortisone sodium succinate (Solu-Cortef), 5 mg per kg per day intramuscularly or intravenously, is given in three divided doses for 1 or 2 days or longer. An equivalent dose of prednisone is then given orally when possible and gradually reduced over a 5 to 8 day period.

Neurologic Complications. Palatal paralysis, the most common and often the only paralysis, usually appears early during the course of dipththeria. Intravenous therapy or nasogastric feeding may be required. Paralysis of respiratory muscles usually appears from 6 to 8 weeks after the onset of pharyngitis. Assisted or controlled ventilation by mechanical means is indicated until the patient can resume spontaneous respiration with satisfactory alveolar ventilation.

ECHINOCOCCOSIS

(Hydatid Disease)

method of
HERBERT B. TANOWITZ, M.D.
Albert Einstein College of Medicine
Bronx, New York

Hydatid disease (echinococcosis) is found in most sheep- and cattle-raising countries of the world. The majority of cases are reported from the Mediterranean Basin, Australia, New Zealand, and Latin America. In the United States most cases are imported, but cases are reported from some western and southern states. Although most often diagnosed in adulthood, hydatid disease is usually acquired in childhood from the close association between children and dogs. The adult worm resides in the intestines of dogs and other carnivores, and ova are found in their stools. The ingested ova eventually penetrate the intestinal wall of humans and larval cysts develop, primarily in the liver (50 per cent) and lung (40 per cent). Virtually any organ can become involved, such as eye, brain, bone, and heart. The presenting signs and symptoms are usually those of an increasing, space-occupying lesion. Untreated hydatid disease may result in several complications, including rupture and dissemination, anaphylaxis, and suppuration. The diagnosis is made by the finding of a space-occupying lesion upon routine radiographic techniques, ultrasound, or CT scan and confirmed by serologic tests.

Treatment

Surgery remains the method of choice for the treatment of a single lesion of the liver or lung. However, in recent years, the introduction of the benzimidazoles, mebendazole (Vermox) and albendazole, has led to a reassessment of treatment. The uncomplicated single hyatid liver cyst or pulmonary cysts caused by *Echinococcus granulosus* is the most common syndrome faced by the clinician. It is best approached by the suction and forceps evacuation of the cyst and its contents (hydatid sand), followed by irrigation of the cavity with scolicidal solutions.

Formalin, once the most common of these solutions, is no longer recommended because it can cause shock as it leaks into the peritoneum. Among the available scolicidal solutions in use today are 20 per cent hypertonic saline, 0.5 per cent silver nitrate solution (final concentration), 5 per cent cetrimide or 0.05 per cent tincture of chlorhexidine. Recently, a suction device with a cryotherm base has been described that can isolate and evacuate the cyst contents. The surgeon must take care not to allow cyst contents to spill into the peritoneal cavity. Therefore, some surgeons actually sew a plastic sheet directly into the wall of the cavity.

In the procedures just mentioned, the area surrounding the cyst may be packed with pads that have been saturated with 20 per cent saline. Before the instillation of irrigant some prefer to first remove a small amount of cyst fluid, especially if there has been an increase in tension. If the cyst has ruptured during surgery the peritoneal cavity can be lavaged with irrigant. In addition, mebendazole (50 mg per kg per day) may be administered for an extended period of time (at least 1 month) in these cases. (Manufacturer's warning: There is no evidence that mebendazole is effective for hydatid disease.) These procedures are followed in simple cases by primary closure of the cysts and surrounding liver tissues. More difficult cases may require procedures such as cystectomy, partial hepatectomy, or marsupialization. Additionally, cystic hydatid lung disease can be managed by extrusion of the cyst through a surgical opening during positive pressure breathing. If this fails, more conventional procedures must be used. The management of extrahepato-pulmonary cystic disease is usually surgical since medical therapy has not proved to be effective in areas such as bone.

Liver or lung involvement caused by alveolar hydatid disease *(E. multilocularis)* is a more difficult management problem. When liver involvement is diagnosed it is often not amenable to resection. Complete excision, when possible, offers the only hope of cure. Palliative measures such as partial resections and various hepatobiliary bypass procedures may be required. Since alveolar hydatid disease is not cystic but rather solid, the risk of peritoneal spillage is low. Alveolar disease of the lung is almost invariably metastatic from the liver. Medical therapy is often needed, either as primary or adjuvant treatment in this particular form.

Medical therapy of echinococcosis is indicated in those patients deemed inoperable because of such factors as general state of health, age, number and location of cysts, alveolar disease (see preceding paragraph), or lack of adequate surgical facilities. If time is not a critical factor, all patients should be given a 3 to 4 week course prior to surgery in an effort to sterilize the cyst. Moreover, in renal hydatid cysts one might consider a course of medical therapy as a possible alternative to nephrectomy.

Mebendazole is not currently approved for this disease by the FDA, and albendazole is an experimental drug. Therefore, appropriate patient consents must be obtained prior to use. Dosage schedules for mebendazole vary. Most authorities suggest 25 to 100 mg per kg per day in two to three divided doses for 1 to 3 months. Some investigators have used up to 200 mg per kg per day. However, there was no advantage of this high dose schedule over the more conventional one. The drug is administered with food, often a fatty meal, to improve absorption. The blood levels are erratic, and it is felt that 80 to 100 ng per ml needs to be maintained for at least 3 months to achieve an effect. Some patients may require repeated treatments. Patients with alveolar disease require treatment for life.

Adverse reactions to mebendazole usually occur within the first month of therapy. These include allergic reactions, alopecia, glomerulonephritis, leukopenia (reversible), prolonged fever, and abnormal liver function tests, especially in patients with pre-existing hepatobiliary disease. Patients with hepatobiliary disease may accumulate higher levels of drug, and as such may be at greater risk for toxicity. In general, most patients show some radiologic evidence of improvement (i.e., reduction in cyst size) within 3 to 6 months. Following therapy, some patients have a decrease in antibody titer, but this should not be used as an indication of cure.

Albendazole, a new experimental benzimidazole, at a dose of 10 mg per kg per day for 28 to 56 days, was found to achieve levels greater than ten times that for mebendazole at 50 mg per kg per day. An experimental protocol is currently being evaluated in which patients are given 800 mg per day in two divided doses for 28 days. Minimal toxicity has been reported with this drug. Tumors have recently been reported in experimental animals treated with albendazole.

The treatment of echinococcosis is still in flux and is probably more an art than a science. The clinician must evaluate each case individually and weigh the relative risks and benefits of surgical and medical therapy, either singly or in combination.

FOOD POISONING

method of
MICHAEL A. POLIS, M.D.,
and GARY L. SIMON, M.D., Ph.D.
George Washington University
Washington, D.C.

DIAGNOSIS

Food poisoning is usually heralded by the acute onset of gastrointestinal symptoms, such as nausea, vomiting and diarrhea, which may be accompanied by systemic or extraintestinal manifestations. To establish an etiologic diagnosis: (1) Define the clinical features of the illness according to incubation period, type and severity of gastrointestinal symptoms, and presence of extraintestinal symptoms. (2) Obtain an epidemiologic history, including the type and preparation of the suspected food, time of year, recent travel, and similar symptoms in companions or family members. In serious episodes, contact the local health department for other related cases. (3) Obtain appropriate specimens for laboratory confirmation, including feces, vomitus, gastric aspirates, blood, and samples of recently ingested food, as indicated by the clinical features of the illness.

TREATMENT

Although specific therapy is occasionally indicated for some patients with food poisoning, most individuals can be adequately cared for by general supportive therapy. This includes careful monitoring of vital signs and neurologic symptoms, adequate hydration, removal of unabsorbed toxin, and symptomatic therapy.

Dehydration may not be immediately evident in acutely ill patients, and pulse and blood pressure should be measured in several positions to demonstrate orthostatic changes. Respiratory status and neurologic symptoms must be followed, and hospitalization is indicated for any patient with signs of neurologic impairment.

Fluid and electrolyte therapy is the mainstay of therapy for most patients with enteric forms of food poisoning. The degree of volume depletion is assessed by examination of skin turgor and mucous membranes and by obtaining a history of urine and diarrheal stool output. Fluid can be administered orally or parenterally, depending upon the severity of the illness, the available facilities, and the patient's ability to tolerate an oral preparation. A standard oral replacement therapy regimen contains 3.5 gm of NaCl, 1.5 gm of KCl, 2.5 gm of $NaHCO_2$, and 20 gm of glucose in 1 liter of boiled water. Sucrose (table sugar) can be substituted for glucose, and one can prepare an oral replacement solution (ORS) by mixing 4 level tablespoons of sugar, 3/4 tablespoon of salt, 1 teaspoon sodium bicarbonate, and 1 cup of orange juice in 1 liter of water. Adequate replacement volume must be given to restore normal intravascular volume, which can be monitored by pulse, blood pressure, and urine output. Individuals who cannot maintain hydration orally should be hospitalized. Since it is difficult to manage hydration therapy in young infants, children, and elderly patients, especially those with cardiovascular disease, hospitalization is indicated.

In some patients with toxigenic food poisoning, unabsorbed toxin may still be present in the gut. Syrup of ipecac, 30 ml orally, or apomorphine, 6 mg subcutaneously, is an effective emetic. These agents should not be employed in neurologically impaired patients, to avoid aspiration of gastric contents. Gastric lavage and administration of a charcoal slurry may help remove toxins. Purgatives may also be useful. Magnesium citrate, up to 300 ml, or sodium sulfate, 15 gm in 300 ml of water, is an effective agent.

Persistent nausea and vomiting can be controlled by the administration of antiemetics. Prochlorperazine (Compazine), 5 to 10 ml orally, 25 mg by rectal suppository, or 10 mg intramuscularly, may be given to adults. Trimethobenzamide hydrochloride (Tigan), 250 mg orally or 200 mg per rectum, is an acceptable alternative. These drugs should not be used in small children.

The use of antidiarrheal agents is controversial. In most patients with food poisoning, diarrhea is brief and self-limited and may help remove toxin. Antidiarrheal agents, such as paregoric, 4 ml every 2 hours; loperamide hydrochloride (Imodium), 4 mg followed by 2 mg after each stool to a maximum daily dose of 16 mg; or diphenoxylate hydrochloride with atropine (Lomotil), 5 mg every 6 hours, reduce peristalis and are contraindicated in patients with fever, fecal leukocytes, or other features that suggest the presence of an invasive pathogen such as *Salmonella, Shigella,* or *Entamoeba histolytica.*

Microbial Agents or Their Toxins

Enterotoxigenic *Staphylococcus aureus* and *Bacillus cereus* cause acute nausea, vomiting, and diarrhea, usually within 8 hours of ingestion of the preformed toxin. Outbreaks of staphylococcal food poisoning are commonly associated with food handler contamination whereas the enterotoxin of *B. cereus* is most often associated wtih reheated fried rice. Both illnesses are generally self-limited and last less than 12 hours. Only symptomatic therapy is necessary, with the major emphasis on restoring intravascular volume. Deaths have been reported rarely with staphylococcal food poisoning.

Clostridium perfringens and long-incubation *B. cereus* food poisoning is caused by toxins produced in vivo, accounting for a longer incubation time, usually 8 to 16 hours. The major symptoms of abdominal cramping and diarrhea generally resolve within 24 hours. Antimicrobial agents have no role in the treatment of these intoxications.

Vibrio cholerae may cause acute diarrheal illnesses with massive fluid loss. Outbreaks of cholera in the United States from contaminated Gulf Coast waters have been described. Treatment is primarily supportive and may require enormous volumes of fluid. Most patients should be hydrated intravenously with Ringer's lactate or Dacca solution (0.5 per cent NaCl, 0.4 per cent $NaHCO_3$, 0.1 per cent KCl). Antibiotics will shorten the duration of illness. Tetracyline, 250 mg every 6 hours, is the drug of choice. In pregnant women ampicillin is an effective alternative. Children should receive ampicillin, 50 mg per kg per day in divided doses. Other antimicrobial agents that can be employed include chloramphenicol, trimethoprim-sulfamethoxazole (Bactrim, Septra), and doxycycline (Vibramycin).

Organisms that produce their effects by tissue invasion, such as *Salmonella, Shigella, Vibrio parahaemolyticus,* and *Campylobacter jejuni,* generally have incubation times greater than 16 hours. The illnesses are characterized by fever, abdominal cramps, diarrhea, and vomiting. Symptoms generally resolve in 1 week. The diagnosis is made by isolation of the organism from stool cultures. (Specific treatment is covered in other sections.) Briefly, antibiotics should be included in the therapy of shigellosis but are not necessary in uncomplicated salmonella enteritis. Antimicrobial therapy is of uncertain utility in *C. jejuni* and *V. parahaemolyticus* food poisoning. Studies of erythromycin therapy in the treatment of campylobacteriosis reveal a shortened duration of microbial carriage without affecting the clinical illness. Recently, a rare *Escherichia coli* serotype, 0157:H7, has been reported to cause a hemorrhagic colitis. Eating hamburgers from a fast food chain was a common factor in affected individuals. The role of antibiotics in the treatment of this illness is unclear. Similarly, a severe hemorrhagic jejunitis and ileitis known as enteritis necroticans or pig-bel has been associated with the ingestion of *Clostridium perfringens* type C.

Traveler's Diarrhea

A number of viral, bacterial, and protozoal agents can cause diarrhea in travelers. Up to 60 per cent of travelers to developing countries may develop acute, watery diarrhea in their first month of travel. The enteric pathogen most frequently isolated is an enterotoxigenic *E. coli* (ETEC); other etiologic agents include many of the pathogens discussed previously as well as rotavirus, which has been identified in 10 to 25 per cent of diarrheal illness in American travelers to Mexico. The incubation time for traveler's diarrhea due to ETEC is usually less than 48 hours, and infection may last 5 to 7 days. Persistent or recurrent diarrhea that develops after a traveler's return is often due to protozoa, usually *Giardia lamblia* or *E. histolytica.*

Traveler's diarrhea can best be avoided by careful attention to diet. Boiled or bottled water, particularly when carbonated, is generally safer than untreated tap water. Raw fruits and vegetables, poorly cooked or cold meats, and dairy products should be avoided.

Most cases of traveler's diarrhea are self-limited, and oral rehydration is generally sufficient. A balanced electrolyte-glucose solution (ORS) as described earlier may be used, but the otherwise healthy adult usually can replace fluids adequately by drinking safe liquids and hot broths.

Prophylaxis has been advocated for the prevention of traveler's diarrhea. Liquid bismuth subsalicylate (Pepto-Bismol), 60 ml four times a day, is effective but the volume required makes its continued use impractical. Doxycycline, 100 mg daily, is also effective against ETEC, but resistance is widespread; sun sensitivity is a common side effect of tetracycline, making it undesirable for vacationers. Trimethoprim (80 mg) and sulfamethoxazole (400 mg), given twice daily, are effective for short periods but the sulfa component induces allergic reactions in up to 5 per cent of individuals.

A more effective approach may be to provide travelers with therapy that can be initiated if and when symptoms develop. Doxycycline, 100 mg daily, or trimethoprim (160 mg) and sulfamethoxazole (800 mg), twice daily for 5 days, can be used.

Botulism

The development of acute gastrointestinal symptoms associated with neurologic dysfunction suggests the diagnosis of foodborne botulism. Most often it is caused by eating contaminated home-processed fruit, vegetables, or meat. The clinical features of botulism are caused by a neurotoxin produced by *Clostridium botulinum.* The most common neurologic manifestations include dry mouth, diplopia, dysphagia, and weakness. Symptoms may appear as early as 6 hours or as late as 8 days after ingestion of contaminated food. Botulism is a medical emergency because neuromuscular paralysis may occur with unpredictable rapidity, and fatality rates approach 25 per cent. All patients with suspected botulism should be hospitalized; the first priority is respiratory support.

A trivalent A,B,E antiserum is available from the Centers for Disease Control against three of the four principal types of botulism. The Centers may be contacted at any time (404/329-3753 days and 404/329-3644 nights, weekends, and holidays) about the treatment, diagnosis, and investigation of suspected cases of botulism.

Infant botulism is caused by the ingestion of *C. botulinum* spores with subsequent production of toxin in vivo. A course of penicillin has been advocated for foodborne cases, but the effectiveness of this treatment has not been established. Guanidine hydrochloride has been used to enhance the release of acetylcholine from terminal nerve fibers but its use is still considered experimental.

Plants

Mushroom Poisoning

There are seven established groups of toxic mushrooms, each elaborating different toxins and producing different clinical syndromes. Five of these clinical syndromes have short incubation periods of 30 minutes to 2 hours; the incubation period of the remaining two syndromes ranges from 6 to 24 hours. Of the short-acting varieties, mushrooms of the *Clitocybe* and *Inocybe* groups elaborate muscarinic compounds and produce an anticholinergic syndrome of sweating, salivation, lacrimation, bradycardia, abdominal cramping, vomiting, retching, and other manifestations of parasympathetic dysfunction. This syndrome may prove lethal and should be treated with atropine sulfate, 1 to 2 mg every 2 to 6 hours, titrated to symptoms, which usually resolve within 24 hours.

Ibotenic acid and other isoxazole derivaties are produced by *Amanita* species and may cause ataxia, dizziness, stupor, and convulsions. Both cholinergic and anticholingeric effects can occur, but specific treatment is usually not indicated. Patients who are severely ill with anticholinergic symptoms may be treated with physostigmine. Barbiturates and benzodiazepines may exacerbate symptoms and should not be employed.

The third group of centrally acting toxins includes psilocybin, psilocin, and other related indoles produced by the *Psilocybe* species. Mood elevation, hallucinations, hyperkinetic activity, and muscle weakness are the major symptoms. Treatment is symptomatic; diazepam (Valium) can be administered intravenously to relieve agitation.

Coprinus species produce a disulfiram-like substance, coprine, which may cause autonomic symptoms following alcohol consumption, with headache, flushing, nausea, vomiting, and paresthesias. Symptoms may recur after drinking alcohol for up to 5 days after mushroom ingestion. Therapy is simply to avoid alcohol.

The fifth short incubation syndrome is that of gastrointestinal symptoms with nausea, vomiting, and abdominal cramping. These symptoms are associated with many different mushroom genera, and only supportive treatment is necessary.

Several species of mushrooms may cause symptoms that do not appear until 6 to 24 hours after ingestion. These syndromes are potentially life-threatening and require hospitalization and supportive and, in some cases, specific therapy.

Various mushrooms in the genus *Amanita* as well as several other genera contain cyclic peptides termed "amatoxins" or "phallotoxins," which are implicated in 95 per cent of fatal mushroom poisonings. A characteristic biphasic illness is associated with this form of intoxication. Symptoms of abdominal pain, vomiting, diarrhea, and fever usually begin 6 to 12 hours after ingestion and resolve within 24 hours, after which the patient appears to be relatively well for 1 or 2 days. Renal and hepatic failure ensue on the third or fourth day. Intensive supportive care is necessary, since the mortality rate approaches 50 per cent. This includes correction of dehydration, electrolyte monitoring, and administration of opiates for relief of pain. Hypoglycemia may occur, and glucose should be administered intravenously with careful monitoring. Gastric lavage and oral administration of charcoal are probably not effective in removing ingested toxin. Similarly, cathartics and enemas appear to be of limited utility. Hemoperfusion may be helpful in removing circulating toxin. For hemoperfusion to be effective, it should be employed early, before organ damage has occurred. Thioctic acid may lower the mortality rate, but its efficacy has not been unequivocally established. It may be obtained through a local poison control center or from Burton Berkson, M.D., Lea Regional Hospital, Hobbs, New Mexico, 505/392-6581.

Mushrooms of the genus *Gyromitra* contain a toxin that, after ingestion, is converted to methylhydrazine, a competitive inhibitor of pyridoxal phosphate. Initial symptoms of nausea and vomiting may be followed by hemolysis with methemoglobinemia, hepatic failure, convulsions, and coma. Specific treatment with pyridoxine hydrochloride, 25 mg per kg, administered intravenously over 15 to 30 minutes, is indicated when neurologic symptoms occur.

Fungi Poisoning

Ergotism is caused by ingestion of alkaloids produced by the fungus *Calviceps purpurea,* which contaminates rye or wheat. Ergot may induce severe vasoconstriction by stimulation of alpha-adrenergic receptors of vascular smooth muscle that leads to ischemic necrosis and gangrene. Symptoms of ergotism include severe abdominal and muscle pain, headache, paresthesias, and convulsions. Treatment of severe cases includes anticoagulation to prevent thrombosis and intravenous sodium nitroprusside, 50 or more μg per minute, to promote vasodilation.

Aflatoxin has been found in commercial peanut butter in the United States. In warmer climates corn and other grains may be contaminated by this mycotoxin. Ingestion of large doses may result in gastrointestinal bleeding, hepatic injury, and hepatocellular carcinoma.

Tricothecenes are heat-stable mycotoxins that occasionally contaminate grains in colder climates. These toxins appear to interfere with nucleic acid and protein synthesis. Ingestion of flour prepared from contaminated grain may result in vomiting, bloody diarrhea, anemia, and leukopenia. Treatment is supportive; avoidance of contaminated foods is the only effective means of preventing mycotoxin-related illness.

Miscellaneous Plant Poisoning

Ingestion of the Italian broad (fava) bean may trigger a hemolytic crisis in patients with glucose-6-phosphate dehydrogenase–deficient red cells. The most severe cases occur in individuals of Mediterranean descent. Episodes of massive hemolysis may require transfusion of packed red cells. Deaths have been reported in severe cases.

Chronic ingestion of sweet peas of the species *Lathyrus sativus* may lead to lathyrism, a slowly progressive spastic paraplegia. Early symptoms of muscle spasm, cramps, and weakness in the legs may be followed by signs of degeneration of the posterolateral tracts of the thoracolumbar spinal cord, with paralysis and incontinence. Large amounts of these peas have been eaten during famines in Asia and Africa. Treatment with subcutaneous neostigmine methylsulfate (Prostigmine), 0.5 mg daily, may be beneficial and should be employed, especially in patients whose symptoms have been present for only a short time.

Oxalic acid poisoning may result from eating rhubarb leaves, beets, spinach, or the houseplants philodendron and dieffenbachia. Hypocalcemic tetany may follow oxalic acid ingestion because of calcium oxalate formation. Treatment is aimed at reducing the oxalate concentration by precipitating calcium oxalate in the gastrointestinal tract. Calcium is given orally in any form such as milk, limewater, or calcium salts. Intravenous calcium gluconate, 10 ml of a 10 per cent solution, should be given if symptoms of hypocalcemic tetany develop. Intravenous fluids and diuretics should also be given to prevent renal tubular damage.

Solanine is a toxin present in the tubers, vines, leaves, and new sprouts of potatoes, the leaves and fruit of the Jerusalem cherry, and in the leaves and stems of tomato plants. The toxin is heat-labile and destroyed by boiling. Solanine may reach humans through the milk of cattle ingesting the jimson weed, which contains the toxin. Symptoms of this intoxication include headache, abdominal pain, diarrhea, and confusion. Treatment is supportive.

Home-brewed teas prepared from foxglove or oleander may produce digitalis intoxication. Treatment is as with any cardiogenic glycoside overdose: maintenance of serum potassium level, electrocardiographic monitoring, and administration of antiarrhythmic drugs or temporary pacing as necessary.

Cyanogenic glycosides or free hydrocyanic acid may be present in the seeds of apples, cherries, pears, peaches, plums, apricots, and cassava and lima beans. Cyanide poisoning may result from ingestion of large numbers of seeds but fortunately is rare. Symptoms may appear within 5 minutes of ingestion and include headache, faintness, anxiety, dyspnea, tachycardia, and a burning sensation in the throat. In extreme cases cyanosis, bradycardia, hypotension, opisthotonus, convulsions, coma, and death may result. Treatment is designed to remove the cyanide anion from intracellular sites by binding it to the ferric ion. Inhalation of amyl nitrate converts hemoglobin to methemoglobin, which binds the cyanide anion. The patient should inhale amyl nitrite capsules for 30 seconds every minute. A new capsule is used every 3 minutes. Intravenous sodium nitrite should be cautiously administered in doses to achieve a methemoglobin concentration of 26 per cent. Excessive nitrite can cause a level of methemoglobinemia that results in a chocolate-brown cyanosis, acidosis, coma, convulsions, and arrhythmias. Sodium thiosulfate may be given to promote excretion of cyanide.

Fish and Shellfish Ingestion

Ciguatera Fish Poisoning

Ciguatera poisoning is the most commonly reported seafood poisoning in the United States, attributed to ciguatoxin, a substance believed to be produced by algae and dinoflagellates. It is concentrated in the food chain so that significant quantities accumulate in the tissues of larger fish. Over 400 species of fish between latitudes 35°N and 35°S have been found to contain ciguatoxin. Most cases in the United States occur in the spring and summer and are reported from Hawaii and Florida, with barracuda, red snapper, amberjack, and grouper most often implicated. The toxin is not affected by heating or freezing, can persist for weeks, and is difficult to detect since it does not alter the taste, color, or odor of contaminated food. Ciguatoxin inhibits red cell cholinesterase activity and reduces the amplitude of the action potential in the frog sciatic nerve.

Symptoms usually develop within 1 to 6 hours of ingestion. Nausea, vomiting, diarrhea, and abdominal pain usually precede neurologic symptoms, which include pruritus, shooting pain in the legs, paresthesias of the perioral region, and a sensation of looseness and pain in the teeth. Dry mouth, myalgias, arthralgias, blurred vision, photophobia, and transient blindness have been reported. In severe cases, cranial nerve palsies, reversal of hot and cold temperature sensation, bradycardia, hypotension, and respiratory paralysis requiring mechanical ventilation may occur.

Treatment is usually symptomatic, but cholinesterase-reactivating drugs may be considered in severe cases. Pralidoxime chloride (Protopam), 1 to 2 gm in 100 ml of saline, is given intravenously over 15 to 30 minutes to patients with life-threatening weakness and low blood cholinesterase concentration. Cathartics and enemas should be given to remove unabsorbed toxin, if not contraindicated by ileus. Death due to ciguatera poisoning is extremely rare. The duration of acute illness is a few days to several months, but pain in the extremities may last for years.

Scombroid Poisoning

Scombrotoxin or "saurine" is produced by decarboxylation of histidine by marine bacteria that infect the flesh of tuna, mackerel, bonito, skipjack, and mahimahi. Symptoms resemble those of a histamine reaction and usually begin 30 minutes after ingestion. These include flushing, headache, nausea, vomiting, pruritus, urticaria, and, in severe cases, bronchospasm. Antihistamines and bronchodilators provide symptomatic relief. Symptoms generally subside within 4 hours.

Puffer Fish Poisoning

Tetrodotoxin is a neurotoxin similar to saxitoxin (see next paragraph) contained in the tissues of the puffer fish. Paralysis of nerve transmission and respiration may require respiratory support after ingestion of improperly cleaned fish.

Paralytic Shellfish Poisoning

"Red tides" are associated with neurotoxin-producing dinoflagellates between May and October in the Northern Hemisphere. Mussels, clams, oysters, and scallops may concentrate the toxin, saxitoxin, but are not affected by it. Saxitoxin ingestion produces paralytic shellfish poisoning, a clinical syndrome characterized by paresthesias of the face and extremities, nausea, vomiting, and diarrhea. In severe cases dysphonia, dysphagia, muscle paralysis, and respiratory impairment may ensue. Symptoms usually appear within 30 minutes of ingestion, although longer incubation periods have been reported. Death may occur from respiratory paralysis within 12 hours. Treatment consists of emptying the gastrointestinal tract of unabsorbed toxin by cathartics and enemas, if no ileus is present, and respiratory support. Duration of the illness ranges from a few hours to a few days. Though red tides commonly signify toxic concentrations of the dinoflagellates, poisoning may occur in the absence of red tides, and not all tides are contaminated. The toxin is heat-stable and is not affected by cooking.

Neurotoxic Shellfish Poisoning

Neurotoxic shellfish poisoning is a syndrome produced by other dinoflagellates that are associated with red tides. Contaminated shellfish are usually harvested from the Atlantic Ocean and Gulf of Mexico near Florida during the spring and fall. The symptoms of neurotoxic shellfish poisoning are similar to those of paralytic shellfish poisoning, but paralysis does not occur. This syndrome occurs within 3 hours of shellfish ingestion and is self-limited.

Miscellaneous

Ingestion of heavy metals like copper, zinc, tin, and cadmium may result in nausea, vomiting, and abdominal pain after an incubation period of 5 to 15 minutes. This most commonly occurs when acid liquids such as citric juices come in contact with metal. Symptoms resolve after removal of the offending agent from the gastrointestinal tract.

Monosodium L-glutamate (MSG) has been implicated in the "Chinese restaurant syndrome." Wonton soup is often found to be the offending food. A burning sensation of the skin, tightness across the face and chest, headache, flushing, and diaphoresis may appear within 10 minutes of ingestion. The syndrome is self-limited and seldom lasts longer than several hours.

NECROTIZING INFECTIONS OF THE SOFT TISSUES, INCLUDING GAS GANGRENE

method of
ROBERT P. HUMMEL, M.D., and
H. STEPHEN BJORNSON, M.D., Ph.D.
University of Cincinnati
Cincinnati, Ohio

A variety of infectious and noninfectious processes can produce the clinical picture of skin or soft tissue necrosis with crepitus. The basis for classification is shown in Table 1. A strict classification of the infectious causes of necrosis with crepitus of the soft tissues is difficult because they are clinical entities rather than specific bacterial infections. Attempts at classification become even more difficult since the clinical findings often overlap.

Necrotizing soft tissue infections are almost always polymicrobic, involving multiple species of gram-positive and gram-negative aerobic, facultative, and anaerobic bacteria (Table 2). The same microorganism(s) can cause infections in different tissue compartments with strikingly different clinical characteristics. The role of anaerobic bacteria in these infections has been better appreciated in recent years with improved techniques for the recovery and identification of these organisms in clinical specimens.

These infections usually occur in areas of trauma, ischemia from vascular insufficiency or atherosclerosis, burns, malignancy, foreign body introductions, or other forms of tissue damage resulting from operative or accidental wounds. Such conditions are thought to cause a local decrease in oxidation-reduction potential of tissues, thereby predisposing the tissue to infection. Necrotizing infections may also originate intra-abdominally, such as at the site of diverticular perforation, and extend along the psoas muscle into the subcutaneous tissues of the thigh or onto the abdominal wall.

Diabetes is present in an impressively large number of patients with necrotizing soft tissue infections. Disease-related vascular insufficiency or depression of host defense mechanisms may predispose the diabetic patient to necrotizing soft tissue infections. In these patients the infection progresses rapidly, with copious gas production and tissue necrosis. Early diagnosis and intervention is mandatory, since reported mortality rates are in excess of 50 per cent.

The necrosis associated with these infections can occur from a number of mechanisms, including pressure necrosis secondary to extensive inflammatory swelling and gas formation. This problem is greatly intensified when the inflammation occurs within closed tissue spaces. Necrosis might also result from thrombosed vessels in the area. Extracellular enzymes or toxins produced by the bacteria may also be a prominent cause of tissue necrosis.

One of the most effective means of preventing polymicrobic soft tissue infections is early and adequate care of traumatic wounds with wide debridement of all devitalized tissue and foreign material. In the case of infected or contaminated elective surgery, every effort should be made to protect the incision from contamination.

The factors that determine the therapy required for necrotizing skin and soft tissue infections are the depth of the involvement of the infection, the presence of tissue necrosis, and the microorganisms involved in the infectious process. Antibiotic therapy effective against aerobes and anaerobes alone may be adequate if tissue necrosis and crepitus are absent. If tissue necrosis is present, these infections must be treated with exploration, aggressive surgical debridement, drainage, and appropriate antibiotic therapy (Tables 3 and 4). In addition, large volumes of fluid are often sequestered in the extravascular space of patients in response to their infection, for which patients require intensive fluid resuscitation (Table 5).

Treatment
(Table 6)

Clostridial Cellulitis. Local trauma or surgery resulting in devitalized tissue and wound contamination by bowel flora can result in necrotizing infections of the subcutaneous tissue caused by *Clostridium perfringens* or other clostridial organisms. Pain is often mild and toxicity minimal, but tissue gas may be extensive and in almost all cases indicates the presence of a necrotizing soft tissue infection. Immediate surgical exploration of the wound is mandatory with inspection of the fascia and muscle. All necrotic tissue must be removed and pus drained. Gram stain of the exudate is required for presumptive bacteriologic diagnosis and initiation of appropriate antibiotic therapy. Thick, gram-positive rods confirm the diagnosis of clostridial cellulitis. High doses of penicillin (10 to 20 million units per day) intravenously are indicated.

Nonclostridial Crepitant Cellulitis. This syndrome often occurs in diabetic patients and is a polymicrobic infection involving a variety of anaerobic and facultative bacteria, including peptostreptococci, *Bacteroides* species, and Enterobacteriaceae. Clinical findings and operative treatment are similar to those of clostridial cellulitis. The Gram stain will show a mixture of gram-positive cocci and gram-negative rods. The antibiotics of choice are clindamycin (Cleocin) or chloramphenicol (Chloromycetin) for the anaerobic component of the infection. Enterobacteriaceae and other gram-negative aerobes are treated with aminoglycosides or a cephalosporin [cefoxitin (Mefoxin) or cefotaxime (Claforan)].

Necrotizing Fasciitis. Acute necrotizing cellulitis, which involves the superficial fascia and subcutaneous tissue and results in extensive undermining infection, is referred to as necrotizing fasciitis. The diagnosis is usually made at operation when the fascia is inspected. Some refer to

TABLE 1. **Classification of Necrotizing Soft Tissue Infections**

	Clostridial Cellulitis	Nonclostridial Anaerobic Cellulitis	Necrotizing Fasciitis	Synergistic Necrotizing Cellulitis	Gas Gangrene	Nonclostridial Myositis	Infected Vascular Gangrene
Predisposing Conditions	Local trauma or operation	Diabetes mellitus; preexisting localized infection	Diabetes mellitus; abdominal surgery, perineal; infection; drug addiction	Diabetes mellitus; cardiorenal disease; obesity; perirectal infection	Local trauma or surgery	Local trauma	Peripheral arterial insufficiency
Swelling	Moderate	Moderate	Marked	Moderate or marked	Marked	Moderate	Moderate or marked
Skin appearance	Minimal discoloration	Minimal discoloration	Erythematous cellulitis	Scattered areas of skin necrosis	Yellow-bronze; dark bullae; green-black patches of necrosis	Erythema	Discolored or black
Exudate	Thin, dark	Dark pus	Seropurulent	"Dishwater" pus	Serosanguineous	Abundant seropurulent	0
Gas	+ + + +	+ + + +	+ +	+ +	+ +	±	+ + +
Odor	Sometimes foul	Foul	Foul	Foul	Variable; slightly foul or peculiar sweet	Slight; "sour"	Foul
Systemic toxicity	Minimal	Moderate	Moderate or marked	Marked	Marked	Only late in course	Minimal
Muscle involvement	0	0	0	+ +	+ + + +	+ + +	Dead

this condition as streptococcal gangrene, but many other organisms besides streptococcus may cause this syndrome. Most cases of necrotizing fasciitis follow trauma or surgery. The infection spreads rapidly along the superficial fascia. Erythema and edema of the skin occur, which may progress to cyanosis, blister formation, and eventually gangrene. The presence of skin crepitus again is an indication for prompt surgical exploration. If crepitus cannot be palpated, surgical intervention may be indicated by a spreading cellulitis despite antibiotic therapy. It is typical of this infection that there is significant undermining of apparently normal skin and subcutaneous tissue. All necrotic fascia and subcutaneous tissue must be widely debrided, and it is not unusual for this condition to require repeated trips to the operating room with extended de-

TABLE 2. **Bacteriology of (Nonclostridial) Deep Soft Tissue Infections**

	Per Cent of Cases with Isolate		
Microorganisms Recovered	**Necrotizing Fasciitis** *(16 Cases)*	**Nonclostridial Crepitant Cellulitis** *(81 Cases)*	**Infected Vascular Ulcers** *(56 Cases)*
AEROBES			
Proteus species	6	41	43
Escherichia coli	25	43	29
Klebsiella species	13	33	16
Enterobacter species	13	0	18
Pseudomonas species	13	12	9
Other gram-negative rods	19	27	9
Staphyloccocus aureus	6	6	38
Enterococcus	25	19	34
β-Hemolytic streptococci	50	15	36
ANAEROBES			
Bacteroides fragilis	13	3	38
Other *Bacteroides*	81	44	32
Fusobacterium species	6	0	7
Peptostreptococcus species	50	57	25
Peptococcus species	25		41
Clostridium species	25	0	28

TABLE 3. **Antibiotic Therapy: Superficial Cellulitis**

Staphylococcus aureus	
Parenteral:	Nafcillin Cephalosporin Clindamycin Vancomycin
Oral:	Cloxacillin Cephalosporin Clindamycin
Streptococci	
Parenteral:	Penicillin G Cephalosporin Clindamycin
Oral:	Cephalosporin Erythromycin Clindamycin

bridements on each occasion. Antibiotic therapy is similar to that described earlier for mixed polymicrobial infections.

Fournier's gangrene was first described in 1883 and is considered a form of necrotizing fasciitis of the perineum and genitalia. Either group A streptococci or mixed bacterial species may be the causative organism(s). This condition often follows anorectal infections, anorectal surgical procedures, or problems associated with the extravasation of urine into the perineal area. This infection may result in extensive gangrene of the scrotum and penis and frequently occurs in obese, diabetic patients. Antibiotic therapy is the same as that for nonclostridial crepitant cellulitis.

Progressive Bacterial Synergistic Gangrene. First described by Meleney, this condition almost always begins at an operative wound site where red, swollen areas develop that gradually evolve into shaggy, gangrenous ulcers. There is usually severe pain but not much systemic toxicity. Chronic burrowing ulcers with excessive undermining develop. *Streptococcus* species *(peptostreptococcus), Staphylococcus aureus,* or Enterobacteriaceae are usually cultured from the ulcers. There is minimal information on the anaerobic bacteriology of this infection. Surgical excision and debridement plus penicillin and aminoglycoside antibiotics are the treatments of choice. Clindamycin may be indicated for coverage of gram-negative anaerobes.

TABLE 4. **Antibiotic Therapy: Deep or Necrotizing Soft Tissue Infections**

Gram-negative bacilli
- Aerobes
  - Aminoglycoside
  - *or*
  - Cephalosporin
- Anaerobes
  - Clindamycin

Gram-positive cocci and bacilli
- Penicillin G
- Nafcillin if Gram stain suggests the presence of *Staphylococcus aureus*

TABLE 5. **Response to Diagnosis of Gas-Forming Soft Tissue Infection**

Immediate IV antibiotics
- aminoglycoside (gentamicin or tobramycin, 5.0 mg/kg/day)
- clindamycin (Cleocin, 600 mg q 6 hr)
- penicillin G (3–4 miilion units q 6 hr)

Emergency surgical debridement and drainage
Obtain Gram stains and cultures (aerobic and anaerobic)
Intensive supportive therapy (blood, electrolytes, pain medication, and so on)
Diabetes control
Hyperbaric oxygen therapy if available
Frequent postoperative dressing changes to inspect wound

Synergistic Necrotizing Cellulitis. This condition generally occurs in patients who are diabetic and obese and have cardiac disease. Cutaneous gangrene with local crepitus is observed in some patients. At the time of incision, extensive fascial and muscle necrosis is observed. The subcutaneous tissue and fascia seem secondarily involved, with the primary problem being the necrotizing infection of underlying muscles. These infections are usually polymicrobial, caused by gram-negative enteric bacilli, peptostreptococci, and *Bacteroides* species. The mortality rate is high. Extensive debridement, including amputation and aggressive antibiotic therapy, along with the treatment of diabetic acidosis will yield occasional survivors.

Clostridial Myonecrosis. This condition is usually

TABLE 6. **Principles of Management of Anaerobic, Necrotizing Infections**

(1) *Prevention,* with employment of proper surgical care that removes all devitalized, contaminated tissue.
(2) *Early recognition* of a developing serious infection that requires prompt surgical attention.
(3) *Gastrointestinal tract* origination; the presence of gas in the tissues is highly suggestive of anaerobic involvement.
(4) Prompt *surgical exploration,* debridement of all necrotic tissue, and wide drainage.
(5) Presumptive *antibiotic therapy.* If clostridial or streptococcal infections are suspected, large doses of intravenous penicillin (3 to 4 million units every 4 hours) are indicated. If polymicrobial infections are suspected, an aminoglycoside (gentamicin or tobramycin), 5.0 mg per kg per day intravenously, and clindamycin (Cleocin), 600 mg every 6 hours intravenously, should be initiated. Further antibiotic therapy is guided by Gram stains at the time of surgery and culture and sensitivity results as they are obtained.
(6) *Hyperbaric oxygen therapy* (100% oxygen at 3 atmospheres of pressure for 1 to 2 hours at 8 hour intervals) may be worthwhile for patients with anaerobic gas-forming infections provided the equipment is accessible without delaying other forms of therapy.
(7) *General supportive therapy,* including component blood transfusions, maintenance of fluid and electrolyte balance, proper surgical dressings, and pain control.

acute, fulminating, and extremely toxic. It occurs in areas of wound trauma, at operative sites, and as a complication of thermal burns. Occasionally, there is no history of antecedent trauma. Pain at the involved site, rapid progression, and extreme systemic toxicity occur. Crepitus is not always detected on physical examination but can often be seen on soft tissue radiographs. A typical bronze discoloration of the tense, swollen skin often develops with bullae formation. Rapid tissue necrosis and systemic toxicity are caused by clostridial toxins and the breakdown of muscle and other soft tissues. *Clostridium perfringens* is the most common species of clostridia causing gas gangrene, but other clostridial species, including *C. septicum, C. novyi,* and *C. hemolyticum,* can also cause this serious syndrome. At the time of operation, the muscle appears friable and edematous and may be brick red in color. It does not bleed, contractility is lost, and gas is often found in the muscle bundles. The treatment of clostridial gas consists of extensive surgical debridement, intravenous penicillin G (10 to 20 million units daily), and supportive measures to maintain renal function and prevent shock and hemolytic anemia. Hyperbaric oxygen may have a role in treatment of gas gangrene but is only supplementary to the other measures mentioned. Other therapy should never be delayed in order to transport a patient to a facility that offers hyperbaric oxygen therapy. The value of polyvalent clostridial antitoxin in the treatment of gas gangrene has never been proved, and this preparation is no longer available.

Nonclostridial Myositis. This form of myonecrosis can be caused by a variety of bacteria, with anaerobic streptococci *(Peptostreptococcus)* being the most common agent. The clinical picture is similar but much less severe than with gas gangrene. Operative findings reveal that the muscle is not dead but bleeds and contracts well. Purulent material is often encountered, and Gram stain reveals gram-positive cocci. Treatment consists of surgical decompression and drainage of purulent material and intravenous penicillin in large doses. In some cases, infections are polymicrobial, including other streptococci and enteric gram-negative bacilli.

Infected Vascular Gangrene. It is not unusual to have serious infections in extremities with peripheral vascular insufficiency. These may be gas-forming infections with gangrenous muscle pain and systemic toxicity. Infections in these cases are polymicrobial in nature but often contain *Bacteroides* species, peptococci, *Staphylococcus aureus,* and even various strains of clostridia. Since these infections are superimposed on ischemic extremities, amputation is usually required.

Noninfectious Causes of Gas in Tissues. Various mechanical conditions may result in the appearance of gas in tissues either by clinical examination or x-ray studies. The mechanical effects of penetrating trauma, which may entrap air under sutured wounds, is a common finding, particularly if the wounds have been irrigated with hydrogen peroxide solution. Occasionally, injuries occur that involve the use of compressed air. When this air under pressure escapes into soft tissues, it may create extensive crepitation.

INFLUENZA

method of
THOMAS R. CATE, M.D.
Baylor College of Medicine
Houston, Texas

Influenza virus infection of the respiratory tract typically causes the rather abrupt onset of dry cough, malaise, myalgias, headache, and feverishness. The acute illness lasts 3 to 5 days, but cough and lassitude often persist 1 or more additional weeks. Other respiratory pathogens can cause similar illnesses, but distinguishing features of influenza virus disease are its occurrence in both children and adults during winter epidemics lasting 4 to 8 weeks. Typical illnesses during such epidemics have a high probability of being due to influenza virus infection. Some patients will have milder illness with only coryza; others in "high risk" groups are more likely to have severe influenza with complications such as pneumonia and a relatively high mortality rate. Included in the high risk groups are persons over 65 years of age and those with chronic heart, lung, or kidney disease; metabolic disease (including diabetes mellitus); severe anemia; or immunosuppression.

The incidence of influenza virus infections each winter increases concomitantly with the proportion of the population susceptible to the current strains. Influenza type A and type B viruses frequently undergo minor changes ("drift") in their hemagglutinin and/or neuraminidase surface antigens. This antigenic drift renders previously acquired immunity less effective and leads to localized epidemics. Major changes ("shift") in one or both surface antigens have been observed only with type A viruses. These shifts occur at 1 to 3 decade intervals and have been associated with worldwide pandemics. Knowledge provided by public health authorities as to which type of influenza is active in the community has implications for prevention and treatment, since the antiviral agent amantadine (Symmetrel) is effective only against type A viruses.

Symptomatic Treatment

Persons with acute influenza should stay home and rest, both for their own benefit and that of others, since transmission of infection is most likely early in illness when the amount of virus in respiratory secretions is greatest. Measures to promote clearance of secretions are helpful in reducing the incidence of secondary bacterial infections, for which one must remain alert. Hydration should be increased using water, fruit juices, or carbonated beverages to the point that urination is necessary every couple of hours. Air humidity should be increased if possible. Use of alcoholic beverages is discouraged since they can increase the viscosity and reduce the clearance of secretions. Smoking also interferes with clearance of secretions by impairing ciliary function and is discouraged.

Fever associated with uncomplicated influenza is not an indication for treatment; in fact, it may aid the body in fighting the virus. An exception is very high fever in young children in whom a danger of febrile convulsions exists. Headache, malaise, and myalgias are often made tolerable by rest. If relief is necessary in order to rest, adults may take acetaminophen in doses of 325 to 650 mg every 4 to 6 hours, not to exceed 4.0 grams per day. The dose of acetaminophen for children is 10 mg per kg every 4 to 6 hours, with the total daily dose not to exceed 50 mg per kg. Alternatively, adults may take aspirin, 650 mg orally every 4 to 6 hours, but aspirin should be avoided in children because of its apparent association with Reye's syndrome. Sponge baths with tepid water may be used to control high fever in young children if acetaminophen is inadequate.

The most troublesome respiratory symptom with influenza is usually cough, which is minimally productive. Fluids, humidified air, and avoidance of irritants like cigarette smoke will provide some relief. Coughing is important for clearing secretions and should not be suppressed any more than is necessary for rest. For the latter purpose, an expectorant-antitussive combination, such as guaifenesin-dextromethorphan (Robitussin-DM) may be given every 6 to 8 hours in doses of 15 ml for adults, 10 ml for children 6 to 12 years old, and 5 ml for children 2 to 5 years old. The pharyngitis associated with influenza may be partially relieved by gargling with saline (one half teaspoonful of table salt to one half glass of warm water) three to four times daily.

Treatment of nasal obstruction and discharge is not generally necessary unless there are symptoms of fullness and pressure in the ears or over the paranasal sinuses. For the latter, pseudoephedrine may be given orally three or four times daily in doses of 30 to 60 mg for adults and 1 mg per kg for children. Forceful blowing of the nose can force secretions into the middle ear or paranasal sinuses and should be avoided. Use of a nasal suction bulb facilitates removal of secretions from young children.

Antiviral Treatment

Treatment with amantadine (Symmetrel) can shorten the duration of fever and symptoms caused by influenza A virus infection. This drug has no direct analgesic or antipyretic effect but works by inhibiting growth of the virus. To be effective, it must be begun within 24 to 48 hours of the onset of illness when large amounts of virus are present. Amantadine is available in 100 mg capsules and as a syrup containing 50 mg per 5 ml. The dose is 100 mg twice daily for persons 10 or more years of age and 3 mg per kg twice daily, not to exceed 150 mg per day, for children 1 to 9 years old. Treatment is continued for 5 days.

Five to 10 per cent of patients experience central nervous system (CNS) side effects such as anxiety, depression, insomnia, or difficulty in concentrating when taking full doses of amantadine prophylactically, but these are usually obscured by influenza symptoms when the drug is used therapeutically. If CNS side effects occur, they are usually mild, may go away while the drug is continued, and always reverse when it is stopped. Amantadine is excreted unchanged in the urine, and its daily dose should be reduced proportionately with any reduction in renal function. It is also excreted in breast milk and should not be given to nursing mothers. Large doses of amantadine have been teratogenic in certain laboratory animals, so risk-benefit ratios must be considered during pregnancy.

Prevention

The major method for preventing influenza is administration of inactivated influenza virus vaccine. The vaccine viruses are grown in embryonated chicken eggs. "Whole virus" vaccines contain purified, inactivated but intact virus particles. "Split virus" or "subvirion" vaccines prepared from disrupted virus particles contain predominantly the viral surface proteins hemagglutinin and neuraminidase, against which protective antibodies are directed. The vaccine potency is adjusted according to micrograms of hemagglutinin per dose. Split and whole virus vaccines have similar reactogenicity and immunogenicity in adults, but only split virus vaccine should be used in patients under 12 years of age because of a lower potential for causing febrile reactions in children.

The formulation, potency, and schedules for influenza vaccine are revised each year by The United States Public Health Service Advisory Committee on Immunization Practices. The aims are to provide the best possible immune response against the type A and type B strains expected from worldwide surveillance to circulate the following winter, and to minimize side effects. About 1 person in 5 will have transient soreness at the site of vaccine injection and about 1 person in 20 will develop headache, malaise, or fever for 1 to 2 days. Acute allergic reactions are extremely rare and are probably due to residual traces of egg antigen. It should not be given to persons who cannot eat eggs without an acute reaction and to those who have previously had severe reactions to influenza vaccine. No association of the Guillain-Barré syndrome (GBS) with influenza vaccine has been detectable since the 1976 swine influenza vaccination campaign, but it is prudent not to vaccinate persons with a history of GBS. Pregnant women may be vaccinated, using the same criteria applied to other persons.

Influenza vaccine should be administered in the fall 1 to 2 months before the influenza season. The antibody response (and protection) can be detected in about 2 weeks and will be near its maximum between 1 and 4 months after vaccination. About a 75 per cent reduction in influenza illness is expected in vaccinees when vaccine strains match those in circulation. Major target groups for annual influenza vaccination are the high risk groups identified previously; personnel involved in the care of high risk patients, to reduce transmission to the patients; and persons who provide essential community services, to minimize disruptions during an epidemic.

Amantadine (Symmetrel) is about equally as protective as vaccine against illness due to type A influenza viruses represented in the vaccine and is also effective against type A strains missed by the vaccine. Protection begins within 1 to 2 days and lasts as long as the drug is taken. Amantadine and vaccine should be given to vaccine target groups that have not been vaccinated when an influenza type A epidemic begins; amantadine can be discontinued after 2 or 3 weeks when vaccine protection begins, or it can be continued throughout the epidemic for additive protection. When the epidemic is due to a type A strain not closely related to one in the vaccine, amantadine will be the major means of protection.

Experience suggests that amantadine is protective at half the dose used for treatment with few side effects (i.e., 100 mg per day for adults), and no more than this should be given to persons 65 years or older because of the normal reduction in renal clearance with age. The drug should be continued for 1 to 2 weeks beyond the last possible exposure when it is the only means of protection. Precautions are described under treatment. Livedo reticularis and ankle edema have occurred during long-term treatment of parkinsonism with amantadine, but these side effects are unlikely with the lower doses used for influenza prophylaxis.

LEISHMANIASIS

method of
PHILIP D. MARSDEN, M.D. (London)
University of Brasília
Brasília, Brazil

Readers are referred to the 7th edition of Conn's Current Diagnosis (1948) for a table showing distribution of the principal *Leishmania* species.

There is no single method for the treatment of leishmaniasis. A protean disease, it has many clinical manifestations, which are classified as visceral (when the parasite is multiplying in the reticuloendothelial system of deep organs), cutaneous (restricted to the skin), or mucosal (when metastasis has occurred from the skin to the facial mucous membranes). No one has practical experience in the treatment of all forms of leishmaniasis.

The course of human infection depends on the host response and the species of infecting parasite. We know most about the latter. One example must suffice to illustrate the current difficulties in treating leishmaniasis. A dermatologist receiving a tourist from South America with a small skin lesion could be examining a patient infected with one of four species of the *Leishmania mexicana* group of parasites, *Leishmania donovani*, or one of four species of the *Leishmania braziliensis* group. In the latter group, metastatic mucosal disease is relatively common. Parasite identification of subspecies is a tedious and lengthy process, the results of which are available only long after treatment has commenced. Many such patients have been treated in the United States with local therapy (e.g., cryotherapy). This is wrong and can result in a protracted illness with recurrences. If there is doubt regarding the infecting species, systemic therapy with pentavalent antimonials is mandatory.

Heavy metals were one of the mainstays of 19th century therapy. All heavy metals can produce cardiac, renal, hepatic, or cerebral injury. The old trivalent antimonials were very toxic and I have seen all these complications with their use. Only the much less toxic pentavalent antimonials (Sb^V) are indicated today for the treatment of leishmaniasis. However, at high dosage, cardiac and renal side effects are not uncommon. Electrocardiographic changes are dose dependent and take the form of changes in the T wave (flattening or inversion) and prolongation of the

TABLE 1. **Treatment of Different Leishmanial Species with Pentavalent Antimonials**

	Easy to Treat	More Difficult to Treat	Most Difficult to Treat
Clinical Form			
Cutaneous	Limited cutaneous lesions *L. tropica* *L. major* *L. m. mexicana* *L. m. amazonensis* *L. peruana*	*L. b. panamensis* *L. b. guyanensis* *L. b. braziliensis* Post-kala azar Dermal leishmaniasis (*L. donovani*)	Diffuse cutaneous leishmaniasis due to *L. aethiopica* *L. m. pifanoi* *L. m. amazonensis* Leishmaniasis recidivans Skin granuloma due to *L. aethiopica*
Visceral or mucosal forms	—	Visceral leishmaniasis (*L. donovani*)	Mucosal leishmaniasis due to *L. b. braziliensis* *L. b. panamensis* *L. b.?*
Dosage (in mg Sb^V/kg/day)	10 mg/kg/day for 10–15 days	10 mg/kg/day for 30 days or 20 mg/kg/day for 20 days	20 mg/kg/day for 30 days

L, Leishmania; L. m., Leishmania mexicana group; *L. b., Leishmania braziliensis* group.
NOTE: Oversimplified, this guide does not take into account the exceptions to the rule. Relapses can occur in individual patients in all categories.

QT interval. The commonest renal lesion occurring at high dosage (20 mg of Sb^V per kg per day for 30 days) is a tubular defect in concentration, which fortunately is reversible in the majority of cases. Rarer is a defect of glomerular function. Even rarer is a hypersensitivity reaction to pentavalent antimony injection with cardiovascular shock. For this reason a test dose of 1 ml should be given intravenously before beginning a course of treatment. Toxic hepatitis can occur after prolonged therapy, but we have not seen cerebral toxicity. In one case, therapy was complicated by peripheral neuritis and exfoliative dermatitis. The daily dose in this patient was miscalculated and over 30 mg per kg per day of Sb^V were given.

Only two pentavalent antimonial preparations are on the market. Pentostam (sodium stibogluconate) is available through the Parasitic Disease Drug Service of the Centers for Disease Control, Atlanta, Georgia. It is marketed in 100 ml flasks; each ml contains 100 mg of pentavalent antimony. Glucantime (meglumine antimoniate) is used in Latin countries, especially Latin America. It is available in 5 ml ampules, each ml containing 85 mg of pentavalent antimony. Such studies as exist suggest that the two compounds are equally efficacious. The precise chemical structure of these compounds is not known. A variation in activity of different batches of drug has been suggested. The mode of action of antimonials on *Leishmania* is not clear.

Both drugs are administered by slow intravenous injection over 5 minutes without diluent. Diluent (20 to 50 ml) has been recommended if venous thrombosis is a problem. Intramuscular injection often has to be used in the field but is more painful. Over 90 per cent of the injected drug is excreted in the urine in a few hours. The little retained is concentrated in the liver and spleen, but the skin antimony content is unknown.

At this time there is no possibility that pentavalent antimonials will be replaced by an easier drug. We need to know more about the formulation, mode of action, and pharmacodynamics of pentavalent antimonials.

The geographic history of a patient is most important, since it gives an indication of the species of *Leishmania* that may have infected the patient. If available, the leishmanin skin test is a simple, valuable test of delayed hypersensitivity. It is negative in diffuse cutaneous leishmaniasis and untreated visceral leishmaniasis. A negative test in mucosal leishmaniasis carries a poor prognosis. Patients with advanced visceral disease or secondary malnutrition associated with mucosal disease must be in the recuperative stage before receiving antimonial therapy. Secondary infections should be treated, severe anemia corrected, and a good diet instituted.

The pentavalent antimonial doses most beneficial in the various forms of leishmaniasis are still under investigation. Treatment problems have been well reviewed in the WHO Technical Report Series 701, Geneva, 1984, on The Leishmaniases. A recent modification has been the abolition of rest periods during treatment with pentavalent antimonials. These were originally instituted for trivalent antimonial treatment, which has a marked cumulative effect because of tissue binding. Pentavalent antimonials are so rapidly excreted in the urine that their cumulative effect is minimal.

Pentavalent antimonial therapy dosages are listed in Table 1. The toxic single dose for patients with normal organ function is 30 mg per kg per day of antimony. In mucosal disease and skin granulomas due to *L. aethiopica,* longer courses may be necessary. Our maximum duration of treatment with 20 mg Sb^V per kg per day to date was 85 days, which cured a patient with mucosal disease unresponsive to conventional antimonial therapy and amphotericin B.

Diffuse cutaneous leishmaniasis is a special case that responds poorly to any drug therapy because the cellular immune response is defective. Daily immersion in hot baths may produce some improvement. For limited skin leishmaniasis in the Old World, cryotherapy or local excision may be effective. This would be reasonable therapy in Israel where only *Leishmania major* exists. No satisfactory trial of local injection therapy with either antimonials or other drugs exists at the time of writing, so this cannot be recommended.

Primary unresponsiveness to antimonials is defined as no clinical or parasitologic improvement after the first course. In visceral leishmaniasis, this occurs in 2 per cent of Kenyan, 5 per cent of Chinese, and 8 per cent of Indian patients. Secondary unresponsiveness occurs during relapse after apparently successful treatment. In both cases, longer, more intensive courses of antimonials are indicated. If this is unsuccessful, then one of the two second line drugs must be employed.

Pentamidine isethionate (Lomidine) is given in a dose of 4 mg per kg intramuscularly three times weekly for 5 to 25 weeks. Intravenous injection is dangerous, producing hypoglycemia and cardiovascular shock. Muscle abscesses and diabetes mellitus may develop with prolonged therapy. Cures in unresponsive *L. donovani* and *L. aethiopica* infections have been achieved with this drug. Amphotericin B (Fungizone) is the usual second line treatment for South American mucosal leishmaniasis. Slow intravenous infusion of 1 mg per kg in 500 ml of 5 per cent dextrose as a maximum single dose on alternate days to a total dose of 2.5 grams is usually effective. The physician must take time to discuss with the patient who otherwise often might not accept the inevitable unpleasant side effects, the necessity for uninterrupted treatment in the hospital. Patients with cardiac disease may do better with amphotericin B; those with renal disease benefit from pentamidine as first line drugs.

It is evident that all three drugs currently recommended for the treatment of leishmaniasis are difficult to administer, especially in field clinics. The young withstand antimonial therapy better than the elderly, who have less cardiac and renal reserve. Periodic electrocardiograms and blood urea, creatinine, and serum transaminase estimations are advised.

The need continues for an orally administered drug. Nifurtimox, benznidazole, cycloguanil pamoate, metronidazole, and rifampin cannot be recommended. Ketaconazole (Nizoral), in a dose of 200 mg twice daily for 1 to 3 months, is currently being tested, but initial results are not promising. Allopurinol derivatives and primaquine analogues are currently being evaluated and could be valuable in the future treatment of leishmaniasis.

Antimonial treatment can be costly due to the long series of injections. For this reason India and China have made their own pentavalent antimonial compounds. Since much still is required in their use and doses may have to be tailored to individual patients, there is an argument for installing leishmaniasis treatment centers in areas where sufficient cases are seen: a situation analogous to the sleeping sickness treatment centers in Africa.

LEPROSY

(Hansen's Disease)

method of
ROBERT R. JACOBSON, M.D.
National Hansen's Disease Center
Carville, Louisiana

Leprosy is a chronic infectious disease, of which the causative agent, *Mycobacterium leprae,* was discovered over 100 years ago. The disease itself has been known since biblical times, but there is still much about it that we do not understand, and treatment is sometimes difficult. Because of the mobility of modern peoples it is seen at least occasionally in nearly every country, but it is common only in a number of Third World countries, in tropical or semitropical areas. The World Health Organization (WHO) estimates that there are about 11 million cases worldwide. The United States now has over 4000 cases, and the number of new cases detected annually in the United States has increased in recent years to approximately 300. This is due entirely to cases among aliens, particularly those from Southeast Asia, Mexico, and the Philippines. Cases among native-born Americans, in fact, have declined in the last few decades, and currently they constitute less than 10 per cent of the total each year.

Leprosy is best viewed not as one disease but as a spectrum of diseases, and the problems encountered in treatment vary considerably from one end of the spectrum to the other. *M. leprae* may be highly infectious but has a low pathogenicity because the overwhelming majority of the population (over 95 per cent) apparently are not susceptible. Those who are susceptible seem to have a defect in their cell-mediated immunity that is relatively specific for *M. leprae*. The exact nature of this defect is uncertain, but considerable research is now under way to delineate it further. Those who are susceptible initially develop indeterminate leprosy. This may be self-healing but, if diagnosed, should always be treated. When self-healing or treatment does not intervene, these patients will eventually develop one of the advanced forms of the disease. Those with the most intact immune response, relatively speaking, keep the infection localized, developing tuberculoid leprosy, which is referred to as polar tuberculoid disease or TT in the Ridley-Jopling classification. On the other hand, those with little or no human response to the infection allow it to become generalized, developing polar lepromatous (LL) disease. Between the two extremes is a broad borderline (dimorphous) region where the disease may be classified borderline-tuberculoid (BT), mid-borderline (BB), or borderline-lepromatous (BL). Accurate classification is important for appropriate overall management of the patient, particularly of the various complications that may arise during chemotherapy.

Treatment

Antileprosy Drugs Currently Available

At present, four drugs are widely used to treat leprosy: dapsone, clofazimine, rifampin, and ethionamide/prothionamide. Dapsone and clofazimine are weakly bactericidal against *M. leprae,* rifampin has very potent bactericidal activity, and ethionamide/prothionamide are intermediate in activity. Other drugs with some activity against *M. leprae,* such as certain aminoglycocides, thiacetazone, thiambutosine, diacetyl diaminodiphenylsulfone (DADDS) (Hansolar), and long-acting sulfonamides, are seldom used because of cost, because of delivery (intramuscular rather than oral administration) or toxicity problems, or because they have only bacteriostatic activity against *M. leprae*. Technically, only dapsone is approved by the Food and Drug Administration for the treatment of leprosy in the United States. Sulfoxone sodium (Diasone) is no longer available. However, rifampin and clofazimine are widely used, and ethionamide/prothionamide are occasionally used both here and throughout the world for this purpose, since there is no question as to the effectiveness of any of these drugs against *M. leprae*. Prothionamide is not available in the United States, and clofazimine is available only from the National Hansen's Disease Center (NHDC) at Carville, Louisiana, or through one of multiple clinics authorized to prescribe it under NHDC IND application. Since *M. leprae* cannot be grown in artificial media, drug sensitivity testing is usually done utilizing the mouse footpad technique. Sensitivity to dapsone, rifampin, clofazimine, and ethionamide is routinely tested at the NHDC.

Dapsone (Avlosulfon). This is available as 25 and 100 mg tablets, and the usual dose is 100 mg daily for adults and 0.9 to 1.4 mg per kg for children. Because of its safety, low cost, and effectiveness it is included in all treatment regimens unless the patient is infected with dapsone-resistant bacilli or has had a serious adverse reaction to it. Its most common side effect is anemia, but except for occasional patients with a G6PD deficiency it is rarely severe enough to require discontinuation of the drug. Gastrointestinal complaints also rarely necessitate its discontinuance with the doses used to treat leprosy. The most serious complications of dapsone therapy are agranulocytosis and the "dapsone syndrome" (infectious mononucleosis–like syndrome). Fortunately, both are relatively rare. Other reported side effects are uncommon and include various skin rashes, peripheral neuropathies, hepatitis, cholestatic jaundice, hypoalbuminemia, the nephrotic syndrome, psychoses, and fever. Methemoglobinemia occurs but is rarely a problem in patients receiving the standard antileprosy doses of dapsone. It may, however, be severe when an overdose is taken and may require the use of supportive measures and methylene blue.

DADDS is the diacetyl derivative of dapsone. Although not obtainable in the United States, it is available elsewhere only as a long-acting parenteral preparation. The usual dose is 225 mg every 11 weeks, which is equivalent to about 2 mg of dapsone daily. Such low doses might encourage the development of dapsone-resistant *M. leprae,* making its use under any circumstances of uncertain efficacy. Certainly, if used it should only be as part of a combinaton drug regimen.

Rifampin (Rifadin). This is available as 150 and 300 mg capsules, and the usual adult dose is 600 mg daily, although in some trials it has been given intermittently at intervals of up to 1 month in doses ranging from 600 mg to 1500 mg. Resistance to rifampin can appear in as little as 3 to 4 years if it is given as monotherapy. It should therefore be used only in combination drug regimens. Its major side effect has been hepatotoxicity, but this is usually not a major problem except when it is used in combination with ethionamide, which is also hepatotoxic. In general, it is discontinued only if the SGPT rises to 2.5 times the upper limit of normal. Thrombocytopenia is occasionally observed among patients taking the drug, but the platelet count rarely drops below 100,000, which would require discontinuing the drug. Rifampin may also produce a reddish orange to reddish brown discoloration of urine, feces, saliva, sputum, sweat, and tears. Other reported side effects include a "flu-like" syndrome, fatigue, drowsiness, headaches, dizziness, pruritus, skin rash, eosinophilia, and, rarely, kidney damage. The drug also affects the metabolism of other medications, decreasing plasma levels of dapsone and corticosteroids and reducing the effectiveness of oral contraceptives.

Clofazimine (Lamprene). This drug is available as 50 and 100 mg capsules from NHDC, Carville, Louisiana. It is extremely useful in the management of leprosy, since it not only treats the disease but also in higher doses suppresses reactive episodes. The usual adult dose for treatment is 50 to 100 mg daily, although doses as high as 300 mg daily may be used to suppress reactive episodes. Only one case infected with clofazimine-resistant *M. leprae* has been reported in spite of its extensive use as monotherapy during the last two decades. Nevertheless, it should be given only in combination with other antileprosy drugs.

The most obvious side effect is pigmentation of the skin. The severity of this is proportional to the dose being given and the extent of infiltration of the skin by the disease process. The color can range anywhere from a reddish hue to a purplish black. It tends to be blotchy, being most pronounced in areas where skin lesions are present. The pigmentation will occur in essentially all patients with active disease, and its absence may indicate that the patient is not taking the drug. As the disease process clears from the skin the coloration will slowly diminish and nearly disappear in patients with inactive disease. Discontinuation of the drug also leads to clearance of most of the pigmentation within 6 to 12 months, although traces of it may remain for several years.

The most serious toxic effect is on the gastrointestinal tract. Patients receiving 50 to 100 mg daily may have mild cramping or burning midabdominal pain, sometimes associated with mild nausea or diarrhea. Patients receiving over 100 mg daily, however, may develop severe cramping abdominal pain, diarrhea, nausea, vomiting, and weight loss, which may progress to symptoms suggesting a partial or complete bowel obstruction. This usually clears rapidly if the drug is discontinued.

Other side effects include anticholinergic activity, which results in diminished sweating and tearing, and phototoxicity reactions, which are uncommon.

Ethionamide. This is available only as 250 mg tablets, and the usual adult dose is 250 to 500 mg daily. Resistance develops rapidly if it is given as monotherapy, and it should therefore be used only in a combination regimen. The most common side effects are various gastrointestinal complaints, such as a metallic taste in the mouth, nausea, vomiting, abdominal pain, diarrhea, anorexia, and hepatotoxicity. These clear rapidly if the drug is discontinued. Giving ethionamide and rifampin together increases the chance of hepatotoxicity considerably, and patients taking this combination must be followed closely, particularly during the first year. The drug is normally discontinued if the SGOT or SGPT rises to 2.5 times the upper limit of normal. Other side effects include postural hypotension, mental depression, drowsiness, peripheral neuropathies, and asthenia.

Treatment Regimens

Newly Diagnosed Patients. Over 80 per cent of newly diagnosed patients in the United States are infected with fully sulfone-sensitive *M. leprae* (no growth in mice tested with 0.0001 per cent dietary dapsone). Bacilli from others show varying degrees of primary resistance to dapsone in mouse footpad testing. Clinically, however, those treated with dapsone monotherapy in the past have shown a normal initial response to standard doses unless their bacilli were fully dapsone-resistant, that is, there was growth in mice treated with 0.01 per cent dietary dapsone. Such resistance represents less than 1 per cent of new cases. Thus dapsone probably remains useful in nearly all newly diagnosed cases. Standard therapy for adult patients seen at the NHDC is 100 mg of dapsone daily until 3 years beyond inactivity in indeterminate and tuberculoid cases, 5 years in borderline tuberculoid cases, 10 years in mid-borderline cases, and indefinitely in borderline lepromatous and lepromatous cases. The dapsone is given in combination with 600 mg of rifampin daily for the first 6 months in paucibacillary patients (indeterminate, TT, and BT) and for the first 3 years in multibacillary patients (BB, BL, and LL). Inactivity (negativity) is here defined as a bacterial index (BI—a semilogarithmic scale for quantifying the number of bacilli seen) of 0 on skin scraping and biopsy for at least a year, and no clinical evidence of activity, such as further sensory or motor loss or reaction, during that period. Since the BI generally falls at the rate of 0.5 to 1 per year, it will require 1 to 2 years for indeterminate and tuberculoid cases to reach an inactive status, 1 to 3 years for borderline tuberculoid patients, 2 to 6 years for mid-borderline patients, and 5 to 10 years for borderline lepromatous and lepromatous patients.

Adding a third drug to this regimen, either daily clofazimine or ethionamide, may further increase its effectiveness. This would also avoid the chance that the patients are infected with dapsone-resistant *M. leprae,* so that in effect they would be receiving only monotherapy with rifampin. Unfortunately, it is often difficult to convince new patients to take clofazimine because of the disfiguring effect of the pigmentation. Giving ethionamide in combination with rifampin also increases the danger of serious hepatotoxicity. Doing mouse footpad studies on all new patients averts the danger that primary dapsone resistance will be missed, but this test is very expensive and is not available to most of those treating this disease. Fortunately, this danger has so far proved more theoretical than real.

Patients Infected with Dapsone-Resistant *M. leprae*. This usually refers to secondary dapsone-resistant infections, i.e., those produced by prolonged intake of dapsone or other sulfones as monotherapy irregularly or in low doses, resulting in relapse with fully dapsone-resistant *M. leprae* 5 to 20 or more years after the start of therapy. Occasionally, as noted above, newly diagnosed patients may also be infected with fully dapsone-resistant bacilli.

The treatment of choice for adult cases is 50 to 100 mg of clofazimine daily, given for the same time intervals as dapsone in newly diagnosed patients, plus 600 mg of rifampin daily for the first 6 months in paucibacillary cases and the first 3 years in multibacillary cases. If the patients will not accept the pigmentation produced by clofazimine, then 600 mg of rifampin with 250 mg of ethionamide daily may be substituted for the clofazimine-rifampin combination. Both the rifampin and the ethionamide are then continued for the same period as the dapsone in newly diagnosed individuals.

WHO Study Group Treatment Regimens. Leprosy control is a major problem in many Third World countries. Patient compliance is frequently poor, case finding and follow-up efforts inadequate, and budgets unrealistically small. Personnel may be poorly trained and motivated and too few in number. Furthermore, the incidence of primary and secondary resistance is often high and steadily rising, creating the possibility that dapsone, which is inexpensive and has proved to be safe and effective for long-term administration, could be lost as a first-line antileprosy drug. This would have a serious adverse effect on most control programs.

In 1981, WHO organized a study group to make recommendations for the "chemotherapy of leprosy for control programs" (WHO Technical Report Series No. 675-1982). The group proposed two regimens. Adult patients with paucibacillary disease should be given 100 mg of dapsone daily, unsupervised, and 600 mg of rifampin, once monthly, supervised, both for a total of 6 months. Therapy is then discontinued. Multibacillary cases should receive 100 mg of dapsone daily, plus 50 mg of clofazimine daily, unsupervised, plus 600 mg of rifampin with 300 mg of clofazimine once monthly, supervised. Therapy is continued for at least 2 years but preferably to a BI of 0, and then discontinued. The once-monthly rifampin and the relatively short period of treatment are controversial. A single dose of 600 mg of rifampin has been shown to have a marked bactericidal effect against *M. leprae* in humans, but whether giving it monthly is as efficacious as daily administration remains uncertain. There is also evidence that shorter periods of treatment may be possible if two or more bactericidal drugs are given to leprosy patients, but the study in question did not consider the use of rifampin given monthly. The WHO regimens, on the other hand, also have certain advantages. Cost is kept relatively low with the use of rifampin only once monthly, and administration can be supervised. Short-term treatment may improve compliance, and if relapse does occur after therapy is discontinued, the *M. leprae* should have the same drug sensitivity pattern as those that originally infected the patient.

Follow-up of Patients on Treatment. Patients are followed at varying intervals depending on the severity of their disease, complications, and the drugs they are receiving. Patients receiving only dapsone with no complications may need to be seen only every 3 months, whereas those with severe reactions may require weekly or more frequent follow-up. It is generally useful to see the patient frequently at first because complications are most likely to occur during the first 1 to 2 years. Later, as the danger of reaction diminishes and the patient has gained an understanding of the disease the visits can be less frequent. Isolation of patients is not necessary because therapy rapidly renders them noninfectious. Also, close contacts have already received maximum exposure prior to the time the diagnosis was established. Pregnancy has little effect on the disease process except for increasing the likelihood of reaction.

Clinically, there will be a gradual clearance of skin lesions. Within 3 to 4 months of the start of appropriate therapy the morphologic index (MI—the percentage of the bacilli that appear viable) should fall to 0, but the BI on skin scrapings or biopsy, as noted, will fall very slowly. Routine follow-up laboratory studies include a complete blood count, urinalysis, and creatinine and liver function tests. These should be done at least every 2 months for those receiving rifampin, particularly in combination with ethionamide. Drug toxicity, however, is uncommon after the first year of treatment, and serious toxicity may manifest itself clinically before it is detected in the laboratory. If available, skin scrapings should be done from several of the most active sites at least every 6 months. Routine follow-up biopsies are not done unless skin scrapings are unavailable.

Reactions

About half of patients with leprosy will have reactive episodes of varying degrees of severity during the course of their disease. Some have them before treatment is started, but most occur during therapy, particularly during the first year. Reaction should not be regarded as a side effect of any drug; rather, it is apparently due to destruction of bacilli by whatever cause and the immune response to bacterial antigens that are released. Chemotherapy should be continued in spite of reactive episodes, and the episodes themselves should be suppressed as needed by other therapy.

Reactions can be broadly divided into two main categories: (1) erythema nodosum leprosum (ENL or type 2 reactions), occurring almost exclusively in BL and LL patients; and (2) reversal (type 1) reactions, occurring throughout the spectrum except for the lepromatous (LL) pole. A third type of reaction known as the Lucio phenomenon may be only an extreme variation of ENL. It occurs in patients from Mexico and some other areas with diffuse lepromatous leprosy. It is occasionally seen in the United States and is managed with corticosteroids. Clofazimine or thalidomide is probably not beneficial here, but experience with these agents is limited. Downgrading reactions are uncommon. They represent inflammation associated with progression of the disease process in untreated patients and are usually managed just by initiation of antileprosy therapy.

Erythema Nodosum Leprosum (ENL or Type 2 Reactions). This usually manifests itself with fever and painful erythematous nodules, but peripheral neuritis, orchitis, lymphadenitis, iridocyclitis, nephritis, periostitis, and arthralgias may also occur. Mild episodes may require no therapy, or symptomatic measures such as aspirin may suffice. Several drugs are useful for the management of severe episodes.

1. *Corticosteroids* are effective in all patients and should always be used if an acute neuritis is present, in order to prevent permanent nerve injury. Usually 60 mg of prednisone daily is sufficient, though patients receiving rifampin may require higher doses. After control is achieved the patient may be tapered off the drug over a period of 2 to 4 weeks. The reactions will often recur, however, and the dose will have to be increased again. If, as often happens, the process becomes chronic and recurs whenever attempts to reduce or discontinue the prednisone are made, prolonged therapy may be needed. In these patients, taper the prednisone to alternate-day therapy first, perhaps eliminating 5 mg from the schedule weekly on alternate days, and slowing the process if the reaction begins to recur. Once an alternate-day schedule is established, continue slowly reducing the dose until either the drug is eliminated or the lowest possible maintenance dose is reached. If the reaction can be controlled with alternate-day steroids, this approach may suffice, but because steroid-associated side effects are often a problem, other forms of therapy should be considered in chronic cases.

2. *Thalidomide,* which is investigational in the United States, is very effective in most patients. They are started on 100 mg four times daily, and the reaction is usually controlled within 48 to 72 hours. The dose is then tapered to a maintenance level (typically 100 mg daily). Short-term therapy may be sufficient, but many patients require prolonged treatment before the drug can be discontinued without recurrence of the reaction. Drowsiness is the only common side effect, but peripheral neuropathies have been reported. It cannot, of course, be given to fertile females because of its well-known teratogenicity. Information regarding procurement of the drug may be obtained from NHDC in Carville, Louisiana.

3. *Clofazimine* is also effective for the control of ENL. A dose of 100 mg two or three times daily will usually bring the reaction under control over a few weeks to a few months, depending on severity. Normally, reaction control is maintained with prednisone in these patients, and the dose of prednisone is gradually diminished as the clofazimine begins to act. As noted previously, gastrointestinal symptoms may develop if the dose is maintained at this level too long, so if possible, reduce the dose to 100 mg daily within a year. Pigmentation from the clofazimine will usually be marked in these patients, and they should be fully cognizant of this before this therapy is started.

Reversal (Type I) Reactions. Clinically, these usually present with fever plus edema and erythema of pre-existing lesions, which may progress to ulceration. Neuritis and adenopathy may also occur. If there is danger of a motor or sensory deficit or of ulceration, high doses of corticosteroids must be used, such as 60 to 120 mg of prednisone daily. The reaction will usually be controlled within 24 to 48 hours, and only a short course of therapy may be necessary if the patient has minimally active disease. Those with higher bacterial counts may require prolonged treatment, however. Patients with chronic disease may be managed with alternate-day steroids as outlined under the treatment of ENL. Clofazimine may also be effective, although it has taken as long as 1 year before the prednisone could be discontinued.

Other Complications. Neuritis may occur independently of any reactive episode. Immediate treatment with high doses of corticosteroids is necessary to avoid permanent injury. The use of a splint or sling to "rest" a nerve, such as the ulnar nerve, may also be useful.

Iridocyclitis is a medical emergency and is probably best managed by an ophthalmologist. Atropine drops and corticosteroid drops must be started at once if permanent damage is to be avoided. Tear substitutes are used in patients with lagophthalmos or decreased lacrimation.

Orchitis may occur with or independent of a reactive episode. It usually responds quickly to corticosteroids, but sterility may result.

Glomerulonephritis or renal amyloidosis may develop in patients with chronic reaction or prolonged active disease. These may progress to renal failure unless the underlying process is controlled.

Injuries are common in all patients with leprosy who have significant degrees of sensory or motor loss. The patient must be taught how to avoid them by frequent inspections of involved skin and the use of protective measures, such as gloves or special footwear. When an injury does occur in an insensitive area, it must be protected from further damage while healing.

Control Measures

Patient education is vital if treatment is to be successful. Compliance with any regimen for many years to life is unlikely unless the patient fully understands the disease and why such prolonged therapy is necessary. The family's cooperation is also important.

Evaluation of contacts in countries of low endemicity, such as the United States, is limited to the household. Contacts should be checked for evidence of the disease at 6 to 12 month intervals for at least 5 years and should know to seek immediate attention if suspicious changes occur. Contact examinations consist of inspection of the skin, palpation of peripheral nerves for enlargement or tenderness, and sensory and motor evaluation.

Possible prophylactic measures include bacille Calmette-Guérin (BCG) and dapsone therapy. The usefulness of BCG remains uncertain, but it probably does not protect against the more severe types of the disease. The Centers for Disease Control, on the other hand, has recommended that all household contacts under the age of 25 years of patients in the BB to LL portion of the leprosy spectrum receive 3 years of full-dose dapsone as a prophylactic measure. Lack of compliance is often a problem here, and it is uncertain whether such prophylaxis will prevent or only delay the onset of the disease in those contacts destined to develop the BL or LL type. Nonetheless, if reasonable compliance can be maintained, it may be worthwhile to give dapsone prophylactically. Because of the uncertainties involved, the use of dapsone or BCG prophylaxis does not, of course, eliminate the need for follow-up contact examinations.

Future Prospects

Considerable research is underway, sponsored by The National Institutes of Health and the NHDC in the United States, and internationally by WHO's Therapy of Leprosy (THELEP) and Immunology of Leprosy (IMMLEP) Scientific Working Groups. Emphasis has been placed on new drug development and improved utilization of existing drugs, cultivation of *M. leprae* in artificial media, antileprosy vaccine development, serodiagnostic tests for the early detection of and follow-up of this disease, and clarification of the immunopathology involved. Considerable progress has already been made. Preliminary trials with antileprosy vaccines are under way, and vaccinotherapy using a mixture of killed *M. leprae* and BCG shows some promise. Serodiagnostic tests to detect very early cases of leprosy also may be available within the foreseeable future.

MALARIA

method of
KIRK D. MILLER, M.D.
and CARLOS C. CAMPBELL, M.D., M.P.H.
Centers for Disease Control
Atlanta, Georgia

Once the diagnosis of malaria is confirmed by the demonstration of intra-erythrocytic protozoa of the genus *Plasmodium* on stained smears of peripheral blood, therapy should be promptly instituted. However, several factors must be considered in choosing an appropriate therapeutic regimen.

Causative Species. Although infections caused by *Plasmodium vivax* and *Plasmodium ovale* may cause acute febrile illness, these infections are generally benign, and recovery can be expected. Therapy of disease caused by these species should take into account that dormant forms of the parasite may persist in the liver and produce multiple relapses for several years unless appropriately treated. *Plasmodium malariae* infections are likewise benign but do not relapse. In contrast to the other three species, infection with *Plasmodium falciparum* does not relapse but can produce severe illness that can be rapidly progressive, culminating in renal and pulmonary failure, shock, encephalopathy, coma, and death.

Immune Status. Persons who have had malaria previously will have some degree of acquired immunity, but only those persons who have recently resided in endemic areas and have experienced chronic or repeated *Plasmodium* infections will have a level of immunity that can be expected to afford substantial protection by limiting the risk of severe illness.

Density of Parasitemia. In nonimmune individuals, the density of parasitemia correlates directly with the severity of the infection and with the probability of complications. Fortunately, the proportion of erythrocytes infected with *P. vivax, P. ovale,* or *P. malariae* rarely exceeds 2 per cent, thereby limiting the severity of the infection. In *P. falciparum* infections, however, the parasite can multiply exponentially, ultimately infecting most of the circulating erythrocytes if unchecked by therapy or acquired immunity. Infection of greater than 5 per cent of erythrocytes constitutes a severe infection with risk of complications.

Area of Acquisition. Although *P. vivax, P. ovale,* and *P. malariae* remain sensitive to chloroquine worldwide, areas with transmission of *P. falciparum* resistant to chloroquine are expanding (Table 1). *P. falciparum* infections in persons with recent exposure in areas with reported chloroquine resistance should be treated as though they had a chloroquine-resistant infection.

Mode of Transmission. Malaria is naturally transmitted by the bite of an infected female *Anopheles* mosquito. Less commonly, transmission occurs by inoculation with infected erythrocytes either congenitally or parenterally by blood transfusion or shared use of hypodermic equipment. *P. vivax* and *P. ovale* infections acquired by one of these less common modes of transmission cannot relapse and therefore do not require therapy to eradicate dormant hepatic forms of the parasite. *P. falciparum* infections are rarely transmitted by such means, but when they occur, the geographic origin of the parasite will usually be unknown. They should therefore be treated as if chloroquine-resistant.

General Care of the Patient

Fever with chills, sweats, and headache are the classic symptoms of malaria. Nausea, vomiting, myalgia, and abdominal or back pain may also be present. Symptomatic treatment of these discomforts with appropriate analgesics, antipyretics, and antiemetics may be instituted unless contraindicated. Additional measures to control high-grade fever (40C, 104F, or greater), such as sponging or the use of a cooling blanket, may be necessary.

Persons with malaria frequently become dehydrated owing to increased insensible water loss and decreased fluid intake. In severely ill patients, fluid management monitored by central pressure measurement is imperative. In the presence of signs of volume depletion, intravenous fluids should be administered to preserve organ perfusion and maintain cardiac output. Care must be taken to avoid fluid overload, which can precipitate acute pulmonary edema, and adult respiratory distress syndrome (ARDS), which are life-threatening complications commonly associated with severe *P. falciparum* infections.

Hemolytic anemia will be present in persons infected with any species of *Plasmodium.* When severe anemia acutely compromises tissue oxygenation, transfusion of packed red blood cells should be undertaken. After the acute attack, most anemias associated with malaria will resolve spontaneously. The anemia of malaria is not associated with iron loss: Therefore, replacement will be helpful only if there was pre-existing iron deficiency. Supplemental folic acid may be beneficial during the recovery period, when there is rapid erythrocyte replacement.

Enlargement of the spleen is a common finding

TABLE 1. **Areas of the World with Reported Chloroquine-Resistant *Plasmodium falciparum****

Africa	Asia	South America
Angola	Burma	Bolivia
Burundi	China (Hainan Island and southern provinces)	Brazil
Central African Republic	Indonesia	Colombia
Comoros	Kampuchea	Ecuador
Gabon	Laos	French Guiana
Kenya	Malaysia	Guyana
Madagascar	Philippines (Luzon, Basilan, Mindoro, Palawan and Mindanao Islands; Sulu Archipelago)	Panama (east of the Canal Zone, including the San Blas Islands)
Malawi	Thailand	Peru (northern provinces)
Mozambique	Vietnam	Surinam
Namibia		Venezuela
Rwanda		
Sudan (northern prov.)		
Tanzania		
Uganda		
Zaire (northeastern)		
Zambia (northeastern)		

Oceania	Indian Subcontinent
Papua New Guinea	Bangladesh (north and east)
Solomon Islands	India
Vanuatu	Pakistan (Rawalpindi)
	Sri Lanka

*Areas of the world with known chloroquine resistance are ever expanding. Physicians are encouraged to contact local or state health departments, or the Malaria Branch of the Centers for Disease Control, Atlanta, Georgia, for the latest information on drug resistance patterns for any particular geographic location.

in patients with malaria and may cause left upper quadrant tenderness and pain. Thrombocytopenia, with platelet counts as low as 10,000 to 20,000, is a frequent manifestation of hypersplenism during the acute attack. However, clinically significant bleeding rarely results, and the platelet count returns to normal promptly after treatment of the infection. Splenic rupture, which is fortunately a very rare complication of malaria, is most commonly associated with *P. vivax* infections. It may either be spontaneous or result from minor trauma, such as splenic palpation. This diagnosis should be considered in any patient with sudden cardiovascular collapse. Prompt recognition, aggressive blood replacement, and expeditious surgical intervention are lifesaving.

The severe complications associated with *P. falciparum* infections (cerebral malaria, renal failure, ARDS, and coagulopathy) carry grave prognoses and can occur precipitously even after therapy has commenced. Therefore, patients with *P. falciparum* infections, especially those with a high-density parasitemia and those who can be expected to have little or no immunity to malaria, should be closely monitored, preferably in a hospital setting.

Chemotherapy of Active Infections

The primary objective of chemotherapy in malaria is to halt multiplication of the parasite and rapidly clear the circulation of infected erythrocytes. This is accomplished by the use of drugs that act rapidly against the asexual erythrocytic stages of the parasite. The two most commonly used drugs for this purpose are chloroquine and quinine.

Mild to Moderate Infections. *P. falciparum* infections can be considered to be mild when the proportion of infected erythrocytes is low (1 per cent or less), *and* there are no complications. Oral chloroquine can be used in treating all *P. vivax, P. ovale,* and *P. malariae* infections, and all mild *P. falciparum* infections, except those acquired in an area where chloroquine resistance is known to occur (Table 2). Because of its long half-life, a course of therapy can be completed in 3 days. Chloroquine therapy is generally well tolerated at the recommended treatment dosage, but occasionally it may cause gastrointestinal disturbance, headache, dizziness, blurred vision, and pruritus. These minor discomforts resolve promptly after therapy is completed and do not necessitate discontinuing the drug's use. Moderate *P. falciparum* infections (proportion of parasitized erythrocytes between 1 and 5 per cent without signs of complications), and mild or moderate *P. falciparum* infections acquired in areas of known chloroquine resistance, should be treated with oral quinine (Table 2). When used in the standard treatment dosage, quinine will often produce an uncomfortable complex of symptoms known as cinchonism (dizziness, tinnitus, visual disturbance, and headache). Because of these side effects, it is recommended that oral quinine therapy for mild or moderate infections be continued only until the patient's symptoms have improved markedly and parasites are no longer detectable on peripheral blood smears. While this will usually be accomplished within 3 days, longer therapy may be required for *P. falciparum* infections acquired in Thailand, where decreased sensitivity to quinine has been observed. Therapy can then be completed with either a single dose of pyrimethamine-sulfadoxine (Fansidar) or a 7-day course of tetracycline (Table 2). Tetracycline is preferred for follow-up treatment of infections acquired in Thailand, Indonesia, Papua New Guinea, and the Amazon basin of Brazil, owing to the possibility of resistance to Fansidar.

Severe Infections. *Plasmodium falciparum* infections in which the proportion of parasitized erythrocytes exceeds 5 to 10 per cent, especialy when signs of complications are present, should be considered severe and should be treated with intravenous quinine dihydrochloride. Although approved for marketing in the United States, this drug is not commercially available owing to limited demand. It must be obtained through the Malaria Branch, Division of Parasitic Diseases, Center for Infectious Diseases, Centers for Disease Control (CDC), Atlanta, Georgia (24-hour telephone number: 404-329-2888). Because intravenous quinine may cause hypotension and cardiac arrhythmia, it must be administered slowly under closely monitored conditions. Treatment with intravenous quinine should continue until the patient's parasitemia falls below 0.5 per cent. If at that time the patient is able to tolerate oral medications, he should be given a single dose of Fansidar or a 7-day course of tetracycline as previously described. If the patient is for any reason unable to tolerate oral medications, intravenous therapy may be continued either with quinine or with a tetracycline (e.g., doxycycline hyclate [Vibramycin] 100 mg every 12 hours) for a total 10-day course of therapy.

Monitoring Response to Chemotherapy

Within 24 to 48 hours of commencing appropriate chemotherapy, the proportion of infected erythrocytes should begin to decrease rapidly and febrile episodes should abate. In *P. falciparum* infections, it is recommended that blood smears be checked every 12 to 24 hours until parasites are no longer detectable (*P. falciparum* gametocytes, the sexual forms that infect anopheline mosquitoes, may persist in the peripheral circu-

TABLE 2. **Drugs of Choice for the Treatment of Malaria**[1]

Clinical Setting	Drug(s) of Choice	Pediatric Dosage	Adult Dosage
Uncomplicated attacks of all malaria, EXCEPT *P. falciparum* acquired in areas of chloroquine resistance	Chloroquine phosphate (Aralen)	10 mg per kg base (up to maximum of 600 mg base), then 5 mg base per kg 6 hrs later, then 5 mg base per kg per day for 2 days	600 mg base, then 300 mg base 6 hours later, then 300 mg base per day for 2 days
Uncomplicated attacks of *P. falciparum* acquired in areas of chloroquine resistance	Quinine sulfate *plus*	25 mg per kg per day in three divided doses for 3 days (up to 650 mg per dose)	650 mg every 8 hours for 3 days
	Pyrimethamine-sulfadoxine (Fansidar)[2] *or*	6 to 11 mos: ¼ tablet 1 to 3 yrs: ½ tablet 4 to 8 yrs: 1 tablet 9 to 14 yrs: 2 tablets >14 yrs: 3 tablets in a single dose	3 tablets in a single dose
	Quinine sulfate *plus*	Same as above	Same as above
	Tetracycline[3]	5 mg per kg four times daily for 7 days (up to 250 mg per dose)	250 mg four times daily for 7 days
Severe illness, or when oral therapy cannot be administered for any reason	Quinine dihydrochloride (intravenous)[4]	25 mg per kg per day (up to 1800 mg per day); give one third over 2 to 4 hours; then repeat every 8 hours until oral therapy can be commenced	600 mg in 300 ml normal saline over 2 to 4 hours; repeat every 8 hours (maximum 1800 mg per day) until oral therapy can be commenced
After treatment of *P. vivax* or *P. ovale* to prevent relapses	Primaquine phosphate[5]	0.3 mg base per kg per day for 14 days (maximum of 15 mg per day)	15 mg base per day for 14 days

[1]Consult experts, including Centers for Disease Control, Atlanta, Georgia, regarding alternative regimens.
[2]Fansidar should not be given to persons with known allergy to sulfonamides.
[3]The FDA considers tetracycline investigational when used for malaria. Physicians must weigh the benefit of therapy against the possibility of known side effects in children under 8 years of age.
[4]In the United States, quinine dihydrochloride is available from the Centers for Disease Control, Atlanta, Georgia.
[5]Primaquine may cause severe hemolysis in G6PD–deficient individuals.

lation but are of no clinical significance). If, in *P. falciparum* infections treated with chloroquine, the parasite density increases or remains constant for a period greater than 48 hours after initiation of therapy, the possibility of drug resistance should be considered, and one should switch to appropriate therapy described previously for such infections. If fever persists despite clearance of parasites from the peripheral circulation, the possibility of another intercurrent illness should be investigated. In *P. vivax, P. ovale,* and *P. malariae* infections, follow-up smears should be checked 7 to 10 days after completion of therapy, to assure adequacy of treatment.

Follow-up Chemotherapy of P. vivax and P. ovale Infections

Drugs used to treat acute malaria infection will have no effect on the dormant hepatic forms of *P. vivax* and *P. ovale,* which can cause periodic relapses for up to 3 to 4 years following the primary infection. Such relapses can usually be prevented by the use of primaquine (Table 2), which can be instituted after the symptoms of the acute attack have subsided.

Primaquine can cause severe hemolysis in persons with glucose-6-phosphate dehydrogenase (G6PD) deficiency, especially in those of Mediterranean and Oriental ancestry. This enzyme defect is also common in blacks, but hemolysis resulting from administration of primaquine in this group tends to be less severe. A screening test for G6PD deficiency should be performed on all individuals prior to prescribing the drug. Primaquine may be administered under close medical supervision at a reduced dosage schedule to certain persons with less severe variants of G6PD deficiency. However, in the presence of the more severe variants, the prudent course is to promptly treat relapse with chloroquine during the 3- to 4-year period during which they can be expected to occur. Primaquine should not be administered during pregnancy. Weekly prophylaxis with chloroquine should be maintained until parturition, after which primaquine may be administered.

Management of Complications of P. falciparum Infections

Acute renal failure, hemoglobinuria, pulmonary edema or ARDS, and sepsis due to secondary bacterial infections are not infrequent complications of severe *P. falciparum* infections. They should be aggressively managed in the same manner as when these entities are caused by other agents.

Cerebral malaria, an encephalopathy caused by sludging of infected erythrocytes within the microvasculature of the central nervous system, is a medical emergency that carries a grave prognosis. Signs of cerebral malaria include abnormal mentation, obtundation, coma, seizures, and focal abnormalities of the neurologic examination. Recent studies indicate that cerebral edema is not the primary pathophysiologic defect in cerebral malaria: Therefore, pharmacologic measures to reduce brain swelling are not recommended. Indeed, dexamethasone has been shown to have an adverse effect on outcome in cerebral malaria. Seizure activity should be controlled by standard antiseizure regimens.

Severe hypoglycemia is a recognized complication of severe *P. falciparum* infections, which may be accentuated by therapy with intravenous quinine. Such patients should have blood glucose levels checked periodically, and whenever there is a sudden deterioration in neurologic status. Treatment consists of immediate administration of a bolus of 50 per cent dextrose, followed by continuous infusion of a 10 per cent dextrose solution, which is then titrated to maintain the patient's blood glucose level in the high normal range.

While controlled clinical trials have yet to be carried out, there is mounting evidence that whole-blood exchange transfusion can prevent and indeed reverse the severe life-threatening complications of *P. falciparum* infections. Many experts now recommend a two-volume exchange as a component of therapy in patients who present with extremely high parasitemias (greater than 10 to 20 per cent) and/or clinical signs of cerebral malaria.

Malaria in Pregnancy

Malaria during pregnancy carries substantial risk to both mother and fetus. Abnormal fetal development and spontaneous abortion may result from placental involvement. The disease demands aggressive therapy, which should not be withheld because of relative contraindications to antimalarials during pregnancy.

Malaria Prophylaxis for Travelers

Of greatest importance for travelers to malarious areas is the assurance that they have been advised of appropriate measures to decrease their likelihood of contracting malaria. These consist of chemoprophylaxis and personal protective measures to decrease contact with mosquitoes during evening and nighttime hours by using insect repellents, wearing protective clothes, remaining in screened areas, using mosquito bednets, and spraying indoor areas with pyrethrum-containing insecticides.

The choice of chemoprophylaxis depends on the risk of contracting malaria in areas to be visited, and whether or not those areas have chloroquine-resistant *P. falciparum*. All travelers at risk of exposure to malaria should take chloroquine phosphate (Aralen), beginning 1 week before arrival and continuing for 6 weeks after leaving the endemic areas. The adult dose is 500 mg (300 mg base) once weekly; for children and infants who weigh less than 50 kg, the dose is 8.3 mg per kg (5 mg per kg base) once weekly.

Travelers to areas of chloroquine resistance in Africa and Oceania (Table 1) are at substantial risk of acquiring malaria. In addition to weekly doses of chloroquine, short-term travelers (less than 3 weeks) should be given a single treatment dose of Fansidar to be taken in the event of a febrile illness when medical care is not available. If the traveler uses Fansidar in this fashion, he should seek follow-up medical care as soon as possible. For longer-term travelers, either the weekly use of amodiaquine (adult dose, 400 mg base weekly) *alone,* or the weekly use of Fansidar (adult dose, 1 tablet weekly) in addition to chloroquine can be considered. Amodiaquine is not available in the United States but is widely available overseas.

In general, travelers to areas of chloroquine resistance in Asia and South America (Table 1) are at much lower risk of acquiring malaria and should use chloroquine alone, unless they expect to have extensive rural evening and nighttime exposure in malarious areas.

Prevention of relapses after travel to areas where *P. vivax* and *P. ovale* are endemic (which includes most malarious areas except Haiti) can be accomplished by the use of primaquine (Table 2) with the precautions discussed previously.

Alternative regimens and full discussion of malaria chemoprophylaxis are available in CDC publications *(Health Information for International Travel 1985)* and are regularly updated in Morbidity and Mortality Weekly Report (MMWR).

BACTERIAL MENINGITIS

method of
STEVEN M. OPAL, M.D.
Fitzsimons Army Medical Center
Denver, Colorado

Bacterial meningitis is an uncommon, yet devastating infectious disease associated with an exceedingly high morbidity and mortality rate. The majority of the deaths and irreversible neurologic injury occurs within the first 24 hours of patients' seeking medical attention. The primary determinant of survival is early and appropriate antimicrobial therapy. The incidence of bacterial meningitis is 10 per 100,000 patients in large population-based studies. This indicates that there are approximately 30,000 cases of bacterial meningitis each year in the United States.

Principles of Antimicrobial Therapy

Antimicrobial therapy must be initiated on an urgent empiric basis during the early evaluation of the patient. The choice of antimicrobial agent is usually based upon the patient's age and predisposing factors. A presumptive microbiologic diagnosis frequently can be made from information gathered from the Gram stain of centrifuged cerebrospinal fluid (CSF). The precise identity of the infecting organism will be determined by bacterial cultures 24 to 48 hours after the initial patient evaluation. Antibiotic therapy can then be modified according to the identification and sensitivity of the etiologic agent isolated from the cerebrospinal fluid.

Initial Antimicrobial Therapy Based on Gram Stain Evaluation (Table 1). A careful Gram stain of centrifuged cerebrospinal fluid has a sensitivity of up to 80 per cent. Although false-positives occasionally occur, the information obtained by Gram stain is generally a reliable guide. Other rapid diagnostic techniques, such as counterimmunoelectrophoresis, latex agglutination testing, and limulus lysate assay, may be useful in specific circumstances, but they have not replaced the Gram stain as the simplest and most reliable rapid diagnostic technique.

Antimicrobial Therapy When Gram Stain Is Negative. The decision as to which antibiotic to use depends upon the patient profile and predisposing factors. The most common etiologic agents in bacterial meningitis vary strikingly with the patient's age. Table 2 lists the guidelines to antimicrobial therapy based on the patient's age and likely infecting organism. The organisms listed in each patient category account for at least 90 per cent of all the bacterial isolates found in each age group. Factors associated with increased susceptibility to bacterial meningitis, and associated pathogenic organisms, are listed in Table 3.

Specific Antimicrobial Therapy

Once the culture and sensitivity of the infecting organism are known, antimicrobial therapy should be modified, considering CSF penetration, relative cost, and drug toxicity. Mortality statistics in the treatment of bacterial meningitis have not changed appreciably in the past 30 years, following the introduction of high dose penicillin. The crucial determinant of therapeutic success or failure is the achievement of adequate bactericidal concentrations of the antibiotic in the patient's cerebrospinal fluid. Therapeutic regimens should achieve levels in the CSF at least eight- to tenfold higher than the minimum inhibitory concentration of that antibiotic against the pathogen.

Not all antimicrobial agents attain adequate levels of bactericidal activity in the cerebrospinal fluid. The CSF penetration by various antibiotics is given in Table 4. Some agents, such as aminoglycosides, do not effectively cross the blood-brain barrier. If clinical circumstances dictate their use, note that aminoglycosides will produce bactericidal activity in the spinal fluid only if given intrathecally or intraventricularly. Direct instillation of the aminoglycosides into the cerebrospinal fluid is most readily accomplished by the use of a ventriculostomy delivery system. If such a system for drug delivery is not available, then the drugs may be given in the intralumbar space or by repeated ventricular taps.

In a recent study of gram-negative bacillary meningitis in the neonate, intraventricular or intrathecal aminoglycoside therapy was not found to be superior to parenteral therapy alone. However, this study has been criticized because of the delivery of the aminoglycosides by repeated ventricular taps. Intraventricular administration of aminoglycosides by a ventriculostomy reservoir may be preferred over ventricular taps. Currently, it is recommended that aminoglycoside therapy by a ventricular reservoir be added if there is any delay in the clinical response to gram-negative bacillary meningitis in the neonate. Monitoring of serum and CSF aminoglycoside levels is recommended in this situation.

Fortunately, newer cephalosporins have diminished, but not eliminated, the need for aminoglycosides in the treatment of meningitis. Expert infectious disease consultation is advised in complicated cases, such as gram-negative bacillary infections.

Dosing schedules for antimicrobial agents are given in Table 5. High concentrations of the antibiotic agent in the spinal fluid are important for a successful outcome in bacterial meningitis. Therefore, the doses of each antibiotic approach the maximum tolerated. In some cases, recommendations may exceed the usual dosage recommended by the manufacturer.

Response to Therapy

Antibiotic therapy for bacterial meningitis is generally continued for 10 to 14 days. Staphylo-

TABLE 1. **Initial Antimicrobial Therapy Based on CSF Gram Stain Findings**

Gram Stain Results	Probable Pathogen	Frequency of Occurrence	Treatment of Choice	Alternative Therapy	Comments
Gram-negative coccobacilli	*Haemophilus influenzae*	common	ampicillin + chlor-amphenicol	chloramphenicol alone, moxalactam, cefotaxime, sulfa-trimethoprim	Ampicillin or chloramphenicol may be used as single agents once susceptibilities of organism are known
Gram-negative cocci, single or in parts	*Neisseria meningitidis*	common	penicillin G	chloramphenicol	Third generation cephalosporins also effective
Gram-positive cocci, in pairs or chains	*Streptococcus pneumoniae, Streptococcus*	common	penicillin G	chloramphenicol	Cefotaxime, vancomycin, sulfa-trimethoprim also effective
Gram-negative bacilli	*Escherichia coli,* other enteric bacilli, or *Pseudomonas* species	uncommon	cefotaxmine + amikacin* ± piperacillin†	amikacin* + piperacillin	Moxalactam, cefotaxmine, cefoperazone may also be effective
Gram-positive cocci, large, in clusters	*Staphylococcus aureus, Staphylococcus epidermidis*	uncommon	nafcillin	vancomycin	Vancomycin preferred initial agent if methicillin-resistant *Staphylococcus* are prevalent
Gram-positive rods	*Listeria monocytogenes*	uncommon	ampicillin	ampicillin + gentamicin or chloramphenicol	Third generation cephalosporins are not effective against this organism

*Amikacin should be the empiric aminoglycoside agent of choice until CSF cultures and sensitivities are known. Gentamicin or tobramycin may be substituted for amikacin if resistance to these agents is infrequent at any given institution.

†Antipseudomonal penicillins such as piperacillin, mezlocillin, azlocillin, or ticarcillin should be added to the empiric regimen if *Pseudomonas* is the potential etiologic agent.

TABLE 2. **Empiric Antimicrobial Therapy Based on Patient Age**

Age	Probable Pathogen	Treatment of Choice	Alternative Therapy	Comments
0–2 months	Group B streptococcus, enteric gram-negative bacilli, *Haemophilus influenzae,* and *Listeria monocytogenes*	ampicillin + moxalactam; or ampicillin + amikacin*	ampicillin + cefotaxime; or amikacin* + chloramphenicol	Amikacin may be given intrathecally or intraventricularly as well as intravenously (see text under specific therapy)
2 months –10 years	*Haemophilus influenzae, Streptococcus pneumoniae, Neisseria meningitidis* (rare)	ampicillin + chloramphenicol	chloramphenicol alone, *or* cefuroxime, *or* cefotaxime	If *Haemophilus influenzae* is present and sensitive to ampicillin, discontinue chloramphenicol and continue ampicillin; if resistant to ampicillin, discontinue ampicillin and continue chloramphenicol
10–60 years	*Streptococcus pneumoniae, Neisseria meningitidis*	penicillin G	chloramphenicol, cefotaxime, or cefoperazone	Rare cases of penicillin-resistant *Streptococcus pneumoniae* may be treated with vancomycin
Over 60 years	*Streptococcus pneumoniae,* gram-negative enteric bacilli	cefotaxime, *or* ampicillin + moxalactam	ampicillin + amikacin*	Intrathecal or intraventricular aminoglycoside therapy may be useful (see text under specific therapy)

*Gentamicin or tobramycin may be substituted for amikacin if incidence of resistance to these organisms is low in your hospital.

TABLE 3. **Predisposing Factors and Likely Pathogens in Bacterial Meningitis**

Predisposing Factor	Probable Pathogens	Treatment of Choice	Alternative Therapy	Comments
Status postneurosurgical procedures	*Pseudomonas aeruginosa*, enteric gram-negative bacilli, *Staphylococcus aureus, Staphylococcus epidermidis*	amikacin* + piperacillin† + cefotaxime	vancomycin + amikacin* + cefotaxime or moxalactam	Intrathecal or intraventricular aminoglycoside therapy may be warranted (see text under specific therapy)
Immunocompromised host	enteric gram-negative bacilli, *Listeria monocytogenes*	ampicillin + cefotaxime *or* moxalactam ± amikacin*	amikacin* + trimethoprim-sulfamethoxazole	If *Pseudomonas* found on culture, addition of piperacillin† and intrathecal amikacin* is warranted
Ventriculoperitoneal or ventriculoatrial shunt	*Staphylococcus epidermidis*, gram-negative enteric bacilli	vancomycin or nafcillin + amikacin*	cefotaxime	Infected ventricular shunt should be removed and replaced if necessary
CSF dural leaks (rhinorrhea or otorrhea)	*Streptococcus pneumoniae*	penicillin G	chloramphenicol	Pneumococcal vaccine indicated to prevent further episodes. Close dural leak surgically if it persists
Late complement component deficiencies	*Neisseria meningitidis*	penicillin G	chloramphenicol or cefotaxime, moxalactam	Meningococcal vaccine may be of some value
Asplenia	*Streptococcus pneumoniae, Neisseria meningitidis, Haemophilus influenzae*	ampicillin	penicillin G, chloramphenicol	Pneumococcal vaccine should be give prior to splenectomy, if possible. Meningococcal vaccine may be of benefit, but this remains unproved.

*Gentamicin or tobramycin may be substituted for amikacin if incidence of resistance to these organisms is low in your hospital.
†Mezlocillin, ticarcillin, or azlocillin may be substituted for piperacillin.

coccal meningitis or gram-negative bacterial meningitis is treated for 3 to 4 weeks. The response to treatment in bacterial meningitis is usually rapid and resolution of fever generally occurs within 72 to 96 hours. Repeated spinal taps are no longer recommended unless the diagnosis is uncertain, the patient fails to respond to appropriate therapy of adequate duration, or the patient has an initial response then subsequently deteriorates. The patient with a microbiologically documented episode of bacterial meningitis who responds to appropriate therapy does not require a follow-up lumbar puncture. Routine follow-up lumbar punctures are currently indicated only for the neonate or patients with persistent decreased levels of consciousness, for assessment of an adequate response. A favorable trend in CSF formulas should occur with appropriate therapy. Isolated CSF abnormalities may persist and, in the absence of supporting clinical data, do not indicate treatment failure.

TABLE 4. **Penetration of Antimicrobial Agents into Cerebrospinal Fluid**

Agent	Per Cent of Blood Level Measured in CSF: *Normal Meninges*	*Inflamed Meninges*
penicillin	<1	3–5
ampicillin	<1	25
nafcillin	<1	15–25
ticarcillin	—	20
mezlocillin	—	20
azlocillin	—	20
piperacillin	—	30
moxalactam	—	15–40
cefotaxime	<1	2–25
cefoperazone	<1	<1–4
TMP–SMX	30–50	50–80
vancomycin	<1	20–25
chloramphenicol	60	75
gentamicin	<1	10–25
tobramycin	<1	10–25
amikacin	10–20	30–50

Failure to respond to therapy, or initial response followed by recrudescent symptoms, necessitates a search for complications of bacterial meningitis, intercurrent illness, or drug fever. Patients may have a parameningeal septic focus, such as a subdural empyema, cerebritis, ventriculitis, or brain abscess. Recrudescent fever may be a manifestation of a nosocomial complication like phlebitis, urinary tract infection, pulmonary infection, or drug fever.

Recurrent Bacterial Meningitis

Recurrent bacterial meningitis is virtually always the result of an anatomic, immunologic, or mechanical abnormality. No patient should ever have more than one episode of bacterial meningitis without undergoing a thorough evaluation to exclude possible causes of recurrent bacterial meningitis. Predisposing factors include (1) late complement component deficiencies; (2) persistent CSF dural leaks; (3) dural sinuses; (4) ventricular shunts; (5) immunodeficiencies; and (6) parameningeal septic foci such as brain abscesses, subdural empyema, or epidural abscesses.

TABLE 5. **Antibiotics Useful in the Treatment of Bacterial Meningitis**

Drug	Pediatric Dose*	Adult Dose	Number of Doses/Day
penicillin G	200,000 units/kg/day	18 to 24 million units/day	6 or 12
ampicillin	200 mg/kg/day	12 to 16 gm/day	6
nafcillin	200 mg/kg/day	9 to 12 gm/day	6
ticarcillin	300 mg/kg/day	16 to 18 gm/day	6
mezlocillin	300 mg/kg/day	16 gm/day	6
azlocillin	300 mg/kg/day	16 gm/day	6
piperacillin	300 mg/kg/day	16 gm/day	6
moxalactam	200 mg/kg/day	12 gm/day	6
cefotaxime	200 mg/kg/day	16 gm/day	4 to 6
cefoperazone	150 mg/kg/day	12 gm/day	3 to 4
trimethoprim-sulfamethoxazole	10 mg/kg/day (trimethoprim component)	10 to 15 mg/kg/day (trimethoprim component)	4 to 6
vancomycin	50 mg/kg/day	2 gm/day	3 to 4
chloramphenicol	100 mg/kg/day	6 to 8 gm/day	6
gentamicin†	7 mg/kg/day	7 mg/kg/day	3
tobramycin†	7 mg/kg/day	7 mg/kg/day	3
amikacin†	15 mg/kg/day	15 mg/kg/day	3
INTRATHECAL OR INTRAVENTRICULAR DOSES			
gentamicin‡	2.5 mg/day	8 mg/day	once
tobramycin‡	2.5 mg/day	8 mg/day	once
amikacin‡	5 mg/day	20 mg/day	once

*Trimethoprim-sulfamethoxazole is contraindicated in infants less than 2 months of age; azlocillin—the manufacturer does not recommend the use of this agent in the neonate; piperacillin—the doses for this drug have not been established by the manufacturer for children under the age of 12 years.

†Aminoglycoside blood and cerebrospinal fluid levels should be monitored during therapy.

‡These drugs should be administered without preservative as a single dose every 24 hours.

General Supportive Measures

All patients with bacterial meningitis should be placed under careful medical and nursing supervision, with monitoring for neurologic complications, drug toxicity, or other septic complications. The patient's cardiovascular and respiratory status must be carefully monitored; supportive therapy with artificial ventilation and pressor agents may be necessary. Frequent neurologic examinations should be performed to exclude local septic complications. Respiratory isolation is unnecessary except for the first 24 hours of treatment in *Neisseria meningitidis* meningitis. Other forms of bacterial meningitis do not require isolation precautions.

Intravenous fluid therapy should be carefully monitored, and free water delivery should be restricted because inappropriate ADH secretion is common. Overly vigorous fluid resuscitation may contribute to hyponatremia, water intoxication, cerebral edema, worsening cerebral perfusion pressure, and cerebral hypoxia. Fluid and electrolyte status needs continuous careful evaluation throughout the course of treatment. Surveillance for concomitant medical illnesses, drug toxicity, or nosocomial infectious complications is also important.

Seizure precautions should be instituted early. Generalized seizures are common sequelae of bacterial meningitis. Treatment with benzodiazepines, phenobarbital, or diphenylhydantoin should be employed as necessary. Focal seizure disorders or status epilepticus suggests a possible septic complication, such as a brain abscess, subdural empyema, or subdural effusions. High dose penicillin therapy may also produce seizures in the pediatric age group or in patients with renal insufficiency. Focal seizures should be evaluated with a head CT scan to exclude focal neurologic complications.

Steroid therapy is currently indicated only in patients who appear in septic shock or have evidence of impending brain stem herniation. Steroid agents are useful in decreasing intracranial pressure resulting from cerebral edema. Steroid therapy may also be indicated in septic shock caused by gram-negative organisms and possible adrenal hemorrhage seen in meningococcal meningitis and meningococcemia. Intravenous mannitol or glycerol therapy may also be useful in the treatment of increased intracranial pressure associated with bacterial meningitis. These treatments are effective but may cause circulatory overload in patients with concomitant renal insufficiency or cardiac decompensation.

Subdural effusions appear to be a frequent

complication of meningitis in the neonatal age group. Such patients tend to have a more prolonged febrile course and may have persistent marked abnormalities on CSF analysis. If evidence of a subdural collection of fluid is noted on CT scan, the fluid should be removed by direct needle aspiration and examined for the presence of bacterial organisms to exclude the possibility of a subdural empyema.

Prophylaxis for Contacts of Patients

No prophylaxis is indicated in pneumococcal, gram-negative bacillary, staphylococcal, or listerial meningitis.

Meningococcal meningitis merits a program of antimicrobial prophylaxis for intimate contacts of the index case (household members, such as spouses, children, or roommates) and for medical personnel who have had direct contact with potentially infectious secretions, as during mouth-to-mouth resuscitation. Casual contacts like classmates and coworkers need not receive meningococcal antibacterial prophylaxis.

The regimen of choice in index case contacts is rifampin, 600 mg orally twice a day for 2 days for adults and 10 mg per kg twice a day for 2 days for children. (Note: Manufacturer's recommended dosage for adults is 600 mg once daily for 4 days; for children, 10 to 20 mg per kg, not to exceed 60 mg per day.) Alternative antimicrobial prophylaxis for adults is minocycline, 100 mg orally twice a day for 5 days; minocycline should not be given to children under 8 years of age.

Some authorities suggest treating the index case of meningococcal meningitis with rifampin as well. This assures eradication of the nasopharyngeal carrier state, preventing the possibility of recurrent meningitis following treatment with penicillin. This also prevents the index case from being a potential, persistent public health hazard to close patient contacts.

Intimate contacts (young family members or playmates in day care centers) of index cases with *Haemophilus influenzae* type B bacterial meningitis who are 4 or less years of age should receive antimicrobial prophylaxis. The dose of rifampin required for hemophilus prophylaxis appears to be higher, 20 mg per kg per day given orally as a single dose for 4 days. Rifampin is available in a pediatric suspension for this purpose. (Manufacturer's note: Data to determine rifampin dosage for children under 5 years of age are not available.)

INFECTIOUS MONONUCLEOSIS

method of
HAROLD A. KESSLER, M.D.,
and STUART LEVIN, M.D.
Rush-Presbyterian-St. Luke's Medical Center
Chicago, Illinois

Infectious mononucleosis (IM) is a clinical syndrome caused by infection with the Epstein-Barr virus (EBV). The classic clinical manifestations consist of a triad of fever, sore throat, and lymphadenopathy. Infection with EBV is exceedingly common. In some communities approximately 50 per cent of children have serologic evidence of infection by the age of 6 years. The prevalence of antibodies to EBV rises to 90 to 95 per cent in adult populations. Infection in the younger age group most commonly results in subclinical or nonspecific illness which is not recognized as caused by EBV. Exposure to and infection with EBV is frequently delayed until adolescence and young adulthood in higher socioeconomic groups and is usually transmitted by oral pharyngeal secretions. This accounts for the recognized peak incidence of IM in the 15 to 24 year old age group. Because of the high prevalence of antibodies in adults, IM in individuals over 40 years of age is uncommon but is seen even in the geriatric age group, in whom the classic symptom of pharyngitis is usually absent.

Complications

Respiratory. Acute upper airway obstruction due to extensive swelling of lymphoid tissue is a rare but life-threatening complication of IM. Associated parenchymal infiltrates have been reported in 3 to 5 per cent of cases; however, their relationship to EBV infection has not been established.

Splenic Rupture. Splenic rupture is another rare but life-threatening complication. The development of abdominal pain, left upper quadrant tenderness, or unexplained hypotension should alert the physician to the possibility of this complication. A history of antecedent abdominal trauma or strenuous exercise may be present in up to one half of cases.

Neurologic. Encephalitis, aseptic meningitis, Guillain-Barré syndrome, transverse myelitis, peripheral nerve palsies, and other neurologic complications have been reported in less than 1 per cent of cases. Although 85 per cent of patients recover without sequelae, neurologic complications of IM are the most common cause of death in otherwise healthy persons.

Hematologic. Mild anemia, granulocytopenia, and thrombocytopenia are seen in up to 50 per cent of cases. Severe autoimmune hemolytic anemia occurs in 0.5 to 3 per cent of cases. Profound thrombocytopenia and granulocytopenia possibly due to autoimmune mechanisms have been reported rarely.

Hepatic. Mild liver function abnormalities are common in acute IM, occurring in 80 to 90 per cent of cases. These abnormalities are usually manifest as mild elevations in serum aminotransferases (two to five times normal), with elevations of alkaline phosphatase and LDH higher than expected from the aminotransferase abnormalities.

Streptococcal Infection. Isolation of group A beta-hemolytic streptococci from the pharynx has been reported in up to 33 per cent of patients with acute IM. The contribution of this finding to the associated pharyngitis is unclear, but antibiotic therapy for 10 days is indicated to prevent poststreptococcal sequelae.

Chronic Mononucleosis. A small number of individuals have recently been described who have chronic or recurrent symptoms of IM lasting over months to years. These symptoms have most commonly been manifested as fatigue, pharyngitis, lymphadenopathy, fever, headaches, arthralgia, depression, dyslogia, and myalgia. These symptoms may cause significant morbidity, resulting in the inability to maintain a normal life style. This syndrome may be distinguished serologically by evidence of ongoing active EBV replication with significantly elevated titers of antibodies to the viral capsid and early antigens. No specific immunologic defects have been noted in these patients.

Severe, Fatal, and Malignant Complications. A specific recessive X-linked immunodeficiency syndrome, Duncan's syndrome, has been described in which affected family members have developed either overwhelming acute EBV infection resulting in death or late complications of the infection manifested as agammaglobulinemia, aplastic anemia, or lymphomas. Patients with other types of immune defects, such as transplant patients and patients with the acquired immune deficiency syndrome, have also developed fatal lymphomas felt to be secondary to uncontrolled proliferation of EBV-infected B lymphocytes.

Treatment

The therapy of uncomplicated symptomatic IM with moderate to severe pharyngitis is largely symptomatic. No specific antibiotic or antiviral therapy has been shown to shorten the course of the illness. Treatment of nonstreptococcal pharyngitis with metronidazole has not been shown to be efficacious. Patients in whom group A beta-hemolytic streptococci are isolated from throat cultures should be treated with a 10 day course of oral penicillin, or erythromycin for the penicillin-allergic patient. Ampicillin, amoxicillin, or the newer combination of amoxicillin/clavulanic acid (Augmentin) should be avoided because of the high incidence of rash in patients with IM who are given ampicillin. The antiviral drug acyclovir has been shown to have in vitro activity against the EBV but has not been shown to shorten the course of the illness in patients hospitalized with moderate to severe IM. Whether antiviral therapy will modify milder forms of the syndrome will require further study.

The usual clinical course of IM runs 2 to 5 weeks, with the most severe symptoms occurring during the first 6 to 10 days of illness. The only medication generally needed is an analgesic and antipyretic to relieve the symptoms of fever, headache, and pharyngitis. Acetaminophen is probably preferable to aspirin, especially in children and adolescents, because of the association between aspirin and Reye's syndrome. In addition, aspirin inhibits platelet function, which may not be desirable if an associated thrombocytopenia is present. Throat gargles or irrigations with warm saline solutions may help relieve the symptoms of pharyngitis.

Activity of the patient as well as resumption of normal activities should be guided on an individual basis. Prolonged bed rest has not been shown to be of benefit. Because of the high incidence of splenic enlargement and the association between splenic rupture and trauma or strenuous exercise, activity should be modified to avoid this potential risk. Specifically, participation in strenuous contact sports such as football, wrestling, gymnastics, basketball, and soccer should be avoided for 3 to 4 weeks. If an individual had symptomatic splenic enlargement—that is, left upper quadrant tenderness or fullness, radiographic evaluation of splenic size may be indicated prior to resumption of full athletic participation.

The role of corticosteroids in the treatment of uncomplicated IM has been controversial. No well-controlled studies have addressed the short-term benefits versus any potential long-term adverse consequences, such as the development of "chronic mononucleosis" or neoplasia. Until such data become available, we do *not* recommend the use of corticosteroids for the usual uncomplicatedcase of IM. However, we do recommend corticosteroids for the treatment of life-threatening complications of severe IM, especially impending airway obstruction, acute neurologic complications, myocarditis, or severe hemolytic anemia, thrombocytopenia, or granulocytopenia. For these complications, initial doses of 40 to 60 mg of prednisone per day or its equivalent for 3 to 5 days, with rapid tapering thereafter, may modify the course of illness.

MUMPS

(Epidemic Parotitis)

method of
BLAISE L. CONGENI, M.D.
Northeastern Ohio Universities
Akron, Ohio

Mumps is generally a benign, self-limited illness. The peak incidence is in children 10 to 14 years of age; less than 15 per cent of cases are seen in adolescents and adults. The patient is contagious from 1 day prior to parotid swelling until the swelling has subsided, usually about 1 week. Thirty to 40 per cent of the cases are subclinical.

The clinical manifestations most often seen with mumps require only symptomatic treatment. Many patients will experience a short prodrome of 1 to 4 days with headache, myalgia, and arthralgia. The patient may then complain of earache, especially after drinking sour liquids. Shortly thereafter the parotid swelling occurs and is unilateral 25 per cent of the time. The swelling is firm, but without overlying erythema. Trismus and dysphagia occur less often.

Treatment of the uncomplicated case usually requires nothing more than mild analgesics such as aspirin or acetaminophen (Tylenol) in doses of 10 mg per kg every 4 to 6 hours. A bland diet or cool compresses may also be used if they afford symptomatic relief.

Complications

Mumps Meningoencephalitis. The central nervous system (CNS) complication most often encountered is mild aseptic meningitis (AM). Frequently the only manifestation of AM is headache and pleocytosis. This complication is seen in 10 to 20 per cent of cases; consequently mumps is one of the leading etiologic agents associated with AM. Mumps may be overlooked as the etiology since 30 to 40 per cent of children with mumps AM have no parotitis. In addition, some cases of AM may precede or follow the parotitis. The child with AM secondary to mumps frequently notes significant improvement in headache following the lumbar puncture.

Almost all deaths seen with mumps are secondary to encephalitis. Most children with CNS involvement have mild disease best characterized as AM. A spectrum of CNS complications occurs, though, and encephalitis is felt to complicate 2.6 per 1000 cases of mumps. The associated fatality rate in these cases is 1.4 per cent. Encephalitis is more commonly seen with increasing age and occurs more commonly in males than females.

The treatment of all CNS complications is symptomatic with analgesics, as previously mentioned. Intravenous fluids or anticonvulsants may also be needed.

Epididymo-Orchitis. The complication that generates the most anxiety in adolescent and adult men is epididymo-orchitis. This complication is seen in 20 to 30 per cent of males and usually occurs as the parotid swelling is subsiding. It is associated with fever, nausea, and vomiting. Tenderness of the testicle is seen in association with swelling and erythema of the scrotum. Associated discomfort is frequently severe, necessitating bed rest. Applications of ice and support of the scrotum with a towel may be of benefit. Because of the severity of the pain, aspirin and acetaminophen (Tylenol) are frequently not effective. Codeine, 0.5 to 1.0 mg per kg per dose given every 4 to 6 hours with a maximum dose of 3 mg per kg per day, or even meperidine (Demerol), 6 mg per kg per day in divided doses with a maximum dose of 100 mg, may be needed for relief. Because of the associated constitutional symptoms, oral intake may be poor, and intravenous fluids may also be beneficial.

During the acute phase, steroids are generally employed to relieve inflammation. An initial dose of prednisone, 1.5 to 2 mg per kg per day in three to four divided doses, is used. This dose is continued until inflammation subsides. Then the dose may be tapered over 1 week and given as a single daily dose in the morning, to prevent adrenal axis suppression. Controlled studies documenting the efficacy of steroids in this condition are lacking, although anecdotal information is available suggesting that they relieve inflammation and pain.

Local infiltration of the spermatic cord with anesthetic agents such as lidocaine is usually not needed. Surgical incision of the tuncia albuginea or the tuncia vaginalis should be avoided.

A major reason for the associated anxiety seen with this complication is fear of sterility or impotence. The patient should be reassured that these complications occur in less than 2 per cent, even with bilateral involvement.

Pancreatitis. Although pancreatitis is uncommon, it should be considered in those patients with persistent nausea, vomiting, and abdominal pain, and marked elevation of the serum amylase. Diagnosis rests on clinical grounds, and patients again are treated symptomatically with intravenous fluids, nasogastric suction, and analgesics. The patient usually recovers without complications.

Presternal Edema. Presternal edema is an unusual manifestation that is seen in 5 to 10 per cent of children with mumps. The swelling usually extends down over the upper half of the sternum and is soft, with mild erythema. Occasionally this complication is confused with a cellulitis. No antibiotics or other specific treatment is needed, and the inflammation usually subsides in 3 to 5 days.

Other Complications. These are encountered even more rarely. Oophoritis is seen in 5 per cent of infected females. Deafness also occurs infrequently and is usually unilateral, although frequently profound. Other uncommon complications include arthritis, ocular complications, myocarditis, thrombocytopenia, and thyroiditis. Only symptomatic treatment is needed for these conditions.

Prevention

Since the licensure of the live mumps vaccine in 1967, the number of reported cases has decreased yearly. The live mumps vaccine is prepared in chick embryo cell culture. A subclinical infection is produced, which is not communicable. After a single dose of vaccine, an antibody response similar to that seen after natural disease is elicited. Seroconversion as well as protection from clinical challenge occurs in over 90 per cent of recipients. Consequently, when the vaccine is administered along with the live rubeola and rubella vaccines (MMR) to children over 12 months of age—usually at 15 months of age—immunization is highly cost effective. Immunization of children prior to their first birthday may be less effective because of maternal antibody; such children should be reimmunized after reaching 1 year of age. Mumps vaccine is available in the monovalent form as well, but when given alone this preparation is less cost effective because of the low morbidity and mortality associated with the disease. The duration of immunity following immunization is unknown, although protection appears complete for at least 15 years.

Use of the vaccine after exposure to natural disease is of unknown value but is not contraindicated. The use of mumps immune globulin or regular immune serum globulin in this situation is not generally recommended.

The mumps vaccine is well tolerated, and adverse effects following immunization are rare. Low grade fever or parotitis are infrequently encountered. A small number of patients have a variety of CNS manifestations within 2 months of immunization. These symptoms generally have resolved, and any possible association with vaccination is felt to be remote.

Contraindications to vaccine administration are those noted with any live viral vaccine and include

(1) Immunocompromised patients (generalized malignancies, T or B cell defects, those receiving immunosuppressant drugs);

(2) Pregnant women;

(3) Patients with marked hypersensitivity (anaphylactic) to vaccine components (e.g., egg, neomycin). Individuals with nonanaphylactic reactions following ingestion of eggs may be immunized; and

(4) Patients who have received whole blood, plasma, or gamma globulin within 8 weeks prior to administration of the vaccine.

Determination of susceptibility may at times be desirable in the unimmunized adolescent or adult male. Since 30 to 40 per cent of cases are subclinical and since most adults have been naturally infected, a negative history is not helpful. Skin test reactivity is also not reliable since control material is not available and because foreign protein reactions may produce false-positive reactions. In addition, false-negative reactions may occur. Serologic study is therefore generally needed to establish susceptibility. Complement-fixing antibody to the soluble "S" antigen of the mumps virus appears early and indicates recent infection. Complement-fixing antibodies to the viral "V" antigen appear late and indicate immunity.

A number of reports have appeared lately describing parotitis in previously immunized children. Evaluation of such children using both culture and serology to establish the etiology should be undertaken. Parotitis in such patients has been noted to occur for any of the following reasons:

1. Initial failure to seroconvert to the live mumps vaccine.
2. Infection with mumps virus even in the face of adequate antibody titer.
3. Parotitis due to alternative viruses.

PLAGUE

method of
BRUCE TEMPEST, M.D., F.A.C.P.
Indian Health Service, U.S.P.H.S.
Gallup, New Mexico

Diagnosis

Yersinia pestis, a bipolar staining coccobacillary gram-negative bacterium, is the cause of plague. Plague remains enzootic in many parts of the world as a circulating bacterial infection among certain relatively resistant wild rodent hosts. Human populations in geographic areas adjoining these enzootic regions are at particular risk. These areas in the United States include especially New Mexico, Arizona, Colorado, and California. Transmission among the natural reservoir of wild rodents is primarily by associated flea vectors. Humans also are most commonly infected by the bite of an infected flea. Certain carnivores play a substantial role as transporters of infected fleas to other rodent populations and to people. Occasionally they serve as direct sources of human *Y. pestis* infection, especially from domestic cats and dogs. The organism can also enter breaks in the skin if a person handles tissues of infected animals.

Regional lymphadenitis is the first clinical response to the infection in most cases, producing exquisitely tender buboes; hence, the name bubonic plague. The lymph nodes most commonly involved are inguinal, followed next in frequency by axillary and cervical nodes.

The organism can then spread hematogenously, occasionally producing a secondary pneumonia and—less commonly—meningeal, cutaneous, pharyngeal, or ophthalmic plague. In about 10 per cent of cases, primary septicemic plague occurs without lymphadenitis. Primary pneumonic plague results from aerosol exposure to *Y. pestis* from infected animals or humans, producing a fulminant, rapidly fatal infection in untreated patients. Fortunately, this form of the disease is rare; the only recent human cases in the United States were transmitted from domestic cats with plague pneumonia. The incubation period for bubonic plague is 2 to 5 days, which is sufficiently long that travelers from endemic areas may have onset of illness in areas where plague does not naturally occur.

Since plague is such a rare disease (12 to 40 human cases diagnosed per year in the United States since 1974), the index of suspicion is low in nonendemic areas. A diagnostic aspirate of the bubo should be made immediately and appropriate smears and cultures performed. Blood cultures should be obtained in all suspected cases.

The Plague Branch, Centers for Disease Control, P.O. Box 2087, Fort Collins, CO 80522, 303/221-6400, will provide guidance for further diagnostic testing, therapy, and epidemiologic investigation.

Treatment

Since mortality rates for untreated plague have been reported as high as 70 per cent, therapy should be instituted promptly in all suspected cases. Streptomycin is the drug of choice. Adults should receive 30 mg per kg of body weight per day; children, 20 to 40 mg per kg per day; and infants, 10 to 20 mg per kg per day. Streptomycin should be administered intramuscularly in two to four divided doses per day. Chloramphenicol and tetracycline are excellent alternative drugs and may be given intravenously as second drugs in hypotensive patients in whom the mobilization of intramuscular streptomycin is compromised. Chloramphenicol should be given intravenously at a dose of 50 to 75 mg per kg per day in four doses to serously ill patients. The same dose may be given orally when tolerated. Concern that aplastic anemia may result from the use of chloramphenicol should not be a factor in withholding treatment from seriously ill plague patients. Because it penetrates the meninges and eye, it is the drug of choice for meningeal and ophthalmic plague.

Tetracycline may be given orally as a loading dose of 15 mg per kg to a maximum of 1 gram, followed by 30 mg per kg per day in four doses. The intravenous dose is 12 to 20 mg per kg per day until oral medication is tolerated. The risk of administering tetracycline to children under 8 years of age or to pregnant women must be weighed against the specific benefit of the drug to such patients. Oral tetracycline can be used to complete a full therapeutic 10 day course after streptomycin or intravenous chloramphenicol have been given for 5 days in the clinic or hospital. Such a switch in antibiotic therapy minimizes the risk of renal and vestibular damage from streptomycin and the risk of aplastic anemia from chloramphenicol.

Other drugs have been used successfully for the treatment of plague, but they are not recommended because the antibiotics listed here have been so highly effective. Ampicillin and amoxicillin have suboptimal efficacy in vivo against *Y. pestis*. Trimethoprim/sulfamethoxazole, gentamicin, and kanamycin have not been used extensively in treating patients with plague and therefore should not be used selectively. The efficacy of doxycycline for this purpose has not been tested; therefore, it is not recommended.

Therapy should be continued for a minimum of 10 days or for 3 or 4 days after the patient has become afebrile and has clinically recovered. The patient's condition may deteriorate during the first 24 hours of therapy, but clinical improvement is usually evident within 1 to 3 days.

Clinical Course

The principal early complications of plague include septic shock, secondary plague pneumonia, adult respiratory distress syndrome (ARDS), consumption coagulopathy, and meningitis. Later complications, in some instances attributable to the early complications or delay in antimicrobial therapy, include cardiac failure, bubo suppuration, and peripheral gangrene. It is frequently difficult to determine whether pulmonic pathology is related to ARDS, to secondary pneumonic plague, or to a combination of the two. Sputum specimens can be stained and cultured to confirm the diagnosis. Mechanical ventilation may be necessary for plague pneumonia or ARDS. Septic shock is best treated with fluid replacement and vasopressors. Pulmonary artery pressure monitoring can be of value in managing the cardiopulmonary complications. Steroids and heparin have no proved value in managing the septic or hematologic complications.

When possible, patients should be treated in an intensive care unit isolation room. After 3 days of antibiotic therapy and supportive care, the patient usually begins to improve: the fever abates, and the hematologic and acid-base abnormalities are corrected. Although the buboes may be enlarged and painful for several weeks and occasionally cause persistent fevers, they usually recede with the continuation of antibiotic therapy; they rarely require surgical drainage. The buboes should be reaspirated and cultured when fever recurs or persists longer than 1 week. Consideration should also be given to other causes of recurrent fever, such as drugs and nosocomial infections. No streptomycin-resistant *Y. pestis* organisms have been isolated from humans.

Prevention

All hospitalized plague patients should be kept in strict isolation for the first 48 hours of antibiotic therapy, after which time the isolation procedures may be terminated if pneumonia or draining lesions have not developed. Since pneumonia is the primary concern regarding communicability from person to person, chest radiographs should be made for all patients being treated for plague. Hospital personnel caring for patients with plague pneumonia should follow respiratory isolation procedures rigorously, and patients should be continued in isolation until 4 days of antibiotic treatment are completed.

Patients with bubonic or septicemic plague but without secondary pneumonic involvement pose no hazard to their family contacts. The family contacts, however, should all be initially evaluated for symptoms and their temperatures measured because of the concern that they may have had exposure to the same source as the patient. Such persons should be evaluated daily for the next 7 days for symptoms and fever.

If hospital staff or family members are exposed to unsuspected or untreated plague pneumonia, prophylactic therapy should be given. Tetracycline, 500 mg orally four times a day for 6 days, is the preferred method of treatment in adults. Trimethoprim/sulfamethoxazole is recommended for children under 8 years of age and pregnant women. Hospital personnel who have observed recommended isolation procedures do not need prophylactic therapy. With such a notorious disease, prophylaxis is frequently an emotionally charged issue. Despite its bad reputation and a 25 per cent incidence of pneumonia in plague patients in the United States since 1974, plague has not been transmitted from one person to another in the United States for over 50 years.

Plague vaccine is available for use in military personnel and persons with significant repeated exposure to plague-infected animals, but it is not appropriate for general use. Suspected or confirmed cases of plague should be reported promptly to the local or state health department so that epidemiologic investigations can be conducted and preventive measures instituted in the community.

PSITTACOSIS

(Ornithosis)

method of
CLARK M. KERR, M.D.
Denver Clinic Medical Centers
Denver, Colorado

Psittacosis is a disease of birds transmissible to humans. Rarely, it may be transmitted human to human. This mode of transmission, however, frequently results in more severe disease. *Chlamydia psittaci,* the causative agent, an obligate intracellular parasite, is considered a specialized bacterium.

Infection occurs via inhalation of dried bird excreta, in which the agent can survive for long periods. Reinfection may occur in humans. The disease is usually mild, ranging from an influenza-like illness to an atypical pneumonia, but it may cause multisystem disease and is included in the differential diagnosis of culture-negative endocarditis.

Diagnosis

The usual presenting features are fever, malaise, headache, and a nonproductive cough. On physical examination, as with certain other intracellular infections (e.g., brucellosis, typhoid), the pulse rate may be slow relative to the height of the fever. Considering the paucity of chest findings, the roentgenographic findings may show remarkable pulmonary involvement.

Differential diagnostic possibilities are protean and include mycoplasma infection, tularemia, legionnaires' disease, influenza, Q fever, and fungal infections. Twenty per cent of cases may have no history of exposure to birds.

When the diagnosis is considered, presumptive therapy with tetracycline is advised, since definitive diagnosis requires isolation of the organism, which can be hazardous, or a fourfold rise or fall in antibody titer. A single titer of 1:32 in a patient with a compatible illness is presumptive evidence of psittacosis. Maximum titers are seen after 3 to 4 weeks of illness; however, early therapy with tetracycline may delay this sequence by several weeks. False-positive titer rises, while uncommon, have occurred in some patients with legionnaires' disease.

General Measures

(1) Hospitalization of patients with dyspnea or with multisystem disease.

(2) Oxygenation depending on clinical status and arterial blood gases. When death occurs, it is usually secondary to pulmonary insufficiency.

(3) Respiratory isolation to prevent potential human to human transmission.

(4) Appropriate fluid and electrolyte replacement.

(5) Symptomatic treatment of fever, headaches, and myalgias.

(6) Notification of the Health Department for initiation of epidemiologic investigation to determine the source of infection.

(7) Observation for complications, especially pericarditis, endocarditis, and myocarditis, all of which have been reported.

Specific Therapy

Tetracycline is the only reliable therapy and should be administered in doses of 2 to 3 grams per day. While a response to therapy usually occurs within 48 to 72 hours, it may be delayed. Chloramphenicol and penicillin have been recommended as second line drugs; however, the efficacy of these agents is uncertain. Rifampin, 600 mg daily, has been reported to be of value in the treatment of psittacosis unresponsive to tetracycline. Therapy should be continued up to 14 days after defervescence, because relapses are common.

Prevention

Every effort should be made to identify the bird that served as the source of infection. Virtually any species of bird can serve as host. Asymptomatic birds may still transmit infection. Prolonged exposure is not necessary to acquire infection.

A decline in cases in the United States is due to (1) the incorporation of tetracycline-medicated poultry food, (2) the requirement that imported psittacine birds be medicated for 30 days prior to entry into this country, and (3) the increase in the domestic parakeet-breeding industry. This, however, is no guarantee that psittacosis will be eradicated in this country as foreign birds may continue to shed the organism for months after illness and remain infectious.

Q FEVER

method of
FREDERICK T. KOSTER, M.D.
University of New Mexico
Albuquerque, New Mexico

Q fever is caused by *Coxiella burnetii,* a rickettsia that is enzootic primarily in sheep, goats, and cattle worldwide. Humans become infected primarily by inhaling dust contaminated with infected products of animal conception, animal excrement, or hides or by direct ingestion of infected milk or meat. Although most infections appear to be asymptomatic, acute influenza-like illness with or without atypical pneumonia is quite common. Cases that follow a chronic course may present an acute, flulike disease or fever and malaise of insidious onset, and manifest as hepatitis or endocarditis, with, rarely, involvement of other organs. Unlike other rickettsia, *C. burnetii* is rarely associated with a rash and does not produce a positive Weil-Felix reaction.

Diagnosis

Diagnosis is made by the fourfold rise in antibody titer measured by complement fixation or microagglutination and can be supported by the finding of characteristic doughnut-shaped granulomas in liver, bone marrow, and other tissues.

Treatment

For acute Q fever, therapy should be initiated after a presumptive clinical diagnosis has been made; that is, in the acute illness characterized by high fever, chills, malaise, headache, and arthralgia, among slaughterhouse workers, farmers, and tourists. In most cases of acute symptomatic infection, the disease is self-limiting: by the time the diagnosis is made, the fever, headache, myalgias, and cough have abated. Antibiotics are likely, but not proved, to lessen clinical symptoms; antipyretics, analgesics, and bed rest are also helpful. Tetracycline begun within the first 3 days of illness results in a clinical response within 48 hours; 500 mg every 6 hours by mouth is continued until the patient has been afebrile for 5 days. Doxycycline, 100 mg every 12 hours by mouth or parenterally, may also be used. Chloramphenicol, another rickettsiostatic agent, is reserved for patients in whom tetracycline is contraindicated (usually because of age or renal status). Antibiotics are not required for patients whose symptoms have abated prior to diagnosis.

Uncommonly, patients will have persistent symptoms, with or without antibiotics, or will recover clinically from the initial illness only to relapse weeks later with malaise and fever. Such patients have chronic Q fever, most commonly Q fever hepatitis, and require tetracycline, 500 mg every 6 hours by mouth for 30 to 60 days. A clinical response may be expected in 5 to 10 days of resumption of therapy.

The rare patient in this group will relapse clinically when the tetracycline is stopped, even after 60 days of therapy. In these cases, the diagnosis of endocarditis can be confirmed by cardiac valvular abnormalities, a phase I complement fixation titer of greater than 1:200, and an in vitro lymphocyte stimulation test demonstrating complete unresponsiveness to *Coxiella* antigen (National Institutes of Health, and Rocky Mountain Laboratory, Hamilton, Montana 59840; phone (406)363-3211). Endocarditis must be treated with long-term suppressive therapy, as there appears to be a specific immunologic defect that prevents cure. In these cases, tetracycline is usually used in combination with rifampin or cotrimoxazole. The duration of antibiotics is controversial but is usually 2 or more years. Antibiotic therapy may be stopped only if valvular insufficiency is insignificant and stable and if the phase I antibody titers have decreased dramatically (<1:200).

Valve replacement is indicated by hemodynamic deterioration or emboli. The lack of extensive clinical experience with Q fever endocarditis necessitates individualized approaches to each patient within the preceding guidelines. There is no evidence that Q fever endocarditis can be prevented. Considering the significant mortality rate of endocarditis, however, I recommend 30 days of tetracycline therapy for patients with documented acute Q fever and pre-existing valvular abnormalities.

Prevention

The extensive enzootic distribution of Q fever makes it a potential problem in slaughterhouses, tanneries, and many animal habitats. Pasteurizing milk, which can transmit Q fever, is an important preventive measure. Unfortunately, the resistance of *C. burnetii* to desiccation and disinfection makes its general elimination from the environment impractical.

Research facilities that use sheep or goats in the study of fetal-placental physiology have experienced outbreaks of Q fever. Guidelines to lessen this risk include serologic evaluation of flocks and personnel and special animal facilities if Q fever is present. Except in designated laboratories, isolation of *C. burnetii* should not be attempted. Although Q fever is not a reportable disease in many states, local health authorities should be notified of cases, since investigation may help identify specific high risk situations amenable to control.

Putative person-to-person spread of Q fever has occurred rarely, primarily in relation to aerosols produced at postmortem examination. Nevertheless, infected patients are usually placed on "secretion precautions" if hospitalized. Vaccines for humans and animals are being studied but are not yet commercially available.

RABIES

method of
RODNEY A. MICHAEL, M.D.,
and C. KENNETH McALLISTER, M.D.
Brooke Army Medical Center
San Antonio, Texas

Because of the almost fatal nature of this disease, each physician should assess carefully the potential risk for the acquisition of rabies in each case. It is of vital importance that state and local health authorities be contacted when the diagnosis of rabies is suspected. When the circumstances of exposure are ambiguous and the potential risk of rabies uncertain, expertise in the management of rabies exposure should be sought. The Centers for Disease Control (404/329-3095 weekdays; 404/329-3644 after office hours) is a source of information should state or local expertise be unavailable.

EPIDEMIOLOGY

Transmission of rabies virus may occur via either unimmunized domestic animals ("urban" rabies) or wild animals ("sylvatic" rabies), including skunks, foxes, raccoons, coyotes, bobcats, and bats. The risk of transmission to humans has been altered in most developed countries by immunization of domestic animals and programs to control stray animals. Such programs initiated in the United States in 1946 have nearly eliminated rabies in dogs and cats. In each year prior to 1950, over 6000 dogs and cats were found to be rabid, contrasted with fewer than 300 per year since 1975. With this decline in domestic animal rabies, human rabies has declined from 22 cases per year prior to 1950 to 2 per year since 1960. In the United States, 85 per cent of animal rabies is now found primarily in wildlife and only 5 per cent in domestic dogs and cats. On the other hand, countries that have not controlled canine rabies still have a significant problem with human rabies. The reported annual incidence of 800 cases of human rabies worldwide reflects the global nature of this disease but probably represents underreporting; estimates of up to 20,000 cases per year are closer to the true incidence.

The state of Hawaii is free of rabies as are the cities of New York and Philadelphia, with the exception of bat rabies for the two cities. Yet eight states have reported more than 200 cases of animal rabies per year. The primary animals affected are raccoons in Virginia and Southeastern states, skunks in the Southwest, Midwest, and California, and foxes in Central Eastern states. Rabid bats are a particular problem in Texas and other Southwestern states but are found throughout the continental United States.

The introduction of rabies into humans is primarily through the bite of a rabid animal whose saliva contains the virus. Although uncommon, human rabies has been acquired without a bite, through entry of the virus into open cuts, wounds, and mucous membranes and from airborne virus in the laboratory. A unique case of human rabies acquisition is described from a bat-infested cave in Texas; aerosolization of bat urine appears to have been the mode of infection. If an individual is bitten by a rabid animal, the risk of acquiring rabies ranges from 15 to 20 per cent and depends upon the location and extent of the bite (head and facial bites being of greater risk), the species of biting animal, and the amount of rabies virus in the animal's saliva.

The incubation period of rabies in humans ranges from 10 days to greater than 365 days but is usually less than 60 days. Extensive bites and those located on the head are associated with shorter incubation periods than bites of the trunk and extremities.

RABIES PREVENTION AND TREATMENT

Indications for Prophylaxis

The principal arguments for prophylaxis are the almost invariably fatal nature of rabies infection (only three survivors known) and the well-demonstrated efficacy of properly administered immunoprophylaxis and wound care. Generally, the most difficult decision faced by the treating physician is whether or not to initiate prophylaxis. This decision depends on the type of exposure, the biting animal, and the circumstances of the bite (Table 1).

Type of Exposure

Bite. A bite exposure is any penetration of the skin by teeth, and thus, presumed wound contamination with infected saliva.

Nonbite. A nonbite exposure is any scratch, abrasion, open wound, or mucous membrane suspected of having been contaminated with infected saliva or other infected tissue or secretions.

Casual. Exposure such as petting without bite or nonbite exposure does not constitute an indication for immunoprophylaxis.

The clearest indications for prophylaxis are bites, but of major concern is the nonbite situation. An individual who carries a potentially rabid bat adjacent to an open wound of the hand should be strongly considered for prophylaxis.

The Biting Animal

Bites and nonbite exposures to skunks, raccoons, foxes, coyotes, bobcats, and bats require postexposure immunoprophylaxis. Once initiated, prophylaxis may be discontinued if the suspect animal is shown to be free of rabies. However, generally the animal is not captured, and no determination of disease is possible. In these circumstances prophylaxis should be completed.

Other wild animals—chipmunks, mice, squirrels, gerbils, guinea pigs and other rodents, and rabbits and hares—almost never are infected in nature and have not been associated with human rabies in the United States. Consultation with local and state public health officials is of major importance in identifying the potentially rabid species in a specific geographic area.

Exposures from domestic (pet) dogs and cats should be evaluated on a case-by-case basis, with specific attention to the animal's immunization status and close observation of the animal when possible. The "in house" pet will have little opportunity for exposure to rabid animals as will the roaming animal.

Circumstances of Bite. An unprovoked bite by any animal is more suspect; however, provocation is subject to interpretation. Generally, any exposure in which the patient was attempting to approach, pet, or feed a strange or unfamiliar but otherwise healthy-appearing animal (especially a wild animal) should be construed as provoked.

Determination of Exposure and Evaluation of Animal

The risk of rabies transmission is greatest when the patient is bitten in an unprovoked attack by a skunk, bat, or raccoon; however, the situation usually involves exposure to a domestic animal in an urban area.

Although human rabies has been acquired from domestic pets that have been vaccinated against rabies, our view is that effectively immunized

TABLE 1. **Management of Rabies Exposure**

	Low Risk	High Risk
I. ASSESSMENT OF RISK OF RABIES FROM EXPOSURE		
Type of exposure	Casual, such as petting; no exposure to secretions of open wounds or mucous membranes; no penetration of skin	Wild animal bite (skunks, bats, raccoons, foxes); bites of face or head; unimmunized cat or dog bite
The biting animal	Rodents (squirrels, chipmunks, etc); rabbits; immunized domestic pets	Skunks, bats, raccoons, foxes, wolves
Circumstances of bite	Provoked	Unprovoked

In cases clearly at high risk for rabies exposure, administer postexposure prophylaxis with both HRIG and human diploid cell vaccine. In most low risk exposures, prophylaxis is not given, but in specific situations domestic pets should be observed.

II. PROPHYLAXIS ± ADMINISTERED—MANAGEMENT OF ANIMAL

1. Quarantine domestic pets for 10 days
   If normal during 10 days of observation by qualified veterinarian, discontinue prophylaxis
   If abnormal behavior compatible with rabies develops, sacrifice animal for brain examination for rabies virus
   1. If positive, complete prophylaxis
   2. If negative, discontinue prophylaxis
2. *Sacrifice stray domestic animals (dog, cat) and wild animals* (if available) for rabies studies of brain*
   If positive, complete prophylaxis
   If negative, discontinue prophylaxis
3. *If the animal cannot be found or immunization status is uncertain, complete antirabies prophylaxis*

*Identification may be impossible; if doubt exists about the animal involved, continue prophylaxis.

domestic animals are virtually incapable of transmitting rabies. However, a number of variably effective animal vaccines are available throughout the United States; when an animal's behavior suggests rabies, a veterinarian should be consulted about the vaccine status. Clearly, rabies vaccine administered by a qualified veterinarian (who can readily document the timing of vaccination and the appropriateness of immunization procedures) is the only admissible animal immunization data. In the absence of such documentation, one should assume the animal is unimmunized.

If the animal involved in the biting episode is an apparently healthy domestic dog or cat, the animal should be confined, observed for 10 days and evaluated by a veterinarian at the first sign of illness (Table 1). Rabies virus is not present in the saliva of dogs and cats for more than 10 days before the onset of clinical illness. Therefore, a dog or cat that remains healthy for at least 10 days will not have transmitted rabies and postexposure prophylaxis is not warranted. If the animal is ill at the time of the exposure or if signs of rabies develop during the observation period, the animal should be humanely killed and the head removed, packed in wet ice (without freezing), and shipped intact for rabies examination by a qualified laboratory designated by the local or state health department. If fluorescent antibody testing of the brain is negative for rabies virus, it can be safely concluded that the animal was not infected, and prophylaxis is not indicated or may be discontinued. Quarantine is not recommended for any animals except domestic dogs and cats; any potentially rabid wild animal that has bitten a person should be killed at once, with submission of the head for rabies examination.

The decision to administer postexposure prophylaxis is clearly a case-by-case determination. Our own experience with animal bites has led to several helpful clinical axioms: (1) When the animal is not found and provocation is unclear, prophylaxis appears prudent. (2) The handling of a bat or bat secretions by an individual with multiple skin lesions or open wounds should be strongly considered as grounds for prophylaxis. (3) When dealing with a small child that has either been bitten or otherwise exposed to a rabid bat, the history may be extremely ambiguous and one should err on the side of administering prophylaxis.

RABIES ANTISERUM AND VACCINE

Rabies antiserum, whether derived from human or equine donors, provides rapid, passive immune protection with a half-life of approximately 21 days. Failure of rabies prophylaxis has been documented in instances when antiserum was not administered as a component of prophylaxis. Rabies immune globulin is administered on day 0 of rabies prophylaxis with the first dose of vaccine.

Human rabies immune globulin (HRIG or RIG) is antirabies gamma globulin harvested from immunized human donors. Because it is obtained from human donors, risk associated with its use is minimal. Since its release in the United States in 1975, there have been no reports of transmitted viral illnesses and no reports of other significant adverse reactions associated with its use. It is supplied in 2 ml (300 international units [IU]) and 10 ml (1500 IU) vials by Cutter Laboratories (Hyperab) and by Merieux Institute (Imogam).

Equine antirabies serum (ARS) is antirabies globulin derived from hyperimmunized horses. As a heterologous antiserum, it is associated with a significant risk of either anaphylaxis or serum sickness. ARS is supplied in 1000 IU vials (approximately 5 ml) by Sclavo (Antirabies Serum).

Rabies vaccine induces an active host humoral immune response that requires 7 to 10 days to develop and that may persist for up to a year or more.

Human diploid cell vaccine for rabies (HDCV) is the only rabies vaccine presently available for use in the United States. It is prepared from inactivated rabies virus grown in human diploid cell culture. As currently produced, the vaccine is immunologically potent, requiring only five 1 ml doses for development of an adequate antirabies antibody titer in all recipients. The vaccine has been shown to be safe with no deaths in over 2 million doses given worldwide. Minor systemic side effects include headache, malaise, fever, lymphadenopathy, nausea, and abdominal pain in up to 20 per cent of patients. Up to 6 per cent may experience an illness suggestive of an immune complex disorder following booster doses of HDCV. The illness is characterized by the onset of generalized urticaria 2 to 21 days after vaccination and may also include arthralgias, arthritis, angioedema, nausea, vomiting, fever, and malaise. Fatal anaphylaxis has not been observed. A Guillain-Barré type of syndrome has been reported in two patients, both of whom recovered. Cause and effect were not established. HDCV is marketed in the United States by Wyeth Laboratories (Wyvac) and by Merieux Institute (Rabies Vaccine) in 1 ml, single dose vials.

Postexposure Prophylaxis

Following the decision for prophylaxis, therapy should not be delayed. Recent data show that in the United States the average interval between exposure and treatment is 5 days. However, even in the event of the passage of days or weeks between exposure and prophylaxis, appropriate prophylaxis should still be initiated with both rabies immune globulin and rabies vaccine. The incubation period for human rabies has been reported as short as 9 days and as long as 19 years, most frequently ranging from 20 to 90 days.

Effective rabies prophylaxis has two goals:

1. To reduce the titer of virus at the local wound site. Thorough cleansing to the full depth of the wound with soap and water solution reduces the risk of rabies infection by up to 90 per cent.

2. To establish immediate and long-lasting neutralizing antibody to rabies virus. This involves the administration of both human rabies immune globulin (HRIG) for early passive immunity and rabies vaccine to stimulate active host production of neutralizing antibody.

Local Wound Care

Vigorous scrubbing with a 20 per cent soap solution, followed by thorough flushing of the wound, is recommended. Both the mechanical and the chemical actions are important in reducing the inoculum of virus. Any soap compound may be used effectively, including the quaternary ammonium compounds and chlorhexidine. Prudent care of animal bites of the hands and feet or other nontrivial bites may include a 5 day course of antibiotics and tetanus prophylaxis when indicated.

Passive Immunization

Human rabies immune globulin (HRIG) is administered only once, upon initiation of prophylaxis. The recommended dose is 20 international units per kg (9 IU per pound) of total body weight. Up to 50 per cent of the total dose should be thoroughly infiltrated in the local wound site, with the remainder given intramuscularly at a site separate from that used for vaccine administration. If HRIG is unavailable, or if for some other reason globulin is not administered on day 0 of prophylaxis, it can and should be given up to 1 week after the first dose of vaccine. Several failures of vaccine used without rabies antiserum have been documented; therefore, even if delayed for up to a week, HRIG is indicated. After 7 days the patient has presumably begun actively producing neutralizing antibody.

If HRIG is not available, equine antirabies serum may be used. However, the high frequency of anaphylaxis and serum sickness reactions with this product make its use undesirable except when HRIG is not available and the risk of rabies infection is high. The dose of equine serums is 40 IU per kg (18 IU per pound); it is administered as is HRIG.

The dose of HRIG or ARS should not exceed the recommended dose because the concomitant administration of antirabies globulin may interfere with active host production of antibody.

Active Immunization

Vaccination with human diploid cell vaccine (HDCV) is initiated in conjunction with HRIG. Vaccine should be administered intramuscularly in five separate 1 ml doses, the first dose as soon as possible after exposure. The remaining four 1 ml doses should be administered on days 3, 7, 14, and 28 after the first dose. Testing for antibody response is indicated only in patients with an immunosuppressive disorder or in those who have received immunosuppressive agents (including glucocorticoids) before or during the period of vaccination. Testing should be performed 2 to 3 weeks after the last dose of vaccine. Consultation with local and state health authorities or with the Centers for Disease Control may be helpful.

Patients who have received pre-exposure prophylaxis with HDCV or who have a documented adequate antibody response for another rabies vaccine require only local wound care and two 1 ml doses of HDCV, one each on days 0 to 3.

Patients who have undergone uncertain vaccination regimens or whose treatment was begun in a foreign country should have an antibody titer determination after the final vaccine dose. A titer of less than 1 to 5 by rapid fluorescent focus inhibition test (RFFIT) is an indication for additional vaccine.

Pre-Exposure Prophylaxis

Pre-exposure immunization with HDCV is recommended for all persons considered to be at high risk for rabies exposure, such as veterinarians, certain laboratory workers, and travelers to areas of the world where rabies may be epizootic. Pre-exposure prophylaxis serves several useful purposes:

1. Protection for patients who may be inapparently exposed, such as laboratory workers who work with live rabies virus or persons working in vaccine production facilities.

2. Early protection for patients whose postexposure prophylaxis may be delayed.

3. Simplification of postexposure prophylaxis by elimination of the need for HRIG and three doses of vaccine.

Pre-exposure immunization with HDCV is given as three 1 ml intramuscular injections on days 0, 7, and 28. Vaccine prepared by the Merieux Institute has also been approved for intradermal use when used for pre-exposure prophylaxis only. The vaccine is administered as three 0.1 ml intradermal injections on days 0, 7, and 28. However, recent experience and study following the death of a Peace Corps volunteer from rabies suggests that postimmunization antibody titers achieved with intradermal immunization may often be subprotective. Therefore, it is now recommended that all patients receiving pre-exposure immunization intradermally have serologic testing 2 to 3 weeks after the third dose. Any vaccine with an antibody titer (by RFFIT) of less than 1 to 16 should receive a booster dose of vaccine and repeat serologic testing in 2 to 3 weeks. Routine serologic testing is not indicated following intramuscular immunization except in the immunocompromised host.

Serologic testing or booster immunization should be performed every 2 years in patients who remain at high risk.

Special Situations

Pregnancy is not a contraindication to postexposure prophylaxis for either the mother or the fetus. Data from immunization experience with women in all stages of pregnancy indicate no association of HDCV with fetal abnormalities.

Immunosuppression does not contraindicate postexposure prophylaxis. All patients who require the use of immunosuppressive agents either during or shortly before the period of immunization should have postvaccination serologic testing.

Infants and children receive immunization similar to that for adults, with identical doses of vaccine and HRIG administered, 20 mg per kg.

Patients exposed to live, attenuated virus vaccine generally do not require postexposure prophylaxis. Rabies infection associated with such exposure has not been reported.

A history of allergy or hypersensitivity requires caution in administering HDCV. Antihistamines may be used concomitantly, and epinephrine should be readily available.

RAT-BITE FEVER

method of
PERRY G. PATE, M.D.
Tulane University
New Orleans, Louisiana

Rat-bite fever is the single name given to two similar syndromes with distinct bacterial etiologies. Infection with *Streptobacillus moniliformis* or *Spirillum minus* is usually acquired following the bite of a rat, mouse, or other rodent, although one cannot always obtain a history of a rodent bite. The disease has a worldwide distribution. Persons most at risk for infection are laboratory animal workers, children, and the urban poor. Streptobacillary disease has followed ingestion of raw milk presumably contaminated by rats (Haverhill fever).

Streptobacillus moniliformis is a nonmotile, pleomorphic, gram-negative rod, which can be isolated from the oropharynges of up to 100 per cent of healthy wild and laboratory rats; it is the principal agent of rat-bite fever in the United States. Streptobacillary rat-bite fever has a relatively short incubation period (usually less than 10 days), and the bite wound heals promptly. Characteristically, the patient experiences the abrupt onsert of an acute, prostrating illness with fever, chills, and myalgias. Polyarticular arthralgias or arthritis and a generalized morbilliform or petechial rash usually follow the onset of fever within a few days. If untreated, the fever may resolve and the disease may assume a relapsing course over weeks to months. The untreated mortality may be up to 10 per cent. Serious complications of infection with *Streptobacillus moniliformis* include endocarditis, pericarditis, pneumonia, and abscess formation. The diagnosis of *Streptobacillus moniliformis* infection is usually made by culturing the organism from blood or other sterile fluids. Of note, up to 25 per cent of infected individuals may have positive nonspecific serologic tests for syphilis.

Spirillum minus is a short, thick, coiled, gram-negative rod common in Asia, where the disease it produces is known as sodoku ("rat poison"). The incubation period is longer than that of *Streptobacillus moniliformis*. Unlike streptobacillary disease, spirillary rat-bite fever is commonly accompanied by inflammation at the bite site, with regional lymphangitis and lymphadenitis as well. Arthritis is uncommon. The rash is usually generalized and composed of large reddish-brown or purple macules. As in streptobacillary disease, untreated spirillary rat-bite fever may assume a relapsing course and may be complicated by endocarditis or other focal infections. *Spirillum minus* cannot be cultivated on artificial media but may be found on dark field examination of material from the local bite area, regional lymphatics, or blood or by inoculation into laboratory animals.

Prophylaxis

It is estimated that infection may occur in as many as 10 per cent of rat-bite wounds. Therefore, it is important that a fresh bite wound be flushed with saline and a local antiseptic. The efficacy of antibiotic prophylaxis in this entity is unknown. However, prophylaxis is at least warranted for patients with a heart murmur or known history of valvular heart disease. Oral phenoxymethyl penicillin in a dose of 500 mg four times a day for 3 days has been used.

Antibiotics

Streptobacillus moniliformis and *Spirillum minus* are both susceptible to penicillin, tetracycline, and streptomycin. Other antibiotics, including intravenously administered clindamycin, have also been used successfully.

For uncomplicated infection, 2 grams per day of oral phenoxymethyl penicillin in divided doses or 600,000 units intramuscularly of procaine penicillin G every 12 hours for 10 days have been successful.

Although penicillin is the drug of choice for infection with these organisms, penicillin-resistant L-forms of *Streptobacillus moniliformis* have been shown to arise in some patients on penicillin therapy. In such patients, or in those with penicillin allergy, tetracycline, 2 grams per day, or streptomycin, 15 mg per kg per day, has been used successfully.

The minimum effective antibiotic dosage regimen for complicated infection with either organism is unknown. However, in endocarditis, most experts recommend a standard "endocarditis dose" of penicillin, such as 12 to 20 million units of penicillin G intravenously daily.

The response to appropriate antimicrobial therapy is usually prompt, with defervescence of fever within 48 hours. The main dilemma for the physician when dealing with this disorder is not in naming the appropriate antimicrobial agent but in making the presumptive diagnosis when a high risk individual is seen with symptoms compatible with the disease.

RELAPSING FEVER

method of
STUART M. POLLY, M.D.
Texas Tech University
El Paso, Texas

Relapsing fever is an acute, infectious disease caused by any of several species of spirochetes of the genus *Borrelia.* The disease is worldwide and is transmitted to humans by lice or ticks. It is characterized by recurrent 3 to 6 day paroxysms of fever followed by week-long afebrile periods. Two or three febrile episodes are seen in louseborne disease whereas up to 13 episodes may occur with the tickborne variety. Louseborne (epidemic) relapsing fever is frequent in some parts of Africa and South America but not in North America. Tickborne disease occurs worldwide and is found in the western United States, particularly among campers, hunters, and fishermen. Relapsing fever is a protean disease with a variety of clinical symptoms, courses, and mortality rates. The tickborne form tends to run a milder, but more prolonged, course than the louseborne type.

Treatment

The goals of patient management are (1) supportive care, (2) eradication of the spirochete, (3) prevention and treatment of the complications of the disease, and (4) attenuation of the Jarisch-Herxheimer reaction that frequently accompanies antimicrobial therapy.

General Measures. Most patients are acutely ill. Hospitalization with bed rest and close observation is essential. Severe dehydration, vascular collapse, and mental confusion may occur precipitously. Proper fluid and electrolyte balance is important. Oral rehydration is preferred, but intravenous fluids may be required. Clinical appearance, blood pressure, pulse, and urine output should be followed. Occasionally, central venous pressure monitoring is necessary.

Nausea and vomiting are common and should be treated with chlorpromazine, 25 mg orally or intramuscularly, every 4 to 6 hours.

Fever need not be controlled unless it exceeds 40°C (104°F) or is poorly tolerated by the patient. Sponging with tepid water is the safest means of lowering the body temperature, but hypothermic blankets may be used in extreme situations. Salicylate antipyretics should be avoided.

Pain may be severe and may be alleviated with nonsalicylate analgesics such as acetaminophen (650 mg every 4 hours), codeine, or meperidine.

Antibiotic Therapy. A number of antibiotic treatment regimens are effective in treating relapsing fever. However, tetracycline is the drug of choice. An oral dose of 30 mg per kg per day in four divided doses is given for 10 days. Most adults can be treated with 500 mg every 6 hours. Children and pregnant women should receive erythromycin, 30 to 50 mg per kg per day in four divided doses. For patients unable to take oral medication, intravenous tetracycline, in a dose of 10 mg per kg per day in three divided doses, may be employed. Chloramphenicol is also effective in a dose of 30 mg per kg per day given intravenously in four equal portions. A single oral dose of 500 mg of tetracycline hydrochloride or erythromycin stearate has been shown to clear spirochetes from the blood in louseborne disease. Therapy is continued for 5 to 10 days to prevent relapse. Penicillin is less effective than tetracycline, although 600,000 units of procaine penicillin G intramuscularly every 6 hours has been used effectively. Another successful regimen includes 300,000 units of penicillin G intramuscularly, followed 24 hours later by 500 mg of oral tetracycline.

The Jarisch-Herxheimer Reaction

The Jarisch-Herxheimer reaction (J-HR) consists of the abrupt onset of chills, fever, apprehension, and cardiovascular changes following the initiation of antimicrobial therapy. It is thought to be due to the rapid destruction of large numbers of spirochetes and the sudden release of spirochetal "endotoxin." It is very similar to, but more severe than, the febrile cycles of relapsing fever. Four phases have been described. The *prodromal phase* is uneventful and lasts about 1 hour. The *chill phase* lasts 10 to 30 minutes, with intense rigors. The *flush phase* brings rectal temperatures to 41 to 43°C (106 to 110°F) with profound peripheral vasodilation and a sharp drop in arterial blood pressure. After 7 to 8 hours, the *phase of defervescence* heralds recovery.

The J-HR occurs regularly during the treatment of relapsing fever but appears to be more profound in louseborne infections. Anticipation is prudent, and treatment should be directed toward the systemic symptoms and complications of the reaction. Hypotension may be controlled by intravenous fluid therapy in most cases, but occasionally vasopressors may be required as well. Digitalization is indicated if heart failure develops. A number of techniques have been tried to attenuate the J-HR. However, the use of slow-release penicillin (PAM), corticosteroids (either before or during the reaction), and antipyretics has had little or no effect on the intensity of the reaction.

Complications

The complications of relapsing fever include hemorrhage, heart failure, hepatic insufficiency, abortion, and splenic rupture. Respiratory and neurologic complications have also been described.

Hemorrhagic phenomena such as epistaxis, petechial skin rash, and rarely hemoptysis, hematemesis, hematochezia, and hematuria generally do not require specific therapy unless severe. Prolonged prothrombin times can be reversed with 10 to 20 mg of vitamin K intramuscularly. Disseminated intravascular coagulopathy (DIC) occurs uncommonly but should be considered when any severe hemorrhage is encountered. Therapy consists of (1) control of the infection with antimicrobial agents, (2) administration of heparin, 600 to 850 USP units per kg every 24 hours, and (3) transfusion (if indicated) with fresh blood, platelet-rich plasma, or platelet concentrates.

Splenic rupture may occur as a result of necrosis of splenic infarcts. Intense abdominal pain, initially in the left upper quarter, coupled with a falling blood pressure should suggest the need for an emergency splenectomy.

Prevention

Prevention of relapsing fever requires control of the arthropod vectors. In louseborne epidemics, mass delousing measures should be instituted. DDT-resistant louse strains have developed, and insecticides such as malathion (1 to 5 per cent powder) may be necessary. For individual use, pediculicides such as pyrethrins and piperonyl butoxide (Rid), malathion (Prioderm Lotion) or lindane (Kwell) are suggested. In areas of endemic tickborne disease, the use of protective clothing and repellents such as diethyl-m-toluamide (Off) may be helpful.

When hospitalized, patients with relapsing fever do not require isolation, but blood may remain infectious outside the body for up to 4 days. Careful needle and syringe handling is essential, and care in the laboratory is prudent.

RHEUMATIC FEVER

method of
AMNON ROSENTHAL, M.D.
University of Michigan
Ann Arbor, Michigan

The serious early and long-term consequences of rheumatic fever are related to the presence and severity of cardiac involvement and not other manifestations of the disease. Because of the lifelong implications of the diagnosis of rheumatic fever to the patient, consultation with a cardiologist is highly desirable during the initial acute phase and if possible prior to the initiation of therapy. New diagnostic techniques such as echocardiography have been particularly useful in detecting and confirming cardiovascular involvement. Pericardial effusion, valvular changes, and mild degrees of myocardial dysfunction and enlargement can be diagnosed by two-dimensional echocardiography. Doppler echocardiography may be helpful in the initial identification of mitral or aortic regurgitation. The important measures in the treatment of rheumatic fever are bed rest, aspirin or steroids or both, eradication and prevention of group A streptococcal infections, and patient and parent education about the disease. Despite numerous national and international cooperative controlled studies, there is no uniformity of opinion or consensus regarding the type, dose, or duration of anti-inflammatory drug used, or the duration of bed rest. Furthermore, there is no evidence that therapy with salicylates or steroids prevents subsequent permanent residual heart disease.

Hospitalization

A patient known to have or suspected of having acute rheumatic fever should be hospitalized for complete evaluation and initiation of therapy. Hospitalization provides an appropriate opportunity to monitor closely signs of rheumatic activity (temperature, sleeping pulse rate, serum phase reactants), therapeutic and potential adverse effects of anti-inflammatory medications, possible progression of valvular regurgitation, or development of congestive heart failure. When carditis with cardiomegaly is present, hospitalization should be at a tertiary care center. The hospital stay for the patient will be between 2 and 12 weeks, rarely longer, depending on the severity of the illness.

Bed Rest and Diet

Bed rest alleviates symptoms and facilitates healing. The required rest and period of ambulation depend to a large extent on the cardiac involvement (Table 1), the patient's age, clinical or laboratory findings, and rheumatic activity. Bathroom privileges should be allowed to all but the most symptomatic patients. Bed rest should be maintained as long as fever (temperature, ≥37.8°C or 100°F), tachycardia (sleeping heart rate, ≥100 per min), elevated sedimentation rate (Wintrobe, ≥20 mm per hr), or a positive serum C-reactive protein is demonstrated. Ambulation should be gradual, limited initially to indoor and subsequently to outdoor activity. Return to school may be achieved within 4 to 6 weeks of the onset of acute rheumatic fever if there is no carditis, 8 to 10 weeks in patients with carditis but without cardiomegaly, and 3 to 6 months in those with cardiomegaly or congestive failure. No special diet is required. A low salt diet may be necessary in those with marked congestive heart failure.

Anti-Inflammatory Agents

Salicylates, steroids, or steroids and salicylates in combination are used to relieve symptoms and reduce the inflammatory process. In general, salicylates alone suffice in the absence of carditis, or when carditis is mild and manifested by hemodynamically insignificant mitral or aortic regurgitation. If cardiomegaly, pancarditis, or congestive heart failure is present, steroids are preferred (Table 1). The response of arthritis to aspirin is excellent and occurs within 24 to 48 hours of the onset of therapy. The response to steroids in the patient with pancarditis or congestive heart failure is often dramatic. For the patient without carditis, salicylates, 100 mg per kg per 24 hours in four divided doses, are begun, and a serum salicylate level of 20 to 25 mg per dl is maintained. A higher dose of 100 to 140 mg per kg per 24 hours is occasionally required in younger children. The total dose should not exceed 10 grams per day. The dose is reduced after 2 weeks to 75 mg per kg per 24 hours and gradually tapered over the next 2 to 4 weeks. If side effects of salicylates develop, such as tinnitus, hyperventilation, nausea, emesis, or hepatic damage, the dose should be adjusted. We occasionally prefer to use enteric-coated tablets or Ascriptin (aspirin with Maalox) because these tend to produce less gastric irritation. The antacid, however, may decrease the effectiveness of the salicylate. When carditis without cardiomegaly is present, a similar initial dose of salicylates is used. After 3 to 4 weeks the dose is reduced to 75 mg per kg per 24 hours for 1 to 2 weeks and then gradually tapered over a 2 week period.

In the presence of cardiomegaly, more severe carditis, or hemodynamically significant mitral or aortic regurgitation, steroids are used. Prednisone is the steroid of choice because of the extensive accumulated experience with the drug, its lower toxicity, and fewer side effects. Initial therapy is 2 mg per kg per 24 hours (not to exceed 60 mg per day) in two divided doses. After 2 weeks the prednisone is reduced to 1 mg per kg per 24 hours, and concomitantly salicylates, 100 mg per kg per 24 hours, are begun. Two weeks later the prednisone is gradually tapered over 1 to 2 weeks while the dose of salicylates is maintained for a full 2 weeks. During the last 2 to 4 weeks of therapy, the patient is off steroids while salicylates are gradually tapered.

When severe carditis, pericarditis, or congestive heart failure is present, prednisone and salicylates are used as indicated for patients with cardiomegaly. However, prednisone in full dose is used for 2 to 4 weeks, in reduced dose (1 mg per kg per 24 hours) from 4 to 6 more weeks, and then gradually tapered over a 1 to 2 week period. Anti-inflammatory therapy should total 3 months, or longer if clinical evidence of conges-

TABLE 1. **General Guidelines for Bed Rest and Anti-Inflammatory Therapy for Patients with Acute Rheumatic Fever**

Cardiac Diagnoses	Bed Rest and Ambulation	Anti-Inflammatory Therapy
No carditis	Bed rest for 2 weeks, slow indoor ambulation for 1–2 weeks	Salicylates for 4–6 weeks
Carditis, no cardiomegaly	Bed rest for 4 weeks, slow indoor ambulation for 2–4 weeks	Salicylates for 6–8 weeks
Carditis and cardiomegaly	Best rest for 6 weeks, slow indoor ambulation for 4 weeks	Prednisone for 6–8 weeks. After 2 weeks reduce prednisone dose and add salicylates. Maintain salicylates for 4–6 weeks
Carditis with congestive heart failure	Bed rest for the duration of heart failure and persistence of rheumatic activity. Slow ambulation over 6–12 weeks	Prednisone for 8–10 weeks. After 2–4 weeks reduce prednisone dose and add salicylates. Maintain salicylates as long as congestive failure is present

tive failure or rheumatic activity persists. Side effects of prednisone therapy may include cushingoid features, emotional lability, peptic ulcer, systemic hypertension, sodium retention, and to a lesser extent loss of potassium. It is therefore important to be alert to the onset of epigastric pain or discomfort, to search for the presence of blood in the stool, and to monitor blood pressure twice daily.

While on steroids, patients are at increased risk of other complications. Contact with chickenpox should be avoided in those without prior infection since it could result in severe disseminated disease. In tuberculin-positive children, steroids are best omitted. In superimposed severe bacterial infection, the steroid dose may need to be reduced or gradually withdrawn.

Clinical and laboratory rebound phenomena may occur when anti-inflammatory therapy is tapered or discontinued. They generally subside spontaneously and rarely require reinstitution of therapy.

Antibiotics

Since rheumatic fever follows a group A streptococcal infection, therapy with penicillin is essential for eradication of the organism. It should be administered after a throat culture is obtained. Benzathine penicillin (Bicillin), 1.2 million units intramuscularly, is the treatment of choice. Oral penicillin V, 0.5 grams four times a day for 10 days, is a less desirable alternative. Patients allergic to penicillin should receive oral erythromycin, 250 mg four times a day (for small children, 40 mg per kg per day) for 10 days. A lower dose of antibiotic is administered after the therapeutic dose to prevent subsequent beta-streptococcal infections.

Congestive Heart Failure

When there is clinical evidence of congestive heart failure, a low sodium diet, mild fluid restriction, and diuretics are utilized. We prefer intravenous furosemide (Lasix), 1 mg per kg, in severe or acute situations when immediate diuresis is desirable. In mild congestive heart failure or after a satisfactory response to furosemide in more severe cases, a combination of oral chlorothiazide (Diuril), 20 mg per kg per day divided in two doses, and spironolactone (Aldactone), 2 mg per kg per day in two divided doses, provide satisfactory diuresis.

Digoxin is helpful in patients with florid congestive heart failure and should be used with caution. As in other forms of myocarditis the heart is most sensitive to digoxin. In children, the digitalizing dose is 0.02 to 0.03 mg per kg, half given immediately and a quarter of the dose 6 to 8 hours later and repeated after 6 to 8 hours. In adults the total digitalizing dose is 1.5 to 2.5 mg given in a similar fashion.

The serum potassium should be monitored since hypokalemia may result from decreased intake of potassium or the use of diuretics and steroids. Afterload reducers such as sodium nitroprusside (Nipride) intravenously, 0.5 to 5 micrograms per kg per minute; prazosin (Minipress) orally, 5 micrograms per kg per dose up to a maximum of 25 micrograms per kg every 6 hours; or hydralazine (Apresoline) orally 0.5 to 2.0 mg per kg per day in three or four divided doses, may also be helpful in patients with severe mitral regurgitation and congestive heart failure. While a patient is on therapy, left ventricular performance should be monitored by periodic echocardiograms or radionuclide studies.

Arrhythmias

These are rare in acute rheumatic fever. Second degree heart block usually responds to atropine. Third degree heart block will require a pacemaker if associated with a slow rate, congestive heart failure, or symptoms; steroids should also be used. Atrial ectopy may require no therapy or, if associated with cardiovascular compromise, can usually be controlled with digoxin. Ventricular ectopy may be secondary to digoxin or myocarditis; therapy will depend on type, severity, and associated symptoms.

Cardiac Surgery

Cardiac surgery, such as aortic value or mitral valve replacement, may be required during the course of therapy for acute rheumatic fever in patients with intractable congestive heart failure or when the illness is complicated by bacterial endocarditis. Cardiac surgical consultation should be obtained if such intervention is anticipated or suspected and before the patient is in extremis.

Preventive Therapy

1. *Prevention of group A streptococcal infection and recurrence of rheumatic fever.* Recurrent episodes of streptococcal infection are associated with recurrence of rheumatic fever. Carditis may develop in those in whom carditis did not occur during the initial episode. To prevent the development or recurrence of carditis, *all patients* with rheumatic fever should be on continuous antistreptococcal antibiotic prophylaxis.

The most effective regimen is 1.2 million units of benzathine penicillin (Bicillin) every 28 days. This regimen should be used in all patients with prior carditis and cardiomegaly and in those in a poor social situation, with questionable compliance and uncertain medical follow-up. In all others, 250 mg of penicillin V (Pen-Vee K) twice a day provides excellent protection. Compliance with oral penicillin therapy may be monitored by urinalysis. Oral penicillin prophylaxis leads to the appearance of resistant alpha-streptococci in the oropharynx whereas intramuscular benzathine penicillin does not.

For patients allergic to penicillin, sulfadiazine, 500 mg twice a day (once daily for children under 30 kg), provides adequate protection. While adverse reactions to sulfonamides are rare, a complete blood count is advisable 2 weeks after the initiation of therapy.

Prophylaxis should be continued to at least age 21 years in those without prior carditis and probably as long as there is a high risk of exposure to streptococcal infections (for example in schoolteachers, nurses, and physicians). In patients with carditis or rheumatic heart disease, prophylaxis is for life.

2. *Antimicrobial prophylaxis for the prevention of bacterial endocarditis.* The antimicrobial prophylaxis used to prevent recurrences of rheumatic fever is not sufficient for prevention of bacterial endocarditis in patients with rheumatic heart disease. *Streptococcus viridans* resistant to penicillin may be present in the oral cavity. The American Heart Association therefore recommends that patients on continuous oral penicillin be given erythromycin for dental procedures that cause gingival bleeding and for other oral and respiratory tract surgery. Erythromycin dosage is 1.0 gram (20 mg per kg for children) 1 hour prior to the procedure and then 500 mg (10 mg per kg for children) 6 hours later. The child's dose should not exceed the adult dose. For those who are on continuous erythromycin or cannot tolerate erythromycin, an oral cephalosporin such as cephalexin (Keflex) or cephradine (Anspor), 1.0 gram 1 hour prior to the procedure plus 500 mg 6 hours later, may be useful. In patients with a prosthetic valve, those at high risk of bacterial endocarditis, and those undergoing genitourinary or gastrointestinal tract procedures, parenteral ampicillin and gentamicin are recommended. Ampicillin, 1.0 to 2.0 grams (50 mg per kg for children) *plus* gentamicin, 1.5 mg per kg (2.0 mg per kg for children) are given intramuscularly or intravenously 0.5 hour prior to the procedure and 8 hours later. In patients at high risk of penicillin allergy, intravenous vancomycin, 1.0 gram (20 mg per kg for children) is given *slowly* starting 1 hour prior to the procedure. A repeat dose is not necessary. Children's antibiotic doses should not exceed the maximum adult dose.

3. *Maintenance of good dental hygiene* to reduce bacteremia and colonization of heart valves. Gingivitis or periodontal infections are associated with increased bacteremia in the absence of any dental procedures.

4. *Periodic follow up and cardiovascular evaluation.* Yearly cardiovascular examinations are advised for all patients, especially those with an initial episode of carditis. Periodic evaluation will detect the subsequent development or progression of rheumatic heart disease and such lesions as mitral stenosis or mitral regurgitation. Periodic noninvasive studies such as an electrocardiogram, chest radiograph, or echocardiogram are recommended for those individuals with definite cardiomegaly or congestive heart failure at the initial episode. During follow-up, any symptoms suggesting a recurrence of rheumatic fever require throat culture, sedimentation rate, antistreptolysin titer, and C-reactive protein studies to exclude recrudescence.

5. *Relatives, especially siblings with streptococcal infections, should receive early and adequate treatment.* Symptomatic children with a sore throat, tonsillitis, or otitis should have a throat culture and be treated with penicillin if acutely ill or if a throat culture is positive for group A streptococcus. If rheumatic fever is to be prevented, treatment should be provided within 5 days of the onset of symptoms.

Patient and Family Education

Since the diagnosis of rheumatic fever has serious lifelong ramifications, the patient and family should be fully informed about the pathogenesis of the disease, the therapy, and the long-term prognosis. Periodic discussions should reinforce the need for preventing streptococcal infections, the possibility of future recurrences, appropriate therapy for streptococcal infections, and the need for different antibiotic prophylaxis for the prevention of bacterial endocarditis. Insurability and employability should also be discussed and the young patient guided toward recreational and vocational goals that can be met and practiced during adult life. Various educational materials may be obtained for patients from affiliates of the local American Heart Association or the national office in Dallas, Texas.

Chorea

Chorea generally occurs as an isolated manifestation of acute rheumatic fever. Despite the often severe neurologic involvement and prolonged course, which may last 3 to 6 months, it is self-limiting and without permanent residua. Anti-inflammatory therapy is usually of little benefit, though in severe cases prednisone has been used. Treatment with penicillin to eradicate streptococcus is required. Sedatives are often helpful in controlling the chorea and making the patient more comfortable. In most cases phenobarbital (15 to 30 mg every 6 hours) is effective. If this is ineffective, oral diazepam (Valium), 0.2

mg per kg per 24 hours, divided every 6 hours (maximum, 0.8 mg per kg), chlorpromazine (Thorazine), or haloperidol (Haldol) may be used. The patient should be in a quiet room and measures taken to protect against self-injury (padded bed railing). Continuous reassurance and support to the patient by the family, nurses, and physicians is required concerning the self-limiting nature of the symptoms.

ROCKY MOUNTAIN SPOTTED FEVER

method of
TIMOTHY W. LANE, M.D.
The Moses H. Cone Memorial Hospital
Greensboro, North Carolina

Rocky Mountain spotted fever (RMSF) caused by *Rickettsia rickettsii* is the most common of the rickettsial infections that occur in the United States and carries the greatest burden of morbidity and mortality. It is recognized in nearly all the contiguous states and is particularly prevalent in southeastern and south central regions of the country. Other rickettsial infections that can be confused with RMSF, even though they have a much lower incidence, include flying squirrel–associated endemic typhus, rare cases of recrudescent endemic typhus, murine typhus, and rickettsialpox. The most important challenge to the clinician is considering the possibility of RMSF and instituting effective antimicrobial therapy early in the course of illness. Accurately differentiating RMSF from other infectious diseases with similar signs and symptoms is frequently impossible, and empiric antibiotic treatment is justified if the clinical presentation is compatible.

Clinical Manifestations. The incubation period after tick bite and before onset of symptomatic RMSF ranges from 3 to 14 days. Most often, symptomatic RMSF follows 6 to 8 days after tick exposure. The typical onset is relatively abrupt over 1 to 3 days. The patient complains of striking malaise, chills, abdominal pain, diffuse myalgias, prominent headache, and high (39 to 40°C, 102 to 104°F) fever. Nausea and vomiting are commonly present, and diarrhea is seen in as many as 25 per cent of patients. The presence of diarrhea may lead to misdiagnosis of a viral or bacterial enteritis and inappropriate therapy. Early in the illness, RMSF may occasionally show a picture compatible with aseptic meningitis with cerebrospinal fluid pleocytosis (10 to 50 mononuclear white blood cells per ml), leading to diagnostic confusion with viral meningitis that has the same seasonal pattern. Cervical and occipital lymphadenopathy, splenomegaly, and nonpurulent conjunctivitis are present in 5 to 15 per cent of patients. Other signs and symptoms seen in less than 5 per cent include jaundice, orchitis, parotitis, and sensorineural hearing loss.

A helpful diagnostic finding is the appearance of the rash of RMSF. Typically the onset is 3 to 6 days into illness; the rash begins on the distal extremities, including the palms and soles, and spreads centrally. Exceptions are common, and in about 20 per cent rash can be diffuse when first noted. The rash begins as faint, small (3 to 5 mm), blanching erythematous macules that can progress to petechial lesions. Ten to 15 per cent of patients with RMSF have no rash at all or develop a late rash after 10 days of illness. These so-called cases of Rocky Mountain "spotless" fever occur disproportionately in elderly adults and are more likely to result in delayed recognition and a fatal outcome. In advanced, untreated cases of RMSF, usually of more than a week's duration, severe manifestations can include pneumonitis, myocarditis with shock, rhabdomyolysis with elevated serum CPK levels, renal failure, gangrene of skin and occasionally the distal extremities, and encephalitis that can be accompanied by coma, seizures, and focal cranial nerve deficits. Rarely, frank, disseminated intravascular coagulation will be evident in severe cases.

Diagnosis. Diagnosis of RMSF usually is based on the clinical presentation, history of tick exposure, and, if applicable, residence in or travel to a highly endemic area. The initial diagnosis is almost always a clinical one since serologic confirmation is not possible until about 2 weeks after onset of symptoms. Definitive diagnosis is made by demonstrating a fourfold or greater rise of specific antibody titers between acute and convalescent specimens. Antibodies to Weil-Felix antigens such as OX-19 are nonspecific, and complement-fixing antibodies are too insensitive to be clinically useful anymore. Currently, more accurate serologic methods include indirect immunofluorescent assays, hemagglutination, and latex agglutination. Rarely are any of these serologic tests positive in the early symptomatic phase of illness, and 10 to 14 days are required after onset for serologic conversion. Treatment, therefore, should never be withheld on the basis of negative or nondiagnostic antibody titers. Rickettsial culture is performed in research laboratories but is too hazardous and costly for widespread use. Biopsy of the skin rash and immunofluorescent rickettsial antibody staining can be rapidly confirmatory, with an overall sensitivity of about 70 per cent, but is limited in availability. False-negative results are common if the skin biopsy is delayed beyond 48 hours after instituting effective antibiotic treatment.

Nonspecific clinical clues can be obtained from routine laboratory tests. For example, about 90 per cent of patients with RMSF have a "left-shifted" white blood count (>5 per cent immature forms of polymorphonuclear leukocytes); 30 per cent have hyponatremia (<135 mMol per liter); and 10 to 15 per cent have thrombocytopenia (<100,000 per ml) in the first few days of illness. Mild to moderate elevations in hepatocellular enzymes are common. Because of the delay in the development of positive antibody titers and the lack of sensitive and specific diagnostic tests, diagnosis relies on clinical judgment and on no single finding. A low threshold for early empiric antibiotic treatment when RMSF is suspected, even in the absence of a typical rash, is defensible. Therapy begun before the seventh day of symptoms usually prevents serious complications and death.

Treatment

RMSF is equally effectively treated with tetracycline or chloramphenicol prescribed for 7 to 10 days. Chloramphenicol should be reserved for pregnant women because of fetal bone abnormalities and an increased risk of maternal hepatitis associated with the use of tetracyclines. Otherwise tetracyclines are preferred to avoid the possibility, although rare, of serious blood dyscrasias caused by chloramphenicol. Doxycycline, 50 mg to 100 mg orally or intravenously twice daily, can be used if azotemia is present. The usual adult dosage of chloramphenicol is 500 mg orally or intravenously every 6 hours. The dosage of chloramphenicol in children is 75 mg per kg per day given orally or intravenously in divided doses every 6 hours. Prolonged or repetitive courses of tetracycline can cause discoloration of permanent teeth in children less than 8 years of age, but an abbreviated course of 7 days at 25 mg per kg per day orally in divided dosages, not to exceed 2 grams daily, can be prescribed without discernible dental staining. Tetracycline is avoided when children require intravenous treatment. Anyone given oral therapy on an outpatient basis should be closely followed to assure that vomiting does not interfere with antibiotic absorption. In mild to moderate cases of RMSF, resolution of the signs and symptoms occurs gradually over 3 to 5 days after beginning antibiotic treatment. It may be longer in more severe cases.

Supportive intensive care is important in the severely ill patient. Particular attention must be paid to volume status. Such patients are often dehydrated, but fluid replacement must be judicious because the diffuse capillary injury of RMSF can result in pulmonary edema. In the critically ill with obtundation, seizures, renal failure, and hypovolemia, intensive care with vital sign monitoring and Swan-Ganz catheter measurement of capillary wedge pressure is often necessary. Pharmacologic doses of corticosteroids in the critically ill have been recommended, but there is no substantial evidence to support their use.

Prevention

Public knowledge of RMSF and its tick vectors is probably the best method of prevention. Avoiding outdoor activities in tick-infested areas is often not practical. An alternative is to recommend frequent and vigilant examination for ticks during warm weather months in persons and especially in children with outdoor exposures. Hairlines, the scalp, and axillae are the usual areas of tick attachment. Any discovered ticks should be carefully removed with a facial tissue or tweezers since RMSF can be transmitted through inapparent cuts on unprotected fingers. Cleansing of the site of attachment with soap and water after removal is prudent. A calender notation of the date of tick removal for possible future reference is recommended. Prophylactic antibiotic treatment after tick bite is unnecessary because of the small likelihood that an individual tick is infected with *R. rickettsii*. Gloves should be worn when manually deticking dogs and other domestic animals. Tick repellents have been advocated but their utility is uncertain. Vaccines have been shown not to be protective and are no longer available.

Vigilance by the physician is crucial for the prevention of serious morbidity and mortality.

RUBELLA AND CONGENITAL RUBELLA

method of
JOHN L. SEVER, M.D., Ph.D.
National Institutes of Health
Bethesda, Maryland

Epidemiology

In the United States, epidemics of rubella formerly occurred at 5 to 7 year intervals. Sporadic cases were present every year, primarily in the spring. The last epidemic was in 1964; following it over 20,000 infants were born with the congenital rubella syndrome (CRS). The vaccine program, begun in the late 1960s, was directed at preschool children and susceptible women of child-bearing age. We now recommend immunization of all children at 15 months of age, along with the simultaneous administration of mumps and measles vaccines. Also, women should be tested for antibody; if negative, they should be immunized for rubella when not pregnant.

The widespread use of the vaccine in this country has changed the epidemiology of the disease. Only a few thousand cases of rubella are now reported each year, and usually fewer than 25 children with the CRS. In recent years most cases have been in older school-age children and in young adults who, because of their age, missed the pre-school immunization programs begun in 1968. Rubella also occurs in certain unimmunized populations, such as illegal aliens, foreign students, and religious groups that refuse vaccines. Immunization results in about a 95 per cent seroconversion rate, and thus occasional vaccinated individuals remain susceptible and may experience the disease.

ACQUIRED RUBELLA

Rubella is a very mild disease, particularly in childhood. About one third of infections are subclinical. The usual findings are slight fever, a macular rash which begins on the face and spreads to the shoulders, back, and arms over a period of 1 to 2 days, and posterior auricular or suboccipital adenopathy. The skin lesions vary in size and tend to coalesce into reddish areas during the second or third day. The patient is usually not particularly ill and responds well to rest and aspirin for the fever. The symptoms last about 3 days.

In older children, adults, and particularly women of child-bearing age, the disease may be more severe. These individuals may experience the additional findings of joint pains, petechiae, and conjunctivitis. There are also extremely rare cases of postrubella encephalitis.

Serology. For the serologic documentation of acute rubella, paired serum specimens can be tested when the first specimen is obtained within 2 days of the onset of the rash and the second specimen taken 2 or more weeks later. A seroconversion will establish the diagnosis. However, we now prefer to use a single IgM rubella antibody test with the specimen taken 7 to 28 days after the rash. The presence of IgM rubella antibody indicates very recent infection. A word of caution: recently, some very sensitive IgM tests have shown low levels of IgM rubella antibody in some cases following re-exposure to rubella or vaccination for rubella. The sensitivity of the IgM rubella test must be considered in evaluating these results.

To distinguish immunity and susceptibility, a single serum specimen should be tested for IgG rubella antibody, using any of the many methods now available. We prefer the newer latex agglutination test because it is very rapid (8 minutes), no pretreatment of the serum is needed, the test is read visually, and it can be performed easily in any laboratory or physician's office.

Treatment

Isolation

The individual with acquired rubella sheds the virus from the nasopharynx for about 1 week before and 1 week after the onset of rash. The virus is also in the blood and urine for 1 week before the rash but disappears from these two sites just after the rash begins. The incubation period is 12 to 21 days (average, 12 to 14 days). Whenever possible, patients should be isolated, particularly from susceptible pregnant women, during the period of virus excretion from the nasopharynx.

Management of Exposed Pregnant Women

Since 15 per cent of women are susceptible to rubella, it is important to test women of child-bearing age for antibody to rubella. The immune pregnant woman should be informed that there is no risk for rubella or congenital rubella. However, if she does not have antibody she must be informed that she could develop rubella, in which the risk for significant fetal damage varies with the month of gestation. The risk is approximately 50 per cent with infection in the first month; 22 per cent in the second month; 10 per cent in the third month; and 6 per cent in the fourth and fifth months. There is no danger after the fifth month. The vaccine is of no value for the exposed patient.

In the past, large doses of gamma globulin (20 ml) were given to exposed women in an attempt to prevent rubella. Some studies showed good protection but others did not. This is no longer recommended except for women who indicate they will not consider a therapeutic abortion if they develop rubella. In those cases, since no other therapy is available, 20 ml of gamma globulin should be offered but the patient should be informed of the questionable value of the procedure.

If infection occurs in a pregnant woman, a therapeutic abortion may be considered based on the aforementioned risks. A recent approach for patients who are considering abortion has been to offer testing of fetal blood for IgM antibody to rubella as a means of identifying infected versus uninfected fetuses. This, of course, requires the availability of a center where in utero fetal blood samples can be obtained. Also, IgM antibody to rubella is not made by the fetus until the fifth month of gestation, and the test and possible abortion must be delayed until that time. There have been a few attempts to isolate virus from amniotic fluid as a method of identifying infected children. While there have been several reports of virus isolations, there is insufficient information to document sensitivity of the test and to correlate this with risks for fetal damage.

CONGENITAL RUBELLA

The transmission of rubella virus to the fetus is by the blood through the placenta. Almost 100 per cent of placentas are infected when maternal infection occurs in the first 5 months of pregnancy.

The most frequent defect of the congenital rubella syndrome is deafness. This may be alone or in combination with other major damage, including cardiac malformations (particularly peripheral pulmonic stenosis and patent ductus arteriosus), cataracts and glaucoma, microcephaly, and mental retardation. In the newborn period there may also be low birth weight, failure to thrive, anemia, thombocytopenia and bleeding, hepatosplenomegaly, jaundice, and radiolucencies in the long bones. Severe disease may result in fetal death; in addition, about one third of children with the CRS die in the neonatal period. Rubella defects associated with infection in the fifth and sixth months are usually limited to deafness and mental retardation.

Serology. To confirm the diagnosis of congenital rubella, virus isolation may be used since the virus persists in the nasopharynx of the child for 6 to 12 months. This study, however, is difficult and expensive, and we now usually use the IgM rubella antibody test for this purpose. IgM rubella antibody is present at birth in the CRS and persists for 6 to 12 months. This simple serum test can be used to document congenital infection. We prefer the ELISA method, but other IgM rubella tests are satisfactory. The presence of IgM rubella antibody in an infant indicates congenital rubella or recently acquired infection.

Management of the Child with Congenital Rubella

Children with the CRS may excrete virus from the nasopharynx for 6 to 12 months. The virus may also be present in the urine, stool, and spinal fluid. Virus has been recovered from cataracts removed surgically 3 or more years after birth. Since the virus from the children is fully infectious, care should be taken to avoid contact with susceptible pregnant women during the first year of life.

No drugs are available to terminate the infection. Supportive therapy may be needed for severely ill children. As soon as possible, the child should be referred to a center for full evaluation by a team of specialists. Multiply handicapped children may require surgery for cataracts and heart defects, as well as special schooling. Hearing should be tested carefully in all CRS children.

Late Effects of Congenital Rubella

Longitudinal studies of children with the CRS have shown that about 20 per cent become diabetic by 20 to 30 years of age, and most of these require insulin. Small numbers of CRS patients may have abnormalities of the thyroid, parathyroid, and pituitary or may become deaf later in childhood. In very rare instances the child may suffer from progressive rubella panencephalitis (PRP). This disease appears in the second decade of life. The illness usually begins with ataxia, myoclonus, and/or mental deterioration. The disability progresses slowly over a period of years, and the outcome is fatal. The disease is due to a persistent and extending rubella infection of the brain, which develops 10 or more years after birth. PRP has also been reported, with rarity, after rubella acquired during the first 2 years of life.

PREVENTION

Use of Vaccine

The rubella vaccine now used in the United States is the live, attenuated RA/27 strain grown in human diploid cultures. More than 95 per cent of vaccinees develop antibody after immunization, and antibody appears to persist for life. All children should receive the vaccine except those with congenital immunodeficiencies or patients receiving immunosuppressive chemotherapy. The vaccine should be given with mumps and measles vaccines in one injection at 15 months of age. Most schools require documentation of immunization or immunity based on serologic tests for antibody. There is a low incidence of side effects with the vaccine, particularly in adults, and these include transient rubella-like rash, fever, joint pains, and petechiae.

Vaccine During Pregnancy

It is specifically recommended that the vaccine not be given to pregnant women, and immunized women should not become pregnant for 3 months. This is because of the theoretic risk that the live vaccine might infect the fetus and cause damage.

Some women have been inadvertently immunized during early pregnancy, and others have become pregnant after vaccination. Epidemiologic data gathered by The Centers for Disease Control (CDC) indicate that the risk for fetal damage in these cases must be very small. In a recent report from the CDC, 216 susceptible women who received the vaccine 3 months before or after conception were followed to term, and none of the children had defects associated with congenital rubella. Statistically, this indicates that the risk for fetal damage caused by rubella in women immunized 3 months before or after conception is less than 2 per cent. Two of the children, however, did have IgM antibody to rubella, indicating that in these cases the vaccine virus crossed the placenta and infected the fetus. In another study of susceptible vaccinated women who elected to have therapeutic abortions, rubella virus was recovered from one of 12 products of conception. This also indicates a low risk for transmission of the vaccine virus to the fetus. At present, only about 10 per cent of susceptible women who are immunized within 3 months of conception elect to have a therapeutic abortion. Because of the possible risk to the fetus, however, we continue to recommend that the vaccine not be given to pregnant women, and immunized women should not become pregnant for 3 months.

Transmission of the Vaccine Virus

Extensive studies have shown that the vaccine virus does not transmit from vaccinated individuals to susceptible contacts, even among members of the same household. Thus, it is safe, for example, to give the vaccine to the children of a susceptible pregnant woman. Also, immunization of women in the immediate postpartum period is recommended. Transmission of the vaccine virus through the milk to the neonate is not of concern. The virus has been found in the milk of some immunized women, but transmission to the child has been reported only in one case. The child developed a brief, mild, rubella-like illness, Thus, even if the vaccine virus is transmitted through the milk in rare instances, the child apparently only develops brief, mild rubella along with a "free" immunization.

MEASLES (RUBEOLA)

method of
NASREEN A. BHUMBRA, M.D.,
and GEORGE A. NANKERVIS, Ph.D., M.D.
Medical College of Ohio
Toledo, Ohio

Measles is a highly contagious viral disease with significant morbidity and mortality. After an incubation period of 10 to 12 days, there is approximately a 4 day prodrome characterized by fever, cough, coryza, conjunctivitis, photophobia, and Koplik's spots (gray-white dots with an erythematous base on the buccal and pharyngeal mucosa). A confluent maculopapular rash then erupts on the face and neck and spreads to other parts of the body. The rash, accompanied by an abrupt temperature rise, resolves within 7 to 10 days with desquamation.

When exposed to wild virus, individuals previously immunized with inactivated measles vaccine frequently develop atypical measles, a severe illness characterized by high fever, pulmonary disease, and a maculopapular or petechial rash. In addition, the administration of live vaccine to these patients has sometimes produced local erythema and induration.

Treatment

The treatment of uncomplicated measles is essentially supportive. Fever may be controlled by the use of 5 to 10 mg per kg of acetaminophen (Tylenol, Tempra) every 4 to 6 hours and use of lightweight clothing. Solid foods are not desired, but adequate intake of fluids should be encouraged. As the fever resolves and the anorexia and malaise subside, normal diet and activity can be resumed. Humidification of the room with cold steam may help the harsh, irritating cough. The cough is usually resistant to common antitussives, but the use of these agents is not contraindicated. Nasal congestion may be treated with normal saline nose drops and suction with a bulb syringe, and dryness and irritation about the nares may be prevented by a local application of petroleum jelly (Vaseline). Dim light may decrease the discomfort of photophobia, but the routine use of antibiotic eye drops or ointment is not recommended.

Complications

If fever persists beyond the third day of rash or recurs after an afebrile period, the possibility of complications should be considered. Most of the secondary complications arise from bacterial invasion.

Otitis Media. This is a frequent complication, particularly in the young, and should be treated according to the suspected bacterial etiology for the age group. In children under 6 years of age, *Streptococcus pneumoniae, Haemophilus influenzae,* and *Streptococcus pyogenes* are the more common agents. In older children, *Haemophilus influenzae* infection is unlikely. Effective 10 day therapeutic regimens include the following:

1. Amoxicillin (Amoxil, Larotid)—40 mg per kg per day in three doses.
2. If a penicillinase-producing *Haemophilus influenzae* is suspected, alternative treatments are suggested.

    Combined erythromycin ethylsuccinate and acetyl sulfisoxazole (Pediazole), 50 mg per kg per day of erythromycin component in four doses.

    Trimethoprim-sulfamethoxazole (Bactrim, Septra), 6 to 8 mg per kg per day of trimethoprim component in two doses.

    Cefaclor (Ceclor), 40 mg per kg per day in three doses.

    Amoxicillin/potassium clavulanate (Augmentin), 40 mg per kg per day of amoxicillin component in three doses.

Pneumonia. Although a less frequent complication of measles than otitis, pneumonia is the leading cause of death in this disease. Pneumonia may result from the viral infection itself or may be secondary to superinfection with *Streptococcus pneumoniae, Streptococcus pyogenes, Staphylococcus aureus,* or *Haemophilus influenzae.* After appropriate cultures, antibiotic therapy for the most likely pathogen should be initiated.

Laryngotracheal Bronchitis. This entity is usually mild but rarely may be a severe complication. Serious cases should be hospitalized and treated with humidification and adequate fluid therapy. If airway obstruction occurs or becomes imminent, endotracheal intubation is necessary.

Encephalitis. Encephalitis is a rare complication. It usually develops between 2 and 6 days after onset of rash and is characterized by fever, headache, lethargy, coma, or convulsions, accompanied by signs of meningeal irritation and pleocytosis. The course is unpredictable and treatment is symptomatic and supportive. Mortality can be as high as 16 per cent. Rarely, the patient may develop subacute sclerosing panencephalitis, a progressive, fatal neurologic disease.

Myocarditis. This complication is infrequent but serious. Supportive therapy is required if myocarditis is accompanied by congestive heart failure.

Tuberculosis Activation. Measles can exacerbate

an existing tuberculous process and render the patient anergic. Appropriate antitubercular therapy should be instituted if this situation arises.

Prevention

Active Immunization

Live attenuated measles vaccine (Attenuvax) produces an antibody response in at least 95 per cent of recipients and should be administered at 15 months of age for maximum protection. It is usually given with the mumps and rubella vaccine (M-M-R-II). The vaccine should also be given to all infants immunized prior to one year of age and to those who have been simultaneously given gamma globulin and live measles vaccine. Other indications for the vaccine include persons previously immunized with killed virus vaccine, as well as unvaccinated individuals on the day of exposure to natural measles. Vaccination of adults is rarely necessary because nearly all are immune, but it is not contraindicated.

Vaccine reactions seem to be no more common in adults than in children. Side effects of the vaccine may be seen 7 to 10 days after administration of live vaccine and may include rash, fever, or both. More severe reactions such as malaise, fever, generalized lymphadenopathy, local erythema, and induration may occur in those previously immunized with killed vaccine. Contraindications to live vaccine administration include immunocompromised patients, persons with possible tuberculosis, pregnant women, and patients allergic to neomycin, eggs, chicken, or chicken feathers.

The spread of vaccine virus to susceptible individuals has not been documented. A 15 year follow-up of vaccinees has revealed a persistence of antibody: therefore, reimmunization is not indicated if the vaccine was properly administered. The protection achieved with killed measles vaccine has been shown to decline rapidly over a period of months, and inactivated virus vaccines are not recommended for routine use.

Passive Immunization

Measles prevention or modification in exposed susceptibles usually requires the administration of immune serum globulin (human). A preventive dose of 0.5 ml per kg of body weight (maximum dose not to exceed 15 ml) of immune globulin should be given intramuscularly to unimmunized children as soon as possible after exposure. Immunocompromised children require larger doses of immune globulin than do normal children. Immunologically competent persons who have been passively immunized should receive the live vaccine at age 15 months, or 3 months after the passive immunization if older than 12 months of age. Late administration of serum globulin will not prevent disease but usually leads to a modified course and reduces complications.

TETANUS

method of
C. KIRK AVENT, M.D.
The University of Alabama
Birmingham, Alabama

Tetanus is a rare disease in the United States: in 1984 64 cases were reported to the Centers for Disease Control. Neonatal tetanus, on the other hand, is a common and fatal disease in developing countries. Worldwide, over 50,000 people die every year from tetanus. The mortality rate for tetanus varies extensively, ranging from 10 per cent in mild disease to 80 per cent for severe tetanus. Prompt and aggressive treatment can significantly improve the chances for survival from this completely preventable disease.

Prevention

Immunization. Both active and passive immunization are used in the prevention of tetanus. The type of immunization given to the patient as prophylaxis is determined by the patient's previous immunization history.

The primary sequence of childhood immunization against tetanus involves four injections of combined diphtheria-pertussis-tetanus vaccine (DPT) at 2, 4, 6, and 18 months of age. A booster injection of DPT is given at age 4 to 6 years. For children more than 7 years old and for adults, immunity against tetanus and diphtheria can be reliably achieved by giving 0.5 ml alum-precipitated tetanus-diphtheria toxoid (Td) in three doses. The second injection is given 2 months after the first, and the third is given 6 months after the second. Lifelong immunity can be maintained by giving boosters of Td every 10 years.

Almost any significant, nonsterile wound should be considered "tetanus prone." If an individual has not received three or more doses of tetanus vaccine prior to the injury, 250 units of human tetanus immune globulin (TIG) are administered intramuscularly. In those parts of the world where TIG is not available, 1500 units of equine tetanus antitoxic serum (ATS) may be given after testing for hypersensitivity by injecting 0.05 ml of antitoxin subcutaneously. The specific recommendations of the United States Public Health Service Immunization Practices Advisory Committee are listed in Table 1.

TABLE 1. **Tetanus Prophylaxis in Wound Management**

History of Tetanus Immunization (*Doses*)	Clean Minor Wounds		All Other Wounds	
	Td	*TIG*	*Td*	*TIG*
Uncertain	Yes	No*	Yes	Yes
0 or 1	Yes	No*	Yes	Yes
2	Yes	No	Yes	No†
3 or more	No‡	No	No§	No

*Patients have developed tetanus following relatively trivial wounds. If a wound appears sufficiently severe to suggest a "tetanus booster," we would recommend that a careful history of immunization be obtained; if immunization is incomplete or dated, TIG should also be administered.

†Yes, if wound is more than 24 hours old.

‡Yes, if more than 10 years have elapsed since last dose.

§Yes, if more than 5 years have elapsed since last dose.

Treatment

Neutralization of Toxin. Tetanospasmin is rapidly bound to nerves. Once the toxin is bound to tissues, its effects cannot be blocked by antitoxin. When the diagnosis is first suspected, therefore, give 500 units of TIG by deep intramuscular injection. If TIG is not available, 10,000 units of ATS may be given with the precautions previously described. Although some authorities recommend the administration of 250 units of TIG intrathecally, this practice has not gained uniform acceptance.

Wound Treatment. Since tetanospasmin is so potent a toxin, the wound associated with tetanus may appear trivial or even be inapparent. If there is an obvious wound, it should be promptly incised, debrided, drained, and packed open. Aqueous penicillin G (1,000,000 units intravenously every 4 hours in adults) given for 5 days will eradicate the toxin-producing vegetative forms of *Clostridium tetani.* Adults allergic to penicillin may be given 500 mg of tetracycline or erythromycin every 6 hours orally or intravenously.

Control of Spasms. The patient should be placed in a quiet, dark room. Pentobarbital in doses of 150 to 250 mg intramuscularly may be used to sedate adults, but the effective dose may vary widely. Diazepam (Valium), 2 to 20 mg intravenously every 2 to 8 hours, may be used to control seizures.

Cardiovascular Complications. One of the most serious complications of tetanus is the syndrome of sympathetic overactivity, manifest by tachycardia, sweating, hyperpyrexia, and labile hypertension. Labetalol (Trandate, Normodyne), given to adults orally in doses of 50 to 100 mg every 6 hours or intravenously by constant infusion in doses of 1 to 2 mg per minute, is particularly useful because of its combined alpha- and beta-blocking properties.

Maintenance of Ventilation. In all cases careful attention must be paid to early signs of respiratory embarrassment. Intubation and mechanical ventilation are frequently required in generalized tetanus because of spasm of laryngeal muscles and the muscles of respiration. Dysphagia is an early sign that endotracheal intubation may be necessary. If the sedation necessary to control spasms produces hypoventilation or if the tetanic contractions themselves interfere with respiration, then endotracheal intubation, curarization, and intermittent positive pressure breathing will be required.

General Patient Support. Meticulous nursing care, enteral or parenteral alimentation, prophylactic heparinization, maintenance of a normal fluid and electrolyte balance, and bladder drainage are important general adjuncts to the specific measures used to treat tetanus.

Immunization. The quantity of tetanus toxin capable of producing clinical disease may not be sufficient to provoke an immune response. As a result, it is important to remember to give the full immunization sequence of three doses of toxoid to patients who have recovered from tetanus.

TOXOPLASMOSIS

method of
HENRY W. MURRAY, M.D.
The New York Hospital–Cornell Medical Center
New York, New York

Toxoplasmosis is a common and worldwide infection caused by the intracellular coccidian protozoa, *Toxoplasma gondii.* After cysts or oocysts are ingested, liberated trophozoites spread hematogenously to virtually every organ, where intracellular replication commences following phagocytosis by tissue macrophages or invasion of parenchymal cells. With the development of an effective immune response, extracellular trophozoites are killed by specific serum antibody, whereas intracellular Toxoplasma are killed or inhibited by T cell–dependent mechanisms. Some organisms, however, survive and form tissue cysts. The brain, retina, myocardium, lung, and skeletal muscle are favored sites for encystment. During the acute stages of toxoplasmosis, most patients remain asymptomatic or develop only nonspecific symptoms. In addition, although all individuals probably remain infected with tissue cysts for life, clinical problems related to chronic toxoplasmosis (other than perhaps reactivated ocular disease) seldom if ever develop in the immunocompetent adult. Thus, in most infected individuals treatment is never required. However, certain groups of patients do warrant specific therapy (see Table 1).

TABLE 1. **Syndromes Caused by *Toxoplasma gondii* Infection**

Toxoplasma Infection	Treatment Appropriate?
Acute	
Asymptomatic	No
Lymphadenitis	Rarely
Laboratory-acquired	Yes
Ocular (retinochoroiditis)	Yes
During pregnancy	Yes
Congenital	
Subclinical	Yes
Overt	Yes
Chronic/Reactivated	
Ocular	Yes
Disseminated	Yes

Antitoxoplasma Therapy

The combination of pyrimethamine plus sulfadiazine is the most effective regimen for the treatment of toxoplasmosis. These agents act synergistically against the proliferative trophozoite form of *T. gondii* but do not eradicate the tissue cysts. Pyrimethamine therapy is initiated with a loading dose of 2 mg per kg (up to 50 mg per day total) for the first 2 days, and thereafter 1 mg per kg (up to 25 mg per day) should be given only every 2 to 4 days because of the drug's long half-life (4 to 5 days). As a folic acid antagonist, pyrimethamine's principal adverse effect is dose-related bone marrow suppression. Although this effect can be reduced to a large extent by simultaneous treatment with 5 to 10 mg of intramuscular or oral folinic acid (calcium leucovorin) given three times per week, patients receiving pyrimethamine still must have complete blood and platelet counts performed at least weekly. Pyrimethamine may also cause headaches and gastrointestinal upset.

Among the sulfonamides, sulfadiazine, sulfapyrazine, sulfamerazine, and sulfamethazine all display activity against *T. gondii* and can act synergistically with pyrimethamine. Thus, either sulfadiazine or trisulfapyrimidine (a mixture of sulfapyrazine, sulfamerazine, and sulfamethazine) are appropriate to use. For both agents, a loading dose of 75 mg per kg (up to 4 grams) is given, followed by 100 mg per kg per day (up to 6 grams per day) in two or three divided doses. The half-life of sulfadiazine is 10 to 12 hours. Adverse reactions to the sulfonamides include fever, rash, leukopenia, thrombocytopenia, anemia, and gastrointestinal upset.

Three other agents have been used to treat patients with toxoplasmosis—spiramycin (not available in the USA), trimethoprim-sulfamethoxazole and clindamycin. For both trimethoprim-sulfamethoxazole and clindamycin, however, there is insufficient evidence to recommend their use. Although not generally available in the United States, spiramycin, a macrolide antibiotic, does appear to be useful in treating acute infection during pregnancy as well as congenital infection. Spiramycin is given at 100 mg per kg per day in two divided doses.

Patients Requiring Treatment

Immunologically Normal Individuals. Seldom do immunologically intact children or adults who develop acute symptomatic toxoplasmosis require treatment. However, with either vital organ involvement or a particularly severe or persistent illness, pyrimethamine plus sulfadiazine can be given for 4 to 6 weeks. Because of unknown virulence and direct inoculation, infections acquired by blood transfusion or laboratory accident probably also should be treated.

Retinochoroiditis. Active ocular toxoplasmosis, which is typically a manifestation of reactivated infection, should always be treated, using pyrimethamine plus sulfadiazine for 4 weeks. About two thirds of the patients show good responses; retreatment with multiple courses may be necessary in the remainder. If vision is threatened, corticosteroids (prednisone, 60 to 100 mg per day) should be employed to reduce the destructive inflammation caused at least in part by the apparent hypersensitivity component of the retinal disease. Although clindamycin is concentrated in the ocular choroid, convincing evidence that this antibiotic is effective in treating ocular toxoplasmosis has not been reported.

Infection in Pregnancy. Two goals in treating the pregnant woman in whom acute *Toxoplasma* infection can be documented and who elects not to undergo therapeutic abortion are (1) reducing the likelihood that the fetus will be infected, and (2) if infection does occur, attempting to treat the fetal infection. Currently available information suggests that treatment does reduce the incidence of fetal infection, but has little beneficial effect on already established infection. Empiric regimens employed in pregnant women from the time of diagnosis of acute toxoplasmosis include (a) repeated cycles of 3 weeks of spiramycin (2 to 3 grams per day) alternating with 2 weeks of no treatment until term, and (b) repeated cycles of 2 weeks of pyrimethamine plus sulfadiazine, alternating with 3 to 4 weeks of no treatment until term. Pyrimethamine should not be used during the first 16 weeks of pregnancy since it is teratogenic. Data are insufficient to know whether pyrimethamine is entirely safe later on in pregnancy or whether sulfadiazine alone is as effective as spiramycin.

Congenital Toxoplasmosis. Although little firm evidence indicates clear benefit from drug treatment of infants born with established neurologic or systemic *T. gondii* infections, therapy for 6 to 12 months is recommended in hopes of limiting further infection or tissue damage and to potentially ameliorate the effects of late sequelae. Infants with both overt and subclinical congenital infections have been treated for a total of up to 6 to 12 months with cycles of 3 week courses of pyrimethamine plus sulfadiazine alternating with 4 to 6 week courses of spiramycin. Usually, no more than four courses of either of these drugs are given in the first year, after which no further treatment is given. Prednisone (1 to 2 mg per kg per day) can be used in the presence of evidence indicating an on-going inflammatory process. For the apparently healthy neonate whose mother acquired acute toxoplasmosis during pregnancy, pyrimethamine plus sulfadiazine for 3 weeks followed by spiramycin alone probably should be given while awaiting laboratory confirmation of possible subclinical congenital infection.

Reactivated Toxoplasmosis

In the immunologically intact individual, reactivated toxoplasmosis seldom if ever occurs in areas other than the retina (see Retinochoroiditis). In the immunocompromised host with suppressed cellular immune responses, however, reactivation of quiescent (cyst) infection with liberation of trophozoites may occur virtually anywhere and result in potentially life-threatening disseminated infection. In patients with the acquired immune deficiency syndrome (AIDS), for example, intracerebral toxoplasmosis has become a major clinical problem. Thus, in any immunosuppressed patient in whom the diagnosis is suspected or proved, therapy should be initiated immediately with pyrimethamine plus sulfadiazine and continued for a minimum of 4 to 8 weeks after resolution of all signs of active infection. In severe infections, the dose of pyrimethamine can be doubled to 50 mg per day and also given every day if clinically warranted. In transplant recipients and AIDS patients (if they survive long enough), therapy is often required for 6 months or more and sometimes is given indefinitely.

TRICHINELLOSIS

method of
MICHAEL L. LEVIN, M.D.
Lutherville, Maryland

The clinical picture of trichinellosis is determined by the worm burden and premorbid health of the patient. The majority of patients consuming infected meat have mild symptoms or are asymptomatic. There is no therapy that rids the intestinal tract of the ingested adult worm. The symptoms require either no treatment or supportive, nonspecific therapy with anti-inflammatory antipyretics (aspirin, 600 mg every 4 hours) until symptoms abate.

A small number of patients with trichinellosis are quite symptomatic and unresponsive to salicylate therapy. Modest, decreasing oral doses of steroids (50 mg daily for 3 days, then decreasing daily doses until completion of course in 10 days) usually suffice to ameliorate symptoms related to the vasculitis and granulomatous response to encystment of *Trichinella* larvae.

For an even smaller number of patients, steroid therapy does not alleviate the severe symptoms. The toxicity related to the central nervous system and cardiac or multiple striated muscle involvement dictates more specific antihelminthic therapy. This may occur in the acute or less common subacute or chronic phase of the illness.

Mebendazole (Vermox) is a safe and effective oral larvicidal agent. It is reported to have limited use for trichinellosis because of alleged poor gastrointestinal absorption. Though not listed in the 1985 Physicians' Desk Reference or the manufacturer's directives for this use, it has provided cures with limited side effects.

The specific dose and duration of mebendazole therapy are unknown for trichinellosis. However, 20 to 25 mg per kg per day, in a divided dosage every 6 hours for several months, appears safe and effective without significant side effects. Laboratory parameters that document improvement include a falling erythrocyte sedimentation rate, decreasing serologic titers, improving electromyograph studies, and if necessary, muscle biopsies demonstrating larval destruction.

A 2 month course of mebendazole has proved effective if relapse occurs.

A Herxheimer-like reaction may occur shortly after initiation of larvicidal therapy such as with mebendazole. Symptomatic treatment with salicylates ameliorates these self-limited reactions.

TULAREMIA

method of
TIMOTHY F. MURPHY, M.D.
*State University of New York at Buffalo,
Buffalo, New York*

Tularemia is caused by *Francisella tularensis*, a small, pleomorphic, gram-negative bacillus. Humans usually acquire infection following contact with tissues or body fluids of an infected rabbit or other mammal, or through the bite of an infected arthropod such as a tick or deerfly. The disease is typically manifested by the abrupt onset of fever, chills, malaise, and fatigue, followed by one of the following six clinical syndromes related to portal of entry: ulceroglandular, glandular, oculoglandular, typhoidal, oropharyngeal, or pneumonic. The ulceroglandular form is the most common and usually occurs as a result of cutaneous inoculation through an inapparent skin lesion. Ulceroglandular tularemia is characterized by a skin ulcer and tender regional lymphadenopathy.

The diagnosis is generally confirmed serologically. A fourfold rise in the tularemia agglutination titer is diagnostic of infection. The organism can be isolated from clinical specimens using specialized media. However, this is not generally recommended because of the risk of infection in laboratory personnel.

Symptoms may persist for weeks to months without appropriate therapy. Prior to the availability of antibiotics, the mortality rate ranged from 5 to 30 per cent. More recently, with proper therapy, mortality is less than 1 per cent.

Treatment

Streptomycin is the drug of choice for all forms of tularemia. The usual adult dosage is 0.5 to 1.0 gram intramuscularly every 12 hours for 10 to 14 days. Children should receive 15 to 20 mg per kg per day in divided doses. In severe illness, higher doses (up to 30 mg per kg per day) can be administered for the first 2 or 3 days. Streptomycin is vestibulotoxic and nephrotoxic, and the dose should be adjusted downward in patients with renal failure. The response to therapy is usually prompt. The fever generally responds within 24 to 48 hours unless suppurative lymph nodes are present. Relapses after streptomycin therapy are unusual; however, if relapse occurs, another course of streptomycin therapy is indicated.

Other agents have been used in treating tularemia. Gentamicin (1.7 mg per kg every 8 hours), an aminoglycoside antibiotic related to streptomycin, is effective, but there is less experience with this agent compared with streptomycin. Tetracycline and chloramphenicol (both 30 mg per kg per day in four divided doses) have been used, but relapses occur frequently with these agents, particularly when administered for less than 2 weeks. Recently, case reports suggest that erythromycin may be effective in tularemia.

Prevention

The risk of acquiring infection can be minimized by avoiding contact with infected rabbits and other wild animals. Wearing gloves while skinning or eviscerating infected animals probably reduces the risk of infection. Measures to protect from deerfly and tick bites will reduce the risk of arthropodborne disease. These include avoiding tick-infested areas when possible, wearing protective clothing including tight-fitting protection around wrists and ankles, and using insect repellents.

A live, attenuated tularemia vaccine is available. The vaccine is effective but does not provide complete protection. Laboratory workers who handle *F. tularensis* and individuals who are repeatedly exposed to wild mammals or infected vectors should be considered for immunization. The vaccine is available from the Centers for Disease Control, Atlanta, Georgia.

SALMONELLOSIS
(Other Than Typhoid Fever)

method of
MARWAN UWAYDAH, M.D.
American University of Beirut
Beirut, Lebanon

The term *salmonellosis* is conveniently used to refer to a wide spectrum of infections caused by organisms belonging to the genus *Salmonella* of the family Enterobacteriaceae. Only three species of *Salmonella* are currently recognized, and they are identified on the basis of biochemical reactions and antigenic differences. Whereas *S. typhi* and *S. choleraesuis* each designate a single serotype, the third species, *S. enteritidis,* comprises the remaining multitude of different serotypes and bioserotypes, exceeding 2000 in number. In contrast to *S. typhi,* of which the human host is its only natural reservoir, other salmonellae may be recovered from a large number of wild and domestic animals; these, together with the human host, constitute an immense source for infection that is practically impossible to eradicate—hence, the worldwide endemicity of salmonellosis other than typhoid fever. The infection is usually acquired by the oral route via contaminated food or drink. Infectivity is enhanced by heavy contamination or by improper storage conditions promoting multiplication of the organism in the vehicle, before it is ingested. Direct person-to-person transmission may occur but is rather uncommon, and exaggerated concern over this mode of transmission is not justified.

Traditionally, salmonellosis occurs in four major clinical forms: gastroenteritis (or enterocolitis), enteric fever (including typhoid and paratyphoid), bacteremia with or without demonstrable extraintestinal tissue localization, and the asymptomatic carrier state. Caution should be exercised in the rigid application of such a broad classification so as not to overlook overlapping syndromes. A presumably self-limited episode of gastroenteritis in patients with serious underlying diseases or predisposing abnormalities may lead to bacteremia and extraintestinal tissue localization, a complication that should be promptly recognized because of important prognostic and therapeutic implications.

Treatment

Not all patients with salmonellosis require antimicrobial therapy. The decision to treat and the choice of an appropriate regimen should be based on a number of considerations related to the site(s) of infection, host factors, species or serotype designation of the pathogen as an indicator of its pathogenic potentials, and the susceptibility of the isolated strain to antimicrobial agents of proven therapeutic efficacy. In this context, only chloramphenicol, ampicillin, amoxicillin, and trimethoprim-sulfamethoxazole have gained general acceptance. The emergence of multiply resistant strains bearing R-factors in many communities emphasizes the need for confirming the in vitro susceptibility of the infecting organism to the selected drug. Antimicrobial therapy is described in accordance with currently accepted guidelines, but I hold the following reservations:

1. Choice options of therapeutic agents have remained surprisingly restricted, despite the rapidly increasing number of available antimicrobial agents.
2. Treatment results, particularly in immunocompromised patients, have not been altogether satisfactory.
3. The full therapeutic potentials of a number of promising antimicrobial agents have not been adequately explored.
4. The widely held opinion that antimicrobial therapy is *contraindicated* in salmonella gastroenteritis is based on a generalization that is open to question. The reported controversial or paradoxic results obtained with certain antimicrobial regimens should not necessarily imply that any other regimen, using the same or different agents, will also fail.

Gastroenteritis (Enterocolitis)

This is the most common symptomatic form of salmonellosis. Relatively few serotypes of *S. enteritidis* are responsible for the majority of cases. One or more pathophysiologic mechanisms related to mucosal invasion and enterotoxin production may involve the colon and the small intestine. After an incubation period of 1 to 3 days, the disease manifests rather abruptly with nausea, sometimes vomiting, diarrhea, fever, and abdominal pain of varying severity. A profuse diarrhea may lead to dehydration, electrolyte depletion, metabolic derangements, and circulatory disturbances. The impact is most profound in infants, the aged, and debilitated patients. Bacteremia may occur but is usually transient, and its true incidence is uncertain. Ordinarily, the disease is self-limited; spontaneous recovery, in the absence of serious complications, should be expected within 3 to 5 days. In the occasional case, but more commonly in patients at the extremes of age and in those with suppressed immune response or serious underlying disorders such as inflammatory bowel disease, malignancy, sickle cell anemia, and schistosomiasis, the illness may run a protracted course with intermittent bacteremia and the development of extraintestinal foci of infection.

Treatment. For previously healthy adults with mild diarrheal illness, relative rest and some dietary restriction, with emphasis on electrolyte-rich beverages, should suffice. In severe cases, and for patients at the extremes of age, further treatment measures will be needed:

1. Blood pressure, urine output, and other vital functions should be closely monitored. Intravenous administration of isotonic saline and glucose solutions should be administered promptly to combat severe dehydration and hypotension. Potassium chloride or sodium bicarbonate additives may have to be used judiciously, as guided by serum electrolyte determinations, to correct electrolyte losses and to restore acid-base balance. Repeated body weight and urine specific gravity measurements provide helpful clues for assessing the state of hydration.
2. If vomiting does not subside spontaneously within a few hours, it may be controlled with prochlorperazine (Compazine), in a dose of 5 to 10 mg, or trimethobenzamide hydrochloride (Tigan), in a dose of 200 to 250 mg, administered orally or intramuscularly three times daily. In children, dosage adjustments and special precautions for use below certain age limits should be observed. Antiperistaltic or constipating agents, such as diphenoxylate hydrochloride with atropine (Lomotil), or opiates are to be avoided because of their possible aggravating effects on the course of the illness.
3. At present, there is a consensus that antimicrobial therapy is not recommended in the uncomplicated case of *Salmonella* gastroenteritis. This attitude has emerged following the reports that such therapy not only fails to reduce morbidity but also prolongs the period of fecal excretion of the pathogen. In my opinion, these conclusions should be related to the specific treatment regimens used and not to antimicrobial therapy in general. Obviously, the full potential usefulness of all currently available antimicrobial agents in this infection is far from being established. Treatment is indicated when the illness is protracted or intermittent bacteremia is demonstrated. Either ampicillin, chloramphenicol, or

trimethoprim-sulfamethoxazole may be used in the dosage regimens outlined below, and after the in vitro susceptibility of the bacterial isolate is confirmed.

Enteric Fever

A number of *S. enteritidis* serotypes may cause paratyphoid fever, which is a febrile bacteremic illness that is clinically indistinguishable from the classic typhoid fever caused by *S. typhi*. Both typhoid fever and paratyphoid fever are collectively referred to as enteric fever. The illness is characterized by high fever, severe headache, dry cough, constipation (more often than diarrhea), mental obtundation, and the apearance of transient rash (rose spots). Relative bradycardia, splenomegaly, hepatomegaly, and leukopenia are frequently noted. If left untreated, the infection persists for several weeks and may lead to serious complications, including intestinal hemorrhage and perforation.

Treatment. Antimicrobial therapy should be instituted as soon as the diagnosis is made. Any of the following regimens may be used, after confirming the in vitro susceptibility of the organism:

1. Ampicillin in a daily dose of 8 to 12 grams (200 to 300 mg per kg in children) to be administered in six divided doses by slow intravenous infusion over 30 to 60 minutes. In the relatively mild case, or when the patient becomes afebrile after initial intravenous therapy, a smaller dose orally may be used. For this purpose, amoxicillin in a daily dose of 4 grams (75 to 100 mg per kg in children) divided every 6 hours is preferred because of its more predictable absorption.

2. Chloramphenicol in a daily dose of 3 to 4 grams (50 to 75 mg per kg in children) to be administered in three or four divided doses by mouth or by slow intravenous infusion. After complete defervescence, the dose is reduced to half and maintained for the rest of the treatment course. It is mandatory that patients receiving this antibiotic be carefully monitored for evidence of bone marrow toxicity.

3. Trimethoprim-sulfamethoxazole (Bactrim, Septra), in a dose of two tablets (each containing 80 mg of trimethoprim and 400 mg of sulfamethoxazole) every 12 hours. More frequent dosing is not necessary because of the prolonged serum half-life of this drug. In children, appropriate adjustment of dosage should be made. (This use of trimethoprim-sulfamethoxazole is not listed in the manufacturer's directive.)

Both chloramphenicol and trimethoprim-sulfamethoxazole are better avoided in neonates and pregnant women. Therapy with any of the proposed agents should be continued for a total of about 2 weeks, or 10 days after complete defervescence. Shorter treatment courses result in high relapse rates. Even after adequate treatment, about 10 per cent of patients relapse within 2 to 4 weeks after therapy is concluded, necessitating another course with the same or another agent. In our experience, cefazolin (Ancef, Kefzol), cefamandole (Mandol), and more recently moxalactam (Moxam) were found effective when the antibiotic was administered in such dosage to maintain the serum drug concentration above the minimal inhibitory concentration of the infecting organism. Although these agents are not to be recommended at present for routine clinical use, they may prove advantageous under special circumstances when alternative therapeutic agents are sought.

The supportive care of the patient should be emphasized. A low-residue diet is allowed as tolerated. Intravenous fluids are indicated if oral intake is judged inadequate, or for the purpose of administering antimicrobial agents. Fever may be alleviated by applying cold compresses over the extremities, but antipyretics should be avoided as they may cause sudden hypothermia and hypotension. The beneficial effects of corticosteroids have not been confirmed and their use, if at all, should be restricted to the severely toxic and rapidly deteriorating patient receiving appropriate antimicrobial therapy and supportive care.

Bacteremia and Focal Infection

Intermittent rather than persistent bacteremia and absence of the characteristic typhoidal features distinguish this entity from enteric fever. Usually, chills and fever are the main presenting symptoms with or without evidence of any focal infection. Possible complications include osteomyelitis, especially in patients with sickle cell anemia, arthritis, empyema, endocarditis, localization in an aortic aneurysm, cholecystitis, and meningitis (predominantly in neonates). Presumably, the disease complicates a primary gastrointestinal infection, but a history of preceding diarrheal illness is not necessarily elicited. Although *S. choleraesuis* has been reported to be the most common cause of this syndrome, any other *Salmonella* serotype may prove to be the etiologic agent.

Treatment. The infecting strain should be properly identified and its susceptibility to antimicrobial agents tested, preferably by quantitative techniques. It is advisable to have the organism kept in the laboratory until treatment is concluded in case further laboratory tests, such as serum antibacterial activity, are deemed necessary for modifying the treatment regimen. Although any of the options proposed for the treatment of enteric fever may be chosen, ampicillin is preferred because of its bactericidal action and relative safety when used in high doses for long periods. Based on our experience, cefazolin, cefamandole, and moxalactam may be used as second line drugs, if the need arises.

Duration of therapy depends on the particular details of the case, including the anatomic site and extent of the focal lesion and the nature and severity of any pre-existing or predisposing conditions. Whereas 2 weeks of treatment are chosen empirically for the patient with bacteremia and absence of extraintestinal tissue localization, 6 or more weeks of intensive intravenous therapy may be required for endocarditis or osteomyelitis. Surgical intervention should be considered for the drainage of an abscess or debridement of necrotic tissues. Careful follow-up is advisable to ensure that the infection is completely eradicated and not simply suppressed into a transiently asymptomatic phase.

Carrier State

Frequently, patients become fecal excreters of *Salmonella* for variable periods of time after recovery from acute gastroenteritis. Unlike individuals infected with *S. typhi,* such convalescent carriers rarely continue to excrete the pathogen beyond 1 year to be called chronic carriers. Patients with schistosomiasis are more prone to become chronic carriers because of the peculiar phenomenon of persistence of the bacterium in the gut of the parasite. A urinary carrier state may complicate *Schistosoma haematobium* infection.

Treatment. Convalescent carriers are completely asymptomatic and thus require no treatment. Nevertheless, they should be instructed to observe strict personal hygiene, particularly if they are food-handlers or if they happen to come in close contact with immunocompromised patients or other individuals at high risk. The carrier state is considered terminated when three consecutive stool cultures, at weekly intervals, are negative. Antimicrobial therapy of the chronic carrier state has not proved to be consistently effective. The commonly proposed regimens include the use of ampicillin (1 to 1.5 grams orally every 6 hours), amoxicillin (1 gram orally every 8 hours), or trimethoprim-sulfamethoxazole (two tablets, each containing 80 mg of trimethoprim and 400 mg of sulfamethoxazole, every 12 hours). Treatment should be continued for a total of 4 to 6 weeks. In patients with cholelithiasis, cholecystectomy may prove curative.

TYPHOID FEVER

method of
FRANCISCO SERAFIN, M.D.
National Autonomous University of Mexico
México, D.F.

Typhoid fever is an acute, systemic disease caused by *Salmonella typhi.* It is characterized by fever, malaise, diffuse abdominal pain, and leukopenia. Bradycardia may occur even in the absence of fever; rash and neuropsychiatric alterations known as "typhoidic status" are also frequent. Extraintestinal localization can be expected. Intestinal bleeding and perforation occur in 3 to 5 per cent of patients. Definitive diagnosis is by blood or marrow culture. Antimicrobial therapy has not decreased the incidence of relapses.

Treatment

Chloramphenicol. This is the drug of choice. The recommended dosage is 3.0 grams per day in adults and 100 mg per kg per day in children divided into four doses and given for 10 to 12 days. Give intravenously if the oral route is impaired. The intramuscular route is not recommended because it produces low and variable serum concentrations. The response to chloramphenicol is not dramatic. Subjective improvement occurs after 48 hours of treatment, and temperature returns to normal 3 to 5 days after the beginning of therapy.

Side effects of chloramphenicol include bone marrow toxicity resulting in suppression of hematopoietic activity, but this is reversible upon cessation of the drug. Aplastic anemia is an exceptional event, occurring in 1 of 40,000 to 50,000 patients.

The important effect of chloramphenicol is its ability to reduce major complications and lethality. Deaths decreased from 12 to 2 to 3 per cent after introduction of the drug.

Since 1972 chloramphenicol-resistant strains of *S. typhi* have been reported from Mexico, Southeast Asia, and India. In these situations alternative drugs such as amoxicillin, furazolidone (Furoxone), or trimethoprim-sulfamethoxazole (Bactrim, Septra) sould be used.

Amoxicillin. This drug has the same spectrum of activity as ampicillin but is more effective in typhoid fever. When given orally it is better absorbed than ampicillin, is not interfered with by meals as is ampicillin, achieves twice the serum levels that ampicillin does, and produces fewer gastrointestinal side effects than ampicillin. The recommended dosage in adults is 4.0

grams per day divided in four doses and in children 100 mg per kg per day. Treatment should be given for 14 days. The clinical response is slower than with chloramphenicol; fever disappears after 7 days of treatment.

Furazolidone. This agent belongs to the nitrofurans group and has been used in intestinal infections different from typhoid fever. The first reports showing its effectiveness came from India in 1967. In 1972 the drug was used with good results in Mexico during an outbreak produced by strains resistant to chloramphenicol. Fever disappeared after 7 days of treatment. Side effects are gastrointestinal discomfort, rash, eosinophilia, and fever.

In our experience furazolidone is similar to other antimicrobial drugs in chloramphenicol-resistant cases and is less expensive (This use is not listed in the manufacturer's directive). The recommended dosage in adults is 800 mg per day divided in four doses and in children, 10 to 15 mg per kg per day for 12 days. (Manufacturer's recommended children's dose is 8.8 mg/kg/day).

Trimethoprim-Sulfamethoxazole. This drug is less effective than the other drugs. The recommended dosage in adults is 160 mg of trimethoprim and 800 mg of sulfamethoxazole every 12 hours and in children, 7 mg of trimethoprim and 35 mg of sulfamethoxazole per kg per day divided in two doses. Treatment must be given for 14 days. In our experience fever disappears after 8 days of treatment; relapses occur in 4.4 per cent of patients. The common side effects are nausea, vomiting, and rash. Major problems are less frequent.

Treatment of Complications

Intestinal hemorrhage and bowel perforation are the most frequent complications and occur in 10 and 3 to 5 per cent of patients, respectively. Both are produced by necrosis of Peyer's patches that extends from erosion to involvement of muscular and serosal layers of the bowel. These complications occur during the second week and involve the distal 20 to 40 cm of ileum. Clinical signs are melena or fresh blood in feces, abdominal pain, and peritonitis. A change from leukopenia to leukocytosis generally occurs.

Hemorrhage is treated with blood transfusion. In patients with bowel perforation or major hemorrhage that is difficult to control, surgical intervention is required. According to the severity, treatment varies from simple closure of the perforation to extensive intestinal resection and ileostomy, and in more severe cases colostomy. Additional antimicrobial therapy, including an aminoglycoside, is required in these cases. Intravenous metronidazole should be used against anaerobic intestinal flora.

Typhoid fever is a septicemic condition and extraintestinal localization of *S. typhi* is possible, producing meningitis, osteomyelitis, arthritis, thrombophlebitis, and pneumonia. In cases of pneumonia, pneumococci may produce secondary infection. Nephritis, myocarditis, orchitis, hepatitis, and intravascular coagulation also can occur. Specific supportive measures and antimicrobial therapy are indicated.

Relapses occur in 5 to 20 per cent of patients, usually 1 to 2 weeks after treatment. The course is usually similar to that of the initial infection, and the antimicrobial therapy is the same.

A chronic carrier state is another peculiar characteristic of typhoid fever. The chronic carrier is symptom-free but after a year is still excreting salmonella in stool. The gallbladder is the common site of infection. Many of these patients have gallstones and gallbladder dysfunction requiring cholecystectomy. Ampicillin is also recommended for 2 or 3 weeks.

Chronic carriers can be treated with ampicillin, 6 grams per day for 6 weeks divided in four doses, in association with probenecid. Amoxicillin, 2 grams three times a day for 4 weeks is an alternative. Due to the increased dosage, gastric discomfort is frequent.

Supportive Treatment

Supportive measures include bed rest, nutritional support, and maintenance of hydration. A hypercaloric diet is recommended. Antipyretics are not recommended because hypothermia and vascular collapse may occur. Some recommend the use of corticosteroids in severe cases of toxicity, but in our experience this measure increases the risk of intestinal hemorrhage, bowel perforation, and secondary infection.

Prevention

The major preventive measure is environmental sanitation and medical education. The currently used vaccine, prepared by acetone extraction with preservation of the Vi antigen, confers protection to 90 per cent of those aged 3 or more years. Parenteral administration of two monthly doses of 0.5 ml is recommended during epidemics and in persons traveling from nonendemic areas. Side effects of this vaccine are fever, local reaction with edema and erythema, lethargy, and malaise.

An oral vaccine produced from a mutant strain of *S. typhi* deficient in galactose-epimerase has been successful in field trials in Egypt and has shown irregular effectiveness in Chile. This vaccine could be a good alternative in the future.

TYPHUS FEVERS

method of
PETER L. PERINE, M.D., MPH
Uniformed Services University of the Health Sciences
Bethesda, Maryland

Typhus fevers are caused by different species of closely related rickettsiae which are transmitted to humans by the bite or infected feces of certain arthropods. Epidemic typhus *(R. prowazekii)* is transmitted by human body lice feces, which contaminate the bites when crushed. This disease will become latent if left untreated and may recrudesce 10 to 25 years later as Brill-Zinsser disease. Louseborne typhus is currently epidemic in the famine areas of East Africa. Human beings are the principal reservoir, but *R. prowazekii* is also present in flying squirrels in the eastern United States. Although the mode of transmission is not known, several human cases are reported each year in Americans whose homes are infested by flying squirrels. Between 60 and 80 cases of murine or rat-flea typhus *(R. typhi)* are reported annually in the United States, usually from Texas and other Gulf Coast states. Infected rats are the reservoir for *R. typhi*, and the disease is transmitted to humans by rat fleas. Scrub typhus *(R. tsutsugamushi)* is found only in the rural areas of southeast Asia. Rodents and small mammals are its reservoir, and human beings become incidentally infected by the bite of infected mites (chiggers).

Epidemic and murine typhus usually presents with fever, headache, and maculopapular rash. Elevated Weil-Felix (Proteus OX-19) serologic titers are characteristic of these diseases, but Weil-Felix antibodies may not appear before the second week of illness, and only specific serologic tests can distinguish epidemic from murine typhus. Scrub typhus is recognized by way of an inflamed eschar where the patient was bitten, together with rash, adenitis, and an elevated titer to Proteus OX-K antigen. All rickettsiae spread systemically and multiply preferentially within vascular endothelial cells of small blood vessels, producing focal or disseminated vasculitis. When this occurs in small arteries, thrombosis leading to gangrene may occur. The release of rickettsiae toxins also increases vascular permeability with extravasation of intravascular fluids into the interstitial spaces, producing hypovolemia that may progress to shock. The principles of treatment are specific antimicrobial therapy and general supportive measures.

Treatment

Although only rickettsiostatic, the tetracyclines or chloramphenicol is the treatment of choice. Doxycycline (Vibramycin) is the most easily administered tetracycline because of its prolonged, effective blood levels. Doxycycline given in a single oral or intravenous dose of 5 mg per kg (200 mg total) is effective treatment for scrub, epidemic, and murine typhus, although it is not proved that such treatment eradicates this organism. Patients usually experience prompt symptomatic improvement and become afebrile within 72 hours after initiation of therapy. Tetracycline hydrochloride (25 mg per kg per day in four divided doses, orally or intravenously) may also be used in any typhus fever. Therapy should be continued until the patient has been afebrile for at least 2 days.

Oral or intravenous chloramphenicol (Chloromycetin) is given in a dose of 50 mg per kg per day in 4 divided doses until the patient has been afebrile for at least 2 days. Infants and children should receive no more than 25 mg per kg per day. Chloramphenicol is more widely available and less costly in Africa and Asia than is doxycycline, and it may be the only drug available to treat epidemics of louseborne typhus. Chloramphenicol should be given preferentially to more seriously ill patients with azotemia or renal failure because it is metabolized by the liver.

Endothelial cell damage is usually widespread in seriously ill patients with epidemic and scrub typhus, and myocarditis and encephalitis are common. In addition to local thrombosis and hypovolemia, disseminated intravascular coagulopathy may occur with hemorrhage, but heparin is not recommended. Hypovolemia can be corrected by intravenous saline or albumin but must be given cautiously to prevent acute pulmonary edema. Confused or comatose patients may require feeding by nasogastric tube or by parenteral alimentation, and patients should be turned frequently to prevent decubitus ulcers. High dose corticosteroids have been given to critically ill patients, but their efficacy has not been proved.

Scrub typhus can be prevented by prophylactic use of oral doxycycline, 100 mg twice weekly, and by avoiding travel in rural areas where the disease is known to be endemic. The same doxycycline prophylaxis is probably also an effective prophylaxis against epidemic and murine typhus. An attenuated strain (E, Madrid) of *R. prowazekii* protects against epidemic typhus, but it is not licensed for use in the United States and is not commercially available elsewhere.

Patients with louseborn typhus should have their clothing decontaminated by boiling and have their hair and skin treated with 1 per cent gammabenzenehexachloride lotion followed by a shower, to rid themselves of body lice. Insecticides such as DDT can also be used to delouse the patient, his or her clothing, and habitat, but human body lice are often resistant to this insecticide in those parts of the world where typhus is epidemic. All suspect typhus fever cases in the United States should be reported to local health departments; here arrangements often can be made to have special diagnostic tests performed on patient sera, for follow-up of patient contacts, and for evaluation of vectors.

WHOOPING COUGH

(Pertussis)

method of
MOSES GROSSMAN, M.D.
University of California, San Francisco
San Francisco, California

Whooping cough (pertussis) is an acute, highly contagious infection of the respiratory tract. It is caused by a gram-negative microorganism, *Bordetella pertussis.* A clinically similar but milder disease may be caused by two related organisms, *Bordetella parapertussis* and *Bordetella bronchosepticum.* Certain adenoviruses also cause a similar clinical illness; *Chlamydia trachomatis* produces an illness in infants under 4 months of age characterized by paroxysmal cough, which might be mistaken for pertussis. The incubation period is 7 to 10 days; the disease is most communicable during the catarrhal stage. The illness then goes on to a paroxysmal stage which may be very severe, particularly in young infants who often have apneic spells following the paroxysm. Mortality occurs essentially only in young infants. Specific diagnosis depends either on culturing the organism from the nasopharynx (using a special Bordet-Gengou media) or on identification by direct immunofluorescent staining. The principal complications of pertussis are pneumonia, hypoxia, apneic spells, convulsive seizures, and encephalopathy.

Pertussis can and should be prevented by active immunization. The vaccine currently in use is accompanied by frequent minor reactions (fever, fussiness) and infrequent severe reactions (convulsive seizures, encephalopathy). A newer form of vaccine is currently being studied in the hope that it will produce fewer reactions.

Treatment

Hospitalization. Infants under 3 months of age should always be hospitalized; those between 3 and 6 months of age should be hospitalized unless their disease is mild. Beyond 6 months of age hospitalization is reserved for children with an unusually severe illness or complications.

Isolation. Pertussis is highly communicable. Parents should protect susceptible playmates and family members from contact with the patient for 3 weeks from the onset of the illness. Children are not immune until after they have received all three injections of pertussis vaccine (or DPT). Hospitalized patients with pertussis should be placed in a private room with respiratory isolation precautions.

General Supportive Care

Monitoring for apnea. Whether in hospital or in the home, the young infant needs to be monitored for the occurrence of apneic spells that may prove fatal or result in permanent sequelae. This can be done by using a cardiorespiratory monitor or by rigorous vigilance by caretakers.

Avoiding paroxysms. Paroxysmal cough is often initiated by cigarette smoke, dust, excessive stimulation, pooled thick secretions, and large feedings. Small feedings, a quiet room, avoidance of smoking, and humidification of inspired air are valuable aspects of therapy.

Fluids and caloric intake should be maintained. On occasion vomiting may necessitate intravenous hydration.

Hypoxia should be avoided. *Pneumonia* is a common complication of pertussis and may require supplemental oxygen.

Cough medications are generally not helpful.

Antimicrobials. Erythromycin, 50 mg per kg per day for 7 to 10 days is recommended. Erythromycin is helpful clinically only during the catarrhal stage. Its administration during the paroxysmal stage will decrease the period of communicability and thus is desirable. If the infant or child cannot tolerate erythromycin, ampicillin is the second choice.

Unproved medications. Pertussis immune globulin and glucocorticoids have both been suggested and used in the management of severe pertussis. There is no scientific basis for using these medications and we do not recommend them.

Management of Exposed Susceptibles. Pertussis is very contagious. Up to 90 per cent of susceptible individuals contract the disease unless protective measures are undertaken. Household and other close contacts who were previously immunized against pertussis should receive a booster dose (preferably DPT). *In addition,* all such contacts should receive erythromycin (50 mg per kg per day) for 10 days. Pertussis immune globulin is of no value in protecting exposed susceptibles.

Section 3

The Respiratory System

ACUTE RESPIRATORY FAILURE

method of
GARY W. WAHL, M.D.,
and WILLIAM J. HALL, M.D.
University of Rochester
Rochester, New York

Three clinically important physiologic categories of acute respiratory failure exist: (1) alveolar hypoventilation, (2) ventilation perfusion (V/Q) mismatch, and (3) intrapulmonary shunt. A few basic physiologic concepts are helpful in differentiating these categories. Their understanding forms the basis for our therapeutic approach. Although these categories are addressed separately, it is important to acknowledge that more than one mechanism may be present in a patient at a given time.

Alveolar Hypoventilation. The $Paco_2$ represents an equilibration between the production of carbon dioxide during cellular metabolism and its excretion from the lungs. This equilibrium is represented by the relationship

$$Paco_2 = K \times Vco_2/Valv$$

where $Paco_2$ is arterial carbon dioxide tension, K is a constant, Vco_2 is carbon dioxide production, and Valv is minute alveolar ventilation. Accordingly, elevation of $Paco_2$ occurs under two conditions. First, a reduction in tidal volume or respiratory rate may occur. This occurs secondary to central nervous system disease (e.g., stroke, anesthesia, drug overdose, trauma), neuromuscular disease (Guillain-Barré, myasthenia gravis), and severe chest deformities (flail chest, severe kyphoscoliosis). Second, if a significant portion of inhaled air ventilates lung regions without blood flow, an increased total ventilation is required to maintain a normal $Paco_2$. This elevation of respiratory "dead space" is seen commonly in lung disorders such as emphysema and chronic bronchitis.

Hypercapnia causes important, but variable, clinical sequelae, depending on its severity and rate of development. The sudden increase of the $Paco_2$ from normal (40 torr) to 80 to 90 torr produces life-threatening respiratory acidosis and may induce central nervous system narcosis. Slowly evolving hypercapnia has no significant neurologic effect, and the acidosis is usually attenuated by renal retention of bicarbonate. An invariable and important consequence of alveolar hypoventilation is a reduction in arterial oxygen tension. As carbon dioxide increases in alveoli, it replaces alveolar oxygen. We can best quantify this relationship by using the alveolar gas equation:

$$PAO_2 = FiO_2\,[Pb - PH_2O] - Paco_2/R$$

where PAO_2 equals alveolar oxygen tension, FiO_2 equals inspired oxygen concentration, Pb equals barometric pressure, PH_2O equals the partial pressure of water at body temperature, $Paco_2$ is the arterial carbon dioxide tension, and R is the respiratory exchange coefficient of the lung (usually 0.8 when breathing room air). The equation may be simplified as follows:

$$PAO_2 = FiO_2\,(Pb - PH_2O) - 1.2 \times Paco_2$$

This equation now states that the alveolar oxygen tension is a function of inspired oxygen concentration minus the corrected $Paco_2$. If no intrinsic lung disease is present, the difference between the calculated alveolar oxygen tension and the measured arterial oxygen tension (the A-a gradient) will be less than 10 torr while breathing room air.

For example, the room air blood gases of a patient suffering from barbiturate overdose may show a PAO_2 of 50 and a $Paco_2$ of 80. In this situation, the PAO_2 is 54 ($0.21 \times (760 - 47) - 1.2 \times 80$), and the A-a gradient normal (4 mm Hg). In this case, the proper treatment of hypoxemia is not necessarily supplemental oxygen. Increased ventilation alone will reduce the elevated $Paco_2$ and raise the oxygen tension.

Except for alveolar hypoventilation, all other clinically important causes of acute respiratory failure are associated with an increased A-a oxygen gradient, implying intrinsic abnormalities of the lung. It follows, therefore, that hypercapnia is not typical in the early stages of respiratory failure except when due to hypoventilation. However, superimposed neuromuscular fatigue may develop in all forms of acute respiratory failure and reduce alveolar ventilation enough to cause the $Paco_2$ to rise. Airway obstruction, stiff lungs, and an increased minute ventilation (increased dead space) increase the work of breathing. The likelihood of respiratory muscle failure is increased when conditions such as anemia, reduced cardiac output, acidosis, malnutrition, or pain that limits diaphragmatic excursion are present.

Ventilation Perfusion Inequality (V/Q). A decreased ratio of ventilation to perfusion is responsible for the majority of conditions leading to acute respiratory failure. For example, pulmonary edema, pneumonia, bronchitis, and asthma all cause hypoxemia to some extent because of low V/Q ratios. This form of hypoxemia is substantially corrected by the administration of supplemental oxygen. It is fairly uncommon that mechanical ventilation is required to correct hypoxemia in this form of respiratory failure. Aggressive therapy of reversible factors such as bronchospasm, airway secretions, and interstitial edema plays an important role in treatment.

Intrapulmonary Shunt. When blood flow continues to areas of lung in which there is no gas exchange, intrapulmonary shunt exists. As a result, mixed venous blood proceeds unaltered through the lung and mixes (venous admixture) with arterialized blood in the pulmonary vein. Because the unsaturated hemoglobin in the shunted blood does not interface with alveolar gas, the hypoxemia of intrapulmonary shunt is refractory to supplemental oxygen administration.

This mechanism of hypoxemia is associated with some of the most serious cases of acute respiratory failure. In the setting of intrapulmonary shunt, there is an important relationship between mixed venous oxygen content and arterial oxygenation. As the oxygen content of mixed venous blood falls, it induces more severe arterial hypoxemia when mixed with the pulmonary blood coursing through normal pathways. Therefore, in the setting of intrapulmonary shunt, not only will the hypoxemia be refractory to supplemental oxygen, but any condition that reduces mixed venous oxygen content also reduces arterial oxygen content. Some of the causes of reduced mixed venous oxygen content are (1) reduced cardiac output, (2) decreased hemoglobin content of the blood, and (3) increased peripheral oxygen consumption.

Treatment

Initial Therapy

Regardless of the underlying cause of acute respiratory failure, the initial goal of treatment is to reverse life-threatening hypoxemia and respiratory acidosis. Therefore, initial management must insure (1) a patent airway, (2) sufficient supplemental oxygen to insure adequate oxygen delivery, and (3) adequate ventilation to control arterial pH. Intensive respiratory care and frequent monitoring of clinical parameters and arterial blood gases are central to care. This is best accomplished in an intensive care unit.

Oxygen Therapy

The goal of supplemental oxygen therapy is to attain a PAO_2 of about 60 torr. This correlates with 90 to 95 per cent saturation of the hemoglobin with oxygen. Higher partial pressures of oxygen can only add very little additional oxygen to the blood, and the risk of lung injury from oxygen administration increases as the FIO_2 reaches 0.55 to 0.6.

A small minority of patients with chronic carbon dioxide retention rely on their hypoxic drive to maintain ventilation. Oxygen administration can remove this drive and lead to respiratory suppression and CO_2 retention. In most cases, the judicious use of low concentrations (24 to 30 per cent) of supplemental oxygen will alleviate hypoxia without causing respiratory suppression. Frequent arterial blood gases are needed to evaluate the therapy of these patients. Despite the risk of respiratory depression, supplemental oxygen should never be withheld from a patient in respiratory distress. If the arterial pH cannot be maintained above 7.30, assisted ventilation may be necessary to allow adequate oxygenation.

Nasal cannulas can be used to administer low flow rates of oxygen (0.5 to 5 liters per minute). This is an inexpensive and well-tolerated method for delivery of 24 to 35 per cent oxygen, but precise control of FIO_2 is impossible. Loose-fitting face masks fitted with a Venturi attachment deliver precise concentrations (24, 28, 32, 35, 40, 50 per cent) of oxygen-enriched air. These should be used when the concern for respiratory suppression is high. Face masks are somewhat uncomfortable and must be removed during meals or for clearance of secretions. Tight-fitting masks with reservoir bags can deliver concentrations of oxygen of from 50 per cent to 80 per cent for short periods but are unreliable for sustained use. They are uncomfortable and poorly tolerated. Various modalities exist for oxygen delivery without intubation, but these are only reliable for extended periods when the required FIO_2 is 0.5 or less. When a prolonged FIO_2 greater than 0.5 is needed, tracheal intubation and mechanical ventilation are frequently required.

Mechanical Ventilation

At times the need for mechanical ventilation may be obvious. Apnea or agonal respirations, as well as respiratory distress in the setting of severe cardiovascular instability, are clear indications for mechanical ventilation. In other situations, the necessity for assisted ventilation will be defined through observation and monitoring of patients over a period of time. Progressive hypoxemia unresponsive to an FIO_2 of 0.5 or greater, progressive CO_2 retention associated with acidosis, inability to clear secretions, increased work of breathing associated with severe medical or cardiovascular instability, and respiratory support during diagnostic procedures in patients with underlying lung disease are some of the more common indications. An endotracheal tube with a high volume, low pressure cuff should be placed by an experienced person either nasally or orally. Sedation should be used with great caution as it may induce sudden respiratory arrest. If possible, intubation should be performed electively, not in the setting of respiratory arrest.

Initial ventilator orders include inspired oxygen concentration, mode of ventilation (control, assist, intermittent mandatory ventilation), minute ventilation, and the amount of positive end-expiratory pressure (PEEP). An important part of any ventilator manipulation is assessment of arterial blood gases 15 to 30 minutes after the modification.

Adequate arterial oxygenation must be assured, so initially an FiO_2 of 0.6 to 0.9 is selected. After measurement of arterial blood gases, the FiO_2 is adjusted to the lowest concentration yielding a PAO_2 of 60 or greater. If an FiO_2 of 0.5 to 0.6 results in unacceptable hypoxemia, the administration of PEEP should be considered, and cardiac output and hemoglobin content should be assessed. Sustained administration of FiO_2 greater than 0.55 to 0.6 can produce a diffuse lung injury similar to acute respiratory distress syndrome. Burning substernal chest pain or cough related to tracheal irritation may be an early sign of oxygen toxicity.

PEEP stabilizes alveolar air spaces and increases the gas-exchanging surface of the lung. It effectively reduces the intrapulmonary shunt in diffuse lung disease and will improve arterial PaO_2. Generally, 3 to 5 cm of water pressure is used initially while careful attention to blood gases, blood pressure, and urinary output is maintained. PEEP is increased by increments of 3 to 5 cm of water until satisfactory oxygen delivery is obtained or unacceptable side effects occur. Cardiac output may fall, probably secondary to the effect of increased intrathoracic pressure on venous blood return. It is possible to improve the PaO_2 but actually reduce oxygen delivery when PEEP causes a drop in cardiac output. Therefore, most patients requiring 7 to 10 cm of water or more of PEEP should have a pulmonary artery catheter placed to determine cardiac output. Inotropic agents, afterload therapy, and intravascular volume adjustments may be needed to maintain both gas exchange and cardiac output. PEEP is generally not effective in unilateral or focal lung disease and may even worsen arterial oxygenation.

The minute ventilation is used to regulate the $PaCO_2$—increasing ventilation will reduce $PaCO_2$. In most situations, a tidal volume of 10 to 12 ml per kg and a respiratory rate of 10 to 15 per min make up an appropriate starting point. Further adjustments are made based on arterial blood gas measurements. The goal is to normalize pH. Patients with chronic CO_2 retention may develop dangerous respiratory alkalosis if their $PaCO_2$ is reduced to "normal."

Three modes of positive pressure ventilation are commonly used. Initially, the *assist control* mode, in which an inspiratory effort by the patient triggers a preset volume to be delivered by the ventilator, is used. A controlled back-up rate is set, which will assure adequate ventilation should the patient become apneic or be heavily sedated from anesthesia or narcotics. The primary benefit of this mode is in allowing the patient to adjust his or her minute ventilation while still being provided with full inspiratory support, thereby reducing the work of breathing. Patients who are agitated or in pain may require sedation to prevent dangerous hyperventilation. Hyperventilation can also be avoided through the use of the *intermittent mandatory ventilation* (IMV) mode. Here, spontaneous respiration is augmented by a preset number of ventilator-assisted breaths. This mode is generally well tolerated but requires spontaneous ventilation to supplement the preset backup. The IMV mode is often used to assist in weaning. The backup rate can be gradually turned down until the patient is breathing spontaneously. In the infrequently used *control mode*, a preset number of ventilator breaths are delivered to the patient. The patient can take no spontaneous or assisted breaths in addition to those that are preset.

Complications related to mechanical ventilation are common and must be anticipated. The risk of lung rupture with resultant pneumothorax or pneumomediastinum increases as pressure required for ventilation increases. Virtually all pneumothoraces occurring during positive pressure ventilation require closed-chest tube drainage. Obstruction of the endotracheal tube with secretions, clotted blood, or a herniated cuff can cause difficulty with ventilation. Migration of the tube into the right main stem bronchus can lead to collapse of the left lung as well as inadequate ventilation. There is a high incidence of gastrointestinal bleeding in ventilated patients: prophylaxis with H_2 blockers or antacids should be ordered. Intubated patients have an increased risk for respiratory infection, often with difficult-to-treat hospital-acquired organisms.

Weaning from Mechanical Ventilation. In patients requiring brief ventilatory support for rapidly improving conditions (postoperative support, drug overdose, pulmonary edema, and so on), weaning can generally be accomplished as the underlying situation stabilizes. If acceptable oxygenation can be attained with less than 5 cm PEEP and an FiO_2 of 0.5 or less, a T tube apparatus is attached to the endotracheal tube. This permits the patient to breathe spontaneously while maintaining airway protection. If the patient is comfortable and Pa_{CO_2} and pH are adequate after 45 to 60 minutes, the tube can be removed after careful suctioning. Humidified air with an F_{IO_2} equal to that administered through the T tube is administered. Deep breathing and cough are encouraged after extubation to remove secretions and prevent atelectasis.

In patients with underlying lung disease or with complicated conditions requiring prolonged ventilatory support, weaning can be a more difficult task. Infection, malnutrition, respiratory secretions and bronchospasm, cardiovascular instability, and anemia must be treated or controlled. When the P_{AO_2} is 55 or greater on an F_{IO_2} of 0.4 to 0.5 and 0 to 5 cm PEEP, we initiate weaning.

Some simple bedside tests can help assess respiratory muscle strength and airway functions. If the maximal inspiratory force is more negative than -20 cm of H_2O and the forced vital capacity greater than 10 to 12 ml per kg, very brief, closely monitored T tube trials can be attempted. These are gradually prolonged until tolerated for 45 to 60 minutes. Alternatively, using the IMV mode, the back-up ventilatory support can be gradually reduced until the patient is breathing spontaneously. If there is no clinical evidence of distress (respiratory rate over 30 per min, pulse over 120 per min, and so on) after 45 minutes of spontaneous respiration, the minute ventilation (MV) and blood gases are measured. If the MV is less than 10 liters and the P_{AO_2} and pH are adequate, extubation can be considered. Frequently, several 2 to 4 hour T tube trials are performed on marginal patients prior to extubation. When weaning occurs over several days, it is important to provide respiratory support at night to allow adequate rest.

Common situations that prevent weaning include resistance from small diameter endotracheal tubes, persistent airway secretions or bronchospasm, and malnutrition.

Specific Forms of Respiratory Failure

Adult Respiratory Distress Syndrome (ARDS). ARDS describes diffuse lung injury that occurs in association with many serious medical conditions. Hypotension, sepsis, bacterial or viral pneumonia, massive trauma, pancreatitis, aspiration, and multiple blood transfusions are some of the more common causes. Central to the syndrome is an increase in permeability of the alveolar capillary membrane, which results in interstitial and alveolar edema. Collapse of terminal airways and alveoli also occurs, probably due to alterations in surfactant production. The lungs become stiff (reduced compliance). These abnormalities produce a large intrapulmonary shunt and an increased respiratory dead space. This combination of injury results in the clinical presentation of marked tachypnea, refractory hypoxemia, and diffuse x-ray infiltration.

Although the mortality of ARDS is over 50 per cent, aggressive, supportive therapy is indicated for virtually all patients. No reliable predictors of outcome exist, but those who do recover attain nearly normal lung function.

As in all forms of respiratory failure, assuring sufficient oxygen delivery to the tissues is a primary goal. The increased dead space and a noncompliant lung frequently prohibit spontaneous maintenance of the large minute ventilation required to maintain pH and Pa_{CO_2}. The large intrapulmonary shunt usually prevents correction of the hypoxemia with supplemental oxygen. Therefore, most patients with ARDS will require intubation and mechanical ventilation early in the course of their illness. PEEP is a mainstay of therapy in ARDS. By increasing resting lung volume and maintaining airway stability, air/blood interface and compliance are increased and shunt reduced. In most cases, adequate arterial oxygenation can be attained with 15 cm of water or less of PEEP. However, regular assessment of cardiac output is required to assure adequate oxygen delivery. We feel that pulmonary artery catheterization, at least initially, is mandatory in patients requiring 7 to 10 cm of water PEEP or more. The "optimal" PEEP is the smallest pressure that provides satisfactory oxygen delivery.

The pulmonary capillary wedge pressure (PCW) is maintained as low as possible without reducing cardiac output. This helps reduce intrapulmonary fluid and shunt. Oxygen delivery is maximized by correcting anemia and supporting cardiac output. Mixed venous oxygen content is maintained by reducing oxygen consumption (e.g., suppress fever, support ventilation, sedation). Nutritional supplementation is initiated early, as prolonged support is often necessary.

No conclusive evidence exists that colloid provides an advantage over crystalloid as fluid replacement. Similarly, there is no conclusive support for the widespread use of steroids in treating ARDS. However, some centers are using large doses (20 to 30 mg per kg per day) of steroids for 48 hours, particularly when ARDS is associated with gastric aspiration or the fat emboli syndrome.

The high pressures required to ventilate these patients results in a significant risk for pneumothorax and pneumomediastinum. All critically ill patients are at risk for gastric bleeding, and prophylaxis with antacids or H_2 blockers should be administered. Emotional support of the patient and family is too often neglected.

Weaning of patients recovering from ARDS is

no different from that described for other long-term ventilator patients. We begin weaning when the patient is stable, with an FIO_2 of 0.5 or less, and PEEP has been reduced to 0 to 5 cm of water.

Exacerbations of Chronic Lung Disease. Acute respiratory failure superimposed on chronic lung disease usually represents acute bronchitis, pneumonia, or exacerbation of bronchospasm. Because the primary pathophysiologic mechanism is V/Q mismatch, supplemental oxygen will correct hypoxemia in most situations. Judiciously used, oxygen therapy rarely suppresses respiration. Intubation and mechanical ventilation can usually be avoided. These patients can be very difficult to wean when ventilatory support is required.

Bronchospasm must be treated aggressively. Intravenous aminophylline is infused at approximately 0.5 mg per kg per hr. If not administered chronically, an initial loading dose of 6 mg per kg is given. Since the metabolism of aminophylline is highly variable, blood levels are determined and the infusion adjusted to maintain a concentration of 10 to 20 micrograms per ml. Inhaled beta-agonists are administered with an oxygen- or air-driven nebulizer. Isoetharine (0.5 ml in 5 ml of saline) and metaproterenol (0.3 ml in 5 ml of saline) are the most commonly used agents. There is no advantage, and some potential danger, to IPPB as a tool for delivery of beta-agonists.

Gram stains and cultures of sputum should be obtained and antibiotic therapy started. *Haemophilus influenzae* is a common pathogen in these patients, so ampicillin or a second generation cephalosporin is generally selected. Postural drainage and percussion are often utilized to help with clearance of secretions, although evidence for their effectiveness is inconclusive. We do not use mucolytics because of their potential for exacerbating bronchospasm.

Steroids, such as methylprednisolone, 0.5 to 1.0 mg per kg every 6 hours are given to most patients with evidence of bronchospasm and respiratory failure. These generally facilitate improvement 12 to 24 hours after initiation. Steroids are rapidly tapered over 7 to 10 days if improvement occurs.

Respiratory Failure Due to Primary Hypoventilation. Drug overdose, cerebral vascular accident, severe chest wall deformity, and neuromuscular disease are the common causes of primary hypoventilation. The A-a gradient is generally near normal unless aspiration or atelectasis is present. Accordingly, ventilation to reduce alveolar CO_2 tension is required if respiratory acidosis occurs. In patients with fluctuating weakness, such as Guillain-Barré syndrome or myasthenia gravis, frequent measurement of vital capacity can predict the need for assisted ventilation. If the vital capacity falls below 800 to 1000 ml, assisted ventilation is likely to be required. If available, ear oximetry or end-tidal CO_2 measurement can be a helpful adjunct in following these patients.

ATELECTASIS

method of
LOREN F. HIRATZKA, M.D.
University of Iowa
Iowa City, Iowa

Atelectasis may be defined as collapse of the lung due to absence of air within the alveoli. It may involve anatomic segments, lobes, or whole lungs but also may be a diffuse miliary process, as in the adult respiratory distress syndrome.

Treatment

The keys to the treatment of atelectasis are the anticipation and prevention of atelectasis in various clinical situations, the recognition and treatment of underlying disease, and the prompt initiation of vigorous treatment once atelectasis is found. Repeated assessment by physical examination (and in critically ill patients by serial chest x-ray views as well) is necessary to determine the presence of atelectasis and its response to treatment.

Compression of lung parenchyma by pleural space collections should be relieved by thoracentesis, tube thoracostomy, or thoracotomy. Decompression of the obstructed or poorly functioning gastrointestinal tract by tube drainage or surgical correction may alleviate diaphragmatic elevation. Surgical excision of intrathoracic mass lesions is usually required for diagnosis or therapy or both. Excision of bullous defects in the lung can be useful in selected patients.

Airway obstruction should be considered in any patient with atelectasis of an anatomic lung division (segment, lobe, or whole lung). Bronchoscopy can be diagnostic in patients with either intrinsic or extrinsic lesions and potentially therapeutic, particularly in patients with foreign body aspiration. When neoplasm is found to be the cause for atelectasis, surgical excision of the lesion and surrounding lung is usually required. Laser fulguration of large airway tumors has been recently successful in reopening obstructed airways.

Hypoventilation due to a central nervous system deficit or respiratory depressant drugs usually requires endotracheal intubation and assisted ventilation. Respiratory depression due to narcotics can be reversed with judicious administration of naloxone, either intravenously or intramuscularly.

Prevention of *postoperative atelectasis* can be aided by preoperative attention. Patients who smoke should be encouraged to stop smoking for one to two weeks prior to elective surgical procedures. Patients with chronic sputum production should be instructed in postoperative techniques such as incentive spirometry, chest percussion, postural drainage, coughing, and intermittent positive pressure breathing (IPPB) for medication delivery. Specific antibiotic therapy should be used if sputum is infected.

Intraoperative measures should be directed toward prevention of atelectasis. In the unconscious patient, the airway must be protected to avoid aspiration. Periodic suctioning may be required to remove secretions. Tidal volumes of 10 to 15 ml per kg with intermittent "sighs" or positive end expiratory pressure may help prevent microatelectasis.

Prevention and treatment of atelectasis center around maintenance of clear airways and restoration of as near normal ventilatory mechanics as possible. The principles are the same for nonoperated patients as well:

1. Inspired air should be *humidified* to avoid inspissation of tracheobronchial secretions. *Supplemental oxygen* may be given to maintain arterial $Po_2 \geq 80$ torr (must accept lower in patients with severe chronic pulmonary disease).

2. Unconscious or sedated patients should be placed in lateral decubitus position to *avoid aspiration,* particularly if the airway is not protected by an endotracheal tube.

3. Patients should be *turned in bed* every hour and encouraged to move about, changing positions to avoid atelectasis in dependent areas of lung.

4. *Early mobilization and ambulation,* if possible, further encourage expansion of different lung segments.

5. *Coughing and deep breathing* aid mobilization of tracheobronchial secretions and improvement of functional residual capacity. *Incentive spirometry* is helpful in cooperative and awake patients. *Endotracheal suctioning and injection of saline* through a small needle or catheter passed through the cricothyroid membrane can be added stimuli to induce coughing in less cooperative or obtunded patients. However, care must be taken to limit endotracheal suctioning to avoid hypoxemia. In addition, either of these more invasive measures can cause significant laryngospasm in some patients.

6. *Chest percussion and postural drainage* should be used, particularly if atelectasis is present with abundant tracheobronchial secretions.

7. *Adequate pain control* usually requires small, frequent doses of narcotic analgesics to permit cooperation with coughing, deep breathing, chest percussion, and postural drainage and to avoid respiratory depression associated with larger doses of these drugs. Epidural analgesia or intercostal nerve blocks or both are helpful, particularly in patients with poor pulmonary reserve for whom narcotic-induced respiratory depression could be detrimental. Transcutaneous nerve stimulation has been described as useful in decreasing incisional pain as well.

8. *Bronchodilators* such as isoproterenol or racemic epinephrine should be administered by nebulizer or IPPB treatments for patients with bronchospasm in whom cardiac disease or arrhythmia is not a problem. Intravenous aminophylline with monitoring of blood levels, or subcutaneous terbutaline, may be used with similar precautions with regard to cardiac disease. The *routine use of IPPB* alone does *not* prevent atelectasis and is not cost effective.

9. *Mucolytic agents* agents such as N-acetylcysteine can be given by IPPB or nebulizer in patients with tenacious secretions.

10. *Bronchoscopy* should be used early in cases of lobar or significant segmental atelectasis and particularly when atelectasis is refractory to other measures. Obstructing mucus plugs and foreign bodies can be removed and inspissated secretions liquified by saline lavage.

11. If secretions are purulent, a *Gram stain and culture* of the sputum should be obtained and specific antibiotic therapy given.

12. *Ventilatory support* with *tracheostomy* may be required for severe, prolonged respiratory insufficiency. Tracheostomy alone may be required for patients with limited respiratory reserve to reduce ventilatory dead space and facilitate direct tracheobronchial suctioning.

The treatment of adult respiratory distress syndrome requires limitation and treatment of the primary inciting factor (such as sepsis, pancreatitis, shock) as well as the aforementioned treatment modalities. In addition, attention should be directed to fluid restriction, diuresis (furosemide, 0.5 to 1.0 mg per kg intravenously every 4 to 6 hours), ventilator support using positive end expiratory pressure to maximize functional residual capacity, and maintenance of adequate cardiac output.

CHRONIC OBSTRUCTIVE PULMONARY DISEASE AND BRONCHIECTASIS

method of
LEE S. NEWMAN, M.D.,
and ROBERT M. TATE, M.D.
University of Colorado
Denver, Colorado

Diagnosis

Chronic bronchitis and emphysema are distinct pathologic entities. However, they overlap clinically to such a large extent that we call them chronic obstructive pulmonary disease (COPD). "Pure" bronchitis or "pure" emphysema is relatively uncommon. Chronic bronchitis is defined by the following clinical history: symptoms of daily cough and sputum production for a minimum of 3 months for 2 consecutive years. Emphysema is an anatomic diagnosis: the pathologic dilatation of terminal airspaces, associated with destruction of alveolar walls. COPD is characterized by predominant, fixed airflow limitation. However, many patients demonstrate partial reversibility of airflow limitation, which can be capitalized upon in COPD management.

Bronchiectasis is defined anatomically: irreversible, pathologic dilatation of the bronchi. Bronchial injury due to infection is the usual basis of bronchiectasis. In a small percentage of cases it will be a manifestation of a specific disorder, such as cystic fibrosis. Bronchiectasis is also associated with airflow limitation, but in the setting of recurrent infection, persistent cough, and copious sputum production. Chest radiographs or bronchography may be diagnostic. Methods of treatment of bronchiectasis overlap with those of COPD.

Principles of Management

Objectives in COPD management are to (1) help prevent its occurrence, (2) treat the reversible components of the disease, (3) anticipate and treat the complications, such as infection, cor pulmonale, hypoxemia, and respiratory failure, (4) provide symptomatic relief through a program of pulmonary rehabilitation, and (5) try to slow the natural progression of disease through oxygen therapy and helping patients stop smoking.

Prevention

Smoking cessation should be a high priority for those interested in reducing the incidence and severity of COPD. Cigarette smoke is the prime etiologic agent. Health professionals should urge all patients to stop smoking, work to strengthen the rights of nonsmokers, help restrict smoking in public areas, including hospitals, and set an example by not smoking. Smoking cessation programs exist in many cities, often as a social service adjunct to a pulmonary rehabilitation program. These yield 1-year success rates of from 25 to 40 per cent. Although not a panacea, nicotine-containing gum (Nicorette) may be a useful crutch for weaning the patient who is already motivated to stop smoking. It should be prescribed judiciously with complete instructions and with adequate physician follow-up, preferably in conjunction with a smoking cessation program. Improper usage of nicotine resin gum (excessive chewing, for example) may result in unpleasant side effects such as lightheadedness and nausea, with consequent discontinuation of the gum.

TREATMENT

Bronchodilators

Because most COPD patients have a reversible component to their airway obstruction, an aggressive trial of bronchodilator therapy is always indicated. Even patients who objectively show no response to bronchodilators during routine pulmonary function testing may derive symptomatic benefit. Three main groups of bronchodilators are available: (1) beta-adrenergic agonists, (2) theophyllines, and (3) anticholinergic agents.

Inhaled beta-agonist aerosols are the logical choice for initial therapy. There are few side effects, and most patients have a good response. Anticholinergic aerosols are useful as a substitute for beta-agonists in some patients. Those with particularly severe disease may benefit from a regimen combining theophylline with alternating aerosolized beta-agonists and anticholinergics. The role of corticosteroids is discussed later.

Beta-Adrenergic Agents

When beta-receptors are stimulated, the activity of the enzyme adenyl cyclase increases. This, in turn, increases production of cyclic AMP, which leads to bronchodilation and inhibits the release of chemical mediators of inflammation. Beta-2 receptors are found primarily in the airways, whereas beta-1 receptors are present elsewhere, including the heart. Thus, there are practical and theoretic reasons for using more beta-2 specific bronchodilators. Table 1 illustrates the evolution of adrenergic agents from the nonspecific beta-agonist isoproterenol (Isuprel) to the currently favored beta-2 selective agents like albuterol (Ventolin, Proventil), terbutaline (Brethaire, Brethine), and metaproterenol (Alupent, Metaprel). Increasing beta-2 selectively is associated with less tachycardia, palpitations, and gastrointestinal upset. Also, there is less chance of patients becoming refractory to the action of these newer agents, compared with isoproterenol. We recommend the use of any of these beta-2 selective agents. They may vary slightly in their effectiveness and side effects for individual patients, so if one agent is a problem, others should be tried.

TABLE 1. **Aerosolized Bronchodilators**

	Activity	Onset	Duration	Usual Dose MDI	Usual Dose Solution
Sympathomimetic Agents					
isoproterenol (Medihaler, Isuprel)	β_1 and β_2	1–5 min	1–3 hr	2 puffs 4–6× daily	0.5 ml (1:200) in 2 ml normal saline over 20 min q 4 hr
isoetharine (Bronkometer, Bronkosol)	$\beta_2 > \beta_1$	5 min	1.5–3 hr	2 puffs 4–6× daily	0.5 ml in 1.5 ml q 4 hr
metaproterenol (Alupent, Metaprel)	$\beta_2 > \beta_1$	5–30 min	1–5 hr	2 puffs 4–6× daily	0.3 ml in 1 ml q 4 hr
albuterol (Ventolin, Proventil)	$\beta_2 > \beta_1$	within 15 min	3–6 hr	2 puffs 4–6× daily	NA
terbutaline (Brethaire)	$\beta_2 > \beta_1$	5–30 min	3–6 hr	2 puffs 4–6× daily	NA
Anticholinergic Agents					
atropine sulfate		within 15 min	4–6 hr	NA	0.025 mg/kg q 4–6 hr
ipratropium bromide (Atrovent)		within 5 min	4–6 hr	2 puffs 4–6× daily	NA

For COPD outpatients, the usual mode of delivery of aerosol is via metered-dose inhalers (MDI)—a typical dose being 2 puffs four times a day, with an additional 1 or 2 puffs acceptable on a prn basis. Remind patients to use the inhaler prior to anticipated increases in activity or exposure to cold or other known provocative stimuli. To improve the effectiveness of the MDI, the health professional must take the time to instruct the patient in proper use and check inhaler technique on subsequent office visits. In an effort to improve delivery of aerosol, several tubelike reservoir chambers have been designed to attach to the MDIs. These do improve delivery and make it possible to prescribe the MDI for some elderly patients who otherwise might have difficulty coordinating their inhalations with aerosol puffs.

Compressor-driven nebulizer units are available for home use, as an alternative to the MDI. While these nebulizers are less convenient, they can deliver a somewhat higher dose over a longer period. Certain patients with severe COPD will benefit more from the use of such devices and may use them in conjunction with the portable MDIs.

For inpatients with exacerbations of symptoms, we routinely use the compressed-air nebulizer treatments in lieu of MDIs. A typical dosing is metaproterenol (Alupent, Metaprel), 0.3 ml in 1.5 ml of normal saline, nebulized every 4 hours and prn. In the hands of a respiratory therapist supervising treatments at the bedside, this affords maximal beta-agonist benefit.

There is no proven benefit to the use of intermittent positive pressure breathing (IPPB) devices in delivery of bronchodilators. However, in rare instances, patients with end-stage COPD may be able to avoid mechanical ventilation by use of IPPB delivery of beta-agonists.

For a comparable amount of bronchodilation, oral beta-agonists have significantly more systemic side effects than do aerosols. We reserve the use of oral forms for patients who are too uncoordinated to manage aerosols. Combining oral and aerosol beta-agents increases side effects without significantly improving bronchodilatation. The use of subcutaneous preparations, such as terbutaline or epinephrine, is reserved for emergency situations and has no role in the routine management of COPD.

Most complications associated with beta-adrenergic agents are due to excessive sympathomimetic effect. Adverse reactions include tachycardia, palpitations, and increased blood pressure. Tremor and nervousness, which may subside after several weeks of use, are fairly common complaints. These medications should be used with caution in patients with hyperthyroidism, diabetes mellitus, hypertension, and coronary atherosclerotic heart disease.

Theophyllines

Although methylxanthines have been in use since 1900, the mechanism by which they cause bronchodilation remains obscure. The phosphodiesterase enzyme that degrades cyclic AMP can be inhibited by theophylline but not at the theophylline concentrations achieved therapeutically. A number of other proposed mechanisms for bronchial smooth muscle relaxation have been proposed, but none are proved. Aminophylline is a potent stimulant of diaphragmatic contractility, both before and after diaphragmatic fatigue. Aminophylline is also a central respiratory stimulant that is capable of improving the ventilatory response to hypoxemia. The dual regimen of theophylline plus beta-adrenergic aerosols is the cornerstone of COPD therapy.

Oral preparations fall into two categories: the older preparations—soluble salt forms of the drug, and the newer, sustained-release anhydrous preparations. The former are well absorbed, with peak levels 2 hours after ingestion. Their disadvantage is that they must be taken every 6 hours to maintain adequate serum levels. This leads to compliance problems. The use of these salts has been supplanted by the sustained-release forms. These have undergone substantial improvement to provide more even blood levels.

It is advisable to monitor theophylline blood levels regardless of the type of preparation or its mode of delivery. The therapeutic range is 10 to 20 micrograms per ml. Many patients will manifest a bronchodilator response below this range. Adverse side effects may be experienced in the subtherapeutic range. There is no benefit in pushing serum levels to the high therapeutic range versus low therapeutic range in chronic outpatient use. Blood levels should be checked 4 to 6 hours after the last dose of sustained-release preparation, or 2 hours after a conventional tablet. These trough levels may be useful in identifying patients with inadequate dosing or rapid clearance.

Dosing with theophyllines for chronic, outpatient use should start low (400 to 600 mg per day for adults), and gradually be increased over the first few weeks. This titration should be based on appearance of side effects, improvement of symptoms, and serial blood levels. The usual final dose will be approximately 800 mg per day, but factors influencing metabolism and volume of distribution will alter this figure. Acute changes in patient status or the addition of medications that interact with theophylline (Table 2) warrants new blood level measurements.

When managing acute exacerbations of COPD, intravenous aminophylline should replace oral theophyllines. In patients not currently using theophyllines, a full loading dose of aminophylline (5.6 mg per kg of ideal body weight) is administered in 100 ml of intravenous fluid over 20 to 30 minutes. Patients already on theophyllines may require a one-half loading dose unless they are already known to have therapeutic levels. The maintenance intravenous dose will vary with the patient and should be adjusted according to blood levels. Recommended starting doses are for healthy nonsmokers, 0.6 to 0.7 mg per kg body weight per hour; healthy smokers, 0.8 to 0.9 mg per kg per hour; elderly patients, 0.4 to 0.5 mg per kg per hour; patients with liver disease, congestive heart failure, or cor pulmonale, 0.3 to 0.4 mg per kg per hour. If rapid theophylline assays are not available, more conservative dosing should be used.

TABLE 2. **Some Conditions That May Affect Theophylline Metabolism**

Increased **Metabolism—May Need to Increase Dose**	***Decreased*** **Metabolism—May Need to Decrease Dose**
Smoking	Heart failure
Children, adolescents	Hepatic dysfunction
Phenytoin (Dilantin)	Cimetidine (Tagamet)
Barbiturates	Erythromycin, clindamycin, troleandomycin
Decrease in dietary methylxanthines	Oral contraceptives
	Infants (< 6 months)
	Old age

Adverse effects of theophyllines include gastrointestinal symptoms (nausea, diarrhea, heartburn) and central nervous system stimulation (insomnia, tremor, anxiety). These can occur at any level of therapy. Seizures and cardiac arrhythmias are two life-threatening complications that occur with greater frequency when levels exceed 35 micrograms per ml. Seizures may occur with no other warning side effects, are quite refractory to therapy, and have a 50 per cent mortality rate. Ventricular ectopy is usually responsive to lidocaine (Xylocaine). At therapeutic dosage levels, there is no evidence that theophyllines increase ventricular ectopy. Theophyllines pose no known risk to pregnant women, fetuses, or breast-feeding infants.

If an overdosage of theophylline is suspected, discontinue the drug immediately. Administration of activated charcoal by mouth or nasogastric tube will double the clearance rate.

Anticholinergic Agents

Anticholinergics are potent bronchodilators, equal to or even superior to the beta-adrenergic aerosols in COPD patients. At the present time, atropine sulfate remains the only available preparation in the United States, although it is anticipated that new atropine-like agents such as ipratropium bromide (Atrovent) will soon be available. This synthetic compound has the advantages of (1) the convenience of a disposable, metered-dose inhaler, (2) fewer side effects than atropine sulfate, and (3) a longer duration of action.

Atropine and the new synthetic agents are both specific inhibitors of the muscarinic actions of acetylcholine. The latter agent is more selective for the bronchial tree. Because it is poorly absorbed, ipratropium bromide stays at the site of deposition and will not cross the blood-brain barrier.

Atropine sulfate is an effective addition to the therapy of hospitalized COPD patients and some highly refractory patients who have home nebulizer units. The usual adult dose is 0.025 mg per kg nebulized in 1.5 ml of normal saline approximately every 6 hours. A typical dose, then, is 1 to 2 mg every 6 hours, usually alternating with a beta-adrenergic agent, although the two can be combined in a single treatment. For ipratropium bromide, the typical dose is 2 puffs four times a day by MDI. Patients should be aware that the onset of action of anticholinergics is slower than with the beta-aerosols—approximately 1 hour.

Toxicity is dose related for all the antimuscarinic agents. Adverse symptoms include dry mouth and dry skin at low dose. Tachycardia and blurred vision due to meiosis occur at an absorbed dose of atropine of 2.0 mg. Higher doses are associated with speech, swallowing, and micturition problems in some patients. Frank confusion or agitation can occur. Atropine sulfate should be avoided in patients with glaucoma or bladder neck obstruction.

The inhaled ipratropium bromide is poorly absorbed and therefore will rarely manifest these side effects, except for dry mouth. It is safe in patients with glaucoma and bladder neck obstruction. While atropine sulfate has been criticized as causing a decrease in mucociliary clearance, this effect is usually not significant nor a deterrent to its use in normal dosage. Ipratropium has no significant effect on mucus clearance, production, or viscosity.

Corticosteroids

Steroids have an important role in the management of severe COPD, but they must be used cautiously because of their significant side effects. They are reserved for patients who are still symptomatic despite maximal bronchodilator therapy, as previously outlined. They may be used chronically or in higher doses during acute exacerbations. Although the action of corticosteroids is obscure, generally they are felt to reduce airway inflammation and augment beta-receptor responsiveness to bronchodilator agents.

When initiating steroids in a refractory outpatient, we begin with prednisone, 40 to 60 mg orally each morning, for 2 weeks. Pulmonary function tests are then repeated to evaluate efficacy. If FEV_1 and the FEV_1/FVC ratio improve, the patient is maintained on the prednisone, but an immediate effort is made to taper to the smallest dose required to maintain clinical benefit. If the patient does not show response on pulmonary function testing to the steroid trial, prednisone is discontinued. Subjective response in itself is not sufficient justification for continuous steroids. Once it is established that a patient benefits from prednisone, at least one effort should be made to place the individual on an alternate-day regimen. Alternate-day schedules produce fewer long-term side effects.

Steroid-dependent patients requiring less than 20 mg of prednisone or its equivalent should also be tried on an inhaled steroid preparation such as beclomethasone diproprionate (Vanceril, Beclovent). These are prescribed as a metered dose inhaler to be used following an inhaled bronchodilator treatment. By using it after a beta-agonist, beclomethasone is less likely to irritate the airway and will have better drug delivery. Inhaled steroids offer the advantage of less systemic absorption, less hypothalamic-pituitary-adrenal axis suppression, and fewer side effects than oral corticosteroids. Even if the patient cannot be tapered off oral prednisone entirely, the beclomethasone is still worthwhile if it allows a partial decrease in the systemic steroid dose. Two new oral aerosol formulations are now available—flunisolide (Aerobid) and triamcinolone acetonide (Azmacort).

While converting from systemic oral preparations to steroid aerosols, remember that it may take 2 weeks for the inhaled form to reach therapeutic effect. Taper the oral preparation slowly to avoid COPD exacerbations. Do not use inhaled steroids during acute exacerbations since they can accentuate bronchospasm. Adverse effects of inhaled corticosteroids are hoarseness and *Candida* or *Aspergillus* infections in the mouth, pharynx, or larynx. Topical antifungal drugs usually suffice to treat this complication. Typical dosing is beclomethasone 2 to 4 puffs four times a day following one-half hour after beta-adrenergic aerosol treatment.

During any exacerbation of COPD or in periods of stress such as surgery, steroid-dependent patients should be given a boost of steroids, usually administered intravenously. A typical dose is methylprednisolone (Solu-Medrol), 60 to 125 mg every 6 to 8 hours for 48 to 72 hours or until symptoms begin to improve. Then it is appropriate to switch back to prednisone, 40 to 60 mg a day, with a gradual taper back to the smallest effective dose.

Other Pharmacologic Agents

Cromolyn sodium (Intal), while having an important place in the treatment of asthma and bronchospasm due to cold exposure or exercise, is not usually used in COPD. The role of calcium channel blockers, such as nifedipine, in treating diseases of airflow limitation is being actively investigated. But to date these agents have not found a place in the routine management of COPD. Mucolytic agents such a *N*-acetylcysteine (Mucomyst) are rarely useful as aerosolized agents. Their efficacy in helping "loosen" secretions has been called into question. However, a rare patient with inspissated secretions may show a clinical response to aerosolized doses of 10 to 20 mg of a 10 to 20 per cent solution. It should be administered with a bronchodilator agent.

Pulmonary Rehabilitation

Selected motivated patients will clearly benefit from a comprehensive pulmonary rehabilitation program. The major goals include breathing training (diaphragmatic breathing; pursed-lip breathing; slow, deep breathing), physical reconditioning, techniques of postural drainage and percussion, and counsel in the activities of daily living. Recently, some patients have appeared to benefit from respiratory muscle training by breathing against expiratory resistance devices. Finally, the rehabilitation team can provide education and encourage compliance with all aspects of care, including the proper use of bronchodilators, oxygen, antibiotics, and corticosteroids.

Preventing Complications and Slowing Progression of Disease

COPD patients are plagued by a number of complications, some of which can be averted. Routine office spirometry may detect early disease and allow for early, effective intervention. Recurrent bronchitis and pneumonia may be prevented by early administration of oral antibiotics. Vaccination against pneumococcus and influenza can reduce the incidence of these particularly common infections. Hypoxemia and pulmonary hypertension respond to the use of low flow oxygen therapy.

Early Treatment of Infection

The COPD patient often will be seen with an increase in chronic cough and dyspnea, as well as with a change in the color and consistency of sputum. A short course of a broad-spectrum antibiotic will usually lead to earlier resolution of symptoms and avert hospitalization. The usual bacterial organisms colonizing the bronchial tree of COPD patients are *Streptococcus pneumoniae* and *Haemophilus influenzae*. The antibiotic choice should be made with this in mind, and with the recognition that as many as 30 per cent of *H. influenzae* isolates will be beta-lactamase–positive in some communities and therefore ampicillin-resistant. Initial antibiotics of choice include ampicillin, tetracycline, and trimethoprim-sulfamethoxazole. These are given on an empiric basis, and unless pneumonia is present, sputum and blood cultures are not indicated. COPD patients with diabetes mellitus, alcohol abuse, bronchiectasis, recent antibiotic use, recent hospitalization, or who live in nursing homes have a much higher risk of infection with gram-negative organisms, such as *Pseudomonas, Klebsiella,* and *Escherichia coli*. In these patients sputum Gram stain and culture should be performed at the time of empiric antibiotic therapy. Note that 20 to 30 per cent of respiratory infections in COPD patients are due to viruses or *Mycoplasma pneumoniae*.

Prevention of Infection

Pneumococcal vaccine should be administered to patients with COPD. The vaccine is given only once and affords some long-term protection, although protection is not complete. Serious pneumococcal infection can still occur.

Influenza vaccine should be routinely administered each fall. If they miss their injection or have a clear contraindication to its use, COPD patients may be placed on amantadine for prophylaxis (200 mg orally daily throughout the period of risk). Should the COPD patient develop early symptoms of true influenza, early treatment with amantadine (200 mg orally daily for the duration of illness plus 48 hours) helps reduce duration of fever and symptoms. Whether it also reduces the incidence of secondary bacterial pneumonia or prevents fatalities in COPD is not known. Side effects occur mainly in older patients and those with renal insufficiency. These include minor central nervous system symptoms such as confusion, dizziness, and headache. Blurred vision also occurs.

Long-Term Oxygen Therapy

Severe hypoxemia is responsible for some of the most serious and insidious complications of COPD. It is a potent stimulus to pulmonary vasoconstriction, resulting in elevations of pulmonary artery pressure and, ultimately, irreversible pulmonary hypertension, increased right ventricular work, hypertrophy, and failure. Oxygen therapy at low rates reduces pulmonary vasoconstriction. When used in properly selected patients and on a continuous basis, oxygen reduces complications and prolongs life in the end-stage COPD patient.

Candidates for chronic home oxygen therapy include stable COPD patients who show persistently low arterial Po_2 levels on room air (less than 55 mm Hg) despite maximal medical therapy. The patient should be stable for approximately 3 weeks and then restudied, since about 25 per cent will no longer require supplementation when evaluated several weeks after hospital discharge while on intensive bronchodilator therapy. There are sound clinical indications for home oxygen use in addition to the absolute arterial oxygen tension value. These are (1) evidence of pulmonary hypertension, cor pulmonale, and right heart failure by radiograph, physical findings, or electrocardiogram; (2) evidence of significant hypoxemia during sleep; (3) hypoxemia during exercise; (4) oxygen-associated improvement in exercise tolerance, even though the Po_2 remains greater than 55 mm Hg; (5) unexplained confusional states or headaches that improve with oxygen supplementation; and (6) otherwise unexplained erythrocytosis.

Chronic oxygen therapy should be used on a continuous basis. Twenty-four hour oxygen is superior to nocturnal oxygen alone. Sufficient oxygen can be delivered by nasal cannula. Objectives should be to maintain the PaO_2 in the 60 to 65 mm Hg range (or oxygen saturation greater than 90 per cent). Usually 1 to 3 liters per minute is sufficient. Flow rates generally need to be increased by 1 liter per minute when the patient is exercising and when sleeping, especially if nocturnal desaturation is seen. The ear oximeter has proved to be a useful measuring tool in these settings, reducing the need for several arterial blood gases.

The three methods of supplying oxygen in the home are compressed gas, liquid oxygen, and an oxygen concentrator. Compressed gas has the advantage of being the least expensive if used at low flow rates and is also widely available. But the tanks are heavy and cumbersome, and frequent deliveries of new tanks are needed. Although portable tanks can be used, these too are quite heavy and offer a relatively small volume of oxygen. Liquid oxygen is the most portable and convenient system. It can be less expensive if it is used for prolonged periods at high flow rates. At low flow rates it is the most expensive. Portable units are easier to handle and offer twice as much oxygen for their weight as the portable compressed-oxygen tanks. However, some patients have difficulty refilling the portable unit from the larger home reservoir. Oxygen concentrators extract O_2 from the air. These units run on electricity, so a back-up system may be needed. Portable units are not available. Since only about 40 per cent oxygen is extracted, the unit can deliver a maximum O_2 flow of approximately 4 liters per minute. It is most attractive for patients who stay home and use continuous low flow. In that setting it is the most economical over the long term.

Measures to Treat Cor Pulmonale

If pulmonary hypertension and right heart failure are recognized early, some of the damage can be reversed. The objective is to reduce right ventricular work. Oxygen is the most effective agent. Its use was just discussed. Diuretics will reduce edema and can decrease pulmonary pressure by decreasing blood volume but must be handled judiciously. Digitalis is probably ineffective in the treatment of right-sided heart failure. It may have more value in biventricular failure, but even this is subject to debate. Bronchodilators, beta-adrenergic agonists, and theophylline do have some beneficial hemodynamic effects and improve gas exchange, thereby reducing hypoxemia.

Some COPD patients demonstrate increased hypoxemia while asleep. These nocturnal oxygen desaturations may be associated with cardiac arrhythmias and can lead to pulmonary hypertension. COPD patients with histories of prominent snoring, morning headaches, impotence, or daytime hypersomnolence may have true sleep apnea and should undergo a complete sleep evaluation. Nocturnal oxygen therapy may abolish the periods of desaturation. Patients already requiring continuous oxygen therapy should increase flow by 1 additional liter per minute at night.

Treating Complications

Despite maximal therapy, complications will still occur. Exacerbations from any cause require quick action to maximize management. Bronchodilator dosages should be increased if possible, sometimes to as often as every 2 hours by nebulizer. Intravenous aminophylline is substituted for oral theophylline, as outlined earlier. If infection is suspected, antibiotics should be started, following the previous recommendations. High dose steroids early in the exacerbation may be life-saving. Respiratory therapy to help clear secretions can be intensified best if the patient is hospitalized. If cor pulmonale is the reason for deterioration, the addition of a diuretic such as intravenous furosemide (Lasix) will help. Oxygen therapy should be instituted to reduce tissue hypoxia and pulmonary vasoconstriction, but arterial blood gases should be carefully monitored, especially in patients with a known history of hypercapnia. High flow oxygen can abolish the hypoxic drive to breathe and precipitate respiratory arrest.

Respiratory Failure and Mechanical Ventilation

When a COPD patient's FEV_1 is 1 liter or less, the 5 year survival is no better than 50 per cent. Although it is a delicate subject, the issue of mechanical ventilation should be discussed with the individual patient while he or she is relatively stable, not in extremis. Patients should be educated and encouraged to verbalize their opinions and directions regarding management of the disease in its final stages.

Surgical Thearpy

In a rare patient with large bullae, or a bulla of increasing size, surgical resection may be indicated. These tension bullae may compress a large portion of comparatively normal lung tissue. Local resection or plication is preferred to lobectomy to help conserve viable lung.

Treatment of Bronchiectasis

The approach to bronchiectasis follows the same principles described for COPD, especially regarding management of infection. The keys to treatment are (1) teaching patients how to clear secretions, using postural drainage and chest percussion, and (2) early recognition of purulent sputum. The use of short courses of antibiotics in rotating fashion, such as ampicillin, tetracycline, or trimethoprim-sulfa, is useful.

Management is further aided by diagnosis of underlying causes of bronchiectasis. Although usually due to past infection, bronchiectasis may be a manifestation of systemic illness, like cystic fibrosis or hypogammaglobulinemia.

A rare patient will have sufficiently localized bronchiectasis to warrant surgical excision of the affected lobe or segment. Bronchography can be performed through fiberoptic bronchoscopy to define local disease. If the area is well circumscribed and the patient is hindered by debilitating infections or hemoptysis, surgical intervention is justifiable.

PRIMARY LUNG CANCER

method of
H. GUNTER SEYDEL, M.D.
Henry Ford Hospital
Detroit, Michigan

It is estimated that 135,000 new cases of bronchogenic carcinoma were diagnosed during 1984 in the United States; approximately 80 per cent were the nonsmall cell type (squamous cell, large cell undifferentiated, or adenocarcinoma) and 20 per cent, small cell undifferentiated (including oat cell) carcinoma. This classification of histopathology was developed by the World Health Organization (WHO) and has been widely accepted. Approximately 117,000 annual deaths are attributed to lung cancer, making it the most lethal malignancy among American men, with a rapidly rising incidence among women. Surgery is the most effective method of treatment for patients without distant metastases. Chemotherapy with or without radiation therapy is effective in small cell undifferentiated carcinoma, whereas it remains investigational in patients with nonsmall cell cancer. Combined modality treatment has the best prospect for improvement in outcome. Staging helps in the selection of patients for treatment; the system of the American Joint Committee on Cancer has been generally accepted (Tables 1 and 2).

Nonsmall Cell Carcinoma

Surgery

Approximately one half of patients with nonsmall cell lung cancer have distant metastatic disease when the diagnosis is first established. About one third of all patients have inoperable disease localized in one hemithorax without distant metastases, and the remaining one sixth may be considered operable with curative intent.

In patients with localized pulmonary lesions and a forced expiratory volume at 1 minute (FEV_1) of more than 1.5 liters, a lobectomy or pneumonectomy should be considered. Patients who cannot climb a flight of stairs without sig-

TABLE 1. **Tumor-Node-Metastasis (TNM) Classification in Lung Cancer**

Primary Tumor (T)	
TX	Tumor either proven by the presence of malignant cells in bronchopulmonary secretions but not visualized roentgenographically or bronchoscopically, or cannot be assessed
T0	No evidence of primary tumor
Tis	Carcinoma in situ
T1	A tumor that is 3 cm or less in greatest diameter, surrounded by lung or visceral pleura, and without evidence of invasion proximal to a lobar bronchus at bronchoscopy
T2	A tumor more than 3 cm in greatest diameter or a tumor of any size that either invades the visceral pleura or has associated atelectasis or obstructive pneumonitis extending to the hilar region. At bronchoscopy, the proximal extent of demonstrable tumor must be within a lobar bronchus or at least 2 cm distal to the carina. Any associated atelectasis or obstructive penumonitis must involve less than an entire lung, and there must be no pleural effusion
T3	A tumor of any size with direct extension into an adjacent structure, such as the parietal pleura or chest wall, the diaphragm, or the mediastinum and its contents; a tumor bronchoscopically demonstrable to involve a main bronchus less than 2 cm distal to the carina; any tumor associated with atelectasis or obstructive pneumonitis of an entire lung or pleural effusion.
Nodal Involvement (N)	
NX	Minimum requirement to assess the regional nodes cannot be met
N0	No evidence of involvement of regional lymph nodes
N1	Metastasis to lymph nodes in the peribronchial or the ipsilateral hilar region, or both, including direct extension
N2	Metastasis to lymph nodes in the mediastinum
Distant Metastasis (M)	
MX	Minimum requirements to assess the presence of distant metastasis cannot be met
M0	No evidence of distant metastasis
M1	Distant metastasis present Specify ________

nificant dyspnea or with prior serious medical problems such as myocardial infarction may be considered inoperable.

Inoperability because of mediastinal lymph node involvement is excluded by chest radiographs, linear or computed axial tomography (CT), or mediastinoscopy. A mediastinotomy is done by some because of better exposure of the mediastinal lymph nodes.

Patients with pathologic stage 1 disease (T1, N0, M0; T1, N1, M0; or T2, N0, M0) have a reasonable survival following resection: 75 per cent may be expected to be alive at 1 year and approximately 50 per cent at 5 years. The preferred procedure is a lobectomy, with pneumonectomy reserved for centrally located operable tumors. When lymph nodes are involved in the specimen (stage 2), the 5-year survival drops to about 30 per cent. For patients with resectable stage 3 disease, 5 year survivals are about 15 per cent and approximately half of patients are dead 1 year after surgery. Operative mortality should not be more than 5 per cent with lobectomy and 10 per cent with pneumonectomy if careful preoperative work-up is carried out.

In stage 1, lung cancer adjuvant treatment is of no value, whether by postoperative radiation therapy or intraoperative or postoperative use of bacille Calmette Guérin (BCG) in the pleural cavity. This is independent of the histologic type. In patients with lymph node involvement (stage 2) or in patients with stage 3 disease with squamous cell carcinoma, postoperative radiation therapy reduces the local recurrence rate, although its influence on survival has not been established. Most centers in the United States will also recommend postoperative radiation therapy for patients with large cell undifferentiated carcinoma and adenocarcinoma with these stages of tumor.

Although some centers recommend chest wall resection for tumors involving the chest wall, this is not generally accepted and is successful only in experienced hands. The use of preoperative radiation therapy has not been shown to be effective as a routine measure, and its value in superior sulcus tumors is advocated only by a few specialized surgeons and radiation oncologists.

Adjuvant postoperative or preoperative chemotherapy is an investigational method of treatment at this time, the value of which remains to be established.

TABLE 2. **Stage Grouping in Primary Lung Cancer**

Occult Stage: TX, N0, M0
An occult carcinoma with bronchopulmonary secretions containing malignant cells but without other evidence of the primary tumor or evidence of metastasis to the regional nodes or distant metastasis

Stage 1: Tis, N0, M0 carcinoma in situ; T1, N0, M0; T1, N1, M0; T2, N0, M0
A tumor that can be classified T1 without any metastasis or with metastasis to the lymph nodes in the peribronchial or ipsilateral hilar region only, or a tumor that can be classified T2 without any metastasis to nodes or distant metastasis
Note: TX, N1, M0 is also theoretically possible, but such a clinical diagnosis would be difficult if not impossible to make. If such a diagnosis is made, it would be included in Stage 1

Stage 2: T2, N1, M0
A tumor classified as T2 with metastasis to the lymph nodes in the peribronchial or ipsilateral hilar region only

Stage 3:
T3 with any N or M
N2 with any T or M
M1 with any T or N
Any tumor more extensive than T2, any tumor with metastasis to the lymph nodes in the mediastinum, or any tumor with distant metastasis

Radiation Therapy

In approximately one third of patients with diagnosed nonsmall cell carcinoma of the lung, disease is localized in one hemithorax without evidence of distant metastases or is inoperable either because of medical problems or because of local tumor extension or mediastinal lymphadenopathy. Radiation therapy is the mainstay of treatment. Recent advances in radiation therapy techniques, including the use of high energy x-ray beams, special shielding devices, and computed dosimetry, including CT scanning, have made possible the administration of high doses of radiation therapy (5500 centigray or more) without undue complications. The majority of these patients are stage T3 or N2, and the survival rate has been shown to reach 50 per cent at 1 year, 15 to 20 per cent at 3 years, and 5 to 7 per cent at 5 years. Waiting for the asymptomatic patient to become symptomatic usually includes significant rapid local progression of tumor, with distant metastases likely, and a decreased likelihood of long-term tumor control and survival. If patients with borderline pulmonary decompensation are excluded, radiation therapy will be tolerated without undue complications. Treatment planning, including optimal limitation of radiation doses to the normal lung, spinal cord, and heart, is a necessary prerequisite for the long-term disease-free and complication-free survival of these patients. This requires special care, expertise, and equipment.

The combination of radiation therapy with chemotherapy before, during, and after irradiation is under investigation; it offers the best likelihood of improvement of the still disappointing survival results. Because the incidence of brain metastases in patients with large cell undifferentiated carcinoma and adenocarcinoma may reach 40 per cent at the time of death, elective irradiation of the brain (2000 to 3000 centigray in 2 to 3 weeks) is now being investigated.

Palliative Treatment

Standard treatment has not been established for patients with distant metastases. Symptomatic treatment includes the use of radiation therapy to the primary tumor and adjacent lymph nodes; the treatment of bone, brain, and lymph node metastases for palliation of present or expected symptoms; as well as the use of chemotherapy combinations that are becoming more effective in producing responses in gross tumor. Although no optimal drug treatment regimen has been established, the use of protocols designed to test new drug combinations offers not only the possibility of a tumor response but also the prospect of an increased symptom-free survival. Drug combinations are myriad; many of them contain cisplatin, doxorubicin (Adriamycin), and cyclophosphamide (such as the CAP regimen), as well as other drugs such as 5-fluorouracil, vincristine, mitomycin C, bleomycin, and others. As with radiation therapy, doses are limited by normal tissue tolerance, such as the limit of 400 mg per M^2 of Adriamycin to prevent cardiac damage. The combination of chemotherapy with radiation therapy is also being investigated.

Although the survival of patients with non-small cell carcinomas remains disappointing, the elimination of gross tumor (complete response to treatment) is a prerequisite for long-term survival. The survival of patients with metastatic disease is usually measured in months and only 7 to 10 per cent of patients can be expected to survive 1 year.

Small Cell Carcinoma

Limited Disease

Limited disease in small cell lung cancer includes tumor located in one hemithorax without distant metastases or involvement of the pleura or of the opposite lung. The TNM staging is less helpful in oat cell carcinoma.

The majority of the patients are treated following completion of a work-up that includes histologic verification of the tumor; CT scanning of the thorax and upper abdomen to exclude metastases to the lung, lymph nodes, adrenals, and liver; liver function tests; bone scan; bone marrow biopsy; and CT scan of the brain. Staging is similar to that of adenocarcinoma of the lung, except that bone marrow metastases are frequent enough to make a bone marrow biopsy a requirement in all patients.

A few patients are found to have small cell carcinoma when a lobectomy or wedge resection is performed for a coin lesion. They should receive chemotherapy or chemotherapy plus radiation as described later for patients with extensive disease. The risk of metastases to the mediastinum is high in these patients, as is the risk of distant metastatic disease.

Standard treatment is a combination of chemotherapy and radiation therapy. A variety of chemotherapy regimens is used, and multidrug regimens have been found superior to single drug treatment. The drugs may be cyclophosphamide, Adriamycin, and vincristine, sometimes combined with alternating regimens including VP-16, nitrosoureas like CCNU, and others.

The combination with radiation therapy is not standardized, but the usual recommendation is radiation therapy to the thoracic lesions and mediastinal and supraclavicular lymph nodes to a dose of no less than 4500 centigray in 5 weeks, as well as elective irradiation of the brain to 3000 centigray in 2 weeks. Whereas treatment with chemotherapy alone has been reported, there is evidence that thoracic relapse is significantly reduced by the combination with radiation therapy. Brain irradiation reduces the incidence of brain metastases, although it has not as yet been shown to prolong life.

More than half the patients show complete disappearance of tumor with this combined treatment, and 50 per cent are expected to survive 1 year while 15 to 25 per cent will survive 2 years. Complete response is a prerequisite for cure. Maintenance chemotherapy over long periods may be of value but has not been shown to provide freedom from relapse nor increase survival.

Extensive Disease

This includes patients with locally advanced tumors, including the chest wall, bilateral mediastinal metastasis, opposite lung involvement, pleural involvement, or distant metastatic disease.

Standard treatment is aggressive multidrug chemotherapy, such as cyclophosphamide, Adriamycin, and vincristine and others. Radiation therapy is reserved for symptomatic or poorly responding areas which may be in the thorax, lymph nodes, or liver. Brain metastases are routinely treated by radiation therapy as the chemotherapy regimens do not penetrate the blood-brain barrier.

Approximately 15 per cent of patients have a complete response, depending on the bulk of tumor; approximately half show significant reduction in tumor size (partial response). Median survival is approximately 6 months, and only 10 to 20 per cent will survive 1 year. Complete response, again, is a prerequisite for long-term survival. Patients in relapse may be treated with second line therapy, usually including VP-16 and cisplatin or other drugs that have not been used in the initial regimen.

Because of the poor results from treating extensive small cell carcinoma, investigational treatment may be used. This includes the use of anticoagulant agents, so-called consolidation radiation therapy of multiple sites that are unresponsive to chemotherapy, large field irradiation including total body or half body radiation, and attempts to eradicate tumor by marrow lethal dose of chemotherapy with bone marrow transplant to prevent death of the host from myelosuppression.

No randomized trials of long-term chemotherapy have been undertaken, but several large, uncontrolled studies show less morbidity and equal efficacy when an induction course of chemotherapy is used. On the other hand, benefit may be obtained if one selects patients with complete response for reinduction chemotherapy at 6 and 12 months, using single cycles of the same chemotherapy program as used initially.

While many treatment modifications have taken place recently, a plateau has been reached in the treatment of small cell carcinoma of the lung using multiple drug chemotherapy and radiation therapy. New approaches are needed for the prognosis in this cancer to improve.

COCCIDIOIDOMYCOSIS

method of
VIRGINIA S. ROWLAND, M.D.
Phoenix, Arizona

Coccidioidomycosis is a systemic fungal infection caused by the organism *Coccidioides immitis,* which is highly endemic in semiarid areas of the southwestern United States. Disease is almost invariably produced by inhalation of dust containing viable arthrospores. On rare occasions, transmission by fomites has been reported, but direct person-to-person transmission does not occur. Accidental laboratory-acquired coccidioidal disease is a serious and well-documented risk.

Over the past 30 years, the rapid growth of permanent and winter populations in the endemic area has heightened the clinical significance of coccidioidomycosis. In unusual areas, the disease should also be considered in undiagnosed individuals with an appropriate clinical picture and travel history.

DIAGNOSIS

Clinical Patterns of Disease

Primary Pulmonary Cocci. Most all patients with acute pulmonary coccidioidomycosis are either asymptomatic or suffer only a mild, flulike illness. These individuals do not seek medical attention but can be identified by a positive coccidioidal skin test.

Symptomatic acute pulmonary coccidioidomycosis is manifested by fever, malaise, cough (usually nonproductive), and chest pain, usually occurring 1 to 2 weeks following exposure. Cutaneous manifestations may include an erythematous macular rash or urticaria, as well as erythema nodosum and erythema multiforme. Arthritis and arthralgias may also occur, most often in adult white women. Chest radiograph findings include pulmonic infiltrates, hilar adenopathy, and pleural effusion.

Persistent Infiltrative and Cavitary Disease. Patients with symptoms or radiographic abnormalities lasting more than 6 to 8 weeks fall into the category of persistent pulmonary coccidioidomycosis. The persistent infection may be evidenced radiographically by continuing or progressive pneumonic infiltration associated with fever, malaise and fatigue, chest pain, and cough.

Other coccidioidal infiltrates may progress to single or multiple cavitary lesions. Diabetic patients have been reported to have a greater tendency to develop persistent cavitary disease. Complications of coccidioidal cavities include pyopneumothorax secondary to bronchopleural fistula, superinfection with either bacteria or fungi, and pulmonary hemorrhage.

Solitary pulmonary nodules (coccidiomas) may evolve from an area of acute coccidioidal infiltrate. These may be considered a form of persistent disease, since spherules can be identified in nearly all surgically excised cases. Solitary pulmonary nodules present a difficult diagnostic dilemma, especially in groups at high risk for bronchogenic malignancy. Smokers, especially with advancing age, must frequently undergo extensive diagnostic testing, such as percutaneous needle biopsy or surgical excision for diagnostic purposes.

Disseminated Disease. Dissemination occurs in less than 1 per cent of symptomatic patients. A propensity to dissemination has been reported in various racial and ethnic groups, including blacks, Filipinos, and native Americans. The influence of race on dissemination may be influenced by such factors as socioeconomic status and extent of exposure. Females in the second and third trimesters of pregnancy also have been reported to be at increased risk for dissemination. In addition, patients who are immunosuppressed by an underlying disease process, such as Hodgkin's disease or lymphoma, or by chemotherapy have a higher incidence of dissemination.

Disseminated coccidioidomycosis generally occurs within a few months of primary infection. Since even subclinical coccidioidal infection may produce dissemination, a history of symptomatic pulmonary disease is lacking in many cases. Virtually any organ system, including skin, bones and joints, meninges, and the genitourinary system, can be involved in coccidioidal dissemination. A lumbar puncture should be performed if any signs or symptoms of central nervous system involvement, however minimal, are present. Titers of complement-fixing antibodies (IgG) above 1:16 to 1:32 tend to occur in disseminated disease; falling titers usually indicate a favorable clinical course. Cutaneous anergy to coccidioidal antigens is frequently seen with dissemination. Although coccidioidin 1:100 has been the standard, the more recently developed spherulin skin test may more often evoke positive reactions in patients with dissemination.

Treatment

Most patients who develop coccidioidomycosis do not require specific therapeutic intervention. Unfortunately, the indications for drug therapy and treatment of this disease are often not clear-cut. When treatment is indicated, the two drugs currently in use are amphotericin B and ketoconazole, both of which are fungistatic in vivo.

Amphotericin B

Amphotericin B has been the standard form of therapy since the 1950s. Acute systemic reactions to infusion of this drug include fever, chills, and nausea. Administration is best tolerated via "rapid infusion" over 0.75 to 1.50 hours rather than with more prolonged infusions over 3 to 4 hours. Aspirin, 600 mg, or acetaminophen, 650 mg orally, with 50 mg of diphenhydramine (Benadryl) 0.50 hour prior to the infusion also minimizes acute side effects. Heparin (1000 to 2500 units) added to the amphotericin solution and the use of a small gauge scalp vein needle decrease the risk of phlebitis. More severe nausea and chilling can often be managed by adding 25 mg of hydrocortisone to the infusion.

Treatment with amphotericin B is initiated in a low dose (1 mg test dose of amphotericin in 100 ml of 5 per cent dextrose solution over 30 minutes) and increased in a step-wise fashion as tolerated until 40 to 60 mg are being administered daily. For maintenance therapy, alternate-day treatment is used in an outpatient setting to enhance patient compliance. Baseline laboratory studies, including complete blood count, creatinine clearance, serum potassium, creatinine, and BUN, should always be obtained prior to initiation of amphotericin therapy. Dosage must be adjusted according to changes in renal function; generally, amphotericin B should be withheld if the creatinine exceeds 2.5 to 3.0 mg per dl or reaches 2.5 times the pretreatment level. Hypokalemia also occurs and requires oral potassium supplementation. Anemia (normochromic, normocytic) is self-limited and resolves spontaneously after cessation of drug therapy. More infrequent side effects of amphotericin therapy include anaphylaxis, bone marrow suppression, and cardiac and hepatic toxicity.

The recommended dose of amphotericin varies according to the severity and type of coccidioidal involvement. Doses of under 1 gram may effect a satisfactory clinical response in cases of severe acute or persistent pulmonary disease.

In chronic cavitary coccidioidomycosis, the clinical course may be quite erratic. Assessing the response to drug therapy is therefore problematic. Spontaneous closure can occur, and uncomplicated cavitary lesions may be followed conservatively. Persistent symptoms or rupture can consistute indications for treatment, with doses ranging from 2.5 to 3.0 grams (total dose, approximately 30 mg per kg of body weight). Therapy is clearly indicated in disseminated disease. Both intrathecal and systemic routes of administration are utilized in the treatment of *Coccidioides* meningitis. The end point of therapy must be individualized, based on clinical improvement, complement-fixation antibody titer response, and return of skin test reactivity.

Ketoconazole

Ketoconazole (Nizoral) is better tolerated than amphotericin B and can be administered orally. Acute side effects of ketoconazole ingestion include gastric distress and nausea. Skin rashes, gynecomastia in men, and idiosyncratic liver toxicity have also been reported. Since deaths have occurred due to hepatotoxicity, baseline liver function studies should be obtained and repeated initially at 2 weeks and then at monthly intervals. Laboratory abnormalities may also include hypertriglyceridemia and acute suppression of corticosteroid synthesis.

Ketoconazole may be of benefit in persistent infiltrative pulmonary disease, but results have been disappointing in chronic cavitary involvement. In disseminated disease, ketoconazole appears to be most effective in the skin and soft tissue form of coccidioidomycosis. Ketoconazole does not penetrate the blood-brain barrier well and should not be used as primary therapy for coccidioidal meningitis. Since this drug is fungistatic, reactivation of infection is not surprising and has been frequently observed.

Ketoconazole dosage is initiated at 400 mg daily in the morning, usually before or with breakfast. Higher doses in the range of 600 to 800 mg per day may prove more efficacious; however, confirmatory clinical studies are not available.

Surgery

Surgical intervention is appropriate for rapidly enlarging coccidioidal cavities, especially those located peripherally with risk of rupture into the visceral pleura resulting in empyema and bronchopleural fistula. Recurrent, severe hemoptysis and symptomatic secondary infection should also lead to consideration of surgical intervention. The use of an amphotericin B "therapeutic umbrella" to reduce postoperative complications is controversial, and no properly controlled series have been reported.

In disseminated coccidioidomycosis, surgical therapy of localized lesions may involve either excision or drainage to facilitate healing. Synovectomy may be necessary in patients with coccidioidal arthritis; curettage and drainage, in patients with osteomyelitis; and simple excision and drainage, in patients with coccidioidal lymphadenitis.

HISTOPLASMOSIS

method of
ROBERT A. GOODWIN, Jr., M.D.
Vanderbilt University
Nashville, Tennessee

The usual infection caused by inhalation of spores of *Histoplasma capsulatum* is known as acute pulmonary histoplasmosis. With ordinary inhalation exposures (by far the majority of cases), the infection is almost entirely asymptomatic. Heavy inhalation of spores causes a nonspecific, self-limiting febrile illness. In both circumstances the infection heals with development of normal acquired immunity. Occasionally, with heavy inoculations and in unusually reactive individuals, complications involving mediastinal structures may develop from enlargement or acute inflammation of mediastinal lymph nodes, or from the fibrous encapsulation of caseous nodes during healing.

Acute Pulmonary Histoplasmosis

As a rule, neither asymptomatic nor symptomatic infections require specific therapy. Bed rest tends to alleviate symptoms, and activity tends to aggravate them. The following circumstances usually require consideration of specific therapy: (1) acute pulmonary insufficiency, (2) risk of disseminated histoplasmosis, and (3) severe symptoms. Experience with antifungal drugs is limited in these uncommon conditions.

The reaction to unusually heavy inhalation inoculation of the lung may result in a critically reduced blood Po_2 requiring prompt use of oxygen, corticosteroids in anti-inflammatory doses (prednisone, 20 mg three times daily), and amphotericin B, 0.6 mg per kg daily. The prednisone may be reduced by 2.5 mg per dose every 3 to 4 days (watching for rebound), and the amphotericin should be needed for only 2 or 3 weeks. Infected immunosuppressed persons and the rare individuals whose illnesses last longer than 3 weeks are at risk of failing to attain immune control of the infection (disseminated histoplasmosis), and support from drug therapy is clearly indicated. We favor the use of amphotericin B (0.6 mg per kg daily or 50 mg three times weekly) for a total dose of 500 to 1000 mg but consider a trial (not fully tested) with ketoconazole (400 mg daily for 3 to 4 months) as quite reasonable. A severe illness in normal hosts may be shortened by a brief course of amphotericin B, but the slow action of ketoconazole is not likely to be helpful.

Complications. In unusually reactive individuals with heavy infections, markedly enlarged and intensely inflamed mediastinal lymph nodes may cause mass effects and not uncommonly induce an acute fibrinous pericarditis. Temporary partial obstruction of the trachea, bronchi, or esophagus may be symptomatic for days, weeks, or occasionally months but ordinarily requires no specific treatment. If particularly troublesome, a short course of amphotericin B might be tried. Only serious obstruction of the trachea in young children is likely to require surgical correction.

Acute pericarditis heals spontaneously, but approximately 15 per cent of patients may later develop cardiac constriction. There is no consensus as to whether the use of antifungal drugs is advisable. I lean toward the use of a short course of amphotericin B (until well) in more symptomatic cases, although proof of benefit is lacking and the rationale is somewhat shaky. Pericardiocentesis in skilled hands is usually adequate management of cardiac tamponade. Rapidly recurring effusion may be treated with high dose corticosteroids (prednisone, 20 mg three times daily) in an attempt to avoid the need for anterior pericardiectomy.

Healed caseous (often calcified) remnants of old infection, usually in lymph nodes, may soften and dissect into bronchi (broncholithiasis) or the esophagus. These problems are usually self-correcting and do not indicate recrudescence of infection; there is no evidence that antifungal agents would be helpful.

Completely caseous lymph nodes heal by fibrous encapsulation. Rarely, certain individuals continue for years to generate fibrous capsule about such a focus, causing the serious and usually fatal entity called mediastinal collagenosis or fibrosis. I am not aware of any successful management when the process is deep in the mediastinum, whether surgery or the use of amphotericin B or corticosteroids. As a rule we also attempt to avoid surgical exploration of the larger "mediastinal granuloma" (encapsulated mass of paratracheal nodes, usually in right paratracheal area), whether or not it causes symptoms of superior vena caval obstruction. In the event of caval obstruction, the development of collateral circulation in most cases will eventually relieve symptoms.

Disseminated Histoplasmosis

Histoplasmosis is actually "disseminated" in the blood stream and reticuloendothelial system from the onset of a normal infection. It is only when this state persists well beyond the time that acquired cellular immunity is expected to develop that the infection is properly classified as disseminated histoplasmosis. All cases of established disseminated histoplasmosis by this definition should be treated with an antifungal drug. We prefer to treat all patients with amphotericin B if it is reasonable to do so but would not hesitate to use ketoconazole (400 mg daily for 9 to 12 months) for cases of mild chronic disease. The more symptomatic and acute the illness, the more critical is the need for amphotericin B in a dose of 0.6 mg per kg daily. If the patient survives the first week, then 50 mg three times weekly for a total of 2 grams is curative in most patients. The dose in children is 1 mg per kg daily for 6 weeks. In adults with endocarditis we give a total dose of four grams unless valve replacement removes the vegetations.

Chronic Pulmonary Histoplasmosis

The actual infection is within pre-existing emphysematous spaces and not in normal tissues where it would be more accessible to drugs. Pneumonic lesions and many thin-walled cavities tend to heal spontaneously. Thick-walled cavities and those that remain symptomatic or apparently active for 3 months or more tend to continue to harbor colonization. It is our practice to watch patients with known recently acquired disease for 2 to 3 months, encouraging reduced activity. If thin-walled cavities persist, if symptoms persist, or if new pneumonic lesions appear, we favor a trial of ketoconazole, 400 mg daily for 9 to 12 months. If the disease is known to be old, if there is a thick-walled enlarging cavity, if pulmonary function is greatly reduced, or if ketoconazole has failed, we give a full course of amphotericin B, 0.6 mg per kg or 50 mg three times weekly until a total dose of 2.5 grams has been attained. Occasionally more than one course of amphotericin B may be required.

Antifungal Therapy

Amphotericin B. Amphotericin B (Fungizone) is a toxic drug requiring intravenous administration. It is the most effective drug in histoplasmosis and is clearly the drug of choice in more severe cases and whenever prompt effect is necessary. Amphotericin B is insoluble in water and is provided with additives that support colloidial suspension in 5 per cent dextrose in water (D5W) in concentrations of less than 0.1 mg per ml. Saline causes precipitation. The usual dose is 0.6 mg per kg when given daily or 50 mg three times weekly administered intravenously in 5 per cent dextrose (1 mg of drug per 10 ml). Drug reactions, anorexia, nausea, vomiting, headache, chills, and fever are common, particularly early in the course.

To develop drug tolerance, it is best to begin with 5 mg the first day and increase the dose by 10 mg a day. However, in critically ill patients it is usually possible to begin with 15 to 20 mg and increase by 10 to 15 mg a day. In all doses the drug is given slowly, at first over 6 hours and later, if well tolerated, over 4 hours. Some patients may later tolerate a 2 hour course. Those slow to develop tolerance may be helped by diphenhydramine (Benadryl), 50 mg, with aspirin or Tylenol a half hour before the infusion. If symptoms are still troublesome, hydrocortisone sodium succinate (Solu-Cortef), 50 mg, or meperidine (Demerol), 50 mg, in the infusion may be tried until better tolerance develops. It is sometimes necessary to reduce the dose of amphotericin and then gradually increase it. The most peripheral veins (hands) should be used first because of a tendency for phlebitis. It may be necessary in the more susceptible patients to add hydrocortisone sodium succinate (Solu-Cortef), 25 mg, to each infusion.

Amphotericin B frequently causes azotemia, anemia, and hypokalemia. These possible effects should be monitored weekly. If the BUN rises above 50 to 60 mg per dl or the creatinine above 3 mg per dl, the dose should be appropriately reduced. Potassium supplements are often necessary.

Ketoconazole. This is a fungistatic drug of fairly low toxicity that can be administered orally and has been shown to be useful in milder cases of histoplasmosis that require treatment. The effect is slow to become manifest. It is our practice to give a single daily oral dose of 400 mg, usually at a meal or at bedtime to reduce nausea. The drug requires gastric acidity for absorption and should not be used in achlorhydria (without added HCl) or with antacid or cimetidine therapy. Mild transient liver function abnormalities occur in 10 per cent of patients. Severe hepatotoxicity is possible but is rare.

BLASTOMYCOSIS

method of
ROBERT W. BRADSHER, JR., M.D.
University of Arkansas for Medical Sciences
Little Rock, Arkansas

Blastomycosis is the systemic infection identified by round, thick-walled yeast in tissue or sputum specimens or after culture of the organisms in the mycelial phase at room temperature. With rare exceptions, the organisms are initially inhaled and the infection can then progress either locally in the lung or by lymphohematogenous routes to other organs. These metastatic foci of infection due to *Blastomyces dermatitidis* are most commonly located in skin, bone, or prostate, but many organs have been reported to be infected. Spontaneous remission of blastomycosis pneumonia is not uncommon and may also occur with cutaneous disease. Relapse of infection at a later date, either with or without previous antifungal therapy, has been reported.

Indications for Therapy

The first consideration for the patient with blastomycosis is whether or not to treat with an antifungal agent. Since resolution of infection without therapy is most likely in patients involved with an epidemic focus of infection, observation of pneumonia for 1 to 2 weeks is reasonable. If deterioration or progression is noted, antifungal therapy should be started. Observation only is also indicated in the patient with acute pneumonia that resolves before the organism is identified by culture. The presence of pleural disease or any extrapulmonary infection during the course of illness requires antifungal treatment. All other forms of blastomycosis should be treated with systemic therapy.

Treatment

The therapy to be considered initially in treatment of blastomycosis is listed in Table 1. If deterioration occurs in a patient being observed or if disease continues, treat with ketoconazole. If a patient treated with ketoconazole has progression of symptoms or signs of involvement, switch to amphotericin B. There appears to be no advantage to the combination of amphotericin B plus ketoconazole in blastomycosis.

TABLE 1. **Initial Antifungal Therapy in Blastomycosis**

Type of Disease	*Mode of Therapy*
Pulmonary	
1. Epidemic exposure to blastomycosis	Observe
2. Culture positive after acute illness has improved	Observe
3. Asymptomatic with abnormal radiograph	Ketoconazole
4. Symptomatic but not life-threatening	Ketoconazole
5. Overwhelming or life-threatening infection	Amphotericin B
Extrapulmonary	
1. Culture positive after acute illness has improved	Ketoconazole
2. Symptomatic but not life-threatening	Ketoconazole
3. Relapse after previous ketoconazole therapy	Amphotericin B
4. Meningitis or intracerebral infection	Amphotericin B
5. Overwhelming or life-threatening infection	Amphotericin B

Amphotericin B. Since the introduction of amphotericin B in 1956, it has become well recognized that this polyene antifungal drug is effective in the treatment of blastomycosis. In five large series, intravenous amphotericin B resulted in cure without relapse in 16 of 19, 21 of 27, 32 of 35, 13 of 15, and 37 of 41 patients when given in a dosage of at least 1.0 gram. A dose of 2 grams has been associated with cure rates of up to 97 per cent. However, in those patients, 71 per cent had a decline in renal function with other significant toxicities, including anemia (53 per cent), anorexia and nausea (53 per cent), fever (49 per cent), hypokalemia (37 per cent) and thrombophlebitis (19 per cent). These side effects resulted in interruption of therapy in 41 per cent and early cessation of amphotericin B in 14 per cent of the patients. Because of the major toxicity of amphotericin B, consideration is given to not treating or postponing treatment of a patient with blastomycosis.

Amphotericin B must be given intravenously, beginning at 1.0 mg in 100 ml of 5 per cent dextrose in water (D5W) over 2 hours as a test dose. If that dose is tolerated without fever, chills, or hypotension, the dose is increased by 10 to 15 mg per day to reach a daily dose of 40 to 45 mg per day (approximately 0.4 to 0.6 mg per kg per day) in a sufficient volume of D5W to be infused in 4 to 6 hours. Some recommend 0.75 to 1.0 mg per kg per day in children. A total of 2.0 grams should be given unless toxicity is a limiting factor. There is no need to protect the amphotericin B solution from light, but the agent must be mixed in dextrose in water rather than saline.

Toxicity should be monitored by measuring creatinine concentrations in serum biweekly. If the serum creatinine goes above 3.0 mg per dl, the drug should be withheld for 48 hours and adequate hydration must be ensured. When amphotericin B is reinstituted, a lower dose is used before returning to the usual daily dose. Hypokalemia is fairly frequent, so electrolyte assessment must be performed biweekly. Blood counts should be monitored at least weekly. Phlebitis is avoided best by frequent changing of peripheral IV sites rather than by the addition of 25 to 50 mg of hydrocortisone to the infusion. Premedication with aspirin or diphenhydramine is useful to decrease the fever and chills with amphotericin B; if rigors do occur, an intravenous dose of 15 to 25 mg of meperidine is often effective in stopping the chill.

Ketoconazole. Ketoconazole is an imidazole antifungal agent with in vitro activity against *B. dermatitidis* comparable to that of amphotericin B. The drug is well absorbed from the gastrointestinal tract and has generally been well tolerated in the treatment of other fungal infections. Adverse effects include rare hepatocellular toxicity and antitestosterone-like effects (gynecomastia, oligospermia) at high dosages (greater than 400 mg per day). More common but less severe adverse effects include nausea and vomiting when taken without a meal, dizziness, pruritus, or headache. Over a 2-year period, we used ketoconazole to treat 44 patients with blastomycosis. Cure without relapse was obtained in 37. Three patients relapsed after therapy was complete, and in two the lesions did not completely resolve, causing them to be considered failures. The remaining two patients had persistent infection but were noncompliant with the therapy. Side effects were minimal.

Ketoconazole is given orally with a meal early in the day at a dosage of 400 mg (two tablets). If no response is noted within 4 weeks, it is my practice to increase the dose by 200 mg increments to a maximum of 800 mg per day (800 mg per day exceeds manufacturer's recommended dosage). Nausea and vomiting are reduced and greater absorption achieved by administering the drug with a meal. Liver transaminase enzymes should be monitored once a month. It has been my practice to continue ketoconazole for at least 6 months. In those with more extensive disease, a total of 1 year of therapy has been given. The relapse rates with ketoconazole have not been as clearly defined as those with amphotericin B, so subsequent infection in a patient treated with ketoconazole should be carefully examined for evidence of blastomycosis.

Miconazole. Miconazole is an imidazole similar to ketoconazole with activity against *B. dermatitidis*. However, the incidence of adverse effects is similar to that with amphotericin B. Because of this, adequate trials in blastomycosis with this agent have not been performed. Consideration of miconazole should be reserved for the patient who cannot tolerate amphotericin B infusions and who cannot take ketoconazole orally.

PLEURAL EFFUSIONS AND EMPYEMA THORACIS

method of
CREIGHTON B. WRIGHT, M.D.,
and DONALD L. MITTS, M.D.
University of Cincinnati
Cincinnati, Ohio

PLEURAL EFFUSIONS

Pleural effusions are a common clinical manifestation of systemic or pleural disease. Because of the diverse potential etiologies, careful investigation as to the cause of this clinical sign is mandatory. Fever, chills, shortness of breath, tachypnea, and other manifestations of cardiorespiratory dysfunction are important in delineating these problems.

Unilateral pleural effusions unassociated with cardiac manifestations may require more thorough investigation. The causes of pleural effusion are numerous, although cardiac dysfunction, local or metastatic mitotic disease, and renal dysfunction are responsible for the greatest number. Other sources include pulmonary infection, post-pericardiotomy syndrome, post-traumatic, pulmonary emboli, and infradiaphragmatic infections. Often diagnostic efforts to evaluate the effusion can alert the physician to other underlying systemic disorders, such as collagen vascular disease or pancreatitis.

Pleural effusions secondary to congestive heart failure often will respond spontaneously with adequate treatment. These effusions are most commonly bilateral but may be unilateral. Usually the size and location of the effusion are identified radiographically by standard posteroanterior, lateral, and decubitus films. Generally 200 to 300 ml of pleural fluid are required to blunt the costophrenic angles on routine radiograms. The more frequent use of computed tomography (CT) scanning has facilitated identification of unsuspected effusions and more accurate localization. CT scanning has also proved beneficial in accurate catheter placement for more complete drainage in complex situations. Finally, after adequate localization and if the etiology of a pleural effusion is still in doubt, diagnostic and/or therapeutic thoracentesis is undertaken.

Thoracentesis. It is our preference to do routine thoracentesis with the patient in a sitting position, with arms and head comfortably resting on a bedstand. The patient is carefully prepped with antibacterial solution and draped with sterile towels. Using the appropriate radiographic landmarks, the most dependent safe area (usually no lower than the seventh interspace, which is one to two interspaces below the scapular tip, in the posterior axillary line) is generously anesthetized with 1 or 2 per cent lidocaine hydrochloride solution. An 18 gauge needle is then introduced over the upper aspect of the rib into the intrapleural space. The first 10 to 20 ml are collected for culture, cell count, and chemical survey, and then the therapeutic aspiration is continued in most cases. In an exceptionally large pleural effusion, a closed Silastic catheter system through an introducer needle is preferred and the catheter directed toward a more dependent position to completely evacuate as much of the effusion as possible. Attempts to tap the paravertebral gutters are fraught with potential problems; one of the worst is penetrating the diaphragm and concomitant intra-abdominal viscera.

With large effusions, a sterile vacuum bottle is used to minimize the duration of the procedure for the patient. Generally, we feel that no more than 1800 to 2000 ml of fluid should be removed acutely at one setting to minimize the chance of hemodynamic instability of the patient. With the small catheter clamped, an hour or so pause is made and then the remaining effusion drained. Having the patient take deep breaths, cough, and lean from side to side during the procedure can also maximize the amount of aspirate. With direct needle technique one must be careful during the last moments of the thoracentesis not to puncture the lung as it expands, by keeping the depth and angle of the needle very secure. The aforementioned newer disposable systems that allow sealed passage of a dull catheter into the pleura are very helpful in avoiding trouble and increasing thorough drainage.

When neoplastic disease is suspected, a closed pleural needle biopsy should be performed at the same setting, using an Abrams or Cope needle. Care must be taken to direct the biopsy needle caudally and laterally rather than cranially to avoid injuring the vascular bundle of the cephalad rib. Pleural biopsies taken in this manner increase the diagnosis of mitotic disease, tuberculosis, and mesothelioma, even in the face of negative cytologic assay of the pleural fluid.

Note is made whether the evacuated fluid is sanguineous, serous, cloudy, or purulent and of the amount; samples are sent to the laboratory for anaerobic and aerobic culture, AFB culture and stain, fungal culture, and cytology. Immediate Gram stain of the fluid can help ascertain suspected pulmonary infections. Aliquots of fluid should be sent for cell count, specific gravity, glucose, pH, LDH, and amylase studies as dictated clinically. Pleural transudates characterized by a low protein content (less than 3 grams per ml) and low specific gravity (less than 1.016) usually indicate major organ dysfunction, such as congestive failure, renal failure, or cirrhosis. In congestive failure or postpericardiotomy syndrome, the pleural effusion often recedes with the treatment of the underlying disorder. However, some patients may have respiratory embarrassment secondary to the volume of effusion, and therapeutic thoracentesis is indicated. Pleural exudates, characterized by a protein content greater than 3 grams per ml of specific gravity greater than 1.016, are more typical of infections, pulmonary emboli, or neoplastic disorders. If one is highly suspicious of a cancerous etiology, an aliquot of pleural fluid can be spun down for cell block cytologic assay in efforts to improve the diagnostic yield.

Thoracostomy. If large nonmalignant or malignant pleural effusion tends to recur at short intervals after relatively complete evacuation and causes significant respiratory symptoms, closed tube thoracostomy with a No. 32 to 36 French chest tube should be done. The chest tube is placed under local anesthesia in the midaxillary line, in the direction for optimal drainage, and placed on water seal (15 to 20 cm) to completely evacuate the effusion and attain apposition of visceral and parietal pleurae. This also allows for re-expansion of all underlying atelectatic lung. In nonmalignant pleural effusions in which the drainage diminishes rather rapidly, this form of treatment will probably be adequate.

Pleurodesis. With recurrent pleural effusion associated with malignancy, chemical pleurodesis should be considered. Many agents have been recommended for pleurodesis: tetracycline, nitrogen mustard, talc powder, and so on. Our preference, in general, has been to use tetracycline. Nitrogen mustard is reserved specifically for effusion associated with bronchogenic cancer.

Pleural instillation is done after premedication with a narcotic and sedative combination (morphine, 6 to 8 mg, and Nembutal, 50 to 75 mg intramuscularly). Tetracycline, 1 gram, is diluted with 100 ml of saline and injected through the chest tube after the effusion has been completely evacuated and chest tube drainage has become minimal. The tetracycline is flushed into the pleural space using an additional 25 ml of saline, and the tube is clamped for roughly 2 hours. The patient is then rotated from side to side and into multiple positions in an effort to disperse the chemical agent throughout the pleural space. The addition of lidocaine hydrochloride has been advocated by some to minimize discomfort, but the mainstay is adequate premedication. The tube is subsequently unclamped, underwater seal drainage is continued for 2 to 3 days, and the tube then removed. It may be removed earlier if the drainage is slight (less than 100 ml per 24 hours).

Thoracotomy. For recurrent pleural effusions with the possible presence of a mass and no apparent diagosis following thoracentesis and pleural biopsy, one should consider thoracotomy. This may demonstrate metastatic pleural implants or mesothelioma, both of which carry a rather grim prognosis. Prompt diagnosis, however, allows for more appropriate management. Either an anterolateral or posterolateral thoracotomy can be used, depending on the location of the fluid or mass.

EMPYEMA

Empyema is an intrapleural infection consisting of variable amounts of fluid, bacteria, and leukocytes, often associated with a parapneumonic process. Other possible causes are lung abscess, aspiration of foreign body, trauma, surgery, esophageal disease and manipulation, pulmonary infarction, and the infrequent extension of subdiaphragmatic processes. Therapy consists of antibiotics appropriate to the organism, adequate drainage of the pleural collection, and re-expansion of the underlying lung. Cultures of the pleural fluid, sputum, and blood may be helpful in identification of the best antibiotic, which is usually administered systemically.

Streptococcal empyema, particularly in children, often can be drained adequately via routine thoracentesis and managed successfully with antibiotics because of its liquid nature. Staphylococcal empyema often creates very viscous, thick pus that requires tube thoracostomy for drainage, or in some cases thoracotomy. However, children with associated staphylococcal pneumatoceles often can be treated more conservatively without tubes and with antibiotics and thoracentesis. Even tuberculous collections, once feared because they produced chronic sinus tracts or bronchopleural fistulas, can be treated successfully by needle aspiration or a tube thoracostomy and antituberculous drugs.

When drainage of acute empyema requires tube thoracostomy, a standard chest tube placement is performed. A No. 32 to 36 French tube is placed in the routine manner, with digital efforts to break down loculations and adhesions. Serial chest radiographs and the patient's clinical course determine whether further tube thoracostomy or other drainage procedures are required. The CT scanner has been valuable in localizing loculated pockets of purulent material and determining whether adequate drainage has been attained. The scans have also been helpful in differentiating collected extrapleural fluid from atelectatic or infiltrated lung, and especially in diagnosing underlying lung abscess. If drainage after tube placement persists over a long period of time and there is no air leak, the chest tube can be cut off close to the skin and gradually withdrawn over a period of months with the patient as an outpatient. These difficult problems may occur when the diagnosis is not made early or drainage is not thorough enough, so that the empyema cavity persists.

If the empyema cavity is chronic, dependent, and localized, it can be converted to an open, externally drained space with resection of one or two overlying dependent ribs and suturing of the epithelial edges to the pleural base, as was described by Eloesser. This may allow gradual re-expansion of the lung, remolding of the pleural peel, and healing. In the case of large persistent empyema cavities, such as those found in trauma patients with large collections of infected hematoma, one should consider early thoracotomy and debridement. Decortication refers to removal of a chronic fibrinopurulent peel from both the visceral and parietal pleura and re-expansion of the underlying lung. Chronic empyema cavity and the need for decortication are now rare.

Postsurgical empyemas are much more difficult to treat because of prior pulmonary resections and concomitant residual unfilled space. These can generally be resolved with multiple chest tubes or decortication or both.

If one is still dealing with an infected space, then thoracoplasty may have a role. Newer plastic surgical procedures involving pectoralis or latissimus dorsi flaps may be applied after the underlying infection has been adequately drained and treated with appropriate antibiosis. Sealing of a bronchopleural fistula can be accomplished with muscle or pleural flaps and sterilization of the cavity using antibiotic or Dakin's solutions, resulting in long-term resolution of the problem. When there is apparent maximum re-expansion of underlying lung and yet persistence of moderate empyema space, thoracotomy and decortication should be considered. When empyemas are found and adequately drained early, the lung can be expected to expand and once again fill the pleural space.

PRIMARY LUNG ABSCESS

method of
EBEN M. RUBIN, M.D.
University of Miami
Miami, Florida

The incidence of lung abscess, once declining with the introduction of antibiotics, is again rising largely because of the increasing number of immune-compromised patients seen in current practice. Anaerobic organisms, usually from the oral cavity, predominate, but lung abscess may be caused by any necrotizing infection reaching the lung via the airways, by hematogenous seeding, or by direct spread through the diaphragm.

Altered states of consciousness, poor airway control, and poor oral hygiene account for the greatest number of patients developing anaerobic abscesses, and the incidence correlates with alcoholism, seizures, anesthesia, and dental procedures. Characteristically, these abscesses are found in dependent areas of the lung. In contrast, abscesses due to opportunistic organisms are often bloodborne and occur with nearly equal frequency in all pulmonary segments. They are commonly seen in drug abusers, transplant recipients, cancer patients, and other immune-compromised patients.

Bacteria of anaerobic abscesses consist of mostly penicillin-sensitive strains, with the significant exception of *Bacteroides fragilis*. Aerobic abscesses are most often caused by *Staphylococcus aureus, Neisseria, Streptococcus pneumoniae, Pseudomonas, Proteus, Escherichia coli,* and *Klebsiella*.

Clinically, patients present with indolent signs of infection, which may include weight loss, anemia, clubbing, and cough. In most cases, a compatible chest radiograph and the presence of putrid sputum productive of large, mixed flora counts on Gram stain, which grows mouth flora on culture, adequately indicates an anaerobic abscess in communication with the bronchial tree. However, the clinical picture may vary and can present as a fulminating process.

A specific microbiologic diagnosis should be made if there is suspicion of a nonanaerobic organism or a poor clinical response to therapy. Transthoracic needle aspiration is the procedure of choice. Transtracheal aspiration is less sensitive, and also has a 13 to 18 per cent incidence of false positives. Fiberoptic bronchoscopy is significantly inferior due to nasopharyngeal contamination.

Antibiotic Therapy

Penicillin G remains the drug of choice for empiric treatment of anaerobic abscesses. It should be given initially in high dosages (2 million units every 4 to 6 hours intravenously) until clinical improvement occurs, then orally in the phenoxymethyl form in doses of 500 mg every 6 hours for 6 to 8 weeks, until radiographic clearing. Since abscesses are often polymicrobial, penicillin is usually effective even if the resistant *Bacteroides fragilis* is present, because eradication of the sensitive organisms is sufficient to permit resolution.

Others suggest clindamycin as the initial drug of choice, because of its greater anaerobic spectrum, including *B. fragilis*. Clindamycin has been successful in penicillin failures and may shorten the duration of treatment. The drug is given intravenously in dosages of 600 mg every 4 to 6 hours. Its major side effect is pseudomembranous colitis. Chloramphenicol (1 gram intravenously every 6 hours) and metronidazole (500 to 750 mg intravenously every 8 hours) are alternate choices.

Drug choice in nonanaerobic infections should be guided by in vitro sensitivity testing. The semisynthetic penicillins oxacillin or nafcillin, given intravenously in dosages of 1.5 to 3 grams every 6 hours, should be used to treat staphylococcal abscesses. Cephalosporins and vancomycin are alternatives. Gram-negative aerobic bacilli should be treated with an aminoglycoside in combination with penicillin. Third generation cephalosporins may also be suitable for mixed aerobic/anaerobic abscesses, particularly if acquired nosocomially. Renal function must be taken into account for the dosing of aminoglycosides, especially since prolonged therapy is usually required.

Adjunctive Therapy

Bronchoscopy is indicated if there is suspicion of neoplasm or other cause of airway obstruction. Drainage is important for any abscess and should be facilitated by cough and posture. Bronchoscopy may promote drainage in selected cases.

Surgery should be considered if the patient is toxic, is poorly responsive to antibiotic therapy, or has a bronchopleural fistula, airway obstruction, massive hemoptysis, or large abscess cavity. The usual procedure is lobar resection, which should be curative. An alternative to open resection, which may be indicated in patients too ill to withstand surgery and which has been advocated to reduce treatment time, is tube thoracostomy with or without rib resection. Posterior abscesses in which the affected lobe is adherent to the pleura may be managed by daily or alternate day thoracentesis with large bore needles, but this procedure should be reserved for highly selected cases. Thoracostomy or thoracentesis when the lobe is not adherent to the parietal pleura may increase the risk of empyema.

OTITIS MEDIA

method of
CHARLES D. BLUESTONE, M.D.
University of Pittsburgh
Pittsburgh, Pennsylvania

Otitis media is the most prevalent disease of childhood after respiratory tract infections. Acute otitis media and otitis media with effusion are the most common forms. Acute otitis media is usually suppurative or purulent. There are many terms for otitis media with effusion, such as serous, secretory, catarrhal, mucoid, nonsuppurative, or allergic. It is often difficult to determine the specific variety of otitis media without a diagnostic aspiration of the middle ear effusion. The complications and sequelae of otitis media represent significant health hazards in children.

Acute Otitis Media

In the usual course, a child suffering an upper respiratory infection for several days suddenly develops otalgia, fever, and hearing loss. Examination with the pneumatic otoscope reveals a hyperemic, opaque, bulging tympanic membrane of poor mobility. Purulent otorrhea may be present. However, earache and fever are not invariably present.

When the diagnosis of acute otitis media is in doubt or identification of the causative agent is desirable, aspiration of the middle ear should be performed. Tympanocentesis should also be considered for children who are seriously ill or appear toxic; for unsatisfactory response to antibiotic therapy; for onset of otitis media in a patient who is receiving antibiotic agents; for suppurative aural, intratemporal, or intracranial complications; and for otitis in the neonate, the very young infant, or the immunologically deficient patient, in each of whom unusual organisms may cause infection.

Most experts agree that infants and children who have the signs and symptoms of acute otitis media should receive antimicrobial therapy; however, several investigators have questioned the need for antimicrobial agents in all cases. Since the rate of suppurative complications has decreased in the antibiotic era, antimicrobial therapy is still the treatment of choice.

Amoxicillin or ampicillin is the currently preferred drug for initial treatment of otitis media; both are active in vitro and in vivo against *Streptococcus pneumoniae* and *Haemophilus influenzae*. Other satisfactory regimens include trimethoprim-sulfamethoxazole, cefaclor, combinations of a sulfonamide with oral penicillin V or erythromycin, and amoxicillin–potassium clavulanate. Oral ampicillin, 50 to 100 mg per kg per day in four divided doses for 10 days, is recommended. Amoxicillin, 40 mg per kg per day, is equally effective, can be given in three divided doses, and has fewer side effects, such as diarrhea. Treatment for 10 days is recommended. If the child is allergic to the penicillins, then a combination of oral erythromycin, 40 mg per kg per day, and sulfisoxazole, 120 mg per kg per day in four divided doses, or trimethoprim-sulfamethoxazole (8 mg of trimethoprim plus 40 mg of sulfamethoxazole per kg per day in two divided doses) is a suitable alternative. If beta-lactamase-producing *H. influenzae* or *Branhamella catarrhalis* is suspected or documented by tympanocentesis, then appropriate choices would be these combinations or cefaclor, 40 mg per kg per day in three divided doses. The combination of amoxicillin and potassium clavulanate is now available (40 mg per kg per day in three divided doses) and is effective when these resistant organisms are present. The clinical efficacy of these antimicrobial agents is summarized in Table 1.

With appropriate antimicrobial therapy, most children with acute bacterial otitis media are significantly improved within 48 to 72 hours. The physician should be in contact with the patient to ascertain that improvement has occurred. If there is persistence or recurrence of otalgia or fever or both, then the child should be re-examined before the completion of the antibiotic course. However, at this time the appearance of the tympanic membrane alone should not determine a change in the treatment. Almost all children will have a persistent middle ear effusion, and even erythema and bulging of the tympanic membrane may still be present. Persistent pain or fever signals the need for surgical intervention or selection of another antimicrobial agent or both. Tympanocentesis with or without a myringotomy is a logical management option in such cases since culture of the middle ear effusion may reveal the presence of an ampicillin-resistant bacterium. Further antimicrobial treatment is based on the results of the culture. If surgery is not feasible, then a new antimicrobial agent is administered.

The new antimicrobial agent should be effective against organisms such as a beta-lactamase-producing *H. influenzae* or *B. catarrhalis*. If ampicillin or amoxicillin was given initially, then the combination of erythromycin-sulfisoxazole or trimethoprim-sulfamethoxazole appears to be effective when these organisms are present or suspected to be present. However, trimethoprim-sulfamethoxazole is apparently not effective when *Streptococcus pyogenes* is the causative organism. Cefaclor is probably effective against all the ampicillin-resistant organisms except possibly some strains of beta-lactamase-producing *B. catarrhalis*.

All children should be re-examined at the end of the course of antimicrobial therapy—that is, after 10 to 14 days. At this time, some children will have a persistent middle ear effusion—approximately 50 per cent of those treated with amoxicillin. Since the presence of a persistent middle ear effusion after a 10 day trial of an antimicrobial agent in an otherwise asymptomatic child is common, this finding alone is not sufficient grounds for performing surgery such as a myringotomy and tympanostomy tube insertion or adenoidectomy.

Additional supportive therapy, including an-

TABLE 1. **Efficacy of Selected Antimicrobial Agents for Common Pathogens in Acute Otitis Media***

Antimicrobial Agents	**Pathogen** *Streptococcus pneumoniae* *(35–40%)*†	*Haemophilus influenzae* *(20%)*	*Branhamella catarrhalis* *(<20%)*	*Streptococcus pyogenes* *(<10%)*	*Staphylococcus aureus* *(<10%)*
Ampicillin or amoxicillin	+	±	±	+	±
Erythromycin and sulfisoxazole	+	+	+	+	+
Trimethoprim-sulfamethoxazole	+	+	+	−	+
Cefaclor	+	+	±	+	+
Amoxicillin–potassium clavulanate	+	+	+	+	+

*Based on available data from clinical trials and laboratory studies.
†Percentages of the cases of acute otitis media caused by each pathogen.
+, effective; ±, effective for strains not producing beta-lactamase; −, not effective.

algesics, antipyretics, and local heat, will usually be helpful. An oral decongestant, such as pseudoephedrine hydrochloride, may relieve nasal congestion, and antihistamines may help patients with known or suspected nasal allergy. However, the efficacy of antihistamines and decongestants in the treatment of acute otitis media has not been proved. Complete clearing of the effusion may take 6 or more weeks. Within 2 to 3 months, the tympanic membrane should be entirely normal. If complete resolution has occurred and the episode represents the only known attack, the patient may be discharged. However, periodic follow-up is indicated for patients who have had recurrent episodes.

Persistent Middle Ear Effusion

If the middle ear effusion persists after the initial 10 days of antimicrobial therapy, one or more of the following treatment options have been advocated to hasten the resolution of the effusion during the next, or subacute, phase:

(1) A course of an antimicrobial agent different from the initial one, based on the hope that if a resistant organism is present the new antimicrobial agent may be effective;
(2) A topical or systemic nasal decongestant or antihistamine, or a combination of these drugs;
(3) Systemic corticosteroids; or
(4) Middle ear inflation (e.g., Valsalva maneuver, politzerization).

Unfortunately, none of these commonly employed methods have been shown to be effective in random controlled trials of children with subacute otitis media with effusion. An oral decongestant and antihistamine were not effective in eliminating persistent middle ear effusion in a study that involved over 500 infants and children. At present, the most appropriate treatment for children who have asymptomatic (except for hearing loss) otitis media with effusion still present after 2 weeks is watchful waiting with re-examination 6 weeks later, i.e., 2 months after the initial visit. At this time, the middle ear should be effusion-free in most children. However, treatment with another antimicrobial, such as cefaclor, trimethoprim-sulfamethoxazole, erythromycin-sulfisoxazole, or amoxicillin–potassium clavulanate, which are effective against possible resistant bacteria, is a reasonable alternative, especially if the child has any signs or symptoms of persistent infection, such as otalgia, or if such organisms have been isolated from subacute effusions in the community. If the child still has persistent otitis media after 2 or 3 months, the condition is chronic and should be treated.

Recurrent Acute Otitis Media

It is not uncommon for an infant to have recurrent bouts of acute otitis media. Some children develop an acute episode with almost every respiratory tract infection, have more or less dramatic symptoms, respond well to therapy, and have fewer episodes with advancing age. Others have persistent middle ear effusion and suffer recurrent episodes of acute otitis media superimposed on the chronic disorder. The child with recurrent acute otitis media whose disease completely clears between episodes may be managed as previously outlined. However, if the bouts are frequent and close together, prevention may be desirable. In many of these children, the underlying cause is not evident, but myringotomy with insertion of middle ear ventilation tubes is frequently helpful. Prophylactic antibiotics (a daily dose of amoxicillin or sulfonamides) have been advocated as an alternative to myringotomy and ventilating tubes. The preventive efficacies of myringotomy with tympanotomy tube insertion, chemoprophylaxis, hyposensitization, and adenoidectomy, with or without tonsillectomy, are not established.

Otitis Media with Effusion

Otitis media with effusion lacks the signs and symptoms of acute infection. Frequently, either a retracted or convex tympanic membrane is seen. The membrane is usually opaque, but when it is translucent, an air-fluid level or air bubbles may be seen and an amber or sometimes bluish fluid may be apparent in the middle ear. The mobility of the eardrum is almost always impaired. The auditory acuity is usually decreased, and although systemic symptoms are usually absent, there may be behavioral disturbances due to the child's inability to communicate adequately. A feeling of fullness in the ear, tinnitus, and even vertigo may be present. Audiometry may be helpful in establishing the diagnosis but is not reliable because some patients, even with thick middle ear effusions, have fairly good hearing. Tympanometry is more reliable.

Most asymptomatic middle ear effusions resolve spontaneously within a few months, but a patient with chronic otitis media with effusion who has not received prior antibiotic therapy should be treated initially as a case of acute otitis media since bacteria are frequently present. The lack of efficacy of decongestant and antihistamine therapy has been established. Corticosteroid therapy, hyposensitization, and middle ear inflation by the Valsalva or Politzer method are popular, but have not proved to be effective in convincing clinical trials. If the effusion persists for 3 or more months or if there have been frequent recurrences of episodes of acute otitis media, the patient requires further evaluation for upper respiratory allergy, adenoid tissue obstructing the nose and nasopharynx, an immunologic disorder (if other organs are involved), or abnormalities such as submucous cleft palate or a tumor of the nasopharynx.

For patients in whom medical management (including a trial with an appropriate antibiotic) has failed, myringotomy with aspiration of the middle ear fluid is indicated if the effusion has persisted for 3 months. Frequently, insertion of a ventilation or tympanostomy tube will be necessary to allow the middle ear mucous membrane to return to normal and to prevent subsequent accumulation of effusion. Ventilation tubes may prevent permanent structural damage and cholesteatoma if a deep retraction pocket develops in the posterosuperior quadrant or in the attic (pars flaccida) portion of the tympanic membrane. Occasionally, troublesome otorrhea develops after the insertion of tympanostomy tubes, which can usually be treated successfully with ear drops containing neomycin, polymyxin, or colistin with hydrocortisone. Since these medications may be ototoxic, some physicians advocate the use of systemic antibiotics without the aural drops. In selected cases, allergic hyposensitization and adenoidectomy, with or without tonsillectomy, may be beneficial; the efficacy of these has not been fully assessed.

Complications and Sequelae of Otitis Media

The intracranial suppurative complications of otitis media are relatively uncommon except in neglected cases. However, those that occur within the aural cavity and adjacent structures of the temporal bone are more common, and awareness of them is essential in management of children with otitis media. The aural and intratemporal complications and sequelae of otitis media are hearing loss, perforation of the tympanic membrane with or without suppuration, acquired cholesteatoma, mastoiditis, petrositis, adhesive otitis media, tympanosclerosis, ossicular discontinuity, facial paralysis, and labyrinthitis.

Hearing loss is the most prevalent complication and morbid outcome of otitis media and may be caused by one or more of the intratemporal complications. To a varying degree, fluctuating or persistent loss of hearing is usually associated with acute or chronic middle ear effusions or high negative pressure within the middle ear in the absence of an effusion. The audiogram usually reveals a mild to moderate conductive loss, but permanent conductive hearing loss can result from irreversible changes secondary to recurrent acute or chronic inflammation, such as adhesive otitis, tympanosclerosis, or ossicular discontinuity. Irreparable sensorineural loss may also occur, presumably as the result of spread of infection through the round or oval window membrane. Although persistent or episodic conductive hearing loss may result in impairment of speech, language, and cognitive and emotional development of children, the degree and duration of the hearing loss required to produce such deficits have not been defined.

BACTERIAL PNEUMONIA

method of
SIMONE SALTZMAN, M.D.
Albert Einstein College of Medicine
Bronx, New York

Bacterial pneumonia, an infectious process involving lung parenchyma, usually causing acute illness, can be classified according to etiologic agent and according to whether the infection is acquired in the community or in the hospital. Patients with bacterial pneumonia generally present with fever, chills, sputum production, tachypnea, rales or signs of consolidation on physical exam, leukocytosis with a left shift, and infiltrates on chest x-ray.

Pneumonia due to *Streptococcus pneumoniae* is the most common cause of community-acquired bacterial pneumonia seen in adults. Frequently these patients complain of pleuritic chest pain and are coughing up purulent or rusty sputum. Up to 25 per cent of them have bacteremia.

Streptococcus pyogenes pneumonia usually follows a viral illness, such as measles or influenza, or may complicate streptococcal infection elsewhere in the body.

Staphylococcus aureus pneumonia may be a primary infection of the lung, occurring especially in elderly, debilitated patients and infants with severe underlying disease, or it may occur as a complication of influenza. In patients who have staphylococcal bacteremia arising from a focus elsewhere in the body, the lungs may become secondarily involved. Indeed, staphylococcal pneumonia (with multiple densities on x-ray in the periphery of both lungs) is a common presenting manifestation of right-sided endocarditis in intravenous drug abusers. In both forms of staphylococcal pneumonia abscess formation and empyema are fairly common. *Staphylococcus aureus* is also responsible for many nosocomial pneumonias, and many of these isolates may be resistant to methicillin.

Aspiration of oropharyngeal contents (predominantly anaerobes) results in a mixed flora anaerobic pneumonia, which usually presents with an indolent clinical course and may progress to abscess and empyema formation. Patients in whom aspiration should be considered are those who have been unconscious, who experience dysphagia, or who have poor dentition or oropharyngeal infections.

Gram negative enteric organisms cause pneumonia in patients with chronic underlying diseases and alcoholism. These orgaisms, along with *Pseudomonas aeruginosa,* are also the main pathogens implicated in nonsocomial pneumonias. Hospital patients and patients with chronic illness are more likely than normals to have pharyngeal colonization with gram negative bacilli (even if they have not received prior antibiotic therapy), and pneumonia probably results from occult aspiration of these organisms. In addition, these organisms are capable of living in moist areas and may contaminate respiratory therapy devices. Patients with tracheostomies usually become colonized with gram negative enterics and *Pseudomonas* species and thus are at increased risk for developing pneumonia due to these organisms. *Pseudomonas aeruginosa* has a predilection for granulocytopenic hosts and thus may cause pneumonia in these patients.

Legionella pneumophila is responsible for both community- and hospital-acquired infection, and several nosocomial outbreaks have been described. Most commonly the organism produces pneumonia that may be severe and progressive, with multisystem disease being a prominent feature of the presentation. *Legionella micdadei* (Pittsburgh pneumonia agent), first described as a cause of pneumonia in immunosuppressed patients, probably produces illness very similar to that caused by *Legionella pneumophila. Francisella tularensis* (tularemia), *Pasteurella pestis* (plague pneumonia), *Bacillus anthracis* (anthrax), and *Pseudomonas pseudomallei* (meliodosis) are rare causes of bacterial pneumonia; however, a history of pertinent travel, residence, or exposure should be sought in evaluating patients with pneumonia so as not to overlook these possible etiologies. Effective antibiotic regimens for the various causes of bacterial pneumonia are listed in Table 1 (adult doses are given).

Treatment

Unlike patients with viral or mycoplasma pneumonia, most patients with bacterial pneumonia should be admitted to the hospital for initial management and observation. It is crucial to obtain sputum for Gram stain in order to correctly identify the causative organism and thus choose the correct antibiotic regimen.

The sputum Gram stain probably provides more useful information about etiology than does the culture of expectorated sputum, which may fail to detect *Streptococcus pneumoniae* or *Haemophilus influenzae* and, in cases of anaerobic infection, can only be expected to show normal oral flora. In addition, various organisms not important in the patient's infection (e.g., mouth contaminants) may be isolated. At least two blood cultures should be part of the initial work-up of a patient with pneumonia, as these may be positive when the sputum culture is negative. If expectorated sputum is unobtainable or is not diagnostic, transtracheal aspiration (by an experienced person) should be considered. This method also has the advantage of bypassing the oropharynx so there is less contamination of the specimen. It is sometimes necessary to perform bronchoscopy to obtain sputum or to do a transbronchial lung biopsy for diagnosis. Bronchoscopy may also be indicated to assess poor response and to evaluate possible obstruction. In patients who are immunosuppressed and have a wide range of diagnostic possibilities and more rapidly progressive illness, open lung biopsy may be the safest procedure with the highest yield.

Uncomplicated bacterial pneumonias are generally treated with 10 to 14 days of antibiotic administration. Legionnaires' disease and gram negative pneumonia, even if uncomplicated, may require longer therapy to prevent relapse. If cavitation or effusion occurs or if there is a slow response to therapy, a longer course is required. Staphylococcal pneumonia usually requires three to six weeks of intravenous antibiotics. Hospitalized patients with pneumonia should be treated initially with parenteral antibiotics; after defer-

TABLE 1. **Antimicrobial Therapy of Bacterial Pneumonia**

Pathogen/Syndrome	Drug	Dose	Route
Gram Positive Cocci			
Streptococcus pneumoniae	Aqueous penicillin G	400,000 U q 4 hr	IV
	Erythromycin	250–500 mg q 6 hr	PO or IV
	(Cephalosporin or vancomycin[1])		
Staphylococcus aureus	Oxacillin or nafcillin	1–3 grams q 4 hr	IV
	Vancomycin[1]	500 mg q 6 h	IV
Streptococcus pyogenes (group A)	Same as for *Pneumococcus*		
Mixed Anaerobic Organisms (Aspiration pneumonia)			
Community-acquired	Aqueous penicillin G	2 million U q 4 hr	IV
	Clindamycin	600 mg q 6–8h	IV
Hospital- or nursing home–acquired	Aqueous penicillin G or clindamycin	As above	
	plus		IM or IV
	Gentamicin[2] or tobramycin[2]	1–1.5 mg/kg q 8 hr	
	(Cefoxitin)		
Gram Negative Bacilli			
Klebsiella pneumoniae	Cephalosporin[3]	Depends on cephalosporin chosen	
	plus		
	Gentamicin[2] or tobramycin[2]	1–1.5 mg/kg q 8 hr	IM or IV
Escherichia coli	Ampicillin or cephalosporin[3]	1 gram q 4 hr	IV
	plus		
	Gentamicin[2] or tobramycin[2]	1–1.5 mg/kg q 8 hr	IM or IV
Pseudomonas aeruginosa	Ticarcillin, piperacillin (or carbenicillin)	3 grams q 4 hr	IV
	plus tobramycin[2]	1–1.5 mg/kg q 8 hr	IM or IV
Proteus mirabilis	Ampicillin plus gentamicin or tobramycin[2]	1–1.5 mg/kg q 8 hr	IM or IV
	(Cephalosporin[3])	Depends on cephalosporin chosen	IV
Proteus species	Same as for *Pseudomonas* (cephalosporin[3])		
Enterobacteriaceae species	Same as for *Pseudomonas* (cephalosporin[3])	Depends on cephalosporin chosen	
	or		
	trimethoprim/sulfamethoxazole	2.5–5.0 mg/kg q 6 hr based on trimethoprim components	PO or IV
Serratia marcescens	Gentamicin[2]	1–1.5 mg/kg q 8 hr	IM or IV
	Cephalosporin[3]	depends on cephalosproin chosen	
	(Ticarcillin)		
	(trimethoprim/sulfamethiazole)		
Haemophilus influenzae	Ampicillin (cephalosporin[3])	1 gram q 4–6 hr	IV
	(Chloramphenicol)		
Legionella pneumophila	Erythromycin	500 mg 1 gram q 6 hr	PO or IV
	(± Rifampin)		
Legionella species	As above		

[1]Vancomycin is indicated for treatment of resistant strains.
[2]Dosage must be adjusted for renal disease.
[3]Newer cephalosporins are only indicated in case of an organism resistant to first or second generation cephalosporin.

vescence and clinical improvement oral antibiotics can be instituted.

Supportive Measures

Patients with pneumonia generally require intravenous replacement of fluid lost as a result of high fever, sweating, and increased respiratory rate. Some patients will develop septic shock and will require vasopressors to maintain blood pressure. If the arterial blood gas reveals hypoxemia, supplemental oxygen is indicated to maintain an arterial pO_2 of greater than 60 torr. Postural drainage and chest physiotherapy may help the patient clear bronchial secretions. Some patients will require intubation and mechanical ventilation to maintain adequate oxygenation and pulmonary toilet. If bronchospasm occurs, bronchodilators should be added to the regimen.

Prevention

The new pneumococcal polysaccharide vaccine contains the 23 capsular types responsible for about 90 per cent of serious pneumococcal infections. It should be given to patients over two years of age who exhibit increased susceptibility to pneumococcal disease. These include patients with chronic cardiorespiratory conditions, diabetes mellitus, impaired or absent splenic function (e.g., sickle cell anemia), alcoholism, and nephrotic syndrome or immunosuppression and all patients over 50 years old.

VIRAL RESPIRATORY INFECTIONS

method of
BARRY FARR, M.D.
University of Virginia
Charlottesville, Virginia

Viral respiratory infections are the most common acute illnesses of mankind and the leading reason for patient visits to physicians in the United States. They also account for a large proportion of industrial and scholastic absenteeism.

The majority of these viral respiratory infections result in the symptom complex known as the common cold. Cold symptoms include nasal obstruction and discharge, sore throat, sneezing, and coughing. Some cold sufferers develop laryngitis. Small children often have fever with a cold, but in adults this is rare.

The common cold is caused by many antigenically distinct viruses, but the colds they produce cannot be distinguished from one another on clinical grounds. The rhinovirus group alone comprises more than 100 serotypes, for which only very limited cross immunity is believed to occur. Other etiologic agents include coronavirus, parainfluenzavirus, respiratory syncytial virus, adenovirus, and even influenza virus, which does not always produce the classic influenza. These cold viruses may cause other clinical syndromes in infants and young children such as bronchiolitis, croup, and pneumonia. These viruses account for about two thirds of all colds, and the remaining third is believed to be due to yet undiscovered viruses.

Influenza is a less common but more severe illness manifested by fever, malaise, myalgias, headache, cough, nasal discharge, chilliness, and occasionally rigors.

Treatment of the Common Cold

The common cold is easily diagnosed clinically, and virologic studies to determine the causative virus are unnecessary. The mainstays of therapy for this self-limited condition remain reassurance, rest, and fluids. Antiviral therapy is not yet available, and antibacterial treatment is not recommended because it does not shorten the duration of the cold and may lead to the development of antibiotic-resistant flora or potentially hazardous side effects.

Treatment is confined to relief of symptoms, but combination cold remedies containing compounds for all possible cold symptoms should be avoided since they expose the patient to a higher risk of unnecessary side effects. Instead, medications should be prescribed to relieve the specific symptoms of the individual patient.

The most frequently required medication is a nasal decongestant. Topical preparations such as 0.1 per cent xylometazoline (Otrivin) or 0.05 per cent oxymetazoline (Afrin) may be administered to adults as intranasal drops or sprays. A less concentrated solution of xylometazoline (0.05 per cent) may be used for children. Sprays are administered upright (one or two sprays per nostril), whereas drops are administered in a recumbent position with the neck extended and the head rotated toward the side being treated (one or two drops per nostril). These preparations should be used regularly every 12 hours for 2 to 3 days until obstructive cold symptoms diminish. The patient should be warned about the hazard of rhinitis medicamentosa, which follows prolonged usage of nasal decongestants. Patients treated with monoamine oxidase (MAO) inhibitors should not use decongestants.

Oral preparations are available such as pseudoephedrine hydrochloride (Sudafed), which may be given three to four times daily at a dosage of 15 mg per dose for children aged 2 to 5 years, 30 mg for those 6 to 11 years old, and 60 mg for those over 11 years old. Oral preparations are probably less effective than topical preparations and may cause a rise in blood pressure, which could be hazardous to patients with prior hypertensive or other cardiac disease.

Antihistamines exert a drying effect on the nasal mucosa due to an anticholinergic side effect, but used alone they do not relieve nasal congestion. The slight possible benefit afforded by adding an antihistamine to a decongestant must be weighed against the antihistamine's prominent side effect of drowsiness, which may impair work performance and automobile driving safety.

Sore throat is usually mild and may be relieved by saline gargles, but occasionally an analgesic is required. Aspirin may be given orally every four hours (adult dose 325 to 650 mg, pediatric dose 10 mg per kg of body weight to a maximum of 650 mg). Acetaminophen (Tylenol, Tempra) may be given orally every four hours to patients unable to take aspirin. The dose of acetaminophen is 60 to 120 mg for children between 1 and 3 years old, 120 mg for those 3 to 6 years old, 240 mg for those 7 to 11 years old, and 325 to 650 mg for those over 11 years old. Severe sore throat, especially with exudate, cervical adenopathy, and fever, should suggest the possibility of streptococcal pharyngitis, which may be confirmed by throat culture. Treatment for this condition is discussed in another article.

Cough does not usually require therapy in the common cold, but moderate to severe coughing may require a suppressant after the possibility of pneumonia has been excluded by history, physical examination, and (if necessary) radiography. Effective cough suppressants include codeine and dextromethorphan hydrobromide (Romilar, Congesprin); either of these drugs may be given orally every four hours at the following doses: 2.5 to 5 mg for a child 2 to 5 years old, 5 to 10 mg for a child 6 to 11 years old, and 10 to 20 mg for those over 11 years old. Patients taking MAO inhibitors should not receive these cough suppressants. Expectorants have not been proven to provide effective cough therapy.

Constitutional symptoms and headache are usually minimal with a cold but occasionally require treatment with one of the antipyretic/analgesics previously listed.

The most frequent bacterial complication of the common cold is otitis media, which occurs in approximately 2 per cent of colds, involving mostly children. Otalgia, or diminished auditory acuity, indicates the need for pneumatic otoscopy. Acute bacterial sinusitis follows about 1 of 200 colds and tends to occur more frequently in adults. It cannot be distinguished from a cold on the basis of purulent nasal discharge, which may occur in the uncomplicated cold owing to the viral infection itself. Persistent nasal obstruction and facial pain suggest the need for sinus transillumination and/or radiography. These bacterial complications require antibiotic therapy as discussed in other articles in this book.

Patients and their families should be instructed that colds are caused by infectious viruses that spread from person to person. Although the mechanism of spread in the natural setting has not been definitively established, experimental evidence suggests that rhinoviruses are spread by hand contact. Hand washing and conscious avoidance of finger-to-nose or finger-to-eye contact (which inoculates the virus) after exposure to a cold sufferer may reduce the risk of transmission.

Ingestion of large doses of vitamin C has not been shown to be effective prophylaxis against or therapy for the common cold. Prospects for a vaccine are poor because of the multiplicity of viral agents. Interferon has shown promising activity as a prophylactic agent but is still undergoing clinical testing.

Treatment of Influenza

The diagnosis of influenza is made on clinical and epidemiologic grounds. As with colds, diagnostic virology is usually unnecessary for management of the patient with influenza, but the practitioner should be aware of reports on influenza activity by the Centers for Disease Control or the state health department. During winter these reports give evidence of the predominant type and frequency of influenza virus isolates in sentinel practices.

The systemic symptoms of influenza are the primary target of therapy. Bed rest and increased fluid intake are necessary. During an influenza A epidemic, amantadine may be considered the drug of choice, being more effective than acetaminophen or aspirin and reducing illness duration by half. The oral dosage for adults is 200 mg initially followed by 100 mg twice daily and for a child 1 to 2 mg per pound of body weight twice daily (not over 150 mg per day). Treatment should continue for three to four days. Its use has been associated with minor and reversible side effects on the central nervous system such as insomnia, difficulty concentrating, and dizziness.

When influenza B predominates in the area, acetaminophen may be prescribed (dosage given previously), since amantadine lacks activity against this virus. Aspirin should not be prescribed for children in view of recent epidemiologic evidence relating Reye's syndrome to salicylate use for influenza or varicella.

Cough is often moderate to severe, requiring prescription of a cough suppressant such as codeine or dextromethorphen (dosage given previously) after the possibility of pneumonia has been excluded. Nasal congestion may warrant a topical decongestant as previously described.

Prevention of influenza is possible by vaccination, which is recommended for those at risk of serious complications and death from influenza. This group includes principally the elderly (above 65 years of age) and those with a chronic disease, especially of the heart or lungs. Persons providing essential services to the community should also be vaccinated. Egg allergy is one of the few contraindications to vaccination.

High risk individuals unable to receive the vaccine may be treated prophylactically with amantadine (at the dosage previously given) during an epidemic of influenza A. If amantadine is begun prophylactically at the time of vaccination, it should be continued for 14 days to allow time for an effective vaccine response.

VIRAL AND MYCOPLASMAL PNEUMONIAS

method of
BRUCE H. HAMORY, M.D.
University of Missouri–Columbia
Columbia, Missouri

Viral Pneumonia

Diagnosis

Viral pneumonias are most commonly diagnosed in the presence of epidemic disease caused by influenza A viruses, respiratory syncytial virus, parainfluenza viruses, or adenoviruses. Widespread recognition of the seasonal nature of these infections, together with increased availability of diagnostic techniques such as direct fluorescent antibody staining of respiratory secretions and viral culture to document the presence of a particular viral strain, has resulted in more frequent recognition of specific agents. This is a necessary prerequisite to the specific treatment of those viruses for which antiviral chemotherapy exists.

In addition to pneumonia associated with epidemics of viral respiratory disease, viral pneumonia may complicate the course of chickenpox (varicella-zoster) and measles in normal hosts, and of cytomegalovirus infection and herpesvirus hominis infection in the immunosuppressed patient. These agents should be considered when a diffuse pneumonia with profound hypoxemia occurs in a patient with cell-mediated immunity, such as high dose steroid therapy, after organ transplantation, or with a lymphoma. Bronchoscopy with biopsy or open lung biopsy is usually required to confirm the diagnosis speedily.

Treatment

Influenza virus infection usually occurs in epidemics in the winter. After cultural documentation of the first few cases in an outbreak, subsequent patients with the same clinical syndrome are presumed to have the same disease. About 5 per cent of these patients will have primary influenza pneumonia, and an additional group will be at high risk for adverse outcome. These patients should receive specific antiviral chemotherapy with oral amantidine, 100 mg twice a day (for adults). The dose for children is 5 mg per kg of body weight (maximum of 15 mg per day for children under 9 years) given in two divided doses. The usual duration of therapy is 7 days. In general, hospitalization is indicated only for the elderly with severe shortness of breath, for those individuals who develop evidence of congestive heart failure, and for those with evidence of bacterial superinfection. The most common pathogens responsible for bacterial pneumonia are pneumococci, *Staphylococcus aureus*, and *Haemophilus influenzae*. Bacterial superinfection is most commonly recognized about the third day of illness when the fever that has begun to diminish increases again.

Respiratory syncytial virus (RSV) and parainfluenza viruses are the premier viral respiratory pathogens of children. RSV usually occurs in the late winter and is heralded by the onset of bronchiolitis in young children. Parainfluenza virus infections usually occur in the spring. Children younger than 4 months of age with lower respiratory involvement should be hospitalized for observation, hydration, and possible treatment of bacterial superinfection. For older children, fluids, bed rest, and frequent follow-up are recommended. Fever may be controlled with acetaminophen when over 38.5C. (102F). No specific chemotherapy is currently licensed for either RSV or parainfluenza virus infection, though experimental evidence suggests that ribavirin administered by small particle aerosol may favorably affect this disease.

Viral pneumonia occurring in an immunosuppressed host should signal hospitalization, together with tapering or the discontinuation of any drugs that may be responsible for the immunosuppressed state (for example, steroids). In any patient who is ill enough to be hospitalized, arterial blood gases should be carefully monitored and oxygen administered to maintain a PaO_2 of at least 80 mm Hg. If the pCO_2 increases above 40 to 50 mm Hg, intubation and mechanical ventilation should be considered.

Adequate hydration by oral fluids should be assured. Cough may be controlled by judicious use of dextromethorphan or terpin hydrate and codeine. Aspirin is helpful to control fever, myalgias, and headache in adults but is contraindicated in children because of the risk of Reye's syndrome. If the patient fails to improve, or starts to improve (defervescence and decreased cough) but then worsens, a bacterial superinfection should be sought.

Mycoplasmal Pneumonia

Diagnosis

Mycoplasma pneumoniae is a common cause of pneumonia in young adults and older children. Though outbreaks are usually recognized in the late summer and fall, the disease may occur at any time of the year. Cough is the most prominent symptom, and the absence of a prominent, nonproductive cough makes the diagnosis unlikely.

Treatment

Treatment with erythromycin, 500 mg orally every 6 hours (2 grams per day) for 10 days, is usually adequate. Tetracycline, 500 mg orally every 6 hours, is an acceptable alternative in adults. Adequate hydration with oral fluids should be assured, and medication for the control of cough is often required. Hospitalization is rarely needed. Complications are relatively uncommon but include otitis media, sinusitis, hemolytic anemia, arthritis, myocarditis, skin rashes, disseminated intravascular coagulation, and a spectrum of central nervous system abnormalities. Occasionally, a relapse of pneumonia occurs and needs retreatment. In those instances, my preference is to use erythromycin therapy for another 10 days.

LEGIONELLOSIS

(Legionnaires' Disease and Pontiac Fever)

method of
PAUL H. EDELSTEIN, M.D.
Veterans Administration
Wadsworth Medical Center
Los Angeles, California

Legionella species bacteria, which are fastidious gram negative bacilli, cause pneumonia, known as Legionnaires' disease, as well as some rare extrapulmonary infections. In addition, there is a strong association between aerosol exposure to *Legionella* organisms and a systemic, febrile, nonfatal illness known as Pontiac fever; this disease may be an intoxication rather than an infection.

Therapy

Therapy of legionella infections is based on anecdotal clinical experience only. No comparative clinical trials have been undertaken for this disease. Erythromycin appears to be effective, as compared with antimicrobials usually used for the treatment of pneumonia, such as penicillins, cephalosporins, and aminoglycosides. There is no information available about antimicrobial treatment of Pontiac fever, but antibiotic therapy is probably not beneficial.

There is very good experimental evidence that drugs other than erythromycin may also be effective in the treatment of Legionnaires' disease. Cotrimoxazole (sulfamethoxazole-trimethoprim) (Bactrim, Septra), doxycycline (Vibramycin) and rifampin (Rifadin, Rimactane) appear to be as effective as erythromycin in the treatment of animal models of the disease. In addition, there are scattered case reports of clinical response to these drugs in patients with Legionnaires' disease. The use of rifampin alone has been discouraged because of the possibility of emergence of resistance to this drug when used by itself. Because rifampin is so active both in vitro and in vivo, many clinicians recommend its use for severe disease in conjunction with another drug, such as erythromycin or doxycycline.

TABLE 1. **Antimicrobial Treatment of Legionella spp. Infection**

Intravenous Administration Until Clinical Response Noted (Usually 2 to 4 days)	
First Choice	Erythromycin 0.5 to 1.0 gram every 6 hr
Second Choices	Doxycycline 100 mg every 12 hr
	Cotrimoxazole 5 mg per kg of trimethoprim component every 6 hr
Follow-up Oral Administration For 18 to 21 Days Total Duration of Therapy	
First Choice	Erythromycin 500 mg every 6 hr
Second Choices	Doxycycline 200 mg once per day
	Cotrimoxazole 3 to 5 mg per kg of trimethoprim component every 6 hr
Special Cases	
Severe Illness	Add rifampin, 600 mg given orally every 12 hr, to erythromycin, doxycycline, or cotrimoxazole as above for the first 1 to 2 weeks of therapy until clinical response noted.
Lung Abscess	Continue therapy until cavities close, add rifampin as above; generally oral therapy is sufficient after initial intravenous therapy.

Therapy should be prolonged, probably for at least 18 to 21 days, because of known relapses after shorter courses of antimicrobial treatment. These relapses are most likely because the intracellular environment that legionella grows in protects the bacterium from extracellular antibiotics. Courses of therapy as long as two to three months are indicated for the treatment of legionella lung abscesses, which should be treated until the cavities close.

Erythromycin is best given intravenously (see Table 1) until a clinical response is documented; it can then be given orally. For very mild cases, initial therapy can be with an orally administered drug. Some patients may relapse when changed from intravenous to oral erythromycin therapy, presumably because of poor absorption. Intravenous erythromycin administration commonly causes phlebitis, local pain, or both; addition of sodium bicarbonate and slow administration of diluted drug are sometimes helpful. In addition, patients with severe renal failure may develop transient deafness when receiving intravenous erythromycin therapy; this seems to resolve after cessation of therapy or reduction in dosage but may be an indication for use of another drug. Diarrhea, abdominal discomfort, and anorexia are occasional side effects of oral erythromycin therapy in some patients; sometimes a change of erythromycin formulation resolves these problems. As with administration of all antimicrobials, prolonged diarrhea is an indication for stopping therapy if possible and consideration of antimicrobial-associated colitis. Administration of rifampin, doxycycline, or cotrimoxazole may also be responsible for gastrointestinal tract side effects; in addition, hepatitis, hematologic abnormalities, and renal disease may occur with some of these drugs as well.

Since rifampin is so active against *Legionella,* it is tempting to use it in every case of Legionnaires' disease. This is probably not necessary in mild cases of the disease, especially since rifampin can cause serious side effects and also because combination therapy has not been studied in clinical trials. It should be used in combination with erythromycin or doxycycline in severe cases of Legionnaires' disease as well as for the treatment of cavitary legionella pneumonia. A one to two week course of rifampin is probably sufficient.

The response to appropriate antimicrobial therapy is usually prompt. Patients generally start to feel better within one to two days after starting therapy but remain febrile for as long as a week. Some severely immunocompromised patients have remained febrile for periods as long as two to four weeks. This makes it important to consider all possible factors, such as appetite, myalgia, breathlessness, and general overall condition, in addition to temperature when assessing response to therapy. Pulmonary infiltrates on chest roentgenograms often continue to worsen despite overall clinical improvement with treatment; these changes should stabilize within a few days and then gradually improve over a period of several weeks to months. A few case reports have demonstrated that some patients will not improve with erythromycin therapy alone but will promptly become afebrile after changing to another regimen, such as combined rifampin and cotrimoxazole. Once the patient has become afebrile for more than 12 to 24 hours, it is very unusual for new fever to appear in uncomplicated cases; patients with recrudescent fever should be evaluated for dual infection, superinfection, mistaken diagnosis, drug reaction, and failure to absorb orally administered antimicrobials.

PULMONARY EMBOLISM

method of
DANIEL A. PIETRO, M.D.,
G. V. R. K. SHARMA, M.D.,
KEVIN M. McINTYRE, M.D.,
and ARTHUR A. SASAHARA, M.D.
Veterans Administration Medical Center
Brockton/West Roxbury, Massachusetts

A comprehensive approach to the therapy of pulmonary embolism must include early recognition, indications for medical and surgical therapy, the treatment of acute cor pulmonale when present, and the recognition and treatment of recurrent pulmonary embolism. Since prevention of pulmonary thromboembolism is certainly preferable to treatment of an acute event, recognition and control when possible of factors predisposing to venous thrombosis constitute the approach of choice to thromboembolism and accordingly deserve special consideration.

Early Recognition—Diagnostic Considerations

The first and most consistently helpful step in the early recognition of pulmonary thromboembolism is the awareness of patient predisposition to deep vein thrombosis. Among the more important predisposing factors are immobilization for trauma (especially hip fracture), the postpartum and postoperative periods, congestive heart failure, chronic venous insufficiency of the legs, obesity, and oral contraceptive agents. Since deep vein thrombosis may be present with no clinical evidence in half the cases, physical signs cannot be relied upon to exclude this diagnosis.

It is important to appreciate that the clinical manifestations of pulmonary thromboembolism may be nonspecific or suggestive. When hemoptysis, pleuritic chest pain, or a pleural friction rub occurs acutely as the result of pulmonary embolism, the diagnosis of embolism can usually be established quickly by the usual studies and treatment instituted promptly. Frequently, however, clinical manifestations are nonspecific: dyspnea, tachycardia, tachypnea, and fever-signs and symptoms consistent with a number of cardiopulmonary processes. When embolism manifests itself in such nonspecific terms in patients with underlying heart or lung disease, embolism as a cause of these symptoms can be easily overlooked. Accordingly, the unexplained development of such symptoms in patients under treatment for symptomatic heart or lung disease should raise the question of superimposed pulmonary embolization. The acute development of nonspecific cardiopulmonary symptoms in a patient with clinically recognizable thrombophlebitis should be considered to be due to thromboembolism until that diagnosis is excluded.

Diagnosis of pulmonary embolism is usually established in the young patient with no prior cardiopulmonary disease by the finding of arterial hypoxemia, signs of pulmonary infarction on chest x-ray, and an abnormal perfusion lung scan. In the patient with prior cardiopulmonary disease, however, all these abnormalities are nonspecific. Lung scanning, with an objective assessment of the leg veins for deep vein thrombosis or selective pulmonary angiogram, should be done to confirm the diagnosis.

Therapy of Acute Pulmonary Embolism

Anticoagulant Therapy: Massive and Submassive Thromboembolism. The primary treatment of acute pulmonary embolism is clearly medical. The use of fibrinolytic agents is an accepted and recommended treatment in *massive* pulmonary embolism and is increasingly utilized for large submassive pulmonary emboli. Although the benefits of the fibrinolytic agents streptokinase and urokinase are well documented, the risk and complications with these agents are greater.

These lytic agents have been shown to lyse fresh clot (less than 5 to 7 days old) and to improve hemodynamics and circulation. Additionally, clot lysis in the deep venous system also occurs, tending to reduce the risk of immediate recurrent emboli, as well as reducing the likelihood that venous changes will result in a source for chronic recurrent thrombi. Prior to the use of thrombolytic agents, it is important that (1) the diagnosis be firmly established; (2) the severity of the clinical problem exceed the risk of complications from the therapy; and (3) there be clear understanding of the details of therapy, including monitoring, management of bleeding complications, and control of subsequent anticoagulation.

The major complication of the systemic thrombolytic agents is bleeding. These agents create a systemic lytic state and will lyse all fresh clot without regard to location. Thus invasive procedures and recent surgery are contraindications because of the risk of bleeding. Any central line should be inserted via an arm vein cutdown, with careful attention to control of bleeding. Arterial blood gas samples should not be obtained from the femoral artery because of the potential for large, unrecognized blood loss in this region. Endotracheal intubation should be considered a contraindication to lytic therapy because of the high risk of tracheal bleeding from the trauma of the endotracheal tube against the lining of the trachea.

In the absence of contraindications, urokinase may be administered intravenously in a loading dose of 4400 units per kg of body weight (2000 units per pound) over 10 minutes, followed by a maintenance dose of 4400 units per kg per hour for 12 hours. Streptokinase is administered in a loading dose of 250,000 units over a 30 minute period, followed by a maintenance infusion of 100,000 units per hour for 24 hours. Prior to streptokinase loading, the intravenous injection of 100 mg of hydrocortisone and 50 mg of Benadryl will reduce the commonly encountered allergic response to the streptococcal antigens. Heparin should be discontinued prior to initiating thrombolytic therapy and restarted after lytic therapy is discontinued and clotting time has returned to normal. During initial infusion of streptokinase or urokinase, the lytic state should be monitored by measurement of the thrombin time (TT) or the whole blood euglobulin lysis time (WBELT). If these studies are not available, the prothrombin time (PT) and partial thromboplastin time (PTT) may be used. Unlike heparin, for which a range of PTT prolongation is recommended, with lytic treatment it is only necessary to demonstrate that a prolongation over the control value is achieved. Greater prolongation does not require a reduction in the usual maintenance infusion of the lytic medication, but inadequate prolongation will require an additional bolus and possibly higher infusion rates. Subsequent anticoagulation with intravenous heparin and warfarin (after completion of lytic treatment) is continued according to conventional methods (discussed subsequently).

In *submassive* pulmonary emboli, the risk of systemic fibrinolysis is often greater than the expected benefit, and the time-tested conventional approach of intravenous heparin is recommended. In the adult patient, a 5000 to 10,000 unit of heparin as an intravenous bolus is followed by an immediate continuous intravenous infusion of 1000 to 2000 units per hour. Adjustment of the infusion rate and the need for additional heparin boluses is determined by the activated partial thromboplastin time (aPTT). The aPTT should be prolonged to 2 to 2.5 times the normal range. Although continuous intravenous infusion is the preferred and standard form of delivery, an intermittent bolus technique may be utilized if an infusion pump is unavailable. A loading dose of 5000 to 10,000 units of heparin is followed by a 5000 to 8000 unit bolus every 4 hours, the dose being adjusted to maintain the aPTT at 2 to 2.5 times control when measured 30 minutes before the next bolus is to be injected.

Anticoagulation with heparin should be maintained for 5 to 7 days, which will allow time for existing thrombus, usually in the deep venous system, to fix firmly to vessel walls, thus reducing the risk of recurrent emboli. It is recommended that bed rest be maintained over this period to minimize the risk of re-embolization. Gradual ambulation may be started at or after the seventh day. Coumarin derivatives may be started several days before ambulation. Heparin therapy can usually be reduced with institution of oral anticoagulants, because the interaction of the latter agents with heparin usually results in a prolonged clotting or partial thromboplastin time. The prothrombin time is usually less affected by combined use. Alternatively, coumarin derivatives may be instituted when heparin is begun, providing a longer period for adjustment or oral anticoagulant dosage.

Effective oral anticoagulant therapy (warfarin) requires achievement and maintenance of a dosage level which will prolong the Quick one-stage prothrombin time to about two times the control level. Warfarin should be given in dosages of 10 to 15 mg per day for 3 days initially and regulated thereafter by the prothrombin time. A loading dose need not be given, because it may excessively depress factor VII and result in bleeding. In addition to a decrease in factor VII, depression of factors II, IX, and X must be achieved to retard coagulation. Depression of these factors requires

3 to 4 days of therapy and may not be hastened by employing a loading dose of warfarin. Before therapy is begun, the patient's medications should be examined for those that interact with warfarin.

Anticoagulation should usually be maintained for at least 3 months and preferably for 6 months, even if the predisposing factor has been eliminated. If the predisposition is chronic, indefinite oral anticoagulation is recommended. When contraindications to anticoagulant therapy are present, including evidence of active bleeding, significant liver disease, independent abnormalities of the clotting system, recent surgery, or unreliability of the patient, consideration must be given to an inferior vena caval interruption.

Treatment of Acute Cor Pulmonale

Although the great majority of patients with massive or submassive embolism can be satisfactorily treated with the medical regimen detailed earlier, a few patients with massive embolism and shock may require intensive medical therapy consisting of oxygen, intravenous isoproterenol (useful for both its inotropic and its vasodilator effects), vasopressors, and heparin. It is recommended that isoproterenol be given by drip (2 to 4 mg per 500 ml of 5 per cent dextrose in water) to increase cardiac output and, ideally, restore systemic arterial pressure. If hypotension persists after isoproterenol administration, dopamine (5 micrograms per kg per minute) may be used. Occasionally, when central venous pressure is low, administration of intravenous fluids may be helpful in improving the hemodynamic status. It is important to treat such coexisting causes of hemodynamic impairment as may be present, e.g., left heart failure, with such agents as digitalis, glycosides, and intravenous diuretics as indicated clinically.

A number of patients with hypotension or shock secondary to massive embolism will quickly stabilize and be candidates for thrombolytic therapy. A few, however, may have persistent hypotension and may require mechanical removal of emboli to survive. Pulmonary embolectomy with cardiopulmonary bypass is indicated in this situation once pulmonary arterial obstruction has been shown by angiography to be massive and to be sufficiently proximal to be surgically accessible. Pulmonary embolectomy carries a high mortality risk and is therefore infrequently employed.

Adjunctive Therapy

Adjunctive therapy plays an important role in acute pulmonary embolism. Since most patients with clinically detectable pulmonary embolism will have some degree of hypoxemia, oxygen therapy is an important adjunct. Since hypoventilation is rarely a cause of hypoxemia in pulmonary embolism, oxygen may be administered comfortably by nasal catheter without fear of suppressing ventilation.

In patients who complain of severe pleuritic pain or who exhibit apprehension, intravenous morphine sulfate administered slowly, 1 mg at a time (up to 5 to 10 mg), may be very helpful. Apprehension is lessened, and ventilation is frequently improved. Codeine sulfate (30 to 60 mg) may be given for lesser pain.

Recognition of Recurrence of Thromboembolism

The recognition of "true" recurrence during the acute phase of pulmonary embolism is a difficult problem that cannot be resolved without the aid of lung scanning or pulmonary angiography. Only by angiography can the distinction between recurrent pulmonary embolism and fragmentation with distal migration of the original clot be made. The importance of this distinction lies in the therapy. Should true recurrence happen during a period when adequate anticoagulation with intravenous heparin has been maintained, the patient may be considered a "heparin failure" and caval interruption indicated. The fragmentation and migration process, on the other hand, requires only continuation of heparin.

If recurrence takes place during well-controlled oral anticoagulation in the recovery period or during long-term anticoagulation, management depends on the cardiopulmonary status of the patient, the magnitude of recurrence, the status of the deep veins, and the nature of the predisposing event. If the underlying cardiopulmonary status is satisfactory, the embolic episode submassive (less than 40 per cent of total pulmonary vasculature affected), the deep veins minimally abnormal, and the predisposing event temporary (e.g., leg trauma), retreatment with intravenous heparin may be carried out, following the same time course as in the initial event. However, if the underlying cardiopulmonary status is unstable, the recurrence massive, the deep veins grossly abnormal, or the predisposing condition chronic (e.g., varicose veins), caval interruption is recommended.

Interruption of Inferior Vena Cava

Currently, the procedure is indicated in the following conditions: (1) presence of contraindications to anticoagulation, (2) recurrence during adequate anticoagulation, (3) septic pelvic thrombophlebitis with embolism, (4) recurrent pulmonary emboli, and (5) as an adjunct to pulmonary embolectomy.

The majority of patients requiring inferior vena caval interruption are those in whom contraindications to anticoagulation exist. These include severe systemic hypertension with Grade III or IV retinopathy; presence of an actively bleeding lesion in the gastrointestinal or genitourinary tract (symptomatic lesions without active bleeding are considered relative contraindications); craniotomy or a cerebrovascular accident within the prior 2 months; evidence of a lesion known or suspected to be associated with intracranial hemorrhage, including malignancy; presence of an uncontrolled hypocoagulable state, including coagulation factor deficiencies, platelet abnormalities, or other spontaneous hemorrhagic or purpuric phenomena; and severe renal or hepatic insufficiency. Relative contraindication must be considered on an individual patient basis, weighing the risk and impact of bleeding against the morbidity of venous interruption.

Although interrupting the inferior vena cava will prevent further embolization in the acute period, recurrences are possible. In addition, the mortality and morbidity of such procedures under general anesthesia have limited their use. The introduction of the inferior vena cava filters, which can be placed under fluoroscopy with local anesthesia, has minimized the hazards of inferior vena caval interruption. The procedure is associated with a negligible recurrence rate and complications.

SARCOIDOSIS

method of
D. GERAINT JAMES, M.D., FRCP,
and M. A. VELLA, M.Phil., MRCP
Royal Northern Hospital
London, England

Sarcoidosis is one member of a large family of granulomatous disorders in which the common denominator is the histology of epithelioid cell granulomas. Like many other members of this loose knit family, its etiology is unknown.

It is a multisystem disorder that most commonly affects young adults, presenting with intrathoracic, dermatologic, and ocular lesions. The diagnosis is most secure when clinicoradiographic findings are supported by histologic evidence of widespread noncaseating epithelioid cell granulomas in more than one system. A positive Kveim-Siltzbach skin test and raised serum angiotensin–converting enzyme (SACE) levels both reflect activity of the disease. There is evidence of depression of delayed type hypersensitivity with impairment of thymus-mediated T cells in the peripheral blood but with increased numbers and activity of T helper cells in lungs and bronchoalveolar fluid and at other sites of activity away from the blood. There is simultaneous evidence of lympho-proliferation with overactivity of B cells, raised serum immunoglobulin levels, elevated lambda and kappa light chains, increased antiviral antibody titers, and autoantibodies. Other common features are circulating immune complexes and hypercalciuria with or without hypercalcemia.

The course and prognosis correlate with the mode of onset; an acute onset with erythema nodosum heralds a self-limiting course and spontaneous resolution, whereas an insidious onset may be followed by relentless progressive fibrosis. Corticosteroids relieve symptoms, suppress the inflammation and granuloma formation, suppress the Kveim-Siltzbach skin test, and normalize raised SACE levels, thereby suggesting a direct action on the epithelioid granuloma.

Corticosteroids are the universal treatment of choice, administered to about one half of those afflicted.

Indications for Steroids

Eyes

The inflamed iris is relieved by local atropine eye drops to maintain a dilated pupil. Topical corticosteroids should always be administered for iridocyclitis in the form of eye drops applied frequently during the day, reinforced with a corticosteroid eye ointment applied at night. If there is no substantial and continuing improvement after one week, then the concentration of corticosteroids in the anterior segment of the eye may be increased by a local subconjunctival depot of cortisone. Oral prednisolone is indicated if local treatment does not lead to a rapid response or if ophthalmoscopy reveals posterior uveitis. The latter is best visualized by fluorescein angiography that demonstrates leakage of dye due to retinal vasculitis. This responds well to oral prednisolone, 40 mg daily. Treatment is continued for about 3 months depending upon the degree of involvement of other systems.

Increased intraocular pressure due to local steroid eye drops is a signal to switch to fluormethalone eye drops, which are least likely to cause a rise in pressure, and also to consider adding Timoptic eye drops, which will return the intraocular pressure to normal.

Involvement

Bilateral hilar lymphadenopathy is likely to subside without treatment, particularly if there is associated erythema nodosum. It has therefore been traditional, worldwide, not to treat stage 1 hilar adenopathy. However, we now know from lung biopsy experience that there are active sarcoid granulomas in the lungs even when they are not evident in the chest radiograph. Increased

SACE levels and radioactive gallium scans disclose their activity. The first must surely be extinguished in these widespread granulomas, for otherwise they may lead eventually to pulmonary fibrosis. Therefore, we treat hilar adenopathy if there is a significantly elevated SACE level.

Pulmonary infiltration that remains static or worsens during the course of three months is an indication for oral prednisolone, again in an effort to prevent eventual irreversible pulmonary fibrosis. Several factors influence the likelihood of resolution of the chest radiograph. The younger the patient, the more likely it is to clear. The presence of chronic skin lesions or bone cysts indicates an unfavorable prognosis, for these are the hallmarks of chronicity. Their presence suggests that the pulmonary lesions are unlikely to subside. Substantial improvement in the chest radiograph is also related to the length of time before treatment is given. Results are considerably better in those treated within 2 years of onset of the disease.

Breathlessness. If this symptom is present, the patient has already reached a stage of irreversible pulmonary fibrosis or disturbed gas transfer. Oral steroids provide symptomatic relief but do not influence the natural history of the disease or its grave prognosis at this irreversible stage.

Upper Respiratory Tract Sarcoidosis. This may involve the pharynx and larynx with edema, hoarseness, and stridor due to laryngeal obstruction. Intravenous steroids may be a matter of urgency, relieving life-threatening stridor. If given sufficiently early, intravenous therapy may be sufficient to avoid tracheostomy.

Skin

Steroid therapy is indicated for unsightly skin lesions such as lupus pernio, involving the nose, lips, eyelids, cheek, or ears. Steroids shrink the disfiguring lesions, but they recur when treatment is discontinued. Methotrexate, in a small dose of 5 mg once weekly, is also most effective in overcoming unsightly lupus pernio. When given with steroids, it allows the dose of prednisolone to be reduced to a minimum. (This use of methotrexate is not listed in the manufacturer's directive.)

Nervous System

Resolution of neurosarcoidosis is more likely to occur in younger patients whose sarcoidosis has an explosive onset. The response to treatment is better in those with accompanying erythema nodosum rather than chronic skin lesions, with acute rather than chronic uveitis, and with hilar adenopathy rather than old diffuse pulmonary infiltration.

Glandular Involvement

This is treated if there is disordered function, for example, dry eyes due to lacrimal gland involvement, dry mouth due to salivary gland enlargement, and hypersplenism due to sarcoidosis of the spleen. The indication for treatment is disordered function rather than anatomic enlargement of the gland.

Heart

It is easy to include involvement of the heart in a theoretical list of indications for corticosteroid therapy but much more difficult, in practice, to recognize myocardial sarcoidosis. It is suspected and treated when a patient with multisystem sarcoidosis develops cardiac arrhythmia or bundle branch block.

Treatment demands prolonged steroids for resolution of the granulomas, chloroquine as an antifibrotic agent, beta blockade, nifedipine as a calcium antagonist, antiarrhythmic agents, and earlier use of cardiac pacemaker.

Bone

Bone cysts cause pain, swelling, and deformity of hands and feet. Steroids provide relief of symptoms, but bone cysts persist despite treatment and symptoms recur when steroids are discontinued. Methotrexate (this usage not listed in manufacturer's directive) or indomethacin is a helpful alternative treatment.

Alternative Routes of Administration

Oral corticosteroids may be reinforced under various circumstances by intravenous or intramuscular administration. Eye drops may be reinforced by subconjunctival or retro-orbital hydrocortisone. Triamcinolone may be injected directly into skin plaques or joints.

Other Drugs

H_2 Antagonists

There may be a relative contraindication to oral prednisolone because of peptic ulceration, and a switch to other lines of treatment may be indicated. However, other drugs are all markedly inferior in the management of sarcoidosis. Consider the use of cimetidine or ranitidine in addition to prednisolone. The combination is effective and safe if used under close medical supervision.

Indomethacin

The active macrophage produces interleukin 1, which, in turn, influences T_4 helper lymphocytes. The macrophage–T lymphocyte feedback axis is prostaglandin-mediated. Indomethacin is a potent inhibitor of prostaglandin synthetase, and this may be its site and mode of action. It should be considered in acute exudative sarcoidosis, particularly acute uveitis, phlyctenular conjunctivitis, sarcoid polyarthritis, and erythema nodosum.

Chloroquine

The way in which chloroquine acts is unknown, but it controls some instances of chronic fibrotic sarcoidosis involving lungs and skin. It is particularly helpful in the management of lupus pernio and pulmonary fibrosis. In view of its ocular toxicity, it should only be given in a dose of 200 mg on alternate days for up to 9 months. (This use of chloroquine is not listed in the manufacturer's directive.)

Methotrexate

This drug is helpful in the treatment of chronic skin lesions, particularly lupus pernio. Since it is known to cause hepatic fibrosis when taken daily for prolonged periods, we restrict it to 5 mg taken once weekly for courses of three months. Patients are soon aware of its value for it shrinks the cosmetically unacceptable lupus pernio effectively. However, when the course of treatment is discontinued, lupus pernio slowly recurs during the following three months. Repeated courses every 6 months, possibly in conjunction with oral steroids or chloroquine and cosmetic camouflage, represent the best regimen. (This use of methotrexate is not listed by the manufacturer.)

Potassium Para-Aminobenzoate (Potaba)

It is known to have an antifibrotic effect in Peyronie's disease, scleroderma, and rheumatoid arthritis. It is worth considering in pulmonary fibrosis and lupus pernio due to sarcoidosis. Two-gram envules should be taken by mouth four to six times daily for several months. This form of treatment is an alternative to corticosteroids, methotrexate, and chloroquine, and giving all four in rotation helps to overcome the undesirable long-term complications of any one drug. (Potaba for sarcoidosis is not listed by the manufacturer.)

Immunomodulation

Transfer factor and *levamisole* were briefly popular but are no longer used. *Azathioprine* and *chlorambucil* are sometimes used in conjunction with steroids, allowing the dose of steroids to be reduced. *Cyclosporine* may find its way into this same category of a steroid-sparing supporter. Thus far, it has proved disappointing in the management of sarcoidosis; it remains an investigational drug for this use.

Special Situations

Abnormal Calcium Metabolism

Disordered calcium metabolism is due to overactivity of calcitriol. The natural form, cholecalciferol (vitamin D_3), is metabolized first in the liver to 25-hydroxycholecalciferol and then a second hydroxy group is added in the kidney to produce the potent highly active 1,25-dihydroxycholecalciferol (calcitriol). Calcitriol, produced by activated sarcoid macrophages, causes increased intestinal calcium absorption, leading to hypercalcemia and hypercalciuria. This can also be induced by sunlight. It is overcome swiftly by steroid therapy.

Persistent hypercalciuria may need calcium chelation by one of the following:

Sodium Cellulose Phosphate. This is indicated for the treatment of absorptive hypercalciuria associated with recurrent formation of renal calculi. It is an ion exchange compound with a particular affinity for divalent cations. It binds calcium ions in the lumen of the stomach and intestine, and the calcium complex is excreted harmlessly in the feces. It is a white to beige fibrous powder. Each 5 gram sachet binds 250 mg of calcium. The usual adult dose is 5 grams three times daily.

Effervescent Phosphate (Sandoz). Each effervescent phosphate tablet provides 500 mg of elemental phosphorus to bind calcium. The daily adult dose is 1 to 2 grams.

Pregnancy

Sarcoidosis is not a contraindication to pregnancy. Indeed, there is usually a most favorable effect. If the pregnant patient is receiving oral steroids then the dose can be reduced and even discontinued. The fetus is unaffected, and normal delivery can be expected. Chest radiography is contraindicated, and instead SACE is useful as a serial monitor of sarcoidosis activity.

Childhood

Sarcoidosis is rare in childhood, but it may be troublesome to manage. Prednisolone is the mainstay of treatment, but prolonged systemic therapy is undesirable. Therefore it is important to restrict treatment to precise and important indications, use topical rather than systemic steroids whenever possible, and consider nonsteroidal anti-inflammatory agents as less toxic alternatives.

SILICOSIS

method of
JAMES H. DAUBER, M.D.
University of Pittsburgh
Pittsburgh, Pennsylvania

Pulmonary disease resulting from the inhalation of dust containing silica was suspected as long as 6000 years ago, but the final chapter in this story was not written until the early 20th century when this association was conclusively documented. Although cause and effect between the deposition of silica in the lung and the development of nodular fibrosis is now universally accepted, the mechanisms by which these particles produce this distinctive reaction remain incompletely elucidated. Even though the clinical manifestations of disease can be prevented by limiting exposure to siliceous dusts, this goal has been achieved in neither the highly industrialized nor the developing nations.

Strictly defined, silicosis is the reaction in the lung to the deposition of crystalline silicon dioxide, often called free silica. Quartz, a component of most classes of rock, is the most abundant form of silica. Two isomers of silica, tridymite and cristobalite, which occur naturally and as a result of industrial processing, are also fibrogenic. Most exposures to respirable size particles (0.3 to 5.0 microns) of silica occur in the work place (Table 1). All these occupational exposures exist today and therefore represent potential causes of silicosis. Exposure through avocations or in the home are unusual. The prevalence of silicosis in the United States is not known. In 1960 it was estimated to be 5.4 per cent in lead-zinc miners in Utah. Although its prevalence appears to be declining as a result of better control measures, outbreaks of silicosis continue to be recognized when protection is inadequate.

The intensity and duration of exposure to silica seem to dictate the rate and severity of the reaction in the lung. When the content of free silica in dust is less than 30 per cent and the level of respirable dust in the air is relatively low, disease will not develop for 20 to 40 years. This form is called chronic silicosis. Accelerated silicosis ensues in 8 to 10 years if the content of free silica in the dust exceeds 30 per cent and the level of dust is several times that causing chronic silicosis. Exposures many times heavier than these produce symptoms in months to a few years. This condition is termed acute silicosis. Although relatively rare, it remains a uniformly fatal disease.

TABLE 1. **Occupations Associated with Exposure to Silica**

Category	*Source of Free Silica*
Mining	Dusts from drilling and cutting hard rock
	Sand used to improve traction on rails
Manufacturing	
Stone dressing	Cutting, grinding, polishing
Abrasives	Crushing quartz
Foundry work	Removing sand from castings
Pottery*	Cleaning surfaces to be enameled
Refractory products	Crushed quartz used in products
Inert fillers	Fine milling makes "silica flour"
Filter materials	Heating diatomaceous earth produces cristobalite
Construction	
Tunneling	Dust from drilling
Road-building	Rock crushed for bedding
Renovation	Dust from drilling in concrete
Steel fabrication	Sand-blasting surfaces
Boiler-scaling	Flue dust may contain silica

The pathologic hallmark of the chronic and accelerated forms is the silicotic nodule. These lesions consist of a core of concentrically arranged connective tissue fibers and a halo of inflammatory cells (primarily macrophages) that form preferentially in the subpleural, paraseptal, and peribronchiolar interstitial space. Up to 30 per cent of individuals with these forms of silicosis develop massive fibrotic lesions, which consist of acellular amorphous hyaline material and exceed 1 cm in diameter. Massive lesions often develop after a superimposed infection with *Mycobacterium tuberculosis* but also occur in uninfected individuals. They have a predilection for the upper lobes. The reaction in the interstitial space is more diffuse and less well organized in acute silicosis. Silicotic nodules may be few or even absent. Alveoli are filled with inflammatory cells and acellular proteinaceous material that appears to be lipoprotein (silicoproteinosis).

Individuals with uncomplicated chronic and accelerated silicosis are usually asymptomatic save for a chronic productive cough that often reflects exposure to cigarette smoke or other dusts encountered in the work place, or both. The onset of dyspnea usually signals the occurrence of progressive massive fibrosis (PMF). The productive cough worsens at this time as well. Sudden onset of severe dyspnea in this setting may be due to pneumothoraces, which tend to be recurrent and refractory to the usual therapy. Fatigue, fever, and weight loss are highly unusual in uncomplicated silicosis. Connective tissue diseases, particularly scleroderma, occur more commonly than expected in this population.

Dyspnea may occur as soon as 6 months after exposure in acute silicosis. Fever, weakness, and weight loss usually herald infection with mycobacteria or fungi but may occur in the absence of documented infection. A lupus-like syndrome has been encountered in some patients. Before the advent of antituberculous therapy, overwhelming tuberculosis was the usual cause of death, but now it is respiratory insufficiency.

Pulmonary function is normal in most cases of uncomplicated chronic and accelerated silicosis. Restriction, obstruction, or a combined impairment occur after PMF has set in. The level of immunglobulin in serum is characteristically elevated, as may be the activity of angiotensin-converting enzyme (30 per cent). The prevalence of autoantibodies (ANA, RF) is also higher than expected.

Treatment

No specific therapy has yet been devised. If disease develops with continuing exposure, the individual should be removed from the contaminated environment, particularly if young and the exposure is heavy, as the disease usually progresses even after exposure ceases. Polyvinyl pyridine-*N*-oxide, a polymer that acts as a hydrogen acceptor, blunts the cytotoxic action of silica on macrophages and lessens the fibrotic response in the lungs of experimental animals. Presumably it binds to the surface of silica particles and prevents interaction between the particle surface and cell membrane. This agent is not approved for use in humans.

Complications

Complications of the disease should be treated vigorously. The obstructive impairment often improves following the type of bronchodilator therapy used in chronic obstructive lung disease. Acute purulent bronchitis should be treated with antibiotics. Since *Haemophilus influenzae* and *Streptococcus pneumoniae* are the most common infecting agents, either ampicillin or tetracycline, 500 mg orally every 6 hours for 7 to 10 days, is usually effective. Vaccination against pneumococci and influenza is indicated.

Although the prevalence of tuberculosis in individuals with silicosis has decreased, their risk of developing active tuberculosis remains greater than normal. Individuals with active disease proved by smear or culture should be treated with isoniazid (INH) 300 mg daily, and rifampin, 600 mg daily, although some experienced physicians recommend triple drug therapy (ethambutol, 15 mg per kg daily). The duration of chemotherapy has not been well defined. Some physicians advocate continuing therapy for 6 months following conversion of sputum culture (minimum of 9 months of therapy), whereas others advocate lifetime therapy since relapse after completion of therapy is not uncommon. Conversion of the tuberculin skin test requires prophylactic therapy with INH, 300 mg daily. In these patients, cultures of sputum or gastric aspirates should be obtained. A suspicion of active disease demands therapy with INH and rifampin. The latter drug may be stopped if cultures are negative. INH is continued for at least 1 year and often longer.

Patients with severe obstruction are candidates for pulmonary rehabilitation programs. Arterial hypoxemia at rest or with exercise improves with supplemental oxygen therapy, which may also relieve dyspnea. Cor pulmonale supervenes in far-advanced disease and should be treated with diuretics and digitalis. Although acute respiratory embarrassment from a pneumothorax responds to insertion of a chest tube, complete reexpansion of the lung is often difficult to achieve.

Corticosteroids have been used in patients with acute silicosis but appear to have no role in the chronic or accelerated forms except when they are complicated by steroid-responsive connective tissue diseases. Because of the dismal prognosis for acute silicosis, heroic therapeutic measures such as whole lung lavage and lung transplantation have been employed. The efficacy of these forms of therapy, however, remains unproved and likely will be difficult to establish because this form of the disease is fortunately uncommon.

HYPERSENSITIVITY PNEUMONITIS

method of
HAL B. RICHERSON, M.D.
University of Iowa
Iowa City, Iowa

Hypersensitivity pneumonitis, also called extrinsic allergic alveolitis, is an allergic inflammation of the lung parenchyma including terminal airways caused by the repeated inhalation by a susceptible host of a variety of etiologic agents including organic dusts and simple chemicals (Table 1). Clinical presentation may be acute, subacute, or chronic, and diagnosis depends on clinical suspicion and a history of exposure to a causative occupational or environmental inhalant, appropriate clinical manifestations, demonstration of serum precipitins to the suspected agent, and clinical improvement with its avoidance. Since effective management depends largely upon avoiding the antigen, identification of the causative agent and its source is obviously important.

Treatment

Management of hypersensitivity pneumonitis involves antigen avoidance, possible use of premedication in instances of unavoidable environmental exposure, and the occasional need for corticosteroid therapy.

Environmental Control

The most effective way to avoid an incriminated agent is to separate the patient from the source. In many instances the source is an area or place of employment, and avoidance requires a job change. This recommendation cannot be given lightly and requires thoughtful consideration of alternatives. The dairy farmer with acute recurrent episodes may be able to avoid areas and activities associated with heavy burdens of respirable thermophilic organisms and may be persuaded to wear protective equipment (masks, respirators, ventilated helmets, filtration devices). The prognosis appears to be good in such patients if acute febrile episodes do not recur. Bird fanciers should avoid exposure completely

TABLE 1. **Examples of Hypersensitivity Pneumonitis**

Disease	Source of Antigen	Antigen
Farmer's lung	Contaminated hay, grain, silage	Thermophilic actinomycetes, *Aspergillus* sp.
Bird fancier's, breeder's, or handler's lung	Parakeet, pigeon, dove, chicken, turkey proteins	Avian droppings
Humidifier or air conditioner lung	Contaminated water in humidification aerosols, vaporizers, sprays, ventilation systems	Thermophilic actinomycetes, *Aureobasidium pullulans,* amoeba, other
Bagassosis	Contaminated bagasse (sugar cane)	Thermophilic actinomycetes
Mushroom worker's lung	Mushroom compost	Thermophilic actinomycetes, other
Vineyard sprayer's lung	Vineyard sprays	Thermophilic actinomycetes
Malt worker's lung	Moldy barley	*Aspergillus fumigatus, A. clavatus*
Maple bark stripper's disease	Maple bark	*Cryptostroma corticale*
Papermill worker's lung	Moldy wood chips	*Aspergillus* sp.
Sauna taker's lung	Contaminated sauna steam	*Auerobasidium pullulans,* other
Sequoiosis	Redwood sawdust	*A. pullulans, Graphium* sp.
Suberosis	Moldy cork	*Penicillium frequentans*
Woodworker's lung	Oak, cedar, mahogany dusts; pine and spruce pulp	Wood dust; *Alternaria* sp.
Coffee worker's lung	Coffee beans	Coffee bean dust
Pituitary snuff taker's lung	Heterologous pituitary powder	Bovine and porcine proteins
Chemical worker's lung	Polyurethane foam and insulation, synthetic rubber manufacturing, meat wrapping and labeling, other	Toluene diisocyanate (TDI), methylene diisocyanate (MDI), phthallic anhydride, vinyl chloride, other

but may demand compromise, and the use of protective equipment may prove useful. Contaminated humidification, air conditioning, and ventilation systems can be removed, replaced, or thoroughly cleaned at intervals. Those systems that generate vapor, particles, or sprays more often cause hypersensitivity pneumonitis than those involving simple evaporation. Other avoidable occupational and environmental hazards are self-evident as listed in Table 1. Recently various chemicals, many known to cause occupational asthma, have been found to cause hypersensitivity pneumonitis. These chemicals are ordinarily encountered in industry but have been reported in bathtub finishers and insulation installers. Protective equipment must be much more elaborate in such situations, since masks and filters do not remove small molecular weight substances.

Recurrence of symptoms demands more drastic measures for complete environmental control. Compromise measures are not recommended except in patients with acute, recurrent, self-limited episodes of hypersensitivity pneumonitis for which clinical monitoring is practical.

Premedication

Recommendations have been made for the use of prednisone (40 mg in one dose) or cromolyn sodium (20 mg by Spinhaler) as premedication prior to single, infrequent exposures to an unavoidable source. Although such premedication may seem effective in preventing acute episodes, the practice may be abused. No controlled trials of long-term results of premedication are available, and suppression of symptoms may not prevent progression of functional impairment.

Corticosteroid Therapy

Acute, recurrent episodes of hypersensitivity pneumonitis are typically self-limited and do not require drug therapy. Severe symptoms or progressive impairment may, however, warrant corticosteroid therapy provided the diagnosis has been established. The use of corticosteroids as a therapeutic trial cannot be recommended, since temporary improvement may result in many interstitial lung diseases and steroids may be harmful in interstitial diseases of infectious origin.

Progressive, subacute hypersensitivity pneumonitis requires corticosteroid therapy. Prednisone 60 mg daily in four divided doses is initiated, continued for 7 to 14 days depending upon the response, tapered over one week to 20 mg daily in a single dose, and gradually reduced unless a relapse occurs.

Patients with chronic disease should gradually improve following avoidance of the antigen source; recovery may take 6 to 12 months. Corticosteroids may be indicated in some cases to expedite recovery if symptoms or impairment warrant it. A regimen similar to that used for subacute disease is appropriate while monitoring the response. In general, corticosteroids are not necessary or recommended in patients with improving mild to moderate disease unless recovery has plateaued despite appropriate environmental control.

SINUSITIS

method of
ROBERT B. STANLEY, JR., M.D., D.D.S.
University of Southern California
Los Angeles, California

The sterility of the paranasal sinuses is usually maintained by the respiratory epithelial cilia, which constantly clear the sinuses of secretions and bacteria. However, viral infections, allergens, airborne pollutants, and vasomotor disturbances may cause cilial hypomotility and lead to bacterial superinfections. Nasal obstruction by polyps, septal deviations, and indwelling nasotracheal or nasogastric tubes may also contribute to this problem. The most common initial event is a viral upper respiratory infection, the "common cold." The virus not only causes mucosal edema in the nose to block the natural sinus drainage pathways but also evades the cilia to enter the sinus and cause mucociliary dysfunction.

It is often difficult to distinguish a prolonged common cold from a bacterial sinusitis and thus to decide which patients are to be treated with antibiotics. The most reliable symptom to indicate the transition from one to the other is a purulent nasal discharge, usually from the area of the middle meatus. Periorbital swelling and facial tenderness are strong but less common indicators. Fever is present in less than one half of patients, most of these being children. Headache, if present, may help localize the sinus with maximum involvement. Radiographs are relied on heavily to document a bacterial sinusitis with air-fluid levels, total opacification, and mucosal thickening of 4 to 5 mm or greater, correlating well with purulence that yields a positive culture. Most often, a pansinusitis is present, and involvement of an isolated sinus should warn the examiner that an unusual infection such as a fungal infection is possible.

The microbiology of sinusitis is variable, but *Streptococcus pneumoniae* and *Haemophilus influenzae* are the most commonly implicated organisms in acute maxillary sinusitis. Other organisms that may be found occasionally include *Branhamella catarrhalis, Staphylococcus aureus, Streptococcus pyogenes,* and miscellaneous anaerobes. Hospital patients with tubes through the nose may develop gram-negative infections. Patients with chronic sinusitis will most likely have facultative or obligate anaerobes, such as *Peptostreptococcus, Fusobacterium,* and *Bacteroides* species.

Treatment

The mainstay in treatment of acute sinusitis is oral antibiotic therapy, with ampicillin (500 mg orally every 6 hours for 10 to 14 days) used because of the high incidence of *Haemophilus influenzae*. Cefaclor (Ceclor) may become the drug of choice if the incidence of beta-lactamase–producing, penicillin-resistant organisms increases. Acceptable alternatives in the penicillin-allergic patient are erythromycin and trimethoprim-sulfamethoxazole. Response to antibiotic therapy should be evident within 48 to 72 hours; if it is not, antral puncture and aspiration for culture should be considered. Nasal cultures are of little help in documenting the causative organism. At the same time, the maxillary sinus can be gently lavaged to speed clearance of the purulence. Supportive therapy to reduce intranasal edema and possibly improve sinus drainage and aeration includes short-term (7 to 10 days) use of decongestant sprays and oral decongestants. The use of the latter is controversial and their effectiveness has not been proved.

Hospitalization and intravenous antibiotics are indicated for cases of acute sinusitis complicated by possible involvement of the orbital or intracranial structures. Although ampicillin alone (1 gram intravenously every 6 hours) is adequate in most of these cases, a later generation cephalosporin should be considered if there is a high incidence of penicillin-resistant *Haemophilus influenzae* in the community. If the maxillary sinus in involved, antral puncture is again helpful in documenting the causative organism. At one time, antral puncture was considered inadvisable without having had the patient on antibiotics for 24 to 48 hours. However, it appears that a diagnostic puncture can be done safely prior to initiating antibiotic therapy. Frequently, these cases will require a drainage procedure before maximum effect of the antibiotic therapy is achieved. Such procedures include creation of nasoantral windows, ethmoidectomy, and frontal sinus trephination. Antibiotic selection for patients with nosocomial infections and immunosuppressed patients with acute sinusitis requires antral puncture as the causative organisms cannot be accurately predicted.

Chronic sinusitis therapy also usually includes surgical management, such as removal of polyps, correction of a septal deviation, or establishment of drainage pathways into the nose. Because of the higher incidence of anaerobic infections, penicillin (Pen-VK, 500 mg orally every 6 hours for 10 to 14 days) is the drug of choice for acute exacerbations. The choice to treat by oral or intravenous administration is based on the same factors as with acute sinusitis.

STREPTOCOCCAL PHARYNGITIS

method of
STANFORD T. SHULMAN, M.D.
Northwestern University
Chicago, Illinois

The management of patients with acute pharyngitis remains controversial. The major issues are (1) the importance of using the throat culture for diagnosis of streptococcal pharyngitis, (2) the risk-benefit ratio of antibiotic therapy for streptococcal pharyngitis in areas where acute rheumatic fever has become rare, and (3) the effectiveness of therapy upon symptoms of streptococcal pharyngitis. Clearly, prevention of rheumatic fever and rheumatic heart disease is the major justification for identification of group A streptococcal pharyngitis.

Throat Cultures

The throat culture is a valuable diagnostic tool because there are no distinctive clinical findings (except for tender anterior cervical nodes or the rash of scarlet fever) that make possible a reasonable accurate clinical diagnosis of streptococcal pharyngitis. It is essential that throat cultures be inexpensive (they should be routinely processed *only* for detection of group A streptococci) and that results be available within 48 hours. The major disadvantage of throat cultures is that they do not differentiate between acute streptococcal infection and chronic streptococcal carriage with intercurrent acute viral pharyngitis. The major value of the throat culture is to identify the large group of culture negative individuals for whom the cost and risks of antibiotic therapy are not justified. Children under three years of age and older adults so rarely develop acute rheumatic fever that routine culturing of throats in these groups is not warranted. Asymptomatic household contacts of patients with streptococcal pharyngitis should not be cultured unless there is a previous history of rheumatic fever.

Definition of the role of rapid techniques for detection of group A streptococcal antigens will require further evaluation.

Therapy

Risk-Benefit Ratio of Therapy

Accurate diagnosis and effective treatment of streptococcal pharyngitis have several benefits, including reducing the risk of acute rheumatic fever (which has become very rare in most areas of the USA and other developed countries); reducing the low risk of suppurative complications such as peritonsillar or retrophryngeal abscesses, suppurative lymphadenitis, and sinusitis; interrupting spread of group A streptococci; and possibly shortening the duration of symptoms. Therapy does not appear to decrease the risk of acute post-streptococcal glomerulonephritis. The potential risks of treatment of acute streptococcal pharyngitis are essentially limited to the cost and the side effects (including allergic reactions) of antibiotic therapy. Parenteral antibiotic therapy (e.g., intramuscular benzathine penicillin) is associated with more serious allergic reactions than is oral therapy. In the USA and other developed countries, parenteral treatment should be limited to selected patients at particularly high risk for rheumatic fever (i.e., with personal past history or strong family history of rheumatic fever). In areas of the world with substantial rates of rheumatic fever, the increased risk associated with parenteral therapy may well be justified for routine use.

Timing of Therapy

Streptococcal pharyngitis is a self-limited illness with symptoms lasting about two to three days without antibiotic therapy. Appropriate antibiotic therapy of streptococcal pharyngitis has at best only a modest effect upon symptoms, shortening fever and sore throat by 12 to 24 hours if at all. Except in the most acutely ill patients with pharyngitis, fever, and tender anterior cervical nodes or in patients with a previous history of acute rheumatic fever, therapy should be instituted after a definite diagnosis of streptococcal pharyngitis is established, i.e., as soon as throat culture results are available. In the exceptional circumstances noted previously, initiation of therapy at the time the throat culture is obtained is appropriate. It is noteworthy that, if effective therapy is instituted as late as 9 days after the onset of pharyngitis, acute rheumatic fever is still preventable. Hence, delaying the onset of therapy until culture results are available presents no significant risk to the patient and may decrease greatly the inappropriate (and expensive) administration of antibiotics for viral illnesses.

Specific Therapeutic Regimens
(Table 1)

Penicillin is the drug of choice for streptococcal pharyngitis, except for patients allergic to this drug. Ten days of therapy are necessary to maximize eradication of group A streptocci and prevention of acute rheumatic fever. In areas of the world (such as across most of the USA) in which acute rheumatic fever has become rare, *oral penicillin V*, 125 to 250 mg twice or four times a day for 10 days is the drug of choice. Oral therapy requires patient and parent cooperation but is associated with fewer allergic reactions than parenteral penicillin.

The slightly greater degree of prevention of acute rheumatic fever afforded by *intramuscular benzathine penicillin G* justifies the use of this

TABLE 1. **Treatment of Streptococcal Pharyngitis: Alternatives**

1. Oral penicillin V, 125 to 250 mg tid or qid or 10 days
2. Intramuscular benzathine penicillin G
   600,000 units ≤ 60 pounds
   1,200,000 units > 60 pounds
3. Oral erythromycin estolate (20 to 40 mg/kg/day) in two to four doses or erythromycin ethyl succinate (40 mg/kg/day) in two to four doses for 10 days

antibiotic in regions with high rates of acute rheumatic fever, in families with a rheumatic individual, in patients with a previous history of rheumatic fever, and in clinical situations with particularly low expected rates of compliance with oral regimens. Preparations containing procaine penicillin in addition to benzathine penicillin G are associated with decreased pain at the injection site; if used, they should contain benzathine penicillin G in the following dose: 600,000 units for patients weighing 60 pounds or less and 1.2 million units for patients over 60 pounds. It appears likely that the combination of 900,000 units of benzathine penicillin G and 300,000 units of procaine penicillin is satisfactory, even for adults.

Antibiotics other than penicillin offer no advantage for treatment of streptococcal pharyngitis and should be limited to penicillin-allergic individuals. The drug of choice for these patients is oral *erythromycin* for 10 days. Erythromycin estolate (20 to 40 mg per kg per day) in two to four divided doses or erythromycin ethyl succinate (40 mg per kg per day) in two to four divided doses for 10 days is effective. The maximum daily dose of erythromycin is 1 gram. Although strains of group A streptococci resistant to erythromycin are prevalent in some areas of the world, they are rare in the United States. *Clindamycin* (10 to 20 mg per kg per day) in two divided doses may be as effective as penicillin or erythromycin but should be restricted to situations in which less toxic antibiotics are contraindicated. Oral cephalosporins such as *cephalexin or cefaclor* (40 mg per kg per day) in three divided doses are acceptable alternatives for the penicillin-allergic patient. However, they are expensive and should *not* be used in patients with *anaphylactic* hypersensitivity to penicillin.

Certain antibiotics have no role in the treatment of streptococcal pharyngitis. Tetracyclines should not be used because of the high prevalence of strains resistant to these agents. The sulfonamides, including trimethoprim/sulfamethoxazole, although effective in the *prevention* of streptococcal infection, are ineffective in *treatment* of streptococcal infection. *Penicillinase-resistant penicillins* have no proven advantage over penicillin, even in patients who harbor staphylococci, and should not be used.

Post Therapy Studies

Patients may be considered noncontagious 24 to 48 hours after initiation of therapy and may return to school or to other activities. Post therapy throat cultures are *not* recommended in routine circumstances, unless the patient remains symptomatic or is from a family that includes a rheumatic individual. The reason for this is that post therapy cultures most often detect chronic streptococcal carriers, who do not represent a risk to their contacts and who are not at risk for development of acute rheumatic fever. Until quite recently, treatment of chronic carriers had been a source of great frustration. However, we have recently reported that intramuscular benzathine penicillin G together with oral rifampin (10 mg per kg twice daily for 4 days) is highly effective in eradicating carriage. This therapy should be reserved for those selected circumstances in which it appears desirable to terminate the carrier state.

Prevention

Special efforts to prevent streptococcal pharyngitis are warranted for patients who have had acute rheumatic fever or rheumatic heart disease. To prevent recurrent rheumatic fever, continuous lifelong antibiotic prophylaxis against streptococcal infection is recommended by the American Heart Association. The options for prophylaxis are (1) benzathine penicillin G, 1.2 million units intramuscularly every 4 weeks, (2) sulfadiazine, 1 gram daily, and (3) penicillin V, 125 to 250 mg twice daily. Erythromycin, 250 mg twice daily, may be used for the exceptional patient who is allergic to both penicillin and sulfonamides.

Tonsillectomy has not definitely been shown to be of great value in the prevention of streptococcal pharyngitis. This procedure should be limited to the very few, severely affected children and is only rarely indicated for recurrent pharyngitis.

Non Group A Streptococcal Pharyngitis

Although not yet proved, there is the impression that beta streptococci of Lancefield groups C, F, and G (which are commonly cultured from throats of symptomatic as well as asymptomatic patients) may cause a self-limited acute pharyngitis. There are few data to indicate that such infections lead to post-streptococcal sequelae. Until additional data are available, routine treatment of patients with non group A streptococcal throat isolates is not warranted.

TUBERCULOSIS AND OTHER MYCOBACTERIAL DISEASES

method of
MICHAEL H. CYNAMON, M.D.
State University of New York
Syracuse, New York

Tuberculosis continues to be an important communicable disease problem in the United States. In 1982 there were approximately 25,500 new cases with a case rate of 11 per 100,000. Extrapulmonary tuberculosis (pleural, lymphatic, bone and/or joint, genitourinary, miliary, meningeal, peritoneal, and others) accounted for 16 per cent of the total cases.

The management of patients with tuberculosis has undergone many changes in recent years. It is now known that the most important factors influencing response to treatment are appropriate chemotherapy and cooperation of the patient in adhering to a particular regimen. The severity of the disease has little effect on the ability of present drug regimens to "sterilize" the sputum. Other factors such as diet, rest, climate, and nursing care do not affect the bacteriologic outcome. The most appropriate regimen at the present time for pulmonary tuberculosis in the United States is isoniazid (INH) and rifampin (RIF) daily for nine months. Alternatively, these drugs can be given daily for one month followed by supervised twice weekly therapy for eight months. There is usually little advantage in adding ethambutol (EMB) or other drugs to this regimen except when primary resistance to either INH or RIF is suspected on epidemiologic or other grounds. There has been considerable interest and satisfactory experience with intensive four to six month regimens consisting of INH, RIF, pyrazinamide (PZA), and streptomycin (SM); however, these are not recommended at this time.

Once a presumptive diagnosis of tuberculosis is established (based on a positive acid fast smear, positive culture, or appropriate clinical setting), the patient can be managed as follows. The public health authority should be notified so that contact investigation can be initiated. Most patients with pulmonary tuberculosis can be treated as outpatients. The indications for hospitalization are complications of their disease (e.g., respiratory failure, hemoptysis), general debilitation, adverse drug reaction, and, occasionally, diagnostic evaluation (bronchoscopy). The presence of a positive acid fast smear, which correlates well with communicability, is *not* an indication for hospitalization since the greatest risk to a patient's contacts is during the period prior to diagnosis and initiation of therapy.

If the patient is hospitalized, respiratory isolation (private room with nonrecirculating ventilation) should be instituted. Infectious droplet nuclei are generated by coughing; therefore the patient should be instructed to cough into a disposable tissue that can subsequently be burned. Chemotherapy should be started with at least two drugs that the patient has not previously used. After treatment has been initiated the standards for discharge are that the patient's condition has improved and that adequate ambulatory care is available.

Drug susceptibility studies should not be performed routinely on pretreatment isolates. The incidence of primary resistance is relatively low in this country. If a patient is at high risk of having primary resistance to INH (e.g., an immigrant, particularly from Southeast Asia) or secondary resistance (e.g., a retreatment patient), then susceptibility studies should be obtained on the pretreatment isolate and the drug regimen should be modified appropriately (see hereafter). Follow-up cultures should be obtained at four, five, and six months after therapy has been initiated. At four months less than 8 per cent of the patients will have a positive culture, and by six months virtually all the patients should have a negative culture. A chest x-ray should be performed at six months and at the conclusion of therapy. If the patient has had a good response to therapy no routine follow-up is needed after the conclusion of the nine month regimen.

THERAPY

Principles of Antituberculous Therapy

The care of patients with mycobacterial disease, particularly tuberculosis, rests on several principles. An effort should be made to isolate the organism by culture. Drug susceptibility studies should be obtained for all patients who are being retreated after a therapeutic failure. Cultural confirmation is especially important in patients with extrapulmonary disease and in patients at high risk of nontuberculous mycobacterial infection. Active disease should be treated with at least two drugs to avoid the emergence of resistant organisms. The use of single drug therapy increases the chance of selecting naturally occurring organisms resistant to that drug. Multiple drug regimens decrease the chance of selecting naturally occurring resistant organisms during the course of therapy.

The treatment of tuberculosis can be considered in two phases. The initial, or intensive, phase is the period during which the host's population of organisms is largest and the multidrug regimens are most important in suppressing the emergence of resistant organisms. The continuation phase is that period, after the population of organisms has been markedly decreased during the intensive phase, when the number of acid fast bacilli is further reduced toward the "sterile" state. If bactericidal drugs are added to INH and RIF during the intensive phase a shorter total duration of therapy can be achieved; conversely, if a bacteriostatic agent is substituted for INH or RIF a longer total duration of therapy will be required for comparable outcomes. The addition of EMB to INH and RIF therapy during the intensive phase adds little to the overall effectiveness of

TABLE 1. **Classification of Antituberculous Drugs**

Bactericidal	Bacteriostatic
Isoniazid (INH)	Ethambutol (EMB)
Rifampin (RIF)	Para-aminosalicylic acid (PAS)
Pyrazinamide (PZA)*	Cycloserine (CS)
Streptomycin (SM)†	Capreomycin
Ethionamide (ETA)	
Kanamycin	

*Active against intracellular organisms.
†Active against extracellular organisms.

the regimen but does provide safety if primary resistance is a consideration. The presence of extensive cavitation does not require a change in these regimens. The drugs used to treat individual patients with tuberculosis can usually be obtained without charge from the county or local health department.

The following drugs are felt to be bactericidal: isoniazid, rifampin, pyrazinamide, streptomycin, kanamycin, and ethionamide (Table 1). Ethambutol, para-aminosalicylic acid, cycloserine, and capreomycin are considered bacteriostatic. Isoniazid and rifampin are thought to be active against both intracellular and extracellular organisms. Pyrazinamide is felt to be active only against the intracellular population of organisms, and streptomycin is only effective against the extracellular population of organisms. The regimen containing INH and RIF provides two bactericidal agents active against both populations of organisms. If PZA, SM, or EMB is substituted for either INH or RIF the regimen will be significantly weakened and an effective course of therapy would require more than 9 months. When PZA and SM are added to the initial phase of therapy with INH and RIF a shorter total duration of therapy has been possible.

Intermittent Supervised Chemotherapy

There has been extensive experience in this country and abroad with various intermittent supervised chemotherapy regimens. The advantage of this approach to chemotherapy is that the irregularity of self-administered oral regimens is avoided owing to greater patient compliance. For many patients who have difficulty adhering to a self-administered regimen, the intermittent supervised regimen provides a high likelihood of cure. The regimen most extensively studied in this country is INH, 300 mg per day, and RIF, 600 mg per day for 30 days followed by INH, 15 mg per kg, and RIF, 600 mg twice weekly for 8 months.

Treatment of Drug Resistant Tuberculosis

If primary resistance is thought to be likely, INH, RIF, and EMB can be used or, alternatively, INH, RIF, SM, and PZA could be used pending susceptibility studies. If secondary resistance develops, previous therapy was inappropriate or the patient did not adhere to the regimen. In all situations in which a self-administered regimen has failed a supervised intermittent regimen should be utilized. The initial drug selection will depend on which agents were previously used and can usually be modified once susceptibility data define the particular pattern of resistance. The initial regimen should always contain two agents (preferably bactericidal) that were not previously utilized such as (1) ethionamide, PZA, and SM, (2) RIF, PZA, and SM, or (3) RIF, PZA, and EMB.

Extrapulmonary Disease

The treatment of extrapulmonary tuberculosis should be approached in a manner similar to that of pulmonary disease. There have been few randomized prospective comparative studies of various regimens in the treatment of extrapulmonary disease. A regimen of INH and RIF daily for nine months should be satisfactory for most extrapulmonary sites, although some clinicians would favor 12 to 18 months of therapy. The optimal treatment of tuberculous meningitis has not been established. I would use INH, RIF, and PZA in standard dosage for one month followed by INH and RIF for a further 8 to 12 months. Corticosteroids should be used if there is a mass effect with evidence of increased intracranial pressure.

TABLE 2. **Drugs Used for the Treatment of Mycobacterial Disease**

Drug	Dosage: *Daily*	Dosage: *Twice Weekly*	Most Common Adverse Reactions	Tests for Adverse Reactions
Isoniazid	300 mg	15 mg/kg	Peripheral neuritis, hepatitis, rash, fever	SGOT/SGPT (not as routine)
Rifampin	600 mg	600–900 mg	Hepatitis, febrile reaction, thrombocytopenia (rare)	SGOT/SGPT, platelet count (not as routine)
Ethambutol	15 mg/kg	45 mg/kg	Optic neuritis (rare at 15 mg/kg), skin rash	Visual acuity, red-green color discrimination†
Pyrazinamide	20–35 mg/kg	4 grams	Hyperuricemia, hepatitis, arthralgia	Uric acid, SGOT/SGPT
Streptomycin	0.75–1.0 gram	0.75–1.0 gram	8th nerve damage (vestibular), nephrotoxicity, rash, fever (rare)	Creatinine† vestibular function, audiograms

*Pyridoxine, 50 mg twice weekly, should be used when INH is given for intermittent therapy.
†Should be determined at the start of therapy.

Antituberculous Drugs (Table 2)

Isoniazid

This drug, the hydrazide of isonicotinic acid, is bactericidal against actively growing tubercle bacilli. It is well absorbed when administered orally and readily diffuses into all body fluids and cells.

The drug is metabolized mainly by enzymatic acetylation in liver microsomes, but a fraction of the drug is hydrolyzed to isonicotinic acid. The relative rate of acetylation of INH is genetically determined. In patients receiving standard daily doses of INH there is no clear evidence of a difference in toxicity or therapeutic efficacy related to the rate of acetylation.

The most frequent adverse reactions to this drug include rash, fever, jaundice, and peripheral neuritis. Pyridoxine (vitamin B_6) in doses as small as 6 mg per day can prevent the development of peripheral neuritis. Pyridoxine supplementation is usually not needed for patients on a normal diet.

The risk of INH-associated hepatitis appears to be age related. Hepatic damage is rare in patients less than 20 years old, rising to 0.3 per cent in those 20 to 34 years old, whereas the incidence increases to 2.3 per cent in those greater than 50 years old. Approximately 10 to 20 per cent of patients receiving INH will experience transient elevation of serum glutamic oxaloacetic acid transaminase (SGOT). If the SGOT in an asymptomatic patient is less than three times the upper limit of normal, the drug can be continued and the enzyme rechecked in a week. If the patient has malaise, fever, nausea, vomiting, or jaundice with a mildly elevated SGOT or is asymptomatic with an SGOT greater than three times normal the INH should probably be discontinued and another drug substituted.

Isoniazid is thought to be safe for use during pregnancy and lactation. Its metabolism is affected little by renal dysfunction, and dosage adjustment is not necessary unless the creatinine clearance is below 5 to 10 ml per minute.

Overdose with INH, either accidental or intentional, is life-threatening and results in metabolic acidosis with tonic and clonic convulsions. Optimal therapy for this intoxication is not established, but the best experience has been with infusions of pyridoxine approximating the estimated ingested dose of INH.

Rifampin

Rifampin is a broad spectrum antibiotic that is active against both multiplying and latent forms of susceptible mycobacteria. It is well absorbed from the gastrointestinal tract and reaches effective concentrations in many body fluids including the cerebrospinal fluid. The drug is metabolized by deacetylation in the liver and enters the bile, where there is subsequent enterohepatic circulation. The deacetylated metabolite retains antibacterial activity. About one third of a dose of the drug is excreted in the urine. Modification of the dosage in patients with renal failure is not necessary. Patients should be forewarned that this agent has an intense orange red color that may be imparted to urine, sweat, saliva, and tears.

Rifampin infrequently causes adverse reactions; the most common are rash, fever, and nausea with vomiting. Hepatitis has been associated with rifampin use but rarely occurs in patients with normal hepatic function. Severe hepatic problems are felt to occur more frequently in patients with chronic liver disease, alcoholism, and old age.

Rifampin causes significant interaction with coumarin type oral anticoagulants, oral contraceptives, glucocorticoids, and methadone.

Ethambutol

This agent is active only against mycobacteria. About 75 per cent of an oral dose of EMB is absorbed from the gastrointestinal tract. About half of an ingested dose is excreted unchanged in the urine, and a small fraction of the drug is metabolized in the liver. Renal failure may require adjusting dosage to avoid toxicity.

Ethambutol in doses of 15 mg per kg per day is usually well tolerated. Retrobulbar optic neuritis, the most serious adverse reaction, is dose related and results in decreased visual acuity and loss of ability to perceive the color green. The decrease in visual acuity may be unilateral or bilateral. Doses less than 25 mg per kg per day have rarely been associated with this problem. Tests of visual acuity and color vision should be obtained prior to starting therapy and periodically thereafter.

Asymptomatic hyperuricemia, due to decreased renal excretion of uric acid, occurs in about half of the patients using this drug.

Pyrazinamide

This pyrazine analogue of nicotinamide is well absorbed from the gastrointestinal tract and widely distributed in tissue and body fluids. It is excreted primarily by the kidney. The drug is bactericidal against the population of intracellular tubercle bacilli. It is not active against extracellular organisms. This agent should be used only for the treatment of infections due to *M. tuberculosis,* since other mycobacteria are not susceptible to it.

The most common serious adverse effect of PZA is hepatic dysfunction. Jaundice with subsequent hepatic necrosis has occurred when the daily dose

TABLE 3. **Categories for INH Preventive Therapy***

1. Household members and other close associates of persons with recently diagnosed pulmonary tuberculosis.
2. Individuals known to have converted their skin test within the previous two years.
3. Positive tuberculin skin test reactors with findings on chest roentgenogram consistent with nonprogressive tuberculous disease in whom there are neither positive bacteriologic findings nor a history of adequate chemotherapy.
4. Positive tuberculin skin test reactors in special clinical situations:
   (a) prolonged therapy with adrenocorticoids,
   (b) immunosuppressive therapy,
   (c) hematologic and reticuloendothelial diseases (e.g., leukemia or Hodgkin's disease),
   (d) diabetes mellitus,
   (e) silicosis, and
   (f) after gastrectomy.
5. Other positive reactors less than 35 years of age.

*In decreasing order of risk.

exceeded 35 mg per kg. Hepatic dysfunction is infrequent when the dose is 20 to 35 mg per kg per day.

Pyrazinoic acid, a metabolite of pyrazinamide, competes with uric acid for excretion by the kidney and causes hyperuricemia and occasionally clinical gout. Other observed side effects include arthralgias, anorexia, nausea, vomiting, and malaise.

Streptomycin

This drug should no longer be used for initial therapy of tuberculosis since its frequency of adverse reactions is greater than is seen with ethambutol. It has a role in evolving short course regimens and the treatment of patients with multiple resistant organisms.

Preventive Therapy of Tuberculous Infection

Isoniazid in a dose of 300 mg per day for adults and 10 mg per kg per day for children (not to exceed 300 mg per day) over a 9 to 12 month period has been demonstrated to reduce the incidence of tuberculosis in infected groups. The reduction in morbidity is approximately 75 per cent during the first year and from 50 to 66 per cent for the duration of follow-up, which exceeded 15 years.

Every positive tuberculin skin test reactor and contact of a person with recently diagnosed pulmonary tuberculosis are at some risk of developing active disease. Preventive therapy would be of theoretical benefit to all these individuals. Since the risk of developing INH-associated hepatitis has been appreciated, priorities for preventive therapy must be based on the relative risk of developing tuberculosis. Categories for preventive therapy in decreasing order of risk of developing tuberculosis are listed in Table 3. The risk of developing tuberculosis is lifelong, and the risk of INH-associated hepatitis is small for individuals less than 35 years of age. In tuberculin reactors less than 35 years of age without other risk factors the benefit of INH preventive therapy outweighs the risk of hepatitis. Since compliance is often poor in asymptomatic patients it is important to carefully select well-motivated patients for INH preventive therapy and to avoid this therapy in patients who are not likely to be compliant (ethanol abusers) or who cannot be adequately supervised. History of previous adverse reaction to INH is a contraindication to INH preventive therapy, as is the presence of acute liver disease of any etiology. Although no harmful effects of INH to the fetus have been observed, it is felt that preventive therapy should be avoided during pregnancy. Isoniazid should be started in the postpartum period when the risk of tuberculosis for the new mother is increased.

Prior to initiation of therapy a chest x-ray should be obtained to rule out active disease. The patient should be evaluated monthly for symptoms of hepatitis (nausea, vomiting, anorexia, or jaundice). The patient should be instructed to contact his physician and to discontinue the INH if these symptoms develop (see INH under Antituberculous Drugs). Routine monitoring of the SGOT is not felt to be necessary in individuals taking INH preventive therapy who are asymptomatic.

When a candidate for INH preventive therapy is a contact of a patient excreting INH resistant organisms the efficacy of INH is unknown. If preventive therapy is indicated, a 9 to 12 month course of RIF, 600 mg per day, with EMB, 15 mg per kg per day, would seem to be more appropriate than INH.

A tuberculin skin test of 10 mm or larger is considered to represent previous infection with *M. tuberculosis*. If a previously BCG-vaccinated individual has a tuberculin skin test of 10 mm or larger INH preventive therapy should be based on the previously discussed criteria.

INFECTIONS WITH NONTUBERCULOUS MYCOBACTERIA

The nontuberculous mycobacteria are being isolated with increased frequency and are often implicated in a clinically significant infectious disease process. These organisms (usually *M. kansasii, M. marinum, M. avium-intracellulare, M. fortuitum,* and *M. chelonei*) have been isolated from the environment, predominantly soil and water, and less frequently from human foodstuffs. Isolation of these organisms from clinical specimens (commonly sputum) usually implies colonization rather than invasive disease. The trans-

TABLE 4. **Nontuberculous Mycobacteria Frequently Associated with Human Disease**

Species	Site Commonly Involved	Suggested Regimen
M. kansasii	Pulmonary	INH, RIF, and EMB
M. avium-intracellulare	Pulmonary	RIF, EMB, SM
	Disseminated*	RIF, EMB, SM, Cycloserine Ethionamide
M. marinum	Soft tissue	Trimethoprim/Sulfamethoxazole Tetracycline
M. fortuitum	Soft tissue	Cefoxitin, Amikacin, Sulfonamide, Doxycycline
M. chelonei	Soft tissue	Cefoxitin, Amikacin Erythromycin

*Particularly in patients with AIDS.

mission of these agents from man to man is extremely rare and occurs only under unusual circumstances. These organisms should be considered opportunistic. Infections have been noted in the increasing number of patients who are immunocompromised on the basis of antineoplastic therapy and immunosuppressive therapy (i.e., transplantation, systemic lupus erythematosus, Wegener's granulomatosis, and so on). *Mycobacterium fortuitum* and *M. chelonei* have been implicated in infections associated with prosthetic devices (e.g., breast implant, prosthetic heart valve). Recently *M. avium-intracellulare* (MAI) has been isolated (sputum, blood, and bone marrow) from patients with the acquired immunodeficiency syndrome (AIDS).

Diagnosis depends on a high index of suspicion and appropriate cultures with biopsy (if indicated). Differential skin testing is not recommended since the current reagents have little ability to discriminate between organisms. If mycobacteria are isolated from a biopsy specimen then an etiologic relationship is usually readily established. The clinical significance of an organism in sputum specimens is more difficult to assess. The nontuberculous mycobacteria are most frequently isolated in sputum from patients with the following underlying pulmonary conditions: pneumoconiosis, chronic bronchitis, previous history of tuberculosis, chronic obstructive pulmonary disease, bronchiectasis, and chronic aspiration from esophageal disease. They can also be isolated from individuals without apparent underlying lung disease or deficiency of cell-mediated immune function. In an appropriate clinical setting (i.e., a symptomatic patient with abnormal chest x-ray) a presumptive mycobacterial etiology can be established if the organism is isolated from sputum on multiple occasions with numerous colonies (≥ 100) on primary culture in the absence of other significant agents. The demonstration of the organism in tissue (e.g., bronchoscopic biopsy specimen) remains the best evidence for establishing etiology in difficult clinical settings.

There is currently no satisfactory standardized method for drug susceptibility testing of nontuberculous mycobacteria. Clinical laboratories usually test the standard antituberculous agents against the nontuberculous mycobacteria. This is of questionable value, and drug susceptibility studies should not be performed routinely with the nontuberculous mycobacteria. Treatment should be based on previous clinical experience with infections caused by these organisms. Improved methods for evaluating drug susceptibility of the slowly growing mycobacteria will likely be developed in the future. An assessment of antimycobacterial activity for the rapid growers *(M. fortuitum* and *M. chelonei)* can usually be accomplished by utilizing modified standard agar or broth dilution susceptibility testing methods.

Therapy

The treatment of nontuberculous mycobacterial infections is based on the cumulative experience at various medical centers (Table 4). There have been retrospective studies but comparative prospective evaluations have not been done. In addition, the natural history of pulmonary MAI infections in non-AIDS patients has not been adequately studied and therefore evaluation of the efficacy of currently suggested regimens is difficult.

Pulmonary infections due to *M. kansasii* have responded well to INH, RIF, and EMB. These drugs, used together for 12 to 18 months, should lead to clinical cure in over 90 per cent of patients. Pulmonary infections in non-AIDS patients caused by MAI are hard to treat. The literature is difficult to evaluate since some patients have apparently done well with INH, RIF, and EMB, whereas others have required intensive therapy with RIF, EMB, SM, ethionamide, and cycloserine. The latter regimen is not well tolerated and has not consistently yielded good results.

Disseminated infections due to MAI have been observed frequently in patients with AIDS. It is not clear what role this organism plays in these patients' complicated disease process. At this point there is probably little to offer these patients using current regimens; however, I would favor the five drug regimen previously described if therapy is undertaken. It is clear that more effective regimens are needed to treat MAI infections.

Soft tissue infections caused by *M. marinum* frequently heal without therapy but may persist for many months if untreated. Tetracycline or trimethoprim/sulfamethoxazole have been used successfully. If these do not result in clinical improvement RIF and EMB should probably be used. A four to six week course of therapy is probably appropriate.

Isolates of *M. fortuitum* are usually susceptible to doxycycline, sulfonamides, amikacin, and cefoxitin. The latter two agents should be used for moderate to severe infections. Cefoxitin and amikacin can usually be used to treat *M. chelonei* infections. Sometimes *M. chelonei* is susceptible to erythromycin and a trial with this agent leads to clinical improvement. If the patient is not responding to the suggested drugs susceptibility studies should be performed.

Section 4

The Cardiovascular System

ACQUIRED DISEASES OF THE AORTA

method of
E. STANLEY CRAWFORD, M.D.,
JOSEPH S. COSELLI, M.D.,
and HAZIM SAFI, M.D.
Baylor College of Medicine
Houston, Texas

The aortic wall is an intrinsically simple structure, and, consequently, acquired diseases of the aorta manifest themselves in only a limited number of ways. In the majority of cases these include aneurysmal dilatation, luminal occlusion, and dissection. The etiology, clinical manifestations, and surgical management vary considerably depending primarily on the anatomic segment of the aorta involved and the disease process.

Treatment

Preoperative Preparation

Patients requiring aortic surgery are usually in an older age group and often have associated heart, lung, kidney, and other diseases. Prior to surgical intervention, these medical problems should be thoroughly evaluated and treated to optimize the patient's condition. Medications should be continued until the time of operation, deleting only those that interfere with coagulation. The effect of coumadin is reversed by vitamin K and fresh-frozen plasma, whereas the antiplatelet effect of Persantine or aspirin requires postponing surgery for 1 week or the administration of fresh platelets during the procedure. Whenever possible, the entire extent of aortic involvement should be determined by total aortography. Since contrast material sometimes depresses renal function, surgery is often delayed until renal function has returned to its preaortogram level. This judgment is based upon serial determinations of serum BUN and creatinine levels.

Preoperatively, patients are prepared with an enema and intravenous fluids the night before. Prophylactic antibiotics (currently we use a cephalosporin) are administered just prior to surgery and are continued for 48 hours.

Anesthesia and Intraoperative Management

Preoperative medications include diphenhydramine (Benadryl), 25 to 50 mg; lidocaine, 20 mg; and diazepam (Valium), 0.1 mg per kg. Anesthesia is induced with fentanyl (Sublimaze), a narcotic with short duration and no myocardial depression. Relaxation is achieved with pancuronium (Pavulon), 0.1 mg per kg. A double lumen endotracheal tube is utilized to permit collapse of the left lung, which reduces injury to the lung and minimizes the adverse cardiovascular effects created by pressure on the heart from retraction of the lung. Anesthesia is maintained with fentanyl and diazepam and relaxation by pancuronium.

Fluid replacement prior to and during aortic clamping is by balanced crystalloid solution with additional fresh-frozen plasma to maintain a colloid osmotic pressure of 15 torr. The hemoglobin is maintained at 9 grams per dl. Fluids are administered to maintain a normal pulmonary wedge pressure and normal cardiac hemodynamics. A few moments prior to release of the aortic clamp, volume replacement is begun through the four intravenous catheters, utilizing 1 unit of fresh-frozen plasma for every 3 units of packed red blood cells in addition to 12 units of platelets. Coagulation profiles are followed and deficits treated appropriately. Fresh-frozen plasma is administered for an elevated prothrombin time, and excessive fibrinolysis is treated with aminocaproic acid (Amicar). Low fibrinogen levels are treated with 4 to 10 units of cryoprecipitate, and platelets are administered to maintain a platelet count of 100,000. Mannitol, in a dose of 25 grams, is given for osmotic diuretic effect by intravenous drip in 200 ml of lactate solution 30 minutes before the aorta is cross clamped. Heparin is not utilized because the problem of hemostasis exceeds that of thrombosis.

During aortic cross clamping, it is important to maintain a normal systemic blood pressure and cardiovascular hemodynamics. Since cross clamping the distal transverse aortic arch or thoracic aorta distal to the subclavian artery increases acutely the cardiac afterload, intravenous nitroprusside (Nipride) is administered continuously to maintain peripheral vascular resistance and blood pressure at normal levels during this interval. Nitroprusside administration is begun just before application of the clamps and continues until a few moments prior to releasing the clamps. Since aortic cross clamping is associated with distal hypoperfusion and subsequent metabolic acidosis, sodium bicarbonate solution is given by drip during the period of aortic clamping to maintain a base excess ranging between 3 and 5.

Ventilation during the operation is aimed at maintaining a pCO_2 within the normal range of 35 to 44 torr. During the period of one lung anesthesia, the right lung is ventilated with 80 per cent of calculated tidal volume, while the respiratory rate is increased by two to four per minute and followed with arterial blood gases every 15 minutes. Since hypothermia is associated with a multitude of coagulation and metabolic aberrations, every effort is made to maintain a normal core temperature.

Since surgical procedures on the ascending aorta and the proximal transverse aortic arch are performed with cardiopulmonary bypass and often profound hypothermia, the anesthetic and perioperative management are similar to those employed in cardiac procedures utilizing cardiopulmonary bypass.

Postoperatively, patients are kept in the intensive care unit for at least 48 hours, with careful monitoring of the electrocardiogram, blood pressure, central venous pressure, pulmonary artery pressure, pulmonary capillary wedge pressure, cardiac output, peripheral vascular resistance, and rectal temperature. Arterial blood gases, serum electrolytes, and hematocrit are monitored every four hours for the first 24 hours and then as needed.

ANEURYSMS

Abdominal Aortic Aneurysms

The most common aortic aneurysms are in the infrarenal abdominal aorta, and the overwhelming majority of these are due to atherosclerosis. The natural history of the disease includes progression to rupture and death in about one half of the patients within a year and in about 90 per cent within 5 years. Elective surgery carries a mortality rate of between 2 and 4 per cent, whereas emergency surgery in the event of rupture carries a mortality rate of up to 50 per cent. Some clinicians feel that aneurysms less than 5 cm in diameter should be treated expectantly; however, one third of ruptured aneurysms have been found to be in this range. Further, ruptures have been known to occur without evidence of expansion. Our opinion is that operation is indicated in the asymptomatic patient when the diameter of the lesion is twice that of the proximal or distal uninvolved aorta. Abdominal ultrasound and computed tomography scans have been useful adjuncts for both the diagnosis and evaluation of abdominal aortic aneurysms.

Ruptured Abdominal Aneurysms

When abdominal aortic aneurysms rupture freely into the peritoneal cavity, death soon follows. Therefore, in most patients treated for ruptured abdominal aortic aneurysms, the rupture is initially contained within the retroperitoneum. Once the diagnosis of ruptured aneurysm is made, the patient is taken immediately to the operating room. Operative treatment is not delayed by extensive resuscitative efforts in the emergency room, the acquiring of radiographs, ECGs, CT scans, or aortograms, or the drawing of blood for routine studies. Blood is drawn for immediate saline typing and cross matching. Satisfactory treatment of the patient's condition requires control of the hemorrhage at the earliest possible moment.

Experience indicates that the technique for control of the abdominal aorta at the diaphragm is likewise helpful in the management of patients who also have juxtarenal abdominal aortic aneurysms or inflammatory aneurysms of the infrarenal abdominal aorta and for patients who require a second operation of the infrarenal abdominal aorta.

Aortoduodenal Fistula

Occasionally an infrarenal abdominal aortic aneurysm will rupture into the duodenum rather than into the retroperitoneum and present as gastrointestinal bleeding. More often a false aneurysm at the proximal anastomosis of a previous abdominal aortic graft replacement will rupture into the duodenum. Patients who have had previous abdominal aortic surgery and who present with gastrointestinal bleeding must be suspected of having an aortoduodenal fistula until proven otherwise and treated appropriately. Treatment consists of control of bleeding, graft replacement of the aneurysm, and repair of the duodenum in layers. Aortic clamping at the subdiaphragmatic level is often very helpful in this situation. Antibiotics are usually given for at least 5 days, after which time graft infections or recurrences have been extremely rare.

Thoracoabdominal Aneurysms

Although the exact frequency of these lesions is not precisely known, they are certainly more common than was once believed. The two most common etiologies include atherosclerosis and medial degenerative disease. Since up to 25 per cent of thoracic aortic aneurysms will be shown to have abdominal extension of the disease process, we strongly recommend that the entire aorta be evaluated by either total aortography or CT scan. Most patients with thoracoabdominal aortic aneurysms fall into an older age group in which heart disease, chronic obstructive pulmonary disease, and marginal renal function are commonly associated medical conditions. A thorough evaluation of medical problems and maximal medical management are associated with an improved surgical result.

Treatment is by graft replacement of the aneurysm, and all symptomatic patients are subjected to surgical intervention. All asymptomatic patients, excluding those with overwhelming medical contraindications, are recommended to undergo elective surgical intervention.

With the lung retracted, the descending thoracic aorta is cross clamped at a level above aneurysmal involvement. The increased cardiac afterload is controlled with a continuous nitroprusside infusion. The thoracic component of the aneurysm is opened laterally with the electric cautery and the edges retracted with stay sutures. The incision is then extended onto the posterior lateral surface of the abdominal component to the most distal level of aneurysmal involvement. Distal clamping of the aorta or iliac vessels is rarely necessary because backbleeding is usually minimal; however, utilization of a cell saver device can be an important adjunct. Backbleeding from visceral vessels is controlled with Fogarty balloon catheters, and small intercostal and lumbar arteries are sutured for hemostasis.

We are currently undergoing evaluation of renal preservation utilizing hypothermic renal artery perfusion. We routinely do not use heparin and believe it to be detrimental because hemostasis rather than distal thrombosis is the significant challenge. An appropriately sized woven Dacron graft is then selected for replacement, and the proximal anastomosis is performed using 3-0 Prolene in a running technique. After checking the proximal anastomosis for hemostasis, previously spared intercostal arteries are reattached to small openings made in the graft by suturing the edge of the openings around the origin of these vessels. Following this, the viscera and renal vessels are reattached to side openings made in the graft using a running 3-0 or 4-0 Prolene suture.

Descending Thoracic Aorta Aneurysms

True aneurysms in this region are usually secondary to atherosclerosis and medial degenerative changes. Since total aortography and CT scans to evaluate the entire aorta have become routine, it has become apparent that the abdominal aorta is involved, either in continuity or as a separate area, in up to 25 per cent of patients who have aneurysmal disease of the thoracic aorta. All symptomatic patients are operated upon urgently regardless of the size of the aneurysm. Asymptomatic patients are subjected to surgery when the diameter of the aneurysm is twice that of either the proximal or distal aorta. Surgery consists of tube graft replacement, utilizing the inclusion technique, between occluding vascular clamps. Routinely a double lumen endotracheal tube is utilized to allow collapse of the left lung. Afterload is controlled with nitroprusside, and blood is conserved by utilizing a cell saver device. Heparin, shunts, and bypass devices are avoided.

Aneurysms of the distal transverse aortic arch have an etiology and treatment similar to those of descending thoracic aortic aneurysms. These aneurysms involve the region of the left subclavian and/or left common carotid artery origins. They are well localized, often sacciform, usually secondary to atherosclerosis, and located on the concave side of the aortic arch. Treatment is by graft replacement utilizing the inclusion technique between clamps. The transverse aortic arch can be clamped between the innominate and left common carotid or between the left common carotid and left subclavian with a separate clamp placed across the appropriate brachiocephalic vessels. Sacciform aneurysms involving less than 50 per cent of the aortic circumference are replaced with a Dacron patch; sacciform aneurysms greater than 50 per cent and fusiform aneurysms are replaced with woven tubular Dacron grafts.

Brachiocephalic vessels are reattached or bypassed.

Ascending and Aortic Arch Aneurysms

Most aneurysms of the ascending and transverse aortic arch are secondary to medial degeneration; other causes include dissection with aneurysmal dilatation of the false lumen and infection. The term *medial degeneration* is used here for mucoid degeneration, myxomatous degeneration, and cystic medial necrosis. Atherosclerotic change, often superimposed on degenerative disease, is virtually never the primary cause of an aneurysm in the ascending aorta. The degenerative process often involves the sinuses of Valsalva with aneurysmal dilatation of all three sinuses. Aortic valvular insufficiency commonly results from annular dilatation. Definitive diagnosis is by aortography, with complete examination of the aorta stressed as being important because of the diffuse nature of the disease process.

When the aneurysmal involvement is limited to the ascending aorta and it is safe to cross clamp proximal to the innominate artery, surgical treatment has consisted of composite valve graft replacement with direct reattachment of the coronary artery openings to the graft as previously described by Bentell and DeBono. This technique requires heparinization, cardiopulmonary bypass, and, usually, arterial cannulation of the femoral artery. It has been our experience that when the valve is replaced and a separate tube graft is used to replace the ascending aorta without including the coronary arteries, there is a significant percentage of cases with progressive aneurysmal dilatation of the sinuses of Valsalva, requiring a more complicated second surgical intervention. Therefore, whenever feasible, these patients are considered for composite valve graft replacement.

Aortic Dissections

The most common catastrophic event occurring in the aorta is acute dissection. Dissection of the aorta can occur in a diseased aorta but occurs most often in a previously normal aorta. The common denominator in virtually all cases is hypertension. The aortic tear originates in the ascending aorta in 65 per cent of patients, in the arch in 10 per cent, and in the proximal descending thoracic aorta in 25 per cent. The blood dissects within the aortic media, creating two lumens, one true and one false, and proceeds distally. Ascending aortic involvement is not only common but also the most lethal aspect of the process. Acute dissection may result in external rupture with exsanguination, rupture into the pericardial sac with tamponade, dissection into the aortic root producing aortic valvular insufficiency, occlusion of the coronary arteries producing acute myocardial infarction, rupture into the right ventricle causing left to right shunt, or compression of the main pulmonary artery causing right-sided heart failure.

A variety of complications evolve from obstruction of major aortic branches. Late complications include recurrence of dissection, with or without aortic valvular insufficiency, and aneurysmal dilatation of the false lumen with rupture. Because of the multitude of fatal complications occurring in the acute phase, dissections involving the ascending aorta are treated surgically. Uncomplicated dissections involving the descending thoracic aorta are initially managed medically.

We immediately admit all patients with aortic dissections to the intensive care unit. Arterial blood pressure, urinary output, central venous pressure, and ECG are monitored continuously. A Swan-Ganz catheter is inserted, allowing measurement of pulmonary capillary wedge pressure and serial cardiac outputs. Nitroprusside is begun as a continuous intravenous infusion to lower the systolic blood pressure to 120 mm Hg, and propranolol (Inderal) is given intravenously to reduce the force of myocardial contraction. After the patient is initially stabilized, total aortography is performed for evaluation of the extent of the dissection process. It has been our recent experience that CT scans are extremely valuable in both the acute and chronic evaluation of these patients.

In acute situations involving the ascending aorta, immediate operative intervention is indicated. The proximal ascending aorta is replaced with a graft to replace the origin of dissection and/or rupture; this averts further dissection and deters recurrence. Simple graft replacement is performed whenever possible. When the dissection involves the juxtacoronary artery segment of the aorta producing aortic insufficiency but the inner layer at the annulus is not disrupted, the valve can be resuspended utilizing Teflon strips. When the proximal intima is disrupted and there is aortic insufficiency, the aortic valve is resected and a prosthetic valve inserted. This often requires a composite valve graft operation with reimplantation of the coronary artery orifices. Obstructed coronary arteries from either dissection or atherosclerosis may require autogenous saphenous vein bypass grafting.

In all cases the distal aorta is handled by sandwiching the two layers between Teflon felt strips, i.e., obliterating the false lumen, prior to performing the distal anastomosis. This maneuver directs blood flow into the true lumen, preventing progression of the dissection by reducing the pressure within the false lumen, and further serves to relieve obstruction of the distal aorta and major branches. In situations involving a previously dilated distal ascending aorta and/or transverse arch or dissections originating in the transverse aortic arch, circulatory arrest may be required.

Patients with dissection of the descending thoracic aorta are maintained on medical management unless faced with impending rupture, continued pain, or obstruction of major aortic branches. In the chronic phase, all patients are followed carefully with serial chest radiographs and CT scans or aortography at least biannually. When dilatation to twice the normal aortic size occurs, graft replacement of the dilated segment is then undertaken on an elective basis. One third of all late deaths have resulted from rupture of late aneurysmal formation in segments of the aorta that had not been replaced.

Occlusive Disease of the Aorta

Atherosclerotic occlusive disease often involves the infrarenal abdominal aorta and iliac arteries, resulting in incapacitating lower limb claudication, rest pain, ulceration, and/or gangrene. Surgical therapy involves re-establishment of satisfactory flow to the superficial femoral and deep femoral arteries. When there is localized involvement of the infrarenal aorta and common iliac arteries, excellent long-term patency rates have been achieved with endarterectomy procedures. Endarterectomy is contraindicated in the face of aneurysmal disease, atretic vessels, and extensive involvement of the external iliac and common femoral vessels. Since contraindications to endarterectomy are common and the patency rates are comparable, it has been our preference to employ prosthetic bypass grafting. Minimal dissection of the infrarenal abdominal aorta is employed, and if the external iliacs and common femoral arteries are suitable, groin incisions are avoided.

ANGINA PECTORIS

method of
CHARLES H. CROFT, M.D., FACC
Southwestern Medical School
Dallas, Texas

Angina pectoris is a clinical syndrome resulting from myocardial ischemia, manifesting as paroxysmal retrosternal pain, usually of a dull aching nature and of short duration, and frequently radiating to the shoulders, arms, or jaw. The anginal syndrome has been subdivided into the following categories: (1) stable exertional angina (angina pectoris of effort), (2) unstable angina pectoris (acute coronary insufficiency, intermediate coronary syndrome), (3) variant (Prinzmetal's) angina, and (4) mixed angina. These subsets differ not only with respect to their clinical presentation but with regard to their underlying pathogenic mechanisms and prognosis. These differences in turn dictate individualized patient management strategy.

General Management

Risk Factor Modification

Effective communication with the patient and an adequate explanation of the underlying cause of his chest pain, treatment options, and reasons for lifestyle modifications are imperative.

Vigorous efforts should be directed toward the control of hypertension, smoking, hypercholesterolemia, and obesity. There is considerable debate about the utility of exercise programs, both in the prevention of ischemic heart disease and in the reduction of complications once clinical manifestations occur. Regular dynamic exercise does, however, have a beneficial effect on cardiac performance, particularly on the conditioning of skeletal muscle, thereby allowing the patient to expend greater physical effort for any given level of total body oxygen consumption.

Identification of Contributing Factors

A careful medical history, physical examination, and laboratory profile should be performed on all patients with the anginal syndrome to detect coexistent factors that may aggravate angina. Congestive heart failure, significant valvular heart disease, anemia, thyrotoxicosis, hypoxemia, and infection all increase myocardial oxygen requirements, thereby precipitating or aggravating angina. Specific therapy to correct these factors should be instituted.

Drug Therapy

Nitrates

Nitrates exert an antianginal effect by virtue of their vasodilatation of both the systemic and coronary circulations. Their predominant mechanism of action is to decrease myocardial oxygen demand by favorably decreasing preload and afterload. Recent evidence from quantitative computer-assisted measurements of coronary arterial diameter suggests that nitrates also cause some vasodilation of stenoses in epicardial arteries. Furthermore, nitrates redistribute blood flow preferentially to the subendocardial ischemic region. The overall effect of nitrate preparations is therefore a combination of a reduction in myocardial oxygen requirements and an increase in oxygen supply to ischemic myocardium.

Sublingual nitroglycerin (0.15 to 0.6 mg) is the drug of choice for the treatment of the acute anginal attack. It is also useful when taken prophylactically just prior to an activity that is anticipated to produce angina. Nitroglycerin has a shelf life of approximately 6 months to 2 years, depending on the amount of exposure to light, and is probably inactive when it fails to elicit a slight burning sensation under the patient's tongue. The commonest adverse reactions include headache, flushing, and hypotension.

Nitroglycerin is also available in an oral form (Nitro-Bid, Nitroglyn, and Nitrospan) in strengths of 2.5 to 9 mg administered at 8 to 12 hour intervals. Clinical experience with this drug is somewhat limited but the available evidence suggests that it is efficacious.

Three long-acting nitrates other than nitroglycerin are available in sublingual, buccal, oral, and topical forms. These include isosorbide dinitrate (Isordil, Sorbitrate), pentaerythritol tetranitrate (Peritrate), and erythrityl tetranitrate (Cardilate). Isosorbide dinitrate is available in 2.5, 5, and 10 mg sublingual tablets; a 10 mg buccal (chewable) form; 5, 10, 20, and 30 mg tablets for oral use; and a 40 mg sustained release capsule. There is no doubt that isosorbide dinitrate is an effective drug for the prevention and relief of angina pectoris. These nitrates, however, undergo rapid hepatic metabolism requiring the administration of large doses (5 to 40 mg) as frequently as every 2 to 3 hours for effective anginal prophylaxis.

Two per cent nitroglycerin ointment applied to the skin (0.5 to 2 inches) is an effective antianginal agent for periods of up to 6 hours. Its relatively long period of efficacy makes it particularly useful for reducing nocturnal angina, but it is also effective when applied every 4 to 8 hours while awake.

Sustained release transdermal nitroglycerin preparations have been marketed since 1982 in an attempt to obviate the messiness and inconvenience of nitroglycerin ointment and, most importantly, to eliminate the requirement for multiple nitrate dosing throughout the day. These nitroglycerin preparations (Transderm-Nitro, Nitrodisc, Nitro-Dur) are attractive in both design and concept. However, recent evidence strongly suggests that transdermal nitroglycerin preparations in standard doses (2.5 to 15 mg over 24 hours) have relatively minor antianginal effects and at moderate or high dosage (15 to 45 mg per 24 hours) do not provide protection 24 hours after application. Moreover, clinical data suggest that sustained high nitrate plasma levels may more readily induce tolerance than intermittent dosing with smaller doses. This may result from counter-regulatory arterial vasoconstriction or a failure of vascular smooth muscle to maintain a response to nitroglycerin for periods beyond 8 to 12 hours.

Though no major "blind" controlled trial has been undertaken, most cardiologists feel that the recent commercial availability of intravenous nitroglycerin formulations is a significant therapeutic advance for patients with refractory unstable angina pectoris. It is most commonly administered by constant intravenous infusion, and its short half-life allows rapid attainment of new steady state blood levels after changes in infusion rates. Intravenous administration is usually started at 5 to 10 micrograms per minute followed by variable increments in the infusion rate every 5 minutes until the systolic arterial pressure falls either *by* 10 to 15 mm Hg or *to* 100 to 110 mm Hg. Further increases in the infusion rate are titrated to the patient's symptoms and adverse hemodynamic reactions.

Beta-Adrenergic Blocking Agents

These agents constitute a cornerstone of therapy for stable angina pectoris of effort. Six beta-blockers are currently available in the United States (propranolol [Inderal], atenolol [Tenormin], metoprolol [Lopressor], nadolol [Corgard], pindolol [Visken], and timolol [Blocadren]). They appear to be equally effective in the treatment of angina but differ in their cardioselectivity, intrinsic sympathomimetic activity, membrane-stabilizing properties, and lipo- or hydrophilic properties. Blockade of noncardiac "beta-2" receptors inhibits catecholamine-induced glycogenolysis and catecholamine-induced vasodilatation of peripheral vessels. The action of noncardioselective beta-blockers on these receptors, thereby tending to impair defenses against both insulin-induced hypoglycemia in those with diabetes and poor extremity perfusion in those with atherosclerotic peripheral vascular disease, may be obviated by the use of a cardioselective beta-1 blocker such as atenolol or metoprolol. In high doses, however, the cardioselectivity of these two drugs may be lost.

The intrinsic sympathomimetic activity of pindolol results in partial agonistic activity, thereby causing little if any slowing of heart rate, depression of atrioventricular conduction, or depression of myocardial contractility at rest. This agent does, however, block the effects of exercise on these parameters. Its partial agonistic activity also induces bronchial dilatation. This agent may, therefore, be the beta-blocker of choice in patients with sinus bradycardia, AV block, left ventricular dysfunction, and bronchospasm. The hydrophilic beta-blockers, i.e., atenolol and metoprolol, tend not to penetrate into the central nervous system and are therefore associated with less mental depression and sleep disturbance than the more lipophilic agents.

Beta-blockers work in angina pectoris predominantly by decreasing the determinants of myocardial oxygen demand, particularly heart rate and contractility. In addition, prolongation of diastole secondary to a reduction in heart rate may allow a greater time for diastolic perfusion of the subendocardium. Some reports have suggested that propranolol may improve oxygen delivery to the myocardium by shifting the oxyhemoglobin dissociation curve to the right. Furthermore, these drugs appear to decrease the enhanced platelet aggregability that has been found in patients with ischemic heart disease.

For optimal results, the dose of beta-blocker should be carefully titrated to the patient's symptoms or the results of exercise testing. The dosage requirement of propranolol in the management of angina pectoris can vary from 40 mg per day to 1 to 2 gm per day (the manufacturer's directive lists the maximum daily dose for treatment of angina as 320 mg). There appears to be a dose-related response in the control of symptoms.

The complications of beta-adrenoreceptor blocking agents are relatively minor. Side effects occur in approximately 10 per cent of patients and serious or life-threatening complications in less than 2 per cent of patients. The most common side effects include sinus bradycardia or AV nodal block, congestive heart failure, bronchospasm, and central nervous system effects such as hallucinations and nightmares.

Calcium Channel Blockers

Three calcium channel blocking agents have been introduced into clinical use in the United States in the last few years. Although these agents (nifedipine [Procardia], diltiazem [Cardizem], and verapamil [Calan, Isoptin]) differ in their potency for peripheral vasodilatation and decreased inotropic, chronotropic, and dromotropic effects on the heart, all three improve blood flow to ischemic myocardium at rest and during exercise and are effective in preventing coronary spasm.

Nifedipine is the most potent vasodilator of the three calcium channel blocking agents. As a result of systemic vasodilation and consequent afterload reduction, nifedipine reduces myocardial oxygen consumption. In addition, it increases coronary blood flow as a result of its coronary dilating effect. Verapamil's major mechanism of action appears to be a reduction in myocardial oxygen demand secondary to its negative inotropic and chronotropic effects. It appears to be as effective as propranolol in the therapy of angina of effort. The actions of diltiazem appear to lie somewhere between those of nifedipine and verapamil. There is also evidence, however, that diltiazem may have a relatively selective vasodilator effect on the coronary vasculature.

The major side effects of nifedipine include headaches, hypotension, leg edema, and flushing. Alternatively, verapamil and diltiazem depress cardiac contractility, heart rate, and AV conduction.

A number of clinical studies have indicated that a combination of a beta-adrenergic blocking agent and a calcium channel blocking agent is superior to either drug alone. The use of nifedipine as the calcium blocker in this setting may be preferable to verapamil or diltiazem, particularly in those patients with occult or overt heart failure or AV nodal disease.

Antiplatelet Agents

Patients with ischemic heart disease appear to have heightened platelet reactivity. A recent study suggests that one buffered aspirin a day as an antiplatelet agent may reduce the incidence of death and nonfatal myocardial infarction by approximately 50 per cent in men with unstable angina pectoris. Low dose aspirin should, therefore, be strongly considered as an adjunct to standard therapy for unstable angina pectoris. (The use of aspirin as an antiplatelet agent is not listed in the manufacturer's directive.)

Anticoagulant Therapy

No controlled trial has demonstrated the efficacy of either heparin or warfarin in the management of patients with angina pectoris.

Intra-Aortic Balloon Counterpulsation Therapy

Intra-aortic balloon counterpulsation has been shown to lower myocardial oxygen consumption and increase coronary blood flow. A significant incidence of vascular complications, which increases with the duration of therapy, has dictated that intra-aortic balloon counterpulsation be reserved for patients who cannot be stabilized on maximum medical therapy. These patients then undergo coronary angiography with a view to urgent coronary revascularization. Nonrandomized studies suggest that the perioperative morbidity and mortality in patients with angina refractory to medical therapy are reduced by intra-aortic balloon counterpulsation.

Percutaneous Transluminal Coronary Angioplasty (PTCA)

The technique of catheter-guided dilatation of coronary stenoses using a small intracoronary balloon was first introduced in 1977. Between 2 and 8 per cent of patients with coronary artery disease are suitable for angioplasty. The ideal candidate for angioplasty fulfills the following characteristics:

1. The patient would otherwise be a candidate for coronary artery bypass surgery.
2. A proximal, discrete, subtotal, relatively concentric, and noncalcified lesion is present in one or two or possibly three coronary arteries.
3. Hemodynamically significant left main coronary artery stenosis is absent.

The overall mortality rate in 3,079 patients enrolled in the NHLBI PTCA Registry was 0.9 per cent. Myocardial infarction resulting from attempted angioplasty occurred in 5.5 per cent, whereas coronary dissection, occlusion, and coronary spasm each occurred in approximately 5 per cent of patients. Coronary events occurred more frequently in women and in patients with unstable angina. The initial success rate of angioplasty was 61 per cent, and 72 per cent of these remained improved at 1 year with no further procedures. Fifty two per cent were entirely asymptomatic at this point without repeat angioplasty or coronary artery bypass surgery. The percentage of patients who were improved and/or asymptomatic at 2 and 4 years was similar. Angioplasty is therefore an effective mode of therapy for selected patients with angina who would otherwise require coronary artery bypass surgery.

Coronary Artery Bypass Surgery

The major indication for coronary artery bypass surgery in the patient with stable angina pectoris of effort is significant disability resulting from moderate to severe angina pectoris that limits the patient's lifestyle despite optimal medical therapy. This broad indication is colored by many considerations, including the underlying coronary anatomy, the patient's age, his level of activity at work, left ventricular function, and side effects resulting from medical therapy. In stable exertional angina, coronary artery bypass surgery would be indicated in patients with significant (greater than 50 per cent) left main coronary artery stenosis, possibly for symptomatic three vessel coronary artery stenosis with impaired left ventricular function, and would be more readily undertaken in young patients with significant coronary artery disease and in patients who genuinely desire to return to a very active lifestyle or work situation.

Coronary artery bypass surgery is also indicated on an urgent basis in patients with unstable angina and operable coronary anatomy who cannot be controlled with standard antianginal therapy.

Guidelines for the Management of Subsets of Patients with Angina Pectoris

Stable Angina of Effort

In situations where pain is highly predictable and infrequent, drug treatment may be simplified by the use of sublingual nitroglycerin just prior to activities that predictably cause angina. With more frequent or severe angina, prophylactic therapy is indicated. Since stable exertional angina is due to intermittent increases in myocardial oxygen consumption, a beta-blocker, which will decrease the determinants of myocardial oxygen demand, is the most logical therapeutic agent. The choice of a beta-blocker depends to some extent on associated conditions, such as bronchospasm, diabetes, peripheral vascular disease, or sinus bradycardia, that may be aggravated by beta-adrenergic blockade. If these agents are clearly contraindicated, then long-acting nitrate preparations or calcium antagonists, which are of proven efficacy in the therapy of stable exertional angina, are useful alternatives. The combination of a beta-blocker and a calcium antagonist such as nitroglycerin is a very effective mode of therapy for patients with chronic angina of effort. Finally, in more resistant cases a combination of nitrates, a calcium antagonist, and a beta-blocker may be indicated.

There is no universal agreement as to when a patient with chronic angina of effort should undergo coronary arteriography. The following subsets of patients should be considered for early arteriography:

1. Patients under 40 years of age,
2. Patients with atypical chest pain,
3. Those with persistent angina despite maximum medical therapy, and
4. Those with a strongly positive exercise test (greater than 1 mm ST segment depression at a heart rate of less than 120).

Patients with left main coronary artery disease and those with angina despite maximum medical therapy should be considered for coronary artery bypass surgery. Patients who fall into this latter category who have single vessel disease with discrete subtotal concentric stenosis would benefit best by percutaneous transluminal coronary angioplasty.

Unstable Angina Pectoris

The syndrome of unstable angina embraces a number of diverse subsets including:

1. Crescendo (accelerated, progressive) angina superimposed on a previous pattern of relatively stable angina of effort,

2. New onset angina brought on by minimal exertion, and

3. The recent onset of angina at rest as well as with minimal exertion in patients with previous stable exertional angina.

Once the diagnosis of unstable angina is suspected, the patient should be admitted to the hospital for evaluation and treatment. Standard hospital therapy includes bed rest, oxygen administration, reassurance, sedation, ECG monitoring, and intravenous catheterization. All patients with unstable angina should probably be treated with one aspirin a day.

Since unstable angina frequently is due to intermittent limitation of coronary blood supply by variable amounts of vasospasm, superimposed on fixed coronary stenoses, a calcium blocking agent or a long-acting nitrate is the drug of choice. If either drug fails, the two can be combined. With continued episodes of chest pain and depending on the frequency and severity of these episodes, a beta-blocker may be added to the regimen. Beta-adrenergic blocking agents do play a major role in the pharmacologic treatment of unstable angina pectoris. Although blockade of the coronary beta-2 receptors may leave alpha-adrenergic activity unopposed, thus enhancing the potential for coronary spasm or dynamic increases in coronary vascular resistance, documented exacerbations of unstable angina due to beta-blockers are uncommon.

With frequent recurrent episodes of unstable angina one or more of the previously mentioned steps may be bypassed and intravenous nitroglycerin substituted. At this point, or alternatively, if intra-aortic balloon counterpulsation is required, the patient should undergo coronary arteriography. Coronary artery bypass surgery is then indicated, provided suitable coronary anatomy is found.

Alternatively, if unstable angina is easily controlled, the patient should undergo submaximal exercise testing during the ensuing several days to stratify his risk. A number of centers are performing coronary arteriography in all patients with unstable angina who have a positive (> 1 mm of ST segment depression) submaximal exercise test.

Percutaneous transluminal coronary angioplasty might be considered in the patient with single vessel disease resulting in uncontrolled angina, although the risks of this procedure in the setting of unstable angina pectoris are higher than in the setting of stable angina.

Variant Angina

Variant, or Prinzmetal's, angina is defined as a syndrome of ischemic pain occurring at rest and associated with ST segment elevations on the electrocardiogram. Because the major mechanism for the onset of chest pain in this syndrome is coronary artery spasm, calcium blocking agents constitute the cornerstone of therapy. The calcium channel blockers have been found to be extremely effective in preventing the coronary artery spasm of variant angina. Alternatively, nitrates are an effective form of therapy in preventing attacks.

In patients with predominant vasospasm and minimal or no coronary artery disease, beta-blockers should probably be avoided. Blockade of beta-2 receptors, which effects coronary dilatation, would theoretically allow unopposed alpha receptor–mediated coronary artery vasoconstriction to occur.

Coronary artery bypass surgery is not indicated in patients with predominant vasospasm, although it has a role in the overall management of patients who have fixed severe coronary artery stenoses and superadded vasospasm.

Mixed Angina

Mixed angina is defined as a form of stable angina caused by a combination of a fixed atherosclerotic lesion and superadded vasoconstriction in the coronary artery. The clinical presentation is typified by episodes of exertional angina with a variable threshold or by a combination of exertional angina and either emotion-induced angina, cold-induced angina, or episodes of angina at rest.

This subset of patients with angina is best managed with a calcium antagonist, which will not only prevent coronary artery vasospasm but diminish myocardial oxygen consumption. Should a calcium antagonist be ineffective, then a beta-blocker and/or a long-acting nitrate preparation may be sequentially added. Failure of medical therapy is an indication for coronary arteriography and a consideration for coronary artery bypass surgery.

CARDIAC ARREST

method of
ARNOLD SLADEN, M.D.
University of Pittsburgh
Pittsburgh, Pennsylvania

Cardiopulmonary Cerebral Resuscitation (CPCR)

CPCR consists of two major components: basic cardiac life support (BCLS) and advanced cardiac life support (ACLS). Loss of cerebral circulation for longer than 4 to 6 minutes can result in gross and irreversible cerebral damage even though some cerebral neurons still remain viable. To attain global cerebral recovery, an effective circulation by artificial means must be provided within 4 to 6 minutes of a cardiac arrest. Because of this time constraint, it is mandatory that BCLS begin within 4 minutes of a cardiac arrest; ACLS must be delivered within 8 minutes.

Basic Cardiac Life Support (BCLS)

BCLS consists of recognizing unconsciousness, alerting the hospital system, positioning the patient, opening the airway, providing mouth-to-orifice respiration, and applying external chest compression.

In the hospital, BCLS is the first line of therapy when cardiac arrest was not witnessed, ACLS is not available, and electrical activity is not known. Outside the hospital, where the lay public usually initiate cardiopulmonary resuscitation (CPR), BCLS is first line defense for all patients with cardiorespiratory arrest. Indeed, if BCLS is not rapidly delivered by the lay public, ACLS offers very little for the patient who has had a cardiac arrest outside the hospital.

Unconsciousness is recognized when the patient fails to respond to the classic "shake and shout," that is, shaking the patient and simultaneously calling out to ascertain whether he or she is "all right." Lack of response is followed by the rescuer's alerting the hospital system, either by calling for assistance or by pressing a call or alarm button. Every hospital department and patient area should have appropriate means for a member of the hospital staff to summon assistance immediately. Next, the patient should be positioned flat on the back. Because the possibility of a cervical spine injury is minimal in hospital patients who sustain a cardiac arrest, protection of the cervical spine during positioning is not essential, but in the prehospital scene, where trauma is suspected or known to have occurred, protection of the cervical spine is essential when turning the patient to the supine position.

A—Airway. Establishing the airway is the first of the three steps in BCLS, which are the ABCs of CPR: airway, breathing, and circulation. There are several techniques for elevating the mandible to open the airway. The most frequently used is the head-tilt maneuver: placing the hand on the patient's forehead and applying firm, backward pressure. This tips the head back and opens the airway. Unfortunately this maneuver may not be performed successfully with one hand, in which case the second hand should be used to produce the addition of either neck lift or chin lift.

Head tilt, neck lift consists of maintaining backward head tilt with one hand while placing the other hand under the neck and lifting it. Beware of this maneuver whenever the possibility of cervical spine trauma exists.

Head tilt, chin lift consists of maintaining backward head tilt with one hand while lifting the chin with the other hand. This is most easily accomplished by placing the tips of index and middle fingers under the tip of the chin and pulling the chin upward and forward. It is essential to keep the tips of the fingers off the soft tissue below the chin, in order not to compress the tissue and thus compromise and not open the airway. An alternative is to place the index, middle, and ring fingers on the lower aspect of the horizontal ramus of the mandible, with the thumb in the sulcus between the lower lip and the angle of the jaw, and lift or pull the jaw upward and forward. This maneuver frequently will open the airway when head tilt, neck lift attempts fail.

If head tilt, chin lift fails to open the airway, displacement of the jaw can be improved with anterior jaw thrust. This is performed by the rescuer's placing the hands on either side of the patient's jaw, including the angle of the mandible. The index through ring fingers should be below the vertical ramus of the mandible, with the thumb above it. In this way the mandible is grasped and displaced forward while the head can be tilted backward.

Jaw thrust without head tilt should be used whenever a cervical spine injury is suspected. The maneuver is similar to jaw thrust with head tilt, except that the neck is not extended.

B—Breathing. After the airway has been opened, the breathing must be assessed. Bend close to the patient's nose and mouth to both feel and hear breathing. If none is detected, try to ventilate the patient artificially. Mouth-to-mouth technique is most frequently used, and to keep the rescuer's exhaled air from escaping it is necessary to pinch off the patient's nostrils. When the head-tilt maneuver is used, the hand not maintaining the backward position of the head pinches off the nose. When the head tilt, neck lift maneuver is used, the hand maintaining head lift is turned so that the heel and palm of the hand maintain head tilt while the fingers are used to pinch off the nose. The rescuer takes a deep breath, seals his or her lips against those of the patient, and exhales fully and rapidly. Without waiting for full deflation of the patient's chest, the rescuer gives an additional three breaths. The absence of adequate exhalation, termed stacking of breaths, is believed to raise lung volume to total lung capacity. This is an attempt to reverse atelectasis by producing a positive end-expiratory pressure (PEEP) effect. External chest compression reduces functional residual capacity and promotes atelectasis. While giving the first deep breath, the rescuer should assess whether the patient is being ventilated. Does the chest rise in exhalation? Subsequently, does the patient's chest fall, can exhaled air be heard, and, finally, is ventilation accomplished with ease?

If any question is answered negatively, the possibility of upper airway obstruction exists. The commonest cause of upper airway obstruction is the tongue. Attempts should be made to reposition the head to establish the airway, followed by mouth-to-mouth breathing. Unless a patient's artificial dentition becomes loose and obstructs the airway, it should be left in place.

In mouth-to-nose ventilation, the rescuer exhales into the patient's nose while closing off the patient's mouth with the rescuer's cheek.

When the head tilt, chin lift maneuver is used, the head-tilt hand should be turned so that the heel and palm of the hand maintain head tilt while the fingers are used to pinch off the nose. Following this, mouth-to-mouth ventilation is given in the usual way.

In the jaw-thrust maneuver, mouth-to-mouth ventilation is given while the rescuer's cheek seals off the patient's nose.

For a patient with a laryngectomy or with a tracheostomy tube in place, mouth-to-stoma or to tracheostomy tube is the first method of providing ventilation when adjunctive equipment is not available immediately.

C—Circulation. After completing four breaths in rapid succession, the rescuer should assess the status of the circulation by palpating one of the major arteries for a pulse, the most accessible being the carotid artery. While the hand on the patient's head remains in position to maintain the airway, the other hand is used to palpate the pulse. The correct technique is to palpate the thyroid cartilage and, with the patient supine, slide the tips of the ring, middle, and index fingers backward into the groove bounded by the omohyoid and thyrohyoid muscles anteriorly and by the sternomastoid posteriorly. Avoid excessive pressure and take ample time—up to 10 seconds—to assess the status of the pulse. When heart block or sinus bradycardia is present, there may be only two pulsations during a 10 second period.

ARTIFICIAL CIRCULATION. Cardiac arrest means no palpable pulse, and artificial circulation must be generated by what has become known as external cardiac compression. Its purpose is to apply rhythmic external compressions to the chest, to increase pressure within the thoracic cavity in relation to the circulation outside the thoracic cavity. It is essential that external compression be carried out without trauma to the patient and with maximal efficiency by the rescuer. The optimal position for manual compression is over the lower half of the sternum, excluding the xiphoid process.

The fingertips of the hand closest to the victim's feet are slid along the costal margin of the rib cage until the middle finger locates the notch between the xiphoid process and the rib cage. The heel of the other hand is then placed on the long axis of the lower half of the sternum, touching the ring finger of the first hand. The hand locating the xiphoid notch then is removed and placed on top of the other hand, interlocking fingers with the lower hand and simultaneously pulling the fingers of the lower hand upward and away from the chest wall. This leaves only the heel of the hand in contact with the patient's sternum and reduces trauma to the rib cage during compression. With shoulders directly over the patient, the rescuer applies sufficient force to depress the patient's sternum by about 1.5 to 2 inches. By concentrating on the hands, the rescuer will easily recognize an adequate depth of sternal depression. After the downward thrust has been completed, the pressure should be released. Rhythmic compression and relaxation should then be continued.

When there is a single rescuer, after 15 compressions have been completed at a rate of 80 per minute the rescuer gives the patient two quick breaths and rapidly returns to chest compression. At a compression rate of 80 per minute, the time required to deliver mouth-to-mouth ventilation and return to compression precludes delivering more than some 60 compressions over a 1 minute period. After four cycles of 15 compressions and 2 ventilations, the rescuer stops to reassess the carotid pulse. If none is found, resuscitation continues.

If a second rescuer is present or when one arrives, external cardiac compression is interrupted and a backboard or tray is placed behind the patient's chest to improve the effectiveness of chest compression. With two rescuers the compression rate is decreased to 60 per minute, and the second rescuer delivers a breath after every fifth compression cycle. It takes considerable practice to develop the appropriate skill to deliver a breath during the relaxation phase of the fifth compression cycle. An attempt to deliver mouth-to-mouth ventilation during the compression phase results in both inadequate ventilation and inadequate compression.

PRIMARY AIRWAY OBSTRUCTION. Sudden and unexpected cardiac arrest from "cardiovascular disease" accounts for about 600,000 deaths annually. During the initial period of resuscitation, establishing an airway may be difficult owing to the presence of foreign material—most frequently gastric material regurgitated into the oral pharynx and occasionally displaced dentures. This usually can be eliminated by the fingers sweeping the mouth and pharynx. Cardiac arrest from hypoxia secondary to foreign body obstruction of the airway is relatively infrequent compared with cardiac arrest from myocardial infarction.

Advanced Cardiac Life Support (ACLS)

Advanced cardiac life support consists of the following components: basic cardiac life support; adjuncts for airway control and ventilation; adjuncts for artificial circulation; electrical monitoring for dysrhythmia recognition; defibrillation and synchronized cardioversion; intravenous lifeline techniques; drugs to reverse cardiac arrest and provide overall support during the postarrest period; and stabilization and transportation of the patient.

Adjuncts for Airway Control and Ventilation

POCKET MASK. The simplest adjunct for ventilation is the pocket mask, a triangular shape with an inflatable collar and a chimney rising from its center, through which the rescuer can ventilate the patient. The base of the triangle fits into the sulcus between the lower lip and tip of the chin, the apex of the inflatable collar over the bridge of the nose. The ring, middle, and index fingers of each hand elevate the mandible and establish the airway, while the thumbs wrap around the lower part of the mask, maintaining a seal between the mask and the face. Mouth-to-chimney respirations are performed as necessary. A nipple on the mask can be connected by a length of plastic flexible tubing to an oxygen source to increase the concentration of oxygen delivered to the patient. The pocket mask is useful during two person resuscitation.

AIRWAYS. Cardiac arrest is associated with loss of muscle tone, which results in prolapse of the tongue into the posterior pharynx.

A plastic or rubber airway can be inserted through either the mouth or the nose into the pharynx, between the posterior pharynx and the prolapsed tongue. Airways are available in a variety of sizes to suit the size of the patient. It is suggested that an airway be used whenever a bag-valve-mask system is used.

OROPHARYNGEAL AIRWAY. As its name implies, this is inserted into the mouth and extends from the lips to the pharynx. It has a passage either in the center or on either side of a central column, which runs the length of the airway. Classically, the oropharyngeal airway is shaped like a "C" with a flange in the front to impinge on the lips or front teeth. Because of the C curve, the oropharyngeal airway should not be inserted directly, or it will push the tongue into the posterior pharynx. First lubricated, then turned upside down, the oropharangeal airway should be inserted into the mouth with the convexity of the C on the tongue and the concavity toward the hard palate. When the airway is almost completely in position, its long axis should be rotated through 180 degrees and advanced into the pharynx. The flange of the oropharyngeal airway should not be taped to the face because this fixes the front of the airway and the backward pressure of the airway may ulcerate the pharynx.

NASOPHARYNGEAL AIRWAY. After lubrication, the nasopharyngeal airway is inserted carefully and gently through the external nares and advanced toward the pharynx. If obstruction is met, no further attempts should be made to advance the airway. It should be removed and passed through the alternate nares. A trumpet-shaped expansion at the nasal end of the airway prevents it from being lost through the nares.

BAG-VALVE-MASK SYSTEM (BVM). The BVM system consists of a manual resuscitation bag, entrainment and reservoir systems for delivery of 100 per cent oxygen, and a mask, preferably transparent, that will cover both the mouth and nose, provide a good seal, and allow delivery of an adequate tidal volume. The first step in BVM use is to connect the oxygen nipple to a hollow flexible tube, which in turn is converted to an oxygen flow meter. The flow meter should be set to deliver either a minimum of 12 liters per minute or, if possible, "flush." The mask is held with the fingers of one hand, usually the middle, ring, and little fingers, under the horizontal ramus of the mandible, maintaining the airway, while the index finger and thumb hold the mask tightly against the face, completing the seal. An inflatable collar assists in maintaining a leak-free system. The other hand squeezes the manual resuscitator bag. Use of the BVM system requires extensive training to develop the correct skills and ongoing training to maintain those skills.

A hazard of the BVM system is failing to maintain the airway by lifting the mandible, instead pressing downward with the mask and thus occluding the airway. If the airway is occluded or partially occluded, with each manual compression of the bag oxygen is pushed into the stomach, causing gastric distention initially and subsequent regurgitation of gastric contents with potential aspiration. More significant is a failure to deliver oxygen and remove carbon dioxide. Unless the rescuer is prepared to develop and maintain the skills necessary to use BVM, a pocket mask with oxygen should be used until personnel skilled in the use of BVM arrive at the resuscitation scene.

ENDOTRACHEAL INTUBATION. Endotracheal intubation is the "gold standard" for securing and maintaining the airway, protecting the lung from aspiration, and providing optimal ventilation and delivery of oxygen. The endotracheal tube is a hollow, plastic (red rubber is hardly ever used today) tube about 30 cm long that has a built-in inflatable balloon-type cuff close to the distal end. The proximal end has a 15 mm standard male connector, which can be inserted into a bag-valve system. Endotracheal tubes are introduced through either the mouth or the nose and advanced through the vocal cords. For correct positioning, the tube should be advanced until the inflatable cuff has completely passed through the vocal cords. This should locate the tip of the tube at the level of the top of the aortic arch, well above the carcina. The endotracheal tube can be advanced blindly, but for the most part is inserted under direct vision using an illuminated laryngoscope. The use of the laryngoscope is not the monopoly of the anesthesiologist, but considerable skill is required plus ongoing training to maintain that skill. Endotracheal intubation must be completed in 30 seconds or less. There is nothing more disastrous during cardiac arrest than the waste of precious time with neither ventilation nor oxygenation while an inadequately trained but self-assured person repeatedly attempts to use a laryngoscope and place an endotracheal tube. Use a single device, i.e., pocket mask with oxygen, until trained personnel arrive.

THE ESOPHAGEAL OBTURATOR AIRWAY (EOA) AND ENDOTRACHEAL INTUBATION. When a patient arrives in the emergency department with an EOA in place, remember to remove only the mask of the EOA, intubate the trachea with an endotracheal tube (preferably under direct vision), and ventilate the patient. Only after this has been completed successfully should the large cuff of the EOA be deflated and the EOA removed. The inflated cuff in the esophagus prevents regurgitation, and if the EOA cuff is deflated prior to intubation of the trachea, massive regurgitation and aspiration can occur. The use of a laryngoscope to insert an endotracheal tube in a patient with an EOA is recommended to provide direct vision of the pharynx and glottis and prevent entwining of the endotracheal tube with the EOA.

TRANSTRACHEAL CATHETER VENTILATION. When upper airway obstruction occurs from trauma (e.g., lacerated tongue, pharynx, or larynx), establishing an airway with the usual techniques may not be feasible. An alternative is to insert a 14 gauge plastic intravenous catheter-needle through the cricothyroid membrane, remove the stylet, and ventilate through the plastic catheter with a hand-operated jet ventilator. To insert the catheter, a catheter-needle is attached to a syringe and the needle is advanced through the cricothyroid membrane, in the midline, backward and caudally at an angle of 45 degrees while traction is maintained on the plunger of the syringe. As soon as air is aspirated, indicating entrance into the trachea, the catheter is advanced into the trachea while the metal needle obturator is removed. The hand-held jet is attached to the hub of the plastic catheter. The total system consists of a connector to the high pressure oxygen wall outlet, a length of high pressure hose attached to a reducing valve and a hand-operated release valve, and intravenous tubing between the release valve and a metal male connector, which is attached to the plastic catheter. Opening and closing the hand-operated release valve delivers intermittent oxygen flow to the catheter and into the lungs. Exhalation is passive, it is hoped through a nontotally obstructed upper airway. If the airway is totally obstructed, it is feasible to insert a second catheter-needle, which can be occluded during inspiration and opened during exhalation.

CRICOTHYROTOMY. If transtracheal catheter ventilation equipment is not available, cricothyrotomy can be performed. A small horizontal skin incision is made over the cricothyroid membrane, the the tip of the scalpel incises the cricothyroid membrane. A small endotracheal tube (4 mm in internal diameter) can be inserted through the opening and, with the 15 mm connector at the proximal end, ventilation can be delivered using a bag-valve system.

Adjuncts for Circulation. Manual external chest compression is tiring, and as the operator tires the efficiency of external chest compression decreases. Admittedly, team members can rotate, but over a long resuscitation period optimal chest compression may not be maintained.

MANUAL CHEST COMPRESSOR. This is a simple, hinged, manually operated mechanical chest compressor. It delivers an adjustable stroke of 1.5 to 2 inches and can be applied rapidly and without considerable interruption in CPR. The main disadvantage is a tendency for the compressor head to shift and for the tightening device to loosen. The result is a change in site position or depth of compression.

AUTOMATIC CHEST COMPRESSORS. These are powered by compressed gas, are large and bulky, and are not usually used for inhospital resuscitation.

Cardiac Monitoring. Electrocardiographic monitoring should be begun as soon as possible, to determine the electrical activity of the heart and to delineate therapy. Unless the patient has a cardiac arrest in a monitored area, portable electrocardiographic equipment usually will be brought on an emergency cart to the patient area. Invariably this will be monitor/defibrillator rather than monitor alone. The monitor/defibrillator is usually a battery-operated model, which when not in use is kept on continuous charge. Most monitor/defibrillators in current use incorporate quick look paddles, both as electrodes to display electrical activity and to deliver countershock.

Satisfactory contact between electrode and skin is achieved by applying a conductive medium to the paddles and giving them a quarter turn in either direction as they are applied to the skin. This technique allows the gel to more effectively penetrate the epithelial cells of the skin and reduce skin resistance.

For optimal monitoring and delivery of countershock, the standard paddle position is used. One paddle is placed on the right side of the chest, just below the clavicle and immediately lateral to the right border of the sternum; the other is placed to the left of the left nipple in the anterior axillary line. Electrical activity is displayed on the small oscilloscope of the defibrillator/monitor, and in addition there may be a paper recording of the rhythm. An alternative to the standard electrode position is the anterioposterior (A-P) position. One paddle is placed anteriorly, over the precardium, and the other posteriorly, behind the heart. The A-P position is not frequently used because correctly positioning and maintaining the electrodes is difficult.

An alternative to using the monitor/defibrillator is connecting the patient to a standard portable electrocardiograph machine, with electrodes applied to the four extremities. A paper recording of a selected lead can display the cardiac rhythm. Lead 2, with polarity from negative (below the right clavicle) to positive (left nipple), is used most frequently. When the electrical activity is displayed, the rescuers should evaluate the waves and complexes; the rate, rhythm, and site of the dominant pacemaker; and the configuration of the P and QRS waves.

CARDIOVERSION—DIRECT CURRENT. As discussed, BCLS is a holding operation, and for the patient with cardiac arrest and absent pulse from ventricular ectopy, electrical countershock is the only effective therapy to restore organized electrical activity and an effective cardiac output.

It is essential to understand that electrical cardioversion (countershock) does not convert ventricular fibrillation or tachycardia into normal sinus rhythm. The goal of electrical cardioversion is to produce simultaneous and mass depolarization of cardiac cells, which, it is hoped, will be followed shortly thereafter by a pacemaker's taking over and producing appropriate electrical impulses to generate effective ventricular contractions. When a pacemaker does not effect any electrical activity, ventricular fibrillation is followed by asystole. When ventricular fibrillation or tachycardia is recognized, electrical countershock should be delivered as soon as possible. When a monitor/defibrillator is in use, countershock can be delivered without delay; when an ECG is used to monitor the rhythm, a defibrillator must be brought to the patient while BCLS is continued.

VENTRICULAR FIBRILLATION. Cardioversion of ventricular fibrillation initially should consist of a delivered electrical energy level of 200 joules. If unsuccessful, countershock should be repeated without increase in "dose." Repeated countershock decreases the electrical resistance across the chest wall and, in fact, delivers more energy across the heart without changing the delivery "dose." Failure of repeated doses at this level is an indication to progressively increase the watt/seconds to a maximum of 360 joules.

When the operator is about to deliver a countershock, he or she should first ascertain that the defibrillator is fully charged to the desired level, then call out for everyone to stand clear, quickly look to see that everyone is away from bed and patient contact, and only then simultaneously press the button on each electrode paddle. Delivery of an adequate countershock is physically demonstrated by diffuse contractions of the patient's musculature. After countershock, the paddles should be kept in place to assess electrical activity.

VENTRICULAR TACHYCARDIA. Unlike ventricular fibrillation, with its totally chaotic rhythm, ventricular tachycardia usually is reasonably organized. It is appropriate to deliver the electrical energy during a specific part of the QRS complex—synchronized countershock. This requires less energy to be effective and produces less dysrhythmia. In turn, it may avoid converting ventricular tachycardia into ventricular fibrillation. Be certain that the cardioverter you plan to use for the patient with ventricular tachycardia can deliver synchronized countershock.

Activate the synchronizer circuit and set the delivered energy level to 200 joules. Remember that this is ventricular tachycardia with cardiac arrest: smaller energy levels may be useless and time-consuming. *Press* and *hold* buttons on the paddles until countershock is delivered. If unsuccessful, resynchronize the circuit and repeat, using the same doses recommended for defibrillation.

If ventricular tachycardia is "cardioverted" to ventricular fibrillation, turn off the synchronizer circuit, charge the defibrillator to 200 to 300 joules of delivered energy, and defibrillate. Remember that if the synchronizer is not deactivated, it will not be possible to cardiovert ventricular fibrillation.

Intravenous Fluid Lifeline. During a cardiac arrest it is usual to have to deliver drugs and fluids.

The venous route is most effective to enter the circulation rapidly and achieve appropriate drug levels (potentially tissue levels). The intravenous fluid lifeline, as it has become known, needs to be inserted by an ACLS team member while others simultaneously are intubating the trachea, ventilating the lungs, observing cardiac activity, and continuing BCLS. Current consensus is that the intravenous line should be central and inserted into the thoracic cavity from major veins, not threaded through the veins in the lower limbs. I am concerned that this statement may give license for external chest compression to be discontinued for longer than 30 seconds while a catheter is inserted into an internal jugular or subclavian vein. It is not possible to gain access to either of these veins while external chest compression is in progress, particularly to avoid penetrating the lung and pleural space, producing a pneumothorax. Insertion of a "long line" into the cephalic vein in the antecubital fossa often results in an inability to thread the catheter through the site of the clavipectoral fascia. Hence, the internal jugular or subclavian vein may have to be selected, but remember that external chest compresion must not be interrupted for longer than 30 seconds.

FLUID INFUSION. Fluid infusion during cardiac arrest depends on the cause of the cardiac arrest. For the patient with sudden arrest, possibly in association with a myocardial infarction, a 5 per cent dextrose solution in moderate volumes is suitable. It lacks sodium and should not potentiate pulmonary edema. When cardiac arrest is the result of trauma or hypovolemia, massive volume replacement is essential. Two or three liters of lactated Ringer's solution should be infused as rapidly as possible, preferably through two large bore, central venous lines. When blood has been lost, patient compatible group blood should be requested. There is considerable argument as to whether colloid solution is more effective in maintaining intravascular volume than crystalloid alone in patients in hypovolemic shock. Certainly the discussants are vehement in their opinions, but without doubt 5 per cent plasma protein derivative (PPD) or 6 per cent hydroxyethyl starch augments the efficiency of crystalloid infusion.

Pharmacology of Drugs Used in Resuscitation. Drug therapy during a cardiac arrest has very limited therapeutic goals. When ventricular fibrillation or tachycardia is present, drug therapy is designed to prepare the heart for countershock so that subsequently a normal sinus rhythm can be established and maintained; when cardiac standstill or electromechanical association is present, drug therapy is designed to stimulate and maintain contractility; and in complete heart block to speed up ventricular rate and augment contractility. Where an effective pulse has been restored, additional drugs can be added to augment blood pressure and myocardial contractility, alter cardiac preload and afterload, and treat pulmonary and cerebral edema and seizure activity.

OXYGEN. Hypoxemia is common and there is often a need to ventilate the patient with 100 per cent oxygen and thus ensure maximum alveolar oxygenation. Many rescuers express concern over the use of 100 per cent oxygen, because of toxicity or the presence of chronic obstructive lung disease. Oxygen toxicity does not develop during the first 24 hours of exposure to 1 atmosphere of the gas, and the concern that the patient with COPD will fail to breathe because of lack of hypoxic drive is not relevant until and unless the patient is resuscitated. Resuscitate the patient, then deal with potential sequelae.

SODIUM BICARBONATE. Reversal of acidosis is essential to the management of resuscitation. Metabolic acidosis does not develop after arrest; reversal of acidosis can be attempted by inducing hypocapnia, a respiratory alkalosis, until an intravenous line can be secured and bicarbonate injected. Respiratory acidosis, or hypercapnia, appears to have a rapid detrimental action. Carbon dioxide easily and quickly diffuses through cell walls and decreases intracellular pH. Therefore meticulous attention must be paid to efficient ventilation for adequate elimination of carbon dioxide.

Dosage of sodium bicarbonate consists of an initial intravenous bolus of 1 mEq per kg, which may be followed by one half of the initial dose, 0.5 mEq per kg, every 10 minutes that spontaneous circulation is absent or as dictated by arterial blood gas determinations. In my experience, arterial blood gas determinations frequently are not available, and even when results are available they usually are not relevant to the moment in time when the results are delivered. In an ICU with its own blood gas laboratory, such determinations may provide pertinent data.

Remember that bicarbonate infusion and its combination with lactic acid produce additional carbonic acid, which in turn requires additional ventilation. After each dose of bicarbonate, the infusion line should be flushed, both to deliver the drug and to remove it from the infusion line. Sodium bicarbonate inactivates catecholamine-type drugs (e.g., epinephrine, dopamine, isoproterenol).

The strict recommendations for dosage arose when it became apparent that excess bicarbonate was being infused. The sequelae of alkalemia are a shift of the oxygen dissociation curve to the left and an increase in affinity of hemoglobin for oxygen, this occurring at a time when every effort is being made to donate oxygen to the tissues. Alkalemia potentiates hypokalemia, which in turn potentiates ventricular dysrhythmias, when one is attempting to reduce and control dysrhythmia. Yet another additional and frequently forgotten complication of sodium bicarbonate therapy is that each milliliter of sodium bicarbonate contains 2 mOsm. During a prolonged resuscitation—perhaps over 60 minutes—a total of 320 ml of sodium bicarbonate may be infused, or 640 mOsm. If spontaneous breathing and circulation are restored but the patient fails to awaken, it may not be possible to determine whether the coma is a sequel to cerebral hypoxia or is hyperosmolar coma, until serum osmolality has been measured.

EPINEPHRINE. Epinephrine is believed to increase the amplitude of the fibrillatory wave in ventricular fibrillation (that is, it converts fine to coarse fibrillation). Coarse fibrillation responds to countershock more easily than does fine fibrillation. To this end, epinephrine is used to prepare the heart for countershock in patients with ventricular fibrillation. Dosage of epinephrine is 0.5 to 1.0 mg intravenously every 5 minutes. Currently, epinephrine is available in prepacked syringes (1:10,000 solution), and 5 to 10 ml is the prescribed dose. Because the half-life of the drug is so short, to be effective it must be repeated at 5 minute intervals. It must be flushed through the infusion line, both for delivery into the vascular compartment and to prevent inactivation by any subsequent injection of sodium bicarbonate.

Nebulized or injected into the tracheobronchial tree, epinephrine rapidly crosses the aveolar-capillary "membrane," enters the pulmonary circulation, and achieves satisfactory systemic blood levels. When an intravenous lifeline is not available, injection of 10 ml of a 1:10,000 solution (i.e., 1 mg) down the endotracheal tube, followed by efficient manual ventilation, is an effective delivery route for this drug. Unless the needle is permanently fixed to the syringe, it should be removed prior to injection of epinephrine into the endotracheal tube.

Direct intracardiac injection of epinephrine is an alternate route when neither an intravenous lifeline nor an endotracheal tube is available. When the intracardiac route is used, access to the cardiac chamber must be ascertained by easy withdrawal of blood prior to injection of epinephrine. Injection of epinephrine into myocardial muscle results in intractable vetricular fibrillation. Other hazards of intracardiac injection include pneumothorax, cardiac tamponade, and coronary artery laceration. There is some speculation that irritation by the needle alone may be a direct stimulus to myocardial contraction in the asystolic heart.

When used as a life-support postresuscitation to support flow, resistance, and pressure, epinephrine should be infused continuously up to 0.04 micrograms per kg per minute. One mg of epinephrine diluted in 250 ml of 5 per cent dextrose in water provides 4 micrograms per ml. Begin the infusion at 0.4 microgram per min (0.006 microgram per kg per min for a 70 kg person) and increase to obtain optimal function. Pay particular attention to the peripheral circulation for compromise of the extemities due to excessive alpha activity.

LIDOCAINE. Indications for lidocaine usage during cardiac arrest are (1) failure to restore or maintain normal sinus rhythm after countershock for ventricular fibrillation, or (2) to prevent return of fatal ventricular ectopy after countershock.

Dosage of lidocaine is 1 mg/kg, which may be repeated every 10 minutes to a total dose of 225 mg. Because of the short half-life of lidocaine, to maintain a therapeutic level an infusion of 2 mg per min must be started immediately after the first bolus. If repeated boluses are required to increase the blood level, it is appropriate simultaneously to increase the infusion dosage.

A satisfactory dosage regimen for a 70 kg person is:

Time	*Bolus*	*Infusion*
—	75 mg	2 mg per min
+10 min	50 mg	3 mg per min
+10 min	50 mg	4 mg per min
+10 min	50 mg	—
TOTAL	225 mg	

If lidocaine was not required prior to countershock therapy for successful cardioversion of ventricular tachycardia or fibrillation, a bolus should be injected and an infusion begun as soon as possible. To suppress ventricular ectopy, a lidocaine blood level of 1.5 to 6.0 micrograms per ml is required. In the presence of low cardiac output (shock) or liver failure, the infusion dosage should be reduced by 50 per cent to prevent the blood level from rising into the toxic range. If an intravenous lifeline is not available, lidocaine, like epinephrine, can be administered through the endotracheal tube.

Complications of lidocaine toxicity primarily affect the central nervous system and can include focal and grand mal seizures. Excessive doses also can produce myocardial and circulatory depression.

PROCAINAMIDE. Procainamide is an antidysrhythmic drug that may be effective when lidocaine has failed. Its activity resembles that of lidocaine in depressing phase-4 depolarization and in terminating re-entry mechanisms by opening blocked Purkinje pathways. Failure to suppress ventricular ectopy after 225 mg of lidocaine and an infusion rate of 4 mg per min is an indication to use procainamide.

Dosage of procainamide is 100 mg per 5 minutes (20 mg per min) until ectopy is terminated or a maximum of 1 gram has been administered. Procainamide should be infused, 1 to 4 mg per min, to maintain a therapeutic blood level. Toxic manifestations—that is, hypotension or widening of the QRS complex—cannot occur in patients with a cardiac arrest from ventricular fibrillation.

BRETYLIUM TOSYLATE. This is a quaternary ammonium compound with postganglionic adrenergic-blocking effects and was previously a therapeutic agent for hypertension. Its side effects and the availability of other improved antihypertensive drugs diminished its use, but it has since been resurrected as a potent antidysrhythmic drug for patients with ventricular tachycardia or fibrillation refractory to countershock after treatment with both lidocaine and procainamide. When lidocaine fails to be effective, procainamide is frequently bypassed for bretylium. Like lidocaine, bretylium elevates the ventricular fibrillation threshold. Dosage of bretylium is 5 mg per kg intravenously, which can be increased in increments of 5 mg every 10 to 15 minutes to a maximum of 30 mg per kg.

CALCIUM CHLORIDE. Calcium ion is essential for muscle contraction. When an electrical impulse reaches a cardiac muscle cell, the permeability of the cell wall changes and calcium ions freely pass into the sarcoplasm of the muscle cell. Calcium previously present in the cell and bound to the sarcoplasmic reticulum is released and migrates adjacent to both the actin and the myosin. Shortening of the myofibrils results in contraction. During relaxation a portion of the calcium is pumped out of the cell, while the remainder is bound to intracellular muscle protein. Calcium chloride is indicated in electromechanical dissociation and may be of value in asystole.

Dosage of calcium chloride in a 10 per cent solution is 5 to 7 ml per kg or about 250 to 400 mg for a 70 kg person; it may be repeated at 10-minute intervals. Prefilled syringes, 10 ml of a 10 per cent solution, hold a total of 1 gram, which contains 13.6 mEq of Ca. Remember to flush any bicarbonate infusion before injecting calcium chloride, and similarly flush the calcium chloride before injecting bicarbonate. Failure to flush will precipitate calcium carbonate "chalk" in the infusion line.

ISOPROTERENOL. This synthetic catecholamine differs from epinephrine in that there is alkyl substitution in the amino group; it increases beta activity. Isoproterenol increases cardiac output by both its chronotropic and its inotropic action and by improved venous return. Because it dilates the peripheral vascular bed, the increase in cardiac output will augment systemic systolic pressure while it reduces diastolic pressure. It may be of value in asystole and in complete heart block resistant to atropine.

Isoproterenol is available in 1 mg vials, which provide a concentration of 4 micrograms per ml when mixed in 250 ml of 5 per cent dextrose in water. Start the infusion at 0.4 microgram per min and increase up to 20 micrograms per min if necessary. The goal of therapy is a heart rate of about 60 beats per min. The drug increases myocardial oxygen consumption, potentiates ventricular ectopy, and certainly can produce ventricular fibrillation.

ATROPINE SULFATE. Atropine is a parasympatholytic drug, inhibiting the action of acetylcholine on structures innervated by postganglionic parasympathetic nerves. The sympathetic and parasympathetic nervous systems carefully balance the cardiac rate, either by increasing the activity of one or by decreasing that of the other—the pendulum is either pushed or pulled. When bradydysrhythmia occurs, and particularly complete heart block without an efficient cardiac output, parasympathetic blockade will allow sympathetic activity to dominate. Therefore, atropine is used to block the vagus at the SA node and, it is hoped, halt and reverse the bradycardia. Atropine also is recommended in asystole that does not respond to both epinephrine and calcium. Dosage of atropine is 0.5 mg intravenously every 5 minutes until a heart rate of 60 beats per min is achieved or a total of 2 mg has been injected. Two milligrams of atropine produce complete vagal blockade, and further dosage is of no value. Concern has been expressed over the increase in myocardial oxygen consumption when atropine is used in patients with acute myocardial infarction. It should be clearly understood that the asystolic heart is dead, and any drug that may "restart" the heart is worthwhile and should be used.

MANAGEMENT OF CARDIAC ARREST

Ventricular Fibrillation

Monitored. Monitored arrests are cardiac arrests that occur when a patient is under ECG monitoring. The patient usually will be in the emergency department or the coronary care unit but might be in any ICU or in an invasive radiographic suite where ECG monitoring is used.

1. Give a precordial thump. This consists of striking the midsternum with the fleshy part of a closed fist.
2. If successful, administer bolus and infuse lidocaine.
3. If unsuccessful AND A DEFIBRILLATOR IS IMMEDIATELY AVAILABLE countershock with 200 joules delivered energy.
4. If this fails, repeat the countershock with the same dose of electrical energy.
5. If ventricular fibrillation is still present, begin BCLS and augment with ACLS as soon as it is available. Follow the protocol for unmonitored arrest beginning with step 3.

Countershock is first line therapy in the witnessed arrest with ventricular fibrillation because it is possible to deliver countershock within the first minute after cardiac arrest. At this time hypoxia and acidosis may not be present, and the results of immediate countershock are very good. The criteria for optimal defibrillation are absence of hypoxia and acidosis and defibrillation performed very shortly following onset of ventricular fibrillation.

Unmonitored. In this situation the patient is not under ECG monitoring, and the defibrillator with "quick look" paddles is not available immediately. In addition, the duration of cardiac arrest may be unknown.

1. Begin BCLS and summon assistance and ACLS.
2. When a defibrillator monitor arrives, apply electrode conductive material and quick look paddles. Stop BCLS and observe the cardiac electrical activity. If ventricular fibrillation is present, continue with BCLS, charge the defibrillator to 200 joules, stop external chest compression and ventilation, and deliver the countershock. Observe the ECG: if fibrillation is still present, continue with BCLS and repeat the countershock procedure.
3. If a palpable pulse is obtained with either of these two countershocks, inject a bolus of lidocaine, 75 mg, and begin an infusion of 2 mg per min.
4. *If two countershocks fail to defibrillate,* each member of the ACLS team follows the designated ACLS procedure. Continue external chest compression. Commence bag-valve-mask ventilation with 100 per cent oxygen and as soon as possible intubate the patient with a cuffed endotracheal tube and continue ventilation with 100 per cent oxygen. Establish an intravenous lifeline, using an infusion fluid of 5 per cent dextrose in water. Inject epinephrine, 0.5 to 1.0 mg, into the line and flush. If an IV line is not attainable, inject the epinephrine into the endotracheal tube. If the elapsed time from the cardiac arrest is believed to exceed 5 to 10 minutes, inject sodium bicarbonate, 1 mEq per kg IV and flush the line. If not in place, apply regular ECG leads.
5. Stop external chest compressions, rapidly review the cardiac electrical rhythm:
   a. If ventricular fibrillation, continue external chest compression and recharge the defibrillator to 300 to 360 joules. When the defibrillator is fully charged, stop ventilation and compression, discharge the defibrillator, and observe the electrical activity.
   b. If there is an organized rhythm *and a palpable pulse,* give an intravenous bolus of lidocaine, 75 mg, and start an infusion of 2 mg per min. Assess ventilation; if present, provide a delivery of high oxygen concentrations to the endotracheal tube. If spontaneous ventilation is absent, continue to support ventilation manually and subsequently mechanically. Measure the blood pressure and transport the patient to a monitored area.
   c. If fibrillation is replaced with asystole or electromechanical dissociation, continue CPR and follow the protocol for asystole or EMD (described later).
6. If ventricular fibrillation persists, continue BCLS, inject lidocaine, 75 mg IV, and start infusion with 2 mg per min. Reattempt countershock, with appropriate stopping and restarting of ventilation and chest compression.
7. If ventricular fibrillation persists, sufficient time will have elapsed to repeat the epinephrine, 0.5 to 1.0 mg IV, and possibly the bicarbonate, 0.5 mEq per kg (half the initial dose).
8. Attempt countershock.
9. Failure to cardiovert ventricular fibrillation is an indication to sample arterial blood for measurement of arterial blood gases and pH, and to continue chemical therapy with lidocaine to a total of 225 mg and an infusion of 4 mg per min, coupled with periodic doses of epinephrine and sodium bicarbonate.
10. If repeated countershock is unsuccessful, proceed to procainamide, to a maximum of 1 gram, and/or bretylium to a maximum of 30 mg per kg. Attempt defibrillation after each additional drug bolus.
11. It is obvious that failure to defibrillate, after a long time period and maximal dosage of drugs, demonstrates intractable ventricular fibrillation. Further resuscitation is futile and should be abandoned by the physician in charge of the resuscitation.

Asystole

Initial drug therapy and respiratory support are identical to that in the management of ventricular fibrillation.

1. As soon as the rhythm is recognized, either begin (monitored) or continue (unmonitored) BCLS. When ACLS is available, replace mouth-to-mouth ventilation with 100 per cent oxygen and perform endotracheal intubation as rapidly as possible.
2. ECG leads should be attached and the rhythm reassessed. As soon as an intravenous lifeline is secured, inject epinephrine, 0.5 to 1.0 mg; if no IV line can be secured, inject the epinephrine down the endotracheal tube. Discontinue external chest compression, palpate the pulse, and observe the ECG. If asystole is still present, continue ventilation and external chest compression.
3. Inject sodium bicarbonate, 1.0 mEq per kg, and flush the line. Reassess the pulse and ECG; if asystole persists, inject calcium chloride, 300 mg, at 10 minute intervals or atropine, 0.5 mg, at 5 minute intervals, in either order. Check the pulse after injecting each drug. Continue with epinephrine and sodium bicarbonate; consider isoproterenol and finally a pacemaker.

The results of treating cardiac arrest with electrical standstill, asystole, are very poor.

Electromechanical Dissociation (EMD)

Treatment is identical to that for asystole, using repeated doses of epinephrine, sodium bicarbonate, and calcium chloride. If EMD persists, an isoproterenol infusion may be of value.

Ventricular Tachycardia

1. Primary therapy for ventricular tachycardia without a pulse is synchronized cardioversion with 200 joules. While awaiting the cardioverter, begin BCLS and ventilate with 100 per cent oxygen. When the ACLS equipment arrives, charge the cardioverter; when the capacitor indicates 200 joules of delivered energy, stop ventilation and external chest compression, then countershock.
2. If cardioversion is successful, inject a bolus of lidocaine, 75 mg, and follow with an infusion of 2 mg per min. If unsuccessful, repeat initially with 200 joules and progressively increase the electrical energy, with ventilation and chest compression continuing between countershocks. Begin the lidocaine protocol if the second cardioversion is unsuccessful.
3. If ventricular fibrillation is produced after countershock, SWITCH OFF SYNCHRONIZER and use the protocol for ventricular fibrillation.

ATRIAL FIBRILLATION

method of
ROBERT B. LEMAN, M.D.
Medical University of South Carolina
Charleston, South Carolina

Atrial fibrillation is one of the more common types of atrial arrhythmias and occurs in about 1 per cent of the general population. It is present in 12 to 14 per cent of adult hospitalized patients. The incidence increases with age and peaks between 50 and 70 years of age. It is uncommon in children. In adults it is noted 20 times more frequently than atrial flutter. Causes of atrial fibrillation are listed in Table 1.

The hemodynamic consequences of atrial fibrillation are multiple. The rapid irregular rates cause marked variations of diastolic filling time for an adequate cardiac output. These changes affect preload and cause a variable decrease in stroke volume, especially in mitral stenosis, which is dependent on the filling time. The loss of atrial contraction eliminates the booster pump effect, and the cardiac output is no longer augmented by 20 to 60 per cent. Noncompliant ventricles, i.e., hypertrophic cardiomyopathies, are dependent on the atrial contraction, and its loss can lead to medical emergencies.

Management

The aim of routine initial management of acute onset of atrial fibrillation is to control the ventricular response. If the patient is tolerating the rapid rate without hemodynamic compromise, the ventricular rate is controlled by rapid digitalization. Digoxin is given at 0.5 mg intravenously initially, followed in 2 to 4 hours by a similar dose. Subsequent doses depend on the ventricular response. Rapid digitalization will convert more than 80 per cent of each acute episode to a regular sinus rhythm.

TABLE 1. **Etiologies of Atrial Fibrillation***

1.	Hypertension
2.	Rheumatic heart disease
3.	Coronary artery disease
4.	Thyrotoxicosis
5.	Alcohol toxicity
6.	Pulmonary disease
7.	Pericardial disease
8.	Atrial septal defect
9.	Cardiomyopathy
10.	Pre-excitation
11.	Toxins
12.	Lone atrial fibrillation

*The first five categories are the most common.

After the ventricular rate is controlled or a regular sinus rhythm occurs, the patient can be studied to determine the cause of the arrhythmia. Emboli can occur in approximately 1 to 2 per cent of patients at cardioversion regardless of whether antiarrhythmic drugs or electrical conversion is used. The incidence of emboli at conversion is four to seven times higher if the patient is not anticoagulated. Therefore, I initially try to anticoagulate all my patients prior to cardioversion, especially if the arrhythmia has been present for more than two weeks. The patient is started on coumadin to try to obtain a one and one half to two times elevation of the prothrombin time. Emboli can occur right at the onset of cardioversion or up to ten days post conversion. Because it takes five to eight days to endothelialize a thrombus, I recommended anticoagulation for two weeks prior to cardioversion. The incidence of return to atrial fibrillation is highest in the first month post conversion, and therefore anticoagulation should be continued for at least one month post cardioversion. Some causes of atrial fibrillation such as hypertrophic cardiomyopathy or mitral stenosis have a higher rate of emboli with cardioversion and anticoagulation is extremely important in patients in this group. Emboli can occur in 17 to 40 per cent of patients in whom cardioversion is not successful and atrial fibrillation persists. The higher incidence is seen in those patients with rheumatic heart disease, ischemic heart disease, and cardiomyopathy. Long-term anticoagulation therapy should be considered in such patients.

Cardioversion should be attempted in all symptomatic patients with acute onset to decrease the risk of emboli and hemodynamic consequences of atrial fibrillation. Certain patients should not be candidates unless significant clinical deterioration is present. Patients with sick sinus syndrome (those with a slow ventricular response during atrial fibrillation off of all medications) tend to have atrial fibrillation as an escape mechanism for sinus node dysfunction, and cardioversion can result in asystole. Patients with digoxin toxicity are at risk of ventricular fibrillation with cardioversion. Patients with a history of chronic atrial fibrillation (greater than one year duration) often cannot be cardioverted or they soon revert after conversion. Patients with an enlarged left atrium (greater than 45 mm as measured by echocardiography) have a low incidence of maintaining a sinus rhythm for greater than six months. Other patients, such as those who are intolerant or are noncompliant to a medical regimen, probably are not candidates for cardioversion.

Chemical cardioversion is initially attempted after digoxin has been administered for rate control and the patient has been fully anticoagulated. Quinidine is the drug of choice for chemical cardioversion. Procainamide and disopyramide are other choices. These drugs should be used only after the ventricular rate has been controlled with digoxin because they may increase AV nodal conduction and further increase the rapid ventricular response. Quinidine is used most often at a dosage of 300 mg every six hours. About 20 per cent of patients will revert to sinus rhythm in up to 48 hours. Quinidine, if not successful, is also helpful in improving electrical cardioversion by decreasing energy requirements and controlling incidental arrhythmias.

Elective electrical cardioversion should only be attempted under intensive care settings. The patient should be moved to the intensive care unit with adequate monitoring and resuscitation equipment. Electrolytes should be in balance, and digoxin, quinidine, and food should be withheld the morning of cardioversion. Optimal management includes anesthesiology for airway management. Sedation can be done with methohexital sodium (Brevital) or diazepam (Valium). After sedation is achieved, cardioversion is attempted at 50 joules with a synchronized defibrillator. If unsuccessful, repeated attempts are used with doubling of energy. Some patients with lone atrial fibrillation, coronary artery disease, preexcitation, or cardiomyopathy are somewhat resistant, and therefore 100 joules is usually the initial dose in these groups. After cardioversion, I monitor the patients for 12 hours for possible development of arrhythmias (return of atrial fibrillation) or pulmonary edema. Those patients who are cardioverted are continued on digoxin and quinidine for the prevention of recurrence of the arrhythmia. It is possible to use just quinidine, but the majority of the patients seem to need digoxin for other reasons.

Complications that can occur with cardioversion are asystole (those having a slow ventricular response off of all medications), ventricular fibrillation (from digoxin toxicity or a nonsynchronizing defibrillator), and pulmonary edema secondary to initiation of right atrial contraction with a delay in resumption of left atrial contraction. The success rate for electrical cardioversion is approximately 90 per cent, but maintenance of sinus rhythm for one year is unfortunately only between 30 and 50 per cent.

If cardioversion is unsuccessful or the patient is not a candidate for cardioversion, then the ventricular response should be controlled. The resting rate should be between 60 and 80 beats per minute, and the exercise rate should not increase to greater than 100 to 120 beats per minute. Large doses of digoxin may be needed and can often cause side effects. The addition of a beta-blocker can often be helpful in controlling the rate. Those patients with thyrotoxicosis as the cause of atrial fibrillation respond better to beta blockade than to digoxin therapy. Propranolol additionally blocks the cardioversion of T4 to T3 and therefore controls the rate through decreasing thyroid stimulation and AV nodal conduction. A dosage of 40 mg every six hours can be used but larger dosages are often necessary. Verapamil is another effective drug for controlling the rate through AV nodal blockade. In an emergency it can be given at 60 to 120 micrograms per kg bolus and then orally beginning at 80 mg every eight hours. Although usually ineffective in cardioversion, verapamil is very effective in rate control. Those patients who have a rapid ventricular response with exercise can sometimes be brought under better control with verapamil alone or with digoxin and verapamil together.

Emergency Problems with Atrial Fibrillation

Patients with pre-excitation can have a rapid conduction of flutter waves because of the loss of the decremental conduction of the AV node and a decrease of the refractory period of the accessory pathway. A rapid ventricular response can range from 160 to 300 beats per minute because of conduction through the accessory pathway. Those patients with a short RR interval (less than 200 msec, meaning a very short refractory period) can have a rapid response and actually degenerate into ventricular fibrillation. This group of patients should not be treated with digoxin because digoxin blocks the AV node conduction, shortens the refractory period of the accessory pathway, and so preferentially will favor conduction through the accessory pathway, possibly speeding up the ventricular response. Quinidine is helpful because it slows conduction and prolongs the refractory period in the accessory pathway.

Inderal can also slow conduction and increase the refractory period in the AV node. Some patients are refractory to routine therapy, and experimental therapy with amiodarone (a class III antiarrhythmic) may need to be tried. This drug slows conduction through the accessory pathway and AV node. It is also helpful in preventing the initiation of atrial fibrillation. Amiodarone can be used in doses of 200 to 400 mg but occasionally may need to be used in larger doses ranging from 600 to 800 mg daily.

Rapid atrial fibrillation can cause serious problems with noncompliant ventricles as seen in idiopathic hypertrophic subaortic stenosis (IHSS) or aortic stenosis. This group of patients needs atrial contraction for the booster pump effect to supply adequate preload for maintenance of sufficient cardiac output. The development of atrial fibrillation in most cases can cause vascular collapse, and rapid D/C cardioversion may be needed.

The rapid ventricular rate of atrial fibrillation can also compromise mitral stenosis because of the decrease in diastolic filling time. Although patients may have normal contractility, pulmonary edema can result from increased left atrial pressure because of decreased flow across a stenotic valve with insufficient flow time. Cardioversion may have to be attempted and can be done as an emergency even in those patients who are pregnant. Prophylactic digitalization is often used in mitral stenosis to prevent this possible complication.

Overall, chronic atrial fibrillation is a common entity that has a variable prognosis depending on the type of organic heart disease involved. The addition of atrial fibrillation in those patients with organic heart disease can increase their mortality and morbidity. Those patients with paroxysmal atrial fibrillation and no organic heart disease, however, do not have an increase in mortality or morbidity from the arrhythmia.

PREMATURE BEATS

method of
MARTIN A. ALPERT, M.D.
University of Missouri
Columbia, Missouri

Premature beats may be classified as atrial premature beats (APBs), atrioventricular (AV) junctional premature beats (JPBs), or ventricular premature beats (VPBs) depending on their site of origin. These arrhythmias occur in both normal individuals and persons with organic heart disease. In deciding which patients with premature beats should be treated, the clinician must determine whether unacceptable symptoms attributable to the arrhythmia are present or whether the patient is at risk for developing more serious ventricular arrhythmias. Successful management of patients with premature beats includes careful clinical assessment and a reasonable attempt to identify underlying causes and precipitating factors, in addition to pharmacologic considerations. The clinical and pharmacologic properties of drugs used to treat premature beats are presented in Table 1.

ATRIAL AND AV JUNCTIONAL PREMATURE BEATS

Causes and Precipitating Factors

Both APBs and JPBs may occur in persons with otherwise normal hearts. Anxiety and fatigue are two common physiologic precipitating factors. Pharmaco-

Text continued on page 183

TABLE 1. **Drugs Used in the Treatment of Premature Beats**

Drugs: *Generic Name*	Drugs: *Brand Name*	Route	Usual Dosage	Usual Dosage Schedule	Therapeutic Serum Level (range)*	Side Effects	Clinically Important Drug Interactions
amiodarone†	Cordarone	Oral	200 mg	5 times/day for 10 days then 2–3 times/day	Uncertain	Cardiac: possibly ventricular fibrillation; Other: pulmonary infiltrates (hypersensitivity?), corneal deposits, bluish gray skin discoloration on sun-exposed areas, nausea, constipation, abnormal liver and thyroid function tests, gait disturbances, proximal muscle weakness	Warfarin compounds, quinidine, procainamide, digitalis
bretylium tosylate	Bretylol	IV	5–10 mg/kg diluted in 50 ml D5W administered over 8 min or 1–4 mg/min	Every 6 hours Continuous infusion	Not routinely done	Cardiac: exacerbation of ventricular arrhythmias; Other: hypotension (supine or orthostatic), dizziness, weakness, vertigo, nausea, vomiting	Digitalis (intoxication)
		IM	5–10 mg/kg undiluted	Every 6 hours			
digoxin	Lanoxin Lanoxicaps	Oral Oral	0.125–0.25 mg 0.1–0.2 mg	Daily Daily	0.7–2.0 ng/ml	Cardiac: ventricular ectopic activity, automatic AV junctional arrhythmias, AV block, atrial tachycardia with block; Other: anorexia, nausea, vomiting, diarrhea, visual disturbances, altered sensorium	Quinidine, verapamil, calcium thyroid supplement, sympathomimetic drugs, antacids, kaolin pectin, sulfasalazine, neomycin, cholestyramine
disopyramide phosphate	Norpace Norpace CR	Oral Oral	150 mg 300 mg	Every 6 hours Every 12 hours	2–5 μg/ml	Cardiac: heart failure, AV block, hypotension; Other: dry mucous membranes, blurred vision, glaucoma, urinary hesitancy or retention, bloating, constipation, impotence, possibly hypoglycemia	Quinidine, procainamide, phenytoin
flecainide acetate†	—	Oral	100–200 mg	Every 12 hours	200–1000 ng/ml	Cardiac: exacerbation of ventricular arrhythmia, heart failure, conduction disturbances; Other: abdominal cramps and distention, constipation, flatulence, dry mouth, nausea, vomiting, tremors, dyspnea	None reported

Table continued on opposite page

TABLE 1. **Drugs Used in the Treatment of Premature Beats** *Continued*

Drugs: *Generic Name*	Drugs: *Brand Name*	Route	Usual Dosage	Usual Dosage Schedule	Therapeutic Serum Level (range)*	Side Effects	Clinically Important Drug Interactions
lidocaine hydrochloride	Xylocaine	Oral	50–100 mg bolus infusion followed by continuous infusion at a rate of 1–4 mg/min		2–5 μg/ml	Cardiac: AV block, sinus bradycardia, subsidiary rhythms; Other: hypotension/vascular collapse, apprehension, dizziness, visual abnormalities, altered sensorium, coma, seizures, respiratory arrest	Beta-blockers, cimetidine
mexiletene†	Mexitil	Oral	200 mg	tid	0.8–2.0 μg/ml	Cardiac: possible depression of sinus node function and ventricular conduction; Other: dyspepsia, nausea, tremor, ataxia, dizziness	None reported
phenytoin sodium	Dilantin	Oral	100 mg or 300–400 mg	tid–qid Daily	10–20 μg/ml	Cardiac: asystole AV block, ventricular fibrillation, hypotension; Other: ataxia, dysarthria, nystagmus, lassitude, tremor, nausea and vomiting at toxic levels, gingival hyperplasia, hirsutism, pseudolymphoma, pseudoxanthomas, megaloblastic anemia, pancytopenia, hypersensitivity rash, erythema multiforme, hepatitis, osteomalacia, hypoglycemia	Warfarin anticoagulants, quinidine, disopyramide tolbutamide, chloramphenicol, phenobarbital, INH, phenylbutazone, alcohol, phenothiazines, diazepam, chlordiazepoxide, halothane, carbamazepine, reserpine, estrogens, vitamin D
		IV	50 mg/min, maximum of 500 mg during first hour; maximum of 1000 mg during first 24 hours				
procainamide hydrochloride	Pronestyl	Oral	375–500 mg	Every 3 hours	8–20 μg/ml including NAPA derivative	Cardiac: AV block, asystole; Other: hypotension (usually with IV administration), positive ANA, SLE-like syndrome, agranulocytosis, anorexia, nausea, urticaria and other rashes, pruritus, angioedema	Quinidine, disopyramide
	Pronestyl SR	Oral	50 mg/kg	Divided doses every 6 hours			
	Procan SR	Oral	50 mg/kg	Divided doses every 6 hours			
procainamide hydrochloride injection	—	IM	500–1000 mg	Every 4–8 hours	8–20 μg/ml including NAPA derivative	See procainamide hydrochloride	See procainamide hydrochloride
		IV	100 mg every 5 min until arrhythmia is controlled up to a total dose of 1000 mg or		8–20 μg/ml including NAPA derivative	See procainamide hydrochloride	See procainamide hydrochloride
			2–6 mg/min	Continuous infusion			

Table continued on following page

TABLE 1. **Drugs Used in the Treatment of Premature Beats** *Continued*

Drugs: *Generic Name*	Drugs: *Brand Name*	Route	Usual Dosage	Usual Dosage Schedule	Therapeutic Serum Level (range)*	Side Effects	Clinically Important Drug Interactions
propranolol hydrochloride‡	Inderal	Oral	10–40 mg	Every 6 hours	40–100 ng/ml	Cardiac: heart failure, AV block, sinus node dysfunction, hypotension. Other: bronchospasm, masks hypoglycemia in patients on insulin, lassitude, depression, impotence, dizziness, parasthesias, nausea and vomiting, diarrhea, Raynaud's phenomenon, arterial insufficiency	Reserpine
quinidine gluconate	Quinaglute Duratabs	Oral	324–648 mg	Every 8–12 hours	2.5–5.0 μg/ml	Cardiac: ventricular tachycardia and fibrillation, AV block, asystole; Other: diarrhea, nausea and vomiting, immune hemolytic anemia, immune thrombocytopenia, hypoprothrombinemia, cinchonism, flushing, vascular collapse, respiratory arrest	Warfarin anticoagulants, thiazides, carbonic anhydrase inhibitors, sodium bicarbonate, anticholinesterase drugs, anticholinergic drugs, procainamide and disopyramide, digitalis, antacids, phenobarbital, phenytoin
	Duraquin	Oral	330–660 mg	Every 8– 12 hours			
quinidine gluconate injection	—	IM	200–300 mg	Every 6 hours	2.5–5.0 μg/ml		
quinidine polygalacturonate	Cardioquin	Oral	275 mg	Every 8–12 hours	2.5–5.0 μg/ml	See quinidine gluconate	See quinidine gluconate
quinidine sulfate	Quinora	Oral	200–300 mg	Every 6 hours	2.5–5.0 μg/ml	See quinidine gluconate	See quinidine gluconate
	Cin-quin	Oral	200–300 mg	Every 6 hours			
	Quinidex Extentabs	Oral	600 mg	Every 8–12 hours			
tocainide	Tonocard	Oral	400–600 mg	Every 8 hours	4–10 μg/ml	Cardiac: depression of ventricular conduction; Other: dizziness, tremors, paresthesias/numbness, visual disturbances, nausea and vomiting, diaphoresis, altered sensorium, leukopenia, hypoplastic anemia, thrombocytopenia, possible pulmonary alveolitis/fibrosis	None reported
verapamil	Calan	Oral	80–120 mg	tid	Not routinely done	Cardiac: heart failure, hypotension, depression of sinus and AV node function; Other: peripheral edema, dizziness, fatigue, headache, abnormal liver function tests	Beta-blockers, vasodilators, nitrates, disopyramide, quinidine
	Isoptin	Oral	80–120 mg	tid			

Notes: IV = intravenous, IM = intramuscular, AV = atrioventricular, CR = controlled release, SR = sustained release, ANA = antinuclear antibody, SLE = systemic lupus erythematosus, NAPA = *N*-acetyl procainamide, tid = three times/day, qid = four times/day.

*Therapeutic range at the University of Missouri Health Sciences Center.

†Investigational drug at the time of writing.

‡Most commonly used beta-blocker for cardiac arrhythmias—uncertain whether other beta-blockers are similarly effective.

logic causes include digitalis intoxication and the use of sympathomimetic drugs, caffeine, alcohol, and tobacco (nicotine). Common pathologic causes include atrial enlargement, distention or thickening (from any cause), congestive heart failure, myocardial ischemia or infarction, hypoxia (from any cause), and acute viral illnesses.

Management

APBs and JPBs require treatment only if they (1) produce symptoms that are unacceptable to the patient or (2) herald protracted paroxysms of atrial tachyarrhythmias. Initially, the clinician should attempt to identify and eliminate reversible precipitating factors. For example, it may be useful to advise the patient to switch to decaffeinated coffee, reduce alcohol consumption, or discontinue over-the-counter medications that contain sympathomimetic drugs (e.g., nose drops, cold capsules). If symptomatic APBs or JPBs remain or if protracted paroxysms of atrial tachyarrhythmias recur despite attention to reversible causes, medical therapy should be considered. Digitalis preparations are frequently effective in controlling APBs and JPBs, particularly in patients with left atrial hypertension. Orally administered beta-adrenergic blocking agents may also be useful, particularly in patients with mitral valve prolapse or when excessive catecholamine release is suspected (e.g., anxiety). Orally administered verapamil may also be effective in suppressing APBs and JPBs. Oral quinidine is highly effective in suppressing APBs and JPBs; however, the potential risks of this drug preclude its frequent use for these relatively innocuous arrhythmias. Procainamide and disopyramide are less effective.

VENTRICULAR PREMATURE BEATS

From a therapeutic point of view it is useful to classify VPBs as infrequent (<30 per hour per 24 hours) or frequent (≥30 per hour per 24 hours). Moreover, certain electrocardiographic patterns may have prognostic significance. These are unifocal VPBs (single morphology), multifocal VPBs (multiple morphologies), VPB couplets (pairs), salvos of ventricular tachycardia (three or more ventricular beats in rapid succession), and early cycle ("R on T") VPBs.

Causes and Precipitating Factors

VPBs occur commonly in persons with no other evidence of heart disease. Physiologic causes include anxiety and exercise. VPBs may also occur during bradycardic periods induced by pathologic or reflex mechanisms. Pharmacologic causes include digitalis intoxication; the use of caffeine, tobacco (nicotine), alcohol, and sympathomimetic drugs; the administration of certain general anesthetics; and glue sniffing. VPBs may occur in association with any form of organic heart disease but are particularly common in patients with ischemic heart disease (acute and chronic), valvular heart disease (including mitral valve prolapse), and various cardiomyopathies. They frequently occur in association with congestive heart failure. Other pathologic causes include hypoxia, acidosis, hypokalemia, severe systemic infections, and myocarditis.

Management

Initial efforts in the management of VPBs should be directed at identifying and eliminating reversible causes and precipitating factors. Such efforts may spare the patient the expense and potential morbidity of long-term antiarrhythmic drug therapy. The clinician should also take reasonable steps to determine whether underlying organic heart disease is present. VPBs warrant treatment if they (1) cause symptoms that are unacceptable to the patient or (2) impose excessive risk for sudden cardiac death.

VPBs that occur in persons without organic heart disease do not impose excessive risk for sudden cardia death. Therefore, treatment of asymptomatic individuals is unnecessary. Symptomatic patients should be reassured of the innocuous nature of their problem and advised that the risk associated with antiarrhythmic drug therapy is probably greater than risk associated with VPBs. If symptoms remain unacceptable despite such advice, then treatment should be initiated. Reasonable choices include orally administered quinidine, procainamide, disopyramide, or tocainide. Beta-adrenergic blocking agents may be useful as first line therapy in anxious individuals or those with exercise-induced VPBs but are more commonly used as adjunctive therapy. Oral phenytoin is occasionally useful in association with other antiarrhythmic agents in suppressing VPBs (see Table 1 for drug interactions).

VPBs are common during the first few days after acute myocardial infarction. In such circumstances it has been customary to initiate treatment if patients develop so-called "warning arrhythmias" (VPB patterns that may herald the onset of sustained ventricular tachycardia or ventricular fibrillation). These include ≥6 VPBs per minute, multifocal VPBs, VPB couplets, "R on T" VPBs, and salvos of ventricular tachycardia. Patients with these arrhythmias should receive an intravenous bolus infusion of lidocaine, followed by continuous intravenous infusion of lidocaine (for 2 to 4 days in most cases). Should lidocaine fail to suppress VPBs, procainamide, administered intravenously or intramuscularly (preceded by an intravenous loading dose) may be used to achieve arrhythmia control. Intravenous administration of bretylium should probably be reserved for patients with VPBs that are known harbingers of ventricular tachycardia or ventricular fibrillation. During the past decade increasing numbers of clinicians have used lidocaine prophylactically during the early phases of acute myocardial infarction. This practice is based on studies showing a high incidence of primary ventricular fibrillation (no premonitory ventricular ectopic activity) in patients with acute myocardial infarction. The therapeutic regimen consists of an intravenous bolus administration of lidocaine on admission to the emergency room or coronary care unit, followed by continuous intravenous infusion of lidocaine for 48 hours. In patients with acute myocardial infarction, VPBs may occur during periods of bradycardia. When such occur, the clinician should take appropriate steps to increase the heart rate (e.g., intravenous atropine, temporary pacing) before considering specific antiarrhythmic therapy.

The presence of VPBs during the early phases of acute myocardial infarction does not necessarily imply the need for long-term antiarrhythmic drug therapy. However, certain VPB patterns observed after the first week appear to be associated with an inordinately high incidence of sudden cardiac death during the ensuing year. Should 24 hour ambulatory electrocardiographic monitoring disclose frequent unifocal or multifocal VPBs, repetitive VPB couplets, "R on T" VPBs, or ventricular tachycardia, then treatment with quinidine, procainamide, disopyramide, or tocainide should be considered. If VPBs persist, the addition of a beta-adrenergic blocking agent may facilitate arrhythmia control in some patients by reducing myocardial oxygen demand. This is a particularly important consideration for patients with exercise-induced VPBs. Phenytoin may rarely be useful as adjunctive therapy. Antiarrhythmic drug therapy should be continued for 3 to 6 months. Ambulatory electrocardiographic monitoring should then be repeated with the patient off drugs to determine the need for long-term antiarrhythmic therapy.

Despite intense investigative interest in the prognosis of patients with chronic ischemic heart disease and VPBs, considerable controversy exists over whom to treat. Infrequent unifocal and multifocal VPBs are associated with negligible risk for sudden cardiac arrest, hence treatment is unnecessary unless unacceptable symptoms are present. There is a progressive increase in the risk for sudden cardiac death in patients with frequent unifocal VPBs, frequent multifocal VPBs, repetitive VPB couplets, short runs of ventricular tachycardia, and "R on T" VPBs. For this reason, a trial of antiarrhythmic drug therapy would seem justifiable in such patients whether they are asymptomatic or symptomatic. Yet many authorities recommend therapy only for patients with VPB patterns associated with the highest risk of sudden cardiac death (VPB couplets, ventricular tachycardia, and "R on T" VPBs).

Orally administered quinidine, procainamide, disopyramide, and tocainide are all reasonable choices for initial therapy of VPBs in patients with chronic ischemic heart disease. The addition of an oral beta-adrenergic blocking agent to the primary antiarrhythmic drug regimen may facilitate arrhythmia control in some cases by reducing myocardial oxygen demand. Phenytoin may occasionally be useful as adjunctive therapy.

Little information exists concerning the risk for sudden cardiac death in patients with other forms of chronic organic heart disease who have VPBs. Until reliable prognostic information becomes available it seems reasonable for the clinician to manage such patients much as he would patients with chronic ischemic heart disease. Possible exceptions to this policy include patients with mitral valve prolapse, hypertrophic cardiomyopathy, or one of the nonacquired delayed repolarization (long QT) syndromes. Patients with mitral valve prolapse or hypertrophic cardiomyopathy and VPBs may derive greatest benefit from therapy with beta-adrenergic blocking agents (very high doses may be required in hypertrophic cardiomyopathy). Quinidine, procainamide, and disopyramide should be considered as alternative or adjunctive therapy in these patients and then only in those with normal corrected QT intervals. The role of tocainide for such patients is uncertain.

In patients with one of the nonacquired delayed repolarization syndromes (Jervell and Lange-Nielsen syndrome, Romano-Ward syndrome) and some patients with mitral valve prolapse, the drug of choice for treatment of VPBs is oral propranolol (whether other beta-adrenergic glocking agents are similarly effective is unknown). Orally administered phenytoin alone or in combination with propranolol may also be effective in such cases. When ventricular tachycardia or fibrillation recurs despite appropriate medical therapy, atrial pacing may be required for arrhythmia prophylaxis. Quinidine, procainamide, and disopyramide are specifically contraindicated in patients with any of the delayed repolarization syndromes, since they may produce inordinate QT interval prolongation and markedly increase the risk for sustained ventricular arrhythmias. The role of tocainide in these patients is uncertain.

The presence of left ventricular dysfunction, with or without clinical congestive heart failure, further increases the risk for sudden cardiac death in patients with ischemic heart disease and VPBs (and presumably in patients with other forms of organic heart disease and VPBs). Moreover, left ventricular dysfunction may actually precipitate ventricular ectopic activity in such patients. Accordingly, treatment with digitalis and other measures aimed at improving left ventricular performance may reduce the frequency and severity of VPBs and thus improve prognosis.

VPBs are observed commonly in patients suffering from digitalis intoxication, frequently occurring in bigeminal or multifocal patterns. Such patients should be hospitalized and should undergo electrocardiographic monitoring. Digitalis should be withdrawn and low serum potassium concentrations should be corrected by oral or intravenous supplementation. Infrequent unifocal or multifical VPBs require no specific therapy. Frequent unifocal or multifocal VPBs, VPB couplets, short salvos of ventricular tachycardia, and "R on T" VPBs all may predispose to sustained ventricular arrhythmias and should therefore be treated.

Intravenous administration of lidocaine (bolus injection followed by continuous infusion) is usually successful in suppressing ventricular arrhythmias associated with digitalis intoxication. Should lidocaine fail to suppress these arrhythmias, then intravenous administration of phenytoin should be considered. If intravenous phenytoin is successful in suppressing the ventricular arrhythmia, then oral phenytoin should be administered until the danger of digitalis intoxication has passed. Intravenous procainamide is less effective than lidocaine or phenytoin in suppressing ventricular arrhythmias in the setting of digitalis intoxication. Therapy with bretylium should probably be reserved for refractory sustained ventricular arrhythmias or VPBs that are known harbingers of such rhythm disturbances.

Enthusiasm for chronic treatment of VPBs is tempered by four major considerations. (1) Conventional antiarrhythmic agents are relatively ineffective in suppressing VPBs. For example, quinidine, the most effective antiarrhythmic drug, significantly suppresses ventricular ectopic activity in only 50 to 60 per cent of those receiving the drug. (2) There is no reliable evidence that conventional antiarrhythmic drug therapy of VPBs reduces the incidence of sudden cardiac death. (3) The incidence of formidable side effects of such drugs is extraordinarily high (see Table 1). (4) The cost of conventional antiarrhythmic drug therapy remains high. These drawbacks force the clinician to critically examine and reexamine the potential risks and benefits associated with antiarrhythmic drug therapy on a case by case basis before initiating treatment.

Three drugs, presently under investigation in the United States, appear to hold promise in the treatment of ventricular arrhythmias: amiodarone, mexiletene, and flecanide (see Table 1). All these drugs are substantially more effective in suppressing VPBs than conventional agents. Amiodarone appears to be more effective than mexiletene, flecainide, or conventional antiarrhythmic drugs in preventing ectopic ventricular arrhythmias and is also useful in suppressing atrial arrhythmias, including those in patients with an accessory conduction pathway. Routine use of amiodarone, however, may be precluded by potentially life-threatening pulmonary side effects (see Table 1). Mexiletene administration is frequently associated with gastrointestinal disturbances (mainly dypepsia and nausea), which usually respond to antacid therapy. Flecainide is relatively free of serious or limiting side effects. Clinical studies are nearing completion on all three drugs, and they will likely be available for general use in the United States by the time of publication. Other drugs currently under investigation for use in patients with ventricular arrhythmias include ajmaline, aprindine, bepridil cibenzoline, encainide, ethmozine, lorcainide, permenol, and propaferone.

Serum drug levels are routinely available for most conventional antiarrhythmic drugs and provide an invaluable tool for efficient and effective control of ventricular arrhythmias. By adjusting drug dosages to achieve therapeutic serum levels the clinician saves time and avoids unnecessary repetition of diagnostic tests.

HEART BLOCK

method of
ALBERT A. DEL NEGRO, M.D., FACC
Georgetown University
Washington, D.C.

Normally, transmission of the sinus node impulse to the ventricle occurs from the high right atrium to the atrioventricular node by way of specialized intra-atrial conduction fibers. This transmission is exceedingly rapid and takes less than 0.05 second. Passage of the electrical wave front through the atrioventricular (AV) node is much slower and takes up to 0.14 second. Once through the AV node, rapid propagation through the bundle of His occurs. This is the final common pathway prior to division into the main left and right bundle branches.

Both halves of the autonomic nervous system ennervate that portion of the conduction system where clinically important heart block may occur. Impulse conduction is in fact modulated by the interplay between these two limbs of the central nervous system, but parasympathetic influences on impulse conduction and automaticity appear to be absent below the human mid bundle of His. Thus, for AV nodal block due to inferior myocardial infarction, default to a relatively reliable junctional (i.e., His bundle) rhythm means that extreme bradycardia, if it occurs at all, may be countered by reducing parasympathetic influences with atropine. In fact, this may entirely relieve the heart block. Bilateral bundle branch block due to anteroseptal myocardial infarction occurs below the level of parasympathetic influence on conduction, and withdrawal of parasympathetic tone will neither speed the idioventricular pacemaker, which thereafter assumes control, nor abolish heart block. Because idioventricular rhythm is ordinarily quite inappropriately slow, it follows that block below the bundle of His is the more clinically dangerous form.

This understanding of the clinical importance of the locus of heart block has led to the designations "proximal," or more benign AV nodal block, and "distal," or more dangerous infra-His block. Commonly, pacemaker therapy is not recommended for proximal block but is almost always required for distal block.

Management

First Degree AV Block

First degree AV block is defined as a PR interval of greater than 0.20 second. Ordinarily, in the absence of second or third degree AV block, first degree block needs no therapy. It is commonly due to an increase in AV nodal conduction time. Excessive use of digitalis, beta-blockers, or verapamil is a reversible iatrogenic cause of first degree AV block owing to the effect these drugs have on prolonging AV nodal conduction time. Alternatively, bilateral bundle branch delay is also a cause for first degree AV block although AV nodal conduction may be normal. This latter form of first degree AV block is indistinguishable from that due to AV nodal delay on the surface electrocardiogram and may be aggravated by the use of drugs such as quinidine or procainamide.

Second Degree AV Block

This form of heart block occurs when some or any of the normal sinus P waves fail to be conducted to the ventricle. Usually, if the block lies in the AV node, it is benign, disappears with exercise, and needs no treatment. If the block lies instead within the bundle branches, gradual progression to higher degrees of AV block, as well as the need for pacemaker therapy, can be expected. Note that both types of second degree AV block, proximal and distal, may initially not be associated with symptoms so that the decision for pacemaker therapy relies on discovering the locus of the block.

One may easily distinguish between proximal and distal second degree AV block on the basis of electrocardiographic patterns. Wenckebach or Mobitz I block associated with a narrow QRS is classically located within the AV node. As indicated previously, this is usually benign and requires therapy only if extreme bradycardia or hemodynamic compromise occurs. Wenckebach patterns with a QRS duration of 0.12 second or greater are also most commonly due to AV nodal block. However, 25 to 30 per cent of patients with this latter pattern may have block in the distal system instead of the AV node. Patients in this group should undergo electrophysiologic study to define the locus of block with certainty.

Mobitz II block refers to 3:2 or lower ratios of AV conduction in which all the PR intervals are the same. The fixed AV conduction times of this type of block are characteristic of the "all or nothing" response of conduction in the distal system. It is no surprise, then, that Mobitz II conduction patterns are seen only in distal block. For this reason, this form of second degree AV block warrants pacing therapy even in the asymptomatic patient, since progression to higher grades of block are expected and are associated with extreme bradycardia.

Finally, any form of second degree AV block associated with symptoms clearly due to bradycardia warrants permanent pacing therapy. This is true irrespective of the locus of block.

Third Degree Heart Block

Without the association of P wave and QRS to describe an AV relationship and so estimate the locus of block, third degree AV block presents a special challenge. Certain decisions can nonetheless be made on the basis of noninvasive assessment. If there is a profoundly slow heart rate, especially in the presence of symptoms of bradycardia, then pacing therapy is clearly indicated. If there are no symptoms, heart rate is usually not profoundly slow, and no therapy may be necessary, especially if appropriate rate acceleration occurs with atropine or exercise. This response predicts that the locus of block is in the AV node. Lack of rate increase with exercise or administration of atropine indicates block in the distal system, usually associated with a ventricular escape mechanism, which is quite slow. Of course, pacing therapy is indicated in this latter case. When symptoms are absent and there is indecision about the significance of the heart block, the issue can be resolved by an intracardiac electrophysiologic study to define the locus of block. A decision regarding therapy may be made based on this study. See Table 1.

Heart Block in Acute Myocardial Infarction

Both acute anterior and inferior myocardial infarction may be associated with heart block.

TABLE 1. **Clinical and Anatomic Correlations in Heart Block**

Locus	AV node (proximal)	Bundle Branches (distal)
Escape mechanism	junctional	Idioventricular
Exacerbating drugs	digitalis β-blockers verapamil	quinidine procainamide lidocaine
Myocardial infarction	inferior	anterior
Clinical course	reversible	progressive
Therapy	atropine, rarely pacemaker	pacemaker

By far, this is more common in inferior infarction where the heart block is commonly due to reflex vagal effects or direct ischemic effects on the AV node. This may be successfully treated pharmacologically with intravenous atropine, 0.5 to 1.0 mg intravenously, or not treated at all if heart rate is not slow and hemodynamics are stable. Only drug-refractory bradyarrhythmias that compromise hemodynamics or encourage ventricular ectopy warrant temporary pacing therapy. Permanent pacing is virtually never required, since recovery of heart block associated with an inferior infarct is the rule.

Heart block in anterior myocardial infarction is due to necrosis in and around the proximal bundle branch system. Such patients will be refractory to atropine, and heart rate is usually profoundly slow. Emergency treatment is required and consists of immediate temporary transvenous pacing. If no recovery from heart block occurs, permanent pacing is performed prior to discharge from the hospital. Even if there is resumption of conduction, many clinicians still perform permanent pacing, since recurrence is common.

Heart block in anterior infarction may be anticipated if there is a new conduction disturbance caused by the infarction. Some investigators predict the risk of at least transient AV block in 40 per cent of patients with acute anterior infarction if a new right bundle branch block is found. Prophylactic temporary pacing is warranted in this situation.

The use of chronotropic stimulants for the bradyarrhythmia of heart block in acute infarction is to be avoided, except as a last resort, because of the known risk of provoking lethal ventricular arrhythmias. Isoproterenol, 1 microgram per minute intravenously, may be used cautiously. It is desirable to avoid antiarrhythmics such as lidocaine or procainamide until pacing therapy is established, since these agents will slow the rate of the escape focus.

Specific Pacing Therapies

Temporary Pacing

Temporary transvenous pacing is performed by the introduction of a temporary pacing electrode percutaneously from the femoral vein, the subclavian vein, or the internal jugular vein. The catheter is passed by fluoroscopic guidance to the apex of the right ventricle. Adequate parameters for ventricular pacing and sensing should be assured. Malposition of the lead in the coronary sinus and down its first tributary, the posterior interventricular vein, is common when the approach is from above. This is detected by right bundle branch block on pacing rather than the expected left bundle branch block of right ventricular pacing. Most patients can adequately be treated by this technique alone; however, hemodynamic compromise is a possible complication because of the loss of the atrial contribution to ventricular filling. Stroke volume may be quite low despite the increase in rate, and hypotension will occur. For patients with this complication, temporary AV sequential pacing may be performed. Lead systems for atrial and ventricular pacing are available with atrial pacing and sensing performed from the right atrial appendage or the coronary sinus. Special AV sequential pacemakers are generally available for temporary pacing.

The spontaneous displacement rate of temporary cardiac pacing leads is as high as 20 per cent. This requires a daily assessment of the integrity of the entire pacing system including threshold measurement and evaluation of sensing. Should the lead become displaced, it must be repositioned or replaced.

The electrical isolation of the temporary pacemaker is of great importance. Sixty cycle currents from improperly isolated electrically operated equipment can be conducted directly to the myocardium and can induce ventricular fibrillation. This is avoided by placing the pacemaker in a surgical glove and sealing it with adhesive tape. Daily wound care can ensure absence of infection, and carefully maintained systems can be used for several days.

Permanent Pacing

Permanent pacing is performed by placing a pacing electrode in the heart by the percutaneous subclavian approach (both atrial and ventricular leads may be simultaneously inserted using a single sheath) or by cephalic or jugular vein cutdown. A subcutaneous pocket of adequate size to accommodate the pulse generator is created adjacent to the initial lead insertion site and parameters for pacing and sensing are obtained. Depending on these parameters, the pulse generator will be programmed for optimal rate, sensing, output, and AV interval if a dual chamber pacer is implanted. Such a procedure obviously requires skill and considerable expertise as well as intimate knowledge of the engineering aspects of the pulse generator used.

Following implantation, observation in a monitored setting is necessary to ensure normal pacer function and lack of arrhythmia. Commonest among postimplantation malfunctions are lack of sensing, mechanically stimulated premature ventricular beats, and loss of cardiac capture. These are most commonly due to lead displacement, but they frequently may be overcome by a programming change if the pulse generator is programmable. This obviates the need for additional surgery and argues for the exclusive use of programmable pacemakers.

Physiologic or "universal" pulse generators are now commonly used. They allow a greater latitude of choices for pacing modes, and their versatility allows one to overcome placing complications, such as undersensing and inducible arrhythmias without the need for repeat surgery. Some newer models even have automatic tachycardia recognition and reversion modes. These generators are quite complex and are capable of their own set of engineering-based complications, such as the induction of a reciprocating tachycardia. Newer models possess a wide range of refractory periods to prevent this complication.

TACHYCARDIA

method of
ERIC N. PRYSTOWSKY, M.D.,
and DOUGLAS P. ZIPES, M.D.
Indiana University
Indianapolis, Indiana

Arrhythmias may be caused by disorders of impulse formation (automaticity), disorders of impulse conduction (re-entry), or combinations of both. Only indirect evidence exists to enable a clinical classification of arrhythmias according to pathogenesis. In addition, an arrhythmia may be initiated and perpetuated by different mechanisms. For example, spontaneous diastolic depolarization (automaticity) may trigger a premature atrial or ventricular complex that initiates an arrhythmia maintained by re-entry. Thus, the clinical classification of tachycardias according to mechanism remains speculative to a degree. Antiarrhythmic agents specifically indicated to treat one mechanism or the other do not yet exist.

Supported in part by the Herman C. Krannert Fund, Indianapolis; by Grants HL-06308 and HL-07182 from the National Heart, Lung and Blood Institute of the National Institutes of Health, Bethesda, Maryland; by the Attorney General of Indiana Public Health Trust and the Roudebush Veterans Administration Medical Center, Indianapolis; and by a Grant-in-Aid from the American Heart Association, Indiana Affiliate, Inc., Indianapolis, Indiana.

SUPRAVENTRICULAR ARRHYTHMIAS

We have divided supraventricular tachycardia (SVT) into three groups based on the therapeutic approach to be taken in each case. It should be noted that the term *paroxysmal atrial tachycardia (PAT)* does not appear in our classification. Many physicians consider PAT to be a specific arrhythmia—for example, AV nodal re-entry—whereas other physicians use the term to designate any SVT that is intermittent and starts and stops suddenly. If the mechanism of a paroxysmal tachycardia is known, such as atrial fibrillation, the arrhythmia should be classified as paroxysmal atrial fibrillation. If the mechanism is unknown, we prefer the term *paroxysmal supraventricular tachycardia (PSVT)*.

Group I

Sinus tachycardia, owing to enhanced discharge of the sinus node, maintains a rate of between 100 and 160 per minute but may be higher with extreme exertion and in infants. The P-P interval may vary slightly from cycle to cycle. P waves have a normal contour but may develop a larger amplitude and become peaked. Carotid sinus massage, the Valsalva maneuver, or other vagal maneuvers gradually slow a sinus tachycardia, which then accelerates to its previous rate. More rapid sinus rates may fail to slow in response to a vagal maneuver. Sinus tachycardia is the normal reaction to a variety of physiologic and pathophysiologic stresses, such as fever, hypotension, thyrotoxicosis, anemia, anxiety, exertion, hypovolemia, pulmonary emboli, myocardial ischemia, congestive heart failure, or shock. Inflammation such as pericarditis may produce sinus tachycardia. Sinus tachycardia is usually of no physiologic significance; however, in patients with organic myocardial disease, reduced cardiac output, congestive heart failure, or arrhythmias may result. Since heart rate is a major determinant of oxygen requirements, angina or perhaps an increase in the size of an infarction may accompany persistent sinus tachycardia in patients with coronary artery disease. Chronic nonparoxysmal sinus tachycardia may occur in otherwise healthy persons, possibly due to increased automaticity of the sinus node or an automatic atrial focus located near the sinus node.

Treatment

Therapy should be directed toward correcting the underlying disease state that caused the sinus tachycardia. Elimination of tobacco, alcohol, coffee, tea, or other stimulants (e.g., sympathomimetic agents in nose drops) may be helpful. If sinus tachycardia is not secondary to a correctable physiologic stress, then treatment with sedatives, beta-adrenergic blockers, and verapamil may be helpful.

Group II

There are two common types of supraventricular tachycardia in which the AV node participates in the re-entrant circuit. In AV nodal re-entry, most, if not all, of the re-entrant circuit utilizes AV nodal tissue for antegrade and retrograde conduction. In patients who have an accessory pathway (Wolff-Parkinson-White [WPW] syndrome), during AV re-entrant tachycardia antegrade conduction occurs most commonly over the AV node and retrograde conduction occurs over the accessory pathway.

In both AV nodal and AV re-entrant tachycardia, the heart rate is usually between 150 and 200 per minute and 1:1 AV conduction is present, although AV block may rarely occur in AV nodal re-entry. In many instances, AV nodal tachycardia cannot be differentiated in an electrocardiogram from AV re-entrant tachycardia. In general, the tachycardia rate usually is faster in AV re-entry ($>$ 175 per minute) than in AV nodal re-entry ($<$ 170 per minute), but considerable overlap is present. Furthermore, patients who have AV nodal tachycardia are usually older and more frequently have associated organic heart disease than do patients with AV re-entry.

None of these variables are specific enough to differentiate between the two arrhythmias. However, three ECG features are diagnostically helpful. First, during the tachycardia, a negative P wave recorded in ECG lead I occurs in some patients who have AV re-entry with retrograde atrial conduction occurring over a left-sided accessory pathway; negative P waves do not occur in lead I in patients who have AV nodal tachycardia. Second, a slower tachycardia rate during functional bundle branch block (i.e., QRS width $>$ 120 ms), compared with the tachycardia rate during normal ventricular conduction, demonstrates that part of the ventricular conduction system is utilized in the tachycardia circuit. This may occur in AV re-entry but not in AV nodal re-entry. Third, the timing of atrial depolarization, determined by atrial electrograms recorded on an esophageal or intra-atrial electrode, in relation to ventricular depolarization may yield important diagnostic information.

During AV nodal tachycardia, atrial and ventricular depolarizations often occur simultaneously. In contrast, during AV re-entrant tachycardia, atrial depolarization must occur after ventricular depolarization, since a requisite amount of time is necessary for conduction to proceed through the ventricle and over the accessory pathway. Therefore, if atrial and ventricular depolarizations occur simultaneously during a tachycardia, AV re-entry is excluded and AV nodal re-entry is suggested.

Acute Treatment

Treatment of the acute attack depends on the clinical situation and the consequences of the arrhythmia, the natural history of the attacks in the individual patient, and the presence of associated disease. For some patients, rest, reassurance, and sedation may be all that are required to abort an attack. Since AV nodal conduction is essential to the maintenance of both AV nodal and AV re-entrant tachycardia, initial therapy is directed at interrupting AV nodal conduction.

1. *Vagal maneuvers.* Carotid sinus massage and the Valsalva maneuver increase vagal tone and may abruptly terminate tachycardia. (Actually, there is often a slight slowing of the tachycardia rate prior to termination.) Before massaging the carotid sinus, one should auscultate the neck to check for carotid bruits; if a bruit is present, it is advisable to massage the opposite carotid sinus. Right and left carotid sinus massage should not be performed simultaneously. Furthermore, carotid sinus massage should be performed cautiously in patients who are taking digitalis because ventricular arrhythmias or asystole or both may occur. If these maneuvers do not terminate the tachycardia, one may immerse the patient's hands or face in ice water for 2 to 5 seconds. Facial immersion is unpleasant and often painful for the patient but may enhance vagal tone significantly. If unsuccessful initially, these maneuvers should be tried again after each pharmacologic approach.
2. *Verapamil* (Calan, Isoptin), 5 to 10 mg intravenously, has become the treatment of choice should simple vagal maneuvers fail. Diltiazem (Cardizem) may also be effective but is still an investigational drug for treating arrhythmias. Intravenous verapamil should not be given to patients with atrial fibrillation who demonstrate antegrade conduction to the ventricle over an accessory pathway.
3. *Cholinergic drugs* prevent acetylcholinesterase from degrading acetylcholine, thereby enhancing vagal tone. Edrophonium chloride (Tensilon), a short-acting cholinesterase inhibitor, may be given initially at a dose of 3 to 5

mg intravenously (investigational for this use), and, if unsuccessful, repeated at a dose of 10 mg intravenously. Its action is rapid in onset and short in duration, with minimal side effects. Edrophonium should be used cautiously or not at all in patients who are hypotensive or who have lung disease, especially a history of asthma.

4. *Propranolol* (Inderal) may be administered to patients who have no contraindications to beta-adrenergic blockade. We give 1 mg intravenously over 15 seconds as a test dose, and if no adverse reactions occur within 1 minute, follow this with additional propranolol (0.15 mg per kg, to a maximal dose of 12 mg) at a rate of 1 mg per minute until the tachycardia ceases or blood pressure falls. The patient's clinical status and blood pressure should be re-evaluated after each 1 mg aliquot of propranolol.
5. *Pressor drugs* may terminate tachycardia by inducing reflex vagal stimulation mediated by baroreceptors in the carotid sinus and aorta when the systolic blood pressure is acutely elevated to levels of about 180 mm Hg. One of the following drugs, diluted in 5 to 10 ml of 5 per cent dextrose and water, may be given intravenously over 1 to 3 minutes: phenylephrine (Neo-Synephrine), 0.5 to 1.0 mg; methoxamine (Vasoxyl), 3 to 5 mg; or metaraminol (Aramine) (investigational for this use), 0.5 to 2.0 mg. Pressor drugs should be used cautiously or not at all in the elderly and in patients with organic heart disease, significant hypertension, hyperthyroidism, or acute myocardial infarction. This potentially dangerous procedure is rarely needed unless the patient is also hypotensive, a situation in which electrical cardioversion should also be considered.
6. *Digitalis.* This drug may be given to patients whose tachycardia is known (e.g., by previous electrophysiologic studies) to be caused by AV nodal re-entry or AV re-entry using an accessory pathway that is incapable of antegrade conduction (concealed accessory pathway). We discourage the administration of digitalis as a single drug to patients who have WPW syndrome, or to patients in whom no previous ECG is available to evaluate the presence of WPW syndrome.

   Digitalis can facilitate antegrade conduction over accessory pathways in some patients, and if the re-entrant tachycardia converts to atrial fibrillation during administration of digitalis, a rapid ventricular response may occur and produce hypotension or even ventricular fibrillation on occasion. If digitalis is used, one of the following regimens may be tried: ouabain, 0.25 to 0.50 mg intravenously, followed by 0.1 mg every 30 to 60 minutes if needed, keeping the total dose less than 1.0 mg within a 24 hour period; digoxin (Lanoxin), 0.5 to 1.0 mg intravenously, followed by 0.25 mg every 2 to 4 hours, with a total dose less than 1.5 mg within a 24 hour period; or deslanoside (Cedilanid-D), 0.8 mg intravenously, followed by 0.4 mg every 2 to 4 hours, restricting the total dose to less than 2.0 mg within a 24 hour period. Oral digitalis administration to terminate an acute attack is generally not indicated. Vagal maneuvers, previously ineffective, may terminate tachycardia after digitalis administration and therefore should be repeated.
7. *Procainamide.* If a patient has re-entrant tachycardia utilizing an accessory pathway, one may give intravenous procainamide (10 to 14 mg per kg, to a maximal dose of 1000 mg) to try to block conduction over the accessory pathway. We give procainamide in 50 mg doses every minute. Before each subsequent dose, the patient's blood pressure, QRS complex, and Q-T interval should be evaluated. Procainamide may also terminate AV nodal re-entry in some patients.
8. *Electrical therapy.* Prior to administering digitalis, propranolol, procainamide, or pressor drugs, it is advisable to reassess the clinical status of the patient and consider whether electrical therapy (atrial pacing or DC shock) should be used at this stage. DC shock, after patients have received excessive amounts of digitalis, may be dangerous and result in serious postshock ventricular arrhythmias. If digitalis has been given, it is preferable to terminate the arrhythmia with atrial pacing using either an esophageal or intra-atrial pacing catheter. If signs of cardiac decompensation occur, DC electrical shock should be considered early. DC shock, synchronized to the QRS complex to avoid precipitation of ventricular fibrillation, successfully terminates AV and AV nodal tachycardia with energies in the range of 10 to 50 watt-seconds; higher energies may be required in some instances. We prefer using short-acting barbiturates like methohexital (Brevital), given intravenously, to provide anesthesia. Dosages must be individualized and in general should be reduced for patients with heart failure, hypotension, or liver disease.

During DC cardioversion, a physician skilled in airway management should be in attendance, an intravenous route established, and all equipment and drugs necessary for emergency resuscitation immediately accessible. Oxygen, 100 per cent, is administered throughout the procedure, employing manual assisted ventilation if required. If DC shock becomes necessary in patients who have received large amounts of digitalis, one should begin with 1 to 5 watt-seconds and gradually increase the energy level in increments of approximately 25 to 50 watt-seconds as long as ventricular extrasystoles do not result. If ventricular extrasystoles occur but can be suppressed with lidocaine or phenytoin, the next higher energy level may be tried.

Chronic Treatment

Prevention of recurrences is often more difficult than terminating the acute episode. Precipitating factors such as smoking, alcohol, caffeine, and excessive fatigue, if identified, should be avoided. Initially, one must decide whether the frequency and severity of the attacks warrant drug prophylaxis. For example, tachycardia associated with minimal symptoms occurring twice yearly in an otherwise healthy patient should probably not be treated chronically.

Choice of therapy also depends on whether tachycardia is due to AV nodal or AV re-entry. In patients with AV nodal re-entry or re-entry using a concealed accessory bypass tract that lacks antegrade conduction, digitalis is our initial drug of choice. In patients with AV re-entry and manifest WPW—that is, the presence of a delta wave in the sinus-conducted QRS complex—we do not recommend digitalis as single drug therapy unless electrophysiologic evaluation has shown that the accessory pathway is *not* capable of rapid antegrade conduction during atrial fibrillation. Digitalis can shorten accessory pathway antegrade refractoriness, and, in patients with rapidly conducting accessory pathways, very rapid ventricular responses may ensue during atrial fibrillation and lead to ventricular fibrillation in some instances. In these patients we recommend starting therapy with quinidine (Cardioquin, Cin-Quin, Duraquin, Quinaglute, Quinidex, Quinora), procainamide (Procan SR, Pronestyl SR) or disopyramide (Norpace, Norpace-CR) (not FDA-approved for use in SVT), with the possible addition of digitalis, propranolol, or verapamil to effect AV nodal conduction. Generally, in patients with AV re-entry we usually begin treatment with disopyramide as a single agent, starting with 400 to 600 mg daily, because disopyramide has a relatively low frequency of side effects and demonstrated efficacy in these patients.

Oral verapamil (not FDA-approved for this use) can effectively prevent recurrence of either AV nodal or AV re-entry, and quinidine, procainamide, and disopyramide can also be used alone or with digitalis, verapamil, or propranolol to prevent episodes of AV nodal re-entry. Propranolol is usually ineffective as a single agent unless the arrhythmia is related to exercise but may be helpful in combination therapy. If more than one drug is used, particular attention should be given to drug interactions—for example, increased plasma digoxin levels during concomitant verapamil or quinidine therapy.

1. *Digitalis*. The speed at which digitalization is achieved is determined by the clinical situation. Using digoxin, rapid oral digitalization can be accomplished in 24 to 36 hours with an initial dose of 1.0 to 1.5 mg, followed by 0.25 to 0.5 mg every 6 hours for a total dose of 2.0 to 3.0 mg. A less rapid oral regimen digitalizes in 2 to 3 days with an initial dose of 0.75 to 1.0 mg, followed by 0.25 to 0.5 mg every 12 hours for a total dose of 2.0 to 3.0 mg. Finally, digoxin administered as a maintenance dose of 0.125 to 0.5 mg daily achieves digitalization in about 1 week. Because of its shorter half-life, digoxin may provide more effective control when administered twice daily. Digitoxin (Crystodigin), which has a longer duration of action, may be used instead of digoxin. Oral digitalization with digitoxin may be accomplished in 24 to 36 hours with an initial dose of 0.5 to 0.8 mg, followed by 0.2 mg every 6 to 8 hours until reaching a total dose of 1.2 mg. A slower approach involves administering 0.2 mg three times daily for 2 or 3 days. Complete digitalization can also be accomplished in about 1 month by simply giving a maintenance dose, 0.05 to 0.2 mg daily.
2. *Propranolol* can be given at 40 to 160 mg daily. Verapamil is usually administered at 80 to 120 mg three to four times daily.
3. *Usual dosages* are 300 to 500 mg four times daily for quinidine sulfate; for long-acting procainamide hydrochloride (Procan-SR; Pronestyl-SR), 500 to 1000 mg four times daily; and for disopyramide phosphate (Norpace), 100 to 200 mg four times daily or 200 to 400 mg twice daily (Norpace CR).
4. *Pacemaker implantation*. In certain carefully selected individuals, pacemaker implantation provides a reasonable, and often preferable, form of therapy. Pacemakers are either automatic or patient-activated. This form of therapy should be considered only after extensive electrophysiologic evaluation has demonstrated pacing to be both effective and safe.

Group III

These arrhythmias are grouped together because the initial therapeutic goal often is to slow the ventricular response of the atrial or junctional tachycardia. If the atrial rate is not rapid (e.g., 100 to 130 per minute) or the ventricular response is slow (e.g., 60 to 100 per minute), no immediate therapy may be necessary. If one decides to decrease the ventricular response, digitalis is usually the drug of choice, provided the arrhythmia has not resulted from digitalis toxicity.

Sinus Nodal Re-Entry

Sinus nodal re-entry is characterized by average atrial rates of 130 to 140 per minute (range, 80 to 200 per minute) associated with P waves that electrocardiographically are identical or very similar to the sinus P wave morphology. AV block may occur without affecting the tachycardia, and vagal meneuvers may slow and then abruptly terminate the tachycardia. Most patients do not require therapy, for the rate of tachycardia often is relatively slow and well tolerated and the episodes are self-terminating. If treatment is necessary, propranolol, digitalis, or verapamil may be tried.

Atrial Tachycardia (With or Without Block)

Atrial tachycardia may be automatic or reentrant. The presence of AV block depends on the rate of tachycardia, the conduction properties of the AV node and His-Purkinje system, and concomitant drug therapy. The atrial rate is usually between 150 and 200 per minute, with a range of 150 to 250 per minute. When caused by digitalis excess, the atrial rate is generally less than 200 per minute and may be noted to increase gradually as the digitalis is continued. The AV block is generally of the Wenckebach variety. Vagal maneuvers may increase the degree of AV block but usually do not terminate the arrhythmia.

A different type of atrial tachycardia, multifocal or chaotic atrial tachycardia, is characterized by atrial rates of 100 to 250 per minute, associated with marked variation in P wave morphology ($\geq$ 3 P wave contours) and totally irregular P-P intervals. This tachycardia occurs commonly in patients with pulmonary disease, especially during acute respiratory failure, and in diabetes mellitus and is rarely produced by digitalis. Eventual development of atrial fibrillation is not uncommon. Therapy for multifocal atrial tachycardia should be primarily directed toward the underlying disease, and antiarrhythmic agents are often ineffective in slowing the atrial tachycardia rate or the ventricular response. In patients with pulmonary disease we prefer to use verapmil instead of digitalis or beta-adrenergic blockers.

Treatment

If the ventricular rate is in a normal range and the patient is asymptomatic, no therapy may be necessary.

1. Very slow ventricular rates may respond to atropine (0.5 mg increments intravenously) or, rarely, may require ventricular pacing.
2. Atrial tachycardia with block in a patient who is not taking digitalis may be treated with digitalis, verapamil, or beta-adrenergic blockers to slow the ventricular rate.
3. If atrial tachycardia with block remains after drug therapy to slow the ventricular response, oral quinidine, procainamide, or disopyramide may be added.
4. The rhythm in some patients may resist termination by pharmacologic means; if digitalis excess is not the cause, DC cardioversion may be tried but is usually ineffective.
5. If atrial tachycardia with block appears in a patient receiving digitalis, it should be assumed initially that the digitalis is responsible for the arrhythmia, especially if the patient has received diuretics, the serum potassium is low, the digitalis dose has been increased, or multiple ventricular extrasystoles are also present, and treatment should be started during continuous ECG monitoring. In such patients, initial therapy includes omission of digitalis and potassium-depleting diuretics, and, if the serum [K^+] is not elevated, the administration of potassium chloride orally (30 to 45 mEq initially, repeated if necessary in 1 hour) or intravenously (0.5 mEq per minute in 5 per cent dextrose and water for a total of 30 to 60 mEq initially). A gradual slowing of the atrial rate with a decrease in AV block usually occurs if the arrhythmia is due to digitalis. Particularly in the presence of advanced AV block, potassium, as well as other antiarrhythmic agents, should be given with great caution under constant ECG monitoring, because it may increase the degree of block. Remember that renal dysfunction, acidosis, and excess digitalis predispose to the development of hyperkalemia, and therefore potassium must be administered cautiously, with frequent ECG and serum potassium checks. Administration of lidocaine, propranolol, or phenytoin may be useful. Of note, the ventricular response often is not excessively fast and withholding digitalis may be all that is necessary.

Atrial Flutter

See pages 239–240.

Atrial Fibrillation

See page 177.

Nonparoxysmal AV Junctional Tachycardia

Nonparoxysmal AV junctional tachycardia is usually of gradual onset and termination, hence the modifier "nonparoxysmal." The rate of discharge is usually between 70 and 130 per minute. The rate may be slowed by enhanced vagal tone, and the atria often are controlled by an independent sinus, atrial or uncommonly a second AV junctional focus. Nonparoxysmal junctional tachycardia occurs most frequently in patients who have underlying heart disease, such as inferior wall myocardial infarction or acute rheumatic myocarditis, and after open heart surgery. Probably the most important cause is excessive digitalis. It is especially important to recognize slowing and regularization of the ventricular rhythm caused by nonparoxysmal junctional tachycardia as an early sign of digitalis intoxication in a patient who has atrial fibrillation.

Treatment

1. If the ventricular rate is rapid, the cardiovascular status is compromised, and the patient is not taking digitalis, digitalization should be the first measure.
2. Uncommonly, in an emergency situation or if the arrhythmia does not respond to digitalization and is clearly not induced by digitalis, electrical DC cardioversion may be employed, although it usually is ineffective.
3. However, if the patient tolerates the arrhythmia well, careful monitoring and attention to the underlying heart disease are usually all that is needed. The arrhythmia most often abates spontaneously.
4. If digitalis toxicity is the causative factor, the drug must be immediately stopped. Potassium may be given (see treatment of atrial tachycardia with block). The ECG should be monitored, because the blocking effects of potassium administration and digitalis are additive in the AV junctional tissue and AV heart block may result. The rate of potassium administration is important, because a rapid infusion of potassium, especially in a potassium-depleted patient, may result in transient cardiac arrest or depression of AV conduction.
5. Lidocaine, propranolol, or phenytoin also may be tried.

VENTRICULAR ARRHYTHMIAS

Premature Ventricular Complexes

See page 183.

Ventricular Tachycardia

The ECG diagnosis of ventricular tachycardia is suggested when a series of three or more bizarrely shaped premature ventricular complexes occur that exceed 120 msec in duration, with the ST-T vector pointing opposite to the major QRS deflection. Depending on the particular type of ventricular tachycardia, the rate ranges from 70 to more than 250 per minute, and the onset may be paroxysmal or nonparoxysmal. The most important question is deciding which patients require therapy and for what length of time. In general, the relative risks of symptoms or sudden cardiac death for each type of ventricular tachycardia determine the course of therapy.

Nonsustained Ventricular Tachycardia. We arbitrarily define nonsustained ventricular tachycardia as tachycardia that is 3 beats to less than 30 seconds in duration. In most patients, recorded runs of nonsustained ventricular tachycardia consist of 6 or fewer consecutive beats and the patients are asymptomatic or have palpitations only. Longer runs of ventricular tachycardia may result in more severe symptoms, such as lightheadedness or syncope. Urgent therapy with intravenous drugs to suppress the arrhythmia is rarely required; treatment, if necessary, can be started with oral preparations of either quinidine, procainamide, disopyramide, or tocainide (see SVT section for dosages).

Most patients have *paroxysmal* episodes of ventricular tachycardia—that is, they occur intermittently. If the patient is asymptomatic and has no obvious structural heart disease, we usually recommend no specific antiarrhythmic therapy. Patients who have coronary heart disease and nonsustained ventricular tachycardia, especially those with substantial left ventricular myocardial dysfunction, appear to be at increased risk for subsequent sudden death in the first 6 to 12 months following acute myocardial infarction. The relative risk of sudden death is not clear in patients with coronary artery disease without acute myocardial infarction or in patients who have other forms of heart disease, such as idiopathic congestive cardiomyopathy. Further, no data to date demonstrate a decrease in cardiac mortality in any patient group that receives antiarrhythmic therapy other than beta blockers. Since antiarrhythmic drugs are also arrhythmogenic and can cause fatal ventricular tachyarrhythmias, the benefit/risk ratio of treatment may not be in the patients' best interests. For this reason we have no "general" rules of therapy; rather, we carefully assess multiple factors in each patient, including type of heart disease, left ventricular function and the presence of an acute precipitating event, and *individualize* therapy for each patient.

Using this approach we might administer antiarrhythmic drugs to patients with nonsustained ventricular tachycardia who had a recent myocardial infarction associated with a left ventricular ejection fraction of less than 30 per cent, or to patients with nonsustained ventricular tachycardia and hypertrophic obstructive cardiomyopathy with a family history of sudden death. Alternatively, we probably would not treat an asymptomatic patient with relatively slow, (e.g., < 170 per minute) nonsustained ventricular tachycardia and a remote (i.e., > 1 year) history of myocardial infarction. It is important to *reemphasize* that prevention of sudden death by quinidine, procainamide, disopyramide, or tocainide therapy is unproved for any patient subgroup. The value of newer techniques such as electrophysiologic testing and signal-averaged electrocardiograms to identify high risk patients is unclear and currently under investigation.

Some patients have a very unusual form of tachycardia, referred to as *repetitive monomorphic ventricular tachycardia* (RMVT). Unlike the paroxysmal form, RMVT often occurs throughout the day and is characterized by groups of usually 3 to 15 ventricular complexes that have a uniform QRS morphology, and the interectopic sinus-conducted complexes have a normal QRS without intraventricular conduction delay or pathologic Q waves. Episodes of ventricular tachycardia may cluster around certain time periods in some patients. Further, patients have no or only minimal structural heart disease, and arrhythmia-related deaths occur infrequently. The prognosis is usually favorable in these patients, and ventricular tachycardia may disappear with time. If patients are asymptomatic, we usually recommend no specific antiarrhythmic drug treatment.

Accelerated Idioventricular Rhythm. The ventricular rate, commonly between 50 and 110 per minute, usually hovers within 10 beats of the sinus rate so that control of the cardiac rhythm may be passed back and forth between these two competing pacemaker sites. Consequently, long runs of fusion beats often appear at the onset and termination of the arrhythmia as the pacemakers vie for control of ventricular discharge. The arrhythmia occurs as a rule in patients with heart disease, such as in the setting of acute myocardial infarction, or as an expression of digitalis toxicity. In the infarct patient, it is transient and intermittent, with episodes lasting a few seconds to a minute, and does not appear to affect seriously the course or prognosis of the patient. Suppressive therapy is rarely necessary, because the ventricular rate is generally less than 100 per minute.

Treatment

1. The best initial therapeutic approach appears to be close observation, rhythm monitoring, and care of the underlying heart disease.
2. Digitalis administration should be discontinued if the drug is implicated in the genesis of the arrhythmia.
3. Atropine (0.5 mg intravenously initially, repeated if necessary to a total dose of 2.0 mg) or atrial pacing may be used to speed the sinus rate and capture the ventricles.
4. Lidocaine may be given to suppress the ectopic ventricular focus. If chronic treatment is required, then quinidine, procainamide, disopyramide, or tocainide may be used.

Sustained Ventricular Tachycardia. Sustained ventricular tachycardia is usually an ominous event, indicative of underlying cardiac disease. The majority of patients have coronary artery disease or cardiomyopathy, but patients with mitral valve prolapse, valvular or congenital heart disease, and primary electrical disease (no recognizable evidence of structural heart disease) may also have sustained ventricular tachycardia. This arrhythmia almost always causes symptoms and requires acute suppressive treatment, most often followed by chronic therapy, to prevent recurrent arrhythmic episodes. Chronic therapy may not be necessary if ventricular tachycardia is caused by a specific, reversible, transient abnormality, such as acute myocardial infarction.

An important and still unresolved issue is how best to define therapeutic efficacy for chronic suppressive drug treatment. Although some investigators advocate that maintenance of a "therapeutic" plasma drug concentration will prevent recurrent ventricular tachycardia, we do not think this technique has acceptable predictive accuracy and discourage its use as a sole method to guide drug efficacy. One must remember that "therapeutic" is actually a retrospective term used in this context, and no matter what the plasma drug concentration is, if recurrence of arrhythmia is prevented the drug plasma level is therapeutic. Furthermore, it is also possible that in some patients the disappearance of spontaneous arrhythmia is unrelated to drug treatment.

Two useful techniques to evaluate drug efficacy are serial electrophysiologic-pharmacologic testing and continuous ECG recordings. Advocates of both methods claim predictive accuracy; no definitive data are available to suggest superiority of one technique over the other. It is stressed that the methods are *not* mutually exclusive, and we employ both tests to judge drug efficacy. For example, we obtain 24 hour ECG recordings before and during drug therapy and perform repeat electrophysiologic testing only during drug trials that demonstrate suppression of spontaneous episodes of ventricular tachycardia for a period of 24 or more hours. If spontaneous arrhythmia occurs infrequently prior to treatment, then electrophysiologic testing per se is used as the sole marker to define drug efficacy.

Treatment

1. Ventricular tachycardia that does not cause substantial hemodynamic decompensation may be treated medically by administering lidocaine intravenously in a bolus of 1 to 2 mg per kg of body weight at a rate of approximately 20 to 50 mg per minute, with a second injection of one half the initial dose 20 to 40 minutes later. If the initial bolus of lidocaine is ineffective, up to two more boluses of 1 mg per kg may be given at 5 minute intervals. If lidocaine abolishes the ventricular tachycardia, then a continuous intravenous infusion of 1 to 4 mg per minute should be given to the patient. Infusion rates should be reduced in patients with liver disease, heart failure, or shock.
2. If maximal doses of lidocaine are ineffective, then intravenous procainamide or bretylium may be tried. We administer procainamide at 50 mg per minute to a total dose of 10 to 14 mg per kg, and if successful a maintenance infusion of 2 to 6 mg per minute can be used. Bretylium is given in doses of 5 to 10 mg per kg diluted in 50 to 100 ml of 5 per cent dextrose in water and administered slowly over 10 to 20 minutes; the maintenance infusion dose is 0.5 to 2.0 mg per minute. Of note, patients who receive several days of bretylium by constant infusion may experience orthostatic hypotension up to a week after discontinuation of therapy, and attempts should be made to prevent orthostatic syncope. Quinidine may be given intravenously but can cause profound hypotension and should be used with great caution.
3. If the arrhythmia does not respond to medical therapy, then cardioversion may be used. However, ventricular tachycardia that precipitates hypotension, shock, angina, or congestive heart failure should be treated promptly with DC cardioversion. Very low energies may terminate ventricular tachycardia; we generally begin with a synchronized shock of 10 to 50 watt-seconds (see treatment of ventricular fibrillation in a later section). Digitalis-induced ventricular tachycardia is best treated medically. After reversion of the arrhythmia to a normal rhythm, it is essential to institute measures to prevent a recurrence.
4. Striking the patient's chest, sometimes called "thumpversion," may terminate ventricular tachycardia by mechanically inducing a premature ventricular complex that presumably interrupts the re-entrant pathway necessary to maintain the ventricular tachycardia. However, this technique also may initiate ventricular fibrillation and therefore should be performed only if back-up DC defibrillation is readily available.
5. Ventricular pacing through a catheter positioned in the right ventricle (the apex is the most stable site) may be tried to terminate tachycardia. Paced runs of three to eight complexes beginning at a cycle length 50 msec shorter than the tachycardia cycle length are more effective than introduction of one or two extra stimuli to terminate ventricular tachycardia, but the former technique is also more likely to accelerate the tachycardia rate or induce ventricular fibrillation. Pacing should be done only when back-up DC defibrillation is present. A new catheter electrode has been developed recently through which synchronized cardioversion can be performed.
6. A search for reversible conditions contributing to the initiation and maintenance of ventricular tachyarrhythmias should be made and the condition corrected if possible. For example, the ventricular arrhythmia related to hypotension or hypokalemia at times may be terminated and recurrences prevented by the use of vasopressors or potassium.
7. Prevention of recurrences is generally more difficult than is terminating the acute episode. Initial preventive drug therapy for recurrent ventricular tachycardia should include quinidine, procainamide, disopyramide or tocainide (see SVT section for dosages). Propranolol or phenytoin may be tried next, although these drugs are usually ineffective unless the ventricular tachycardia is related to ischemia, catecholamine stimulation, or digitalis toxicity. Combinations of drugs with different mechanisms of action may be successful when single drug therapy fails. A trial of ventricular or atrial pacing, combined with antiarrhythmic drugs if necessary, may be tested; however, unless ventricular tachycardia is initiated by significant bradycardia, for example a ventricular rate < 40 per minute, "overdrive" pacing to prevent ventricular tachycardia is usually ineffective.
8. Surgery may be used to abolish ventricular tachycardia in selected patients. A variety of operations have been proposed, and the selection of a particular procedure depends on the

underlying anatomic abnormality and the skill of the surgeon in the various techniques. Whenever possible, the site of ventricular tachycardia should be identified by electrophysiologic mapping techniques prior to and during surgery.

Ventricular Flutter and Ventricular Fibrillation

Ventricular flutter and ventricular fibrillation represent severe derangements of the heart beat that usually terminate fatally within 3 to 5 minutes unless they are promptly stopped. Ventricular flutter resembles a sine wave in appearance, with regular, large oscillations occurring at a rate of between 150 and 300 per minute—usually about 200 per minute. Ventricular fibrillation is recognized by the presence of irregular undulations of varying contour and amplitude. Distinct QRS complexes, S-T segments, and T waves are absent. The differentiation between rapid ventricular tachycardia and ventricular flutter may be difficult and is usually of academic interest only.

Treatment

Ventricular flutter and ventricular fibrillation are totally unphysiologic, life-threatening arrhythmias for which immediate electrical (nonsynchronized) DC cardioversion, using 200 to 400 watt-seconds, is the only reliable treatment. When ventricular tachycardia produces the same hemodynamic response as does ventricular flutter or fibrillation, it also must be immediately cardioverted. Cardiopulmonary resuscitation is employed only until defibrillation equipment is readied.If the patient is not monitored and it cannot be established whether asystole or ventricular fibrillation has caused the cardiovascular collapse, the electric shock should be administered without wasting precious seconds attempting to record the ECG. The DC shock may cause the asystolic heart to begin discharging and may terminate ventricular fibrillation if present. If the circulation is markedly inadequate despite return to sinus rhythm, closed-chest massage with artificial ventilation as needed should be instituted. Pressor agents and often sodium bicarbonate may be needed and should be given when appropriate.

It is now known that ventricular fibrillation not related to an acute myocardial infarction is usually preceded by rapid ventricular tachycardia. In these patients, prevention of recurrent attacks of ventricular fibrillation should begin with prevention of recurrent episodes of ventricular tachycardia (see Sustained Ventricular Tachycardia section).

Torsade de Pointes

Torsade de pointes is a syndrome of a specific form of ventricular tachycardia that occurs in patients with prolonged QT intervals during sinus rhythm. Tachycardia is characterized by QRS complexes of changing amplitude that appear to twist around the isoelectric line (which may be noted only in certain ECG leads) and occur at rates of 200 to 250 per minute. It is important to emphasize the associated prolonged QT interval, because polymorphic ventricular tachycardia may resemble torsade de pointes yet the approach to treatment may be markedly different for these two arrhythmias.

Treatment

Although many predisposing factors have been identified, the most common are severe bradycardia, hypokalemia, and drugs such as quinidine, procainamide, and disopyramide. The most effective initial therapy to suppress ventricular tachycardia is temporary atrial or ventricular pacing, usually at rates of 80 to 120 per minute. Isoproterenol can be tried until pacing is instituted. At the same time correction of underlying causes should be done, such as administering potassium if the patient is hypokalemic or discontinuing previous antiarrhythmic therapy. Recently, intravenous infusion of magnesium sulfate has been suggested as acute treatment of torsade de pointes, but its effectiveness in a variety of pathophysiologic mechanisms remains unclear. (Patients with idiopathic long QT syndrome are discussed separately.)

Long QT Syndrome (LQTS)

The upper limit for the duration of the normal QT interval corrected for heart rate (QTc) is stated to be 0.44 second, although the rate correction formulas used to derive this figure are imperfect and may not be applicable in the presence of certain drugs or alterations of autonomic tone. Delayed repolarization (QTc interval > 0.44 second) can be acquired and caused by multiple factors such as antiarrhythmic drugs (see torsade de pointes), or it can be *primary* or idiopathic. The primary form is a congenital, often familial, disorder that may be associated with deafness. Symptomatic patients with LQTS develop ventricular tachycardias that in many instances are due to torsade de pointes. However, sudden death may occur in this group of patients and may be caused by torsade de pointes progressing to ventricular fibrillation. Electrocardiograms should be obtained from all family members when the propositus presents with symptoms.

Treatment

Therapy of patients with congenital LQTS is determined by the clinical situation. No therapy is recommended for patients with LQTS who have no syncope, complex ventricular arrhythmias, or family history of sudden cardiac death. In asymptomatic patients with complex ventricular arrhythmias or a family history of premature sudden cardiac death, maximally tolerated dosages of beta blockers are recommended. Patients with syncope are treated with phenytoin, phenobarbital, or both, in addition to beta blockers at maximally tolerated dosages. Recurrent syncope during triple drug therapy may respond to left-sided cervicothoracic sympathetic ganglionectomy.

Bidirectional Ventricular Tachycardia

This uncommon ventricular tachycardia, most often but not exclusively caused by digitalis excess, is characterized by QRS complexes with a right bundle branch block pattern seen in ECG lead V_1 and alternating polarity in the frontal plane from -60 to -90 degrees to $+120$ to $+130$ degrees. If excessive digitalis administration is suspected, drugs such as lidocaine, potassium, phenytoin, and propranolol may be useful, although the overall prognosis is poor. The usual approach to ventricular tachycardia is suggested, as in other patients.

CONGENITAL HEART DISEASE

method of
LARRY T. MAHONEY, M.D.
University of Iowa
Iowa City, Iowa

The incidence of congenital heart disease in the United States is about 8 per 1000 live births. Of an estimated 35,000 infants born annually with congenital heart disease, approximately 25 per cent require immediate medical attention within the first several months of life. Eighty per cent of infants who die from congenital heart disease and its complications do so during the first year of life. The most critical factor in determining overall mortality is the primary physician's accurate diagnosis of congestive heart failure and central cyanosis and referral of the symptomatic infant to a cardiac care center.

ACUTE MANAGEMENT OF THE NEONATE

After deciding to transport the critically ill neonate to a pediatric cardiac center, time and safe transport remain the important considerations. Most centers have a ground transport vehicle and helicopter or fixed wing aircraft services. Certain principles are basic to transporting the neonate.

Equipment. Since hypothermia further compromises the stressed neonate, the infant should be placed in a transport incubator, which provides a proper thermal environment. Respiratory support may include either a bag and face mask or endotracheal intubation for administering continuous positive airway pressure or assisted ventilation. A heart rate monitor and emergency cardiac medications are also essential.

Personnel. Many centers will provide a transport team consisting of paramedical personnel and pediatric nurses accustomed to caring for the seriously ill neonate. A pediatrician also may accompany the team. These individuals should have considerable knowledge and skill in resuscitation and critical care medicine.

Stabilization. A variety of conditions that relate to the existing structural heart defects may respond to interventions available only at a cardiac care center. Therefore, the team should identify abnormalities of cardiac rate, acid-base status, hypoxia, hypoglycemia, anemia, and respiratory insufficiency and initiate appropriate therapy with expediency to facilitate transport.

Cyanosis

Cyanosis in neonates may be classified as (1) peripheral cyanosis, which is assumed to be secondary to decreased cardiac output and increased tissue oxygen extraction, or (2) central cyanosis, which is apparent when the arterial blood contains 5 grams of desaturated hemoglobin. Anemia will make it difficult to detect cyanosis. Central cyanosis may result in a patient with structural heart disease who has diminished pulmonary blood flow and a right to left shunt, intracardiac admixture of pulmonary and systemic venous blood, or congestive heart failure with pulmonary edema and decreased uptake of oxygen. Noncardiac processes may also cause central cyanosis. These may include decreased respiratory effort due to neuromuscular disease, abnormalities in oxygen-hemoglobin binding, or primary pulmonary disease caused by alveolar hypoventilation, ventilation perfusion mismatch, or intrapulmonary shunting. Pulmonary diseases are usually associated with an arterial carbon dioxide partial pressure ($PaCO_2$) over 50 torr. However, this is a variable and nondifferential factor. Management of the cyanotic infant varies depending on the underlying pathophysiology.

Hyperoxic Test

To distinguish heart disease from pulmonary disease, the physician should evaluate the response of the patient's arterial oxygen partial pressure (Pa_{O_2}) in 100 per cent oxygen. This extremely safe test consists of (1) obtaining an arterial blood gas from the right radial artery while the infant is breathing room air, (2) placing the infant in 100 per cent oxygen for 10 minutes, (3) repeating the arterial blood gas measurement (an increase in Pa_{O_2} of less than 10 torr suggests cardiac disease, whereas an increase of greater than 30 torr suggests pulmonary disease), and (4) obtaining a lower P_{O_2} from a postductal site via an umbilical arterial catheter, which suggests that the right to left shunting is through a patent ductus arteriosus.

Specific Causes

1. *Cyanosis associated with diminished pulmonary blood flow and an intracardiac right to left shunt.* Many structural heart defects require patency of the ductus arteriosus to allow adequate perfusion of the pulmonary circulation from the aorta. Prostaglandin E_1 (0.05 to 0.1 mcg per kg per min) maintains patency of the ductus arteriosus. Prostaglandin may precipitate apnea, bradycardia, or hypotension, and thus one should be prepared to ventilate a baby given this agent.

2. *Cyanosis associated with hypercyanotic spells.* Classically the young patient with tetralogy of Fallot may become irritable, severely cyanotic, hyperpneic, and often syncopal. A period of somnolence follows the spell. If severe, hypercyanotic spells result in acidosis and may be life-threatening.

Initial treatment consists of physical maneuvers, such as placing the infant into a knee-chest position or at least placing the legs up under the abdomen. Supplemental oxygen is administered by face mask unless this further agitates the infant. Morphine sulphate, 0.1 to 0.2 mg per kg, reduces hyperventilation and may specifically relieve right ventricular infundibular spasms. Acutely increasing the systemic vascular resistance with a medication such as methoxamine, 0.25 mg per kg per dose intramuscularly or 0.1 mg per kg per dose intravenously, may reduce the intracardiac right to left shunt. For resistant spells, administer propranolol, 0.1 to 0.15 mg per kg per dose, intravenously slowly over 5 minutes and repeat the dose every 20 minutes for a maximum of four doses, or 1 mg per kg per dose orally four times daily (correcting the associated acidosis with sodium bicarbonate, 0.3 mEq × kg × unit of base deficit, is most important). (The safety and efficacy of propranolol for use in children have not been established.)

3. *Cyanosis associated with pulmonary edema.* Refer to the discussion on congestive heart failure.

4. *Cyanosis accompanying persistent elevated pulmonary vascular resistance.* In some newborn infants persistence of fetal pulmonary vascular resistance results in pronounced right to left shunting through a patent foramen ovale and ductus arteriosus. It may occur with or without apparent pulmonary disease. A PaO_2 difference between the distal aortic and right radial artery confirms the ductal shunting. The diagnosis requires exclusion of structural heart disease by echocardiography.

Maintaining an adequate pH and PaO_2 reduces pulmonary vasoconstriction. This may require one or more of the following: (1) assisted ventilation at respiratory rates greater than 50 per min, (2) supplemental oxygen up to 100 per cent to maintain a PO_2 in excess of 60 torr, (3) paralysis of an infant with pancuronium bromide, 0.06 to 0.15 mg per kg per dose, or (4) administration of tolazoline, a vasodilator, either as a single bolus of 1 to 2 mg per kg infused over 10 minutes or as a continuous infusion of 10 to 30 mcg per kg per min.

5. *Cyanosis associated with polycythemia.* The newborn, having received a maternal-fetal transfusion, may present with an elevated hematocrit (Hct) over 65 per cent. Symptoms of respiratory distress, hypoglycemia, or lethargy necessitate lowering the hematocrit to 55 per cent. A partial exchange transfusion should be performed according to the following calculation:

$$\text{Volume of blood to be removed} = (\text{wt [kg]} \times \text{newborn blood volume [ml/kg]}) \times \frac{\text{actual Hct} - \text{desired Hct}}{\text{actual Hct}}$$

As the patient's blood is slowly being withdrawn, replace the removed volume with a colloid solution.

Acidosis

Acid-base abnormalities often accompany cyanosis and congestive heart failure in the neonate and small infant. The basic approach to therapy depends upon the patterns of acid-base imbalance.

1. *Metabolic acidosis (decreased pH and normal or decreased Pa_{O_2} and Pa_{CO_2}).* Hypoxemia and impaired tissue perfusion associated with a decreased cardiac output may cause metabolic acidosis. With increasing acidosis, the infant hyperventilates and produces a compensatory respiratory alkalosis.

Hypothermia compounds metabolic acidosis by shifting the oxygen dissociation curve to the left and altering peripheral blood flow. Therefore, the skin temperature should be maintained above 36.5 C. Hypoglycemia (serum glucose less than 45 mg per dl) further compromises the infant and requires immediate infusion of 2 ml per kg of 25 per cent glucose in water and then maintenance fluids of 10 per cent glucose in water. In an anemic infant, the hematocrit should be raised above 40 per cent with whole blood at 10 ml per kg or packed red cells at 5 ml per kg over 2 to 3 hours.

To correct metabolic acidosis, administer sodium bicarbonate as follows: mEq of sodium bicarbonate = base deficit × 0.3 × weight (kg). Too rapid an infusion may result in hypernatremia and possibly an intracranial hemorrhage. Slowly infusing the calculated bicarbonate dose over 5 minutes avoids a rapid increase in plasma osmolarity.

In the presence of hypernatremia or an ineffective response to bicarbonate infusion, use THAM as follows: ml THAM = base deficit × weight (kg). Infuse half the calculated dose over 30 minutes and the remainder over the subsequent 1 to 2 hours. Since hypoglycemia occurs frequently, infuse 10 per cent glucose in water concomitant with THAM. Other side effects associated with THAM include apnea, hypotension, and vomiting.

2. *Respiratory acidosis (decreased pH, increased* $PaCO_2$*, and normal or decreased* PaO_2*).* These data indicate inadequate ventilation secondary to pulmonary disease, central hypoventilation, pulmonary venous obstruction, or volume overload due to congestive heart failure. A combination of causes may also occur (e.g., pneumonia aggravating previously compensated congestive heart failure).

Therapy is directed at improving the airway. The nurse caring for the patient should frequently percuss the chest and suction the oropharynx or trachea to maintain patency of the airway. Ventilation should be improved with tracheal intubation and mechanical support. After determining the primary etiology, institute specific therapy, either pharmacologic or surgical.

Repeated arterial blood gas determinations during attempts to correct metabolic or respiratory acidosis will prevent either overcorrection of the imbalance or failure to recognize further deterioration.

Congestive Heart Failure

With congestive heart failure, the circulation inadequately sustains the physiologic needs of the patient. Heart failure commonly occurs in neonates and small infants. Patients feed poorly and demonstrate inadequate weight gain. They present with a respiratory rate greater than 50 per minute, a heart rate greater than 160 beats per minute, hepatomegaly, gallop rhythm, and, in extreme cases, peripheral edema. The chest x-ray demonstrates cardiomegaly.

Vigorous therapy should begin immediately after recognizing the condition. Therapy consists of increasing myocardial contractility, improving peripheral perfusion, and decreasing pulmonary and systemic vascular congestion.

Supportive Measures

Provide humidified oxygen in an initial concentration of 30 to 40 per cent. Monitor the arterial blood gases for evidence of hypoxemia and acidosis. Placing the patient in an infant seat or semi-Fowler's position may improve the cardiorespiratory system and reduce the preload. In a restless and agitated patient, administer parenteral morphine sulphate, 0.1 to 0.2 mg per kg. Although its beneficial effects result from reducing both preload and afterload, morphine sulfate may compromise respiration and cause respiratory failure. Restrict fluid administration to 60 to 70 per cent of maintenance. Attend to any laboratory evidence of hypocalcemia, hypoglycemia, or anemia. In severe cases, placing the infant on a respirator with a moderate continuous positive airway pressure of 4 to 8 cm of water will not only correct respiratory failure but decrease the metabolic work required for breathing.

Diuretics

Since many infants have obvious signs of increased extracellular fluid, promoting diuresis will decrease preload. Administer furosemide 1 to 2 mg per kg per dose, or chlorothiazide, 20 to 50 mg per kg per day. Parenteral furosemide has a rapid peak effect and will enhance fluid excre-

TABLE 1. **Digoxin Dosages for Infants and Children***

Total Digitalizing Dose (TDD) by Age	IM/IV mg/kg
Premature	0.02–0.03 (20–30 micrograms)
Term Infant to 2 Years	0.04 (40 micrograms)
Over 2 Years	0.03 (30 micrograms)
Maximum: 1.0 mg (1000 micrograms)	
Initial: ½ TDD	
Subsequent: ¼ + ¼ TDD at 6–8 hour intervals	
Maintenance Digoxin Dose	
¼ to ⅓ TDD per day orally q 12 hr	
Digoxin Preparations:	
Digoxin (Lanoxin) elixir, 0.05 mg/ml (50 micrograms/ml)	
Digoxin for injection, 0.10 mg/ml (100 micrograms/ml)	

*Caution: Digoxin is a potentially toxic drug. Dosages should be calculated carefully by two individuals and orders written in milligrams (micrograms) and milliliters for added safety.

tion. Since potassium may become depleted with vigorous diuresis, use either a potassium supplement, 1 to 2 mEq per kg per day, or a potassium-sparing mild diuretic such as spironolactone, 2 to 4 mg per kg per day, in conjunction with the diuretic therapy.

Digitalis

This drug, which increases myocardial contractility, remains a primary pharmacologic agent in the treatment of congestive heart failure. Digoxin has a predictable onset of action, duration of effect, and rate of renal excretion. Table 1 lists the dosages commonly used in infants and children. Since digoxin has a small margin of safety, two people should individually calculate the dose. For added safety, write the order in milligrams (micrograms) and milliliters. Modify the dose in the presence of increased myocardial sensitivity with myocarditis or decreased renal excretion with renal insufficiency. Electrolyte disturbances, such as hypokalemia, may predispose to toxicity.

Since the critically ill infant has decreased cardiac output and poor peripheral perfusion, administer digoxin intravenously. In a mildly asymptomatic infant with adequate peripheral perfusion, intramuscular administration is acceptable. Administer maintenance digoxin orally or parenterally.

Digitalis toxicity results primarily from overdosage and manifests in a variety of ways. One must consider arrhythmias occurring during digoxin administration as evidence of toxicity until proven otherwise. These include bradyarrhythmias; supraventricular or ventricular tachycardias; atrial, junctional, or ventricular ectopy; and conduction disturbances. Prolonged P-R interval, ST segment depression, and T wave inversion do not indicate either adequate digitalization or digitalis toxicity. Gastrointestinal or central nervous system symptoms less reliably indicate toxicity. A digoxin level in excess of 5 ng per ml usually signifies overdosage. A level less than 2 to 3 ng per ml suggests an adequate therapeutic range; however, signs of toxicity may occur in this range if hypokalemia exists. Many infants will have an elevated level of 3 to 5 ng per ml without overt signs of toxicity.

Treatment of digitalis toxicity includes (1) withdrawal of digoxin, (2) and administration of intravenous potassium chloride, 0.5 mEq per kg per hour to a maximum total dose of 2 mEq per kg; do not use potassium in the presence of a conduction disturbance, since it may further depress atrioventricular conduction, (3) phenytoin (this use of phenytoin is not listed in manufacturer's directive), 10 to 15 mg per kg as an intravenous loading dose divided into two to three doses and each increment given over a 5 minute period, and (4) other agents (see section on arrhythmias).

Other Drug Therapy (Table 2)

Patients with a markedly decreased cardiac output refractory to the previously mentioned measures may respond to catecholamines or vasoactive drugs. These potent drugs have a potential for toxicity and should be administered in an intensive care unit. Each nurse caring for the patient must accurately check the rate of infusion and concentration. Administer the drug by a constant infusion pump. Carefully monitor urine output, arterial blood pressure, and, if possible, central venous pressure and left atrial or pulmonary capillary wedge pressure to assess the effectiveness of treatment.

Sympathomimetic drugs have a positive inotropic effect in addition to a peripheral vascular action. Dopamine, 2 to 20 micrograms per kg per min, also acts to increase renal blood flow and enhance urine production (safety and efficacy for use in children have not been established). Epinephrine and isoproterenol, 0.1 to 1.5 micrograms per kg per min, should not be used in combination.

Vasodilator therapy increases cardiac output by decreasing afterload, thus reducing myocardial oxygen consumption. Although frequently used in adults, these drugs currently are being evaluated in the pediatric patient. Since the indications for vasodilator therapy have not been established, their use should be restricted to the cardiac center. Nitroprusside is a drug commonly used for acute management. Infuse 1 to 12 mcg per kg per min by constant infusion in 5 per cent glucose in water. Since it is light sensitive and deteriorates, do not expose the solution to light. Cover the infusion syringe and tubing with aluminum foil. If the patient must be managed by chronic afterload reduction, give hydralazine, 1.7 to 3.5 mg per kg per day divided into four doses.

Premature infants with respiratory distress syndrome and a patent ductus arteriosus may present with congestive heart failure. Although the previously mentioned methods for treating congestive heart failure are often successful, a trial of a prostaglandin inhibitor may prove effective in constricting the ductus. Give indomethacin, 0.1 to 0.2 mg per kg orally, and if necessary repeat the dose in 8 to 12 hours. Contraindications to indomethacin include decreased renal function, bleeding diathesis, hyperbilirubinemia, and gastrointestinal distress. (This use of indomethacin is not listed by the manufacturer.)

The infant of a diabetic mother with a form of hypertrophic cardiomyopathy may develop congestive heart failure from subaortic obstruction.

TABLE 2. **Dosage Schedules**

Drug	Supplied	Route	Dosage
atropine sulfate	Vial: 0.04 mg/ml	IV,IM	0.01–0.03 mg/kg q 4–6 hr
calcium gluconate	Ampule: 10 ml; 100 mg/ml	IV	40–80 mg (0.4–0.8 ml)/kg/dose
chlorothiazide (Diuril)	Suspension: 250 mg/5 ml Tablet: 250, 500 mg	PO	20–50 mg/kg/day
dopamine hydrochloride* (Intropin)	Vial: 200 mg/5 ml	IV	2–20 mcg/kg/min
epinephrine (Adrenalin)	Ampule: 1 ml, 1:1000 (1 mg)	IV IV	Bolus (1 amp in 9 ml saline): 0.1 ml/kg/dose (10 mcg/kg/dose) Infusion: 0.1–1.5 mcg/kg/min
furosemide (Lasix)	Ampule: 2 ml, 10 ml; 10 mg/ml	IV,IM,PO	1–2 mg/kg/dose
hydralazine (Apresoline)	Ampule: 1 ml; 20 mg/ml Tablet: 10, 50 mg	IV,IM,PO	0.2–0.5 mg/kg/dose q 4 hr
indomethacin (Indocin)	Suspension: 25 mg capsule in 250 cc sterile water	PO	0.1–0.2 mg/kg/dose; repeat dose in 8–12 hr
isoproterenol (Isuprel)	Ampule: 1 ml, 5 ml; 0.2 mg/ml	IV	0.1–1.5 mcg/kg/min
lidocaine (Xylocaine)	Ampule: 50 mg/5 cc; 200 mg/10 cc Vial: 2 gm/50 cc	IV	Bolus: 1 mg/kg Infusion: 20–40 mcg/kg/min
methoxamine (Vasoxyl)	Ampule: 1 ml; 20 mg/ml	IM IV	0.25 mg/kg/dose 0.10 mg/kg/dose
morphine sulfate	Ampule: 1 ml; 10, 15 mg/ml	IV,IM	0.1–0.2 mg/kg/dose
nitroprusside (Nipride)	Vial: 50 mg/5 ml	IV	1–12 mcg/kg/min
pancuronium bromide (Pavulon)	Vial: 10 ml; 1 mg/ml	IV	0.06–0.15 mg/kg/dose
phenytoin (Dilantin)	Ampule: 2, 5 ml; 50 mg/ml Suspension: 30, 125 mg/5 ml Capsule: 30, 100 mg	IV PO	10–15 mg/kg divided into 3 doses 2–4 mg/kg bid
potassium chloride	Vial: 20 ml; 2 mEq/ml Syrup: 20 mEq/15 ml	IV PO	0.5 mEq/kg/hr 1–2 mEq/kg/day
procainamide (Pronestyl)	Vial: 10 ml; 100 mg/ml	IV	Bolus: 1 mg/kg, repeat q 5 min to total of 15 doses Infusion: 1–4 mg/kg/hr
propranolol* (Inderal)	Ampule: 1 mg/ml Tablet: 10, 20, 40 mg	IV PO	0.01–0.15 mg/kg/dose over 5 min 0.25–2.0 mg/kg q 6 hr
prostaglandin E_1 (Prostin VR)	Ampule: 500 mcg/ml	IV	0.05–0.1 mcg/kg/min
quinidine sulfate*	Tablet: 100, 200 mg	PO	7–12 mg/kg q 6 hr
sodium bicarbonate	Syringe: 5 mEq/10 ml Vial: 44.6 mEq/50 cc	IV	dose in mEq = base deficit × 0.3 × weight (kg)
spironolactone (Aldactone)	Tablet: 25 mg (must be made into suspension)	PO	2–4 mg/kg/day
tolazoline (Priscoline)	Vial: 10 ml; 25 mg/ml	IV	Bolus: 1–2 mg/kg over 10 min Infusion: 10–30 mcg/kg/min
Tris-buffer (THAM)	IV container; 500 ml, 0.3 M	IV	ml THAM = base deficit × weight (kg)
verapamil hydrochloride (Isoptin)	Ampule: 2 ml; 2.5 mg/ml	IV	75–150 mcg/kg/dose; may repeat dose in 30 min

Note: See text for additional details.
*Safety and efficacy for use in children have not been established.

Digoxin may further aggravate this obstruction. Propranolol, 0.25 to 2.0 mg per kg dose every 6 hours, may effect relief of the obstruction but should be used in patients with heart failure only with great caution as judged by echocardiography. The beta-blocker may be discontinued when the septal hypertrophy diminishes.

Arrhythmias

Although dysrhythmias uncommonly occur in the pediatric practice, abnormalities of heart rate and rhythm may cause cardiovascular compromise. The physician must differentiate benign arrhythmias from potentially life-threatening arrhythmias. Structural heart disease, hypoxia, or acidosis may exacerbate the dysrhythmia. Effective therapy of the dysrhythmia may depend upon recognition and concurrent treatment of the associated abnormalities.

Sinus Node Function

A phasic or periodic variation of the heart rate, sinus arrhythmia, usually occurs with low basal heart rates. It occurs in premature and full term infants as well as older children. It should be considered a normal phenomenon. Sinus bradycardia and tachycardia usually result from noncardiac conditions. A failure of impulse formation lasting for a few beats, sinus pause, occurs frequently in premature and full term infants, especially in association with sinus bradycardia. A symptomatic patient with bradycardia usually responds to atropine, 0.01 to 0.03 mg per kg, or isoproterenol, 0.1 to 1.5 mcg per kg per min.

Supraventricular Tachycardia

Premature atrial or junctional contractions occur in many healthy newborns. The majority do not cause any cardiovascular compromise and generally resolve during the first weeks of life. However, they may occasionally trigger supraventricular tachycardia (SVT). SVT is the most common symptomatic arrhythmia in the newborn and young child. Infants with paroxysmal SVT, including atrial flutter, have heart rates in excess of 220 beats per minute. If the tachycardia persists for greater than 12 hours, cardiovascular compromise may occur. In the symptomatic patient, DC electrical cardioversion with 0.25 to 1.5 Watt-sec per kg should be initially employed. Children over one year of age require sedation prior to cardioversion. In the patient with minimal or no symptoms, intravenous digoxin is highly effective in converting the arrhythmia and providing maintenance therapy (see Table 1). Propranolol, 0.25 to 2.0 mg per kg per dose every 6 hours, may be used as an alternative to or in combination with digoxin. Single drug therapy is preferential, but in refractory cases multiple drug therapy may be essential. In such cases, the patient should undergo an intercardiac electrophysiologic study to determine the most effective drug regimen.

Recently, the efficacy of verapamil, 75 to 150 mcg per kg per dose, intravenously over 2 minutes, repeated if necessary in 30 minutes, has been demonstrated in patients with SVT. Its cardiovascular effects include a negative chronotropic effect in the sinoatrial node, delayed conduction in the atrioventricular node, a negative inotropic effect, and arteriolar vasodilation. Verapamil is contraindicated in congestive heart failure, hypotension, atrioventricular block, and sick sinus syndrome and with beta-blocker usage. Monitor the electrocardiogram and blood pressure during treatment. If adverse reactions occur, treat with calcium gluconate, 40 to 80 mg (0.4 to 0.8 ml) per kg per dose, catecholamines, atropine, or cardiac pacing.

Ventricular Dysrhythmia

Premature ventricular contractions require no therapy if they have the following characteristics: uniform, fixed coupling, disappear with exertion, no couplets, and unaccompanied by structural heart disease or prolonged QT intervals on the electrocardiogram. Although not universally accepted as criteria for initiating therapy, the following characteristics have led many physicians to begin suppressive drug treatment: multiform, occurring in runs of three beats or more, increasing with exercise, associated with heart disease or prolonged QT syndrome, and causing symptoms.

A patient on digitalis may have toxicity manifesting as premature ventricular contractions, which requires discontinuing the drug (see section on digitalis). On the other hand, congestive heart failure manifesting with premature ventricular contractions may respond to digitalis therapy with a decrease or disappearance of the ectopy.

Before initiating drug therapy, treat possible acute causes such as hypoxia or an abnormally placed intracardiac catheter. Acute drug interventions include the use of (1) phenytoin, 15 mg per kg intravenously divided into three doses, (2) lidocaine, 1 mg per kg intravenous push, which can be repeated every 5 minutes for a total of three doses or followed by a continuous infusion of 20 to 40 mcg per kg per min, or (3) procainamide, 1 mg per kg intravenously repeated every 5 minutes to a total of 15 doses or a continuous infusion of 1 to 4 mg per kg per hour. Chronic maintenance therapy includes the use of (1) phenytoin, 2 to 4 mg per kg twice daily, (2) propranolol, 0.25 to 2.0 mg per kg every 6 hours, or (3) quinidine sulfate, 7 to 12 mg per kg every 6 hours.

In addition to the previously mentioned therapy for premature ventricular contractions, ventricular tachycardia may be managed with synchronized DC electrical cardioversion of 0.5 to 1.5 Watt-sec per kg or rapid ventricular pacing. Propranolol, 0.01 to 0.15 mg per kg, may be repeated every 10 minutes for a total of four doses. Use an intercardiac electrode catheter when giving intravenous propranalol in case immediate treatment of bradycardia becomes necessary.

Congenital Complete Atrioventricular Block

This conduction defect commonly occurs in association with congenital heart disease or myocarditis. Also, infants born to mothers with systemic lupus erythematosus are at high risk for heart block. Drugs with a positive chronotropic effect, such as atropine or isoproterenol, may affect temporary treatment. Indications for surgical placement of a permanent pacemaker in an infant include (1) a ventricular rate of less than 50 beats per min, (2) unresponsiveness of the ventricular rate to atropine, (3) an atrial rate greater than 150 beats per min with a slow ventricular response, (4) cardiomegaly and other signs of congestive heart failure, especially in the presence of structural heart disease, and (5) demonstration of the block distal to or within the His bundle. This may indirectly be assumed by the presence of a wide QRS ventricular morphology or directly demonstrated by an intracardiac electrophysiologic study. In the older child, syncope or signs of congestive heart failure are accepted criteria for a permanent pacemaker. Temporary pacing may be indicated in the presence of severe infection, during induction of anesthesia, or while awaiting placement of a permanent pacemaker.

Cardiac Arrest

Cardiac arrest results from ventricular asystole or as the end result of ventricular fibrillation or electromechanical dissociation. In addition to basic cardiac life support with optimal ventilation and chest compression, begin the following: (1) sodium bicarbonate, (2) epinephrine 1:10,000 solution, 0.1 ml per kg per dose, (3) calcium gluconate, 40 to 80 mg per kg per dose, (4) atropine, 0.01 to 0.03 mg per kg per dose, (5) isoproterenol, 0.1 to 1.5 mcg per kg per min and in persistent asystole, and (6) transvenous or transthoracic temporary pacing.

The administration of additional bicarbonate should be based on subsequent arterial pH and $Paco_2$ determinations or clinical judgment if they are not available. Epinephrine is ineffective at a low pH. Since calcium gluconate precipitates in the presence of sodium bicarbonate to form an insoluble substance, avoid administering these drugs simultaneously.

After restoration of palpable pulses and relatively normal cardiac rhythm, transfer the patient to an intensive care unit. Further diagnostic and supportive measures usually are required.

CHRONIC MANAGEMENT OF THE CHILD AND YOUNG ADULT WITH CONGENITAL HEART DISEASE

Diet and Exercise

The growing child with congenital heart disease has a greater need for calories than does an adult. When symptoms of congestive heart failure or cyanosis are present, inadequate weight gain occurs secondary to either inability to consume sufficient calories or an elevated metabolic expenditure. Management consists of (1) more frequent feedings, (2) increased caloric content of the feeding, such as 24 calories per ounce of formula plus adding medium-chain triglyceride oil, or (3) adding solids to the diet if the infant has difficulty sucking or swallowing liquids.

The older child with heart disease should be made aware of proper nutrition and ideal weight gain. Obesity may add a further burden to an already stressed myocardium. Therapy of chronic congestive heart failure may include restriction of salt intake.

The physician should discourage a sedentary life style and encourage physical activity in programs such as physical education but stress with school personnel that the child should be allowed to rest when fatigued. An exercise stress test directly measures the patient's exercise tolerance and provides valuable information regarding advice for level of activity. The child with a dilated heart or significant left or right heart obstructive lesions should not participate in competitive athletics. Participation in such organized sports as baseball, golf, or bowling may be acceptable.

A child may have significant absenteeism from school due to chronic illness or frequent hospitalizations for diagnostic or surgical procedures. Every effort by parents, physicians, and school personnel should be made to provide a tutorial service during these situations. The child should attend regular classes when possible. Occasionally, this requires special adjustments to overcome physical limitations, e.g., inability to climb stairs. The main emphasis is allowing the child to lead as normal a life as possible.

If the child or family is having difficulties coping with the heart defect, parent and child support groups are often beneficial. Many cardiac centers are encouraging the organization of such groups, which can provide educational, emo-

TABLE 3. **Bacterial Endocarditis Prophylaxis**

Prophylaxis for Dental Procedures and Surgical Procedures of the Upper Respiratory Tract	
REGIMEN A—Penicillin	
1. Oral	
Adults:	Penicillin V 2.0 grams 1 hour prior to the procedure and then 1.0 gram 6 hours later.
Children:	Penicillin V 1.0 gram 1 hour prior to the procedure and then 500 mg 6 hours later.*
2. Parenteral	
Adults:	Aqueous penicillin G 2 million units IV or IM 30–60 minutes prior to the procedure and 1 million units 6 hours later.
Children:	Aqueous penicillin G (50,000 units/kg) IV or IM 30–60 minutes prior to the procedure and (25,000 units/kg) 6 hours later.*
REGIMEN B—For Patients Allergic to Penicillin	
1. Oral Erythromycin	
Adults:	Erythromycin 1.0 gram 1 hour prior to procedure and then 500 mg 6 hours later.
Children:	Erythromycin (20 mg/kg) 1 hour prior to procedure and then (10 mg/kg) 6 hours later.*
REGIMEN C—For Patients with Prosthetic Valves and Others With Highest Risk of Endocarditis	
1. Parenteral Ampicillin and Gentamicin	
Adults:	Ampicillin 1.0–2.0 grams plus gentamicin (1.5 mg/kg) both IV or IM one half hour prior to the procedure followed by 1.0 gram oral penicillin V 6 hours later.
Children:	Ampicillin (50 mg/kg) plus gentamicin (2.0 mg/kg) both IM or IV one half hour prior to the procedure followed by 1.0 gram oral penicillin V 6 hours later.*
REGIMEN D—For High Risk Patients Allergic to Penicillin	
1. IV Vancomycin	
Adults:	Vancomycin 1.0 gram IV slowly over 1 hour starting 1 hour prior to procedure.
Children:	Vancomycin (20 mg/kg) IV slowly over 1 hour starting 1 hour prior to procedure.*
Prophylaxis for Gastrointestinal and Genitourinary Tract Surgery and Instrumentation	
REGIMEN A—For GU and GI Tract Procedures	
Adults:	Ampicillin 2.0 grams IM or IV plus gentamicin (1.5 mg/kg) IM or IV given one half to one hour before procedure. One follow-up dose may be given 8 hours later.
Children:	Ampicillin (50 mg/kg) IM or IV plus gentamicin (2.0 mg/kg) IM or IV given one half to one hour before procedure. One follow-up dose may be given 8 hours later.*
REGIMEN B—For Patients Allergic to Penicillin	
Adults:	Vancomycin (1.0 gram) given IV slowly over 1 hour plus gentamicin (1.5 mg/kg) IM or IV 1 hour prior to procedure. These doses may be repeated once 8–12 hours later.
Children:	Vancomycin (20 mg/kg) up to 1 gram given IV 1 hour prior to procedure plus gentamicin (2.0 mg/kg) IM or IV 1 hour prior to procedure. These doses may be repeated once 8–12 hours later.*
REGIMEN C—Oral Regimen for Minor or Repetitive Procedures in Low Risk Patients	
Adults:	Amoxicillin 3.0 grams orally 1 hour before procedure and 1.5 grams 6 hours later.

*Smaller antibiotic dosages are for children less than 60 lb (27 kg) and should not exceed the maximum adult dosages. Taken from Prevention of Bacterial Endocarditis, Circulation Vol. 70, 1984 with compliments from the Division of Pediatric Cardiology, University Hospitals, Iowa City, Iowa.

tional, and personal support not usually provided by health professionals.

Employers will often deny jobs to patients with congenital heart disease. Job counseling and vocational training are often available through state rehabilitation agencies, which assess patients' abilities and help them seek appropriate career goals.

Noncardiac Surgery

General anesthesia often causes concern in a patient with congenital heart disease. When giving anesthesia, maintain oxygenation and prevent hypotension. Monitor the intraoperative electrocardiogram, blood pressure, and arterial blood gases during major procedures. The choice of anesthetic agent will depend on the existing physiology of the cardiac defect. Agents that lower systemic resistance (thiopental, halothane, and spinal anesthesia) will enhance right to left shunting in patients with tetralogy of Fallot; conversely, an agent that raises systemic resistance (ketamine, cyclopropane, and nitrous oxide) may be favorable. Anesthesia risk is high in patients with pulmonary hypertension. Cyclopropane and ether will increase pulmonary vascular resistance and thus should be avoided.

Prophylaxis Against Bacterial Endocarditis

During dental or surgical manipulations, bacteremia may occur. A child with structural heart disease should receive antibiotic prophylaxis to prevent the uncommon complication of endocarditis. Table 3 lists the American Heart Association's recommended antibiotic prophylaxis schedule. Sterile procedures, e.g., cardiac catheterization, do not require antibiotic prophylaxis. Children with congenital heart disease should not receive continuous antibiotic prophylaxis to minimize infections, since this may produce resistant strains of bacteria.

Cerebral Vascular Accidents

Children with cyanotic heart disease may develop a cerebrovascular accident. Marked arterial desaturation combined with relative iron deficiency anemia is often present. Closely monitor hemoglobin, hematocrit, and red blood cell indices. If relative anemia is present, begin oral iron supplementation. The older child may present with polycythemia, which may produce cerebral ischemia and thrombotic infarction.

A child with right to left shunting who develops signs of an infection and an expanding brain mass should be considered to have a brain abscess until proved otherwise. Treatment consists of antibiotic therapy and surgical drainage.

Pregnancy and Contraception

Women with mild to moderate acyanotic congenital heart disease usually tolerate pregnancy and come to term without any difficulties. Pregnancy in a female with cyanotic congenital heart disease may pose many problems. Besides the threat to her own health, the mother may not realize the danger to the fetus; the rates of miscarriage and stillbirth are higher than in normal women. If pregnancy might result in a severe disability or even a potential fatality, a tubal ligation should be considered. The physician should ensure that the patient fully understands sexual physiology and methods for contraception. Such methods as intrauterine devices or birth control pills are contraindicated in patients with significant heart disease. The physician may advise the use of a condom and a diaphragm with spermicidal gel or foam.

Insurability

Most children with structural heart defects can obtain life insurance. The exception include patients who have tetralogy of Fallot, aortic stenosis, and preoperative coarctation of the aorta or patent ductus arteriosus. Many insured patients will have the standard premium rating or only a mild rate increase.

MITRAL VALVE PROLAPSE

method of
H. CECIL COGHLAN, M.D.
The University of Alabama
Birmingham, Alabama

The therapy of mitral valve prolapse (MVP) cannot be discussed without a recognition of its heterogeneity, as well as a keen awareness that, in spite of the "explosion" of literature on the subject, there are fundamental gaps in our knowledge. Ignoring its complexity, equating it simply to other causes of mitral regurgitation, or accepting the oversimplified and probably naive view that MVP syndrome is merely "neurosis" leads to poor patient care, complacency that considers our task fulfilled by merely putting a label on our patients, and incapacitating and expensive patient despair.

We have not found that showing appropriate interest and concern, attempting to explain the nature of the problem, and discussing honestly the possible psychogenic components, when present, have led to the much-feared iatrogenic disease. On the contrary, patients seem often to wander from one physician to another when they detect what they view as lack of interest, often reinforcing their fear that their condition has not been recognized or is not susceptible to treatment. Documenting the abnormal physiology without resorting to excessively costly tests and explaining it to the patient in a manner that attempts to teach the patient how to cope with, and if possible, overcome the handicaps, have helped our symptomatic patients make adjustments in life style and plan activities more productively and with less anticipatory anxiety about the "effect on their condition." Open and frank discussion that acknowledges that we do not know everything about MVP in general has promoted patient confidence and compliance to a greater degree than advice to merely ignore their disease or "learn to live with it" but without our help.

Heritable connective tissue disorders in which auscultatory and echocardiographic MVP may be present (Marfan syndrome, Ehlers-Danlos syndrome, pseudoxanthoma elasticum, and osteogenesis imperfecta) should be differentiated, as these have specific defects and natural history that are not determined by the MVP and are not part of the MVP syndrome. Muscular dystrophies with echocardiographic MVP should also be ruled out, as well as endocrine and neurologic diseases that may cause similar symptoms and could fail to be recognized because of the findings of a "coincidental" MVP.

Asymptomatic Patients

It is likely that a large subset of patients are asymptomatic ("anatomic MVP" of Wooley). Very thorough population studies carried out in Framingham showed no difference in the incidence of symptoms often associated with MVP in subjects with and without echocardiographic MVP. Clicks and murmurs were notoriously infrequent in those subjects, a fact that differs markedly from clinical series and has made some investigators suggest that a large percentage of those subjects represented "anatomic variants" of normal. An increased incidence of arrhythmias and endocarditis has already been recognized in that population. If (increasingly rare) errors from transducer position, and conditions leading to abnormally reduced end-diastolic volume of the left ventricle (such as hyperdynamic circulation from hyperthyroidism, anemia or extreme anxiety, and hypertrophic cardiomyopathy) are excluded and if mitral leaflets appear thickened in a high resolution two-dimensional echocardiogram, we prefer to explain the finding, emphasize that a large percentage of patients are not symptomatic and need not become so, and encourage regular physical activity to maintain conditioning that promotes the best possible autonomic regulation in patients. Also, we strongly discourage smoking and use of caffeinated beverages and refined sugars.

Patients with repolarization changes in a resting electrocardiogram are best evaluated with Holter monitoring to try to detect unrecognized arrhythmias that are potentially threatening. We reassure the patient about the generally favorable prognosis and very low probability of complications. Follow-up examination every 2 years with two-dimensional echography to evaluate chamber size, check aortic root dimensions and point of coaptation of aortic leaflets, and carefully listen for significant mitral and aortic regurgitation is advisable and reassuring to patients. It becomes especially important in patients beyond the age of 60 years who should be seen more frequently, as they are more prone to develop atrial fibrillation and congestive failure secondary to mitral regurgitation and have an increased incidence of coronary disease.

These presentations occur in the later decades even in subjects who have been apparently asymptomatic. We explain the small but proved risk of endocarditis, as well as the fact that the exact risk is not defined, and advise endocarditis prophylaxis, following the recommendations of the American Heart Association, in all patients who are not allergic (with particular care if regimens with parenteral penicillin are to be used). We do not exclude patients with "click but no murmur."

Symptomatic Patients ("MVP Syndrome")

The exact percentage of symptomatic patients with idiopathic MVP is debated. Some internists feel that the overwhelming majority of patients with classic MVP seen in the practice of internal medicine do not have cardiovascular symptoms. Other clinical series report that 16 to 20 per cent are asymptomatic. Symptoms may be mild, but in certain patient subsets severe and incapacitating symptoms occur.

The exact pathogenesis of symptoms is not totally elucidated. Extensive study of autonomic regulation in such symptomatic patients has led us to believe that imbalance or dysregulation (dysautonomia, without structural neural disease) may play an important role. This has therapeutic implications. We echo Jeresaty in his important quote of Dr. Halberstam: "This is not to indicate despair at the state of modern medicine, only to recall how much mystery remains. Because of this, physicians will continue—must continue—to apply partially understood therapies to barely understood illness. It is foolish for critics of medicine to puff up righteously about unproven therapies." Admitting that much investigation is still needed to elucidate the various aspects of this interesting yet poorly understood syndrome, it is important to analyze what can be attempted to try to help symptomatic patients. The main symptoms and their possible therapies are best discussed separately, even though they may clearly occur simultaneously in varied combinations of severity or sequence.

Chest Pain. Coinciding with Dr. Jeresaty's valuable observations, we have seen pain unrelated to activity and particularly frequent following effort, and most especially after accumulation of fatigue in 82 per cent of patients; exertional, in 9 per cent; and both exertional and at rest, in 9 per cent. The last two types are often very difficult to differentiate from stable and unstable angina. In effort pain, because of the frequency of ischemic ST-T changes on graded exercise tests in MVP, a normal ^{201}Tl exertional myocardial scintigram may be required to exclude coronary artery disease (provided an adequate level of exertion is achieved). In doubt, coronary arteriography is necessary, as in patients who present with rest pain.

A minority of patients have classic variant or vasospastic angina. Migraine headaches and Raynaud-like discomfort are more frequent in these patients. The mechanism of "noncardiac pain" is debated. We have found this symptom particularly in patients who exhibit clear hyperadrenergic responsiveness or in those with mixed hyperadrenergic and hypervagal reactivity. An exaggerated heart rate and respiratory response to exercise (or to central stimuli such as emotions) may lead to abnormal contracture of chest wall muscles that is painful, particularly in subjects like MVP patients who appear to be hypersensitive to pain and other sensory inputs. The frequently associated dyspnea (not necessarily hyperventilation) may have a similar pathogenesis.

Chest pain and dyspnea have been documented to result from dyskinesis of respiratory muscles in patients with extrapyramidal disorders. Maekawa documented tetanic contraction in chest wall muscles during pain in patients with "neurocirculatory asthenia." We noted similar findings with simpler and less extensive recordings. There is probably a component of "mechanical" stimulation of chest wall muscles due to the tapping of a hyperdynamic heart against a chest wall of abnormal proximity caused by the frequently narrow anteroposterior chest diameter or pectus excavatum.

Beta blockers have been the mainstay in the literature. Like Jeresaty, we have found that MVP patients frequently complain of increased fatigue, particularly when using lipid-soluble drugs like propranolol (Inderal). Occasional patients respond well to nadolol (Corgard), 20 to 40 mg twice daily; atenolol (Tenormin), 25 to 50 mg every morning; or metoprolol (Lopressor), 25 to 50 mg twice daily. Lipid-soluble drugs also have shown a definite tendency to produce or accentuate depression and sleep disturbances. We have had particularly gratifying results with the cautious use of clonidine (Catapres). We titrate the dose carefully to avoid hypotension and drowsiness, starting with 0.05 mg at bedtime and increasing to twice daily and three times daily according to tolerance and response. This therapy has been particularly helpful in patients with excessive peripheral vasoconstriction (cold feet with slow capillary filling in the absence of arterial obstructive disease and cold hands with or without Raynaud's disease).

Patients who do not tolerate clonidine or do not get adequate relief have responded very well to calcium antagonists. We choose verapamil (Isoptin, Calan) 80 mg two or three times a day, or diltiazem (Cardizem), 30 to 60 mg three times a day, rather than nifedipine because with the latter patients complain of weakness and tachycardia (hypotensive effect with exaggerated reflex response in MVP patients). We are beginning to use labetalol (Trandate, Normodyne) in small doses (150 mg once or twice daily), as its combined alpha and beta blocker effect may prove very helpful in patients with vasoconstriction. Strong reassurance, with diligent and convincing exclusion of coronary disease, is valuable and necessary.

Esophageal motility disorders account also for a minority of the rest pains. Diffuse esophageal spasm is uncommon, but esophageal contractions of exceedingly long duration and high amplitude in the distal esophagus are more frequent and may respond dramatically to calcium antagonists or nitrates. (The latter do not relieve the other types of noncardiac pain and also may cause discomfort from venous pooling in dysautonomic MVP patients.) Reflux must be corrected as it may cause pain from secondary motility disorder.

The exact mechanism of the effect of clonidine and calcium antagonists is the subject of ongoing research. The former reduces (centrally) efferent sympathetic traffic and peripheral norepinephrine release. Diltiazem attenuates baroreflex sensitivity in humans, in addition to local effects on muscle contraction.

Dyspnea and Fatigue. Both occur frequently. Both have been attributed merely to neurosis. We believe the problem is more complex. Sixty per cent of our patients who had remained moderately active had a 20 per cent reduction of effort tolerance on treadmill testing, and 25 per cent had a reduction of 50 per cent or more. These symptoms occur in hyperadrenergic patients, associated with inappropriate sinus tachycardia on standing and with minimal activity. Respiratory drive also appears excessive for the level of exercise. There may be an abnormal buildup of serum lactate with exertion, possibly related to excessive levels of catecholamines, which also contribute to fatigue. The excessive respiratory drive is perceived as increased work of breathing manifested as dyspnea during or following exertion. Few patients have psychogenic hyperventilation. The hypervagal patients manifest abnormal regulation of the capacitance system, with excessive venous pooling in the lower body during standing and inadequate rise in cardiac output during exercise. Postural hypotension is frequent in this subset and almost certainly accentuates the feeling of fatigue during upright activity.

Reduction of excessive adrenergic tone by clonidine or beta blockers may prove helpful and may permit beneficial conditioning exercises after pharmacologic therapy becomes effective. Hypervagal patients generally respond to small doses of oral phenobarbital, 15 to 30 mg at bedtime, or two or three times a day. Experimental work has shown significant reduction of vagal tone (we believe centrally). It may be necessary to add fludrocortisone (Florinef), 0.05 to 0.1 mg every morning. Such small doses sensitize arterioles to catecholamines without fluid retention, in our experience. Syncope with features of vasovagal syncope may occur in these patients.

Palpitations and Arrhythmias. Palpitations may represent either the awareness of a hyperactive heart, or sinus tachycardia inappropriate for the circumstances (not correlated with dysrhythmias on Holter monitor) or true dysrhythmias that occur frequently in patients with MVP. Holter monitor evaluation is essential to identify the minority of patients with threatening complex arrhythmias. Patients with infrequent premature ventricular or atrial contractions that are isolated, not associated with ST-T changes on resting electrocardiogram (ECG), and without increase or induction of complex arrhythmias on exercise testing require only reassurance; these contractions often become controlled with measures to reduce sympathetic tone. Ventricular couplets, bigeminy, and short or more sustained self-terminating ventricular tachycardia require careful evaluation as they may be life threatening. These may respond well to beta blockers. If the QT is prolonged, type I antiarrhythmics may be associated with a risk of torsade de pointes, even at therapeutic serum levels.

Experimental drugs like aprindine have been necessary in a minority of patients. Ethmozine appears to hold special promise. Patients with sustained supraventricular tachycardias need special evaluation as they may have abnormal (left-sided) bypass tracts. If they conduct antegrade, atrial flutter and especially paroxysmal atrial fibrillation may be very dangerous and cause ventricular fibrillation. Careful Holter monitoring will generally allow the diagnosis initially and permit the selection of the patients requiring specialized electrophysiologic studies.

Neurologic Symptoms. Syncope may be due to arrhythmia, orthostatic hypotension, or vasovagal reactions. Transient ischemic attacks, strokes in young patients without atherosclerotic vascular disease or other cause of emboli, and transient visual disturbances from retinal emboli have been well documented. Platelet emboli from the abnormal valve have been implicated. Standard therapy with anticoagulants, followed by antiplatelet agents is required. Barnett's group has reported a 16 per cent recurrence in spite of such treatments over an 8 year follow-up. Endocarditis must be carefuly ruled out, as well as atrial arrhythmias that increase the risk. Syncope may also result from partial complex seizure disorder (temporal lobe seizures) and from intermittent heart block. EEG and Holter monitor are essential, in addition to a thorough neurologic evaluation.

Psychiatric Manifestations. These have often been emphasized as an almost constant component of the MVP syndrome. Extensive investigation in our population with personality inventories has not shown an incidence of psychopathology different from that of the general population. Anxiety is frequent, and panic attacks do occur in some patients. Most patients feel "anticipatory anxiety" secondary to symptoms they have experienced. Psychotherapy without attempts to carefully define the abnormal physiology and try to correct it has been notoriously unsuccessful. Our patients have often received treatment for depression before the diagnosis, with distressing increase of their discomfort and enhancement of their anxiety and despair. Patients with MVP are very sensitive to drugs, and the vagolytic effect of tricyclics makes them far more symptomatic. There is a propensity to depression and decreased ability to cope. An understanding team approach, with a psychologist or psychiatrist when indicated, without ignoring the patients' total syndrome or allowing them to feel that they are being referred to the specialist out of lack of interest or desire to try to help them, has been very useful.

Often patients will respond to 25 to 50 mg at bedtime of desipramine (Norpramin), maprotiline (Ludiomil), or doxepin (Sinequan). Patients should be warned that the effect will take time and that some degree of tachycardia is likely to occur. Trazodone (Desyrel) 25 to 50 mg at bedtime, has fewer autonomic effects but, unfortunately, often causes uncomfortable sedation. We have found useful on short-term therapy small doses of lorazepam (Ativan), 0.5 to 1 mg two or three times a day, and alprazolam (Xanax), 0.25 to 0.5 mg two or three times a day.

We emphasize to patients that depression is common in the syndrome (60 per cent in a large study), possibly related to partially defined imbalances in neurotransmitters of the brain, which are likely to improve with the medications. We do not want to make them feel they are mental patients who have to "pull themselves together" and overcome their distressing symptoms on their own. True panic attacks require expert psychiatric therapy, as does severe depression with feelings of hopelessness or self-depreciation, which we have found infrequently. Attention to the emotional aspects is fundamental, as the biologic reactions of fight-or-flight and conservation-withdrawal exert profound influences on circulatory and autonomic regulation in general through the central controls located in the limbic system.

Reassurance and gradual progressive physical conditioning as soon as cardiovascular symptoms begin to improve are particularly important to build confidence and allow better cardiorespiratory performance, and will reassure patients by making it possible for them to perform activity more reliably.

We initiate exercise therapy with recumbent exercises in patients with significant weakness or orthostatic hypotension, to achieve physical conditioning without having to adjust also to the orthostatic stress. Swimming, with due precautions (lifejacket), is an excellent exercise. Speedwalking, after gradually building up, is also very good. We discourage isometric exercises or those involving jumping (acceleration-deceleration stress) until there has been significant improvement.

Questions Regarding Inheritance

Patients are becoming increasingly worried about the mode of inheritance. They should be told that all the facts are not known and that there may be autosomal transmission, but with strong emphasis on the varying expressivity and the fact that MVP is a spectrum of severity such that significant disease need not occur in their offspring.

A positive, reassuring, and genuinely interested attitude, with careful attention to identification of subsets of greater risk and due recognition that patients older than age 60 years should be watched more closely, has been rewarding in this fascinating and partially understood syndrome. We should "watch Salome drop her veils," as Dr. Melvin Cheitlin stated, but should maintain a calm and positive attitude.

CONGESTIVE HEART FAILURE

method of
MARTIN J. FRANK, M.D.,
and ABDULLA M. ABDULLA, M.D.
Medical College of Georgia
Augusta, Georgia

Heart failure is defined as that state in which the ventricles are unable to pump sufficient blood to meet the ordinary metabolic demands of the body tissues. The term congestive heart failure is frequently used because so many of the clinical manifestations of heart failure result from accumulation of interstitial fluid. Since both sides of the heart are in circuit, it is obvious that with time, failure of the left ventricle will result in failure of the right ventricle. Heart failure is produced by inadequacy of the myocardial contractile mechanism, occurring either as a primary problem (cardiomyopathy) or secondary to conditions such as coronary, hypertensive, or valvular disease. Myocardial failure may also be aggravated by factors such as hypoxia, hypercapnia, acidosis, hyperkalemia, arrhythmias, uncontrolled hypertension, excess fluid intake, beta-adrenergic blockers, and antiarrhythmic drugs such as disopyramide phosphate.

Treatment

Asymptomatic patients with mild left ventricular dysfunction probably do not require immediate drug treatment. Patients with heart failure who require treatment include those in the following diagnostic subsets: (1) acute pulmonary edema, (2) pulmonary and visceral congestion and peripheral edema, and (3) low cardiac output states.

Pulmonary Edema. Pulmonary edema is a medical emergency that requires immediate and intelligent therapy. It results from conditions that produce an abrupt elevation in pulmonary capillary pressure. This causes congestion, primarily due to fluid accumulation in the interstitial tissues (including the pulmonary lymphatics) and in the air passages. Pulmonary congestion may result from noncardiac causes that alter capillary permeability. These include smoke inhalation, narcotic overdose, salicylate overdose, and septicemia. Treatment of noncardiac pulmonary edema includes large doses of corticosteroids, whereas treatment of pulmonary edema of cardiac origin is based primarily on measures that reduce pulmonary capillary pressure and improve left ventricular performance. Patients are best treated in a bed with the head elevated to about 45 degrees to reduce venous return to the lungs and improve breathing. Oxygen via a 40 to 60 per cent Venti-mask should be started. Morphine sulfate is probably the most important drug for this condition, since it alleviates anxiety, reduces the oxygen cost of breathing, and lowers left atrial pressure by venodilation. It may also improve cardiac output by its sympatholytic effect, which decreases peripheral vascular resistance. Morphine sulfate is best administered in a dilute solution (1 mg per ml) and given intravenously at a rate of approximately 1 mg per minute in a dose of 3 to 5 mg. This dosage can be repeated as needed at 15 minute intervals to a total dose of 10 to 15 mg, depending on the patient's size. This drug should be used with caution in the hypotensive patient and in those not felt to have a large preload, since it may cause an abrupt fall in the systemic blood pressure if effective circulating blood volume is reduced. It must also be used with great caution in patients suspected of having impaired pulmonary function. Respiratory depression is best corrected by naloxone, 0.4 mg given intravenously, repeated at 2 to 3 minute intervals as necessary.

Probably the second most useful drug is furosemide, a potent "loop" diuretic, which should be begun intravenously at a dose of 20 mg. Substitute 25 mg of ethacrynic acid for patients with known hypersensitivity to sulfonamide diuretics. In addition to their diuretic effect, "loop" diuretics cause venodilation that provides almost immediate hemodynamic improvement and also enhances lymphatic drainage of pulmonary edema fluid. Indeed, resolution of pulmonary edema may occur in the absence of a significant diuresis. The initial use of large doses of furosemide should be strongly discouraged, particularly in patients who develop pulmonary edema in the presence of a normal circulatory volume without preceding chronic heart failure. Under these circumstances the loss of one third or more of the blood volume into the lungs as a consequence of pulmonary edema, followed by a large diuresis after an excessive dose of furosemide, commonly results in hypotension, the "pseudo-shock" of congestive heart failure. It is therefore preferable to give a second, larger dose if the desired degree of diuresis and clinical improvement is not seen within 30 minutes. Most patients will note dramatic improvement of dyspnea within 10 minutes. If this does not occur, sublingual nitroglycerin, as a 0.4 to 0.6 mg tablet, may be beneficial, since it will intensify the venous pooling effect of morphine and furosemide and rapidly reduce pulmonary capillary pressure. Nitroglycerin, morphine (as described previously), and furosemide, 20 to 80 mg, may be repeated if dyspnea is not controlled and hypotension is not provoked. Patients with a marginal effective blood volume who are refractory to or develop hypotension with morphine, furosemide, and sublingual nitroglycerin may benefit from intravenous nitroglycerin, since the dosage may be adjusted more precisely. A 50 mg ampule diluted in 500 ml of 5 per cent dextrose solution yields a concentration of 100 micrograms per ml. Start the infusion at 0.5 to 1 μg per kg per minute (35 to 70 μg per minute). The infusion is best delivered using a pump, with adjustment of the dosage upward until the desired therapeutic effects are obtained. Unless a Swan-Ganz catheter is employed, effects should be limited to a blood pressure reduction of no more than 10 to 20 mm Hg to avoid a fall in arterial oxygen content and a potential decrease in coronary perfusion. It is also important to remember that intravenous nitroglycerin may prolong the effects of narcotics and barbiturates, potentiate the anticholinergic and hypotensive effects of tricyclic antidepressants, and enhance the effects of other potentially hypotensive agents such as propranolol.

Patients not responsive to the foregoing protocol, particularly those who have persistent hypertension following administration of morphine (diastolic pressure 110 mm Hg or greater), are candidates for an arteriolar and venous vasodilator. Our preference is for sodium nitroprusside because of its very short half-life. It is supplied as a lyophilized powder in a 50 mg vial to be diluted in 5 per cent dextrose and water *only*. A micro-drip regulator is mandatory, and a constant infusion device is highly desirable. The required dosage varies widely, from 0.5 to 8 μg per kg of body weight per minute. Infusion is best begun at 20 μg per minute and increased as needed, taking care to avoid an excessive fall in blood pressure. The average dose is approximately 3 μg per kg per minute, but lower doses may be required for patients receiving other antihypertensive medications. Administration of sodium nitroprusside must be accompanied by frequent blood pressure measurements. An intra-arterial line and a Swan-Ganz catheter are highly desirable. The systolic pressure should not be allowed to fall below 100 mg Hg, and this level may prove to be too low for patients presenting initially with severe hypertension. If mental confusion develops or urinary output falls, the blood pressure should be allowed to rise to a more acceptable level. When signs of significant symptomatic and hemodynamic improvement are apparent, the infusion rate should be tapered and finally discontinued. Hypertensive patients should be started on oral agents during intravenous therapy to reduce the time that nitroprusside is required.

Digitalis, long the mainstay of therapy in chronic heart failure, is of little benefit in the first few hours of acute pulmonary edema since it does not reach its maximum effect for several hours. Therefore, it should follow, rather than precede, administration of the triad of morphine, furosemide, and nitroglycerin. When indicated, digoxin, 0.5 to 0.75 mg, should be given slowly intravenously to patients who have not previously received the drug and are in sinus rhythm. This should be followed by a daily oral maintenance dose of 0.25 mg. Patients with renal failure should, of course, receive a lower maintenance dose (0.125 mg daily or on alternate days), as dictated by the degree of renal insufficiency. Other inotropic agents, such as dopamine and dobutamine, may be employed when patients have acute pulmonary edema complicated by marked myocardial dysfunction with hypotension and signs of low cardiac output. The classic setting for this situation is following a large myocardial infarction. Although both drugs are potent inotropic agents, we prefer dobutamine because it has less vasoconstrictive effect and is less likely to increase left ventricular work. The increase in cardiac output results from an enhanced stroke volume rather than from an accelerated heart rate. Dobutamine, 250 mg, is mixed in 250 ml of dextrose and water and begun at a dose of 1 μg per kg per minute, increasing gradually to 10 μg per kg per minute, or until the desired response has occurred.

Intravenous aminophylline, 250 to 500 mg, may be infused over 15 minutes every 4 hours to patients with pulmonary edema who have considerable wheezing despite the use of more conventional forms of treatment. The drug relieves bronchospasm and increases cardiac and urinary output. However, its tendency to provoke cardiac arrhythmias indicates that it must be employed with caution. External phlebotomy (withdrawing 300 to 500 ml of blood) is rarely indicated because of current availability of powerful venodilating agents. The technique of rotating tourniquets has lost popularity for similar reasons and also because it tends to trap blood centrally rather than in the extremities. Patients with renal failure and marked volume expansion may benefit from peritoneal dialysis or ultrafiltration.

Patients with significant respiratory embarrassment ($P_{O_2} < 50$ mm Hg or $P_{CO_2} > 50$ mm Hg) despite optimal oxygen supplementation should undergo endotracheal intubation and mechanical ventilation. Positive end-expiratory pressure (PEEP) may improve oxygenation and lower pulmonary capillary pressure by reducing venous return. However, PEEP may cause significant hypotension in patients with marginal or low circulating blood volumes and pulmonary capillary pressure.

Tachyarrhythmias, particularly ventricular tachycardia associated with or provoking acute pulmonary edema, require urgent corrective therapy in the form of electrical cardioversion followed by appropriate antiarrhythmic drug therapy. When using antiarrhythmic drugs, remember that quinidine sulfate, procainamide, and disopyramide phosphate have a negative inotropic effect. This effect is more pronounced with disopyramide, particularly when the dose is not appropriately reduced in patients with renal insufficiency. Moreover, all three agents have an anticholinergic effect on the atrioventricular node during the early phase of administration and may produce an increase in heart rate in patients with atrial fibrillation or flutter. In such cases, these drugs should not be used until the ventricular rate has been reduced to below 90 per minute by digoxin. In patients with advanced ventricular dysfunction, quinidine has less negative inotropic effect than procainamide or disopyramide, while tocainide has the least. (Mexiletine and amiodarone also have minimal, if any, negative inotropic effects but are not approved by the Food and Drug Administration.) Quinidine increases the serum level of digitalis because of reduced renal clearance and decreased tissue binding. Toxicity is avoided by reducing the dosages of digoxin by approximately one half.

After resolution of acute pulmonary edema, the patient is treated in a manner similar to that described below.

Pulmonary and Visceral Congestion and Peripheral Edema. Patients usually develop symptoms and signs of congestion and edema in the pulmonary, splanchnic, and systemic circulation because of an inappropriate increase in filling pressure and preload of one or both ventricles and an expanded intravascular volume. It is important to identify the cause and to recognize and correct reversible factors. A reduced salt intake and bed rest will reduce the work of the heart and reverse normal orthostatic antidiuresis. Indeed, significant diuresis and improvement are often noted with this modality alone. Strict bed rest is discouraged because of an increased risk of pulmonary thromboembolism. Patients confined to bed for several days should be treated with "minidose" heparin (5000 units subcutaneously every 8 to 12 hours). If no contraindications exist, oral anticoagulants are desirable for chronic failure. Digoxin, 0.25 mg, should be started on a daily basis. This program usually achieves its maximum effect in 7 to 10 days. Large initial doses of digoxin are seldom indicated in chronic failure and should be reserved for patients with atrial tachyarrhythmia. Patients with renal insufficiency require proportionately smaller doses of digoxin (as described earlier). Digitoxin (in a dose of 0.1 to 0.15 mg per day) is preferred by one of us because of better and more predictable oral absorption of the drug and its lack of dependence on the kidneys for clearance. However, its longer duration of action prolongs digitalis toxicity when this occurs. Thiazide diuretics and related drugs produce a direct inhibition of sodium resorption in the cortical diluting segment of the loop of Henle and have a moderate potency. The usual dose of hydrochlorothiazide is 50 mg daily. It will promote sodium and water excretion and reduce intravascular volume and systemic and pulmonary congestion. We use furosemide (40 to 240 mg per day) in patients resistant to thiazides, those with severe failure, and those with renal insufficiency (creatinine $>$ 2.5 mg). Furosemide acts on the medullary diluting segment. It has a steep dose-response curve, a short duration of action, and a proportionate increase in diuresis with stepwise increments in dosage. A single daily dose is preferable, since it is less likely to produce hypokalemia. Recent experience with metolazone (2.5 to 10 mg per day) suggests that it is a very useful adjunct to furosemide in patients with refractory failure and severe fluid retention, since it markedly potentiates the action of the latter. Also, it may produce diuresis when the glomerular filtration rate is as low as 20 ml per minute.

Patients with pulmonary congestion due to mitral stenosis who remain in sinus rhythm benefit from diuretic therapy. Digitalis offers little help in the absence of atrial tachyarrhythmias. Propranolol in small doses (10 to 20 mg two to four times daily) may be beneficial by reducing an inappropriately rapid heart rate response to effort and thereby increasing the duration of left ventricular filling. This will reduce the left atrial pressure rise during exercise and decrease the tendency toward pulmonary congestion. Hypertrophic cardiomyopathy is another cause of congestive heart failure for which propranolol in conjunction with the cautious use of diuretics (rather than digitalis) is the treatment of choice for those who remain in sinus rhythm.

Diuretics may induce hypokalemia and increase the risk of digitalis arrhythmias, unless oral potassium supplements or potassium-sparing diuretics (spironolactone, amiloride, or triamterene), which act on the distal convoluted tubules and early collecting ducts, are added. Although distal tubular drugs have a weak diuretic action when given alone, they potentiate the effect of other diuretics by enhancing sodium excretion. Commercially available salt substitutes have a high potassium content and are a relatively inexpensive source of oral potassium. Other potential problems associated with chronic diuretic therapy, particularly when a combination of furosemide and metolazone is necessary, include hyponatremia, hypophosphatemia, hypomagnesemia, hyperglycemia, and hyperuricemia. These side effects may increase sensitivity to digitalis, worsen heart failure, or aggravate pre-existing diabetes or gouty arthritis. Also, excessively vigorous diuresis may reduce the effective circulatory volume and result in hypotension and azotemia.

When failure persists despite optimal therapy with digitalis and diuretics, the use of nitrates as venodilator drugs is often helpful. We use oral isosorbide dinitrate, 10 to 80 mg four or more times daily, or a topical nitroglycerin patch. Dosage should be titrated to an orthostatic blood pressure fall of less than 20 mm Hg to avoid an excessive reduction in left ventricular filling pressure. Nitrate-induced headaches should be treated with aspirin or acetaminophen. Headaches usually subside in a week or two, but a reduction in dosage or discontinuation of the drug may be required. Nitrate therapy should be delayed in patients with severe peripheral edema, since it may be ineffective because of reduced venous distensibility. The use of indomethacin should be avoided, since its prostaglandin-inhibiting effect may interfere with venodilatation. When congestive heart failure is associated with a reduced left ventricular ejection fraction and symptoms of easy fatigability, the use of arteriolar dilators should also be considered (see below).

Low Cardiac Output States with or without Associated Congestive Heart Failure. When congestive heart failure is a result primarily of an increased preload with secondary changes in the afterload and contractile state, conventional therapy with digitalis and diuretics is usually adequate, although some patients will require nitrates because of their venodilator action. Such patients have a normal or only moderately reduced stroke volume, and the positive inotropic effect of the digitalis glycosides is adequate. However, when congestive heart failure results from a loss of the contractile mechanism (as in primary cardiomyopathies or following acute myocardial infarction) or with secondary myocardial failure (as in progressive ventricular dilatation due to chronic valvular regurgitation), stroke volume is severely depressed and afterload is significantly increased because of the high systolic wall tension required for ventricular emptying. Under these circumstances, digitalis has only limited benefits. Diuretic therapy, with or without the use of nitrates, may be effective in controlling the symptoms of pulmonary and peripheral congestion, but a chronic low cardiac output state will still be manifested as easy fatigability and tachycardia. If there is progressive loss of the contractile mechanism, azotemia and mental confusion may develop.

In the absence of persistent congestive heart failure, depletion of the effective circulatory volume should be suspected, particularly in patients with impaired ventricular compliance due to massive hypertrophy or in those with ischemic heart disease but a normal cardiac size. This situation is best identified by measurement of orthostatic changes in blood pressure and blood volume and noninvasive determination of left atrial pressure (JAMA *243*:1539, 1980). However, when evidence for a depleted circulatory volume is absent, the use of vasodilator drugs should be considered. The rationale is based on the fact that an elevated systemic vascular resistance depresses left ventricular myocardial function profoundly in the presence of left ventricular contractile failure. Under these circumstances, a drug that acts specifically on arteriolar smooth muscle, such as hydralazine, will be of benefit by reducing aortic impedance and thereby improving left ventricular emptying, with a consequent increase in stroke volume. Hydralazine should be started with a test dose of 25 mg and continued only if a fall in blood pressure does not occur. It is best given initially at 6 hour intervals with an increase of 25 mg every second dose to a total dose of 600 to 800 mg per day or until maximum improvement has occurred. (This dose may be higher than that stated in the manufacturer's official directive.) On this program, since the fall in peripheral resistance is countered by an increased stroke volume, blood pressure is not significantly lowered and may even increase. Urinary output often improves, and azotemia is corrected.

In patients with signs of persistent pulmonary congestion, a venodilator, such as oral isosorbide, will be of benefit. Prazosin is an alternative dilator drug that has the property of a combined arteriolar and venous effect. The latter obviates the need for additional management with oral nitrates. Prazosin is particularly useful when hydralazine is contraindicated because of a positive antinuclear antibody. It should be begun with a test dose of 1 mg at bedtime. If orthostatic hypotension does not develop, it is unlikely to occur subsequently, and dosage may be increased gradually to a maximum of 5 to 7.5 mg every 6 hours. Prazosin may cause an increase in plasma renin, and the need for diuretics may increase because of fluid retention. Moreover, the drug has a flat dose-response curve, whereas hydralazine has a steep one. Nevertheless, significant clinical improvement is maintained both at rest and during physical effort in many patients treated with prazosin, and long-term side effects are less severe than with hydralazine, which may induce the lupus syndrome when used chronically at a daily dose of above 400 mg.

Nifedipine, a calcium channel blocker, may prove to be very useful in the management of congestive heart failure and the low cardiac output state of ischemic cardiomyopathy. It is a powerful coronary vasodilator and also dilates systemic resistance vessels. Nifedipine may be particularly useful in patients with significant angina and/or associated hypertension. Sublingual placement of punctured capsules, repeated at 10 to 30 minute intervals, has proved highly effective in the emergency management of hypertensive crisis. Captopril is a vasodilator that acts by angiotensin-converting enzyme inhibition. It has combined arteriolar and venous dilating effects and is unlikely to produce reflex tachycardia (except in volume-depleted patients). Captopril may be of particular benefit when congestive heart failure is associated with high renin-angiotensin activity and has proved to be effective when used in conjunction with other vasodilator drugs. Start with 6.25 or 12.5 mg three times daily. Increase the unit dosage stepwise while carefully monitoring effects until maximum benefit is obtained. The maximum unit dose needed is rarely more than 50 mg. Initially, serum creatinine should be checked weekly, since captopril may induce azotemia. Patients with poor renal function are also at increased risk of neutropenia.

In summary, vasodilators may be useful as supplemental therapy when congestive heart failure is refractory to conventional management. Drugs that have a positive inotropic effect when taken orally are also under investigation, but none are of proven chronic benefit. There is evidence that currently available drugs improve the quality of life. However, the long-term benefits of these drugs to the morbidity and mortality of congestive heart failure remain to be demonstrated.

INFECTIVE ENDOCARDITIS

method of
MELVIN D. CHEITLIN, M.D.,
and REMO L. MORELLI, M.D.
University of California
San Francisco, California

Infective endocarditis, untreated, is almost invariably fatal. Often, the diagnosis must be suspected and treatment begun before the identification of the organism is available. A useful rule is that any patient with unexplained fever for more than 7 to 10 days and an organic murmur (pansystolic murmur, diastolic or continuous murmur) may be presumed to have endocarditis and be started on treatment after three separately drawn blood cultures are obtained. The exception to this rule is the intravenous drug abuser with a fever for more than 24 hours with or without an organic murmur and any patient with staphylococcal septicemia without an obvious source, such as indwelling catheter, recognized abscess, or infection such as osteomyelitis. If the blood cultures are sterile and fever has resolved, the antibiotics can be stopped after 7 to 10 days and the patient observed for recurrence of fever. If fever returns, blood for cultures should be redrawn and the patient kept on appropriate antibiotics for a 4 to 6 week period.

Others in whom the clinical picture can be atypical and a high index of suspicion for infective endocarditis must be entertained are the debilitated patient, the immunologically compromised patient, and the elderly patient. In these patients an unexplained fever, anemia, uremia, or change in cerebral function—such as the new onset of dementia or change in mentation—should be thought as possibly due to infection. Where no site is obvious, endocarditis should be suspected and blood cultures obtained.

TREATMENT

Antibiotics

The choice of antibiotics and duration of treatment are dictated by the organism or organisms cultured from the blood. Since organisms are constantly shed from the site of infection, the septicemia is constant and blood cultures, properly obtained, with few exceptions will identify the organism. Although changes in the type of causative organisms have occurred over the years, the most common organism seen in infective endocarditis is still the streptococcus, especially *Streptococcus viridans,* because of its universal presence in the oral cavity and the importance of dental manipulation as its portal of entry. *Enterococcus* is also commonly seen, its entry usually from the gastrointestinal and contaminated genitourinary tracts. *Staphylococcus aureus* is also common, especially in intravenous drug abusers, and is the predominant organism in tricuspid endocarditis in these patients.

Because of the special requirements of certain organisms, both aerobic and anaerobic cultures should be obtained. Certain organisms, such as fungi and the microaerophilic streptococcus, may take several weeks to grow. Therefore, cultures should be maintained for at least 2 to 4 weeks before being reported as showing no growth. When there is a problem identifying the organism, it is important to involve the microbiologist in the care of the individual patient; frequently, he or she may suggest special preparation and collection of blood to give the fastidious organism, such as *Gonococcus,* fungus, or *Rickettsia,* every chance of being cultured. Rarely, more than one organism may be isolated. In general, in less than 5 per cent of infective endocarditis patients, their blood cultures fail to grow an organism.

In the patient with aortic valve involvement and the patient who is very septic, it is frequently necessary to start treatment before the organism is identified. The clinical situation can frequently give important clues that can determine the choice of antibiotics to be started empirically. For instance, in patients with recent dental manipulation or with poor dentition or dental infection, *Streptococcus viridans* is the most likely infecting organism. In patients with GI or GU infection or instrumentation, *Enterococcus,* and even gram-negative organisms, are more common. In intravenous drug abusers, *Enterococcus* and *Staphylococcus aureus* are most likely, although these patients have a higher incidence of infection with unusual organisms, such as *Serratia marcescens, Pseudomonas aeruginosa,* and fungi than the nonaddict. Prosthetic valve infection occurring early after surgery has a higher incidence of infection with *Staphylococcus epidermidis (albus)* and other more unusual organisms, whereas in patients with prosthetic valve infection occurring 2 months or longer after surgery, causative organisms are similar to those that infect the native valve. Patients with indwelling catheters in the hospital are more likely to have *Staphylococcus aureus* or even fungi as causative organisms. Finally, patients with colonic carcinoma have a propensity to develop infection with *Streptococcus bovis.* More frequently, unsuspected carcinoma of the colon is found when the patient is discovered to have *Streptococcus bovis* endocarditis.

The dose and route of administration of the antibiotic are best judged by the sensitivity of the organism, and an attempt is made to achieve a killing serum level of the antibiotic in at least a one-to-eight dilution of the patient's serum. This knowledge is most valuable when fever recurs during the course of the treatment and a decision has to be made concerning changing the type of antibiotic. In general, if the type and amount of antibiotic given result in appropriate killing levels, this is the best evidence that proper treatment is being delivered and other reasons should be sought for continuation of fever. Close collaboration with the microbiologist is essential for the verification of appropriate cidal levels of antibiotics. It is also important to retain the organism or culture for the entire 4 to 6 week period of therapy to determine cidal levels and to monitor adequacy of antibiotic dosage.

General Approach

Because damage to the valve is, in part, related to the duration of infection, it is important to start antibiotic treatment as soon as possible. When endocarditis is suspected, therefore, treatment should be started after three separate blood cultures are drawn. Table 1 lists the recommended antibiotics, dosage, and duration of treatment according to the infecting organism.

The patient should be followed carefully, several times per day, with blood pressure, pulse, and temperature monitoring. Physical examinations several times daily may be necessary to detect the appearance of or changes in murmurs, signs of increasing volume overload, development of congestive heart failure, or signs of systemic emboli. In aortic valve involvement, one of the first signs of valvular incompetence may be the drop in diastolic blood pressure, a result of valve rupture.

Although complications such as congestive heart failure and systemic emboli are usually associated with symptoms, at times these events are detected first by physical examination. For instance, pericardial friction rub, Roth spots, Janeway lesions, absent arterial pulses, motor weakness, and abnormal reflexes or changes in mentation can be present without the patient complaining of symptoms.

Daily electrocardiograms are valuable. Since the conduction system is close to the aortic ring, one sign of extravalvular infection is the development of AV block. This can be clinically unsuspected and identified only by electrocardiogram.

Red cells in the urine can indicate either antigen-antibody glomerular nephritis or, at times, renal infarction secondary to emboli.

Chest radiographs are helpful in judging cardiac size, pulmonary vascularity, and congestion; they are essential in patients with tricuspid valve or right-sided endocarditis to detect pulmonary infiltrates and evidence of pulmonary emboli.

A two-dimensional echocardiogram should be obtained since most patients with endocarditis will develop identifiable vegetations on the valve. The echocardiographic absence of identifiable vegetations does *not* exclude the diagnosis of endocarditis. In general, the patients with large (greater than 1 cm) vegetations by echocardiogram have a greater incidence of complications, such as severe congestive heart failure, emboli, and, in our experience, recurrence of endocarditis. The echocardiogram can be repeated at intervals to detect the appearance or progression of vegetations or change in the hemodynamic status, as reflected by chamber volumes or wall motion.

TABLE 1. **Antibiotic Treatment of Infective Endocarditis**

Infecting Organism	Regimen of Choice[1]	Duration (Weeks)	Alternate Regimen[1]	Duration (Weeks)
STREPTOCOCCI				
Penicillin-Sensitive				
α-Streptococci (*S. viridans*)	1. Penicillin G	4	1. Vancomycin	4
nonenterococcal group D streptococci	2. Penicillin G or procaine penicillin	4	2. Cefazolin or cephalothin[3]	4
β-streptococci (Groups A, B, C, E, F, H, etc)	and streptomycin	2		
S. pneumoniae	3.[2] Penicillin G or procaine penicillin	2		
	and streptomycin	2		
Relatively Penicillin-Resistant				
α-streptococci in setting of rheumatic fever prophylaxis (e.g., *S. mitis, S. sanguis*)	1. Penicillin G	4	1. Vancomycin	4
S. bovis	2. Penicillin G or procaine penicillin	4	2. Cefazolin or cephalothin	4
Nutritionally deficient variant *S. viridans*	and streptomycin	2		
Penicillin-Resistant				
enterococci (*S. faecalis*)[4]	1. Penicillin G or ampicillin	6	1.[5] Vancomycin	6
	and streptomycin or gentamicin	6	and streptomycin or gentamicin	6
STAPHYLOCOCCI				
Penicillin-Sensitive				
S. aureus	1. Penicillin G	4–6	1. Vancomycin	4–6
S. epidermidis (albus)			2. Cephalothin or cefazolin	4–6
Penicillin-Resistant				
Methicillin-Sensitive				
S. aureus	1. Nafcillin	4–6	1. Vancomycin	4–6
S. epidermidis	2. Oxacillin	4–6	2. Cephalothin or cefazolin	4–6
	3. Methicillin[6]	4–6		
Methicillin-Resistant				
S. aureus	1. Vancomycin	4–6	1. Cephalothin or ceptazolin	4–6
S. epidermidis				
Tolerant Staphylococcus				
S. aureus	1. Higher doses of semisynthetic penicillin ± vancomycin	4–6	1. Vancomycin and rifampin	4–6 4–6
S. epidermidis	2. Semisynthetic penicillin	4–6	2. Cephalothin or cefazolin and rifampin or gentamycin	4–6 4–6
	and rifampin or gentamicin	4–6		
GRAM-NEGATIVE BACILLI				
Haemophilus parainfluenzae	1. Ampicillin	4–6		
	and gentamicin or tobramycin ± chloramphenicol	4–6		
Other *Haemophilus* sp.	1. Penicillin[7] and streptomycin	3–4	1. Penicillin-allergic patients may require desensitization, followed by a course of penicillin or ampicillin	3–4
	2. Ampicillin[7]	3–4		
Pseudomonas aeruginosa	1. Carbenicillin[8]	6		
	and tobramycin or gentamicin or amikacin	6		
Serratia marcescens	1. Carbenicillin[8] or cefoxitin or trimethoprim-sulfamethoxazole	6		
	and tobramycin or gentamicin	6		

Table continued on following page

TABLE 1. **Antibiotic Treatment of Infective Endocarditis** *Continued*

Infecting Organism	Regimen of Choice[1]	Duration (*Weeks*)	Alternate Regimen[1]	Duration (*Weeks*)
Other Gram-Negative Bacilli	Therapy depends on antimicrobial sensitivity testing—combination antimicrobial therapy often required	4–6		
MISCELLANEOUS CAUSES				
Neisseria sp.	1. Aqueous penicillin G	4–6	1. Penicillin-allergic patients will require desensitization followed by course of penicillin 2. Erythromycin or cefoxitin	4
Corynebacterium sp.	1. Aqueous penicillin G and gentamicin 2. Vancomycin for gentamicin-tolerant *Corynebacterium*	4–6 4–6 4–6	1. Vancomycin	
Diphtheroids	1. Vancomycin	4–6		
Anaerobes				
Bacteroides fragilis	1. High dose penicillin if penicillin-sensitive 2. Metronidazole			
Other	1. High dose penicillin			
Candida sp.[9] *Torulopsis* sp.[9]	1. Amphotericin B and 5-fluorocytosine and surgery	for 6 weeks after surgery		
Aspergillus sp.[9]	1. Amphotericin B and 5-fluorocytosine or rifampin and surgery	for 6 weeks after surgery		

1. Dosages given assume the patient has normal hepatic or renal function; appropriate dosage adjustments must be made where there is significant functional impairment:

amikacin	5 mg/kg IV q 8 hr	gentamicin	1 mg/kg IM or IV q 8 hr
amphotericin B	1.5–3 grams IV total dose (0.75–1.25 mg/kg/day)	methicillin	12–16 gm/day IV
ampicillin	12–18 grams/day IV	metronidazole	750 mg q 8 hr, PO or IV
aqueous penicillin G	10–20 million units/day IV continuously, or in frequent, divided doses	nafcillin	8–12 grams/day IV
		oxacillin	8–12 grams/day IV
cefoxitin	1–2 grams IV q 6 hr	procaine penicillin	1–2 million units IM q 6 hr
carbenicillin	30–40 grams/day IV	rifampin	300–600 mg/day PO (single dose)
cefazolin	2 grams IV q 6–8 hr	streptomycin	10 mg/kg (not to exceed 500 mg) IM q 12 hr
cephalothin	2 grams IV q 4–6 hr	tobramycin	1 mg/kg IM or IV q 8 hr
chloramphenicol	3–6 grams/day IV	trimethoprim-sulfamethoxazole	10–20 mg/kg trimethoprim (with appropriate sulfamethoxazole equivalent) IV per day in divided doses
erythromycin	500 mg IV q 6 hr	vancomycin	10 mg/kg (not to exceed 500 mg) IV q 6 hr
5-fluorocytosine	150 mg/kg/day PO in divided doses		

2. Not recommended for complicated patients with shock, extracardiac foci of infection, prosthetic valve endocarditis, or infection with nutritionally deficient variant *S. viridans*.
3. For minor penicillin allergy (e.g., rash). There is not enough experience with the 2 week therapy with cephalosporins.
4. Although therapy for 6 weeks is commonly recommended for enterococcal endocarditis, 4 weeks may be used in mitigating circumstances, such as unacceptable drug toxicity, and if the course is otherwise uncomplicated.
5. Cephalosporins should not be used for enterococcal endocarditis.
6. Because of the risk of methicillin-associated nephritis, its use is not recommended.
7. Beta-lactamase production may require use of second and third generation cephalosporins.
8. Other ureidopenicillins (ticarcillin, mezlocillin, piperacillin) may be substituted. May require concomitant colistin or polymixin B.
9. Surgery should be considered early.

Complications

The treatment of the patient with endocarditis, in addition to eradicating the infection with antibiotics, consists of dealing with the complications. Those conditions leading to operation are listed in Table 2.

Congestive Heart Failure

Congestive heart failure in infective endocarditis can occur slowly as a result of gradually increasing valvular insufficiency or acutely as a result of sudden rupture of the aortic or mitral valve itself or the chordae tendineae of the mitral valve.

Acute Aortic Insufficiency. Acute rupture of the aortic valve is an indication for immediate surgical replacement of the valve. This is usually manifested by a sudden drop in diastolic blood pressure, collapsing carotid pulse, a soft first heart sound, an S_3 gallop, and, frequently, pulmonary edema. The chest film will usually show pulmonary edema or pulmonary congestion. Frequently, there is early closure of the mitral valve on echocardiogram. In the intervening period before surgery, intravenous nitroprusside and Lasix to lower the impedance and decrease the venous capacitance is very effective in increasing forward cardiac output, decreasing pulmonary artery wedge pressure, and alleviating symptoms.

Sudden death is not uncommon in this group of patients because of the marked increase in wall tension due to the volume overload, leading to an increase in myocardial oxygen demand, together with impairment of diastolic myocardial blood flow and subsequent subendocardial myocardial ischemia. Such patients do poorly when treated medically and, in most series, 90 per cent die or are in severe congestive heart failure within 1 year. For this reason, once the clinical picture of acute aortic insufficiency is seen and the patient started on appropriate antibiotics for 12 to 24 hours, surgery should be performed as soon as possible. There is sufficient evidence now that once appropriate antibiotic blood levels are achieved, there is minimal danger of infecting the new prosthetic valve, while the consequences of delay are so devastating that immediate surgery is unquestionably indicated.

Acute Mitral Insufficiency. In this state a sudden volume overload of the unprepared left ventricle within a noncompliant, normal pericardium also occurs, resulting frequently in acute pulmonary edema. There is no isovolumic contraction period; the left ventricular volume decreases immediately upon contraction, delivering the blood back to the left atrium before the aortic valve opens. In this way the increase in left ventricular wall tension is minimized, and the ventricle frequently can accomodate by hypertrophy to reduce wall stress and maintain this new volume load. Immediate treatment consists of intravenous furosemide, 20 to 40 mg, to reduce preload, and intravenous nitroprusside to reduce afterload, starting with 20 micrograms per min and increasing by 5 micrograms per min every 5 minutes until pulmonary edema is relieved or systolic blood pressure falls below 100 mm Hg. This can markedly decrease left atrial pressure and improve forward effective stroke volume. The patient can also be started on intravenous digoxin, 0.75 to 1.0 mg slowly, followed by maintenance digoxin, 0.25 mg per day. In our experience about half the patients respond very well to this therapy and maintain this good response for long periods of time. With time, the left ventricular wall stress is returned toward normal by hypertrophy of the left ventricular wall. The patient now behaves like a patient with chronic mitral insufficiency. If there is poor response to medical therapy, corrective surgery should be performed.

Chronic Aortic and Mitral Insufficiency. If the patient gradually develops hemodynamically significant mitral or aortic insufficiency, medical management is indicated with digoxin and diuretics to control symptoms. If the patient is

TABLE 2. **Indications for Surgical Intervention in Infective Endocarditis**

Hemodynamic consequences of valvular insufficiency: the most common indication with or without emboli, in at least 85 per cent of the cases.
Acute aortic insufficiency
Acute mitral insufficiency not responding to medical management
Chronic severe aortic or mitral insufficiency, symptomatic with ordinary activity while on medical management, or with lesser degrees of symptomatology if systolic function is decreasing (increasing end-systolic and/or end-diastolic volume or decreasing ejection fraction to 50 per cent or less)
Tricuspid insufficiency and severe right heart failure not responding to medical management
Embolization as a primary indication (unusual as sole indication without congestive heart failure)
Mitral or aortic valve involvement with repeated macroemboli, especially with echocardiographic vegetation 1 cm or larger
Tricuspid vegetation with multiple continued pulmonary emboli in spite of anticoagulation. Debridement and valvuloplasty, if at all possible
Special Circumstances
Presence of extravalvular ring abscess, usually with aortic valve endocarditis
Valvular infection with resistant organisms such as *Serratia, Pseudomonas,* or fungi
Prosthetic valve endocarditis with resistant organism
Infection with implanted prosthetic material, such as intracardiac patches, conduits, or pacemakers
Small VSD with repeated endocarditis
Extracardiac infective endarteritis, such as that involving AV fistulas, patent ductus arteriosus, or infection in an aortic aneurysm

symptomatic on ordinary activity (functional class III) in spite of medical management, surgery should be considered.

Valve replacement should be recommended only after careful consideration. The surgical perioperative mortality of 5 to 10 per cent with valve replacement, the subsequent 2 to 3 per cent per year late mortality rate, and the morbidity due to embolization, valve disruption, and prosthetic valve infection make it necessary to balance these risks against the risks of medical management of the unoperated patient. The left ventricular systolic fuction in these patients should be monitored by periodic echocardiography. We use echocardiography to make serial measurements of the left ventricular diastolic and systolic diameters as well as left atrial size. Echocardiograms can be obtained yearly or every other year in the absence of change in symptoms or physical examination. If the end-systolic or end-diastolic volume increases or the ejection fraction begins to fall, the patient should be monitored more frequently, every 3 to 6 months. Once a trend is evident, then the patient should be repaired surgically, even if the patient is only functional Class II. In our experience, by the time this occurs most of the patients are already in functional Class III, but, occasionally, we see a patient who may not admit to symptoms or functional impairment. In these instances, an objective treadmill exercise test evaluating exercise tolerance and observing the development of diastolic gallops or pulmonary congestion can be helpful. In any case, if the left ventricular ejection fraction falls to 50 per cent or below, the patient should be considered for surgery in spite of lack of severe symptoms.

Tricuspid Insufficiency. Infection of the tricuspid valve is mainly a problem seen in the intravenous drug abuser, although occasionally endocarditis in patients with an interventricular septal defect can involve the tricuspid valve or even the right ventricular outflow tract or pulmonary valve. In the presence of a normal pulmonary vascular resistance, the patient tolerates the hemodynamic consequences of severe acute or chronic tricuspid insufficiency well for a long period of time. For this reason, in our experience tricuspid valve surgery is rarely indicated. In fact, we have performed tricuspid valve replacement in only three patients in the last 10 years. These patients usually do quite well with medical management alone, even when residual severe tricuspid insufficiency is present.

Of more importance are the consequences of multiple pulmonary emboli and infarctions, with lung destruction and impairment of pulmonary function, eventually hypoxemia, and respiratory failure. In the presence of continued pulmonary embolization we have, on occasion, treated these patients with anticoagulants once the acute infection is controlled, to decrease the frequency of embolization, although the results have been equivocal at best. In patients with large vegetations, we have at times recommended valvular debridement with removal of the infected portion of the valve and valvuloplasty. Every attempt should be made to salvage the valve, even leaving the patient with moderately severe tricuspid insufficiency, since tricuspid valve replacement has poor long-term results and should be avoided whenever possible. However, tricuspid valve replacement is necessary for severe tricuspid insufficiency with elevated total pulmonary arterial resistance. Even with a tissue graft, the long-term results are still poor.

Embolic Phenomena

Macroemboli are most frequently seen during the first few weeks of the infection but can occur even after therapy is complete and the infection eradicated. This is best seen in intravenous drug abusers, in whom emboli to the lungs are almost universal. It is not unusual to see evidence of repeated embolization on serial chest radiographs, at times without clinical symptoms. When arterial obstruction involves a sufficiently large vessel, for instance the popliteal, femoral, or brachial artery and there is ischemia of the limb, immediate embolectomy is indicated. If resting ischemia is not present, it is often possible to treat this condition without emergency embolectomy.

Although unusual, recurrent embolization without severe hemodynamic valvular insufficiency can be an indication for valvular surgery. This is especially true when the echocardiographic vegetation is larger than 1 cm. Although no good evidence supports this approach, the larger and more mobile the vegetation on echocardiography, the more compelling is the desire to surgically excise the vegetation or replace the valve. Because of the significant perioperative mortality associated with valve replacement, as well as the high incidence of late mortality and morbidity, including embolization, even after what appears to be successful valve replacement, such a course of action should be undertaken only after great consideration when the indication for surgery is embolization alone. In the absence of embolization we do not recommend surgery, even with a large vegetation.

With embolization, the question of anticoagulation is raised. Animal experiments indicate that the growth of vegetations can be markedly reduced by anticoagulants although the spread of infection in the tissue may be enhanced in these animals. The probability of converting a bland embolic cerebral infarction into a larger hemorrhagic infarction discourages the general use of anticoagulants except in patients with prosthetic valve endocarditis already anticoagulated. In these cases, the Mayo Clinic experience strongly suggests that the patients fare better when continued on anticoagulants. In patients without prosthetic valves, in whom cerebral embolization occurs, we recommend a computed tomography scan. In the absence of identifiable hemorrhagic infarction, anticoagulants may be started. This approach may decrease the risk of the anticoagulants.

Special Circumstances

Intravenous Drug Abusers. Intravenous drug abusers are frequently noncompliant with therapy and tend to sign out against medical advice before completion of their course of antibiotics. Preliminary data suggest it may be possible to treat those with uncomplicated tricuspid endocarditis with parenteral nafcillin and tobramycin for 2 weeks. Less than half the intravenous drug abusers presenting with infective endocarditis would be eligible for this form of therapy, excluding those patients with endocarditis complicated by congestive heart failure or shock or significant hepatic or renal dysfunction or who have preexisting or known mitral or aortic valvular in-

TABLE 3. **Prophylaxis for Infective Endocarditis**

Procedure	Regimen of Choice	Alternate Regimen
Dental Procedures or Upper Respiratory Tract Manipulation		
Dental manipulation, dental prophylaxis Endoscopy with rigid instruments Endoscopy with biopsy	1. Aqueous penicillin G, 1 million units, and procaine penicillin, 600,000 units IM 30–60 min prior to procedure, followed by penicillin V, 500 mg PO q 6 hr for 8 doses 2. Penicillin V, 2 grams PO 30–60 min prior to procedure, followed by penicillin V, 500 mg q 6 hr for 8 doses 3. Aqueous penicillin G, 1 million units, and procaine penicillin, 600,000 units IM, and streptomycin, 1 gm IM 30–60 min prior to procedure, followed by penicillin V or erythromycin, 500 mg PO q 6 hr for 8 doses 4. Amoxicillin, 3 grams PO 60 min prior to procedure 5. Ampicillin, 1 gram IM 30–60 min prior to procedure	1. Vancomycin, 1 gram IV 30–60 min prior to procedure, followed by erythromycin, 500 mg PO q 6 hr for 8 doses 2. Erythromycin, 1 gram PO 90–120 min prior to procedure, followed by erythromycin, 500 mg PO q 6 hr for 8 doses
Prosthetic valve	1. Aqueous penicillin G, 1 million units, and procaine penicillin, 600,000 units IM, and streptomycin, 1 gram IM 30–60 min prior to procedure, followed by penicillin V or erythromycin, 500 mg PO q 6 hr for 8 doses	1. Vancomycin, 1 gram IV 30–60 min prior to procedure, followed by erythromycin, 500 mg PO q 6 hr for 8 doses
Gastrointestinal or Genitourinary Procedures		
Urethral instrumentation or catheterization Prostatectomy Gastrointestinal instrumentation or surgery	1. Aqueous penicillin G, 2 million units or ampicillin, 1 gram IV or IM 30–60 min prior to procedure and gentamicin, 1.5 mg/kg (not to exceed 80 mg) or streptomycin, 1 gram IM 2. Ampicillin, 1 gram IM or IV, and tobramycin, 1.5 mg/kg (not to exceed 80 mg) IM or IV 1 hr prior and 12 hrs after procedure	1. Vancomycin, 1 gram IV 30–60 min prior to procedure, followed by erythromycin, 500 mg PO q 6 hr for 8 doses, and streptomycin, 1 gram IM 30–60 min prior to procedure
Skin Conditions		
Incision and drainage of abscess Debridement of burns	1. Vancomycin, 1 gram IV, and tobramycin, 1.5 mg/kg (not to exceed 80 mg) IM or IV 30–60 min before and 12 hr after procedure	

sufficiency or endocarditis. At our institution so far 17 patients have been treated with this regimen with the only recurrence of endocarditis in a patient who in retrospect had concomitant mitral valve involvement.

When valve replacement is indicated, because of these patients' unreliability in maintaining chronic anticoagulation, tissue valves are used. Aspirin, 0.3 gram per day, and Persantine, 50 to 75 mg three times daily, can be given to those with mitral valve replacement in an attempt to decrease the incidence of embolization (this use of aspirin and Persantine is not listed in the manufacturer's directive). Patients with aortic tissue valves may do equally well without anticoagulation.

Prosthetic Valve Endocarditis. If the infecting organism is very sensitive to antibiotics in those without severe hemodynamic dysfunction, a single attempt to eradicate the infection should be made with medical management. If the infection recurs, or if the organism is not very sensitive to antibiotics, appropriate antibiotics should be started for 24 to 48 hours, the infected tissue debrided as much as possible, and the valve replaced. In spite of this approach, mortality in late prosthetic valve endocarditis is still 30 to 50 per cent.

Extravalvular Infection. The development of aortic or mitral ring abscess, myocardial abscess, or purulent pericarditis indicates extension of the infection, either through direct local spread outside the confines of the valve leaflet itself or through septic myocardial emboli. A frequent sign of local invasion of the infection into the periaortic area is the development of varying degrees of AV block owing to the proximity of the AV node and His bundle to the aortic ring. The development of AV block heralds the possibility of high degree or complete AV block and is an indication for temporary pacemaker placement, catheterization, and early surgical intervention. The surgical approach to ring abscess is to debride the necrotic muscle and attempt to obliterate the abscess. At times, seating of the prosthetic valve is made impossible in this circumstance, and in these cases removal of as much as possible of the infected valve and necrotic tissue is done, together with placement of a valved Dacron graft for the ascending aorta. The coronary arteries are then bypassed to the graft above the prosthetic valve. This operation has had limited success in these high risk patients.

Endarteritis is associated with infection in extracardiac sites, such as patent ductus arteriosus, arteriovenous fistulas, and aortic-pulmonary arterial shunts, and requires surgical correction after medical treatment of the infection. Endarteritis of aortic aneurysms, frequently with *Salmonella* infection, requires immediate surgical correction, since rupture of the aneurysm is highly likely to occur, even with appropriate antibiotics.

Multivalvular Infection. Polyvalvular involvement occurs in about 5 per cent of the cases of infective endocarditis. Most commonly, the mitral valve is infected through the regurgitant jet from the infected, leaking aortic valve. In intravenous drug abusers we have seen involvement of the mitral or aortic valve together with the tricuspid valve. Mortality in these cases is higher than with single valve involvement and consideration for surgery should be based on the hemodynamic effect of the combined lesions on the patient.

Prevention of Infective Endocarditis

In the animal model of endocarditis, it is possible to show that the incidence of infection of the valve can be decreased by the prophylactic use of appropriate antibiotics in correct amounts given at the time of bacteremia. For this reason, prophylactic antibiotics are recommended in the dose and time schedule in Table 3 in all patients deemed at risk of endocarditis undergoing procedures known to cause a transient bacteremia. Because of the problem of compliance with such a complicated dosing regimen as recommended by the American Heart Association, simplified regimens have been suggested for endocarditis prophylaxis, such as the use of a single dose of amoxicillin in patients undergoing dental procedures or upper respiratory tract manipulation.

HYPERTENSION

method of
RAY W. GIFFORD, JR., M.D.
The Cleveland Clinic
Cleveland, Ohio

Selection of Patients for Treatment

Whenever diastolic blood pressure is consistently ≥90 mm Hg, treatment is indicated—nonpharmacologic, pharmacologic, or both. The higher the blood pressure, the greater the risk and the more urgent the indication for bringing it down. Moreover, the 1984 Report of the Joint National Committee (JNC) on Detection, Evaluation, and Treatment of High Blood Pressure has identified a "high normal" group with diastolic blood pressures of 85 to 89 mm Hg who are at intermediate risk. Pharmacologic treatment is not indicated for this high normal group; nonpharmacologic treatment, especially dietary sodium and obesity control as well as exercise, may be advisable for those who have family histories of hypertension with premature cardiovascular disease.

Most authorities now agree that drug treatment is indicated (1) for patients with diastolic blood pressures of ≥100 mm Hg, and (2) for those with diastolic blood pressures of 95 to 99 mm Hg if nonpharmacologic treatment fails to reduce it to <90 mm Hg after 3 to 6 months.

There is still debate about the advisability of drug therapy for patients with diastolic blood pressures of 90 to 94 mm Hg in the absence of target organ disease and other major risk factors for cardiovascular disease (hyperlipidemia, cigarette smoking, family history). I prescribe antihypertensive drugs for this group if they do not respond to dietary sodium restriction, obesity control, and isotonic exercise programs after 6 months. I believe that the Hypertension Detection and Follow-up Program (HDFP) has shown conclusively that the mortality rate can be reduced for these patients when drugs are used.

More and more physicians are prescribing antihypertensive agents for patients with isolated systolic hypertension (systolic blood pressure of ≥160 mm Hg and diastolic blood pressure of <90 mm Hg) even though no controlled clinical trials have been done to demonstrate that this reduces the increased risk for cardiovascular disease that these patients are acknowledged to have. I concur with this practice, although age plays a role in my decision. In the absence of target organ disease I usually do not use antihypertensive drugs for patients older than 70 years of age until the systolic blood pressure is ≥170mm Hg, provided diastolic blood pressure is normal.

The ideal time to treat hypertension is before target organ disease develops. Once there is evidence of cerebrovascular disease, atherosclerotic heart disease, left ventricular hypertrophy, congestive heart failure, or renal insufficiency, the mortality rate is 3.5 times higher than it would have been without such evidence, even with effective antihypertensive treatment. Nevertheless, if the patient does not come under medical supervision until target organ disease is present, it is still worthwhile to treat the hypertension aggressively, because cardiovascular events can thereby be reduced and life prolonged.

Nonpharmacologic Treatment

The fear of adverse effects of antihypertensive drugs is not justified by the facts. Nevertheless, it is always desirable to avoid pharmacologic agents if the same thing can be accomplished by nonpharmacologic means.

No long-term clinical trials have been done to establish that a low sodium diet, obesity control, exercise, and other nonpharmacologic measures will reduce cardiovascular morbidity and mortality to the same extent that drug therapy has done when tested under controlled conditions. It is more difficult for most patients to comply with changes in life style than to take one or two pills a day. Too often the patient and physician are willing to settle for less than optimal control of hypertension on a nonpharmacologic regimen rather than to add an antihypertensive drug.

TABLE 1. **Indications for Selection of Step One Drug**

Diuretic
Black patients
Elderly patients
Isolated systolic hypertension in the elderly
Chronic renal failure
Congestive heart failure
Contraindications to beta blocker (e.g., heart block, asthma, peripheral occlusive arterial disease)
Beta Blocker
Young patients
Evidence of hyperkinetic circulation (resting tachycardia, cardiac awareness, wide pulse pressure, flow murmur at left sternal border)
Angina pectoris
Postmyocardial infarction
Migraine
Gout

Ineffective nonpharmacologic therapy is thus used as an excuse to delay the prescribing of more effective drug treatment.

I tell patients at the outset that if the hygienic measures fail to control blood pressure adequately after 3 to 6 months I will recommend medication. Often this admonition will motivate patients to greater compliance with their diets; at the same time it prepares them for the eventual use of drugs should this become necessary. On the other hand, some patients indicate that they will not or cannot adhere to dietary restrictions, and so I prescribe drug therapy immediately.

Dietary Sodium Restriction

Limiting dietary sodium to less than 2 grams daily (equivalent to 5 grams of sodium chloride or 85 mEq of sodium) has been shown to reduce blood pressure in mild hypertension. To achieve maximal compliance, it is important for a dietitian to instruct the patient and the food preparer regarding foods to avoid, how to prepare appetizing recipes using nonsodium flavoring substitutes, and how to select foods when eating away from home. Measurement of a 24 hour urine specimen for sodium gives an objective estimate of compliance and should be used not so much to chastize a noncomplier as to decide whether a low sodium diet is going to be effective in controlling blood pressure, and to help a compliant

TABLE 2. **Attributes of Ideal Step One Drug**

Effective as monotherapy
Inexpensive
Long-acting (one dose daily preferred)
Easy titration (flat dose-response curve)
No pseudotolerance
Well tolerated (few symptomatic adverse effects)
Augments action of other antihypertensive drugs
Safe

patient discover whether there are unsuspected sources of sodium in the diet. Even though a low sodium diet may not control the hypertension adquately, it may minimize the doses of antihypertensive medications needed for optimal control. Consequently, the 1984 JNC report recommended that all patients be advised to curtail sodium in their diets, either as primary treatment or as an adjunct to drug therapy.

Weight Control

Several controlled trials have shown that a weight loss of 10 or more pounds will reduce blood pressure in hypertensive patients. In general, the greater the weight loss, the greater the fall in blood pressure. In my opinion, weight control for the definitely obese hypertensive patient is even more effective than sodium control in reducing blood pressure but is more difficult to achieve and maintain. Most obese patients who are able to lose large amounts of weight gain it back within 24 months. Nor are there any long-term studies to show that blood pressure remains controlled once weight loss has been accomplished and isocaloric diets are resumed. I strongly advise my obese hypertensive patients to reduce, whether or not I plan to initiate drug treatment immediately, but even with intensive dietary counseling my success has been discouraging.

Other Dietary Measures

There is great interest at this time in the role of dietary calcium and, to a lesser extent, potassium and magnesium as treatment for hypertension. While there may be some theoretic validity to this, clinical studies are inconclusive and conflicting and I do not subscribe to the use of calcium, potassium, or magnesium in the treatment of hypertension.

Alcohol

Consumption of more than 2 or 3 ounces of alcohol daily increases blood pressure. It has been postulated that excessive alcohol intake may be the most prevalent form of potentially curable hypertension in the United States. Any nonpharmacologic approach to the management of hypertension should include moderation of alcohol consumption.

Exercise

Short-term studies have shown that regular isotonic exercise (walking, cycling, swimming, jogging) has a modest beneficial effect on blood pressure of hypertensive individuals. The data are less convincing than for low sodium and low caloric diets. Nevertheless, it is my opinion that judicious exercise should be an integral part (along with diet) of a nonpharmacologic regimen for hypertension. Isometric exercise (weight lifting, push-ups) should be avoided because it raises blood pressure and does not bring about cardiovascular conditioning.

Behavioral Modification

Biofeedback, relaxation response, transcendental meditation, yoga, and stress management have their advocates for management of hypertension, but the meager data on the effectiveness of these modalities are equivocal, usually poorly controlled and short-term. I consider these methods to be investigational at this time.

Tobacco

Although smoking temporarily increases blood pressure for some individuals, there is no evidence that tobacco has any long-term detrimental effect on blood pressure. Nevertheless, cigarette smoking is a potent, independent risk factor for coronary disease, especially sudden death, and it should be emphatically discouraged.

Pharmacologic Treatment

Numerous controlled clinical trials have demonstrated the effectiveness and safety of drug treatment for hypertension. The classes of antihypertensive drugs are (1) diuretics, (2) adrenergic blocking agents, (3) vasodilators, (4) converting enzyme inhibitors, and (5) calcium slow channel blocking agents.

Stepped-Care Approach

The 1984 JNC report has endorsed the stepped-care approach but has recommended that some adrenergic blocking agents, especially beta blockers, be considered as alternatives to diuretics as step one in certain patients (Table 1). The attributes of the ideal step one drug are listed in Table 2. Both diuretics and beta blockers possess these attributes more than do some of the other adrenergic blocking agents and the vasodilators. However, it is possible that the converting enzyme inhibitors and perhaps the slow channel calcium blocking drugs may eventually have a role as step one agents.

In selecting a step one drug it must be remembered that many of the nondiuretic antihypertensive agents, especially the adrenergic blocking agents (except for beta blockers) and the vasodilators, can cause subtle retention of sodium and water when prescribed as monotherapy. This eventually leads to a loss of antihypertensive effectiveness—a phenomenon known as "pseudotolerance" because the original effectiveness can be restored by adding a diuretic to the regimen. This has been demonstrated for methyldopa, re-

TABLE 3. **Oral Diuretic Drugs Useful as Antihypertensive Agents**

	Trade Name	Usual Daily Dose *(mg)**	Side Effects
Benzothiadiazine derivatives			
chlorothiazide	Diuril	250–500	Unpleasant taste, dry mouth GI irritation Sexual dysfunction (male) Skin rash Photosensitivity (except ethacrynic acid) Pancreatitis Hyperuricemia (with or without gout) Hypokalemia Hyperglycemia Hypercalcemia Hypercholesterolemia Azotemia Marrow depression (rare) Hypochloremic alkalosis
hydrochlorothiazide	HydroDiuril Esidrex Oretic	25–50	
hydroflumethiazide	Saluron	50–100	
bendroflumethiazide	Naturetin	2.5–5	
trichlormethiazide	Naqua Metahydrin	2–4	
methyclothiazide	Enduron	2.5–5	
benzthiazide	ExNa Aquatag	25–50	
polythiazide	Renese	1–4	
cyclothiazide	Anhydron	2–4	
Phthalimidine derivative			
chlorthalidone	Hygroton	25–50	
Quinazoline derivatives			
quinethazone	Hydromox	50–100	
metolazone	Zaroxolyn Diulo	2.5–5	
Indoline derivative			
indapamide	Lozol	2.5–5.0	
Metamilamide derivative			
bumetanide	Bumex	0.5–4.0†	
Anthranilic acid derivative			
furosemide	Lasix	40–200†	
Phenoxyacetic acid derivative			
ethacrynic acid	Edecrin	50–200†	
Distal tubular diuretics (potassium-sparing)			
spironolactone	Aldactone	50–200	Skin rash, GI irritation, hyperkalemia, azotemia, hyponatremia, dry mouth Spironolactone only: gynecomastia, hirsutism, lethargy, and menstrual irregularity
triamterene	Dyrenium	50–200	
amiloride	Midamor	5–10	

*Given once daily unless otherwise indicated.
†Loop diuretics and given twice daily.

serpine, and guanethidine but is probably true for most of the other adrenergic inhibiting agents, with the exception of beta blockers. The converting enzyme inhibitors do not cause salt and water retention because they inhibit aldosterone production. While edema is a recognized side effect of slow channel calcium blocking agents, especially nifedipine, this may be a local phenomenon and not a reflection of volume expansion.

There is no particular virtue in trying to control hypertension with a single agent. Indeed, one of the advantages of the stepped care approach is to minimize side effects by using small doses of two or more agents that have a complementary action.

If the drug selected as step one fails to control hypertension, the physician may choose to withdraw it and try another step one drug. Similarly, if one of the adrenergic blocking agents chosen for step two is ineffective, another step two agent can be substituted rather than going on to step three. Indeed, there is great flexibility in the stepped-care concept.

When hypertension is mild (diastolic blood pressure of 90 to 104 mm Hg) and uncomplicated, therapy should begin with only one drug. A second agent should not be added until it is obvious that the response is suboptimal after 6 to 12 weeks of monotherapy, during which time the dose can be increased if necessary. When diastolic blood pressure is ≥115 mm Hg, it is unlikely that monotherapy with any drug will be effective, and so I start treatment for such patients with two drugs simultaneously, usually a diuretic and a beta blocker.

When hypertension is severe (diastolic blood

TABLE 4. **Beta Blockers**

	Trade Name	Dose *(Mg/Day)**	Side Effects
propranolol	Inderal	80–480§	Bradycardia
	Inderal LA	80–420	Congestive heart failure (in patients with diminished cardiac reserve)
metoprolol†	Lopressor	50–450	
nadolol	Corgard	40–360	Bronchospasm (in patients with propensity for asthma), skin rash
pindolol‡	Visken	10–60§	
timolol	Blocadren	20–60§	AV block
atenolol†	Tenormin	25–100	Vasospasm (Raynaud's syndrome)
acebutolol†,‡	Sectral	200–800	Worsening of intermittent claudication
			Ischemia of toes (in patients with pre-existing chronic occlusive arterial disease)
alpha and beta labetalol	Normodyne	200–1200§	Sexual dysfunction (male)
	Trandate		Fatigue, bone marrow suppression (rare)
			Purpura (rare), gastrointestinal irritation

*Once daily unless otherwise indicated.
†Cardioselective.
‡ISA (intrinsic sympathomimetic activity).
§BID dosage.

pressure of ≥130 mm Hg) I often initiate treatment with three drugs simultaneously, usually a diuretic, beta blocker, and vasodilator.

Inherent in stepped care is to "step down" after hypertension has been well controlled for a year or more. This implies a gradual reduction in dosage or even elimination of one or more drugs in a multidrug regimen. This must be done with close and prolonged observation because it sometimes takes weeks or months for blood pressure to rise again after step down. Rarely is it possible to eliminate drugs altogether without return of hypertension.

Diuretics (Table 3)

An oral diuretic alone will normalize blood pressure for up to two thirds of patients with mild hypertension.

When there is no special indication for a beta blocker as step one (Table 1) and no contraindication for a diuretic, I usually elect to start treatment with an oral diuretic. I prefer one of the kaliuretic thiazide or thiazide-like compounds, most of which can be given once daily, which enhances compliance. The loop diuretics are more potent than conventional thiazide com-

TABLE 5. **Other Adrenergic Blocking Drugs**

	Trade Name	Oral *(Mg/Day)**	Side Effects
$Alpha_1$-blocking agent			
prazosin	Minipress	1–30†	First dose syncope, orthostatic hypotension, weakness, headache, nausea, tachycardia, sexual dysfunction (male)
Central $alpha_2$-agonists			
clonidine	Catapres	0.1–2.4†	Drowsiness, dry mouth, sexual dysfunction (male), constipation, withdrawal hypertension (methyldopa only: hepatitis, positive Coombs' test, drug fever)
methyldopa	Aldomet	500–2000†	
guanabenz	Wytensin	4–42†	
Neuroeffector blockade			
Rauwolfia			
reserpine (single alkaloid)	Serpasil	0.05–0.25	Lethargy, drowsiness, depression, nasal congestion, laxation, activation of peptic ulcer, sexual dysfunction (male), bradycardia
	Sandril		
whole root extract	Raudixin	100–300	
alseroxylon fraction	Rauwiloid	2–4	
Guanethidine	Ismelin	10–200	Nasal congestion, orthostatic hypotension, diarrhea, bradycardia, sexual dysfunction (male)
Guanadrel	Hylorel	10–200†	

*Given once daily unless otherwise indicated.
†BID dosage.

pounds but have a short duration of action, requiring two or three doses daily, and offer no advantage in the management of hypertension unless renal function is impaired, in which case they become the diuretics of choice.

The 1984 JNC report recommended small doses of diuretics (Table 3) because it has been shown that daily doses as low as 12.5 mg of hydrochlorothiazide have an antihypertensive effect and that exceeding 50 mg daily of either hydrochlorothiazide or chlorthalidone increases the metabolic side effects without much, if any, additional antihypertensive effect.

A diuretic should be used as step two for patients who receive a beta blocker or another type of drug as step one.

The indications for preventing or treating diuretic-induced hypokalemia are cardiac arrhythmias, concomitant digitalis therapy, an abnormal resting electrocardiogram, evidence of cardiac disease, symptomatic hypokalemia, and a serum potassium level below 3 mEq per liter. Prescribing smaller doses of the kaliuretic diuretics (Table 3) will minimize potassium loss in the urine, as will a low sodium diet. Increasing dietary intake of potassium is unreliable, and using potassium chloride tablets or elixirs in doses large enough to be effective in treating or preventing hypokalemia (60 to 100 mEq daily) is often met with noncompliance. Consequently, the most effective and reliable way to deal with this problem is to use a potassium-sparing diuretic (triamterene, spironolactone, or amiloride, Table 3), in combination with a thiazide. The potassium-sparing diuretics are not potent and by themselves do not have much antihypertensive effect.

Most of the studies that have related an oral diuretic to an increase in serum cholesterol or triglycerides have been short-term (< 6 months). Long-term observations for a year or more have not shown any increase in cholesterol or triglycerides. Diabetes is not a contraindication to the use of an oral diuretic unless it increases blood glucose enough to disturb control, which is distinctly unusual.

Asymptomatic hyperuricemia does not require treatment and is not a potent risk factor for coronary disease. If the patient has or develops gout, an appropriate antiuricemic regimen should be introduced, using either probenecid or allopurinol. For this reason, I prefer to use a beta blocking drug as step one for patients with gout.

Adrenergic Blocking Agents

Beta Blockers (Table 4). Approximately 50 per cent of patients with mild hypertension will become normotensive on a beta-adrenergic blocking drug as monotherapy. Beta blocking drugs are as well tolerated as diuretics and produce less male sexual dysfunction. The most troublesome symptomatic side effects of beta blockers are lethargy and fatigue. Theoretically the hydrophilic beta blockers (atenolol, nadolol) should not penetrate the blood-brain barrier and therefore should produce fewer of the central nervous system side effects, but this has not been the case clinically.

Absolute contraindications to beta blockade are asthma, second or third degree heart block, and congestive heart failure. Sinus bradycardia is not a contraindication. Relative contraindications are insulin-dependent diabetes mellitus and chronic occlusive arterial disease.

From my own experience I have not been impressed that beta blockers will obscure warning signs and symptoms of hypoglycemia in insulin-dependent diabetics, although I would recommend a cardioselective beta blocker for such patients because nonselective beta blockers may

TABLE 6. **Direct Vasodilators**

	Usual Dose	Side Effects
hydralazine (Apresoline)	Oral: 20–300 mg/day* IM: 10–50 mg or IV: 10–20 mg	Headache, palpitations, skin rash, tachycardia, fluid retention, GI irritation, psychosis (rare), LE type illness (>300 mg/day)
minoxidil (Loniten)	Oral: 5–40 mg/day*	Headache, palpitations and tachycardia, fluid retention, GI irritation, pericardial effusion, hirsutism
sodium nitroprusside (Nipride, Nitropress)	IV: 0.5–10 μg/kg/min continuous infusion	Restlessness, agitation, cutis anserina, nausea, vomiting, hypotension, toxic psychosis (when thiocyanate level is >10 mg/dl)
diazoxide (Hyperstat)	100 mg bolus IV every 5–10 min	Hypotension, palpitations and tachycardia, restlessness, nausea, vomiting, flushing, hyperglycemia, hyperuricemia
nitroglycerin Tridil Nitrostat Nitro-BID nitroglycerin injection	IV 5 μg/min to 100 or more μg/min	Headache, palpitations, nausea, vomiting, hypotension, restlessness, abdominal pain

*Usually divided and given twice daily.

TABLE 7. **Converting Enzyme Inhibitors**

	Trade Name	Usual Dose *(Mg)*	Side Effects
captopril	Capoten	12.5 bid to 150 tid on empty stomach	Skin rash; GI irritation, hypotension, dysgeusia (reversible), neutropenia (in patients with autoimmune-collagen disorders), proteinuria (rare at recommended doses); acute renal failure in patients with bilateral renal artery stenosis or severe stenosis in artery to solitary kidney
enalapril	Vasotec	10 to 40 once daily	Acute renal failure in patients with bilateral renal artery stenosis or severe stenosis in artery to solitary kidney; skin rash (rare), headache, dizziness, fatigue, diarrhea, nausea, hypotension

prolong insulin-induced hypoglycemia by delaying the release of glycogen.

Beta blockers tend to increase serum cholesterol and triglycerides and to reduce HDL cholesterol. This effect is more prolonged than it is for diuretics. Beta blockers can also increase blood glucose. Nevertheless, they are effective antianginal drugs and they have a cardioprotective effect in patients who have had a myocardial infarction, reducing the risk of reinfarction and sudden death and improving overall survival for at least 30 months after the infarction. Consequently, I select a beta blocker as step one for hypertensive patients who have angina pectoris or who have had a myocardial infarction.

Labetalol has both beta- and alpha-adrenergic blocking properties. Usually it has a greater effect on standing than on supine blood pressure, but symptomatic orthostatic hypotension is unusual. Given intravenously, it has a prompt antihypertensive action for management of hypertensive crisis, but orally it is no more effective than conventional beta blockers.

Alpha-Adrenergic Blocking Drugs (Table 5). Phentolamine (Regitine), phenoxybenzamine (Dibenzyline), and prazosin (Minipress) are alpha-adrenergic blocking drugs, but only prazosin has been used for management of primary hypertension, usually as a step two or step three agent. Unlike the other two, prazosin is a selective $alpha_1$-receptor blocker; it does not block the $alpha_2$-receptor on the sympathetic nerve ending and therefore does not interfere with the feedback mechanism that turns off norepinephrine release from the sympathetic nerve terminal. This may be why it is less likely to cause tachycardia than the nonselective alpha blockers.

Prazosin can cause orthostatic hypotension, especially after the first dose, and patients should be warned about this possibility. The effective dose range is wide, varying from 1 to 10 or 15 mg twice daily, often requiring numerous visits for titration of dosage. It does not cause metabolic disturbances such as hyperlipidemia or hyperglycemia. It is particularly indicated in managing hypertension for patients with pheochromocytoma or congestive heart failure. For the latter it reduces preload and afterload. It must be given at least twice daily.

Centrally Acting $Alpha_2$-Agonists (Table 5). Methyldopa (Aldomet), clonidine (Catapres), and guanabenz (Wytensin) all have a high side effect profile, especially of drowsiness and dry mouth. They are used as step 2 drugs, usually with a diuretic, and must be given twice daily. I have found that a small dose of clonidine (e.g., 0.2 to 0.4 mg) at bedtime has been very helpful in managing severe and resistant hypertension when added to a triple drug regimen consisting of an oral diuretic, a beta blocker, and hydralazine. Abrupt cessation of any of these drugs, especially clonidine, can cause a severe hypertensive crisis owing to release of norepinephrine.

Clonidine is available for transdermal administration in impregnated patches that are applied once weekly. The patches contain 2.5, 5.0, or 7.5

TABLE 8. **Calcium Channel Blocking Agents**

	Dosage	Side Effects
verapamil (Isoptin) (Calan)	80 mg bid–160 mg tid	GI irritation, constipation, skin rash, headache, hypotension, dizziness, myocardial depression, congestive heart failure, heart block, fluid retention
diltiazem (Cardizem)	30 mg bid–90 mg tid	GI irritation, headache, skin rash, palpitation, fluid retention
nifedipine (Procardia)	10–30 mg tid	Flushing, edema, constipation, GI irritation, headache, palpitations

TABLE 9. **Management of Hypertension with Complications**

Complication	Drugs of Choice	Drugs to Be Used with Caution If at All
Azotemia	furosemide, ethacrynic acid, bumetanide, indapamide, or metolazone hydralazine beta blocker methyldopa clonidine guanabenz minoxidil prazosin reserpine diazoxide sodium nitroprusside	Oral diuretics except furosemide, ethacrynic acid, bumetanide, indapamide, and metolazone Guanethidine
Congestive heart failure	oral diuretic hydralazine captopril nifedipine prazosin methyldopa clonidine guanabenz sodium nitroprusside nitroglycerin	beta blocker minoxidil verapamil
Ischemic heart disease	oral diuretic beta blocker methyldopa guanadrel clonidine guanabenz reserpine calcium channel blocker sodium nitroprusside nitroglycerin	hydralazine guanethidine diazoxide
Cerebrovascular insufficiency	oral diuretic methyldopa clonidine guanabenz beta blocker hydralazine reserpine sodium nitroprusside	guanethidine guanadrel prazosin diazoxide

mg of clonidine, delivering 0.1, 0.2, or 0.3 mg daily. This unique dosage form seems to be as effective as the oral route with fewer side effects. Unfortunately, about 20 per cent of patients develop cutaneous reactions at the site of application, requiring discontinuation.

Peripherally Acting Adrenergic Inhibitors (Table 5).

RESERPINE. This is one of the oldest antihypertensive drugs. It is used as step two with a diuretic. Recently the tendency is to use small doses (0.05 to 0.1 mg daily) to minimize side effects, which have been a deterrent to its use. These include lassitude, sedation, depression, nasal congestion, and activation of peptic ulcer.

GUANETHIDINE. This drug is largely reserved for step four because it is so potent and frequently produces side effects such as orthostatic hypotension, especially in the morning, diarrhea, and male sexual dysfunction.

GUANADREL. This agent is similar to guanethidine but is less potent, is shorter-acting, and produces similar but less severe side effects. It is a step two drug and must be given twice daily.

Vasodilators (Table 6)

Hydralazine and minoxidil act directly to dilate the peripheral arterioles and reduce peripheral resistance. They are step three drugs because, given without an oral diuretic and a sympathetic depressant, they cause fluid retention and reflex tachycardia. They must be given twice daily.

Hydralazine in doses of more than 300 mg daily can cause a lupus-like syndrome. Minoxidil is probably the most potent antihypertensive agent available but causes hirsutism, which is unacceptable to most women. Sometimes the fluid retention associated with minoxidil requires large doses of a loop diuretic.

TABLE 10. **Hypertensive Emergencies**

	Preferred Drugs	Drugs to Avoid or Use with Caution
Hypertensive encephalopathy	sodium nitroprusside diazoxide trimethaphan camsylate labetalol	reserpine methyldopa ester
Acute intracranial hemorrhage	sodium nitroprusside trimethaphan camsylate	all others
Acute cerebral infarction	sodium nitroprusside trimethaphan camsylate nitroglycerin	all others
Acute left ventricular failure	sodium nitroprusside nitroglycerin trimethaphan camsylate diazoxide* hydralazine hydrochloride*	labetalol
Acute coronary insufficiency	nitroglycerin sodium nitroprusside labetalol trimethaphan camsylate reserpine methyldopa ester nifedipine (SL)	hydralazine hydrochloride diazoxide
Dissecting aneurysm	reserpine + trimethaphan camsylate + guanethidine (PO) + beta blocker (PO) or sodium nitroprusside + propranolol (IV)	diazoxide hydralazine hydrochloride nitroglycerin
Eclampsia	hydralazine hydrochloride methyldopate ester diazoxide	trimethaphan camsylate reserpine sodium nitroprusside
Catecholamine crisis: Pheochromocytoma Monoamine oxidase inhibition Clonidine or guanabenz withdrawal	phentolamine mesylate sodium nitroprusside prazosin (PO)	all others
Head injury	sodium nitroprusside trimethaphan camsylate hydralazine hydrochloride	reserpine methyldopate ester diazoxide
Extensive body burns	sodium nitroprusside diazoxide labetalol hydralazine hydrochloride reserpine methyldopate ester	
Malignant hypertension	diazoxide labetalol sodium nitroprusside hydralazine hydrochloride reserpine nifedipine (SL)	
Postoperative hypertension	methyldopate ester sodium nitroprusside nitroglycerin reserpine hydralazine hydrochloride labetalol diazoxide nifedipine (SL)	trimethaphan camsylate

*Concomitant administration of venodilator (e.g., isosorbide dinitrate) to reduce preload.

I prefer to use hydralazine as step three unless hypertension is severe and resistant.

Converting Enzyme Inhibitors (Table 7)

Captopril and enalapril are the first of a new class of drugs that block the enzyme that converts angiotensin I to angiotensin II. While these agents are particularly useful in patients with angiotensin II–dependent hypertension, they are also effective in primary hypertension as step one or step two agents. An oral diuretic enhances their effectiveness. They have also been used as step three drugs along with an oral diuretic and a beta blocker.

I do not use these agents routinely but reserve them for patients with resistant hypertension who have not responded to standard triple drug therapy with an oral diuretic, a beta blocker, and hydralazine. (Enalapril is an investigational drug not yet approved by the F.D.A.)

Calcium Slow Channel Blocking Agents (Table 8)

Hemodynamically, these agents behave as direct vasodilators and reduce blood pressure by decreasing total peripheral vascular resistance. They are usually used as step two agents with an oral diuretic, although they may ultimately be useful as step one drugs. Verapamil, and to a lesser extent diltiazem, have a negative inotropic effect; they should not be used in patients with second or third degree heart block and should be used cautiously with a beta blocker, which has similar effects. On the other hand, verapamil is useful in treating supraventricular paroxysmal tachycardia. Nifedipine has no significant cardiac effect, and for this reason it can cause reflex tachycardia as do hydralazine and minoxidil.

Calcium channel blocking drugs seem to be especially useful in elderly patients with isolated systolic hypertension, either as step one or step two agents.

Management of Hypertension with Complications

Sometimes the presence of cardiovascular complications calls for alterations in the regimen to include certain drugs that are especially indicated or to avoid drugs that may be relatively contraindicated. Table 9 lists some of the complications and the drugs to use or avoid under these circumstances.

Hypertensive Emergencies

At times prompt reduction of blood pressure by parenteral administration of appropriate antihypertensive drugs can be lifesaving or prevent serious sequelae. For this purpose, one of the direct vasodilators (diazoxide, sodium nitroprusside, or nitroglycerin) or the alpha and beta blocking drug labetalol can be given intravenously. Nifedipine given sublingually is effective and convenient for managing some emergencies. Some of the hypertensive emergencies and the agents of choice for their management are listed in Table 10.

Compliance

It has been estimated that up to 50 per cent of hypertensive patients either drop out of treatment entirely or do not take their medications as prescribed. Frequently this is the fault of the health care system. The following are tips on ways to enhance compliance:

—Explain the nature of hypertension, its potential complications, and the benefits of treatment.

—Keep the regimen simple; once a day dosage is preferable when possible.

—Combination tablets incorporating two different drugs can be helpful in gaining compliance, but these should be prescribed only after titration with individual drugs has demonstrated the need for two drugs in the ratio provided by the combination tablet.

—Teach the patient to take and record his or her blood pressure at home.

—Minimize side effects by altering the regimen when necessary.

—Always give an appointment for the next visit before the patient leaves the office.

—Follow-up with phone calls to patients who do not keep appointments.

—Minimize waiting time.

—Use each office visit to answer questions and to reinforce the message to "keep taking your pills." A nurse or physician's assistant can be as effective as the physician in this role.

ACUTE MYOCARDIAL INFARCTION

method of
JOSEPH R. BENOTTI, M.D.
University of Massachusetts
Worcester, Massachusetts

The therapy of acute myocardial infarction (AMI) has evolved dramatically within the past 20 years. The establishment of coronary care units (CCU), where patients with AMI are cared for and continually monitored in specially designated areas staffed by nurses trained in critical care and advanced cardiac life support, has resulted in a dramatic decline in the incidences of arrhythmia-related sudden deaths. Similarly, the period of hospitalization after uncomplicated AMI has been abbreviated from approximately 6 weeks to 10 to 14 days.

Treatment of AMI is premised on the facts that survival is determined by the extent of coronary artery disease, by the cumulative amount of irreversible myocardial injury (cellular death), and by the presence of complicated ventricular tachyarrhythmias in the late, hospital convalescent phase. Extensive coronary artery disease portends the development of angina, myocardial infarction, and sudden cardiac death (usually resulting from ischemia-induced ventricular tachycardia/ventricular fibrillation (VT/VF). Extensive cumulative myocardial injury with ventricular dysfunction presages sudden (arrhythmic) cardiac death and congestive heart failure.

AMI therapy is directed at reducing the ultimate size of the infarct through measures designed to ensure the survival of ischemic yet viable myocardium. The jeopardized zone of myocardium may reside in the same vascular distribution area served by the acutely occluded (thrombosed) coronary artery responsible for myocardial infarction, along the perimeter of the infarct zone. In patients with multivessel coronary disease, however, it is not uncommon for ischemia to manifest itself in one or more coronary artery perfusion zones anatomically distinct from the occluded coronary vessel responsible for the initial infarction. This finding may be a consequence of the catecholamine-mediated increase in myocardial contractility and compensatory hyperkinesis in the myocardial region distinct from the infarct zone, as it assumes a greater hemodynamic burden, and its requirement for aerobic metabolism outstrips the ability of the diseased coronary artery to deliver oxygenated blood. The principle of therapy is to reduce the oxygen demand of the myocardium and to increase the capability of the diseased coronary circulation to satisfy these oxidative demands. Myocardial oxygen demand is minimized by such measures as bed rest; effective analgesia for the pain of myocardial infarction, pericarditis, or recurrent myocardial ischemia; light sedation to alleviate anxiety; rapid detection, diagnosis, and institution of effective therapy for bradyarrhythmias or tachyarrhythmias; aggressive treatment of pyrexia; and routine use of beta-blocking agents to reduce heart rate and myocardial contractility. Measures designed to increase the ability of the diseased coronary circulation to satisfy myocardial oxidative requirements include administration of oxygen; correction of anemia; treatment with calcium channel–blocking agents and nitrates for coronary vasodilation; intra-aortic balloon counterpulsation for improved coronary perfusion; thrombolytic therapy with streptokinase to dissolve the intracoronary thrombus proximately responsible for AMI; and angioplasty or coronary artery revascularization surgery, or both.

Emergency Room Treatment

All patients with suspected or proven AMI should immediately undergo the following interventions:

1. Administration of oxygen at 2 L/min via nasal cannula. This is designed to correct mild to moderate arterial hypoxemia consequent to the ventilation to perfusion imbalance, resulting from minor elevations in mean left atrial and pulmonary arterial pressure consequent to AMI.
2. Placement of an 18 to 21 gauge plastic intravenous cannula into a reliable vein in the nondominant upper extremity. After blood specimens for diagnostic laboratory evaluations (complete blood count, blood urea nitrogen, creatinine, glucose, electrolyte, and cardiac enzyme levels) are obtained, intravascular access is maintained with 5 percent dextrose at a rate of 10 ml/hr. Reliable vascular access is important for administration of narcotic analgesics, anti-arrhythmic drugs, and vasopressor medications should the need arise.
3. The patient should be immediately connected to a portable ECG monitor capable of continuous oscilloscopic display. This monitor permits the physician to rapidly detect, diagnose, and treat potentially life-threatening arrhythmias.
4. The patient should be positioned with the head and thorax elevated approximately 45 degrees above the horizontal plane to minimize gravitational propensity for the development of pulmonary congestion.
5. Analgesia is best provided with the judicious intravenous administration of morphine sulfate or nalbuphine hydrochloride, 3 to 5 mg intravenously every 5 to 10 min, adjusted to achieve satisfactory pain relief without producing significant hypotension (systolic blood pressure < 90 to 100 mmHg), respiratory depression (arterial $P_{CO_2} > 45$ mmHg), and excessive obtundation.

The CCU staff is notified immediately of the patient's admission and impending transfer to their unit. If there is clear-cut electrocardiographic evidence of transmural myocardial infarction or ventricular premature beats (VPBs), or both, it is prudent to administer lidocaine intravenously as a slow bolus to a total dose of 1 to 2 mg/kg and to begin simultaneously an intravenous infusion of lidocaine at 2 mg/min. Such prophylactic therapy has been shown to reduce the incidence of primary ventricular fibrillation in the first 24 to 48 hr after myocardial infarction.

The patient is transferred to the CCU under the supervision of a physician or a nurse skilled in advanced cardiac life support. It is prudent to have the assistance of an orderly, also skilled in basic life support, to help with patient transport. Lidocaine, 100 mg, and atropine, 2 mg, drawn up in syringes and prepared for immediate administration should be conspicuously labeled and taped to the ECG oscilloscope, available for immediate administration should VT/VF or bradyarrhythmia, or both, develop.

Thrombolytic Therapy

Two years ago streptokinase and urokinase, administered directly into the occluded coronary artery, were approved for use by the Food and Drug Administration to digest the coronary artery thrombus that is proximately responsible for acute transmural myocardial infarction in about 80 percent of patients. It is anticipated that the rapid restoration of coronary arterial perfusion into the zone of myocardial infarction will tip the scales in favor of greater survival of the majority of myocytes that are ischemic but not yet infarcted so that over the next several days regional wall motion in the zone of myocardial infarction will recover, and the cumulative volume of myocardial infarction will be reduced by thrombolytic therapy. Intracoronary administration of streptokinase reperfuses the infarct-related coronary artery in approximately 60 to 80 percent of the cases. Clearly, restoration of coronary arterial flow with intracoronary streptokinase has been associated with improved myocardial uptake of thallium^{201} in the equilibrium phase and with improved regional ventricular wall motion, suggesting that this therapy, when successful, reduces myocardial infarction size. In AMI patients receiving intracoronary streptokinase, comparison between patients in whom coronary artery reperfusion has been re-established and maintained over the duration of hospitalization and patients in whom the infarct-related coronary artery remains totally occluded despite intracoronary streptokinase or in whom the coronary artery, initially reperfused, subsequently re-occluded during hospitalization reveals that reperfusion is associated with improved regional wall motion and improved hospital survival rate. It appears that intracoronary streptokinase might be particularly beneficial to patients with high risk myocardial infarctions, including infarctions of the anterior wall and those associated with heart failure or cardiogenic shock. In terms of clot dissolution and myocardial salvage, intracoronary thrombolytic therapy with streptokinase or urokinase is likely to be most successful if coronary artery and myocardial reperfusion can be established within 4 to 6 hr of the time at which the patient first develops symptoms of myocardial infarction.

Administration of intracoronary thrombolytic therapy within the time required for restoration of coronary arterial patency and myocardial salvage imposes several limitations. The first is that for patients to undergo successful coronary thrombolysis within 4 to 6 hr requires that they arrive at the emergency room within 1 to 2 hr after they first experience myocardial infarction symptoms. This allows additional time for catheterization and institution of intracoronary thrombolytic therapy so that clot dissolution and coronary artery flow can be re-established within 4 to 6 hr.

Most patients with chest pains suggestive of myocardial infarction procrastinate to some degree as a result of denial and of delay in making contact with the family physician. Further valuable time elapses if the physician attempts to advise treatment over the telephone before recommending that the patient come to the office or to the emergency room for an ECG. Probably less than 30 percent of patients with AMI present to a hospital emergency room within the time interval in which intracoronary thrombolytic therapy might be of benefit. A much greater limitation of intracoronary thrombolytic therapy is that it requires round-the-clock availability of an “angiographic suite” and a highly skilled cardiac catheterization team. Fewer than 10 percent of hospitals in the United States have the capability for cardiac catheterization and coronary arteriography.

Thrombolytic therapy with a high dose (1.5 million units), short term (90 min) of streptokinase or high dose (2 million units), short term (15 min) of urokinase establishes coronary artery reperfusion in only approximately 35 to 60 percent of patients and carries a small but significant risk of bleeding. Intravenous streptokinase or urokinase has been approved for use by the Food and Drug Administration as a therapy designed to dissolve the coronary thrombi causing AMI. Tissue plasminogen activator (t-PA) is a serine protease synthesized by vascular endothelial cells that selectively dissolves only fibrin thrombi without producing a systemic thrombolytic state or increasing the risk of hemorrhage. It can be synthesized in large quantities using recombinant DNA technology. When administered intravenously to patients with AMI consequent to thrombotic coronary occlusion, t-PA establishes antegrade coronary arterial flow in previously occluded vessels in approximately 65 to 75 percent of cases.

Intravenously administered t-PA is as effective as intracoronary streptokinase in the dissolution of coronary artery thrombi causing acute myocardial infarction. Because t-PA can be administered intravenously without the potential for hemorrhagic complications associated with nonspecific thrombolytic agents such as streptokinase or urokinase, it is anticipated that t-PA could be administered to the majority of patients within the first few hours of suspected myocardial infarction by emergency room personnel under the supervision of emergency room physicians or even by ambulance personnel after the diagnosis of transmural myocardial infarction has been confirmed by ECG obtained on the scene by paramedics and telemetered to the emergency room physicians. Studies are currently underway to determine if intravenous thrombolytic therapy with t-PA can reduce the size of myocardial infarction, improve overall ventricular performance, and increase survival following myocardial infarction.

Uncomplicated Myocardial Infarction

Treatment

The patient with uncomplicated myocardial infarction requires careful observation in the CCU for the first 24 to 48 hr to ensure rapid diagnosis and treatment of recurrent chest pain, arrhythmias, and heart failure. A mild sedative (diazepam 5 mg qid or lorazepam 2 to 3 mg bid or tid) is routinely prescribed to allay anxiety and promote relaxation. A sleep-inducing medication, flurazepam (Dalmane), 15 or 30 mg, is routinely prescribed to be taken at night. The use of mild tranquilizers, sedatives, and hypnotics is minimized in the patient with chronic obstructive pulmonary disease and better avoided if carbon dioxide retention is a possibility. A stool softener promotes elimination and minimizes straining. It is best to allow patients to use commodes with assistance if they are capable, as the energy expended in using bedpans exceeds that in using commodes. For the first 3 or 4 days of hospitalization, intravenous access is maintained through a plastic cannula carefully secured into a reliable vein of the nondominant upper extremity. This cannula provides immediate intravascular access for the administration of antiarrhythmic or vasopressor medication, or both. Oxygen, 2 to 4 L, by nasal cannula is also routinely administered to assure adequate oxygenation of the arterial blood.

For the first 12 to 24 hr, the patient is maintained on clear liquids in order to minimize the likelihood of nausea or vomiting caused by reflux ileus or narcotic analgesics. Subsequently, meals are given as 4 or 5 small ones, with a total of 1200 to 1500 calories daily in order to minimize the postprandial increase in cardiac output and myocardial oxygen consumption consequent to the specific dynamic action of food and to the increased activity of the digestive tract. If obesity is a problem, the patient's caloric intake is restricted. It is appropriate to select a diet that has fish and poultry as primary protein sources, along with green, leafy vegetables (a low-saturated fat and cholesterol diet). It is best for the patient to avoid foods high in cholesterol and saturated fats, such as whole milk; cheese; ice cream and other dairy products; eggs; red meat; and hydrogenated fats and oils.

Heparin, 5000 units subcutaneously every 8 to 12 hr, is routinely administered in order to reduce the likelihood of venous thromboembolic disease during the period of bed rest. This treatment is not associated with a detectable derangement in the coagulation mechanism and does not increase the risk of bleeding. Subcutaneous heparin should be discontinued as soon as the patient is transferred out of the CCU and begins regular physical activities (ambulation).

Beta-blocking agents have been shown to reduce the incidence of sudden cardiac death following myocardial infarction. This reduction may be related to the protection afforded against recurrent myocardial ischemia as a result of the reduction in heart rate, systolic wall tension, and myocardial contractility (myocardial oxygen consumption), resulting from a beta-adrenergic receptor blockade. This finding has been demonstrated for timolol (Blocadren), atenolol (Tenormin), metoprolol (Lopressor), and propranolol (Inderal). The precise mechanism for protection against sudden cardiac death has not been clarified. Though this protection has not been shown for other beta-blocking agents, it is likely that reduction in the frequency of cardiac morbidity following myocardial infarction is related to a nonspecific beta-adrenergic receptor blockade and not to the unique chemistry of any particular formulation. In patients with reactive airway disease, insulin-requiring diabetes and attacks of hypoglycemia, congestive heart failure consequent to systolic ventricular dysfunction (left ventricular ejection fraction <0.35), ischemic limb discomfort despite bed rest, and other contraindications to beta-blocking agent therapy, timolol (Blocadren) 10 to 20 mg bid, metoprolol (Lopressor) 50 to 100 mg bid, atenolol (Tenormin) 50 to 100 mg once daily, or propranolol (Inderal) 20 to 80 mg qid may be prescribed. This therapy can be instituted immediately with metoprolol or within the first 24 to 72 hr following hospital admission. Since the protective effect of beta-blocking agents has been demonstrated for as long as 3 years following AMI, therapy is continued for at least 2 years following AMI, if well tolerated.

The patient sustaining a first inferior wall myocardial infarction who is free of previous ischemic symptoms and who does not develop angina, evidence of myocardial ischemia during an exercising or resting thallium^{201} scintography, or evidence of ventricular dysfunction during a radionuclide ventriculography (ejection fraction exceeding 0.50) has an excellent, short-term survival expectancy (97 to 99 percent, 1 year following myocardial infarction). It is unlikely that prophylactic beta-blocking agent therapy, with a goal toward prevention of sudden cardiac death, is likely to benefit such a patient. Patients at high risk following myocardial infarctions include those with infarctions of the anterior wall resulting from occlusion of the left anterior descending vessel, angina, and myocardial ischemia as shown by exercise stress testing in the late convalescent phase of myocardial infarction or sustained ventricular arrhythmia in the late convalescent phase. Such patients are at high risk for recurrent angina or myocardial infarction and have a cumulative mortality of 12 to 15 percent during the first year after hospital discharge. Prophylactic treatment with beta-blocking agents to prevent sudden cardiac death is clearly indicated. Moreover, it should certainly be instituted prior to hospital discharge, since the risk of cardiac morbidity is greatest within the first several weeks after discharge and declines substantially thereafter.

Complications Following Myocardial Infarction

Pain. Patients with AMI characteristically present with rather severe squeezing, sharp, oppressive, or burning retrosternal anterior chest discomfort radiating into one or both arms, neck, or jaw, or all of these areas, which is often described as the worst pain in their lives. Such discomfort typically is not relieved by nitroglycerin (Nitrostat); in fact, complete relief within 3 to 5 min following the administration of sublingual nitroglycerin is often used as a test virtually pathognomonic of reversible myocardial ischemia, i.e., angina. When the diagnosis of AMI is clearly established, it is reasonable to assume that the pain is consequent to ongoing myocardial necrosis and inflammation as well as to resistant ischemia. It is best not to rely solely on nitrates, beta-blocking agents, or calcium channel–blocking agents to provide relief, rather, it is better to completely alleviate the patient's discomfort with the judicial, intravenous administration of morphine or nalbuphine. In addition to their potent analgesic properties, morphine and nalbuphine reduce sympathetic outflow thereby reducing left ventricular end diastolic volume (preload), afterload, and the force of myocardial contraction, while effecting no change or decrease in the heart rate. The net effect is to reduce myocardial oxygen demand and, it is hoped, to limit the size of the myocardial infarction. When morphine or nalbuphine is administered in 3 to 5 mg intravenous bolus doses every 5 to 10 min, adjusting the amount to the point of satisfactory pain relief, respiratory depression and hypotension are usually avoidable. However, these complications still may occur. Hypotension results from a redistribution of blood volume from the central thoracic to the peripheral venous system. Patients with reduced intravascular volume due to pyrexia, diaphoresis, or vomiting are exquisitely sensitive to the hypotensive effects of morphine. Significant respiratory depression may result in CO_2 retention. Hypotension is treated by administering crystalloids and by placing the patient in Trendelenburg's position with the legs elevated well above the level of the chest. If respiratory depression eventuates in unresponsiveness or CO_2 retention, or both, it should be promptly corrected with naloxone (Narcan), a narcotic antagonist, in a dose of 0.4 to 2 mg intravenously.

With cases of transmural myocardial infarction, it is reasonable to assume that for the first 18 to 24 hr most residual chest discomfort is the result of active cell death and inflammation rather than the result of myocardial ischemia. The exception would be new and dramatically worsening discomfort associated with the re-elevation of the S-T segments in 2 or more subadjacent leads on the ECG, reflecting the initial infarct zone. This sign suggests reversible myocardial ischemia consequent to coronary arterial spasm or thrombotic re-occlusion of the infarct related coronary artery. Recurrent angina associated with the S-T segment depression in 2 or more subsequent leads, anatomically distinct from the region of initial infarction (e.g., leads II, III, and AVF in an anterior wall infarction), suggests more remote subendocardial ischemia, i.e., "ischemia at a distance," and correlates with the presence of severe multivessel coronary disease. These syndromes of "ischemia in the infarct zone" or "ischemia at a distance" should be managed with anti-anginal drugs (nitrates and calcium channel–blocking agents or beta-blocking agents) in addition to parenteral narcotic agents. In general, however, for patients with clear-cut AMI pain administration of morphine is preferential to a therapeutic trial of a narcotic or nitroglycerin. It is sometimes suggested that the pain associated with inferior wall myocardial infarction (IMI) is best treated with meperidine (Demerol) because it has less vagotonic effects. It is also expected that meperidine would be likely to provoke less bradyarrhythmia and heart block, rhythm disturbances to which the patient with IMI is predisposed. Meperidine can be administered in a dose of 20 to 50 mg intravenously with the dose repeated every 5 to 15 min until adequate analgesia has been achieved. The risks of narcosis, hypotension, and respiratory depression are similar with meperidine. Because of the possibility of circulatory insufficiency or reactive ileus, orally administered narcotics are unreliably absorbed and should be avoided. Likewise, intramuscular injections are not to be given, since release of enzymes into the blood stream after skeletal muscle trauma negates the specificity of elevations in the total creatinine phosphokinase serum concentrations in the laboratory evaluation of myocardial infarction and the estimation of its size.

Before ascribing any discomfort to myocardial necrosis and inflammation, it is the physician's duty to exclude other causes of chest pain from the differential diagnosis, such as the pericardial inflammation of adjacent epicardial necrosis and inflammation and pericardial friction rub. It is important to promptly recognize pericarditis complicating transmural myocardial infarction because it responds promptly to indomethacin (Indocin), 25 to 50 mg tid, to other nonsteroidal, anti-inflammatory drugs, and to aspirin (650 mg qid). Of equal importance is that patients with post-myocardial infarction pericarditis, in contrast to patients with ongoing myocardial ischemia and pain, have good prognoses. In those with pericarditis complicating myocardial infarction, it is advisable to avoid or to terminate full doses of anticoagulant therapy with heparin, as the risk of hemorrhagic effusion with tamponade may be increased.

Another cause of chest pain in the patient with myocardial infarction is recurrent angina (reversible myocardial ischemia) or myocardial infarct extension. Recurrent angina is usually associated with correctable electrocardiographic S-T segment depressions or elevations in 2 or more subadjacent leads in the distribution of the infarct related artery (ischemia around the zone of infarction). It may also be associated with S-T segment ECG shifts in leads that monitor the myocardium perfused by a coronary artery not involved with the initial thrombotic process, reflecting "ischemia at a distance." Angina is usually relieved with sublingual nitroglycerin or another nitrate preparation. More importantly, this symptom identifies the presence of viable myocardium at risk for subsequent infarction. It is likely that the patient with angina appearing as "ischemia at a distance" after myocardial infarction has severe multivessel coronary disease in which life expectancy might be prolonged by coronary artery revascularization.

Should infarct extension occur, treatment is the same as that for the initial myocardial infarction. The exception is the high risk patient in whom the recurrent ECG reflects the injury that is immediately detected; there is a high likelihood of effecting thrombolysis with intracoronary streptokinase or more permanent reperfusion with coronary angioplasty or bypass surgery. If catheterization is available, immediate coronary arteriography with an aim toward intracoronary thrombolytic therapy with streptokinase or urokinase, with angioplasty, or with bypass surgery might be undertaken. Infarct extension is best avoided by vigorous therapy of post-infarction myocardial ischemia (post-infarction angina).

Another cause of chest pain in cases of suspected AMI, particularly of the inferior wall, is aortic dissection. Though rare, dissection of the ascending aorta is worthy of diagnostic consideration, certainly to the extent that a good posterior-anterior chest x-ray be obtained, particularly when there is no infarct pattern on the patient's ECG at admission. In my experience, 2-dimensional echocardiography has occasionally helped document type I (proximal) aortic dissection in this circumstance, when it was otherwise totally unsuspected. Should any mediastinal widening or abnormality of the ascending aorta be evident, urgent aortography is indicated to confirm or exclude this diagnosis.

Fever. For the first 1 to 4 days following myocardial infarction, the patient may have a temperature as high as 101 to 103°F consequent to myocardial necrosis and the inflammatory reaction. There may be moderate leukocytosis (12,000 to 18,000/mm^2) and an elevation in the erythrocyte sedimentation rate. When the fever first develops, it is always prudent to obtain blood cultures, a urine culture if there is pyuria or other symptoms of a urinary tract infection, and a sputum stain and culture if there is clinical evidence of chest infection. The patient is then treated with aspirin or acetaminophen (Tylenol or Panadol) every 4 to 6 hr to maintain normal or near normal body temperature. This treatment is important because antipyretics reduce the increases in cardiac output and myocardial oxygen consumption that are part of the cardiovascular system's response to fever. After 48 to 72 hr, antipyretics are discontinued. Although aspirin and acetaminophen are equally effective, if there is evidence of pericarditis aspirin should be avoided to minimize the likelihood of hemorrhagic effusion and tamponade. When clinical or microbiologic evidence of infection is present, appropriate antibiotics are prescribed.

Hypertension. Following myocardial infarction, some patients may have arterial systolic pressure consistently in excess of 140 mmHg, which is possibly the first manifestation of an underlying genetic hypertensive diathesis; more commonly, this manifestation represents an elevation in the cardiac output and arterial resistance, resulting from an exaggerated sympathetic nervous system response to myocardial infarction. Hypertension following myocardial infarction must be vigorously treated in order to reduce myocardial oxygen demand and myocardial infarct size. Because of its analgesic and central sympatholytic effects, intravenous morphine (3 to 5 mg every 10 to 15 min) is very effective. Similarly, nitroprusside (Nipride) (0.5 to 1 microgram/kg/min, increased by 5 or 10 micrograms every 10 min) or nitroglycerin (5 micrograms/min, increased by 5 to 10 micrograms every 5 minutes), both very rapidly acting parenteral vasodilator agents, is adjusted to lower the systolic blood pressure to the range of 110 to 130 mmHg. Simultaneously, furosemide (Lasix) (10 to 40 mg IV) and propranolol (20 to 60 mg po) are administered to allow a sustained reduction in blood pressure over the next 12 hr so that parenteral antihypertensive therapy can be discontinued. A diuretic (furosemide (Lasix) 20 to 40 mg/day or hydrochlorothiazide (Hydrodiuril) 50 mg qid) and a beta-blocking agent (propranolol (Inderal) 20 to 80 mg bid, nadolol (Corgard) 10 to 40 mg qid, metoprolol (Lopressor) 50 to 100 mg bid, or atenolol (Tenormin) 50 to 100 mg qid) usually are effective in maintaining the blood pressure within a physiologically normal range.

Arrhythmias. Within the first 48 to 72 hr, the myocardial infarction patient is at risk for the development of ventricular and, less commonly, supraventricular arrhythmias. Intravenous antiarrhythmic therapy for arrhythmia complicating myocardial infarction is summarized in Table 1 and oral therapy in Table 2. Following myocardial infarction, the ventricle is electrically unstable and there is propensity to develop automatic and re-entrant ventricular arrhythmias. Although of highest risk within the first minutes to hours after infarction, the risk of developing VPBs/VT/VF declines exponentially over the next 24 to 48 hr. The critical time for continuous monitoring of the patient's cardiac rhythm is within the first 72 hr following myocardial infarction. It was initially thought that VPBs heralded the development of VT/VF, but this is not the case and, indeed, as many as 50 percent of patients with AMI may have primary VF unaccompanied by premonitory ventricular arrhythmias. Furthermore, it has been shown that lidocaine (Xylocaine) administered prophylactically when myocardial infarction is first diagnosed, reduces the frequency of spontaneous ventricular fibrillation. Hence, it is advisable to treat the patient prophylactically with lidocaine as soon as the diagnosis of myocardial infarction has been made. This treatment is continued for the first 24 to 48 hr. Prophylactic lidocaine therapy for the prevention of primary VF in patients with AMI is administered as a slow intravenous bolus (1 to 2 mg/kg) followed by a continuous intravenous infusion at 2 mg/min.

Should the patient experience VPBs or unsustained VT, lidocaine is administered at a similar bolus and infusion dose. If after 3 to 5 min of lidocaine infusion VPBs are not completely abolished, another slow intravenous bolus of 50 to 75 mg may be administered and the infusion dose increased to 3 to 4 mg. The rate of lidocaine infusion should not exceed 5 mg/min for any length of time. In the elderly and in those with primary hepatic disease or impaired hepatic perfusion as a result of a low cardiac output, the lidocaine infusion should not exceed 2 to 3 mg/min for any long period. The therapeutic plasma lidocaine level is 1.4 to 6.0 micrograms/ml.

Sustained ventricular tachycardia is treated according to its hemodynamic consequences. If the patient is conscious, mentating appropriately, and has a systolic blood pressure exceeding 80 mmHg, a lidocaine bolus (1 to 2 mg/kg) is administered. If this approach terminates the arrhythmia, a lidocaine infusion is instituted at 2 mg/kg. If the patient experiences symptomatic hypotension or if the patient is unconscious, the treatment is immediate, synchronous DC-cardioversion at a low energy level (10 to 50 watt seconds). While the patient is being prepared for cardioversion, lidocaine is administered, the airway is protected, and 100 percent oxygen via a mask and bag is given. It is important to administer diazepam (Valium), 5 to 10 mg IV, to the conscious patient prior to synchronized cardioversion, even when this is an urgent procedure. Effective sedation provides amnesia for the discomfort of cardioversion, and the amount of time required to prepare the patient for cardioversion permits parenteral diazepam administration without delaying the urgent and potentially life saving therapy of cardioversion.

Ventricular arrhythmias following myocardial infarction that fail to respond to lidocaine can be treated with procainamide (Pronestyl). This is administered as an intravenous loading dose of 10 to 12 mg/kg at a rate not to exceed 25 mg/min in order to avoid hypotension. Simultaneously, an infusion is started at a rate of 1 to 4 mg/min. The effective plasma procainamide level is 4 to 8 micrograms/ml. Procainamide is frequently successful in terminating ventricular arrhythmias not responsive to maximally therapeutic doses of lidocaine. Procainamide can be given as an oral preparation when chronic arrhythmia suppression therapy is indicated. It is available as an oral preparation that must be administered every 4 hr to maintain effective serum levels. However, a sustained release preparation (Procan SR), which can be administered every 6 hr, has recently been approved.

Toxic manifestations of excessive lidocaine serum levels include agitation, hallucinations, bizarre behavior, and seizures. These manifestations are associated with plasma lidocaine levels exceeding 6.0 micrograms/ml. Aside from causing hypotension consequent to vasodilatation, during excessively rapid bolus administration, procaina-

TABLE 1. **Guide for Rapid Intravenous Administration of Anti-arrhythmic Drugs**

Drug	Dosage	Plasma Level	Side Effects	Comments
Lidocaine	200 mg IV bolus over 20 min followed by 2–4 mg/min constant infusion. Half the normal loading and maintenance doses are given for patients with pulmonary edema, shock, and hepatocellular disease.	1.4–6.0 micrograms/ml	Focal seizures, grand mal seizures, respiratory arrest, dizziness, heart block (usually associated with pre-existing abnormal His-Purkinje conduction), sinoatrial arrest.	Significant reduction in dose in patients with heart failure; moderate reduction in dose in patients with hepatic disease; no oral form available; no significant myocardial depression; toxicity usual at high plasma levels; toxicity at low plasma levels may be caused by metabolites.
Procainamide	10–12 mg/kg IV slowly (25 mg/min).	4–8 micrograms/ml	Hypotension, prolonged AV, and His-Purkinje conduction.	Myocardial toxicity usually occurs only at high plasma levels or after rapid administration.
Propranolol	1 mg/min IV up to 10 mg.	40–85 ng/ml	Hypotension, bradycardia, prolonged AV conduction and heart block, myocardial depression, bronchospasm.	Should probably not be considered in the presence of heart failure; many of the side effects corrected by large doses of isoproterenol.
Phenytoin	50–100 mg IV slowly (50 mg/min) every 5 min up to 1000 mg. Additional 500 mg on following day.	10–18 micrograms/ml	Hypotension, 1:1 conduction in atrial flutter, respiratory arrest, idioventricular rhythm, ventricular fibrillation, asystole.	IM administration provides erratic blood levels; toxicity usual only after rapid administration.
Atropine	0.6–1.0 mg IV as a rapid bolus.	—	Sinus tachycardia, glaucomic crisis, urinary retention, psychosis.	Occasionally precipitates paradoxical slowing of heart rate or ventricular tachycardia.
Bretylium tosylate	5–10 mg/kg loading dose over 10 min followed by maintenance infusion of 1–2 mg/min.	—	Hypotension, nausea, vomiting, transient increase in heart rate and blood pressure.	Dose should be reduced in patients with renal failure; response may be better when drug is used alone rather than with other anti-arrhythmic drugs.
Verapamil	5–10 mg (0.075–0.15 mg/kg) as an intravenous bolus over 2 min. Repeat as a 10 mg (0.15 mg/kg) dose 30 min after the first dose if the initial response was inadequate.	—	Hypotension; rapid ventricular response and ventricular fibrillation in patients with atrial flutter or fibrillation and an accessory A-V nodal pathway (Wolf-Parkinson-White syndrome); bradycardia; asystole; worsening heart failure.	Do not combine intravenous verapamil with intravenous beta-blocking agents, as combined use may provoke severe myocardial depression. There is no known adverse reaction with other anti-arrhythmic drugs.

Modified from Alpert, J. S., and Francis, G. S.: *Manual of Coronary Care,* 2nd ed. Boston, Little, Brown and Co., 1981.

mide may cause conduction disturbances and repolarization abnormalities, appearing as prolongation of the QRS and QT intervals. In fact, the administration of procainamide should be terminated if the QRS interval is longer than 1.5 times its control value. QT interval prolongation may be associated with or may herald emergence of polymorphic ventricular tachycardia (torsade des pointes). Therapy for this complication requires withdrawal of the offending type I anti-arrhythmic agent (quinidine, procainamide, or disopyramide) and correction of any associated electrolyte disturbances, particularly hypokalemia and hypomagnesemia. In refractory cases administration of isoproterenol, as a temporary measure to increase the sinus rate 5 to 20 beats above baseline value followed by temporary atrioventricular or ventricular overdrive pacing, is usually required to abolish the drug-induced repolarization abnormalities responsible for emergence of the re-entrant circuit causing polymorphic VT.

An equally appropriate anti-arrhythmic drug for VT/VF complicating AMI is bretylium tosylate (Bretylol). This drug initially depletes catecholamine stores from the autonomic nerve endings in the heart and ganglia. Subsequently, it

TABLE 2. **Long-term Oral Administration of Anti-arrhythmic Drugs**

Drug	Usual Total Daily Dose	Frequency	Plasma Level (micrograms/ml)	Half-life (hr)	Side Effects	Comments
Propranolol	80–320 mg	q6h	40–85 nanograms	3–4.6	Myocardial depression, prolonged AV conduction and heart block, bradycardia, bronchospasm, fatigue and depression, peripheral vascular insufficiency, hyperglycemia, hypoglycemia, alopecia, gastric distention.	Active metabolites may play a role in clinical effect; dose chosen empirically should be tapered slowly in patients with angina; caution needed in patients with cardiac function dependent on sympathetic tone.
Procainamide	2–6 gm	q3–4h	4–8	3–4	Nausea, vomiting, agranulocytosis, lupus-like syndrome, myocardial depression, prolonged A-V and His-Purkinje conduction.	Toxic myocardial effect, usually only at toxic plasma levels; half-life markedly prolonged in renal failure or alkaline urine.
Procainamide (sustained release)	2–6 gm	q6h	4–8			
Phenytoin sodium	300–400 mg	Once daily	10–18	22	Nystagmus, ataxia, lethargy, nausea, vertigo, rash, pseudolymphoma, megaloblastic anemia, peripheral neuropathy, hyperglycemia, seizures.	Half-life longer at higher doses; rate of metabolism affected by many drugs; clinically significant decrease in plasma binding in azotemia and hypoproteinemia; initiate therapy with 1 gm loading dose.
Quinidine	1.0–2.4 gm	q6h	2.3–5.0 (using double extraction assay; higher for precipitation assay)	—	Hypotension, nausea, vomiting, diarrhea, tinnitus, vertigo, prolonged His-Purkinje conduction, rash, fever, thrombocytopenia, hepatic dysfunction, hemolytic anemia, ventricular arrhythmias.	Minor gastrointestinal side effects controlled with symptomatic therapy; clinically significant decrease in plasma binding in hypoproteinemia and hepatic disease; myocardial toxicity usually only at toxic plasma levels; accumulation of metabolites in renal disease.
Disopyramide	400–800 mg	q6h	2–5	—	Myocardial depression, hypotension, prolonged AV conduction and heart block, glaucoma, urinary retention, "drug mouth," constipation, blurred vision, nausea, anorexia.	Half-life 7 hr; reduced dosage in hepatic and renal insufficiency; hypotension can occur in patients with myocarditis or cardiomyopathy, or both; 300 mg loading dose advised in patients with life-threatening arrhythmias.
Tocainide	1200–1800 mg	q8h	4–10	—	Confusion, lightheadedness, ataxia, lethargy, nausea.	Reduce dose by 33 percent in patients with hepatic or renal dysfunction.

Modified from Alpert, J. S., and Francis, G. S.: *Manual of Coronary Care,* 2nd ed. Boston, Little, Brown, and Co., 1981.

blocks re-uptake of catecholamines effecting a "pharmacologic sympathectomy." For ventricular fibrillation or hemodynamically unstable ventricular tachycardia, the dose is 5 mg/kg administered undiluted as a rapid intravenous injection. If cardioversion is unsuccessful, bretylium tosylate is administered at 10 mg/kg and repeated as necessary. For continuous arrhythmia suppression, bretylium tosylate is given intravenously at a 5 to 10 mg/kg loading dose over 10 minutes followed by 1 to 2 mg/min maintenance infusion. Adverse effects of bretylium tosylate include hypertension during initial administration resulting from catecholamine release from nerve endings. Thereafter, hypotension may develop; however, it is usually responsive to elevation of the legs and volume replacement administration.

The development of VPBs/VT/VF during the first 72 hr following myocardial infarction does not adversely affect the patient's prognosis. These arrhythmias are usually a consequence of transient electrical instability of the infarcted and ischemic myocardium. The propensity for the development and perpetuation of arrhythmias seems to subside in time. In the first several hours following AMI these arrhythmias, particularly accelerated idioventricular rhythms, sometimes result from reperfusion of the infarct zone, as a result of spontaneous or streptokinase-mediated lysis of the fibrin clot responsible for the AMI. Though sometimes causing hypotension and therefore requiring specific therapy, they are usually self-limiting and carry no adverse long-term effect on prognosis.

Complicated ventricular tachyarrhythmias occuring after the first 3 days of hospitalization for AMI frequently reflect substantial myocardial infarction with an advanced degree of left ventricular dysfunction. Accordingly, patients with this condition carry a far more ominous prognosis. The goal of anti-arrhythmic therapy is to prevent VT and to eliminate VPBs occurring as couplets, as pairs, or as multiples. Not only is it difficult to abolish all VPBs in patients following AMI, but it has not been shown that therapy to abolish all VPBs improves the patient's prognosis. More important is the fact that all drugs effective in arrhythmia suppression have very high incidences of side effects.

Episodic VT that does not resolve spontaneously after intravenous anti-arrhythmic therapy requires suppression with oral anti-arrhythmic therapy. Appropriate drugs include quinidine sulfate in a dose of 200 to 600 mg qid, titrated to maintain a trough plasma quinidine level between 2.3 and 5.0 micrograms/ml. Equally effective is procainamide in a dosage of 50 mg/kg over 24 hr, administered every 4 hr and adjusted to maintain a trough plasma level of 4 to 8 micrograms/ml. An available sustained release procainamide preparation permits a more convenient 6 hr interval between doses, with continuous maintenance of effective plasma levels.

Adverse effects of quinidine are diarrhea, bradyarrhythmias, heart block with sick sinus syndrome, and QRS and QT prolongation with syncope consequent to ventricular tachycardia. Quinidine also reduces the renal clearance and distribution volume of digoxin (Lanoxin). A patient maintained on a stable dose of digoxin may develop a 30 to 60 percent increase in the serum digoxin level in conjunction with the institution of quinidine therapy. Accordingly, it is advisable to reduce the daily digoxin dose empirically by 30 to 50 per cent when beginning quinidine therapy and to make subsequent adjustments in the daily digoxin dose according to serum digoxin levels. Diarrhea as a side effect of quinidine may be managed with a variety of antidiarrheal preparations. It is anticipated that the patient will become tachyphylactic to this adverse effect. If this is not the case, this unpleasant side effect may be managed by changing therapy from quinidine sulfate to one of many quinidine gluconate preparations with adjustments in the total daily dose, according to the clinical response and the trough plasma level.

The side effects of procainamide include bradyarrhythmia and heart block with sick sinus syndrome, QRS prolongation, and QT prolongation with or without ventricular tachycardia. Additionally, long-term procainamide therapy has been associated with the development of a lupuslike syndrome characterized by fever, pleuritis, skin rash, arthritis, and elevations in the antinuclear antibody titer values. This development is not associated with nephritis and resolves promptly with discontinuation of procainamide. Particularly disabling symptoms, e.g., pleural effusions and arthritis, may be treated with a 7 to 10 day course of adrenocortical steroids in a regimen of tapering doses.

Disopyramide (Norpace), another effective type II antiarrhythmic taken orally, may be useful in the long-term treatment of ventricular arrhythmias. This drug, marketed as the phosphate salt, comes in capsules containing 100 or 150 mg of base. In adults, a loading dose of 300 mg is followed by a maintenance dosage of 150 mg every 6 hr. In patients with heart failure, hepatic or renal failure, and in patients weighing less than 50 kg, the dose should be reduced. In healthy individuals, the peak serum concentration level occurs 2 to 3 hr after administration, and the serum half-life is approximately 7 hr. The therapeutic serum level for disopyramide is 2 to 5 micrograms/ml with a considerable risk of toxicity when serum level exceeds 7 micrograms/ml.

In patients lacking clinical evidence of ventricular dysfunction in whom rapid control of ventricular arrhythmia is essential, an initial loading dose of disopyramide, 300 mg, is administered followed by the appropriate maintenance dosage, which is usually 150 mg every 6 hr. The adverse effects of disopyramide include the development of heart failure and hypotension consequent to its negative inotropic properties. This medication should be avoided in patients with clinical evidence of congestive heart failure caused by systolic ventricular dysfunction (ejection fraction <0.40). Likewise, QRS widening may occur, and if in excess of 25 percent over the control value, disopyramide should be discontinued. Like other type II anti-arrhythmic preparations (quinidine and procainamide), disopyramide may cause prolongation of the QT interval with worsening of ventricular arrhythmias, even with the development of ventricular tachycardia or ventricular fibrillation. If QT prolongation in excess of 25 percent over control value is observed or if ventricular arrhythmias persist, or both occur, the patient should be monitored closely, and this drug should be discontinued. Because of the negative inotropic effect of disopyramide, it should not be used in conjunction with propranolol or other beta-blocking agents. Owing to its anticholinergic effects, disopyramide should not be used indiscriminantly in patients with glaucoma, myasthenia gravis, or urinary retention.

In 1984, tocainide hydrochloride (Tonocard) was approved for the treatment of symptomatic ventricular arrhythmias. This compound is an amine analog of lidocaine that does not undergo hepatic first-pass metabolism following oral administration and therefore has nearly 100 percent bioavailability. Its electrophysiologic properties are similar to those of lidocaine and dissimilar to those of quinidine, procainamide, and disopyramide. Tocainide does not produce significant sinus node dysfunction, does not prolong the effective refractory period of cardiac conduction tissues, does not delay intercardiac conduction, does not prolong the QRS duration, and does not lengthen the QT interval. Therefore, tocainide is a theoretically appealing drug in the treatment of ventricular arrhythmias associated with prolongation of the QT interval and has minimal myocardial depressant effects. In patients with compensated congestive heart failure, it produces some depression in the rate of isovolumic left ventricular pressure generation; however, it does not change the cardiac index or the pulmonary artery wedge pressure, neither does it exacerbate congestive heart failure. Its myocardial depressant effects may be additive to those of beta-blocking agents to further lower the peak positive rate of left ventricular isovolumic, left ventricular pressure generation, thereby reducing cardiac index and elevating pulmonary artery wedge pressure to a clinically significant degree. Accordingly, therapy with both tocainide and a beta-blocking agent is to be avoided in post-myocardial infarction patients with evidence of impaired ventricular performance. Based upon similarities in electrophysiologic effects, it was anticipated that the arrhythmias that had been corrected by lidocaine would be corrected by tocainide. Likewise, when lidocaine was ineffective in arrhythmia suppression, tocainide would also be ineffective. Though this rule holds in the majority of patients, there are exceptions so that suppression of ventricular arrhythmia by lidocaine does not guarantee that tocainide will be as effective in each patient. Equally important is the fact that in some patients in whom ventricular arrhythmias are not fully controlled with lidocaine, ventricular arrhythmias are fully controlled with tocainide.

Like all other anti-arrhythmic drugs, tocainide should not be used in patients with symptomatic ventricular arrthymia and underlying second-degree or third-degree heart block unless a pacemaker is in place. Tocainide is also contraindicated in patients who are hypersensitive to lidocaine or other local anesthetics. The usual adult dosage of tocainide is 1200 to 1800 mg daily given in 3 divided doses. Therapy is instituted at 400 mg every 8 hr. The effective plasma tocainide level is 4 to 10 micrograms/ml. Tocainide is metabolized by the liver and by the kidney so that approximately 40 percent of the administered dose is excreted unchanged in the urine. In patients with evidence of renal or hepatic impairment, the daily dose should be reduced by approximately 33 percent. Side effects are significant: lightheadedness and dizziness (15 percent), and anorexia, nausea, and vomiting (15 percent). In patients receiving long-term tocainide for ventricular arrhythmia suppression, approximately 20 percent ultimately discontinue the medication because of adverse central nervous system or gastrointestinal effects. There is no known interaction between tocainide and digoxin.

Atrial arrhythmias resulting from myocardial infarction are far less frequent than ventricular arrhythmias. They usually result from substantial myocardial infarction with left ventricular dysfunction, pericarditis, or atrial infarction. Atrial fibrillation with a rapid ventricular response (when associated with angina, pulmonary edema, or hypotension) is optimally treated with synchronized DC-cardioversion at an energy level of 50 to 100 watt seconds. Synchronized DC-cardioversion does not carry increased risk in fully digitalized patients; however, it may produce life threatening ventricular tachyarrhythmias in patients who have been excessively digitalized. If atrial fibrillation is otherwise well tolerated because of a more normal physiologic ventricular rate, digoxin may be administered at 0.25 mg intravenously, every 4 to 6 hr, for a total loading dose of 1.0 to 1.5 mg over 24 hr. This usually effects satisfactory slowing of the ventricular response to a range of between 70 and 90/min. When full digitalization does not achieve satisfactory control of the ventricular response, a modest dose of propranolol (Inderal), 10 to 40 mg every 6 hr, may be added to further depress atrioventricular conduction and to slow the ventricular response. At this point, quinidine may be started in a dose of 300 mg every 6 hr in order to effect pharmacologic cardioversion. If the patient remains in atrial fibrillation for more than a few days, 2 weeks of full anticoagulation therapy is indicated prior to electrical cardioversion to minimize the risk of systemic embolization. In cases in which atrial fibrillation is consequent to acute atrial distention associated with elevation in diastolic ventricular pressure resulting from heart failure, therapy should also include a modest dose of a diuretic (furosemide, 10 to 30 mg intravenously) to lower the left atrial pressure and to reduce the propensity for atrial fibrillation.

Atrial flutter may be a result of heart failure consequent to myocardial infarction or a result of pulmonary complications, such as atelectasis, pneumonia, pleural effusion, chronic obstructive airway disease, and pulmonary embolism. Immediate synchronized DC-cardioversion at an initial low energy setting of between 10 and 25 watt seconds is the best treatment. Because the flutter rate of the atria approximates 300/min and in untreated cases there is 2:1 A-V block, the flutter rate of the ventricles is usually around 150/min; this arrhythmia is commonly associated with hemodynamic embarrassment (hypotension; pulmonary congestion or myocardial ischemia with chest pain, or both; S-T segment depression or ventricular premature beats, or both). Accordingly, atrial flutter is usually best managed with prompt definitive therapy; low energy (starting at 10 to 25 watt seconds) synchronized DC-cardioversion rather than the more time consuming pharmacologic titration with digoxin, propanolol, verapamil, or other anti-arrhythmic drugs.

Paroxysmal A-V node re-entrant tachycardia, a relatively rare complication of myocardial infarction, is treated with verapamil, 5 mg, by slow intravenous push. This can be repeated 1 or 2 times. Verapamil should be avoided when the morphology of the re-entrant tachycardia (P waves distinct from the QRS complex) suggests macro re-entry due to a concealed atrioventricular nodal bypass pathway. Here propranolol, up to 0.1 mg/kg given intravenously over 30 to 45 min, is usually effective in converting tachycardia to sinus rhythm. If tachycardia is accompanied by hemodynamic compromise (symptomatic angina, hypotension, manifestations of congestive heart failure, shock) immediate, low energy synchronized DC-cardioversion is the preferred therapy. Intravenous verapamil effects cardioversion to sinus rhythm in over 90 percent of cases. If therapy with verapamil has been attempted, intravenous propranolol should not be used because of the significant myocardial depressant effects of these drugs in combination. When the rhythm is particularly fast, is refractory to verapamil, or is associated with hemodynamic compromise or myocardial ischemia, the treatment of choice is immediate synchronized DC-cardioversion with an initial low energy setting of 10 to 50 watt seconds.

Heart Block. Heart block consequent to ischemia, edema, or infarction of the A-V node and the His-Purkinje system may occur within the first 1 to 4 days after myocardial infarction. Inferior myocardial infarction, commonly associated with excessive vagotonia (sinus bradycardia, nausea, and vomiting) may be complicated by the development of second degree A-V block (Mobitz I, otherwise known as Wenckebach block or Mobitz type II block). Mobitz II or complete A-V block may complicate anterior wall myocardial infarction whether or not there is fascicular block. Treatment of heart block is individualized according to the hemodynamic consequences of the bradyarrhythmia and the clinical setting in which it occurs. First-degree heart block occurring as a complication of inferior wall myocardial infarction does not require specific therapy. Mobitz type I second-degree A-V block in this situation, if associated with hypotension, VPBs, or a ventricular rate below 40/min, requires treatment with atropine to improve conduction through the A-V node and to speed up the heart rate. This drug is administered as a 0.5 mg bolus intravenously every 2 to 3 min until a total dose of 2 mg has been administered. If the arrhythmia does not respond to atropine or isoproterenol, 1 ampule, in 200 or 400 ml of dextrose and water, is slowly infused and adjusted to increase the ventricular rate to 70 to 90/min. Symptomatic heart block (irrespective of the clinical setting) that requires atropine or isoproterenol for immediate stabilization should be managed by inserting a temporary transvenous pacemaker. Heart block resulting from inferior wall myocardial infarction usually reflects edema and ischemia of the proximal region of the A-V node and resolves in 3 to 5 days, at which time the temporary transvenous pacemaker can be removed.

With anterior wall myocardial infarction, high grade A-V block may develop precipitously or may be heralded by the appearance of a right bundle or left bundle branch block pattern as recorded on the ECG. Similarly, high grade A-V block may be presaged by a left anterior fascicular or left posterior fascicular block pattern. The development of heart block following anterior wall myocardial infarction generally reflects substantial ventricular septal damage with severely compromised residual ventricular function. The patient's prognosis is guarded. Prophylactic insertion of a temporary pacemaker is appropriate, though it has not been shown to improve the prognosis. The sudden appearance of high grade A-V block in this case is treated with atropine and isoproterenol followed by temporary ventricular pacemaker insertion as outlined earlier. Patients with high grade A-V block complicating anterior wall myocardial infarction usually require insertion of a permanent ventricular pacemaker.

In cases of heart block complicating AMI, the clinician must be certain that drugs such as digoxin, type I anti-arrhythmics (quinidine, procainamide, disopyramide), and tocainide are not aggravating the conduction abnormality. If a patient with any degree of renal insufficiency has been maintained on a full dose of one or more of these medications, there is a possibility that heart block may be a manifestation of drug toxicity. If heart block is associated with increased atrial or ventricular ectopic activity and if the patient is receiving digoxin, excessive digoxin administration must be considered as a contributing factor. It is advisable to measure the serum digoxin level and withhold this medication temporarily even if the digoxin level is only within the high therapeutic range (1.5 to 2.0 ng/ml).

Additionally, the serum potassium level should be maintained at or above 4.2 mg/L with supplementation. Hypokalemia and hypomagnesemia are risk factors for the development of VT/VF following myocardial infarction. This fact is particularly important in the patient receiving concomitant diuretic therapy for hypertension or heart failure. Even when the serum potassium level is in the "normal" range, these kaluretic preparations can cause profound depletion of the total body potassium stores. Type I anti-arrhythmic drugs may cause heart block syndromes when administered to excess. The patient with sick sinus syndrome may develop heart block as a consequence of anti-arrhythmic drug administration even when the serum drug concentration is within therapeutic range. If anti-arrhythmic drug therapy is required for supraventricular tachycardias or for ventricular arrhythmias in a patient with sick sinus syndrome manifested by long sinus node pauses (>1.5 sec), insertion of a temporary transverse ventricular demand pacemaker should be considered prior to institution of pharmacotherapy. For ventricular arrhythmias in these cases, intravenous lidocaine, tocainide, or diphenylhydantoin (Dilantin) rather than a type I anti-arrhythmic preparation may be more appropriate, since these other compounds have little or no effect on conduction within the A-V node of the His-Purkinje system.

Pericarditis. Pericarditis frequently occurs within the first few days following transmural myocardial infarction. This is important to recognize; though the pain of pericarditis may be severe, it responds promptly to aspirin or nonsteroidal anti-inflammatory drugs. Unlike recurrent myocardial ischemia or infarct extension from which pericarditis must be differentiated, the patient's prognosis is not adversely affected by the development of post-myocardial infarction pericarditis. This development is usually a self-limiting process, requiring no more than 7 to 10 days of anti-inflammatory therapy. Pericarditis usually manifests as a sharp stabbing chest pain aggravated by coughing or any moving of the trunk, such as deep breathing or changing to the recumbent position. It is often alleviated somewhat by sitting up and leaning forward. There may be basilar rales consequent to splinting and atelectasis with a pleural rub. The hallmark of pericarditis is a three component friction rub best characterized as a very scratchy superficial multifrequency sound with discrete systolic, early diastolic, and presystolic components. Though there is usually insufficient pericardial fluid to cause gross enlargement of the cardiac silhouette on the chest roentgenogram, an echocardiogram often demonstrates pericardial effusion. Tamponade may occasionally complicate post-myocardial infarction pericarditis if the effusion is particularly large or if it accumulates rapidly, particularly when there is bleeding from the inflamed visceral and parietal pericardia. When pericarditis is evident, it is prudent to avoid full doses of prophylactic anticoagulation agents to minimize the risk of hemorrhagic effusion or hemopericardium complicated by cardiac tamponade. Likewise, acetaminophen should be substituted for aspirin to avoid pericardial bleeding due to platelet dysfunction.

Dressler's syndrome, an auto-immune pericarditis related to sensitization against antigenic substances released by the injured myocardium, may occur 10 to 14 days following myocardial infarction. The clinical appearance is identical to that of pericarditis immediately following myocardial infarction. However, there is often a distinct recrudescence of fever and an elevation in the erythrocyte sedimentation rate. Immediate pericarditis associated with transmural myocardial infarction and with Dressler's syndrome has similar characteristics and treatments. However, Dressler's syndrome may recur weeks to months after the initial episode. Therapeutic management is with aspirin or with other nonsteroidal anti-inflammatory compounds as outlined previously. Very occasionally, Dressler's syndrome may be complicated by the rapid accumulation of pericardial effusion of sufficient magnitude to cause cardiac tamponade. In this circumstance, the treatment is pericardial drainage followed by a tapering course of prednisone for 10 days to 2 weeks. Chronically recurrent pain and pericardial effusion may mandate pericardiectomy.

Post-infarction Angina. Approximately 50 per cent of patients who have had myocardial infarction develop angina. Angina occurs more frequently days to weeks following AMI as the patient resumes normal activities, but unstable angina may develop at any time during the initial hospitalization. The discomfort of angina is characteristically retrosternal, oppressive, or squeezing in nature, and radiates to the arms, neck, or jaw. Though similar in quality to the pain of myocardial infarction, it is usually not as intense. Occasionally, the pain may appear as retrosternal burning, jaw pain, or "indigestion." In fact, unstable angina must be considered in the differential diagnosis of any discomfort that develops between the forehead and the umbilicus in the patient convalescing from AMI.

During an anginal episode, the physical examination may reveal hypertension, diaphoresis, and tachycardia consequent to enhanced sympathetic nervous outflow. If patients do not respond promptly to nitroglycerin, 0.4 mg given sublingually every 3 to 4 min for a total of 3 doses, they should be given morphine sulfate, 2 to 5 mg intravenously, for immediate pain control and should be transferred to the CCU. At this point, it is crucial to monitor the ECG continuously and to ensure that myocardial infarction has not recurred by evaluating the cardiac enzymes levels (creatinine phosphokinase, lactate dehydrogenase and serum glutamic-oxaloacetic transaminase) and the ECG every 8 hr for the next 24-hr period. Transfer of the patient to the CCU also facilitates the safest and most effective use of intravenous morphine for prompt pain control. It also facilitates controlled institution and upward adjustment of anti-anginal medications.

The treatment of post-myocardial infarction angina includes general medical measures directed at reducing the demand of the myocardium for oxygen: correction of anemia, suppression of fever, sedation to alleviate anxiety, analgesia for pain, and the identification and treatment of more occult processes, e.g., thyrotoxicosis that might contribute to the severity of myocardial ischemia. Additionally, oxygen supplementation at 2 L/min via nasal cannula should be administered to maximize arterial oxygen saturation.

Post-myocardial infarction angina may result from supraventricular tachyarrhythmias including atrial flutter, atrial fibrillation, and A-V junctional tachycardia. Recording of the 12-lead ECG and continuous monitoring of the ECG is required for rapid diagnosis and therapy. The treatment of atrial flutter or fibrillation associated with angina in the post-myocardial infarction patient is best accomplished with immediate synchronous DC-cardioversion. Flutter requires a low starting energy setting at 10 to 50 watt seconds, while atrial fibrillation requires 50 to 200 watt seconds. AV-node re-entrant tachycardia converts to sinus rhythm in more than 90 percent of patients treated with intravenous verapamil, administered as a 5 mg slow intravenous push and repeated 1 or 2 times every 5 min for a total dose of 15 mg. If this treatment is unsuccessful, synchronous DC-cardioversion with an initial energy setting at 10 to 25 watt seconds is required. Cardioversion should be always performed with the patient under light anesthesia with diazepam or with a rapidly acting barbiturate. If high energy (over 150 watt seconds) is likely to be required in a nonemergency case, more effective anesthesia is provided with a rapidly acting barbiturate administered under the supervision of an anesthesiologist whose skills help guarantee adequate ventilation and airway protection.

Medical therapy for angina following the post-myocardial infarction period includes one of a variety of long-acting organic nitrate preparations and calcium channel–blocking agents or beta-blocking agents.

In addition to these measures, patients with unstable angina may benefit by aspirin administration in an attempt to reduce platelet adhesion, aggregation, and release of vasoconstrictive substances within the diseased epicardial coronary arteries, a mechanism that may be very important in the genesis of the increase in coronary vascular resistance responsible for unstable angina. The effectiveness of therapeutic anticoagulation with full doses of heparin in controlling unstable angina in more refractory patients has not been established. However, many patients with left main or multivessel coronary disease and unstable angina are more effectively controlled following therapeutic heparinization, particularly during the interval between cardiac catheterization and coronary artery revascularization surgery.

Organic Nitrates

Nitroglycerin is the active ingredient in several preparations including sublingual, oral, and topical preparations administered every 4 to 6 hr or in impregnated patches that need be applied only once a day (Table 3). All nitrate preparations alleviate angina by reducing the oxygen requirement of the myocardium and by improving oxygen delivery, possibly through dilatation of atherosclerotic vessels or through improved delivery of coronary blood via collateral sources, or both. Nitrates effect venous dilatation to reduce ventricular preload and effect a mild to moderate arteriolar dilatation to reduce afterload. Preload and afterload are important determinants in the magnitude of ventricular tension during systole. This parameter in turn is directly related to myocardial oxygen consumption. Myocardial oxygen demand is reduced by nitrates by lessening ventricular tension development. There is evidence to suggest that many patients acquire partial tolerance to the hemodynamic and anti-ischemic effects of nitrates, particularly when these nitrates are administered continuously by the transcutaneous route (patch or ointment).

Adverse effects of nitroglycerin preparations are extensions of their therapeutic effects. Arterial hypotension consequent to a decline in ventricular diastolic filling pressure (preload) and systemic vascular resistance (afterload) may occur, especially if the patient has been previously depleted of salt and water because of dietary restriction, nausea, and vomiting, or because of natruresis that accompanies bed rest for any length of time. The treatment of hypotension is directed at restoring ventricular preload by elevating the patient's lower extremities above the level of the right atrium and by administering intravenous crystalloid solution. Nitrates characteristically may provoke severe headaches as a

TABLE 3. **Nitrate Preparations**

	Route	Dose	Onset	Peak Effect	Duration
Nitroglycerin (Nitrostat)	Sublingual (0.3, 0.4, 0.6 mg tablets)	0.3–0.6 mg every 15 min, 2–3 times	1–2 min	3–5 min	<30 min
Isosorbide dinitrate (Isordil)	Sublingual	2.5–10 mg every 4 hr	Within minutes	1–2 hr	3–4 hr
	Oral	20–60 mg every 4–6 hr	½ hr	1–2 hr	4–6 hr
Nitroglycerin ointment (Nitrol)	Topical	½–3 in every 4–6 hr	½ hr	1–2 hr	4–6 hr
Organic nitrate (Nitrodisc Patches)	Topical	20–40 mg	½ hr	Sustained antianginal effect	12–24 hr
Nitroglycerin solution	Intravenous	Start at 10–20 micrograms/min and increase by 10–20 micrograms/min every 5 min until anginal relief or hypotension.	Immediate	Sustained	Effect terminated immediately upon disconnection of infusion because of short half-life.

result of cerebral vasodilatation. This effect usually can be managed by the concomitant administration of acetaminophen. Fortunately, most patients become tachyphylactic to this unpleasant side effect in a short period of time. Nitroglycerin preparations include the following:

1. *Sublingual nitroglycerin (Nitrostat)*. This is available in a 0.3, 0.4, or 0.6 mg dose. Its onset of action is within 1 to 2 mins, the peak effect occurs within 3 to 5 min, and the duration is approximately 1/2 hr. For angina, 1 tablet is administered sublingually every 3 to 5 min; this can be repeated 2 to 3 times.

2. *Isosorbide dinitrate (Isordil)*. This is administered as a 2.5 to 10 mg sublingual dose or as a 20 to 60 mg oral dose every 6 hr. With oral administration, the onset of action is within 1/2 hr; the peak effect occurs at 1 to 2 hr and persists for approximately 4 to 6 hr. When administered sublingually, the onset of action is within minutes, the peak effect occurs at approximately 1 to 2 hr, and the duration of effect is 3 to 4 hr. There is also a chewable nitrate preparation (Cardilate).

3. *Nitroglycerin ointment (Nitrol Ointment)*. This is administered in an amount of 1/2 to 3 inches topically every 4 to 6 hr. Topical nitroglycerin has a time to onset and peak effect similar to that of orally administered isosorbide dinitrate, and its duration of effect is similar at 4 to 6 hr. The major disadvantage of the ointment is the inconvenience and mess associated with transcutaneous application.

4. *Organic nitrate (Nitrodisc patches)*. These are available as 5 to 10 mg organic nitrate impregnated on a matrix that causes sustained nitrate release so that it is absorbed continuously through the skin over a 24-hr period. The theoretical advantage of this preparation is that it is administered only once a day. Though Nitrodisc patches have been shown to maintain an "effective" organic nitrate level in the blood for as long as 24 hr, the anti-anginal effect of these preparations has been clearly documented for only 8 to 12 hr. However, the hemodynamic effect (reduction in cardiac preload) of Nitrodisc patches in patients with heart failure may be sustained over the 24-hr interval. The cumulative nitrate dose applied in the patch formulation required for effective anti-anginal protection over 8 to 12 hr ranges between 20 and 40 mg. This therapy is very expensive.

5. *Intravenous nitroglycerin*. For the treatment of unstable angina refractory to oral, sublingual, or topical nitrates, intravenous nitroglycerin is very effective. Therapy is started at 10 to 20 micrograms/min, and the dose is increased by 10 to 20 micrograms/min every 5 to 10 min, adjusting the amount to produce anginal relief. The blood pressure must be measured every few minutes during dose titration. The complications of intravenous nitroglycerin include arterial hypotension consequent to its potent preload and afterload reducing effects. Arterial hypotension is managed by reducing the dosage by 10 to 20 micrograms/min, by elevating the patient's legs, and by rapidly administering crystalloid to the patient with no clinical evidence of congestive heart failure. For the patient with clinical evidence of congestive heart failure due to severe ventricular dysfunction complicating myocardial infarction, it is advisable to measure the pulmonary artery wedge pressure with a pulmonary artery catheter whenever evaluating hypotension. This allows for judicious administration of crystalloid, with less risk of provoking pulmonary congestion and pulmonary edema. There may be

TABLE 4. **Oral Calcium Channel Blocking Agents**

	Dose	Arterial Vasodilatation	Coronary Vasodilatation	Myocardial Depression	Sinus Bradycardia	Depressed A-V Nodal Conduction
Nifedipine (Procardia)	10–30 mg every 6–8 hr	+ + +	+ + +	0	0	0
Diltiazem (Cardiazem)	30–120 mg every 8 hr	+ +	+ +	0–½ +	½ +	½ +
Verapamil (Calan, Isoptin)	40–120 mg every 8 hr	+	+	+	+	+ +

some question as to the routine need for intra-arterial blood pressure monitoring when administering intravenous nitroglycerin. If the systolic blood pressure is consistently more than 105 mmHg, is easily obtainable by the cuff method, and is more than 100 mmHg as the intravenous nitroglycerin dose is increased, it is not necessary to insert a cannula into the radial artery for continuous arterial blood pressure monitoring. However, if the systolic blood pressure declines to less than 90 to 100 mmHg in response to nitroglycerin administration and cannot be promptly restored to a level consistently more than 100 mmHg following volume administration, the radial artery should be prepared with a cannula to continuously monitor the intra-arterial blood pressure on an oscilloscope, as the patient receives intravenous nitroglycerin.

In comparison with oral and topical nitrate preparations intravenous nitroglycerin may not be as effective in controlling unstable angina. However, because the onset and offset of action are so very prompt, the dose is easily adjusted. Intravenous nitroglycerin can be rapidly escalated in conjunction with the blood pressure response so that the desired therapeutic effect of complete pain relief can be more rapidly achieved.

Calcium Channel–Blocking Agents

The pivotal role of calcium conductance across the cell membrane in the mechanism of myocardial and smooth muscle contraction has recently been recognized. Drugs that block the calcium flux across the cell membrane during the period of diastolic depolarization (phase III of the action potential) uniformly depress the force of contraction in myocardial and vascular smooth muscle cells. The effect of direct myocyte depression is somewhat negated by compensatory sympathetic nervous system activity. However, as a consequence of smooth muscle relaxation in the vasculature, vasodilatation of veins, arterioles, and coronary arteries ensues. Myocardial preload, afterload, systolic wall tension, contractility, and oxygen consumption decline while coronary blood flow improves. Thus, drugs with this property of calcium inflow blockade are particularly effective in the treatment of angina pectoris. Properties of the 3 calcium channel–blocking agents approved for use in the United States are summarized in Table 4.

1. *Nifedipine (Procardia)*. Nifedipine is a very potent arterial and venous dilator that decreases myocardial oxygen consumption by reducing preload and afterload so as to lessen ventricular systolic tension development. Likewise, it improves myocardial delivery of oxygen through coronary arterial vasodilatation or reversal of coronary arterial spasm, or both. The net effect is to bring the oxygen requirement of the metabolizing heart in line with the limitations in myocardial oxygen delivery imposed by coronary atherosclerosis and to alleviate any component of coronary vasospasm. Nifedipine does not depress conduction into the AV node. For the treatment of postinfarction angina, it is administered in a dosage of 10 to 40 mg tid or qid. Adverse effects, actually extensions of therapeutic effects, include hypotension, flushing, palpatations, tachycardia, and dependent edema consequent to an elevation in capillary hydrostatic pressure associated with dilatation of the precapillary arterial sphincters. Edema can be managed with hydrochlorthiazide (HydroDiuril) 50 mg qid. In those patients with an intrinsically slow sinus rate; in those receiving a beta blocking agent; and in those with atrioventricular, intraventricular conduction delays, nifedipine is very effective.

2. *Diltiazem (Cardiazem)*. Though not as potent a vasodilator as nifedipine, diltiazem is very effective in the management of post-infarction angina. Diltiazem is an intermediate agent between nifedipine and verapamil in its propensity to slow the rate of the sinus node and to depress A-V nodal conduction; however, it very rarely slows the heart rate or lowers the blood pressure to excess. Diltiazem does not seem to cause dependent edema and is administered in a dosage of 30 to 120 mg every 8 hr.

3. *Verapamil (Calan, Isoptin)*. Verapamil likewise has arterial, venular, and coronary artery vasodilator properties but is not nearly as potent as nifedipine in this regard. It also has the capability of significantly depressing sinus node activity and conduction of the cardiac electrical

impulse through the A-V node. It may improve coronary blood flow slightly, but verapamil improves angina primarily through the lowering of myocardial oxygen consumption by reducing preload, afterload, and heart rate. Verapamil also reduces myocardial oxygen demand by decreasing contractility. By lowering the heart rate, myocardial contractility, and systolic wall tension, verapamil is very effective in lowering myocardial oxygen demand and alleviating angina. Its depressant effect on A-V nodal conduction makes verapamil a very effective agent in the treatment of supraventricular tachycardia, particularly paroxysmal A-V nodal re-entrant tachycardia. Because of verapamil's myocardial depressant effect it should not be used in conjunction with a beta blocking agent for control of supraventricular tachycardia. It there is no heart failure or conduction system disease and if ventricular function is normal, verapamil can be safely used in conjunction with a beta blocking agent for control of angina. Because verapamil can slow the sinus rate, one must use it cautiously in conjunction with a beta blocking agent, as a symptomatic sinus bradycardia or a sinus rate of less than 40/min would require reduction in the dose of one or the other agent.

Beta Blocking Agents

Drugs that block the influence of epinephrine and norepinephrine on the myocardial adrenergic (beta) receptor reduce the heart rate, depress the force of myocardial contraction, and slow the velocity of impulse conduction in the A-V node and His-Purkinje system. A decrease in heart rate, systolic wall tension, and myocardial contractility lowers the myocardial oxygen demand. This is indeed a primary goal in the treatment of patients with unstable angina. Competitive antagonists of norepinephrine and epinephrine bind to the myocardial beta receptors and do not activate them. They prevent transmission of impulses from the post-ganglionic synapse to the myocardium via norepinephrine release.

One beta blocking agent, pindolol (Visken) has intrinsic sympathomimetic activity (ISA) properties. Pindolol competes favorably with norepinephrine for binding at the beta receptor; however, in contrast to norepinephrine, pindolol effects minimal activation of the beta receptor. The result is depression of myocardial contractility and heart rate and prolongation of conduction of the cardiac impulse through the A-V node and His-Purkinje system only under conditions of increased beta adrenergic myocardial stimulation (exercise or emotional upset). Pindolol may cause a slight increase in heart rate because of ISA under baseline conditions. Drugs that block the beta receptor are usually effective antihypertensive and antianginal agents even though their use has not been approved specifically for that purpose. Beta blocking agents that are currently approved by the Food and Drug Administration for use are summarized in Table 5.

1. *Propranolol (Inderal).* This drug, the first beta blocking agent available in the United States, is effective in the treatment of hypertension and angina pectoris. When administered in a dosage sufficiently high to consistently maintain the resting heart rate below 70/min and to prevent a rise in heart rate in excess of 20 percent above control value in response to moderate exercise, propranolol is very effective in the alleviation of angina. The administration of other beta blocking agents is similarly adjusted in relation to the resting heart rate and its response to moderate exercise in the treatment of angina pectoris. The usual propranolol dosage effective in angina is between 160 and 480 mg/24 hr, administered tid or qid. Adverse effects include the precipitation of bronchospasm in patients with asthma, the development of congestive heart failure in patients with compromised ventricular function in whom the force of myocardial contraction is more dependent upon sympathetic tone, and the neuropsychiatric dysfunction characterized by depression, extreme fatigue, and nightmares. The autonomic response to insulin-induced hypoglycemia may be lessened in insulin-dependent diabetics, resulting in profound hypoglycemia without any premonitory manifestations. Rarely, patients may develop Raynaud's phenomenon or worsening limb claudication consequent to inhibition of beta receptor–mediated arterial vasodilatation, leaving alpha-adrenergic vasoconstriction unopposed. Possibly by a similar mechanism in the coronary vascular bed, propranolol may aggravate Prinzmetal's variant angina owing to predominant coronary artery spasm in which there is little or no underlying atheromatous coronary artery obstruction.

Propranolol is a short-acting beta blocking agent, and a dosing schedule of every 6 or 8 hr is required for effective antianginal therapy. Its short half-life is an advantage in the post-myocardial infarction patient who may require beta blockade for angina or arrhythmia control. If propranolol is not tolerated, the drug can be discontinued, and its pharmacodynamic effect should dissipate in 4 to 6 hr.

2. *Metoprolol (Lopressor).* Originally developed as a beta blocking agent to be more selective in inhibiting the myocardial beta receptor, this agent in effective antianginal doses usually causes nonselective beta blockade but may provoke asthma in susceptible patients. It can be administered on a regimen of 50 to 200 mg bid.

Intravenous followed by oral metoprolol may

TABLE 5. **Beta Blocking Agents: Comparative Product Features**

	Propranolol (Inderal)	Metoprolol (Lopressor)	Atenolol (Tenormin)	Nadolol (Corgard)	Timolol (Blocadren)	Pindolol (Visken)
Dosage	BID–QID	BID	Once Daily	Once Daily	BID	BID
Plasma Half-Life	2–3 hr	3–4 hr	6–9 hr	20–24 hr	4–5 hr	3–4 hr
Approved for Hypertension	Yes	Yes	Yes	Yes	Yes	Yes
Approved for Angina	Yes	No	No	Yes	No	No
Hydrophilic	No	No	Yes	Yes	No	No
Cardioselective	No	Relative	Relative	No	No	No
*Effect on RBF**	Reduced	Reduced	Reduced	Maintained or improved	?	No effect
Metabolized by Liver (first pass)	99 % first pass	50 %	5 to 10 %	None	50 %	Minimal
Active Metabolites	Yes	?	Yes	Not Metabolized	No	N/A
Food affects Bioavailability	Yes	No	Yes, 20 %	No	Yes, 20 %	N/A
ISA†	No	No	No	No	No	Yes
MSA‡	Yes	No	No	No	No	Slight
Available Strengths	10, 20, 40 and 80 mg	50 and 100 mg	50 and 100 mg	40, 80, 120 and 160 mg	10 and 20 mg	5 and 10 mg
Pharmacist's Cost/100 tablets (as of 4/1/83)	10— $5.73 20— $8.05 40—$11.61 80—$19.36	50—$15.59 100—$28.06	50—$33.55 100—$50.32	40—$24.29 80—$33.33 120—$43.08 160—$47.92	10—$17.75 20—$32.75	5—$15.60 10—$23.34

*RBF: renal blood flow.
†ISA: intrinsic sympathomimetic activity.
‡MSA: membrane stabilizing activity.

be useful in the treatment of hemodynamically stable patients with definite or suspected AMI to reduce cardiovascular morbidity. Early treatment of myocardial infarction should be initiated in the CCU as soon as the patient's hemodynamic condition has stabilized. It begins with the administration of 3 bolus injections of 5 mg of metoprolol. The injections should be given at approximate 2 min intervals, with careful continuous monitoring of heart rate, blood pressure, and the ECG. The patient should tolerate the full intravenous dose (15 mg). Metoprolol tablets, 50 mg every hr, should be initiated 15 min after the last intravenous treatment and continued for 48 hr. Thereafter, the maintenance dosage is 100 mg, twice a day. In patients in whom there is a contraindication to treatment during the early phases of suspected or definite myocardial infarctions or in patients in whom the full, early metoprolol treatment is not tolerated, and in patients in whom the physician wishes to delay treatment for any reason, metoprolol can be instituted at 100 mg bid as soon as clinical conditions allow. Metoprolol therapy should be continued for at least 3 months. Although the efficacy of this therapy beyond 3 months has not been conclusively established, data from studies with other beta blocking agents suggest treatment should be continued for 1 to 3 yr.

3. *Nadolol (Corgard)*. This water soluble, long-acting beta blocking agent can be administered in a single daily dose of 40 to 120 mg. It may have fewer adverse neuropsychiatric effects in comparison with propranolol.

4. *Timolol (Blocadren)*. Timolol was the first beta blocking preparation that was shown to be effective in the prevention of recurrent myocardial infarction and sudden cardiac death in the 2 years following myocardial infarction. It is administered in a dosage of 10 to 20 mg bid or tid.

5. *Atenolol (Tenormin)*. This water soluble, long-acting beta blocking agent, approved only for the treatment of hypertension, is administered as a single dose of 50 to 200 mg. It may also have less adverse neuropsychiatric effects when compared with propranolol.

6. *Pindolol (Visken)*. This lipid-soluble, short-acting beta blocking agent, approved only for the treatment of hypertension, is, in and of itself, a weak beta agonist and therefore has ISA. In comparison with other beta blocking agents, pindolol lowers blood pressure by reducing peripheral vascular resistance, the elevation of which is the fundamental hemodynamic derangement in long-standing, essential hypertension. Other beta blocking agents lower blood pressure by reducing cardiac output, while peripheral resistance is unchanged or slightly increased. It has been suggested that because of ISA, pindolol should cause less myocardial depression. The clinical significance of ISA, as related to reduction of systemic resistance in antihypertensive therapy and maintenance of ventricular compensation in patients at risk for developing heart

failure in response to beta blockade, has not been established.

Treatment

Arterial Counterpulsation

The postmyocardial infarction patient with angina refractory to combined maximal medical therapy with a beta blocking agent, a nitrate preparation, and a calcium channel blocking agent in effective dosages is a candidate for arterial counterpulsation therapy. The principle of counterpulsation therapy is to pressurize the aorta in diastole in order to increase coronary perfusion pressure and to improve coronary blood flow. The aorta is rapidly decompressed just prior to the onset of mechanical systole, which lowers the impedance to ventricular ejection and reduces the myocardial oxygen requirement. The net effect is improvement of myocardial oxygen delivery and reduction of the oxygen demand of the working myocardium, which assists left ventricular function and alleviates ischemia.

Counterpulsation therapy is most commonly accomplished by inserting a balloon catheter into the descending thoracic aorta via percutaneous femoral artery entry or direct cutdown. This requires the skills of a vascular or cardiac surgeon, and one is not usually available in hospitals lacking cardiac catheterization or open heart surgery facilities.

Upon insertion of the intra-aortic balloon, the patient is treated with a full dose of heparin or with low molecular weight dextran to maintain the partial thromboplastin time at 2.5 times control. This treatment prevents coagulation or reduces platelet adhesiveness to retard thrombus formation or platelet aggregation on the intra-aortic balloon catheter.

External counterpulsation is effected by encasing the lower extremities in a fluid-filled medium. Treatment is synchronized with the ECG, and the tank holding the fluid is intermittently pressurized after aortic valve closure and depressurized just prior to the onset of ventricular systole. The effect is to elevate aortic diastolic pressure and to improve coronary perfusion. External counterpulsation is less effective than intra-aortic counterpulsation, however. The rapid alternate compression and decompression of the lower extremities is somewhat disconcerting to the patient. Though less effective and somewhat more uncomfortable than intra-aortic balloon counterpulsation, it is somewhat effective and is not associated with the vascular and infectious complications of intra-aortic balloon counterpulsation: limb ischemia, gangrene, aortic dissection, and infection, which occur in approximately 5 to 15 percent of patients so treated. Patients with angina responsive only to arterial counterpulsation nearly always require mechanical revascularization with coronary artery angioplasty or bypass surgery.

Coronary Artery Revascularization Surgery

Postmyocardial infarction angina not responsive to antianginal medication is managed with coronary artery revascularization surgery, if coronary arteriography demonstrates coronary artery pathoanatomy suitable for revascularization. Coronary artery revascularization surgery for angina in the immediate post-myocardial infarction period can be performed with an acceptable operative mortality rate of <5 percent in most major medical centers. It is imperative that the patient with angina following myocardial infarction not easily controlled with an effective dose of one or more antianginal medications be promptly transferred to a major medical center, where the staff possesses expertise in intra-aortic counterpulsation, cardiac catheterization, and cardiovascular surgery. These various diagnostic and therapeutic options should be available around the clock.

Congestive Heart Failure

Diagnosis

Myocardial infarction involves the necrosis of myocytes, resulting from a critical reduction in regional blood supply. The amount of remaining viable and functional myocardium is inevitably reduced. Furthermore, as a result of myocardial infarction there is almost invariably a region of myocardial ischemia, the so-called border zone, the survival of which is optimally ensured by measures to reduce the demand of the myocardium for oxygen and to improve myocardial oxygen delivery through the jeopardized coronary circulation. The overall impact on the zone of infarction and its surrounding zone of myocardial ischemia is an impairment in the pumping capability of the heart, that is, an impairment in ventricular systolic function, the magnitude of which is initially determined by the aggregate size of the zone of ischemia and infarction. The ultimate determinant of the adequacy of ventricular function following myocardial infarction is the overall mass of viable myocardium surviving the insult and the adequacy of its regional blood supply.

Myocardial infarction of lesser magnitude is characterized by impaired diastolic ventricular dysfunction. The heart pumps an adequate or nearly adequate volume of blood per beat; however, in order to fill the heart to this volume at end diastole, an inordinate elevation in diastolic pressure is required, that is, the stiffness of the myocardium is increased or the compliance (change in volume per unit change in pressure) is decreased.

Mild heart failure after a small to medium sized myocardial infarction commonly results from diastolic dysfunction leading to increased myocardial stiffness. The consequence is that a higher ventricular filling pressure is required to generate a satisfactory stroke volume. Cumulative myocardial injury of a greater magnitude also compromises the ability of the heart to generate tension and to shorten ejection of blood during systole; systolic function is impaired. The most sensitive overall noninvasive indicator of myocardial systolic dysfunction is a reduction in the global ejection fraction of the left ventricle (<50 percent) as assessed by radionuclide ventriculography.

Treatment

The pharmacotherapy of congestive heart failure and shock complicating myocardial infarction is summarized in Table 6. The treatment of mild congestive heart failure following myocardial infarction includes measures to reduce the salt and water content of the lungs. Furosemide (Lasix) in a dose of 20 to 40 mg intravenously or ethacrynic acid (Edecrin) in a dose of 25 to 50 mg intravenously causes prompt diuresis to reduce left atrial (pulmonary capillary) pressure and pulmonary congestion. Because of the kaluretic effects of these diuretics, potassium chloride supplementation should be provided (25 to 100 mEq/day), particularly if the patient is receiving concomitant digoxin therapy. Other measures effective in reducing venous return and pulmonary capillary wedge pressure are positioning of the patient with the head and torso elevated at least 45 degrees above the horizontal plane so as to reduce venous return. Nitrate preparations enhance venous capacity by a venodilatory effect that causes redistribution of blood from the central thoracic volume to the peripheral venular pool. This redistribution alleviates pulmonary

TABLE 6. **Guide to Intravenous Administration of Drugs Employed in the Treatment of Heart Failure or Shock**

Drug	Dosage	Therapeutic Plasma Level	Side Effects	Comments
Digoxin (Lanoxin)	0.25 mg IV q8h for 2 days and then 0.25 mg qid	1.0–2.0 (ng/ml)	GI toxicity, cardiac arrhythmias, AV conduction disturbances, insomnia, visual disturbances	May be given PO at same dose and rate of administration; should not be given IM
Furosemide (Lasix)	20–40 mg IV (or more) as needed	—	Ototoxicity, hypokalemic metabolic alkalosis, dehydration	Ethacrynic acid is an acceptable alternative
Nitroprusside (Nipride)	15–200 micrograms/min by gradually increasing a continuous IV infusion	—	Hypotension, anemia, hypothyroidism, encephalopathy due to thiocyanate toxicity in patients with impaired hepatic disease	Direct arterial pressure monitoring may be required
Dopamine (Intropin)	Start with 3–5 micrograms/kg/min; increasing to a maximum of 50 micrograms/kg/min	—	Cardiac arrhythmias, gangrene of extremities	Direct arterial and pulmonary artery pressure monitoring is advised; beware of subcutaneous injection of infusate
Norepinephrine	2–8 micrograms/kg/min; start with a low dose, gradually increasing every 3–4 min	—	Cardiac arrhythmias, acute tubular necrosis, ganrene of extremities	Direct arterial and pulmonary artery pressure monitoring is advised; beware of subcutaneous injection of infusate
Dobutamine (Dobutrex)	3–10 micrograms/kg/min, occasionally as high as 40 micrograms/kg/min	—	Cardiac arrhythmias, nausea, headache	Direct arterial and pulmonary artery pressure monitoring is advised; has a less positive chronotopic effect than does dopamine
Amrinone (Inocor)	0.5 mg/kg IV over 5 min; then 5–10 micrograms/kg/min; may repeat loading dose and double infusion rate to attain satisfactory hemodynamic response	—	Reduction in platelet count, nausea, amnesia, hepatic dysfunction	Direct arterial and pulmonary artery pressure monitoring is advised; hemodynamic effectiveness similar to that of dobutamine

Modified from Alpert, J. S., and Francis, G. S.: *Manual of Coronary Care,* 2nd ed. Boston, Little, Brown, and Co., 1981.

congestion to lessen dyspnea and improve pulmonary gas exchange. For acute pulmonary edema, morphine (3 to 5 mg IV every 15 to 30 min) alleviates dyspnea by a similar mechanism. Nitroprusside (Nipride), an arterial and venous dilator, reduces afterload and preload to improve left ventricular function, to improve left ventricular compliance, and to reduce venous return. The net results are increased cardiac index and decreased left ventricular filling pressure, providing rapid, substantive improvement in the patient with pulmonary edema. Intravenous nitroglycerin, a potent vasodilator, reduces preload (left ventricular diastolic pressure) and improves ventricular function by relieving myocardial ischemia. It is similarly useful in pulmonary edema complicating myocardial infarction, although it is not as potent as nitroprusside in reducing afterload.

Even though cardiac glycosides exert a modest inotropic effect, their use in the treatment of congestive heart failure following myocardial infarction in patients with sinus rhythm is somewhat controversial. However, if systolic ventricular dysfunction is prominent, that is, there is clear-cut evidence of cardiomegaly, a third heart sound, and pulmonary congestion with an ejection fraction less than 0.40, it is reasonable to treat the patient with digoxin (Lanoxin). This may be administered in a dosage of 0.25 mg by slow intravenous bolus every 4 to 6 hr until a total of 1 to 1.25 mg has been administered over a 24-hr interval. After intravenous digitalization has been achieved, the daily maintenance dose of digoxin is determined by the patient's renal function (serum creatinine level), since digoxin is excreted by glomerular filtration. The maintenance dose of digoxin is usually 0.25 mg qid in the adult with normal renal function. Downward adjustment is determined by the severity of renal impairment as measured by the serum creatinine level. The daily digoxin requirement in a hemodynamically stable patient can be reliably estimated according to the serum creatinine level, but it is prudent to confirm the validity of this estimate by measuring the serum digoxin level. The usual therapeutic range is approximately 1 to 2 ng/ml.

Dobutamine (Dobutrex) administered intravenously at a dosage of 5 to 15 micrograms/kg/min elevates cardiac output and may reverse manifestations of hypotension and shock (oliguria, decreased mentation, cool moist skin, acrocyanosis).

Amrinone (Inocor) is a vasodilator and inotropic drug that may be administered intravenously to improve cardiac performance. In a dose-dependent fashion, it will increase cardiac index, reduce pulmonary wedge and right atrial pressure, and lower systemic vascular resistance. Mean arterial pressure usually declines insignificantly or does not change, and heart rate may increase. Amrinone has hemodynamic characteristics that are virtually identical to dobutamine and may be useful in cases of myocardial failure following myocardial infarction. As with the sympathomimetic agents (dopamine and dobutamine), amrinone has not been specifically approved for the treatment of advanced cardiac dysfunction following myocardial infarction. However, the salutary hemodynamic and myocardial oxygen consumption sparing effects of amrinone and preliminary experience in the treatment of patients with pump dysfunction caused by myocardial infarction suggest that amrinone may be safe and effective. It is administered as a loading dose of 0.5 mg given by slow intravenous bolus over 5 min, followed by a continuous infusion at 5 to 10 micrograms/kg/min. If the desired hemodynamic effect is not observed within 15 to 30 min of instituting therapy, the patient may receive a second 0.5 mg/kg intravenous bolus with the infusion rate increased to 15 or 20 micrograms/kg/min.

STRUCTURAL COMPLICATIONS OF MYOCARDIAL INFARCTION

Ventricular Septal Rupture

Diagnosis

Septal necrosis consequent to infarction of the inferior or, more commonly, the anteroseptal region may eventuate in perforation of the ventricular septum with the development of a left to right shunt. Commonly occurring within the first 3 to 5 days after infarction, ventricular septal rupture is heralded by the appearance of hypotension or congestive heart failure, or both, and with a new harsh holosystolic murmur loudest midway between the apex and the lower left sternal border. The diagnosis of ventricular septal rupture is confirmed by catheterization of the pulmonary artery with careful measurement of the oxygen concentration of blood in the right atrium, right ventricle, and pulmonary artery, as the catheter is progressively advanced. An increase in the blood oxygen concentration exceeding 1 volume percent in the right ventricle and pulmonary artery in comparison with that in the right atrium helps confirm the diagnosis of ventricular septal rupture.

Treatment

Treatment includes pharmacotherapy with nitroprusside that, as an arterial vasodilator, reduces the impedance to ventricular ejection. This action favors the forward ejection of blood from the left ventricle into the aorta rather than retrograde movement of blood across the septal perforation into the right ventricle. Nitroprusside reduces the volume of the left to right shunt, improves effective cardiac output, and may lower the pulmonary wedge pressure through venodilatation.

Transfer of the patient to a medical center with intra-aortic counterpulsation therapy and full cardiac catheterization and surgical facilities is mandatory, as soon as the diagnosis of ventricular septal rupture is established. Urgent cardiac catheterization is required to assess the severity of ventricular functional impairment and the adequacy of the coronary anatomy for bypass grafting, in addition to confirming the presence of ventricular septal rupture. It is prudent to attempt to medically stabilize such patients so that healing and fibrosis of the infarcted segment can occur. However, if shock cannot be corrected by maximal pharmacologic and intra-aortic counterpulsation therapy over 8 to 16 hr, urgent corrective cardiac surgery is required. In addition to ventricular septal repair with a patch or with primary closure, coronary artery revascularization, myocardial infarctectomy, and if necessary mitral valve replacement may be undertaken with a reasonable likelihood of patient survival (40 to 50 percent).

Mitral Regurgitation

Mitral insufficiency of a clinically insignificant magnitude consequent to transient papillary muscle dysfunction occurs in approximately 50 percent of patients with AMI. As a consequence of anteroseptal infarction or, more commonly, of inferoposterior infarction, there may be more substantial necrosis of the anterior or posterior papillary muscle heads. Rupture of an entire papillary muscle head results in the precipitous development of cardiogenic shock and acute pulmonary edema. The abrupt and catastrophic appearance of this complication precludes definitive diagnosis and successful surgical outcome. Partial rupture of a papillary muscle head with detachment of the distal papillary muscle segment and one or more attached cordae tendenae causes tumultuous mitral regurgitation. However, with prompt diagnosis and mitral valve replacement there is a reasonable likelihood for survival.

Mitral regurgitation, resulting from papillary muscle disruption, is heralded by the development of worsening congestive heart failure or shock, or both, usually 3 to 5 days following AMI. The diagnosis of mitral insufficiency may be suggested by pulmonary artery catheterization with measurement of the pulmonary artery wedge pressure. The mean wedge pressure is elevated, and tall "regurgitant waves" in the pulmonary artery wedge pressure exceed the mean pulmonary artery wedge pressure by at least a factor of 2 and are almost pathognomonic of severe mitral insufficiency. These appear with the T wave on the ECG. However, regurgitant waves may be small or virtually absent in the pulmonary artery wedge pressure recording when the patient with acute severe mitral insufficiency has been appropriately treated with diuretics and vasodilators. Likewise, very large "V" waves may be seen in patients with heart failure, ventricular septal rupture, or severe reversible myocardial ischemia (angina) in the absence of severe mitral insufficiency. Concomitantly, the absence of an oxygen "step-up" from right atrium to right ventricle, as measured by sampling atrial and ventricular blood during catheter insertion, excludes the diagnosis of ventricular septal rupture as a cause of the new systolic murmur and clinical decompensation.

Treatment

The treatment of acute mitral insufficiency consequent to myocardial infarction involves the use of dobutamine to improve the force of myocardial contraction in order to improve total ventricular output. Nitroprusside, a potent venous and arteriolar smooth muscle relaxant, promotes reduction in preload and afterload to lower mean pulmonary artery wedge pressure and systemic vascular resistance. This effect results in an alleviation of pulmonary congestion and an improvement of effective cardiac output, as the impedance to the ejection of blood into the aorta is lowered. Forward flow across the aortic valve rather than systolic retrograde flow into the left atrium across the incompetent mitral valve is favored. Should these pharmacologic measures fail to promptly correct oliguria, to improve cutaneous perfusion, to assist mentation, and to reduce other signs of shock, intra-aortic counterpulsation therapy is instituted. If the patient can be stabilized medically, mitral valve replacement is deferred for as long as possible to permit adequate healing and fibrosis in the zone of myocardial infarction. Otherwise, urgent cardiac catheterization is performed to confirm the presence of hemodynamically severe mitral insufficiency and to assess the adequacy of ventricular function and coronary pathoanatomy. In addition to mitral valve replacement, definitive surgical management often requires concomitant coronary artery revascularization and, possibly, myocardial infarctectomy, if dyssynergy is likely to be contributing significantly to the overall state of hemodynamic decompensation.

Right Ventricular Infarction

As a consequence of inferior wall infarction there may be substantial involvement of the right ventricular free wall with relative sparing of the left ventricular myocardium. This is usually caused by thrombotic occlusion of the right coronary artery proximal to the takeoff of the marginal branches responsible for right ventricular perfusion. The patient often presents with hypotension, shock, and evidence of distended neck veins (central venous pressure exceeding 8 mmHg) but with little or no evidence of pulmonary congestion in the setting of an inferoposterior AMI. Bradycardia and heart block may be prominent consequent to ischemia and edema of the A-V node and proximal His-Purkinje systems. There may be inspiratory increases in the central venous pressure and pulsus paradoxus—findings suggestive of cardiac tamponade.

The absence of echocardiographic evidence of pericardial effusion excludes the differential diagnosis of tamponade. The hemodynamic findings pathognomonic of right ventricular infarction include elevations in right atrial pressure and right ventricular diastolic pressure, normal or near normal right ventricular systolic and pulmonary artery pressures, and reduced cardiac output. The mean normal right ventricular and pulmonary artery systolic pressures similarly implicate right ventricular infarction rather than massive pulmonary embolism as a cause of acute right-sided heart failure.

Treatment

Treatment includes vigorous volume administration (sometimes several liters of crystalloid are required over a few hours) in order to increase right atrial preload and to improve the pumping capability of the right ventricle. Additionally, dobutamine may be required to enhance right ventricular systolic function. As this hemodynamic derangement resolves spontaneously in 2 to 4 days, vasopressor therapy is weaned and the patient frequently recovers uneventfully.

Bradyarrhythmias and heart block often complicate right ventricular infarction. They should be treated with a temporary, atrioventricular sequential pacemaker. The impaired and mechanically ineffective right ventricle is exquisitely dependent on an appropriately timed atrial systole for preload augmentation and adequate compensation by the Frank-Starling mechanism. Pacing with a ventricular pacemaker entails disruption of synchronous atrial contraction and frequently causes precipitous hemodynamic deterioration. Conversely, A-V sequential pacing optimizes right ventricular preload and cardiac output. An atrioventricular sequential pacemaker is clearly the pacing modality of choice in a patient with bradyarrhythmias and heart block complicating right ventricular infarction.

Cardiogenic Shock

Cardiogenic shock is defined as profound systolic dysfunction consequent to extensive cumulative myocardial injury. An excess of 25 to 30 percent of the total ventricular myocardium usually has been irreversibly damaged. Cumulative injury to the myocardium exceeding 40 percent of total muscle mass is incompatable with survival; it is clear that myocardial reserve is marginal and the patient's prognosis is guarded.

Treatment

Treatment consists of dobutamine to maintain effective cardiac output by stimulating myocardial contractility. If the patient does not respond satisfactorily to dobutamine, amrinone may be effective. When hypotension is a problem, dopamine at a starting dosage of 8 to 12 micrograms/kg/min is preferred. If blood pressure is adequate, nitroprusside is administered to reduce preload, therefore relieving pulmonary congestive symptoms and improving gas exchange. It also reduces afterload to improve effective cardiac output. When these pharmacologic measures do not promptly improve cardiac output and urine flow and correct the shock syndrome, intra-arterial counterpulsation therapy is instituted. Its purpose is to correct shock and to stabilize the patient so that cardiac catheterization and coronary arteriography can be performed. In cases of extensive coronary artery disease amenable to myocardial revascularization or of an extensive aneurysmal segment of infarcted myocardium that is impairing mechanical ventricular efficiency, it is reasonable to proceed with emergency coronary artery revascularization surgery and, possibly, myocardial infarctectomy. The prognosis of patients in cardiogenic shock treated medically is dismal, with a mortality rate exceeding 75 to 80 percent in most series. Aggressive management with emergency catheterization and myocardial revascularization with or without myocardial infarctectomy may save an additional 10 to 20 percent.

Late Convalescence

Following uncomplicated myocardial infarction, the patient is progressively ambulated, usually under the supervision of an experienced cardiac rehabilitation team. During supervised exercise, these paramedic personnel carefully observe the patient for excessive fatigue, dyspnea, and the development of angina or arrhythmia. Such untoward effects implicate advanced degrees of left ventricular dysfunction or easily provokable angina consequent to extensive coronary disease with jeopardized myocardium. These findings delineate a population of post-myocardial infarction patients (15 to 25 percent) who need coronary artery revascularization. Early cardiac catheterization and coronary arteriography may be indicated in such patients so that myocardial revascularization surgery can be offered after a reasonable period of convalescence (at least 3 weeks following myocardial infarction). If the patient has had a substantial myocardial infarction, it may be appropriate to obtain a 24-hr recording of a continuous ECG prior to discharge. In hospitals that have reliable continuous ECG monitoring as the patient convalesces in a step-down unit bed following his or her discharge from the CCU, a 24-hr continuous ECG may be unnecessary, as malignant ventricular arrhythmias occurring during this period should be adequately detected.

Extensive myocardial infarction increases the likelihood of malignant ventricular arrhythmias in the patient's late hospitalization phase. Antiarrhythmic therapy is prescribed for multiform, frequent ventricular premature beats or episodic (nonsustained) ventricular tachycardia, and it is hoped that this may reduce the risk of sudden death consequent to ventricular arrhythmia. If antiarrhythmic therapy is prescribed for complicated ventricular arrhythmias, it is important to obtain follow-up ambulatory 24-hr monitoring of the ECG and exercise testing results to ensure that the anti-arrhythmic agent is effective and to ensure that it is not associated with adverse changes in impulse generation and conduction that might be harbingers of arrhythmogenic side effects or sudden cardiac deaths (QT prolongation, short bursts of polymorphic ventricular tachycardia). Though invasive electrophysiologic testing as a means of eliciting and choosing effective anti-arrhythmic therapy for malignant and refractory ventricular arrhythmias is a very exciting and promising diagnostic and therapeutic modality, its exact role in the detection and management of patients at risk for sudden cardiac death, whether or not they have complicated ventricular premature beats in the post-myocardial infarction convalescent phase, has not as yet been established. Exercise testing with thallium^{201} myocardial scintography enhances the sensitivity and specificity of the detection of residual myocardial ischemia, particularly in patients convalescing from interior wall myocardial infarction.

In a patient with an uncomplicated late convalescence, it is reasonable to perform an exercise test according to a modified Bruce protocol just prior to hospital discharge. The purpose of this test is as follows: 1. to demonstrate to the patient that he or she is capable of moderate exercise following discharge. This improves self-image and self-confidence. 2. To objectively determine the patient's exercise capacity and to make a rational outpatient exercise prescription on this basis. 3. To detect angina or objective evidence of myocardial ischemia, or both; untoward events will suggest the patient is at an increased risk for a morbid cardiac event (recurrent angina, myocardial infarction, or sudden death) in the weeks to months following discharge. In this group, it is appropriate to recommend early cardiac catheterization, ventriculography, and possibly coronary artery revascularization surgery.

During a modified exercise test, patients exercise until they experience the determined target heart rate of approximately 120 beats/min, until a certain duration of exercise has been achieved, or until the patients experience symptoms of undue fatigue, lightheadedness, dyspnea, or angina, at which point the test is terminated.

CARE AND REHABILITATION AFTER MYOCARDIAL INFARCTION

method of
CARTER NEWTON, M.D.
University of California
Los Angeles, California

Many who have had their first myocardial infarction (MI) recover and get back to a state of health which is in fact better than that prior to their illness. This is no paradox: For most, the actual incident was the result of a lifetime of progress of atherosclerosis, ignorance of or ambivalence to warning signs, and the maintenance of a life style of "coronary risk," such as by smoking cigarettes.

Surviving the myocardial infarction, overcoming the inevitable depression of the event, resuming work, and taking on a healthier life style (regular exercise, stopping smoking, losing weight, controlling blood pressure, and eating sensibly) are all expected outcomes. The post-MI patient has just entered a new era in his or her life and the doctor must lead the patient through the following: (1) acute intensive hospital management, (2) convalescence and in-hospital rehabilitation management, (3) 3 months' postdischarge management, and (4) long-term management. With some sound principles to follow, good communication, and common sense, patients can be guided to the various treatment options and benefit from the falling cardiac mortality that is at last a feature of medicine in the 1980s.

Acute Management

Interventions

Many centers utilize intravenous or, if a catheterization laboratory is available, intracoronary streptokinase and are offering balloon angioplastic dilatation of a narrowed coronary artery in the setting of acute myocardial infarction. If either or both are performed early (6 hours or less), there is good evidence that the size of the myocardial infarction can be reduced. Patients in this category must be maintained on heparin and subsequently make a transition to oral antiplatelet agents, such as aspirin in combination with dipyridamole (this use of aspirin and dipyridamole is not listed by their manufacturers). Most protocols also administer nitrates and calcium channel blockers after the procedure. A history of a bleeding ulcer should preclude the use of streptokinase, and physicians should be aware of the risk of spontaneous central nervous system hemorrhage, which is small (less than 1 per cent) but rises with age. Nitrates and calcium channel blockers can lead to hypotension, and these drugs should be withdrawn if the blood pressure is less than 100 mm Hg systolic.

Intensive Care Unit

Here a patient is put to bed in privacy with continuous electrocardiographic (ECG) monitoring. A low flow of nasal oxygen is given and an intravenous line established. The nursing staff should be reassuring and confident. Patients need to see that the situation is under control and that recovery and rehabilitation *will* occur. They should be made as comfortable as possible and should receive an oral or intramuscular tranquilizer like diazepam (Valium) (normally 2 to 5 mg every 4 hours) for relief of anxiety.

Persistent Pain

If chest discomfort persists, sublingual nitroglycerin, 0.4 mg, should be given in up to three doses spaced 5 minutes apart, not allowing the blood pressure to go under 100 mm Hg. If this medication improves the situation, then topical nitroglycerin (0.5 to 1 inch every 6 to 8 hours) should be applied. This drug should be removed upon severe headache or hypotension. If there is no relief with nitroglycerin, morphine sulfate in repeated 2 mg boluses, up to 15 mg every 3 hours, may be necessary. Pain that persists for greater than 6 hours or recurs and responds to nitroglycerin suggests that the infarction will enlarge or that other areas of heart muscle are endangered. Such patients should be managed more aggressively with stronger application of nitrates and consideration of early coronary arteriography.

Congestive Heart Failure

If signs of congestive heart failure (pulmonary rales, diastolic gallop, tachycardia) are noted, intravenous furosemide should be given along with potassium orally. If a clearly favorable trend is not apparent in 1 to 2 hours, a balloon-tipped pulmonary wedge catheter should be placed to direct fluid management and the use of intravenous unloading agents, such as nitroprusside. These patients are the most critically ill, since their infarction has been a large one, and they should be graduated to rehabilitation activities more cautiously and slowly.

TABLE 1. **Phased Postinfarction Activity Levels**

Level I.	Bed rest May feed self Out of bed permitted for bedside commode Deep breathing exercises every 2 hours while awake Partial self-bath (hands, face, and personal hygiene) May brush teeth, comb hair, shave, put on makeup Passive range of motion of arm and leg joints
Level II.	All previous activities, plus Sit in chair for 20 minutes twice a day Active range of motion of arm and leg joints twice a day
Level III.	All previous activities, plus Sit in chair 20 minutes three times a day Partial bath, including arms and legs Eat meals while seated in chair
Level IV.	All previous activities, plus Walking 1/16 mile in 3 minutes twice a day Begin dietary instruction for home diet Side bends times three, trunk rotations times three
Level V.	All previous activities, plus May dress self Sit in chair two to three times a day for 30 to 60 minutes Side bends times five, trunk rotations times five, once a day Walking 1/8 mile in 6 minutes twice Stroll as desired
Level VI.	All previous activities, plus Side bends times ten, trunk rotations times ten Walking 1/4 mile in 10 minutes once Shower while seated
Level VII.	All previous activities, plus Side bends times fifteen, trunk rotations times fifteen Walking 1/4 mile in 10 minutes twice Walk up and down on flight of stationary stairs Wash hair in shower with assistance Evaluate home activities with telemetry

Ventricular Arrhythmias

If ventricular ectopic complexes occur, lidocaine as a bolus, followed by continuous infusion, should be given for 48 hours. If this is ineffective, procainamide as a bolus with subsequent infusion should be tried. The routine use of lidocaine frequently leads to central nervous system side effects and therefore is not recommended for arrhythmia prophylaxis alone. Before leaving a monitoring situation, the antiarrhythmic drug should be stopped to allow assessment of ectopic tendencies when the patient is off medication. If complex or frequent premature ventricular contractions are noted, monitoring should be continued until control is attained by oral agents such as quinidine or procainamide.

Initiation of Rehabilitation

Once the patient has demonstrated clinical stability, that is, there are no signs of congestive heart failure, pain and discomfort are not occurring at rest, and potentially serious ventricular arrhythmias have been controlled, activity can be increased in stages under supervision and monitoring; also a period of education begins.

Inpatient Recovery and Rehabilitation Management

Table 1 illustrates the phased activity levels that patients may progress to every 1 or 2 days, provided they remain clinically stable and show no evidence of further myocardial ischemic activity. The principle is to begin activity as soon as it is safe and progress gradually to minimize the inevitable deconditioning that will occur with bed rest and lack of exercise. If a patient is able to complete all the activities at one level without provoking cardiac symptoms, experiencing an inappropriate tachycardia (greater than 110 beats per minute), or experiencing a fall in blood pressure (greater than 30 mm Hg), then he or she may progress to the next activity level the following day. Vital signs should be checked before and after each activity session and recorded in a special section of the nursing notes so that the doctor can assess from the heart rate and blood pressure responses how taxing the activity was. The patient with a tendency to develop signs of left ventricular failure or an effort-related arrhythmia can thereby be identified and the therapy modified.

By the time patients reach cardiac level VI, they should be nearing time for discharge. At this point a low level stress test should be performed with ECG monitoring on a walking treadmill. The patient should be able to get to an activity level that comfortably exceeds the activities expected when going home. This should take into account whether or not there are stairs at home and what the neighborhood environment and terrain are as patients graduate to more and more activity out of doors. Our low level stress test protocol is illustrated in Table 2.

Equally as important as the supervised activity increments in the week post-MI is a period of education. Patients should be taught about their own anatomy, what has happened to their coronary artery circulation, and how to check their own pulse and, if possible, blood pressure. This is a period of time when depression is inevitable, and in addition to support from the medical staff, education about their problem is essential. They should receive nutritional instructions about the correct number of calories needed to achieve an ideal weight and how to limit their daily fat intake to not more than 30 per cent of those calories. Foods high in cholesterol should be limited and excessive use of salt discouraged. Inpatients need to be optimistically instructed about rehabilitation: keeping their weight and blood pressure under control, exercising correctly, and learning the warning signs of cardiac problems to bring to the attention of their physicians. It is also essential that an all-out effort to discourage smoking take place during this time. The patient is ready for discharge when a low level exercise test has been completed without difficulty and when the patient and his or her spouse have completed educational and counseling sessions on activity, diet, warning signs, and the dose schedule for medication.

TABLE 2. **Low Level Stress Test**

Three minutes walking 1.5 MPH, level
Three minutes walking 1.5 MPH, 10 per cent grade
Three minutes walking 2 MPH, 10 per cent grade

Test conclusion at 9 minutes or when heart rate of 120 is reached, unless ischemic signs or symptoms occur.

Management Three Months Postdischarge

The 3 month period following a heart attack is one of emotional adjustment, initial recovery, return to work, resumption of sexual activity, and the establishment of life style habits, some of which may be very new and difficult to maintain. The key element here is that the physician and rehabilitation support staff, if one is available, show the patient that he or she is making progress and *can* accomplish something favorable about heart disease by sticking to a rehabilitation program. More and more hospitals and now even some recreational facilities are developing organized programs of monitored cardiac rehabilitation. There is no question that such centers provide a better overall environment and means of speedy recovery if they are economically feasible for the patient and conveniently located. Ideally, the outpatient rehabilitation program over the 3 month postmyocardial infarction is constructed in two phases:

Preconditioning/Educational Phase. One to two weeks are spent at a rehabilitation center "learning the ropes." Patients make the acquaintance of the nursing staff and support personnel, and they meet other patients involved in different levels of the rehabilitation program. They learn how to attach themselves to a telemetered ECG monitor, they learn how to use the exercise equipment (treadmill, stationary bicycle, arm ergometer, and wall pulleys), they learn how to check their own pulse, and how to limber their muscles in a warm-up and cool-down interval. They then have monitored walking sessions at a low work level initially but progressing slowly in speed and duration as tolerated. During this phase the patient gains familiarity with how to exercise correctly and is surrounded by skilled personnel to answer questions about symptoms, nutrition, life style changes, and cardiovascular physiology as they wish. It is also a time when early problems with walking or other associated medical problems, such as diabetes or lung disease can be brought to the attention of the private physician by the nursing staff. Patients may resume sexual relations when they have demonstrated an exercise capacity during walking that exceeds the effort used during intercourse. A general guideline is resumption of relations after 3 weeks and after a heart rate of 130 can be achieved without untoward symptoms.

Phase II/Physical Conditioning. Four to six weeks following an acute myocardial infarction, a stress test should be performed. A stress test following one of many available protocols provides the basis of a safe training exercise prescription. The exercise test, whether it be by stationary cycling or walking, should be sufficiently strenuous to raise the heart rate to greater than 85 per cent of the maximum predicted by age or bring the patient to 3+/4+ symptom limitation (leg fatigue, dyspnea, and so on). Provided the stress test is "passed" without signs of potential clinical instability, a 12-week interval of regular aerobic training should begin. The patient should exercise three to four times per week, preferably with continuous ECG monitoring, for sessions of approximately 30 minutes' duration. Patients in general should exercise at a "target heart rate," which should be 20 beats per minute less than the maximum achieved on their stress test. It is important that patients learn to count their pulse by feeling their own radial pulse for a period of 15 seconds and then multiplying it by four. Patients should teach themselves or be shown by the rehabilitation staff when they have exceeded their target heart rate and should cut back on their intensity until they again drop below the target zone. During this time physicians are kept informed of their patient's progress, specifically regarding exercise-related arrhythmias, blood pressure, weight loss, attitude, and compliance with such life style changes as smoking abatement. In the monitored setting changes in antiarrhythmic therapy and antihypertensive therapy can be observed, and patients can be taught to use nitroglycerin prophylactically if angina is present during their exercise sessions. At the conclusion of a 12-week period of monitored training, a maximal stress test is repeated by the same protocol used initially. The data from this test can be used to show patients improvements in their conditioning and blood pressure responsiveness, and these data can be used as markers of stamina for them to maintain over the ensuing months and years.

Postrehabilitation Maintenance Program

Once patients have completed 12 weeks of exercise training, most can graduate to a nonmonitored home program. It is important that regular contact between the patient and physician be maintained, however, to try to insure compliance with the life style change elements that have been gained at this point. Patients should continue an exercise habit in a walking program at a minimum of four times a week. Many rehabilitation centers offer their "graduates" the use of their facilities without ECG monitoring in classes where friendships and habits that were learned can be maintained. Patients should see their doctors at least at 3-month intervals, and they should have repeat stress testing at least yearly, with 6-month intervals probably preferable. Regular exercise testing is an additional incentive to keep up the acquired athletic habits.

At this point ideal patients have reached a healthy body weight, blood pressure is controlled either by avoidance of salt or by a minimum of antihypertensive medications, cardiovascular physiology is understood both by patients and physicians, they are not smoking cigarettes, and are eating a diet prudently low in cholesterol and animal fat.

If at any point during phased rehabilitation or thereafter the patient develops new or worsening angina, warning symptoms of arrhythmias, or signs or symptoms of overt heart failure, the management plan should change either to stabilize this problem or to proceed to diagnostic coronary arteriography. Most physicians have different thresholds in proceeding to cardiac catheterization in the course of management of their post-infarction patients; however, at a point 3 months following myocardial infarction and after a rehabilitation program, the physician is in an optimal position to make a decision about whether angiographic information is needed for long-term planning.

The following factors seem most consistently to play a role in determining whether or not a patient should proceed to cardiac catheterization: (1) age of patient, (2) intolerance of antianginal medication, and (3) objective signs of myocardial ischemia at less than high cardiac workloads. The improvement in both survival statistics and in operative mortality and morbidity during bypass surgery, and the promising successes with single and multiple vessel coronary angioplasty techniques, are all promising elements to patients with coronary artery disease. However, the maintenance of habits learned in a rehabilitation program and close medical follow-up with a physician, with regular stress testing at yearly intervals, remains permanently a treatment of atherosclerosis for many.

PERICARDITIS

method of
CHARLES A. BUSH, M.D.
Ohio State University
Columbus, Ohio

Pericarditis may be an isolated disease process affecting the pericardium alone or, more commonly, may occur secondary to or in association with another disease process. Early recognition and an accurate diagnosis of related disease are essential to appropriate treatment. Pericarditis is frequently idiopathic. It may be secondary to an infectious process most commonly, viral, bacterial, or tuberculous. Frequently it is associated with acute myocardial infarction or dissecting aortic aneurysm or occurs following myocardial infarction. It is often associated with collagen vascular diseases, including rheumatic and rheumatoid disease and systemic lupus erythematosus. Drugs, irradiation, and thoracic surgery are also important secondary causes, and it is commonly associated with chronic renal disease and various neoplastic diseases.

Manifestations of Pericarditis

These include the signs and symptoms of acute pericardial inflammation, frequently involving pain or cardiac arrhythmias. Pericardial fluid may be of little or no hemodynamic significance, may moderately impair cardiac filling, or may be of major hemodynamic significance in the form of cardiac tamponade. Chronic inflammation and fibrosis of the pericardium may result in pericardial constriction which may be occult or overtly manifest in inability to fill the heart. It is exceedingly important to recognize that individual manifestations or a combination may occur in any specific patient.

Treatment

Acute Inflammation

Pain is the most common symptom. Acute inflammatory pericarditis may be best managed with anti-inflammatory agents. In general, the severity of the symptoms dictates whether to use aspirin, indomethacin, or corticosteroids as the initial anti-inflammatory approach. Failure to achieve an appropriate therapeutic response within 48 hours by relief of pain, fever, and other signs of acute inflammation is an indication to increase dosage or proceed with additional anti-inflammatory agents. Occasionally, a patient with acute inflammatory pericarditis or recurrent bouts of acute inflammation will require pericardiectomy because of failure to control acute inflammation or because of side effects of prolonged medication.

Arrhythmias

The most common rhythm disturbances associated with pericarditis are sinus tachycardia and atrial arrhythmias, including premature atrial contractions, atrial flutter, and atrial fibrillation. In general, the rhythm disturbances resolve with anti-inflammatory therapy. Digitalis or propranolol may be indicated for the management of the patient with a rapid ventricular response to atrial fibrillation or atrial flutter. There is little if any indication for the use of other antiarrhythmic agents, and the use of electrical cardioversion for atrial arrhythmias is not advisable.

Pericardial Effusion

The hemodynamic significance of fluid in the pericardial space is a major determinant of the treatment. Small asymptomatic pericardial effusions of known etiology, most commonly diagnosed by echocardiography, either may be treated by anti-inflammatory agents or not treated. The presence of a pericardial effusion of unknown etiology that is of minor hemodynamic significance should be approached from a combined diagnostic and therapeutic approach. The safest and most complete approach is subxiphoid pericardial drainage and biopsy. This permits drainage of the fluid with simultaneous diagnostic studies being performed on the fluid and the pericardial tissue. Frequently a drainage procedure alone is curative for chronic pericardial effusion. In patients with marked hemodynamic compromise from pericardial effusion (those with cardiac tamponade) drainage is urgent and subxiphoid pericardiotomy is the best procedure. The decision to proceed with needle pericardiocentesis versus a subxiphoid drainage with fluid analysis and biopsy should be based upon experience and the availability of support facilities. In general, needle pericardiocentesis has a higher inherent risk of complication than does a subxiphoid drainage procedure. Needle pericardiocentesis should be performed only by experienced individuals and only when subxiphoid drainage procedures are not readily available.

Patients with hemodynamically significant pericardial effusion and life-threatening cardiac tamponade may be treated acutely with aggressive intravenous fluid administration and a potent cardiac inotrope. In patients with cardiac tamponade, atrial filling occurs only during ventricular systole. Therefore, potent inotropic agents such as isoproterenol and dopamine, which increase ventricular contractility, actually serve to augment atrial filling. Aggressive intravenous fluid administration increases atrial filling pressure and allows more fluid to enter the atrium that is impaired in its filling by tamponade. It is emphasized that the combined use of fluids and inotropic agents is a temporizing treatment only. However, such an approach may be lifesaving while a more definitive drainage procedure is readied.

Occasionally pericardiectomy is warranted for the patient with chronic effusive pericardial disease. When pericardiectomy is performed, pericardial effusive disease is cured; the underlying cause is frequently identified by the appropriate diagnostic studies on fluid and tissue.

Pericardial Constriction

Depending upon the hemodynamic significance of pericardial constriction, pericardiectomy is generally the treatment of choice. Occasionally, however, patients with pericardial constriction have occult hemodynamic findings and few symptoms. Such patients can be followed without specific therapy and may have a stable disease process that does not require pericardiectomy. Diuretic therapy and volume depletion must be carefully avoided in patients with constrictive pericardial disease. A reduction in resting cardiac output or an inadequate cardiac output response to exercise is the result of an inappropriate intravascular volume in such patients. Pericardiectomy is definitive treatment for patients with constrictive pericardial disease but is not required until symptoms become disabling or there are overt hemodynamic manifestations.

Pericarditis Secondary to Specific Disease Processes

In patients with pericarditis secondary to another disease, the primary disease is treated. If this does not alleviate the pericarditis, then specific management of the pericarditis is indicated, as discussed. Likewise, if the acute hemodynamic manifestations of pericarditis are life-threatening, appropriate relief of those hemodynamic findings must be instituted on an emergency basis prior to a definitive diagnosis.

PERIPHERAL ARTERIAL DISEASE

method of
JOHN A. SPITTELL JR., M.D.
Mayo Medical School
Rochester, Minnesota

Peripheral arterial diseases are common clinical problems since atheroclerosis is the major cause of occlusive arterial disease and arterial aneurysms. Both these types of atherosclerotic arterial disease are readily diagnosed in their early stages when they are often asymptomatic and most effectively treated. The nonatherosclerotic types of occlusive peripheral arterial disease are less frequent but nonetheless important because they often affect young persons and, if recognized before ischemic complications occur, can be effectively treated.

The vasospastic disorders, when mild, may be considered only a nuisance by patients when in reality they may be an early manifestation of some underlying disorder. In addition, pharmacologic advances have provided more effective agents for relief of vasospasm, it must also be remembered that certain commonly prescribed drugs may aggravate or produce vasospastic symptoms as side effects. As such, vasospastic symptoms should be a standard part of the medical inquiry or review of symptoms.

Arteritis can be seen in persons of all age groups. Its clinical presentation can be confusing because of its protean manifestations, but keeping it in mind is rewarding to the alert clinician since corticosteroid therapy may avert complications and control its activity.

Aortic dissection warrants special attention because it so commonly mimics other catastrophic illnesses, and current therapeutic approaches significantly improve the formerly dismal prognosis.

Chronic Occlusive Arterial Disease

Regardless of the etiology (Table 1) and location of occlusive peripheral arterial disease or any specific therapy selected for it, certain general measures have so much to offer that every patient should become familiar with them.

Tobacco in any form has a vasoconstrictive effect on the peripheral arterial circulation so should be interdicted. Stopping smoking may seem an impossible task for the veteran smoker, but when the adverse effect of smoking on prognosis for limb survival is made clear, most patients realize the benefit is worth the effort. Vasoconstrictive agents that may be prescribed

TABLE 1. **Etiology of Chronic Occlusive Peripheral Arterial Disease**

Arteriosclerosis obliterans
Thromboangiitis obliterans
Trauma
Blunt trauma
Chronic occupational occlusive arterial disease in the hand
Arterial compression or entrapment
Thoracic outlet compression
Adductor tendon compression of superficial femor artery
Popliteal artery entrapment
Arteritis
Connective tissue disorders
Giant cell (temporal) arteritis
Takayasu's arteritis

for associated hypertension or coronary artery disease (beta blockers) or for migraine (ergot preparations) are best avoided in the patient with occlusive peripheral arterial disease, particularly since alternative therapy is available.

A significant number of amputations result from some type of preventable trauma. Patients with occlusive peripheral arterial disease should be made aware of this and instructed not only in the local care of the skin of their ischemic limb but in protection of it from chemical, thermal, and mechanical trauma. Properly fitting and protective footwear should be stressed.

A walking program also has much to offer the patient with occlusive peripheral arterial disease, particularly if intermittent claudication is a complaint. Whether a walking program increases collateral circulation or merely conditions muscles or both is not settled, but significant improvement in the walking distance may occur with a walking program followed regularly for 2 to 3 months. Walking—to the point of limb discomfort, then standing until relief occurs before resuming walking again—for a period of 30 minutes several times each day is a convenient program for most patients except, of course, for those whose exertion is limited by angina pectoris or whose walking is limited by musculoskeletal or neurologic disability. Weight reduction in the obese patient, aided by a walking program, may help improve the walking distance.

More specific therapeutic measures for occlusive peripheral arterial disease include pharmacologic agents, restoration of pulsatile flow, and sympathectomy. The selection of one of those modalities is an individual decision for each patient based on the degree of ischemia, the disability it is causing, the risk of limb loss, and any associated health problems that might adversely affect surgical risks or longevity. Restoration of pulsatile flow to the limb is elective because it does not (a) affect longevity, or (b) ameliorate coronary or cerebrovascular disease; the incidence of severe ischemia is relatively low; runoff should be adequate; complications of the procedure, though infrequent, do occur; and reocclusion may occur.

Arteriography is not performed (except when the etiology of the occlusive arterial disease is in doubt) unless an attempt to restore pulsatile flow is being considered. While the development of digital subtraction angiography (DSA) allows arterial imaging without arterial puncture, resolution may not be adequate for surgical decisions, and the hazards associated with using contrast media remain.

An estimate of the degree of ischemia can be obtained at the bedside or in the office by the elevation-dependency tests (Table 2), which take only a few minutes to perform. The availibility of noninvasive technique adds an objective dimension to evaluation, and when supine systolic brachial and ankle pressures are done before and after standard exercise, a good estimate of functional impairment of occlusive arterial disease can be obtained (Table 3) to provide a baseline for evaluating therapy.

TABLE 2. **Elevation-Dependency Tests**

Grading of Elevation Pallor

(Elevation of extremity at angle of 60° above the level)

Grade of Pallor	*Duration of Elevation*
0	No pallor in 60 seconds
1	Definite pallor in 60 seconds
2	Definite pallor in less than 60 seconds
3	Definite pallor in less than 30 seconds
4	Pallor on the level

Color Return (CR) and Venous Filling Time (VFT)

	Time for CR (Sec)	*VFT (Sec)*
Normal	10	15
Moderate ischemia	15–25	20–30
Severe ischemia	40+	40+

(From Spittell JA Jr: Recognition and management of chronic atherosclerotic occlusive peripheral arterial disease. Mod Concepts Cardiovasc Dis *50*:19, 1981. With permission of the American Heart Association, Inc.)

While the restoration pulsatile flow in the nondiabetic patient with only intermittent claudication is elective, as just noted, when the patient is diabetic or has ischemic rest pain or ischemic ulceration, restoration of pulsatile flow is indicated if feasible. This is because the incidence of limb loss is relatively high without treatment; it may permit a lower level of amputation; and the risks of the procedure are less than is the risk of amputation. Percutaneous balloon angioplasty (PTA) can restore pulsatile flow in selected patients with reduced morbidity, mortality, and cost compared with arterial surgery, but best results are obtained with focal iliac or femoropopliteal stenoses that are neither complete occlusions nor heavily calcified. Restenosis remains a problem with both PTA and bypass grafts, particularly at the femoral or more distal levels; the incidence of both early and late restenosis or graft occlusion may be lessened with antiplatelet therapy if the good results reported with the use of dipyridamole and aspirin after coronary artery surgery carry over to peripheral arterial procedures.

Interest in the role of hemorrheology in intermittent claudication has been stimulated by the recent release of pentoxifylline (Trental), a methylxanthine, for the treatment of intermittent claudication. This agent is alleged to improve the microcirculation by lowering blood viscosity and increasing erythrocyte deformabililty, both of which have been reported to be abnormal in atherosclerosis. The drug may actually have

TABLE 3. **Noninvasive Laboratory Assessment of Arterial Insufficiency of the Legs**

Degree of Arterial Insufficiency	Standard Exercise		Systolic Blood Pressure Index*	
	Claudication	*Duration (Min)*	*Before Exercise*	*After Exercise*
Minimal	0	5	Normal to mildly abnormal	Abnormal
Mild	+	5	>0.8	>0.5
Moderate	+	<5	<0.8	<0.5
Severe*	+	<3	<0.5	<0.15

*Often patients have a systolic ankle blood pressure of less than 50 mm Hg, in addition.

+, Systolic pressure index is obtained by dividing the systolic ankle blood pressure by the systolic brachial blood pressure, both taken in the supine position (normal 0.95 or greater).

(From Spittell JA Jr: Recognition and management of chronic atherosclerotic occlusive peripheral arterial disease. Mod Concepts Cardiovasc Dis *50*:19, 1981. With permission of the American Heart Association, Inc.)

other effects on platelet aggregability and vascular smooth muscle that could favorably influence intermittent claudication. A multicenter trial in this country indicated that there is a significant increase in claudication distance over a period of 6 weeks with the use of pentoxyfylline in a dose of 400 mg three times a day orally.

Other presently available oral vasodilating drugs have not been shown to increase muscle blood flow during exercise and thus would be expected to improve intermittent claudication. Antithrombotic therapy in the form of either coumarins or antiplatelet agents has not been shown to have any benefit for patients with peripheral arterial disease unless recurrent thrombotic arterial occlusion is a problem, and then either may be worth a trial.

Surgical sympathectomy to increase cutaneous vasodilation is used to aid healing of ischemic ulceration in the rare patient whose occlusive arterial disease is not amenable to restoration of pulsatile flow by surgery or balloon angioplasty. Since sympathectomy, like oral vasodilators, does not increase muscle blood flow, it does not relieve intermittent claudication.

TABLE 4. **Acute Arterial Occlusion**

- Thrombotic arterial occlusion
  - Arterial disease
    - Arteriosclerosis obliterans
    - Thromboangiitis obliterans
    - Arteritis
  - Arterial trauma
    - Penetrating
    - Blunt
  - Hematologic disease
    - Polycythemia vera
    - Thrombocytosis
    - Hypercoagulability
- Embolic arterial occlusion arising from thrombi of:
  - Cardiac origin
  - Proximal arterial disease
    - Arterial aneurysm
    - Atherosclerotic plaques
- Miscellaneous causes
  - Arterial spasm
    - Ergotism
    - Secondary to trauma
  - Aortic dissection
  - Foreign bodies

Acute Arterial Occlusion

Since sudden and complete occlusion of a peripheral artery can be caused by thrombosis of a diseased artery, thrombosis secondary to systemic diseases, or an embolus from the heart or a more proximal arterial lesion (Table 4), both survival of the patient and limb salvage must be considered in management decisions. Emergent measures include pain relief and protection of the ischemic limb—avoiding local heat, cold, and elevation. Intravenous heparin is useful to protect collateral circulation while general evaluation and preparations for definitive management are underway. Arteriography is indispensable in evaluating acute arterial occlusion and planning its management. Surgical embolectomy utilizing a Fogarty catheter has been a major advance; when the arterial occlusion is thrombotic there are several options for management, depending on the size of the artery occluded and its duration when diagnosed. Arterial patency may be restorable by surgical thrombectomy or thrombolytic therapy if the arterial occlusion is seen early and the patient's general condition permits; if either is not possible or contraindicated, one may temporize with anticoagulant therapy and general measures in the acute case and hope for a more favorable opportunity for surgical treatment.

Arterial Aneurysm

Since atherosclerosis is the most common cause of aortic and peripheral arterial aneurysms, coronary artery disease is commonly associated; hence, when evaluating the patient with an aneurysm for surgery, particular attention should be paid to cardiac status, including an assessment of exercise tolerance.

Hypertension is also a frequent finding in patients with arterial aneurysms; it is an important factor favoring surgical treatment and an equally

TABLE 5. **Clinical Features Suggestive of Type I or Type II Dissecting Aneurysm**

Initial pain in anterior chest
Decreased or absent pulses and blood pressure in the right arm
Decreased right carotid artery pulsation
Aortic diastolic murmur
Pericardial friction rub
Evidence of myocardial ischemia or infarction on the electrocardiogram

(From Spittell JA Jr: Clinical aspects of aneurysmal disease, in Harvey WP, et al (eds): Current Problems in Cardiology. © 1980 by Year Book Medical Publishers, Inc., Chicago.)

important therapeutic consideration after successful surgery.

Thoracic aortic disease is commonly first discovered on a chest roentgenogram and is often confused with nonvascular masses. Computed tomography is particularly useful in diagnosing thoracic aortic aneurysm. The indications for surgery in thoracic aortic aneurysm are: it is 6 cm in diameter or larger in size; it is enlarging under observation; it exerts pressure on surrounding structures; there is associated hypertension; or it is secondary to trauma (incomplete aortic rupture). Incomplete aortic rupture as a result of sudden deceleration may result in aneurysm formation at the isthmus of the aorta; since the stabililty of these aneurysms is unpredictable, surgical resection is advisable.

The risk of rupture is low if an abdominal aortic aneurysm is smaller than 4.0 cm in diameter, but when the diameter is 5 cm or greater the risk of rupture increases progressively. Thus, in a good risk patient surgical resection is indicated for an abdominal aortic aneurysm 4.5 cm in diameter or larger. In the patient who is a poor surgical risk, 5 cm aneurysms can be observed closely with ultrasound measurement every 3 or 4 months. When an aneurysm exceeds 5 cm in diameter or becomes symptomatic, surgery should be advised for any but the poorest risk patient.

Aneurysms of the femoral or popliteal arteries are fairly common and are ideally treated surgically before complications, usually thromboembolic, occur.

TABLE 6. **Pharmacologic Treatment Program for Acute Dissecting Aneurysm**

Hypertensive patients
Trimethaphan intravenously until the following oral drugs control blood pressure:
Reserpine, 0.25 mg two to four times daily
Propranolol, 20 mg four times daily
Guanethidine, 25 to 50 mg per day
Normotensive patients
Propranolol, either 2 mg intramuscularly every 4 to 6 hours or 20 mg orally every 6 hours

(From Spittell JA Jr: Clinical aspects of aneurysmal disease, in Harvey WP, et al (eds): Current Problems in Cardiology. © 1980 by Year Book Medical Publishers, Inc., Chicago.)

Surgical treatment of renal artery aneurysms is indicated only when they are symptomatic, are greater than 2 cm in diameter, or occur in pregnant patients.

Aortic Dissection

Since the prognosis and management may differ, depending on the location of the primary tear, it is important to localize it. Some clinical findings suggest that the tear is in the ascending aorta (Table 5), and computed tomography coupled with injection of contrast media may demonstrate the dissection, but definitive localization usually requires aortography.

Management needs to be individualized. Pharmacologic therapy (Table 6), designed to decrease the force of ventricular contraction and to control any hypertension, is indicated in all patients as soon as the diagnosis of aortic dissection is made. Most centers prefer prompt surgical treatment when the primary tear is in the ascending aorta because of the high risk of rupture in this type. When the initial tear is in the descending aorta beyond the left subclavian artery, some prefer continued pharmacologic treatment as long as the patient is stable whereas others advocate surgical treatment.

Vasospastic Disorders

Although Raynaud's phenomenon, primary (Raynaud's disease) and secondary, is the most frequent and well known vasospastic disorder, several other conditions (primary and secondary livedo reticularis, acrocyanosis, chronic pernio), characterized by intermittent change in color and temperature of the skin, are due to spasm of dermal arterioles.

Other than often providing an early clue to some underlying disorder, the vasospastic disorders are important to recognize because there are new and effective measures to lessen or relieve vasospasm. All patients should avoid cold exposure and any drugs that may accentuate cutaneous arteriolar vasospasm, such as beta blockers, ergot preparations and clonidine.

Prazosin hydrochloride (Minipress) in very modest doses (1 mg once or twice a day) has been effective in many patients with a vasospastic disorder (this use is not listed in the manufacturer's directive). Nifedipine (Procardia), 10 mg three times a day, has been useful in some patients also. When it is desirable to avoid pharmacologic therapy, biofeedback has been used successfully to normalize responses to decreased environmental temperature changes and lessen vasospasm. Sympathectomy is best reserved until other therapeutic modalities have been given an adequate trial; best results are obtained in patients with Raynaud's disease.

Arteritis

In addition to thromboangiitis obliterans, certain arteritides, principally giant cell (temporal) arteritis and Takayasu's arteritis, may involve extremity arteries.

Giant cell (temporal) arteritis, since it involves persons older than 55 years of age, may be confused with atherosclerotic occlusive disease when symptoms or signs of peripheral occlusive arterial disease are present.

Takayasu's arteritis is less common and more distinctive in that it typically affects persons less than 40 years of age.

In both giant cell and Takayasu's arteritis the cornerstone of therapy is prednisone in adequate dose for adequate periods to control the activity of the disease.

THROMBOPHLEBITIS

method of
RAYMOND H. ALEXANDER, M.D.
University Hospital of Jacksonville
Jacksonville, Florida

Thrombophlebitis is a unique disease in our society in that, as far as can be ascertained, most cases occur within the hospital setting, and more specifically, during operative therapy. The disease kills approximately 50,000 individuals in the United States every year. Its sequela, venous insufficiency, disables over 850,000 individuals per year. Thrombophlebitis is also unique in the fact that clinical diagnosis of the disease is inaccurate: 50 per cent of the individuals with traditional signs and symptoms of thrombophlebitis have other causes for their symptoms, whereas approximately 50 per cent of individuals having thrombophlebitis exhibit no symptoms whatsoever.

The backdrop for therapy, therefore, rests on two premises: (1) Since thrombophlebitis occurs in a controlled hospital situation, every effort should be made to prevent the disease through prophylactic measures. (2) Patients should be monitored carefully for presence of the disease, using objective methods to make this diagnosis.

Prophylaxis

When thrombophlebitis occurs, its first symptom may be a life-threatening or life-taking pulmonary embolism. Once the disease has established itself in the deep veins of the legs, destruction of venous valvular function, leading to venous insufficiency, lymphedema, and ulceration, may occur. Therapy for venous insufficiency is basically symptomatic and is usually only partially successful.

Prophylactic therapy falls into two categories, drug therapy and compressive therapy. Drug therapy consists of therapeutic regimes of low dose heparin and dextran administration. Both have been shown, statistically, to decrease the incidence of thrombophlebitis perioperatively. Although aspirin has been advocated as a prophylactic measure, there are no conclusive studies showing its efficacy in this disease. Low dose heparin, although quite effective, has several limitations. Increased intraoperative bleeding has been shown to occur. In addition, the wound complication rate, particularly from wound hematomas, appears higher. The use of dextran has associated problems, also. Difficulty in crossmatching of blood, allergic anaphylactic reaction, renal shutdown—particularly in low flow states, and bleeding diathesis due to coating of the platelets with the negatively charged material make many physicians reluctant to consider dextran for prophylaxis routinely.

Compressive measures include intermittent compression with a boot stocking and the use of support stockings in the perioperative period. Such mechanical therapy also has its limitations. External compressive devices are uncomfortable for the awake patient and unwieldy for the interoperative patient. The equipment required for a patient is expensive and bulky and requires special expertise to use. The use of compressive stockings has also been advocated and in some studies they have been shown to be effective. Their effectiveness has been attributed to "forcing" blood from the superifical to the deep system, thereby increasing volume flow.

Rather than routinely using some type of prophylactic therapy, our approach has been to identify the high risk patients. The significant risk factors in this disease appear to be age greater than 60 years, previous history of documented thrombophlebitis, or evidence of venous insufficiency. The type of operative procedure also appears to influence the risk of thrombophlebitis. Studies of patients undergoing orthopedic operations indicate that as many as 50 per cent have evidence of thrombophlebitis postoperatively by radioactive fibrinogen scanning. The extremely high risk of thrombophlebitis in hip fractures is well known and fully appreciated by orthopedic surgeons. Major vascular operations, such as aneurysmectomy and femoropopliteal bypass, have been studied at this institution and the risk of thrombophlebitis after these operations is quite high. General abdominal operations, in which the major intra-abdominal veins (vena cava and iliac) undergo some type of dissection, appear to place the patient at greater risk for thrombophlebitis. On the other hand, multivariant studies, as well as our own data, show that chest operations, in particular coronary artery bypass, have an extremely low incidence of this disease. In patients with hip fractures, drug therapy with low dose heparin does not appear to be effective, and full anticoagulation with heparin or warfarin (Coumadin) is necessary for prophylaxis in these cases. Our recommendations, therefore, are as follows:

1. In low risk patients, that is, those with coronary bypass, abdominal operations not involving large veins, and so on, compressive stockings perioperatively should be used, particularly if interoperative time is greater than several hours.

2. In patients with documented thrombophlebitis or having physical signs of venous insufficiency, prophylactic therapy with low dose heparin is indicated, as detailed in Table 1. In such patients, compression therapy is also indicated if facilities exist. In patients undergoing operations in which a significant amount of bleeding might occur and, in particular, operations requiring the use of porous vascular grafts, we do not advocate the use of low dose heparin. We have seen several serious significant bleeding diatheses as well as increased interoperative blood loss in these patients and feel the risk of this therapy is too great. In such cases, intermittent compression or "prophylactic surveillance," i.e., postoperative daily monitoring by Doppler or other noninvasive means, should be used.

3. In patients having major orthopedic operations involving the lower extremity or hip, if other conditions allow, full heparinization or dicumarol (Coumadin) should be used as prophylaxis for the high incidence of thrombophlebitis that may occur.

TABLE 1. **Heparin Administration for Thrombophlebitis**

	Low Dose	Therapeutic
Loading dose	None	100 U/kg body weight
Maintenance	5000–10,000 units q 6–12 hr	750–1500 units to maintain PTT or clotting time 2 to 2.5 × normal
Site	Deep subcutaneously	Intravenously
Monitoring	None	Clotting time or PTT
Duration	2 hr preop. until fully ambulatory	10–14 days

Treatment

Anticoagulation

Because of the great inaccuracy in the clinical diagnosis of thrombophlebitis, some objective test should confirm the diagnosis before the various treatment modalities are instituted. Once diagnosed, most cases of thrombophlebitis respond to therapeutic heparinization. Although administration of heparin in thrombophlebitis has run the gamut of subcutaneous administration to intravenous bolus therapy and then to continuous heparinization, currently continuous heparinization is the most acceptable route. If continuous heparin is used, it should always be administered by infusion pump, and the doses should maintain the partial thromboplastin time or clotting time at two to two and one-half times the normal range (see Table 1). The partial thromboplastin time should be checked at least once, and preferably several times a day to monitor the anticoagulant effect of the heparin after a therapeutic dose has been ascertained. Initially, the partial thromboplastin times should be obtained every 4 hours, to tailor the dose of heparin to the therapeutic range desired.

Most physicians experienced in the treatment of thrombophlebitis usually continue the patient on oral anticoagulant therapy, namely dicumarol (Coumadin), for a period of 3 to 6 months after treatment with heparin. Studies have shown that the risk of recurrent thrombophlebitis peaks approximately 2 weeks after the initial case, and the risk of recurrence stays at a peak level for 3 months and only then begins to decline. Therapeutic levels of dicumarol should be obtained before the heparin is tapered and finally discontinued. Ten to twenty mg of dicumarol are administered orally each morning until the prothrombin time is two to two and one-half times normal, after which the heparin dose is decreased gradually over 12 to 24 hours.

Traditionally, patients have been maintained at strict bed rest while being treated for thrombophlebitis, for fear that a clot would dislodge if the patient were allowed to ambulate. My feeling is that bed rest does not contribute a great deal to either the therapy of thrombophlebitis or the prevention of emboli during treatment. Bed rest may prevent swelling, which occurs with venous obstruction; however, this could be prevented by the use of support stockings. I advocate limited ambulation during the treatment of thrombophlebitis for possible prevention of venous stasis with prolonged bed rest.

Bleeding from heparinization appears to be far more common in middle-aged women; therefore, the clinician must use great caution in this group. Recently a syndrome of hypersensitivity to the heparin molecule, which results in rampant intravascular coagulopathy, has been described and observed. This is a devastating syndrome that results in clotting of small vessels and massive tissue necrosis. In addition, associated clotting of the coronary vessels, resulting in massive myocardial infarction, cerebrovascular occlusion resulting in stroke, as well as other systemic manifestations, are described. This phenomenon is a true hypersensitivity that is not dose-related, and once it occurs can be triggered by a small amount of heparin in a heparin flush. Cardinal signs of the syndrome are diffuse coagulopathy, failure of large doses of heparin to create prolongation of the clotting time or PTT, and rapid decrease in platelet count. In such a situation, the heparin should be stopped immediately and all contact with heparinized products discontinued.

The use of dicumarol (Coumadin) has also been associated with bleeding diathesis. A very common manifestation is a retroperitoneal hematoma. The patient should be carefully monitored.

Dicumarol has been used in the past as a primary treatment of thrombophlebitis. From a theoretic and practical viewpoint, this agent has fallen out of favor for the acute phase.

Thrombolysis

A recent treatment modality for thrombophlebitis is thrombolytic therapy. Most commonly, streptokinase is the agent of choice (Table 2). Urokinase may also be used, but its use is limited somewhat by its extraordinary cost and its relative unavailability. Streptokinase therapy is administered systemically by an intravenous infusion. Initially, a 250,000 unit "loading dose" is given, followed by 100,000 to 200,000 units of streptokinase per hour intravenously by infusion pump. During therapy, clotting parameters should be monitored on a 4 to 6 hour basis. Bleeding occurs frequently, most commonly from the infusion site. Should systemic bleeding occur, the drug must be stopped.

TABLE 2. **Thrombolytic Therapy**

	Amount	Vehicle
Streptokinase		
Loading dose	250,000 IU	Normal saline or D5W
Maintenance dose	100,000 IU/hr for 24–72 hr	
Urokinase		
Loading dose	4400 IU/kg	15 ml normal saline over 10 min
Maintenance dose	4400 IU/kg/hr	15 ml solution/hr × 12 hr
Monitoring		
Thrombin time		2 × control
Partial thromboplastin time		Not sensitive but obtained for follow up
CBC		Stable
Platelet count		Stable
Fibrinogen level		>30% baseline
Fibrin split products		Greatly increased if therapy out of control

The effectiveness of thrombolytic therapy should be monitored by objective parameters, usually venography. The appeal of this therapy is that, if the clots are dissolved rapidly, valvular function in the leg will be maintained and the sequela of thrombophlebitis, venous insufficiency, will not occur. Because of such a rationale, thrombophlebitic therapy is not particularly efficacious in a well-established case of thrombophlebitis in which one surmises that the valvular function has already been compromised. That, coupled with decreased effectiveness of the thrombolysis in "old clot," makes it unwise to run the risk of this therapy in established cases more than 72 hours old.

Surgery

In the past, venous embolectomy has been used in acute cases, particularly when such cases involve the iliofemoral segment. Venous thrombectomy, in general, has been unsuccessful because in most cases the vein will rethrombose afterward. Indications for venous thrombectomy, therefore, must be kept rather rigid. Thrombectomy can be used in cases of severe venous obstruction resulting in the syndrome of phlegmasia cerulea dolens. In this situation, clotting of the extremity is massive and involves both the deep veins and superficial collaterals. If heparinization does not reverse this process, then lack of venous outflow will eventually cause loss of viability to the extremity because of limitations of arterial inflow. Venous thrombectomy can then be done, particularly if the disease has existed less than 72 hours. Unfortunately, many thromboembolized veins reocclude soon after operation.

Fasciotomy in venous disease is seldom required. In phlegmasia cerulea dolens, in which venous outflow is obstructed, increased back pressure on the capillary bed results in leaking of fluid and increases the intracompartmental pressure. Lack of attention to this problem can produce neurogenic loss in the extremity as well as muscle necrosis caused by the increased pressure causing shutdown of the arteriolar beds. Compartmental pressures can be a guide to such a diagnosis; kits containing the materials to measure compartmental pressures are available. A simple method of introducing a needle into the compartment, measuring its pressure by manometry, may not be accurate. I would be reticent to trust this evaluation. If in doubt, fasciectomy should be carried out, at least on clinical suspicion.

Superficial Thrombophlebitis

In most cases, superficial thrombophlebitis is a disease that has none of the implications of the deep vein disease. It can be diagnosed clinically by thrombosis, inflammation, and pain in superficial veins of the legs. Very often, the disease occurs in patients with varicose veins. Varicosities allow stagnation and clotting of the blood in these structures. The treatment is purely symptomatic. Phenylbutazone (Butazolidin), 100 mg three or four times per day, or one of the other nonsteroidal anti-inflammatory drugs such as ibuprofen (Motrin), 400 mg every 4 to 6 hours, along with moist heat and elevation of the extremities, is the treatment of choice. When occasional cases do not respond to this therapy, the use of heparin, either in low doses or in full heparinizing doses, will produce excellent results. Heparin appears to have thrombolytic as well as anti-inflammatory properties.

In recurrent cases of superficial thrombophlebitis in the same set of veins, localized stripping may be necessary to prevent further attacks.

Chronic Venous Insufficiency

The sequela of thrombophlebitis, chronic venous insufficiency, is the result of edema in the legs produced by venous hypertension owing to loss of valvular competence. This edema leads eventually to lymphedema and subcutaneous scarring with obstruction of the lymphatics. Diagnosis is made by observing deeply pigmented, leathery, swollen skin over the distal extremities, particularly severe in the so-called gater areas above the medial malleolus. Ulceration may occur in later stages of the disease because of poor nutrition of the swollen skin, coupled with a most insignificant traumatic event. Chronic venous insufficiency is treated best at the present time by support stockings. Some type of graduated compression stockings (such as Parke-Davis support stockings) is useful in preventing the swelling that initiates the other changes. Patients should put on the stockings before arising from bed in the morning and wear them during the day. It is also helpful for them to plan a time during the day to elevate the legs for 15 to 30 minutes. In men, knee length stockings are most effective, for full length stockings require a constrictive band or tend to roll, creating a constrictive band. In women, panty hose are clearly superior to other options. In no case should the stocking have a constrictive band at the top, which would produce a tourniquet effect increasing the potential for venous hypertension.

Section 5

The Blood and Spleen

APLASTIC ANEMIA

method of
BRUNO SPECK, M.D.
Universitätskliniken, Kantonsspital
Basel, Switzerland

Diagnostic Considerations

Aplastic anemia usually reflects a failure of all cell lines of the bone marrow. In most instances it presents as a pancytopenia. Sometimes it starts with isolated anemia, thrombocytopenia, or granulocytopenia. Mild and moderate forms of the disease occur, but they usually progress to severe aplastic anemia. The severe form is characterized by the following blood criteria: granulocytes less than 500 per cubic mm, thrombocytes less than 20,000 per cubic mm, and reticulocytes less than 20,000 per cubic mm. In addition, a hypoplastic bone marrow with predominance of lymphoid elements proven by biopsy is required.

Most cases of acquired aplastic anemia are idiopathic. Sixty nine to 76 per cent are idiopathic, 9 to 15 per cent induced by drugs or chemicals, 9 to 10 per cent virus-associated, 0 to 5 per cent pregnancy-associated, 1 to 5 per cent congenital, and 0 to 6 per cent unclassified.

For a long time chloramphenicol was the drug most frequently associated with aplastic anemia. Other medications that have been reported to induce aplastic anemia in relatively large numbers of patients are the butazones, gold compounds, anticonvulsants (in particular methylphenylethylhydantoin and trimethadione), and quinacrine. With these drugs the mechanism of induction of aplasia is usually dose-related. Rare cases of aplastic anemia have also been reported with antimicrobials (tetracyclines, penicillins, sulfonamides, and antifungal agents), antithyroid drugs, analgesics, orally administered antidiabetic drugs, and cimetidine.

Several viral infections can cause aplastic anemia. Most common is posthepatic aplastic anemia. It is seen most frequently after non-A, non-B hepatitis, and the symptoms appear several months after hepatitis. We have also seen aplastic anemia in association with infectious mononucleosis, and it has also been described after dengue virus, cytomegalovirus, rubella virus, and herpesvirus infection.

Cytostatic agents, ionizing radiation, benzene, and inorganic arsenicals induce marrow aplasia in a dose-related fashion.

Laboratory Findings

Usually there is pancytopenia, but the lack of one cell line can predominate. It is very important to always combine bone marrow cytology and histology. If the marrow is not completely aplastic it is important to rule out preleukemia. In the differential diagnosis of these two disorders cultures of hemopoietic precursor cells are very important: in aplastic anemia there is usually no growth at all. In leukemic disorders there are many small colonies (clusters). Furthermore the cytogenetic examination of the marrow can give important clues to the existence of a leukemic disorder.

THERAPY

Androgens are active in only a small percentage of patients. Oxymetholone (Anadrol) has the most experience worldwide. Usually a dose of 2 to 3 mg per kg per day is given orally. It acts relatively slowly, and hematopoietic improvement takes 1 to 3 months. The main side effect is hepatotoxicity, which can range from slightly disturbed liver function tests to peliosis hepatis and hepatomas. Other side effects are virilization, decreased potency, amenorrhea, and disturbed growth in children.

We use norethandrolone, 0.5 to 1.0 mg per kg per day orally, because in our experience it has fewer side effects than other androgens. We have used other androgens, but in our experience they have neither important therapeutic advantages nor fewer side effects. In prospective randomized studies in patients with *severe* aplastic anemia no value of androgens could be demonstrated.

SUPPORTIVE CARE

In most instances long-term cell substitution is necessary. Whole blood should not be transfused.

Red Cell Transfusions

The aim is to control symptoms of anemia. In general we keep the hemoglobin above 10 grams per dl. The main problem with normal red cell transfusions is that they are relatively rich in leukocytes and therefore cause marked sensitization to leukocyte and platelet antigens. We therefore use one of the following three types of red cell transfusions.

Leukocyte-Poor Erythrocytes. Leukocytes are removed by repeated centrifugations or by adhesion to nylon fibers (e.g., Leukopak).

Leukocyte-Poor Washed Erythrocytes. In addition to having the leukocytes removed, the red cells are washed in physiologic saline.

Cryopreserved Erythrocytes. The erythrocytes are frozen with a cryopreservative (e.g., glycerol) and kept at −80 C.

Problems of Red Cell Transfusions

Iron Overload. Approximately 300 mg of iron are given per transfusion. This can eventually result in organ siderosis. Sensitization occurs against leukocyte antigens and plasma proteins. This can be followed by a lack of transfusional platelet increments and allergic transfusion reactions. Transmission of viruses, in particular hepatitis and cytomegaly, is a problem with all transfusions. All donors should be serologically screened. The allergic and infectious problems are almost nonexistent with cryopreserved red cells. Unfortunately, this type of transfusion is the most cumbersome and most expensive.

Thrombocyte Transfusions

The number of thrombocytes, not the hemorrhagic diathesis, is the deciding factor for thrombocyte transfusions. Platelets are transfused when platelet values fall below 20,000 per cubic mm. Thrombocyte concentrates as produced by standard procedures in blood banks are no longer used. They are produced from four to six different donors, resulting in a four- to sixfold immunization and a four- to sixfold risk of infection.

Thrombocytes are substituted from healthy single donors. Cell separators such as the FENWAL CS-3000 are used. This machine can extract the platelets from four liters of blood within 1½ hours. Another standard blood cell separator for this purpose is maufactured by HAEMONETICS. With single donors the risk of sensitization can be kept at a minimum. All donors are serologically tested for hepatitis and cytomegaly.

Granulocyte Transfusions

Granulocytes are transfused only if there is agranulocytosis or severe granulocytopenia complicated by septicemia. Healthy single donors are used. With modern cell separators it is relatively easy to isolate more than 10^{10} granulocytes. The transfusions must be repeated daily until the septicemia is under control. In general at least four daily granulocyte transfusions are required.

For patients who are candidates for bone marrow transplantation, no family blood products should be given because of a high risk of sensitization and marrow rejection.

Antibiotics

If the patient has fever of over 38.5 C, antibiotic administration is started immediately to avoid septic shock. In our experience the best empiric combination is a cephalosporin (e.g., Cephacetril, 3 grams every 8 hours intravenously), an aminoglycoside (e.g., tobramycin, 80 mg every 8 hours intravenously), and a ureidopenicillin (e.g., Azlocillin, 5 grams every 8 hours intravenously) daily. With positive blood cultures and known bacteriology, the antibiotics are changed according to the antibiogram.

With candidiasis or aspergillosis, we start amphotericin B in a total daily dose of 10 mg intravenously, increasing to 0.5 mg per kg intravenously daily. For viral infections of the herpes varicella type we start acyclovir (Zovirax), 5 to 10 mg per kg every 8 hours as 1-hour intravenous infusions. For cytomegalovirus infections we use human hyperimmune serum.

ANTILYMPHOCYTE GLOBULIN (ALG)/ ANTITHYMOCYTE GLOBULIN (ATG)

At present this is the best available treatment for patients with severe aplastic anemia who do not qualify for bone marrow transplantation. The exact mechanism of action is unknown. With this type of therapy we are able to induce remissions in over 80 per cent of patients with severe aplastic anemia. (In the United States, these are investigational agents.)

Preparations

We use ALG from horses immunized with human thoracic duct lymphocytes. The purified IgG fraction is given in a dose of 40 mg per kg in 300 ml of physiologic saline as a 3-hour intravenous infusion on each of 4 successive days. This is a xenogeneic serum, and anaphylactic complications can occur. Arterial hyper- and hypotension are relatively common complications, and careful monitoring of the cardiovascular system is indicated. We use prophylactic intravenous antihistaminics (e.g., 1 ampule of Sandosten-calcium containing Ca-gluconolactobionate 1.375, thenalidine maleinate 0.05 or another antihistamine). ALG also has a marked thrombocytopenic action.

Therefore we give a thrombocyte transfusion before and again 2 hours after the ALG infusion.

Other active preparations also produced from horses are the ATG manufactured by Upjohn and Merieux. Remission rates with these two preparations are between 40 and 65 per cent. ATG's from rabbits and goats are also available. About 50 per cent of the patients develop serum sickness approximately 10 days after ALG infusion. It responds to low dose glucicorticosteroids. We give 0.5 mg per kg per day orally until the symptoms subside.

One of the problems with ALG is that the restoration of marrow function is relatively slow. On the average, 3 months are required until the patients are self-sustaining and independent of transfusions. During this period, intensive supervision and supportive care are required. About 10 per cent of the patients will have a relapse, which usually responds to a second course of ALG. Occasionally patients later develop clonal disorders. Among 100 patients we have observed frank paroxysmal nocturnal hemoglobinuria four times and leukemia once.

In our experience androgens have a synergistic action if combined with ALG. We give norethandrolone, 0.5 to 1.0 mg per kg per day orally, and reduce the dose as soon as hematopoietic functions improve. The minimal maintenance dose is 1 10-mg tablet 3 times weekly.

In the last 30 patients we have seen we combined high dose methylprednisolone with ALG. This resulted in a remission rate of 90 per cent and a shorter supportive care period. We gave methylprednisolone–sodium succinate, 20 mg per kg, as a 24-hour continuous intravenous infusion for 4 days parallel to the ALG followed by 10 mg per kg as a 24-hour intravenous infusion the next 4 days. The following week the patients were given 2 mg per kg prednisone orally and the next week 1 mg per kg orally. This was followed by a total dose of 5 mg per day for the next 2 weeks. ALG was infused as previously outlined. Some centers have reported good results with high dose methylprednisolone alone.

BONE MARROW TRANSPLANTATION

Bone marrow transplantation is possible if a syngeneic or HLA-identical sibling is available as a marrow donor. The results are very good in children and young adults. In untransfused young patients it is possible to achieve 80 per cent cure rates.

In polytransfused patients marrow rejection is a major problem. Transfusions from family members should be absolutely avoided because they make this problem even worse. Other inherent risks of allogeneic bone marrow transplantation are acute and chronic graft-versus-host disease and, to a lesser extent, interstitial pneumonia.

Preparations

For bone marrow transplantation the marrow is removed from the donor with multiple punctures at the pelvis. The aim is to obtain more than 2×10^8 nucleated marrow cells per kg body weight of the recipient. The marrow is infused intravenously. To condition the recipient we use cyclophosphamide, 50 mg per kg intravenously, on each of 4 successive days. To ensure engraftment we give donor buffy coat from 4 units of blood on each of 5 successive days following marrow transplantation.

For prophylaxis against graft-versus-host disease we use cyclosporin A, starting the day before transplantation with 20 mg per kg as a 24-hour continuous intravenous infusion. The dosage over the next 5 days is 10 mg per kg as a 24-hour continuous infusion, followed by 5 mg per kg continuous intravenous infusion for the next 5 days. The oral maintenance dose is 12.5 mg per kg once daily. This dose is adjusted to the kidney function, as measured by serum creatinine and creatinine clearance, and the whole blood cyclosporin A trough level. After 6 months the cyclosporin A dosage is gradually reduced and is then stopped after 1 year. Forty per cent of the patients develop signs of graft-versus-host disease upon dose reduction or cessation. For them we continue cyclosporin A in a dose of 1 to 3 mg per kg.

Bone marrow transplantation has the advantage that, so far, neither relapses nor clonal diseases have been reported. Its disadvantages are that an HLA-identical sibling is required and that the upper age limit in most centers is 40 years. Even above the age of 30 the results are rather poor. Chronic graft-versus-host disease used to be an enormous problem in at least 20 per cent of the long-term survivors. We think that cyclosporin A has been a major breakthrough, and we have not had any patients with severe chronic graft-versus-host disease since we began using it. Even in polytransfused patients our cure rates are approximately 70 per cent.

PROGNOSIS

Severe aplastic anemia has a poor prognosis. With conventional therapy approximately 50 per cent of the patients die within 6 months. Less than 20 per cent have spontaneous hematopoietic reconstitutions. Mild and moderate forms of the disease have a slightly better prognosis.

IRON DEFICIENCY

method of
JAMES A. STOCKMAN, III, M.D.
Northwestern University Medical School
Chicago, Illinois

Despite a wealth of information regarding the causes and prevention of iron deficiency, it remains the most common nutritional deficiency in the United States. It is particularly common in children and in women of menstruating and child-bearing age. There are only two principal reasons why iron deficiency may occur—inadequate intake and absorption of iron, and losses of iron from the body in excess of amounts ingested. Dietary iron deficiency is the more prevalent cause.

Diagnostic Considerations

Iron deficiency should not be equated with iron deficiency anemia. The depletion of body stores of iron occurs well in advance of the onset of anemia. Iron is an essential component of many enzyme systems. It has been shown, for example, that the systemic effects of iron deficiency can, and often do, precede the onset of anemia. Such signs and symptoms can include koilonychia, pagophagia, decreased exercise tolerance, irritability, stomatitis, small bowel mucosal alterations, beeturia, and poor school performance, often seen in association with hyperactivity. Iron deficiency can be present with one or more of these signs and symptoms in the absence of anemia. For these reasons, a high index of suspicion concerning the presence of iron deficiency should exist whenever one deals with a population that is at high risk for nutritional deprivation or gastrointestional bleeding. It has been suspected that metabolic alterations resulting from iron deficiency result in abnormal catecholamine, serotonin, and 5-hydroxytryptamine metabolism. Recognition of these nonhematologic manifestations of iron deficiency is critical since therapy that stops at the point of correction of anemia is unlikely to increase iron stores and sustain correction of these metabolic derangements.

Treatment

The management of dietary iron deficiency is essentially the same as for that resulting from blood loss. However, if the cause of the iron deficiency is not determined, the condition will recur after a period of time. In other words, the best treatment is prevention. In early childhood, this includes the avoidance of whole cow's milk, which contains only 0.3 to 0.8 mg per liter of iron. The introduction of whole cow's milk into the diet before 6 months of age frequently also causes gastrointestional mucosal alterations resulting in bleeding. Although human milk contains only 0.1 to 1.3 mg of iron, the enhanced absorption of iron from breast milk usually is sufficient to ward against iron deficiency until a child is 6 to 12 months of age. If solid foods are introduced into the diet in the first year of life, they should be enriched with iron or a vitamin with iron should be prescribed. Formulas enriched with iron (on the average, 12 mg per liter) are ubiquitous in this country and have been demonstrated to prevent or slowly correct iron deficiency. It has been recommended that the term infant receive approximately 1 mg per kg per day of iron in the diet during the first year of life. After this, the diet should be designed to provide 10 to 15 mg of iron per day.

The four highest iron-containing foods per serving are clams (4.2 mg of iron per 2 ounces), beef kidney (4.7 mg of iron per 2 ounces), raw oysters (3.2 mg of iron per 2 ounces), beef liver (4.7 mg of iron per 2 ounces). The highest iron-containing foods expressed per 100 grams of dry weight are cocoa powder (11.6 mg of iron), soy bean flour (13 mg of iron), and brewer's yeast (18.2 mg of iron). Additionally, lean meats, leafy green vegetables, egg yolks, meats in general, dry peas and beans, dried fruits, dark molasses, whole grain bread and cereals, nuts, and certain fruits (apricots, prunes, peaches, and raisins) are satisfactory dietary sources of iron.

Oral Iron Therapy

A wide variety of salts of iron may be given to treat iron deficiency. Ferrous sulfate is the most commonly administered salt, although ferrous gluconate, ferrous fumarate, and ferrous lactate are approximately equivalent to the ferrous sulfate salt. Ferric salts may be given, but the percentage absorbed will be less. These salts are available in both liquid and tablet forms. The elemental iron content of these preparations determines the amount of biovailable iron. Attention should be paid to the exact element iron content, which varies among preparations, especially when dealing with small children in whom intoxication with iron is always a possibility.

The usual approach to iron therapy in adults is to prescribe a single tablet of ferrous sulfate (40 to 60 mg of elemental iron) three times daily. Remember that when iron salts are taken with food, the bioavailable iron will be reduced by more than half. It is better, therefore, to recommend ingestion of medicinal iron between meals—at midmorning, midafternoon, and bedtime—if it is tolerated. Many over-the-counter preparations of iron contain ascorbic acid. Ascorbic acid facilitates iron absorption, and with its use at any given dose of iron a greater quantitative amount may be absorbed. The use of such preparations may or may not be desirable and has been noted by some to increase the frequency of gastrointestinal complaints.

In infants and younger children, the medicinal dose of iron utilized must be carefully calculated. It is recommended that 2 to 3 mg of elemental iron be administered per kg three times daily (again recalling that ferrous sulfate preparations are usually 20 per cent elemental iron). Once this quantity of iron approximates the amount that would normally be given to adults (20 to 60 mg of elemental iron three times daily), the adult recommendations may be followed. Liquid iron preparations may cause a dark discoloration of the teeth. Children taking liquid preparations must brush their teeth or drink a liberal amount of liquids following the iron administration. Iron poisoning is one of the most common forms of intoxication in young children. Adults should be warned to keep their iron prescriptions out of the reach of children.

Controversy exists about the frequency of gastrointestinal complaints related to iron ingestion. These seem to be more prevalent in adults. Complaints such as mild diarrhea or constipation may occur and appear to be unrelated to the amount of iron given. Abdominal cramping, dyspepsia, and epigastric discomfort are the most troublesome side effects; these usually occur within 2 hours following the administration of oral iron. These seem to dose-related and can be reduced by diminishing the therapeutic amount of iron given at any one time. The side effects can also be ameliorated by giving iron with meals, recognizing that the amount of bioavailable iron is diminished. There is no harm in this approach to the management of side effects of medicinal iron. The course of iron therapy will have to be lengthened, however.

In children, it has never been conclusively documented that iron preparations or the use of formulas enriched with iron causes side effects similar to those noted in adults. Delayed-release iron preparations are available and have been advocated for management of gastrointestinal side effects. However, because iron is absorbed in the upper part of the gastrointestinal tract, enteric-coated preparations significantly impair iron absorption. Their use should be restricted to patients who seem intolerant of the aforementioned maneuvers.

Expected Responses to Iron Therapy

The changes observed after iron therapy follow a sequential evolution. In 24 to 48 hours the nonhematologic manifestations of iron deficiency begin to be corrected. During this time, one might notice the disappearance of irritability and anorexia. Some patients have noted a significant feeling of energy, despite the fact the hemoglobin has not yet begun to rise. In 48 to 72 hours, the first hematologic evidence of a response to iron therapy will be seen, characterized by a rise in reticulocyte count. Maximum reticulocytosis is usually noted at about 10 days following the institution of therapy. Beginning at 3 days from the institution of iron therapy, the hemoglobin will begin to rise; the rise is indirectly proportional to the severity of the anemia when treatment starts. The hemoglobin may rise as little as 0.1 to as much as 0.35 gram per dl per day, again based on the magnitude of the original anemia. With such a response, it would be rare to see a period of greater than 6 to 8 weeks for full correction of anemia.

Once the anemia has been corrected, iron therapy should be continued for 1 to 3 months to replenish body iron stores. In an adult, this would be at least approximately 500 mg. Since correction of anemia is not an indication of the adequacy of iron store replenishment, full treatment can be verified by a determination of the serum ferritin level. Serum ferritin roughly approximates the amount of storage iron: 1 microgram per liter of serum ferritin is roughly equivalent to 10 mg of stored iron. In adults, it has been recommended that iron therapy be continued until the serum ferritin rises above 50 micrograms per liter. Specific recommendations in children have not been made.

The use of serum ferritin values also gives an indication of early recurrence of iron deficiency. Patients adequately treated for iron deficiency who are following prescribed iron-rich diets should not have recurrence; if this occurs, evidence of blood loss should be sought.

Causes of Failure to Respond to Oral Therapy

There are many reasons why iron-deficient individuals do not respond to oral iron therapy: the wrong diagnosis, the presence of a combined deficiency, failure of compliance, improper administration, improper dosage, malabsorption of iron, poor iron utilization, and iron losses in excess of the amount of therapeutic iron being given. Several disorders mimic iron deficiency, one of the most common being the presence of beta-thalassemia trait. The anemia of chronic disease may also mimic iron deficiency. Neither of these may respond to the administration of oral iron if the patient is not iron-deficient to begin with. Combined iron and folic acid deficiency may result in failure to completely respond to iron therapy alone. In these cases, hematologic correction of microcytosis may be seen. The patient then will give evidence of the macrocytic (the folate component) portion of the anemia.

Failure of compliance is one of the most frequent causes of nonresponsiveness to iron. This can be suspected if the patient's stools have not darkened during the course of iron therapy. Simple tests that determine the presence of inorganic medicinal iron in the stool are available if one wishes to verify that a patient has been noncompliant. Improper administration of iron is usually the result of taking it with food substances that tend to significantly block iron absorption. The most commonly ingested food substance that will do this is whole cow's milk, and tea is also potent chelator of inorganic iron, reducing iron absorption by as much as 95 per cent. If a patient appears to be nonresponsive, a careful history should be obtained to determine how the iron is administered and the exact dose that was given. Improper dosage is quite common, especially when patients readily attribute gastrointestinal side effects to the medicinal iron.

Some patients with iron deficiency may actually malabsorb iron. As noted previously, iron is an important constituent of many cellular systems. It has been estimated that up to 5 per cent of severely iron-deficient individuals have gastrointestinal dysfunction resulting in poor absorption of iron. These patients will continue to respond poorly to oral iron administration; other routes of therapy are desirable in these unusual cases. Finally, if a patient with iron deficiency fails to respond to appropriate doses of iron, a search for continuing blood loss should be undertaken.

Malabsorption, caused by small bowel disease, such as celiac disease, can be detected by use of an oral iron absorption test. In adults, this is done by administering 100 mg of elemental iron in the fasting state, followed by serum iron measurements at 1 and 2 hours. In an iron-deficient individual capable of absorbing orally administered iron, the increase in the serum iron level will be at least 100 micrograms per dl. In children this test can be performed using the same parameters by giving 1 mg per kg of elemental iron in the fasting state. Adults who have undergone partial gastrectomy may have a defect in the absorption of iron because of failure to acidify portions of the upper bowel.

Parenteral Iron Therapy

Parenteral iron therapy should be restricted to very specific circumstances. It is recommended when a patient is noncompliant; it may be necessary in patients who fail to absorb adequate amounts of orally administered medicinal iron. Some patients with underlying systemic disorders that impair iron absorption may respond to parenteral iron therapy. If a patient has ongoing blood loss, the amount of iron made available by the oral route may not be sufficiently tolerated to keep up with the rate of hematopoiesis. In these cases, parenteral iron is indicated and may be necessary on multiple occasions if the cause of blood loss cannot be determined or corrected. Examples of these are patients with hereditary hemorrhagic telangiectasias or uncontrolled inflammatory bowel disease with blood loss. Parenteral iron administration carries a greater risk than does oral iron therapy, and its use must be restricted to these specific circumstances. All other things aside, parenteral iron administration is not expected to produce a greater rise in hemoglobin than orally administered medicinal iron.

The commonly used form of parenteral iron in the United States is iron dextran (Imferon). This preparation consists of a complex of ferric hydroxide and dextran resulting in a molecular weight of approximately 6000 daltons. This preparation may be given intramuscularly or intravenously. When given intramuscularly, the iron dextran complex is removed from the injection site by the lymphatic circulation over several days to a week. The dextran moiety is split from the iron by the reticuloendothelial system; iron is then bioavailable for hematopoiesis. Serum iron may reach extraordinarily high levels soon after administration of iron dextran. This does not produce toxicity since iron is still complexed in a relatively nontoxic moiety. It is the reticuloendothelial cell that disengages the iron, allowing it to be transferred by serum transferrin to the hemoglobin-synthesizing bone marrow cell. If the intramuscular route is utilized, the drug must be administered by a deep zig-zag intramuscular injection. Iron dextran deposited in the upper layers of the skin will produce a tatoo, which the zig-zag administration is designed to prevent.

It has recently become apparent that the most efficient way to administer iron dextran preparations is by the intravenous route. Iron dextran contains 50 mg elemental iron per ml. It should be diluted substantially. In adults, the optimal approach is the total dose infusion method, in which the calculated dose of iron dextran is diluted in 500 ml of saline. Adverse reactions certainly may occur. Anaphylaxis has been noted. To minimize this risk, at the start of the infusion a small test dose should be given over 10 minutes (10 drops per minute). If no adverse reactions are noted, the remainder of the iron can be infused over 4 to 6 hours. Presumably, the risk of anaphylaxis increases with repetitive administrations of iron dextran. For these reasons, whenever the drug is administered resuscitative equipment should be available. Most reactions are seen in patients who have never previously been given iron dextran, and some feel that the risk does not increase with repeated injections.

The amount of iron administered via the parenteral route may be calculated from the following formula:

$$\text{Total iron (mg)} = \frac{\Delta Hb}{100} \times \text{blood volume} \times 3.4$$

With this formula, hemoglobin deficit (ΔHb) is expressed as grams per dl and the blood volume may be estimated by multiplying the weight of the patient times 75 ml per kg. The value 3.4 is the number of milligrams of iron contained in 1 gram of hemoglobin. To the amount of iron calculated in the formula should be added approximately 500 mg of "storage iron" for adults. A lesser amount of stored iron may be used for infants and small children. Other iron complexes are available for use as an alternative to iron dextran.

In other parts of the world, iron sorbitol–gluconate complex has undergone preliminary trials. This agent seems to have a lower risk of anaphylaxis. Iron sorbitol–citric acid complex also is associated with fewer anaphylactic side effects. However, the complex is much less firmly bound and results in higher levels of free iron over short periods of time. This may result in headache, hypotension, flushing, and shock. This drug is given by daily intramuscular injections. For all the reasons noted, iron dextran seems to remain the favored drug when indications are present for the parenteral administration of iron.

AUTOIMMUNE HEMOLYTIC ANEMIA

method of
LESLIE E. SILBERSTEIN, M.D.,
and DOUGLAS B. CINES, M.D.
University of Pennsylvania
Philadelphia, Pennsylvania

GENERAL PRINCIPLES

In most cases, autoimmune hemolytic anemia (AHA) is a chronic disorder, caused by antibodies directed at the patient's own erythrocytes. The approach to the management of AHA depends, in part, on whether the disease is primary or secondary to disorders such as B cell malignancies and systemic lupus erythematosus (SLE). Other factors that determine the initial therapy include the temperature at which the antibody binds to the red cell (cold or warm-reactive) and the isotype (IgG versus IgM) of the autoantibody.

The goal of therapy is the alleviation of symptomatic anemia while minimizing the complications of the therapy itself. When AHA accompanies SLE or a malignant lymphoma, therapy of the underlying disorder may be sufficient to control the rate of hemolysis. In addition to the specific therapy to be detailed, patients with most forms of chronic hemolytic anemia are often advised to take folate, 1 mg orally daily, in view of possible additional requirements imposed by the accelerated rate of hematopoiesis.

The end point of therapy is not the normalization of the direct antiglobulin test (DAT). Patients may have positive direct antiglobulin tests without hemolysis or without anemia. This is often the case with the autoantibodies that develop following methyldopa (Aldomet) or L-dopa administration and antibodies of the IgG_4 subclass. Occasional patients with AHA may demonstrate well-compensated hemolysis with symptomatic anemia only following episodes of infection. Furthermore, occasional patients may have symptomatic AHA with a negative DAT. Finally, the most common forms of therapy, detailed below, may raise the level of hemoglobin whereas the DAT may remain positive.

WARM AHA

Corticosteroids

For adult patients with either the idiopathic or the secondary forms of warm AHA, corticosteroids are the initial therapy of choice. Therapy is initiated with prednisone, at a dosage of 1 to 2 mg per kg per day, depending on the severity of the anemia and the rate of hemolysis. Approximately 70 to 80 per cent of patients will respond to this dosage; a somewhat higher dose may be required in an additional 10 to 20 per cent of patients. An occasional patient will show complete resistance to prednisone at any dose. The reticulocyte count begins to fall between the 5th and 14th days of therapy, but sometimes a fall may occur within the first 2 days. In the usual case, the hemoglobin level rises at a rate of 2 to 3 grams per week. Over 90 per cent of responses to corticosteroids will occur within the first 3 weeks of therapy.

The initial clinical response to corticosteroids results primarily from their effect on tissue macrophages, which become less efficient in clearing IgG or C3-coated cells. In some cases, corticosteroids also may impair the binding of red cell antibodies to the erythrocyte. Only following several weeks of therapy is a significant fall in antibody production observed. Therefore, the initial response to prednisone often is not accompanied by a corresponding fall in the degree of sensitization of the red cells with IgG antibody.

Among adults, permanent remissions of AHA are observed in less than 20 per cent of the cases. Therefore, subsequent therapy is based on the presumption that clinical relapse is likely to occur. Following the initial clinical response, the schedule with which steroids are tapered depends, in part, on the severity of the initial presentation and the severity of side effects from therapy. In the absence of significant contraindications, prednisone is continued at the initial dose until the hemoglobin reaches a level of 10 grams per dl. Prednisone is then gradually tapered to 20 mg over the next 4 to 6 weeks and further tapered as tolerated over the next 3 to 4 months. The results from large series have shown that about half the patients will require 5 to 20 mg of prednisone per day to maintain a relatively normal level of hemoglobin. An additional 15 to 20 per cent of patients prove dependent on prednisone at even higher doses. Even patients who are well compensated may develop rapidly worsening hemolysis and a falling reticulocyte count during intercurrent viral or bacterial infections. Increased prednisone may be required at this time.

Splenectomy

The subsequent therapeutic decisions in warm AHA are based on the need to maintain an adequate level of hemoglobin and the need to avoid the complications of long-term steroid administration or immunosuppression. In the elderly patient who is mildly anemic, therapy with prednisone at a dose of 10 mg daily for an indefinite period of time may be the best alternative therapy. In contrast, in most young patients with idiopathic AHA, serious consideration must be given to splenectomy at some point during the illness. There is a 1 to 2 per cent risk of developing the overwhelming postsplenectomy sepsis syndrome immediately following surgery, but bacterial infections occur long after the postoperative period as well. These risks may be reduced by the use of pneumococcal and meningococcal vaccines and by the prompt use of antibiotics for each febrile illness. The morbidity of splenectomy may be increased in elderly patients and in those with the secondary forms of AHA.

Indications for splenectomy include failure to respond to prednisone, dependence on prednisone dosages that exceed 10 to 20 mg per day, or intractable steroid-related side effects. The preoperative criteria of age, presence or absence of an underlying B cell disorder, the serologic profile of the DAT, response to prednisone, or pattern of sequestration of ^{51}Cr-labeled red cells cannot be used alone to predict the response to splenectomy. Patients whose red cells are less heavily sensitized with IgG may be more likely to show a complete response to steroids and to splenectomy, although there are exceptions to this generalization. The role of splenectomy in patients with mixed IgG, IgM, or mixed cold and warm reactive IgG antibodies requires further definition. The spleen functions both as a major site of red cell sequestration and as a significant source of antibody synthesis. Approximately 50 to 60 per cent of patients will have a good to excellent initial response to splenectomy and will require less than 15 mg of prednisone a day to maintain an adequate level of hemoglobin. Late relapses do occur, presumably caused by enhanced antibody synthesis and hepatic sequestration. Little information is available regarding the presence or clinical significance of accessory spleens in warm AHA.

Immunosuppressive Therapy

The use of immunosuppressive therapy should be considered only for symptomatic patients (1) who fail to respond to splenectomy or who relapse following splenectomy, (2) for whom splenectomy represents an unacceptable medical risk, or (3) who have serious side effects from corticosteroids. Most published data in warm AHA have been obtained using 6-mercaptopurine (80 mg per M^2 per day) or cyclophosphamide (60 mg per M^2 per day) (this use is not listed in the manufacturer's directive). The latter drug has gained favor in several other hematologic disorders caused by autoantibodies. These initial doses must be carefully adjusted depending on the neutrophil and platelet counts. Therapy should be continued as tolerated for at least 3 months to insure maximal inhibition of antibody synthesis. Approximately 40 per cent of patients respond with a rise in the hemoglobin that can be maintained at significantly reduced doses of prednisone. This response rate may be overly optimistic since it may be based on the publication of series with more favorable results.

In addition to the depression of hematopoiesis, the long-term use of these drugs may impair the normal immune response, with an increased risk of certain infections and neoplasia. The use of cyclophosphamide, an alkylating agent, is also associated with the risk of developing hemorrhagic cystitis and the potential to develop myeloid leukemia. Because of concerns with the long-term side effects of these drugs, their initial use should be restricted to severe cases and attempts should be made to discontinue their use gradually in the responsive patient.

Additional Forms of Therapy

Plasma Exchange. This lowers the serum level of IgG in normal individuals and has proved to be effective in a number of disorders mediated by IgG antibodies, such as myasthenia gravis and Goodpasture's syndrome. However, the efficacy of exchange is limited in warm AHA (WAHA) by the continuous antibody production and the large extravascular distribution of IgG. Experience with plasma exchange has been gained in isoimmune hemolytic anemia of pregnancy. Mothers whose children are at risk for isoimmune hemolytic disease have serum levels of IgG antibody of between 10 and 100 micrograms per ml. In most cases, a weekly plasma exchange of 1 to 1.5 plasma volumes is effective in lowering the level of antibody by at least 50 per cent. There is far less information in WAHA, where most autoantibody is present on the cell itself rather than in the plasma as in isoimmune hemolytic anemia. In addition, upon cessation of therapy the return to preapheresis levels of antibody will depend on the rate of autoantibody production. However, occasional dramatic responses have been reported in patients who are being prepared for surgery or as a temporizing measure following the initiation of immunosuppressive therapy.

Vinca Alkaloids. Vincristine (Oncovin) and vinblastine (Velban) have been effective in about a third of patients who produce antiplatelet antibodies, presumably by interfering with the ability of macrophages to bind or ingest IgG-coated cells. Responses in a few patients with WAHA have been reported following infusion with vincristine-laden, IgG-coated platelets as a vehicle for delivery of the drug to the macrophage. Reported responses have been of long duration and associated with a delayed fall in the titer of the DAT. In idiopathic thrombocytopenic purpura (ITP), weekly intravenous injections of vincristine (1 to 2 mg) or intravenous infusions of vinblastine (5 to 10 mg over 4 to 6 hours) also have been efficacious, although there is limited information about the response rate for either drug in WAHA, when given in this manner. (This therapeutic use of vinca alkaloids is not listed in the manufacturer's directive.)

Other Modalities. Danazol (Danocrine), an attenuated synthetic androgen, also has proved efficacious in patients with idiopathic thrombocytopenic purpura when given in a dose of 400 to 600 mg orally daily and has proved to be of benefit in some patients with refractory WAHA. Remission durations of up to 1 year associated with a fall in the titer of the DAT have been reported. Intravenous gamma globulin (400 mg per kg daily for 5 days) also has been shown effective for managing subacute emergencies in idiopathic thrombocytopenic purpura. It is possible that the drug may bind to Fc receptors on macrophages and thereby increase the life span of circulating cells coated with IgG antibody. Therefore, this drug may prove to have an adjunctive role in the management of WAHA as well. In view of the relatively low risk of long-term side effects, danazol may be used in the future with increasing frequency in the management of steroid-dependent patients. However, additional experience will be necessary to determine both the duration of therapy and the proper role of this drug in WAHA.

Transfusions

Transfusion therapy represents a special hazard in patients with warm AHA. The patient's red cells are coated with immunoglobulin, precluding a direct analysis of their surface antigens. Furthermore, since most of the clinically significant antibodies in WAHA are "panagglutinins," the serum of these patients cannot be directly evaluated for the presence of alloantibodies that could initiate severe hemolytic transfusion reactions.

Therefore, transfusions must be reserved for the acute therapy of patients with anemia of life-threatening severity. Symptoms requiring transfusion include angina or neurologic disturbances, which often begin as lethargy, but which may progress to coma. Symptomatic patients should be maximally oxygenated while placed at rest; more definitive therapy must begin coincident with transfusions. Blood should always be transfused slowly under direct supervision, and signs and symptoms of accelerated hemolysis should be watched for. The amount of blood transfused should be guided by the alleviation of symptoms rather than by seeking to establish a specific level of hemoglobin. Transfusion of as little as 100 to 200 ml of blood may be sufficient for symptomatic relief of patients with moderate rates of hemolysis and well-compensated anemia. Furthermore, many patients are in a partially compensated state of high output congestive heart failure prior to receiving transfusions. Patients who receive the additional intravascular colloid load of transfusion may develop pulmonary edema.

In the acute circumstance, blood must be found that carries the least risk for producing acute intravascular hemolysis which may be caused by a coexisting alloantibody. The presence of an alloantibody should be suspected when the indirect Coombs' test shows a stronger reaction than the direct antiglobulin test. To identify the "least incompatible unit," warm autoantibodies can be eluted from the patient's erythrocytes by one of several established techniques. If the patient has not received a recent transfusion, the patient's red cells can then be used to absorb residual warm autoantibodies from his or her own serum. Following several steps involving autoabsorption, the patient's serum will no longer place IgG on autologous cells. This serum can then be evaluated for the presence of alloantibodies in the conventional manner.

Following elution of the autoantibodies by this

technique, the phenotype of the patient's red cells can also be directly evaluated, using conventional antigen-specific typing sera. This information allows the blood bank to provide red cells whose antigenic phenotype closely matches that of the patient. Additional information about the antigenic phenotype also can be obtained by incubation with antisera of known specificity. Following incubation, the residual antisera can be retested against a panel of normal typing cells and evaluated for loss of reactivity.

The "differential absorption" test is another test that can be used. It is predicated on the fact that a relatively small number of pre-existing serum alloantibodies are responsible for most clinically severe acute hemolytic transfusion reactions. Therefore, it is most important to detect warm-reactive antibodies against the Rh, Kell, Kidd, and Duffy antigens. Serum from patients with WAHA is first incubated with an excess of erythrocytes that lack the antigen in question (i.e., Jk^a-negative cells) in order to absorb out the panagglutinins. The serum is then tested for residual antibody using the antigen positive (Jk^a-positive) cell. For occasional patients, the panagglutinin itself may have a "relative specificity" within the Rh system, allowing cells lacking the corresponding Rh antigen to be used for further transfusion.

In vivo tests of compatibility have been developed based upon the survival of an aliquot of ^{51}Cr-labeled red cells from a prospective unit which is to be transfused. While a normal 1 hour survival of these cells indicates that there is little risk of severe hemolysis, a relatively shortened survival time has not been shown to preclude successful transfusion of that unit of blood.

Some patients have been reported to show a better response to red cells that have been washed free of plasma complement, although this has not been found to be of sufficient benefit in most cases to warrant the additional time, expense, and risks of infection associated with routinely preparing red cells in this manner.

We wish to emphasize that all red cells transfused to a patient with WAHA are incompatible to a varying degree and will have a reduced intravascular survival. Although additional serologic tests (i.e., autoabsorption) may detect a coexisting alloantibody, the transfusion of erythrocytes lacking the corresponding antigen does not necessarily guarantee a longer survival. The tests that can easily be done and should be performed when at all possible before transfusion include determination of the patient's red cell phenotype and the relative specificity of the autoantibody within the Rh system. Therefore, transfusion of symptomatic patients should not be delayed for the sole reason of performing additional serologic tests.

COLD AGGLUTININ SYNDROMES

The preferred therapy for the cold agglutinin syndromes depends upon the severity of the symptomatology, the serologic characteristics of the autoantibody, and the nature of the underlying disease, if present. The extent of hemolysis primarily depends on the thermal amplitude of the antibody. For example, cold-reactive antibodies that develop after viral or mycoplasmal infection usually do not show significant reactivity above 30 C regardless of their titer at 4 C; therefore, most patients do not hemolyze and are occasionally adequately treated simply by keeping them warm. In contrast, significant hemolysis occurs frequently in patients having low titers of antibodies that retain reactivity above 30 C, and remaining in a warm environment may be insufficient in these cases.

Three questions must be addressed when a patient has symptomatic cold autoimmune hemolytic anemia (CAHA): (1) Does the patient have idiopathic CAHA or the secondary form, which is often associated with an underlying malignancy? (2) Can the rate of hemolysis be decreased with steroids or splenectomy, as in warm AHA? (3) When and how should the patient be transfused?

Patients with idiopathic CAHA often have moderately severe, partially compensated anemia. Periods of fatigue and malaise are the major symptoms in most patients. Prolonged survival is common, and the disease may show spontaneous remissions and exacerbations. In almost all cases, chronic idiopathic cold agglutinins are IgM kappa monoclonal proteins directed at the "I" antigen. In contrast, antibodies that contain lambda light chains and specificities outside the "I" region occur more commonly in the secondary forms of the disorder. Furthermore, patients with idiopathic CAHA as a rule do not have lymphadenopathy or splenomegaly. As many as 25 per cent of cold agglutinins may be cryoprecipitable. This finding may relate to the development of acrocyanosis, Raynaud's phenomenon, ischemic digital infarcts, or ulcers, which occasionally dominate the clinicial symptomatology in either form of disease.

Medical therapy of idiopathic CAHA is generally unsatisfactory. Having the patient remain in a warm environment may be sufficient when the antibody shows minimal activity at 30 C. Steroids have been successful in occasional patients with cold agglutinins when the antibody has a high thermal amplitude but is present only in low titer, or when an IgG cold-reactive antibody is found. Consequently, steroids are not efficacious in most patients with idiopathic CAHA, although this has not been adequately evaluated. Similarly, splenectomy is not usually effective, presumably because the liver is the dominant site of sequestration of red cells heavily sensitized with C3. Chronic administration of oral alkylating agents helps many patients with the secondary forms of CAHA but is only occasionally successful in patients with the idiopathic form of the disease who have high titers of circulating IgM antibody. Plasma exchange may be effective in acute situations and can be considered as a temporary measure. The use of "inline" blood warmers is advisable; and more elaborate measures to perform the entire exchange process at 37 C are occasionally required.

When the presence of cold agglutinins is part of an established B cell malignancy, such as a lymphoma, Waldenström's macroglobulinemia, or chronic lymphocytic leukemia, the severity of hemolysis often waxes and wanes in parallel with the underlying process. Therapy for the malignancy with prednisone and an alkylating agent is often sufficient to control the rate of hemolysis as well. Occasionally, splenectomy or other therapy directed specifically toward the CAHA is required. The advanced age of the patients and underlying illnesses limit the therapeutic goals and options in this group, and rarely can the control of hemolysis be obtained without control of the malignancy. In a recent series, the median survival was 2 years in patients with CAHA and lymphoma, 2.5 years in those with CAHA and Waldenström's macroglobulinemia, and 6 years in patients with CAHA and CLL.

Since most of these therapies have little practical impact on the management of CAHA, patients with mild, compensated anemia are often not treated for long periods of time or may require only episodic transfusions. The routine use of washed red cells has also been recommended to limit the infusion of complement, which may augment the clearance of transfused red blood cells. Cross-matching is technically less difficult in cold AHA than in warm AHA since few cold agglutinins are reactive when the cross-match is performed at 37 C. Residual IgM activity can be removed with 2-mercaptoethanol. Because of the limited responsiveness of CAHA to current therapy, a trial of danazol (Danocrine) may benefit some patients. During transfusion the patient should be kept warm and the blood should be administered through an inline warmer.

NONIMMUNE HEMOLYTIC ANEMIA

method of
BERNARD J. DREILING, M.D.,
and MARTIN H. STEINBERG, M.D.
Veterans Administration Hospital
Jackson, Mississippi

There is no completely satisfactory classification of the hemolytic diseases. Traditionally they are grouped into disorders in which the red cell itself is at fault (intracorpuscular defects) and those in which the cell environment plays the major role (extracorpuscular defects). The former are generally inherited, the latter acquired. Another, more useful classification is based on the primary site of red cell destruction. In the more common extravascular hemolysis, red cells are removed by cells of the reticuloendothelial system, whereas in intravascular hemolysis the cells are lysed in the blood. Because proper treatment depends on accurate identification of the cause of hemolysis, an understanding of the laboratory manifestations of intravascular and extravascular hemolysis is essential (Table 1). The clinical conditions associated with primary intravascular and extravascular hemolysis are listed in Table 2.

TREATMENT

Acquired Disorders

Erythrocyte Fragmentation Syndromes. Mechanical destruction of red cells in the circulation is seen in several circumstances, the diagnostic feature being found in the blood smear in the form of irregularly contracted or schistocytic red cells.

The most common of the fragmentation syndromes is probably traumatic cardiac hemolysis. Though reported to occur with calcific aortic and tight mitral stenoses, most cases have been associated with a leaking artificial aortic valve. Iron supplements are needed and are best given as ferrous sulfate, 300 mg three times daily. Because of the demands of increased cell turnover, folic acid, 1 mg daily, is also beneficial. Since the degree of hemolysis is dependent on cardiac output, reduction of physical activity, bed rest, and transfusion with packed red cells may be appropriate. Replacement or correction of the defective valve is sometimes required.

Though mechanical destruction of red cells may occur in marching soldiers, distance runners, bongo drummers and martial artists, most often it is mild and unrecognized. Adequate protection of pressure areas is advised when hemolysis is significant.

TABLE 1. **Laboratory Manifestations of Hemolytic Disease**

Evidence of increased red cell production		
	Polychromasia	
	Reticulocytosis	
	Marrow erythroid hyperplasia	
Evidence of increased red cell destruction		
	Extravascular hemolysis	
		Elevated carbon monoxide
		Unconjugated bilirubinemia
		Increased fecal and urinary urobilinogen
		Elevated plasma lactate dehydrogenase
	Intravascular hemolysis	
		Haptoglobin depletion
		Hemoglobinemia
		Hemoglobinuria
		Hemopexin depletion
		Methemalbuminemia
		Hemosiderinuria
Direct evidence of shortened red cell survival		
	Decreased radiochromium red cell half-life	

Microangiopathic Hemolytic Disorders. The common denominator is an abnormality of the vascular endothelium of small blood vessels. When clotting occurs, red cells must pass through fibrin-filled vessels. The force of the flowing blood causes the cell to fragment and schistocytes appear in the blood. Disseminated intravascular coagulation and thrombotic thrombocytopenic purpura are discussed elsewhere. The closely related hemolytic-uremic syndrome, formerly thought to be primarily a pediatric problem, is now seen as a constellation of clinical and laboratory findings resulting from a variety of unrelated causes. In addition to the classic form seen in young children, postinfectious, hereditary, and immunologic forms and forms related to pregnancy and the use of oral contraceptives have been described in adults. Plasma infusion, plasmapheresis, and exchange transfusion are currently in vogue and have led to a marked decrease in the hematologic and renal manifestations, but the prognosis, especially in the puerperal type, is still grave.

Hypersplenism. Any disease that causes splenomegaly can result in hypersplenism. It should be considered whenever cytopenia occurs in the presence of an enlarged spleen because splenectomy may be curative. Characteristics of the syndrome are splenomegaly, anemia, thrombocytopenia, and neutropenia, or any combination thereof, in association with generalized bone marrow hyperplasia. Because of the frequent association with other disorders, the underlying cause of the hypersplenism needs to be identified.

Treatment of the underlying illness may shrink the spleen and cure the hypersplenism. When splenectomy is contemplated, it must be kept in mind that life-threatening thrombosis or bleeding may occur and prophylaxis with platelet disaggregating agents or anticoagulants may be necessary. The risk of overwhelming infection, mentioned later in this section, is a relative contraindication. Though the pancytopenia accompanying portal hypertension is readily reversible with splenectomy, this is usually not necessary. Blood counts are rarely low enough to place the patient at significant risk for bleeding or infection. In fact, the risk of surgery usually outweighs the benefit of splenectomy.

Paroxysmal Nocturnal Hemoglobinuria (PNH). Though not common, this is a fascinating acquired disease, resulting from clonal production of abnormal stem cells that produce red cells, granulocytes, and platelets with both membrane and enzyme defects. The red cell abnormality results in excessive binding of the third component of complement, with intravascular lysis of the cell. For reasons still obscure, cell lysis may be greatest at night and may be paroxysmal, sometimes associated with infections. In most patients hemolysis is perpetual, resulting in chronic hemosiderinuria and iron deficiency.

In the anemic iron-deficient patient with PNH, oral doses of iron may permit rapid proliferation of complement-sensitive cells and an increase in the severity of hemolysis. Hypertransfusion prior to or prednisone (60 mg daily) during the initial 1 to 2 weeks of iron therapy will prevent this. Transfusions should always be given carefully and as washed packed red cells, since plasma has been known to precipitate hemolysis. Thrombotic complications are common in patients with paroxysmal nocturnal hemoglobinuria, and hepatic vein thrombosis is one of the major causes of death. Though there are reports of exaggerated hemolysis with heparin therapy, the risk is small and full dose intravenous heparinization is warranted. Hemolysis in PNH patients can often be ameliorated by every other day prednisone therapy in a dose of 20 to 50 mg. The response is often abrupt and sustained. In patients with relative bone marrow hypoproliferation, oxymethalone in a daily dose of 150 to 200 mg may be of benefit. Because of thrombotic complications, surgery and pregnancy are poorly tolerated and are best managed with hypertransfusion and alternate day corticosteroids. Though still too risky a procedure for most patients, the ideal treatment

TABLE 2. **Conditions Associated with Hemolysis**

Intravascular	
	Fragmentation hemolytic disorders
	Paroxysmal nocturnal hemoglobinuria
	Paroxysmal cold hemoglobinuria
	Acute G6PD hemolysis
	ABO incompatibility reactions
	Unstable hemoglobinopathies
	Clostridium welchii sepsis
	Severe burns
Extravascular	
	Hereditary spherocytosis
	Most hemoglobinopathies
	Autoimmune hemolysis
	Hypersplenism
	Erythrocyte enzymopathies
	Delayed transfusion reactions

for PNH would be bone marrow transplantation, replacing the abnormal clone with normal ones. The terminal event in some patients may be acute granulocytic leukemia.

Other Acquired Hemolytic Disorders. Anemia is common in patients with *liver disease* and is multifactorial. Among the several mechanisms of hemolysis are splenic sequestration, spur cell anemia, stomatocytosis, impaired red cell metabolism, acute phosphate depletion, and Zieve syndrome. Except for phosphate repletion in the hypophosphatemic patient, treatment is directed at the underlying liver disease. Though the anemia of *renal failure* has a hemolytic component, marrow suppression by as yet undefined myelotoxic and erythropoietin-related factors are of greater significance.

Inherited Hemolytic Disorders

Hemolytic anemia can be associated with genetically determined disorders of the hemoglobin molecule, of erythrocyte metabolism, and of the erythrocyte membrane. The most prevalent of the hemoglobin disorders, sickle cell diseases and the thalassemias, are covered elsewhere. At our present level of knowledge, no therapeutic approaches to these disorders directly alter the basic gene mutation. We are left with the following options: (1) Population screening, heterozygote detection, and prenatal diagnoses, most applicable and useful in the thalassemias and sickling disorders. (2) Avoiding agents or situations in which hemolysis may be instigated or intensified. Avoiding "oxidant" drugs in G6PD deficiency and unstable hemoglobin disorders exemplifies this option. (3) Transfusion, when the anemia becomes symptomatic. (4) Splenectomy, when removal of this major site of erythrocyte destruction has been associated with prolongation of red cell life, as in hereditary spherocytosis. (5) General attention to preserving good health, nutrition, and folic acid sufficiency. If hemolysis is severe and chronic, then folic acid, 1 mg daily, is recommended.

Hemoglobinopathies Other Than Sickle Cell Disease and Thalassemia. Some clinical features of the common hemoglobinopathies are shown in Table 3. Heterozygotes for HbE or HbC are virtually normal. The HbAE individual has mild microcytosis. This is due to the HbE gene, and in the absence of coexistent iron deficiency, it does not respond to iron supplementation. Homozygotes for HbC may be mildly anemic and have splenomegaly. This requires no therapy because the degree of hemolysis is mild. Homozygotes with HbE have microcytic erythrocytes but, in the absence of complicating problems, have minimal anemia and require no therapy. HbE and HbC are extremely common hemoglobin variants. By themselves they are innocuous; however, when they coexist with β-thalassemias or sickle cell hemoglobin they can be associated with severe anemia and other problems. For this reason, some have advocated screening for these disorders and educating carriers in populations where their prevalence is high.

Unstable hemoglobins occur sporadically in the world's population, often are the result of a new mutation, and are associated with hemolytic anemia of varying severity. In some patients, hemolysis is prompted by drugs. The spleen may be enlarged, and some patients' anemia improves following splenectomy. This response is far from uniform, and the degree of anemia in many patients does not warrant this operation. Patients should be cautioned to avoid "oxidant" drugs like sulfonamides and certain antimalarial drugs.

The M hemoglobins result from amino acid substitutions that permit heme iron to remain in its Fe^{+++} form. Ferric heme cannot participate in oxygen transport, and patients have cyanosis that begins at birth or within the first half year of life. They are, however, asymptomatic. Treatment is not needed, and it is important that therapeutic misadventures not be embarked upon in an attempt to reverse this irreversible cyanosis.

Erythrocyte Enzymopathies. In numerous instances a deficiency or abnormality of one of the enzymes of glycolysis, the pentose phosphate pathway, glutathione metabolism, nucleotide metabolism, or other erythrocyte metabolic pathway has been associated with hemolytic anemia. None of these genetic abnormalities are curable, and the treatment available consists solely of splenectomy in selected instances, transfusion (rarely indicated), and the avoidance of drugs that might provoke or intensify hemolysis. Fortunately, hemolysis is most often mild and needs no treatment, and most of the enzymopathies are very rare.

G6PD Deficiency. Erythrocyte glucose-6-phosphate dehydrogenase (G6PD) deficiency is one of the most prevalent genetically determined human disorders. Numerous varieties account for several different clinical syndromes—congenital hemolytic disease, favism, chronic hemolytic anemia, and drug-induced hemolytic anemia. The variety of G6PD deficiency common in populations of the Mediterranean basin is associated with favism and chronic hemolysis. G6PD deficiency in blacks is characterized by hemolysis only when provoked by "oxidant" drugs or some other "stress."

There is no treatment for any of the types of G6PD deficiency. Fortunately, the disease is rarely serious and is frequently asymptomatic. Patients should be cautioned to refrain from tak-

TABLE 3. **Hemoglobinopathies and Hemolysis**

Disorder	*Distribution*	*PCV*	*Clinical Features*
HbAE	Southeast Asia	Normal	Mild microcytosis
HbEE	Southeast Asia	Normal—slightly reduced	Target cells and microcytosis
HbAC	Africa	Normal	Target cells
HbCC	Africa	Slightly reduced	Target cells, spherocytes, splenomegaly
Unstable hemoglobin	Sporadic	Normal to reduced	Hemolyic anemia, drug-induced
HbM	Sporadic	Slightly reduced	Cyanosis

ing drugs known to provoke hemolysis. The commonest of this group are some antimalarials, sulfonamides, and nitrofurantoins. When hemolysis occurs in black men with G6PD deficiency, it is almost never severe. At times, if continuation of the drug that is presumed to have led to hemolysis is deemed critical to the patient's well-being, it may be continued and the hemolysis will abate as the blood is repopulated by a cohort of young erythrocytes that have higher enzyme levels. Occasionally neonates with hemolytic disease require exchange transfusion. Otherwise, transfusions are rarely needed in the hemolysis of G6PD deficiency, nor is splenectomy advocated.

Pyruvate kinase (PK) deficiency may be the most prevalent enzymopathy after G6PD deficiency, but it is a rare disorder. The anemia may be severe, and splenectomy has been effective in raising the hemoglobin level. Transfusions are occasionally needed, especially in children, and their use can be eliminated, or drastically reduced, by splenectomy. There is some indication that salicylates may injure PK-deficient cells; these should be avoided.

Disorders of the Erythrocyte Membrane. Hereditary spherocytosis constitutes a group of disorders caused by qualitative or quantitative abnormalities of one or another of the proteins that make up the erythrocyte membrane skeleton. The variable proportion of spherocytes present and the degree of hemolysis reflect, in all likelihood, the heterogeneous nature of the molecular abnormality. Some individuals have no anemia, minimal hemolysis, few spherocytes, and only a small population of osmotically sensitive cells. These patients rarely need treatment, and splenectomy is probably not indicated. Patients with more intense hemolytic disease may benefit clinically from splenectomy. When the spleen is removed, the reticulocyte count falls to nearly normal levels as the erythrocyte lifespan rises toward normal. This may relieve the patient from the considerable metabolic burden that the body assumes, since in some instances of hereditary spherocytosis the production of erythrocytes is nearly ten times normal, or about 200 ml daily. Return of anemia following splenectomy may indicate the presence of functioning accessory spleens. Cholelithiasis is common in individuals with chronic hemolytic anemia and may occur at remarkably young ages. Splenectomy, by eliminating hemolysis, curtails the development of gallstones. When stones are already present, and if they are asymptomatic, it may be best to observe the patient and not perform a cholecystectomy, although there are few data upon which to base a firm recommendation.

As in any chronic hemolytic anemia, temporary cessation of erythropoiesis can rapidly lead to profound anemia. These aplastic crises, apparently caused by human parvovirus infection, often require prompt transfusion with packed erythrocytes. Other than these sporadic episodes, transfusions are rarely needed.

The decision whether to perform a splenectomy in hereditary spherocytosis must weigh the following: the severity of hemolysis, upon which is predicated the likelihood of severe aplastic crisis and development of cholelithiasis, and the intra- and perioperative complications of the operation, the most serious of which is possible fulminant postsplenectomy sepsis. When possible, splenectomy should be delayed until the patient reaches age 6 or more years.

Hereditary Elliptocytosis and Pyropoikilocytosis. Like hereditary spherocytosis, these disorders are quite heterogeneous and are due to a number of different molecular causes. They may not produce detectable hemolysis, and the blood film may contain elliptocytic erythrocytes. Rare patients may have marked hemolysis and bizarre red cell morphology. In patients with hemolytic disease of sufficient severity to cause significant anemia, splenectomy may be useful, although it less reproducibly abolishes hemolysis, as is the case in hereditary spherocytosis.

PERNICIOUS ANEMIA AND OTHER MEGALOBLASTIC ANEMIAS

method of
ROBERT J. JACOBSON, M.B.
Georgetown University
Washington, D.C.

The electronic particle counters in common use today in hematology laboratories routinely determine the red blood cell mean corpuscular volume (MCV) of patients and alert physicians to the possibility of megaloblastic anemia. An elevated MCV may not always be due to macrocytic red cells, and correlation with the peripheral blood smear is essential. A prominent reticulocytosis and cold agglutinins are two examples of situations causing an elevated MCV without macrocytosis. For the most part, however, an elevated MCV is produced by macrocytic red cells, and it is important to determine whether megaloblastosis is present in the marrow erythroid precursors. Macrocytosis often without megaloblastosis can be found in association with liver disease, myelodysplastic syndromes, and acute and chronic leukemias, and following therapy with cytotoxic drugs. The clinical history, physical examination, and other striking blood and bone marrow findings, particularly in leukemia and preleukemic syndromes, contribute to establishing these diagnoses. In adults the commonest causes (over 90 per cent) of megaloblastic anemias are deficiencies of vitamin B_{12} or folic acid.

While the blood and bone marrow morphology cannot be used to distinguish vitamin B_{12} (cobalamin) deficiency from folic acid deficiency, neurologic abnormalities, particularly of the posterior and lateral columns, point to a vitamin B_{12} deficiency. A history of alcoholism or pregnancy indicates the megaloblastic anemia is most likely due to a dietary lack of folic acid. Laboratory studies offer the most reliable means of diagnosing vitamin B_{12} and folic acid deficiency. When patients present with megaloblastic anemia, determination of serum vitamin B_{12} and folic acid should be obtained immediately. A Schilling test, which shows correction of vitamin B_{12} malabsorption when intrinsic factor is added, and serum intrinsic factor antibody are diagnostic of pernicious anemia. (It is important to note that the flushing dose of vitamin B_{12} [usually 1000 μg] administered at the start of the Schilling test is therapeutic.) The availability and reliability of serum vitamin measurements and the other diagnostic tests have made 7 to 10 day therapeutic trials with small doses of either vitamin B_{12} or folic acid virtually unnecessary. Because of the hematologic responsiveness (albeit not complete) of either vitamin B_{12} or folate deficiency to large doses of the other vitamin, "shotgun" therapy must be avoided. Not only does it diagnostically mislead the physician but also of particular concern is that *in cobalamin-deficient patients, 100 μg or more of folic acid may improve the hematologic picture, but neurologic manifestations can progress and may become irreversible.*

Patients with vitamin B_{12} deficiency occasionally present severe neurologic features out of proportion to their mild anemia. In many of these patients megaloblastosis and hypersegmented neutrophils are evident in the blood and bone marrow. These patients may give a history of eating a diet rich in folate-containing foods, such as fruit and vegetables. Patients with folic acid or vitamin B_{12} deficiency also may have an anemia without macrocytosis (MCV < 100 fl). Physicians should be aware that combined iron deficiency, α- and β-thalassemia trait, chronic infection, or inflammation all can mask macrocytosis of the erythrocytes. The clue to the megaloblastic nature of the anemia in these patients can be be found in the white blood cells. Neutrophil hypersegmentation and giant metamyelocytes persist.

Therapy of Vitamin B_{12} Deficiency Pernicious Anemia

Initial Therapy

Patients with pernicious anemia are treated with parenteral vitamin B_{12}. Intramuscular or subcutaneous injections are the preferred routes of administration. Since after injection significant amounts of the vitamin are excreted in the urine, the initial therapy should be several large doses (1000 μg) of vitamin B_{12}. Injections spaced more than a day apart are retained better than daily injections. No established regimen appears to work better than all others. As long as vitamin B_{12} is given parenterally, the immediate goals of therapy—correction of the deficiency and replenishing the stores—will be achieved.

My approach is to treat patients initially with six or seven intramuscular injections of 1000 μg of vitamin B_{12} every other day over a 2 week period. This can be easier achieved in hospitalized rather than ambulatory patients. Some patients (or family members) readily learn to inject the vitamin B_{12} themselves, and the opportunity to learn this skill should be offered. It is most important to fully educate the patient about the disease and the lifelong need for vitamin B_{12} therapy. I continue with weekly injections of vitamin B_{12} for the next 4 weeks to ensure replenishment of the vitamin stores. In patients with severe neurologic damage, such as subacute combined degeneration of the cord, vitamin B_{12} may be required weekly for up to 3 months.

While hospitalization is expensive and not all patients with pernicious anemia are acutely ill, several advantages are offered by initially evaluating and treating the patient in hospital. Diagnostic studies can be performed in a more controlled environment (urine collection for the Schilling test is often mishandled), the physician can ensure that the initial large doses of vitamin B_{12} are administered, and the response to therapy can be monitored. The patient's response to vitamin B_{12} is often dramatic and predictable as far as the hematologic manifestations are concerned. Within 1 to 2 days of the first injection, patients describe a general feeling of improvement; within a week, appetite returns, the mood is brighter, and glossitis resolves. A reticulocyte response is first noted after 3 days, and the hematocrit and red cell count begin to rise 5 to 7 days after treatment. Macrocytic red cells take up to 3 weeks to disappear from the peripheral blood. On the other hand, the neurologic deficits respond far more slowly and less predictably and indeed may not completely recover.

The two forms of vitamin B_{12} available for therapy are cyanocobalamin and hydroxocobalamin. Cyanocobalamin is the most widely used form of vitamin B_{12} in the United States. It is inexpensive and in the body is converted to the physiologic forms of cobalamin. Hydroxocobalamin is a more physiologic form and is retained longer than cyanocobalamin. It is more costly than cyanocobalamin and in the United States does not have as common a use as it has in the United Kingdom and Europe. Injections of vitamin B_{12} are well tolerated and are associated with virtually no toxicity. Rare patients may have allergic reactions to the injections, and this appears to be directed more against the preservative than the actual vitamin.

Serum potassium should be measured in patients during the initial week of therapy. Hypokalemia may occur as a result of plasma potassium entering the proliferating hematopoietic cells that are responding to vitamin B_{12}. I administer oral potassium to those patients with hypokalemia, to patients with heart failure, and to those receiving diuretic therapy. Another effect of the proliferating and differentiating cells is an increase in uric acid excretion. In patients with a history of gout or hyperuricemia, an acute attack of gout may occur on the 6th or 7th day after therapy is begun.

Maintenance Therapy

Patients can be maintained in remission with 1000 μg of cyanocobalamin given every month by intramuscular injection or 1000 μg of hydroxocobalamin administered every 3 months. Patients who administer the vitamin themselves and patients who receive the injections by a nurse should see a physician at least once or twice a year. My patients have an annual or biannual evaluation, at which time they have a clinical examination and complete blood count. There is a 2 to 3 per cent risk of carcinoma of the stomach in patients with pernicious anemia. Radiologic and endoscopic studies should be confined to patients who have suggestive symptoms, such as weight loss or abdominal pain. The routine investigation of asymptomatic patients has not yielded any earlier detection of this gastric tumor. Patients with pernicious anemia also manifest other autoimmune diseases, particularly of the thyroid and adrenal glands.

Unfortunately, relapse in pernicious anemia is seen all too often. For a variety of reasons, patients may discontinue maintenance treatment and in periods varying from 12 months to 10 years present again with frank megaloblastic anemia. Physicians must stress the need for lifelong therapy.

Therapy of Other Causes of Vitamin B_{12} Deficiency

Patients who have had a total gastrectomy or ileal resection require parenteral vitamin B_{12} for the rest of their lives. I give these patients 1000 μg of hydroxocobalamin or cyanocobalamin every 3 months. Patients with blind loop syndrome, ileal disease, or tropical sprue also require vitamin B_{12} injections indefinitely, unless the underlying disease is medically or surgically corrected. Vegetarians who have cobalamin deficiency can be treated with oral cyanocobalamin, 25 μg daily, or they can be given 1000 μg of intramuscular vitamin B_{12} every 6 months. Infants born of and breast-fed by strict vegetarian mothers have been reported to have severe neurologic abnormalities. They should be treated with 1000 μg of vitamin B_{12} intramuscularly daily for 4 to 5 days. Most important is the education of vegetarian mothers of the need for vitamin supplementation during pregnancy and when breast-feeding infants.

Therapy of Folic Acid Deficiency

The daily requirements of folic acid are 100 to 200 μg; since body stores (8 to 12 mg) are sufficient for only about 4 months, deficiency can readily occur. Dietary deficiency is the commonest cause of folic acid deficiency. I treat patients with megaloblastic anemia due to dietary folate deficiency with 1 mg of folic acid by mouth daily for 3 months. Thereafter, if most patients have been instructed about the need for folate-rich foods—fresh vegetables and fruit—the deficiency does not recur. Since folic acid is a heat-labile vitamin, boiling, steaming, or even canning these foods greatly reduces the amount of vitamin. Adolescents or young adults who mainly eat in "fast food" restaurants or who have unusual diets or food faddism may have little or no folate in their diets. From puberty on, the growth spurt in teenagers is accompanied by a greater need for folate, and their diet may be insufficient in folic acid to meet this need. Educating them about their physiology and correct dietary practice goes a long way in resolving this and other dietary deficiencies.

Pregnancy is another physiologic condition in which there is an increased utilization of and requirement for folic acid. To prevent and treat megaloblastic anemia in pregnancy, 1 mg of oral folic acid daily is administered throughout the pregnant state and period of lactation. In alcoholic patients, folic acid deficiency often accompanies the overall poor nutritional state. Lack of compliance and interest makes these patients susceptible to recurrent deficiency. I treat them initially with large doses of folic acid, 5 mg daily, because maintenance therapy is often difficult and unpredictable.

An increased need for folic acid occurs in patients with chronic hemolytic anemias (sickle cell anemia and thalassemia) and patients requiring long-term hemodialysis. Folic acid, 1 mg daily by mouth, is sufficient to prevent deficiency. Patients who have developed folate deficiency while taking anticonvulsants (particularly phenytoin) or oral contraceptives can be continued on these drugs if they take 1 mg of folic acid daily. In patients with malabsorption (sprue) syndromes, folic acid in daily doses of 2 to 5 mg should be administered. Megaloblastic anemia in patients with tropical sprue is treated with both folic acid and vitamin B_{12}. If the malabsorption syndrome is uncorrectable, then the patients are maintained indefinitely on folic acid, 2 mg per day, and intramuscular vitamin B_{12}, 1000 μg every 6 months.

Intravenous folic acid is indicated in patients with folic acid deficiency who are unconscious or unable to take oral medication or poorly absorbing folic acid, as with severe malabsorption. Five mg administered intravenously twice weekly is sufficient to correct megaloblastic anemia. Oral folic acid is begun when the patient's clinical condition allows. Folinic acid (citrovorum factor) is a metabolically active form of folic acid which is also administered by intravenous or intramuscular injection. Folinic acid is used in preventing the toxicity from the drug methotrexate, which blocks the folic acid reducing enzyme dihydrofolate reductase.

Therapy of Coexisting Iron Deficiency

Iron deficiency may be combined with the vitamin B_{12} lack in patients with pernicious anemia or after gastrectomy and may be associated with folic acid deficiency in pregnancy and in alcoholics. The absence of bone marrow iron may mask the development of macrocytes, but the white cell precursors will show megaloblastic features and the neutrophils will have hypersegmentation. Patients with combined deficiency respond to oral iron (325 mg of ferrous sulfate three times a day) and vitamin B_{12} or folic acid, depending on which vitamin is lacking. Iron deficiency should also be suspected in patients who do not fully respond to vitamin B_{12} or folate therapy. These patients have marginal iron stores which become depleted when hematopoiesis increases with the specific vitamin therapy. One of the values of performing a bone marrow aspirate in megaloblastic anemia is the assessment of the iron stores.

Therapy of Severely Anemic or Acutely Ill Patients

In most patients with megaloblastic anemia, the gradual decrease in red blood cell count has enabled them to compensate and not manifest circulatory disturbances. If they are severely anemic, with hematocrit counts under 20 per cent, and have no signs of cardiac failure or other distress, I confine the patients to bed and obtain the appropriate diagnostic studies. It is *not* necessary to immediately start these patients on both vitamin B_{12} and folic acid or to consider transfusion therapy. Within a few days the specific deficiency is identified and the therapy begun.

Rare patients present with a markedly decreased hematocrit count, under 15 per cent, and not showing signs of circulatory distress, yet any delay in therapy is deemed ill advised. At the very least, diagnostically, a small volume of blood for serum vitamin determinations should be obtained and then the patient treated with both 1000 μg of intramuscular vitamin B_{12} and 1 mg of oral folic acid per day until the diagnosis is established. Patients with deteriorating neurologic manifestations or altered mental status should also be immediately started on vitamin B_{12} therapy. If there is a history of alcoholism or poor dietary intake, I also administer folic acid, 5 mg intravenously. It is stressed that in emergency situations in which megaloblastic anemia and neurologic dysfunction are found, folic acid should not be administered alone but together with vitamin B_{12}.

There are a few indications for transfusion therapy such as patients with megaloblastic anemia and signs of circulatory distress. Elderly patients particularly may have angina pectoris, cardiac failure, or cerebral dysfunction with even moderate degrees of anemia (hematocrit counts above 25 per cent) and require a more rapid rise of their blood count than that provided by vitamin therapy alone. After obtaining a blood sample for the vitamin measurement, I transfuse such patients *slowly* with 1 or 2 units of packed red cells and also administer a diuretic and replacement potassium as indicated. Patients with a megaloblastic anemia coexisting with another disease (such as hepatic or renal failure, gastrointestinal bleeding, or respiratory insufficiency) that requires immediate treatment with blood transfusion are managed the same way. Plasma volume overload is a problem in patients with megaloblastic anemia; careful monitoring, especially for pulmonary edema, is necessary when transfusing patients. In my experience, when megaloblastosis is associated with leukopenia and thrombocytopenia, the administration of either vitamin B_{12} or folic acid is sufficient to correct these abnormalities, and no other therapeutic agent or transfusion is necessary.

THALASSEMIA

method of
RUSSEL E. KAUFMAN, M.D.
Duke University
Durham, North Carolina

The thalassemias are disorders of hemoglobin synthesis characterized by decreased production of normal alpha- or beta-globin chains of hemoglobin. This abnormality results in the production of erythrocytes with a low hemoglobin content and a tendency to undergo destruction in the marrow and spleen. In the most severe form, beta-thalassemia major, greatly decreased synthesis of beta-chains produces a severe, life-threatening anemia. Less severe forms of the disease result from a moderate reduction of beta-chain synthesis (beta-thalassemia minor) or alpha-chain synthesis (alpha-thalassemia). The simultaneous occurrence of alpha- and beta-thalassemia, or thalassemia and another hemoglobinopathy such as sickle cell disease, produces a wide spectrum of clinical disorders.

Diagnosis

Alpha-Thalassemia. The alpha-globins are the products of four alpha-globin genes per diploid genome. Four distinct clinical syndromes are associated with defects involving one or more of these genes. These syndromes range in clinical severity from a silent carrier state to a severe intrapartum anemia that results in stillbirth (hydrops fetalis). Intermediate clinical syndromes include alpha-thalassemia minor, a mild microcytic anemia, and hemoglobin H disease, a more severe microcytic anemia in which beta-globin tetramers (HbH) can be identified by hemoglobin electrophoresis or brilliant cresyl blue staining of erythrocytes. The silent carrier condition (alpha-thal-2) cannot be detected by morphologic or routine laboratory analysis of peripheral blood. For all practical purposes, alpha-thalassemia minor is diagnosed by exclusion of iron deficiency and beta-thalassemia. If essential, diagnosis can be established by globin synthetic studies or alpha-globin gene mapping.

Beta-Thalassemia. The beta-thalassemia syndromes vary widely in clinical severity; the most common forms are thalassemia minor and major. Beta-thalassemia minor or trait produces a mild to moderate microcytic hypochromic anemia with frequent targeting of the erythrocytes. The HbA2 level is moderately elevated (3.8 to 8 per cent) in most cases, while increased levels of fetal hemoglobin (1 to 10 per cent) occur in approximately half the cases. Beta-thalassemia major is a severe anemia characterized by markedly hypochromic erythrocytes, which have numerous inclusions and show marked variations in size and shape. Fetal hemoglobin usually constitutes a large percentage of the total hemoglobin. The diagnosis can be confirmed by measuring beta-globin chain synthesis in the reticulocytes, although the presence of beta-thalassemia minor in both parents is usually adequate evidence to support the diagnosis when the clinical picture is appropriate.

Alpha-globin chains are synthesized during fetal and adult development for incorporation into fetal hemoglobin (alpha-2, gamma-2) and hemoglobin A (alpha-2, beta-2). Since alpha-globin chains are a component of fetal and adult hemoglobins, deficient synthesis is manifest during fetal and adult life. Defective beta-chain synthesis, on the other hand, is not clinically apparent until 3 to 6 months after birth, when hemoglobin A replaces fetal hemoglobin. Patients with beta-thalassemia major then develop a progressively severe anemia, with hemoglobin values usually falling to less than 7 grams per dl. Blood transfusion is required to maintain a hemoglobin adequate for even minimal activity. Impaired growth and development and susceptibility to serious infections characterize the first several years of life for these children. By the age of 5 years, long-term complications become apparent. The spleen becomes progressively enlarged in response to the large burden of thalassemic and transfused erythrocytes. Transfusion requirements gradually increase as the first signs of hypersplenism become apparent. Eventually most patients will require splenectomy as thrombocytopenia and leukopenia become additional manifestations of the hypersplenism.

The severe anemia associated with beta-thalassemia is a potent stimulus for erythroid marrow proliferation. Marrow expansion fills most of the marrow space and causes extensive skeletal changes. Long bones become osteoporotic and are easily broken, while cranial bones thicken and produce disfiguring facial changes. Extramedullary marrow proliferation can produce spinal cord compression or visceral masses, which are sometimes painful or interfere with other organ functions.

An additional response to the severe anemia is increased gastrointestinal iron absorption. This contributes to the already great transfusional iron burden and may play a significant role in the eventual severe iron toxicity. Iron overload is the greatest threat to the individual with beta-thalassemia major. Iron deposition in the heart produces cardiac failure and life-threatening arrhythmias. Chronic damage by iron to hepatocytes results in cirrhosis and altered hepatic function. Likewise, endocrine gland function, especially that of the pituitary and adrenals, may be impaired and lead to serious metabolic disturbances, which may be recognized only at times of stress such as surgery or serious infection.

The tissue iron toxicity is probably mediated in part by free radical damage. The highly reactive free radicals produced by ionized iron are scavenged by the antioxidants vitamin E and ascorbic acid, resulting in low serum and tissue levels of these vitamins.

Treatment

Beta-Thalassemia Minor

No therapy is required for the mild anemia associated with beta-thalassemia minor. Iron therapy should not be given in this condition unless the patient has proven iron deficiency. Moreover, treatment should least only until iron stores are re-established. Supplemental vitamin administration likewise has no benefit for the patient who lacks evidence of dietary inadequacy, except for folic acid, which is metabolized at a high rate in patients with increased erythropoiesis.

Beta-Thalassemia Major

The goals of therapy are to maintain the most beneficial hemoglobin level and prevent or delay long-term complications. This requires an individualized program of transfusions, iron chelation, and careful attention to the possible development of skeletal, endocrine, and cardiac abnormalities. Most of the guidelines applied to beta-thalassemia major also can be applied to a milder form of homozygous beta-thalassemia termed beta-thalassemia intermedia. These patients may not be dependent on transfusions but can still develop many of the complications associated with thalassemia major, particularly skeletal changes. The decision to transfuse depends in large part on the patient's capacity to undertake the comprehensive program to be described here.

Transfusion Therapy. Transfusion schedules prior to the 1960s were predicated on the goal of limiting iron accumulation since this complication was the major factor of early mortality. Hemoglobin values were generally maintained between 8 and 10 grams per dl. Studies in the 1960s demonstrated that hypertransfusion programs, in which the hemoglobin values were kept above 10 grams per dl, resulted in more normal growth and development and limited the skeletal changes. More frequent transfusions were required, however, and the iron burden increased. Coupled with iron chelation therapy, more aggressive transfusion programs were initiated, which maintained hemoglobin above 12 grams per dl. These "supertransfusion" programs generally required no great increase in the rate of transfusion once the patient was transfused and maintained at the higher hemoglobin level. This is probably explained by the reduction of the greatly expanded blood volume seen prior to initiation of "supertransfusion." Gastrointestinal iron absorption is also suppressed. Most centers use an aggressive transfusion program, although numerous factors can affect this decision.

To reduce the frequency of febrile and urticarial transfusion reactions, we recommend the use of washed, frozen, thawed packed cells when available. Accurate records of transfusion requirements will help document the development of hypersplenism. The desired hemoglobin level can usually be obtained by transfusion on an outpatient basis two to four times per month. The anticipated transfusion requirement for most supertransfusion programs is less than 250 ml per kg per year for an individual after splenectomy or without hypersplenism. Requirements can increase greatly following the development of hypersplenism. Experimental programs using new apheresis and separation techniques allow the infusion of blood enriched with young erythrocytes (neocytes) and depleted of aged erythrocytes. Such efforts are designed to reduce total transfusion requirements by extending the survival of transfused cells. The transfusional iron burden is also reduced owing to the removal of aged erythrocytes, which have a short survival time following transfusion. These programs remain largely experimental but are being utilized in centers treating large numbers of patients.

Iron Chelation Therapy. It is now clear that aggressive iron chelation therapy can prevent heavy iron loading and probably prevent many of the associated complications. There is little evidence, however, that cardiac damage from iron loading can be reversed, although chelation therapy may prevent or slow progression of the disease. Effective iron excretion can be achieved by the daily subcutaneous continuous infusion of desferrioxamine (Desferal) administered by a small portable pump. Patients with significant iron stores excrete 15 to 60 mg of iron daily when given 20 to 40 mg per kg per day of the drug. Children started on the program at age 3 years can be maintained in negative iron balance even with supertransfusion therapy. We begin therapy for most children at the age of 5 years when they can be taught to self-administer the drug by subcutaneous infusion to the abdomen or thigh via a 27 gauge "butterfly" needle. Infusions last 10 to 12 hours and can be continued overnight. Pruritus, swelling, and pain at the injection site jeopardize the chance of long-term compliance. This can be prevented in many cases by adding 0.1 mg of hydrocortisone to each ml of Desferal at the time of infusion. Use of cold towels or Benadryl cream can reduce the discomfort once the local reaction has developed.

Excretion of iron is enhanced by the administration of ascorbic acid along with desferroxamine. When ascorbic acid is administered in high doses cardiotoxicity frequently develops; therefore, the dose of ascorbic acid should be less than 100 mg per day. Vitamin E is also a potent antioxidant that is frequently present in low amounts in the serum of transfused thalassemic individuals. Replacement therapy has not been demonstrated to reduce the toxicity of iron overload. Furthermore, in this disease replacement therapy does not have any significant effect on erythrocyte survival, although it may reduce the rate of desferrioxamine-induced iron excretion. Studies are in progress to determine the role of vitamin E in iron chelation therapy.

Splenectomy. Hypertransfusion programs have greatly reduced the incidence of hypersplenism in early childhood and the need for early splenectomy. After the age of 6 years transfusion requirements are less for splenectomized patients. While arguments have been made for splenectomy to reduce iron burden, there is no evidence that these patients will have less iron toxicity. Furthermore, they are at much greater risk from serious infections. We prefer to perform splenectomy only when the blood requirements are twice normal or if significant leukopenia or thrombocytopenia develops. In general, splenectomy should be delayed until after the child is 5 years old. Occasionally the spleen becomes large and painful in the absence of overt hypersplenism and may require removal. In all cases, splenectomy should be preceded by immunization with polyvalent pneumococcal vaccine. Some clinicians advise documenting a rise in antibodies in response to the vaccine and repeat vaccination if no response was observed. The role of booster vaccinations has not been established. Daily postsplenectomy prophylactic administration of pencillin V (125 mg daily) is encouraged if compliance can be assured. In the event of unexplained fever in the splenectomized patient, parenteral administration of broad-spectrum antibiotics is indicated because of the serious threat of overwhelming sepsis.

Complications of Iron Overload

Cardiac Complications. Histologic studies on cardiac tissue from patients with iron overload in beta-thalassemia have indicated that early deposition of iron is in the pericardium and myocardium. This pattern parallels the clinical events. Pericarditis is a frequent and early event. Atrial arrhythmias are frequent complications of the pericarditis. Within several years of the onset of pericarditis, most patients develop ventricular ectopy, including ventricular tachycardia. Cardiac rhythm disturbances usually herald the onset of myocardial contraction dysfunction and a poor prognosis. Echocardiography and radionuclide cineangiography of patients without clinical evidence of pump failure demonstrate thickening of the ventricular wall and impaired ejection fractions with exercise. Symptoms of cardiac failure usually develop within 2 to 3 years of the onset of cardiac signs unless the iron loading is reversed.

The treatment of these conditions is primarily symptomatic and is chosen from those approaches and drugs that constitute good general medical treatment. Pericarditis is best managed with bed rest, analgesics, and anti-inflammatory drugs such as indomethacin or ibuprofen. Atrial arrhythmias can be suppressed with digoxin, propranolol, or calcium channel–blocking drugs. Ventricular arrhythmias are more difficult to manage and may be impossible to eliminate. In such cases we aim to suppress ventricular premature beats to a level that is symptomatically tolerable to the patient. Agents of choice are those active against ventricular arrhythmias in other conditions. However, therapy must be highly individualized and monitored by portable monitoring devices. In addition, combinations of quinidine, propranolol, digoxin, and disopyramide (Norpace) may be needed and in high doses.

The onset of congestive heart failure is ominous. In the early stages, symptoms of volume expansion and pulmonary congestion can be managed with salt restriction, diuretics, and digoxin. In later stages of heart failure, pulmonary congestion may decrease, but the patient may complain of severe fatigue and experience wasting of skeletal muscle in a pattern typical of biventricular cardiac failure. These patients are prone to develop ascites since they have coexisting hepatic disease. In some patients, agents that produce afterload reduction have been successful.

Hepatic Complications. Most patients who have beta-thalassemia and are on a transfusion program will have some degree of hepatomegaly. Hepatic enzymes may be mildly elevated chronically and are greatly increased only with hepatitis or other cause of significant hepatocyte damage. The synthetic capacity of the liver is impaired only after extensive iron damage has occurred, although prothrombin times may be moderately prolonged. This can usually be corrected with injections of vitamin K. It appears that iron chelation therapy is effective in reversing many of the hepatic complications of iron loading. Unlike the heart, the liver has remarkable regenerative capacity. As in most hemolytic anemias biliary disease from the formation of pigmented stones in thalassemia is an almost certain complication and should be managed surgically when appropriate.

Endocrine Complications. Virtually all endocrine glands accumulate iron when total body iron stores increase; however, the amount of endocrine dysfunction is highly varied. Failure of sexual maturation is often the first sign of iron overload. This is due to impaired gonadotropin release rather than target organ failure. Early iron deposition in the adrenals is in the zona glomerulosa, although mineralocorticoid regulation is seldom impaired. Later in the course of disease, the corticosteroid response to ACTH becomes blunted and the patient takes on a slate gray appearance typical of that seen with ACTH hypersecretion. Adrenal crisis can occur during times of severe stress unless adrenal insufficiency is recognized and appropriate replacement therapy given. Pancreatic endocrine function is frequently impaired late in the illness and usually requires insulin therapy to treat the diabetes mellitus. Subclinical deficiencies of thyroid and parathyroid function have been reported but are usually not a problem. The most important aspect of the endocrine abnormalities is early recognition. Therapy in all cases is by appropriate replacement.

Bone and Skeletal Disease

For patients with beta-thalassemia, serious facial disfiguration is frequently their greatest concern. Fortunately, this has become much less a problem since the initiation of aggressive transfusion programs. Experimental programs using vitamin D and calcium are underway in attempts to prevent the osteoporosis. Extramedullary hematopoiesis can have serious consequences in patients with the thalassemic syndromes, especially when it occurs in the spinal canal and causes spinal cord compression. If the proliferation of erythroid tissue cannot be controlled with transfusion therapy, local radiation therapy may prove useful.

Experimental Therapy

Bone Marrow Transplantation. Experience with marrow transplantation in children with aplastic anemia and leukemia has generated enthusiasm for the correction of other hematologic disorders, including the thalassemias and hemoglobinopathies. Marrow transplantation can only be considered if the appropriate donor is available and if the patient is young; the treatment otherwise would have a low chance of success. The extensive transfusion history of most of the patients may make graft rejection a serious problem. Currently, marrow transplantation will be limited primarily to individuals who are unable for some reason to participate in the usual programs described earlier.

Genetic Manipulation. Recent studies of gene organization and regulation have provided new ideas about the treatment of these diseases. The principal goals of genetic manipulation are to replace adult hemoglobin synthesis with fetal hemoglobin synthesis, or to replace the dysfunctional beta-globin gene with a normal beta-globin gene. Studies in progress have recently reported attempts to stimulate fetal hemoglobin synthesis using hydroxyurea or the pyrimidine analogue 5′-azacytidine. In the reported cases, fetal hemoglobin synthesis increased adequately to make the patients temporarily transfusion-independent. This therapy should be considered experimental and only used in centers authorized to perform these studies since the long-term effectiveness of these potent agents has not been established. Additional ethical questions have been raised by such studies, which must be considered seriously before this type of therapy becomes routine and generalized.

Prevention of Beta-Thalassemia

In general, parents at risk for having a child with thalassemia major can be easily identified by simple laboratory measurement of erythrocyte parameters. In the past, such parents had few options other than limiting the size of their family. Recent developments allowing detection of hemoglobin variants and thalassemias in utero stress the importance of the recognition of beta-thalassemia minor and the need to properly inform individuals with this condition of their risk of having a child with beta-thalassemia major. Many couples at risk have chosen to reduce the chance by antenatal diagnosis and termination of pregnancy when the fetus is deemed likely to have beta-thalassemia major. This approach has been limited in the past because of the unacceptable fetal wastage associated with the need to sample fetal blood. Recently developed techniques have reduced the risk to the fetus and increased the accuracy of the diagnostic method. These techniques require direct examination of DNA derived from fetal cells present in the amniotic fluid. Markers linked to the defective beta-globin gene on the chromosomal DNA of the parents can be used to determine whether the beta-thalassemic globin gene has been transmitted to the fetus. The pattern of the markers can be used to predict the genotype of the fetus. This technique is applicable in more than 95 per cent of the fetuses at risk and can be performed with less than 0.1 per cent chance of inadvertent fetal wastage.

In developed parts of the world, use of these techniques should lead to a great reduction of the incidence of the severe form of the disease. Simplification and standardization of these techniques are essential to make them applicable to underdeveloped regions of the world in which thalassemia is common.

SICKLE CELL DISEASE

method of
CHRISTINE A. JOHNSON, M.D.
Bowman Gray School of Medicine
Winston-Salem, North Carolina

The sickle cell syndromes include all the conditions in which a gene for S hemoglobin production is combined with another abnormal gene for β globin chain synthesis. The most common of these in the United States is homozygous sickle cell disease (SS), occurring in about 1 per 600 American blacks and rarely in individuals of other ethnic backgrounds. S-β^0 thalassemia, seen less frequently, is a doubly heterozygous sickle cell state in which no A hemoglobin is synthesized, resulting in a condition clinically indistinguishable from SS disease. All other doubly heterozygous states tend to be less severe than SS, including S-O Arab, S-D, S-C, and S-β^+ thalassemia, listed in order of decreasing clinical severity. There is a marked range of clinical severity with SS disease itself, although all the reasons for moderation of clinical symtoms are not known. The concurrence of α thalassemia, the level of fetal hemoglobin within sickle-containing erythrocytes, and the inherent adhesive potential of the sickle erythrocyte have all been implicated as possible modifiers of disease, but the exact relationships between these phenomena and clinical symptoms are still under investigation.

Diagnostic Considerations

The clinical problems in sickle cell disease result from the combination of a moderately severe hemolytic anemia and the more specific defects caused by recurrent vaso-occlusive crises in major organs. In older children and adults, the baseline hemoglobin level typically ranges from 6 to 8 grams with a reticulocytosis of 5 to 20 per cent and an average leukocytosis of 15,000 per cubic mm. The bilirubin level ranges from 1 to 3 mg per dl. Most patients with this degree of anemia also exhibit cardiomegaly and exercise intolerance. Cardiomegaly may be severe, with mitral valve incompetence resulting. Chronic hemolysis leads to the formation of bilirubin stones in approximately 50 per cent of all patients over age ten. Children with SS, because of heightened erythropoiesis, generally exhibit frontal and maxillary skeletal hyperplasia. It is also common for these youngsters to be troubled with tonsillar and adenoidal hypertrophy, occasionally leading to night apnea from airway obstruction.

Recurrent vaso-occlusive crises in major organs result in clinical problems that are more specific to the individual with sickle cell disease. Autoinfarction of the spleen, with irreversible functional asplenia, occurs in all patients with SS, generally by age five to six. All adult patients also have some measurable renal parenchymal damage from recurrent infarcts. Recurrent pulmonary infarcts, often with superimposed infection, are also common, leading to microatelectasis, chronic pulmonary artery hypertension, and a decrease in vital capacity.

Less frequently, as a result of recurrent infarction or infection, there may be baseline abnormalities in liver function tests (observed in 30 per cent of adult patients) or aseptic necrosis of the humoral or femoral head (10 to 15 per cent of patients with SS and 20 to 70 per cent of patients with SC). Retinal vessel infarction may be associated with peripheral neovascularization, vitreous hemorrhage, or traction retinal detachment. Sixty to 90 per cent of adults develop peripheral vascular ulcers, which are often refractory to conventional therapy.

TREATMENT

Acute Problems

Traditionally the acute problems or complications of SS disease have been referred to as the sickle cell crises: vaso-occlusive, hypoplastic, and hemolytic.

Vaso-occlusive Crisis

Vaso-occlusive crisis is the most characteristic and most common of the acute complications of sickle cell disease. Most frequently, it presents as a pain crisis that may be mild or may severely disable the patient. Infarction from aggregated sickle cells may occur in the extremities, abdomen, or chest, and severe ischemic pain, along with local tenderness, heat, and swelling, is experienced. Because of these findings, often there is difficulty in differentiating infarct from infection. The pain of infarct is generally more diffuse than that expected with infection. The body temperature is usually not as high and the leukocytosis not as impressive. When infarct pain occurs in the skeletal system, the patient often requests local heat or massage, in distinct contrast to the patient with septic arthritis or osteomyelitis, who chooses not to be touched.

If infection can be excluded, pain crisis can be managed symptomatically with rest, adequate hydration, and effective analgesia. Narcotics may be required to control the more severe painful attacks. In young children, morphine sulfate can be given intramuscularly in a dose of 0.1 mg per kg every 3 to 4 hours (not to exceed 15 mg per dose). Older children and adults can be treated with hydromorphone (Dilaudid), 2 to 4 mg per dose every 4 to 6 hours. Oral medication is well absorbed. The availability of a 3 mg hydromorphone suppository is an added convenience. Phenothiazines are relatively contraindicated, since they decrease the threshold for seizures.

When pain crisis begins to improve, the patient should be weaned from narcotics gradually, reducing the dose of medication rather than extending the frequency of administration. Recurrent, severe pain crises occur in a select subpopulation (20 to 30 per cent) of the patients with SS disease or S-β° thalassemia. These patients are subject to repeated hospitalizations, disruption of normal daily life, and narcotic withdrawal and dependency. They demand a great deal of psychosocial support as well as educational counseling, vocational-rehabilitation training, and financial aid.

Vaso-occlusive crises that involve massive infarction of major organs demand particular attention. Central nervous system infarction is not rare, reportedly occurring in 6 to 15 per cent of the patients with SS disease. Children are apparently at greater risk for stroke than adults. Strokes often present dramatically with a sudden onset of hemiparesis, but severe headache, localized weakness, visual problem, or other neurologic signs and symptoms should be seriously evaluated in patients with this disease. The immediate management of stroke is partial exchange transfusion to reduce the level of sickle hemoglobin to less than 40 or 50 per cent. The long-term management, chronic transfusion with packed cells, is designed to keep the bone marrow suppressed (reticulocytes less than 5 per cent) and the hemoglobin near normal range (10 to 13 grams).

There is controversy regarding the ideal duration of transfusion treatment after strokes, some clinicians believing that they should be discontinued in three to five years to avoid the risk of iron overload. Others, citing the high recurrence rate of stroke (60 to 70 per cent in most reported series) and the data suggesting that hypertransfusion fails to reverse the anatomic abnormality observed in the cerebral vessels, believe that transfusions should be continued for life. If this approach is taken, iron chelation therapy should be offered before iron overload becomes clinically evident. These problems are best managed through a comprehensive sickle cell center.

Another important site for major infarction is the lung. Acute pulmonary infarct may be mild, resulting in chest pain, dyspnea, and typical radiographic findings. Less commonly, massive infarction may occur, a complication carrying a high risk of mortality. Although clinicians have sought a definitive test to clearly distinguish pulmonary infarction from infection in sickle cell disease, such an aid is not available. Since pulmonary infection is very common and treatable, the symptomatic patient with fever and radiographic infiltrates should be given antibiotics. In children, a good starting choice is ampicillin, 100 mg per kg per 24 hours intravenously divided into 4 to 6 doses. In adults, intravenous penicillin is the drug of choice if there is no history of allergy. After 24 to 48 hours of antibiotics, certain clinical findings are suggestive of pulmonary infarction rather than infection. These would include continued or new chest pain, progressive radiographic changes, an increase in serum bilirubin, and the appearance of blister cells or poikilocytes in the peripheral blood. Pulmonary vascular occlusion, when suspected in a very ill patient, should be aggressively treated with rapid exchange transfusion to reduce S hemoglobin levels.

Adolescent or postpubertal males may experience priapism, and this vaso-occlusive crisis unfortunately tends to be recurrent. It is best treated with packed cell transfusion designed to increase the level of circulating hemoglobin to 13 or 14 grams. Transfusions must be given slowly over the course of several days. Successful treatment usually does not result in the immediate return of complete flaccidity to the penis, and treatment may be discontinued as soon as the patient is pain-free. Most hematologists feel that surgical intervention is contraindicated because of the risk of subsequent impotence or postoperative necrosis.

Hypoplastic Crisis

All patients with impressive hemolysis become rapidly more anemic if the elevated reticulocyte count is not maintained. If erythropoiesis is suppressed completely for just a few days, baseline hemoglobin levels may fall from 7 to 3 or 4 grams. Recently human parvovirus infection has been linked to hypoplasia in sickle cell disease. Other viral infections could have a similar effect on red cell production. The etiology of the sudden anemia is readily confirmed with a reticulocyte count of less than 5 per cent. A more gradual fall in hemoglobin levels may be seen when either iron or folate deficiency is superimposed on SS disease. Patients with reticulocytopenia should be treated based on symptoms not the absolute level of hemoglobin. If the SS patient in hypoplastic crisis has significant tachycardia, a small packed cell transfusion (3 to 5 ml per kg) should be administered slowly to prevent circulatory overload. Otherwise, hospital observation is adequate.

Hemolytic Crisis

Hemolytic crisis is best described as an acute event that causes either an elevation of bilirubin or a decrease in hemoglobin not associated with marrow hypoplasia. The prime consideration in this hemolytic state is superimposed bacterial infection. Pneumonia, urinary tract infections, and hepatitis are special considerations in the patient with sickle cell disease. The clinician must also consider the possibility of cholecystitis or common duct obstruction from bilirubin stones. A more severe and serious possibility to be considered is hepatic infarction.

Special Problems

Pregnancy

Female adolescents with sickle cell disease pose special problems for the practitioner. These young women should receive counseling about birth control methods, emphasizing the increased risk of serious thrombotic complications in women with sickle cell disease using conventional birth control pills. Intrauterine devices are also relatively contraindicated because of the increased risk of infection in women with SS disease. Barrier methods are excellent for women and their partners who express willingness to comply. Genetic counseling should also be encouraged at this age.

Young women should be advised to seek medical care at the first suspicion of pregnancy, and, when confirmed, referral to high risk obstetric care is indicated. The untreated pregnant sickle cell patient faces a 40 per cent risk of fetal wastage or perinatal mortality from placental insufficiency. Maternal morbidity and mortality have been reported as high as 10 to 25 per cent. The pregnant woman is at much increased risk for urinary tract infection, and, in SS disease, 30 per cent of women with urinary tract infection develop sepsis.

There is currently no uniform approach to management of the pregnant patient with SS disease. For women with a past history of significant clinical problems, we recommend chronic transfusion support from the time of detection through delivery. The risk of hepatitis to the patient and infant can be reduced by maternal immunization with hepatitis B vaccine.

Every effort should be made to obtain hemoglobin electrophoresis results on prospective fathers as early in pregnancy as possible. Mothers and partners should be aware that newer restriction endonuclease methodology provides an accurate means of diagnosing sickle cell disease in almost all fetuses from amniotic fluid samples, which can be obtained between the 14th and 16th weeks of pregnancy. The DNA analysis, however, must be done in conjunction with samples from both parents to eliminate errors due to polymorphism.

Infant and Child

Sickle cell screening is recommended for all nonwhite newborn infants. Since sickle hemoglobin is present in the affected neonate, screening by qualitative hemoglobin electrophoresis can be accomplished accurately on small blood samples. The trait can be distinguished from the doubly heterozygous sickle cell states. If newborn screening cannot be accomplished, a quantitative hemoglobin electrophoresis should be obtained between three and six months of age to establish diagnosis prior to onset of any serious complications of disease.

Natural history studies have shown that the earliest clinical manifestations in the infant are likely to be recurrent abdominal colic and the so-called hand-foot syndrome of dactylitis, in which painful swellings of the hands and feet occur owing to infarction in the small bones of the extremities. Both problems can be treated conservatively with good hydration and mild analgesia.

The major concern in the infant and young child with sickle cell disease is the markedly increased risk of pneumococcal pneumonia, meningitis, and sepsis. The individual child's risk for meningitis is 5 per cent, with an additional 4 per cent risk of sepsis. As compared with the general population, the youngster with sickle cell disease has a 300 × increased risk of developing pneumonia and a 600 × increased risk of developing meningitis. Still more important is the high mortality rate (30 per cent) associated with these infections in children with sickle cell disease due to their inability to opsonize pneumococci prior to phagocytosis and to effectively kill phagocytized organisms in the reticuloendothelial system. These high risks have led hematologists to recommend pneumococcal prophylaxis of all children with sickle cell disease. Specific recommendations vary, but most centers treat with oral prophylactic doses of penicillin (125 mg 3 times daily) from the time of diagnosis until age two or three, at which time pneumococcal vaccine is known to be effective in 80 to 90 per cent of immunized children. Since the risk of serious pneumococcal disease markedly diminishes by age eight to ten, most pediatricians are currently not reimmunizing their youngsters with SS disease. Physicians with responsibility for children with this disease agree that unexplained temperatures of significant degree (38.9 to 39.4 C [102 to 103 F]) and all known pneumococcal infections (otitis media or pneumonia) necessitate aggressive treatment with intravenous antibiotics to reduce the risk of mortality from overwhelming pneumococcal sepsis or meningitis, even in those children receiving appropriate prophylaxis.

There are several other complications of the disease that are exclusive to the child. The most serious of these is acute splenic sequestration, reported in children with SS and S-β° thalassemia from ages five months to six years. Although the pathophysiology of this complication is not fully understood, the clinical manifestations are protean. The child suddenly becomes pale or lethargic with gross enlargement of the spleen, which traps 20 to 30 per cent of the circulating blood volume. Severe tachycardia, hypotension, and collapse may result. The hallmarks of the condition are massive enlargement of the spleen, marked decrease in hemoglobin, and marked increase in reticulocytosis. Mortality in acute sequestration is 30 per cent. Treatment should be rapid but cautious owing to the compromised cardiovascular status. Slow replacement with packed cells and partial exchange transfusion seem to be equally effective. These patients, within 24 to 48 hours, will autotransfuse themselves with the cells sequestered by the spleen, so overly aggressive transfusion is not necessary. Recurrent splenic sequestration is an indication for splenectomy.

Children with SS and S-β° thalassemia are known to be small for their age. By two to three years, these youngsters generally begin to exhibit a subnormal linear growth and weight gain. Endocrinologic, metabolic, and nutritional studies to date have failed to yield a definite etiology for this observed phenomenon. Adolescence is also delayed for both girls and boys. The mean age of menarche for girls is 15.4 years, and the adolescent male growth spurt and pubertal changes may be similarly delayed by two to three years. Once sexual maturation begins, however, it progresses in normal fashion, and adolescents should be reassured that they will eventually be a competitive match for their peers.

Special Precautions

Surgery and anesthesia pose certain risks for the patient with SS disease because of the possibility of hypoxia, acidosis, or hypothermia. We recommend gradual exchange transfusion prior to any elective surgery and a partial exchange transfusion prior to any emergency surgery.

Hypoxia from high altitude may increase the risk of sickling, and patients should be cautioned not to fly in unpressurized aircraft. Patients should avoid prolonged activity in excessive heat or cold, both of which tend to bring on vaso-occlusive crises.

NEUTROPENIA

method of
DAVID HARMON, M.D.,
and THOMAS STOSSEL, M.D.
Harvard Medical School
Boston, Massachusetts

Neutropenia means an absolute blood segmented and band neutrophil count 2 or more standard deviations below the mean (i.e., less than 1500 per microliter for white adults). The blood neutrophil count is an inaccurate window into what is physiologically most important, the neutrophil turnover—the transit of neutrophils from bone marrow to blood to the tissues where neutrophils fight infection. When a fall in blood neutrophils below 1000 per microliter parallels a reduction in turnover, as in bone marrow failure, infection becomes an increasing threat; below 500 per microliter, "severe neutropenia" or "agranulocytosis" creates a marked risk. Moderating that risk are the marrow's neutrophil reserves, the duration of neutropenia, and the health of the body's other defenses—the integument, mucous membranes, monocytes, lymphocytes, antibodies, and complement.

A period of observation is usually required to determine whether any treatment at all is indicated because some persons having chronic neutropenia suffer few infections despite counts below 200 per microliter. Many blacks and some Yemenite Jews "normally" have counts half those of normal Caucasians without ill effects. Presumably their neutrophil turnover is not reduced.

The evaluation of neutropenia involves identifying correctable causes, assessing the risk of infection, and finding the nature of any infection. Therefore, the history focuses on possible etiologic agents—especially drugs and toxins (Table 1), frequency and duration of infections, associated diseases, and family background. The physical examination looks for infection, lymphadenopathy, and hepatosplenomegaly. Laboratory studies define the neutropenia's severity, duration, periodicity, and responsiveness to stress. Bone marrow aspiration and biopsy help diagnose leukemia and other malignant diseases as well as aplastic or megaloblastic anemia. Serum levels of vitamin B_{12} and folic acid reveal treatable deficiencies. Tests for rheumatoid factor and antinuclear, antierythrocyte, and antineutrophil autoantibodies characterize complex rheumatologic and specific immunologic causes of neutropenia. Rarely, a study of neutrophil mobilization in response to prednisolone or a formal indium-111 leukokinetic study can help establish the mechanism of neutropenia and its likely response to various therapies. Unfortunately, the latter test is difficult to perform and evaluate in neutropenic individuals.

Treatment

Protective Environment. Since most infections in neutropenic patients arise from endogenous flora,

TABLE 1. **Agents Occasionally Causing Neutropenia**

Analgesics/antipyretics—carbamazepine, ibuprofen, indomethacin, phenylbutazone
Antibiotics—cephalosporins, chloramphenicol, semisynthetic penicillins, sulfonamides, vancomycin
Antihistamines
Antithyroid agents—methimazole, propylthiouracil
Cardiovascular drugs—captopril, procainamide, quinidine
Diuretics—thiazides
Hypoglycemic agents
Sedatives—chlordiazepoxide, diazepam, phenothiazines
Miscellaneous—allopurinol, ethanol, solvents

protective isolation usually plays a limited role. However, it may be reasonable to restrict patients with counts below 500 per microliter to private rooms, require strict handwashing, use masks, and exclude from contact people with obvious infections. Where available, maximal isolation (laminar flow sterile environments) can be used for patients likely to be severely neutropenic for extended periods but who have a prospect for recovery. Good oral hygiene and avoidance of rectal trauma are essential.

Antibiotics. In most neutropenic patients the prophylactic use of antibiotics probably does little more than select for resistant organisms (although in childhood acute lymphocytic leukemia Bactrim prophylaxis may reduce infections, and for "dirty" procedures brief antibiotic coverage may be protective). However, in any patient with fewer than 1000 neutrophils per microliter, fever (above 38 C) or other evidence of infection demands emergency evaluation and empiric treatment with broad-spectrum antibiotics. Infections of the skin, pharynx, middle ear (in children), lungs, anorectal region, blood, and urine are common in neutropenic hosts but may produce fewer signs and symptoms of inflammation than usual so should be sought with cultures and radiographs. Even if no source of fever is evident, therapy should start immediately and cover the most common isolates: *Staphylococcus aureus, Pseudomonas aeruginosa, Escherichia coli,* and *Klebsiella pneumoniae.*

Recommended initial empiric therapy consists of an intravenous aminoglycoside such as gentamicin, 1 to 2 mg per kg every 8 hours (adjusted according to serum levels and creatinine), and a semisynthetic penicillin such as nafcillin, 25 mg per kg every 4 hours. Where resistant *Pseudomonas* spp. are common, one might choose tobramycin, 3 to 5 mg per kg per day, and ticarcillin, 45 mg per kg every 4 hours. In some settings cephalosporins are preferred, e.g., cefoperazone (Cefobid), 30 mg per kg every 6 hours. More appropriate regimens can be devised if a likely source emerges, and specific therapy can be prescribed if the pathogen is isolated.

Therapy should continue for at least 2 to 3 weeks except in the briefest periods of neutropenia and fever. Mycostatin mouthwash is given to prevent superinfection with fungus. However, if fever does not respond after 7 days of antibacterial therapy, evidence of fungal infection is sought with repeated cultures and biopsy of suspicious skin lesions. In hospitals having a high incidence of fungal infection, amphotericin is added empirically, following a test dose, at 0.5 mg per kg per day to a total of 25 mg per kg or until fever subsides and neutrophils return. In extreme cases with continued bacteremia despite 48 hours of appropriate antibiotics, the administration of leukocyte transfusions daily for at least 3 days is practical in some medical centers. Cell separators presently employed yield approximately 10^{11} leukocytes per day. This number cannot raise the neutrophil count appreciably in septic adults but might provide the minimum number of phagocytes to contain an infection, especially in small children. Most studies have failed to show a benefit of prophylactic leukocyte transfusions.

Stop Medications. Drugs are the commonest cause of acute severe neutropenia. Unless the cause of neutropenia is known, all nonessential drugs must be discontinued immediately and substitutes found for essential ones. Predictable dose-related neutropenia accompanies most cytotoxic chemotherapy, but many other drugs such as the phenothiazines suppress the marrow on an idiopathic basis. As well as suppressing marrow, antibiotics (especially semisynthetic penicillins) may act immunologically, while antiarrhythmics (procainamide) can produce a lupus-like syndrome.

Replacement Therapy. Vitamin B_{12} and folic acid are curative for the neutropenias caused by their respective deficiencies.

Bone Marrow Stimulation. Androgens and lithium occasionally raise neutrophil counts, but side effects limit their role to occasional therapy of aplastic anemia (androgens) and Felty's syndrome (lithium).

Splenectomy. Although it removes another host defense, splenectomy reportedly raises the neutrophil count and reduces infection in two thirds of patients with Felty's syndrome, especially those with high antineutrophil antibody levels. In many case reports of idiopathic neutropenia, however, splenectomy has no lasting benefit. Lymphoma-associated and idiopathic autoimmune neutropenia often respond to splenectomy, but although counts may also improve in systemic lupus erythematosus, an increased risk of vasculitis lessens splenectomy's value. Removing the spleen is an effective treatment for the neutropenia of hairy cell leukemia and occasionally for that due to other malignancies but is rarely required for hypersplenism due to benign causes.

Corticosteroids. Prednisone, 1 to 2 mg per kg per day for up to 3 weeks, elevates neutrophil levels dramatically in some patients with immunologically mediated neutropenia. Corticosteroids can then be tapered slowly occasionally, providing a lasting remission as in immune thrombocytopenia. Detecting antineutrophil antibodies in the serum predicts responsiveness of neutropenia in autoimmune diseases, lymphoma, infectious mononucleosis, and Graves' and Felty's syndromes. Some patients with cyclic neutropenia are treated effectively with chronic low dose corticosteroids, but since corticosteroids inhibit neutrophil function, they may not reduce infections despite improving counts.

Plasmapheresis. Removing antineutrophil antibodies in idiopathic, isoimmune, and drug- or lymphoma-associated neutropenia can have a dramatic although often temporary benefit.

Intravenous Gamma Globulin. Infusing 400 mg per kg per day of intravenous gamma globulin for 3 days is expensive but has induced remissions in immune neutropenia of infancy.

Antithymocyte Globulin. For severe neutropenia as part of aplastic anemia, antithymocyte globulin has been surprisingly beneficial in over half the cases. For isolated neutropenia its use is experimental.

Immunosuppression. Vincristine, cyclophosphamide, and similar agents are sometimes useful for immune neutropenia. Gold and danazol also may help.

Bone Marrow Transplantation. Bone marrow transplantation may be justified for severe aplastic anemia and severe congenital or hereditary neutropenia.

HEMOLYTIC DISEASE OF THE NEWBORN

(Erythroblastosis Fetalis)

method of
DAWN G. MUELLER, M.D.,
FAY O. REDWINE, M.D.,
and HAROLD M. MAURER, M.D.
Medical College of Virginia
Richmond, Virginia

A number of disorders may produce hemolytic disease of the newborn (HDN). Major causes include fetal-maternal red blood cell incompatibility with isoimmunization due to a variety of red blood cell antigens; congenital (hereditary) defects of the red blood cell membrane, enzymes, or hemoglobin; infection; disseminated intravascular coagulation; drugs and toxins; and metabolic abnormalities. Isoimmune HDN is the most common cause of anemia with hyperbilirubinemia. It occurs when maternal antibodies stimulated by incompatible fetal red cells in the maternal circulation cross the placenta and bind to antigenic sites on the fetal red blood cell, precipitating hemolysis. There is subsequent compensatory production of nucleated red blood cells in the bone marrow, liver, and spleen. Hemolysis leads to anemia, hypoproteinemia, anasarca, heart failure, and, ultimately, fetal death in severe cases. This picture of fetal hydrops also can be caused by more than 50 nonimmunologic disorders including congenital intrauterine infections; congenital abnormalities of the lungs, kidneys, or gastrointestinal tract; and vascular and cardiac anomalies. Although fetal-maternal ABO incompatibility is more common, the most serious cause of HDN is fetal-maternal Rh incompatibility. Additional antibodies that can cause HDN are C, E, Kell, Duffy, Kidd, MNSs, and others. The principles of managing HDN are similar regardless of cause. This discussion will focus on Rh isoimmunization.

The development of anti-D globulin (RhoGAM) in 1967 significantly decreased the incidence of Rh HDN by preventing maternal sensitization to the D antigen. However, maternal sensitization is still seen for the following reasons: failure to obtain or laboratory error in determining a pregnant woman's blood type; failure to obtain or accurately type the newborn infant's blood; clerical error in recording the mother's blood type; failure to administer anti-D globulin when indicated, e.g., following amniocentesis, placenta previa, abruptio placenta, ectopic pregnancy, or spontaneous abortion; failure to administer anti-D globulin at 28 weeks gestation in all Rh negative unsensitized women; and failure to respond to the standard dose of anti-D globulin administered post partum because of an excessive fetal-maternal transfusion.

MANAGEMENT

Antepartum Diagnosis

All women should undergo blood typing and antibody screening (indirect Coombs' test) at the beginning of each pregnancy. The diagnosis of isoimmunization is made by detecting and then identifying the antibody during prenatal testing. If the antibody titer is equal to or less than 1 to 8, the test must be repeated monthly. In most centers a titer of greater than 1 to 8 signifies that the fetus is at risk for HDN, and more precise fetal evaluation through amniotic fluid analysis must be undertaken.

Amniocentesis is performed under real time ultrasound guidance. The amniotic fluid bilirubin concentration is measured by spectrophotometric analysis at 450 millimicrons ($m\mu$). The result is reported as the difference between the measured and control optical densities (Δ OD 450). The δ OD 450 is then plotted on a semilogarithmic graph (Liley graph) that depicts degrees of sensitization (zones 1 to 3) (Figure 1). The timing of the first amniocentesis for Δ OD 450 depends on the severity of isoimmunization. If sensitization is noted with the first pregnancy, the initial amniocentesis should be done between 26 and 28 weeks gestation. If a woman has had a baby who suffered an intrauterine death from Rh HDN or a previous child with severe HDN or fetal hydrops, the first amniocentesis should be done at 24 weeks and, in unusual cases, perhaps as early as 20 weeks.

If the initial Δ OD 450 is in zone 1, amniocentesis should be repeated every two to three weeks.

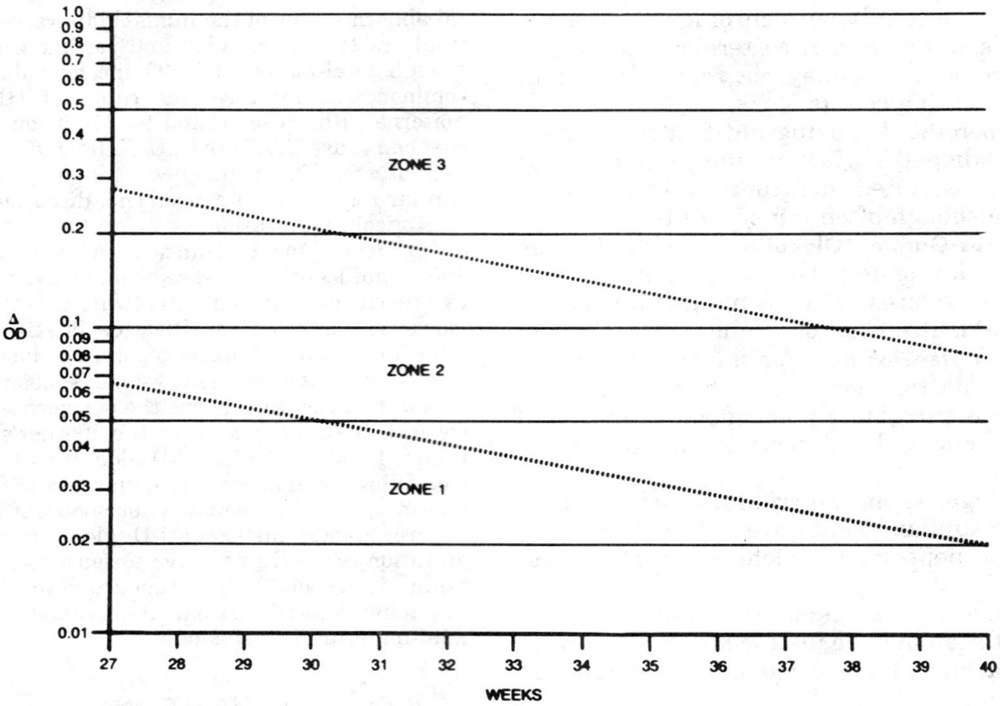

Figure 1. Modified Liley graph depicting degrees of sensitization.

If the initial Δ OD is in zone 2, amniocentesis should be repeated in seven to ten days. For the fetus whose Δ OD 450 is in zone 3 or in zone 2 but rapidly rising toward zone 3, intervention in the form of either an intrauterine transfusion or premature delivery is indicated. Prior to 32 to 34 weeks gestation the fetus should be managed with intrauterine transfusions. Beyond 34 weeks delivery should be considered. All decisions should be based on gestational age as well as on the results of amniotic fluid studies for fetal lung maturity (lecithin/sphingomyelin [L:S] ratio and the presence of phosphatidyl glycerol). The mode of delivery depends on the inducibility of the cervix and the presentation of the fetus. If labor is to be induced, the fetus should be carefully monitored with a continuous heart tracing. Prompt delivery by cesarean section should be performed if there is evidence of fetal distress. Selection of the optimal date for delivery requires a joint obstetric-pediatric decision weighing the risk of continued hemolysis in utero versus the risk of severe respiratory distress syndrome following birth.

Intrauterine Transfusion

The fetus who is remote from maturity and has a rapidly rising Δ OD 450 in zone 2 or a Δ OD 450 in zone 3 should receive an intrauterine transfusion. Real time ultrasonography has revolutionized this procedure, and with skilled operators the fetal loss rate per transfusion is less than 5 per cent. Cytomegalovirus negative, O negative washed packed red blood cells, guided by ultrasound imaging, are infused into the peritoneal cavity of the fetus. The procedure requires sterile conditions and at least two skilled operators; one to perform continuous ultrasonography and the other to place the catheter. A 16-gauge radiopaque catheter is used for this procedure. With ultrasound, a suitable entry site into the uterus is selected with attempts made to avoid the placenta and, more importantly, the umbilical cord insertion on the placenta. The entry point into the fetal abdomen is selected to avoid the liver, umbilical cord insertion, and bladder. The tip of the catheter is prominently displayed with ultrasound and therefore can be precisely positioned. Once the catheter is in place, the needle is removed, leaving the plastic catheter in the fetal peritoneal cavity. While one operator continuously monitors the fetal heart rate, the other operator slowly infuses the blood. The volume of blood to be instilled is calculated by the following formula: (weeks of gestation $-$ 20) $\times$ 10 $=$ ml of packed red blood cells required. The procedure is discontinued if fetal tachycardia or bradycardia is encountered or if a rise in fetal intraperitoneal pressure is perceived by the operator. At the end of the transfusion, the catheter is removed, and the mother is observed for 6 hours at bed rest before being allowed to ambulate.

Intrauterine transfusions are repeated every two to three weeks depending on the condition and gestational age of the fetus. The transfused red blood cells are absorbed by the fetal lymphatic system, and approximately 90 per cent of the red blood cells are subsequently incorporated into the fetal intravascular circulation. An intrauterine transfusion may have limited success in a fetus who is grossly hydropic because the red blood cells are poorly absorbed from the abdominal cavity. Investigators in England have perfected a direct intravascular intrauterine transfusion technique involving catheterization of the umbilical vein under ultrasound guidance. In the future, this procedure may gain acceptance as the preferred method for intrauterine transfusion, especially in cases of massive fetal hydrops.

The overall perinatal survival rate for infants requiring intrauterine transfusions is approximately 75 per cent. This technique, however, treats fetal hemolysis rather than the underlying immunologic disorder. Over the past 15 years, other treatment modalities for the severely sensitized patient have been investigated. These include intensive plasmapheresis of the mother to reduce circulating anti-Rh antibody, immunosuppression with corticosteroid or promethazine hydrochloride (Phenergan) therapy, and attempts at maternal desensitization through oral administration of Rh positive red cell membranes. The use of these immunologic treatments to prevent Rh sensitization has not consistently improved outcome. Because therapy with these methods remains controversial, they are not recommended.

Delivery

A pediatrician should be in attendance at the delivery of all severely Rh-sensitized infants. Although many infants will be born with a mild anemia, the severity of the disease cannot always be accurately predicted on the basis of amniotic fluid bilirubin levels. The child should be assessed quickly for evidence of pallor, hepatosplenomegaly, edema, and ascites. Jaundice, even with significant in utero hemolysis, is rarely evident on the initial exam. Cord blood should be sent immediately to the laboratory for hemoglobin and hematocrit assessments, reticulocyte count, blood typing, direct Coombs' testing, and bilirubin determination.

If a moderately or severely affected infant is anticipated, the neonatal team should be notified so that advanced planning can be done. Delivery room personnel must be prepared to aggressively manage asphyxia, respiratory distress, shock, profound anemia, and congestive heart failure. Respiratory insufficiency secondary to ascites or pleural effusion may require paracentesis or thoracentesis. A team of physicians and nurses should be assigned to the infant. Following delivery, the child is rapidly dried off, suctioned, and placed under a radiant warmer. One physician is responsible for airway management, while the others are free, if necessary, to undertake external cardiac massage, insert the umbilical arterial and venous lines, and perform paracentesis or thoracentesis. An umbilical venous catheter (UVC) is inserted first for administration of medications, removal of blood for laboratory studies, and facilitation of transfusion. The umbilical arterial catheter (UAC) is inserted to facilitate monitoring of oxygenation, ventilation, and pH during resuscitation. The nurses must have all resuscitation medications readily available and must be able to assist with various procedures.

In such circumstance, O negative packed red blood cells less than five days old should be available for use in the delivery room. If the hematocrit is less than 30 per cent, a partial exchange transfusion with packed red blood cells is performed to rapidly correct the anemia and increase the total blood oxygen carrying capacity. This procedure also avoids the danger of volume overload that may occur if a simple transfusion is used. We have found that a partial exchange transfusion of 40 ml per kg will raise the infant's hematocrit by approximately 10 points. In this procedure the blood is warmed to near body temperature. The exchange transfusion is carried out through the UVC, which has been inserted 5 to 10 cm (depending on the size of the infant), until good flow is obtained with blood withdrawal. The partial exchange transfusion is then performed over 15 to 30 minutes, utilizing 5 to 20 ml aliquots based on the infant's weight. With profound shock an additional 10 ml per kg of packed red blood cells should be directly infused following completion of the partial exchange.

Central venous pressure measurements can be helpful in assessing the blood volume. However, such readings in the delivery room are frequently in error because the UVC may be positioned within the portal system. Elevated readings may be indicative of the increased abdominal pressure seen in association with ascites or hepatosplenomegaly rather than hypervolemia. For this reason, central venous pressure values should not form the basis for clinical management decisions until the UVC position is documented radiographically to be above the diaphragm at the junction of the inferior vena cava and the right atrium. Furthermore, recent studies have shown that after correction of the asphyxia and acidosis seen in hydropic or nonhydropic severely Rh-sensitized infants, central venous pressure measurements fall to normal without blood volume manipulations. Contrary to previously held beliefs, many Rh-affected infants are normovolemic or hypovolemic at birth.

Once the infant's respiratory and cardiovascular systems have stabilized, transfer to the newborn intensive care unit can be accomplished safely.

Neonatal Intensive Care

Management after transfer from the delivery room is based on the infant's initial presentation. In some cases, anemia and hyperbilirubinemia will be the only concerns. In others born prematurely with significant hemolytic disease, the physician is faced with the challenge of caring for an infant who also has asphyxia, severe respiratory distress syndrome, and congestive heart failure. Such infants require aggressive respiratory support and careful fluid management. Radiographic documentation of line placements should be obtained immediately after admission. Central venous and aortic pressure measurements are utilized in assessing the infant's cardiovascular status. Normal central venous pressure values range from 1 to 8 cm water pressure, or 1.5 to 6 torr. Mean arterial pressure measurements are directly related to weight and range from a normal of 25 torr in 1-kg infants to 45 torr in 3- to 4-kg infants. Echocardiography may be helpful in assessing cardiac function and the need for inotropic drugs. The urine output should be measured and furosemide (Lasix), 1 to 2 mg per kg per dose, used to assist with fluid mobilization.

Exchange Transfusion

By effectively removing sensitized red blood cells and reducing potentially toxic levels of bilirubin, exchange transfusion remains the treatment mainstay in preventing the development of kernicterus in HDN. In a double volume exchange transfusion, approximately 85 per cent of sensitized infant cells are removed. The serum bilirubin falls to 50 per cent of the pre-exchange concentration after the procedure but rebounds to 75 per cent of the original level as tissue-bound bilirubin re-enters the circulation within a few hours of completion of the procedure. The first double volume exchange transfusion removes the majority of sensitized cells. Subsequent exchange transfusions, when needed, effectively lower serum bilirubin levels.

Infants with Rh HDN have a fairly predictable incidence of hemolysis. Criteria for performing an exchange transfusion are based on these projected trends. In addition, one can generally assume that if intrauterine transfusions have been required, the affected infant will most likely need at least one exchange transfusion after birth. Infants with cord bilirubin levels greater than 4 to 5 mg per dl (normal 0.4 to 2.7 mg per dl) and cord hematocrits less than 35 per cent should receive an exchange transfusion as soon as blood can be set up. In full term or near full term infants, additional indications for the initial exchange transfusion include serum bilirubin levels greater than 10 mg per dl in the first 24 hours, greater than 15 mg per dl in the second 24 hours, and equal to or greater than 20 mg per dl after 48 hours of age. In low birth weight infants in whom the risk of kernicterus is aggravated by asphyxia, hypoxia, acidosis (pH less than 7.25), hypothermia, sepsis, and hypoalbuminemia, the levels are lower (Table 1). The level of indirect-reacting (unconjugated) bilirubin is the basis for determining the need for treatment. In some infants with severe HDN, the level of direct-reacting (conjugated) bilirubin can rise sharply in the first few days of life, presumably owing to in utero hepatocellular dysfunction. Although some centers have utilized various bilirubin binding studies (e.g., HBABA, salicylate saturation index) to formulate exchange transfusion criteria, these studies are ancillary at best. After the first exchange transfusion, subsequent exchange transfusions are done if the rate of rise of serum bilirubin is greater than 0.5 mg per dl per hour.

Technique

All exchange transfusions should be performed through a No. 5 or 8 French catheter. Because of the risk of emboli mobilization with the use of an umbilical artery catheter, this line should only be used for an exchange transfusion when there is no access to the umbilical vein. If blood cannot be withdrawn easily through the UVC despite manipulations, one can withdraw blood slowly through the UAC and infuse blood via the UVC. Maintenance intravenous fluids should be infused through a peripheral intravenous line or UAC while the exchange transfusion is in progress. We reprep the UVC and abdomen and drape the patient prior to starting the exchange transfusion because the UVC may require manipulation during the procedure to maintain good blood flow. The operator wears a cap, mask, gown, and gloves. A second operator records vital signs and the blood warmer temperature every 15 minutes and monitors the glucose level every 30 minutes using a glucose reagent test strip. All this information is recorded in chronologic order, along with a notation of each volume increment exchanged with a cumulative running total. A

TABLE 1. **Indications for Exchange Transfusion in Low Birth Weight Infants by Level of Total Bilirubin (mg per dl) and Birth Weight**

	<1000 grams	1000–1249 grams	1250–1499 grams	1500–1999 grams	2000–2500 grams	>2500 grams
No risk factors	10	13	15	17	18	20
Risk factors for kernicterus*	8	10	13	15	17	18

*Asphyxia, hypoxia, acidosis (pH < 7.25), hypothermia, sepsis, hypoalbuminemia.

Pharmaseal Sterile Exchange Transfusion Tray (Pharmaseal Laboratories, Glendale, California) is used. In our institution, citrate-phosphate-dextrose-adenine (CPD-A_1) O negative packed red blood cells less than five days old are utilized. The cells are then reconstituted with group specific (for the infant) or AB fresh frozen plasma to a final hematocrit of 50 to 60 per cent. For a double volume exchange transfusion, 160 to 180 ml per kg up to a maximum of 500 ml of whole blood is used. The total volume ordered should include an additional 60 to 100 ml of blood to fill the tubing. Generally, the infant should be given 1 gram per kg of 25 per cent albumin 60 to 90 minutes prior to the procedure to mobilize tissue-bound bilirubin. This "albumin priming" is contraindicated if there is pre-existing edema or significant anemia (hematocrit less than 35 per cent), since the volume produced by the albumin may precipitate congestive heart failure.

The blood is warmed to 37 C (98.6 F) using a Fenwal Blood Warming Bag and Blood Warmer (Fenwal Labs, Deerfield, Illinois). The volume aliquots used for the exchange transfusion are dependent on weight; they range from 5 ml in the infant less than 1000 grams to 20 ml per exchange volume in infants greater than 3000 grams. To allow adequate time for cardiovascular stabilization, the total time for performing the procedure should be 1 to 1½ hours. Following completion of the exchange transfusion, an additional 10 to 20 ml of blood may be directly infused if the infant was significantly anemic at the outset or had an abnormally low central venous pressure measurement. Pre-exchange transfusion laboratory studies should include blood culture, complete blood count with differential, platelet count, and total and direct-reacting bilirubin. Post–exchange transfusion studies include the aforementioned along with serum electrolytes and calcium. A blood sample should be sent to the blood bank in anticipation of a subsequent exchange transfusion.

After completion of the exchange transfusion, vital signs and blood pressure should be measured every 15 minutes for one hour and every 30 minutes for an additional two hours before resuming routine monitoring. Glucose levels must also be followed closely for the first few hours after the procedure. Although it is a good practice to remove the UVC after completion of the procedure, we generally leave the catheter in place until the trend of subsequent bilirubin levels has been determined. Hematocrit and bilirubin determinations should be obtained three hours post–exchange transfusion and every four to six hours thereafter. In the more critically ill infant, the UVC is left in place to continue central venous pressure monitoring. Because of the risk of gastrointestinal ischemia, infants should not be fed while a UVC is in place. Feedings are withheld for 12 hours after removal of the line.

In experienced hands, the mortality rate from exchange transfusion is less than 0.5 per cent. Complications, although infrequent, still can occur. Associated electrolyte and metabolic abnormalities include hyperkalemia (generally not significant if blood less than four days old is used), reactive hypoglycemia due to the high dextrose concentration in the CPD anticoagulant, and, infrequently, acidosis. Hypocalcemia also is a concern because of the postulated increase in calcium-citrate binding. Although some centers advocate routinely giving supplemental calcium gluconate at periodic intervals during the exchange transfusion, we only infuse this drug at a dose of 100 mg per kg slowly over 5 minutes if the infant develops tachycardia or increasing irritability or jitteriness or if a prolonged ST segment is noted on EKG monitoring. Arrhythmias secondary to catheter placement in the right atrium, hypothermia, sepsis, air or blood emboli, and thrombosis also have been reported. Thrombocytopenia is common and may become a significant problem if repeated exchange transfusions are necessary.

Phototherapy

Phototherapy is an *adjunctive* treatment in the management of HDN. In mild cases this may be the only therapy required. The mechanism of action appears to be a light-induced conversion, or photoisomerization, of unconjugated bilirubin to geometric isomers (termed photoisomers or photobilirubin), which are water soluble, and thus excreted by the liver without further transformation. The effective wavelength of light is

420 to 470 nanometers (nm). The light waves act primarily on the portion of bilirubin deposited in the skin. For phototherapy to be effective, as much of the body surface area as possible must be exposed to the light. As a general rule one should consider starting phototherapy when the serum bilirubin concentration is 5 to 10 mg per dl below the established exchange transfusion level. Because of the predictable and rapid hemolysis seen in Rh disease, affected infants generally require early therapy. An exchange transfusion should not be delayed for a trial of phototherapy.

Known complications of phototherapy include dehydration from either an increase in insensible water loss or diarrhea. Maintenance fluids are increased 10 to 20 per cent for infants undergoing phototherapy. Lactose-free formulas are used if the diarrhea is severe. Hyperthermia, irritability, and a transient rash also can be seen. To prevent retinal damage, the eyes are patched. Improper placement of these patches may be responsible for corneal damage, and if the nares are obstructed apnea may occur. Tanning of the skin may be seen, as the light can induce melanin synthesis. In addition, some infants requiring phototherapy for greater than 48 hours develop the "bronze baby" syndrome. This brown pigmentation of the skin occurs following the abnormal accumulation of photoproducts and pigments that are not efficiently excreted from the liver in patients with hepatocellular dysfunction.

Phototherapy should be discontinued when a progressive decline is noted in the bilirubin and the serum level is greater than 5 to 8 mg per dl below the exchange level. If there is a significant elevation in the direct-reacting fraction of bilirubin (greater than 3 to 5 mg per dl), phototherapy also should be stopped. A slight rebound in the bilirubin level within 8 to 12 hours of discontinuing therapy can be expected. Serum hematocrit and bilirubin determinations should be monitored for an additional 12 to 36 hours.

Phenobarbital is known to increase bilirubin excretion from the liver by enhancing hepatic microsomal enzymes. Oral agar and other binding agents are somewhat effective in lowering serum bilirubin concentration by blocking enterohepatic recirculation of bilirubin. Both of these treatment modalities have limited clinical applicability and should not be used in managing HDN.

Other Problems

In addition to the reactive hypoglycemia that may develop following an exchange transfusion, infants with Rh HDN may have a more protracted problem with hypoglycemia. The release of amino acids during red cell hemolysis in utero (specifically alanine) is felt to stimulate pancreatic islet cell hyperplasia and subsequent hyperinsulinism in the fetus. After birth such infants may require dextrose infusions as high as 15 to 20 per cent and steroids to enhance gluconeogenesis in an effort to maintain normal blood glucose levels. In conjunction with abnormal levels of direct-reacting bilirubin, some infants with HDN may have elevated liver enzyme values. These infants frequently have required in utero transfusions and more often develop the "bronze baby" syndrome. The liver enzyme values generally return to normal within four to six weeks.

Late Anemia

With milder forms of HDN, phototherapy may be the only treatment required. However, because an exchange transfusion was not employed, circulating maternal antibodies can cause a slow, steady hemolysis. These infants may require a simple transfusion with packed red blood cells (15 mg per kg) within the first week of life, or they may be noted to be anemic at four to six weeks of age. Although most infants with anemia at this age are well compensated, the child with persistent tachycardia, sweating, poor feeding, or other signs of congestive heart failure may require a simple transfusion. Because of the frequent occurrence of a late anemia, hemoglobin or hematocrit and reticulocyte levels must be monitored closely following discharge.

HEMOPHILIA AND RELATED CONDITIONS

method of
EDWARD H. ROMOND, M.D.
University of Kentucky
Lexington, Kentucky
and JOHN A. PENNER, M.D.
Michigan State University
East Lansing, Michigan

Plasma Products and Other Agents Used to Treat Bleeding (Table 1)

One unit of any clotting factor activity is defined as the coagulant activity found in 1 ml of fresh normal plasma.

Plasma. Fresh frozen plasma (FFP) contains about 200 units of clotting factor activity in each bag of 225 to 250 ml. This is slightly less than the foregoing definition of one unit per ml since about 10 to 20 per cent of the clotting activity is

TABLE 1. **Agents for Treatment of Hemophilia**

Product	Dose	Complications	Factor Deficiency Indications
Plasma	10 ml/kg	Congestive heart failure, hepatitis, isoagglutinin hemolysis	Fibrinogen, factor V, factor VII, factor VIII (mild), factor IX (mild), factor X, factor XI, factor XIII
Cryoprecipitate	2 bags/10 kg	Isoagglutinin hemolysis, hepatitis	Hemophilia A, VWD, fibrinogen
Factor VIII concentrates	10–30 units/kg	Hepatitis,* AIDS*	Hemophilia A
Prothrombin complex concentrates	30–100 units/kg	Hepatitis,* AIDS,* thrombosis†	Hemophilia B, factor VIII inhibitor, VII, X
Anti-inhibitor protease concentrates	30–100 units/kg	Hepatitis, AIDS, thrombosis†	Factor VIII—high inhibitor, hemophilia A
EACA	30–50 mg/kg	Thrombosis	Hemophilia A, VWD
DDAVP	0.3 μg/kg	Tachycardia	Mild hemophilia A, VWD—Type I, IIa

*Markedly reduced in heat-treated products.
†Reduced in heparin-containing products.

lost during freezing and thawing. FFP is used to treat bleeding when the deficient clotting proteins needed for hemostasis are labile coagulation factors, when the quantity of needed factor is small, or when the needed factor is one for which there are no prepared concentrates. It is, therefore, the product of choice for replacing deficiencies of factors V and XI and may also be used to replace factor VIII in mild hemophilia A when only small amounts of factor VIII:C are needed. Also, because of the hepatitis risk of nonheat-treated factor IX concentrates, plasma (not necessarily fresh) continues to be used for some patients with mild hemophilia B.

Cryoprecipitate. If plasma is frozen and then slowly thawed, a precipitate forms in the bottom of the bag. This cryoglobulin, when separated from the rest of the plasma, has a volume of about 20 ml and contains over half the factor VIII:C, von Willebrand factor, and fibrinogen of the original unit of plasma. It also contains factor XIII. Cryoprecipitate contains 80 to 120 units of factor VIII:C per bag and, compared with FFP, has the advantage of supplying an equivalent amount of factor VIII:C in about 15 per cent of the volume. Also, since it is made from single donor units of plasma, the chance of transmitting hepatitis and probably acquired immune deficiency syndrome (AIDS) is much less likely than with factor VIII concentrates. The main disadvantages of cryoprecipitate are that it must be stored at −25 C and that it takes time to reconstitute and administer. Because of the von Willebrand factor activity and fibrinogen content (0.25 gram per bag), cryoprecipitate is the treatment of choice for significant bleeding in von Willebrand's disease and hypofibrinogenemia.

Commercial Factor VIII Concentrates. Lyophilized concentrates of factor VIII:C form the cornerstone of treatment for most patients with severe hemophilia A. The concentrates can be reconstituted, drawn up in a syringe, and administered intravenously by the patient or by parents. Concentrates are manufactured from large pools, each containing plasma from several thousand donors. Even though plasma is screened for hepatitis B surface antigen, the size of the plasma pool results in some risk for both hepatitis B and non-A, non-B hepatitis. Indeed, about 90 per cent of hemophiliac patients regularly treated with concentrate eventually develop hepatitis B antibodies, and in about half liver function tests are chronically abnormal. The large number of plasma donors for each lot of concentrate also may be a factor in the transmission of AIDS to hemophiliacs. A heat-treated concentrate of factor VIII is now commercially available and is associated with a greatly reduced risk of hepatitis. In addition, data are now available to indicate that transmission of AIDS virus is probably eliminated in heat-treated products. In contrast to cryoprecipitate, lyophilized factor VIII concentrates have less von Willebrand factor activity and, therefore, are not used in the treatment of von Willebrand's disease.

Prothrombin Complex Concentrates (PCC). Preparations containing the vitamin K–dependent clotting factors (prothrombin, VII, IX, and X) are available from three commercial sources in the United States under the product names Konyne, Proplex, and Profilnine. These products contain small amounts of activated factors VIIa, IXa, and Xa as well and are the treatment of choice for patients with moderate or severe hemophilia B. Heat-treated PCC, which poses less risk of transmitting hepatitis and AIDS, is now available. In the near future a purified concentrate of factor IX with low levels of the other vitamin K–dependent factors will be available for treatment of hemophilia B.

Anti-Inhibitor Protease Concentrates. The hypothesis was set forth several years ago that a product containing activated factors, especially factor Xa, could "bypass" the need for factor VIII in the clotting sequence and might therefore be useful in treating patients with inhibitors (antibodies) to factor VIII. In vitro studies as well as clinical trials with patients have shown that prothrombin complex concentrates are able to control bleeding in patients with factor VIII and factor IX inhibitors. Two prothrombin complex concentrates with a high level of *activated* factors (Autoplex and FEIBA) now are available for the treatment of patients with factor VIII inhibitors. At a cost of several thousand dollars per dose, treatment with these anti-inhibitor protease concentrates should be limited to patients with high titer inhibitors who fail to respond to nonactivated products. All the prothrombin complex concentrates carry a risk of hepatitis and, because of the content of activated clotting factors, there is a significant risk of iatrogenic thrombosis, including disseminated intravascular coagulation and pulmonary embolism. Confirmed thrombotic complications, however, have been observed only with those products that do not contain heparin. The thromboembolic risk is greatest in patients with liver dysfunction or those undergoing surgery.

Epsilon-Aminocaproic Acid (EACA, Amicar). This agent inhibits lysis of clots by preventing activation of plasminogen. It has no effect on coagulation per se but helps stabilize clots once they are formed. As such, it is a helpful adjunct to cryoprecipitate or factor VIII concentrate in patients with hemophilia A or von Willebrand's disease. It is particularly useful as a means of controlling bleeding resulting from dental extractions or to decrease menorrhagia in women with von Willebrand's disease. Administration immediately before an extraction permits the incorporation of the agent into the forming clot and is most effective in preventing activation of the fibrinolytic system. In patients with mild or moderate deficiencies of clotting factors, EACA may be effective in controlling minor bleeding even when used alone. Because of increased risk of thrombosis, it should *never* be used in conjunction with prothrombin complex concentrates or in patients with hematuria.

Deamino-D-Arginine Vasopressin (DDAVP). This is a synthetic analogue of antidiuretic hormone that will increase a patient's circulating factor VIII:C or factor VIII:VWF level from two- to sixfold following intravenous administration. The higher levels of factor VIII can be maintained for about 48 hours. DDAVP, therefore, is recommended for patients with mild hemophilia A or type I or IIa von Willebrand's disease when short-term treatment is deemed sufficient to control moderate bleeding. In these patients it is recommended that a test dose of DDAVP be given (measuring predose and postdose factor levels) during an asymptomatic period, to determine the individual dose response that might be expected in the event of bleeding. DDAVP should be given at a dose of 0.3 micrograms per kg of body weight slowly over a 20 minute period to avoid tachycardia. Water retention has not been a problem with this drug.

HEMOPHILIA A

Comprehensive Care

The two most important developments in the treatment of hemophilia are the availability of factor VIII and factor IX concentrates for replacement therapy and the introduction of home care. At comprehensive care centers in five regional areas of the United States, teams of health care personnel provide medical and dental evaluation, orthopedic services, physical therapy, educational and emotional support, and vocational and genetic counseling. Because of these comprehensive care programs and the educational activities of the National Hemophilia Foundation, many hemophiliac patients are knowledgeable about their disease and participate actively in decisions about their health care. Thus, it is especially important for emergency care providers to discuss openly with patients or their parents the reasons behind diagnostic or treatment decisions.

The comprehensive care approach in concert with provision for home care has made it possible for hemophiliac patients to live virtually normal lives. Self-treatment at home and at school or work has markedly reduced the delay between injury and treatment.

Treatment of Bleeding Episodes

It is important to keep in mind that not all symptoms in hemophiliac patients are due to bleeding and not all of their bleeding is due to the hemophilia. Patients with gastrointestinal bleeding usually have an underlying pathologic lesion, such as a peptic ulcer. When bleeding occurs, however, from whatever cause, patients with hemophilia usually require treatment with factor VIII concentrate or cryoprecipitate. A convenient rule of thumb for estimating the appropriate dose of factor VIII is that the immediate postinfusion level of factor VIII:C (measured as a per cent of normal factor VIII:C activity) is about twice the numeric dose in units per kilogram of body weight. Thus, for example, a dose of 25 units per kg will result in an immediate post-transfusion factor VIII:C level of 50 per cent of normal (0.50 unit per ml). The half-life of factor VIII:C in plasma is approximately 8 to 12 hours but may be shorter if antibodies (inhibitors) to factor VIII are present.

Effective analgesia is an important part of treatment, and the best way to reduce pain from bleeding is to treat early. For mild or moderate bleeding a few doses of acetaminophen (with or without codeine) or propoxyphene usually are effective. For severe bleeding initial treatment with oxycodone or meperidine may be needed and can be prescribed for up to 24 hours. The intramuscular route of drug administration should be avoided. Although aspirin-containing drugs should never be used (discussed subsequently), some patients find significant relief from arthritic symptoms without a noticeable increase in bleeding tendency by using nonsteroidal anti-inflammatory agents. Narcotics should not be used for chronic pain because of the risk of addiction.

Hemarthroses. Bleeding into joints, especially knees, ankles, and elbows, is the most common form of acute bleeding in patients with hemophilia. Ice or cold packs applied immediately to the joint for 30 to 60 minutes help decrease pain and swelling and in cases of mild injury may obviate the need for factor replacement. In all but very mild injuries, however, the rule is to treat as early as possible (within 30 minutes) with concentrate or cryoprecipitate. When children with joint bleeding come to hospital emergency departments, they should be evaluated and treated immediately since a delay of only 30 minutes may cause sufficient build-up of pressure to produce severe pain, greater destruction to the joint, and a need for several days of treatment. Bleeding into the hip joint especially is important to diagnose and treat aggressively since it could produce aseptic necrosis of the femoral head. Inflammation in the hip joint can be distinguished from hematomas of the psoas and groin muscles by internally rotating the leg, which usually will elicit severe pain if the joint space is involved.

In general, the initial dose should raise the plasma factor VIII to a level of 20 to 30 per cent—that is, 10 to 15 units per kg. With more severe hemarthroses, including suspected episodes of hip bleeding, higher doses of 20 to 25 units per kg should be used, and in these cases, a lower dose of 15 units per kg should be repeated every 12 hours for 2 to 3 days.

Because bleeding and the resulting inflammation increase the vascularity of a joint, patients with recent hemarthroses are at significant risk for recurrent bleeding in the same joint. It is important, therefore, to immobilize the injured joint for a few days until inflammation has subsided and healing is well under way. Hiking boots for stabilizing ankles, slings for elbows, and splints for knees and wrists are helpful. Crutches should be used when weight-bearing joints are involved. However, prolonged continuous immobilization is not advisable, since this will result in muscle atrophy and further instability of the joint.

If frequent, recurrent joint bleeding does occur, consideration should be given to continuing treatment with factor replacement at 10 to 20 units per kg on a daily or every other day schedule for at least 3 to 4 weeks. Patients given prophylactic treatment also can be given EACA at a dose of 50 mg per kg every 3 to 6 hours for 7 to 10 days. When any episode of joint bleeding has resolved, it is important that a physiotherapy program be followed to restore maximum joint mobility and muscle strength.

Muscle and Soft Tissue Hemorrhage. Hemorhage into a muscle is less common than joint bleeding in patients with hemophilia. The symptoms include pain, swelling, and limitation of motion. Mild episodes of muscle bleeding may be treated with doses of concentrate or cryoprecipitate similar to those used for joint bleeding. More severe bleeding should be treated with higher doses of factor VIII at 20 to 50 units per kg every 8 to 12 hours for several days until pain has resolved. Bleeding into closed fascial compartments of the forearm, wrist, hand, or lower leg may cause vascular or neurologic compromise and may require surgical decompression if pain and neurologic function do not improve with factor replacement and elevation of the limb.

The amount of hemorrhage into large muscles of the thigh or abdomen may be much greater than clinically apparent. Blood loss dissecting along fascial planes may be massive enough to produce hypotension and shock. Retroperitoneal bleeding into the iliopsoas muscle may extend caudally to compress the femoral nerve, resulting in loss of sensation over the anterior thigh and loss of strength in the quadriceps muscle. The groin pain in psoas bleeding is exacerbated by extension of the hip but is not significantly increased by internal rotation. An abdominal x-ray view or an ultrasound study may demonstrate lateral displacement of the kidney and ureter. Psoas bleeding or any expanding hematoma, regardless of size, that may potentially compromise vascular, neurologic, or respiratory function is an indication for hospitalization, close observation, and frequent factor replacement in the doses mentioned previously.

Oral Bleeding. Bleeding in the pharynx, neck, or sublingual region constitutes an emergency because soft tissue swelling in these areas may occlude the airway. Hospitalization, with factor replacement at 30 units per kg every 8 hours, is indicated. Because clots on the tongue are so easy to dislodge, small children who bite their tongues often require hospitalization, frequent factor replacement for 4 to 5 days, and nutritional maintenance with intravenous fluids. For stabilization of clots, epsilon-aminocaproic acid (EACA) also is useful and should be continued for 5 to 7 days after bleeding has stopped. Minor gingival bleeding often can be controlled with topical thrombin, followed by several days of oral EACA.

Hematuria. About one of five hemophiliac patients at some time develops hematuria. When gross hematuria occurs as a result of trauma, treatment with cryoprecipitate or concentrate is indicated. Frequently, however, the cause of hematuria is not apparent. In these cases, as long as secondary causes such as infection have been ruled out, it is reasonable simply to force fluids and to treat with one or two doses of factor VIII at 10 units per kg. Epsilon-aminocaproic acid should not be used in patients with hematuria, since clots that form may produce an obstructive uropathy. Excretory urography may be performed as long as compression of the ureters is avoided.

Central Nervous System (CNS) Bleeding. CNS bleeding is a common cause of death in hemophilia. Any patient with moderate or severe head trauma should receive immediate factor VIII replacement therapy at 30 to 50 units per kg. After relatively minor trauma such as a fall, however, it may take hours or even days for symptoms to develop. Therefore, any patient who develops unexplained symptoms referable to the brain or spinal cord—such as lethargy, headache, or new peripheral neuropathy—should be given initial factor replacement in the same dose as for severe trauma while the problem is being evaluated. Lumbar puncture, if indicated, should be done only by an experienced physician and only after factor VIII levels have been raised to over 50 per cent and a computed tomography scan of the brain shows no space-occupying hematoma. If symptoms of spinal cord compression are present, it may be necessary to consider surgical intervention.

Prevention of Bleeding

Aspirin should never be used by patients with hemophilia since it produces irreversible platelet dysfunction by inhibiting platelet cyclo-oxygenase. The fact that so many proprietary drug combinations contain aspirin requires careful education of each hemophiliac so that he learns to recognize and avoid the myriad preparations that contain this ingredient. Antihistamines, phenothiazines, and nonsteroidal anti-inflammatory drugs also inhibit platelet function to a degree and should be avoided if alternative agents are effective.

Dental care is an important part of hemophilia preventive care. Daily attention to oral hygiene and regular check-ups are the best way to avoid the need for major dental work, such as tooth extractions. Local anesthesia should not be used without adequate factor replacement. Before any surgical procedure, including dental extraction, the patient should be evaluated for the possible presence of an inhibitor. If none is found, he should then receive concentrate or cryoprecipitate at 30 units per kg immediately before the procedure, and doses should be repeated every 12 hours for 2 to 3 days. EACA should also be given at about 30 mg per kg every 6 hours for 10 days.

Prevention of bleeding through a daily program of exercise that does not involve trauma to the joints or muscles should be strongly encouraged. Swimming, bicycle riding, and isometric exercises are excellent for strengthening muscle groups that support and stabilize synovial joints.

For patients who have had repeated episodes of joint or soft tissue bleeding, a program of prophylactic every-other-day replacement therapy may be considered. The potential benefit of such an approach, however, must be balanced against the cost and the increased risks of hepatitis, development of an inhibitor, and possibly AIDS. In general, we advocate such a program only in patients in whom all other approaches have failed; we continue the prophylaxis for a predetermined period of 6 to 12 weeks.

Surgery

Once adequate clotting factor replacement has been established, and provided the patient does not have an inhibitor, the risks of uncomplicated surgery for a patient with hemophilia are the same as those for a patient without hemophilia. Because of the potential for intraoperative or postoperative complications, however, major elective surgery should be performed only under the care of physicians experienced in hemophilia management and with the support of a coagulation laboratory capable of performing accurate factor and inhibitor assays on demand. A sensitive screening assay always should be performed preoperatively to exclude the presence of an inhibitor to factor VIII. Within 1 hour before surgery, 30 units per kg of factor VIII should be administered, followed by a continuous intravenous infusion of 3 units per kg per hour during the first 24 to 48 hours, depending on the extent of surgery. If the patient remains clinically stable, the same dosage (30 units per kg) should be continued at 8 hour intervals for 3 to 5 days, after which the interval can be increased to every 12 hours for an additional 5 to 7 days. Following major orthopedic procedures, it may be important to continue factor replacement for several weeks. Physical therapy, if needed, should be arranged

TABLE 2. **Other Inherited Coagulation Factor Deficiencies**

Factor	Clinical Features	Lab Studies	Treatment	Comments
Fibrinogen	Dysfibrinogen: Uterine bleeding and/or thrombosis	PT, TCT, prolonged	FFP, cryo	Anticoagulate if thrombosis
	Afibrinogen: joint hemorrhage, epistaxis	PT, TCT, bleeding time prolonged	FFP, cryo	Homozygous state, rare
V	Menorrhagia,* epistaxis, bruising	Prolonged PT and PTT	FFP, platelet concentrates	PT not corrected by RVV
VII	Menorrhagia,* mucous membrane bleeding, gastrointestinal bleeding	Prolonged PT, normal PTT	FFP, PCC	PT corrected by RVV
X	Variable: bruising, menorrhagia,* hemarthrosis	Prolonged PT and PTT	FFP, PCC	PT corrected +/− by RVV
XI	Menorrhagia,* epistaxis, bruising	Prolonged PTT on fresh plasma	Plasma	Jewish ancestry, New York City, Los Angeles
XII, Fitzgerald, Fletcher	No known bleeding disorders	Prolonged PTT	None	
XIII	Ecchymosis, hematomas, poor wound healing, intracranial hemorrhage, spontaneous abortion	PT, PTT, TCT, all normal	Plasma, cryo	Clot soluble in 5M urea

*Birth control pills decrease menorrhagia.

Cryo, cryoprecipitate; FFP, fresh frozen plasma; PCC, prothrombin complex concentrate; PT, prothrombin time; PTT, partial thromboplastin time; RVV, Russell's viper venom; TCT, thrombin clotting time.

so that it is given after scheduled doses of factor replacement. If possible, a predose plasma level of factor VIII activity should be checked daily for several days.

Activated partial thromboplastin time (APTT) assay also may be obtained daily to monitor therapy but cannot substitute for the availability of an accurate factor VIII activity assay (APTT may be normal when factor VIII levels are at 15 to 20 per cent). If the APTT becomes more prolonged or if the factor level decreases, the presence of an inhibitor should be suspected. If an inhibitor is confirmed, the factor dose should be increased, and if this is not effective, anti-inhibitor protease concentrates should be used.

In patients with blood types A, B, or AB who receive frequent large doses of factor VIII concentrate, the development of spherocytes on the blood smear, a rising serum lactate dehydrogenase level, or an increased indirect bilirubin level may indicate the development of a Coombs-positive hemolytic anemia caused by anti-A or anti-B isoagglutinins in the concentrate. For these patients type-specific concentrate should be used. Note also that factor VIII concentrates contain significant amounts of fibrinogen and that the large doses of factor required for surgery may produce a striking increase in fibrinogen with subsequent hemolytic anemia.

Treatment of Patients with Inhibitors

About 10 per cent of the patients with hemophilia develop antibodies or inhibitors to factor VIII. The level of inhibitor, measured in Bethesda units, may be thought of as the number of milliliters of normal plasma that can be reduced to 50 per cent factor VIII:C activity by 1 ml of patient plasma. Sometimes in patients with inhibitors treatment with factor VIII does not stimulate or increase the inhibitor titer. In these patients, whose plasma usually has less than 8 Bethesda units, factor VIII concentrate is effective if given in doses sufficient to override the inhibitor. However, most patients characteristically develop an anamnestic response to treatment, in which the initially low inhibitor level rises rapidly 4 to 6 days after exposure to factor VIII. When the inhibitor titer measures less than 40 Bethesda units, plasmapheresis over a several day period may decrease the antibody level and thereby the dose of concentrate needed for treatment. With higher levels of inhibitor or when the anamnestic response has occurred, prothrombin complex concentrates (PCC) or anti-inhibitor protease concentrates should be used. Inhibitor patients with less than severe bleeding may respond to doses of 50 to 100 units per kg of PCC administered at 8 to 12 hour intervals. If the patient does not improve after two or three doses, continued treatment with nonactivated products is seldom effective, and activated concentrates should be considered in doses of 30 to 100 units per kg. Because of serious problems that may arise, patients with inhibitors who require extended treatment for any reason should be managed by a hemophilia center.

Treatment and the Risk of AIDS

Even though the acquired immune deficiency syndrome (AIDS) in hemophiliac patients is undoubtedly associated with a retrovirus transmitted through the use of factor VIII concentrates, the National Hemophilia Foundation has stated quite clearly that patients should not delay or avoid treatment of bleeding because of fear of AIDS. To minimize the risk of AIDS, however, the following guidelines have been set forth: (1) Physicians should strongly consider prescribing heat-treated concentrates for patients with severe hemophila. (2) For newborn infants, children under 4 years of age, and newly identified patients with severe hemophilia never previously treated with concentrates, heat-treated factors VIII and IX are the preferred products. (*Note:* Hepatitis B vaccination should also be administered to these patients.) In areas where the incidence of AIDS in the general population is low, however, cyroprecipitate (for hemophilia A) or fresh-frozen plasma (for hemophilia B) may still be preferable for these young patients. (3) DDAVP should be used whenever possible in patients with mild or moderate hemophilia. (4) Elective surgical procedures should be cautiously evaluated with respect to the possible advantages and disadvantages of a delay.

HEMOPHILIA B

About 20 per cent of all patients with hemophilia have factor IX deficiency with clinical symptoms indistinguishable from those of classic hemophilia. The principles of treatment for hemophilia B and hemophilia A are essentially the same; the main difference in treatment is in the products and dosages used. For mild hemophilia B and for minor bleeding, plasma is the treatment of choice. For moderate or severe hemophilia B, prothrombin complex concentrate (PCC) is needed. One bag of plasma contains about 200 units of factor IX. The factor IX content of PCC is indicated on the package for each preparation. Since the factor IX molecule is much smaller than the factor VIII complex and is more easily distributed in the extravascular space, the dose needed to achieve a given plasma level of factor IX is about twice that used in estimating a dosage of factor VIII. Thus, 25 units per kg will raise the plasma factor IX level by approximately 25 per cent. On the other hand, because of the longer half-life of factor IX compared with factor VIII, replacement may be given less frequently. In most instances, PCC at a dose of 20 to 30 units per kg of PCC every 24 hours is sufficient to control bleeding.

Elective surgery in hemophilia B must be considered carefully with respect to the potential thrombogenicity of PCC. When surgery is necessary and PCC must be used, it should be administered preoperatively at 40 units per kg. For nonheparinized products, about 500 units of heparin should be added to accelerate the clearance of activated clotting factors. Subsequent doses of PCC should be split over the course of the day (10 units per kg every 8 hours) to minimize the risk of thromboembolic complications. The fibrinogen, platelet count, and fibrin degradation product level should be followed daily to detect early disseminated intravascular coagulation. Some information also may be obtained by checking the antithrombin III level. If it is decreased, fresh frozen plasma should be administered to replenish antithrombin. Epsilon-aminocaproic acid should never be used concurrently with PCC because of the enhanced risk of thrombosis. Postoperative immobilization also increases the thrombogenic risk, and, therefore, early physical therapy and ambulation are strongly encouraged.

VON WILLEBRAND'S DISEASE

Because platelet adhesion is secured by VW factor and is an initial step in controlling bleeding from open surfaces, patients with von Willebrand's disease (VWD) most often are seen with mucocutaneous bleeding. A history of bleeding after dental extractions or tonsillectomy is typical. Fortunately, most patients with VWD do not experience the severe spontaneous bleeding that is characteristic of hemophilia. Certain situations, however, require specific attention.

Surgery in patients with VWD requires enough von Willebrand factor (factor VIII:VWF) to correct the hemostatic defect. Fresh frozen plasma (FFP) at 10 ml per kg or cryoprecipitate at 1 bag (80 to 100 units) per 10 kg usually will provide adequate hemostasis even though the bleeding time may not become completely normal. Repeated doses of FFP or cryoprecipitate need to be administered every 8 hours. Paradoxically, in patients with severe VWD and associated low levels of factor VIII:C, administration of FFP or cryoprecipitate stimulates the release of factor VIII:C from storage sites and stabilizes it in the circulation so that blood levels of the coagulant portion of the factor VIII complex may remain near normal for many hours.

In minor bleeding, replacement with blood products should not be done because of the small but real risk of hepatitis. Epistaxis usually can be controlled by local pressure. If this is not effective, the nostrils should be packed with gauze coated with petroleum jelly. Prophylaxis against nosebleeds includes use of a humidifier and, of course, avoidance of aspirin-containing drugs. In patients with mild VWD who are having dental extractions, use of cryoprecipitate often can be omitted by raising the factor VIII level with DDAVP. Epsilon-aminocaproic acid (EACA) also should be used before and continued for a week after dental extractions. Severe nosebleeds likewise should be treated with EACA for 1 week.

DDAVP may be used effectively in type 1 (classic) VWD in which there is a low but not absent level of functional protein. In type IIa VWD, the protein is present in normal amounts but is dysfunctional and the effectiveness of DDAVP is variable. In type IIb VWD, the protein is present in normal or increased amounts and there is hyper-responsiveness to platelet-aggregating agents. In this uncommon type of VWD, DDAVP is contraindicated. In type III VWD, there is total absence of protein, and therefore cryoprecipitate must be used.

Women with VWD who have menorrhagia may benefit from taking estrogen-containing birth control pills, since these compounds usually increase factor VIII:VWF activity in plasma. Similarly, the hormonal changes of pregnancy usually produce a spontaneous rise in the factor VIII level which lasts throughout delivery. Indeed, if the bleeding time and factor VIII:VWF have become normal at the end of pregnancy, a normal vaginal delivery should be planned. Cryoprecipitate should be on hand in case excessive bleeding occurs in the postpartum period. When the bleeding time and factor VIII:VWF do not become normal, cryoprecipitate should be administered during labor and continued after delivery.

OTHER INHERITED COAGULATION FACTOR DEFICIENCIES

These, along with treatment, are presented in Table 2.

PLATELET-MEDIATED BLEEDING DISORDERS

method of
JOHN G. KELTON, M.D.
McMaster University
Hamilton, Ontario

The hemostatic system limits the amount of blood lost when blood vessels are cut. Hemostasis requires the interaction of the blood vessels, platelets, and coagulation factors. A minor defect or deficiency in one of the components by itself will not cause bleeding; however, severe defects in a single component or minor defects in two or more can lead to bleeding. Thus a mild defect in platelet number or function will not result in bleeding, unless it is accompanied by a coagulation or vascular defect. Platelet-mediated hemostatic defects are usually quantitative (thrombocytopenia) but can be qualitative (defective platelet function). The hallmark of either is spontaneous microvascular bleeding that ranges in severity from petechiae and purpura to overt bleeding. Occasionally, the first evidence of a platelet function defect is excessive bleeding at surgery. In this situation, a hemostatic defect that otherwise would be trivial is exacerbated by vascular damage.

Thrombocytopenia (Quantitative Defects)

It is important to determine whether the thrombocytopenia is due to underproduction or increased destruction, since the treatment of each is different. Hematopoietic cells originate from a common stem cell; therefore, most patients with thrombocytopenia caused by reduced platelet production (aregenerative thrombocytopenia) have a reduction in the other blood cells, especially the leukocytes. In contrast, isolated thrombocytopenia usually is due to the destruction of platelets following their release from the bone marrow (consumptive thrombocytopenia) (Table 1). Patients with consumptive thrombocytopenia produce normal or increased numbers of platelets but are thrombocytopenic because the platelets are prematurely destroyed. Consequently, they have increasd numbers of platelet precursors (megakaryocytes) in the bone marrow. Because their platelets have a shortened lifespan, those platelets remaining in the circulation tend to be large, "young" platelets.

The first step in the investigation of a patient with thrombocytopenia is to confirm that the patient in fact is thrombocytopenic. Pseudothrombocytopenia must be excluded by examination of a stained blood film.

Consumptive Thrombocytopenia

After consumptive thrombocytopenia is diagnosed, the underlying cause is identified and corrected and the bleeding treated. The sudden development of thrombocytopenia in a hospitalized patient often is due to drug-induced thrombocytopenia, septicemia, or disseminated intravascular coagulation (DIC). The "well patient" who seeks medical attention because of isolated thrombocytopenia often will have idiopathic thrombocytopenic purpura (ITP). Less commonly, the patients will have drug-induced platelet destruction.

Septicemic Thrombocytopenia. Thrombocytopenia often is the first sign of gram-positive or gram-negative bacterial septicemia. Some patients

TABLE 1. **Investigation and Management of Patients with Thrombocytopenic Bleeding**

	Typical Peripheral Blood Findings	Typical Bone Marrow Findings	Other Investigations	Specific Treatment	Platelet Transfusions: *Prophylactic*	Platelet Transfusions: *Therapeutic (For Serious Bleeding)*
CONSUMPTIVE THROMBOCYTOPENIA						
Immunologic						
Idiopathic thrombocytopenic purpura	Isolated thrombocytopenia	Increased megakaryocytes	Thyroid function, ANA, platelet-associated IgG	Adults: corticosteroids, splenectomy, immunosuppressive agents	No	Yes
Drug-induced thrombocytopenia	Isolated thrombocytopenia	Increased megakaryocytes	Exclude other causes	Discontinue the drug	Yes	Yes
Post-transfusion purpura	Isolated thrombocytopenia	Increased megakaryocytes	Platelet typing, platelet-associated IgG	Corticosteroids, plasmapheresis	No	Uncertain
Secondary immune thrombocytopenia (sarcoidosis, lymphoproliferative disorders, SLE, etc)	Isolated thrombocytopenia	Increased megakaryocytes	Depends upon suspected underlying disorder, e.g., lymph node biopsy for lymphoproliferative disorder	Treat the underlying disorder	Yes	Yes
Immunologic plus nonimmunologic						
Septicemia	Thrombocytopenia plus leukocytosis		Blood cultures	Antibiotics	Yes	Yes
Nonimmunologic						
DIC	Isolated thrombocytopenia	Increased megakaryocytes	Coagulation screens (APTT, TCT, FDP, PT, protamine sulfate)	Coagulation replacement and treat underlying disorder	Yes	Yes
AREGENERATIVE THROMBOCYTOPENIA						
Chemotherapy	Pancytopenia	Pancytopenia plus residual malignant cells			Yes	Yes
Marrow infiltration (leukemia)	Thrombocytopenia plus malignant cells	Malignant cells		Chemotherapy	Yes	Yes
Idiosyncratic drug reactions	Isolated thrombocytopenia alone or more frequently pancytopenia	Reduced megakaryocytes alone or more frequently pancytopenia	Confirm the diagnosis in vitro	Stop all medications	Yes	Yes
Megaloblastic anemia	Macrocytic anemia, pancytopenia	Megaloblastic changes	B_{12}, red cell folate	B_{12}, folate	Yes	Yes
Aplastic anemia	Pancytopenia	Pancytopenia	Excludes secondary causes	Support (bone marrow transplantation, antilymphocyte globulin)	No	Yes

have clinical or laboratory evidence of disseminated intravascular coagulation but most do not, and the thrombocytopenia is an isolated finding probably due to immune mechanisms. Septicemic thrombocytopenia must be considered in any patient at risk, and the diagnosis is confirmed by positive blood cultures.

Treatment includes appropriate parenteral antibiotics. At my center, we give platelet transfusions if the platelet count falls to less than 20,000 per μl because one cannot predict that the platelet count will not continue to fall. The transfused platelets will have a shortened survival, but they may have a hemostatic effect prior to being removed from the circulation.

Drug-Induced Thrombocytopenia. Drug-induced thrombocytopenia, like septicemic thrombocytopenia, is a diagnosis of exclusion. Drugs most frequently associated with drug-induced thrombocytopenia include heparin, quinidine, gold, and the sulfa antibiotics. Heparin-induced thrombocytopenia is common and can develop in patients receiving heparin by any route. Usually it is not serious, but rarely it can be complicated by acute arterial thrombi in the brain, heart, and limbs. This complication of heparin therapy often results in significant morbidity and can be fatal.

Treatment includes the immediate discontinuation of the suspected causative drug. If the drug was used to treat a life-threatening condition—for example, heparin in the treatment of pulmonary embolism—then alternate therapy must be given. We administer platelet prophylactic transfusions to those patients with severe drug-induced thrombocytopenia (platelet count less than 20,000 per μl). We do not give prophylactic platelet transfusions if the patient has heparin thrombocytopenia plus thrombosis.

Disseminated Intravascular Coagulation (DIC). Patients with DIC have consumptive thrombocytopenia caused by thrombin. DIC is a laboratory diagnosis based on abnormal coagulation tests. The investigation of a patient with DIC does not stop with the diagnosis. DIC is always due to an underlying condition that must be treated before the hemostatic abnormalities will correct. Patients with DIC are managed by correcting the cause of the DIC while replacing the depleted coagulation factors and platelets.

[See next article for full discussion of DIC.—Ed.]

Post-Transfusion Purpura (PTP). Thrombocytopenia in patients with PTP develops precipitously about 1 week following the transfusion of blood or a blood product. The patient, usually a woman lacking the platelet-specific antigen Pl^{A1}, develops severe, isolated thrombocytopenia that can be fatal. The platelet destruction is caused by antibodies against the patient's own platelets. The diagnosis is confirmed by demonstrating that the patient has antiplatelet antibodies and lacks the platelet-specific antigen Pl^{A1}. Since these tests are performed at few institutions, the diagnosis is usually one of exclusion. The optimal treatment is uncertain, but most physicians recommend plasmapheresis, to remove the antibody, and corticosteroids, to suppress further antibody production. Platelet transfusions are contraindicated in these patients unless there is life-threatening bleeding.

Other Consumptive Thrombocytopenic Disorders. Hospitalized patients can develop consumptive thrombocytopenia from other causes, such as preeclampsia and cardiopulmonary bypass, among others. Usually, the cause of the thrombocytopenia is obvious, and the hemostatic defect is minor and does not require treatment.

Consumptive Thrombocytopenia in an Otherwise Well Patient

These patients seek medical attention because of clinical evidence of a hemostatic defect.

Idiopathic Thrombocytopenic Purpura (ITP). This common autoimmune disorder is caused by an antiplatelet antibody that binds to the patient's platelets, causing their destruction by the spleen. The two forms of ITP are childhood and adult. Childhood ITP often follows an infection, and the thrombocytopenia usually resolves spontaneously in several weeks. Depending upon the severity of the patient's symptoms, some clinicians do not treat these children. Others administer corticosteroids (prednisone, 1 mg per kg). In contrast to childhood ITP, the majority of adults with ITP will not have a spontaneous resolution of their illness. Adult ITP occurs predominantly in young or middle-aged women and can present abruptly or develop insidiously. The patients seek medical attention because of easy bruising. Laboratory investigations are usually normal except for thrombocytopenia. The physical examination is normal except for cutaneous evidence of thrombocytopenia. Splenomegaly virtually excludes the diagnosis of ITP. Other investigations to be performed include bone marrow aspiration, antinuclear antibody tests, and thyroid function tests. A bleeding time test is useful to assess the clinical impact of the hemostatic defect. We do not treat an asymptomatic patient whose bleeding time is normal, irrespective of the platelet count.

The initial treatment for a severely thrombocytopenic patient with ITP is corticosteroids (prednisone, 1 mg per kg). The platelet count rises in most patients in 5 to 10 days, and once the platelet count is at normal or near-normal levels, the corticosteroids can be reduced over the next month. The majority of patients will relapse when the corticosteroids are tapered, and more definitive therapy is indicated. Splenectomy will result in a long-term remission for two thirds of all patients with ITP. Prior to splenectomy, the patient should receive an antipneumococcal vaccination. Many patients with systemic lupus erythematosus have immune thrombocytopenia, but these patients are less likely to respond to splenectomy than are patients with ITP.

Patients with ITP often continue to have antiplatelet antibody in their circulation even after their platelet count has returned to normal. Pregnant patients with active ITP or a past history of ITP require careful management, since the antiplatelet antibody is IgG and crosses the placenta potentially, causing thrombocytopenia in the infant.

Other Immune Thrombocytopenic Disorders. Immune thrombocytopenia can complicate systemic lupus erythematosus, sarcoidosis, infectious mononucleosis, and certain lymphoproliferative disorders, including Hodgkin's disease and chronic lymphocytic leukemia. Many of the patients have splenomegaly. Treatment is directed at managing the underlying disorder. Corticosteroids may be indicated for some patients.

Aregenerative Thrombocytopenia

Thrombocytopenia due to underproduction of platelets is termed aregenerative thrombocytopenia. Because the red cells, white cells, and platelets all originate from a common stem cell, cytopenia due to underproduction usually affects more than one cell line. Aregenerative thrombocytopenia is characterized by reduced numbers of platelets, a normal or near-normal platelet survival, and reduced numbers of megakaryocytes in the bone marrow. Most hospitalized patients with aregenerative thrombocytopenia have received chemotherapy as a treatment for malignancy. Less commonly, patients can have aregenerative thrombocytopenia caused by an infiltration of their marrow by neoplastic cells (leukemia), an idiosyncratic drug reaction, deficiency of B_{12} or folate, aplastic anemia, or a severe infection such as tuberculosis.

Aregenerative Thrombocytopenia Due to Chemotherapy. Chemotherapeutic agents induce pancytopenia in a dose-dependent fashion, and aregenerative thrombocytopenia due to chemotherapy is probably the most common cause of thrombocytopenia in the hospitalized population. Treatment is supportive (platelet transfusions, discussed subsequently).

Aregenerative Thrombocytopenia in the Patient Not Receiving Chemotherapy. Marrow infiltration by malignant cells (leukemia) and systemic infections (tuberculosis) can result in aregenerative thrombocytopenia.

The sudden development of aregenerative thrombocytopenia in a hospitalized patient is unusual and can be secondary to acute megaloblastic anemia (folic acid deficiency) or can be an idiosyncratic drug reaction producing aplastic anemia (such as occurs with chloramphenicol).

Certain patients with aplastic anemia present isolated aregenerative thrombocytopenia. The investigation and management of these patients is discussed elsewhere. Platelet transfusions for these patients should be avoided if possible since alloimmunization can result.

Rationale for Platelet Transfusions

Platelet transfusions are given to prevent bleeding *(prophylactic platelet transfusions)* and to control bleeding *(therapeutic platelet transfusions)*. The usual dose of random donor platelets (collected from different individuals) is 6 to 8 units per transfusion, and this dose will raise the platelet count by 30,000 to 60,000 per μl provided the platelets are not destroyed in the patient's circulation. All platelet transfusions should be followed by a 1 to 2 hour post-transfusion platelet count to ensure that the patient has had a rise in the platelet count. The lack of a post-transfusion platelet increment may mean that the patient has a destructive component to the thrombocytopenia, such as septicemia or hypersplenism. It may also indicate that the patient has alloantibodies against the transfused platelets and hence should receive HLA-matched or platelet cross-matched single donor platelets.

Therapeutic platelet transfusions should be given to any patient with life-threatening bleeding caused by any quantitative or qualitative platelet defect. Possible exceptions to this rule include patients with post-transfusion purpura and thrombotic thrombocytopenic purpura. These disorders may be worsened by platelet transfusions.

The decision to administer prophylactic platelet transfusions is more difficult and is made after the clinician has weighed the relative risks and benefits. For example, platelet transfusions can transmit infection, especially hepatitis. Of greater concern is the development of antiplatelet antibodies. Approximately two thirds of all patients who receive long-term random donor platelet support will form alloantibodies against platelets and will not respond to random donor platelet transfusions. Consequently, one must remember that any prophylactic platelets given to prevent a bleeding episode could stop the patient from responding to therapeutic platelet transfusions in the future. For this reason, we give platelet transfusions after considering the patient's bleeding risk and the probable duration of the thrombocytopenia. For example, patients with lifelong quantitative or qualitative platelet defects should not receive prophylactic platelet transfusions because they will develop alloantibodies.

Certain patients have an acute transient thrombocytopenic episode that occurs once and will not recur. Such patients include those with thromobocytopenia secondary to septicemia and idiosyncratic drug reactions. We administer prophylactic platelet transfusions to these patients when their platelet count falls below 20,000 per μl.

Another consideration is the mechanism of the thrombocytopenia. Transfused platelets have a near-normal survival in the circulation of nonimmunized patients with aregenerative thrombocytopenia. In contrast, all transfused platelets have a reduced lifespan in patients with a consumptive thrombocytopenia, because the transfused platelets, like the patient's own platelets, are destroyed by the process causing the thrombocytopenia. Patients with chronic consumptive thrombocytopenia usually are not given prophylactic platelet transfusions because the platelets will circulate for only a short time, yet the process causing the platelet consumption (for example, idiopathic thrombocytopenic purpura) may persist for a long time.

Hypersplenism

Patients with splenomegaly can be thrombocytopenic because the platelets are trapped in the large spleen, a condition termed hypersplenism. About one third of all platelets are found in the spleen in healthy individuals, but as the spleen increases in size in certain diseases, more and more platelets become trapped within it. Most patients with hypersplenism have depression of other cells besides the platelets. Since the thrombocytopenia of hypersplenism tends not to be severe, definitive treatment—splenectomy—is seldom required. The diagnosis can be confirmed by platelet survival studies; patients with hypersplenism have a markedly reduced platelet recovery, but the platelets remaining in the circulation have a normal survival.

Patients with certain disorders associated with splenomegaly, such as systemic lupus erythematosus, sarcoidosis, and lymphoproliferative disorders, have immune thrombocytopenia that can be confused with the thrombocytopenia of hypersplenism.

Qualitative Platelet Defects

Qualitative platelet defects are less common than quantitative defects, and the hemostatic defect tends to be less severe. Platelet function defects can be congenital or acquired. Bernard-Soulier syndrome is caused by a congenital absence of the platelet membrane glycoprotein Ib; patients with this disorder have a prolonged bleeding time and defective ristocetin-induced platelet aggregation. Glanzmann's thrombasthenia is caused by a congenital absence of the platelet glycoproteins IIb and IIIa and is characterized by a prolonged bleeding time and absent platelet aggregation to all aggregating agents except ristocetin. These disorders of platelet function are exceptionally rare, and currently there is no known treatment. Platelet transfusions should not be administered unless the patient has life-threatening bleeding.

An acquired disorder of platelet function should be suspected if the patient has signs of a platelet-type hemostatic defect (petechiae and purpura) and a prolonged bleeding time with a normal or near-normal platelet count. Patients undergoing cardiopulmonary bypass can develop a transient platelet function defect despite relatively mild thrombocytopenia (platelet nadir of 75,000 to 150,000 per μl). These patients can have profound bleeding. Treatment, if required, consists of platelet transfusions.

Some patients with uremia have a prolonged bleeding time, abnormal platelet aggregation, and adhesion. Treatment includes dialysis or infusions of cryoprecipitate. Platelet transfusions usually are not effective.

Many drugs interfere with platelet function, but it is uncommon for drug-induced platelet dysfunction by itself to result in bleeding. However, when the platelet dysfunction is accompanied by a secondary defect of hemostasis, such as a coagulation or vessel wall abnormality, then bleeding can occur. Drugs that have been associated with platelet dysfunction include aspirin, other nonsteroidal anti-inflammatory agents, and the semisynthetic penicillins.

DISSEMINATED INTRAVASCULAR COAGULATION

method of
ALAN R. GILES, M.D.
Queen's University
Kingston, Ontario

Disseminated intravascular coagulation (DIC) or consumption coagulopathy is, in its severest form, a fulminating, life-threatening failure in the hemostatic mechanism. Alternatively, it may be recognized only following the careful scrutiny of sensitive laboratory tests of the coagulation mechanism. The laboratory and clinical abnormalities are a function of the consumption of platelets and coagulation factors, particularly factors V and VIII and fibrinogen, following the initiation of intravascular coagulation by varying thromboplastic stimuli. The resulting hemostatic defect is further compromised by the generation of fibrin (fibrinogen) degradation products, resulting from fibrin(ogen)olysis, which interfere with fibrin polymerization and platelet function. In some cases, the latter may play a primary role in the bleeding tendency that results, i.e., pathologic fibrinolysis. DIC is encountered against a wide spectrum of clinical situations. Certain conditions, however, have a particular propensity for being associated with this complication. In some, such as sepsis and obstetric pathology, this relates to an increased risk of the generation of intravascular thromboblastic activity whereas in others, such as liver disease, it apparently relates to deficiencies in mechanisms responsible for inhibiting inappropriate activation of the hemostatic process.

Diagnosis

The diagnosis of DIC rests on careful clinical observation and the application of appropriate laboratory screening tests in those patients known to be at risk of developing the complication. A fall in platelet count associated with features of microangiopathic anemia on the blood smear should suggest DIC in such patients until proved otherwise. Screening tests of coagulation such as the prothrombin time (PT), activated partial thromboplastin time (APTT), thrombin clotting time (TCT), fibrinogen, and measurement of FDP provide additional support of the diagnosis but occasionally may be misleading. For example, fibrinogen and factor VIII levels are elevated during pregnancy, and this may be reflected by the finding of a normal APTT despite other evidence of significant consumption. Similarly, levels of fibrin/fibrinogen degradation products (FDP) are frequently elevated in conditions likely to be complicated by DIC. To accommodate these difficulties, frequent testing is indicated when clinical suspicion suggests DIC, in order to document the progressive nature of the condition. The TCT is an important test in this context due to its simplicity and sensitivity both to fibrinogen levels and elevation in FDP.

Treatment

The keystone of successful treatment of DIC is to direct management to the underlying mechanism responsible and supplement this as necessary by blood component replacement and occasionally by anticoagulant or antifibrinolytic therapy.

Treatment of the Precipitating Cause. In many cases of DIC, successful treatment of the primary medical condition, such as aggressive treatment of sepsis with appropriate antibiotics or the removal of the dead fetus in intrauterine death, results in its resolution. Additional supportive therapy, such as correction of fluid or electrolyte imbalance, may be required. Corticosteroids may be indicated in the treatment of the underlying disease or associated shock but have no role in the treatment of DIC itself.

Replacement Therapy. Blood component replacement therapy is indicated when significant bleeding is occurring, when the underlying condition cannot be rapidly or predictably corrected, and to facilitate surgical procedures required to treat the underlying cause, such as removal of a dead fetus. The primary component used is cryoprecipitate. This provides both factor VIII and fibrinogen. Although the dose required can be calculated on the basis of the deficit recorded and the approximate fibrinogen and factor VIII content of a bag of cryoprecipitate (250 mg and 80 units respectively), the consumptive nature of the disorder requires that the response should be closely monitored by clinical observation of bleeding and appropriate repetitive laboratory testing. The TCT is particularly useful for this purpose. Fibrinogen concentrates are no longer recommended owing to the high incidence of viral hepatitis attending their use. Other blood components, such as stored or fresh-frozen plasma, may be added to the regimen as required to correct deficiencies of other clotting factors, red cell concentrates and crystalloids given to replace blood loss. Platelet concentrates should be available but may not be required in all patients because of the significant thrombopoietic reserve of the bone marrow. They should be given to patients known to have bone marrow suppression—for example, patients on chemotherapy. Vitamin K deficiency frequently complicates the management of patients in intensive care, particularly those receiving broad-spectrum antibiotic therapy. Vitamin K supplements should be given to all patients with DIC in this category.

Anticoagulant-Antifibrinolytic Therapy. In some patients, the use of heparin is indicated. The rationale for its use is to prevent, in concert with antithrombin III, further activation of coagulation. Unfortunately, its use is complicated by difficulty in monitoring the dose to be used. The laboratory monitoring tests customarily used (APTT and TCT) are already abnormal due to DIC. Similarly, the clinical indicator of overanticoagulation (bleeding) may already be present. These difficulties restrict its use but, when the precipitating cause cannot be predictably corrected or when adequate replacement cannot be achieved, it may be life-saving. The dose used is arbitrary, but an initial dose of 500 to 1000 units per hour by continuous infusion in a 70 kg patient is suggested. Where available, heparin assays should be used to adjust the dose to achieve plasma heparin levels of 0.2 to 0.3 units per ml.

Although fibrinolytic activity is probably increased in most patients with DIC, the use of antifibrinolytic agents such as epsilon-aminocaproic acid (EACA) is rarely indicated and, in most situations, is actually contraindicated. Their use may enhance the likelihood of ischemic damage occurring in vital organs from failure to remove intravascularly deposited fibrin. DIC associated with prostatic surgery is the one exception to this observation. The high concentration of plasminogen activator in prostatic tissue is thought to be responsible for the pathologic fibrinolysis that may occasionally complicate prostatic surgery. Other causes of DIC, such as sepsis, must be excluded.

THROMBOTIC THROMBOCYTOPENIC PURPURA

method of
ALAN R. GILES, M.D.
Queen's University
Kingston, Ontario

Thrombotic thrombocytopenic purpura (TTP) is a serious disease of unknown etiology characterized by a process of platelet consumption and platelet thrombi formation in the absence of any other observable abnormality in the hemostatic mechanism. Until recently, the condition was invariably fatal, with death occurring from hemorrhage and system failure induced by ischemia consequent to the widespread formation of platelet thrombi in the microvascular circulation. Clinically, the presenting features are those of cerebrovascular and renal insufficiency, bleeding, and abdominal pain. The laboratory features are severe thrombocytopenia and a microangiopathic blood picture associated with no abnormalities of the usual screening tests of coagulation, such as the prothrombin time, activated partial thromboplastin time, and thrombin clotting time. There is apparently some overlap between this condition and the hemolytic uremic syndrome.

Treatment

A significant improvement in the prognosis of this condition has occurred with the demonstration of benefit from plasma infusion with or without plasma exchange. Previously, the use of anticoagulants, platelet suppressant therapy, immunosuppression, and splenectomy had been shown to be of little, if any, benefit.

The use of intensive plasma exchange (IPE) results in a response rate of over 90 per cent, although some patients may relapse acutely or chronically. At the present time, it is uncertain whether plasma exchange is required merely to accommodate the infusion of sufficient quantities of replacement normal plasma or whether it results in the removal of an agent or agents responsible for initiating the condition. Although plasma infusion alone has been shown to be efficacious, plasma exchange facilitates the therapeutic process, particularly in avoiding the difficulties of fluid overload in patients acutely ill with widespread system failure. Although not supported by controlled clinical trials, case reports suggest that replacement by physiologic fluids other than plasma is ineffective.

The precise protocol recommended is largely empiric. Plasma exchange should be initiated early, as treatment failures in the main have been reported in patients in whom IPE was instituted as a last resort. Single plasma volume exchanges (3 liters in a 70 kg patient) should be carried out on a daily basis and repeated as required, with the platelet count and clinical observation (such as level of consciousness and urine output) serving as indicators of therapeutic response. Acute relapse may be handled by IPE 2 or 3 days per week. The use of an automated cell separator greatly facilitates treatment. If plasma replacement is effected by fresh frozen plasma, associated coagulation abnormalities due to clotting factor depletion usually do not occur.

It is not clear whether platelet suppressive therapy augments the efficacy of intensive plasma exchange. Clinical trials of this aspect of therapy are currently underway. It is suggested that, when IPE is apparently ineffective or relapse is a persistent feature, such therapy may be added to the regimen. The choice rests between aspirin, 600 mg every 12 hours; dipyridamole, 150 mg every 6 hours; and sulfinpyrazone, 200 mg every 6 hours. The use of such drugs is considered investigational since their efficacy in thrombotic thrombocytopenic purpura has not been established by controlled clinical trial with or without intensive plasma exchange.

The use of steroids, although of no proved benefit in the treatment of the primary condition, may be indicated in some patients as part of general supportive therapy. The latter should also include renal dialysis in patients with significant renal failure. Platelet transfusions are ineffective and may actually exacerbate the condition. Case reports of increased fatality following platelet transfusions have been reported. Red cell transfusions are indicated when necessary as general replacement therapy.

As the etiology of this condition remains uncertain, management will remain empiric. Recent research observations have suggested that patients with TTP have an abnormality in the synthesis or release of prostacyclin (PGI-2) by endothelial cells. Case reports of apparent benefit following the infusion of prostacyclin require further confirmation by appropriate clinical trial. Similarly, the possible relationship of disease activity to the premature release of abnormal forms of von Willebrand factor from damaged endothelial cells may offer some explanation of the benefit accruing from intensive plasma exchange. Such observations may result in the development of more specific approaches to the therapy of this condition in the near future.

HEMOCHROMATOSIS

method of
WALTER G. FREY, M.D.
Dartmouth Medical School
Hanover, New Hampshire

Hemochromatosis is an autosomal recessive disease of unappreciated frequency characterized by increased absorption of dietary iron. Since there are no compensatory excretory channels, this excess iron gradually accumulates in the liver and other organs at a rate of 2 to 5 mg per day. Eventually, massive tissue overload with iron adversely affects organ function, particularly the liver, pancreas, heart, pituitary, and joints.

If the patient so afflicted is not anemic, there is only one acceptable form of therapy—repeated phlebotomies. However, before embarking on this simple but time-consuming approach, the physician needs some understanding of the pathogenesis and inheritance of hemochromatosis and must also be armed with the most crucial diagnostic information—a liver biopsy specimen properly analyzed histologically and quantitatively for iron. Once this confirmatory information is in hand, the physician is in a position to estimate the severity of the overload and the urgency with which treatment need be pursued.

Since 1 ml of red blood cells contains about 1 mg of iron, the removal of 1 unit of whole blood (500 ml) will extract 250 mg of iron from the patient. Most symptomatic patients have accumulated an excess of at least 20 grams of dangerous storage iron and may require over 80 phlebotomies for removal. Frequency of blood lettings must be individualized. There is clearly some urgency in the treatment of a symptomatic middle-aged man. Many patients can tolerate the removal of 500 ml of blood as often as three times a week without exceeding the capacity of the bone marrow to increase its output (often six times normal). For others, one phlebotomy each week may suffice.

This initial deironing process requires many months to accomplish. As the patient's iron stores are depleted, they may be less readily mobilized. At this point, the hemoglobin concentration may fall but returns to normal as the rate of phlebotomies is slowed. When the hemoglobin concentration drops and stabilizes at 10 grams per dl for a month without phlebotomy, the iron overload has probably been corrected. Monitoring of therapy by other laboratory tests, such as serum iron or serum ferritin, is not necessary and may be misleading. Of course, final confirmation of therapeutic success could be obtained by repeating the liver biopsy but again is usually not necessary.

Once the patient is deironed, the physician should not lose sight of the fact that the patient's basic metabolic abnormality of increased dietary iron absorption remains. To prevent reaccumulation in the treated patient, a prophylactic phlebotomy program during which the patient is bled 500 ml every 2 to 3 months is maintained indefinitely. The cooperation of Red Cross bloodmobile programs has been achieved in many sections of the country, since there is no reason why this blood should not be used for transfusions.

In the symptomatic patient, therapy may improve cardiac function, decrease insulin requirements, reverse liver function abnormalities, and restore a sense of well-being. However, it would be unwise to expect reversal of joint symptoms or testicular atrophy. Patients treated before the development of hepatic cirrhosis may have the same survival as do nonhemochromatotic controls. The risk for development of hepatocellular carcinoma (a leading cause of death in hemochromatosis) may persist in those deironed after the development of cirrhosis. Even those treated after the development of cirrhosis have much improved survival statistics when compared with those untreated. In some patients the actual cirrhotic process has been reversed, after years of phlebotomy therapy.

Although managing an individual hemochromatotic patient through months of therapy requires skill as a phlebotomist, perseverance, maintenance of flow sheets, and encouragement, the treating physician's responsibilities are not over. Other family members similarly afflicted, who may or may not be symptomatic, must be sought. There is some disagreement as to what constitutes adequate screening tests. Most agree that serum iron, transferrin saturation, and serum ferritin levels should be obtained in siblings, parents, and children of symptomatic hemochromatotic patients. Because the hemochromatosis gene is located close to the HLA locus on chromosome 6, HLA typing of siblings may identify others at risk for hemochromatosis. Liver biopsy is the definitive test; it should be performed when screening tests are abnormal or signs and symptoms consistent with iron overload are uncovered. Asymptomatic relatives with demonstrable iron deposition in hepatocytes should also have therapeutic phlebotomies. Unlike most other recessively inherited diseases, hemochromatosis has often been found in successive generations in the absence of marital consanguinity. This reflects the fact that there is an extraordinarily high frequency of the heterozygote state in the general population (perhaps 8 to 10 per cent).

Iron overload may also complicate anemic patients with hemolysis and repeated transfusion requirements. If confined to the reticuloendothelial system, this excess iron is insignificant. However, with time, redistribution of a massive transfusional iron overload can damage the liver and heart. In this situation, there may be a role for an iron-chelating agent, deferoxamine (Desferal). Unfortunately, this drug must be administered parenterally and its use is costly and complex.

Dietary restrictions are unnecessary in an identified patient with iron overload because phlebotomy therapy is so efficient in removing the absorbed excess iron. However, indiscriminate fortification of the diet with iron supplements may put at risk unidentified hemochromatotic patients in the population.

Finally, the patient may benefit from being put in touch with Iron Overload Diseases Association, Incorporated, organized to support and encourge patients with hemochromatosis and their families.

HODGKIN'S DISEASE: CHEMOTHERAPY

method of
NICHOLAS J. ROBERT, M.D.
and RICHARD A. RUDDERS, M.D.
New England Medical Center
Boston, Massachusetts

The demonstration of the curative role of combination chemotherapy in widespread Hodgkin's disease has been one of the more successful chapters in the short history of medical oncology. With current treatment regimens, approximately half the patients with advanced disease treated with chemotherapy achieve durable remissions. However, a significant number of patients with advanced disease are not cured, and new approaches to improve this situation are needed.

Treatment

Limited Disease (Stages I and II) (Table 1)

TABLE 1. **Hodgkin's Disease: Ann Arbor Staging System**

Stage I	Involvement of a single lymph node region (I) or of a single extralymphatic organ or site (IE).
Stage II	Involvement of two or more lymph node regions on the same side of the diaphragm (II) or localized involvement of extralymphatic organ or site and of one or more lymph node regions on the same side of the diaphragm (IIE).
Stage III	Involvement of lymph node regions on both sides of the diaphragm (III), which may be accompanied by localized involvement of extralymphatic organ or site (IIIE), or by involvement of the spleen (IIIS), or both (IIISE).
Stage IV	Diffuse or disseminated involvement of one or more extralymphatic organs or tissues with or without associated lymph node enlargement. The reason for classifying the involvement as Stage IV should be identified further by defining the site by symbols.
Note:	Fever > 38 C (100.5 F), night sweats, and/or weight loss >10 per cent of body weight in the 6 months preceding admission are defined as systemic symptoms and denoted by the suffix letter B. Asymptomatic patients are denoted by the suffix A.

Patients with Hodgkin's disease in early stages without "B" symptoms (see Table 1) are conventionally treated with radiotherapy alone. This group represents patients in stages IA, IAE, IIA, and IIAE. Although chemotherapy has been shown to be an effective alternative for this group, radiotherapy is standard treatment. However, one subset of patients requires chemotherapy in addition to radiotherapy—patients with large mediastinal masses, defined as greater than one third of the cardiothoracic diameter on chest roentgenogram. This group has been shown to have a high relapse rate if treated by conventional radiotherapy alone. Our recommendation is to treat initially with combination chemotherapy, followed by mediastinal radiotherapy.

Patients in early stages who have associated B symptoms represent a controversial group in terms of treatment recommendations. The concern is that the patient's symptoms indicate systemic disease not disclosed by the staging studies, including a staging laparotomy. The intent of this procedure is to perform a splenectomy as well as take liver biopsies and multiple lymph node biopsies from the various regions of the abdomen. It should be stressed that splenectomy (especially in younger patients) significantly increases the risk of life-threatening infections with encapsulated bacteria such as *Haemophilus influenzae* and *Diplococcus pneumoniae*. The use of both pneumococcal and meningococcal vaccines is recommended and should be administered prior to the splenectomy in order to be effective. Radiotherapy alone does not seem to have the same curative success as combined radiation and chemotherapy, although long-term side effects are an additional risk if a combined modality approach is used.

Advanced Disease (Stages III and IV)

Patients are classified as IIIA1 if the disease is limited to the upper abdomen—for example, spleen or splenic, celiac, and porta hepatis lymph nodes. Patients are termed stage IIIA2 when involvement extends more inferiorly to include mesenteric, para-aortic, or iliac nodes. IIIA1 patients have been successfully treated with radiotherapy alone although there is a higher relapse rate compared with a combined modality approach. The survival rate in both groups is the same because of the subsequent successful "salvage" with chemotherapy in patients treated with radiotherapy who later relapse. In IIIA2 patients, combined modality should be used initially since salvage with subsequent chemotherapy has not been as successful as in the IIIA1 patient group. In patients with extensive splenic involvement (five or more nodules) regardless of the substage of IIIA, combined modality treatment appears to be necessary. An alternative has recently been suggested by Lister of St. Bartholomew's Hospital, London, who has demonstrated that chemotherapy alone produces comparable results in all stage IIIA patients. This observation requires further confirmation.

Patients in stages IIIB, IVA, or IVB are uniformly treated with combined chemotherapy. In some cases an argument can be made to treat patients subsequently with radiotherapy to bulky sites of initial disease although the evidence is not conclusive that this is beneficial.

Other Factors Influencing Treatment Decisions

In addition to stage, other factors that may influence prognosis include the patient's age and the specific histologic subtype of Hodgkin's disease. Pediatric patients may be better treated with chemotherapy to avoid the need for laparotomy and splenectomy and the problems associated with growth retardation in radiotherapy. On the other hand, patients over 70 years of age do less well with chemotherapy and must be treated extremely carefully. It is important to decide initially whether the patient is truly a candidate for full dose chemotherapy, remembering that chemotherapy in this setting is given with the intent to cure, not only to palliate. Another factor is the histologic subtype, stage notwithstanding. The lymphocyte depletion type appears to carry a poorer prognosis; more aggressive treatment has been suggested for these patients. Also, nodular sclerosis, particularly with bulky masses, as in the mediastinum, tends to have a higher relapse rate with chemotherapy alone and patients may require combined modality treatment.

Chemotherapy Programs

MOPP: The Gold Standard

The MOPP regimen consists of four drugs: nitrogen mustard (Mustargen), vincristine (Oncovin), procarbazine (Matulane), and prednisone (Table 2). Prednisone is usually given only in the first and fourth cycles. This program has become the standard chemotherapy treatment for Hodgkin's disease. A review of 198 patients who have received this treatment disclosed an 80 per cent response rate. Fifty-five per cent of the treated patients remain free of disease and thus are cured! It is important to remember that although many patients will promptly go into remission and require only six cycles of treatment, some will require additional treatment to achieve complete remission. Thus patients should get at least two cycles of treatment after complete remission and should achieve a minimum of six cycles. This approach has been described as the flexible MOPP program. Therefore, it is mandatory that all initial sites of disease be monitored closely for evidence of response.

MOPP: Alternatives

Numerous additional combinations of drugs have been tested clinically in an attempt to improve on the results obtained with MOPP (Table 3). One approach has been to replace some of the drugs in the MOPP program with other drugs. This has usually led to substituting drugs of a similar class for nitrogen mustard or vincristine or both. The results generally appear to be comparable to those with the original MOPP. However, these alternative programs may be better tolerated and elicit fewer side effects such as nausea, vomiting, and chemical phlebitis.

Another approach has been to try to improve on the results of MOPP by cycling another regimen with MOPP. The most encouraging example is from the Bonadonna group in Milan, Italy, who use MOPP alternating with a noncross-resistant regimen called ABVD, which consists of doxorubicin (Adriamycin), bleomycin (Blenoxane), vinblastine (Velban), and dacarbazine (DTIC). Further studies are under way to compare the efficacy of MOPP and MOPP-like regimens with this eight drug program. We reserve this type of alternating regimen for patients with advanced disease who are at high risk of relapse.

Second Line or "Salvage" Treatment

Another important development in the chemotherapeutic treatment of Hodgkin's disease is the development of "salvage" or secondary treatment in patients who are either refractory to initial treatment or relapse. If the disease-free interval has been long ($>$ 1 year) the initial regimen may be used again to induce remission. An alternative is to use drugs that are different from those in MOPP or MOPP-like regimens. The ABVD combination is such an example. In the treatment of MOPP failures with ABVD, the response rate has been variable, ranging from 29 to 62 per cent. Other programs have used drugs such as streptozocin (Zanosar) and CCNU, but results have

TABLE 2. **MOPP Regimen***

nitrogen mustard	6 mg/M^2 intravenously	Days 1 and 8
vincristine	1.4 mg/M^2 intravenously	Days 1 and 8
procarbazine	100 mg/M^2 orally	Days 1 through 14
prednisone	40 mg/M^2 orally	Days 1 through 14
		Cycles 1 and 4 only

*Cycle is to be repeated every 28 days

Dose Modifications

WBC Count	*Platelet Count*	*Dose Adjustment*
>4000/mm^3	>100,000/mm^3	100% all drugs
3000–4000/mm^3	>100,000/mm^3	100% vincristine 50% nitrogen mustard 50% procarbazine
2000–3000/mm^3	50,000–100,000/mm^3	100% vincristine 25% nitrogen mustard 25% procarbazine
1000–2000/mm^3	>50,000/mm^3	50% vincristine 25% nitrogen mustard 25% procarbazine
<1000/mm^3	<50,000/mm^3	no therapy

also varied. However, relatively few patients to date achieve long-term remissions with second line treatment. Exceptions are patients who relapse following a long disease-free interval, and particularly when relapse is confined to lymph nodes rather than viscera. Such patients may achieve durable remissions with either MOPP or ABVD.

Complications

The short term side effects of chemotherapy are well known and include nausea, vomiting, hair loss, chemical phlebitis, and myelosuppression. The latter requires close follow-up so that blood transfusions can be given for anemia, platelets for thrombocytopenia, and broad-spectrum parenteral antibiotics for the development of fever associated with neutropenia. Although peripheral cytopenias resolve following completion of chemotherapy, varying degrees of bone marrow compromise may persist.

A number of specific toxicities related to drugs commonly used in the treatment of Hodgkin's disease should be borne in mind. Bleomycin (Blenoxane) may cause hypersensitivity pneumonitis and pulmonary fibrosis. The incidence of this complication is acceptable at recommended total dose levels. Doxorubicin (Adriamycin) is potentially cardiotoxic; care must be exercised to stay below a total administered dose of 450 mg per M^2. Vinca alkaloids such as vincristine (Oncovin) and vinblastine (Velban) are neurotoxic and may cause severe disabling neuropathy if dose levels are maintained in the face of persistent neurologic symptoms or signs. The toxicities of the other drugs commonly used in combined regimens are more or less predictable and not necessarily distinctive. All drugs may cause gastrointestinal disturbance, alopecia, and mucositis.

Other long-term effects are significant and are often not reversible. A common problem is infertility, usually seen in male patients. Prepubertal patients appear to be less affected. In women, the use of oral contraceptives during treatment may protect the ovary from the effects of chemotherapy, but this needs further study. In men, sterility may occur in as much as 80 per cent. Current studies are focusing on the use of luteinizing hormone–releasing factor analogues to prevent sterility. For specific chemotherapy regimens that may be less disruptive for gonadal function, evidence suggests that ABVD when given alone may be less toxic than MOPP. However, this combination regimen contains Adriamycin, providing additional risk for cardiotoxicity.

Last and most important is the potential risk of developing a second episode of malignant disease as a consequence of treatment. Two specific cancers are of concern: acute nonlymphocytic leukemia and non-Hodgkin's lymphoma. Other cancers appear at a much lower frequency. The risk of developing acute leukemia is increased when the patient is treated with both chemotherapy and radiotherapy. The actuarial risk has been estimated to be as high as 7 per cent at 7 years post-treatment and it appears to be even higher in patients over the age of 40 years. The time

TABLE 3. **Alternatives to MOPP**

ABVD			
Doxorubicin (Adriamycin)	25 mg/M²	intravenously	Days 1 and 15
Bleomycin (Blenoxane)	10 U/M²	intravenously	Days 1 and 15
Vinblastine (Velban)	6 mg/M²	intravenously	Days 1 and 15
Dacarbazine (DTIC)	375 mg/M²	intravenously	Days 1 and 15
Repeat every 28 days			
B-DOPA			
Bleomycin (Blenoxane)	4 U/M²	intravenously	Days 2 and 5
Dacarbazine (DTIC)	150 mg/M²	intravenously	Day 1 through 5
Vincristine (Oncovin)	1.5 mg/M²	intravenously	Days 1 and 5
Prednisone	40 mg/M²	orally	Day 1 through 6
Doxorubicin (Adriamycin)	60 mg/M²	intravenously	Day 1
Repeat every 21 days			
BVCPP			
BCNU (BiCNU)	100 mg/M²	intravenously	Day 1
Vinblastine (Velban)	5 mg/M²	intravenously	Day 1
Cyclophosphamide (Cytoxan)	600 mg/M²	intravenously	Day 1
Procarbazine (Matulane)	100 mg/M²	orally	Day 1 through 10
Prednisone	60 mg/M²	orally	Day 1 through 10
Repeat every 28 days			
CVPP			
Chlorambucil (Leukeran)	6 mg/M²*	orally	Day 1 through 14
Vinblastine (Velban)	6 mg/M²*	intravenously	Days 1 and 8
Procarbazine (Matulane)	100 mg/M²	orally	Day 1 through 14
Prednisone	40 mg/M²	orally	Day 1 through 14
Repeat every 28 days			
CVB			
CCNU (Lomustine)	100 mg/M²	orally	Day 1
Vinblastine (Velban)	6 mg/M²	intravenously	Days 1 and 8
Bleomycin (Blenoxane)	15 U/M²	intravenously	Days 1 and 8
Repeat every 28 days			
CVPP			
Cyclophosphamide (Cytoxan)	300 mg/M²	intravenously	Days 1 and 8
Vinblastine (Velban)	10 mg/day	intravenously	Days 1, 8, and 15
Procarbazine (Matulane)	100 mg/M²	orally	Day 1 through 15
Prednisone	40 mg/M²	orally	Day 1 through 15 (cycles 1 and 4 only)
Repeat every 28 days			
SCAB			
Streptozocin (Zanosar)	500 mg/M²	intravenously	Day 1 through 5
CCNU (Lomustine)	100 mg/M²	orally	Day 1
Doxorubicin (Adriamycin)	45 mg/M²	intravenously	Day 1
Bleomycin (Blenoxane)	15 U/M²	intravenously	Days 1 and 8
Repeat every 28 days			

*Do not exceed 10 mg

interval to development of leukemia is usually 2 to 8 years after treatment. Patients may first develop unexplained cytopenia, sometimes associated with an abnormal-appearing bone marrow and abnormal chromosomes on cytogenetic analysis, which then transforms into clear-cut leukemia. Unfortunately, these leukemic patients do poorly with aggressive treatment, showing low remission rates and short survival compared with patients with de novo leukemia. This potential complication has been described in the different types of chemotherapy programs, including ABVD. The risk of non-Hodgkin's lymphoma, which is of high grade type, also appears to be higher with combined modality treatment. The actuarial risk has been estimated to be as high as 4.4 per cent at 10 years post-treatment.

HODGKIN'S DISEASE: RADIATION THERAPY

method of
RICHARD T. HOPPE, M.D.
Stanford University
Stanford, California

Treatment

The concepts that form the foundation of the curative radiotherapy treatment programs for patients with Hodgkin's disease include the use of a tumoricidal dose of irradiation; the prophylactic treatment of clinically uninvolved sites adjacent to sites of known involvement; the design of large fields that encompass multiple lymph node regions; the use of megavoltage equipment to provide skin sparing and permit the treatment of large fields at extended distance; and the use of field simulation and verification during treatment.

When we use irradiation alone, we treat to a dose of 4000 to 4400 rad in 150 to 200 rad fractions to all initially involved sites. Protective lead blocks are placed within these fields to limit the dose to sensitive structures. For example, when the mantle field is treated, blocks are used routinely to limit the dose to the spinal cord, larynx, humeral heads, and portions of the heart. The use of these blocks can be varied according to individual clinical circumstances.

In the prophylactic treatment of uninvolved lymphoid regions, we utilize a dose of at least 3600 rad in 150 to 200 rad fractions. Organs such as the lungs or liver may be considered at high risk for involvement in the presence of disease in the ipsilateral pulmonary hilum or spleen, respectively. However, a dose of 3600 rad cannot be delivered safely to these organs. In these situations, we utilize "partial transmission lead blocks" to provide low dose irradiation to these organs. A 37 per cent transmission block permits lung irradiation to 1650 rad during the time that the mantle field receives 4400 rad. A 50 per cent transmission block facilitates hepatic irradiation to 2200 rad during the time required to treat the para-aortic nodes to 4400 rads.

When irradiation is combined with chemotherapy, the doses utilized may be less. In adults we treat involved sites to at least 3600 rad even when combined modality therapy is planned. In growing children, we deliver only 1500 to 2500 rad to involved regions when chemotherapy is combined. Higher doses may have adverse effects on growth and must therefore be restricted to sites of initially bulky disease.

The large radiation fields, such as the mantle or inverted Y, are shaped to conform to the patient's anatomy and designed to treat multiple contiguous lymph node regions. This minimizes the risk of either "overlap" or "underdosage," which could result in serious normal tissue toxicity or inadequate treatment if small "patchwork" fields are used adjacent to each other. Field blocking is provided by individually contoured cerrobend or lead blocks.

To treat these large fields, a machine capable of treating at an extended distance is required. This capability is available primarily with contemporary linear accelerators. We use a 6-MeV linac. This beam provides substantial skin sparing, since the maximum ionization occurs at a depth of about 1.5 cm.

Essential to treatment accuracy and reproducibility is the use of field simulation and verification. We design fields using a dedicated simulator since this permits precise tumor and normal tissue localization using a diagnostic quality x-ray beam. Routine beam verification or "port" films confirm that the desired areas are being treated and facilitate adjustment of the blocks.

The *mantle field* is designed to treat the cervical, supraclavicular, axillary, infraclavicular, mediastinal, and pulmonary hilar lymph nodes. These lymphoid regions may be involved or at high risk for involvement in most patients with Hodgkin's disease. We treat this field by an evenly weighted anteroposterior opposed technique to 4400 rad in 5 to 6 weeks. Unless otherwise indicated, the larynx is protected anteriorly throughout the course of treatment. In the posterior field, a block is placed over the cervical spinal cord throughout treatment and over the thoracic spinal cord at a dose of 2000 rad. The infraclavicular lymph nodes are treated only by the anterior field and therefore must be "boosted" anteriorly with orthovoltage (low energy) x-rays or electrons, if involved. In the absence of mediastinal disease, the apex of the heart is protected throughout treatment. When the mediastinum is involved, the entire cardiac silhouette is treated initially. A block is then inserted over the apex of the heart at 1500 rad and over the subcarinal portion of the heart (two vertebral bodies below the carina) at 3000 to 3500 rad. When the pulmonary hilum is involved, the ipsilateral lung is treated by a partial transmission (37 per cent) lung block.

The design of the mantle field is often modified during therapy. As enlarged mediastinal lymph nodes regress, wider lung blocks may be cut to protect more of the lungs (shrinking field technique). If the initial mediastinal mass is large, treatment is given slowly, i.e., only 150 rad per day to a total dose of 1500 rad. Therapy is then interrupted for 7 to 10 days to permit regression of the mediastinal adenopathy and design of larger lung blocks. In appropriate patients, low dose mantle irradiation is completed *prior* to staging laparotomy to avoid problems with intubation or anesthesia.

The *Waldeyer field* utilized in Hodgkin's disease is actually intended in most instances to treat the preauricular lymph nodes. We treat this region with opposed lateral fields, matching the inferior border to the superior edge of the mantle field. Xerostomia often accompanies treatment to this area, so prophylactic irradiation (3600 rad in 4 weeks) is restricted to patients being treated with irradiation alone who have high cervical lymphadenopathy (above the level of the thyroid notch). Occasional patients have bulky involvement of the jugulodigastric, submandibular, or high cervical lymph nodes. We treat these nodes through larger opposed lateral fields, matching to a mantle field in the *low* neck, inferior to the sites of bulky disease. Since the oropharynx and larynx cannot be shielded with this technique, after 2000 rad the treatment is often changed to a standard mantle (upper border near the edge of the mandible) and small Waldeyer (preauricular) field.

The *spade field* and *the inverted Y field* are designed to treat subdiaphragmatic sites. These fields are matched to the mantle in the midplane, and a skin "gap" is calculated based upon field size, beam divergence, and patient thickness. In the design of these fields, the location of the kidneys is important. Normal kidney position is confirmed by pretreatment staging studies, such as a computed tomography scan or intravenous pyelography. The subdiaphragmatic field is treated by the anteroposterior opposed technique, 4 days a week, at a dose of 150 to 200 rad per day, depending on the field size and patient tolerance.

When the spleen is intact, the subdiaphragmatic field includes the entire spleen. Careful localization of the left kidney is required in these cases, and no more than the upper one third of the left kidney is included in the treatment field. In patients with a risk of liver involvement (documented splenic involvement) who are being treated by irradiation alone or in patients with hepatic involvement being treated with combined modality therapy, the subdiaphragmatic field includes the right lobe of the liver, which is treated by means of a partial thickness (50 per cent) block.

The spade field includes the para-aortic nodes, common iliac nodes, and splenic hilum. The inverted Y field includes these same areas but also extends down into the pelvis to encompass the external iliac and inguinal-femoral nodes. A generous-sized midline block is utilized in the pelvis to protect the bladder and rectum, unless there is bulky pelvic lymphadenopathy. In women, a double-thickness midline pelvic block provides protection for the ovaries, which were transposed to the midline during laparotomy.

Total lymphoid irradiation (TLI) implies sequential treatment to the mantle and inverted Y fields. *Subtotal lymphoid irradiation* (STLI) indicates treatment to the mantle and spade fields. After completion of irradiation to one field (i.e., mantle) and before treating the next, a "split" (break) is provided to permit hematologic recovery. These splits average 10 days to 2 weeks. When the subdiaphragmatic field is an inverted Y, especially if the intact spleen or liver is being irradiated, this large field is divided into two portions at the level of the iliac crests. These two fields are then treated sequentially.

Combined Modality Treatment Programs

When combined with chemotherapy, the techniques and dose of radiation may be modified. In most combined modality programs the sequence we utilize is an alternating approach in which chemotherapy (usually two cycles) is administered first, followed by irradiation to one of the major fields, followed by two more cycles of chemotherapy, and so on until six cycles of chemotherapy have been administered and all the fields to be irradiated have been treated. In combined modality programs, we do not irradiate prophylactically the preauricular nodes, lungs, or liver. However, if there is known involvement of those sites they are irradiated. The dose of irradiation that we use in combined modality programs varies from 1500 rad (in children) to 4400 rad (in adults with initial bulky sites of disease). In most situations, we utilize a dose of at least 3000 rad to uninvolved lymphoid regions and 3600 rad to initially involved lymphoid sites.

Recommendations and Outcome
(Table 1)

Stage I-IIA. (The Ann Arbor staging classification for Hodgkin's disease is given in Table 1 of the preceding article.) We treat most stage I-IIA (supradiaphragmatic) patients with STLI. Stage I-IIA (subdiaphragmatic) patients are treated with TLI, often with only 3000 rad to the uninvolved mediastinum. For lymphocyte-predominant Hodgkin's disease limited to the high neck or Hodgkin's disease limited to intrathoracic sites, mantle irradiation alone is probably adequate, but we often also treat the para-aortic nodes and splenic hilum (or spleen if no prior splenectomy).

Stage I-IIB. We use TLI.

Stage IIEA-B. We treat the same as the IIA-B, but extralymphatic sites of involvement are treated to at least 3600 rad.

Large mediastinal masses in Stage I-II. The maximum width of the mediastinal mass is compared with the maximum intrathoracic width. If the ratio exceeds one third, the mass is considered large. The patients are managed individually, since irradiation alone may not control bulky disease. We usually initiate treatment by slowly administering a dose of 1500 rad in 2 weeks to the mantle. We then interrupt treatment for 1 to 2 weeks and assess the patient's response. If the response is good, we continue irradiation (with a shrinking field technique) to at least 4400 rad.

TABLE 1. **Recent Results Treating Hodgkin's Disease at Stanford University**

Stage	Treatment	5 Year Survival (%)	5 Year Freedom from Relapse (%)
I–IIA	STLI or TLI	98	82
I–IIB	TLI	95	89
IIEA–B	STLI/TLI	100	83
I–II Large mediastinal mass	Combined modality	83	80
IIIA S^- or S^+ minimal	TLI	91	80
IIIA S^+ extensive	Combined modality	87	86
IIIB	Combined modality	88	80

STLI, subtotal lymphoid irradiation; TLI, total lymphoid irradiation.

We may boost the dose to the mediastinum to 5000 rad. A staging laparotomy is often done during the 1 to 2 week rest period, or it may be done after completion of the entire course of mantle therapy. Final treatment decisions are based upon the laparotomy findings. In patients who have inadequate response to 1500 rad, we initiate chemotherapy, planning to use a split course or alternating combined modality approach. In this situation we do not perform a staging laparotomy, but base our treatment program only on the clinical staging studies.

Stage IIIA or IIISA with minimal splenic involvement (fewer than five nodules). We use TLI. Low dose irradiation is given to the liver if the spleen is involved.

Stage IIISA with extensive splenic involvement (five or more nodules). These patients have a high relapse rate if treated with irradiation alone. Therefore, we use alternating chemotherapy and irradiation. One field is often irradiated prophylactically, i.e., para-aortic nodes if disease was restricted to spleen and splenic hilar region, pelvic nodes if disease involved para-aortic nodes.

Stage IIIB. Same treatment as IIISA with extensive splenic involvement.

Stage IV, marrow uninvolved. Same as Stage IIIB.

Stage IV, marrow involved. Radiotherapy is restricted to involved regions to permit optimal chemotherapy administration.

Special Considerations

Staging and treatment of older patients should follow the same general guidelines as outlined earlier. A worse prognosis has been associated with older age (>40 or >60 years), but this often reflects inadequate staging or therapy rather than a different biologic behavior of the disease. Older patients in good general condition are able to tolerate the programs already outlined for Stages IA-IIIA. The tolerance for more aggressive treatment programs, however, is not as good as in younger patients. In combined modality programs for patients over 60 years of age, radiation doses may be lower (i.e, 2500 to 3600 rad), except for initial bulky sites of disease, which should be treated to at least 4000 rad, and the radiation fields may be limited to involved sites.

In children, a major concern is the effect of irradiation on growth. Normal growth of the musculoskeletal system may be impaired by doses in excess of 2500 rad. Since a dose this low is inadequate for reliable control of all sites of involvement, we utilize combined modality treatment for all stages of disease in children. In Stage I-II, involved field irradiation is followed by six cycles of chemotherapy. In Stage III-IV, alternating programs of chemotherapy and irradiation are employed, with radiation limited to involved sites.

Palliation

The modest dose of irradiation required for initial treatment permits retreatment for palliation in selected patients. After initial treatment with 4000 rad, individual sites may be treated later for palliation with total doses as high as 2000 to 2500 rad when careful consideration is given to toxicity of adjacent organs. Palliative irradiation in the patient with advanced recurrent disease is frequently useful in ameliorating symptoms and should not be withheld unnecessarily.

Complications

Constitutional symptoms such as anorexia and fatigue often develop during treatment. The rate of recovery is variable and is age-dependent, but an average of 6 to 12 months is required for patients' energy level to return to normal. *Nausea,* occasionally with vomiting, may occur during therapy. It is most common at the outset of treatment and may diminish thereafter, even without specific therapy. Nausea and vomiting usually respond well to simple oral antiemetic agents such as prochlorperazine (Compazine). *Mild xerostomia* may accompany treatment to the mantle field. This problem is more severe and prolonged when the periauricular nodes are treated. Because of the alteration of salivary secretions and the attendant increase in dental caries, patients are carefully instructed in proper oral hygiene, including regular dental check-ups, flossing, and fluoride treatment. Many patients develop *mild pharyngitis* more than halfway through the course of mantle therapy. Rarely does this evolve into a patchy or confluent mucositis requiring interruption of therapy. Usually symptomatic measures suffice in its management.

Skin reactions in the treatment fields are minimal with megavoltage irradiation. Reactions may be noted on the lateral aspects of the neck and shoulders, where the beam passes tangentially to the body contour. Topical steroid creams are used for significant erythematous reactions. Topical emollients should be used after erythema has subsided to relieve dryness. *Epilation* occurs in the irradiated fields and is most noticeable in the suboccipital region (where the upper part of the mantle field enters and exits through the posterior scalp).

Adverse *hematologic effects* may be observed during therapy. Hemograms and platelet counts are obtained weekly. Most commonly, difficulties are encountered during treatment of the second radiation field, especially if the patient has received prior chemotherapy. Blood counts are obtained more frequently than weekly if there is evidence of significant depression of the white blood cell or platelet count. Interruption of therapy as a result of granulocytopenia or thrombocytopenia is based upon the rate of decline in the counts, the point in the patient's overall treatment program, and the volume of marrow being irradiated. In some instances the field being treated (i.e., the inverted Y) may be divided into two portions and treatment restricted to one half of the field, with completion of the second half later. Occasionally, a slight lowering of the daily dose permits better hematologic tolerance. In any case, we rarely continue treatment if the total white blood cell count is less than 2000 per mm^3 or the platelet count is less than 50,000 per mm^3. Hematologic recovery gradually becomes complete even after TLI, and normal peripheral counts are almost always present within 3 months after the completion of therapy. *Lymphocytopenia* may be observed for a year or more after therapy, and evaluation of T cell subsets reveals an excess of suppressor/cytotoxic cells compared with helper/inducer cells, thereby reversing the normal ratio of these cell populations.

Radiation pneumonitis may occur within 3 months of completion of mantle irradiation. Symptoms and signs include cough, mild shortness of breath, dyspnea on exertion, pleuritic chest pain, fever, and an infiltrate on chest roentgenogram that may conform to the design of the radiation portals. The likelihood of developing radiation pneumonitis is related to the volume of lung irradiated, the total dose, and the dose rate. In the treatment programs outlined earlier, radiation pneumonitis occurs in less than 5 per cent of patients, and only a small proportion of these develop symptoms severe enough to require treatment. The preferred therapy is high dose corticosteroids (e.g., prednisone, 60 mg per day) with the dose very *gradually* tapered over a period of at least several weeks. A more rapid taper may cause exacerbation of the pneumonitis. Most patients treated with mantle irradiation develop long-term paramediastinal fibrosis which is evident on routine chest radiograph. The administration of high doses of corticosteroids followed by sudden withdrawal in any patient who has received mantle irradiation may result in the development of a latent radiation pneumonitis.

Symptoms and signs of *radiation pericarditis* may include fever, pleuritic chest pain, pericardial friction rub, pericardial effusion, low voltage changes on electrocardiogram, and pericardial tamponade. The onset is usually within the first year after mantle irradiation but may be delayed as long as several years after treatment. Occasionally radiation pericarditis may progress to cause a chronic pericardial effusion or constrictive pericarditis. The likelihood of developing pericarditis is correlated with the volume of heart irradiated, the total dose, and the dose rate. The majority of cases of radiation pericarditis are evident only as small pericardial effusions on routine post-treatment radiographs. Large pericardial effusions may cause tamponade and require pericardiocentesis. Chronic constrictive pericarditis with hemodynamic compromise may necessitate pericardial stripping. Fewer than 5 per cent of patients treated with standard mantle fields develop radiation pericarditis requiring therapy. It can be avoided completely utilizing the mantle techniques described (including the subcarinal block after 3000 rad). As in radiation pneumonitis, radiation pericarditis may be induced by sudden withdrawal from high dose corticosteroid therapy.

Occasional *infectious complications* of staging and treatment may be identified. In the asplenic patient there is an increased risk of infection with gram-positive, encapsulated organisms, especially *Streptococcus pneumoniae*. The infections may occur even many years after staging and treatment. Routine presplenectomy vaccination with Pneumovax does not provide complete protection, since several serotypes of *S. pneumoniae* are not included in the vaccine, antibody titers may not be elevated sufficiently in long-term follow-up, and *Haemophilus influenzae* remains a potential problem. Patients who have undergone splenectomy and treatment for Hodgkin's disease should be advised of this risk and should be evaluated carefully by a physician when they develop symptoms of an upper respiratory infection, especially when associated with fever, and appropriate cultures and antibiotic coverage should be provided. Approximately 15 per cent of patients will develop localized herpes zoster (shingles) within 18 months of completion of therapy for Hodgkin's disease. In 5 per cent of these cases cutaneous dissemination occurs, and in less than 1 per cent visceral infection develops. Treatment consists primarily of symptomatic measures, including appropriate analgesics. Treatment with acyclovir may limit the duration or severity of the infection.

Although it is partially protected by the larynx block, the *thyroid gland* receives a significant dose of irradiation. Nearly two thirds of patients treated with a mantle field develop thyroid dysfunction documented by an elevated thyroid-stimulating hormone (TSH) level with normal or low T4 levels. We recommend thyroid replacement therapy if the TSH is elevated even if the T4 value is normal. If physical examination reveals palpable thyroid abnormalities, these should be assessed further with appropriate studies.

Reproductive complications are not a concern unless irradiation includes treatment to the pelvic lymph nodes. A testicular shield should be used in men who want to preserve reproductive capability. With the lead shield we utilize, the testicular dose is only 0.75 per cent of the dose to the inguinal-femoral nodes. In women who have undergone oophoropexy, the midline protective block limits the dose of irradiation (by scatter) to 8 per cent of the dose to the pelvic nodes. Despite this low dose, many women do experience transient menstrual abnormalities during therapy. However, in at least half, normal menses return. The recovery of menstrual function is related to age at the time of therapy. More than two thirds of patients under the age of 20 years at the time of treatment experience a return of normal menstrual function, but less than 20 per cent of patients over the age of 30 years do.

Secondary malignant change is a potential complication of therapy in Hodgkin's disease. Such diseases include leukemia (acute nonlymphocytic), non-Hodgkin's lymphoma, and solid tumors. The occurrence of acute nonlymphocytic leukemia is generally limited to patients who receive chemotherapy that includes an alkylating agent or procarbazine. The latent period before development of leukemia is generally 3 to 5 years, and the actuarial risk for patients treated with chemotherapy may be as high as 5 per cent at 7 years. The secondary non-Hodgkin's lymphomas that occur are generally high grade. They occur less commonly than leukemia does but may be observed in patients treated initially with irradiation alone. Common secondary solid tumors include malignancies of the breast, lungs, and gastrointestinal tract. The latent period to their development is quite long (usually at least 10 years) and they also may be seen after any type of initial therapy.

Follow-Up

We see patients every 2 months during the first year, every 3 months during the second year, every 4 months during the third year, every 6 months during the fourth and fifth years, and annually thereafter. On each visit, we complete a relevant history and physical examination, obtain a hemogram and platelet count, erythrocyte sedimentation rate, and serum copper, alkaline phosphatase, and chest and abdominal x-ray studies. Serum T4 and TSH levels are determined annually. In patients whose pelvic lymph nodes have been unirradiated, a lymphogram is usually repeated during the second year of follow-up, unless there is adequate residual opacification of pelvic lymph nodes to permit their continued observation for 3 years after completion of therapy.

Abnormalities brought to light by any of the aforementioned examinations or studies should lead to appropriate further evaluation. Suspected relapses are almost always documented pathologically. Surveillance for potential complications of therapy, especially secondary malignancy, is continued throughout the follow-up period.

ACUTE LEUKEMIA IN ADULTS

method of
ERNEST BEUTLER, M.D.
Scripps Clinic and Research Foundation
La Jolla, California

Although cures are still relatively uncommon, there has been dramatic improvement in the outlook for adults with acute leukemia in the past 2 decades. This change is due to the availability of more effective chemotherapeutic agents and bone marrow transplantation, on the one hand, and on the development of supportive measures that make it possible for patients to survive a degree of bone marrow failure today that formerly would have been lethal.

First Steps When the Diagnosis Is Established

Although definitive chemotherapy usually should be started within a few days of the diagnosis of acute leukemia, some steps need to be taken from the outset to maximize the chances of at least temporary success and to minimize discomfort and anxiety of the patient. To learn that a diagnosis of acute leukemia has been established is a devastating experience. In imparting this information to the patient and family, the physician must try to blend realism with hope. Patients must soon endure the discomforts and hazards of induction therapy and should be forewarned of the probability of infection with fever, and of bleeding. They will then be much less fearful when these expected complications occur.

Patients with blast counts of over 100,000 per μl require urgent attention. Such counts represent an immediate hazard, since fatal central nervous system bleeding is quite common in this subgroup of patients. Reduction of the white count is best achieved by repeated leukapheresis on a cell separator. At the same time, the patient should be given 6 to 8 grams of hydroxyurea orally daily until the white count comes under control. This may be done concurrently with the administration of induction chemotherapy, which may be undertaken immediately or delayed for a few days while essential baseline information is being collected. Induction chemotherapy can wait, but cytoreduction in patients with high white counts should have first priority in patient management.

Extensive pretreatment laboratory examinations do not serve a useful purpose, but it is prudent to obtain, in addition to the routine blood count and bone marrow examination, a baseline blood chemistry panel, chest radiograph, and electrocardiogram. If the bleeding manifestations seem out of keeping with the degree of thrombocytopenia, or if the cytologic characteristics of the bone marrow suggest that the leukemia may be progranulocytic, evaluation of hemostasis is indicated as well.

Patients are well served by placement of a right atrial catheter before induction therapy is started, particularly if treatment consists of continuous infusion. Providing this type of access to the venous system greatly facilitates the administration of chemotherapeutic agents, blood products, and antibiotics and the obtaining of blood samples for the laboratory, thus minimizing patient discomfort.

Since they will be quite susceptible to infection, patients undergoing induction therapy are best hospitalized in a single room. Strict isolation precautions are not essential even when severe neutropenia is present, and their enforcement tends to isolate the patient from the medical and paramedical staff in a counterproductive manner. It is prudent, however, to instruct the staff to wash their hands and to wear a gauze mask when entering the rooms of patients whose granulocyte counts have fallen below 200 per μl. Allopurinol (Zyloprim) should be given to those patients who have a very high white count or those whose bone marrow is packed with blasts. Three hundred mg per day is a suitable dose, which should be started before chemotherapy is initiated. Indiscriminate use of this drug in patients undergoing chemotherapy is unwise, since the skin eruption that commonly occurs in patients receiving allopurinol cannot be distinguished from that caused by administration of antibiotics and other drugs, therefore creating a possible therapeutic dilemma. Because of its effect on platelet function, aspirin is contraindicated.

The therapy of acute leukemia is hazardous and should be undertaken only by physicians with experience in the care of such patients and in the administration of the drugs that are used.

Induction Therapy

General Considerations

In the choice of induction therapy, it is sufficient to classify the leukemia as acute lymphoblastic (ALL) or as acute myeloid leukemia (AML). In adults I generally approach acute undifferentiated leukemia (AUL) as I do AML. The subclassification of AML is not important from a therapeutic point of view.

Since complete remission rates in acute leukemia approach 70 per cent and are only slightly lower even in the elderly, most patients with acute leukemia should be treated with the goal of inducing remission. Some patients, however, become frankly leukemic only after a prolonged prodrome of marrow dysplasia and mixed types of pancytopenias. If the general health and functional status of such patients are fairly satisfactory with supportive therapy, such as periodic red cell transfusion and treatment of infections with antibiotics, I tend to delay institution of induction therapy. Other exceptions to prompt initiation of induction chemotherapy include patients who are in such poor physical condition, either from the complications of their leukemia or from pre-existing disease, that they seem unlikely to survive induction. Refusal of therapy by patients to whom it has been properly explained is quite rare in our experience. It is generally unwise to delay institution of therapy by more than a day or two because of cytopenia or infection. Over the long run these will be brought under control only if the patient achieves remission, and delay in beginning treatment usually proves to be counterproductive.

Induction Therapy in Patients with AML

A continuous infusion of cytosine arabinoside at a dose of 100 mg per M^2 of body surface per 24 hours is given for 7 days. On the first, second, and third days of treatment, single doses of daunorubicin, 45 mg per M^2 are given.

If the patient is not pancytopenic before induction therapy is instituted, he or she will become so within a few days. Prophylactic antibiotics are not given, but when the patient becomes febrile, cultures of urine, blood, and if present sputum and a chest radiograph are obtained, and antibiotic therapy is begun without waiting for the results of the cultures. Intravenous administration of a cephalosporin antibiotic such as cefazolin (Ancef), an aminoglycoside such as tobramycin (Nebcin), and a semisynthetic penicillin such as ticarcillin (Ticar) is given. If fever persists for several days, the administration of amphotericin (Fungizone) should be considered, even in the absence of a proven fungus infection.

Most patients will require red cell transfusions and some degree of platelet support. The latter type of therapy should be given when the bleeding occurs as a result of thrombocytopenia. The routine administration of platelets when the count falls below 20,000 per μl that is followed in some centers is in my view unnecessary and undesirable. Rather, I prefer to administer platelets only when clinical evidence of bleeding is present. If the platelet count declines to under 5000 per μl, then platelet transfusions are usually needed. Granulocyte transfusions are expensive and subject donors to some discomfort and risk. Fortunately, they are needed only under unusual circumstances. We consider the implementation of granulocyte support only in patients with granulocyte counts under 200 per μl who have life-threatening infections unresponsive to antibiotics for at least 2 days.

About 7 days after completion of the treatment course, careful re-evaluation of the patient's hematologic status is required to decide whether or not a second course of therapy should be given immediately. If substantial numbers of leukemic blasts persist in the periphery, then it is clear that treatment has been insufficient to achieve a remission. If no blasts are present in the blood, then a bone marrow examination is performed. If the marrow is hypoplastic, then remission may be around the corner, and no immediate additional chemotherapy is given. If, on the other hand, large numbers of blasts persist, cytosine arabinoside for 5 days and daunorubicin for 2 days are given at the same daily dosage as before.

If the course of treatment is not repeated, then the patient's hematologic status is observed carefully. An increasing platelet count and the appearance of normal leukocytes in the peripheral blood indicates that a remission may be occurring. On the other hand, sometimes blasts reappear in the periphery, even when the marrow was free of blasts immediately after the first induction course. If this occurs, a second course of cytosine arabinoside and daunorubicin should be initiated.

We do not usually give patients more than two courses of this type in the initial attempt to induce a remission. However, if the patient has not entered a complete remission but shows substantial improvement after a second course, a third course may be administered. Subsequently, attempts to induce remission are either abandoned, or a second type of induction therapy is given.

What to Do If Remission Is Achieved

Once a remission is achieved in a patient with acute myeloid leukemia, one must face the sobering reality that with or without additional chemotherapy the very best that one may hope for is a 25 per cent chance of prolonged remission or cure. Only allogeneic bone marrow transplantation offers much better prospects, and unfortunately many patients are not suitable candidates for this treatment.

The first step, then, after achieving remission is to identify those patients who are suitable candidates for transplantation. In 1985 the criteria are simple and, unfortunately, rather restrictive. The patient must have an HLA-matched sib who is willing and able to donate bone marrow. The patient should also be under 35 years of age. Between the ages of 35 and 45 marrow transplantation may also be carried out, but the advantage over chemotherapy is not nearly so clear-cut as in the younger patients because of the increasing incidence of fatal graft-versus-host disease in the older patient group. Patients over 45 years of age are poor candidates for bone marrow transplantation.

Patients in Remission Who Are Not Candidates for Bone Marrow Transplantation

Although very critical to the welfare and possible survival of the patient with acute leukemia who enters remission, no reliable data exist with respect to further management. By analogy with the treatment of acute leukemia of childhood, a variety of maintenance programs have been tried. These range in aggressiveness from the monthly administration of subcutaneous cytosine arabinoside to severely myelosuppressive monthly regimens, each representing therapy virtually as myelosuppressive as the original induction. Such therapy is sometimes designated as "consolidation." The weight of evidence suggests that such aggressive early treatment of patients who achieve remission may indeed increase the percentage of patients who are cured. However, such an advantage can hardly be considered cheaply bought; the morbidity from such treatment is considerable.

A relatively simple consolidation program that has been used with considerable success in a limited number of patients consists of the administration of 3 grams of cytosine arabinoside per M^2 of body surface via a 1 hour intravenous infusion every 12 hours for 12 doses, followed by rapid intravenous infusion of daunorubicin, 30 mg per M^2 of body surface once daily for 2 days. A single course of this very aggressive therapy has resulted in long remission in about one half the patients treated.

Management of Patients with Relapsed AML

The success rate in achieving remission in patients after failure of initial induction therapy or in those who have relapsed is much lower than that of patients undergoing their first induction therapy. Yet, some 25 per cent of such patients may enjoy complete remissions with alternative modes of therapy. Although such remissions are usually brief and may be purchased at high cost, an attempt to achieve remission in such patients may often be worthwhile. In other patients, such as those who have already failed to achieve a good response with an attempt at remission reinduction, or those whose physical or mental condition precludes further intensive therapy, other means of treatment must be sought.

Remission Reinduction

When a patient has enjoyed a fairly prolonged remission after induction therapy with cytosine arabinoside and daunorubicin, readministration of the same schedule is worthwhile. If the patient has failed this type of induction therapy, however, the administration of high dose cytosine arabinoside may prove to be useful. Three grams of the drug per M^2 are administered intravenously over a 3 hour period for six doses given at 12 hour intervals. The administration of 6000 IU of L-asparaginase per M^2 3 hours after conclusion of the last dose seems to be promising. Even patients who have failed to respond to standard doses of cytosine arabinoside may achieve remission with this kind of treatment. A second method of reinducing induction that has sometimes been successful is administration of the acridine derivative m-AMSA (available from National Cancer Institute, Bethesda, MD: 301–496-5223). Five hundred to 700 mg of the drug are administered per M^2 over a period of 5 to 7 days.

Management of Patients in Whom Remission Induction Is Not to Be Attempted

While it is clear that there is no real substitute for a prolonged complete remission in the management of patients with acute leukemia, it is unfortunately a fact that most patients with this disease reach a stage in their clinical course in which an attempt to induce a remission is no longer to their advantage. But the length of life of such patients, too, can be prolonged and the quality enhanced by judicious treatment. Supportive therapy is of major importance. It is futile, and probably counterproductive, to attempt to maintain the platelet count with repeated platelet transfusions. Administration of platelets should be reserved for bleeding episodes. The hematocrit should be maintained by providing red cell transfusions as needed. Antibiotics are given to control infections. Occasionally the chronic administration of trimethoprim/sulfamethoxazole (Bactrim) may be useful.

Patients in this stage of AML have a poor prognosis whatever is done to help them. Thus, the patient should be spared extensive diagnostic studies. A pragmatic approach to management of complications is justified. A rising blast count may be controlled by the administration of either cytosine arabinoside, hydroxyurea, or 6-thioguanine. Cytosine arabinoside is used in doses much smaller than those employed when attempting remission induction. The administration of 5 mg per M^2 of cytosine arabinoside subcutaneously (subcutaneous use is not listed in the manufacturer's directive) every 12 hours for 3 to 5 days may be useful if the platelet count is not too low. Alternatively, 3 to 6 grams of hydroxyurea daily for a few days, followed by a maintenance dose of 0.5 to 2.0 grams per day, to control the white count may be useful. 6-Thioguanine at 90 mg per day may also be employed. Unfortunately, these drugs all produce thrombocytopenia and cannot be given if the patient already has a low platelet count. Intermittent doses of 1 mg of vincristine may be helpful and may be used in patients who are severely thrombocytopenic. Given alone or in combination with these drugs, the administration of prednisone in doses between 10 and 80 mg per day may improve the patient's sense of well-being and may improve the peripheral blood counts.

Induction Therapy in Patients with ALL

Remission induction in ALL is achieved using a combination of Oncovin (vincristine), prednisone, L-asparaginase, and daunorubicin (Cerubidine). This is much less rigorous for the patient than induction therapy for AML; pancytopenia is usually less severe and less prolonged than that observed with treatment with cytosine arabinoside and daunorubicin. Yet the incidence of complete remission is quite high, especially in those patients whose leukemic cells are of the "null" variety with the common ALL antigen.

An induction program that has been found quite successful consists of three weekly intravenous injections of 2 mg of vincristine; 45 mg of daunorubicin per M^2 on days 1, 2, and 3; and prednisone, 40 mg per M^2 daily for up to 35 days. Starting on day 16, a 10 day course of L-asparaginase, consisting of 5000 units per M^2, is given. Once remission is achieved, the peripheral granulocyte count is permitted to rise to over 1500 per cu mm and the platelet count to over 125,000 per cu mm. If remission is achieved, bone marrow transplantation offers the best opportunity of cure to suitable candidates. Others should be given consolidation therapy and placed on maintenance for a period of about 2 years. To effect consolidation, 6-mercaptopurine, 500 mg per M^2 per day (this dose is higher than recommended in the manufacturer's directive), and methotrexate, 15 mg per M^2 per day, are given intravenously as two 5 day courses spaced 2 weeks apart. Younger patients with ALL should also receive prophylactic cranial irradiation of 2400 rad and five spaced doses of 12 mg of intrathecal methotrexate over a period of at least 3 weeks.

Maintenance therapy is usually given to adults with ALL, mainly in analogy with the proved benefit of such treatment in children. Multiple drug combinations are employed, and these generally contain methotrexate and 6-mercaptopurine. A relatively simple program that appears to be as effective as more complex schedules consists of the administration of 6-mercaptopurine, 90 mg per M^2 orally every day, plus methotrexate, 20 mg per M^2 weekly.

Unfortunately, in contrast to circumstances in children, the relapse rate in adult ALL is as high or higher than that observed in AML. As in children, the prognosis of patients whose blasts contain T cell or B cell markers is very poor.

Bone Marrow Transplantation

Transplantation should be performed in a center that has both the facilities and the experience that help minimize the risks of the procedure. Although transplantation carried out in hematology/oncology services that only occasionally perform this procedure may be successful, it is best to carry out transplantation in a center that performs at least 20 allogeneic transplants per year. The chances of success do not seem markedly influenced by the mode of preparation used for transplantation. In almost all cases, 1000 rad of total body irradiation given as a single dose or 1200 rad given in fractionated doses is employed. In addition to radiation, cyclophosphamide is usually employed, and cytosine arabinoside is also administered.

ACUTE LEUKEMIA IN CHILDHOOD

method of
WILLIAM A. SMITHSON, M.D.,
and GERALD S. GILCHRIST, M.D.
Mayo Clinic
Rochester, Minnesota

There are two major forms of acute leukemia in childhood—lymphocytic and nonlymphocytic. It is possible to cure children with acute leukemia, especially those with the lymphocytic form. At present there is no one standard method of treatment; most children in the United States are treated on research protocols that incorporate the best-known therapy but also include innovative therapy that can be evaluated in a research setting. The treatment programs we utilize are based on those developed over the past 25 years in the Children's Cancer Study Group. They may vary in some details from those employed by other cooperative groups or pediatric cancer centers, but the same basic principles underlie all the treatment regimens currently in use.

Acute Lymphocytic Leukemia (ALL)

Lymphocytic leukemia is subclassified in four ways: (1) by the findings on physical examination and routine laboratory values, (2) by morphologic criteria using standard microscopic techniques, (3) immunologically, and (4) cytogenetically. At the present time therapy can be planned based on the first two sets of criteria. Leukemic blasts can be shown to correspond to lymphocyte subsets, but with the exception of the membrane receptor for sheep erythrocytes (E-rosette receptor), these subclasses have not yet proved to be independent variables in determining prognosis, using results from trials begun 5 to 10 years ago with relatively "standard" regimens. Cytogenetic findings are emerging which may identify children with greater and lesser chances of long-term survival.

All children with acute lymphocytic leukemia die if they are not treated. The terms good, intermediate, and poor prognosis refer to relative chance of remission at 5 years (and presumed cure) when children are treated by standard treatment protocol.

Induction

Standard treatment for children with leukemia begins with induction of remission with intravenous vincristine (Oncovin), oral prednisone, intramuscular L-asparaginase (Elspar), and intrathecal methotrexate. Renal function and serum uric acid should be normal or improving before treatment is started. Correction of anemia and treatment of infection should also be well under way before specific antileukemic therapy begins. Prednisone in a dose of 40 mg per M^2 per day in three divided doses is given by mouth for 28 days; vincristine, 1.5 mg per M^2 (maximal dose; 2 mg) intravenously every 7 days for four doses; and L-asparaginase, 6000 international units per M^2 intramuscularly beginning on the third day of treatment and continuing at three doses per week for a total of nine doses. The dose of intrathecal methotrexate is adjusted according to the age of the child: less than 2 years, 8 mg; 2 to 3 years, 10 mg; and 3 years and over, 12 mg. This is given on the first day of treatment and again on Day 14.

Consolidation

Remission is achieved when the bone marrow no longer contains leukemic blasts, extramedullary involvement has resolved, and peripheral blood counts are normalizing. At this point treatment is directed to eradicating occult disease of the central nervous system, which is assumed to be present in most children. Intrathecal methotrexate is given weekly for four additional doses. Children in the intermediate and poor risk groups receive cranial irradiation (1800 rad in 10 fractions) whereas children in the good prognosis group do not. Attempts are being made to eliminate cranial irradiation without an unacceptable increase in the incidence of central nervous system relapse. Younger children (under 3 years of age) are thought to be at greater risk for central nervous system toxicity related to the radiation.

Maintenance

Maintenance chemotherapy is part of every ALL protocol. A standard program includes vincristine, 1.5 mg per M^2 (maximal dose, 2 mg) administered intravenously once every four weeks. Prednisone, 40 mg per M^2 orally in three divided doses, is given for 5 days starting the day the vincristine is administered. 6-Mercaptopurine (Purinethol), 75 mg per M^2 orally, is given once daily and methotrexate, 20 mg per M^2 orally, once weekly. Intrathecal methotrexate is administered every 12 weeks if children have not received cranial irradiation. Treatment is continued for 2 to 3 years from the time of diagnosis. Routine bone marrow studies during remission are not absolutely indicated since most relapsing children will exhibit changes in the peripheral blood count or show some other indication of relapse. Treatment of relapse is not jeopardized by delay of a few weeks in diagnosis.

Routine examination of the cerebrospinal fluid after cytocentrifugation is indicated every 12 weeks since central nervous system leukemia is best treated before it becomes symptomatic. A testicular biopsy should be done on boys before treatment is stopped. If occult testicular leukemia is present, treatment should be continued, with testicular irradiation added.

Additive Therapy

Children with an intermediate or poor prognosis are usually treated in clinical trials that attempt to identify therapy that represents an improvement over standard treatment. These protocols are characterized by the addition of drugs such as cytosine arabinoside (Cytosar), daunorubicin (Cerubidine), doxorubicin (Adriamycin), and cyclophosphamide (Cytoxan). In induction, consolidation, and remission, these drugs produce greater toxicity and are associated with an increased likelihood of infectious and other complications, particularly during induction. Whether an individual child should be treated on such a protocol and randomly assigned to a standard or innovative regimen is a difficult issue that should be thoroughly explored with the family.

Infants have had a very poor prognosis with standard therapy, and all are treated in a more intensive fashion. Children with lymphomatous features are currently being treated with innovative programs which should be undertaken in a research setting. Burkitt's cell leukemia is currently treated in the same way as Burkitt's cell lymphoma.

Relapse on Treatment

Bone Marrow Relapse. If bone marrow relapse occurs while the child is on maintenance therapy, the prognosis is very poor. A variety of chemotherapeutic approaches has produced few long-term survivors following this type of relapse. One of the best reported regimens utilizes a standard reinduction with the addition of daunomycin, 30 mg per M^2 intravenously weekly for three doses. For maintenance, methotrexate, 100 mg per M^2 intravenously, is given, followed 24 hours later with L-asparaginase, 15,000 units per M^2 intramuscularly. This two day cycle is given every 10 days as tolerated until relapse or unacceptable toxicity occurs or for three years of continuous remission. Alternatively, if the child has relapsed on a standard regimen, the use of one of the additive programs could be considered.

Central nervous system prophylaxis should be repeated after relapse because the CNS is a frequent site of subsequent relapse. If there is a suitable donor, bone marrow transplantation is indicated for the child who relapses while on therapy, since this has produced long-term survival in approximately 30 per cent of children so treated.

Central Nervous System Relapse. This should be treated with craniospinal radiation, intrathecal methotrexate, systemic reinduction, and prolongation of the period of treatment, with intrathecal chemotherapy included in the maintenance phase. Repeated relapse is an indication for the addition of cytosine arabinoside and hydrocortisone to intrathecal therapy. A second course of cranial irradiation should be avoided if the child is a marrow transplant candidate.

Testicular Relapse. This is treated with radiation to the scrotum (usually 2400 rad), systemic reinduction, and prolongation of the period of treatment.

Relapse Off Treatment

Relapse after the child has finished a standard period of maintenance therapy has a better prognosis. It is treated in substantially the same manner as relapse occurring on treatment, except that bone marrow transplantation is not currently recommended for children who relapse after being off treatment more than 6 months.

Acute Nonlymphocytic Leukemia (ANL)

Standard therapy for nonlymphocytic leukemia has produced far fewer cured patients than treatment for lymphocytic leukemia, nor have prognostic factors been clearly defined. Almost all children with nonlymphocytic leukemia are treated in similar fashion. This situation will probably change soon because of the emerging differences based on FAB morphologic classification and cytogenetic analysis.

The standard induction therapy consists of cytosine arabinoside (Cytosar), 100 mg per M^2 per day by continuous intravenous infusion for 7 days; daunomycin (Cerubidine), 45 mg per M^2 is given by intravenous push daily for the first 3 days. Cytosine arabinoside is given intrathecally to treat occult central nervous system disease, which is recognized with approximately the same frequency as in lymphocytic leukemia. The dose of intrathecal cytosine arabinoside is 20 mg for children under 1 year of age, 30 mg for children 1 to 2 years old, 50 mg for children 2 to 3 years old, and 70 mg for children over age 3 years.

There is no standard approach following induction and, in fact, the value of maintenance therapy remains a valid research question. In recent years, many children have undergone bone marrow transplantation in lieu of conventional chemotherapy. The advantage of this approach in children remains to be confirmed. Another promising approach is very intensive chemotherapy following the induction of remission. Very high dose cytosine arabinoside is currently under investigation for this purpose.

A standard maintenance regimen for children that has yielded the best reported results consists of five drugs given in 28 day cycles. 6-Thioguanine (Tabloid), 75 mg per M^2 orally, is given daily throughout the maintenance period. Vincristine (Oncovin), 1.5 mg per M^2 (maximal dose, 2 mg), is given on the first day. Cytosine arabinoside, 75 mg per M^2 intravenously; 5-azacytidine (investigational drug), 100 mg per M^2 intravenously; and cyclophosphamide (Cytoxan), 75 mg per M^2 intravenously, are given daily for 4 days. The whole cycle is repeated every 28 days.

The duration of treatment for ANL is for 2 years from the time of remission. Relapse of nonlymphocytic leukemia in the bone marrow is virtually always fatal when treated with conventional chemotherapy. It is a definite indication for bone marrow transplant if it is possible.

INITIAL MANAGEMENT

This section applies to both types of acute leukemia (Table 1).

Anemia

In transfusing packed red cells to correct anemia, we use the same criteria for transfusion as in other patients. In the presence of cardiovascular compromise, fever, and a hemoglobin level less than 6 grams per dl, more urgent transfusion will be required. If possible, the blood products should be irradiated to 2000 rads to prevent graft-versus-host disease. Red cells should be given only to correct symptomatic anemia in children with hyperleukocytosis. For other children, packed cells in a volume of 10 ml per kg over 1 to 2 hours are usually tolerated without cardiovascular compromise. Several small transfusions may be necessary to raise the hemoglobin level to 8 to 9 grams per dl.

TABLE 1. **Initial and Emergency Measures**

Finding	Management
Diagnosis of leukemia	Inform family and reassure (see text)
WBC > 100,000	Cranial irradiation
Congestive heart failure and/or hemoglobin < 5.0 gm/dl	Transfuse packed red cells, 10 ml per kg (if WBC < 100,000)
Bleeding	Transfuse platelets, 1 unit/M^2 per 10,000 increment desired; determine whether DIC is present
Infection	Blood cultures. Antibiotics for both gram-negative and gram-positive organisms
Hyperuricemia Hyperkalemia Renal failure	Allopurinol Hydration Urinary alkalinization

Fever

Fever in the newly diagnosed child may be secondary to the leukemia or to infection. If the child is febrile, blood for cultures should be drawn. Culture all local sites of infection since even a small skin infection may lead to sepsis in these immunocompromised children. At this stage, if the child is not clinically septic antibiotics can be withheld pending culture results. Fever often resolves within hours of starting specific antileukemic therapy.

If antibiotics are started, coverage for gram-negative organisms and penicillin-resistant staphylococci should be included. We use oxacillin in a dose of 200 mg per kg per day in six divided doses, gentamycin (Garamycin) in a dose of 3 to 7 mg per kg per day in three divided doses, and mezlocillin in a dose of 200 to 300 mg per kg per day in six divided doses. Fungal and other opportunistic infections are less likely to occur, and infections with common bacterial pathogens are more common at the time of diagnosis.

Bleeding

Bleeding is usually caused by thrombocytopenia, although disseminated intravascular coagulation may be a contributing factor. One unit of platelets per M^2 produces an average increment of 10,000 per microliter. Platelet counts of 50,000 per microliter will usually produce normal hemostasis. In parallel with platelet transfusion, local measures to stop bleeding are usually indicated (for example, packing the nose for control of epistaxis).

Hyperleukocytosis

If the total white cell count is over 100,000, there is a significant risk of cerebral hemorrhagic infarction as a result of leukostasis. We have successfully prevented this complication by cranial irradiation in a single dose of 400 rad on the day of diagnosis. This should be done in consultation with a radiation therapist experienced in the treatment of childhood leukemia. Leukapheresis should be considered, particularly if the white blood cell count is over 300,000 per microliter. Red cell transfusion to above 6 grams per dl should be avoided until the blast count is subsiding because the increased hematocrit will increase viscosity and the danger of hemorrhagic infarction.

Metabolic Stabilization

Newly diagnosed children are at risk for developing hyperuricemia, which can result in renal failure, hyperkalemia, and hypocalcemia. Measurements of uric acid, creatinine, sodium, potassium, calcium, and phosphorus should be obtained immediately and monitored closely during the initial management period. Allopurinol (Zyloprim), in a dose of 50 to 100 mg orally three times daily, should be started as soon as diagnosis is made. Hydration should be maintained with intravenous fluids. In the absence of renal failure, we use fluid containing 5 per cent dextrose, 0.2 per cent sodium chloride, 20 to 40 mEq per liter of potassium chloride, and sodium bicarbonate in a dose of 2 mEq per kg per day. The goals of this hydration are to keep body weight stable, urine output up to 100 ml per M^2 per hour, urine pH over 7, and serum sodium and potassium within normal limits. Usually, 3000 ml per M^2 per day is adequate. Hypocalcemia and hyperphosphatemia occur because of the inability of the renal tubules to handle the large phosphate load from the lysis of leukemia cells. Replacing calcium is not always necessary and should be undertaken with great care because it is possible to cause nephrocalcinosis. If renal infiltration with leukemia is contributing to renal failure, irradiation of the kidneys should be considered, but it is not always necessary. Renal dialysis is occasionally required.

Psychosocial Stabilization

The family and child with the diagnosis of leukemia are extremely vulnerable. The physician can offer realistic support by assuring the family that every child with the diagnosis has the potential for cure (the actual percentage in numerical terms ranges widely and can be predicted more accurately when other clinical features are taken into account). In addition, it is reassuring to families to know that most children will enter a period of remission (70 to 95 per cent, depending on the type of leukemia). Assuring the family that they have done nothing to cause the disease, that it will not likely affect siblings, and that it could not have been prevented helps allay much of their anxiety. We point out that other family members should not be neglected in spite of the enormous attention that will be directed to the child with leukemia. Referral to financial counselors and early identification of the need for financial assistance should be done during the first week. Published material, such as the book by Lynn S. Baker, *You and Leukemia* (2nd ed., W. B. Saunders Company, Philadelphia, 1978), provides accurate information in understandable language and can enable the family to begin to frame their questions about how this disease will affect them. Other materials are available from the National Cancer Institute and American Cancer Society. After the initial interview, further conferences with the parents will be necessary to

TABLE 2. **Drugs Used to Treat Acute Lymphocytic Leukemia**

	Commonly Encountered Adverse Reactions
vincristine (Oncovin)	Alopecia, neuritic pain, constipation, difficulty in walking, peripheral neuropathy, leukopenia, severe cellulitis if extravasated
prednisone (Deltasone)	Immunosuppression, increased appetite and weight gain, Cushing's syndrome, myopathy, mood changes, diabetes mellitus, relative adrenocortical insufficiency in times of stress
L-asparaginase (Elspar)	Anaphylactic reactions, decreased protein synthesis (including coagulation factors), pancreatitis and diabetes mellitus
6-mercaptopurine (Purinethol)	myelosuppression, hepatotoxicity, immunosuppression
methotrexate (Low dose, oral)	Stomatitis, myelosuppression, immunosuppression, photosensitivity, hepatic fibrosis
doxorubicin (Adriamycin)	Myelosuppression, cardiac toxicity, alopecia, nausea and vomiting, stomatitis, gastrointestinal ulceration, severe cellulitis if extravasated, hypersensitivity reactions
daunomycin (Cerubidine)	Myelosuppression, cardiac toxicity, alopecia, nausea and vomiting, stomatitis, gastrointestinal ulceration, severe cellulitis if extravasated, hypersensitivity reactions
cyclophosphamide (Cytoxan)	Myelosuppression, nausea and vomiting, hemorrhagic cystitis, decreased gonadal function, alopecia
cytosine arabinoside (Cytosar)	Myelosuppression, nausea and vomiting, stomatitis

reinforce material discussed earlier. Most parents are unable to assimilate all the facts while still coming to grips with the diagnosis of a potentially fatal disease in their child.

It is our policy to explain the diagnosis, the nature of the disease, and the prognosis to both patient and parents. We ensure that the child feels comfortable asking questions of parents, nurses, social workers, and physicians. Principles of treatment are also covered in an early session. Answers to questions always start with an assessment of the child's information level in asking it. The reaction of many parents to "protect" their child from this type of information must be resisted. But the child can be protected from details he or she is not ready to handle by answering questions directly and concretely after first assessing what the patient already knows.

MANAGEMENT DURING REMISSION

If leukemia remains under control, the result should be a child emotionally and physically capable of participating in a full range of normal activities in a healthy family environment. Prevention and therapy should be available for most problems that could endanger this outcome.

Psychosocial Management

Children in remission will usually be in school and enjoying the normal activities of childhood. Athletics and other extracurricular activities are to be encouraged. Discipline both at school and at home should not be different for the child with leukemia. Siblings of the patient should receive adequate recognition to prevent those problems that occur when children feel they are secondary in the family's concerns.

A social worker familiar with the psychosocial effects of childhood cancer is an important member of the treating team. In addition to evaluating the child's and family's emotional resources, the social worker can assist in determining whether the family is eligible for assistance through various state or federal programs. Other support from the Leukemia Society of America and the American Cancer Society is available. Nonmedical expenses incurred by the family are often a greater burden because they are not covered by medical insurance. Facilities such as the Ronald McDonald Houses are available to reduce the cost of living away from home. The Leukemia Society of America may pay some travel costs. Car pooling may be possible. Certain costs are tax deductible.

Local support groups assist many families in dealing with problems associated with diagnosis of a potentially fatal disease. Many groups are affiliated with the Candlelighters Foundation (Suite 1011, 2025 Eye Street Northwest, Washington, DC 20006; 202/659–5136).

Some couples may need referral for marriage counseling. Every relationship in the family will be strained by the occurrence of leukemia in a child, and asking about these problems should become a routine part of medical care.

Infection During Remission

Fever. Infection when the neutrophil count is over 1000 per microliter may be handled just as it would be for a child without leukemia. That is, specific infections are treated whereas undifferentiated illnesses may be assumed to be viral and self-limited unless they take a different course.

If there is neutropenia (particularly if the count is under 200 per microliter), fever alone may be an indication for blood cultures and initiation of

TABLE 3. **Treatment of Chemotherapy Extravasations**

Vincristine (Oncovin)

1. Stop administration of drug immediately if extravasation is suspected
2. Inject hyaluronidase (Wydase) locally. Use a 25 gauge needle and multiple injections subcutaneously to include the entire erythematous area. Amount of hyaluronidase will vary depending on the size of the infiltration
3. Apply moderate heat to the area to help disperse the drug and decrease local tissue destruction
4. Hydrocortisone sodium succinate or other steroid cream can be used following administration of hyaluronidase

Steps for Other Vesicant Antineoplastic Agents

1. Inject hydrocortisone sodium succinate (Solu-Cortef), 100 mg through the IV tubing before removing the needle
2. Remove the needle
3. Inject hydrocortisone sodium succinate (Solu-Cortef), 50–100 mg subcutaneously. Use a 25 gauge needle and multiple injections, being sure to include the entire erythematous area. Dosage of Solu-Cortef will vary depending on the size of the infiltration
4. Apply a film of steroid cream, cover the skin with sterile gauze, and secure with paper tape
5. Apply ice packs to the area for 24 hours
6. Have the patient apply steroid cream twice daily until all the erythema has disappeared, more often if tension in the area. Encourage exercising the affected hand or arm; do not allow pain to restrict full range of motion. Use heat to the area as tolerated by the patient to relieve inflammation

triple antibiotics. Clinical judgment must be used to differentiate which children need antibiotics and which should be observed.

***Pneumocystis carinii* Pneumonia.** This formerly fatal complication can be prevented by the use of prophylactic trimethoprim-sulfamethoxazole (Bactrim, Septra), 5 mg per kg per day have in two doses. If the disease occurs, it should be treated with trimethoprim-sulfamethoxazole intravenously. If this fails, pentamidine should be used. Respiratory failure is often a complication of this type of pneumonia, so a child should be treated in a facility capable of ventilatory support.

Varicella. If patients have had chickenpox prior to the diagnosis of leukemia, they will remain immune. If they have not had chickenpox and are exposed through a sibling or playmate (physical contact), then they are at risk for fatal complications of chickenpox. Varicella zoster immune globulin (VZIG) in a dose of 1 vial per 10 kg is given intramuscularly within 96 hours of exposure. This product is available through Red Cross blood banks. VZIG may attenuate chickenpox and not prevent it completely. If the disease occurs, most children will require specific antiviral treatment along with discontinuation of all chemotherapy until resolution. Both acyclovir (Zovirax) and Ara-A (Vira-A) are effective for the treatment of varicella.

Immunization. All live virus vaccines (measles, mumps, rubella, and polio) should be avoided while a child is on treatment and for 6 months thereafter. DPT immunizations may be given safely and have recently been shown to give effective antibody levels, even while chemotherapy is continued. Immunizations may be administered on schedule to siblings. Although children with malignancies who are on chemotherapy develop appropriate antibody responses to influenza vaccines, we do not recommend their routine use.

Myelosuppression

During remission on standard treatment, it is unusual for major myelosuppression to occur in other than the granulocyte series. The more intensive regimens currently in use, however, may produce significant thrombocytopenia and anemia. These complications should be managed with appropriate transfusion support. Persistent pancytopenia may herald the onset of relapse, and a bone marrow examination is indicated if recovery is not prompt. Modification of doses of maintenance drugs may be necessary to prevent severe myelosuppression.

Drug-Related Toxicities

The institution where therapy is planned should provide the treating physician with information about the toxicities of the specific drugs a patient is to receive. Problems of alopecia, constipation, hypercortisonism, and myelosuppression are common to all treatment programs. Most of the drugs used in childhood leukemia treatment are reviewed in the Physician's Desk Reference (Medical Economics Company, Oradell, New Jersey, 1984). Table 2 is a partial list of drug toxicities; Table 3 outlines a method for treating extravasation of vesicant drugs.

THE CHRONIC LEUKEMIAS

method of
STEPHEN A. CANNISTRA, M.D.,
and GEORGE P. CANELLOS, M.D.
*Dana-Farber Cancer Institute
Boston, Massachusetts*

The chronic leukemias comprise a group of slowly progressive neoplasms of diverse hematopoietic cell origin. Malignant transformation at the level of the pluripotent stem cell is responsible for chronic myelocytic leukemia, whereas transformation of early lymphoid precursor cells is responsible for the chronic lymphocytic and hairy cell leukemias.

CHRONIC MYELOCYTIC LEUKEMIA

Chronic myelocytic leukemia (CML) usually progresses through three distinct phases, each differing in its clinical characteristics, response to treatment, and prognosis. These phases are known as chronic or stable phase, accelerated phase, and blastic transformation or blast crisis.

Diagnosis

The chronic phase is commonly asymptomatic, although mild constitutional symptoms may be present, and an occasional patient may present with left upper quadrant discomfort and early satiety due to splenic enlargement. The disease is often incidentally detected on routine blood count analysis, which usually reveals granulocytosis with varying degrees of anemia and thrombocytosis. The granulocytosis comprises the entire spectrum of myeloid differentiation, from promyelocyte to polymorphonuclear leukocyte, and occasional blast forms (approximately 1 to 3 per cent) may also be observed. The median duration of chronic phase is approximately 36 to 44 months in most series, although patients who present earlier in the natural history, with only low grade leukocytosis and minimal splenomegaly, may anticipate a longer chronic phase averaging five to six years.

The development of accelerated phase disease may be heralded by gradual resistance to previously effective chronic phase treatment. The accelerated phase may be characterized by fever, weight loss, refractory splenomegaly, myelofibrosis, progressive anemia, thrombocytopenia, and refractory leukocytosis composed of increasing numbers of basophils and circulating blasts. The duration of accelerated phase disease is variable, although the development of frank blastic transformation usually follows in a matter of months.

Blastic transformation is characterized by the development of an acute leukemia and represents expansion of an undifferentiated clone of either myeloid (60 per cent), erythroid (10 per cent), or lymphoid (30 per cent) origin. This acute leukemic phase is most refractory to treatment, with median survival after blastic transformation being less than six months.

Treatment of Chronic Phase

The goal of treatment during chronic phase is to decrease the proliferating tumor burden as manifested by leukocytosis, thrombocytosis, splenomegaly, and constitutional symptoms. With the exception of allogeneic or isogeneic bone marrow transplantation, however, most therapy for CML is palliative. For this reason, appropriate candidates for bone marrow transplantation (see hereafter) should be identified early in the course of chronic phase, since the effectiveness of this treatment modality is markedly reduced when it is attempted during either accelerated phase or blastic formation.

Drug Therapy

Hydroxyurea (Hydrea) and busulfan (Myleran) are the most commonly used drugs in the treatment of chronic phase disease. Hydroxyurea has the advantages of rapid reduction in leukocytosis (initial effects in 12 to 24 hours), short duration of myelosuppression once the drug is stopped (three to five days), low incidence of side effects (nausea, skin rash, hyperkeratosis of palms and soles), and minimal risk of prolonged pancytopenia. Busulfan has been successfully used in the treatment of chronic phase for many years, but it has a number of potential disadvantages, including delayed onset of action (10 to 14 days), prolonged duration of myelosuppression, and very rare pulmonary toxicity due to fibrosing alveolitis ("busulfan lung"). Because of its radiomimetic properties, busulfan has the potential to interfere with future bone marrow transplantation by increasing the incidence of pulmonary complications (e.g., interstitial pneumonitis) after total body irradiation.

Treatment for chronic phase disease is usually initiated if the patient is symptomatic in the setting of an evolving leukocytosis and/or thrombocytosis. In view of its ease of administration and low potential for serious side effects, hydroxyurea is preferred by the authors as initial therapy for chronic phase CML. It is begun at a dose of 1 gram orally twice daily, and the patient's response is followed with weekly blood counts. Allopurinol at a dose of 300 mg orally daily should begin 24 hours prior to the institution of hydroxyurea. When the white count reaches 20,000 per cu mm, hydroxyurea may be decreased to 1 gram daily, and allopurinol should be discontinued if the serum uric acid is not elevated. Thereafter, the dose of hydroxyurea may be adjusted to maintain the white count between 15,000 and 20,000 per cu mm or a level that maintains normal hemoglobin and platelet counts. Blood counts may be obtained every three to four weeks once a stable hydroxyurea dose has been achieved (usually 1.0 to 1.5 grams per day). Future dose increments may be necessary, depending on blood count measurements, although long-term control of chronic phase disease with hydroxyurea is usually possible.

Busulfan therapy may be reserved for patients who are poorly controlled by hydroxyurea or who are not candidates for future marrow transplantation. Despite the disadvantages mentioned previously, it is very effective in controlling chronic phase disease and may be initially administered in an intermittent fashion, making it more convenient to the patient. The usual starting dose of busulfan is from 4 to 6 mg orally daily, with concurrent allopurinol administration as previously described. The white count should be determined at weekly intervals, and the busulfan dose should be halved when the white count reaches 50 per cent of the initial level. The dose should be decreased in this fashion and discontinued when the white count reaches 20,000, which usually occurs during the third or fourth week of treatment. In view of its potential for long-term myelosuppression, it is also advisable to discontinue busulfan if the platelet count suddenly drops to 100,000 per cu mm during the first two weeks of therapy.

After discontinuation of busulfan therapy, it is not uncommon to observe continued decreases in the blood counts for two to three weeks as well as slow resolution of splenomegaly over three to six months. Blood counts should be monitored on a weekly basis until stability occurs and then monthly therefter. Many patients may remain clinically stable for 6 to 12 months after one course of busulfan treatment, with the administration of subsequent courses dictated by rising leukocyte and platelet counts, enlarging spleen, and recurrence of constitutional symptoms. As the disease progresses, it is not uncommon for the interval between treatment courses to shorten considerably, often making maintenance therapy with busulfan a necessity. The maintenance dose is adjusted by weekly blood counts and may vary between 4 mg once a week and 2 mg daily. Progressive disease in the face of a previously effective busulfan dose will rarely improve with additional dose increments and may herald the onset of blastic transformation. If the patient becomes resistant to busulfan in the absence of overt blastic transformation, a trial of hydroxyurea may prove beneficial in controlling the leukocytosis and thrombocytosis of the accelerated phase.

In addition to the previously noted side effects, including prolonged myelosuppression and fibrosing aveolitis, busulfan commonly produces amenorrhea after two to three months of treatment, and about one third of patients develop increased skin pigmentation after two to three years of chronic therapy. Busulfan may also cause dysplasia of sputum or urine cytology, which should not be confused with malignancy.

Other agents, such as mercaptopurine, thioguanine, melphalan, and cyclophosphamide, are effective in controlling the proliferative component of the chronic phase but are usually not necessary in view of the high response rates observed with either hydroxyurea or busulfan.

Splenectomy

Removal of an enlarged spleen in chronic phase CML may provide useful palliation for selected patients. For instance, an occasional patient may develop progressive thrombocytopenia with busulfan that becomes a dose-limiting toxicity despite persistently elevated leukocyte counts and constitutional symptoms. If the degree of thrombocytopenia is severe, prolonged, associated with hemorrhage, and unresponsive to multiple platelet transfusions, or if prolonged thrombocytopenia in the setting of progressive chronic phase disease precludes administration of chemotherapy, it may be reasonable to perform splenectomy to remove a large reservoir of platelet sequestration. Many patients in this situation will respond favorably with an increased platelet count that will be maximal within one to two months after surgery. Since the risks of splenectomy include hemorrhage, splenic vein thrombosis, and subdiaphragmatic abscess formation, the procedure should be reserved for those selected patients who may derive long-lasting palliation. For example, a patient with thrombocytopenia resulting from bone marrow failure during blastic transformation would not be expected to benefit significantly from splenectomy, and the poor prognosis associated with this phase of CML would rarely justify the risks of this procedure. Splenectomy may also be useful for the treatment of symptomatic hypersplenism (pain, early satiety) in chronic phase patients whose splenomegaly has become refractory to drug therapy. Patients with refractory, symptomatic hypersplenism who are not surgical candidates may be treated with local radiotherapy, althought the results are short-lived and the radiation dose is limited by intestinal and bone marrow toxicity.

Allogeneic or Isogeneic Bone Marrow Transplantation

The technique of bone marrow transplantation offers the only potential for cure in chronic phase CML. Several patients with identical twins have undergone isogeneic bone marrow transplantation in chronic phase with apparent ablation of the Philadelphia chromosome positive clone, and the procedure has been extended to allogeneic bone marrow transplantation with encouraging results. Enthusiasm for this approach must be tempered by the following: (1) relatively short follow-up of most ongoing transplantation trials; (2) approximately 30 per cent complication rate from allogeneic bone marrow transplantation, including death, graft-versus-host disease, opportunistic infections, and interstitial pneumonitis; and (3) increased risk of developing complications of bone marrow transplantation in "older" patients (greater than 30 to 40 years old). It should also be noted that only 25 per cent of patients have an HLA–identical sibling match, and approximately 0.5 per cent have an identical twin. Furthermore, a procedure with a 30 per cent serious complication rate must be weighed against the fact that 20 per cent of chronic phase patients may survive with minimal or no symptoms for five years before undergoing blastic transformation. Once frank blastic transformation has occurred, however, the results of allogeneic or isogeneic BMT have been poor, the major difficulty being total eradication of the leukemic clone (Table 1).

In view of these considerations, it is reasonable to explore the possibility of allogeneic or isogeneic bone marrow transplantation in patients with newly diagnosed chronic phase CML who are less than 40 years old. HLA typing of the patient and potential bone marrow donors should be performed, and if a suitable match exists the risks and potential curative benefits of a bone marrow transplantation should be discussed with the patient. Once the decision to undergo transplantation is made, current evidence suggests that younger patients with matched donors should receive transplants as early as possible in the chronic phase, in view of the high relapse rate following bone marrow transplantation in accelerated or blast phase CML.

Blastic Transformation

Treatment

The treatment of acute blastic transformation has been unsatisfactory owing to the low remission rates obtained with agents that are usually effective in the remission induction of de novo acute leukemia. It is useful to identify the lymphoblastic variant of blast crisis by biochemical, morphologic, and immunologic techniques since it may respond well to a combination of vincristine and prednisone (or similar induction regimens for adult acute lymphoblastic leukemia). Such treatment regimens have resulted in unexpected and significant neutropenia in some cases of lymphoblastic transformation prior to the re-establishment of a stable phase marrow. Maintenance therapy with hydroxyurea or methotrexate may prolong the remission, but it is often short-lived. The treatment of myeloblastic transformation has been much less successful in the past, although varying degrees of blast cell control and occasional remissions have been observed with the use of high dose cytosine arabinoside. Nevertheless, a satisfactory treatment regimen with predictable benefit is lacking for nonlymphoid transformation.

A potentially more effective (albeit palliative) approach to the treatment of blastic transformation is ablative therapy followed by autologous transplantation of cryopreserved stem cells. It is well established that chronic phase peripheral blood has adequate numbers of pluripotent stem cells that are fully capable of bone marrow engraftment. Current trials using intensive chemotherapy followed by reinfusion of autologous, chronic phase peripheral blood mononuclear cells have shown that in most patients it is possible to re-establish the chronic phase morphology in both marrow and peripheral blood. The major difficulty with this approach, however, has been the short duration of blast cell suppression, obviously reflecting inadequate ablation prior to transplantation. Some patients have survived for 12 months or longer after autologous transplantation for the blastic phase, demonstrating the potential utility of this approach. As more effective ablative regimens using high dose combination chemotherapy become available, the effectiveness of this approach may increase. For this reason, chronic phase peripheral blood from selected, newly diagnosed cases of CML is collected and cryopreserved in some institutions for future autologous transplantation during the accelerated or blast phase.

TABLE 1. **Allogeneic Transplantation in CML**

Group	Phase	No. of Patients	Survivors	Duration (Months)
1. Seattle (Fefer et al, ASCO Proc. #C-800, 1984)	Chronic	32	18 (15 NED,* 3 relapsed)	12+ – 54+
	Accelerated/Blast		8	15+ – 69+
2. Hammersmith (Goldman et al, Blood *62*:223a, 1983)	Chronic	29	23	1+ – 30+
	Accelerated/Blast	6	3	1+ – 2+
3. UCLA (Champlin et al, Blood *60*:1038, 1982)	Chronic	4	4	3+ – 20+
	Accelerated/Blast	4	2	5+ and 14+

*NED, No evidence of disease.

Unique Complications of Blastic Transformation

Patients with elevated peripheral blast counts, usually greater than 75,000 to 100,000 per cu mm, may develop life-threatening leukostasis in the cerebral, retinal, or pulmonary microvasculature. This medical emergency should be treated with intravenous cyclophosphamide (20 mg per kg) or oral hydroxyurea (75 mg per kg) together with aggressive hydration (with careful attention to fluid balance) and allopurinol administration to prevent hyperuricemia. Cranial irradiation may be added if central nervous system signs or symptoms are present. These measures are usually effective within 12 to 24 hours, although leukapheresis may be added if progressive deterioration occurs during the first 6 to 12 hours of treatment.

With more effective treatment of blastic transformation, especially of the lymphoblastic variant, an occasional patient may live long enough to develop meningeal leukemia. This may respond well to intrathecal methotrexate (12 mg total dose) or intrathecal cytosine arabinoside (40 mg total dose) administered every four days until clearing of leukemic blasts from the cerebrospinal fluid is observed. The dosing interval may then be gradually lengthened until a maintenance dose of intrathecal therapy is administered at monthly intervals.

In a minority of patients, extramedullary collections of blast cells may precede systemic blastic transformation. These myeloblastomas may present as skin, lymph node, or bone lesions and are very responsive to low dose irradiation.

CHRONIC LYMPHOCYTIC LEUKEMIA

The most common type of chronic lymphocytic leukemia (CLL) represents neoplastic transformation of an early B lymphocyte precursor, although greater utilization of immune marker studies has revealed that a minority of patients have a T lymphocyte cell phenotype. CLL is a disease of the older age group, with a median age of 60 years at diagnosis.

Diagnosis

Patients may present with constitutional symptoms, lymphadenopathy, or abdominal discomfort due to splenomegaly, although the diagnosis is often made after the incidental finding of lymphocytosis in the peripheral blood. Hypogammaglobulinemia is present in at least 50 per cent of patients, becoming more severe as the disease progresses. The combination of hypogammaglobulinemia and progressive neutropenia due to bone marrow infiltration makes infection a leading cause of death in this disease. The development of a clinical staging system with prognostic value in CLL has resulted in better identification of patients who are at greater risk of dying from their disease (Table 2).

TABLE 2. **Clinical Staging for CLL***

Stage	Clinical Characteristics	Median Survival (mo)
0	Lymphocytosis of peripheral blood (15,000/cu mm or greater) and bone marrow (30 per cent or more lymphocytic infiltration)	150
I	Lymphocytosis plus enlarged lymph nodes	101
II	Lymphocytosis plus enlarged spleen and/or liver	71
III	Lymphocytosis plus anemia (hemoglobin less than 11 grams per dl)	19
IV	Lymphocytosis plus thrombocytopenia (platelets less than 100,000/cu mm)	19

*Adapted with permission from Rai KR, Sawitsky AN, Cronkite EP, et al.: Clinical staging of chronic lymphocytic leukemia. Blood *46*:219, 1975.

Treatment

Drug Therapy

Drug therapy most likely does not alter the natural history of CLL. The disease may be quite indolent and affects an older patient population whose survival is often dictated by comorbid medical problems. Nevertheless, in view of the poor prognosis associated with stage III or IV disease, treatment is generally indicated in an attempt to improve hematopoiesis by reducing the extent of bone marrow tumor infiltration. Stages 0 and I are usually not treated, in view of the favorable survival associated with these stages as well as the lack of evidence to suggest that therapy prolongs survival. Stage II disease in an asymptomatic, older patient with significant cardiovascular disease may never contribute to either the morbidity or mortality of that individual, obviating the need for immediate therapy that may be potentially harmful. In contrast, stage II disease in a younger individual has the potential to progress to a more advanced stage that is associated with a less favorable prognosis and is more difficult to treat owing to bone marrow compromise by tumor. In view of these considerations, it is generally reasonable to treat stage II CLL, especially in the younger patient who has no major comorbid disease, although the ultimate long-term survival benefit is unknown.

The combination of chlorambucil (Leukeran) and prednisone administered in an intermittent fashion for the treatment of CLL yields the highest response rates in most series. Chlorambucil may be given as a single dose of 0.4 mg per kg orally on day 1, along with prednisone at a dose of 80 mg orally daily on days 1 to 5. This cycle is repeated every two weeks, and the chlorambucil dose may be slowly increased to 0.8 mg per kg if bone marrow function is adequate. The intermittent nature of this treatment reduces the myelosuppressive effects of chlorambucil and the immunosuppressive effects of prednisone. When significant bone marrow failure has occurred as a result of progressive stage III or IV disease, a trial of prednisone alone, administered at a dose of 1 mg per kg daily orally for three to four weeks with a slow taper over two weeks, may result in hematologic improvement and may allow the patient to better tolerate subsequent intermittent chlorambucil/prednisone therapy as outlined. The potential for steroids to result in mood changes, hyperglycemia, fluid retention, hypokalemia, and immunocompromise should always be kept in mind.

In the elderly patient with slowly progressive disease who has contraindications to steroid therapy (e.g., diabetes, congestive heart failure, hypertension), it may be preferable to omit prednisone and simply treat with intermittent chlorambucil, 0.4 mg per kg orally every two weeks, with gradual dose escalation as necessary for disease control. Alternatively, it may be simpler for some patients to follow a daily oral schedule of chlorambucil administration at a dose of 0.1 to 0.2 mg per kg. When treatment for CLL is initiated, it is also advisable to begin allopurinol at a dose of 300 mg orally daily, especially if the serum uric acid is initially elevated or if there is coexistent renal insufficiency. Allopurinol may be discontinued after approximately two weeks if the serum uric acid is within normal limits.

Blood counts should be carefully followed, initially on a weekly basis, to assess response to therapy and to adjust the chlorambucil dose. The initial response to treatment, as measured by a decrease in lymphadenopathy and splenomegaly as well as improvement in peripheral blood counts, is usually seen within three to four weeks. Treatment may be continued as long as clinical improvement is noted, although a treatment break is advisable when bone marrow reserve becomes diminished as a result of chronic chlorambucil administration. It is not uncommon for a four to six month period of drug therapy to be associated with long periods of disease inactivity or slow, asymptomatic progression of lymphadenopathy requiring no therapy.

Alternative Treatment

The treatment of CLL is difficult once resistance develops to chlorambucil or prednisone. A trial of cyclophosphamide (Cytoxan) is reasonable under these circumstances, although other drugs, such as vincristine or antimetabolites, have no proven effectiveness. Occasional patients with splenomegaly who have splenic sequestration of platelets in the absence of autoimmune thrombocytopenia or bone marrow failure may benefit from splenectomy. Finally, radiotherapy may provide very effective palliation for localized areas of painful lymphadenopathy.

Complications

Autoimmune Phenomena

A course of daily, high dose steroids is indicated for treatment of autoimmune thrombocytopenia or autoimmune Coomb's positive hemolytic anemia, which may sometimes occur in association with CLL. Steroid treatment is usually effective in controlling these autoimmune complications, with most patients eventually being tapered off steroids without recurrence. Occasionally, the rate of hemolysis may be brisk and unresponsive to steroids, requiring emergency splenectomy as a lifesaving measure.

Infection

The patient with CLL is susceptible to serious infection by both common pathogens and opportunistic organisms, in part because of hypogammaglobulinemia and immunosuppressive treatment regimens. Unexplained fever should not be attributed to CLL unless an aggressive and comprehensive search for a possible infectious etiology has been performed. Prophylactic administration of pneumococcal and influenza vaccinations is a reasonable measure, although their effectiveness in the immunocompromised patient is uncertain.

Richter's Syndrome

This unusual complication represents a highly aggressive transformation of CLL into a malignant disease that histologically resembles diffuse histiocytic lymphoma. Immunologic marker studies usually confirm that this transformation occurs at the level of the malignant CLL cell. Patients may initially present with a rapidly enlarging peripheral lymph node, back pain due to rapid expansion of retroperitoneal lymphadenopathy, or nonspecific constitutional symptoms such as fever and decreased appetite. This complication is particularly refractory to chemotherapy owing to the development of drug resistance. The course is one of rapid deterioration, with the median length of survival being approximately four months after diagnosis.

Prolymphocytic Transformation

CLL may rarely transform into a blastic leukemic phase, with immature cells resembling prolymphocytes infiltrating bone marrow, peripheral blood, and lymph nodes. This complication, like Richter's syndrome, may have immunologic surface marker characteristics similar to those of the original CLL cell. Treatment is generally unsatisfactory, although transient responses to doxorubicin have been observed. Progressive tumor growth usually leads to death secondary to bone marrow failure.

Second Malignancies

There may be a higher incidence of other nonhematopoietic malignancies in the CLL patient, including melanoma, sarcoma, and lung cancer. Detection of an early malignancy by careful follow-up may be lifesaving, especially in view of the potential chronicity of uncomplicated CLL.

HAIRY CELL LEUKEMIA

The most common cell of origin in hairy cell leukemia (HCL) is the B lymphocyte, as evidenced by the presence of immunoglobulin gene rearrangement as well as expression of multiple heavy chain isotypes on the tumor cell membrane.

Diagnosis

The clinical features of HCL, also known as leukemic reticuloendotheliosis, are pancytopenia, splenomegaly without lymphadenopathy, and a propensity for developing serious infections, including pulmonary involvement with atypical mycobacterial species. The patient is usually male and may present with an infectious complication, or he may be totally asymptomatic and have evidence of pancytopenia on routine blood count determination.

Examination of the peripheral blood smear may reveal circulating tumor cells characterized by irregular borders and "hairy" projections representing long, villous extensions of the cell membrane. The diagnosis is confirmed by demonstrating the presence of tartrate-resistant acid phosphatase in the malignant cells. Bone marrow aspiration is usually unsuccessful owing to the presence of associated myelofibrosis, although bone marrow biopsy is virtually pathognomonic of the disease and should be performed to establish the diagnosis and to exclude other causes of pancytopenia.

Treatment

Many patients with serious pancytopenia or with progressive disease respond well to splenectomy as initial therapy. Splenectomy is most effective when splenomegaly is present and when the bone marrow function is not severely compromised. The response to splenectomy is usually manifested by partial resolution of pancytopenia and decreased numbers of circulating tumor cells, with complete responses being unusual. After splenectomy, patients may do well for prolonged periods of time without further treatment. Splenectomy represents palliative treatment and is of no proven benefit in the asymptomatic patient with acceptable bone marrow function and minimal splenomegaly.

If no response is obtained with splenectomy, or if an initial good response is followed by progressive pancytopenia, it is reasonable to attempt a trial of low dose chlorambucil (0.1 mg per kg per day orally) in an effort to decrease the bone marrow tumor burden. A beneficial response to this therapy may require four to six months. Chlorambucil may also be useful for the control of excessive numbers of hairy cells in the peripheral blood. In patients refractory to chlorambucil, other cytotoxic agents have rarely been successful owing to their myelosuppressive effects in the presence of extensive marrow involvement. Corticosteroids have no proven value in the treatment of this disease and may exacerbate the degree of immunocompromise associated with HCL. Investigational agents that are currently undergoing active study include pentostatin (2′-deoxycoformycin) and alpha interferon. Both these agents represent an interesting approach to the treatment of HCL and have been successful in achieving hematologic improvement following failure of splenectomy and chlorambucil therapy.

NON-HODGKIN'S LYMPHOMAS

method of
BENJAMIN KOZINER, M.D.
and BURTON J. LEE, M.D.
Memorial Sloan-Kettering Cancer Center
New York, New York

Treatment

Therapeutic alternatives for non-Hodgkin's lymphomas (NHL) are many, ranging from involved field (IF) to total body irradiation (TBI), from single agent chemotherapy to aggressive multidrug treatment protocols. One must be careful to balance the harm of the treatment with the good it is likely to provide. If none of the therapeutic modalities is superior to the others in regard to survival span, the less toxic and carcinogenic modality should be adopted. Of utmost concern is the recent awareness of secondary malignant disease, mostly acute nonlymphocytic leukemia unresponsive to conventional therapy, developing in patients treated with combination chemo- and radiotherapy.

Radiation

Patients with stage I disease (see Table 1 in Hodgkin's Disease: Chemotherapy, page 311, for the Ann Arbor staging system) who have only local residual tumor suspected after initial surgery and thorough staging evaluation should be treated with IF irradiation at a tumoricidal dose (3500 to 4500 rad, depending on histologic type). IF or extended field radiation therapy can also be used as primary treatment in patients with stage II disease, although it should be recognized that they probably have generalized disease. Further treatment with total lymphoid irradiation (TLI), single agent or combination chemotherapy in "low grade" NHL, or combination chemotherapy in "intermediate grade" NHL should follow (Table 1). TLI alone to a total dose of 4000 rad in stage III low grade nodular lymphoma has resulted in remission durations of up to 10 years in 40 per cent of patients and actuarial survival of 37 per cent at 15 years. Similar results have been reported with the use of TBI to a total dose of 100 to 250 rad.

Because of their biologic features and aggressive natural history, there seems to be no primary role for radiation therapy in "high grade" NHL. For all histologic types of NHL, adjunct radiotherapy (2000 rad plus "boost") to areas of original bulky involvement appears to have the merit of preventing local recurrences. However, this approach only applies to patients considered to have responded to systemic chemotherapy and without bone marrow involvement. For all forms of radiotherapy (mostly those involving the treatment of axial nodal chains), irradiation of the bone marrow should be of concern, since it will penalize the future administration of chemotherapy and other systemic modalities.

Emergency radiotherapy could be quite effective in correcting (1) symptoms and neurologic signs from spinal cord compression by epidural lymphoma; (2) facial swelling and venous engorgement of the superior vena cava syndrome from mediastinal lymphoma; (3) anuria and azotemia from ureteral obstruction and kidney involvement by lymphoma; and (4) cranial nerve palsies that result from lymphomatous meningitis of the base of the brain. However, all the described situations will also require the administration of systemic chemotherapy, since in all likelihood evidence of progressive disease elsewhere could be found. The treatment of lymphomatous meningitis should also include the frequent administration (twice weekly for 5 weeks) of intrathecal chemotherapy with methotrexate (6.5 mg per M^2) or cytosine arabinoside (30 mg per M^2) through on Ommaya reservoir.

TABLE 1. **Classification of Non-Hodgkin's Lymphomas**

Low Grade	
	Small lymphocytic (SL)
	Follicular, predominantly small cleaved cell (FSC)
	Follicular mixed, small cleaved and large cell (FM)
Intermediate Grade	
	Follicular, predominantly large cell (FL)
	Diffuse, small cleaved cell (DSC)
	Diffuse mixed, small and large cell (DM)
	Diffuse large cell, cleaved/noncleaved (DL)
High Grade	
	Large cell, immunoblastic (IBL)
	Lymphoblastic convoluted/nonconvoluted (LBL)
	Small noncleaved cell (SNE)

Chemotherapy

The single drugs of greatest use are alkylating agents, especially cyclophosphamide (Cytoxan) and chlorambucil (Leukeran). Only patients with low grade lymphomas will be responsive to this conservative and nontoxic systemic modality of treatment. For the more aggressive non-Hodgkin's lymphomas, although clinical responses are seen with single chemotherapeutic agents the majority of these responses fall into the partial remission category. It is now well established that patients who attain a complete remission live longer than those who achieve a partial remission or fail to respond to therapy. More recently, considerable progress in the treatment of these lymphomas has resulted from the progressive use of combination chemotherapy (Table 2). MOPP and C-MOPP treatment demonstrated that extended disease-free survival could be seen in patients with advanced stages of diffuse large cell lymphoma upon achievement of a complete response. Following these results, several combinations, most of which employed Adriamycin and bleomycin (CHOP, BACOP, CHOP-Bleo) showed varying complete remission incidences of 40 to 70 per cent with 40 to 50 per cent prolonged survival. More recently, programs such as PRO-MACE-MOPP and M-BACOD have shown complete remission rates of over 70 per cent and a more than 60 per cent probability of disease-free survival. However, these last two regimens are very intensive and should be administered by chemotherapists experienced with their respective toxicities. Although the original recommended dose of methotrexate in M-BACOD was 3 grams per M^2, similar therapeutic results now have been reported with the same regimen in which the methotrexate dose was reduced to 300 mg per M^2. In general, at least six to eight cycles of the different combination chemotherapy programs are administered; some patients might require more prolonged treatment. Since the median time for achievement of a complete remission is approximately 3 months, it has been estimated somewhat arbitrarily that at least three more cycles are required for consolidation of response.

Periodic monitoring of the blood counts is mandatory before administration of each intravenous dose of chemotherapy. The doses should be ti-

TABLE 2. **Chemotherapy Programs for Non-Hodgkin's Lymphomas**

Regimen	Drugs	Dose (mg/M²)	Administration	Cycle Frequency	Complete Remission Rate in Diffuse Lymphomas
CVP	cyclophosphamide	400	days 1 to 5	q 21 days	41
	vincristine	1.4	day 1		
	prednisone	100	days 1 to 5		
MOPP, C-MOPP	nitrogen mustard *or*	6	days 1 and 8	q 28 days	41
	cyclophosphamide	650	days 1 and 8		
	vincristine	1.4	days 1 and 8		
	procarbazine	100	days 1 to 14		
	prednisone	40	days 1 to 14		
COMLA	cyclophosphamide	1500	day 1	q 91 days	55
	vincristine	1.4	days 1, 8, 15		
	methotrexate	120	day 22, then weekly × 7		
	leucovorin	25 (total)	24 hrs after methotrexate q 6 hr × 8 times		
	cytosine arabinoside	300	day 22, then weekly × 7		
HOP	Adriamycin	80	day 1	q 21 days	60
	vincristine	1.4	day 1		
	prednisone	100	days 1 to 5		
CHOP	cyclophosphamide	750	day 1	q 21 days	67
	Adriamycin	50	day 1		
	vincristine	1.4	day 1		
	prednisone	100	days 1 to 5		
BACOP	cyclophosphamide	650	days 1 and 8	q 28 days	48
	Adriamycin	25	days 1 and 8		
	vincristine	1.4	days 1 and 8		
	bleomycin	5 units	days 15 and 22		
	prednisone	60	days 15 and 22		
CHOP-Bleo	cyclophosphamide	750	day 1	q 28 days	69
	Adriamycin	50	day 1		
	vincristine	1.4	days 1 and 5		
	prednisone	60	days 1 to 5		
	bleomycin	15 units	days 1 to 5		
M-BACOD	methotrexate	3000	day 14	q 21 days	78
	leucovorin	10 (total)	days 15 to 17, q 6 hr		
	bleomycin	4 units	day 1		
	Adriamycin	45	day 1		
	cyclophosphamide	600	day 1		
	dexamethasone	6	days 1 to 5		
PRO MACE-MOPP	prednisone	60	days 1 to 14	q 28 days	74
	methotrexate	1500	day 14		
	leucovorin	10 (total)	days 15 to 17, q 6 hr		
	Adriamycin	25	days 1 and 8		
	cyclophosphamide	650	days 1 and 8		
	VP-16	120	days 1 and 8		
	(MOPP is given for a variable number of cycles after achievement of a remission)				

trated according to the results of blood counts taken prior to every dose of intravenous medication. Marrow reserve in patients with NHL is very unpredictable. It is always wise to err on the low side of any projected dose at the start of therapy, unless sophisticated support facilities are available. Proper hydration should be used with the administration of cyclophosphamide (Cytoxan) to avoid the risk of hemorrhagic cystitis and uric acid nephropathy. Uric acid nephropathy can also be avoided by giving the patient allopurinol. Tumor lysis is a feared complication of the treatment of rapidly proliferating, high grade NHL, mainly the small noncleaved variety that includes Burkitt's lymphoma. It should be anticipated and watched for when treating patients with bulky abdominal masses and an elevated serum LDH level. Tumor lysis syndrome is characterized by abrupt elevations of uric acid, potassium, and phosphorus levels and a concomitant drop in serum calcium. Forced intravenous hydration, alkalinization of the urine, and allopurinol (300 mg orally, three times daily) should be used for prevention in high risk patients. If the tumor lysis syndrome is not controlled by these measures, either peritoneal dialysis or hemodialysis is necessary. The administration of Adriamycin and bleomycin requires periodic monitoring with radionuclide heart scan and pulmonary function tests, respectively. Adequate urinary output and monitoring the level of creatinine clearance are prerequisites to the administration of high (1 to 3 grams per M^2) and moderate (300 to 500 mg per M^2) doses of methotrexate. This should be followed by folinic acid (leucovorin) rescue.

Choices of Therapy

Low Grade Lymphomas

Regardless of stage, if symptoms are lacking and there is no evidence of progression of lymphomatous disease after an adequate period of observation (1 to 3 months), the "watch and wait" approach should be continued. Conversely, if disease progression is documented by monitoring of physical findings and radiologic abnormalities, several therapeutic alternatives are to be considered.

For stage I, tumoricidal radiation (3500 to 4000 rad) to an involved field (IF) seems sufficient. For stages II, III, and IV (without bone marrow involvement), the therapeutic alternatives range from the use of single alkylating agents (oral cyclophosphamide or chlorambucil), combination chemotherapy (CVP), total lymphoid irradiation or total body irradiation. In a prospectively randomized study, no differences in the complete remission rate (single agent, 64 per cent; CVP, 88 per cent; and TBI, 71 per cent) and survival (84 per cent alive at 4 years) were observed among these three different treatment modalities. For stage IV with bone marrow involvement, similar comments regarding therapy could be made. However, radiation therapy is not indicated unless it is used for palliation of symptoms or prompt resolution of mechanical problems, such as ureteral, gastrointestinal, or epidural compressions.

Recently, therapeutic responses to human and recombinant leukocyte A interferon have been reported in a proportion of patients with low and intermediate grade NHL. This biologic modifier, and the in vivo use of monoclonal antibodies to B cell antigens and immunoglobulin idiotypes, are new and experimental therapies of promise.

Our recommended approach, mainly when sophisticated radiotherapy is not available, includes the initial administration of oral chlorambucil (Leukeran), at 4 to 6 mg orally daily or 30 mg per M^2 orally every 3 weeks, until disappearance of signs and symptoms of disease. Alternatively or upon failure of single alkylating therapy, a regimen of CVP as described in Table 2 could be used periodically until achievement of a complete remission. The prolonged administration of oral chlorambucil or combination CVP chemotherapy as maintenance should be discouraged, because of its myelotoxic and carcinogenic potentials. Furthermore, the same chemotherapeutic modality could be restarted and expected to be effective upon disease recurrence. In the event of failure to respond to the previously described therapies or transition to a more aggressive histology, a new line of more intensive polydrug programs (HOP, CHOP, CHOP-Bleo, BACOP, COMLA) could be administered.

Intermediate Grade Lymphomas

The therapy of choice in patients with stage I of nodal presentation remains controversial. If only tumoricidal (4500 rad) radiation therapy to the site of lymphomatous involvement is to be delivered, a thorough staging evaluation that might include exploratory laparotomy will be in order. However, most centers are now enrolled in clinical trials to establish the effectiveness of adjuvant chemotherapy (mostly CHOP and CHOP-Bleo) to radiotherapy in localized cases. Preliminary results tend to confirm the soundness of this approach. Similar good results with identical chemotherapy as the sole treatment modality have also been reported. The treatment of stage I extranodal presentation varies widely according to the structure or organ involved (gastrointestinal, breast, skin, bone, gonads, kidney, thyroid, and so on), escaping the formulation of fixed guidelines. These cases could benefit from discussion at multidisciplinary Tumor Boards or referral to cancer centers in consultation.

For the remaining stages II, III, and IV, "good" and "poor" prognosis patients could be defined who will require different treatment approaches. Patients with poor prognosis—less than a 40 per cent estimated 2 year survival—include those with bulky tumor masses, serum LDH levels of more than 500 units per liter, or retroperitoneal, mediastinal, and extranodal (bone marrow or gastrointestinal tract) involvement. Although PROMACE-MOPP, M-BACOD, and other intensive chemotherapy combinations represent reasonable treatment alternatives, preliminary evidence suggests that a program of high dose chemotherapy with or without TBI, followed by transplantation of cryopreserved autologous marrow, might represent a more definitive modality of treatment. However, this treatment program can be carried out only in cancer research centers with experience in this modality and for patients without evidence of bone marrow involvement. The group of patients with good prognosis is defined by absence of the features previously

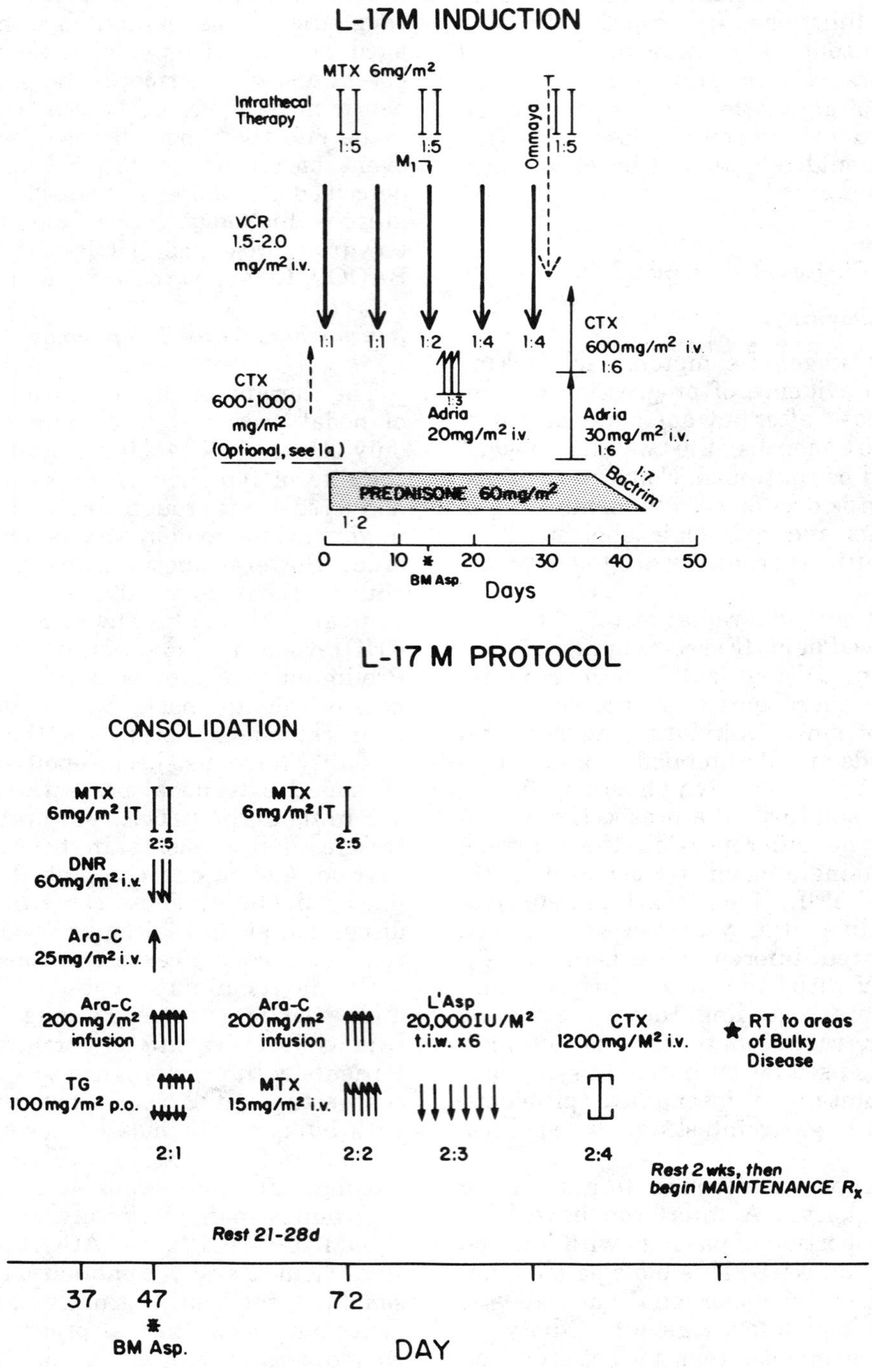

Figure 1. L-17M protocol: Induction and consolidation phases for the treatment of acute lymphblastic leukemia and lymphoblastic lymphoma. With this regimen and preceding programs (L-2, L-10, L10M), a remarkable improvement in prognosis, with an estimated 50 per cent disease-free survival at 3 years, has been observed at Memorial Sloan-Kettering Cancer Center.

Adria, Adriamycin; ARA-C, cytosine arabinoside; CTX, cyclophosphamide; DNR, daunomycin; L'Asp, L-asparaginase; MTX, methotrexate; RT, radiotherapy; TG, thioguanine; VCR, vincristine.

described (LDH levels below 500 units per liter without bulky tumor masses and retroperitoneal, mediastinal, bone marrow, or gastrointestinal tract involvement). Since chemotherapy with combinations containing Adriamcyin (CHOP, CHOP-Bleo, BACOP) provides for a higher than 80 per cent chance of prolonged survival, the use of other more intensive and toxic regimens like M-ABCOD and PROMACE-MOPP might not be necessary. Furthermore, since most relapses in this histologic category occur within the first year after chemotherapy, prolonged survival might be equivalent to "cure."

High Grade Lymphomas

Because high grade NHL is different from previously discussed histologic categories, the Ann Arbor staging system is irrelevant to therapeutic considerations. All patients, including those presenting with a single site of disease, should be treated with the intensive systemic treatment to be described.

Lymphoblastic Lymphoma

This lymphomatous type has been recently recognized as a distinct subgroup of NHL, clinically and cytologically similar to acute lymphoblastic leukemia (ALL). Most patients formerly became frankly leukemic before death, which occurred at a median of 9 to 12 months, when conventional chemotherapy regimens (MOPP, C-MOPP) were used. These patients should be referred now to cancer centers for proper documentation of diagnosis and initiation of chemotherapy on an anti-ALL type of program, including intensive induction and consolidation and prolonged maintenance chemotherapy. Chemoprophylaxis of central nervous system disease with intrathecal chemotherapy (methotrexate or cytosine arabinoside or both) should be part of the regimen. Figure 1 depicts the L17M program in use at Memorial Sloan-Kettering.

Diffuse Large Cell, Immunoblastic, and Small Noncleaved Cell (Burkitt-Like) Lymphomas

The classic description of Burkitt's lymphoma applies to African children with bulky extranodal tumors involving the jaw bone and abdominal viscera that are extremely responsive to cytotoxic chemotherapy (cyclophosphamide). A nonendemic form of Burkitt's lymphoma has been recognized worldwide.The American Burkitt's lymphoma has a predominantly intra-abdominal (mostly small intestine) presentation, with more frequent involvement of bone marrow and meninges than in the originally described African type.

Recently, an increased incidence of small, noncleaved Burkitt-like lymphomas has been noted in immunodeficient homosexual men. The development of NHL has been observed not only in patients with acquired immunodeficiency syndrome (AIDS) but also in homosexual men without the syndrome but who have laboratory markers of immunodeficiency and epidemiologic backgrounds similar to those of patients with AIDS. Characteristically, these lymphomas run a very aggressive course, with shortened survival and a predilection for central nervous system involvement. More recently, hemophiliac patients receiving factor VIII concentrate developed Burkitt's lymphoma, raising concern about the possibility of this neoplasm occurring in other populations at risk. Another type of NHL seen in patients with AIDS is large cell lymphoma of the brain without involvement of other organs, as previously reported in cases of IgA deficiency, ataxia telangiectasia, Wiskott-Aldrich syndrome, organ transplantation, and acquired immune suppression, which indicates that there is a pathogenetic role for immunosuppression in some stage of lymphoma development. Pertinent to this observation is the increased incidence of secondary NHL, mostly of high grade histology, after combined modality treatment for Hodgkin's disease.

Although improved results for both large cell immunoblastic and small noncleaved NHL have been observed with recently described chemotherapy combinations (PROMACE-MOPP and M-BACOD), because of the extremely poor prognosis of these rapidly proliferating neoplasms our preference has been to recommend their treatment with the new program of autologous bone marrow infusion preceded by intensive cytoreductive therapy with high dose chemotherapy and TBI.

CUTANEOUS T CELL LYMPHOMAS (CTCL): MYCOSIS FUNGOIDES AND THE SÉZARY SYNDROME

method of
STANFORD I. LAMBERG, M.D.
The Johns Hopkins University
Baltimore, Maryland

Mycosis fungoides (MF) and its variant, Sézary syndrome (SS), are lymphomas of thymus-derived helper lymphocytes. Males are affected twice as often as females, and races are affected equally. The average age of onset is 55, although cases in young adults do occur. Occupational exposure to heavy manufacturing or chemicals is associated with an increased risk of

CTCL, and family members of patients appear to have a higher than expected frequency of other leukemias or lymphomas.

Diagnosis

Most cases begin with clinically suggestive and pathologically diagnostic lesions. However, about 20 per cent have a premycotic phase that either resembles a common benign disorder, such as psoriasis or atopic eczema, or appears with one of the following distinctive clinical patterns: poikiloderma atrophicans vasculare, characterized by patches of combined telangiectasias, atrophy, and pigmentation resembling radiation dermatitis; alopecia mucinosa, with hair loss associated with an inflammatory mucinous infiltrate around hair follicles; or large plaque parapsoriasis, seen as scaly, pink to dusky, sometimes slightly infiltrated patches. The individual lesion characteristic of MF is a thickened, reddish brown, annular or serpiginous plaque. The first lesions appear most commonly on the lower part of the trunk. Most patients with CTCL have pruritus; itching is especially severe in SS. Patients with SS have widespread erythroderma, and atypical lymphocytes comprise more than 5 per cent of the circulating lymphocytes.

The tests recommended for the routine evaluation and staging of patients with MF and SS are listed in Table 1. These procedures should be performed as soon as a skin biopsy diagnosis is confirmed.

The TNM (Tumor-Node-Metastasis) classification system of the American Joint Committee for Cancer Staging, modified to record the extent of CTCL, has been used widely (Table 2). The only clinical variables found to be significantly associated with survival in CTCL are the extent of T (skin) and N (peripheral lymph node) involvement. The staging classification, based on T and N, also is used to assign patients to treatment. In advanced disease, histologically proven extracutaneous lymphoma in blood (B) or viscera (M) indicates further shortening of survival and may affect treatment selection.

TABLE 1. **Recommended Evaluation Procedures**

1. History and physical examination
2. Skin biopsy
3. CBC and platelet count
4. Absolute lymphocyte count and per cent of atypical convoluted and blastlike lymphocytes
5. Serum chemistries, liver function tests, renal function tests, uric acid, Ca, PO_4
6. Chest roentgenogram
7. Lymph node biopsy*
8. Liver biopsy†
9. Bone marrow biopsy†
10. Scans and/or biopsies of organs when history or physical exam suggests abnormalities
11. Abdominal ultrasound and CT scans are investigational until their value can be determined

*Palpable node from an area draining cutaneous lesions with priority to cervical before axillary before inguinal or femoral. If no palpable nodes, "blind" biopsy may be performed with the same area priorities.

†Liver and bone marrow biopsies are not routine but are obtained to assess abnormal function or size. Multiple directed liver biopsies obtained at peritoneoscopy and bilateral bone marrow biopsies are more sensitive than single biopsies.

TABLE 2. **TNM Classification of Cutaneous T Cell Lymphomas (CTCL)**

Classification	Description
T: *Skin**	
T0	Clinically and/or histopathologically suspicious lesions
T1	Limited plaques, papules, or eczematous patches covering less than 10 per cent of the skin surface
T2	Generalized plaques, papules, eczematous patches covering 10 per cent or more of the skin surface
T3	Tumors, one or more (three or more according to the MFCG)
T4	Generalized erythroderma
N: *Peripheral Lymph Nodes*†	
a) Clinical	
N0-8	The number of sites of palpable peripheral lymph nodes.
b) Combined Clinical and Pathological:	
N0	No clinically or palpably abnormal peripheral lymph nodes, pathology negative for CTCL
N1	Clinically abnormal peripheral lymph nodes, pathology positive for CTCL
N2	No clinically abnormal peripheral lymph nodes, pathology positive for CTCL
B: *Peripheral Blood*	
B0	Atypical circulating cells not present or less than 5 per cent
B1	Atypical circulating cells present in 5 per cent or more; total WBC, total lymphocyte counts and number of atypical cells per 100 lymphocytes recorded
M: *Visceral Organs*	
M0	No involvement of visceral organs
M1	Visceral involvement (must have confirmation of pathology; organ involved should be specified)

*Pathology of T1-4 is diagnostic of a CTCL. When characteristics of more than one T exist, all are recorded and the highest is used for staging, e.g., T4(3).

†Cervical (left + right = 2), epitrochlear (1), submandibular (1). Total possible = 8.

TREATMENT

The optimal therapy for CTCL has not yet been established. Controversy still exists as to whether patients with "early" disease, apparently confined to the skin, should be treated aggressively with multimodal topical and systemic therapy or conservatively with topical therapy alone. It is clear that patients with extensive areas of skin involvement (greater than 10 per cent of the skin surface), particularly with palpable lymphadenopathy, even if negative for CTCL histologically or with tumors or erythroderma, have a significantly shorter survival and shorter duration of remission after therapy. Long remissions and possible cures have been induced in patients with early disease, but present modes of treatment are not curative for patients with visceral involvement.

Development of optimal schedules for present therapies and investigation of new forms of therapy cannot occur unless patients with CTCL are entered into ongoing treatment protocols whenever possible. Most studies permit the referring physician to participate in the continuing care of the patient. Information on studies in progress can be obtained by calling the Cancer Information Service, National Cancer Institute, Bethesda, MD, at 1–800–4CANCER.

General Measures

Pruritus is a common, sometimes overwhelming problem for patients with MF and SS. Moderate relief may be gained by the use of systemic antihistamines, such as hydroxyzine, 25 mg orally every 4 hours as needed, and topical emollients, such as Eucerin, or topical corticosteroids, such as betamethasone, fluocinonide, or triamcinolone, in either cream or ointment form applied as needed or overnight under plastic wrap occlusion. Ultraviolet light (A) combined with oral psoralen (investigational for this use) suppresses early thin lesions; however, cures of patients with histologically proven MF are unlikely with this therapy alone, and such patients usually require light treatments every few days to maintain control. Psoralen and UV (A) light appears to cure some patients with the large plaque form of parapsoriasis.

Specific Measures

Early MF Apparently Confined to the Skin: T_1 and N ($_{any}$) or T_2 and N_{0-1} (M_0)

The relative effectiveness of topical chemotherapy as compared with superficial radiation or a combination of the two has not yet been clarified by ongoing randomized trials. Electron beam therapy is associated with acute and chronic complications and may be difficult for the older person to accept. Electron beam therapy followed by long-term topical application of nitrogen mustard appears no more effective than electron beam therapy alone.

Topical Mechlorethamine (Nitrogen Mustard, HN2). Topical application of nitrogen mustard can yield excellent response rates (60 to 90 per cent) and long-term "cures" are claimed, although sustained remissions probably require continued use of the agent. Although there is no bone marrow suppression or other systemic toxicity associated with topical HN2, epidermal neoplasms occasionally appear after many months of use. (This use of this agent is not listed in the manufacturer's directive.)

INSTRUCTIONS. The metal cap of a 10 mg vial of nitrogen mustard is pried off by the patient and the contents mixed just before use in 1 to 2 oz of distilled water, purchased from a grocery or drug store by the gallon. After bathing to remove surface lipids and after the skin is dry, the patient applies the solution from head to toe with a 2 inch nylon brush, reserving a small volume for intertriginous areas. To minimize irritation, the reserved solution should be further diluted before application to those areas. Nighttime use is best, as the skin often feels dry and itchy following the application; a teaspoonful of glycerin may be added to the solution to ease the dryness. Patients may apply an emollient, such as Eucerin, on arising.

Treatment is carried out daily until complete clearing, which may take three to six months; then the frequency may be reduced to every other day, but the patient should be told to plan on using the medication for several years. Unfortunately, allergic reactions to the drug develop in up to 40 per cent of patients after long-term use. Desensitization can be accomplished in about half the patients who develop allergy by graded increases of diluted HN2, generally managed by dermatologists with prior experience with the agent. Tumors may respond to intralesional injection with 100 micrograms per ml of HN2 in isotonic saline.

Topical Carmustine (BCNU). Topical BCNU appears to be an effective alternative to HN2; allergic reactions are uncommon but local irritation and persistent telangiectasias may develop. Because the drug is absorbed, reversible bone marrow depression may also develop. (This use of this agent is not listed in the manufacturer's directive.)

INSTRUCTIONS. The pharmacist dissolves a 100 mg vial of BCNU powder in 50 ml of 95 per cent or absolute ethyl alcohol. This stock solution is refrigerated by the patient. For treatment, 5 ml of the stock is added to about 60 ml of distilled water; this solution is applied once daily to the entire body, as with HN2. The solution may be further diluted when used in the intertriginous areas to minimize irritation. Treatment should continue for six to eight weeks, depending on the degree of irritation. Steroid cream may be used topically if excessive irritation develops. After a six week rest period, the course may be repeated. If the response is incomplete, the concentration may be doubled (10 ml stock per 60 ml water) for another six to eight weeks. During rest periods residual lesions may be treated with the full strength alcoholic stock solution, up to twice daily for up to six weeks not exceeding 70 mg (35 ml of stock) per week.

Complete blood counts, including platelet

counts, should be obtained every two to four weeks during and for six weeks after BCNU applications. The cycle of treatment may be repeated as necessary to suppress visible lesions.

Electron Beam Radiotherapy. MF is radiosensitive and conventional orthovolage radiation therapy has been used for decades. Electron beam radiation has a distinct advantage over orthovoltage radiation; the penetration of electrons, being particles, can be controlled to reach depths as shallow as a few millimeters, whereas orthovoltage wave form radiation passes deeply into tissues. Thus, a relatively large surface dose can be given with electron beam radiotherapy without deep tissue injury or bone marrow suppression. Therapy is fractionated over six to ten weeks to a total of about 3000 to 3600 rads. All portions of the body must be treated; a higher recurrence rate is found in patients who elect scalp shielding to prevent hair loss. Acute side effects, which usually subside in one month, include skin edema, fissuring, and erythema. Late effects are radiodermatitis, hair loss, nail loss, and dry skin from loss of eccrine function. Hair, nails, and sweat gland function usually return in three to six months. This treatment is costly ($5000 to $10,000), although insurance generally covers most or all of the expense. Most large cities have medical centers capable of electron beam radiotherapy.

Later Stage MF with Poorer Prognostic Signs, Although Apparently Confined to the Skin: T_2 and N_{2+} or T_3 (M_0)

Such patients respond poorly to topical chemotherapy and tend to relapse quickly if electron beam therapy is used alone. Generally electron beam therapy is used to induce cutaneous remission and systemic chemotherapy to maintain remission. Effective single drug chemotherapies include methotrexate, systemic nitrogen mustard, cyclophosphamide, and chlorambucil. The Mycosis Fungoides Cooperative Group uses an attenuated CHOP protocol after electron beam radiation for such patients (day 1 cyclophosphamide 500 mg per square meter, intravenously; doxorubicin 40 mg per square meter, intravenously; vincristine 1.4 mg per square meter, intravenously; and, on days 1 to 5, prednisone 60 mg per square meter, orally, repeated every 21 days for a maximum of six courses).

Late Stage MF with Visceral CTCL, Failure of Previous Therapy, or SS

Methotrexate with Citrovorum Factor. Moderate to high doses of methotrexate (120 to 500 mg per square meter) followed by citrovorum factor (25 mg every 8 hours for six doses) have been used to induce remissions, although resolution of cutaneous tumors usually requires radiotherapy as well. Remissions may be maintained with lower doses, generally 25 to 75 mg per week of methotrexate, orally or intramuscularly.

Combination chemotherapies used most frequently include methotrexate, cyclophosphamide, and prednisone; cyclophosphamide, vincristine, and prednisone; mechlorethamine, vincristine, procarbazine, and prednisone; cyclophosphamide, vincristine, and prednisone with or without bleomycin; Ara-C and doxorubicin; and chlorambucil and predisone. Additional drugs being studied for effectiveness in CTCL include VM-26, V-16, ICRF-159, gallium nitrate, methyl-GAG, 2′-deoxycoformycin, synthetic forms of retinoic acid, acyclovir, and cimetidine.

Experimental Approaches

Other attempts to control or cure CTCL include topical application of a wide variety of agents known to be useful for other lymphomas and leukemias when used systemically, antithyrocyte globulin, monoclonal antibodies directed against T lymphocytes or CTCL cell surface markers, leukapheresis for removal of circulating atypical Sézary cells, and interferon.

MULTIPLE MYELOMA

method of
ROBERT A. KYLE, M.D.
Mayo Clinic
Rochester, Minnesota

Diagnosis

If myeloma is suspected, in addition to a complete history and physical examination the patient should have determinations of hemoglobin, hematocrit values, and leukocyte, differential, and platelet counts; measurements of serum creatinine, calcium, phosphorus, alkaline phosphatase, and uric acid; roentgenographic survey of bones including humeri and femurs (bone scans with technetium-99m are inferior to conventional roentgenograms; computed tomography may reveal lytic lesions when roentgenograms are normal); serum protein electrophoresis including immunoelectrophoresis or immunofixation; quantitation of immunoglobulins and tests for cryoglobulins and viscosity; bone marrow aspiration and biopsy; routine urinalysis; and electrophoresis and immunoelectrophoresis or immunofixation (or both) of an adequately concentrated aliquot from a 24 hour urine specimen.

Minimal criteria for diagnosis include a bone marrow specimen that contains more than 10 per cent abnormal plasma cells or histologic proof of an extramedullary plasmacytoma and at least one of the following: monoclonal (M) protein in the serum (usually greater than 3 grams per dl), M-protein in the urine, or osteolytic lesions. Connective tissue diseases, chronic infections, carcinoma, lymphoma, and leukemia may simulate some of the characteristics of myeloma and should be excluded unless other features make the diagnosis of multiple myeloma clear.

One should not treat patients who have monoclonal gammopathy of undetermined significance (benign monoclonal gammopathy) that is characterized by an M-protein level of less than 3 grams per dl in the serum, fewer than 5 per cent bone marrow plasma cells, no anemia or osteolytic lesions, normal serum albumin, either no or small amounts of M-protein in the urine, and no evidence of progression. Most patients who fulfill the diagnostic criteria of myeloma have symptoms or findings that require therapy. Some, however, have smoldering myeloma (serum M-protein level higher than 3 grams per dl, more than 10 per cent plasma cells in the bone marrow but no anemia, renal insufficiency, or skeletal lesions), and these patients should not be treated but must be re-examined at 3 to 6 month intervals. A plasma cell labeling index is helpful in differentiating patients with smoldering myeloma from those with overt myeloma. It should be emphasized that all clinical and laboratory features must be considered before treatment is given. If there is no progression, continued observation with repeated evaluation is indicated.

Treatment

Hypercalcemia. Hypercalcemia occurs in one third of the patients with myeloma and must be suspected in the presence of anorexia, nausea, vomiting, polyuria, increased constipation, weakness, confusion, stupor, or coma. Hypercalcemia often leads to renal insufficiency, so prompt treatment is essential. Because dehydration frequently accompanies hypercalcemia, the patient should be hydrated. Isotonic saline solution is the agent of choice. After hydration has been achieved, furosemide (Lasix) may be helpful. During diuretic therapy the electrolytes must be monitored closely. In addition to hydration, prednisone should be given in an initial dosage of 25 mg four times daily. The prednisone dose must be reduced when the serum calcium level decreases and should be discontinued as quickly as possible. If the calcium level does not decrease, mithramycin should be given intravenously in a dosage of 25 micrograms per kg. Its effect is produced within 24 to 48 hours, but hypercalcemia often recurs after 2 to 3 days, and qualitative or quantitative platelet abnormalities may occur. Calcitonin has been used with some success. If hypercalcemia recurs after an initial response, inorganic phosphate (Neutra-Phos) may be used on an outpatient basis but must not be given if renal insufficiency or hyperphosphatemia is present. Since prolonged bed rest often contributes to hypercalcemia, patients with myeloma should be encouraged to be as active as possible.

Renal Insufficiency. More than 50 per cent of patients with myeloma will have renal insufficiency. Hypercalcemia, protein casts in the proximal and distal tubules (myeloma kidney), hyperuricemia, deposition of amyloid, pyelonephritis, and infiltration of the kidney with plasma cells all may contribute to renal insufficiency. Intravenous pyelography or preparation for barium enema may precipitate renal failure, but these can be performed with little risk if dehydration is avoided. The maintenance of a high fluid intake (greater than 3 liters per 24 hours) is important in preventing renal failure. If hyperuricemia occurs, allopurinol, 300 mg daily, provides effective therapy. If the patient is allergic to allopurinol, sodium bicarbonate, 0.6 to 0.9 gram three or four times daily, and acetazolamide (Diamox), 250 mg at bedtime, can alkalinize the urine adequately.

Acute renal failure must be recognized and treated promptly with alkalinization and maintenance of fluid and electrolyte balance. If these measures are not successful, hemodialysis or peritoneal dialysis is indicated. Long-term hemodialysis can prolong life provided the multiple myeloma is controlled. Renal transplantation for myeloma kidney has been followed by prolonged survival.

Infections. Bacterial infections are more common in patients with myeloma than in the normal population. The period of greatest risk for infection is in the first 2 months after the initiation of chemotherapy. Gram-negative infections are now more common than are gram-positive infections. Significant fever is an indication for appropriate cultures, radiography, and consideration of antibiotic therapy. The selection of antibiotics can be made more specific once the results of the cultures are known. There is considerable doubt about the efficacy of injections of gamma globulin. Gamma globulin may be given intravenously, but it is very expensive. Occasionally, in patients with multiple myeloma and recurrent, severe gram-positive infections, penicillin has been used prophylactically and the results have been good. Although antibody response is impaired in myeloma, pneumococcal vaccine should be given.

Skeletal Lesions. Bone lesions manifested by pain and fractures constitute a major problem. Although bone lesions may heal with chemotherapy, this rarely occurs. Frequently, a brace or supporting garment is helpful, but avoidance of trauma is more important because even mild stress may result in multiple fractures. Nevertheless, the patient should be encouraged to be as active as possible because confinement to bed increases demineralization of the skeleton. Analgesics should be given to control pain so that the patient can be ambulatory. Long bone fractures or large lytic lesions in weight-bearing bones may be treated effectively with an intramedullary rod and methacrylate. Theoretically, fluoride (which stimulates osteoblastic activity), calcium (which calcifies the osteoid tissue), and oral diphosphonates (which reduce osteoclastic activity) may prove to be of value in the treatment of myeloma bone disease.

Anemia. Almost every patient with multiple myeloma eventually becomes anemic. An increase of plasma volume from the osmotic effect of the M-protein may produce hypervolemia and spuriously lower the hemoglobin or hematocrit concentration. Transfusion of packed red cells remains the cornerstone of therapy. A hemoglobin concentration of 8 to 10 grams per dl is adequate in most patients, unless there is significant coronary artery disease or cerebrovascular insufficiency. Successful therapy of the primary disease often restores erythropoiesis. Androgens may raise the hemoglobin level in some patients, but the results generally have been disappointing.

Hyperviscosity Syndrome. The symptoms of hyperviscosity may include oronasal bleeding, blurred vision, neurologic symptoms, and congestive heart failure. Most patients have symptoms when the relative serum viscosity reaches 6 to 7 centipoises (cp), (normal, less than 1.8), but the relationship between serum viscosity and clinical manifestations is not precise. Hyperviscosity is more common in IgA myeloma than in IgG myeloma. Vigorous plasmapheresis with a cell separator will relieve the symptoms, but treatment with alkylating agents is necessary for long-term benefit.

Extradural Plasmacytoma. In the patient with multiple myeloma who states that his legs are weak or he has difficulty in voiding or defecating, the possibility of extradural myeloma must be considered. The sudden onset of severe thoracic pain or the presence of a paraspinal mass is suggestive of compression of the spinal cord. If any of these occur, neurosurgical consultation is urgently needed and myelography is essential. Radiation therapy in a dose of approximately 3000 rad is beneficial. To reduce the edema, dexamethasone should be administered daily during radiation therapy. If the neurologic deficit worsens during the course of irradiation, one must proceed with surgical decompression and then resume radiotherapy.

Chemotherapy

Chemotherapy is the preferred initial treatment for overt, symptomatic multiple myeloma. In most instances, analgesics combined with chemotherapy can control the pain. This combination is preferred to local irradiation because pain frequently recurs at another site since irradiation does not benefit systemic disease. Although irradiation may be repeated, its use ultimately is limited by the development of leukopenia or thrombocytopenia because the bone marrow reserve of many patients is reduced. For persistent, disabling pain that is clearly the result of a well-defined focal process, palliative radiation in a dosage of 2000 to 2500 rad is helpful. The myelosuppressive effects of radiotherapy and chemotherapy are cumulative; therefore it is best to complete the palliative irradiation therapy 3 weeks before starting chemotherapy and to determine the leukocyte and platelet counts.

The major controversy in the chemotherapy of multiple myeloma is whether melphalan and prednisone or a combination of alkylating agents should be used. Although combinations of chemotherapeutic agents produce a greater number of objective responses, significant differences in survival have not yet been proved. Furthermore, a combination of intravenously administered chemotherapeutic agents is more inconvenient and more costly, produces more side effects, and reduces the therapeutic options for future treatment.

The oral administration of melphalan (Alkeran) and prednisone is standard chemotherapy and produces objective response in 50 to 60 per cent of patients. Melphalan may be given orally in a daily dose of 0.15 mg per kg for 7 days (this amounts to between 8 and 10 mg daily for an average-sized patient and between 56 and 70 mg per course) with 20 mg of prednisone given three times daily for the same period. This regimen should be repeated every 6 weeks. The patient should avoid alcohol and caffeine-containing products and take antacids while receiving the prednisone. Leukocyte and platelet counts should be measured every 3 weeks after the start of chemotherapy. The dose of melphalan must be calculated on the basis of the patient's ideal body weight and altered until modest midcycle cytopenia occurs. Melphalan should be given while the patient is fasting because the absorption is delayed and reduced to about one half after food is eaten. If the leukocyte and platelet counts are low at 6 weeks, chemotherapy should be delayed and the counts repeated at weekly intervals until they increase. If the leukocyte and platelet counts remain low or if the counts obtained at 3 weeks are unduly low, the melphalan dose in the next 7 day course must be reduced accordingly. At least three courses of melphalan and prednisone are advised before this therapy is discontinued, unless there are significant toxic effects or the disease progresses rapidly despite adequate therapy. Maximal improvement may not be achieved for several months.

Because of the obvious shortcomings of melphalan and prednisone therapy, various combinations of chemotherapeutic agents have been tried. The best known combination, the M-2 protocol, includes melphalan, cyclophosphamide (Cytoxan), carmustine (BCNU), vincristine (Oncovin), and prednisone. In a randomized trial comparing the M-2 protocol with a combination of melphalan and prednisone, objective response was noted in 74 per cent and 53 per cent, respectively. However, the median survivals of 33 and 29 months, respectively, were not significantly different.

The ideal duration of chemotherapy is unknown. Cessation of treatment usually results in relapse, whereas continued chemotherapy may be associated with a myelodysplastic syndrome or overt acute leukemia. Chemotherapy probably should be continued for 2 years and then discontinued, provided the M-protein levels in the serum and urine have been stable for at least 6 months and the patient has no other evidence of active disease. The patient must be followed closely and chemotherapy reinstituted when relapse occurs.

If there is no response to melphalan or if the patient becomes resistant after responding, a combination of carmustine (BCNU), 30 mg per M^2, doxorubicin (Adriamycin), 30 mg per M^2, vincristine, 2 mg—all given intravenously on day 1—and prednisone (20 mg) three times daily for 5 days every 3 to 4 weeks has produced some benefit in 40 per cent of patients. Doses of carmustine and doxorubicin can be increased in 10 mg increments every 3 to 4 weeks if leukopenia or thrombocytopenia does not develop.

A continuous infusion of vincristine and doxorubicin accompanied by large doses of dexamethasone produced response in 70 per cent of patients resistant to alkylating agents. High doses of cyclophosphamide, vindesine (investigational drug), high dose cytosine arabinoside, cisplatin, bleomycin, and interferon have all produced limited benefit. Hemibody irradiation has produced decrease of pain and myeloma cell mass but at the expense of hematologic toxicity.

New considerations of therapy include large intravenous dose of melphalan, small doses of alkylating agents, hydroxyurea plus alkylating agents, interferon combined with chemotherapy, and autologous bone marrow transplantation.

Criteria for response to therapy include (1) decrease of serum M-protein by 50 per cent or more, (2) decrease of urinary M-protein by 50 per cent or more if the initial value was 1 gram or more per 24 hours, (3) increase of hemoglobin concentration by 2.0 grams per dl from an initial value of less than 11.0 grams per dl without transfusion, (4) decrease of plasma cells in bone marrow by 50 per cent or more, (5) recalcification of skeletal lesions and absence of new bone lesions, and (6) increase of performance and decrease of pain by two grades or more.

Variant Forms of Myeloma

Solitary Plasmacytoma (Solitary Myeloma) of Bone. The diagnosis is based on histologic evidence of a plasmacytoma. In addition, complete skeletal roentgenograms must show no other lesions of myeloma, the bone marrow aspirate must contain no evidence of multiple myeloma, and immunoelectrophoresis or immunofixation of the serum and concentrated urine should show no M-protein. There are exceptions to the last criterion, but therapy for the solitary lesions should result in the disappearance of the M-protein. Treatment for solitary plasmacytoma consists of irradiation in the range of 4000 to 5000 rad. Electrophoresis, immunoelectrophoresis, and immunofixation of serum and urine are helpful in following the course of the patient who has solitary plasmacytoma. In most instances, widespread multiple myeloma eventually develops.

Extramedullary Plasmacytoma. These plasmacytomas arise outside the bone marrow. The upper respiratory tract, including the nasal cavity and sinuses, nasopharynx, and larynx, is the most frequent location of lesions. Epistaxis, rhinorrhea, and nasal obstruction are the most common symptoms. The diagnosis is made on the basis of a plasma cell tumor in an extramedullary site and the absence of multiple myeloma. Irradiation in a dose of 4000 to 5000 rad is the most satisfactory treatment for localized disease. Extramedullary plasmacytomas usually spread locally and infrequently develop into typical multiple myeloma.

Osteosclerotic Myeloma. The major clinical feature is a chronic inflammatory-demyelinating polyneuropathy with predominantly motor disability. Single or multiple osteosclerotic bone lesions are characteristic. In contrast to that in multiple myeloma, the hemoglobin level is usually normal and erythrocytosis may occur. Thrombocytosis is common. The bone marrow aspirate usually contains less than 5 per cent plasma cells, while hypercalcemia and renal insufficiency rarely occur. Most patients have a small M-protein of the lambda type. Hepatosplenomegaly, hyperpigmentation, gynecomastia, edema, digital clubbing, hypertrichosis, atrophic testes, and impotence may occur. The diagnosis is confirmed by biopsy of an osteosclerotic lesion. Radiation of solitary osteosclerotic lesions benefits neuropathy in most patients. Chemotherapy is usually less effective.

Plasma Cell Leukemia. These patients have greater than 20 per cent plasma cells in the peripheral blood and an absolute plasma cell content of at least 2000 per mm^3. In two thirds of the patients, the leukemia occurs before multiple myeloma is recognized. Treatment is generally unsatisfactory, but melphalan and prednisone have produced impressive responses. There also have been responses with combinations of cyclophosphamide, vincristine, doxorubicin, and prednisone. Plasma cell leukemia as the preterminal phase of multiple myeloma rarely responds to chemotherapy.

Psychologic Factors

Any patient with a serious disease such as multiple myeloma or related disorders has psychologic problems and needs substantial, continuing emotional support. The approach must be positive. The physician must have confidence in his or her ability to cope with the patient's problems, and the patient should be able to sense this confidence. Potential benefits of therapy should be emphasized. It reassures the patient to know that some patients survive for 10 years or more. The physicians caring for patients with myeloma must have the interest and capacity to deal with incurable disease over a span of months to years with assurance, sympathy, and resourcefulness.

POLYCYTHEMIA VERA AND OTHER POLYCYTHEMIC CONDITIONS

method of
STEPHEN A. LANDAW, M.D., Ph.D.
Veterans Administration Medical Center
Syracuse, New York

Polycythemia vera is a malignant disorder of the pleuripotent stem cell that is associated with an absolute increase in circulating red cells as well as varying degrees of leukocytosis and thrombocytosis. Average survival is in the range of 10 to 15 years and, for PV patients treated with radioactive phosphorus (^{32}P), is similar to that of an age- and sex-matched normal U.S. population. Late in the disease the patient may develop an enlarging spleen and variable degrees of cytopenia due to myelofibrosis/myeloid metaplasia, which can be extremely difficult to treat. A variable number of patients will develop acute leukemia, which is usually unresponsive to intensive chemotherapy.

Treatment has always been controversial, although it has long been known that the survival of untreated patients averages two years, with death secondary to thrombotic or hemorrhagic complications. The major controversy in the 1960's centered on the place of myelosuppression. The Polycythemia Vera Study Group (PVSG) attempted to answer this and other questions through a prospective randomized long-term clinical trial comparing phlebotomy alone, phlebotomy plus ^{32}P, and phlebotomy plus chlorambucil (Leukeran). More than 400 patients were enrolled, and current follow-up is longer than ten years. The most interesting finding is that the choice of therapy has less effect on survival than it has on the complication suffered by the patient. Thus, patients treated with Leukeran suffered from an excess incidence of early leukemia, and this arm of the study was discontinued. Patients undergoing treatment involving both myelosuppressive arms showed an increased incidence of malignancy, including leukemia, whereas those involved with the phlebotomy arm showed an increase in thrombotic events.

Prepared, in part, with aid from USPHS Grant # CA-10728 from the National Cancer Institute to the Polycythemia Vera Study Group (PVSG).

Diagnosis

PV is not the most common cause of an elevated hematocrit level; thus appropriate studies must be performed to rule out other causes. The history should include questions about gout, pruritus, cardiopulmonary disorders, and thrombotic and hemorrhagic symptoms. A family history of polycythemia should be sought as well as a medication history, including the use of androgens, diuretics, tobacco-containing products, and caffeine-containing beverages (colas, tea, coffee, and so on). A blood volume study should independently measure both red cell mass and plasma volume to determine whether there is absolute (increased red cell mass) or relative (decreased plasma volume) polycythemia or both. Ancillary tests may include liver spleen imaging, renal imaging, determination of the P_{50} of hemoglobin, 2,3-DPG levels, blood carboxyhemoglobin (preferably near the end of the day), and a directly measured arterial O_2 saturation (not calculated from the pO_2). Less commonly, one might obtain serum erythropoietin levels or determine the presence of "endogenous" erythroid colonies in culture. The leukocyte alkaline phosphatase is elevated in 70 per cent of PV patients, which makes this the most valuable ancillary test for PV. More than 90 per cent of PV patients are iron deficient when first seen and usually present with a low red cell mean corpuscular volume (MCV).

Relative polycythemia poses fewer diagnostic problems, as most cases are due to cigarette smoking, use of diuretics, or excessive caffeine ingestion. Occasionally, pheochromocytoma or other endocrine abnormalities may be involved.

Treatment

Phlebotomy

Patients with an increased blood volume and hematocrit usually have symptoms related to sluggish blood flow. Cerebral blood flow is reduced when hematocrits are in excess of 45 per cent. Headache, flushing, tinnitus, dizziness, pressure behind the eyes, and the like usually respond promptly to venesection. It is important to restrict venesection to patients with an elevated total blood volume. All patients with relative polycythemia have normal or low total blood volume, which would only be made worse by venesection. Patients with chronic lung disease may be in balance with an expanded volume and may tolerate phlebotomy poorly. Thus in these patients, as well as in the elderly, first phlebotomies should be 250 to 300 ml and should be performed slowly. Subsequent phlebotomies should be done only if the patient has obtained symptomatic relief. The hematocrit level should be kept at 40 to 45 per cent, although there are no data correlating hematocrit with symptoms or complications. Initial treatment goals for PV are to reduce hematocrit to about 45 per cent with 500 ml phlebotomies performed two to three times per week.

Phlebotomy works by producing a state of chronic iron deficiency, and low serum iron, low MCV, and low ferritin levels are to be expected. Treating such patients with iron will lead to an exacerbation of the polycythemia and should be avoided. If symptoms of iron deficiency are intolerable or if thrombocytosis is exacerbated, then myelosuppression may be indicated. Phlebotomy alone appears to be contraindicated in older PV patients with prior thrombosis. Such patients are at risk for a fatal thrombotic event within the subsequent two years if treated only with phlebotomy and are best treated with myelosuppressive agents.

Myelosuppression

Radioactive phosphorus (^{32}P as the phosphate, given intravenously) has been used as a treatment for PV for more than 40 years and has an initial success rate of 80 to 90 per cent. It is a strong beta emitter and works by irradiating mitotically active cells of the bone marrow (both directly by isotope uptake and indirectly through uptake by surrounding bone). Initial treatment should be 2.7 mCi per square meter intravenously (total dose less than 5 mCi). If after 12 weeks there has been insufficient control, a second treatment can be given at a 25 per cent dose escalation (total dose not to exceed 7 mCi). The goal should be a reduction of symptoms, thrombocytosis, and/or spleen size.

Supplemental phlebotomies are always indicated to aid in controlling the hematocrit. With this regimen, a third injection of ^{32}P at 24 weeks is usually not necessary. However, if control is not achieved after the third dose, then another agent should be used. A typical PV patient will be controlled at 12 weeks following a single injection, resulting in a remission lasting 12 months or more. Supplementary phlebotomies are then performed on an as-needed basis, reserving a repeat dose of ^{32}P for reappearance of thrombocytosis or symptoms. Because absorption from the gastrointestinal tract is erratic, ^{32}P should not be given orally. The usual doses of ^{32}P may produce profound myelosuppression when given to a patient with renal failure and phosphate retention.

Alkylating Agents

Myelosuppression can be achieved through the use of oral agents such as cyclophosphamide (Cytoxan), busulfan (Myleran), or chlorambucil (Leukeran). The PVSG experience with Leukeran resulted in an unacceptably high incidence of leukemia, occurring earlier than that expected after ^{32}P. Thus, the PVSG no longer recommends oral alkylating agent therapy as first line treatment. The European literature suggests that busulfan may be less leukemogenic when given as "pulses" rather than in continuous low dose, but this has not been tested in the United States.

Hydroxyurea (Hydrea)

This agent inhibits DNA synthesis and induces a megaloblastic blood picture (this use of the agent is not listed in the manufacturer's directive). It is about 60 to 80 per cent effective in previously untreated PV. Because it uniformly increases the size of the red cell (often to MCV levels in excess of 110 femtoliters), there may only be modest reduction of the hematocrit. Thus, supplemental phlebotomies are the rule with this agent. Initial doses should be 15 mg per kg per day orally, best given as a single dose on an empty stomach. Giving a loading dose of 30 mg per kg per day for 1 week often leads to leukopenia and thrombocytopenia in subsequent weeks, prompting most physicians to stop the drug at that point. However, blood counts revert to their pretreatment levels if treatment is stopped for as little as 10 to 14 days. To avoid this "roller coaster" effect, it is best to use the lower dose (15 mg per kg per day), to escalate the dose slowly if needed, and to wait at least 2 weeks between dose changes. The goal should be control of symptoms, a white blood cell count in excess of 3,500, and platelet counts in the range of 100,000 to 500,000 with the typical patient taking about 7 to 18 capsules (500 mg each) *per week*.

This agent requires frequent blood counts and visits and excellent patient compliance. Megaloblastic RBC and WBC changes are expected, and folic acid and/or B_{12} supplementation is neither necessary nor recommended. Because hydroxyurea is a metabolic inhibitor of DNA synthesis, it theoretically should not be carcinogenic. Current follow-up of PV patients treated solely with this agent is not sufficiently long to prove or disprove this point, but no early cases of leukemia, such as that seen after chlorambucil, have been noted to date. Toxicity is minimal and has been limited to skin rash, gastrointestinal intolerance, fever, and minimal alopecia.

Antiplatelet Agents

Thrombocytosis is seen in over 60 per cent of PV patients, and counts in excess of 1 million are common, often in association with hemorrhagic and/or thrombotic symptoms and complications. The most rapid lowering of platelet counts can be achieved with platelet pheresis, which can be especially valuable in emergencies. To avoid rebound thrombocytosis, myelosuppressive agents should be started simultaneously. Nitrogen mustard (Mustargen) or cytosine arabinoside (Cytosar) in the usual single agent doses acts the most rapidly to reduce platelet count (three to seven days), hydroxyurea usually takes an intermediate time (10 to 14 days), and the alkylating agents and ^{32}P may take up to six weeks for maximum effect.

Since platelet function may also be abnormal in PV, aspirin with or without dipyridamole (Persantine) may be used to prevent or control thrombotic symptoms. Aspirin, 325 mg orally 3 times a day, plus dipyridamole, 75 mg orally 3 times a day, did not reduce the incidence of thrombotic events in PV patients treated with phlebotomy alone. (This use of aspirin and dipyridamole is not listed by their manufacturers.) Moreover, all patients with platelet counts over 1 million had significant hemorrhagic complications. However, there is a considerable body of anecdotal information that suggests that much smaller doses of aspirin (such as ¼ to 1 tablet per day) may be extremely effective in reducing transient ischemic events in the digital and cerebral circulation.

Treatment of Pruritus and Gout

Postshower or -bath pruritus may be a disabling symptom in PV. Relief is often obtained, at least in part, when the disease is treated with myelosuppression. Cyproheptadine (Periactin), 4 mg orally 4 times a day, may give additional relief; similarly, cimetidine (Tagamet), 300 mg orally 3 or 4 times a day, may also be effective. A few patients may require treatment with both agents, and some may respond to hydroxyurea where other drugs have failed.

Hyperuricemia and gout are common in PV. Allopurinol (Zyloprim), 300 mg orally daily, will effectively lower the serum uric acid concentration. However, in patients with a prior history of gout, this may exacerbate an acute attack. For such patients, initial treatment with maintenance doses of colchicine (0.5 mg orally twice daily) should be given prophylactically before allopurinol is started and should continue for a number of weeks thereafter.

Surgery, Splenectomy, and the Spent Phase of PV

Elective and emergency surgeries in patients with uncontrolled PV are associated with unacceptably high morbidity and mortality. For elective operations, it has been recommended that the disease be under control for at least six months, with the hematocrit 40 to 45 per cent and platelet counts under 600,000. Acute phlebotomy (with possible storage of the removed blood for use at the time of surgery) may raise the platelet count, often requiring short-term myelosuppression or platelet pheresis for control.

Splenectomy is contraindicated in *early* PV, since it may be associated with uncontrollable thrombocytosis and fatal thrombotic complications. However, late in the disease, when myelofibrosis/myeloid metaplasia occurs, the spleen may enlarge greatly, with attendant problems of cytopenias, splenic infarction, early satiety due to gastric compression, and portal hypertension with esophageal varices due to increased splenic blood flow. The care of such patients is exceedingly complex. Low dose splenic irradiation (50 to 150 rads delivered at a dose rate of 50 rads per session) may give relief, but this is often temporary. Trials of folic acid, vitamin B_{12}, and vitamin B_6 with or without steroids have been generally unsuccessful. Androgens are of value when anemia is prominent. Fluoxymesterone (Halotestin), 10 mg orally 3 times per day; oxymetholone (Anadrol), 2.5 mg per kg per day orally in divided doses; or testosterone enanthate (Delatestryl), 600 mg intramuscularly per week, may be tried. Responses usually take three to six months to become evident, and patients failing to respond to one agent may respond to another.

Ultimately, the choice for the patient with an enlarging spleen is surgery or myelosuppression. Low doses of hydroxyurea (starting at a total daily dose of 500 mg per day orally and escalating slowly as tolerated) may be particularly effective, although careful monitoring of blood counts is essential. For potential splenectomy candidates, care must be taken to exclude those with low grade disseminated intravascular coagulation, as these patients have complicated perioperative courses. The surgeon must pay meticulous attention to hemostasis and to the immediate postoperative recovery period. Hydroxyurea should be considered as adjuvant therapy to prevent both thrombocytosis and the often fatal complication of liver failure due to increasing hepatic myeloid metaplasia.

At any stage in the disease, surgery may be associated with perioperative bleeding, even in the absence of abnormalities of routine coagulation tests, and at a time when the platelet count may be normal or elevated. The transfusion of 10 units of platelet concentrate intravenously every 12 hours may dramatically restore hemostasis by serving as a source of normally functioning platelets.

Acute Leukemia

Approximately 1 to 2 per cent of PV patients treated with phlebotomy alone and about 10 to 20 per cent of patients treated with myelosuppressive agents will develop acute leukemia, usually abrupt in onset. A small percentage will have classic acute lymphoblastic leukemia and will respond to vincristine and prednisone combinations with or without anthracycline. The majority will develop a nonlymphoblastic variant that will not respond to vincristine/prednisone combinations. Because of their advanced age, prior history of a myeloproliferative disorder, and possible prior treatment with myelosuppressive agents, they usually respond poorly to combination chemotherapy. However, partial and complete remissions are possible with aggressive therapy, which can be attempted in suitably informed patients with a good performance status. Patients can often be kept comfortable for many months with periodic transfusions of red cells and platelets, and this remains a reasonable alternative for those who are unwilling or unable to receive chemotherapy.

Choice of Therapy

Polycythemia Vera

Although each patient presents a unique combination of clinical circumstances, there are some general principles learned from the PVSG studies.

1. Patients with indolent PV or isolated erythrocytosis and those under age 40 are best managed with phlebotomy alone. Low doses of aspirin (1 tablet per day or less) may be added to prevent thrombotic complaints. (This use of aspirin is not listed in package inserts.)

2. Patients over the age of 40 with a prior thrombotic event or a large phlebotomy requirement should receive myelosuppression. Those closer to age 70 or those who are unreliable or unable to return for frequent follow-up should receive ^{32}P; those closer to age 40 are candidates for hydroxyurea.

Other Polycythemic Disorders

Phlebotomy should be performed only if the total blood volume is increased. First phlebotomies should be performed slowly and in limited volume for the elderly and those with chronic lung disease. When smoking, use of diuretics or androgens, or excessive caffeine intake is responsible for the polycythemia, there is no reasonable treatment other than removal of the offending agent.

THE PORPHYRIAS

method of
KENNETH E. L. McCOLL, M.D.
MICHAEL R. MOORE, Ph.D.
and ABRAHAM GOLDBERG, M.D.
University of Glasgow
Glasgow, Scotland

The porphyrias are predominantly inherited disorders resulting from individual enzyme deficiencies in the pathway of heme biosynthesis. Each enzyme defect results in a different pattern of overproduction of porphyrins and precursors that is characteristic of that type of porphyria.

Clinically the porphyrias can be classified as the *acute porphyrias,* in which there are attacks of neurovisceral dysfunction associated with the overproduction of the porphyrin precursors delta-aminolaevulinic acid (ALA) and porphobilinogen (PBG), and the *nonacute porphyrias,* in which there is overproduction of only formed porphyrins and neurovisceral dysfunction does not occur. Cutaneous photosensitivity due to the interaction of light with porphyrins in the skin is a feature of each type of porphyria, except acute intermittent porphyria, in which there is only overproduction of porphyrin precursors.

THE ACUTE PORPHYRIAS

Acute Intermittent Porphyria

Acute intermittent porphyria is the commonest and most severe form of acute porphyria. It is an autosomal dominant disorder in which there is deficiency of the enzyme porphobilinogen deaminase. Subjects with the genetic trait are at risk of developing acute attacks of neurovisceral dysfunction but do not experience cutaneous photosensitivity.

Diagnostic Considerations

The clinical features of the neurovisceral attacks of acute intermittent porphyria are similar to those of hereditary coproporphyria and variegate porphyria. Abdominal pain, the most frequent complaint, is usually accompanied by nausea, vomiting, and severe constipation. Peripheral neuropathy predominantly affecting the motor nerves may be the presenting feature, and it complicates more than 50 per cent of attacks. Paralysis may progress rapidly, resulting in bulbar weakness and respiratory failure necessitating assisted ventilation. Sensory neuropathy may also occur. Psychiatric manifestations are also a common feature of the acute attack and may result in the patient's being misdiagnosed as suffering from a primary psychiatric disorder. Agitation, mania, depression, auditory and visual hallucinations, and schizophrenic-like behavior may occur. Grand mal convulsions are not uncommon at the height of an attack and in some patients may persist between attacks.

Tachycardia and hypertension are usually present, and hypertensive encephalopathy may develop. Severe postural hypotension resulting in syncope may also be seen. The hypertension and postural hypotension may persist to some extent between attacks. Other manifestations of autonomic dysfunction such as profuse sweating, pallor, and pyrexia may also occur. Severe hyponatremia due to inappropriate secretion of antidiuretic hormone complicates a proportion of attacks and sometimes presents as convulsions or deterioration in the conscious level. All the features of the acute attack are believed to be secondary to neurologic dysfunction involving the central, peripheral, and autonomic nervous systems. The precise relationship between the neurologic dysfunction and the underlying disorder of heme biosynthesis has yet to be eluciated.

Precipitating Factors

Various factors may precipitate acute attacks of porphyria in subjects with the genetic trait, and great care must be taken to prevent exposure to them. Drugs are the most common precipitating agents. Although most of the incriminated drugs are lipophilic and inducers of the hepatic mixed function oxidase system, it is impossible to reliably predict from the drug's chemical structure whether it will be safe in patients with porphyria. A list of drugs generally believed to be unsafe in patients with acute porphyria is given in Table 1. A list of drugs thought to be safe is given in Table 2.

Other factors that may trigger attacks include alcohol ingestion, reduced caloric intake due to fasting or dieting, and infection. Hormones are also important. Attacks are more common in females and rarely occur before puberty or after menopause. Pregnancy and oral contraceptives may also precipitate attacks, and some women experience regular attacks commencing in the week prior to the onset of menstruation.

Management

An acute attack of porphyria still carries a significant mortality of around 10 per cent. A successful outcome largely depends on early diagnosis, removal of precipitating factors, and provision of intensive supportive therapy. On first diagnosing an attack, a careful search should be made for any precipitating factors. When possible, these should be removed. The patient's current drug therapy should be scrutinized and a careful search made for any underlying infection. When appropriate, a pregnancy test should be performed.

Steps should be taken to ensure that the patient has an adequate carbohydrate intake. Most patients suffer from nausea and vomiting during an attack, and their poor carbohydrate intake aggravates the disease process. This cycle must be broken. In mild attacks this may be done by ensuring an adequate oral intake of glucose polymer drinks such as Caloreen (Roussel) or Hycal (Beecham Products). In more severe cases 2 liters of 20 per cent dextrose should be infused every 24 hours into a large peripheral vein or via a central venous line. In patients experiencing frequent attacks and in whom venous access becomes difficult, the constant slow infusion of Caloreen via a fine bore Teflon nasogastric tube may be helpful.

Pain. This is a feature of the majority of attacks. When mild, pain may be adequately controlled with aspirin, paracetamol, or dihydrocodeine. For more severe pain, pethidine (meperidine), morphine, or diamorphine may be required. Buprenorphine, which may be administered either sublingually or intramuscularly, is also useful. More constant pain relief may be achieved by the continuous intravenous infusion of analgesics. There is a danger of addiction in patients experiencing frequent attacks who require large amounts of narcotic analgesics; every attempt should be made to withdraw all narcotic drugs between attacks.

In a few unfortunate patients the pain is refractory to even very large doses of narcotic analgesics, and signs of respiratory and cardiovascular system depression appear before pain relief is obtained. Many of our patients report that the only time the pain goes away is when they are asleep. This observation may be used to advantage by encouraging sleep for several hours by combining chlorpromazine or promazine with the analgesics and leaving the patient relatively undisturbed in a darkened room.

Some patients continue to complain of chronic abdominal pain unaccompanied by any other symptoms between attacks. This can be very difficult to manage, and the risk of narcotic addiction in these patients is high. Although in some cases a psychological overlay may be a factor, in others the pain is clearly genuine and presumably a manifestation of residual neurologic damage.

Nausea and Vomiting. These frequently occur and may be controlled with chlorpromazine, promazine, or prochlorperazine. As the narcotic analgesics used in controlling the pain may often aggravate the nausea and vomiting, it is often helpful to administer the antiemetics along with or shortly before the analgesics. In addition to their antiemetic effects, chlorpromazine and promazine are useful in controlling the agitation and other psychiatric manifestations of the attack. In our experience a number of porphyria

TABLE 1. **Drugs Unsafe for Use in Acute Porphyria**

alcuronium	diethylpropion	lignocaine	phenacetin
*alphaxalone/alphadolone	*dihydroergotamine	lofepramine	phenelzine
aluminum preparations	mesylate	lysuride maleate	phenobarbital
amidopyrine	dimenhydrinate		phenoxybenzamine
aminoglutethimide	dixyrazine		phensuximide
(amitriptyline)	doxycycline	mephenezin	*phenylbutazone
(amphetamines)	drotaverine	mepivacaine	phenylhydrazine
antipyrine		*meprobamate	phenytoin
apronalide		mercaptopurine	piritramide
azapropazone	enflurane	mercury compounds	piroxicam
	*ergot compounds	mestranol	*primidone
	erythromycin	methohexitone	probenecid
*barbiturates	*estrogens	methotrexate	*progesterone
*bemegride	ethamsylate	methoxyflurane	(promethazine)
bendrofluazide	*ethanol	methsuximide	(propanadid)
benoxaprofen	*ethchlorvynol	*methyldopa	*pyrazinamide
busulphan	ethinamate	*methyl sulfonal	pyrrocaine
	ethionamide	*methyprylone	
	ethosuximide	metoclopramide	
carbamazepine	ethotoin	metronidazole	quinalbarbitone
*carbromal	etidocaine	metyrapone	
*carisoprodol	etomidate	minoxidil	
(cephadrine)			rifampicin
(cephalexin)			
(cephalosporins)	flucloxacillin	nalidixic acid	
chlorambucil	*flufenamic acid	*nikethamide	sodium aurothiomalate
*chloramphenicol	flunitrazepam	nitrazepam	sodium oxybate
*chlordiazepoxide	flurazepam	(nitrofurantoin)	†sodium valproate
chlormezanone	fluroxene	norethynodrel	spironolactone
chloroform		novobiocin	stanozolol
*chlorpropamide			succinamides
chloroxazone	*glutethimide		*sulfadimidine
(cimetidine)	glymidine	*oral contraceptives	*sulfonal
cinnarizine	gramicidin	orphenadrine	*sulfonamides
clemastine	*griseofulvin	oxanamide	sulfonylureas
(clobazam)	guaiphenesin	(oxazepam)	sulthiame
clomipramine		oxazolidinediones	
†(clonazepam)		oxycodone	
(clonidine)	*halothane	oxymetazoline	terfenadine
colistin	*hydantoins	oxyphenbutazone	*tetracyclines
crystal violet	hydralazine	oxytetracycline	theophylline
cyclophosphamide	hydroxyzine		*thiopental sodium
cycloserine	hyoscine butyl bromide		tilidate
		paramethadione	tolazamide
		pargyline	*tolbutamide
*danazol	*imipramine	*pentazocine	tranylcypromine
*dapsone	iproniazid	*pentylenetetrazole	troxidone
(dextropropoxyphene)	isometheptene mucate		
†(diazepam)	isoniazid		
dichloralphenazone	isopropylantipyrine		viloxazine
diclofenac sodium			

*Reported association with acute attacks of porphyria.
†See section on epilepsy.
These drugs have been classified as "unsafe" because all have been shown to be porphyrinogenic in animals or in vitro systems. Drugs within parentheses have conflicting experimental evidence of porphyrinogenicity.

patients develop extrapyramidal side effects with phenothiazines, necessitating substitution with cyclizine hydrochloride.

Tachycardia and Hypertension. These are features of the majority of attacks. They are thought to be the result of sympathetic overactivity and should be controlled with propranolol. The dose can be titrated against its effect on the cardiovascular system, and frequently very large doses are required. The pulse and blood pressure should be closely monitored, as they tend to be labile and hypertensive encephalopathy may develop. Postural hypotension leading to syncope may occur when a patient sits upright even when the patient has been hypertensive in the supine position. When postural hypotension does occur the supine blood pressure should still be adequately controlled with propranolol, taking care when moving the patient. Paroxysmal cardiac arrythmias sometimes leading to collapse may also occur and are sometimes precipitated by the patient's suddenly sitting upright. Whenever there

TABLE 2. **Drugs Thought to be Safe for Use in Acute Porphyria**

acetazolamide	desferrioxamine	labetalol	procaine
acetylcholine	dexamethasone	lithium salts	prochlorperazine
adenosine monophosphate	(dextromoramide)	(lorazepam)	promethazine
adrenalin	diamorphine		propantheline
alclofenac	diazoxide	magnesium sulfate	propranolol
allopurinol	diethyl ether	(mebendazole)	proxymetacaine
alpha tocopherol acetate	digoxin	mecamylamine	pyridoxine
amethocaine	dimercaprol	meclozine	pyrimethamine
ampicillin	(diphenhydramine theoclate)	mefenamic acid	
ascorbic acid	disopyramide	(melphalan)	quinine
aspirin	domperidone	metformin	
atenolol	doxorubicin	methadone	(ranitidine)
atropine	droperidol	(methotrimeprazine)	reserpine
		methylphenidate	resorcinol
beta-carotene	ethacrynic acid	metipropranolol	
biguanides	ethambutol	mianserin	sodium bromide
bumetanide		morphine	sodium calcium edetate (EDTA)
bupivacaine	fenoprofen		sodium fusidate
buprenorphine	fentanyl	naproxen sodium	streptomycin
butacaine	flurbiprofen	neostigmine	sulindac
	folic acid	nitrous oxide	suxamethonium
canthaxanthin	(frusemide)		
chloral hydrate		oxybuprocaine	(thiazides)
(chlormethiazole)	gentamicin	oxytocin	thiouracils
(chloroquine)	glafenine		thyroxine
chlorpheniramine	guanethidine	(pancuronium bromide)	tolazoline
chlorpromazine		paracetamol	triamterene
clofibrate	heparin	paraldehyde	trichlormethiazide
cloxacillin	hexamine	penicillamine	trifluoperazine
(cocaine)	(hydrochlorothiazide)	penicillins	tripelennamine
codeine phosphate		pentolinium	tubocurarine
colchicine	ibuprofen	pethidine	
(corticosteroids)	indomethacin	phenoperidine	(vincristine)
corticotrophin (ACTH)	insulin	phentolamine mesylate	
coumarins		pirbuterol	warfarin sodium
cyclizine	(ketamine)	(prazosin)	
cyclopropane	(ketoprofen)	prednisolone	zinc preparations (topical)
		(prilocaine)	
		primaquine	

Drugs within parentheses have conflicting evidence of experimental porphyrinogenicity, occasionally positive, but mainly negative. None of the drugs in this list has been associated with human porphyric attacks.

is evidence of cardiovascular instability, continual ECG monitoring should be performed and full resuscitative facilities kept at hand.

Convulsions. These are not infrequent at the peak of an attack. Their onset may be a sign of hyponatremia due to inappropriate antidiuretic hormone secretion, and plasma osmolality and electrolyte values should be checked. If hyponatremia is the underlying cause it should be corrected by restricting fluid intake to not more than 700 ml. The onset of convulsions may also be a sign of hypertensive encephalopathy, and the blood pressure should be checked. Convulsions occurring during the attack usually disappear as the attack resolves, and therefore therapy should be aimed at treating the underlying disease process. Some patients, however, continue to suffer from convulsions outside of the acute attack.

The management of epilepsy in the porphyric patient causes particular problems. Phenobarbital, primidone, phenytoin, and carbamazepine all increase cellular heme utilization by inducing the synthesis of hepatic monoxygenases and are contraindicated. The benzodiazepines and sodium valproate are not inducers of the monoxygenases, and although they have been shown to be porphyrinogenic in experimental models of porphyria, there is limited evidence that they are porphyrinogenic in man. Status epilepticus in our own experience has been treated successfully with intravenous diazepam. Seizure prophylaxis can be undertaken as a calculated risk with clonazepam or sodium valproate if this is essential, although sporadic clinical reports of porphyrinogenicity do exist. Sodium bromide and magnesium sulfate are safe but generally outmoded anticonvulsants.

Neuropathy. All patients should be examined for evidence of developing peripheral neuropathy. This may progress rapidly, leading to quadriplegia and bulbar and ventilatory paralysis. The latter is heralded by weakening of the voice. When signs of peripheral neuropathy are present the expiratory peak flow rate should be monitored. If there is any reduction in this rate the blood gases should be checked and the patient nursed in an intensive care unit with facilities for assisted ventilation. Even in patients in whom there is widespread paralysis requiring assisted ventilation for many months, good functional recovery can still be expected. Attention should be given to splinting of the joints and appropriate physiotherapy in the paralyzed patient.

Fluid and Electrolyte Balance. Various disturbances of fluid and electrolyte balance may be seen during the acute attack. Dehydration may occur owing to persistent vomiting. Hyponatremia secondary to inappropriate antidiuretic hormone secretion may also occur, sometimes first becoming apparent after commencing intravenous fluids. The hyponatremia can usually be controlled by restricting fluid intake. In order to maintain adequate carbohydrate intake while restricting fluid intake, it may be necessary to use higher concentrations of glucose administered via a central venous line.

Hematin Therapy

The discussion so far has concentrated on treating the acute attack by correcting any factors that may have precipitated it and providing adequate supportive therapy while the attack spontaneously resolves. It is also possible to treat the underlying disease process more directly by administering the end product of the deranged pathway in the form of intravenous hematin. The hematin binds to hemopexin and albumin in the plasma and is taken up by the liver. Here it is thought to supplement the depleted intracellular free heme pool, thus repressing the activity of the initial and rate-controlling enzyme of heme-biosynthesis, ALA synthase, and thereby reducing the overproduction of porphyrins and precursors formed prior to the enzyme block. In an acute attack of porphyria the intravenous administration of hematin consistently reduces both the plasma concentration and the urinary excretion of porphyrin precursors.

The clinical response to the therapy is more difficult to assess. There has been no controlled clinical trial of hematin therapy, and in a disease characterized by spontaneous relapses and remissions it is difficult to be sure whether improvement is the result of therapy or just the natural course of the disease. Our current practice is to use hematin only if there is evidence of progressive neuropathy unresponsive to the removal of precipitating factors and the intravenous administration of dextrose.

No major side effects have been reported with hematin when used in the standard doses. Phlebitis around the injection site occurs in a proportion of patients and is sometimes accompanied by fever and leukocytosis. This can be prevented by injecting the solution into a large peripheral vein or via a central venous line or possibly by administering the hematin together with human albumin solution, to which it will bind. During hematin therapy there is a mild disturbance of coagulation with prolongation of the prothrombin and partial thromboplastin times and a slight reduction in the platelet count. This reverts to normal on completion of the hematin course and has only very rarely resulted in hemorrhagic complications. The aforementioned coagulation indices and the platelet count should be monitored during therapy, and hematin should not be used in conjunction with anticoagulant therapy.

Transient acute renal failure has been reported in one patient who received a bolus intravenous injection of 1000 mg of hematin. However, no renal complications have occurred with the standard recommended dosages, and even patients with renal insufficiency appear to tolerate hematin well, although it is probably wise to reduce the dosage slightly as an added precaution. As hematin is prepared from human blood there is also the possibility of the transmission of infectious agents.

Two disadvantages of hematin therapy are the need for intravenous administration and the lack of readily available hematin solution. Hematin is prepared from hepatitis B surface antigen negative expired human blood by crystallization and recrystallization. Approximately 1,800 mg hematin is obtained from 250 ml packed red blood cells. Pyrogen testing of the final preparation should be performed. The crystals can be stored at 4 C. When required to treat an attack, the crystals are dissolved in 0.25 per cent Na_2CO_3 and the pH adjusted to 7.8 to 8. The solution is made up to contain 6 to 7 mg hematin per ml. The final solution should be stored in the dark at 4 C and used within five days. It should be removed from the refrigerator 30 minutes before use. The appropriate volume is then drawn up into a plastic syringe through a 5 μm aspiration needle filter and injected via a 0.22 μm filter (Millex Millipore) into the rubber bung of a slowly running intravenous infusion of physiologic saline. The generally recommended dose per infusion is 4 mg per kg body weight. For an acute attack one dose is usually given every 12 or 24 hours for 3 to 5 days.

Most centers with a special interest in the porphyrias have stocks of hematin and will provide the solution for use by other physicians as required. Because of concern regarding the stability of the hematin solution, it may be worth lyophilizing the final solution and reconstituting it immediately prior to use. A commercially available lyophilized hematin preparation (Panhematin, Abbott Laboratories) has recently been marketed in the United States.

Prevention of Attacks

Patients who have experienced a clinical attack of porphyria should be carefully counselled concerning the avoidance of precipitating factors. They should be encouraged to maintain a regular diet and to abstain completely from alcohol. In addition, they should be warned about the dangers of certain drugs and given a booklet indicating which drugs are safe and which are unsafe to take (See Tables 1 and 2). It is also important to ensure that the patient's family doctor is fully informed about the disease and also given advice about prescribing drugs. Patients should be reminded to inform any medical attendant that they suffer from porphyria. As an added precaution, they should wear a bracelet or necklace indicating that they have porphyria to prevent the administration of dangerous drugs or anesthetics in the event of an accident or other emergency.

Some women experience regular attacks in the week prior to the onset of menstruation. These are assumed to be initiated by the hormonal fluctuations, and various attempts have been made to prevent them. In some cases merely increasing the carbohydrate intake at the appropriate time of the month is found to be helpful. Interfering with the hormonal fluctuations has produced varying results. Some patients have been reported to benefit from the suppression of ovulation using various oral contraceptive hormone preparations. However, in our own experience as well as that of several other centers, the contraceptive pill has usually precipitated attacks. Dr. Karl Anderson and colleagues in Rockefeller University Hospital, New York, have reported a single patient in whom regular premenstrual attacks were prevented with the use of a long-acting analogue of luteinizing hormone–releasing hormone (LHRH). This preparation inhibits the release of luteinizing hormone (LH) and follicle-stimulating hormone (FSH), thus reducing endogenous hormone levels. The LHRH analogues, however, have an initial stimulatory effect that could precipitate an acute attack. Dr. Joel Lamon and colleagues of the NIH, Bethesda, successfully prevented premenstrual attacks in a 33-year-old woman by the prophylactic administration of hematin in a dosage of 3.3 mg per kg injected intravenously over 15 minutes once each week. Little information is available regarding possible adverse effects of the chronic administration of hematin.

Pregnancy and Acute Porphyria

Pregnancy may precipitate acute porphyria, with attacks being most common in early pregnancy and during the puerperium. In females the first attack often occurs during pregnancy. In patients with the genetic trait who have normal porphyrin excretion and who have never experienced a clinical attack, pregnancy is usually uneventful. If vomiting is a problem in early pregnancy, the patient should be admitted to the hospital at an early stage and dextrose administered intravenously to prevent the reduced dietary intake from inducing an attack. Dextrose should also be administered intravenously during labor. Patients who have had clinical attacks of porphyria and have increased urinary excretion of porphyrins and precursors are likely to experience attacks during pregnancy. We advise such patients not to consider pregnancy until they have been free of symptomatic attacks for at least 18 months. When attacks do occur during pregnancy they should be treated in the usual manner as already described.

As there is insufficient information about the effect of hematin on the fetus, this therapy should be avoided unless the condition of the mother demands it. Most attacks of porphyria during pregnancy settle with adequate supportive therapy, resulting in a successful outcome for both mother and child. We only rarely consider therapeutic termination of pregnancy in patients with acute porphyria and then only in very severe attacks occurring in early pregnancy. In addition to the possible risks of pregnancy, many patients question the advisability of bearing children likely to inherit a genetic disorder. It should be explained to the patient that although each child will have a 50 per cent chance of inheriting the trait, it will remain clinically latent throughout life in the majority. When affected individuals decide to delay or avoid pregnancy they should be warned about the dangers of oral contraceptives and advised about other forms of contraception.

Anesthetics

Provided appropriate precautions are taken, most patients with acute porphyria can tolerate surgery and general anesthesia. However, patients experiencing frequent attacks of porphyria will be at risk of developing complications, and the indications for surgery should be carefully examined. Care must be taken in selecting safe anesthetic agents. Atropine and morphine may be used as premedication. Intravenous ketamine has been found to be a safe alternative to thiopental as an anesthetic-inducing agent. Cyclopropane and ether are safe inhalation agents with respect to the porphyria, but they suffer the disadvantages of being potentially explosive and inducing postoperative vomiting. Nitrous oxide used in conjunction with intravenous narcotics and muscle relaxants may be a more acceptable alternative. Suxemethonium and D-tubocurarine can be used as muscle relaxants and diamorphine, morphine, pethidine, or fentanyl is a suitable narcotic for controlling postoperative pain. In some situations epidural anesthesia may be preferable to general anesthesia, in which case bupivacaine is the local anesthetic of choice. To prevent an attack being induced by fasting, an intravenous infusion of dextrose should be commenced prior to surgery and continued until the patient is able to take an adequate diet.

Hereditary Coproporphyria

Hereditary coproporphyria is inherited in an autosomal dominant fashion and is due to partial deficiency of the enzyme coproporphyrinogen oxidase. This results in accumulation of coproporphyrin and its precursors uroporphyrins PBG and ALA. The coproporphyrin is excreted in increased amounts in both urine and stool, whereas the uroporphyrins ALA and PBG appear only in the urine. Hereditary coproporphyria may present clinically with acute attacks identical to those seen in acute intermittent porphyria. These may be provoked by the same precipitating factors, and patients should be managed in the same way as patients with acute intermittent porphyria.

Because of the overproduction of formed porphyrins, patients with hereditary coproporphyria may also develop cutaneous photosensitivity. The occurrence of skin lesions depends on the degree of porphyrin overproduction and the amount of exposure to sunlight. Skin lesions should be treated by removing any inducing factors, such as drugs, alcohol, or inadequate diet, that may increase the porphyrin overproduction and by shielding the skin from sunlight (see hereafter).

As patients with hereditary coproporphyria are also at risk of developing life-threatening attacks of porphyria, their relatives should be screened for the disorder. The majority of affected relatives show abnormalities of porphyrin excretion in either the urine or feces, but in a small proportion this will be normal. Detection will depend on demonstrating decreased activity of coproporphyrinogen oxidase together with increased activity of the rate-controlling enzyme delta-aminolaevulinic acid synthase in peripheral leukocytes.

Variegate Porphyria

Variegate porphyria is inherited in an autosomal dominant fashion and is thought to be due to a partial deficiency of the enzyme protoporphyrinogen oxidase, although ferrochelatase activity may also be reduced. There is overproduction of protoporphyrin and, to a lesser extent, coproporphyrin, both of which are excreted in the stool, and also of ALA and PBG, which appear in the urine. As with acute intermittent porphyria and hereditary coproporphyria, patients with acute variegate porphyria are at risk of developing acute life-threatening attacks of neurovisceral dysfunction. Consequently, they should be advised about avoiding precipitating factors. If attacks occur they should be treated in the same way as the other acute porphyrias. Relatives should also be screened by examining urine and stool, which will detect most affected subjects, although some will have normal excretion of porphyrins and precursors and will only be detected by measuring the activity of protoporphyrinogen oxidase and delta-aminolaevulinic acid synthase in peripheral blood cells. Patients with variegate porphyria may also experience cutaneous photosensitivity. There are a few reports of a reduction in the skin photosensitivity with the use of β-carotene in variegate porphyria. This form of treatment is discussed in more detail under erythropoietic protoporphyria.

THE NONACUTE PORPHYRIAS

Cutaneous Hepatic Porphyria (Porphyria Cutanea Tarda, Symptomatic Porphyria)

Diagnostic Considerations

Cutaneous hepatic porphyria is the commonest form of porphyria. Patients present with cutaneous photosensitivity. Attacks of neurovisceral dysfunction are not a feature of the condition. The skin lesions are encountered on exposed areas such as the scalp, face, neck, and backs of hands and forearms. They usually start with erythema, progressing to vesicles that become confluent to form bullae. Hemorrhage may occur into the bullae, which heal leaving scars. Increased skin fragility is an important feature and in less severe cases may be the only sign. Hyperpigmentation also occurs, and women often complain of hirsutism.

In the majority of patients presenting with cutaneous hepatic porphyria, acquired factors contributing to the development of the disease will be found. Chronic alcohol ingestion is the commonest and is usually associated with mild alcoholic liver disease and evidence of iron overload. The disorder may also be seen in association with other forms of liver disease. Certain drugs, of which estrogens are the most important, may induce cutaneous hepatic porphyria. Cutaneous hepatic porphyria may present in women on the contraceptive pill and in male patients receiving stilbestrol for prostatic carcinoma. The oral hypoglycemic agents chlorpropamide and tolbutamide have also been incriminated as well as the antimalarial agent chloroquine when used in full dosage. Exposure to certain chemicals is also important and may produce the disorder even in the absence of any genetic predisposition. The disorder has been observed in patients on hemodialysis for chronic renal failure. Other diseases in which there is an increased frequency of cutaneous hepatic porphyria include diabetes mellitus, systemic lupus erythematosus, and hepatocellular carcinoma.

Treatment

Contributing factors should be looked for in all patients presenting with cutaneous hepatic porphyria and will be found in most. Patients should be carefully questioned about alcohol intake. Relatively small quantities of alcohol seem to be capable of precipitating the disorder, and patients should be advised to stop drinking completely. A careful drug history should also be obtained including direct questioning about the use of the contraceptive pill, which some patients do not consider to be a drug or medicine. Enquiries should be made about exposure to any chemicals, either at work or in the home. In most cases discontinuing alcohol or drug usage will be followed by clinical and biochemical remission.

Iron overload is usually present, and correction of this by venesection considerably hastens improvement. Five hundred ml of blood should be removed every second week until clinical remission is achieved or the hemoglobin concentration falls below 12 gram per dl. The iron stores are usually increased by only 1 to 2 grams, and removal of 2 to 4 liters is usually adequate. Prolonged remission is usually achieved following this, but patients may relapse if they resume drinking, in which case a further course of venesection will be required.

Low dose chloroquine therapy has also been shown to result in biochemical and clinical remission in cutaneous hepatic porphyria (this use of chloroquine is not listed by the manufacturer). It is thought to have this beneficial effect by mobilizing tissue-bound porphyrins, forming a molecular complex with them and facilitating their excretion in the urine. Chloroquine is administered orally in a dosage of 125 mg twice per week, and treatment needs to be continued for several months. Although retinal complications are unlikely at such a low dose, visual acuity and fundal appearance should be monitored. Chloroquine therapy does not correct the hepatic iron overload or improve liver histology. As with venesection, a proportion of patients will suffer relapses and require further courses of chloroquine treatment.

There is some evidence that combining venesection and chloroquine therapy can result in earlier remission than can be achieved with either treatment alone. The choice of treatment depends on the individual patient. Patients with evidence of liver disease and iron overload should probably be treated by venesection either alone or combined with chloroquine rather than chloroquine alone. In elderly patients suffering from cardiovascular disorders venesection is not without its risks, and chloroquine may be the better option.

The treatment of cutaneous hepatic porphyria in patients on renal hemodialysis is more difficult. They should be advised to completely abstain from alcohol, and any of the incriminated drugs should be withdrawn. The patient's iron status should be checked and iron supplements discontinued where appropriate. Venesection is clearly precluded by the secondary anemia of chronic renal failure. Because chloroquine exerts its main effect by increasing the renal clearance of porphyrins, it is unlikely to be helpful and is probably associated with increased side effects in the presence of chronic renal failure. The relative inability of hemodialysis to clear porphyrins from the plasma further complicates treatment. We recently attempted treating such a patient by using an activated charcoal hemoperfusion column in series with the hemodialysis column, but this also proved ineffective in clearing uroporphyrin. There are a few conflicting reports of the value of plasmapheresis in treating cutaneous hepatic porphyria associated with renal hemodialysis.

Erythropoietic Protoporphyria

Diagnostic Considerations

Erythropoietic protoporphyria (erythrohepatic protoporphyria) is an autosomal dominant disorder that presents with cutaneous photosensitivity. Symptoms often appear in childhood and usually consist of stinging, burning, and swelling of the skin during or shortly after sun exposure. Repeated exposure results in waxlike linear scars on the bridge of the nose and on the bony prominences of the backs of the hands. Cutaneous photosensitivity is usually the sole manifestation, but a few patients also develop hepatobiliary complications. Gallstones rich in protoporphyrin may occur. A small minority of patients develop liver disease, which may progress rapidly to cirrhosis and hepatic failure.

Treatment

Large clinical studies have confirmed a beneficial effect of β-carotene in reducing cutaneous photosensitivity in erythropoietic protoporphyria. No toxic side effects have been noted with this therapy other than the occasional loose stool. Carotenodermia, a yellow orange discoloration of the skin due to the cutaneous deposition of the drug, develops in all cases. This discoloration may be converted to a more cosmetically pleasing brown tanned color by the simultaneous oral administration of canthaxanthin. The dosage of β-carotene required varies from patient to patient but is usually between 60 and 180 mg per day. Some patients may require higher doses.

Hepatic Features

Although the liver complications of erythropoietic protoporphyria are rare, when they occur there may be rapid progression to fulminant hepatic failure. In most patients with erythropoietic protoporphyria who have died from liver failure death has occurred within a few months of the onset of jaundice. It is important to attempt to identify patients liable to this fatal complication and initiate preventive therapy. Fecal protoporphyrin excretion has not been correlated with the potential to develop liver damage, but the erythrocyte protoporphyrin level has been very high in those patients who develop cirrhosis and liver failure. Liver function tests should be checked at regular intervals and liver biopsy performed at the first sign of any disturbance.

The treatment of liver disease in erythropoietic protoporphyria is aimed at depleting hepatic protoporphyrin stores and diminishing the amount of protoporphyrin delivered to the liver for excretion. Iron deficiency increases protoporphyrin synthesis in erythropoietic tissue and should be corrected. A good dietary intake should also be maintained, as fasting increases fecal protoporphyrin excretion in erythropoietic protoporphyria, probably owing to increased production of protoporphyrin. Alcohol should be avoided completely, as this may further increase hepatic protoporphyrin production and adversely affect liver function. It is also wise to avoid drugs that are potentially hepatotoxic and especially those that may have a cholestatic effect, such as the contraceptive pill. The hepatic protoporphyrin load may be depleted by interrupting its enterohepatic circulation by the oral administration of cholestyramine, which binds protoporphyrin in the gut.

Congenital Erythropoietic Porphyria (Gunther's Disease)

DIAGNOSTIC CONSIDERATIONS

Congenital erythropoietic porphyria is an extremely uncommon disorder that is inherited in an autosomal recessive fashion. It usually presents in early life with severe and often mutilating photosensitive skin lesions. Hypertrichosis also occurs, and the photosensitivity results in sclerotic changes, which may resemble scleroderma. Porphyrins are deposited in most body tissues and result in a reddish brown discoloration of the teeth (erythrodontia) and bones. Erythrocytes are laden with porphyrins consisting mainly of type I isomers of uroporphyrin and coproporphyrin. There is also increased urinary excretion of uroporphyrin I and coproporphyrin I and increased fecal excretion of coproporphyrin I.

Hematologic abnormalities are an important feature of congenital erythropoietic porphyria. The bone marrow is the major site of porphyrin overproduction, and its porphyrin-laden cells fluoresce strongly in ultraviolet light. Anemia is frequently found, due to ineffective erythropoiesis and reduced red blood cell survival. The bone marrow reveals normoblastic hyperplasia, and the peripheral blood film shows a normocytic normochromic anemia with polychromasia. Splenomegaly and hypersplenism resulting in leukopenia and thrombocytopenia may also occur.

Treatment

The treatment of congenital erythropoietic porphyria remains unsatisfactory. Patients must be protected from sunlight and strong daylight. Shielding the skin with light-opaque celluloid may be helpful. β-carotene should also be tried.

Splenectomy has been shown to be beneficial in some patients by improving red blood cell survival and thus reducing the stimulation to red cell production and porphyrin overproduction by the bone marrow. Splenectomy is most likely to be helpful when there is markedly reduced red blood cell survival, with the spleen being the major site of removal of the erythrocytes.

Regular blood transfusion resulting in polycythemia can also reduce the porphyrin overproduction by depressing the bone marrow activity, although secondary iron overload may be a problem. The subcutaneous administration of desferrioxamine has recently been found to be useful in preventing iron overload in patients with thalassemia major requiring frequent blood transfusions, and such therapy may also be applicable in patients with congenital erythropoietic porphyria in whom blood transfusions are found to be useful. Treatment with low dose chloroquine (125 mg twice weekly) (not listed by manufacturer) has shown to be helpful in some cases, reducing erythrocyte fragility and diminishing photosensitivity. In some patients prednisolone improves both the anemia and the thrombocytopenia.

Intravenous hematin therapy was studied in one patient with congenital erythropoietic porphyria by the late Dr. Cecil Watson and his coworkers in Minneapolis. After three days of treatment, decreases in plasma, erythrocyte, and urine porphyrins were observed. The hematin, however, resulted in a transient reduction in the number of circulating normoblasts, suggesting some marrow suppression. This marrow effect is of some concern, as congenital erythropoietic porphyria can be complicated by periods of bone marrow hypoplasia with worsening of the anemia. Alkalinization of the urine can increase the clearance of coproporphyrin but not uroporphyrin, but this has not been associated with clinical improvement. As the bone marrow is the predominant tissue involved in this form of porphyria, bone marrow transplantation should be beneficial. This has not been performed to date but could be considered in patients with severe and life-threatening disease.

Congenital erythropoietic protoporphyria can be diagnosed prenatally by amniocentesis. The amniotic fluid has a red brown discoloration due to the presence of porphyrins and fluoresces on exposure to ultraviolet light.

THERAPEUTIC USE OF BLOOD COMPONENTS

method of
THOMAS H. PRICE, M.D.
Puget Sound Blood Center
Seattle, Washington

Advances in medicine and in blood banking procedures over the last 15 to 20 years have resulted in a greatly increased demand for the use of blood components. Components are routinely prepared from most units of blood within several hours of donation.

Components Containing Red Cells

Whole Blood and Packed Red Cells

A unit of whole blood contains approximately 450 ml of blood and 63 ml of anticoagulant. Transfusion of whole blood provides the recipient with coagulation factors and blood volume expansion as well as with oxygen-carrying capacity. The level of coagulation factors in the plasma of a unit of whole blood depends on the method of preparation and on the length of time that the unit has been stored. At our institution, most of the whole blood is modified whole blood, meaning that platelets or cryoprecipitate has been harvested from the unit. At the time of preparation, units from which cryoprecipitate has been made contain less than 15 per cent of factor VIII and approximately 50 per cent of the fibrinogen present in the original unit of blood. Other coagulation factors (II, V, VII, IX, X, and XI) are present in normal amounts. The effect of storage on the levels of these factors depends on the factor. The most labile of the coagulation factors, factor VIII, drops to 50 per cent of its initial value after 1 to 2 days of storage. Since the initial level of factor VIII in modified whole blood is less than 15 per cent normal, the levels in modified whole blood after 1 to 2 days' storage will be 5 to 10 per cent of normal, levels which would not be expected to be adequate for hemostasis. The next most labile factor, factor V, declines nearly linearly with storage, reaching values of 20 to 30 per cent of normal after 3 weeks, values which are probably still high enough to be hemostatic. The other coagulation factors—II, VII, IX, X, XI, and fibrinogen—do not decline substantially from their original values during the 5 week shelf life of whole blood.

Packed red cells are collected as whole blood, but most of the plasma is removed during component preparation. The final preparation contains approximately 200 to 250 ml of red cells and 75 ml of plasma, although these figures vary with the amount of blood drawn, the hematocrit of the donor, and the extent of plasma removal. In comparison with whole blood, packed cells are identical in their ability to supply oxygen-carrying capacity, but they lack the volume-expanding capabilities of whole blood. Because so little plasma is present, packed red cells do not provide significant amounts of coagulation factors.

Several characteristics are common to both whole blood and packed red cells. The usual anticoagulant is CDP-A1, a citrate-phosphate-dextrose solution to which adenine has been added. Both products can be stored for 35 days at 4 C, the red cells in both products exhibiting similar changes with storage. These changes include decreases in red cell 2,3-DPG and ATP, leakage of potassium from the red cells into the plasma, and loss of viability of approximately 30 per cent of the red cells over the 5 week storage period. The clinical significance of these changes in terms of most transfusion recipients is probably minimal. Adequate levels of 2,3-DPG are important in facilitating the release of oxygen from hemoglobin in the tissues. Although low levels of red cell 2,3-DPG are seen in blood stored more than 10 days, these levels increase rapidly in vivo, reaching levels of 50 per cent of normal 4 hours after transfusion. This temporary defect in red cell 2,3-DPG is of concern only in patients requiring immediate maximal oxygen-delivering capacity; in these patients it may be appropriate to provide blood less than 10 days old. Potassium loss from red cells during storage may result in plasma potassium levels as high as 30 mEq per liter in the stored unit. Hyperkalemia in recipients of such blood does not appear to be a significant problem, with the possible exception of neonates undergoing exchange transfusion. The problem can be avoided in these infants by providing blood less than a week old.

Neither whole blood nor packed cells contain significant numbers of functioning platelets or neutrophils. Administration of either component is through a 170 micron filter designed to trap platelet and leukocyte debris as well as small clots. If circulatory overload is not a likely problem, normal saline may be added to packed red cells to improve the flow rate. No other solutions or drugs should be added directly to blood.

Choice of Red Cell Product

Whether to give a patient whole blood or packed red cells is usually a simple decision based on the blood volume status of the patient. If the patient requires oxygen-carrying capacity but does not have a reduced blood volume, packed red cells should be provided. Administration of whole blood to such a patient, particularly if the patient is elderly or has an increased blood volume, may result in circulatory overload. On the other hand, if the patient requires both volume and oxygen-carrying capacity, whole blood is appropriate. If whole blood is not readily available, such patients may be transfused with packed red cells along with adequate amounts of salt solutions or colloids. In massive transfusion, however, it is desirable to use whole blood since coagulation factors are provided, and the need to supplement red cell components with fresh frozen plasma (and thereby expose the recipient to additional donors) is avoided. Exceptions to this general rule include patients who are normovolemic but who require coagulation factors as well as red cells; in such patients it makes sense to administer whole blood.

Chronic Anemia

Patients with chronic anemia usually have a normal or increased blood volume and should be given packed red cells rather than whole blood. When to transfuse a patient with chronic anemia is a question that cannot be answered simply in terms of the degree of anemia. Issues such as the purpose of the transfusion, the stability of the hematocrit, the etiology of the anemia, the clinical condition of the patient, and the risks of transfusion all need to be considered. In general, the indication for transfusion is the development of symptoms attributable to decreased oxygen-carrying capacity in a patient whose anemia cannot be corrected by more specific therapy such as iron. The symptoms may actually be present or may be ones the physician knows that the patient will develop if not transfused. If the hematocrit is greater than 30 per cent, symptoms are not likely to be attributable to anemia. Patients who are otherwise healthy may be asymptomatic with hematocrits as low as 15 to 20 per cent, and many patients with chronic anemias of this severity are able to function adequately without transfusion.

Most patients with chronic anemia develop symptoms such as fatigue, dizziness, dyspnea on exertion, or headaches at hematocrit levels in the low 20s. Patients with underlying cardiovascular disease may develop angina or congestive heart failure at levels in the mid 20s. Since 1 unit of blood represents about 10 per cent of the circulating red cell mass of a normal-sized individual, an average patient can be expected to increase his or her hematocrit approximately 3 to 4 per cent for each unit of blood transfused.

Acute Blood Loss

Although acute blood loss involves the loss of both oxygen-carrying capacity and blood volume, the symptoms are primarily those of hypovolemia. Most patients will experience no symptoms after a loss of 10 per cent of their blood volume, an amount similar to that lost by a donor during the blood donation process. Orthostatic changes in heart rate and blood pressure are noted after loss of 20 per cent of the blood volume, and clinical shock appears after a loss greater than 30 per cent. Whereas these larger losses in blood volume, if halted, can be managed by fluid replacement without transfusion, continued blood loss usually requires transfusion. Since blood volume is usually just as important as oxygen-carrying capacity in this situation, the component of choice for transfusion is whole blood. It is important to point out that in acute blood loss, the hematocrit is an unreliable indicator of the degree of blood loss or of the need for transfusion. Change in the hematocrit as a result of blood loss alone is a 2 to 3 day process involving re-equilibration of the extracellular fluid. Rapid change in the hematocrit during the acute episode reflects the degree of replacement with salt solutions and colloids more than it does the extent of the bleeding. If replacement fluids have exactly matched the hemorrhage, the fall in hematocrit will correspond to the amount of blood lost.

A number of special concerns relate to the transfusion of red cell–containing components in acute blood loss. The first has to do with pretransfusion testing. Although it is desirable that compatibility testing be completed before the administration of any transfusion, in emergencies there may not be adequate time to accomplish this. In this case, type-specific blood (blood which is the same ABO and Rh type as that of the patient) should be administered. Although the chance of incompatibility or a subsequent hemolytic transfusion reaction is low in these circumstances, particularly if the patient has not been pregnant or previously transfused, it is not zero. In more urgent situations in which the patient is exsanguinating, type 0 Rh negative packed red cells may be administered at the same time that the patient's blood is being typed.

The second concern is that of hemostatic abnormalities arising during massive transfusion as a result of replacing the recipient's blood with blood from the blood bank. The expected defect will depend on whether there were pre-existing hemostatic abnormalities in the recipient, the number of units of blood transfused, and the component used. On the basis of the data presented earlier, if the component used for replacement is whole blood or modified whole blood, even if it has been stored for a prolonged period one would expect to encounter abnormalities only with factor VIII and with platelets. It turns out that factor VIII levels are usually adequate for hemostasis in massively transfused patients, presumably due to mobilization of factor VIII from endogenous stores. By contrast, dilutional thrombocytopenia is a common problem with large volume transfusions. One should consider the possibility of clinically significant dilutional thrombocytopenia after the administration of 1 to 1.5 blood volumes of blood within a several hour period. If whole blood is not available and one uses packed red cells to support a massively bleeding patient, coagulation factor dilution will occur, most factors reaching levels of 20 to 30 per cent of normal after 1 to 1.5 blood volumes' replacement.

Although these general guidelines may be helpful, it is important to emphasize that identification and proper management of these hemostatic abnormalities depend on the availability of laboratory information. Microvascular bleeding in the face of massive transfusion should always prompt laboatory evaluation in the form of a coagulation screen, although one may administer components on the basis of likelihood while awaiting results. Laboratory results may reveal other pathogenetic mechanisms such as disseminated intravascular coagulation, necessitating a change in plans for component support.

Another issue occasionally raised in large volume transfusion is that of citrate toxicity. Citrate is the anticoagulant used by blood banks and works by chelation of calcium necessary for clotting. The concern is that in massive transfusion, the accompanying large citrate load may depress the recipient's ionized calcium levels to such an extent that cardiac arrhythmias may occur. Definitive studies are difficult to find, but it appears that, because of the rapid metabolism of citrate by the liver, clinically significant depression of serum calcium occurs only if the rate of blood administration exceeds 1 liter every 10 minutes. If this rate is exceeded, the administration of supplemental calcium may be appropriate.

Miscellaneous Red Cell Products

Leukopoor Red Cells. These are packed red cells from which most white blood cells have been removed. A variety of centrifugation or filtration procedures may be used for this purpose, most resulting in the removal of 90 to 98 per cent of the white cells in the original unit. With centrifugal procedures there is commonly an associated loss of approximately 20 per cent of the red cells, an important point to remember since patients may require more units of leukopoor cells to raise the hematocrit a given amount. If the preparation of this product requires entry into the closed blood bag system, these cells must be transfused within 24 hours of preparation. The only solid indication for the use of leukopoor red cells is in the transfusion of patients with a history of more than one nonhemolytic febrile transfusion reaction. Patients who have experienced only one febrile transfusion reaction have a low likelihood of experiencing another such reaction and are not candidates for leukopoor red cells.

Washed Red Cells. These have been washed one or more times with saline to remove plasma. Methods for doing this vary somewhat and include both manual and automated centrifugal washing procedures. Some preparations will also be leukopoor and, if so, will contain 20 per cent less red cells. Since the washing procedure requires entering the closed blood bag system, these products must be transfused within 24 hours of preparation. Indications for the use of washed red cells are not clearly defined. Reasonable candidates for washed red cells include patients with repeated severe immunologic reactions to plasma proteins, including IgA, and patients with immune hemolytic anemia in which complement-fixation may be important pathophysiologically and in which it may be desirable to avoid administration of additional complement. Washed leukopoor cells are sometimes advocated for patients with paroxysmal noctural hemoglobinuria to avoid any antigen-antibody reaction that may activate complement.

Frozen Red Cells. Red cells may be combined with a cryopreservative, glycerol, and frozen for up to 3 years. For transfusion these cells are thawed, deglycerolized, and washed. The washing and freezing procedure renders these cells essentially free of other cellular or plasma contamination. It has been claimed that transmission of viral disease by frozen cell preparations may be less than by standard products, but this has not been proved. The principal use of frozen cells is in inventory control and in storing cells of rare blood type. The primary disadvantage is that frozen cells are much more expensive to prepare than are standard products.

Fresh Whole Blood. One occasionally encounters requests for blood that is so fresh that all hemostatic components (and even undefined elements) are present in normal amounts. Such a product does not exist in modern blood banking. In the first place it is unnecessary; there is no known factor in fresh whole blood that cannot be obtained in one of the routinely available components. Second, it would be wasteful in that components not needed by the patient would be unavailable to other patients. Third, such a product would be unsafe since providing so fresh a product would preclude completion of normal blood processing and viral screening procedures.

Red Cell Substitutes. A number of nonred cell–containing oxygen-carrying substances are currently under investigation as possible red cell substitutes. These compounds, which include synthetic perfluorocarbons and stroma-free hemoglobin, are currently of interest for their potential use in emergency resuscitation, particularly under battlefield conditions, and as blood substitutes for patients objecting to transfusion on religious grounds. These substances are not licensed and are not currently available in the United States.

Components for Hemostasis

Platelets

Platelet concentrates are prepared from routinely donated units of blood. Platelet-rich plasma, generated by centrifugation of whole blood at moderate speed, is transferred to a satellite bag and centrifuged again at high speed. The resulting platelet pellet is resuspended in 50 to 75 ml of plasma. This concentrate, which contains 80 to 90 per cent of the platelets present in the initial unit of blood, can be stored for up to 7 days with agitation at room temperature without substantial loss of platelet viability. Platelets should not be refrigerated since they rapidly lose viability at 4 C. For adult recipients, platelets are pooled into transfusion doses of 4 to 8 units. Once pooled and removed from the controlled storage environment, they should be transfused within 2 to 4 hours. Transfusion is through a standard 170 micron blood filter, although physically smaller filters of the same mesh size are often used to minimize loss of the component in the tubing.

Ideally, platelets should be selected to be ABO-matched and Rh(D)-compatible with the recipient. There are several reasons for this. First, there is some evidence that ABO-incompatible platelets survive less well in the recipient than ABO-compatible platelets. Type A platelets given to a type O recipient, for example, may exhibit a 10 to 15 per cent smaller post-transfusion increment than would type O platelets. Second, there is the remote possibility that antibodies in the donor plasma (e.g., anti-A) could cause a hemolytic reaction in an ABO-incompatible recipient. Although these concerns direct our action in ideal circumstances, they are not major concerns, and it is frequently necessary, for inventory reasons, to administer ABO-incompatible platelets. More important than ABO matching is the necessity of providing Rh-negative platelets to Rh-negative recipients, particularly female recipients of child-bearing age. There are enough red cells in a platelet concentrate to result in sensitization of an Rh-negative patient.

The principal indication for platelet transfusion is treatment of bleeding due to thrombocytopenia. The level of thrombocytopenia at which bleeding is likely to occur depends upon the clinical situation. In an otherwise healthy individual, microvascular bleeding ordinarily does not occur until the platelet count has fallen below 5000 per microliter, reflecting the fact that the platelets, although decreased in number, are functionally normal. In patients with platelet dysfunction, bleeding may occur at platelet counts as high as 30,000 to 50,000 per microliter. Such platelet dysfunction may be seen in patients with malignancy, sepsis, DIC, and obstetric complications, and in those on a variety of antibiotics that may compromise platelet function. Patients with disrupted vessels (e.g., trauma victims or those undergoing surgery) may require platelet counts as high as 80,000 to 100,000 per microliter for adequate hemostasis, particularly if there is any associated platelet dysfunction. In patients undergoing cardiac bypass operations, platelets are rendered dysfunctional by the bypass pump, and thrombocytopenic bleeding may occur at platelet counts above 100,000 per microliter. Thus in considering platelet transfusion therapy for thrombocytopenic patients, it is important to understand the effect of the underlying clinical situation on platelet plug formation.

Platelet transfusion is indicated in patients who are bleeding and in whom the bleeding is considered, on the basis of the preceding considerations, to be due to thrombocytopenia. The exception to this is the patient with immune-mediated thrombocytopenia in whom platelet transfusions are usually not useful; in these patients transfusion is generally reserved for situations in which there is life-threatening bleeding. Increasing evidence is accumulating, however, that platelet survival in many patients with immune thrombocytopenia may not be so short as to preclude at least a transient beneficial effect of transfusion.

There is some controversy surrounding the proper use of prophylactic platelet transfusions. In patients with transient thrombocytopenia who are not bleeding, it is standard practice in most institutions to administer prophylactic platelet transfusions for platelet counts in the 10,000 to 20,000 range. Although the rationale in this sort of approach is to prevent life-threatening bleeding, particularly intracranial bleeding, very few patients develop intracranial bleeding in the absence of any other abnormal bleeding, and this practice has not been proved to be beneficial. In general, prophylactic transfusions should be given to patients with moderate to severe thrombocytopenia (50,000) who are about to undergo an invasive surgical procedure. In patients with long-term thrombocytopenia, alloimmunization is a significant problem, and the use of prophylactic transfusions should be much more conservative. Many patients with aplastic anemia, for instance, may have platelet counts below 2,000 to 3,000 and experience little if any bleeding.

If 1 unit of platelets is transfused into a normal-sized adult patient, the platelet count can be expected to increase by about 10,000 cells per microliter. Thus, depending on the clinical situation, 4 to 8 platelet concentrates are pooled to serve as a transfusion dose. Response to platelet transfusion is most appropriately assessed by obtaining a platelet count 1 hour after the transfusion. Suboptimal responses may be seen in patients with disorders associated with increased platelet consumption, and persistent bleeding can usually be successfully treated by the administration of additional platelets. Some patients may not respond at all, which is defined at our institution as failing to increase the 1 hour post-transfusion platelet count by 5,000 per microliter after 6 units of platelets on two consecutive occasions. This refractory state may be seen in patients with sepsis or splenomegaly or in patients who have become alloimmunized to random donor platelets.

Keeping in mind that alloimmunization occurs only in patients who have been previously sensitized by transfusion or pregnancy, patients who are refractory to random donor platelets and who might be alloimmunized may benefit from a trial of more closely matched single donor platelets. Matched donors may come from the patient's family or from available pools of HLA-typed community pheresis donors. If feasible, it is desirable to document alloimmunization by lymphocytotoxicity or platelet antibody testing. Collection of platelets from single donors requires that the donor be attached to a cell-separating machine for 1 to 2 hours. One ordinarily collects the equivalent of 6 units of platelets by this technique. The procedure for monitoring the success of platelet transfusions from these matched donors is identical to that for random platelet transfusions—that is, by determining the 1 hour post-transfusion platelet count.

Cryoprecipitate

Cryoprecipitate is prepared by rapidly freezing plasma to −70 C. The plasma is then warmed to 4 C and allowed to thaw. A small amount of precipitate forms, is separated from the bulk of the plasma, and is stored at −80 C as cryoprecipiate. Cryoprecipitate contains approximately half the factor VIII and one third of the fibrinogen that was in the original unit of plasma. It is thus essentially a factor VIII, fibrinogen concentrate and is primarily used to treat patients with deficiencies in these clotting proteins. For transfusion it is thawed and resuspended in the residual plasma or in saline, and the appropriate number of bags is pooled for transfusion. A transfusion dose for an adult usually consists of 10 to 20 bags.

The principal use of cryoprecipitate is in the treatment of patients with hemophilia A (factor VIII deficiency). It is the product of choice in the treatment of bleeding in patients with von Willebrand's disease. Patients with mild hemophilia and certain patients with von Willebrand's disease may be adequately treated with the synthetic vasopressin DDAVP and thus avoid the risks associated with the administration of any blood product. Cryoprecipitate is also used to treat bleeding due to fibrinogen deficiency, usually in patients with DIC with fibrinogen levels less than 100 mg per dl.

Fresh Frozen Plasma

Fresh frozen plasma is plasma that has been frozen immediately after centrifugal separation from the red cells during initial processing of blood. It can be stored for 1 year and contains all the coagulation factors in normal amounts. With few exceptions the only indications for the use of fresh frozen plasma are for documented deficiencies of clotting factors that are not more specifically treated with other components. In our institution the most common uses of fresh frozen plasma are (1) treatment of congenital deficiencies of coagulation factors, (2) rapid reversal of warfarin anticoagulation, (3) treatment of bleeding or potential bleeding (i.e., anticipated surgical procedure) in patients with factor deficiencies due to liver disease and in whom bleeding is not severe enough that replacement with whole blood will replenish these factors, and (4) massive transfusion when whole blood is not available. When fresh frozen plasma is indicated, it is important to give enough. One unit of plasma in a normal-sized adult recipient can be expected to raise the level of most coagulation factors by 2 to 3 per cent. Thus in most circumstances, 4 units of fresh frozen plasma is an appropriate adult dose. The optimal dose will obviously depend on the patient's pretransfusion factor levels, the patient's plasma volume, and the desired factor level to be obtained.

Factor Concentrates

Lyophilized factor VIII is a commercially prepared concentrate and provides support for most of the hemophilia A patients in the country. Although it is somewhat easier to use than cryoprecipitate, it is more expensive and carries a much higher risk of hepatitis, since it is prepared from pools of tens of thousands of units of plasma.

Prothrombin complex concentrate is a commercially prepared concentrate of factors II, VII, IX, and X. As with factor VIII concentrate, it is made from large pools of plasma and carries a high risk of post-transfusion hepatitis. These concentrates are used primarily for the treatment of patients with hemophilia B (factor IX deficiency) in whom the factor requirements are such that they cannot be met by fresh frozen plasma. They are also used with variable success to treat patients with hemophilia A who have factor VIII inhibitors. Presumably, small amounts of activated factors in these preparations bypass factor VIII–requiring steps in the coagulation cascade and allow clotting to occur. Prothrombin complex concentrates would seem an ideal preparation for the treatment of bleeding due to deficiencies of vitamin K–dependent factors, e.g., liver failure to warfarin anticoagulation. These concentrates should not be used for this purpose, however, because of the high risk of hepatitis and because intravascular clotting has been reported as an adverse reaction to these products, particularly in patients with liver disease.

Choice of Hemostatic Component

When faced with a patient with abnormal bleeding, deciding which blood components are needed, if any, obviously requires knowledge of the patient's history and physical findings. The most important information, however, usually comes from the laboratory. In general, adequate evaluation of the patient's hemostatic competency requires a complete coagulation screen to include prothrombin time, partial thromboplastin time, thrombin time, fibrinogen, and platelet count. The importance of including a measurement of fibrinogen is threefold. First, the fibrinogen level, along with the platelet count, is an important measure of the degree of DIC. Second, it is important to know whether the principal abnormality is hypofibrinogenemia, since proper therapy of this abnormality would be cropprecipitate rather than fresh frozen plasma. Third, if the fibrinogen level is less than 50 mg per dl, the amount of fibrinogen will be limiting in the other clotting tests, and any abnormalities seen in the prothrombin time and the partial thromboplastin times will be uninterpretable. Inclusion of the thrombin time is essential to rule out the possibility of heparin contamination of the sample. The thrombin time is very sensitive to small amounts of heparin that may be present—for example, if the sample is drawn out of an arterial line. It is critical to be able to detect this contamination and not administer blood components on the basis of artifactually prolonged coagulation tests. If significant microvascular bleeding is present and definite abnormalities in the coagulation screen are identified, it is usually possible to make an intelligent choice of blood components based on the knowledge of the contents of each component.

Frequently the question is whether or not the coagulation abnormalities are severe enough to warrant any blood component therapy. In most laboratories, prolongation of the prothrombin time by 2 to 3 seconds or the partial thromboplastin time by 5 to 10 seconds does not represent enough of an abnormality to suggest that component therapy is required. Significant hemostatic abnormalities are usually associated with prolongation of these tests to 1.5 times the control values. The sensitivity of these tests varies from one laboratory to another, however, and the proper interpretation of test results depends on adequate communication between the physician and the coagulation laboratory.

Other Products

Granulocytes

In a normal adult the turnover of neutrophils is approximately 65×10^9 per day. Values for patients with infection are not well defined but may be substantially higher. By contrast, the number of neutrophils in a unit of whole blood is on the order of 2×10^9. Thus, adequate doses of neutrophils for clinical transfusion can be obtained only if cell concentrates are prepared. This concentration is normally accomplished by leukapheresis of a normal donor, a procedure requiring that the donor be attached to a cell separator for 3 hours while approximately two blood volumes are processed. Adequate separation of neutrophils from red cells requires the addition of a red cell sedimenting agent to the donor's blood. Hydroxyethyl starch is generally used for this purpose. In addition, to achieve maximum yields of neutrophils donors are routinely premedicated with corticosteroids to mobilize marrow neutrophil reserves and thereby raise the circulating neutrophil count. One of the most effective premedication schedules involves the administration of 20 mg of prednisone 17, 12, and 3 hours before donation. With this regimen, an average of 30×10^9 neutrophils are collected per donation. Neutrophil concentrates prepared in this way contain 200 to 400 ml of plasma and 2 to 8 units of platelets, depending on the details of the collection procedure. Neutrophils should be kept at room temperature for any necessary storage period, but they should be administered as soon as possible after collection. After 24 hours' storage their function is severely impaired.

Neutrophils should be administered through a routine blood filter over 1 to 2 hours. Adverse effects of neutrophil transfusions include febrile and other allergic reactions; pulmonary adverse effects have been variably reported. Some studies have suggested that serious pulmonary reactions may occur in patients simultaneously receiving amphotericin, but most investigators have not confirmed this finding. It may be important to provide matched neutrophils for alloimmunized patients, but identification of these patients and matching procedures remain controversial. Because of the fact that neutrophil concentrates are heavily contaminated with red cells, however, neutrophil donors and recipients must be ABO-compatible.

Although the number of patients receiving neutrophil transfusions has deceased recently, in part because of improvement in antibiotic therapy, the indications for neutrophil transfusion remain the same as they have been for a number of years. In general, patients should be severely neutropenic (<200 cells per microliter at our institution). They should have a documented systemic infection (positive blood cultures) or a highly probable localized infection, such as pneumonia. Unexplained fever alone is not an indication for neutrophil support. In addition, patients should have failed to adequately respond to 24 to 48 hours of appropriate antibiotic therapy. Once the decision is made to provide neutrophil support, the usual approach is to provide daily transfusions until the patient recovers his or her own neutrophil count or until he has been free of all evidence of infection for several days.

A separate category of patients is that of newborn septic infants with depletion of marrow neutrophil reserves and often neutropenia. Such patients have been shown by some studies to benefit from neutrophil transfusions. In this clinical situation speed is important, and neutrophils should be provided within a few hours if possible. Usually only one transfusion is necessary. Our policy has been to collect neutrophils for these patients by the same leukapheresis procedure that we use for adults, except that we process only half the usual amount of blood and we do not premedicate the donor with corticosteroids. Neutrophil yields on the order of 5×10^9 are obtained by this technique. Some have advocated obtaining neutrophils for these neonates by centrifuging recently donated units of whole blood, but these techniques have not been rigorously shown to result in cells that function as well as those obtained by conventional leukapheresis.

Irradiated Blood Products

Graft-versus-host disease may occur as the result of immunocompetent lymphoid cells' being transfused into immunocompromised patients. Irradiation of lymphocyte-containing blood products with 1500 to 2500 rad inhibits the ability of the lymphoid cells to divide and eliminates the clinical problem. Only patients with severe immunodeficiency appear to be at significant risk for this complication, so it appears reasonable to provide irradiated blood products to premature infants, children with immunodeficiency syndromes, and patients undergoing bone marrow transplantation.

ADVERSE REACTIONS TO BLOOD TRANSFUSION

method of
R. BEN DAWSON, M.D.
University of Maryland
Baltimore, Maryland

Since this subject was addressed comprehensively by the American Association of Blood Banks in 1976, two procedures have greatly reduced the occurrence of hemolytic transfusion reactions and febrile and allergic transfusion reactions. The first is the use of a uniquely numbered armband and attached labels and tags for the sample drawn exclusively for blood typing and transfusion of a patient. The difference between "wrong-hung" units at university hospitals where no system is used and where the Fenwal Typenex system is used is 20 to none per year. The other development that greatly reduces rates of troublesome allergic and febrile transfusion reactions is the use of premedication with diphenhydramine (Benadryl) or acetaminophen (Tylenol) for a patient who has previously had a reaction. An equally effective approach to these common reactions is to supply washed red cells, although this is much more expensive. Thus, in a decade we have gone most of the way toward solving problems of acute hemolytic reactions and allergic and febrile reactions. The only other way to solve the "wrong-hung" units problem seems to be to establish a team of transfusion nurses and let no one else hang blood units, but this has been carried out only in a few hospitals.

The remaining serious and often unrecognized immunologic complication of blood transfusion is the delayed hemolytic transfusion reaction. There were references to it 10 years ago and it is being referred to again in the 1980s as an all too common, but often unrecognized, transfusion complication. Our estimate is approximately 10 cases per year when 30,000 red cell units are given to 10,000 patients.

The major infectious disease transmitted by transfusion continues to be hepatitis, but the most serious one clearly is acquired immune deficiency syndrome (AIDS). Early in 1983 we began disqualifying donors in the United States who were in any of the high risk groups for AIDS. At the time we did not know the magnitude or many details of the transfusion-transmitted AIDS problem, as the long incubation period of usually 2 years had revealed only a few cases. By 1984 it was obvious that 70 transfusion-associated AIDS patients had not been members of high risk groups. On the average, these had received five times as much blood as other transfused patients; of those whose blood sources had been traced, almost all had at least one blood donor who belonged to a high risk group. Thus, the action early in 1983 of disqualifying AIDS risk group members from blood donation may have almost stopped the occurrence of transfusion-transmitted AIDS. Since the high risk AIDS groups are also high risk hepatitis groups, we may also have greatly reduced transfusion-transmitted hepatitis. A warning is in order, however: these predictions are more hopes than expectations. An example of the need for such a warning is the hepatitis antigen testing of blood donations that began in 1972 that had only a modest effect on reducing post-transfusion hepatitis. There is no question that it reduced transmission of hepatitis B virus, but it revealed the hardly expected presence of other, non-A, non-B hepatitis viruses. In the United States, in 1985 compulsory testing began of all blood units for antibody against the AIDS virus, HTLV-III.

Immediate Complications

IMMUNE Hemolytic Reactions

As little as 100 ml of incompatible blood can lead to the death of a recipient during or several hours after the transfusion. Immune lysis of the infused red cells is the most severe complication of a blood transfusion because it may be followed by shock, acute renal failure, or a hemorrhagic diathesis secondary to disseminated intravascular coagulation (DIC).

Clerical or administrative errors by those certifying compatibility and by personnel performing the transfusion are the main cause of this complication.

Red cell lysis results when naturally occurring patient anti-A or anti-B antibodies react with incompatible transfused red cells. Salvage of the patient requires prompt recognition of the problem and treatment.

The critical signs, not all of which may be present, are shock, hemoglobinuria, oliguria, and bleeding, any of which is an absolute indication for terminating the transfusion and instituting therapy. Although subsequent laboratory studies may be useful, the immediate detection of adverse effects and institution of prompt treatment must depend primarily upon clinical evidence. The clinical signs in the anesthetized surgical patient may be overlooked inadvertently; these signs include variable degrees of shock and generalized blood loss or oozing from all surgical wound surfaces owing to accelerated (disseminated) intravascular coagulation.

Additional signs and symptoms of incompatible blood transfusion include chills, fever, flank pain, diaphoresis, and a burning sensation at the site or in the arm receiving the transfusion. The patient also may have tachycardia, tachypnea, hypotension, and, in massive reactions, vascular collapse. Management of uncontrollable hypotension during acute hemolytic reactions should be of utmost concern since it is now considered the most frequent cause of death in the United States from incompatible transfusion.

Management

1. Stop the transfusion, but maintain venous access with an infusion of isotonic saline solution.
2. Consult the blood bank immediately and ascertain whether the right unit was administered to the right patient. Then determine whether the test for compatibility was actually performed on the correct patient's blood sample with the correct donor blood sample. Finally, determine whether two patients have been involved. If so, attempt to prevent the transfusion of the second patient.
3. Blood and urine samples should be obtained and sent to the laboratory. With respect to technique, the most significant error to be avoided is the artificial induction of hemolysis in the first post-transfusion specimen of blood. This can be prevented only through careful venipuncture following minimal stasis and probing and by the use of chemically clean and dry equipment.
4. Table 1 describes the major laboratory findings. These are comparison of hemoglobin in the patient's carefully drawn pre- and post-transfusion plasma samples, and the direct antiglobulin (Coombs') test (DAT). Clear plasma and a negative DAT give assurance that hemolysis, if present, is not great.
5. Table 2 provides supportive laboratory find-

TABLE 1. **Major Laboratory Findings in Transfusion Reactions**

Comparisons for Hemoglobin
Pre- and post-transfusion samples
1. Visual examination
Normal plasma Hb is 2 to 3 mg per dl
Pink plasma indicates Hb concentration of at least 20 mg per dl
Red plasma indicates Hb concentration in range of 30 mg or more per dl
2. Crosby-Furth test on negative suspect plasma
Detection of Red Blood Cells Coated with Antibody in Vivo
Patient's post-transfusion red blood cell sample
Direct antiglobulin (Coombs') test gives a positive reaction with donor cells coated with incomplete antibody from patient's serum

TABLE 2. **Supportive Laboratory Findings in Transfusion Reactions**

Detection of Hemoglobinuria
Post-transfusion urine specimen
Visual examination (pink, red, or brown urine) indicates presence of free hemoglobin ruled in or out microscopically
Detection of Bilirubinemia
Pre- and post-transfusion samples
1. Visual examination
Light yellow color with normal plasma
Intense yellow from increased bilirubin following hemolysis by 4–6 hr
Peak concentration reached in 5 days
2. Perform usual quantative determinants

ings. In addition, coagulation studies should be considered along with blood urea nitrogen and creatinine.

Should this early schema of testing (plasma hemoglobin and direct antiglobulin test) prove positive and confirm an acute hemolytic reaction, therapy should be directed toward prevention of shock, renal complications, and disseminated intravascular coagulation. Consultation with a nephrologist, pathologist, and hematologist is indicated.

If shock is present, maintenance of renal blood flow and prevention of renal shutdown should be attempted by the following measures:

1. Mannitol, administered promptly in an initial dose of 12.5 to 25 grams intravenously in a 20 per cent aqueous solution, will prevent and in some cases reverse early renal shutdown. The initial dose may be followed by additional 25 gram doses as necessary (up to 150 grams daily) to provide a urine flow of at least 50 ml hourly. If, despite 25 grams of mannitol and adequate hydration, sufficient urinary flow has not resulted, one must consider the addition of furosemide.
2. Give 40 to 80 mg of furosemide (Lasix) intravenously as an initial dose. This dose may be repeated once. Lack of a diuretic response in 2 or 3 hours indicates the presence of acute renal failure, and renal dialysis should be considered. The pediatric dose of furosemide is 1 to 2 mg per kg.
3. When furosemide is used, the danger of excessive diuresis contributing to reduced blood volume and circulatory collapse must be anticipated by appropriate hydration. This is accomplished by administering 1000 ml of 5 per cent dextrose in 0.45 per cent saline solution or 1000 ml of isotonic saline solution in a 1 hour period. An additional 500 ml may be given if within the first hour urine output has not reached 1 to 1.5 ml per kg per hour. Fluid loading should be performed with caution. If no diuretic response is observed within 2 hours, further fluid and diuretic administration is unlikely to be effective and may be harmful. The patient should be treated for acute tubular necrosis.

Disseminated Intravascular Coagulation (DIC). This can occur after an acute hemolytic reaction resulting from incompatible blood transfusion, especially ABO incompatibility. DIC leads to the production of degradation products of fibrin which interfere with platelet function and result in generalized bleeding. Coagulation studies are critical. The presence of fibrin degradation products in the patient's plasma associated with generalized bleeding warrants the consideration of prophylactic heparinization. Heparin may be effective in preventing further DIC or lessening its intensification. Further red cell destruction may be prevented through its anticomplementary effect. Heparin therapy is not without risk and should be restricted to those patients in whom an acute hemolytic reaction has been confirmed.

Prophylactic heparinization for an adult patient—continuous intravenous infusion of heparin with 5000 units as a loading dose, followed by 1500 units per hour. Once instituted, heparin therapy should be continued for at least 6 to 24 hours until the likelihood of DIC has passed.

Depleted blood components can be replaced with platelet concentrate or cryoprecipitates for factor VIII and fibrinogen to counter bleeding attributable to deficiencies of these during the administration of heparin.

Prophylactic heparinization should be withheld if its use in patients with exposed surgical fields poses a complication in the management of hypotension and shock.

The primary concern in patients with DIC, except in rare cases, is not bleeding but clotting. When bleeding occurs, there has already been massive intravascular clotting, enough to have consumed significant quantities of critical clotting factors.

Febrile Transfusion Reactions. In patients who have been previously transfused or are pregnant, a reaction often is observed during or following transfusion of blood or blood components, caused by platelets or leukocytes. The reaction may include fever, fatigue, malaise, chills, headache, and tachycardia. Red cell lysis does not cause fever, but, if red cells have been transfused, visual examination of plasma for hemoglobin should be performed to rule out a hemolytic reaction occurring as well.

Febrile reactions are caused by reactions of preformed recipient alloantibodies with donor leukocytes and platelets that carry allotype antigens.

Treatment is symptomatic with the use of antipyretics, but aspirin should be avoided if bleeding or thrombocytopenia is a problem. Acetaminophen (Tylenol) is the usual drug.

These reactions can be reduced by the use of leukocyte-poor red blood cells or HLA-compatible platelets. More effective, however, is the elimination of platelets, leukocytes, and plasma proteins by red cell washing. Sometimes the use of frozen, deglycerolized red blood cells is necessary.

Granulocyte transfusions are associated with an increased frequency of reactions which include chills, fever, and hypotension. Reactions have been reported associated with HLA-specific leukocyte antigens in donor plasma and in the serum of patients. In addition to the symptoms mentioned, leukocyte antibody-induced reactions produce pulmonary infiltrates seen on chest radiographs, suggesting pulmonary edema.

Allergic and Anaphylactic Transfusion Reactions. Allergic reactions were a consistent problem with reusable glass bottles and rubber donor sets, running as high as 40 to 60 per cent of all transfusions given. With the advent of plastic bags and integral donor and recipient tubing, the incidence of urticaria has decreased to 1 to 3 per cent. If fever is present, a hemolytic reaction should be ruled out by immunologic laboratory tests, even though red blood cell lysis may not be apparent. Once this rule-out testing confirms a simple allergic or urticarial reaction, patients may be treated as follows:

1. Antihistamines such as diphenhydramine (Benadryl). Give 50 to 100 mg intramuscularly or intravenously.
2. If bronchospasms occur, 125 to 250 mg of aminophylline may be given intravenously over 5 minutes. If indicated, provide oxygen.
3. In severe cases, it may be necessary to give hydrocortisone, 200 mg intravenously, or adrenergic drugs.

Prevention of allergic reactions in patients who have repeated episodes may be accomplished by the use of packed red blood cells or, if necessary, washed red cells; in extreme cases, frozen-thawed-deglycerolized red cells which are free of plasma may be given.

IgA Reactions. Anaphylactic transfusion reactions occur dramatically and rapidly following the initial infusion of blood or plasma. Symptoms include marked dyspnea, wheezing, flushing, and hypotension, and death can occur. Anaphylactic reactions are attributed to anti-immunoglobulin sensitization and are particularly associated with the formation of anti-IgA antibodies. These reactions can occur in patients with no history of transfusion or pregnancy. Patients with clinical IgA reactions to transfusion fall into two general groups: (1) those people congenitally deficient in IgA who have developed an anti-IgA and manifest an anaphylactic response to transfusion of blood products containing IgA globulins. These anti-IgA antibodies have a broad reactivity and have been termed class-specific; and (2) those who receive multiple transfusions—they have weaker anti-IgA titers and have reactions characterized by urticaria and by anaphylactoid symptoms. These anti-IgA antibodies are described as having a limited specificity.

TREATMENT. 1. Stop the transfusion immediately; maintain intravenous access with a saline infusion; administer no blood products until the cause of the reaction has been determined. 2. Administer 0.5 ml of 1:1000 epinephrine and 250 to 500 mg of hydrocortisone intravenously. 3. Oxygen may be required.

Prevention of such reactions depends on the avoidance of IgA in future transfusions. The sensitized patient will react to even trace amounts of the immunoglobulin. It has been estimated that safe donors for these patients (IgA-deficient donors) occur about 1 in 700 donors in the United States. A registry of blood donors lacking serum IgA has been established at the University of California Medical Center, San Francisco. Suitable donors may be identified through the rare donor files of the American Association of Blood Banks and the American Red Cross Blood Services. These patients should be told the nature of the problem and be issued "medical alert" information.

Pulmonary Hypersensitivity. Transfusions with granulocytes cause this reaction, which is characterized by dyspnea, cyanosis, and chest radiographs showing patchy pulmonary infiltrates. The reaction is currently attributed to antileukocyte antibodies due to passively transfused antibodies reacting with the recipient's autologous leukocytes, or to recipient alloimmunity to granulocyte transfusions. Treatment consists of epinephrine, steroids, and standard measures for pulmonary edema.

NONIMMUNE Immediate Reactions

Air Embolism. From the inadvertent introduction of air by vein, air embolism causes chest pain, cough, and dyspnea. The patient should be positioned head down on the left side, and, if necessary, the right heart should be aspirated to remove the air.

Circulatory Overload. This is a common complication of whole blood transfusion, especially in treating infants or elderly patients. Congestive failure resulting from circulatory overload is easily recognized. The transfusion should be stopped, the patient placed in a sitting position, and the need for phlebotomy considered. Tightly packed red blood cells, rather than whole blood, are less likely to cause circulatory overload, especially when the patient is transfused in a sitting position. In unusual circumstances it may be necessary to administer small amounts of packed red blood cells (1 ml per kg per hour).

Contaminated Blood and Septicemia. Plastic bags and closed tubing systems of harvest and transfer have greatly reduced this problem. Gram-negative organisms, such as *Pseudomonas, Enterobacter, Citrobacter, Serratia,* and *Escherichia,* do cause transfusion reactions, and some capable of growing at refrigerator temperature are classified as cryophilic. As little as 50 ml of blood contaminated with endotoxin from bacteria can cause hypotension, fever, shaking chills, and death.

Wright's stain and Gram stain smears should be performed to identify the bacteria, with immediate administration of appropriate antibiotics intravenously. Supportive therapy for shock caused by sepsis should include consultation with a physician experienced in septic shock treatment. A further complication could be a bleeding diathesis caused by DIC secondary to the sepsis.

Other Sequelae of Massive Transfusion. POTASSIUM TOXICITY (HYPERKALEMIA). The potassium level of plasma in stored whole blood normally is found to be 4 mM at 4 C. Blood stored for more than 5 days has elevated levels of plasma potassium as intracellular potassium continues to leave the red blood cells. However, potassium reenters the red cells after transfusion and warming in vivo, sometimes resulting in hypokalemia. The major concern of potassium toxicity is for patients in renal failure and neonates receiving exchange transfusions for whom red cells or whole blood less than 5 days old is recommended. Alternatively, patients with a critical potassium level can be given frozen-washed, packed red cells and carefully monitored.

CITRATE TOXICITY (HYPOCALCEMIA). The anticoagulant solution of citrate-phosphate-dextrose (CPD) contains approximately 4.7 mM of citrate which ensures anticoagulation but is not sufficient to lower the serum calcium level of a normally transfused recipient. The exceptions to this, however, are patients with severe liver disease, those receiving massive transfusions, and infants treated by exchange transfusion. These patients should receive packed red cells or frozen-deglycerolized cells. There is a reported relationship between citrate toxicity, a fall in the ionized calcium level, changes in the serum pH, and potassium levels. Citrate toxicity is generally characterized by electrocardiographic changes and muscle tremors. The prophylactic use of calcium in patients receiving massive transfusions but not complicated by hypocalcemia has been associated with the production of ventricular arrhythmias and is not recommended. Should the patient have EKG changes (prolonged ST and QT segments) or laboratory-demonstrated hypocalcemia, therapy consists of 5 to 10 ml (adult dose) of 10 per cent calcium gluconate given intravenously. It should be considered prophylactically in massive transfusion when whole blood is given at a rate greater than 100 ml per minute but is not necessary when packed red cells or additive solution red cells are used with colloids and crystalloids.

HYPOTHERMIA. Patients receiving large volumes of 4 C stored blood have experienced lowered body temperature, cardiac arrhythmia, and arrest. During the past decade and a half, a number of maneuvers have been tried to warm the blood before transfusion. These include passing the blood through coils submersed in 37 C water baths and electronic heating devices. As currently as 1980, such practices have at times caused the red cells to completely hemolyze, resulting in death of the recipient, especially infants undergoing exchange transfusion. Blood warming in infants and in massive transfusion should be done when necessary by using an approved warming device equipped with an alarm that will sound if the temperature exceeds 38 C.

DILUTIONAL EFFECTS OF STORED BLOOD: COAGULOPATHY CAUSED BY DILUTION OF PLATELETS AND LABILE PLASMA COAGULATION FACTORS. Collins and associates in 1967–1968 reported that transfusion of combat casualties is accompanied by dilutional coagulation defects compatible with the level of coagulation factors in stored bank blood. Whereas during transfusion platelet levels fall to hemostatically compromising levels of less than 100,000 per cu mm, the prothrombin times, partial thromboplastin times, and fibrinogen levels are less severely affected. Significant operative bleeding is not encouraged in conjunction with these mild dilutional coagulation changes. A partial return of the coagulation factors toward normal is accomplished by administration of stored whole blood to casualties who develop coagulation defects secondary to shock. With the exception of factors V and VIII, all coagulation factors are present in significant amounts in banked whole blood. Fresh-frozen plasma contains normal levels of all clotting factors and is the only source for all factors. The minimum concentration of clotting factors needed to maintain hemostasis is relatively low, about 30 per cent of normal for factors VIII and IX, fibrinogen, and prothrombin and probably 10 per cent for factors V, VII, X, XI, XII, and XIII.

Patients with bleeding problems following massive transfusion of blood and resuscitative fluids (dilutional effect) who demonstrate thrombocytopenia, by count or smear, usually respond to the administration of sufficient platelet concentrates to correct the thrombocytopenia, often 4 to 8 units.

If bleeding persists after platelet therapy, the other causes of bleeding must be ruled out: acute hemolytic transfusion reaction; heparin; and DIC.

The exclusion of these factors strengthens the case for the cause of bleeding being dilutional coagulopathy other than thrombocytopenia, especially with prolonged activated partial thromboplastin time and thrombin time. Therapy would then consist of fresh-frozen plasma and occasionally cryoprecipitates as a source of concentrated factor VIII and fibrinogen.

OTHER COMPLICATIONS OF BLOOD TRANSFUSIONS. 1. Microaggregates are only a theoretic complication of infusing whole blood or red cells that have been stored for longer than 7 days. By this time microaggregates develop and then can be removed by any one of several special "microaggregate filters," which have pore sizes of 20 to 40 microns. The standard blood filter with a pore size of 170 microns is sufficient and is used in all transfusions of blood cells. There is no clinical evidence for the efficacy of "microaggregate filters;" thus, they are not recommended.

2. Metabolic characteristics of stored red cells include depletion of 2,3-diphosphoglycerate (DPG) by 14 days after blood collection. This defect in older, transfused red cells is corrected by the recipient in 6 to 12 hours. It is of no consequence to most patients receiving supplemental augmentation of their red cell mass. Further, most blood units will be less than 14 days old upon transfusion. However, for some, in whom immediate correction of a deficiency in oxygen transport is essential, provision of red cells with normal hemoglobin-oxygen affinity (normal DPG levels) is assured by giving units that are not over 10 days old or by treating older units with a licensed rejuvenation solution.

Delayed Complications

Hemolytic

Delayed hemolytic transfusions occur several days to weeks following a compatible transfusion and result in hemolysis and anemia. The sequence of events involves a patient sensitized to blood group antigens by previous transfusion or pregnancy. At the time of cross-match, the antibodies in the patient's serum were too low to be detected by antigens on the donor's red blood cells when tested by current required procedures, including the antihuman globulin test. An anamnestic response following transfusion of the incompatible red cells results in hemolysis of the transfused cells some time later. Death can also result from delayed reactions, therefore the same protocol should be used as in the case of a suspected acute hemolytic reaction. Since many delayed transfusion reactions are subclinical, the reaction can easily go unnoticed. The few signs are a mild transient hyperbilirubinemia, a brief fall in hemoglobin and hematocrit, and the development of one or more atypical red blood cell antibodies.

Post-Transfusion Purpura. In this syndrome, profound thrombocytopenia develops approximately 1 week after a transfusion in association with the formation of platelet alloantibodies. The antigen Pl^{A1}, located on the platelets of 98 per cent of the population, produces in some individuals with Pl^{A1}-negative platelets a potent complement-fixing antibody. When a Pl^{A1}-negative patient with an anti-Pl^{A1} antibody receives a further transfusion stimulus, profound thrombocytopenia may develop. The antibody developed has such a broad reactivity that not only transfused platelets but also the patient's own platelets are destroyed. The syndrome may be life-threatening and lasts 1 or more weeks. The transfusion of small amounts of plasma (10 ml) to normal individuals containing potent platelet alloantibodies can produce profound thrombocytopenia. It is the one clear situation in which a single, one plasma volume–plasma exchange reverses the clinical manifestations and is thus curative for the episode.

Graft-Versus-Host (GVH) Reaction. This represents the clinical and pathologic sequela of the reactions of immunocompetent cells (lymphocytes or their precursors) in a graft against the cells of the histoincompatible and immunodeficient recipient.

The main features are severe diarrhea, dermatitis, fever, and lymphadenopathy. The mortality is high. GVH disease has occurred in children with immunologic deficiency states following transfusion of whole blood from normal donors. In addition, GVH disease has resulted when patients received white cell transfusions from normal donors and those with chronic myelogenous leukemia. Prevention is currently attempted by irradiation with 1500 rad prior to infusion of blood components containing lymphocytes, such as whole blood, packed red blood cells, platelet concentrates, and granulocyte concentrates when such products are to be transfused to patients with primary or acquired immunodeficiency states. Some transfusion services irradiate with as high as 3000 rad.

Transfusional Hemosiderosis. Hemosiderosis, increased iron deposits in tissues, is often seen in nonbleeding patients after multiple transfusions. The body normally excretes 1 mg of iron per day. Each unit of whole blood and packed red blood cells represents about 225 to 250 mg of elemental iron. In transfusion hemosiderosis the serum iron concentration is raised and the iron-binding capacity of the serum is fully saturated. The serum ferritin level is the best index of the body stores. Therefore, large numbers of transfusions in an individual may lead to high tissue iron concentrations and severe complications. These complications in patients who have long-term chronic transfusion needs, such as in thalassemia major, have been treated with deferoxamine (Desferal), a compound that chelates iron. However, whether constant subcutaneous infusion of deferoxamine, achieved by an infusion pump, will be successful in preventing the life-threatening complications of severe iron overload, such as cardiomyopathy, is not determined.

Current therapy includes the use of fresh red blood cells or frozen-deglycerolized red blood cells to minimize transfusional hemosiderosis and, where available, "neocytes"—specially collected young red cells with a nearly two times longer lifespan than ordinary blood bank red cells.

Disease Transmission. The most common and clinically important diseases transmitted by transfusion are hepatitis, malaria, and syphilis. Although uncommon, acquired immune deficiency syndrome (AIDS) has become the most severe disease transmitted by transfusion.

HEPATITIS. The Centers for Disease Control reported in 1979 that 1 million cases of viral hepatitis infection of all types occur each year. This includes both clinical and subclinical infections. During this period, 26,000 cases of confirmed or suspected infections with hepatitis B virus (HBV) and 31,000 cases of infections with hepatitis A virus (HAV) were reported.

The CDC then estimated that 5 to 15 per cent of all transfused patients will suffer hepatitis damage after being transfused. Individual differences depend on whether the source of blood is volunteer or paid, as well as on the number of units the patient receives. The CDC further estimated that 200,000 cases of transfusion-associated hepatitis occur each year. In the United States, non-A, non-B post-transfusion hepatitis (PTH) accounts for approximately 90 per cent of cases. Since 1970, when HBsAg screening began, the risk of hepatitis B associated with transfusion has dropped from 4.8 to 0.8 per cent. The major form of PTH is not associated with HAV and HBV but rather non-A, non-B. Control of PTH now requires the elimination of carriers of hepatitis B and non-A, non-B as blood donors.

Avoidance of blood products of concentrated coagulation factors made commercially from large pools of donor plasma should be standard procedure when the risk of PTH is under consideration; rather, multiple units of single donor components should be considered. The exception is for those products prepared from plasma pools that are without risk of PTH; these include albumin, gamma globulin, and plasma protein fraction (PPF). The same principles about PTH transmission apply to AIDS transmission.

MALARIA. Although rare, malarial parasites can be transmitted in liquid blood stored at 4 C and in red cells stored at much lower (frozen) temperatures. Parasites involved are *Plasmodium vivax, P. malariae,* or *P. falciparum.* The disease, marked by fever that is typically recurrent, occurs within 7 days of the infecting transfusion and is amenable to specific therapy.

SYPHILIS. Syphilis resulting from blood transfusion has an incubation period of 4 to 18 weeks (average, 9 to 10 weeks). The patient exhibits a typical secondary eruption. The problem is observed more often following the use of very fresh components such as platelets. The donors are usually seronegative because spirochetemia is more likely in the absence of demonstrable serum antibody. Blood stored at 4 C for 4 days, frozen red cells, frozen plasma, or frozen plasma components are least likely to contain viable treponemes. Diagnosis and treatment are as with other cases of syphilis.

OTHER BLOOD-TRANSMITTED DISEASES. These include brucellosis, trypanosomiasis, bartonellosis, cytomegalic viral disease, and infectious mononucleosis. Also reported are Chagas' disease, salmonellosis, typhus, and Rocky Mountain spotted fever.

Section 6

The Digestive System

BLEEDING ESOPHAGEAL VARICES

method of
ALBERT J. CZAJA, M.D.
Mayo Clinic
Rochester, Minnesota

Although bleeding from esophageal varices accounts for only 10 per cent of all cases of gastrointestinal hemorrhage, it has the highest immediate mortality. Death occurs in 30 to 80 per cent of the cases after the first episode of bleeding, usually within 6 weeks. Of survivors, bleeding recurs in 70 per cent, commonly within 6 weeks after the first hemorrhage; the mortality of each recurrence averages 50 per cent.

The principal objective of treatment is to restore and maintain hemodynamic stability. Mortality increases markedly after 48 hours of continuous bleeding, and treatment efforts must be vigorous within this period. Fortunately, bleeding can be controlled rapidly in 90 per cent of patients by nonoperative measures. Variceal hemorrhage, however, commonly recurs. The most effective form of long-term management remains controversial. The severity of the underlying liver disease rather than the specific method of preventing rebleeding seems to be the most important determinant of longevity.

MANAGEMENT

Resuscitation

Clinical Assessment

A systolic blood pressure of less than 100 mm Hg and a pulse rate of greater than 100 beats per minute connote at least a 20 per cent reduction in blood volume. An orthostatic blood pressure drop of more than 10 mm Hg reflects a blood loss of at least 1 liter and correlates more closely with volume changes than the pulse rate. Under such circumstances, intravenous replacement therapy is essential to preserve renal perfusion and minimize liver cell anoxia. Too vigorous resuscitation, however, may be hazardous, especially in the elderly patient with precarious cardiac function. Additionally, the portal pressure is influenced by changes in blood volume, and overexpansion may prolong the bleeding episode or precipitate rebleeding.

Volume Replacement

Intravenous access must be established immediately, and a large bore catheter is preferred. Since the mean number of blood transfusions during the first 24 hours is 3.8 and the mean total during hospitalization is 11, preparations should be made for the delivery of large volumes of blood. At least three units of stored bank blood should be available at all times. The placement of an additional intravenous line is wise in the unstable patient.

Crystalloid solutions (isotonic saline or Ringer's lactate) are appropriate until blood typing and cross matching are completed. Initial blood studies should include hemoglobin level, platelet count, creatinine level, prothrombin time, activated partial thromboplastin time, electrolyte levels, and glucose concentration.

Monitoring Mechanisms

Blood replacement should be guided by hemodynamic assessments rather than hematocrit determinations. Arterial blood pressure and urine output should be monitored closely and a central venous pressure line placed if bleeding is active. If hemodynamic instability is evident, renal function is impaired, or cardiac failure is imminent, a Swan-Ganz catheter should be positioned to assess pulmonary artery and wedge pressures, cardiac index, and peripheral vascular resistance. When the blood pressure is restored to low normal and urine output is increased to 50 ml per hour, the volume of intravenous infusions can be reduced to match losses. A hematocrit between 30 and 35 is adequate for oxygen transport.

Hemostasis

Stored bank blood will provide factors VII, IX, X and prothrombin, but transfusions of fresh blood, fresh frozen plasma, or platelets may be necessary to restore the more labile factors. Two units of platelets and one unit of fresh frozen plasma should be administered after every transfusion of five or more units of stored whole blood or packed red blood cells. For severe hypoprothrombinemia, two to three units of fresh frozen plasma should be infused over a 3 hour period and vitamin K_1 (phytonadione), 10 to 25 mg intramuscularly, should be given.

Supportive Measures

Manifestations of respiratory distress or aspiration justify placement of an endotracheal tube. This should be done in patients with active bleeding who require gastric lavage, endoscopic examination, or balloon tamponade. Additionally, efforts to treat or prevent hepatic encephalopathy should be instituted. Purgation of the gastrointestinal tract with cleansing saline enemas will reduce protein catabolism and ammonia production. After the bleeding has subsided, lactulose (Cephulac), 60 to 120 ml daily, can be given in divided doses by mouth or nasogastric tube. If severe encephalopathy is unimproved, solutions containing high concentrations of branched chain amino acids and low levels of aromatic amino acids (Hepatamine) can be administered intravenously. Approximately 25 calories per kilogram body weight should be provided daily, mainly as an intravenous glucose infusion.

Control of Bleeding

Gastric Lavage

A nasogastric tube should be placed and the stomach lavaged with iced saline or tap water. The contribution of lavage to hemostasis is uncertain, but over 30 per cent of patients stop bleeding during this manuever. Lavage permits assessment of bleeding activity and prepares the upper gastrointestinal tract for endoscopic examination. Vigorous bleeding justifies passage of an orogastric tube (36 French Edlich tube) to evacuate large clots. Tube placement has not been shown to aggravate the varices or perpetuate the bleeding.

Endoscopic Examination

Emergency fiberoptic examination of the upper gastrointestinal tract is essential to establish the site of bleeding and target further therapeutic activities. Portal hypertension predisposes to erosive gastritis as well as to esophageal varices, and as many as 50 per cent of patients with cirrhosis and esophageal varices bleed from a nonvariceal site.

The overall diagnostic accuracy of endoscopic assessment is 67 per cent. Identification of the bleeding site is most likely if the examination is performed within three hours. If vigorous hemorrhage precludes immediate passage of the instrument, the procedure can be deferred until the bleeding abates during the period of lavage and transfusion or after administration of intravenous vasopressin. Gastroesophageal tamponade should never be attempted without endoscopic confirmation of variceal bleeding. If a diagnosis cannot be established because of brisk hemorrhage, emergency visceral angiography should be performed.

Vasopressin (Pitressin) Infusion

Vasopressin should be administered as a continuous intravenous infusion (0.2 to 0.4 units per minute) if bleeding continues after resuscitation and lavage. The drug reduces portal pressure by lowering portal vascular resistance and decreasing splanchnic blood flow. Additionally, vasopressin may diminish flow through the varices by contracting the esophageal musculature. A continuous infusion reduces the wedged hepatic vein pressure by 29 per cent and terminates bleeding in 50 to 86 per cent of patients. Peripheral intravenous administration is as effective as selective intra-arterial infusion and more effective than intermittent intravenous bolus therapy.

Complications of vasopressin infusion reflect mainly the drug's systemic circulatory effects. Reductions in hepatic blood flow and cardiac output may provoke hepatic ischemia, abdominal cramps, bowel ischemia, cardiac arrhythmia, or myocardial infarction. Enchancement of peripheral vascular resistance may increase arterial blood pressure and reduce heart rate, whereas tissue extravasation of the drug may produce a gangrenous extremity. Hyponatremia is usually a consequence of excessive antidiuretic activity.

Side effects can be minimized if vasopressin is administered in low dose under close supervision to adequately resuscitated patients. Continuous electrocardiographic monitoring is advisable during the infusion, and the drug should never be given to patients with myocardial ischemia or shock. Adjunctive use of sublingual nitroglycerin (Nitrostat, 0.4 mg) may improve the hemodynamic response.

Other pharmacologic approaches requiring further assessment and of limited availability include the use of a vasopression analogue (triglycyl lysine vasopressin) and somatostatin. The former drug can be given every 6 hours as a 2 mg intravenous bolus; a more prolonged vasomotor action and fewer side effects than the conventional vasopressin infusion are potential advantages. The latter drug reduces regional splanchnic blood flow and portal pressure in a highly selective fashion when infused intravenously at a constant rate of 7.5 micrograms per minute. Additionally, somatostatin strongly inhibits gastric acid secretion.

Bleeding is usually controlled soon after the institution of vasopressin therapy. The infusion, however, should be maintained for an additional 6 to 12 hours before tapered discontinuation over a 6 hour period.

Balloon Tamponade

Bleeding that originates from esophageal varices and that has not stopped during the first 2 hours after intravenous vasopressin infusion requires balloon tamponade. The triple lumen Sengstaken-Blakemore tube has been used most commonly for this purpose but it necessitates passage of a small nasogastric tube above the inflated esophageal balloon to aspirate secretions. Quadruple lumen tubes, such as the Minnesota tube, permit removal of secretions above the esophageal balloon, thereby reducing the risk of pulmonary aspiration.

Although the multiple lumen tube can be introduced through the mouth, it is better tolerated through the nasal passageway. Placement in the stomach can be verified by auscultation over the area after air insufflation, and the gastric balloon can then be partially inflated with 50 ml of air. After confirmation of appropriate positioning by chest roentgenogram, the gastric balloon can be inflated to its capacity and drawn up tightly against the gastroesophageal junction. Strong traction is not necessary and may be harmful. The tube can be adequately secured by taping to the nose, face mask of a football helmet, or split tennis ball. If bleeding continues, the esophageal balloon should be inflated to the minimal pressure that exceeds variceal pressure (25 to 40 mm Hg). A pair of scissors should be taped to the bedpost for rapid transection of the tube and deflation of the balloons if pulmonary distress develops.

Balloon tamponade stops bleeding in 70 to 88 per cent of cases, especially if instituted within 6 hours after onset. Control is obtained more frequently after the first bleed than after recurrences. Although permanent hemostasis may be achieved after one to three treatments, rebleeding after deflation is common (24 to 64 per cent) and the mortality is 60 per cent. Complications occur in 9 to 39 per cent of patients and include aspiration, esophageal rupture, pressure necrosis, esophageal stenosis, and respiratory obstruction.

Tamponade should not be sustained for more than 36 hours. After bleeding has been controlled for at least 24 hours, the esophageal balloon should be deflated. Deflation of the gastric balloon is warranted if stability is documented over the next 6 hours. Removal of the tube is justified after an additional 24 hours of observation. Vasopressin infusions should be discontinued in a tapered fashion during the period of tamponade.

Emergency Endoscopic Sclerotherapy

Active variceal bleeding despite balloon tamponade is unusual. The position and condition of the balloons should be immediately assessed by inspection and chest roentgenogram. If the tube is correctly positioned and functioning, the possibility of another bleeding source must be excluded by repeat endoscopic examination. In the rare instance where continued bleeding from esophageal varices is confirmed, emergency injection of the varix via the fiberoptic endoscope can be attempted. The sclerosing agent (ethanolamine oleate, sodium morrhuate, or sodium tetradecyl sulfate) is usually introduced directly into the varix, although paravariceal injection is effective and frequently unavoidable. Compression of the varices after injection can be accomplished by balloon tamponade, but its value is controversial. Injection of varices during active bleeding is hazardous and the procedure requires a highly experienced endoscopist.

Percutaneous Transhepatic Variceal Obliteration

In patients with variceal bleeding that is recalcitrant to conventional forms of therapy, hemostasis can be achieved by the selective injection of embolic or sclerosing substances into the variceal tributaries. The left gastric or coronary vein and the short gastric veins that communicate with the gastoesphageal varices can be catheterized using the percutaneous transhepatic route, and the vessels can be occluded by the instillation of gelatine foam, autogenous blood clots, sodium tetradecyl sulfate, thrombin, steel coils, metal clips, or synthetic polymer (isobutylcyanoacrylate). The procedure takes 2 to 5 hours to complete, but varices are obliterated in 80 per cent of cases. Unfortunately, rebleeding occurs in 65 per cent of patients within 5 months and the procedure cannot be repeated long-term. Portal vein thrombosis, which precludes liver transplantation and reduces shunt options, develops in 36 per cent. Collateralization eventuates in 76 per cent of patients and this may enhance hepatofugal blood flow and further compromise liver function. The complications and impermanence of transhepatic variceal obliteration warrant its restriction to patients with recalcitrant bleeding and poor hepatic functional reserve (Child's class C) whose Child's classification can be improved prior to a shunt procedure.

Emergency Nonshunting Procedures

When nonoperative measures fail to halt variceal hemorrhage, surgical options must be considered. Direct intervention at the level of the bleeding vessels has been advocated as a stabilizing step prior to an elective shunt procedure. Transesophageal ligation of varices through a left thoracotomy has a high operative mortality (30 per cent), disappointing rebleeding rate (33 per cent), and dismal one year survival expectation (5 per cent). Transabdominal esophageal transection and devascularization of the lower esophagus have had better success, although prospective randomized comparisons have not been made. The American EEA stapler and Russian SPTU stapling gun simultaneously resect a ring of esophageal wall and reanastomose the esophagus (mucosa-to-mucosa) by means of 12 to 14 tantalum staples. When the procedure is combined with ligation of the left gastric vein and periesophageal collaterals, the one year rebleeding rate can be reduced to 20 per cent and the one year survival increased. Operative mortality, however, in the emergency situation exceeds 30 per cent. Attempts by US surgeons to duplicate the success of Japanese surgeons who perform emergency esophageal transection in conjunction with meticulous devascularization of the stomach and esophagus (Sugiura procedure) have been unsuccessful. In patients with reversible hepatic decompensation who are candidates for an elective shunt operation, esophageal transection and stapling with lower esophageal devascularization can control life-threatening hemorrhage without disruption of hepatic blood flow and subsequent hepatic encephalopathy.

Emergency Shunts

Emergency portacaval anastomosis is the most effective method of lowering portal pressure acutely. Operative mortality, however, is fivefold greater than that of an elective procedure, and a highly individualized benefit risk analysis is required before undertaking the procedure. The risk of surgery must be balanced against the probable life expectancy after the operation. In patients with adequate hepatic functional reserve (Child's classes A and B), the operative mortality of 20 per cent may be an acceptable risk for the years of life that may be gained. In patients with poor hepatic reserve (Child's class C), the surgical procedure with its mortality of 87 per cent may not offer any advantages over the nonoperative approaches.

Most commonly, an end-to-side portacaval shunt or interposition mesocaval shunt is constructed. Shunt selection is determined by the surgical experience, vascular anatomy, hepatic functional reserve (Child's class), and direction of portal vein blood flow. Visceral angiography is necessary in all patients to assess patency and size of the portal, splenic, and renal veins. Additionally, the portahepatic pressure gradient can be measured and the direction of portal blood flow determined. A normal wedged hepatic vein pressure suggests portal vein thrombosis or isolated splenic vein thrombosis. In the latter instance, the portal hypertension can be cured by splenectomy.

In patients of Child's class C, a mesocaval or interposition shunt is preferred since these side-to-side anastomoses are associated with less ascites postoperatively and they can be ligated if severe encephalopathy develops. A side-to-side anastomosis will also avoid intractable ascites in patients with hepatofugal blood flow. In patients with minimal hepatopetal flow, an end-to-side portacaval shunt is possible, whereas in patients with frank hepatopetal flow, a distal splenorenal shunt should be considered to preserve portal perfusion of the liver.

Emergency portacaval shunts stop bleeding in 95 per cent of cases. Complications in survivors include encephalopathy (40 per cent) and shunt thrombosis (10 to 24 per cent).

Prevention of Rebleeding

There is no best method of preventing rebleeding, and controlled clinical trials are necessary to define the most effective long-term therapy. The appropriateness of any approach is determined mainly by the condition of the patient and the available expertise.

Propranolol (Inderal)

Propranolol in divided doses sufficient to reduce the resting heart rate by 25 per cent (dose range, 20 to 180 mg twice daily) has been shown to decrease the frequency of recurrent bleeding from esophageal varices or gastritis in patients with good hepatic functional reserve (Child's class A). (This use of propranolol is not listed by the manufacturer). Since the portal vein has only alpha adrenoreceptors, beta blockade in decompensated cirrhosis may intensify the alpha effect of vasoconstriction on the portal vein and not lower portal pressure. The frequency of rebleeding has not been reduced in patients with severely impaired liver function, and a reduction in hepatic blood flow may precipitate hepatic encephalopathy. Additionally, resuscitation may be more difficult in the bleeding patient with beta blockade. Discontinuation of propranolol therapy should be in a tapered fashion.

Endoscopic Sclerotherapy

Endoscopic variceal sclerosis can obliterate varices after a median of four sessions in 90 per cent of the patients. New varices develop, however, in 67 per cent, and rebleeding from these varices occurs in 19 per cent, usually within 12 months after initial obliteration. To prevent recurrence, endoscopic examinations are necessary every three months for one year after obliteration and then annually thereafter. Although the frequency of rebleeding is reduced by this method, the morbidity of the procedure (fever, chest pain, pleural effusion, injection ulcers, bacteremia, esophageal stricture, and pneumonitis) averages 9 per cent per procedure and 19 per cent per patient (mortality, 0.7 to 2 per cent). Two studies have indicated improved survival after sclerotherapy, but other experiences have been contradictory. Gastric varices are usually not amenable to this form of treatment, and successful obliteration of the esophageal varices may increase the propensity for the fundic varices to bleed.

Distal Splenorenal Shunt

The distal splenorenal shunt separates the splanchnic circulation into portomesenteric and gastrosplenic components, which in selected patients has the advantage of preserving portal vein perfusion of the liver and decompressing the esophageal varices. In experienced hands and well-chosen patients, operative mortality is low. Rebleeding occurs in 10 per cent; hepatic encephalopathy develops in less than 15 per cent; and shunt occlusion occurs in less than 10 per cent. A successful procedure requires an intact spleen, favorable renal and splenic veins, hepatopetal portal blood flow, and absence of ascites. Additionally, patients with nonalcoholic liver disease seem to fare better. Unfortunately, progressive systemic collateralization occurs in time, converting the selective shunt to a total shunt. Hepatic portal perfusion can be maintained in only 42 per cent of patients, and the complications of liver failure and hepatic encephalopathy may develop later.

Liver Transplantation

Bleeding from esophageal varices is a manifestation of portal hypertension usually secondary to advanced liver disease. In these patients, long-term survival is related to hepatic functional reserve, and liver transplantation may be the best mechanism to improve this reserve. If transplantation is a consideration, the methods used to control bleeding in the acute and convalescent periods should be chosen so as not to jeopardize portal vein patency or complicate the transplantation effort. Endoscopic sclerotherapy is preferred under these circumstances.

CHOLELITHIASIS AND CHOLECYSTITIS

method of
THOMAS R. GADACZ, M.D.
Baltimore Veterans Administration Medical Center
Baltimore, Maryland

Cholelithiasis is a common medical problem in the United States. It is estimated that 20 per cent of all adults over the age of 40 have gallstones, and a half million operations are performed for gallbladder or bile duct disorders every year. Eighty five per cent of the people in the United States with stones have cholesterol stones; i.e., the stone contains 60 per cent or more cholesterol. The remaining 15 per cent have pigment stones, and these patients have a hemolytic anemia, such as sickle cell disease, or cirrhosis.

GALLSTONE DISEASE

Approximately 30 per cent of patients with gallstones are not troubled by the stones. They have no significant symptoms, and the changes in the gallbladder are unremarkable. This disease is best characterized as primary gallstone disease. At times these patients are discovered to have gallstones when sonography is undertaken for an unrelated problem. The clinician is then faced with a dilemma as to what to advise the patient who has asymptomatic gallstones. Usually these patients can be observed and warned that they may require an operation if they become symptomatic or their gallbladder becomes diseased. The usual indications for a cholecystectomy in a truly asymptomatic patient include the following:

Diabetes Mellitus and Sickle Cell Disease. For both these diseases the risk during an episode of cholecystitis is significantly greater than in patients without these diseases. An elective cholecystectomy should be performed during a quiescent period to minimize the operative risks.

Nonvisualization of the Gallbladder. This usually indicates significant gallbladder disease and subclinical episodes of cholecystitis.

Stones 2 Cm or More in Diameter. Large stones usually erode and cause more problems than smaller stones.

Calcification of the Gallbladder Wall. This is the only cancer risk in patients with biliary tract disease. It is important to distinguish between calcified stones and calcification of the gallbladder wall; the latter represents an increased risk of cancer of the gallbladder.

Treatment

Patients who have cholesterol stones, typified on oral cholecystography as small floating stones, can be treated with chenodeoxycholate (Chenix or chenodiol). This is a primary bile salt, and 6 months to 4 years are required for complete dissolution of stones. Once dissolution occurs, the patient must be maintained on the bile salt to keep the bile desaturated. The gallbladder must be functioning and the stones must be cholesterol. The National Cooperative Gallstone Study reported a 14 per cent success rate for complete dissolution of stones when patients were treated with chenodeoxycholate, 750 mg daily, for 2 years. This relatively low success rate has significantly decreased the enthusiasm for using this drug. In this study several problems were associated with the use of chenodeoxycholate, including diarrhea and hepatotoxicity.

Another bile salt, ursodeoxycholate, has also been reported to successfully dissolve cholesterol stones, and the toxicity associated with this bile salt may be less than that reported with chenodeoxycholate. The success rates are similar. Patients with asymptomatic stones should be assessed of the presence of the stones, and when symptoms occur cholecystectomy should be advised. It is unwise to delay treatment until the patient's symptoms become worse. If the operation is unduly delayed, the patient usually presents with a significant complication.

GALLBLADDER DISEASE

Ninety five per cent of the patients with cholecystitis have gallstones. The remaining 5 per cent have acalculous cholecystitis, usually associated with such conditions as trauma, burns, stress, and sepsis. Gallbladder disease in patients with gallstones results from episodes of obstruction of the cystic duct by the gallstones.

DIAGNOSIS

The diagnosis of cholecystitis will depend upon the activity of the disease. In patients with acute symptoms, ultrasonography and Tc-IDA radionuclide scanning will confirm the diagnosis. These two modalities are complementary. The sonogram establishes the presence of stones in the gallbladder and provides anatomic information regarding the gallbladder and biliary tract. The technetium scan visualizes the bile ducts and gallbladder, providing functional information.

When there is acute inflammation of the gallbladder, the bile ducts but not the gallbladder will be visualized and contrast will be seen in the small intestine. Nonvisualization of the gallbladder in an asymptomatic patient indicates chronic cholecystitis. It is important to know the serum bilirubin level and the type of IDA compound used for imaging. The HIDA compound will visualize the biliary tract and gallbladder when the serum bilirubin level is 6 mg per cent or less. If the bilirubin in higher, other compounds such as PIPIDA or DISIDA should be used.

In patients recovering from an attack of acute cholecystitis or those suspected of having chronic cholecystitis, oral cholecystography is still an excellent test. This provides not only structural information about the gallbladder but also determines function. Following an acute illness an oral cholecystogram may not reveal changes for several weeks and the appropriate precautions in interpretation must be taken. The diagnosis should be confirmed early in a patient suspected of having cholecystitis so that prompt operative treatment can be given if the patient's condition deteriorates.

Treatment

In a small percentage of patients (5 to 10 per cent) the obstruction of the cystic duct is not relieved and emergency surgery is required. Most patients (70 per cent) with cholecystitis will have a cholecystectomy early in the course of the disease. The timing of the cholecystectomy is not as crucial as once thought, and several reports have now demonstrated that there is no "golden period" for surgery. In general, the patient should be operated on as soon as possible to decrease morbidity and the costs associated with hospitalization. Cholecystectomy is usually performed within 48 to 72 hours of hospitalization following an acute episode. Cholecystectomy in the remaining 20 to 25 per cent of patients is performed at a later date because of associated diseases. Patients with diabetes should be operated on as soon as possible since they may clinically deteriorate rapidly; these patients have a significantly higher mortality and morbidity.

Cholecystectomy

In general patients with acute or chronic cholecystitis should undergo cholecystectomy. An intraoperative cholangiogram usually should be performed to ensure that there are no stones in the common duct and that the common duct is normal. The gallbladder bed is usually drained. The type of drainage (open versus closed) is probably not as critical as the timing of the drain removal. If there is no significant drainage, the drain should be removed within 48 to 72 hours to reduce the risk of infection. In patients who undergo cholecystectomy for chronic cholecystitis drainage may not be necessary.

The outcome of cholecystectomy is related to several factors. Elderly patients (65 years or older), especially those with multiple associated diseases, have a mortality rate of 5 per cent. Patients under 65 who have no associated medical diseases have a mortality rate of 0.6 per cent or less. Exploration of the common duct will increase the mortality rate by 5 to 8 per cent.

The morbidity associated with the operation is due to inadvertent injury to one of the portal structures, usually the common bile duct. About 5 per cent of the patients will have diarrhea following cholecystectomy, but this is usually transient and resolves within a matter of weeks. Patients with persistent diarrhea (usually due to bile salts) can be treated either with cholestyramine (Questran) or magaldrate (Riopan).

COMMON BILE DUCT DISEASE

Treatment

If stones are detected in the common bile duct at the time of cholecystectomy, a choledochotomy should be made and the stones removed. Generally a T-tube is inserted into the common bile duct to provide drainage for the common bile duct and to obtain a postoperative study to ensure that no residual stones are present. At operation stones are best detected manually by palpation; other modalities include intraoperative cholangiography and preoperative sonography or percutaneous transhepatic cholangiography. Stones from the gallbladder and common bile duct should be saved and analyzed for cholesterol. This is best done by incubating the stones in monooctanoin (Moctanin) for 5 days. If they dissolve, the cholesterol content is sufficiently high to ensure dissolution of the stones by monooctanoin.

If stones are discovered on the postoperative cholangiogram, several options are available. If there is no leak from the choledochotomy site and no distal obstruction, the T-tube can be irrigated with monooctanoin and the stones will generally dissolve within 3 to 7 days. If the monooctanoin is not available or if the stones are pigment the options include extraction of the stones through the T-tube tract and endoscopic papillotomy. Extraction through the T-tube tract must be delayed for 6 to 8 weeks after the operation until a fibrous tract is established between the abdominal wall and the choledochotomy. The T-tube is removed and either a Dormia basket is used to extract the stones under fluoroscopy or a choledochoscope can be passed and the stones extracted under direct visualization. This technique does require some expertise.

Endoscopic papillotomy is the other option, but it requires considerable expertise. This technique employs a side-viewing duodenoscope and papillotome that enlarges the ampullary area and allows the passage of stones. A balloon can be passed through the endoscope into the common bile duct and the stones pushed out of the common bile duct. Other techniques that have been used in more complicated conditions include percutaneous transhepatic cholangiography with infusion of monooctanoin through the transhepatic stent. Nasobiliary tubes have also been used to infuse monooctanoin to dissolve retained or primary cholesterol stones.

If at the original operation multiple stones are present in the common bile duct and residual stones are suspected, a choledochoduodenostomy should be performed. The stones will then pass spontaneously and no additional treatment will be required. If the common bile duct is normal in size, a sphincteroplasty is preferred.

Patients who present with acute cholangitis (right upper quadrant discomfort, jaundice, fever, chills, and a high leukocytosis) may be difficult to distinguish from patients with gangrenous cholecystitis. Cholangitis may be suspected by detecting a dilated duct with stones by sonography. Treatment consists of decompression of the common bile duct and antibiotics.

The safest and standard way of decompressing the common bile duct is to operatively insert a T-tube or a cholecystostomy if the cystic duct is patent. Other techniques that have been reported to be successful include percutaneous transhepatic decompression of the common bile duct followed by an elective operation when the patient has stabilized. Endoscopic papillotomy has been used to decompress the common bile duct; however, it does not have a role in decompressing the gallbladder, especially if the cystic duct is obstructed with a stone. The success of these treatment modalities depends upon adequate drainage of the common bile duct. Sometimes this cannot be accomplished through a small transhepatic tube.

Cholecystostomy

Occasionally a patient will be extremely ill with cholecystitis and associated medical problems. A cholecystostomy can be effective and is best done as a planned procedure under local anesthesia, although it is important to have an anesthesiologist support the patient during the procedure. Cholecystostomy is a limited procedure whereby the gallbladder is opened, stones are extracted, and the gallbladder is decompressed with a large catheter. This is usually a temporizing procedure; the patient will require a cholecystectomy at a later date, since stones usually reform in the gallbladder and continue to be a source of trouble.

CIRRHOSIS

method of
K. RAJENDER REDDY, M.D., FACP,
and EUGENE R. SCHIFF, M.D., FACP
Veterans Administration Medical Center
Miami, Florida

CIRRHOSIS

Cirrhosis is a pathologic state of the liver characterized by fibrosis, regenerating nodules, and often ongoing necrosis. The liver involvement is generalized, resulting in distortion of the normal architecture. The pathophysiologic consequences of cirrhosis are both functional and mechanical. Once cirrhosis is established, it is irreversible, but progression is dependent in part on the underlying etiology and whether there is continuing necrosis.

In the Western world alcohol is responsible for most cases of cirrhosis, whereas viral hepatitis, particularly type B, is the leading cause worldwide. Other etiologies for cirrhosis include drugs (e.g., methyldopa, isoniazid, nitrofurantoin, and methotrexate), hereditary metabolic disorders (Wilson's disease, hemochromatosis, alpha-1 antitrypsin deficiency, galactosemia, tyrosinemia, glycogen storage diseases), chronic active hepatitis, chronic nonsuppurative destructive cholangitis (primary biliary cirrhosis), venous outflow obstruction (right-sided heart failure, constrictive pericarditis, Budd-Chiari syndrome), extrahepatic biliary obstruction, and cystic fibrosis. Cryptogenic cirrhosis evolves insidiously and is of unknown etiology, but many of these cases probably represent postnecrotic cirrhosis secondary to non-A non-B hepatitis. Morphologically, cirrhosis can be classified as macronodular, micronodular, or mixed, but there is a lack of good correlation with etiology.

The clinical manifestations of cirrhosis are generally a result of functional and/or mechanical compromise. These include portal hypertension with bleeding esophageal and gastric varices, ascites, spontaneous bacterial peritonitis, encephalopathy, and coagulopathy; each of these has significant morbidity and mortality. In addition, the terminal event may take the form of hepatorenal syndrome or may be a consequence of hepatocellular carcinoma, which frequently occurs in cirrhosis, particularly that resulting from chronic B infection. However, primary cancer of the liver may be seen in conjunction with nonviral forms of liver disease, such as alcoholic cirrhosis or hemochromatosis.

Treatment

Ideally treatment should be directed at the underlying cause of the cirrhosis and toward interfering with progressive fibrosis and nodule formation regardless of etiology. Unfortunately the therapy of alcoholic liver disease rests on abstention, which is difficult to accomplish. Chronic viral hepatitis requires a safe and effective antiviral treatment, which has not yet been developed, and there is no proven means to block the evolution of hepatic fibrosis and nodule formation. In patients with Wilson's disease, penicillamine therapy is effective in reducing copper stores to normal and must be continued throughout life. Primary hemochromatosis is successfully managed with serial phlebotomies and then maintenance phlebotomies to control the iron overload, but, once established, the cirrhosis remains. If the underlying heart disorder can be reversed or corrected, cardiac cirrhosis may improve. Treatment of cirrhosis therefore focuses on management of the complications and prevention of further liver necrosis. In addition, careful evaluation and management of the nutritional status are important in these often debilitated patients.

HEPATIC ENCEPHALOPATHY

Hepatic encephalopathy is a metabolic encephalopathy seen in acute and chronic liver disease and is characterized by an altered mental state and neuromuscular dysfunction.

The term portal-systemic encephalopathy is most often applied to that form of chronic hepatic encephalopathy seen in cirrhosis, wherein there is both intra- and extrahepatic shunting of portal blood rich in enteric protein products, which eventually exert a toxic effect on the central nervous system. This form of encephalopathy may have permanent residual neurologic deficits and contrasts with the acute encephalopathy seen in massive necrosis of the liver, in which complete neurologic recovery can be anticipated if the patient survives the fulminant hepatic failure. The definitive pathogenetic mechanisms involved in hepatic encephalopathy are not clearly understood.

Treatment

In the initial approach to a patient with hepatic encephalopathy, it is important to exclude other causes for this neurologic disorder such as drug overdose, acute alcoholism, delirium tremens, subdural hematoma, or a cerebrovascular accident. Once the diagnosis of hepatic encephalopathy has been established, the initial step in management is to identify and avoid any precipitating factors. Specifically, sedatives, tranquilizers, and narcotics must be discontinued; gastrointestinal bleeding and electrolyte abnormalities, if any, should be recognized promptly and treated appropriately. If a patient is comatose, intravenous nutrition and establishment of an airway are essential.

The protein intake should be markedly restricted initially, depending on the level of encephalopathy. In the patient who is in frank coma, protein should be completely eliminated and gradual increments of 10 to 20 grams every 3 to 5 days to a maximum of 60 grams may be made according to the patient's response. It is important to provide at least 1,500 calories per day to prevent tissue catabolism that might contribute to ammonia production. Vegetables are a preferred source of protein, and foods that include large amounts of preformed ammonia such as cheese, gelatin, peanut butter, commercial hamburgers, and some frozen meats should be eliminated.

Purgatives and gut-cleansing enemas are most effective in the initial stages of therapy, especially if the patient has been constipated or has gastrointestinal bleeding. Lactulose, a synthetic dissaccharride that is neither absorbed nor metabolized in the upper intestinal tract, is a good cathartic. In addition, lactulose therapy will lower blood ammonia levels. This pharmacologic effect is a result of bacterial degradation of lactulose leading to the generation of a lower colonic pH, which enhances ammonia utilization by the bacteria. It is given orally or via a nasogastric tube initially in a dose of 15 to 30 ml every hour until loose bowel movements are produced and then 3 to 4 times a day in an attempt to produce two to three soft stools daily. In the comatose patient, lactulose can be given as a retention enema (300 ml of lactulose in 700 ml of tap water) and can be repeated every 8 hours until the patient is alert enough to take it orally or via a nasogastric tube.

Neomycin, a poorly absorbed aminoglycoside, is an alternative form of therapy; in the patient who cannot tolerate or is unresponsive to lactulose therapy, it can be used either alone or in conjunction with lower doses of lactulose. Although only 3 per cent of neomycin is absorbed, there are potential risks of nephrotoxicity, ototoxicity, and intestinal malabsorption. If there is no impairment of renal function, it can be given orally in divided doses of up to 2 grams per day or as retention enemas 2 or 3 times a day by adding 1 to 2 grams to 100 to 200 ml of isotonic saline. If a patient is being treated for an infection with systemic antibiotics such as a cephalosporin, ampicillin, metronidazole, or sulfonamides, it is unnecessary to use lactulose or neomycin for treatment of encephalopathy.

L-Dopa and bromocriptine have been used in hepatic encephalopathy with equivocal results. The rationale for the use of these agents has been based on their presumed ability to displace so-called false neurotransmitters from nerve endings in the brain. These drugs are not generally recommended unless the patient is refractory to the standard therapy. The intravenous and oral administration of amino acid mixtures high in branched chain amino acids and low in aromatic amino acids has been used with varying degrees of success. Branched chain amino acid mixtures have been successful in achieving a positive nitrogen balance without precipitating, and possibly improving, existing encephalopathy and are recommended in the catabolic patient who cannot tolerate increments in dietary protein. The recommended dose for parenteral hyperalimentation is 80 to 120 grams of amino acids, such as Hepatamine, per day.

ASCITES

The pathogenetic mechanisms operating in the formation of ascites include portal hypertension, especially the postsinusoidal block, which is largely responsible for increased lymph production and subsequent escape into the peritoneal cavity via surface lymphatics; decreased plasma colloid oncotic pressure due to hypoalbuminemia, facilitating loss of the free fluid into the peritoneal cavity; and a diminished "effective" plasma volume, leading to avid renal retention of sodium and water.

Clinical examination is unreliable in the detection of subtle ascites. Ultrasonography and computed tomography are sensitive and specific in detecting small amounts of fluid and should be done in cases of uncertainty. A diagnostic paracentesis is recommended in all patients with new onset ascites. However, in the cirrhotic with ascites who has developed varying degrees of unexplained fever, abdominal pain, or encephalopathy, paracentesis should be performed in search of bacterial peritonitis. Uncomplicated cirrhotic ascites usually has a protein of less than 2.5 grams per cent with less than 300 WBC per cu mm, mostly mononuclear cells, in contrast to spontaneous bacterial peritonitis, where the ascitic fluid white count exceeds 500 WBC per cu mm with more than 50 per cent being polymorphonuclear leukocytes.

Treatment

Complications of cirrhotic ascites include hydrothorax, large umbilical and inguinal hernia, elevation of the diaphragm producing respiratory distress, and increased abdominal pressure causing abdominal pain, anorexia, and gastroesophageal reflux. It is for these reasons that therapy of ascites is recommended. The patient should be hospitalized if tense ascites interferes with breathing and eating, marked ascites with umbilical hernia is present, there is evidence of overt or impending renal failure, or there are electrolyte abnormalities.

The initial management of ascites should include bed rest and salt restriction. A well-balanced low sodium diet, preferably containing no more than 500 mg (22 mEq) of sodium per day, is recommended. Fluid intake is temporarily restricted to 1000 to 1200 ml per day if the patient has hyponatremia, i.e., serum Na^+ less than 130 mEq per liter. In patients with tense ascites and impending rupture of an ulcerated umbilical hernia or respiratory embarrassment due to diaphragmatic elevation, there is an urgent indication for therapeutic paracentesis of 2 to 3 liters of ascitic fluid. Repeated paracentesis should be avoided.

To minimize the length of the hospital stay it is prudent to start diuretics immediately, even though 10 per cent of patients will spontaneously diurese. Spironolactone, an aldosterone antagonist, is an ideal diuretic and has the advantage of potassium sparing. The initial dose is 50 mg twice daily. Diuresis should be controlled to avoid intravascular volume depletion; this is best accomplished by aiming for a ½ to 1 lb weight loss per day. Patients with ascites and peripheral edema are more likely to respond with vigorous diuresis and are less prone to volume depletion. If the patient fails to adequately diurese in 3 to 4 days, the dose of spironolactone should be raised by increments of 50 to 100 mg every 4 days until a satisfactory diuresis or a total daily dose of 300 mg is achieved.

Unresponsiveness at this stage should prompt the physician to evaluate the patient's compliance regarding salt and fluid restriction. In the compliant patient, furosemide can be added up to a maximum of 80 mg per day, carefully following the BUN and electrolyte levels. Some experts have recommended higher doses of either diuretic before considering the patient to be refractory to medical treatment. Other diuretics may be preferred and include bumetanide and the potassium-sparing amiloride. Caution should be exercised in patients receiving high doses of diuretics, since they frequently develop azotemia and electrolyte abnormalities necessitating discontinuation of the medication.

In refractory ascites, the urine sodium is generally less than 10 mEq per liter concomitant with azotemia and hyponatremia. In such cases, peritoneovenous shunting (Leveen or Denver shunt) is recommended and has proven to be effective in selected cases. Contraindications are infected ascites, recent variceal bleeding, severe coagulopathy (PT $>$ 4 sec over control), hyperbilirubinemia (total bilirubin $>$ 5 mg per cent), intrinsic renal disease, and cardiac failure. A peritoneovenous venous shunt is surgically placed subcutaneously, establishing a communication between the peritoneal cavity and the superior vena cava via a Silastic tube. A pressure-sensitive unidirectional valve in the middle of the tubing allows ascitic fluid to flow into the venous system when the pressure gradient is greater than 5 cm H_2O. Complications include shunt thrombosis, disseminated intravascular coagulation, precipitation of variceal bleeding, and local or systemic infection. Overt disseminated intravascular coagulation is life-threatening but may be prevented to a large extent by removing a large volume of ascites at the time of surgery and by giving subcutaneous heparin (5000 units every 12 hr) during the first postoperative week.

In patients with tense ascites and prerenal azotemia, rapid diuresis can be achieved medically by a regimen of fresh frozen plasma or albumin, furosemide, and mannitol. Fresh frozen plasma is preferable if the prothrombin time is prolonged. Two units of fresh frozen plasma or 500 cc of 5 per cent albumin are infused over a 2 hour period followed by 20 to 60 mg of intravenous furosemide and, subsequently, 50 grams (250 cc of 20 per cent) mannitol over 45 minutes. If the response is good, this regimen can be repeated, if necessary. The rationale for this therapy is to expand volume and to deliver more sodium and water to the kidneys to enhance the action of furosemide and mannitol in achieving an effective diuresis. It is important to stress that this is a temporary form of therapy and is most valuable in patients with acute reversible liver injury who have developed refractory ascites. In addition, it may also be helpful in patients with underlying chronic liver disease who have either a superimposed acute liver injury or are awaiting placement of a peritoneovenous shunt.

A side-to-side portacaval shunt is the procedure of choice in a patient who has intractable ascites and has bled from varices.

SPONTANEOUS BACTERIAL PERITONITIS

The cirrhotic patient with ascites is predisposed to the development of spontaneous bacterial peritonitis (SBP), a life-threatening complication occurring in approximately 8 per cent of hospitalized patients with cirrhosis. In addition to ascites, a majority of the patients have clinical evidence of jaundice, esophageal varices, and hepatic encephalopathy. Most often they present with fever, abdominal pain, and worsening of encephalopathy. Hypotension, absent or hypoactive bowel sounds, and abdominal rebound tenderness may also be present. Infrequently a patient may be totally asymptomatic.

The diagnosis of SBP is based on the laboratory characteristics of the ascitic fluid and is confirmed by positive cultures. Analysis of the peritoneal fluid typically demonstrates a white blood cell count of greater than 500 per cu mm with greater than 50 per cent polymorphonuclear leukocytes and a protein concentration of less than 2.5 grams per cent. An ascitic fluid pH of less than 7.3 or an arterial–ascitic fluid pH gradient greater than 0.1 is reported to be a valuable diagnostic parameter. If the ascitic fluid white blood cell count is greater than 5000 per cu mm with predominance of polymorphonuclear leukocytes and the protein concentration is greater than 2.5 grams per cent, one should be alert to the possibility of secondary bacterial peritonitis often due to cholecystitis, appendicitis, or perforation of an abdominal viscus.

Treatment

When the diagnosis of SBP is suspected, antibiotic therapy should be started even prior to receiving the results of the cultures. The commonest causative organism is *Escherichia coli*, an enteric gram negative rod, followed by *Pneumococcus* and *Streptococcus* sp.; anaerobes seldom cause SBP. The recommended therapy is a third generation cephalosporin, e.g., intravenous doses of cefoxitin, 2 grams every 6 hours for 14 days. The dosage must be adjusted in renal failure, and the antibiotic may have to be changed once the results of ascitic fluid cultures and sensitivity studies are available. Aminoglycosides should be avoided because of the demonstrated increased risk of nephrotoxicity in patients with cirrhosis. Serial paracentesis, to determine effectiveness of therapy, is advisable. Successful therapy results in a decrease in the ascitic fluid WBC count and negative cultures.

FUNCTIONAL RENAL FAILURE (HEPATORENAL SYNDROME)

The hepatorenal syndrome, a functional renal impairment, is seen in chronic liver disease with ascites and is usually a terminal event. It is characterized by slow onset and progressive azotemia in the presence of good tubular function. Sodium is avidly reabsorbed by the renal tubules and fluid accumulates; this is evidenced by a urine to plasma osmolality ratio of greater than 1.0, urine to plasma creatinine ratio of greater than 30, and a urine sodium concentration of less than 10 mEq per liter. The serum sodium is usually less than 120 mEq per liter. Intravascular volume depletion, a potentially reversible disorder, mimics but may also precipitate hepatorenal syndrome. Vigorous diuresis, large volume paracentesis, and diarrhea are common causes of volume depletion in the cirrhotic. Pathogenetic mechanisms operating in hepatorenal syndrome have not been precisely defined.

As the syndrome advances, encephalopathy, hypotention, and progressive oliguria evolve. Death is due to liver failure, and survival is dependent on the reversibility of the liver disease.

Treatment

The initial approach should be directed toward correcting any component of intravascular volume depletion. Fresh-frozen plasma or 5 per cent albumin can be used with careful monitoring for signs of volume overload. The placement of a peritoneovenous shunt should be considered in selected cases if the total bilirubin is less than 5.0 mg per cent and the prothrombin time is less than 4.0 seconds over the control. Hemodialysis is not indicated unless there is clinical evidence of potentially reversible intrinsic renal disease.

Nonsteroidal anti-inflammatory drugs inhibit prostaglandin synthesis and may decrease natriuresis as well as induce renal failure in cirrhosis; they are best avoided, particularly in the presence of ascites. Demeclocycline has been found to be effective in treating patients with inappropriate antidiuretic hormone syndrome and theoretically could be useful in correcting hyponatremia and ascites, but it has been associated with the development of severe renal failure and death in cirrhotics and therefore is contraindicated.

COAGULOPATHY

The liver is the site of synthesis of all of the coagulation factors except factor VIII. Plasminogen and certain physiologic inhibitors of hemostasis are also produced by the liver. Furthermore, activated coagulation factors are cleared from the circulating blood and metabolized in the liver. The synthesis of factors II, VII, IX, and X is partly dependent on vitamin K, which in turn is dependent on adequate concentrations of intraluminal bile salts for absorption from the gastrointestinal tract. Thrombocytopenia is commonly found in patients with cirrhosis and most often is a result of splenic sequestration, but marrow suppression due to acute alcoholism and, frequently, folic acid deficiency also contributes. Finally, abnormal platelet aggregation can occur owing to intravascular coagulopathy in severe hepatic failure.

Alteration in at least one hemostatic factor is found in the majority of patients with cirrhosis and can occur as a result of qualitative or quantitative abnormalities in one or more of several factors; the type and severity are dependent on the nature of the liver disease. Objective evidence for altered hemostasis includes a prolonged prothrombin time, low plasma fibrinogen level, low platelet count, prolonged bleeding time, and an increase in fibrin degradation products.

Treatment

Vitamin K should be given to all patients with a prolonged prothrombin time. It is prudent to give vitamin K, 10 mg daily, for 3 days as a subcutaneous injection using a small gauge needle. If the prolongation is the result of vitamin K deficiency secondary to intestinal bile salt deficiency, malnutrition, or antibiotic therapy, the prothrombin time should correct. If the prolonged prothrombin time does not correct with vitamin K, fresh frozen plasma can be administered if necessary. It is indicated in active gastrointestinal bleeding and prior to an invasive procedure such as a liver biopsy if the prothrombin time is prolonged more than 4 seconds. Platelet transfusions are rarely necessary and are indicated in cases of severe bleeding if the platelet count is less than 50,000 per cu mm. Disseminated intravascular coagulation is usually mild but can be particularly severe following a peritoneovenous shunt. The primary approach is to correct the underlying precipitating cause, if possible, and give fresh frozen plasma. The careful use of heparin, preferably as subcutaneous injections of 5,000 units every 12 hours, is also recommended.

CIRRHOSIS AND NUTRITION

The liver plays a primary role in the digestion, storage, and metabolism of nutrients. Nutritional deficiency is multifactorial and may be due to a combination of one or more factors, including decreased intake, decreased absorption, decreased storage, abnormalities in metabolism, or the increased requirement for nutrients. Decreased intake contributes significantly to the catabolic state, particularly in the alcoholic patient. There are deficiencies of water-soluble vitamins, thiamine, riboflavin, nicotinic acid, pyridoxine, folic acid, and vitamin B_{12}. Impaired digestion and absorption may be noted in alcoholics or may be associated with cirrhosis alone. Pancreatic dysfunction may compound the alcoholic liver disease, adding to maldigestion. Malabsorption is common in cirrhosis and is largely a result of a decreased concentration of intraluminal bile salts in the proximal small bowel. Drugs such as neomycin and cholestyramine are frequently used in chronic liver disease and can cause malabsorption and steatorrhea, further adding to the malnutrition. A spectrum of metabolic abnormalities and deficiencies of protein, carbohydrates, lipids, vitamins, and minerals also occur in liver disease. Notable are the alterations in the plasma concentration of amino acids.

Most patients with cirrhosis of the liver are in negative nitrogen balance and relatively catabolic. Unfortunately, although they need dietary protein, some cannot tolerate adequate amounts because of a predisposition to develop hepatic encephalopathy. In the absence of signs or symptoms of encephalopathy, dietary protein need not be restricted, but when a restriction is necessary, the addition of lactulose or neomycin will permit a greater intake of protein.

In patients who must be maintained on less than 40 gm of dietary protein, daily enteral supplements of modified amino acid preparations high in content for the essential branched chain amino acids are indicated but may be prohibitively expensive. The recommended dose is 15 to 30 grams daily in divided doses as a supplement taken between meals. A greater emphasis on vegetable sources for dietary protein may permit an increased intake of protein without precipitating encephalopathy. It is also prudent to restrict sodium intake in most cirrhotics even if ascites and fluid retention are not evident. Minimally the patient should be counselled not to add salt as a seasoning to food, but greater degrees of salt restriction are necessary (to 2 grams or less daily) once fluid retention has developed.

It is judicious to give a multivitamin supplement to all cirrhotics, but in the alcoholic additional supplements of thiamine (100 mg per day) and folic acid (1 mg per day) are indicated. It may also be necessary to give supplements of zinc, magnesium, and selenium. Patients with cholestatic forms of cirrhosis, such as primary biliary cirrhosis, will require water-soluble supplements of the fat-soluble vitamins A, D, E, K, and calcium in advanced stages of the disease. Monthly parenteral replacement of vitamin A (100,000 units) and vitamin D_2 (100,000 units) coupled with oral supplements of vitamin D (50,000 units 3 times per week), vitamin E (200 IU per day), and vitamin K (5 mg per day) should suffice. Caution should be exercised in establishing the dose for vitamin A supplements, since vitamin A hepatotoxicity can compound the underlying liver disease. Oral vitamin A should not be given in a dose greater than 10,000 units daily. Oscal, taken 3 times daily with meals, should provide adequate supplements of calcium in the chronic cholestatic patient.

DYSPHAGIA AND ESOPHAGEAL OBSTRUCTION

method of
JEAN K. HADDAD, M.D.
University of California, San Francisco
San Francisco, California

The term *dysphagia* refers to any difficulty in swallowing and may be associated with pain (odynophagia). True dysphagia (as opposed to globus hystericus) always indicates a pathologic process and requires investigation to determine its cause. Dysphagia may be due to mechanical obstruction, inflammation, or a disorder of esophageal motility. The difficulty may be localized as oropharyngeal (transfer dysphagia), involving the esophageal body (transport dysphagia), or at the lower esophageal sphincter (entry dysphagia).

In evaluating the patient who complains of difficulty in swallowing, one must initially exclude globus, which is a functional complaint and is not associated with a true swallowing disorder. Such patients can swallow normally but complain of a "lump" in the throat or neck that is fairly constant and not related to the act of swallowing. This is a diagnosis of exclusion, and such symptoms must often be carefully investigated before the diagnosis is certain. Globus is treated by satisfying the patient that serious conditions have been ruled out and by reassurance and counseling.

Investigation of dysphagia requires a careful history. Often the patient will localize the site of obstruction.

The site will always be at the level pointed to by the patient or distal to it, but never proximal to it.

CONGENITAL DISORDERS

Esophageal Atresia. This lesion is often associated with a tracheoesophageal fistula. Treatment is directed at the prevention of aspiration until definitive surgery can be performed.

Esophageal Stenosis. This lesion may be dilated if stenosis is partial, but surgical treatment is required if stenosis is complete.

Dysphagia Lusoria. An abnormal origin of the right subclavian artery results in its passage behind the esophagus, causing extrinsic pressure and dysphagia. When it is severe, surgical correction of this vascular abnormality may be necessary.

OROPHARYNGEAL (ENTRY) DYSPHAGIA

Difficulty in propelling the food bolus from the mouth into the upper esophagus may be caused by a variety of disorders. Neuromuscular diseases are responsible for approximately 80 per cent of the cases. Central nervous system disorders such as stroke, Parkinson's disease, multiple sclerosis, amyotrophic lateral sclerosis, and brain stem tumors as well as peripheral neuropathies (diabetes) may be responsible. Myasthenia gravis and disorders of skeletal muscle such as dermatomyositis, muscular dystrophy, or metabolic myopathy (thyroid disease) may also cause oropharyngeal dysphagia.

Treatment

Treatment is not always effective and varies depending on the cause. Medical treatment may be of benefit in selected conditions. Examples include L-dopa (Laradopa) for Parkinson's disease, cholinesterase inhibitors (Mestinon) for myasthenia gravis, and steroids for polymyositis. Some structural lesions will respond to dilatation (bougienage). Dilation of the upper esophageal area is not without risk and must be performed only by those experienced in these techniques.

Many cases of oropharyngeal dysphasia can benefit from cricopharyngeal myotomy. Such treatment is reserved for patients with progressive weight loss or significant pulmonary aspiration. This procedure can be effective in reducing upper esophageal sphincter pressure and, thereby, facilitating the swallowing mechanism. Patients with severe gastroesophageal reflux due to an incompetent lower esophageal sphincter should not undergo this procedure because of the increased danger of aspiration.

The results of surgical myotomy are good in patients who can initiate a swallow normally (normal sensation and voluntary tongue movement). When a Zenker's diverticulum is present, myotomy is often performed with diverticulectomy. Little can be done for patients with bulbar abnormalities who may not have normal sensation or who may not be able to initiate a swallow. In some, feeding gastrostomy and careful oral suctioning are all that can be offered.

MOTOR DISORDERS (TRANSPORT DYSPHAGIA)

Achalasia

Achalasia, a disease of unknown cause associated with a defect in cholinergic innervation, results in dysphagia of insidious onset. The absence of normal esophageal peristalsis and incomplete relaxation of a hypertensive lower esophageal sphincter with swallowing result in functional obstruction to the passage of food. The esophagus eventually becomes dilated with retained food and liquid, which passes into the stomach only by gravity or by the Valsalva maneuver, often performed unconsciously by the patient. In some, high pressure, nonpropulsive contractions occur in the esophagus (vigorous achalasia) and may cause chest pain. Bronchopulmonary aspiration and recurrent pulmonary infections may occur, particularly at night, because of the retained esophageal contents.

Evaluation of patients with achalasia should include endoscopy to exclude those infrequent cases caused by a malignant lesion of the gastric cardia. After confirmation of the diagnosis by radiographic, endoscopic, and manometric techniques, a trial of medical management can be initiated.

Treatment

There is no treatment currently available for the aperistalsis. The goal of treatment, either medical or surgical, is to reduce lower esophageal sphincter pressure so that food may pass into the stomach more easily. Nitrates and calcium channel blockers such as nifedipine (Procardia) may give temporary relief by reducing the lower esophageal sphincter pressure. Long-term results, however, tend to be disappointing. Dilatation with mercury-filed bougies is not effective in this condition. Prevention of nocturnal aspiration and treatment of pulmonary infections may be necessary.

Pneumatic dilatation and surgical myotomy (Heller myotomy) are equally effective means of therapy; both reduce the lower esophageal sphincter pressure. I prefer, in most instances, to initially perform pneumatic dilatation and reserve surgery for those situations where dilatation has not been effective. Following endoscopic visualization, pneumatic dilatation can be performed under fluoroscopic control. I use the Rider-Moeller pneumatic dilator, which comes in several different circumferential sizes. The patient is premedicated with meperidine (Demerol) and atropine and is given diazepam (Valium) intravenously at the time of the procedure.

With the aid of a guide wire, the pneumatic dilator is passed and the balloon centered at the cardioesophageal junction under fluoroscopic observation. The balloon is then inflated under direct obstruction. The pressures used and the time of balloon inflation vary depending on the balloon used. I usually inflate the balloon to 160 to 200 mm mercury for approximately 30 to 60 seconds and may repeat once after deflating. The lower pressure is safer, and the procedure can always be repeated at a higher pressure if necessary. The narrow waist of the balloon can, at times, be seen to widen as the sphincter is dilated. Patients experience pain during inflation, but with the proper use of diazepam often have amnesia for the procedure. Blood is usually present on the balloon when it is removed, since the procedure causes mucosal and muscular tears (medical myotomy).

The patient is observed closely for possible perforation and is not allowed anything by mouth until he has been observed for at least 24 hours and until he has had a contrast study using a water-soluble medium (Gastrografin) performed. The patient is observed for the presence of fever, chest pain, or pleural effusion. Most have an excellent symptomatic improvement. Occasionally a patient may require one or more repeat dilatations. Failure to respond is usually an indication for surgical myotomy.

Long-term results and complication rates are similar for both medical and surgical treatment. Pneumatic dilatation is easier, less expensive, and requires shorter hospitalization. The primary complication is perforation, which usually requires prompt surgical repair. Surgical myotomy requires a thoracotomy and may be associated with significant gastroesophageal reflux.

Patients with achalasia, especially those with longstanding esophageal dilatation, are at increased risk for the development of squamous carcinoma and should have periodic screening endoscopic examinations. Those with achalasia due to a fundal malignancy (adenocarcinoma, lymphoma) are treated either surgically or by radiation therapy. Successful treatment has been reported to result in reversal of the features of achalasia.

Symptomatic Idiopathic Diffuse Esophageal Spasm

This is a poorly defined motor disorder of the esophagus causing dysphagia and chest pain. It is characterized by repetitive, forceful, nonpropulsive esophageal contractions. Some normal peristalsis is usually present, and the lower sphincter usually functions normally. It has been suggested that symptomatic idiopathic diffuse esophageal spasm is related to achalasia. In some cases, the syndrome may result from gastroesophageal reflux. The diagnosis can usually be confirmed by radiographic and manometric methods.

Treatment

Treatment should initially be directed at removing stimuli that may precipitate symptoms such as emotional stress; ingestion of hot, cold, or carbonated beverages; and eating rapidly without proper mastication. It is important to counsel patients to eat slowly in a relaxed atmosphere. Nitrates and calcium channel blockers as well as hydralazine (Apresoline) may be of some benefit. On occasion mild tranquilization with a benzodiazepine may be helpful, as are counseling and reassurance as to the benign nature of the condition.

In those patients with gastroesophageal reflux, antireflux treatment with elevation of the head of the bed, antacid administration, and avoidance of gastric irritants may be effective in relieving the esophageal spasm. In rare instances pneumatic dilatation or Heller myotomy may be required because of severe intractable symptoms. Some of these patients have an associated lower esophageal sphincter dysfunction (hypertensive, poorly relaxing sphincter) and may have hypertrophy of the distal esophageal musculature with resultant diverticulosis. Myotomy in such cases may be the only effective form of therapy.

Indeterminate Motor Abnormalities

There is a group of poorly defined syndromes with esophageal motor abnormalities that demonstrate some, but not all, features of achalasia. In addition, some cases show features intermediate between achalasia and symptomatic idiopathic diffuse esophageal spasm. Treatment of these conditions will depend on the findings seen with manometric studies.

"Nutcracker" Esophagus

A syndrome of dysphagia and chest pain associated with high amplitude distal esophageal peristaltic contractions has recently been reported. Treatment with calcium channel blockers appears to be effective in this subgroup of patients.

Miscellaneous Motor Disorders

Diabetes mellitus and alcoholism may result in neuropathy and disordered esophageal peristalsis. Thyrotoxic myopathy may cause disorders of peristalsis and dysphagia. Treatment is directed at the underlying disease process. Presbyesophagus refers to the peristaltic defects seen in the aged and may be caused by a variety of metabolic disorders and both central and peripheral nervous system disease seen in this age group.

Scleroderma Esophagus

Scleroderma esophagus refers to the smooth muscle disturbance seen in patients with scleroderma, systemic lupus erythematosus, rheumatoid arthritis, and other collagen vascular diseases. Raynaud's phenomenon is often associated with this disorder and may be a part of the cirrhosis–Raynaud's disease–scleroderma –telangiectasia syndrome. Absence of peristalsis in the distal two thirds of the esophagus (smooth muscle portion) and loss of lower esophageal sphincter function result in severe reflux, poor esophageal acid clearing, severe esophagitis, esophageal ulcers, and stricture formation. Esophagitis is severe and is more resistant to treatment than the usual cases of gastroesophageal reflux. Endoscopy should be performed to exclude malignancy.

Treatment

Antireflux treatment includes elevation of the head of the bed on 6 inch blocks and the use of frequent antacids (see gastroesophageal reflux, at top of next column). Stricture formation is common, and periodic bougienage, using tapered mercury-filled rubber (Maloney) dilators, is usually necessary. If the patient initially presents with a very tight stricture, other methods described hereafter will be required. Metoclopramide (Reglan) and bethanechol (Urecholine), which are beneficial in some patients with gastroesophageal reflux, are not usually effective in scleroderma esophagus. Antireflux surgery is usually not recommended for this condition.

INFLAMMATION

Esophagitis is an inflammation of the esophagus most commonly due to gastroesophageal reflux associated with an incompetent lower esophageal sphincter. A hiatal hernia may be associated but is not necessary for reflux to occur. Other causes of esophagitis include caustic burns, infections (*Candida,* herpes simplex) and pill-induced esophageal ulcers.

Esophageal inflammation, in addition to the usual symptoms of heartburn and regurgitation, may also cause dysphagia and odynophagia, even in the absence of stricture. Severe inflammation with associated edema and spasm can result in a sensation of dysphagia. The exact cause of the esophageal inflammation must be determined. Endoscopic examination is usually necessary.

Gastroesophageal Reflux

The treatment of gastroesophageal reflux has been described in the section on scleroderma esophagus. Elevation of the head of the bed prevents nocturnal acid contact with esophageal mucosa. Frequent antacid ingestion (every 2 hours while awake), often with the addition of an H_2 blocker such as cimetidine (Tagamet) or ranitidine (Zantac) at bedtime, both suppresses and neutralizes gastric acid secretion. I usually reserve treatment with bethanecol (Urecholine), which improves lower esophageal sphincter function, and metoclopramide (Reglan), which also improves gastric emptying, for those instances where the basic treatment program has not been effective.

Xanthines (theophylline, coffee, tea, chocolate, cola drinks), nicotine, alcohol, fats, anticholinergics, and female hormones may all potentiate lower esophageal sphincter dysfunction and should be avoided. Patients should not eat within several hours of going to bed and should avoid the use of tight corsets or braces. I also instruct patients to avoid certain straining maneuvers and heavy lifting.

When patients are truly refractory to medical management, are severely symptomatic, and have documented persistent reflux, consideration should be given to antireflux surgery. The Nissen fundoplication procedure currently appears to be the most effective in controlling reflux.

Caustic Burns

Caustic burns are usually accidental in children and the result of suicide attempts in adults. Ingestion of either strong acid or alkali agents severely injures the esophagus and causes extensive stricturing. Prompt endoscopy is mandatory to determine the extent and severity of the corrosive injury. A pediatric endoscope can be used to minimize the risk of perforation. The patient should not be allowed anything by mouth and should be observed closely for signs of perforation and mediastinitis. A water-soluble contrast (Gastrografin) swallow is performed, and, if perforation is present, prompt surgical treatment is required. When there is evidence of severe esophageal injury, treatment with a corticosteroid such as prednisone (60 to 80 mg per day in adults) is initiated promptly and tapered over 2 to 3 weeks. Antacids are given frequently while the patient is awake. Antibiotics may also have a place in the early treatment of severe injury.

Periodic esophageal dilatation is usually necessary except in the mildest of injuries. Dilatation with mercury-filled rubber dilators (Hurst or Maloney) is usually started within 4 to 7 days after the injury and repeated at least several times a week. Initially the dilatation should be performed under fluoroscopic observation. The frequency of dilatation is variable and may, in part, be determined by the degree of resistance experienced by the operator at the time of passage. The interval between dilatations can be gradually increased and eventually the procedure can be discontinued. Subsequent periodic endoscopy is necessary because of the increased incidence of squamous carcinoma in these patients.

Infections

The recent increased incidence of the acquired immune deficiency syndrome has resulted in a greater number of esophageal infections. Infections with *Candida* and herpes simplex are the most commonly seen and may present with dysphagia. Less common infections of the esophagus include tuberculosis and sarcoidosis. Monilial esophagitis may be seen in debilitated, very sick patients and in those with poorly controlled diabetes. Control of diabetes and other supportive measures to control the underlying illness are beneficial. Oral doses of nystatin (Mycostatin), 100,000 units, or clotrimazole (Mycelex) troches are given every 2 hours and are usually effective. Systemic therapy with ketoconazole (Nizoral), 200 to 400 mg per day, is also effective. Herpes simplex infection in immunocompromised patients can be treated using acyclovir (Zovirax), 5 mg per kg intravenously (over 1 hour) every 8 hours if renal function is normal. Treatment should be continued for 7 days.

Pill-Induced Esophageal Ulcers

Certain antibiotics, especially doxycycline and tetracycline, as well as other pills (potassium chloride, ferrous sulfate, quinidine, and ascorbic acid), when swallowed with insufficient liquid, may lodge in the esophagus, causing an ulcer. The presence of an esophageal motor disorder or the act of swallowing while prone (as seen in certain hospitalized patients) increases the risk of this occurrence. Dysphagia is usually temporary and antacid therapy is usually sufficient.

MECHANICAL CAUSES

Causes of mechanical esophageal obstruction may include extrinsic pressure as well as intrinsic lesions. Extrinsic obstruction may be caused by a number of processes anywhere along the length of the esophagus. Intrinsic obstruction can be caused by stricture, tumors, webs, rings, or foreign bodies.

Stricture

Strictures are usually peptic in origin and are a sequela of chronic inflammation due to reflux. They are most commonly seen in the distal esophagus. Barett's columnar-lined epithelium can cause ulcerations and stricturing in the esophagus. Although such strictures are often seen high in the esophagus, near the squamocolumnar junction, distal esophageal ulcers (gastric ulcers) and distal strictures are not uncommon. Caustic ingestion and prolonged nasogastric intubation can result in stricture formation. Chronic strictures from prior caustic ingestion tend to be long and narrow and are particularly difficult to dilate.

Patients with strictures usually require endoscopic evaluation to determine the size and pliability of the narrowing as well as to assess the state of the surrounding mucosa both visually and with biopsy and cytology evaluation. Some dilatation of the stricture can, at times, be performed with the endoscope itself, depending on the instrument used and the diameter of the stricture. I prefer to use tapered mercury-filled (Maloney) dilators whenever possible because of their safety and acceptability by patients.

After topical pharyngeal anesthesia with either Cetacaine spray or benzonatate (Tessalon) (200 mg dissolved on the back of the tongue), peroral passage with the patient in the sitting position is usually easily accomplished. Difficult strictures should initially be dilated under fluoroscopic guidance. Progressive dilatations with bougies of increasing diameter are usually well tolerated without pain. On occasion meperidine (Demerol), 50 mg intramuscularly, is given prior to dilating a very tight stricture.

The tapered tip of the Maloney dilator facilitates passage through the stricture. The weight of the dilator itself promotes passage, and usually very little force is necessary. A sensation of passing through the stricture can be felt at times, and only experience dictates how much force should be used. The initial size of dilator used depends on the diameter of the stricture. I use Maloney dilators of varying sizes from French number 26 to 50. Progressively larger dilators are passed, often at one sitting, depending on the resistance encountered. Dilatation up to the 50 French dilator is usually adequate to ensure normal swallowing. Depending on the cause, periodic dilatations should be continued, the frequency depending on the degree of restricturing that occurs.

Such blind dilatation should not be performed when a foreign body is present or a piece of food is impacted in the esophagus. In such circumstances endoscopic removal of the foreign body or the piece of food is necessary. If an underlying stricture is present, it can be treated subsequently.

Some strictures are particularly difficult to dilate because of a location very high in the esophagus, because they are very narrow or lengthy, or because of associated esophageal diverticula. Under such circumstances, dilatation should be performed under fluoroscopic observation. Again, Maloney dilators are my preference if possible. At times a small Maloney will not pass through the tight stricture and will buckle. I then try a larger dilator and wedge the tip in the stricture and apply some force. Because of its greater weight (more mercury) and diameter, it tends to buckle less and the tapered tip initiates the dilatation. I can then go back and use a smaller dilator effectively.

If this is not feasible, I use Eder-Puestow olive metal dilators. These olive dilators vary in size from French number 21 to 45 and are passed on a flexible rod over a guide wire. The guide wire is usually passed through the stricture under fluoroscopic guidance. When multiple diverticula surround the stricture, the guide wire is best passed under direct vision through the biopsy channel of an endoscope and then left in place as the instrument is withdrawn. Once adequate dilatation with progressively larger olive dilators has been accomplished, I use Maloney dilators.

Recently, small inflatable balloon dilators have become available for use. They come in diffferent sizes (4 to 20 mm diameter) and may become useful in dilating tight strictures. They are expensive, however, and not usually reusable.

Tumors

Tumors of the esophagus are usually malignant and often present with dysphagia. Most are squamous carcinoma except those that arise from Barrett's epithelium or at the cardioesophageal junction, which are adenocarcinoma. Squamous carcinoma of the upper and midesophagus is usually treated with radiation therapy. More distal lesions, when deemed operable, can be surgically resected. Radiation may be beneficial for some adenocarcinomas. Dilatation with Eder-Puestow or Maloney dilators can be safely performed either prior to or during radiation therapy. An esophageal prosthesis may be necessary when the lesion progresses and may provide a certain measure of temporary improvement in dysphagia.

Webs and Rings

Upper esophageal webs occur in the Plummer-Vinson syndrome and can often be easily torn with the endoscope. Lower esophageal (Schatzki) rings are usually seen at the squamocolumnar junction in association with a hiatal hernia. If the diameter is small, they can cause dysphagia. Dilatation can sometimes be accomplished with one of the larger endoscopes or with a Maloney dilator. Other techniques include balloon dilatation, use of endoscopic cutting instruments, and electrocautery.

Foreign Bodies

Foreign bodies, such as chicken and fish bones, can cause dysphagia and odynophagia. Such sharp objects pose a danger of esophageal perforation and mediastinitis. These and other ingested objects should be removed using endoscopic techniques with either rigid or fiberoptic instruments, depending on the nature of the object swallowed and its degree of impaction in the esophagus.

Food impaction may occur, especially in the presence of an underlying esophageal motor disorder or stricture. Removal of the retained piece of food with a fiberoptic endoscope or breaking it up endoscopically and then forcing it into the stomach can usually be accomplished. Treatment of the underlying cause of obstruction is necessary to prevent recurrence.

DIVERTICULA OF THE ALIMENTARY TRACT

method of
JAMES L. A. ROTH, M.D.
Presbyterian-University of Pennsylvania Medical Center
Philadelphia, Pennsylvania

Because of the increases in population and longevity, diverticulosis will become an increasingly common clinical problem in the future. The colon is the most common site of diverticula in the alimentary tract, followed, in order of frequency, by the duodenum, jejunum, ileum, and stomach.

HYPOPHARYNGEAL DIVERTICULUM

A hypopharyngeal diverticulum, better known as Zenker's pouch, is an acquired outpouching of the posterior hypopharyngeal wall. The symptoms of hypopharyngeal diverticulum include initially an irritation of the throat, the sensation of a foreign body, and a gurgling sound with swallowing liquids, and later postprandial or nocturnal regurgitation of mucus and food. If the pouch becomes very large, it may compress the esophagus, giving rise to dysphagia and eventually obstruction to swallowing.

Treatment

Some palliation may be achieved by chewing bland food thoroughly, flushing out the sac by drinking water after meals, and postural drainage or dilatation of the esophagus at the level of the diverticulum. However, persistent symptoms eventually require surgical therapy.

In an early stage when it is technically difficult to excise the diverticulum, a simple cricopharyngeal myotomy may suffice by correcting a pharyngoesophageal motor disorder. However, motility changes following this procedure for symptomatic Zenker's pouch have not yet been reported. When the diverticulum becomes 5 or 6 cm in diameter, most surgeons consider a diverticulopexy with cricopharyngeal myotomy or a one stage diverticulectomy with or without cricopharyngeal myotomy. A rigid esophagoscope or an Ewald tube is passed into the esophagus prior to amputation of the sac and serves to prevent narrowing or stricture with closure of the esophagus.

If the diverticulum is very large or complicated, some surgeons still prefer a two-stage procedure—mobilizing the sac and sewing it under the skin in an inverted position. When granulation tissue has sealed off the neck in 7 to 10 days, the skin is reopened and the sac excised. In the older debilitated patient who cannot tolerate an open operation, the Dohlman procedure may be selected. This consists of the endoscopic division of the cricopharyngeus and the "common party wall" between the esophagus and diverticulum.

Repair of the Zenker's pouch might result in certain complications. A pharyngocutaneous fistula usually undergoes spontaneous closure during nasogastric tube feeding along with local wide drainage and packing of the wound with zinc peroxide and hydrogen peroxide paste to increase oxygenation and promote granulation. Preoperative endoscopic cleansing of the diverticulum, meticulous closure of the pharyngeal wall, and the postoperative use of antibiotics prevent wound infection as a rule. However, if infection develops, drainage through the original incision and down to the prevertebral fascia is mandatory to prevent involvement of the mediastinum.

Injury to the left recurrent laryngeal nerve may give rise to transient or permanent laryngeal paralysis, manifest by hoarseness and aspiration of liquids with swallowing. Spontaneous recovery of laryngeal and glottic function may gradually occur in three to six months, but if it does not, consideration should be given to injecting the paralyzed vocal cord with Teflon. If hypopharyngeal stricture develops, despite use of the indwelling esophagoscope, Ewald tube, or large nasogastric tube as a stent during closure as recommended, an adequate lumen can be restored gradually by periodic dilatation with Maloney-type bougies. Inadequate excision of the diverticulum may result in a recurrence, and, as a preventive measure, many surgeons advocate an associated cricopharyngeal myotomy.

ESOPHAGEAL DIVERTICULUM

Because of the wide mouths and absence of necks in these diverticula, they seldom are symptomatic, for they empty readily. Occasionally (0.4 per cent) dysphagia or substernal pain associated with swallowing is attributed to these pouches. Temporary relief may be obtained from sublingual nitroglycerin (0.3 mg) or inhalation of amyl nitrite (0.2 ml). If esophagoscopy reveals concomitant esophagitis, management should be instituted (frequent small bland feedings, hourly liquid antacids between feedings, no food 2 hours before retiring, elevation of the chest 8 to 10 inches at nighttime, cimetidine). Anticholinergic drugs have not prevented symptoms. Because of the location of these diverticula, surgery may be inadvisable and is seldom required. Some have advocated a long esophageal myotomy to relieve distress from esophageal spasm. However, a midesophageal diverticulum very rarely may ulcerate and perforate into the trachea, bronchus, lung, or mediastinum.

Epiphrenic diverticula, projecting more commonly on the right side just above the lower esophageal sphincter, are associated frequently with hiatal hernia, diffuse esophageal spasm, or achalasia. However, the diverticula are rarely responsible for symptoms. In conjunction with achalasia, stretching the constricted area usually relieves the dysphagia, indicating that it was due to the achalasia rather than the associated epiphrenic diverticulum. Because of the associated conditions, esophagoscopy, although it may be hazardous, is frequently required in the evaluation of these patients. If reflux esophagitis is encountered, the medical measures previously mentioned for midesophageal diverticula should be given a thorough trial.

Operative intervention may become necessary if symptoms cannot be controlled or because of the associated conditions (stricture, obstructing lower esophageal ring). Good results have been reported with esophagomyotomy, relieving the associated motor disorder of either achalasia or diffuse esophageal spasm. If refractory gastroesophageal reflux is demonstrated, an antireflux procedure (Belsey or Nissen) may be required.

GASTRIC DIVERTICULA

Diverticula of the stomach are rare and occur most commonly high in the posterior wall of the stomach

(75 per cent) and in the prepyloric region (15 to 18 per cent). Patients with gastric diverticula may complain of postprandial epigastric fullness or substernal pain, heartburn, nausea, vomiting, and, occasionally, dysphagia. Since most gastric diverticula are asymptomatic, some other cause for these symptoms must be sought. This is particularly true of the prepyloric diverticula. Nevertheless, large juxtacardiac diverticula may be responsible for discomfort after meals, when the patient is recumbent, and especially if relief is obtained by a change in position that seems to favor emptying the sac.

Treatment

Treatment is conservative unless complications develop. The medical measures to be tried are reassurance, bland diet, liquid antacids, and especially postural drainage if fluoroscopy reveals an optimum position for emptying the diverticulum. Surgical intervention is indicated when symptoms are severe and relief cannot be obtained by medical measures, when peptic ulcer complications or malignancy cannot be excluded, or when the diverticula become complicated by massive hemorrhage, perforation, torsion, or invagination into the esophagus with resultant intermittent dysphagia. The procedure of choice is local excision, but the juxtacardiac diverticulum may require a thoracoabdominal approach and splenectomy to permit adequate exposure. A partial gastrectomy may be the better solution to complications of diverticula in the prepyloric region.

SMALL INTESTINAL DIVERTICULA

Diverticulum of Duodenum

Duodenal diverticula may be single or multiple, vary in size from 0.5 to 10 cm, and project from the inner concave (pancreatic) border of the duodenal loop. The majority of these diverticula are within 3 cm of the ampulla of Vater. This location accounts for the symptom patterns ascribed to the diverticula, but most of them are asymptomatic. In approximately 10 per cent of patients with duodenal diverticula, they are considered a possible cause of longstanding symptoms that may simulate peptic ulcer or biliary tract or pancreatic diseases. Diverticulitis, ulceration with perforation or hemorrhage, obstructive jaundice, blind loop syndrome, and pancreatitis have been reported as complications of duodenal diverticula. Hypotonic duodenography, duodenoscopy, and endoscopic retrograde cholangiopancreatography have greatly helped in the clinical evaluation of duodenal diverticular disease.

Treatment

In the absence of a complication, initial treatment should be conservative, namely, gastroduodenal rest (a strict ulcer regimen, peroral jejunal feedings, or intravenous hyperalimentation depending on the severity of associated inflammation) and periodic postural drainage if fluoroscopy reveals a position that best empties a retentive diverticulum. Since duodenal diverticula are rarely responsible for the patient's symptoms, the temptation to attribute them to the diverticula should be resisted as well as an attempt at surgical intervention.

Surgery may be indicated if any of the complications of duodenal diverticula develop, such as diverticulitis, hemorrhage, perforation, abscess formation, or peritonitis; secondary inflammation of the biliary tract, pancreas, or retroperitoneal tissues; and superimposed malignant disease. Although excision of the sac is the preferred procedure, the anatomic circumstances may only permit inversion of the sac or a side-tracking operation. Operation on diverticula in the second portion of the duodenum entails considerable risk because of its retroperitoneal position and proximity to the common bile duct, pancreatic duct, and large blood vessels. When multiple diverticula are present and surgery is necessary, excision or inversion procedures should be limited to the diverticula most likely responsible for symptoms, i.e., those that are large, retentive, inflamed, and near the ampulla. When a duodenal diverticulum is responsible for obstruction to the common bile duct, a choledochoduodenostomy or Roux-en-Y choledochojejunostomy is safer than excision of the diverticulum.

Diverticulum of Jejunum and Ileum

The majority of diverticula of the mesenteric small bowel are multiple, occur in the jejunum, and are hernias of mucous membrane protruding through the muscular wall of the intestine at a point of locus minoris resistentiae, a gap caused by the entrance of blood vessels at the mesenteric border. These diverticula are usually asymptomatic and are discovered accidentally by x-ray examinations in patients over 40 years whose complaints were due to other causes.

Although not characteristic, certain symptom patterns have been attributed to small bowel diverticula, particularly those in the jejunum: (1) chronic mild indigestion with postprandial colicky pain, audible borborygmi, and anorexia; (2) varying degrees of chronic nonmechanical ileus, so-called jejunal dyskinesia (Altemeir), associated with hypertrophy of the jejunum in the segment of multiple diverticula; (3) blind loop syndrome (Badenoch) due to stasis and bacterial overgrowth with resultant megaloblastic anemia (B_{12} deficiency) and/or steatorrhea (deficiencies of vitamins A, D, and K); and (4) the symptoms of an acute abdominal catastrophy due to complication of the diverticula.

Treatment

Before treatment is directed toward the small bowel diverticula, other causes of gastrointestinal complaints must be ruled out. Medical management is the treatment of choice as long as symptoms are not incapacitating and complications do not develop. Medical measures to be considered are (1) diet, surgical liquids to bland foods depending on the symptoms and objective manifestations; (2) anticholinergics, loperamide (Imodium), or diphenoxylate (Lomotil) may be helpful for diarrhea or discomfort; (3) a hydrophilic preparation (psyllium seed) if there is no evidence of obstruction; and (4) if malabsorption of fat or vitamin B_{12} due to a blind loop syndrome is documented, treatment is directed toward reduction of bacterial overgrowth and replacement of nutrients. A 7 to 10 day therapeutic trial with broad spectrum antibiotics (250 mg tetracycline or ampicillin 1 hour after meals and at bedtime) will confirm the diagnosis with subsidence of diarrhea and improvement in fat absorption. Prolonged intermittent antibiotic therapy for 10 days out of every 6 weeks for years may be necessary to maintain the therapeutic response; this therapy has been reported without adverse side effects.

Although useful in the management of the blind loop syndrome, lincomycin and clindamycin, both of which are effective against anaerobic organisms, carry an increased risk of diarrhea or enterocolitis. Until the antibiotic therapy becomes effective, the diet should be low in fat content (40 to 50 grams per day) to reduce steatorrhea, flatulence, and abdominal discomfort. Initially, nutritional deficits will need to be repleted: (1) vitamin B_{12}—100 micrograms parenterally, monthly; (2) vitamin D—50,000 units daily; (3) calcium gluconate—4 to 8 grams daily; (4) vitamin K-phytonadione (AquaMephyton)—10 mg parenterally daily; and (5) if iron deficiency has resulted from chronic blood loss, ferrous gluconate—320 mg 3 times daily after meals.

Surgery may become indicated for complications, such as acute mechanical obstruction; diverticulitis with abscess formation, fistulization, perforation, or generalized peritonitis; hemorrhage; rupture of a diverticulum; foreign bodies; or superimposed neoplastic disease. Because of the risk of perforation, large diverticula that retain barium for long periods of time probably should be removed. Excision of the pouch and invagination of the stump with a pursestring suture is the usual procedure. However, if multiple diverticula are present, resection of the involved segment with an end-to-end anastomosis may be necessary, provided the length of bowel is short. If diverticula are present in a major portion of the intestine, resection should be limited to only that segment in which the largest sacs are located or in which obvious complications are seen.

Meckel's Diverticulum

Failure of complete obliteration of the intra-abdominal portion of the vitelline duct (yolk stalk) gives rise to the most common congenital anomaly in the gastrointestinal tract, Meckel's diverticulum. Unless a complication develops, Meckel's diverticulum is symptomless because of its wide mouth. The complications that produce clinical manifestations are obstruction, most commonly due to intussusception or volvulus; peptic ulceration, with resultant hemorrhage, perforation, or cicatricial stenosis; diverticulitis, with a clinical picture almost indistinguishable from that of acute appendicitis; and occasionally foreign body perforation.

Treatment

Treatment is local excision of the sac and closure of the bowel wall in the transverse axis to prevent stenosis. If the adjacent ileum is affected by peptic ulceration, inflammation, or strangulation, it should be resected along with the diverticulum. When a Meckel's diverticulum is encountered as an incidental finding at laparotomy, the morbidity resulting from excision of an asymptomatic diverticulum makes this intervention unwise.

DIVERTICULAR DISEASE OF THE COLON*

Diverticular disease is probably the most prevalent affliction of the colon in the United States. Approximately one third of the population over age 45 and three fifths over age 70 are estimated to have colonic diverticulosis. When diverticula are demonstrated in a barium enema study, it must be decided whether the patient's symptoms are due to diverticulosis.

Asymptomatic Diverticular Disease

Since diverticulosis of the colon is frequently found during routine investigations or in the evaluation of the irritable colon syndrome, it is not surprising that for many years uncomplicated diverticulosis was not implicated in symptom production. However, sigmoid manometric studies have indicated that patients with diverticulosis have a muscular motor disorder similar to that demonstrated in the irritable colon syndrome. In both conditions there is the tendency for hyperreactivity in response to food ingestion or emotional stimuli, with a marked increase in the amplitude of circular muscle contractions. As a consequence intraluminal pressure is increased, the bowel wall is stretched, pain

*Portions of this presentation have been published in *Current Concepts in Gastroenterology* 2:19, 1977, and are included with permission of the editor.

is experienced, and, it is postulated, mucosal herniation (a diverticulum) through a weak point where blood vessels penetrate the wall eventually occurs. Thus, the irritable colon syndrome maybe a precursor of colonic diverticulosis.

In patients with uncomplicated diverticulosis, symptoms are nonspecific and reflect changes in motility and intraluminal pressures of the colon rather than the presence of diverticula per se. Indeed, a single diverticulum or even simple massed diverticulosis is usually asymptomatic. Colonic diverticulosis should be suspected if a patient over 40 years of age complains of lower abdominal pain, constipation or diarrhea or both, and increased flatulence. The diagnosis depends upon the roentgenographic demonstration of the presence of diverticula. In the absence of any other demonstrable lesion, the colonic symptoms can be attributed to disordered activity of the sigmoid colon, associated with either the irritable colon syndrome or diverticulosis.

Treatment

No therapeutic regimen has been proved to alter the natural history of diverticulosis or to prevent its complications (Table 1). Current theory ascribes the pathogenesis of diverticulosis and diverticulitis to increased intraluminal pressure within the colon. Some investigators have suggested lack of bulk (unrefined fiber) in the diet of Western peoples as the cause of increased pressure. The speculation is based on the infrequency with which diverticular disease is encountered in Africa and Asia, where the diet is high in fiber content.

Although distention of the colon with bulk foods (or hydrophilic agents) reduces intracolonic pressure, there are no controlled, long-term prospective studies to prove that a high fiber diet prevents the development of diverticulosis or diverticulitis. Nor is there sufficient evidence to support the use of a low fiber diet, which has been advocated in the treatment of diverticulosis in the past. Furthermore, emotional stress may be of equal or even greater importance in producing increased intracolonic pressures and is probably more common in so-called Western civilization.

If the lack of fiber in the diet predisposes to the development of diverticulosis or diverticulitis, then it is reasonable to increase dietary roughage. A high fiber diet increases bulk in the stool by absorption of water by the fibers, reduces pressure against the colonic wall since muscular contractions exert pressure longitudinally when colon contents are bulky, and prevents constipation and straining. The high fiber diet produces softer as well as bulkier stools and thus there is less likelihood of hard scybala lodging in diverticula. Blocking the mouth of a diverticulum may increase pressure within it, causing a microperforation and diverticulitis. Therefore, undigestible roughage that might block the mouths of diverticula should be avoided (see Table 1). Increased stool bulk may be achieved from the high fiber content of unrefined wheat, certain fruits, and vegetables (Table 2). Although dietary fiber may do some good, there are circumstances when it should be forbidden, e.g., when acute abdominal pain is associated with inflammation and especially if there is organic narrowing of the bowel lumen.

If the high fiber diet does not prevent constipation or straining, additional dietary fiber, stool bulk formers, or stool softeners may be required. *Bran* (the inner husk of wheat kernel) has been promoted as an efficient dietary source of fiber. Unprocessed or miller's bran is inexpensive but unpalatable and not readily available. Two teaspoonsful may be added to cereals, one to three times daily as tolerated and needed. However, not all patients with the irritable colon syndrome tolerate bran initially, experiencing increased

TABLE 1. **Management of Asymptomatic Diverticular Disease**

1. No therapeutic regimen has proven to alter natural history of diverticulosis or to prevent its complications
2. High fiber diet to increase stool bulk
   a. Unrefined wheat (bran cereals, whole wheat bread), fruit (bananas, peaches, pears, apples, oranges, seedless grapes or raisins, prunes), and vegetables (carrots, turnips, lettuce)
   b. Avoid undigestible roughage: nuts, corn, popcorn, seeds (tomato, cucumber, grapes, figs, strawberries, raspberries, blueberries, sesame, poppy, or caraway), and raw celery
3. Prevent constipation
   a. Supplements of unprocessed bran or processed bran cereals
   b. Hydrophilic colloids: Konsyl, Metamucil, Instant Hydrocil
   c. Stool softeners: Colace or Surfak
4. Understanding the pathogenesis and significance of change in symptoms

TABLE 2. **Relatively High Fiber Foods***

Cereals/Breads	Vegetables	Fruit
Bran	Green peas	Blackberries
Shredded Wheat	Parsnips	Raspberries
Grape Nuts	Winter squash	Figs
Ry-Krisp	Broccoli	Pears
Whole wheat bread	Brussels sprouts	Strawberries
Whole rye bread	String beans	Huckleberries
Graham crackers	Sweet potatoes	Blueberries
Oatmeal	Artichokes	Apples
Puffed Wheat	Lima beans	Tangerines
Wheatina	Carrots	Prunes

*In order of decreasing fiber content.

flatulence and cramping lower abdominal pain. The amount may need to be gradually increased over several weeks. Processed bran cereals are generally more acceptable, but the fiber content varies considerably (all per ounce): 3.0 to 3.6 grams in unprocessed bran; 1.8 to 2.3 grams in Kellogg's All-Bran or Bran Buds; 1.4 grams in Purina's Bran Chex; 0.8 to 1.1 grams in 40 per cent Bran Flakes or Raisin Bran; 0.3 to 1.0 grams in Shredded Wheat, Puffed Wheat, Total, or Krumbles; and 0.4 to 0.7 grams in Farina, Quaker Rolled Oats or Wheatina. Bran may also be incorporated in muffins or cookies.

Hydrophilic colloids can be used to increase stool bulk and are usually well tolerated. Psyllium seed absorbs 15 ml of water per gram of fiber compared with bran, which absorbs only 3 ml of water per gram of fiber. One heaping teaspoonful of Konsyl or Instant Hydrocil or 2 teaspoonsful of Metamucil stirred in half a glass of lukewarm water or juice followed by a full glass of water every morning has been recommended by the author for many years in the management of the irritable colon syndrome or diverticular disease.

If, despite the foregoing measures, the stool remains hard, a stool softener (dioctyl sodium or calcium sulfosuccinate) in a dose of 1 or 2 capsules after the evening meal may be added to the regimen. Occasionally a patient may need a mild laxative such as milk of magnesia or mineral oil in the initial phase of establishing regularity in stool habit. However, loose stools should be avoided, as this will result in increased intracolonic pressures.

The patient with diverticulosis should understand the pathogenesis of the condition. This is most effectively achieved by use of a diagram, explaining the roles of stool bulk and intracolonic pressures. The importance of adhering to the therapeutic measures should be emphasized. Although reassurance is desirable, the patient must be aware of the significance of a change in bowel habit, more severe abdominal pain, the appearance of blood-tinged mucus, fever, and associated urinary symptoms. He should be instructed to notify the physician at once if such a change in the pattern of symptoms develops. This policy will permit early recognition and appropriate treatment of complications.

Painful Diverticular Disease

If, in addition to nonspecific symptoms, the patient experiences more severe recurrent abdominal pain, so-called painful diverticular disease should be considered. The pain is cramp-like or colicky and may be so intense as to force the patient to sit down or go to bed. Although usually localized in the left lower quadrant, the pain may be referred to the hypogastric area or right lower quadrant if a redundant pelvic colon lies in the right iliac fossa. As a result of the gastrocolic reflex, the pain often follows a meal. Relief may occur with passage of flatus or bowel movement, but the latter may be associated with increased pain. The attack may be accompanied by constipation or diarrhea. A tender, freely movable, rope-like mass, similar to that encountered in the irritable colon syndrome, is frequently palpable. However, the signs of localized or generalized peritonitis are absent and the temperature, white blood count, and sedimentation rate are normal. Some abdominal distention may be present, but bowel sounds are normal and survey x-ray films reveal no evidence of adynamic ileus or obstruction.

Treatment

Treatment of painful diverticular disease is directed toward the relief of painful bowel spasm and diverticulosis (Table 3). The measures previously discussed for diverticulosis are recommended, including a high fiber diet, avoidance of undigestible roughage, bran supplements, hydrophilic colloids, and stool softeners as needed. Intraluminal pressure measurements in the sigmoid have demonstrated a marked increased in the amplitude of circular muscle contractions in response to food ingestion or emotional stress in this disorder. Muscle spasm may be relaxed by local application of heat and antispasmodics.

Anticholinergics inhibit normal segmental sigmoid contractions and thus may relieve cramping abdominal pain. Propantheline (Pro-Banthine), 15 or 30 mg, or dicyclomine hydrochloride (Bentyl), 20 mg, ½ hour before meals is commonly prescribed for this purpose. However, caution should be exercised to avoid excess anticholinergic effect, which would aggravate constipation. Anticholinergics have not proved to be clinically effective in painful diverticular disease. Recently, crystalline glucagon has become available, and its inhibition of bowel motility has promptly relieved severe painful spasm. Further critical evaluation of its use is necessary before it can be recommended.

Although *sedatives* do not have a direct pharmacologic action on the colonic muscle, they may alleviate tension and anxiety, which have been shown to increase the amplitude of sigmoid mus-

TABLE 3. **Management of Painful Diverticular Disease**

1. Same as for asymptomatic diverticulosis: high fiber diet, avoidance of undigestible roughage, bran supplements, hydrophilic colloids, and stool softener
2. Relieve colonic spasm
   a. Local heat
   b. Antispasmodics: anticholinergics, glucagon
3. Sedatives or tranquilizers
4. Nonopiate analgesics: Tylenol, Darvon-N

cular contractions. Phenobarbital or butabarbital, 15 to 30 mg, or chlordiazepoxide (Librium) or diazepam (Valium), 5 to 10 mg, may be used 2 to 3 times per day for this purpose. Nonopiate *analgesics* such as acetaminophen (Tylenol) or propoxyphene napsylate (Darvon-N) may be necessary every 3 to 4 hours to relieve pain. More potent analgesics are required in some instances, but glucagon given parenterally has obviated this need in preliminary reports.

Diverticulitis

The acute exacerbation of irritable colon syndrome can be easily mistaken for diverticulitis. Conversely, mild attacks of diverticulitis may go unnoticed or may be assumed to be flare-ups of the irritable colon syndrome. When abdominal distention and marked local tenderness are encountered in painful diverticular disease, a palpable sigmoid loop may be mistaken for an inflammatory mass due to diverticulitis. On barium enema study, narrowing of the sigmoid, irregularity of the luminal contour, and even a saw toothed marginal outline can occur in diverticulosis, and these findings are no longer considered indicative of diverticulitis. Thus, in a patient known to have diverticulosis, the diagnosis of diverticulitis is based upon clinical features: a tender mass, fever, leukocytosis, elevated erythrocyte sedimentation rate, and sometimes bloody mucus or microscopic pyuria.

Treatment

When the diagnosis is not in doubt and the *attack is mild,* the patient may be treated at home as outlined in Table 4. Since diverticulitis results from a microperforation with infection outside the colon (pericolitis) and not within the colonic lumen, a systemically effective antibiotic must be administered. A broad spectrum antimicrobial drug should be selected, one that may be expected to be effective against the colon flora (*E. coli, Bacteroides*). Ampicillin or Keflex, 250 to 500 mg orally every 6 hours, or tetracycline may be used, if the patient is allergic to penicillins. If there is any deterioration in the patient's general condition or if pain worsens and fever mounts, immediate hospitalization is mandatory.

If the attack is more severe and fulminant with intense pain or a tender left lower quadrant mass, fever, and leukocytosis, the patient should be hospitalized without delay to permit close clinical observation. Upon admission, the surgeon should be consulted to permit his participation in the decisions and timing of diagnostic procedures and surgery if needed. Sometimes a persistent marked elevation of the erythrocyte sedimentation rate is the only residual clue to an unsuspected abscess. Sigmoidoscopy should be performed gently and without air insufflation to exclude other diagnostic possibilities (e.g., carcinoma, Crohn's disease of the colon, ulcerative colitis, amebiasis) and to demonstrate the suitability of the rectosigmoid distal to the diverticulitis for an anastomosis in the event of surgical intervention.

TABLE 4. **Management of Acute Diverticulitis**

A. Mild attack, diagnosis not in doubt
  1. May be treated at home with bed rest, liquid diet, anticholingerics, nonopiate analgesics, ampicillin
  2. Immediate hospitalization if pain worsens, fever mounts, or general condition deteriorates

B. Severe, fulminant attack or diagnosis uncertain
  1. Hospitalize at once to permit close clinical observations
     a. Surgical consultation on admission
     b. Vital signs every 4 hours, frequent abdominal examinations, serial survey films of abdomen
     c. Chest x-ray, EKG, urinalysis, periodic WBC and ESR, blood cultures
     d. Sigmoidoscopy without air insufflation
  2. Colonic "rest": bed rest, NPO, nasogastric suction, IV fluids, glucose and electrolytes
  3. Parenteral broad spectrum antibiotics: ampicillin or cephazolin; cefoxitin and amikacin or penicillin G (HD), clindamycin and gentamicin if gram negative septicemia
  4. Demerol (not morphine) for pain relief

C. Attack has subsided
  1. Stepwise advance of diet to solid foods
  2. Continue oral broad spectrum antibiotics until parameters of inflammation have subsided
  3. Resume other measures for asymptomatic diverticulosis
  4. Diagnostic studies: BE, IVP, ? fiberoptic sigmoidoscopy or colonoscopy (caution!), mesenteric arteriography

The objectives of therapy in acute diverticulitis are to put the bowel at "rest" and to combat infection. "Colonic rest" is achieved by bed rest, permitting nothing by mouth, nasogastric suction if nausea and vomiting are present, and appropriate intravenous fluids, glucose, and electrolytes. If mechanical obstruction develops, most often due to adherence of pelvic small bowel loops to a sigmoid inflammatory mass, a long intestinal tube may become necessary for decompression.

Since septicemia due to gram negative organisms (*E. coli* or anaerobic *Bacteroides*) is a possible hazard in diverticulitis, blood cultures should be obtained routinely. If a significant growth is recovered, appropriate therapy may be instituted once the organism has been identified and its antibiotic sensitivity determined. Nonabsorbable oral sulfonamides are not used since the inflammatory process is extracolonic, a peridiverticulitis due to micro- or macroperforation. A broad spectrum antibiotic should be administered *parenterally*. Ampicillin, 0.5 gram every 6 hours, or cephazolin (Ancef or Kefzol, 4 mg per kg per day) may be given at the outset until reports on the blood cultures are available.

If a gram negative septicemia is present, prompt and vigorous therapy is necessary. The preferred combination of intravenous antibiotic therapy is cefoxitin (Mefoxin), 2 grams every 6 to 8 hours, and amikacin (Amikin), 7.5 mg per kg every 12 hours intravenously over 30 to 60 minutes; or penicillin G, 10 to 12 million units per day, clindamycin (Cleocin), 300 to 600 mg every 6 hours, and gentamicin (Garamycin), 1 to 1.5 mg per kg per day (adjusting to serial creatinine determinations). The course of antibiotic therapy is continued for 7 to 10 days, even though a prompt response is obtained.

When pain is severe, the analgesic of choice is meperidine hydrochloride (Demerol), 50 to 75 mg intramuscularly every 3 hours as circumstances may require, because it inhibits segmental contractions of the colon. However, opiates (morphine) are contraindicated since they have been shown to increase intraluminal colonic pressure. Anticholinergics probably should not be used in the presence of diverticulitis because of the possibility of aggravating an ileus or prostatism. The role of glucagon is relieving pain due to peridiverticulitis remains to be established by further experience.

With the foregoing treatment, symptoms and signs of the peridiverticulitis usually begin to subside in 3 or 4 to 7 days. A liquid diet can then be started with progressive advance gradually to solid foods, and ambulation is permitted. Until abdominal pain and tenderness, fever, and leukocytosis have disappeared and the elevated erythrocyte sedimentation rate becomes nearly normal, the broad spectrum antibiotics should be continued orally. When the acute attack has subsided, the maintenance dietary and other measures recommended for asymptomatic diverticulosis are resumed. Diagnostic studies may be pursued when the acute attack has subsided. Barium enema is postponed in the presence of acute peridiverticulitis but is necessary to detect residual changes of a confined abscess, fistula, or associated disease, particularly carcinoma. An intravenous pyelogram should be obtained to exclude asymptomatic urinary tract obstruction. Fiberoptic sigmoidoscopy or colonoscopy may be helpful in selected instances to exclude carcinoma as the cause of persistent narrowing in the sigmoid. Extreme caution must be exercised in performing this examination, however, because of the risk of perforation when the sigmoid is angulated and fixed by inflammation.

Although massive hemorrhage with melena (cecal diverticula) or, more commonly, hematocopria may occur in 5 to 27 per cent of patients with noninflamed diverticular disease, the most common cause of lower gastrointestinal massive hemorrhage is bleeding colonic diverticulosis. The hypertensive, elderly patient with arteriosclerotic vascular disease is most vulnerable. Barium enema has been credited with stopping the bleeding by tamponade effect or hemostatic action of barium sulfate. Mesenteric arteriography may localize the site (if the rate of bleeding is 700 ml per day or more) and permit control of the hemorrhage with selective intra-arterial infusion of vasopressin or embolization of the bleeding vessel or may guide the surgeon in carrying out a selective resection.

The majority of hemorrhaging diverticula have been demonstrated by arteriography to be in the ascending colon. The bleeding frequently subsides spontaneously with conservative measures (bed rest, sedation, blood replacement), but total colectomy and ileoproctostomy may be necessary when bleeding is uncontrollable. Even though the hemorrhage subsides spontaneously (80 per cent) or is controlled by vasoconstrictive action of the vasopressin or selective mesenteric arterial embolization, recurrent bleeding may be massive in 20 to 25 per cent of patients, warranting elective resection. That decision depends upon whether the site of bleeding has been identified, the probability of recurrent hemorrhage (increases to 50 per cent or more after a second hemorrhage), and the estimated risk of operation.

Surgical Management

Complications, such as perforation, abscess, fistula, obstruction, or hemorrhage, occur in 20 per cent of patients with acute diverticulitis. With multiple attacks, the chance of a complication developing is increased threefold. Furthermore, recurrence increases the likelihood that surgical intervention will be necessary. For these reasons, we at the Presbyterian-University of Pennsylvania Medical Center have adopted the policy of performing a prophylactic resection in patients who have had two or more attacks of bona fide diverticulitis (a tender mass, fever, leukocytosis, elevated erythrocyte sedimentation rate, and sometimes bloody mucus or microscopic pyuria), especially if they are under 40 years of age.

Before certain patients develop a serious complication, elective one-stage resection and anastomosis is also advised for the following circumstances: (1) after subsidence of a first attack associated with a persistent palpable tender mass; (2) first attack with a confined microperforation and extravasation of barium outside of the colon; (3) recurrent partial obstruction with narrowing of the lumen and proximal slight distention of the colon; (4) recurrent urinary tract symptoms (dysuria, aggravation of left lower quadrant, or suprapubic pain with micturition) following an episode of diverticulitis; (5) recovery from one or more serious rectal hemorrhages due

TABLE 5. **Surgery for Complications of Diverticulitis**

1. PERFORATION
   a. Free perforation with spreading peritonitis: emergency resection, proximal end colostomy, distal end closed or mucous fistula; systemic antibiotics; delayed second-stage restoration of bowel continuity
   b. Free perforation with established peritonitis and extreme risk: three-stage procedure—proximal colostomy and drainage; resection and anastomosis; restoration of bowel continuity
   c. Perforation with large abscess: three-stage procedure—proximal transverse colostomy and extraperitoneal drainage in left lower quadrant; resection with anastomosis; closure of colostomy
   d. Confined perforation with small abscess: one-stage resection and drainage of the site
2. FISTULA
   a. Colovesical
      (1) Majority: primary resection and closure of bladder fistula
      (2) Extensive inflammation, large abscess or obstruction: three stages—diverting transverse colostomy; resection and closure of fistula; closure of colostomy
   b. Colovaginal: one-stage resection with anastomosis and drainage of pelvis
   c. Coloenteric
      (1) Majority: prompt resection of sigmoid and adherent small bowel en bloc with reanastomosis of two bowel components
      (2) Severe local sepsis: two-stages—resection of involved bowel en bloc, anastomosis of small bowel and proximal colostomy; delayed closure of colostomy
3. OBSTRUCTION
   a. First attack with acute obstructive symptoms: bowel rest, antibiotics, nasogastric suction
   b. Previous episodes of partial obstruction with progressive narrowing of lumen: elective one-stage resection and anastomosis
   c. Almost complete or complete (? associated carcinoma) obstruction: two-stages—decompressive transverse colostomy; subsequent bowel cleansing and preparation; resection and anastomosis several weeks later
   d. Adherent small bowel obstruction: decompression with Miller-Abbott, Cantor, or Joel-Baker tubes, small bowel freed from inflamed sigmoid, diverticulitis treated appropriately
4. BLEEDING (exclude other causes, e.g., carcinoma, angiodysplasia, etc.)
   a. Diverticulosis localized to sigmoid or descending colon: segmental resection and anastomosis
   b. Arteriography demonstrates a bleeding site: resection of appropriate segment
   c. Diverticulosis generalized and bleeding site cannot be identified: colectomy with ileorectal anastomosis

to diverticulosis, particularly if generalized; and (6) when underlying carcinoma cannot be excluded, especially with recurrent episodes of slight bleeding.

A one-stage resection and anastomosis may not always be carried out in these situations. A final decision regarding the most appropriate operative procedure can only be made at the operating table. It is essential for safe healing of the anastomosis that there be no free pus or inflammation of the proximal and distal lines of resection. The hypertrophic muscular segment of the sigmoid and rectosigmoid should be removed. If the severity of the local inflammatory process precludes a safe primary anastomosis, a two-stage or sometimes three-stage procedure should be performed. The various procedures used in the surgical management of the complications of diverticulitis are summarized in Table 5. In recent years mortality and morbidity have been greatly reduced by the multiple-stage procedures, but the recognition of those patients who are vulnerable to further recurrences or complications has prevented the need for emergency surgery by earlier elective prophylactic resections.

CROHN'S DISEASE

method of
GEORGE B. RANKIN, M.D.
The Cleveland Clinic
Cleveland, Ohio

Since the etiology of Crohn's disease remains unknown, treatment of this underlying inflammatory disease remains empiric. Experience has shown that medical regimens must be individualized depending upon the age of the patient and the location and severity of the disease.

Management

Dietary and Nutritional Support

There remains much confusion in practice and the literature regarding the dietary management of Crohn's disease. Strict dietary restrictions are not routinely used. However, in some patients residue restrictions may reduce gaseousness, abdominal discomfort, and diarrhea, and the avoidance of bowel stimulants such as coffee, tea, and carbonated beverages may be beneficial. A food symptom diary is sometimes helpful for identifying poorly tolerated foods. The routine practice of restricting milk and dairy products for all patients with Crohn's disease is unnecessary and should be applied only to those patients with a clear-cut history of lactose intolerance. The majority of the patients who need restriction are those with extensive small bowel involvement or those within that small percentage of the population that clearly have an inherited lactose intolerance. Supplemental lactase preparations (LactAid) are available.

In those patients with hypoproteinemia due to

mucosal loss, malabsorption, or malnutrition, it is prudent to increase the oral intake of protein, if tolerated, and, when necessary, to supplement the diet with one of the available protein supplements (Sustacal, Ensure, and high protein Jello). A reasonable protein intake of 100 grams or more per day is recommended. The use of free elemental diets may be helpful in some patients with diarrhea as they require minimal digestion and thus help to reduce the stool volume. Such dietary preparations include Criticare, Travasorb-HN, and Precision High Nitrogen.

Hyperalimentation. In some patients, especially those who require surgical intervention, peripheral or central hyperalimentation may be extremely helpful in the preoperative correction of severe nutritional deficits, which can be adequately determined by appropriate nutritional assessment. When possible, oral alimentation should be used in these patients; however, when oral alimentation is not possible, the intravenous route is indicated. When resorting to the intravenous route or central venous catheter, concentrated glucose, nitrogen as protein hydrolysates or pure L-amino acids, and lipids are infused along with the required vitamins and trace minerals. When using the central venous catheter, extreme care must be utilized to prevent infection and thrombotic complications. Other complications that one must watch for include hyperglycemia, hypoglycemia, osmotic dehydration, essential fatty acid deficiency, trace metal deficiencies, and hypophosphatemia.

Treatment of the Inflammation

Corticosteroids and Adrenocorticotropin. The use of corticosteroids continues to be the preferred medical treatment of active Crohn's disease, especially when there is small bowel involvement. The dosage regimens vary widely; the starting dosage of prednisone or the equivalent is 25 to 100 mg daily. Oral doses of steroids are usually tapered over several weeks to months depending on the patient's response. The intravenous administration of corticosteroids or adrenocorticotropin has been shown to be effective in hospitalized patients with severe Crohn's colitis. The alternate day use of corticosteroids may help to decrease side effects, but not all patients seem to be well controlled on this type of regimen. The topical application of steroids, as well as retention enemas and rectal suppositories, may be helpful in some patients with Crohn's disease involving the rectosigmoid colon.

Sulfasalazine. Sulfasalazine (Azulfidine) has been clearly shown to be an effective form of therapy in active Crohn's disease, especially when there is colonic involvement. The usual starting dosage is 4 to 6 grams daily, and, as with steroid treatment, the dosage may be tapered over several weeks to months depending on the patient's response. The common side effects of sulfasalazine (nausea, vomiting, and headaches) are usually dose-related. Male infertility may be a side effect of the drug but is completely reversed upon discontinuation of the medication. Severe hypersensitivity reactions are extremely rare. Desensitization programs have been used successfully in some patients.

Metronidazole. Metronidazole (Flagyl) is effective in some patients with colonic involvement as well as some patients with perianal complications, although the medication has not been approved for this use by the Federal Drug Administration. Some patients with Crohn's colitis respond to metronidazole when they have not shown improvement on sulfasalazine. The usual dosage is 20 mg per kg per day. Peripheral neuropathy is a well recognized complication of metronidazole and may last for some weeks after the medication is discontinued. Patients must refrain from using alcohol while on treatment.

Immunosuppressives. Both azathioprine (Imuran) and 6-mercaptopurine (Purinethol) have been used in patients with extensive Crohn's disease, especially when other forms of treatment have failed. Successful healing of fistulae and management of other complications have been reported in patients treated with these drugs, although the Federal Drug Administration has not approved these drugs for this use. The immunosuppressive agents are usually added to the medical regimen after patients have failed to respond to the more conventional treatment. All patients on immunosuppressive therapy need to be monitored carefully for side effects, especially bone marrow suppression.

Symptomatic Treatment

Symptomatic control is an important aspect of the treatment of patients with Crohn's disease. Antidiarrheal agents such as diphenoxylate with atropine (Lomotil) in a dosage of 2.5 mg tablets, 1 or 2 every 6 hours, and loperamide (Imodium) 2 mg capsules, 1 to 2 every 6 hours, and a variety of opiates are commonly used to control diarrhea. The cautious use of these drugs in patients with severe Crohn's colitis is indicated, as there is evidence that in such patients these drugs may precipitate toxic megacolon. (The same caution applies to the use of antispasmodics.) Hydrophilic colloids (Metamucil, Effersyllium, and Hydrocil) are generally well tolerated and add bulk, which is necessary to increase stool formation. Antispasmodics such as belladonna (Donnatal) and dicyclomine hydrochloride (Bentyl) are usually effective in controlling abdominal cramps and spasms. The use of cholestyramine (Questran) or colestipol (Colestid) should be considered in patients with small bowel resections (less than 100 cm) who develop a choleretic-type diarrhea. These patients should also be placed on a low fat diet.

General measures commonly used in the treatment of patients with Crohn's disease include treatment of the anemia after the etiology has been established. Iron deficiency anemias are common in patients with active Crohn's disease, and in those patients with extensive small bowel disease or previous small bowel resections, vitamin B_{12} deficiency should be looked for. Folic acid deficiency is less common in patients with Crohn's disease and occurs occasionally in patients with proximal small bowel Crohn's disease or secondary to the use of sulfasalazine. Intravenous fluids with appropriate electrolyte concentration and mineral replacements (especially calcium, magnesium, and zinc) are often necessary in severely ill patients, especially those with extensive small bowel disease, previous resections, or excessive diarrhea.

Emotional Support

Most patients with Crohn's disease require some form of emotional support, which is usually given by the primary physician; however, nurses, aides, stomal therapists, and others may play a strong supportive and sympathetic role. Tranquilizers are commonly used to relieve anxiety tension states, and antidepressants are often needed to treat mild depressive reactions. Severe emotional disturbances should be managed by psychologists or psychiatrists. Current evidence suggests that Crohn's disease is not caused by psychological stress, but the psychiatric disturbances are the result of the nature of the symptoms and the chronicity of the disease.

Medical Treatment Failure

The failure of a patient to respond to optimal medical treatment (i.e., to attain a satisfactory quality of life) should be considered an indication for surgical intervention. The most common indications for surgery in Crohn's disease are obstruction, hemorrhage, perforation, or the presence of internal fistulae, abscess, or perianal complications that fail to respond to medical treatment. The type of surgical procedure performed is determined by the degree and location of the disease as well as the type of complication, which is recognized either preoperatively or at the time of surgery. Current evidence suggests that maintenance medical treatment after the diseased tissue has been resected or the disease has gone into remission does not prevent recurrence.

HEMORRHOIDS, ANAL FISSURE, AND ANORECTAL ABSCESS AND FISTULA

method of
HENRY W. EISENBERG, M.D.
Cleveland, Ohio

Hemorrhoids

Symptoms of hemorrhoids are among the most common complaints of mankind. The most frequent symptoms are bleeding, pain, prolapse, and discharge. The traditional teaching is that hemorrhoids are masses (piles) of dilated varicose veins located in the anal canal. The newer concept is that hemorrhoids are vascular cushions composed of arterioles and venules communicating in a stroma of fibrocollagenous supporting tissue. These vascular cushions are normal structures and do not cause symptoms until there is degeneration of the fibromuscular supporting tissue in the mucosa above the cushions, which allows a sliding-down process of the vascular cushion to occur. At that time, the vascular cushion (hemorrhoids) prolapse, become congested, enlarge, and bleed. Early symptoms should be treated and progression of the disease prevented by simple methods such as elastic band ligation, sclerotherapy, or cryotherapy.

Hemorrhoids are classified as internal or external, according to their relation to the dentate line, but they communicate with each other across that line to form an internal and external (mixed) hemorrhoidal complex.

Hemorrhoidal bleeding is characteristically bright red, on the surface of the stool, on the tissue paper or in the toilet bowl. Anemia is a rare complication.

Pain does not occur generally unless there are complications, such as acute thrombosis, or associated lesions, such as anal fissure or fistula. Itching is rarely due to hemorrhoids except when there is mucous discharge from prolapsing hemorrhoids. Hence, bleeding, protrusion, discharge, and pain are the principal symptoms.

Patients presenting with these symptoms should be examined carefully, first by inspection, followed by digital examination, anoscopy, and sigmoidoscopy. Flexible sigmoidoscopy has gained widespread acceptance and offers important advantages—namely, examination of the entire sigmoid colon to 60 cm with much greater comfort for the patient. Since flexible sigmoidoscopy allows the entire sigmoid to be examined, the diagnostic yield for finding polyps and neoplasms is greatly increased.

Treatment

Conservative Management. Mild symptoms are usually well controlled by conservative measures such as regulation of bowel habits. Increase in the bulk of the diet with raw vegetables, fruit, and whole grain cereals is useful. Bulk-producing laxatives such as psyllium seeds are also useful. The patient should be cautioned to avoid prolonged straining at stool. Although suppositories and ointments are widely used in the treatment of hemorrhoids, their efficacy is often not clear.

Elastic Band Ligation. This is the ideal method of treatment for bleeding, prolapsing internal hemorrhoids. The advantages of this technique are many. It is an ambulatory office procedure, can be done quickly, is virtually painless, and does not require anesthesia. The results of elastic band ligation are highly satisfactory, and the recurrence rate is low. Contraindications to ligation are few and include principally the presence of an anal fissure, abscess, or fistula. The principal limitation of this method is that it has no effect on external hemorrhoids.

TECHNIQUE. The patient is positioned on a proctologic examining table, a well lubricated anoscope is inserted, and the largest internal hemorrhoid selected for treatment first. Alligator forceps are employed to grasp the internal hemorrhoid into the Barron ligator barrel while an assistant holds the anoscope in place. Several types of ligating instruments are available, and all consist of a ligator with a distal drum onto which the latex band is stretched with a special loading cone. The band is applied to the hemorrhoid above the dentate line to minimize pain. If the patient has discomfort, the ligated site may be injected with lidocaine for local anesthesia. It is best not to use any anesthetic for this procedure.

The elastic band and ligated hemorrhoid usually slough 5 to 7 days after the procedure. Subsequent ligations are performed at 2 week intervals. It is usually sufficient to perform three or four ligations, depending on the extent of the hemorrhoidal disease. Following rubber band ligation, most patients require no pain medication and have no disability. Sitz baths and a mild laxative are usually advised. The incidence of profuse hemorrhage after elastic ligation is approximately 1 to 2 per cent.

Injection Treatment. Sclerosing injection of hemorrhoids is an old procedure that was widely used by many of the senior proctologists in this country. Sclerotherapy has been largely replaced by elastic band ligation. Nevertheless, it is a useful technique for selected patients. The principal advantage of injection is prompt control of bleeding. A solution of 5 to 7 per cent phenol in oil or quinine is used. Injection should be directed into the submucosa where it initiates a mild, inflammatory reaction that results in subsequent fibrosis. Bleeding usually stops. Among the principal disadvantages of this method of treatment are the high rate of recurrence of symptoms within 6 months to 2 years. Another concern with injection therapy is the occasional abscess that may develop.

Cryohemorrhoidectomy. This utilizes liquid nitrogen probes for eradication by freezing of internal or external hemorrhoids. Usually local anesthesia is necessary for this technique. The principal advantage of cryohemorrhoidectomy is its application as an outpatient procedure. It has been successfuly combined with elastic ligation and freezing of the ligated hemorrhoid. This may be the best utilization of this technique. Principal disadvantages of cryosurgery have been the necrosis of normal tissue, which results in sloughing and discharge associated with often foul drainage for several weeks. For this reason many proctologists have abandoned this procedure.

Operative Hemorrhoidectomy. While the total number of operative hemorrhoidectomies is diminishing because of widespread use of the elastic ligation technique, many patients still require operative hemorrhoidectomy. The presence of an anal fissure associated with large hemorrhoids, the failure of ligation treatment, and the presence of a large amount of prolapsing mucosa are all indications for operative hemorrhoidectomy. Choice of anesthesia includes a local anesthetic utilizing bupivacaine with epinephrine (Marcaine) or hyaluronidase (Wydase). Spinal and general anesthesia are also suitable. The closed hemorrhoidectomy technique, in which the operative incisions are closed with running sutures of chromic catgut, offers several advantages. Wound healing is much faster and incisions are usually healed by the end of 3 weeks. There is also relatively less pain, and more perianal skin can be preserved by this technique. The most frequent complication after operative hemorrhoidectomy is urinary retention. Anal stricture can be reduced by selective use of sphincterotomy. Postoperative hemorrhage has been greatly reduced by the use of Surgicel gauze placed in the anal canal following surgery.

Thrombosed External Hemorrhoids. Among the most common hemorrhoidal disorders and one that causes a patient to seek medical attention without delay is the acute thrombosed external hemorrhoid. Sudden in onset, often occurring after vigorous physical activity or severe diarrhea or constipation, it is characterized by a hard, tender, painful lump resulting from a small vessel rupturing under the skin, causing a hematoma with formation of a clot. The pain is throbbing in nature and usually reaches a peak at 24 to 36 hours. After this time the hematoma begins to resolve and will reabsorb without treatment, although this usually leaves a skin tag.

During the acute phase when the patient has severe pain, the thrombosed external hemorrhoid may be treated as a relatively simple office procedure. Incision and evacuation of the clot may be adequate in some instances. However, the wound edges may agglutinate and the hematoma reaccumulate with recurrent symptoms. The preferred technique is to inject a small amount of local anesthesia with a fine gauge syringe needle. Inject slowly and then insert the needle through the wheal and inject close to the lesion. By means of an elliptic incision the entire clot usually can be evacuated by gentle pressure. Bleeding should be controlled by pressure for a few minutes. No suture is necessary. The patient should be observed for a few minutes to be certain that bleeding has stopped.

Following excision of the acutely thrombosed external hemorrhoid, relief of pain will be immediate. Mild analgesics and sitz baths are prescribed. Subsequent sigmoidoscopic examination is indicated.

Anal Fissure

An anal fissure is a tear or ulcer involving the perianal skin and very distal mucosa of the anal canal. This lesion causes pain much greater than one would expect from its size. Fissures may be caused by passage of hard stools, severe diarrhea, foreign bodies, and infection. This is an extremely common condition and occurs in all ages. The symptoms are primarily severe pain following defecation. There is usually bleeding associated with this. Acute fissures may be small and superficial. The chronic anal fissure is usually deeper, is associated with an external hemorrhoid called a sentinel pile, and usually has exposed anal sphincter fibers at the base of the ulcer. Examination of patients with anal fissure is very difficult because of the severe pain with spasm of the anal sphincter mechanism. The diagnosis can usually be made by inspection, particularly when a posterior sentinel pile is present. The most frequent location for anal fissures is in the posterior midline. Less often the fissure will be found in the anterior midline. Sigmoidoscopy may be difficult or impossible to do without injection of local anesthesia. Consideration must be given to more serious systemic illness in patients with anal fissure. The principal disease entities to be considered are Crohn's disease, squamous carcinoma of the anus, syphilis, leukemia, and tubercular ulcers.

Treatment

Conservative Management. For acute anal fissures, conservative treatment will often be successful. The mainstay of conservative treatment is the use of a high fiber diet, allowing bowel regulation with avoidance of both constipation and diarrhea. Frequently, a stool softener will be helpful in this regard. Heat in the form of hot packs and warm sitz baths is prescribed. Topical analgesic ointment and cortisone cream are also useful. Suppositories are of no value and may be harmful for anal fissures because they must be inserted too deeply in the rectum, often traumatizing the fissure. Two weeks is sufficient time for conservative treatment in anal fissure. In the majority of cases, if healing is to occur it will have occurred by the end of 2 weeks.

Lateral Sphincterotomy and Excision of Anal Fissure. When conservative measures fail to give relief and the anal fissure is chronic and symptomatic, lateral sphincterotomy and excision of anal fissure can be done as an ambulatory procedure. This provides dramatic relief of pain and allows healing of the fissure. The technique is relatively simple. Local anesthesia is used. In the left lateral position, the internal involuntary sphincter is partially divided, using a small incision. Hemostasis is achieved and after excising the fissure the incision is closed with 3-0 chromic catgut. Sphincterotomy alone will allow healing of the fissure. However, if the fissure is left in place many patients will subsequently develop an anal fistula and require subsequent surgery. Patients who have large hemorrhoids in conjunction with anal fissure should have operative hemorrhoidectomy.

Anorectal Abscess and Fistula

Anorectal abscesses and fistulas most frequently have their source in the cryptoglandular tissue of the anal canal. Anal fistulas are usually easily diagnosed and treated. However, considerable controversy and misunderstanding exist regarding the complexity of the tracts, high recurrence rate, the necessity for multiple operations, and the danger of incontinence following surgery. Sound understanding and appreciation of proctologic anatomy will prevent most of these problems.

Both abscesses and fistulas result from infection in an anal crypt. Hence, the primary opening of the majority of anal fistulas lies near the dentate line. Anorectal abscesses are usually classified as perianal (more superficial), intersphincteric extending into the anal sphincter muscle, or ischiorectal when there is extension into the ischiorectal fossa.

Treatment

The principal consideration in treatment of anorectal abscess is prompt drainage, which often can be done as an office procedure, using local anesthesia. Antibiotics have a secondary role in the treatment of these patients. Surgical drainage should be done promptly and completely. Delay causes spread of infection, which is often anaerobic and allows the danger of potential necrotizing infections in the perineum. When there is suspicion of either intersphincteric abscess or ischiorectal abscess, hospital admission and surgical drainage in the operating room is indicated. Approximately two thirds of patients with anorectal abscess have an associated fistula.

The fistula can be excised at the time of initial drainage in the hospital or will have to be done at a subsequent time.

Complex anal fistulas and recurrent fistulas require surgical treatment in the hospital with adequate anesthesia. Some complex fistulas involve the anal sphincter mechanism. In these cases a satisfactory method of protecting the anal sphincter is the use of a seton. The seton is used to divide the fistula in a controlled manner and it is removed in a subsequent office visit. Essential considerations for surgery in anal fistula are the proper identification of both the primary internal opening and all secondary fistulous tracts. A second important consideration is saucerization and the avoidance of overhanging edges. Finally, to prevent recurrence and promote proper healing, patients should be seen at 1 to 2 week intervals until the entire wound has healed. Postoperative wound healing varies from 3 to 8 weeks, depending on the extent of the fistula.

GASTRITIS

method of
KEVIN J. IVEY, M.D.
University of California, Irvine
Long Beach, California

Gastritis refers to damage to the gastric mucosa, manifested histologically by hyperemia, surface cell damage or acute inflammatory cells, or endoscopically by erythema, hemorrhages, or erosions. Regrettably, the two do not necessarily correlate. Gastritis also may be classified into erosive, nonerosive, and specific types.

Erosive Gastritis (Acute Hemorrhagic Gastritis; Stress Erosions; Stress "Ulcers")

Drug-Induced. This is the commonest form of gastritis of clinical significance. The commonest cause of this condition is aspirin and other nonsteroidal anti-inflammatory agents (NSAI) used in the treatment of rheumatic disorders. Practically all such agents may cause much damage including indomethacin, phenylbutazone, sulindac, ibuprofen, naproxen, fenoprofen, tolmetin, piroxicam, and even newer agents.

Clinically, endoscopic mucosal damage ranging from erythema to ulcers is present in nearly 100 per cent of subjects taking aspirin. The evidence is lower with other NSAIs. Patients may have no symptoms, symptoms of gastric upset ranging from dyspepsia to peptic ulcer, or symptoms of iron-deficiency (blood loss) anemia.

Treatment is avoidance of the damaging drug when possible, substitution of a less damaging drug such as acetaminophen (Tylenol), or substitution of a safer form of a drug. For short-term pain relief, aspirin (2 tablets) should be taken mixed with one third to one half a teaspoonful of sodium bicarbonate (ordinary baking soda) in a glass of water or as the commercial equivalent, Alka-Seltzer. For therapy longer than 2 to 3 days, enteric-coated aspirin such as Ecotrin should be used. Ecotrin bypasses the stomach and does not produce gastric erosions. Enteric-coated aspirin preparations take 2 to 6 hours to be absorbed from the small intestine and to produce analgesic blood levels after the first dose.

Aspirin and other NSAIs should be taken only with plentiful water and preferably after meals. Because of the risk of esophageal damage, aspirin and NSAI tablets should not be taken immediately before retiring at night. For the same reasons they should not be taken whole by patients with esophageal varices but in solution or crushed in suspension and washed down with lots of water.

With all NSAIs the number of gastroduodenal erosions and amount of damage increase proportional to dose. Because of its prolonged half-life (80 hours), phenylbutazone should not be given in doses greater than 400 mg per day especially during the first 3 weeks of therapy; after this, metabolism of the drug is enhanced. Similarly, when possible, the dose of prednisone should be limited to less than 20 mg per day.

Therapy consists of recognition of the syndrome and the offending drug as the cause of the patient's lesions, stomach symptoms, or anemia. With cessation of the drug the lesions and symptoms will disappear. Treatment by any of the standard antiulcer regimens is effective: 30 ml of liquid antacids or 2 antacid tablets four times a day between meals and at bedtime, or H_2 blockers such as cimetidine, 300 mg every 6 hours; ranitidine, 150 mg morning and night; or sucralfate, 1 gram tablet 1 hour before meals and at bedtime.

For symptomatic patients with rheumatic diseases who must continue NSAI drugs, enteric-coated aspirin plus cimetidine, 300 mg every 6 hours (with or without antacids), has been found to heal gastroduodenal ulcers and prevent ulcer recurrence.

Alcoholic Gastritis. Acute exposure to concentrated alcohol as in whiskey, gin, and vodka may produce acute erosive gastritis, and it is probable that binge drinking of alcohol of any type will also produce such lesions. The damaging effect of most other agents including aspirin is enhanced by alcohol. Gastric mucosa develops tolerance to alcohol long-term so that alcohol per se is not a cause of peptic ulcer disease. *Treatment* consists of cessation of alcohol and use of the measures for aspirin gastritis.

Potassium-Induced Gastritis and Esophagitis. Prospective endoscopic studies in normal volunteers indicate that potassium chloride tablets (as Slow-K in a wax matrix) produce esophageal, gastric, or duodenal lesions in 60 per cent of subjects. Damage is greater (100 per cent) in the presence of gastric stasis induced by anticholinergics. Potassium chloride tablets of any type have the potential to produce erosive gastritis and hemorrhage, but this appears less with microencapsulated crystals. In susceptible patients with a history of ulcer disease or gastrointestinal bleeding, use of liquid preparations or effervescent potassium tablets is recommended.

Treatment consists of recognition of the existence of the syndrome, cessation of potassium therapy, or replacement of it by the less damaging liquid form or effervescent tablets, as well as the therapeutic measures listed under aspirin gastritis.

Acute Hemorrhagic Gastritis (Stress Erosions or Stress Ulcers). Occasionally, severe overt bleeding may result from some drugs. Recognition of the cause and cessation of the offending drug, replacement of blood, and therapy with antacids such as 30 ml of concentrated antacid hourly for 24 to 48 hours; or cimetidine, 300 mg every 6 hours; or ranitidine, 150 mg every 12 hours generally are sufficient. Bleeding will usually stop in 24 to 48 hours. If it does not, diagnostic endoscopy is needed to confirm the diagnosis and rule out drug-induced chronic peptic ulceration or underlying conditions such as esophageal varices, which predispose drug-induced damage to produce greater bleeding.

A potentially more difficult management problem is hemorrhagic erosive gastritis occurring in acutely ill patients in intensive care units, suffering from severe trauma, sepsis, burns, or medical illness. The gastric lesions are multiple, may involve the body or antrum, and histologically usually do not penetrate beyond the muscularis mucosae. Bleeding is usually diffuse from multiple shallow ulcers. It is usually painless and occurs typically 3 to 7 days after the precipitating event, such as burns or major trauma.

The first step in therapy is to correct the underlying predisposing condition. Hypovolemic shock must be treated by establishing adequate intravascular volume. Sepsis, often intra-abdominal or pulmonary, must be treated by surgical drainage or appropriate antibiotic therapy or both. Nasogastric intubation with a large bore tube decompresses the stomach, reducing the risk of vomiting and aspiration. It also yields information about the rate of bleeding and allows iced saline lavage. If this controls bleeding, as it will in 80 per cent of patients, the tube or a smaller diameter nasogastric tube may be left in place for antacid instillation. Keeping the gastric luminal pH at 7 with nonabsorbable antacids by infusion of 30 ml hourly reduces the incidence of rebleeding once it is initially controlled. The H_2 blocker cimetidine, 300 mg every 6 hours intravenously, is equally effective. The combination of the two, however, is necessary to maintain the pH at 7 and is recommended in patients with severe or persistent bleeding. In the intensive care setting when other medications such as theophylline are also being given and in the confused elderly or hepatic-encephalopathic patient, ranitidine, 50 mg every 6 to 8 hours intravenously, may be preferred over cimetidine.

In patients bleeding from erosive gastritis but with known portal hypertension or associated esophageal varices, vasopressin (Pitressin), 0.2 to 0.4 unit per minute in a 70 kg man, may be infused intravenously for 6 to 24 hours, in an intensive care unit setting if the preceding methods fail (investigational). Warning: coronary artery vasoconstriction can occur so vasopressin should be used only with extreme caution, if at all, in patients with coronary artery disease.

Surgical therapy has a high mortality rate of around 50 per cent and is best avoided if possible. It must be considered, however, if a patient loses more than 6 units of blood per 24 hours or continues to bleed heavily for more than 48 hours. Surgery ranges from vagotomy and pyloroplasty with oversewing of lesions to total gastrectomy. Only total gastrectomy will completely prevent rebleeding. In the patient with underlying portal hypertension, portal decompression may be necessary.

Because of the high mortality associated with severe bleeding in this condition, prophylaxis with antacids or H_2 blockers should be considered in all patients in intensive care units prone to such bleeding.

Corrosive Gastritis. Ingestion of concentrated alkalis or acids produces esophageal or gastric damage. In the *acute stage* shortly after corrosive ingestion, the gastric wall is edematous with marked hemorrhagic erosions or ulcerations on endoscopic examination. *Mucosal gangrene* with full thickness necrosis is diagnosed whenever black discoloration is seen. In the late stages, the distal part of the stomach, which bears the brunt of the damage, is narrow and rigid, with clinical and radiologic signs of *stenosis and obstruction.* Management consists of general supportive measures. After massive doses, time is a critical factor and in most cases damage will already have been done. If this is suspected, as in a patient with severe abdominal pain, nothing should be given by mouth. In intermediate cases, *immediately after ingestion* dilution of gastric contents may be tried; the safest diluent is water in large volumes. Weak alkalis such as nonabsorbable antacids or several cups of a solution of household baking soda (sodium bicarbonate: 1 teaspoonful gives 100 mEq of neutralizing capacity per cupful of water) may be given for acids. Weak acids such as 500 ml of equal parts of vinegar (acetic acid) or lemon juice and water may be given for alkali. Nasogastric intubation is best avoided until after endoscopic examination, if used at all. Early, careful fiberoptic endoscopy is recommended. Frank gangrene demands termination of the procedure and urgent surgical resection, as does clinical or radiologic evidence of perforation. In the late stages, elective resection may be required for antral stenosis.

Supportive measures are most important and include maintenance of airways, volume and blood replacement intravenously, sedation, and possible parenteral hyperalimentation. Antibiotics (a cephalosporin) and steroids (prednisone, 40 to 60 mg daily, intravenously) are given for circumferential contiguous injury involving submucosal or muscular layers of the esophagus or antrum.

Bile Reflux Gastritis. After partial gastrectomy, a degree of gastric mucosal atrophy takes place which is characterized by a nonspecific, nonerosive gastritis. In addition, especially after Billroth II anastomosis, there may be a superimposed erosive "bile reflux" gastritis around the immediate area of the stoma. Endoscopically, this lesion is characterized by marked erythema and occasional lesions ranging from superficial erosions to deeper (anastomotic) ulcers.

Patients with symptoms, asymptomatic ulcers, or multiple erosions should be treated with aluminum hydroxide-containing antacids as aluminum binds harmful bile salts. Because of rapid gastric emptying, these may need to be given hourly in severe cases while the patient is awake. The H_2 blocker cimetidine (300 mg every 6 hours) or ranitidine (150 mg twice daily) may also be given because of both its acid-reducing action and a cytoprotective action in the absence of acid. Sucralfate (Carafate) is an alternative. It should be given alone 1 hour before meals and at bedtime. If these fail, the bile salt–binding agent cholestyramine (Questran), 4 grams in juice, milk, or water as preferred, may be tried 1 hour before meals and at bedtime. If this does not help, it too may need to be given in smaller doses hourly. With prolonged therapy, however, fat malabsorption may develop. Finally, metoclopramide (Reglan), 10 mg on waking and 2 hours after each meal, may help prevent reflux of bile from the duodenum if disturbed motility is the problem. As a last resort, surgical establishment of a long loop Roux-en-Y gastroenterostomy with a gastric limb 70 to 75 cm long to prevent bile reflux may be tried.

Radiation Gastritis. Doses of 1600 rad to the stomach produce endoscopic changes of erosive gastritis. Secondary irradiation gastric injury may occur if doses exceeding 4500 rad are applied to the abdomen. The antral region of the stomach is most affected; ulcers may perforate or produce gastric outlet obstruction. Patients should be treated as for peptic ulcer with antacids, H_2 blockers, or sucralfate.

Idiopathic Chronic Erosive Gastritis (Varioliform Gastritis). This *rare* condition is not associated with any of the other conditions. Clinical symptoms range from nondescript dyspepsia to severe anorexia (uncommon), weight loss, and upper gastrointestinal bleeding. While the superficial erosions occasionally can be demonstrated by double-contrast radiography, the diagnosis is made by endoscopy. Biopsy is needed to rule out *specific* forms of erosive gastritis and underlying lymphoma or diffuse carcinoma. The lesions may wax and wane for months or years, and the natural history of this rare disease is unknown. There is no specific therapy, so treatment as for peptic ulcer is recommended.

Non-Erosive Gastritis

Chronic Nonerosive Gastritis. This condition is part of the normal aging process, and as such no specific symptoms or therapy should be attached to it. The diagnosis is by histologic assessment of gastric biopsy. Chronic gastritis is classified as chronic superficial gastritis, chronic atrophic gastritis, and gastric atrophy, the latter being rare and characteristic of pernicious anemia. Only the latter is associated with inability to produce or utilize (due to intrinsic factor antibodies) intrinsic factor, and therefore a deficiency of vitamin B_{12} occurs. Such patients require monthly injection of vitamin B_{12} for the rest of their lives. There is no specific treatment for the gastric atrophy. Unfortunately, there is a 10 per cent incidence of gastric cancer, so such patients need to be followed periodically.

Specific Gastritis

Gastritis Due to Infections. If infectious gastritis is suspected, a specific diagnosis requires special stains and culture of gastric biopsy material including viruses, fungi, tuberculosis, syphilis, tissue smears, and aspirates of gastric fluid via endoscopy. Standard histology is usually insufficient. Treatment of the underlying infectious condition is of primary importance. Symptomatic treatment of the gastritis may be given by any antiulcer regimen. Phlegmonous gastritis is a rare purulent bacterial inflammation of the stomach wall that is usually fulminating. It requires vigorous antibiotic coverage for sepsis of unknown cause and prompt laparotomy and gastric resection.

ACUTE AND CHRONIC VIRAL HEPATITIS

method of
GEOFFREY M. DUSHEIKO, M.D.
University of the Witwatersrand
Johannesburg, South Africa

Three major categories of viral hepatitis are recognized: A, B, and non-A, non-B. Serologic tests distinguish type A from type B; when markers of hepatitis A and B are not present and other causes of hepatitis are absent, non-A, non-B hepatitis is diagnosed by exclusion. Infection by hepatitis A virus (HAV), B virus (HBV), or non-A, non-B virus (NANB) may be followed either by mild illness without clinical evidence of hepatitis (anicteric hepatitis) or overt disease.

Hepatitis A is caused by a 27 nm RNA enterovirus. The disease is generally mild and self-limited and often anicteric, particularly in children, but may rarely be fulminant. HAV infection does not lead to a chronic carrier state. Type B hepatitis is caused by a unique 42 nm DNA virus. Hepatitis B surface antigen (HBsAg) is the diagnostic marker of hepatitis B infection. Hepatitis B e antigen (HBeAg) is an integral part of the viral core protein and correlates closely with the presence of Dane particles in serum. HBeAg positive chronic HBV carriers therefore have "replicative" hepatitis B infection and are more likely to be infectious and have chronic active hepatitis. The outcome of hepatitis B infection is variable, but there are four general patterns of infection: acute icteric hepatitis, subclinical infection, fulminant hepatitis, and chronic infection.

A third form of viral hepatitis exists to account for cases of post-transfusion hepatitis. Evidence has accumulated to suggest that, like hepatitis B, non-A, non-B hepatitis may be transmitted by both parenteral and inapparent parenteral spread; epidemic forms of the disease have also been described. Non-A, non-B infection may lead to the subsequent development of chronic hepatitis. Despite intensive research efforts and several claims to this effect, a single unique virus particle has not been reliably detected and the diagnosis of non-A non-B hepatitis awaits the development of an unequivocal serologic test for the agent(s) responsible for this disease

TREATMENT

Uncomplicated Acute Viral Hepatitis

Acute viral hepatitis is usually a self-limited disease. No specific therapy for acute hepatitis A, B, or NANB effectively alters the outcome of the disease.

Rest

Malaise and disinterest in strenuous exertion occur in the symptomatic phase of acute hepatitis, but nonetheless patients should avoid vigorous or prolonged exertion during the acute illness. Rigid bed rest is unnecessary. Bed rest with bathroom privileges is usual if there is an exacerbation of symptoms. During convalescence a graded return to normal activity is encouraged and subsequent exercise is permitted within the limits of fatigue. Patients may return to work when the serum aminotransferase (ALT and AST) levels are less than twice the upper limit of normal.

Diet

No special dietary supplements, such as vitamins given orally, are necessary. The diet should be made as palatable as possible, since certain foods, usually those high in fat content, may be unappetizing.

Drugs

Potentially hepatoxic medications may complicate the diagnosis and aggravate the hepatic injury and should be discontinued if not essential. Antiemetics can usually be avoided. Oral contraceptives are probably not contraindicated during acute viral hepatitis. For an uncomplicated case of acute hepatitis, corticosteroids are contraindicated. (+)-Cyanidanol-3 (Catergen) has been reported to hasten biochemical and serologic recovery in acute hepatitis B, but this drug is not in wide use and is not available in the United States.

Alcohol

Alcohol is contraindicated during acute viral hepatitis. Conservative hepatologists recommend complete abstinence for 6 months.

Hospitalization

Most patients can be effectively cared for at home unless the illness is particularly severe. Indications for hospitalization include unusually severe vomiting, an inability to maintain a caloric intake of 2000 calories per day, a prolongation of the prothrombin time by more than 2 seconds, the development of ascites, neuropsychiatric changes, and spontaneous bleeding.

Isolation

HAV infection is spread primarily by the fecal-oral route. Excretion of HAV in feces is greatest during the preicteric (late incubation period) and early symptomatic phases. Careful attention should be paid to personal hygiene. If the patient is elderly, incontinent, or a young infant, it is desirable to isolate him in a private room. HBV is spread by parenteral and inapparent parenteral spread. Concentrations of HBsAg are highest in blood, but the virus is also found in urine, saliva, sweat, semen, and vaginal secretions. Kissing should be avoided. Patients usually notice a disinclination for sexual intercourse during the acute symptomatic period, but the use of condoms may be advised to prevent possible infection of the spouse. Particular attention is paid to the cleanliness of food utensils used by the patient. In uncomplicated cases, strict isolation is probably unnecessary. All blood specimens are labeled and handled as potentially infectious. The same recommendations apply for patients with NANB hepatitis.

Investigations

Throughout the course of acute viral hepatitis, total and direct serum bilirubin, alkaline phosphatase, ALT and AST, and prothrombin time values are regularly measured, for example, twice weekly. In uncomplicated acute viral hepatitis, liver biopsy is not usually necessary.

Posthepatitis Syndrome and Relapses

Malaise and nonspecific symptoms may persist for many months after the initial phase of acute viral hepatitis; relapses, characterized by an increase in ALT levels, may occur in a proportion of patients. Rest is encouraged. Exacerbations characterized by elevated serum aminotransferase levels constitute part of the clinical course of acute NANB hepatitis. The possibility of progression of acute HBV and NANB hepatitis to chronic hepatitis must be considered, and prolonged follow-up is necessary if the patient remains HBsAg positive.

Cholestatic Hepatitis

Deep and prolonged jaundice (cholestatic hepatitis) usually follows HAV infection. Ultrasonography may be required to exclude extrahepatic cholestasis. Steatorrhea is usually adequately controlled by a 40 gram fat diet. Bruising is usually corrected by administering 10 mg of vitamin K intramuscularly. Distressing pruritus may occur. Although controlled trials are lacking, a short course of corticosteroids is likely to be effective in relieving the pruritus and rapidly lowering the serum bilirubin concentration. Prednisolone in a dose of 30 mg daily would be appropriate initially. Thereafter it is usually possible to reduce the dose gradually and discontinue the drug altogether in less than a month. The short-term use of steroids in this clinical setting is the only currently acceptable usage of corticosteroids in acute viral hepatitis.

Subacute Hepatic Necrosis

The major manifestations of subacute hepatitis necrosis—ascites, hepatic encephalopathy, and bleeding from the upper gastrointestinal tract—are managed along conventional lines. Hepatic transplantation may improve survival in this distressing condition.

Fulminant Hepatitis

Severe hepatocellular dysfunction accompanied by encephalopathy, coagulopathy, and multiple organ failure may rarely occur in acute viral hepatitis. The prognosis is better for hepatitis A than for B or non-A, non-B. Current treatment is insufficient in the majority of patients with fulminant hepatic failure and grade 3 to 4 encephalopathy.

The patient should be transferred promptly to an intensive care unit. Continuous assessment of vital signs, fluid intake and output, ECG, EEG,central venous pressure, and the clinical neurologic status is essential. The urinary bladder should be catheterized, a nasogastric tube passed, and a central venous catheter inserted. Well recognized complications of hepatic failure, including hypoglycemia, upper gastrointestinal hemorrhage, cerebral edema, hypotension, respiratory arrest, pulmonary edema, electrolyte imbalances such as hypokalemia, acid-base disturbances, hypoxemia, renal failure, cardiac arrhythmias, pancreatitis, and bacterial infections, should be sought and treated vigorously. Liver biopsy carries a risk of serious complications in patients with fulminant hepatic failure. Sedative hypnotic drugs should be avoided.

The patient's colon should be evacuated by administering a high magnesium sulfate enema and subsequently washing the colon twice daily with 1 per cent dextrose. Neomycin 1 gram and lactulose 15 to 30 ml every 6 hours (or ampicillin 500 mg if renal function is impaired) may be administered by a nasogastric tube. No protein or amino acids are given. Caloric intake is maintained by infusing 10 per cent dextrose into a central vein. Hypokalemia is corrected by adding potassium chloride to intravenous fluids. Calcium and magnesium supplementation of intravenous fluids may also be required. Hemodialysis may be required to correct electrolyte imbalance and acid-base disturbances or to manage renal failure. Hypoxemia, anemia, and shock are indications for oxygen by face mask. Respiratory arrest and pulmonary edema are indications for positive end expiratory ventilatory support. Currently available therapies for cerebral edema are unsatisfactory, but mannitol (1 gram per kg of 20 per cent solution by intravenous infusion) may be administered. Administration of branched amino acids (40 grams per day) will partially correct the amino acid imbalance. Acid pepsin–provoked hemorrhage from the upper gastrointestinal tract can probably be reduced by administering cimetidine 150 mg intravenously. Prophylactic infusions of blood products are not given, but for overt hemorrhage, fresh blood, fresh frozen plasma, and platelet concentrates may be infused in an attempt to achieve hemostasis.

The relevant data at this time suggest that steroid therapy is not indicated in the management of fulminant hepatitis and may indeed by harmful. Controlled trials of interferon are required before the use of this antiviral agent in fulminant viral hepatitis can be advocated. Currently no method of providing temporary hepatic support, including exchange blood transfusion, plasmapheresis, conventional or polyacrylonitrile membrane hemodialysis, and hemoperfusion over microencapsulated charcoal, has been shown unequivocally to improve survival in fulminant viral hepatitis. In the future, patients with fulminant viral hepatitis may be candidates for auxiliary transplantation of the liver.

Chronic Viral Hepatitis

Hepatitis A

There is no convincing evidence that HAV infection leads to chronic hepatitis or cirrhosis.

Chronic Hepatitis B

Five to 10 per cent of adults exposed to hepatitis B develop chronic infection, the so-called hepatitis B carrier state. Infants and children are more predisposed. Chronic hepatitis B is a complex disease and the carrier state may lead to chronic persistent hepatitis, chronic active hepatitis, cirrhosis, and hepatocellular carcinoma (HCC). Integrated HBV DNA sequences have been detected in hepatocytes in longstanding chronic carriers, in HCC cell lines in culture, and in HCC tumor tissue.

There is no indication that major restrictions should be imposed on the life style of patients with compensated chronic type B hepatitis. Exercise is permitted within the limits of fatigue, a normal diet is encouraged, and, although the drinking of hard liquor is discouraged, small quantities of beer or wine can be drunk occasionally. All unnecessary medication should be discontinued. The patient is advised against donating blood. There is evidence suggesting that chronic hepatitis B may be transmitted by sexual contact, and regular sexual partners and spouses of patients with chronic type B hepatitis should receive HBV vaccine. Serum total and direct bilirubin, alkaline phosphatase, and ALT and AST levels should be regularly measured, and HBsAg, HBeAg, anti-HBe, and, where possible, HBV DNA polymerase status should be monitored at monthly to trimonthly intervals. This policy will distinguish patients with predominantly "replicative" (HBeAg positive) infection from those with "nonreplicative" (anti-HBe positive) chronic HBV infection and will ascertain the activity of the chronic hepatitis. The patient should be monitored for exacerbations of chronic hepatitis, characterized by elevations of serum ALT levels.

The natural history of chronic HBV infection is variable. Prospective studies of patients with chronic type B hepatitis indicate that approximately 10 to 20 per cent of HBeAg positive carriers spontaneously seroconvert from HBeAg to anti-HBe per year. This transition from predominantly replicative to nonreplicative infection is usually associated with a significant improvement in symptoms, a fall in the concentrations of serum ALT and AST, and an improvement in histologic disease activity. The factors that influence this apparently favorable outcome are unknown. Spontaneous clearance of HBeAg may be accompanied by an abrupt elevation of serum ALT concentrations in some patients. Loss of HBsAg, however, is rare. Spontaneous reactivation of HBV replication, characterized by the reappearance of DNA polymerase or HBeAg in serum and renewed activity of the chronic hepatitis, has been described. Superinfection by the Delta agent, a defective RNA virus, may also exacerbate the chronic hepatitis.

A gradual decrease in the serum albumin concentration suggests progression of chronic hepatitis to cirrhosis. Liver biopsy is desirable in the patient with chronic type B hepatitis. Needle biopsy of the liver is not undertaken when the platelet count is below 80,000, the prothrombin time is more than 2½ seconds prolonged, or there are other specific contraindications. Biopsies are helpful, not only in establishing the presence of chronic hepatocellular disease but also in classifying the lesion and assessing disease activity. Follow-up biopsies may be performed at intervals of 2 to 5 years to assess progression or resolution of the lesion. The prognosis of chronic active hepatitis and cirrhosis is worse than that of chronic persistent hepatitis. Large prospective studies have indicated that as many as 40 per cent of (male) HBV carriers may die of either cirrhosis or hepatocellular carcinoma.

Patients with chronic HBV hepatitis should be monitored for the complications of cirrhosis, particularly ascites, esophageal varices, and encephalopathy, which should be managed along conventional lines. The role of propranolol in the prophylaxis of variceal hemorrhage is attractive but is of unproven efficacy in this group of patients. Particular attention should be paid in this high risk group to the early detection of HCC by frequent (every 4 months) real time ultrasonographic examinations and determinations of serum alpha-fetoprotein. A sustained increase in the serum alpha-fetoprotein concentration or a concentration greater than 200 ng per ml is suspicious. The survival of selected patients after segmental resection of small carcinomas detected by screening may be improved, but the cost effectiveness and overall benefit of mass screening programs in endemic areas of HBV infection in developing countries remain to be tested.

Corticosteroids

Data relating to the natural history of chronic persistent hepatitis indicate that there is no sound foundation for advocating corticosteroid therapy in patients with HBV chronic persistent hepatitis. Retrospective analysis of large trials of corticosteroid therapy of chronic active hepatitis indicates that HBsAg positive chronic active hepatitis is more commonly associated with treatment failures and a high mortality rate than is HBsAg negative chronic active hepatitis. A recent analysis indicated that steroid therapy was not beneficial in HBsAg positive chronic active hepatitis, and there was an appreciable incidence of severe side effects of corticosteroid therapy. Viral replication may be increased by steroid therapy; for this reason, less reliance is placed on long-term prednisolone therapy. The role of limited steroid administration and its subsequent withdrawal is being evaluated.

Antiviral Therapy

The treatment of HBeAg, DNA polymerase positive chronic HBV infection with several antiviral agents is being intensely investigated. Adenine arabinoside, a purine nucleoside, and its congener adenine arabinoside 5′-monophosphate have been evaluated in controlled trials. Despite a demonstrable inhibitory effect on HBV replication, in the majority of carriers adenine arabinoside does not effect permanent inhibition of viral replication. Its use for longer than 1 month has been limited by toxicity—the drug causes a distressing "neuropathic pain syndrome." Although acyclovir is a less toxic compound, it likewise does not appear effective.

Human leukocyte (alpha) interferon has been shown to inhibit HBV replication. The availability of recombinant leukocyte interferons has guaranteed an adequate supply and improved purity of these powerful antiviral and immune-modulating glycoproteins. Suppression of HBV replication and even clearance of HBsAg have been observed in small trials of both recombinant and lymphoblastoid alpha interferons, particularly in patients with severe chronic active hepatitis. Given the number of patients entered into controlled trials worldwide, it should be possible to ascertain in the near future whether interferon is indeed a therapeutic option in at least a subgroup of carriers.

Non-A, Non-B Hepatitis

Chronic hepatitis occurs with disturbing frequency in patients with transfusion-related non-A, non-B hepatitis. The subsequent course is clinically insidious but is characterized by relapses and remissions. Histologic cirrhosis may occur, and regular supervision is required for these patients. The principles of management are the same as those for chronic hepatitis B. However, the absence of reproducible serologic markers precludes monitoring of viral replication in this disease, and the spontaneous fluctuations in ALT levels in these patients make interpretation of the effects of specific therapeutic measures, such as corticosteroids, difficult. Prednisolone cannot be advocated automatically, but patients with aggressive disease may warrant a trial of 3 to 6 months treatment with corticosteroids to assess responsiveness.

PREVENTION

Hepatitis A

Passive Immunoprophylaxis

The effectiveness of human serum immunoglobulin (ISG) in preventing type A hepatitis is established. Anti-HAV titers vary among immunoglobulin lots, and the minimum effective dose has not been ascertained. Recommendations for post- and pre-exposure prophylaxis are summarized in Table 1. Disease is most likely to appear

TABLE 1. **ISG for Prevention of Type A Hepatitis**

Type	Circumstance	Dose	Frequency
Postexposure	Household contact with persons with type A hepatitis.	0.02 ml/kg	Once
Pre-exposure	Workers with imported primates. Travellers to tropical and developing countries.	0.06 ml/kg	Every 4–6 mo
	Visit less than 4 mo	0.06 ml/kg	Once
	Visit more than 4 mo	0.06 ml/kg	Every 4–6 mo

in persons who have close personal contact with a patient who has or is incubating hepatitis A, and spread is also enhanced under conditions of poor sanitation. The use of ISG more than 2 weeks after exposure is not recommended. ISG probably confers protection by passive active immunization and attenuation of the illness. Prophylaxis is not recommended for casual contacts of a single case in schools, offices, factories, or hospitals unless an obvious epidemic exists. Pre-exposure prophylaxis is recommended for travelers from developed countries journeying to areas of the world where hepatitis A is endemic, particularly if the stay is longer than 2 weeks and the traveler intends to deviate from the usual tourist routes. Pre-existing anti-HAV precludes the need for ISG.

Vaccination

HAV has been serially propagated in cell cultures, and candidate live attenuated vaccines provide protection. Clinical trials in a small number of human subjects have begun, with reasonable promise.

Hepatitis B

Postexposure Prophylaxis

Human serum immunoglobulin with known anti-HBs titers is used (HBIG). HBIG induces passive active immunity and thereby attenuates the disease. Postexposure prophylaxis recommendations of the Immunization Practices Advisory Committee are tabulated in Table 2. Pre-existing anti-HBs and anti-HBc preclude the need for HBIG. (In unimmunized persons, the presence of anti-HBs alone may not be protective in all exposed persons.) In HBV immunized anti-HBs positive subjects, a positive P/N RIA ratio of greater than 10 may be regarded as protective. Because health care workers are at continuing risk and the response to hepatitis B vaccine is not impaired by concurrent administration of HBV vaccine, HBIG combined with vaccine is a reasonable recommendation for postexposure prophylaxis. Infants born to HBsAg carrier mothers or to HBsAg positive mothers as a result of recent infection should receive prophylaxis with HBIG (administered intramuscularly, preferably within 12 hours after birth) combined with vaccine, as a recent study has demonstrated the enhanced efficacy of HBV vaccine combined with a single dose of HBIG in preventing perinatal transmission from HBsAg carrier mothers. Prophylaxis of infants from all HBsAg positive mothers is recommended regardless of the mother's HBeAg/anti-HBe status.

Two doses of HBIG should be given to sexual contacts of patients with acute type B hepatitis. Continued sexual contacts of an HBV carrier should receive HBV vaccine after screening for HBV markers.

Vaccination

The currently licensed vaccine is prepared from excess circulating 22 nm viral coat particles obtained from plasma of chronic carriers, (Heptavax B, Merck, Sharp and Dohme) and is subjected to extensive inactivation procedures and safety testing. Other plasma-derived vaccines have been developed in Europe and the Far East. Three injections of 20 micrograms at 0, 1, and 6 months are prescribed, but smaller doses may be as effective. Significant protection against HBV infection is conferred, and despite initial concerns there is

TABLE 2. **Recommendations for Postexposure Prophylaxis of Hepatitis B**

Exposure	HBIG Dose	HBIG Timing	Vaccine Dose	Vaccine Timing
Perinatal	0.5 ml intramuscularly	Within 12 hr of birth	0.5 ml (10 μg) intramuscularly	Within 7 days, repeat at 1 and 6 mo*
Percutaneous	0.06 ml/kg body weight intramuscularly or 5 ml for adults	Single dose within 24 hr	1.0 ml (20 μg) intramuscularly†	Within 7 days, repeat at 1 and 6 mo*
	or‡			
	0.06 ml/kg intramuscularly or 5 ml for adults	Within 24 hr, repeat at 1 mo	—	—
Sexual	0.06 ml/kg intramuscularly or 5 ml for adults	Within 14 days of sexual contact	§	—

Note: Postexposure prophylaxis is recommended only when there is percutaneous contact with blood or blood products known to contain HBsAg, as occurs through direct needle stick or an open cut or through mucosal contact (mouth, eye).

*The first dose can be given at the same time as the HBIG dose but at a separate site.

†For persons under 10 years of age, use 0.5 ml (10 μg).

‡For those who choose not to receive hepatitis B vaccine.

§Vaccine is recommended for homosexually active men and for regular sexual contacts of chronic hepatitis B virus carriers.

¶From the Immunization Practices Advisory Committee, Centers for Disease Control, Atlanta, Georgia.

no evidence for transmission of AIDS. Somewhat lower response rates have been observed in those in the older age groups, hemodialysis patients, immunosuppressed persons, and alcoholics. Fortunately, HBV vaccine is immunogenic in neonates. The cost of the current vaccines has delayed universal neonatal HBV immunization in endemic regions, but potentially cheaper recombinant DNA vaccines constructed in yeast, mammalian cells, and viruses are being tested in humans.

NANB Hepatitis

ISG may be partially effective in preventing icteric NANB hepatitis but is not of proven efficacy. It may be prudent to administer 5 ml of ISG after needle stick exposure to a patient with HBsAg, HAV negative hepatitis. A vaccine for prevention of NANB hepatitis is not available.

THE MALABSORPTION SYNDROMES

method of
GARY M. LEVINE, M.D.
Albert Einstein Medical Center
Philadelphia, Pennsylvania

The proper treatment of the malabsorption syndromes presumes that a definite diagnosis has been established. For the sake of our discussion, we will assume that malabsorption has been proven and differentiated from diarrhea (defined as an increase in stool volume) and incontinence (defined as an inability to retain stool until defecation can occur). "Malabsorption" includes a variety of diseases with maldigestion or malabsorption of nutrients and may be a generalized (e.g., gluten sensitive enteropathy) or isolated (e.g., lactase deficiency) phenomenon. Since a large number of diseases with varying pathogenesis cause malabsorption, it is extremely important to properly treat the disorder. "Shotgun" therapy with dietary supplements, antimotility drugs, and antibiotics is discouraged because these efforts are usually futile and occasionally dangerous.

The malabsorption syndromes can be conveniently grouped as diseases of generalized maldigestion, isolated maldigestion, generalized malabsorption, or isolated malabsorption.

Patients with generalized maldigestion and malabsorption usually present with weight loss and constitutional symptoms such as fatigue, lethargy, and decreased libido. In addition, they have many signs of multiple nutritional deficiencies such as easy bruisability (vitamin K deficiency), anemia (iron, folic acid, or vitamin B_{12} deficiency), bone pain (calcium and vitamin D deficiency), and edema (secondary to hypoproteinemia) as well as abdominal pain, bloating, and distention.

GENERALIZED MALDIGESTION

Pancreatic Insufficiency

After approximately 90 per cent of the pancreas' secretory capacity is destroyed by chronic inflammation (as occurs after prolonged alcohol ingestion or in patients with cystic fibrosis) or blockage of the pancreatic duct (by a tumor or pseudocyst), impaired digestion of fat, protein, and carbohydrate ensues. If patients with alcoholic chronic pancreatitis also have associated liver disease, they may have additional defects in bile secretion causing malabsorption.

Treatment

Alcoholic chronic pancreatitis is the most common cause of pancreatic insufficiency. Pancreatic enzyme replacement is the mainstay of therapy. A variety of commercial preparations are available including pancrelipase (Cotazym-S, Pancrease) and pancreatin (Viokase). In the author's experience, most patients can be successfully treated with from 4 to 8 tablets of pancreatic extract with each meal. Since gastric acid can destroy lipase at a pH of less than 3.5, it is often necessary to neutralize gastric acidity to maximize lipolytic activity. Sodium bicarbonate, 1 to 2 grams with meals, or an aluminum hydroxide antacid, 30 ml with meals, will suffice. The dosage of pancreatic extract necessary for each patient must be individualized.

Variations in acid production, rate of gastric emptying, tablet dissolution, and intestinal motility preclude a fixed dosage schedule. In the author's experience, enteric-coated preparations such as Pancrease or Cotazym-S have not proven superior to conventional tablets or capsules. Furthermore, H_2 inhibitors such as cimetidine (Tagamet) or ranitidine (Zantac) have variable results since these drugs may not reliably increase the gastric pH above 3.5, particularly in patients with normal to above average acid secretory rates.

Even though patients with pancreatic insufficiency have severe steatorrhea, it is unnecessary to seriously restrict fat intake, since steatorrhea does improve with enzyme replacement and fat contains a greater number of calories (9 versus 4 per gram) than carbohydrate or protein. In addition, low fat diets are often unpalatable and difficult to follow.

In addition to pancreatic enzyme replacement, it is important to correct any other deficiencies that have occurred as a result of pancreatic insufficiency. Malabsorption of fat-soluble vitamins (A, D, K) should be considered in addition to the malabsorption of calcium, magnesium, and zinc. Malabsorption of vitamin D and calcium often leads to osteoporosis with pathologic fractures. Zinc and vitamin A deficiencies can cause night blindness, making night driving very hazardous for these patients. At presentation, patients with chronic pancreatic insufficiency also may be vitamin B_{12} deficient because of an inability to neutralize dietary vitamin B_{12} binding proteins. However, once treatment is begun, vitamin B_{12} absorption should normalize.

The most difficult aspect of treating patients with chronic pancreatic insufficiency is management of the pain. Many patients become addicted to narcotic drugs. Severe unremitting pain may prompt a recommendation for pancreatic surgery. Recently the natural history of chronic pancreatic insufficiency has bcome clearer. Three to five years after the development of chronic pancreatic insufficiency, a majority of the patients become painfree as the inflammatory process "burns out." Unfortunately, once pancreatic insufficiency occurs, it is permanent unless some surgically reversible cause is found.

Postgastrectomy Maldigestion

One of the most common causes of malabsorption and maldigestion encountered in clinical practice is gastric surgery. The most common setting for this type of maldigestion is the patient who has undergone vagotomy, partial gastrectomy, and Billroth II reconstruction for the treatment of peptic ulcer disease. However, other types of gastric surgery such as truncal vagotomy and pyloroplasty, superselective vagotomy, or vagotomy with antrectomy and gastroduodenostomy (Billroth I operation) can cause nutritional problems. Although the use of gastric surgery for peptic ulcer disease is decreasing, many thousands of patients undergo these operations each year and are at risk for developing maldigestion.

Treatment

The treatment of gastric maldigestion depends on the cause. For patients who exhibit "dumping" syndrome (hypotension or delayed hypoglycemia caused by the rapid emptying into the bowel and rapid absorption of a meal), treatment should consist of small frequent feedings and limitations on the amount of liquids ingested with the solid portion of the meal. It is preferable to advise the patients to eat their solid foods first and use minimal amounts of liquids to "wash down" food. Liquids should be ingested between meals, and the patient should avoid hypertonic liquids such as carbonated beverages, fruit juices, and highly sweetened coffee and tea.

For patients who have gastric maldigestion as a consequence of bacterial overgrowth, treatment with antibiotics is appropriate (see hereafter). However, if the patient has overgrowth because of a long, stagnant, poorly emptying afferent loop, reoperation may be necessary. Patients usually have to be treated with antibiotics on an intermittent basis; this therapy is largely empiric and must be individualized for each patient.

Patients who have maldigestion predominantly because of poor mixing and motility disturbances are the most difficult to treat. It is usually helpful to perform radionuclide gastric emptying scans in these patients to determine the rates of liquid or solid emptying. In patients with delayed solid emptying, it may be advisable to include a pancreatic enzyme preparation with meals since the delay in solid food entering the intestine will result in poor mixing with endogenous pancreatic secretions. In the author's experience, prokinetic motility drugs such as metoclopramide (Reglan) have not been helpful in this situation.

In addition to correcting the cause of maldigestion, these patients usually require iron, fat-soluble vitamin, and calcium supplementation. Many patients with subtotal gastric resections or bacterial overgrowth will become vitamin B_{12} deficient over time, since there is a decrease in the amount of intrinsic factor available for binding vitamin B_{12} and increased numbers of intraluminal bacteria bind the vitamin, making it unavailable for ileal absorption. It may take 3 to 5 years following surgery for vitamin B_{12} deficiency to become apparent.

If patients do not respond to therapy directed at the specific cause of their maldigestion, it is useful to employ antimotility drugs such as diphenoxylate (Lomotil) or loperamide (Imodium). These agents may slow transit of meals through the intestine and allow more time for digestion and absorption. The dose of medication varies. One should start by prescribing 1 to 2 diphenoxylate tablets or 1 loperamide capsule before each meal and increase the dose to tolerance (diphenoxylate contains atropine, which may cause symptoms if a large number of tablets are administered daily). The author's preference is to use loperamide, up to 2 tablets 4 times a day, before abandoning this form of therapy.

Diet therapy should not be overlooked in these patients, as many become sensitive to lactose, especially if rapid emptying of liquids from this gastric pouch occurs. Lactase levels in the intestine are marginal for adequate lactose digestion, and when a large volume of lactose enters the bowel in these abnormal states diarrhea can occur. Many patients have found it helpful to use milk that has been treated with a commercially available lactase enzyme (LactAid).

Intestinal Resection—"Short Bowel Syndrome"

Resection of more than 100 cm of terminal ileum (most commonly encountered in the surgical treatment of Crohn's disease) or the loss of more than 200 cm of more proximal bowel (as occurs after mesenteric infarction or following severe radiation injury) results in severe maldigestion and malabsorption. The terminal ileum is the major site of active bile salt reabsorption. If a significant portion of the ileum is removed, bile salts escape reabsorption and are lost in the stool. As a result, the total bile salt pool declines, so that the intraluminal bile salt concentration resulting from gallbladder emptying and biliary secretion is below that required for forming micelles. Since fatty acids are absorbed poorly without being transported to the mucosal surface by micelles, severe fat malabsorption results.

Treatment

The treatment of this type of maldigestion is threefold. First, malnutrition must be corrected prior to specific medical and dietary therapy of the underlying condition. For example, a patient with extensive Crohn's disease who has undergone surgery or a patient who has recently suffered a mesenteric infarction with resection of a large portion of the intestine may have become marasmic as a result of active inflammation, surgical stress, and preceding malabsorption. Usually a course of parenteral nutrition is needed in the perioperative period to allow wound healing, prevent infections, and restore body composition. Most patients with the short bowel syndrome should be supported with parenteral nutrition while an enteral feeding regimen is instituted. Often it is helpful to begin refeeding through a small bore (8 to 10 French) nasoduodenal feeding tube.

In patients with massive bowel loss, a chemically defined diet (such as Critcare, Vivonex, Precision, Vital) should be constantly infused beginning at 25 ml per hour. It may be necessary to initially dilute these hypertonic formulas 1:1 with water if the osmotic load causes excessive diarrhea. Attempts should be made to limit fecal losses to 1 to 1½ liters per day. The strength and volume of the diet are gradually increased until the patient's caloric and protein needs are met. Some patients can tolerate casein/soy protein–based diets (such as Isocal, Osmolite, Ensure, Travasorb, or Sustacal). Patients who have undergone massive bowel resection usually tolerate an isotonic tube feeding formula well. It is important to remember that enteral infusion allows intestinal adaptation to occur so that oral intake can begin and parenteral nutrition can be discontinued or tapered.

The second principle of treatment of the patient with an intestinal resection is tailoring an oral diet. Many patients benefit from a reduced intake of conventional (long chain) dietary fats. Many patients can reduce the normal long chain triglyceride intake to 40 to 50 grams a day without too much difficulty. Diets containing less than 40 grams a day impose severe dietary restrictions on patients. It is necessary to accurately measure intake and fecal output to determine the effects of various dietary manipulations. If additional calories are needed in the diet, medium chain triglyceride oil (MCT), containing fatty acids with 8 to 10 carbons instead of the 16 to 18 carbons found in long chain fatty acids, is advised. MCT oil can serve as a substitute for conventional vegetable oils used in cooking, salad dressings, baking and so on. MCT oil is also available combined with milk powder (Portagen). Portagen can be mixed with water and ingested directly or used as an additive in cooking. Four ounces of MCT oil a day provide approximately 1,000 calories.

It is important to monitor the success of the reduction in dietary long chain fat intake. Under the best of circumstances, reduction of fat intake leads to a decrease in steatorrhea and diarrhea, since excessive amounts of fatty acids are no longer passed into the colon where they have a "castor oil–like" effect. Some individuals with an intestinal resection can tolerate normal fat intake, although they absorb only half of the dietary fat ingested. In these patients, steatorrhea does not cause excessive diarrhea, although it does decrease calcium, magnesium, and fat-soluble vitamin absorption.

Patients with intestinal resection and a short bowel also require supplementation of fat-soluble vitamins (A, D, and K) as well as minerals (calcium, magnesium, and zinc).

The third principle of therapy is minimization of fecal losses. Drugs such as diphenoxylate (Lomotil), loperamide (Imodium), paregoric, and tincture of opium are usually administered to these patients. The author prefers loperamide, beginning at a dosage of 2 to 4 mg with each meal up to a maximum dose of approximately 16 mg per day. Some patients who do not respond to these dosages should be instructed to open the capsules and mix the powder in liquid rather than ingest the capsules intact. Another therapeutic modality that should be considered is the use of either cimetidine (Tagamet), 300 mg 4 times a day, or ranitidine (Zantac) 150 mg twice daily. The rationale for the use of these drugs is the fact that, following bowel resection, many patients have gastric hypersecretion, which contributes to their maldigestion and malabsorption.

Patients with lesser degrees of intestinal disease or resection (less than 100 cm) usually have normal fat absorption, and their treatment is discussed elsewhere.

Gastrinoma

Patients with an gastrin-secreting islet cell tumor often have steatorrhea and diarrhea. Excessive concentrations of gastrin cause gastric hypersecretion. The enormous acid load entering the duodenum irreversibly inactivates lipase and leads to a defective fat digestion. In addition, a low pH leads to precipitation of bile salts.

Treatment

Treatment of this rare form of maldigestion is directed at reducing gastric acid secretion. Most patients with gastrinomas are treated medically with either cimetidine (Tagamet), 1.2 to 4.8 grams per day, or ranitidine (Zantac), 600 mg to 2.4 grams per day in divided doses.

ISOLATED MALDIGESTION

Lactase Deficiency

In some ways, it is unrealistic to label lactase deficiency (i.e., lactose intolerance) as a disease, since the majority of the world's peoples have genetically determined low levels of intestinal lactase. High lactase levels are present only in predominantly northern European stocks and result from natural selection related to the domestication of dairy animals. However, since milk products make up such an important part of the American diet, the inability to digest lactose is the most common maldigestion problem encountered in clinical practice. In addition, lactose intolerance can be acquired if the intestine is affected by mucosal disease. For example, following a bout of viral or bacterial enteritis, the level of lactase activity in the intestine falls and may take several weeks to recover. During this period, dairy products will produce symptoms. Chronic intestinal diseases such as gluten-sensitive enteropathy, tropical sprue, and Crohn's disease can also produce an acquired type of lactase deficiency. The inability to break down lactose into its constituent sugars, galactose and glucose, leads to diarrhea, intestinal cramps, and gaseousness. Maldigested lactose acts as an osmotic laxative, holding fluid in the intestine. When lactose reaches the lower bowel and is digested by bacteria, additional osmotically active particles and gas are produced.

Treatment

The usual treatment for lactase deficiency is a lactosefree diet. However, milk and dairy products contain high quality protein, calcium, and vitamin D, so it may be preferable to recommend that patients purchase lactosefree milk, cheese, and ice cream, produced by many dairies throughout the United States. If lactosefree milk is unavailable, the patient may purchase a preparation of semipurified yeast lactase (Lact-Aid). This preparation is added to milk; within 24 hours, a majority of the lactose will be converted to galactose and glucose.

Patients who prefer to restrict their milk intake or who do not enjoy dairy products should be urged to ingest adequate quantities of vitamin D and calcium. This advice is particularly important for middleaged postmenopausal women, who have the highest predilection for osteoporosis. These patients should be treated with calcium carbonate, 500 mg 2 to 3 times daily, and vitamin D, 400 units daily.

GENERALIZED MALABSORPTION

Generalized malabsorption results most commonly from a failure of the intestinal epithelium to absorb nutrients (e.g., gluten sensitive enteropathy). However, in certain conditions, malabsorption occurs because absorbed nutrients do not leave the intestine (e.g., A-beta lipoproteinemia, lymphangectasia). Steatorrhea is the hallmark of malabsorption, although the relative degree of steatorrhea may be less than that seen with the maldigestion syndromes.

Intestinal Disease

Gluten Sensitive Enteropathy—Celiac Disease

Gluten sensitive enteropathy is the "classic" cause of generalized malabsorption. This disorder is caused by an allergic reaction to components of gluten resulting in immunologic destruction of the enterocytes. Intestinal villi are lost and the mucosa is often flat, especially in the proximal gut. Because of the loss of surface area, there is considerable malabsorption of nutrients; in particular, patients are usually deficient in calcium, iron, and folic acid.

Gluten sensitive enteropathy should never be diagnosed solely on clinical grounds. A small bowel biopsy is imperative, since treatment consists of a lifelong glutenfree diet. Since gluten is present in high concentrations in most common cereal grains such as wheat, rye, barley, and oats, this disease requires abstention from most ordinary starches. However, if the diagnosis is substantiated by a small bowel biopsy (villous atrophy, crypt cell hyperplasia, and chronic inflammation of the lamina propria), a course of gluten withdrawal should be attempted. The patient must be closely counseled by the physician as well as the dietitian to avoid both obvious sources of gluten (commercial breads, cookies, cakes, breakfast cereals) and "hidden" sources of gluten. Starches are used as thickening and flavoring agents in a number of prepared foods that do not seem to contain starch. However, a close reading of the label or reference to a list of gluten-containing products will inform the patient of this hazard.

Patients with gluten sensitive enteropathy can benefit from membership in the Celiac-Sprue Society (45 Gifford Avenue, Jersey City, New Jersey 07304). This society will make available a list of glutenfree products as well as products that appear safe but contain gluten. The following is a partial list of prepared foods that present a hazard to patients with gluten sensitive enteropathy as they are made with wheat: commercial soups, ketchup, salad dressing, gravy, some types of ice cream, alcoholic beverages (beer, hard liquor such as scotch, bourbon, and vodka), prepared meals in a can such as meatballs, prepackaged hamburgers, and "junk foods."

Treatment

The overwhelming majority of patients with gluten sensitive enteropathy respond dramatically to a glutenfree diet. Within several days to several weeks, the patient's sense of well being improves, diarrhea abates, and weight gain begins. There is probably no more satisfying diagnosis to make in clinical gastroenterology in the author's experience. The benefits of a glutenfree diet are so dramatic and immediate that it is self-reinforcing.

In place of gluten-containing starches, the patient must use flour made from potatoes, soybeans, and rice. Corn meal is also acceptable, although it does contain a small amount of gluten.

Some patients with gluten sensitive enteropathy are so malnourished and ill that a short course of corticosteroids is indicated at the time diagnosis is made. Prednisone may be prescribed at a dose of 0.5 mg per kg per day in a single dose. Steroids should be continued for approximately 2 to 4 weeks. If a clinical response occurs within that time, the dosage may be quickly tapered over 7 to 10 days. It is also important for the physician to prescribe medications to help replete the patient's multiple deficiencies. Calcium carbonate, 500 mg twice daily, iron sulfate, 300 mg 3 times a day, and folic acid, 5 mg daily, should be prescribed. In addition, some sprue patients may be B_{12} deficient, and a single dose of vitamin B_{12}, 1000 micrograms intramuscularly, is often necessary. The physician should also prescribe a complete multivitamin preparation.

Patients with gluten sensitive enteropathy should also be cautioned to avoid a high intake of dairy products, since the villous atrophy and the loss of enterocyte mass reduce intestinal lactase activity and produce milk intolerance. Many of these patients, even if not genetically lactase deficient, will continue to suffer from milk intolerance because the sprue lesion may never completely revert to normal.

The long-term management of patients with gluten sensitive enteropathy centers around several issues. First, patients should maintain a lifelong abstinence from gluten, since continued exposure will produce subclinical exacerbation of the disease and may lead to subtle development of metabolic bone disease from the long-term malabsorption of calcium and vitamin D. Second, patients with gluten sensitive enteropathy who do not adhere to their diet are at a higher risk than those in the normal population for the development of lymphomas (particularly of the gastrointestinal tract) and solid tumors of the colon, breast, and lung. Therefore, most specialists recommend that patients be maintained on as rigid a glutenfree diet as possible. It is obvious that there will be certain "indiscretions," but patients should be aware that their long-term health depends on following the diet.

Occasional patients with gluten sensitive enteropathy either do not respond initially to therapy or relapse. Most often, a poor response or flare-up is due to purposeful or inapparent ingestion of gluten-containing food. Patients should be re-evaluated and a complete dietary diary obtained. In addition, a search for a complication of gluten sensitive enteropathy such as cancer or the development of collagenous sprue (a situation in which dense collagen is laid down in the lamina propria and submucosa of the bowel) should take place.

Tropical Sprue

Tropical sprue is a chronic illness that may result following a bout of acute infectious enteritis. The acute infection damages the small bowel and allows colonization of the intestinal lumen by gram negative enteric bacteria. These bacteria probably produce toxins and metabolic byproducts that impair gut function, especially of the proximal intestine. As its name implies, tropical sprue is found throughout the warmer parts of the world, especially in areas where sanitation is poor, leading to contamination of foodstuffs with enteric organisms. Not only do residents of tropical countries suffer from this disease, but tourists who spend as little as 1 to 2 weeks in a tropical environment can also contract this disease. Tropical sprue leads to villous atrophy, which should be documented by small bowel biopsy.

Treatment

The treatment of tropical sprue is directed toward altering the intestinal luminal environment to eliminate the offending microorganisms. Most patients respond to tetracycline, 500 mg 4 times daily, or sulfamethoxazole-trimethoprim, 1 double strength tablet twice daily (Bactrim, Septra). Patients who contract this disease in the tropics and return to the temperate zone may need treatment for several weeks. Patients living in tropical areas may need continued antibiotic suppression for 6 months or longer.

In addition to antibiotics, these patients should receive supplemental folic acid, 5 mg orally daily. Many of the symptoms and signs of the disease are related to folic acid deficiency and quickly respond to therapy. Patients who have recently contracted the disease do not require any other vitamin or mineral supplements. However, patients who live in the tropics or who have been ill for long periods of time may need supplemental vitamin B_{12}, iron, calcium, and magnesium replacement. Diarrhea can be treated symptomatically with either diphenoxylate (Lomotil), 1 to 2 tablets three times daily, or loperamide (Imodium), 2 to 4 mg three times daily. If symptoms continue despite these measures, other causes of diarrhea such as concomitant parasitic infection with *Giardia lamblia, Strongyloides*, or hookworm should be investigated.

Whipple's Disease

Whipple's disease is a rare affliction causing malabsorption, particularly in middle aged men. Associated symptoms include arthritis, fever, adenopathy, and central nervous system involvement. The etiology is presumed to be a small bacillus, which is found within macrophages throughout the lamina propria of the intestine as well as in other parts of the body. The diagnosis must be established by biopsy showing the characteristic PAS positive organisms within macrophages.

Treatment

Several antibiotics are effective treatment of this condition including tetracycline, 250 mg 4 times a day, and procaine penicillin, 600,000 units intramuscularly twice daily for 10 days, followed by penicillin V, 250 mg 4 times a day. Antibiotic therapy must be continued for at least 6 months, and adequacy of treatment should be verified by repeat small bowel biopsy.

In addition to antibiotics, these patients may require administration of iron, folic acid, calcium, and magnesium, all of which may be poorly absorbed through the involved bowel.

Eosinophilic Gastroenteritis

Eosinophilic gastroenteritis is a disorder in which eosinophils infiltrate any of the three layers of the intestinal wall (mucosa, muscularis, or serosa). The diagnosis is made by either peroral or operative biopsy. It is not usually possible to identify an etiology, but it may be a hypersensitivity reaction to some undefined food protein.

Treatment

Treatment with corticosteroids (prednisone 0.25 to 0.5 mg per kg per day) produces a dramatic response. Many of these patients relapse when steroids are stopped and require alternate day therapy with low doses of prednisone (10 to 15 mg every other day).

Lymphangiectasia

Destruction or congenital absence of the intestinal lymphatics leads to malabsorption, particularly of fat. In addition, this condition is often associated with a protein-losing enteropathy when obstructed lymphatics become overdistended with fluid and rupture, leaking protein and lymphocytes into the intestinal lumen.

Treatment

Treatment of intestinal lymphangiectasia depends on the etiology. Patients with primary or congenital lymphangiectasis are best treated by a low sodium (less than 2 to 3 grams per day), low fat diet (less than 40 grams per day) and the use of diuretics such as furosemide (Lasix), 40 to 80 mg daily as necessary. Since these patients malabsorb fat, provision must be made for administering fat-soluble vitamins in an aqueous form (Aquasol). Medium chain triglycerides or Portagen should be added to the diet to provide sufficient calories.

In patients with acquired lymphangiectasia, a search for a treatable cause should be considered. For example, some patients with abdominal lymphoma develop lymphangiectasia as a result of enlarged neoplastic lymph nodes. These patients will experience regression when treated with chemotherapy or radiation therapy. Occasionally, patients with severe constrictive pericarditis will develop lymphangiectasia, which responds to pericardial surgery.

Bacterial Overgrowth Syndromes

Many different conditions can lead to an increase in small intestinal flora, causing malabsorption and maldigestion. The absence of gastric acid (achlorhydria), delay in intestinal transit, internal fistulization of the intestine, and resection of the ileocecal valve all produce overgrowth. The advent of breath analysis has made it easy to determine the presence of excessive intestinal bacteria by measuring the abnormal breakdown of orally administered substrates to either hydrogen (following lactulose administration) or $^{14}CO_2$ (following ^{14}C-xylose administration). Recent studies suggest that bacterial overgrowth is a much more common condition than previously considered.

Treatment

The therapy of bacterial overgrowth is straightforward. If any surgically correctable lesion exists, it should be corrected. For example, following a Billroth II gastrectomy, some patients may have a very long, stagnant afferent loop, or a patient with Crohn's disease may have a fistula between the colon and proximal small intestine. However, for the most part, bacterial overgrowth is amenable to treatment with broad spectrum antibiotics. Both aerobic and anaerobic bacteria colonize the small bowel, but the relative contribution of different bacteria to the disease is uncertain, so treatment is somewhat empiric. The author prefers to treat proven bacterial overgrowth with both tetracycline, 250 mg 4 times daily, and metronidzole (Flagyl), 250 mg 3 times daily, for 7 to 10 days. Most patients with bacterial overgrowth respond to this regimen and may not need retreatment for weeks to months. Some may require continued therapy with either tetracycline or metronidazole to keep bacterial flora under control. Another useful drug in treating this condition is chloramphenicol. It should be administered in 4 divided doses not to exceed 50 mg per kg per day. Both the aerobic and anaerobic flora respond nicely to chloramphenicol, but the widespread fear about the rare occurrence of aplastic anemia limits its use.

Parasitic Infections

Although hundreds of species of parasites and worms can infect the human intestine, clinical malabsorption and maldigestion is very uncommon in most parasitic infections. Giardiasis is the most common parasitic infection in the United States. Although many *Giardia* infections are short-lived, some people develop chronic infection with symptoms of diarrhea, intestinal pain, and distention. The diagnosis is usually made by either finding the *Giardia* cysts in the stool or by recovering the trophozoites by aspiration and/or biopsy of the upper intestine.

Treatment

Giardiasis is effectively treated with metronidazole (Flagyl) in a dose of 250 mg 4 times daily for 10 to 14 days. Some patients relapse and may need a second course of prolonged therapy (21 to 28 days).

The roundworm *Strongyloides stercoralis* can also produce malabsorption, espcially in heavily infected patients. Treatment consists of administration of thiabendazole, 25 mg per kg twice a day for 5 days.

Recently it has been recognized that other unusual parasites can produce the malabsorption syndrome. Members of the order Coccidia (*Isospora, Cryptosporidium*) have been found to infect man. These parasites are usually recognized only by examining a small bowel biopsy specimen. Although most of these infections are self-limited, patients with either congenital or acquired immune deficiencies will be affected by these parasites. Unfortunately, a good treatment is not yet available for these infections.

ISOLATED MALABSORPTION

Several defects in absorption of a single nutrient have been described. Fortunately, these are rare conditions usually encountered in neonates and children.

Glucose Galactose Malabsorption

In this condition, the active transport carrier that moves glucose and galactose from the intestinal lumen into the enterocyte is defective. These children usually develop diarrhea when switched from breast milk or lactose-containing formulas to normal foodstuffs containing sucrose and other carbohydrates. Treatment is centered around reducing the amount of glucose- and galactose-containing carbohydrates and substituting fructose wherever possible.

Amino Acid Transport Defects

These syndromes are extremely rare conditions in which the amino acid carrier for one or more amino acids is defective. One of the conditions encountered is Hartnup disease, in which the intestine does not actively transport phenlalanine, histidine, and tryptophan. Another condition occasionally encountered is cystinuria, in which the ability to transport basic amino acids such as arginine, ornithine, lysine, and cystine is defective.

ACUTE PANCREATITIS

method of
JOHN L. CAMERON, M.D.
The Johns Hopkins Hospital
Baltimore, Maryland

During the 1940s, the primary management of acute pancreatitis shifted from operative to nonoperative. Subsequently, a variety of treatment modalities have been suggested, most of which were aimed at decreasing pancreatic secretion or "splinting" the pancreas. During this interval hospital mortality for acute pancreatitis dropped from 25 per cent to 5 per cent. In an effort to determine which of the treatment parameters was responsible for decreasing hospital mortality, in the 1970s a series of prospective randomized studies were performed. These studies failed to demonstrate any clear benefit for any of the treatment parameters. Thus, currently we have no specific therapy for acute pancreatitis. The disease in most patients is an acute, inflammatory, nonseptic, disorder that is self-limited. With excellent supportive care, most patients with acute pancreatitis will survive. Until more specific information is gathered concerning pathogenetic mechanisms, it is unlikely that more specific therapy will be developed.

Management

Patients with mild, acute pancreatitis can be managed safely on the ward. However, patients with a severe episode should be managed in an intensive care setting. Most patients with acute pancreatitis will be somewhat distended, nauseated, and vomiting and should be given nothing by mouth. Since the disease is an inflammatory disorder, sequestration of large volumes of extracellular fluid takes place in the peripancreatic area, the retroperitoneum, the mesentery, and the bowel. Therefore, aggressive intravenous fluid administration is essential. The disease is usually painful, and analgesia is indicated. Because of the risk of overlooking early signs of respiratory failure, all patients admitted to the hospital with acute pancreatitis should have arterial blood gas determinations performed every 12 hours for the first 3 days.

Intravenous Fluids. Patients with mild episodes

TABLE 1. **Ranson's Prognostic Signs**

On Admission
Age > 55 years
WBC > 16,000
Blood glucose > 200 mg per dl
LDH > 350 IU/L
SGOT > 250 units per dl
Markedly elevated amylase
During Initial 48 Hours
Hct ↓ of > 10%
BUN ↑ of > 5 mg per dl
Serum Ca^{++} < 8 mg per dl
Arterial Po_2 < 60 mm Hg
Base deficit > 4μg/L
Fluid sequestration > 6 L

of acute pancreatitis may have only minimal losses of extracellular fluid. These patients can be maintained on 2 liters of D5.2S per day, plus 40 mEq of potassium. However, patients with severe episodes sequester large volumes of extracellular fluid and require close monitoring of their intravascular volume and aggressive fluid replacement. These patients should have a central venous pressure line or, if severely ill, a Swan-Ganz catheter inserted. A Foley catheter should be inserted for monitoring urinary output, which is the most accurate of all the indirect means for monitoring cardiac output. Vital signs should be closely monitored in an intensive care setting. Intravascular volume should be maintained with aggressive administration of Ringer's lactate solution (extracellular fluid) to maintain a urinary output in excess of 30 ml per hour, adequate vital signs, and a central venous pressure or a wedged pulmonary capillary pressure in the normal range.

Analgesia. Patients with acute pancreatitis have severe epigastric pain, often radiating through to the back. Analgesia is almost always required. Because morphine is more apt to cause ampullary spasm than Demerol (meperidine), Demerol is the preferred drug.

Nasogastric Suction. Patients with moderately severe and severe acute pancreatitis are often distended, nauseated, and vomiting. For these patients, as for those with any other abdominal disorder resulting in distention and vomiting, nasogastric suction is indicated to eliminate the annoyance of vomiting and decrease the possibility of aspiration. However, at least four well-controlled prospective randomized studies have failed to demonstrate any benefit of nasogastric suction in shortening or modifying the course of acute pancreatitis. Therefore, in patients who are not markedly distended and who are not vomiting, nasogastric suctioning is not indicated.

Antibiotics. Two prospective randomized studies have been carried out evaluating the routine use of antibiotics in acute pancreatitis. Both studies failed to demonstrate any benefit. This was primarily because the incidence of pancreatic abscess formation in acute pancreatitis is low, between 2 and 8 per cent. However, by utilizing Ranson's criteria (Table 1), one can select a group of patients with a significantly higher risk of developing a pancreatic abscess (Table 2). These patients should have broad-spectrum antibiotic coverage. This coverage should include an aminoglycoside, a high-dose penicillin or ampicillin, and either metronidazole (Flagyl) or clindamycin.

Cimetidine. Because many people still feel that acid-induced secretin release followed by secretin-initiated hypersecretion of the pancreas is an important etiologic pathway in initiating acute pancreatitis, cimetidine has been proposed as a treatment parameter. Two prospective randomized studies, however, have failed to demonstrate any benefit of cimetidine in influencing the course of acute pancreatitis. In some severely ill patients cimetidine might be useful in preventing or treating upper gastrointestinal hemorrhage. However, there is no evidence that the course of the acute pancreatitis itself is modified by cimetidine administration.

Atropine, Glucagon, and Aprotinin (Trasylol) Administration. Hypersecretion of the pancreas and ampullary spasm previously were felt to be important etiologic factors in all patients with acute pancreatitis, and the use of atropine and glucagon seemed logical. Atropine decreases pancreatic secretion and relaxes the ampulla, whereas glucagon is one of the most potent depressants of pancreatic secretion. However, prospective randomized studies have failed to demonstrate any benefit from either drug. Also, Trasylol is a protease enzyme inhibitor and theoretically should be of benefit in acute pancreatitis. Most studies evaluating Trasylol, however, have failed to demonstrate benefit, and therefore this drug also is not indicated.

Peritoneal Dialysis. Most patients with acute pancreatitis, given supportive care as outlined, will improve within 24 to 48 hours. Approximately 10 per cent of patients, however, will not improve, and further treatment and supportive measures will be necessary. In these patients, peritoneal dialysis should be considered. The peritoneal dialysis catheter can be inserted under direct vision through a small midline incision

TABLE 2. **Identification of Patients at High Risk for Pancreatic Abscess**

Number of Ranson's Prognostic Signs	*Incidence of Pancreatic Abscess (%)*
< 3	3
3–5	32
> 5	50

midway between the umbilicus and pubis. Peritoneal dialysis should be carried out with an isotonic electrolyte solution containing 15 grams per liter of dextrose. Heparin and ampicillin may be added to the dialysate fluid. Two liters are infused into the peritoneal cavity, allowed to remain for 30 minutes, and then drained by gravity. This cycle is repeated hourly, usually for 24 to 72 hours. Although most patients will show marked clinical improvement following peritoneal dialysis, it is less clear whether the long-term outcome is modified.

Surgery. In 1925 Lord Moynihan advocated routine surgical intervention in all patients with acute pancreatitis. Subsequently in the 1940s and 1950s surgery was throught to be detrimental and was avoided unless an abscess developed. Full cycle occurred when in the late 1960s and early 1970s once again some surgeons advocated surgical intervention for patients with severe acute pancreatitis. Most physicians currently feel surgery is indicated only in two instances: (1) When there is some doubt of the diagnosis of acute pancreatitis, and other abdominal catastrophes are felt possible, diagnostic laparotomy is indicated; and (2) when pancreatic sepsis develops. If a patient develops a pancreatic abscess, early laparotomy, débridement, and drainage are mandatory.

Complications

Hypocalcemia. Hypocalcemia occurs in approximately 30 per cent of all patients with acute pancreatitis. In many instances it is secondary to depression of the albumin-bound calcium fraction, because of the hypoalbuminemia that is often present. However, less frequently the ionized calcium can be depressed, and calcium infusion is necessary. This is best determined not by the serum calcium level but by following the Chvostek and Trousseau signs. If these signs become positive, calcium chloride or calcium gluconate should be administered slowly IV.

Abscess. Sepsis is the most common cause of death in patients with acute pancreatitis. This results from necrosis of portions of the pancreas, with suprainfection of the necrotic gland, surrounding blood protein, and fibrinous exudate. The earlier a patient is explored and undergoes drainage and débridement, the more likely the patient is to survive. The computed tomographic (CT) scan is currently the most accurate means of detecting a pancreatic abscess early. Small amounts of mottled air, not discernible on the plain x-ray film, can often be detected on the CT scan, as well as small areas of liquefaction necrosis in the pancreas. When there are peripancreatic fluid collections, the differentiation between a sterile fluid collection and an abscess is more difficult. In these instances aspiration with a skinny needle is perfectly safe and may at times help differentiate between the two. Bacteriologic evidence of pancreatic sepsis, such as a positive blood culture, also should lead to early exploration.

The surgical management of a pancreatic abscess includes wide débridement through the lesser sac, kocherization of the duodenum so that the posterior aspect of the head of the pancreas can be examined, and mobilization of the right and left colon so that the lateral gutters can be explored. Following débridement, wide drainage with soft Silastic sumps and Penrose drains should be carried out. Recently some have advocated that the abdominal incision be left open and open packing into the lesser sac performed. The patient is then taken back to the operating room every 48 hours, and under general anesthesia, the old packs are removed, further débridement carried out, and new packs inserted. This is performed until either the open packing can be performed on the ward or the surgeon is convinced that it is safe to close the abdomen with drains left in place. Preliminary data suggest that the open packing method of treating pancreatic abscess is capable of lowering the hospital mortality rate from 50 to about 15 per cent.

Respiratory Failure. Respiratory failure is the second most common cause of mortality in acute pancreatitis. The etiology has been ascribed to lecithinase release by the pancreas, with resultant destruction of pulmonary surfactant, or free fatty acid release in the pulmonary circuit with capillary injury. The respiratory failure in acute pancreatitis appears to be secondary to an increase in pulmonary capillary permeability, with a resultant increase in extravascular pulmonary water. Therefore, one has to be careful early in the course of acute pancreatitis that extracellular losses are not over-replaced, resulting in extravasation of fluid into the pulmonary parenchyma and alveolar spaces. This is perhaps the reason that respiratory failure is often not evident within the first 24 or 48 hours after admission, during which time the patient is hypovolemic and undergoing restoration of intravascular volume. By 24 to 48 hours, when this volume has been replaced and perhaps over-replaced, the leaky pulmonary capillaries lead to a marked increase in extravascular pulmonary water, a decrease in pulmonary compliance, and the development of respiratory failure. An increase in inspired oxygen may suffice in early mild respiratory failure. Patients who develop severe respiratory failure will require endotracheal intubation, maintenance on a respirator, and often the use of 5 to 15 cm of positive end-expiratory pressure (PEEP). Once the patient's cardiovascular system is stable, the use of diuretics may be helpful in hastening the mobilization of the extravascular pulmonary water. Even though albumin therapy has appeared to be effective in mobilizing extravascular pulmonary water experimentally, there is as yet no evidence that albumin is of benefit clinically.

Pseudocyst Formation. The formation of an acute pseudocyst in a severe episode of acute pancreatitis, manifest on CT scan or sonography by a peripancreatic fluid collection, is common. However, in most instances these acute peripancreatic fluid collections will resolve as the patient improves. In other patients, however, true pseudocysts will form secondary to a pancreatic duct disruption. This will occur in from 2 to 5 per cent of patients with episodes of acute pancreatitis. Patients who develop pseudocysts following an episode of acute pancreatitis should be managed as follows: (1) If the patient is symptomatic and cannot eat or drink or has gastric outlet obstruction, he or she needs to be kept in the hospital and given hyperalimentary feedings intravenously for a 6 week period. Then if the patient is asymptomatic and can eat and drink pain-free, discharge from the hospital for follow-up with sonography or CT scan is indicated. However, if symptoms persist after the 6 week period of intravenous hyperalimentation, surgical drainage should be carried out. (2) If the patient improves, becomes pain-free, and does not have gastric outlet obstruction, the patient can be discharged from the hospital and the pseudocyst followed periodically by sonography or CT scan for a minimum of 6 weeks to 6 months. Forty to 50 per cent of these pseudocysts will resolve spontaneously. If the pseudocyst does not resolve, surgical drainage is indicated.

Hemorrhage. A drop in hematocrit secondary to peripancreatic hemorrhage is common in severe acute pancreatitis. This hemorrhage is almost always controlled in the retroperitoneum, and the need to perform a laparotomy to control bleeding is rare. A more common cause of hemorrhage is the formation of a pseudoaneurysm in the wall of a pseudocyst. Patients will have signs of hypovolemia and at exploratory laparotomy will be found to have a pseudocyst filled with blood. Control of the bleeding point by suture ligature and external drainage of the pseudocyst is the treatment of choice. If the diagnosis is suspected prior to laparotomy, angiography often will demonstrate this pseudoaneurysm and allow the initial option of control by embolization through an intra-arterial catheter.

CHRONIC PANCREATITIS

method of
JAMES L. AUSTIN, M.D.,
and HOWARD A. REBER, M.D.
Harry S Truman Memorial Veterans Hospital
Columbia, Missouri

Chronic alcoholism accounts for at least 90 per cent of all cases of chronic pancreatitis in this country. Other causes include hyperparathyroidism, hereditary pancreatitis, and pancreatic duct obstruction. The manifestations of chronic pancreatitis are variable, but malabsorption, diabetes, and pain are the major problems that cause patients to consult their physicians. All three may complicate chronic pancreatitis in an individual patient, but usually one or two predominate.

DIAGNOSTIC CONSIDERATIONS

Patients with alcoholic *chronic* pancreatitis frequently present first with one or more episodes of *acute* pancreatitis. There is often a history of considerable alcohol intake over at least 6 to 8 years. A history of intermittent abdominal pain is common, but the presenting episode is often the most severe the patient can remember.

In most patients after multiple episodes of *acute* pancreatitis over a period of years, pancreatic calcifications eventually develop and pancreatic exocrine or endocrine insufficiency appears. As the disease progresses, the severity and frequency of the acute attacks diminish. Then chronic abdominal pain frequently becomes a persistent problem, and it is present on a daily or even continuous basis. About 20 per cent of the patients may not present acutely and have no pain. The disease is usually diagnosed because of symptoms of severe exocrine or endocrine insufficiency or because of the presence of radiographically visible pancreatic calcifications.

All patients with chronic pancreatitis regardless of etiology have some impairment of exocrine function. This can usually be demonstrated with one of the pancreatic function tests (e.g., Lundh test, secretin-cholecystokinin stimulation test). Nevertheless, because 85 to 90 per cent of pancreatic function must be lost before there is *clinical evidence* of pancreatic insufficiency, i.e., changes in the frequency and character of the stools from fat malabsorption, many patients are not symptomatic. It is generally stated that early in the course of the disease about one third of patients suffer from steatorrhea (fecal excretion of 7 grams of fat per day on a 100 gram fat per day diet). As the disease progresses, the proportion of patients with significant steatorrhea increases to approximately 75 per cent. Patients with calcifications are more likely to suffer from significant steatorrhea than those without them.

Endocrine function may be more sensitive to the inflammatory process in chronic pancreatitis than is exocrine function. Thus at any stage of the disease patients are more likely to experience endocrine insufficiency. Whereas only one third of patients have steatorrhea early in the course of the disease, approximately two thirds of the patients are diabetic. There is some evidence that endocrine function continues to deteriorate as the disease progresses. The development of insulin-requiring diabetes is a significant event in patients with chronic alcoholic pancreatitis, especially if alcohol abuse continues. Appreciable morbidity and mortality are associated with mismanagement of the diabetic state in patients who continue drinking.

Management

Malabsorption

Treatment of malabsorption secondary to pancreatic insufficiency is required in patients with chronic pancreatitis when the lipase and trypsin output of the pancreas is reduced below 10 per cent of normal. Apart from the nutritional disturbances that pancreatic insufficiency causes, the diarrhea secondary to this fat malabsorption is the chief symptom for which the patient desires relief. Creatorrhea (due to protein malabsorption) is less important because other nonpancreatic peptidases still allow for the hydrolysis and absorption of some dietary protein and creatorrhea by itself does not produce symptoms.

In practice it has been found impossible to completely eliminate steatorrhea. However, oral pancreatic enzyme replacement may decrease steatorrhea and improve fat absorption. The commercial preparations available for pancreatic exocrine replacement are of two main types, pancreatin and pancrealipase. Pancreatin preparations are generally alcoholic extracts of hog pancreas that are standardized for amylase and trypsin activity but not for lipase activity. This is a significant deficiency because lipase is the most labile enzyme and the one that is the most important to replace. One type of pancreatin, Viokase, is prepared by desiccation instead of alcoholic extraction and is a reasonable source of lipase (approximately 6,500 units per tablet). A number of preparations of pancrelipase are standardized for the lipase they contain. Examples are Cotazym (8,000 units of lipase per capsule) and Pancrease. Pancrease contains approximately 4,000 units of lipase per capsule. Additionally, enteric coating may allow the enzymes, especially lipase, to resist destruction by gastric acid.

Regardless of the enzyme preparation chosen, the quantity of pancreatic enzymes that reaches the proximal intestine in active form is very small compared with normal. Acid destruction of lipase in the stomach may be limited by the addition of H_2 receptor antagonist therapy to the enzyme replacement. For example, cimetidine, 300 mg ½ hour before meals, along with oral enzymes taken during the meal is usually effective. Cimetidine is generally more effective than antacid administration. More complete correction of creatorrhea can usually be achieved because trypsin is more resistant to acid digestion than lipase and because of nonpancreatic peptidases in an active state.

There is no evidence that hourly administration of enzymes is better than enzyme administration with meals. The latter approach is preferred because it is more convenient. Whichever preparation is chosen, sufficient replacement therapy should be prescribed to provide 30,000 to 50,000 units of lipase to be taken with each of 4 meals. Although a reduction of fat in the diet may be necessary, a normal diet with as much as 100 grams of fat per day is tolerated by most patients. If diarrhea continues to be troublesome, a reduction in dietary fat may help.

In general, these patients should be placed on diets with liberal amounts of carbohydrate (400 grams or more) and protein (100 to 150 grams) and as much fat as can be tolerated without the production of diarrhea. It is important to recognize that even when an optimal treatment regimen has been established, fat malabsorption and steatorrhea will continue. This is satisfactory, provided that diarrhea is controlled and adequate nutrition can be maintained. Medium chain triglycerides, which are absorbed directly without further digestion, occasionally help in refractory patients, and vitamin supplements may also be useful.

Diabetes Mellitus

The management of diabetes in patients with pancreatic insufficiency and chronic pancreatitis may be complicated by irregularities in food intake, malnutrition, and decreased fat absorption. In alcoholic patients with chronic pancreatitis, the situation is made more difficult by their frequent unreliability. Effective management of all these problems improves diabetic control and must be an integral part of the treatment regimen. Although occasional patients with diabetes and pancreatic insufficiency can be managed with oral hypoglycemic agents, most require 20 to 40 units of insulin a day. There is a tendency to hypoglycemia in these patients, which may be due to inadequate glucagon release from the islets or insufficient hepatic glycogen stores. To minimize the chances for hypoglycemia, blood glucose should not be rigidly controlled. Serum glucose concentrations of 150 to 250 mg per dl and mild glycosuria are acceptable. Although ketoacidosis is less frequent than in patients with idiopathic diabetes, it can occur.

Pain

The natural history of pain in patients with chronic pancreatitis is receiving increasing attention. This is because surgical procedures for pain relief might be avoided in some patients if more accurate information were available about the likelihood of spontaneous pain remission. It has been widely accepted that abstinence from alcohol decreases the frequency and severity of painful attacks in patients with alcoholic pancreatitis. However, the relationship between continued ethanol abuse and pain is not so clear. Indeed, there are numerous examples of patients who continue to consume alcohol and have no abdominal pain as well as those who have stopped alcohol consumption in whom pain continues to be a significant problem. There is evidence that continued ethanol ingestion induces pain in patients with chronic pancreatitis as long as there is appreciable residual pancreatic function. However, patients with more advanced pancreatic insufficiency may reach a stage where alcohol may be taken without precipitating pain.

Although it seems reasonable to advise against alcohol consumption in these patients, it is difficult to predict the effects of cessation on the episodes of abdominal pain in individual cases. A beneficial effect may be more likely in those with early disease. In patients with far advanced disease (pancreatic calcifications, severe exocrine insufficiency), alcohol withdrawal is less likely to influence the pain pattern. On the other hand, the likelihood of spontaneous pain relief is greater. Unfortunately, these considerations are of little value in individual patients suffering with severe pain and in need of more immediate assistance.

The principles of pain management consist of abstention from alcohol, consumption of frequent small meals, and use of non-narcotic analgesics. Recent evidence suggests that oral pancreatic enzyme replacement, even in patients who do not have overt steatorrhea, may also decrease pain. About 50 per cent of patients will obtain partial or total relief of their pain when these principles are adhered to.

Unless a complication of chronic pancreatitis is present (e.g., pseudocyst, bile duct obstruction), most patients undergo a period of medical management before surgery for pain relief is considered. Those patients whose pain continues should be considered for surgery. Frequently the decision for surgery in these patients is difficult because the physician and patient both delay operation, hoping for a remission and spontaneous pain relief. However, in general it is best to operate before patients become dependent on narcotics and are seriously depressed by the chronicity of their disease.

When operation is considered under these circumstances, endoscopic retrograde cholangiopancreatography (ERCP) should be done preoperatively. This study delineates the anatomy of both the biliary and pancreatic ducts and may also provide information about a pseudocyst. Should preoperative ERCP be unavailable or unsuccessful, then intraoperative pancreatography must be done. This may be obtained through direct puncture of the duct or by its cannulation in the head or tail of the gland. Information about the size and configuration of the duct is essential for intelligent planning of the operative procedure.

In most cases, the surgical treatment of pain in chronic pancreatitis involves a procedure that either (1) facilitates drainage of a dilated main pancreatic duct or (2) resects diseased pancreatic tissue. Indirect operative procedures such as neurectomy or ductal ligation have been found to be unsatisfactory.

A dilated main pancreatic duct is found in about three fourths of patients with chronic pancreatitis. In these cases, drainage of the duct with a longitudinal pancreaticojejunostomy (Puestow operation) is the procedure of choice. An anastomosis at least 10 cm long is desirable, since there is evidence that its length is directly proportional to long-term patency and perhaps to pain relief. Pain relief is obtained about 80 per cent of the time, and none of the remaining endocrine or exocrine function of the pancreas is sacrificed. Other operations, such as sphincteroplasty or distal pancreaticojejunostomy, are unlikely to be successful and should not be done.

Unfortunately, the long-term results with the Puestow operation are less satisfactory. After 5 years pain may return in about one third of patients. Morbidity and operative mortality are less than 5 per cent. Successful rehabilitation is enhanced by abstention from alcohol and the withdrawal of narcotic medications.

In the absence of a dilated main pancreatic duct, pancreatectomy is the most successful procedure to relieve pain. Other indications include the failure of a previous pancreaticojejunostomy to provide pain relief and extensive disease localized to one part of the pancreas. A significant drawback of major pancreatic resection is that many patients will require insulin postoperatively. Therefore, continued alcoholism is a strong contraindication to extensive resection because such patients are unable to manage the diabetic state. Surgeons may be more willing to recommend resections in patients who are already diabetic from their disease.

Sometimes the extent of resection can be determined from the preoperative ERCP. If the disease is localized to either the distal or the proximal portion of the gland, then resection of the involved portion frequently is the best approach. However, diffuse disease often involves the entire gland, and in this situation subtotal (95 per cent) pancreatectomy is usually preferred. In this procedure a small remnant of the head of the gland is left attached to the duodenum. Total pancreatectomy may be indicated in those patients whose severe symptoms persist after subtotal resection. Total pancreatectomy with islet cell transplantation or segmental autotransplantation of the pancreas may be another option. However, at the present time these procedures are still experimental.

In general, pancreatic resection can be done with an operative mortality of 5 per cent or less. Pain relief is obtained in about 80 per cent of patients. However, major pancreatic resections frequently result in pancreatic functional insufficiency. With limited resections of less than 50 per cent, this is not a problem. However, after more extensive resections, at least 75 per cent of patients will require insulin for diabetes, and all patients will require exocrine replacement therapy. Subtotal (95 per cent) or total pancreatectomy should be reserved for the few patients who already exhibit manifestations of pancreatic insufficiency and who are excellent candidates for rehabilitation.

Using these guidelines to determine surgical therapy, about 50 per cent of patients will benefit with long-term pain relief. This is more likely to be true for patients with calcific pancreatitis and those patients who abstain from further alcohol intake.

PEPTIC ULCER

method of
PHILLIP M. BERMAN, M.D.
University of Illinois
Chicago, Illinois

It is possible to promote the healing of peptic ulcers by three different types of medical treatment: neutralization of acid by antacids, suppression of acid secretion with H_2 blockers, and mucosal protection with antipeptic polysaccharides. Each of these modalities has been shown to be significantly superior to placebo (Table 1).

Other agents used elsewhere but not available nor approved for use in the United States for peptic ulcer therapy will not be discussed. These include carbenoxolone, tricyclic agents, bismuth compounds, and prostaglandins. (At this writing, misoprostol, a prostaglandin E_1 analog, has been approved by the G. I. Advisory Board of the FDA but has not been marketed in the United States.)

Acid Neutralization

The administration of 30 to 60 ml of most commercially available liquid antacids taken 1 and 3 hours after meals and at bedtime will neutralize approximately 1000 mEq of acid. This maintains the intragastric pH above 3.5, the point at which pepsin is denatured and acidity is reduced to promote healing of uncomplicated peptic ulcers. Although antacids are safe and effective, side effects are recognized. Magnesium-containing antacids cause diarrhea. They are well tolerated in patients with normal renal function but not recommended in large doses for those with renal insufficiency. Aluminum-containing antacids cause constipation and phosphorus depletion, particularly in alcoholic patients. Calcium products cause constipation and if absorbed may cause an elevated serum or urinary calcium level. Elevated serum calcium levels have occurred with rebound gastric acid secretion. The sodium content varies among the different antacid formulas. The concomitant administration of antacids with cimetidine, tetracycline, isoniazid, iron, and digoxin may interfere with absorption of these drugs. Other disadvantages include the need for multiple doses, monotonous taste, and expense.

TABLE 1. **Relative Healing Rates in Peptic Ulcer Treatment**

	Healed in 4–6 Weeks (Per Cent)
Duodenal Ulcer	
Placebo	40
Antacids	80
Cimetidine	80
Ranitidine	80
Sucralfate	80
Gastric Ulcer	
Placebo	30
Antacids	40
Cimetidine	70
Ranitidine	70
Sucralfate	70

Antisecretory Agents

The secretion of acid can be markedly reduced by blocking the gastric H_2 receptors for histamine. Cimetidine (Tagamet) and ranitidine (Zantac) are currently available in the United States. (Other agents are being studied.) Both have been shown to improve healing of duodenal and gastric ulcers. Although ranitidine is a more potent inhibitor of gastric acid, the healing rates between the two are not significantly different. Ranitidine differs chemically from cimetidine by having a furan ring instead of the imidazole configuration found in cimetidine and histamine. The greater potency of ranitidine allows a dose of 150 mg twice a day to achieve the same therapeutic effect as cimetidine given 300 mg four times a day.

Adverse reactions to cimetidine in controlled studies and in postmarketing surveys have been few. The most frequent involve the gastrointestinal tract and the central nervous system. The gastrointestinal side effects are diarrhea, nausea, constipation, dry mouth, and bloating.

The central nervous system symptoms of somnolence, confusion, lethargy, agitation, hallucinations, and slurred speech may be seen more frequently in older and younger patients, often in those with multisystem disease such as renal or hepatic insufficiency. This may be due to an increase in the cerebrospinal/plasma ratio, with blockage of H_2 neuroreceptors in the brain. These symptoms are reversible within 4 to 5 days of discontinuing cimetidine.

Leukopenia, thrombocytopenia, and pancytopenia have been reported. The incidence of aplastic anemia is no greater than that seen spontaneously in the general population.

Gynecomastia has been reported in men after prolonged, often large doses of cimetidine. The reports of impotence and loss of libido are largely anecdotal. The effect on sperm count has varied in different studies.

Cimetidine inhibits the cytochrome P450 mixed function oxidase microsomal enzyme system in the liver. This inhibitory effect is felt to result from a pharmacologic action separate from H_2 blockage and may be intrinsic to the drug's imidazole structure. Increased blood levels and delayed excretion of substances utilizing this system as a major metabolic route may occur. It may be necessary to reduce the dose of drugs having this interaction, such as warfarin, theophylline, phenytoin, lidocaine, chlordiazepoxide, diazepam, propranolol, and cyclophosphamide. Reports of decreased hepatic blood flow have varied.

Other rare adverse effects are pancreatitis, myalgia, drug fever, raised prolactin levels with and without galactorrhea, paroxysmal tachycardia, and reversible renal and liver changes.

The worldwide experience with ranitidine has not been as extensive as that with cimetidine; however, both agents seem remarkably safe. Headache is the most common side effect of ranitidine. Gynecomastia is less common. Cimetidine-associated gynecomastia has reversed after a switch to ranitidine. There are recent reports of hepatic injury, and the concomitant use of ranitidine with acetaminophen may increase the risk of hepatotoxicity.

Ranitidine has a lesser effect on the hepatic cytochrome P450–mediated drug metabolism, but there are conflicting reports of interaction with warfarin, benzodiazepine, fentanyl, metoprolol, nifedipine, and acetaminophen.

In the first few days of therapy, some patients find that antacids, taken as needed, reduce pain. If pain persists, consider the complications of posterior penetration, obstruction, and inadequate reduction of acid. The combination of antacids with H_2 blockers is unnecessary. When used, they increase the cost of therapy and increase the incidence of side effects. Antacids also decrease the absorption of H_2 blockers.

Mucosal Protection

Sucralfate (Carafate) is the aluminum salt of sucrose octasulfate which neither reduces secretion nor neutralizes gastric acid. In an acidic environment, the compound becomes a negatively charged paste material, which binds with positively charged proteins such as albumin, fibrinogen, damaged mucosal cells, and dead leukocytes found at the base of an ulcer. Because it is poorly absorbed, sucralfate exerts its effect locally upon the gastric intestinal mucosa, perhaps by the stimulation of prostaglandin production.

Several controlled studies show that sucralfate, 1 gram four times a day on an empty stomach, is superior to placebo and is as effective as intensive antacids or H_2 blockers in healing duodenal and gastric ulcers. It is not approved for the Zollinger-Ellison syndrome, reflux esophagitis, or peptic ulcer prophylaxis.

The incidence of side effects has been extremely low and symptoms, minor. Constipation is the most common. Other nonspecific gastrointestinal symptoms have been reported. Sucralfate may bind other drugs such as tetracycline and reduce the bioavailability of phenytoin. Simultaneous administration with food may impair its effectiveness. Therefore, it is recommended that other medications be given 1 hour before sucralfate, and that food be taken 1 hour after its administration. It should not be used in combination with antacids or H_2 blockers.

Maintenance Therapy

The recurrence rate for healed duodenal ulcer is approximately 70 per cent within 1 year and 90 per cent within 2 years of cessation of therapy (Table 2). This figure can be drastically reduced by the administration of cimetidine, 400 mg, or ranitidine, 150 mg, at bedtime. The period of maintenance therapy is controversial. I recommend 1 year's maintenance therapy for all patients with healed duodenal and gastric ulcers. Therapy should be continued indefinitely for

TABLE 2. **Relative Recurrence Rates of Peptic Ulcer**

	Within One Year (Per Cent)
Duodenal Ulcer	
Placebo	70
Cimetidine, 400 mg h.s.	10
Ranitidine, 150 mg h.s.	10
Gastric Ulcer	
Placebo	56
Cimetidine, 400 mg h.s.	20
Ranitidine, 150 mg h.s.	20

those without side effects who have a history of recurrent ulcers, have complicated ulcers with bleeding, had surgery for perforated ulcer without an acid reduction procedure, and are poor surgical risks.

Failure to Heal

Although approximately 80 per cent of patients with duodenal ulcer heal in 6 weeks with one of the single agents mentioned earlier, some fail to heal. The first consideration must be whether there is compliance with the therapy prescribed. Cigarette smoking should be eliminated, because smoking decreases healing rates with all modalities of treatment. Hypersecretory states, such as the Zollinger-Ellison syndrome, should be evaluated by serum gastrin levels and gastric acid analysis. The use of ulcerogenic agents like alcohol, aspirin, and nonsteroidal anti-inflammatory agents should be discontinued, especially in patients with a gastric ulcer. Patients with nonhealing gastric ulcer should be restudied endoscopically with cytologic and biopsy evaluation. Switching from one H_2 blocker to another may improve healing. The addition of an anticholinergic drug may further decrease acid secretion in those with hypersecretory states.

The recurrence rate after gastric resection for ulcer is about 2 per cent. When marginal ulcers occur, the patient must be evaluated for hypersecretion of acid by a gastrinoma or retained antrum. A trial of medical management with H_2 blockers and perhaps anticholinergic agents is recommended in an attempt to avoid further surgery.

The goals of ulcer therapy—reduction of pain, promotion of healing, and prevention of complications—can be achieved with antacids, H_2 blockers, and mucosa protection. The costs of these therapies are similar; adverse reactions are few; and the efficacy is established. Selection of treatment is based upon patient compliance, concomitant medical problems, the need for administration of other medications, and side effects encountered.

TUMORS OF THE STOMACH

method of
E. GEORGE ELIAS, M.D., Ph.D.
University of Maryland
Baltimore, Maryland

A variety of tumors arise from different histologic tissues that constitute the wall of the stomach. These lesions can be silent and are found incidentally at surgery or autopsy or can become symptomatic and are diagnosed clinically. The symptoms may vary from mild epigastric discomfort to pain, bleeding, obstruction, and loss of weight. The availability of fiberoptic gastroscopy and special upper gastrointestinal radiologic series allow visualization of the exact location and extent of the lesion in over 90 per cent of cases and permit biopsy of the tumor. Computed tomographic (CT) scanning of the abdomen has been helpful in establishing the extent of the disease—especially outside the stomach, such as retroperitoneal invasion or liver metastases—prior to surgical intervention. A CT scan also can be used in follow-up of the patients and for controlled needle biopsy to establish a tissue diagnosis. Some of these tumors may produce tumor markers such as alpha-fetoproteins, but mainly they produce carcinoembryonic antigen (CEA). Such markers can be utilized for the follow-up of these patients by periodically comparing the preoperative levels with the postoperative values.

Serosal Tumors

(1) *Peritoneal mesotheliomas* are rare. The visceral peritoneum of the stomach can be the site of benign solitary ones or involved in the diffuse malignant type. Surgical resection should be carried out if at all possible. Doxorubicin (Adriamycin) is being tried in the treatment of advanced malignant mesotheliomas with varying results.

(2) *Metastatic carcinomas* also can invade the gastric serosa as part of generalized peritoneal spread. This is commonly encountered from ovarian, breast, and lung cancers and melanoma. Such tumors can invade the stomach wall and penetrate it throughout its thickness. Surgery is indicated for palliation, but the primary therapy is directed to control the primary disease.

(3) *Desmoid tumors* also may invade the stomach. These should be resected with safety margins in the hope of preventing recurrences. Multiple recurrent tumors that are not resectable can be treated by Adriamycin.

Serosal tumors can deeply invade the stomach wall, displacing the mucosa, which may later ulcerate intraluminally.

Intramural Tumors

Tumors that originate within the stomach wall proper can be categorized according to their origin.

(1) *Smooth muscle tumors.* Leiomyoma is the most common benign tumor. Sometimes it cannot be differentiated from malignant leiomyosarcoma and leiomyoblastoma. These tumors tend to protrude intraluminally with stretching of the overlying mucosa. Small tumors are treated by wedge resection with 2 to 3 cm margins. Larger tumors are treated by partial gastrectomy. The malignant variety is treated by radical partial gastrectomy. Metastases are usually bloodborne and are treated mainly by chemotherapy: doxorubicin

(Adriamycin), actinomycin-D (Cosmegen), and vincristine (Oncovin) or a combination of these.

(2) *Malignant lymphomas.* These may be primary tumors of the stomach or secondary to lymphomas of lymph node origin, with direct invasion from neighboring lymph nodes or by metastases. These usually protrude intraluminally, causing stretching of the mucosa: later they ulcerate and invade the mucosa. The primary lymphomas of the stomach are usually histiocytic or of poorly differentiated lymphocytic type, i.e., non-Hodgkin's type. Lymphomas of the stomach should be surgically resected, and it is essential to remove the regional lymph nodes to establish their involvement. Complete staging laparotomy is carried out during the same setting to establish the extent of the disease. Surgery is indicated to eliminate the site of gastric lymphoma prior to the initiation of radiation therapy or chemotherapy. This is to avoid sloughing of the tumor site that may result in bleeding or perforation and peritonitis. *Pseudolymphoma* is a benign lymphoid hyperplasia that should be differentiated from lymphoma and plasmacytoma of the stomach, which is a malignant systemic disease.

(3) *Lipomas.* These are rare tumors and are treated by local excision.

(4) *Carcinoid tumors.* These are usually argyrophilic, are a derivative of the foregut carcinoids, and can be associated with multiple endocrine adenomatosis. They can be single or multiple. Some of these tumors are secretors giving rise to clinical symptoms of the carcinoid syndrome. Such tumors are yellow or tanned submucosal nodules. Surgery is the primary treatment for these tumors even in the presence of metastases. Small tumors of up to 1 cm can be locally resected. Tumors greater than 1 cm should be treated as carcinoma in the absence of metastases. Patients with metastases who have the syndrome can be treated symptomatically according to the clinical presentation.

Carcinoid tumors of the stomach may be associated with peptic ulcers or diarrhea. Flushing is common and usually occurs after meals as a vivid red that is patchy and then becomes confluent. Flushing can be controlled by alpha-adrenergic blockers such as phenoxybenzamine (Dibenzyline): 10–20 mg per day to block kinins. Also, prednisone, methyldopa (Aldomet), chlorpromazine (Thorazine), and antiprostaglandins such as aspirin and indomethacin (Indocin) have been beneficial. Actual tumor control by chemotherapy with 5-fluorouracil (5-FU) and streptozotocin (Zanosar) or cyclophosphamide (Cytoxan) and streptozotocin gives a 30 per cent response rate for a short duration.

(5) *Glomus tumors.* These are rare benign tumors formed of fibroneural tissue and are treated by local excision.

(6) *Ectopic pancreatic tissue.* These are usually present in the pyloric region and may cause obstruction. They are treated by surgical resection.

Mucosal Tumors

(1) *Polyps* are the most common benign mucosal lesions, especially common in the elderly. There are two main varieties: the regenerative type, also known as hyperplastic or inflammatory, which comprises 75 per cent of gastric polyps. These are usually multiple and correspond to Ménétrier's disease. The other type is the adenomatous polyp, which is usually single, large, and located in the antrum. Almost 60 per cent of these patients have a coexisting carcinoma. A single polyp can be snared via endoscopy and thoroughly studied histologically. The patient has to be observed for recurrence and cancer. Multiple polyps must be treated by gastrectomy. If the disease is localized, partial gastrectomy is performed; however, if it is widespread throughout the stomach or is persistent Ménétrier's disease, total gastrectomy is in order.

(2) *Carcinoma.* Adenocarcinoma is the most common malignant gastric tumor. The most common precancerous lesions are severe dysplasia of the mucosa, atrophic gastritis, intestinal metaplasia, and severe adenomatous dysplasia. Among the risk factors are duodenogastric reflux of over 10 years, nitrosocompound intake in the diet, adenomatous polyps, achlorhydria, and immunologic gastritis as in pernicious anemia. It is more common in the 6th decade of life and more common in men, with a male to female ratio of 2:1. Endoscopy and detailed upper GI series examinations have yielded a 5 per cent rate of "early carcinoma," located in the mucosa down to the submucosa only with no lymphatic spread. Surgical cure is over 90 per cent in those cases. The primary treatment of all gastric carcinoma is surgery: radical subtotal gastrectomy or total radical gastrectomy. Palliative gastrectomy plays a role in prolonging survival.

Two chemotherapy programs have been claimed to be effective in metastatic disease. These include 5-FU + Adriamycin + mitomycin-C (FAM), and 5-FU + cytosine arabinoside (AraC) + mitomycin-C, with a 20 to 50 per cent response rate of 20 to 30 weeks' duration. Adjuvant chemotherapy, administered 4 weeks after curative surgery to prevent or delay recurrences and metastases, utilizing 5-FU plus methyl-CCNU, showed some improvement in survival in one study, and no benefit in another.

Finally, squamous cell carcinoma is usually encountered at the cardioesophageal junction and is of esophageal origin, with secondary invasion of the proximal end of the stomach.

TUMORS OF THE COLON AND RECTUM

method of
DAVID J. SCHOETZ, Jr., M.D.
Lahey Clinic Medical Center
Burlington, Massachusetts

With approximately 130,000 new cases reported per year, cancer of the colon and rectum is currently the most common visceral malignancy in the United States. Despite advances in surgery, radiation, and chemotherapy, the overall 5 year survival rate has not improved in the past several decades. Obviously, the greatest impact on survival would be achieved by the detection of cancer at an early stage of development, thus permitting greater surgical success in eradicating the cancer. This is based on the fact that the most important single variable in determining long-term survival is the pathologic stage of the tumor at the time of operation.

Advances in fiberoptic technology have provided insight into the polyp-cancer sequence and have facilitated aggressive therapy of potentially premalignant lesions affecting the large intestine. With the widespread use of colonoscopy, 10 to 20 per cent of persons in the United States are now known to harbor neoplastic polyps in the colon. The percentage of these existing polyps that will undergo malignant transformation never will be known accurately, but few would dispute the fact that most colorectal cancers arise in polyps. Removal of these polyps can be expected to decrease the incidence of subsequent cancer in a carefully monitored population of patients with neoplastic polyps.

Although the majority of tumors of the large bowel are either neoplastic polyps or adenocarcinomas, a number of other benign and malignant tumors may occur as well (Table 1). All these lesions generally are found either incidentally during evaluation of nonspecific abdominal complaints or as a result of specific evaluation for complaints of rectal bleeding or a change in bowel habits.

TABLE 1. **Classification of Tumors of the Colon and Rectum**

Malignant
Adenocarcinoma
Epidermoid carcinoma (anus)
Lymphoma
Carcinoid
Melanoma (anus)
Leiomyosarcoma
Benign
Neoplastic polyps
Lipoma
Leiomyoma
Carcinoid

Every evaluation of colonic complaints should include a complete physical examination, digital rectal examination, testing of the stool for occult blood, anoscopy, and proctosigmoidoscopy. Double-contrast barium enemas should be performed when indicated, and the addition of air appreciably improves diagnostic accuracy for small mucosal abnormalities. Total colonoscopy should be reserved for those individuals in whom a diagnostic abnormality requires tissue diagnosis or when evaluation fails to reveal the cause of a complaint that may be of colonic origin.

Management

Cancer

Surgery is the definitive therapy for colorectal cancer. The overall cure rate is 50 per cent; however, lesions can be cured in the earlier stages in approximately 80 per cent of patients. Even when the tumor has metastasized beyond the limits of conventional colonic resection, palliative resection should be performed to prevent obstruction and persistent bleeding.

Preoperative evaluation of the patient with colorectal cancer should be limited to the complete colonic survey outlined. Liver function tests, particularly determinations of serum alkaline phosphatase and serum carcinoembryonic antigen, should be carried out. Radionuclide scans of the liver and computed tomographic scans should be reserved for those rare patients in whom documentation of the liver metastases would alter radically the operative approach. Intraoperative assessment of the liver and peritoneal cavity with biopsy of suspicious lesions is the most accurate diagnostic modality, and resection can be performed during the same period of anesthesia. Chest radiography should be routine; metastatic disease in the lungs may alter the operative procedure.

All patients facing permanent or temporary colostomy should be evaluated preoperatively by a trained enterostomal therapist for counseling and marking of the most appropriate stomal site. Thorough mechanical cleansing of the bowel and perioperative antibiotics should be employed whenever possible to minimize postoperative septic complications.

Radiotherapy is of use in several specific situations. If preoperative clinical assessment of a rectal cancer indicates that fixation and invasion of surrounding tissues make curative resection impossible, a full course of radiotherapy should be administered based on the premise that 50 per cent of such lesions will become clinically resectable. The risk of pelvic recurrence is appreciable after excision of rectal cancer when the perirectal fat or local lymph nodes are involved. Under these circumstances, a full course (4500 to 5000 rad) of postoperative radiotherapy is recommended to reduce the risk of local recurrence. On the other hand, no evidence exists to support radiotherapy for cancer of the intraperitoneal colon if the resection is believed to be curative.

Chemotherapy has never been shown statistically to be of benefit as adjuvant treatment in colorectal cancer. At present, chemotherapy should be recommended only for documented metastatic disease that cannot be removed surgically.

Follow-up of Cancer Patients. Even after presumed curative resection, regular follow-up of patients is necessary. To detect regional or distant metastatic disease, abdominal examination and determinations of carcinoembryonic antigen and alkaline phosphatase should be carried out every 3 months for the first 18 months. Thereafter, examinations take place every 6 months for the next 18 months. Finally, examinations are performed annually for life. Chest radiography is obtained yearly.

Examination of the remaining colon must be vigorous. If an anastomosis has been performed, visualization of the suture line should be achieved within the first year after operation to preclude the presence of an anastomotic recurrence. When preoperative assessment of the entire colon has been inadequate for exclusion of the presence of synchronous lesions, such as may occur with obstructive left-sided colonic cancer, total colonoscopy should be performed 3 to 6 months after resection. Metachronous lesions may develop in 3 to 8 per cent of patients who have had one resection for cancer. Therefore, complete visualization of the colon by either colonoscopy or air-contrast barium enema is performed every 3 years. Testing for fecal occult blood and flexible sigmoidoscopy should be carried out annually for life in those patients at high risk for subsequent development of cancer.

Metastatic disease that is discovered by these methods should be investigated thoroughly. Liver and lung metastases are best treated by surgical resection if evaluation reveals that operation can be performed with a reasonable expectation of cure.

Other Malignant Tumors

Epidermoid carcinoma arising in the colon and rectum is rare. On the other hand, cancer arising in the anal canal is most often of squamous cell origin. The recent introduction of combined chemotherapy and radiation therapy for squamous cell cancer of the anus has obviated the need for abdominoperineal resection in the majority of patients.

Lymphoma is an unusual tumor of the large intestine. When present, it is most often found in the rectum. Before definitive surgical therapy, a complete evaluation must be undertaken to exclude the presence of systemic lymphoma. If the lymphoma is of primary colorectal origin, resection plus adjuvant chemotherapy or radiation or both is the treatment of choice.

Carcinoid tumors are submucosal lesions most often arising in the rectum. Histopathologic diagnosis of malignancy is difficult and depends primarily on the size of the lesion. Lesions less than 2 cm in diameter usually are benign and are treated by local excision. If lesions are larger than 2 cm in diameter or arise in the intraperitoneal colon, surgical resection should be performed.

Melanoma of the anus and rectum is rare. Although surgical resection is the treatment of choice, long-term survival is less than 25 per cent.

Leiomyosarcoma is a submucosal lesion that is best treated by wide surgical resection. Debulking of nonresectable lesions should be performed to palliate symptoms. Metastases should be treated with a combination of radiotherapy and chemotherapy, although these tumors frequently are resistant to both treatment modalities. The overall 5 year survival rate for this lesion is approximately 50 per cent.

Polyps

Many benign lesions of the colon and rectum may appear as polyps (Table 2). Once the diagnosis of polyp has been established, histologic examination must be performed to determine the exact nature of the lesion. Patients with neoplastic polyps must be followed at regular intervals because they are a population at risk for the development of cancer.

A polyp usually can be removed completely endoscopically in combination with the use of electrosurgical techniques. Sometimes a large rectal polyp can be removed transanally in the operating room. For lesions in the more proximal colon, colonoscopy with piecemeal excisions of sessile lesions greater than 2 cm in diameter can be performed by a skilled endoscopist, thus avoiding the need for laparotomy. The removal of large

TABLE 2. **Benign Polyps of the Colon and Rectum**

Neoplastic
Tubular adenoma
Villous adenoma
Tubulovillous adenoma
Non-Neoplastic
Hyperplastic
Juvenile
Inflammatory pseudopolyps

lesions, however, carries a substantial risk of perforation and bleeding even in the most experienced hands. In addition, multiple colonoscopic sessions are frequently required to assure adequate extirpation of the lesion. In most instances, resection of the segment of colon with the large polyp affords more accurate pathologic examination and acceptably low rates of morbidity and mortality.

The risk of cancer in a neoplastic polyp is a function of size and histologic type. Tubular adenoma, the commonest neoplastic polyp, has a 1 per cent incidence of invasive cancer at 1 cm in size, but the incidence increases to 10 per cent at 2 cm. Villous adenomas of equivalent sizes carry about four times these cited risks of invasive cancer. If a resected polyp has carcinoma in situ, defined as cancer not breeching the muscularis mucosa, endoscopic polypectomy is sufficient treatment. On the other hand, when invasive cancer is present in the head of the polyp, resection should be performed if the patient is a reasonable operative risk, although the risk of regional lymph node metastasis is small.

Once the entire colon has been cleared of neoplastic polyps, yearly screening with fecal occult blood testing and flexible sigmoidoscopy should be performed. Colonoscopy should be repeated every 3 to 5 years.

Hyperplastic polyps are benign proliferations of normal colonic epithelium. Most frequently situated in the rectum and distal sigmoid colon and most often found on screening sigmoidoscopy, these are not premalignant lesions. Biopsy should be performed to distinguish them from small adenomatous polyps. Therapy with electrocoagulation is sufficient.

Juvenile polyps are actually hamartomas that most often present with rectal bleeding in patients aged 12 years or younger. The bleeding occurs because these lesions lack a muscularis mucosa and can twist and detach at the base. Removal of these polyps should be performed only for histologic diagnosis.

Inflammatory pseudopolyps represent collections of granulation tissue and regenerated epithelium that are the result of long-standing inflammatory bowel disease. These lesions are seen in both ulcerative colitis and Crohn's disease. Removal is required only to distinguish them from adenomatous polyps when confusion is apparent. Usually the clinical picture and endoscopic appearance are sufficiently diagnostic that the pseudopolyp need not be removed. These lesions do not undergo malignant degeneration.

Other Benign Tumors

Lipomas of the colon are submucosal tumors that are more often found on the right side than on the left. Discovery of these lesions, even if they have achieved considerable size, is usually incidental because their presence is rarely accompanied by symptoms. When symptoms are present, they are those of partial obstruction. Rarely, a lipoma may surface as a cause of intussusception. Confirmation of the benign nature of the lesion can be achieved with colonoscopy. Smaller pedunculated lipomas may be removed with the colonoscope. Surgical removal is indicated only in the presence of symptoms or if the clinical diagnosis is uncertain.

Leiomyomas of the colon are also benign submucosal tumors that can achieve remarkable size. Symptoms are those of either partial colonic obstruction or bleeding. Surgical removal is required to exclude the presence of malignancy.

Screening Programs

Because early detection of colorectal cancer offers the greatest likelihood for improvement in overall survival, efforts to design effective screening programs have increased. Identification of the appropriate population for screening allows application of available techniques with the greatest possible diagnostic yield. Factors that identify a population at high risk are age over 50 years, previous history of colonic neoplasm, family history of colonic neoplasm, polyposis syndromes, and longstanding ulcerative colitis. The most important single factor in defining an at risk population of asymptomatic patients is age. If symptoms are present that may be due to colorectal cancer, complete evaluation should be performed regardless of risk factors.

Recent observations of the changing distribution of cancer of the large bowel, with more right-sided lesions and fewer rectal lesions, have resulted in an increased reliance on fecal occult blood testing for screening. The expectation that a digital rectal examination is sufficient for screening is no longer acceptable. Similarly, the widespread availability of flexible fiberoptic sigmoidoscopy is slowly supplanting rigid sigmoidoscopy as a screening tool because of the marked increase in diagnostic yield with flexible instruments.

Air-contrast radiography and colonoscopy are not cost-effective modalities for screening except for patients with long-standing ulcerative colitis who should undergo regular total colonoscopy with mucosal biopsies in an attempt to document the presence of dysplastic changes in the epithelium. The presence of mucosal dysplasia identifies the patient at appreciable risk for the development of carcinoma, and appropriate surgical therapy should be recommended.

The most reasonable screening program that currently can be offered to patients is annual fecal occult blood testing, supplemented by flexible sigmoidoscopy every 3 years. If a polyp is discovered, air-contrast barium enema and colonoscopy should be performed, and then flexible sigmoidoscopy is performed yearly until the colon has been cleared conclusively of polyps. The regular screening program is then reinstituted.

INTESTINAL PARASITES

method of
MARTIN S. WOLFE, M.D.
George Washington University
Washington, D.C.

Intestinal protozoa and helminths cause some of the major disease problems worldwide. They are ubiquitous and must always be considered in dealing with the disease problems of populations in both developing and developed countries. In the United States several groups are at risk for contracting intestinal parasites: campers and hikers drinking untreated stream water; those served by certain small community water supplies; children in day care centers; male homosexuals; and institutionalized individuals. Imported infections can be present in Americans returning from travel or residence in developing countries and in immigrants and refugees from developing countries. It is important to entertain the possibility of an intestinal parasitic infection in such persons before embarking on a time-consuming and costly medical work-up.

TREATMENT

Most of the drugs described here are licensed and commercially available in the United States. Some are presently licensed for some indications but not for others. A few foreign-made drugs are not approved in the United States but may be obtained from the Parasitic Disease Drug Service of the Centers for Disease Control in Atlanta, Georgia (404-329-3670).

Summaries of drug therapies for intestinal protozoa and helminths are given in Tables 1 and 2.

Protozoan Infections

Giardia lamblia

This is the most common pathogenic intestinal protozoa diagnosed in the United States, and it has also been contracted in both temperate and tropical areas worldwide. Although not all those infected are symptomatic, others may have diarrhea, flatulence, distention, weight loss, fatigue, and malabsorption.

The most effective drug is quinacrine hydrochloride (Atabrine). Cure rates of 90 to 95 per cent are usually reported. Common side effects include gastrointestinal discomfort, headache, and dizziness. Less frequent, but more disturbing, side effects include yellow discoloration of the skin and sclerae, vomiting, fever, exfoliative dermatitis, and toxic psychosis. Tolerance in young children may be improved by placing the ground up portion of the tablet required in a gelatin capsule.

Metronidazole (Flagyl) remains an unapproved drug for giardiasis in the United States but is frequently prescribed. It is somewhat less effective than quinacrine but is generally better tolerated. Side effects may include nausea, metallic taste, dark urine, possible *Candida* overgrowth on the skin and mucus membranes and in the intestine, and a disulfiram-like effect when taken with alcohol. Recent reviews consider the risk to humans of carcinogenicity and mutagenicity to be low, if not negligible, but have recommended that physicians decide whether benefit from the drug outweighs the potential risk.

Furazolidone (Furoxone) is an antibiotic whose major indication for use in the United States is giardiasis. It is the only one of the three available anti-*Giardia* drugs produced in suspension form, making it particularly useful in young children. Cure rates have ranged from 77 to 92 per cent. Side effects may include vomiting, diarrhea, nausea, fever, and skin rash. Furazolidone can produce a disulfiram-like reaction with alcohol; it is a monoamine oxidase inhibitor; and it may cause mild hemolysis in glucose-6-phosphate dehydrogenase deficiency.

Tinidazole (Fasigyn) is not available in the United States, but in trials in Finland a single 2 gram dose has been found to be more effective and better tolerated than metronidazole, a related imidazole product.

Dientamoeba fragilis

Formerly thought to be an amoeba, *D. fragilis* has recently been considered an amoeba-like flagellate occurring only in a labile trophozoite form. Although considered a nonpathogen by some, in recent years correlation has been found with infection and intermittent diarrhea, abdominal pain, anorexia, and, in some cases, eosinophilia. It is being increasingly recognized in diagnostic parasitology laboratories in the United States. Tetracycline and iodoquinol are often mentioned as the drugs of choice, but careful scrutiny of the literature indicates that cure rates are not high with these drugs. Paromomycin (Humatin) may be more effective, although this drug may cause intestinal side effects or diarrhea.

Balantidium coli

This ciliated parasite has a worldwide distribution and infection is particularly common in

TABLE 1. **Drug Therapy of Intestinal Protozoan Parasites**

Parasite	Drug	Adult Dose*	Pediatric Dose*	Availability
Giardia lamblia	metronidazole or	250 mg tid × 7 days	5 mg/kg tid × 7 days	Flagyl (Searle) (tablets)
	quinacrine HCl or	100 mg tid × 7 days	2 mg/kg tid × 7 days	Atabrine (Winthrop) (tablets)
	furazolidone	100 mg (tablet) qid × 7 days	1.25 mg/kg qid × 7 days (suspension)	Furoxone (Norwich-Eaton) (tablets and suspension)
Dientamoeba fragilis	paromomycin or	500 mg tid × 7 days	30 mg/kg/day in 3 divided doses × 7 days	Humatin (Parke-Davis) (capsules)
	iodoquinol or	650 mg tid × 20 days	40 mg/kg/day in 3 divided doses × 20 days	Yodoxin (Glenwood, Inc.) (tablets) Amebaquin (U.S. Product, Inc.) (tablets)
	tetracycline	500 mg qid × 10 days	10 mg/kg qid × 10 days (max 2 grams/day)	
Balantidium coli	iodoquinol or tetracycline	As per *D. fragilis*	As per *D. fragilis*	
Isospora belli	trimethoprim/ sulfamethoxazole or	160 mg TMP/800 mg SMX qid × 10 days, then bid × 3 weeks	—	Bactrim (Roche) (tablets) Septra (Burroughs Wellcome) (tablets)
	furazolidone	As per *G. lamblia*	As per *G. lamblia*	
Cryptosporidium	spiramycin†	3 grams/day in divided doses for 2 to 4 weeks	—	Rovamycin (Rhone-Poulenc/Montreal) (tablets)
Blastocystis hominis	iodoquinol	As per *D. fragilis*	As per *D. fragilis*	

*All recommended drugs given by mouth.
†Not approved in the United States. Permission to use this drug must be obtained from the U.S. Food and Drug Administration.

pigs, which are the main reservoir of infection to man. *B. coli* infection is rarely diagnosed in the United States. The drugs of choice are tetracycline and iodoquinol.

Isospora belli

This sporozoan parasite also has a worldwide distribution but is rarely reported in man. It has recently been recognized as an opportunistic infection in immunosuppressed individuals and in male homosexuals. No effective drug treatment had been available, but in recent years trimethoprim-sulfamethoxazole has been found to be curative. Furazolidone may also be useful.

Cryptosporidium

This coccidial parasite has in recent years been increasingly recognized as a cause of diarrhea in humans. It is a cause of a highly lethal fulminant diarrhea in patients with the acquired immunodeficiency syndrome. *Cryptosporidium* has also been recognized in immunologically normal children and adults in various parts of the world, in travelers, and in children in day care centers in the United States. In these individuals infections are either asymptomatic or self-limited after 5 to 10 days. An effective treatment has not yet been identified. Two patients have been reported who had relief of diarrhea, negative stool examinations, and negative upper intestinal biopsy at the end of a 4 week course of spiramycin. Permission to use this drug must be obtained from the Food and Drug Administration. Treatment of immunosuppressed patients is primarily symptomatic and includes adequate fluid and nutritional support. A few cases of successful intervention have occurred when the underlying immune deficiency has been reversed.

Blastocystis hominis

This organism had been considered a nonpathogenic yeast, but recent evidence indicates that it is a protozoan that, when present in human stools in large numbers, may cause some degree of diarrhea. Treatment with iodoquinol has been found to improve diarrhea in persons with heavy *B. hominis* infections and no other recognized pathogens.

Nonpathogenic Protozoa

A number of nonpathogenic amoebae and flagellates are frequently found on stool examination, indicating fecal contamination of the host. If intestinal symptoms are present, further search should be made for recognized pathogens. These nonpathogens include *Entamoeba hartmanni,*

TABLE 2. **Drug Therapy of Intestinal Helminths**

Parasite	Drug	Adult Dose*	Pediatric Dose*	Availability
Ascaris lumbricoides	mebendazole or	100 mg bid × 3 days	Same as adult dose (> 2 years)	Vermox (Janssen) (tablets)
	pyrantel pamoate or	11 mg/kg single dose (max 1 gram)	Same as adult dose (max 1 gram)	Antiminth (Pfipharmecs) (suspension)
	piperazine citrate	75 mg/kg/day (max 3.5 grams) × 2 days	Same as adult dose (max 3.5 grams)	Antepar (Burroughs Wellcome) (syrup)
Trichuris trichiura	mebendazole	As per *Ascaris*	As per *Ascaris*	
Hookworm *Necator americanus*	mebendazole or	As per *Ascaris*	As per *Ascaris*	
Ancylostoma duodenale	pyrantel pamoate†	As per *Ascaris*	As per *Ascaris*	
Enterobius vermicularis	mebendazole or	100 mg single dose; repeat in 2 weeks	Same as adult dose	
	pyrantel pamoate or	11 mg/kg single dose; repeat in 2 weeks	Same as adult dose	
	pyrvinium pamoate	5 mg/kg single dose; repeat in 2 weeks	Same as adult dose (max 250 mg)	Povan (filmseals)
Strongyloides stercoralis	thiabendazole or	25 mg/kg bid × 2 days (max 3 grams/day)	Same as adult dose	Mintezol (Merck, Sharp and Dohme) (suspension)
	mebendazole† or	As per *Ascaris*	As per *Ascaris*	
	pyrvinium pamoate†	5 mg/kg once daily × 7 days (max 250 mg/day)	Same as adult dose	
Trichostrongylus sp.	thiabendazole† or	As per *Strongyloides*	As per *Strongyloides*	
	pyrantel pamoate† or	As per *Ascaris*	As per *Ascaris*	
	mebendazole†	As per *Ascaris*	As per *Ascaris*	
Tapeworms *Taenia saginata*	niclosamide	Single dose/4 tabs (2 grams) chewed thoroughly	11–34 kg: Single dose/2 tabs (1 gram) > 34 kg: Single dose/3 tabs (1.5 grams)	Niclocide (Miles) (tablets)
Taenia solium *Diphyllobothrium latum* and *pacificum*	or paromomycin† or	1 gram q 15 min × 4 doses	11 mg/kg q 15 min × 4 doses	Humatin (Parke-Davis) (capsules)
Dipylidium caninum	praziquantel†	15 to 20 mg/kg once	Same as adult dose	Biltricide (Miles) (tablets)
Hymenolepis nana	niclosamide	Single 2 grams/dose × 6 days	As above for other tapeworms, single dose daily × 6 days	
	or praziquantel†	15 to 20 mg/kg once	Same as adult dose	
Cerebral cysticercosis cellulosae	praziquantel†	50 mg/kg/day in 3 divided doses × 14 days	Same as adult dose	
Schistosomiasis *Schistosoma mansoni*	praziquantel† or	60 mg/kg in 3 div doses for 1 day	Same as adult dose	Biltricide (Miles) (tablets)
	oxamniquine	Caribbean & S. Am. strains: 15 mg/kg single dose African strains: 15 mg/kg bid × 2 days	Same as adult dose	Vansil (Pfipharmecs) (tablets)

Table continued on next page

TABLE 2. **Drug Therapy of Intestinal Helminths** *Continued*

Parasite	Drug	Adult Dose*	Pediatric Dose*	Availability
Schistosoma japonicum	praziquantel	As per *S. mansoni*	As per *S. mansoni*	
Schistosoma mekongi	praziquantel	As per *S. mansoni*	As per *S. mansoni*	
Schistosoma intercalatum	praziquantel	As per *S. mansoni*	As per *S. mansoni*	
Schistosoma haematobium	praziquantel	40 mg/kg single dose or 20 mg/kg bid for 1 day	Same as adult dose	
Intestinal flukes				
Fasciolopsis buski *Heterophyes heterophyes*	praziquantel or	25 mg/kg tid for 1 day	Same as adult dose	
Metagonimus yokogawai	tetrachlorethylene	0.1 ml/kg single dose (max 5 ml)	Same as adult dose	Nema worm capsules, Veterinary (Parke-Davis)
Liver flukes				
Clonorchis sinensis *Opisthorchis viverrini*	praziquantel†	25 mg/kg tid for 1 day	Same as adult dose	
Fasciola hepatica	praziquantel† or	25 mg/kg tid for 1 day	Same as adult dose	
Paragonimus westermani	bithionol† (capsule)	30 to 50 mg/kg on alternate days × 10 to 15 doses	Same as adult dose	Parasitic Disease Drug Service, CDC, Atlanta, Georgia

*All recommended drugs given by mouth.
†Considered an investigational drug for this purpose by the U.S. Food and Drug Administration.

Entamoeba coli, Endolimax nana, Iodamoeba bütschlii, Chilomastix mesnili, Trichomonas hominis, Enteromonas hominis, and *Retortamonas intestinalis.*

Helminthic Infections

Ascaris lumbricoides *(Roundworm)*

A number of safe and effective drugs are available for this infection. Mebendazole (Vermox) for 3 days is well tolerated and approximately 98 per cent effective. Pyrantel pamoate (Antiminth) in a single dose is also highly effective, but side effects may be more common. Piperazine citrate (Antepar) in a 2 day course is a third choice. Piperazine should be administered in the morning before breakfast, whereas the other two can be taken without regard to meals. When *Ascaris* is present with another intestinal helminth it should preferentially be treated first, as some drugs can cause *Ascaris* worms to migrate to aberrant locations.

Trichuris trichiura *(Whipworm)*

This is perhaps the commonest intestinal helminthic infection and is often associated with *Ascaris.* Most infections seen in the United States are asymptomatic, but all infections can be treated with mebendazole. Cure rates are about 70 per cent, but there is a 98 per cent egg reduction rate.

Hookworm Infections

A distinction must be made in temperate areas between hookworm infection or carrier state and the less common hookworm disease with anemia. Hookworm infection may be treated with anthelminthic drugs alone, but hookworm disease with anemia must also be treated with iron supplements and in severe anemia with transfusions. Mebendazole for 3 days is effective against both common species of hookworm, *Necator americanus* and *Ancylostoma duodenale.* Pyrantel pamoate is an alternative.

Enterobius vermicularis *(Pinworm)*

This is a cosmopolitan infection, found more commonly in middle class children in the United States than in children in developing countries. Although pinworm infection is usually a scourge of children, adults, particularly parents of infected children, can also be infected. Single dose treatments, repeated in 2 weeks, with mebendazole, pyrantel pamoate, or pyrvinium pamoate (Povan), are highly effective and well-tolerated. Care must be taken with pyrvinium pamoate, a cyanine dye, as it can stain clothes; this drug also colors stools red. It is acceptable practice to treat the entire family when at least one member is known to be infected. Attempts should be made to prevent reinfection by keeping nails short, showering every morning, and wearing snug-fitting undergarments. More heroic measures, such as boiling or soaking night clothes and bed linen in ammonia and scrubbing or disinfecting floors and toilet seats, are usually doomed to failure owing to the hardiness of the eggs and their frequent reintroduction into the household.

Strongyloides stercoralis

This parasite can live for 30 to 40 years in an infected host because of its unique autoinfection cycle leading to self-perpetuating infection. The continued presence of this parasite poses a potential threat of lethal dissemination by hyperinfection if the infected individual becomes immunosuppressed or is treated with cancer chemotherapy, radiation therapy, or corticosteroids. *S. stercoralis* must be considered in anyone who has been in an endemic area and has an otherwise unexplained eosinophilia or periodic diarrhea and intestinal discomfort, urticaria, creeping eruption in the area of the buttocks and thighs, and possibly pulmonary complaints. The present available treatment of choice is thiabendazole (Mintezol) in a 2 day course. Although highly effective, this drug is often not well-tolerated, particularly in adults, and can cause nausea, vomiting dizziness, and, rarely, angioneurotic edema. Mebendazole is an alternative treatment that is better tolerated but less effective. Another alternative is pyrvinium pamoate (Povan) in a 7 day course. Albendazole, a newer broad spectrum anthelminthic (not yet available in the United States) has shown some good effect against *S. stercoralis* in studies elsewhere. In disseminated strongyloidiasis, thiabendazole should be continued for at least 5 days.

Trichostrongylus *Species*

This parasite is particularly common in Iran, Korea, and Indonesia and may be the cause of a high eosinophilia and gastrointestinal symptoms in some of those infected. Thiabendazole, in doses used for strongyloidiasis, is the drug of choice. Pyrantel pamoate and mebendazole are alternative drugs.

Tapeworm Infections

Taenia saginata (the beef tapeworm), *Taenia solium* (the pork tapeworm), *Diphyllobothrium latum* and *pacificum* (fish tapeworms), and *Dipylidium caninum* (the dog tapeworm) are best treated with a single dose of niclosamide (Niclocide). An alternative drug is paromomycin (Humatin). Praziquantel (Biltricide) is an effective single dose treatment but is not yet approved in the United States for use against tapeworms. *Hymenolepis nana* (the dwarf tapeworm) and the much less common *Hymenolepis diminuta* (the rat tapeworm) require a 6 day course of niclosamide.

Tissue invasion of the brain or muscles with cysticercosis cellulosae of *T. solium* can now be treated with praziquantel on an investigational basis. Corticosteroids may be given concomitantly to decrease any increased cerebral pressure due to destruction of cysts. Praziquantel is not recommended for ocular cysticercosis.

Schistosomiasis

The most common form of intestinal schistosomiasis seen in the United States is *Schistosoma mansoni*. Rare cases of *S. japonicum* from East Asia, *S. mekongi* from Southeast Asia, and *S. intercalatum* from Central Africa may also be seen. The treatment of choice for all these species, as well as for urinary schistosomiasis (*S. haematobium*), is praziquantel (Biltricide) in a single day course. This drug is now approved in the United States for treatment of all forms of schistosomiasis; it is effective and well-tolerated, and all those with an active schistosomiasis infection should be treated. Oxamniquine (Vansil) is an alternative drug for *S. mansoni*. Somewhat higher doses of oxamniquine are required for the African versus the Caribbean strain.

Intestinal Flukes

Fasciolopsis buski, Heterophyes heterophyes, and *Metagonimus yokogawai* are very rare parasites in the United States. All can be treated with praziquantel, which is presently an investigational drug in the United States for these parasites. Tetrachlorethylene, available only as a veterinary product (Nema worm capsules) is an alternative; this should be given on an empty stomach.

Liver Flukes

Clonorchis sinensis and *Opisthorchis viverrini* infections are not uncommon in refugees from and natives or residents of the Far East and Southeast Asia. *Fasciola hepatica* is rarely reported in the United States. Eggs of *Paragonimus westermani*, the lung fluke, may be found in the stool, and this parasite may rarely cause cerebral lesions. Praziquantel, also investigational in the United States for these parasites, is the drug of choice. Bithionol is an alternative investigational drug for these flukes.

Follow-up Examinations

In all those receiving treatment for intestinal parasites, three stool examinations for ova and parasites should be examined by direct and concentration methods approximately 4 weeks after completion of treatment as a check for cure.

ULCERATIVE COLITIS

method of
BERTRAM FLESHLER, M.D., F.A.C.P
The Cleveland Clinic
Cleveland, Ohio

About 20 years ago, I wrote the article on ulcerative colitis for this book. On being invited to contribute to the current volume, I thought it would be interesting to review that now somewhat ancient manuscript, to determine what progress had occurred and to review present concerns. Somewhat to my astonishment, I found that in some important areas few or no changes have taken place. Ulcerative colitis remains a disorder of unknown etiology, a chronic disease with which the patient, family, and physician must continue to grapple over virtually the patient's entire lifetime. The major "specific" therapeutic agents continue to be steroids and sulfasalazine (Azulfidine), and resective surgery, either total or subtotal colectomy, remains the final and frequent therapeutic option.

However, in a number of areas present concerns and knowledge differ from those of the past. For example, Crohn's colitis was a poorly recognized entity 20 years ago. Today we are aware of that disease, and the differential diagnosis is an important one. The use of fiberoptic endoscopic instrumentation has tended to supplant, to a considerable degree, the routine use of barium x-rays and has enabled the clinician to be more precise regarding both the diagnosis of disease and its extent. Although growth retardation as a major manifestation of ulcerative colitis in children and adolescents and toxic megacolon as a potential life-threatening complication were recognized 20 years ago, awareness of these aspects of the disease has certainly increased. The use of parenteral nutrition, either as an attempt to suppress an acute episode or in preparation for surgery, was unknown and has added to the available therapeutic armamentarium. Cancer of the colon as a complication of prolonged disease and the problems of surveillance in relatively asymptomatic patients are currently major focuses of medical attention.

Over these two decades progress in the treatment of ulcerative colitis has been incremental as compared with dramatic advances in therapy of such other gastrointestinal diseases as peptic ulcer. The major therapeutic challenge in ulcerative colitis continues to be the management of chronic, lifelong disease with continued threats to health, life style, and indeed life itself in terms of acute complications and the danger of cancer of the colon.

DIAGNOSIS

Ulcerative colitis presents as a disorder of altered bowel function, usually diarrhea, and a discharge of blood and pus. This may be accompanied by cramps, malnutrition, and a variety of extraintestinal manifestations. There are no specific diagnostic criteria, and the diagnosis is made on a combination of history and physical findings, especially the appearance, both gross and microscopic, of the colonic mucosa.

Ulcerative colitis may present in various forms. It may involve the whole colon (pancolitis) or parts thereof. Characteristically the rectum (ulcerative proctitis) or a variable extent of bowel up from the rectum is involved. The disease tends to affect all of the involved mucosa uniformly with no skip areas. When the disease involves only the rectum or the rectosigmoid, diarrhea may not be a feature and the patient may actually be constipated because of rectal tenesmus and associated preserved colonic fluid absorptive function.

Differentiation from Crohn's disease, a major mimicking illness, is easy when the small bowel is involved. When only the colon is involved in Crohn's disease, differentiation may be difficult. Here the use of fiberoptic instrumentation has resulted in considerable advances in diagnostic certainty. In Crohn's disease the rectum frequently is spared or only moderately involved, skip lesions are seen, and the ulcerations tend to be linear in nature. Histologic appearance is also different.

Although these generalizations are true in most patients, there are a small number of patients (perhaps 10 per cent or so) in whom differentiation is difficult. It can be argued that the attempt to make a precise differential diagnosis is of little significance because the approach to medical therapy, at least in the acute situation, is quite similar in the two disorders. Prognosis, however, differs greatly, and the threat of cancer is a major problem in ulcerative colitis. Furthermore, whereas colectomy is curative in ulcerative colitis, it may be of less certain therapeutic value in Crohn's disease. Certainly the attempt to make the differential diagnosis seems worthwhile.

There are a number of other disorders that can be confused with ulcerative colitis, especially when the disease has only been present a short time. In patients with new disease stools should be examined for ova and parasites, especially *Entamoeba histolytica*, cultured for bacteria, especially *Yersinia*, and assayed for *Clostridium difficile* toxin under appropriate circumstances. Endoscopic evaluation and biopsies are of great help. Clearly, in these various other diarrheal disorders, therapy and prognosis differ.

MANAGEMENT

Specific Medical Therapy

As was the situation 20 years ago, only two classes of drugs can be identified as useful in patients with ulcerative colitis—sulfasalazine (Azulfidine) and steroids in their various forms.

Sulfasalazine

Sulfasalazine (Azulfidine) is a combination of sulfapyridine and 5-amino-salicylic acid. The drug travels through the stomach and small intestine virtually intact. The sulfapyridine acts to protect the molecule from degradation until it reaches the colon. There, colonic bacteria split the bond linking sulfapyridine and 5-amino-salicylic acid. The sulfapyridine is absorbed and metabolized in the liver. The 5-amino-salicylic acid is largely unabsorbed, remains within the lumen, and appears to be the active moiety. The exact mechanism by which the drug is effective remains controversial. Currently it is thought that 5-amino-salicylic acid inhibits mucosal prostaglandins and affects prostaglandin metabolism. Prostaglandins are an important constituent of the inflammatory reaction. Attempts are under way to develop drugs that will deliver more 5-amino-salicylic acid (or even 4-amino-salicylic acid) to the colon, either through a peroral or a rectal route. These agents may prove to be more effective, delivering greater concentrations with fewer side effects.

Sulfasalazine is used in both acute and chronic states. When used in the acute state, it usually is combined with steroids, since these act more rapidly to reduce inflammation and induce clinical remission. Sulfasalazine can then be used to effect a more chronic suppression of the inflammatory process. By current standards, the dosage of sulfasalazine recommended 20 and more years ago was intolerably high. Attempts were made to have the patient ingest as much as 8 to 12 grams per day. The incidence of side effects was very high and limited the drug's usefulness. It has now been demonstrated that doses in the range of 2 to 4 grams are effective, at least in terms of keeping the disease in remission. Because of side effects, it is common practice to start drug therapy with a dose of 0.5 gram twice daily and to gradually build up tolerance, adding 0.5 gram per day every 2 to 3 days until a dose of 4 grams has been reached. If side effects occur they usually can be handled by decreasing the dose by 1 tablet per day. Common side effects include headache, gastric irritation, and anorexia.

Once clinical remission is achieved, the patient is maintained on sulfasalazine therapy for a prolonged period. The definition of "prolonged" is uncertain and an individual problem. Certainly any patient who has had an acute attack of ulcerative colitis and is in remission should be maintained on 2 to 4 grams of sulfasalazine for at least 1 year and probably longer. Patients can be maintained for many years on such a regimen with no side effects and with apparent reasonable clinical remission.

Corticosteroids

Corticosteroids, in one of the various forms, continue to remain the mainstay of therapy in ulcerative colitis. Although not all patients with ulcerative colitis need to take steroids at all times, clearly patients with enough symptoms to require hospitalization or whose symptoms are severe enough to interfere with a normal life style judged by school attendance and performance, work ability, and ability to participate in normal recreational and extracurricular activities should be considered prime candidates for such therapy. Patients with weight loss, growth retardation, anemia, continued blood loss, nocturnal awakening with bowel movements, and other symptoms that continue for more than either very brief or episodic periods should be treated with steroids. The special case of patients with disease limited to the rectum and the sigmoid (ulcerative proctitis) will be considered hereafter.

Some physicians believe that the way to initiate steroid therapy is to start with a low dose, assess the effects of therapy, and then increase the dose as needed. This approach is an attempt to avoid the undesirable toxic side effects of steroid therapy. I disagree with this approach. It is my practice to start patients requiring steroids on fairly high doses. Thus, the question cannot arise as to whether the patient is not responding to steroid therapy because of inadequate dose, and therapeutic efforts can then be directed to other modalities. If one starts with a low dose, building up gradually, the period of sickness and uncertainty as to whether steroid therapy is going to be effective is prolonged. I thus recommend that patients be started on prednisone, 40 to 60 mg per day in divided doses as initial therapy. When a response occurs, it is usually evident within 10 days to 2 weeks and the dose can be decreased quite rapidly.

Once an initial response is evident, the dose can be lowered by 10 mg per week from 60 mg to 30 mg per day and then by 5 mg per week to 20 mg per day. At that level, decreases should be carried out more slowly and over longer periods of time. Based on the patient's response, I decrease the dosage by 2.5 mg approximately every 2 weeks to 10 mg per day. The dose can then be lowered by 2.5 mg every month to 5 mg a day and then switched to an alternate day regimen (7.5 mg every other day). The dose can then be gradually reduced and discontinued over the next 2 months. This schedule permits adequate judgment as to whether steroids are effective, reduces steroid dosage fairly rapidly to levels where toxicity is reasonably low, and prolongs use of the lower dose sufficiently to secure a remission. This schedule, as outlined, should not be interpreted too rigidly. Many patients at any one of the dose levels may have an exacerbation. In those cases it may not be possible to reduce the steroid level further. Many patients can be maintained on relatively low doses of steroid, that is, 15 mg of prednisone or less per day, especially when combined with sulfasalazine. I initiate the two drugs virtually simultaneously whenever practical in the sick patient requiring drug therapy. Repeated efforts are then made to decrease and, if possible, eliminate the steroids altogether, relying on sulfasalazine for continued remission. As indicated, however, this is not possible in many patients and both drugs are required to keep the patient in satisfactory remission. This is an acceptable state as long as one can keep the steroid dose, on the whole, in the lower ranges. Since prednisolone is the active moeity to which prednisone is converted in the body, some have advocated prednisolone as a better agent, but most experience has not borne this out.

There are a number of patients in whom, because of nausea, vomiting, cramps, severe diarrhea, or the need to use total parenteral nutrition, initial steroid therapy has to be undertaken using intravenous preparations. In these patients, sulfasalazine usage should be withheld until the patient is able to start eating. Intravenous hydrocortisone, 100 to 400 mg per day in divided doses, is potent therapy. Patients who do not respond probably need surgery.

The use of ACTH, instead of steroids, remains controversial. There are no definitive data to indicate that ACTH is beneficial in very sick patients, although some of us, on an anecdotal basis, believe this to be so. In some very sick patients then, ACTH can be given intravenously in a dose of 40 units in 1,000 cc of 5 per cent dextrose in water slowly over 8 hours. This is administered for 16 hours a day, resulting in a total dose of 80 units intravenously slowly over each 24 hour period. After 3 to 4 days, the dose is decreased to 40 units over 8 hours and then can be switched to 40 units administered intramuscularly every 12 hours.

At that point, a decision can be made whether to continue ACTH therapy as maintenance therapy or switch to oral steroids. Some patients prefer taking intramuscular ACTH and learn to use it just as diabetics use insulin. A dose of 40 units once a day usually maintains satisfactory remission in those patients. Most, obviously, prefer to switch to oral steroids, and certainly such an effort should be made.

Treatment of Ulcerative Proctitis

In patients with disease either limited to the rectum or with a line of demarcation clearly evident in the sigmoid and whose symptoms appear to be mainly local in nature, local therapy may be undertaken. These are patients with usually well-maintained nutrition and in whom the disease manifests itself primarily with symptoms of urgency, bleeding, and tenesmus but without weight loss, severe cramps, malnutrition, extraintestinal manifestations, or anemia. Local steroid therapy in such patients may be very effective, and the absorption of steroid is low as compared with steroids administered either intravenously or orally. Thus the danger of side effects from steroid therapy is decreased.

Two commonly used preparations are hydrocortisone retention enemas (Cortenemas) and methylprednisone enemas (Medrol Enpaks). These can be delivered as retention enemas just before bedtime. The patient should be advised to be totally ready for sleep, lie on his left side with the legs slightly elevated and instill the enema very slowly over 10 to 15 minutes. He should then attempt to retain the enema indefinitely. As rectal inflammation decreases, this becomes more and more possible. Such therapy is usually begun as a once a night treatment and continued for 2 to 3 weeks until remission is clearly evident. At that point, therapy can be decreased to an alternate night basis for 3 to 4 weeks and then to twice a week for another 4 to 6 weeks.

In some patients it may be necessary, or convenient, to substitute or add other preparations to those already indicated. Proctofoam-HC is an aerosol preparation containing hydrocortisone that can be instilled and retained without the patient having to go to bed. Steroid suppositories (Hydrocortisone, Cort-Dome 15 or 25 mg) can be utilized as an additional supplement for daytime use along with the steroid enemas at night. A suppository composed of neomycin (15 mg) and hydrocortisone (50 mg) used 1 to 3 times per day has also proved useful in the initial stages of treatment, as a supplement to the nocturnal enemas, or for maintenance once these symptoms are under control.

Belladonna (0.25 gram) and opium (1 gram) suppositories are useful for the relief of tenesmus. In some patients with only rectal or rectosigmoid disease, sulfasalazine can also be used to maintain remission. In most patients, however, treatment as indicated previously will result in satisfactory remission, either without the need for a long-term therapy or with the use of minimal agents such as Cortenemas twice a week or steroid suppositories.

Immunosuppressive and Antibacterial Drugs

Although immunosuppressives have been tried in patients with ulcerative colitis, evidence as to their effectiveness has been lacking. Their use is not recommended except in clinical research settings. Antibiotics have also been frequently used in ulcerative colitis. There is no evidence to indicate that they favorably affect the course of disease. This is not to indicate, obviously, that antibiotics should not be used when there are bacterial complications of ulcerative colitis or in such special situations as toxic dilatation of the colon. They have no role, however, in primary therapy.

"Nonspecific" Aspects of Medical Therapy

Psychotherapy and the Patient-Doctor Relationship

The specific causative role of emotional factors remains in dispute, but it is clear that many patients with ulcerative colitis have severe emotional problems. Formal psychiatric therapy, however, is usually not helpful; in some patients it may be associated with an exacerbation of disease. The patients frequently are hostile, manipulative, and demanding and may sorely tax the physician's own emotional resources. Doctors should be gentle, kind, and firm in all relationships with patients, but the need is particularly great with these patients. The emotional disturbance is part of the disease and should be approached with the same calmness and objectivity with which one deals with the need for blood transfusions or fluid replacement. Discussing the situation with a psychiatrist may aid the physician in understanding the dynamics underlying the various reactions the patient displays and enable him to cope with these reactions and with his own responses to such stimuli. Specific environmental factors may at times be related to attacks of colitis. Temporarily removing the patient from his difficult environment by putting him in the hospital is often helpful.

Rest

The virtues of rest have been extolled, but evidence that rest per se makes a significant contribution to therapy is lacking. A common sense approach to this aspect of therapy, largely governed by the patient's self-assessment of his ability to carry out normal activities, should be pursued. Patients with mild disease and those in remission require little or no limitations. The patient having many bowel movements, who is weak because of nutritional deficiency, fluid loss, toxicity, and anemia, is best cared for in the hospital on a program of restricted activity. All gradations between these extremes occur, but, in general, the patient's activities should be curtailed as little as possible. The tendency toward invalidism in this chronic disease is great and should not be encouraged unnecessarily.

Diet, Vitamins, and Parenteral Fluids

As in the case of rest, evidence is lacking for a beneficial effect of many of the severe dietary restrictions that are traditionally imposed. Patients who feel well will not, in most instances, adhere to a very circumscribed diet. It is best that the patient cooperate in the elimination of a modest number of foodstuffs and eat a normally nutritious diet rather than make adherence to a strict dietary regimen the subject of friction. Because some patients may be intolerant to lactose and there is the belief, not entirely substantiated, that "milk allergy" may be a factor, the intake of milk and milk products should be decreased. This is easily managed in the adult. Even in the child or adolescent, other sources of proteins and vitamins can be substituted. The avoidance of foods generally believed by both layman and physician to produce diarrhea or other bowel symptoms is indicated. Such foods include prunes, prune juice, figs, cabbage, and baked beans. Foods that contain hulls or seeds or are high in crude fiber, such as corn, celery, and grapes, are poorly digested, conceivably might further irritate the inflamed mucosa, and should be eliminated. There is no necessity to eliminate some of the minor amenities, such as coffee, alcohol, and carbonated beverages, when taken in usual amounts.

A constant loss of calories, nitrogen, and electrolytes occurs in patients with diarrhea. The threat to the general nutritional status imposed by these losses is made worse by the anorexia that frequently is present. In such circumstances, although the dietary restrictions listed should be followed if possible, the important thing is that the patient eat. Thus, if milk is the food preferred it is better to allow milk and improve the nutritional status than to worry about some possible damaging effect to the colonic mucosa. The aid of a sympathetic and imaginative dietitian may be extremely helpful. The benefits of dietary restrictions are largely unproven, whereas the threat of nutritional deficiency in the patient with severe active disease is real and immediate.

Specific vitamin deficiency is rare in ulcerative colitis, and there is no need for vitamin supplementation if the patient is eating a reasonably balanced diet. In the patient taking a substandard diet because of continued anorexia, multivitamins in amounts sufficient to provide for daily vitamin requirements should be used (e.g., Decavitamin, 1 capsule daily).

During acute and severe exacerbations, patients may require fluid replacement. The kind of fluid used is based on determinations of serum sodium, potassium, chloride, and carbon dioxide and quantitative estimations of the volume of stool and urine lost. Patients with diarrhea lose large quantities of potassium. Although volume loss and electrolyte deficiency can be corrected by proper intravenous fluid therapy, adequate replacement of calories and protein by this route is impossible. Thus, oral alimentation should be encouraged as soon as feasible. There is little evidence that "bowel rest" by eliminating oral intake is beneficial except in the patient with possible perforation or toxic megacolon, and the nutritional consequences in the already depleted patient may be severe.

Tranquilizers and Anticholinergic and Antidiarrheal Agents

Tranquilizers and other psychotherapeutic agents have no specific role in the treatment of ulcerative colitis. The indications for their use should be the same as in any other patient. Their use and the use of any other agent not absolutely needed should be minimized, since the question of multiple drug use in patients with chronic illness may become a problem.

Anticholinergic agents are helpful in patients with abdominal cramps, frequent bowel movements, and nocturnal defecation. There are some risks involved in their use, since they may predispose to toxic megacolon. Nevertheless, they are frequently helpful adjunctive agents. A variety of anticholinergic agents can be used with apparently equal efficacy. Simply out of habit, and with no thought of recommending that this is the single most useful agent, I normally use dicyclomine HCl (Bentyl), 10 to 20 mg 3 to 4 times a day. As indicated previously, however, the use of any anticholinergic should be restricted as much as possible.

Antidiarrheal agents are extremely useful for patients with cramps and, especially, incapacitating diarrhea. As with the anticholinergic agents, they carry the risk of predisposing to toxic megacolon and their use should be minimized. The two agents currently in use are loperamide hydrochloride (Imodium) and diphenoxylate with atropine (Lomotil). These drugs can be given as 1 to 2 tablets every 4 to 6 hours. Habituation or addiction does not appear to be a problem, and there is no clear indication that one agent is more useful than another. There exists some individual variation, so that patients who do not do well with one agent might be tried on the other.

Special Considerations

Parenteral Nutrition

When total parenteral nutrition became technically feasible, there was considerable hope that a prolonged period of bowel rest accompanied by improved nutrition would result in remissions of ulcerative colitis. This hope has not, in the main, been realized. There are occasional patients in whom a period of total parenteral nutrition, perhaps for a period of 2 to 3 weeks, coupled with use of specific anti-inflammatory agents results in a remission of sufficient length so as to make this a helpful form of therapy. Such an attempt may at times be useful in young people with growth retardation in whom one hopes to avoid surgery and in others in whom surgery is not yet an acceptable alternative. In most patients, however, parenteral nutrition is useful largely in preparation for definitive surgery. That is, by the time one considers this prolonged and expensive form of therapy, the patient has usually had enough recurrences or complications that definitive surgery should be the recommended mode of therapy.

Toxic Megacolon

Toxic megacolon is a potentially life-threatening complication of ulcerative colitis. It may occur spontaneously or may be precipitated by the preparation and performance of endoscopic procedures, barium enemas, or the use of anticholinergic and antidiarrheal agents. Once the diagnosis is suspected, the patient should be hospitalized and treated as an acute emergency. This complication requires close cooperation with the surgeon. The patient should be treated with a program of nothing by mouth, parenteral hydration, and high doses of steroids or ACTH. Antibiotics are indicated, although the specific choice of antibiotic and their exact role is unclear. If there is no improvement within 24 to 48 hours, surgery should be urgently considered. Improvement should involve not only diminution in the size of the colon by x-ray examination but signs of decreasing toxicity, including defervescence, decreasing white cell count, and decreasing tenderness. Standard surgical therapy for toxic megacolon has been the performance of a subtotal colectomy. At this institution, our surgeons often perform a loop ileostomy and diverting colostomy. The acute surgical results are very good with less than 1 per cent mortality. Most patients will need to have definitive surgery, but this can be accomplished when the patient is in better health. In a small number of patients it may be possible to re-establish continuity of the bowel and permit normal bowel function for an indefinite period of time.

Extraintestinal Complications

There are a number of manifestations of the disease that occur outside the gastrointestinal tract. These include arthritis, iritis, uveitis, ankylosing spondylosis, pyoderma gangrenosum, and a variety of hepatic problems such as pericholangitis and sclerosing cholangitis. The activity of these problems may not always run parallel with the intestinal manifestations of disease. Treatment is directed primarily toward treatment of the colitis itself, although nonsteroidal anti-inflammatory agents may be helpful in some patients with arthritis and topical steroids may be of aid in ocular manifestations. The liver problems tend to run a course independent of disease and may persist or worsen even after total colectomy.

Growth Retardation

This is a special manifestation of ulcerative colitis in children and adolescents. Patients in this age group should be monitored carefully to ascertain whether they are continuing in their expected growth curve. A decline in the growth curve can be a manifestation of the disease even without severe intestinal symptoms. Control involves greater therapeutic efforts toward the disease itself, extra attention to nutrition, at times the use of parenteral nutrition, and, if all else fails, colectomy. Definitive therapy should not be withheld for too long, since the optimum time of growth may be missed and the patient may then wind up as a permanently short statured individual.

Cancer

It is now well-recognized that mucosal ulcerative colitis is a serious premalignant condition. The incidence of carcinoma of the colon begins to diverge from a control population as the disease approaches a 10 year period, and the divergence increases thereafter. Carcinoma of the colon occurs not only in patients with continuing severe manifestations of disease but in those with relatively quiescent symptoms who, perhaps, are not receiving any anti-inflammatory treatment because of the relative lack of symptoms. It thus has become important that surveillance programs be carried out on all patients as they approach or exceed 10 years of disease. Surveillance is best carried out by routine colonoscopy coupled with biopsies of any manifest lesion and "multiple biopsies." The appearance of mucosal dysplasia necessitates either a recommendation for colectomy, virtually immediately if the dysplasia is in multiple sites and is of high grade, or, if low grade dysplasia is present, of closer surveillance at 3 to 6 month intervals. If no dysplasia is found, present recommendations are that the patient be re-examined with colonoscopy and multiple biopsies at 2 year intervals.

Surgery

The major indications for surgery in ulcerative colitis are intractability, hemorrhage, extraintestinal manifestations that threaten to become disabling and are uncontrollable, fulminant disease, perforation, toxic megacolon, and the risk of cancer. With the exception of the hepatic manifestations of disease, which may, as indicated previously, continue to progress even after surgery, total colectomy can be considered as curative. Thus the standard operation against which all others should be measured is a total proctocolectomy with conventional ileostomy. Performed at the proper time, this leaves the patient in a healthy state. Because of the undesirable aspects of a permanent ileostomy, a number of other surgical options have emerged. Each of these needs to be considered carefully in the individual patient and measured against the promise of good health of the standard procedure. Other operations that are now being done include proctocolectomy with continent ileostomy (Kock pouch), proctocolectomy with ileoanal anastomosis, colectomy with ileorectal anastomosis and proctocolectomy, and ileoanal anastomosis with construction of an ileal reservoir. These procedures all require more complicated surgery, usually lengthen the perioperative period, are associated with a number of local complications, and may not result in satisfactory continence. Nevertheless, in patients in whom these various modified operations are successful, the return to reasonably normal bowel function is clearly gratifying and beneficial as compared with standard ileostomy.

The United Ostomy Association and the National Foundation of Ileitis and Colitis help by enabling the patient to share experiences with others with similar illness and surgery, provide psychological and material help for the patient and physician in terms of learning materials and aids in controlling the disease, and play a valuable role in promoting research and education in the area of inflammatory bowel disease.

Section 7

Metabolic Disorders

BERIBERI

(Thiamine [Vitamin B_1] Deficiency)

method of
NEVIN S. SCRIMSHAW, Ph.D., M.D.
Massachusetts Institute of Technology
Cambridge, Massachusetts

Classic beriberi, once the scourge of the rice-eating countries of Asia and common among low income populations of the United States as recently as the 1930s, is now rare. Symptoms of beriberi are still seen in alcoholic street people and some individuals with malignancies and other chronic wasting diseases whose nutrient intake is inadequate. It can also occur with malabsorption syndromes and hyperthyroidism. Infantile beriberi is due to inadequate thiamine in the breast milk of mothers subsisting primarily on rice.

Prevention

The adult maintenance requirement of thiamine is approximately 0.5 mg per 1000 calories, that is, in the range of 1.0 to 1.5 mg per day depending on the source and amount of food energy. The requirement for thiamine is greater during pregnancy and lactation and in certain diseases, including hyperthyroidism and infections. For young children, recommended dietary intakes range from 0.3 mg at 6 months to 0.9 mg at 4 to 6 years of age and over 1.0 mg for older children.

The prevention of beriberi requires an increase in the intake of thiamine. There is no substitute, however, for a diet that contains thiamine-rich foods, such as legumes, fresh vegetables, nuts, and meats. Beef, chicken, organ meats, and especially pork are good sources. Ten grams of dried yeast per day will also provide enough thiamine. Dietary change toward less rice and more of other foods has been the major factor in the virtual disappearance of beriberi in areas where it was once common. Parboiling causes the thiamine to enter the endosperm so that it is not lost with polishing; thus populations using parboiled rice do not develop beriberi. Another technically effective measure is the fortification of cereals with synthetic thiamine, although its application has been limited. Synthetic thiamine in oral and parenteral dosage forms is widely used and has probably had some influence on the decline of beriberi in former endemic regions. Thiaminases in raw fish and thiamine antagonists in tea and coffee decrease thiamine availability. Machine milling of rice also removes more thiamine than home pounding.

Diagnostic Considerations

In mild and chronic cases there may be few or no physical signs, and the diagnosis must be inferred from vague symptoms of anorexia and malaise and a diet primarily of polished rice or other refined cereal. The most important neurologic feature is symmetric foot and wrist drop, associated with great tenderness of muscles. A mild disturbance of general sensation over characteristic areas of the outer aspect of the legs, the thighs, and in patches over the abdomen, chest, and forearms is also present. Sometimes there is sensory loss in the lips. Absence of ankle jerks, pains and discomfort in the feet, muscle cramps, and paresthesias are common in beriberi but also have other causes. Some degree of cardiac change is almost universal, but persistent tachycardia may be the only evidence. Beriberi may be sufficiently severe to produce aphonia from laryngeal paralysis and even deafness.

At any time this chronic form may develop into one of the more severe forms. In wet beriberi, edema is the most prominent feature and may involve the face and trunk as well as the extremities. Palpitation and breathlessness are marked and anorexia and dyspepsia are common. The calf muscles are frequently tense and slightly swollen. The pulse is generally fast.

In dry beriberi the muscles become progressively wasted and weak, and walking becomes difficult or impossible. Bedridden patients and those with severe cachexia are very susceptible to terminal infections. When the critical stage of severe thiamine depletion is imminent, sudden death from cardiac failure may occur.

The polyneuropathy seen in chronic alcoholics is commonly due to moderately severe dietary restriction with resulting thiamine deficiency, but it may be complicated by another deficiency, such as that of niacin, and by other constituents of cheap alcoholic drinks, such as arsenic and lead. The foot and wrist drop best identify the alcoholic neuropathy as due to beriberi. With dietary restriction, as in a person who has literally lived on alcohol for 2 or 3 weeks, the outcome is Wernicke's encephalopathy. Wernicke's encephalopathy is usually combined with various degrees of neuropathy depending on past dietary and disease history. These symptoms can also occur with severe recurrent vomiting associated with pregnancy or pyloric obstruction. In the more chronic stages, or after repeated episodes of Wernicke's syndrome, nerve cell changes become general.

Infantile beriberi occurs almost exclusively in the first year of life, with the first to fourth month being the most dangerous. In this period the acute cardiac or fulminating forms are most likely to occur. Early symptoms are vomiting, restlessness, pallor, anorexia, and insomnia. Depending on the chronicity and severity of material depletion and other factors not well understood, three more serious forms are recognized. The subacute form shows vomiting, puffiness, oliguria, abdominal pain, dysphagia, aphonia, and convulsions. It may progress through this form to an acute or to a chronic stage with cyanosis, dyspnea, and tachycardia. In the chronic form there is vomiting, inanition, anorexia, aphonia, neck retraction, opisthotonus, edema, oliguria, constipation, and tympanites in varying degrees.

Treatment

In beriberi with edema, treatment should be started as soon as possible with 25 mg of thiamine given intramuscularly twice daily for 3 days. Thereafter, an oral dose of 10 mg two or three times a day should be continued until convalescence is assured, although there is no doubt that smaller doses are also effective. In early mild and in dry beriberi, 5 to 10 mg intramuscularly daily for 2 to 3 days followed by equal amounts orally for 2 weeks will be sufficient. For the longer term, adequate thiamine-containing foods should be made part of the diet, and attention should be paid to any coexisting nutrient deficiencies. Whenever vomiting or gastrointestinal pathology complicates oral therapy, the parenteral route should be employed.

Infantile beriberi is an acute emergency, but even a moribund child responds promptly to thiamine administration by any route. Since such infants are being breast-fed, treatment should be in part through the mother's milk. The mother should receive 10 mg of thiamine orally twice daily. In addition, the infant should be given thiamine doses of 10 to 20 mg intramuscularly once a day for 3 days followed by 5 to 10 mg orally twice a day. With severe heart failure or convulsion and coma, the initial dose may be increased to 25 to 50 mg given intravenously very slowly.

HYPO- AND HYPERVITAMINOSIS A

method of
VINODINI REDDY, M.D.
National Institute of Nutrition
Hyderabad, India

Vitamin A deficiency is a major public health problem in many developing countries and is an important cause of preventable blindness, especially in young children. Inadequate dietary intake of vitamin A is the major factor responsible for this deficiency disease. Chronic diarrhea and malabsorption can also lead to hypovitaminosis A.

Vitamin A is obtained through the diet as preformed vitamin A or as its precursor, β-carotene. Preformed vitamin A is present in animal foods such as milk, eggs, and liver, whereas green leafy vegetables and fruits like papaya are rich sources of β-carotene. Adequate amounts of these foods shoud be included in the diet for the prevention of vitamin A deficiency. Daily requirements of vitamin A are about 300 μg for children and 750 μg for adults. For β-carotene, the requirement is four to six times greater, since only a part of it is absorbed and converted to vitamin A.

Treatment

Conjunctival Lesions

Night blindness, conjunctival xerosis, and Bitot spots represent signs of mild vitamin A deficiency. They respond to relatively small doses of the vitamin.

1. Oral administration of 5000 to 10,000 IU of vitamin A daily for about 10 days is sufficient to reverse the changes. In a great majority of subjects, these signs disappear within 1 to 2 weeks, but in some cases, chronic Bitot spots persist despite administration of large amounts of vitamin A.

2. Instead of small daily doses, a single massive dose of 200,000 IU of vitamin A can be used for the treatment of xerophthalmia. In addition to bringing about a cure, this dose will help to build up the liver stores and prevent recurrence. This method is now being practiced on a large scale in many Southeast Asian countries for the prevention of vitamin A deficiency. Children between 1 and 5 years of age who are at risk of developing keratomalacia and blindness are given 200,000 IU vitamin A orally, once every 6 months.

Corneal Lesions

Severe deficiency of vitamin A involving the cornea is seen mostly in children less than 5 years of age and is frequently associated with protein-energy malnutrition and infection. Corneal xerosis constitutes a medical emergency since it progresses rapidly to keratomalacia, resulting in loss of vision.

1. All patients with corneal lesions should be treated promptly with an intramuscular injection of 100,000 IU of water-miscible vitamin A. This will result in a rapid elevation of plasma vitamin A levels. Oral administration of vitamin A is also effective, but the parenteral route is preferable as a majority of children have associated gastroenteritis.

Oil-soluble vitamin A should never be injected intramuscularly because the vitamin is liberated extremely slowly from the site of injection. If a water-miscible preparation is not available, oil-soluble vitamin A can be given orally.

2. This should be followed by an oral dose of 200,000 IU of vitamin A a week later to build up the liver stores and prevent recurrence.
3. To control infection, antibiotic eye ointment should be applied locally until the eye lesions clear up.
4. As most of the children have associated protein-energy malnutrition, they should be treated with adequate dietary protein and calories.
5. Gastroenteritis and other associated infections should receive appropriate therapy.

With this form of therapy, the eye lesions show a dramatic improvement. Corneal xerosis clears up rapidly and vision is restored to normal within 2 or 3 days. In more advanced cases of keratomalacia, scar formation is inevitable.

Hypervitaminosis A

Hypervitaminosis A is associated with an excessive intake of vitamin A. The dose required to produce toxic manifestations shows wide individual variations. Some children develop toxic symptoms with as little as 300,000 IU, whereas others can tolerate much larger doses.

Acute vitamin A toxicity manifests as malaise, headache, irritability, vomiting, and, in infants, bulging of the fontanelle. These symptoms are caused by raised intracranial tension. Withdrawal of vitamin A intake results in rapid recovery.

Prolonged ingestion of large doses of vitamin A leads to chronic vitamin A toxicity. The main symptoms are anorexia, weight loss, alopecia, skin changes, and bone and joint pains. The plasma vitamin A level is elevated, although it does not always correlate with the clinical picture. X-ray films reveal periosteal thickening and cortical hyperostosis. Discontinuation of vitamin A will eliminate these signs and symptoms, but the process is a slow one.

DIABETES MELLITUS IN ADULTS

method of
KENNETH KREINES, M.D.
Cincinnati, Ohio

The treatment of diabetes is attracting increasing attention within the medical community because methods to improve the outlook are finally available. Approximately 5.5 million Americans are afflicted with diabetes and the prevalence is rising. Diabetes increases the risks of heart disease and stroke at least twofold and accounts for 300,000 deaths, 25 per cent of all cases of end-stage renal disease, and 20,000 lower limb amputations each year. It is the most important cause of blindness in adults and a major contributor to fetal mortality and birth defects. The financial burden of diabetes exceeds 8 billion dollars annually.

Eliminating the Symptoms of Uncontrolled Diabetes

The symptoms of uncontrolled diabetes are rapidly eliminated when the abnormal metabolic state is reversed. The methods available to accomplish this include diet, exercise, insulin, and oral hypoglycemic agents. If the diabetes is sufficiently out of control to cause symptoms, I prefer to add insulin immediately. This is done regardless of whether the patient has insulin-dependent (type I) diabetes or noninsulin-dependent (type II) diabetes.

During the initial few days, the patient is seen daily and instructed in essential "survival skills," such as the rudiments of diet, blood or urine testing, and injection technique. Almost all insulin-requiring patients are taught self-monitoring of blood glucose. Of the many reagent strips currently available, I prefer those with a double color pad, such as Chemstrip or Visidex II. Most patients can read these strips without an electronic meter, even if the strips are cut in half lengthwise to reduce the cost.

Depending on the time of day and the blood glucose level, an initial dose of 15 to 30 units of lente or NPH insulin is given. The patient is then instructed to increase or decrease the number of units injected each morning by 10 per cent, depending on whether the glucose level before supper is greater than 180 or less than 80 mg per dl. If the glucose level is greater than 240 mg per dl, the patient is to take an additional dose of 6 to 12 units of fast-acting insulin at that time. When compliance with diet is adequate, the insulin dose typically climbs for about 1 week, levels off at 40 to 60 units, and then declines. Frequently it is possible to discontinue injections by the fourth week. If one waits to add insulin or an oral agent, until a trial of diet is unsuccessful, the process will take much longer. In addition, some patients are less receptive to treatment with insulin if it is added later.

Reducing the Risk of Chronic Complications

For patients to have the best chance of avoiding the chronic complications of diabetes, those factors that cause them to be at high risk must be eliminated. In addition to hyperglycemia, "risk factors" include hypertension, cigarette smoking, obesity, hypercholesterolemia, and hypertriglyceridemia. The recommended biochemical indices of metabolic control are shown in Table 1.

Patient Education

Long-term control requires that the patient have a thorough understanding of the nature of the disease and actively participate in its day-to-day management. If the patient is sufficiently ill to require hospitalization, patient education begins there with instruction in "survival skills." Following improvement, the patient is referred to an outpatient diabetes education program for the remainder of the training. National Standards of Diabetes Patient Education Programs are currently being implemented by the National Diabetes Advisory Board.

Diet

Diet is the most important element of treatment because approximately 75 per cent of the patients with type II diabetes can be adequately controlled by diet alone. The diet prescription should be highly individualized, taking into account the patient's occupation, age, build, habits, and life style. For example, although the usual distribution of calories among breakfast, lunch, supper, and evening snack is 1/6—2/6—2/6—1/6, it is more important that the patient eat regularly, even if the pattern differs.

The American Diabetes Association nutritional recommendations for nonobese patients with diabetes are shown in Table 2. Nonobese patients are assigned diets containing 25 to 35 kcal per kg per day, but the typical patient with type II diabetes, who is overweight, is usually started on a hypocaloric diet of only 15 to 25 kcal per kg per day.

The types of carbohydrates selected can also be of importance. Some starches, such as in bread and potatoes, have a greater glycemic response than others, such as pasta and lentils. Small amounts of sucrose and alcohol are permitted if the calories are calculated in the meal plan and the alcohol is taken with food. The non-nutritive sweeteners saccharine and aspartame are safe if used in moderate amounts.

Exercise

Exercise is an important adjunct to diet therapy. It increases glucose utilization and insulin sensitivity, decreases the risk of coronary heart disease by increasing the level of HDL-cholesterol, improves work capacity and a general sense of well-being, and may improve compliance with diet. Although exercise is most effective when performed at least three times per week, the mode and amount should be selected with great care since the patient may have complications such as arthritis, coronary heart disease, peripheral neuropathy, or proliferative retinopathy. For otherwise healthy individuals, a vigorous exercise program at a community center or spa is suitable. For those with a history of cardiovascular disease, referral to a cardiac rehabilitation program may be better, and for older patients, regular walking in the protected environment of an indoor shopping mall might be best.

Oral Hypoglycemic Agents Versus Insulin

If diet and exercise are inadequate, the addition of insulin or an oral hypoglycemic agent should be considered. There is still considerable controversy regarding the choice between the two, but in general, the indication for oral agents grows stronger with increasing age and weaker with

TABLE 1. **Biochemical Indices of Metabolic Control: Top Limits**

Biochemical Index	Normal	Acceptable	Fair	Poor
Fasting plasma glucose	115	140	200	>200 mg/dl
Postprandial plasma glucose	140	175	235	>235 mg/dl
Glycosylated hemoglobin	6	8	10	>10%
Fasting plasma cholesterol	200	225	250	>250 mg/dl
Fasting plasma triglyceride	150	175	200	>200 mg/dl

Adjust for normal values of laboratory.
Increase limits for elderly patients.
(Reprinted by permission from The Physician's Guide to Type II Diabetes (NIDDM): Diagnosis and Treatment. New York, American Diabetes Association, 1984, p 25.)

TABLE 2. **Recommended Nutritional Allowances for Nonobese Patients with Diabetes**

Total calories	25–35 kcal/kg/day
Protein	12–20%
Carbohydrate	50–60%
Fat	≤30%
Cholesterol	<300 mg/day
Dietary fiber	10 grams/day

increasing levels of blood glucose. My own practice is to employ oral agents sparingly because most patients with type II diabetes potentially can be managed by diet and exercise alone. Obese noncompliant patients with type II diabetes should be given oral agents or insulin only in amounts sufficient to achieve reasonable control of the glucose level and relieve symptoms. Further "chasing" of the glucose level might actually be harmful because it encourages more obesity. All available hypoglycemic agents are sulfonylurea derivatives. While the "second generation" agents glipizide and glyburide may reduce the insulin resistance that is a major problem in these patients, there are still insufficient clinical data to justify their routine use for that purpose.

Orally administered drugs are not as predictably effective as insulin. Approximately 20 per cent of patients fail to respond initially, and an additional 20 per cent lose their responsiveness each year thereafter. To guard against the prescription of unnecessary medication, the physician should periodically reduce the dose and observe the blood sugar response. Although the second generation oral agents are more potent on a weight basis than are the first generation agents, they have not been proved to be significantly more effective. Prescribing information for the available sulfonylurea agents is shown in Table 3.

Much has been written regarding the possible cardiovascular toxicity of oral agents. In 1971, the University Group Diabetes Program (UGDP) reported significantly more cardiovascular deaths among patients treated with tolbutamide plus diet than among those treated with diet alone. In addition, the UGDP investigators found no evidence of a beneficial effect of tolbutamide on vascular complications. The report sparked vigorous debate in which the critics cited deficiencies in the design and performance of the study. On the other hand, the Biometrics Society and the Food and Drug Administration conducted independent reviews and concluded that the problems were not sufficient to negate the results of the study. The FDA later ordered that a warning statement be included on each package insert. I cannot see how the prudent physician can completely disregard that warning and agree that the possibility of increased risk must be weighed in the therapeutic balance. We should be reminded, however, that tolbutamide was the sole sulfonylurea studied by the UGDP and it is not definitely known that the UGDP conclusions should be extended to the other agents.

The time course of action of the available insulins is shown in Table 4. Numerous regimens have been proposed for the clinical use of these preparations, ranging from one daily injection of a single insulin to multiple injections of mixtures. As a general rule, the simplest regimen that achieves the desired result is best and in the majority of adults, that means a single injection of NPH or lente insulin once daily, before breakfast. The dose is adjusted by the patient each day according to the "10 per cent" rule. Self–blood glucose monitoring is performed before supper and, periodically, at various other times of the day in addition. If the glucose level is consistently excessive before breakfast, a second injection of intermediate-acting insulin is added before supper. If the glucose level is still excessive before lunch or the evening snack, fast-acting insulin is added before breakfast or supper, respectively. The typical patient who follows this regimen takes approximately two thirds of the daily dose before breakfast and one third before supper, with the ratio of intermediate- to short-acting insulin 2:1 in the AM and 2:1 to 1:1 in the PM.

Highly purified pork and biosynthetic human insulins are less antigenic than the older beef-

TABLE 3. **Time Course of Action of Oral Sulfonylurea Agents**

Generic Name	Brand Name	Daily Dosage Range (*Mg*)	Duration of Action (*Hr*)
tolbutamide	Orinase	500–3000	6–12
chlorpropamide	Diabinese	100–500	60
acetohexamide	Dymelor	250–1500	12–18
tolazamide	Tolinase	100–1000	12–24
glyburide	Diabeta Micronase	2.5–30	up to 24
glipizide	Glucatrol	5–40	8–12

TABLE 4. **Time Course of Action of Insulin Preparations**

	Onset of Action	Peak Action	Duration of Action
Short-acting			
Regular Iletin II (crystalline-zinc)	15–30 minutes	2–4 hours	5–7 hours
Actrapid	30 minutes	2.5–5 hours	8 hours
Velosulin	30 minutes	2–5 hours	8 hours
Humulin	30 minutes	2–5 hours	6–8 hours
Intermediate-acting			
Lente	1–2 hours	6–12 hours	18–24 hours
NPH	1–2 hours	6–12 hours	18–24 hours
Monotard	2.5 hours	7–15 hours	18–24 hours
Humulin	1–2 hours	6–12 hours	14–24 hours
Novolin	1.5 hours	4–12 hours	18–24 hours
Long-acting			
Ultralente	2–6 hours	18–24 hours	32–36 hours

pork preparations and are useful for the treatment of insulin allergy, lipoatrophy, and insulin resistance.

Management of Hypertension

Hypertension rates special attention because it is a complication of diabetes as well as a risk factor for vascular damage. There is evidence that lowering elevated blood pressure to under 160/90 mm Hg improves the prognosis for accelerated atherosclerosis, retinopathy, and diabetic kidney disease. The general approach is to begin with a treatment program that includes sodium restriction, weight reduction, exercise, and stress management. Diuretics and antihypertensive medications are then systematically added as needed.

Several complications of hypertension treatment are of special importance in diabetes. These include increased hyperglycemia by diuretics, particularly in the presence of hypokalemia, impotency and orthostatic hypotension in patients with autonomic neuropathy, and the precipitation of gangrene by beta-blockers in patients with peripheral vascular disease.

Management of Obesity

Most authorities agree that the current treatment of obesity is inadequate and that even the "best" programs have long-term success rates no better than 20 per cent. Anorexigenic agents and classic psychotherapy are usually not helpful, but new approaches, particularly those that employ behavioral modification techniques, are promising.

Intermittent short-term fasting is useful for selected patients with uncontrolled type II diabetes, particularly if they demonstrate significant resistance to insulin. Our experience has been that, by the end of 1 week, the average patient has lost 3 to 5 pounds and no longer requires insulin. At the end of 1 year, a third of the patients fail to return, presumably because they have gained weight, a third continue to lose weight, and the weight is stable in the remainder. Almost all who remain in the program continue to be managed with diet only.

Hyperlipoproteinemia

The elevated lipid levels that are common in uncontrolled diabetes can be primary or secondary to the insulin insufficiency. Therefore, the diabetes should be controlled for a period of 2 to 3 months and the patient encouraged to lose weight before more specific dietary modifications or lipid-lowering pharmacologic agents are added.

Cigarette Smoking

Smoking increases the risks of coronary heart disease and intermittent claudication four- to sixfold and should not be tolerated. Patients often feel that since they have been smoking for many years, stopping would be of no help. To the contrary, evidence shows that cessation of smoking is beneficial even if complications are already present.

Reducing Morbidity from Diabetes Complications

Early diagnosis and treatment can reduce morbidity from chronic complications. This principle is of particular importance since approximately 20 per cent of patients with type II diabetes already have evidence of vascular damage at the time of diagnosis. Each patient should be evaluated for complications at the outset and at least yearly thereafter, with a thorough history and physical examination, electrocardiogram, blood counts, complete urinalysis, blood chemistry profile, and serum lipid determinations. Additional tests, such as a treadmill electrocardiogram and noninvasive studies of the carotid and leg arteries, are obtained if clinically indicated.

Macrovascular Disease

Coronary heart disease, obliterative peripheral vascular disease, and stroke are the major causes of mortality and morbidity in adults with diabetes. While the ready availability of highly sophisticated diagnostic and therapeutic methods has led to much earlier and more effective treatment, it is equally important to retard progression of the complications by correcting hypertension, obesity, and hyperlipoproteinemia and motivating patients to discontinue cigarette smoking.

Approximately one third of patients with type II diabetes develop intermittent claudication by the tenth year after diagnosis, but since gangrene develops in only 1 per cent, surgical intervention is indicated only if disabling symptoms are not relieved by conservative means.

Diabetic Retinopathy

Retinopathy is detected in approximately 50 per cent of patients after 10 years of known diabetes. Although there is overlap, the retinopathy of type II diabetes, characterized by microaneurysms and hard exudates (background retinopathy), follows a more benign course than that of type I diabetes, which is characterized by cotton wool exudates, macular edema, vitreous or retinal hemorrhages, and neovascularization. Untreated, 25 per cent of patients with preretinal hemorrhage, vitreous hemorrhage, or neovascularization progress to serious loss of vision within 2 years. There is convincing evidence, however, that early treatment with photocoagulation reduces that risk by 60 per cent. Although some ophthalmologists elect to photocoagulate background retinopathy as well, the benefit of this treatment is still uncertain. All adults with diabetes should be seen by an ophthalmologist annually for screening for cataract and glaucoma as well as retinopathy.

Diabetic Kidney Disease

Mild impairments of renal function are already noted in many patients with type II diabetes at the time of diagnosis, and by the twentieth year, 5 to 10 per cent have serious kidney damage. To retard progressive kidney damage, meticulous attention must be given to treatment of hypertension, infection, and anatomic or neurogenic obstruction of the urinary tract. Patients with renal disease should be referred to a nephrologist for advice regarding dialysis or kidney transplantation when the serum creatinine exceeds 3 mg per dl.

Diabetic Neuropathy

The diabetic neuropathies involve the somatic as well as the autonomic nervous systems. Somatic neuropathy can affect any of the peripheral nerves, including the cranial nerves, and results in muscle weakness, anesthesia, dysesthesia, and pain. Painful neuropathy is treated with rest, minor analgesics, and mild sedation to which carbamazepine (Tegretol), 200 to 600 mg daily in divided doses and amitriptyline (Elavil), 50 to 200 mg at bedtime, can be added as needed. Aldose reductase inhibitors are promising but still experimental. The most hazardous complication of somatic neuropathy is painless foot ulcer that is neglected and allow to progress to abscess formation, osteomyelitis, and gangrene. These neuropathic foot ulcers often can be managed for extended periods by conservative means and must be distinguished from ischemic ulcers that may require revascularization or extensive amputations. Patients with peripheral neuropathy must be taught to protect their feet from injuries that can lead to ulceration and are provided with special orthopedic shoes when necessary. Even the smallest break in the skin should be immediately reported because prompt treatment with antibiotics and avoidance of weight-bearing can prevent a potential amputation.

Other Pathology

Orthostatic hypotension is hazardous because it causes syncope. The postural fall in blood pressure can be accentuated by commonly prescribed antihypertensive and psychotropic medications, by diuretics, and by any condition that leads to loss of extracellular fluid. It is treated by eliminating the offending agent and cautiously expanding the extracellular space with fluids or the sodium-retaining steroid 9-alpha-fluorohydrocortisone, given in a dose of 0.1 to 0.3 mg daily.

Gastroparesis causes nausea, vomiting, and poor diabetes control and can contribute to diabetic diarrhea. If the condition fails to respond to metoclopramide, 10 to 20 mg four times daily, the patient should be hospitalized for several days of intravenous feeding, followed by gradual refeeding.

Diabetic diarrhea can often be prevented by a broad-spectrum antibiotic, such as tetracycline, 250 mg once daily by mouth, but when the attacks occur, frequent doses of paregoric, Lomotil, or codeine phosphate are required.

Neurogenic bladder can lead to serious urinary tract infection and irreversible renal damage. Bladder emptying is usually improved by bethanechol (Urecholine), 25 to 100 mg four times daily by mouth, or 2.5 mg four times daily by subcutaneous injection. Intermittent catheterization is indicated if the volume of residual urine cannot be decreased to less than 150 ml by these means.

Impotency is a frequent problem in diabetic men, but neuropathy is not the sole cause. Antihypertensive medications and psychologic factors can play an equally important role and must be dealt with before the physician recommends penile implant surgery.

The acute metabolic complications of diabetes, ketoacidosis, hyperosmolar-nonketotic coma, and hypoglycemia, are almost always preventable by careful day-by-day management as described in the previous section. The patient and family must be thoroughly familiar with "sick day" rules to be followed at times of illness. These include frequent monitoring of the blood sugar and urine ketones and the administration of extra-fast-acting insulin every 4 hours until the emergency has passed. The dose of fast-acting insulin is generally equal to approximately 20 per cent of the usual total daily insulin dose. If the blood sugar and urine ketone levels do not improve within 4 hours or other complicating circumstances such as vomiting or high fever arise, the patient should immediately call his or her physician. The treatment of ketoacidosis, hyperosmolar coma, and hypoglycemia are not discussed in this article.

Coping with Diabetes

The caring physician is as concerned with the psychosocial as with the metabolic adjustment to diabetes. The emotional problems associated with diabetes are lifelong, and it is the physician's responsibility to help the patient cope. The first few days following diagnosis are the most important. The patient is extremely impressionable at that time and liable to develop attitudes that will permanently influence compliance. The physician should seize that brief opportunity to instill confidence by acting decisively as well as compassionately. An example is administration of the initial insulin injection by the patient at the very first visit under the personal guidance of the physician.

Long-term patient compliance is also related to the complexity of the treatment program. Superfluous instructions are avoided and the patient should clearly understand the justification for each task that she or he is requested to perform. Reinforcement is given at frequent follow-up visits, preferably by the same physician. Compliance is enhanced if the physician takes adequate time to communicate, has a positive and encouraging attitude, and strives to adapt the treatment regimen to the patient's life style rather than vice versa. Further encouragement is obtained from the patient's family and from support groups such as those organized by many hospitals or the local American Diabetes Association chapter.

DIABETES MELLITUS IN CHILDREN AND ADOLESCENTS

method of
DOROTHY J. BECKER, M.B, BCh.,
FCP (Paed)
Children's Hospital of Pittsburgh
Pittsburgh, Pennsylvania

Diabetes mellitus is one of the most common chronic disorders of childhood and adolescence, affecting approximately 1 in 600 children under the age of 18 years in the United States with an incidence of 14.5 per 100,000 per year. In the child, the most common form of diabetes is insulin-dependent diabetes mellitus (IDDM) or type I diabetes mellitus, which is associated with complete or almost complete beta cell destruction with concomitant insulin deficiency. It appears that the younger children have the most complete beta cell destruction with very low or negligible insulin levels at presentation. Approximtely 3 per cent of patients have other types of diabetes such as noninsulin-dependent diabetes (NIDDM) occurring almost exclusively in obese teenagers, or maturity onset diabetes of youth (MODY) when patients have relatively more endogenous insulin and are not obese but have a strong family history of diabetes with a dominant inheritance pattern. Transient insulin-dependent diabetes can be diagnosed in the neonatal period.

MANAGEMENT

The long-term management of IDDM is extremely complex, requiring the cooperation of the child and family with the health care team. Few other disorders of childhood or adulthood require as much self-management and decision-making by the patient. A vast amount of knowledge and understanding is required by patients, which they obtain by many hours of teaching. Probably the most important advance in the treatment of IDDM is the development of the team approach: participants are the patient and family, the pediatrician or family doctor, the diabetologist, the teaching nurse, the dietitian, the social worker, the psychologist, and psychiatrists. Unfortunately, this type of team is not available in all centers but should be utilized whenever possible.

Diabetic Ketoacidosis

Diabetic ketoacidosis (DKA) may be part of the initial presentation of IDDM or represent a treatment failure in the child with known IDDM. It is the most common cause for rehospitalization in the child with IDDM. DKA is a serious, life-threatening metabolic complication of IDDM. It is our impression that the frequency of DKA is declining, both as the presenting feature of IDDM and as a later recurring problem. With greater awareness and earlier recognition of IDDM in childhood, many patients present with ketosis without acidosis, and the treatment is altered accordingly. Despite improved therapy, DKA remains a major cause of death in IDDM, and it is the most common cause of death in the patient under the age of 20 years. With prompt therapy and constant vigilance, the mortality rate has declined in our center over the past 10 years. Death is usually due to the unexplained complication of cerebral edema.

Fluids

The development of DKA is usually relatively slow, and it should be corrected relatively slowly. The only indication for very rapid correction is impending or actual shock. Because a major feature of DKA is water loss associated with that of electrolytes, rehydration is the cornerstone of therapy. We routinely rehydrate our patients for approximately 1 hour prior to the administration of insulin, while awaiting laboratory results. The initial fluid to be used is normal saline, without the addition of potassium until urine excretion has been confirmed and the serum potassium level is available. This initial hour of rehydration allows one to assess the degree of dehydration and the rate of blood glucose decrement associated with volume expansions rather than insulin action. The fluid deficit is calculated according to either body weight or surface area. This deficit is corrected over a 24 hour period, with half the correction effected over the first 8 hours. Regardless of the initial calculated deficit, it is extremely important to continue to reassess water balance in the patient with measurements of urine output as well as that of total fluid infused or taken orally. The initial intravenous hydration should be at a rate of 10 to 20 ml per kg per hr. Unless severe hyperosmolarity persists after the first hour, the rehydration fluid is changed to half normal saline in order to supply maintenance fluid and correct the deficit with replacement of continual urine losses. Maintenance and fluid volumes are calculated with allowances made for age.

Most of the hydration treatment should be administered intravenously, and oral fluids should not be given to the very ill patient initially, especially if there has been prior vomiting. Even if oral fluids are tolerated, gastrostasis and ileus may prevent rapid absorption of fluids and make it difficult to calculate actual delivery into the intravascular space. It is mandatory to reassess the fluid status on a regular basis and recalculate the fluid requirements as necessary. The composition of the rehydration fluid depends upon the patient's serum sodium and potassium levels and serum osmolarity. In general, one should attempt to rehydrate at least initially with isosmolar solutions, and as the serum osmolarity diminishes, some free water should be administered. Solutions that do not contain sodium should not be used. An example of the calculation of replacement and maintenance fluids is given in Table 1.

Insulin

The use of low dose insulin therapy is now well accepted and is the treatment of choice in children with DKA, achieving its goal in the majority of cases. Occasionally, a patient appears to have a greater than usual degree of insulin resistance, requiring slightly higher doses. Initially, insulin should be given as crystalline or regular insulin in all patients with DKA. The choice of the insulin delivery route depends upon the condition of the patient and the facilities available. If DKA is mild with minimal acidosis and dehydration, the subcutaneous route of insulin delivery is convenient and effective, especially if the patient does not require intravenous rehydration. The dosage regime is approximately 0.25 units per kg given every 4 to 6 hours, if possible prior to meals. Remember that crystalline insulin given subcutaneously has a half-life of approximately 4 hours, with a duration of action of about 6 hours at the most. Therefore, patients must receive insulin at least every 6 hours, even during the night.

If the patient is significantly dehydrated, subcutaneous insulin is poorly and irregularly absorbed. Under these circumstances, the use of the intravenous route is preferred by means of a continuous infusion of 0.1 unit per kg per hr after an initial loading bolus of 0.1 unit per kg. This insulin should be delivered in a fairly concentrated solution (approximately 1 unit per ml of normal saline) with infusion controlled by a syringe pump or IVAC Pediatric Pump through a line connected by piggyback to the rehydration intravenous infusion set. A change of the syringe or infusion bag every 4 to 5 hours and the use of concentrated solutions of insulin minimize the problems of insulin adherence to the plastic of the infusion system. Although some centers successfully mix insulin in the rehydration fluid, we feel this is dangerous, because the delivery rate will depend upon the rate of rehydration rather than that of insulin need. In addition, this results in dilution of insulin, which causes instability of

TABLE 1. **Calculation of Fluid Replacement in Diabetic Ketoacidosis**

	Maintenance Fluid		**Deficit (10% Dehydration)**
Fluid:	100 ml/kg	for first 10 kg	100 ml/kg
	50 ml/kg	for second 10 kg	
	20 ml/kg	for 20 kg	
Na	3 mEq/kg		6 mEq/kg
K	2 mEq/kg		5 mEq/kg

Thus, a 30 kg patient with 10 per cent dehydration would need:

	Maintenance	**Deficit**	**Total**
Fluids	1700 ml	3000 ml	4700 ml
Na	90 mEq	180 mEq	270 mEq
K	60 mEq	150 mEq	210 mEq

Fluids could be given according to the following procedure:

Hour	**ml/kg/hr**	**Fluid Composition**	
1st	15	normal saline	
2nd	10	half/normal saline plus 40 mEq KCl/liter	Add 5%
3rd–8th	8	half/normal saline plus 30 mEq KCl/liter	glucose when
9th–24th	5	quarter/normal saline plus 20 to 30 mEq KCl/liter	necessary

(From Becker DJ, Drash AL: Diabetic ketoacidosis, *in* Dickerman JD, Lucey JF (eds): The Critically Ill Child. Philadelphia, WB Saunders, 1985.)

its structure and loss onto the surface of the infusion apparatus. The advantage of the intravenous route of insulin delivery is the smooth pattern of circulating levels achieved, in addition to the physician's ability to rapidly increase or decrease the amount delivered with immediate effects.

It is important to remember that the patient requires the same degree of vigilance from a clinical and biochemical standpoint whether insulin is infused intravenously or given subcutaneously. The use of intravenous insulin boluses should be discouraged, as this results in intermittent supraphysiologic levels alternating with subphysiologic levels, with rapid changes possibly stimulating abnormal secretion of counterregulatory hormones. Intramuscular insulin delivery with a loading dose of 0.25 unit per kg, followed by injections of 0.1 unit per kg per hr, has been used with the same success as that of the continuous intravenous route. However, the disadvantage of this mode of therapy is the repeated pain of intramuscular injections.

Insulin therapy should be tailored to drop the blood glucose level by approximately (but no more than) 100 mg per dl per hr. If the blood glucose level drops more rapidly than this initially, the insulin dose should be reduced; if the decrease is less than 75 mg per dl per hr, the insulin dose should be increased. However, when the blood glucose falls below 300 mg per dl per hr, glucose should be added to the intravenous solution to control further delivery. Initially, this should be 5 per cent dextrose in water and half/normal saline; if necessary, this can be increased to 10 per cent dextrose in water solution to provide calories. The reason for adding glucose to the regimen at this stage is to prevent cerebral edema, which may have as part of its pathogenesis a very rapid drop in blood sugar, particularly to levels of less than 250 mg per dl.

This mode of therapy should be continued until the acidosis is corrected, hyperglycemia is under control, and ketonemia is virtually absent. Ketonuria will persist for some time after correction of the metabolic acidosis because of slow conversion of beta-hydroxybutyrate to acetoacetate, which is excreted. If the patient is able to eat meals prior to achievement of these goals, a small increment of insulin should be given to cover the anticipated hyperglycemia. When these goals are achieved, the patient should be given approximately 0.25 unit per kg of insulin every 4 to 6 hours subcutaneously, with the next 24 hours being used to evaluate the dose requirements. Thereafter, the regime of intermediate-acting (e.g., NPH or lente) plus short-acting insulin can be started, with the total intermediate-acting insulin dose being approximately three fourths of the previous day's insulin requirement and the remainder as regular insulin given to cover breakfast.

Electrolytes

During therapy, the electrolyte balance should be maintained, with continued biochemical evaluation approximately every hour initially. Potassium should be given with the insulin unless severe hyperkalemia is present. Potassium is given prophylactically to prevent hypokalemia, a pervasive cause of death in DKA. Even when a patient is rehydrated orally, potassium replacement is necessary in the form of fruit juices and diet sodas. In the dehydrated patient, potassium should be given at the rate of 20 to 40 mEq per liter of rehydration fluid. This may need to be increased if serum potassium levels continue to fall below 3.5 mEq per liter. Electrocardiographic monitoring is quite useful for indicating hyper- or hypokalemia by demonstrating peaked T waves in the former and U waves in the latter. Under most circumstances, it is best to deliver the potassium in the form of potassium chloride unless the patient is found to be severely hypophosphatemic. In that event, we usually deliver half the potassium as potassium chloride and the other half as potassium phosphate. The use of phosphate supplements is highly controversial, as excess dosage can induce tetany and hypocalcemia. We add phosphate to the regimen only in very dehydrated, severely ill patients after a serum phosphorus level below 2.5 mEq per liter has been documented. Preferably, phosphate should be given independent of potassium needs, as a sodium phosphate solution in a dose of approximately 4 mmols per kg over a 12 hour period. However, it is more convenient to use potassium phosphate with very careful monitoring of serum phosphorus levels. Although magnesium is lost in the urine together with potassium and phosphate, there is no evidence that it is required in the rehydration fluids. However, severe magnesium depletion in some cases can be associated with transient hypoparathyroidism and hypocalcemia.

Bicarbonate

Bicarbonate administration is one of the most controversial areas of the therapy of DKA. Some physicians feel it should never be used. It is our position that children do not tolerate severe acidosis well, and we usually use bicarbonate very carefully in a patient whose pH is less than 7.2. The amount replaced is initially calculated to correct the serum bicarbonate level to 15 mEq per liter and is given over 4 to 6 hours without any bolus administration. Bicarbonate therapy is discontinued as soon as the venous bicarbonate level has reached 15 mEq per liter, even if the calculated amount has not yet been delivered. To calculate the amount needed, one subtracts the actual serum bicarbonate level from 15, multiplies that by the weight in kilograms and a correction factor of 0.6.

Supportive Measures

If the patient is extremely acidotic and in shock, the administration of oxygen for a short time may improve peripheral oxygenation delivery. Catheterization of the bladder is rarely necessary and carries with it the risk of infection. If the patient is unconscious, nasogastric suction is necessary to prevent inhalation of vomitus. During therapy, continuous clinical and biochemical monitoring is mandatory. Initial hourly measurements should be made of the biochemical profile as well as urine output and fluid intake. In addition, the level of consciousness and evaluation of optic discs should continue hourly into the first 12 to 16 hours of therapy and longer if necessary.

LONG-TERM MANAGEMENT

The long-term management of diabetes in childhood should be based on specific goals. These goals include (1) elimination of symptoms of diabetes—that is, polydipsia, polyuria, polyphagia; (2) prevention of DKA; (3) avoidance of hypoglycemia; (4) maintenance of normal growth and pubertal development with the prevention of obesity; (5) maintenance of emotional well-being with prevention of emotional disorders; this includes the maintenance of as normal a life style as possible within the constraints of the management issues of diabetes; (6) the prevention of chronic complications of diabetes. As we still do not understand the mechanisms of the development of complications of diabetes, we remain uncertain how to prevent them. Although there is some suggestive epidemiologic and clinical evidence that glycemic control plays a role, with supportive research in animal models, this is by no means proved. A rational approach in childhood appears to be to attempt to achieve the best glycemic control possible for that patient, using objective measurements for monitoring; (7) prevention of hypercholesterolemia; and (8) early detection of associated disorders, such as autoimmune hypo- or hyperthyroidism.

The most important aspect of diabetes management is education. This includes education of the diabetes management team as well as the patient and the family. This takes a great deal of time and should continue beyond the time of initial presentation.

Insulin Therapy

Conventional insulin therapy includes the administration of an intermediate-acting insulin with or without a short-acting (crystalline or regular) insulin. Most patients require both forms of insulin. The decision regarding the proportion of each type of insulin depends upon blood or urine glucose measurements at appropriate times of the day. It is important to remember that the duration of action of both the short- and intermediate-acting insulins is modified by the presence of insulin antibodies (presumably) and may vary from patient to patient according to the duration of the IDDM. It is, therefore, important to tailor the appropriate form of therapy to each individual patient. In general, most patients require insulin in a dose of 1 unit per kg per day after the remission period. However, during adolescence, up to 1.5 units per kg per day (occasionally more) may be required for the rapid growth rate. Children can be treated with either one insulin injection in the morning or a split dose, with approximately two thirds of the long-acting insulin given in the morning and one third in the evening prior to dinner. Occasionally, the long-acting insulin is given later in the evening to provide adequate insulinization in the early hours of the morning. We have found this latter regimen to be helpful only in a few patients.

Many clinicians believe that all children should be given two insulin injections per day from diagnosis to obtain adequate insulinization. However, our experience has been that a number of patients do very well on a single dose in the morning, presumably because of some endogenous insulin secretion or a depot of insulin that is provided by insulin antibodies. In patients who do well on one injection per day, our studies have shown no improved effect when they are switched to two injections per day. However, a large proportion of patients cannot be controlled by one injection per day, and in these patients the dose should be split. This is almost invariable in the very young child less than 3 years of age and the adolescent patient, and in patients whose dose increases beyond 1 unit per kg per day. Under these circumstances, the same dose of insulin given in a split dose often controls glycemia. There are other specific indications for two injections daily—for example, a patient who has hypoglycemia before dinner or in the early hours of the morning with hyperglycemia at the other times.

Intensive insulin therapy has become a more prominent feature of the treatment of diabetes in the past few years as home blood glucose monitoring has become available. This was initially achieved by the use of an insulin infusion pump with the delivery of a basal rate of insulin plus a premeal bolus subcutaneously, with the amount of the bolus depending upon the ambient blood sugar at the time. A similar insulin delivery profile can be achieved using multiple dose injections with long-acting insulin, such as ultralente, or two injections of lente or NPH insulin providing the basal rate and regular insulin premeals given subcutaneously. Although this form of therapy has been shown to be highly successful in achieving near-normal glycosylated hemoglobin values in adults, this degree of control has been found to be very difficult to achieve in the child and adolescent with diabetes. In fact, only a few workers have shown an advantage in using intensive insulin therapy in the pediatric population.

Our experience has been that subcutaneous insulin infusion (SCII) can result in improved control but not normoglycemia in a certain population of adolescents extremely carefully selected. These patients should be very highly motivated and be prepared to put in a tremendous amount of work. In addition, the physician who is taking care of the patient needs to put in a large proportion of time and effort. Our position is that insulin infusion pumps and multiple dose injections should be used in only a minority of our patient population. Specifically, insulin infusion pumps do not improve control in difficult patients with persistent hyperglycemia or ketoacidosis. In fact, some of the complications of pump therapy include increased episodes of ketoacidosis, infection at the injection site, and an increased frequency of hypoglycemic episodes.

In many patients, we can achieve equally improved control with a great deal of patient attention by the health care team and consistent monitoring on two injections per day. In our experience, most adolescents, whatever the selection criteria, are unable to comply with the rigorous demands required to make CSII safe and effective. Our data do not support the widespread use of CSII in adolescents unless they have unusual maturity and motivation. It is stressed that this form of therapy requires an enormous time expenditure on the part of both the patients and the professional health care team. This form of therapy should be attempted only if such a support system is available.

A recent change in insulin therapy is the availability of highly purified animal insulin as well as human insulin. As a result, there are a number of insulins on the market provided by different drug companies. The theoretic advantage of purified pork insulin and human insulin is a decreased production of insulin antibodies. It is suggested in relatively short-term studies that this antibody production is even less with the use of human insulin than with the use of purified pork insulin. The efficacy and time course of action of purified pork insulin appear to be almost identical to that of the previously used mixed beef-pork preparations. However, human insulin is different in both the onset and duration of action of both regular and intermediate-acting insulin, in that the onset is more rapid and the duration of action of the intermediate insulin is shorter. It is important that the physician should be aware of these differences when using human insulin, as the proportions of regular and intermediate-acting insulins need to be adjusted differently from that used with animal insulins. Particularly in younger patients under the age of 5 years, we have had some difficulty in preventing early morning ketonuria without producing hypoglycemia with human insulin treatment. However, this issue remains to be proved in controlled studies. In the United States, the purified pork insulins and human insulins are more expensive than conventional insulin, and some patients cannot afford the higher price.

There are some very specific indications for using pure pork or human insulin, such as patients using insulin infusion pumps, patients with lipoatrophy, and the rare event of intermittent insulin use. Lipohypertrophy is not related to insulin purity and cannot be improved by switching insulin, only by using alternative injection sites. In addition, some patients may have allergies to specific forms of insulins and may require a different form. When using lente with regular insulin, the injection should be given within 5 minutes of mixing these insulins in the syringe because the regular insulin becomes a semi-lente insulin beyond this time.

Diet

Good nutritional therapy plays a major role in achieving metabolic control in the patient with IDDM. It is important to use the term "good nutrition" rather than "diet" in the child to prevent the connotation of cutting calories, as is usually the case in an obese adult. The nutrition plan must include enough calories to meet all the requirements for growth and physical activity in the child. Under these circumstances, calorie restriction usually leads to hypoglycemia and growth failure. The child's appetite is usually the best indicator of the total calorie requirement and varies from day to day according to the amount of exercise activity. The situation is very different in the adolescent girl who is usually very inactive and often tends to become obese. Under these circumstances, calorie restriction is important, and good metabolic control should be achieved by manipulating the diet rather than the insulin dose.

The distribution of calories throughout the day should be planned to minimize hypoglycemia while preventing excessive glycemic excursions postprandially. A meal or snack every 3 hours during the day with an occasional additional snack to cover exercise is usually prescribed. Most of our very young patients require a morning snack, but this is not necessary as they grow older. Our dietary recommendations include an estimate of the calories based on age and activity; 50 to 60 per cent of the total calories is derived from carbohydrate, of which at least 70 per cent is from complex carbohydrates, the remainder consisting of lactose, fructose, and sucrose. Approximately 30 to 35 per cent of the calories is derived from fat, with a polyunsaturated to saturated fat ratio of at least 1 and a total cholesterol intake not exceeding 300 mg per day. The protein content of the diet is 15 to 20 per cent of the total calories, most of the protein being obtained from low fat sources such as fish, poultry, and vegetables. In general, children are unable to comply with rigid dietary regimes that require daily weighing of food. However, a scale can be used for teaching and reinforcement of assessment of portion size. There are a number of methods for teaching patients how to assess food components, such as exchange systems and points systems. None have been proved to be better than another, but each can be used as a teaching tool. The concept of a low fat diet is relatively new in many diabetes care clinics and has now been adopted as a recommendation by the American Diabetes Association.

There is a great deal of interest in the so-called "glycemic index" resulting from a re-evaluation of glycemic excursions induced by complex carbohydrates, compared with disaccharides and simple sugars. It is suggested that foods with a high fiber content have a decreased glycemic effect compared with cooked starches such as bread and potatoes. At this time, the evidence is not clear enough to change our recommendations for nutritional treatment in children with diabetes. However, as more studies are available, it may be possible that we will concentrate on high fiber diets and possibly liberalize restrictions on "free sugar." In our experience, it has been extremely difficult to get children to consume high fiber diets because of abdominal bloating and a general distaste possibly related to societal influences.

Exercise

Regular exercise improves glycemic control, and physical fitness is associated with a lower insulin requirement in patients who have very good glycosylated hemoglobin levels. Experiments show that vigorous physical activity results in increased glucose utilization with an improved efficiency of insulin action, possibly related to an increase in insulin receptor activity. It is interesting that long-term studies have not been able to prove that chronic increases in exercise improve metabolic control in cross-over studies. However, because of anecdotal clinical experience, regular exercise is recommended in the treatment regimen for all our patients. This is particularly important in the adolescent girl to prevent obesity. However, this recommendation is not often followed. One situation in which exercise should be discouraged is in the patient who is underinsulinized with ketonuria, when acute exercise results in an increase in blood sugar with the frequent induction of ketoacidosis. Patients should be taught how to handle exercise in relationship to their insulin dose and food intake. In general, in the normal-weight patient we tend to cover exercise with an extra snack or increased meal preceding the activity. However, in the overweight patient, it is more efficient to tailor the insulin dose to the physical activity. In some circumstances, both maneuvers are necessary.

Monitoring of Metabolic Control

Home Glucose Monitoring

This can be achieved by measuring glucose either in the urine or the blood. Urine glucose measurements have been the mainstay of home glucose monitoring for many years with steady improvement of the semiquantitative techniques available. Until recently, we used Clinitest tablets, which read glucose from a range of 0 to 5 per cent and can be used to assess 24 hour urine glucose excretion at home. The recent introduction of accurate strips for urine glucose testing has made this far easier for all our patients. If urine testing is used, we ask our patients to test a second voided specimen in the morning and a first voided specimen at least two other times during the day, distributing the testing times between premeal and evening snack.

We aim for a minimum of 50 per cent of the urine tests being negative (without associated hypoglycemia) and under 1 per cent 80 to 90 per cent of the time. We feel that a total abandonment of urine testing in childhood is a mistake, particularly as there is no other method yet available for the measurement of ketosis. Our patients routinely test their morning specimen for ketones to detect underinsulinization or nocturnal hypoglycemia. Quantitative measurements of glucose in a 24 hour or 6 to 8 hour urine collection are often useful in evaluating periods of hyper- or potential hypoglycemia. We aim at a maximum 24 hour glucose excretion of less than 5 to 7 per cent of the daily dietary carbohydrate intake.

It is undoubted that the measurement of blood sugar is more accurate for moment-to-moment assessment of glycemic control than that of urine glucose. In addition, the measurement of blood glucose is the only way to diagnosis hypoglycemia, which may be present with or without symptoms. It is a very useful technique to ascertain whether symptoms thought to be due to hypoglycemia are really associated with low blood sugar. Home blood glucose monitoring is essential in the patient who attempts intensive insulin therapy in order to make decisions regarding each insulin dose. However, our cross-over studies and those of other workers have not shown that blood glucose monitoring improves glycemic control, as measured by glycosylated hemoglobin, any more efficiently than regular urine glucose monitoring in patients receiving frequent telephone advice. In addition, the introduction of home glucose monitoring in our clinic population has not resulted in a significant decrease in glycosylated hemoglobin, and there is no difference in the degree of control in those patients who use blood glucose monitoring compared with those who use urine glucose testing. Presumably, blood glucose monitoring is only useful in patients who are prepared to use the numbers they see in order to manipulate all aspects of therapy. We find that this is most likely to occur in the very young child whose parents are in charge of the regime.

All our patients are taught blood glucose monitoring, performed three to four times daily, fasting in the morning and premeal and before the evening snack or as often as can be tolerated. In this situation, we ask the patients to test the first voided urine in the morning for both glucose and ketones. Omission of urine testing for ketones can result in ketoacidosis because the situation is not detected early enough. Goals for blood glucose measurements are as good as the patient can achieve. Ideally, fasting blood sugar levels should be between 80 to 120 mg per dl and postprandial values less than 200 mg per dl. However, few patients are able to achieve these levels consistently and become frustrated at their inability to do so. Therefore, we ask patients to keep fasting blood sugar levels between 70 to 150 mg per dl and preprandial values around the same level. Acceptance of blood sugar testing is surprisingly good in most of our patients. If they are going to test at all, they very often will test their blood. However, a significant number of patients prefer urine testing, and in those patients we use blood sugar monitoring to detect hypoglycemia only. It should be stressed that even with meters, accurate blood sugar testing is not easy, and patients require intensive training to read values within 10 per cent of the actual blood sugar level. They should be checked frequently to assess continued accuracy of their techniques.

Glycosylated Hemoglobin

The availability of this test to measure long-term glycemic control may be one of the most important advances in diabetes care in the past decade. For the first time, physicians have an objective measure to assess long-term glycemic control in their patients and do not have to rely on self-report, which is often not performed at all or not done accurately. However, the value of the measurement of glycosylated hemoglobin depends upon the accuracy of the laboratory in which it is performed. Different methods give different results, which are not comparable across laboratories. Glycosylated hemoglobin should be measured in patients at least three to four times annually, regardless of the clinical assessment. It is difficult to know what the goals for the level of glycosylated hemoglobin should be, but a reasonable approach is to aim at a level that is less than the mean in the clinic. In our population, the mean stable glycosylated hemoglobin value is 10.5 per cent, with a normal range of 4.8 to 7.5 per cent. Most of our poorly controlled patients, particularly adolescent girls, have values of between 14 and 17 per cent. However, approximately 3 per cent of our patients, most of whom are in the remission phase, have values within the normal range.

Serum Cholesterol

Because insulin is important in lipid metabolism as well as carbohydrate metabolism, hyperlipidemia is common in the underinsulinized patient. This is often associated with hypercholesterolemia, which is frequently seen in diabetic populations. We measure the serum cholesterol annually in all our patients in order to maintain levels that are normal for age.

Thyroid Function

Because hypothyroidism and thyrotoxicosis are more common in the diabetic population than in normal children, we monitor T_4 and thyroid-stimulating hormone annually. Thyroid disorders affect insulin requirements prior to any other manifestation and are usually detected biochemically before overt clinical symptoms occur.

Sick Days

Ketosis

Any intercurrent illness can result in insulin resistance. Under these circumstances the usual insulin dose is not sufficient to prevent hyperglycemia and ketosis. It is important to remember that ketones will be produced earlier than severe hyperglycemia. When this occurs, patients should be in immediate contact with the health care team and extra regular insulin should be given as indicated every 4 to 6 hours or more frequently if necessary. Usually a regular insulin dose of 10 per cent of the total daily dose is sufficient to control ketosis. In addition, the patient should be asked to drink large amounts of fluid containing potassium and sodium—for example, diet sodas—to replace the fluid and electrolytes lost with hyperglycemia and ketosis. If the patient is vomiting, small sips of sugar-containing fluids at frequent intervals should be tried. However, if a patient vomits more than three times or is unable to keep down any calories, he or she should be seen in the hospital and possibly receive intravenous fluids. A patient with any change in respiration rate, evidence of dehydration, or change in level of consciousness should be brought immediately to the hospital.

Hypoglycemia

Mild symptoms of hypoglycemia can be treated with a small starch snack. More severe symptoms such as dizziness, severe tremor, or change in level of consciousness should be treated with a glucose tablet or 4 to 6 ounces of a sugar-containing drink such as orange juice. This should be followed by a snack of complex carbohydrates. If the patient is unconscious and cannot drink, an injection of 1 mg of glucagon should be given subcutaneously immediately. All families should keep a glucagon kit in their refrigerator for such emergencies. As soon as the patient wakes up, they should be offered sugar-containing food or drink followed by a carbohydrate snack. It should be remembered that glucagon often makes patients vomit, and this must be dealt with. The health care team should always be consulted when a severe hypoglycemic episode occurs. The reason for the episode should be sought and corrective measures undertaken.

Surgery

Patients with insulin-dependent diabetes should not have general anesthesia or skip meals without the advice of a physician. Our routine is to arrange surgery early in the morning. We start an intravenous infusion of dextrose in water up to 6 hours prior to the anesthetic. The insulin dose depends upon the complexity of the surgery anticipated. For minor surgery, we give two thirds of the usual intermediate-acting insulin dose, and regular insulin only if the blood sugar level is high. We then cover the remainder of the day according to the blood sugar measurements, with regular insulin given every 4 to 6 hours if necessary until the patient is able to eat. In situations of complex, long duration surgery, we use regular insulin given intravenously in the same fashion as that given during treatment of ketoacidosis. If at all possible, a patient should not be anesthetized if ketosis is present. Under all circumstances, the patient's blood sugar should be monitored at regular intervals, usually hourly, either using the central laboratory or one of the reagent strips, with maintenance of the blood sugar level between 100 and 200 mg per dl.

Prevention

Recent research has raised the issue of possible prevention of insulin-dependent diabetes or amelioration of hyperglycemia very soon after the onset of the disorder. Our current state of knowledge does not allow us to predict the development of IDDM with certainty in any patient. Thus, preventive therapy is at this stage very strictly a research procedure. There has been a great deal of interest in the use of cyclosporine in the newly diagnosed patient with IDDM, with the goal of elimination of insulin requirement. Although pilot studies appear promising, treatment of the newly diagnosed patient with cyclosporine should only be part of a very strictly controlled research program.

HYPERURICEMIA AND GOUT

method of
MICHAEL A. BECKER, M.D.
The University of Chicago
Chicago, Illinois

The term *gout* refers to a heterogeneous group of diseases in which tissue deposition of monosodium urate or uric acid crystals from supersaturated extracellular fluids results in one or more of a limited array of clinical events. The range of expression of the gout syndrome includes recurrent attacks of acute gouty arthritis; articular, osseous, soft tissue, and cartilaginous crystalline deposits (tophi); renal impairment (gouty nephropathy); and uric acid urolithiasis. Hyperuricemia (a serum urate concentration more than 2 SD above the mean established in the individual laboratory for the sex of the patient) reflects the metabolic derangement in extracellular fluid predisposing to gout and is, in fact, the pathogenetic common denominator through which diverse etiologic influences (heredity, drugs, toxins, diet) give rise to clinical manifestations. Although hyperuricemia is necessary, it most often is not sufficient for expression of gout. It is important to distinguish between the disease state (gout) and the chemical aberration (asymptomatic hyperuricemia) to avoid unwarranted and potentially hazardous treatment of the latter. Recent years have witnessed increasing conservatism in the management of gout and hyperuricemia, particularly in the form of more restricted use of hypouricemic therapy among asymptomatic individuals and patients who have experienced only one or several attacks of gouty arthritis.

A commonly used clinical classification categorizes gout into four periods: asymptomatic hyperuricemia; acute gouty arthritis; intercritical gout; and chronic tophaceous gout. This scheme provides a convenient framework for discussing available management modalities but does not imply either inexorable progression of asymptomatic hyperuricemia into a clinical disease state or a qualitative distinction among the three categories of clinical involvement.

TREATMENT

Asymptomatic Hyperuricemia. The incidence of gouty arthritis among previously asymptomatic persons increases with increasing severity of hyperuricemia and may be as much as 100-fold greater at serum urate levels higher than 9 mg per dl than at 6 mg per dl. Similarly, an increased risk of urolithiasis (both uric acid and calcium stones) is well documented among patients with asymptomatic hyperuricemia. Despite the risks for these clinical events, conservatism in the treatment of asymptomatic hyperuricemia is advisable. First, the estimated lifelong incidence of gouty manifestations among the high proportion (5 to 10 per cent) of the population that is hyperuricemic is less than 20 per cent. Second, the initial attack of acute gouty arthritis and the first urinary tract stone, although painful, are treatable events very unlikely to be attended by serious consequences. Third, effective long-term control of hyperuricemia usually requires lifelong adherence to medication and can be attended by toxic reactions, sometimes severe, to the drugs employed. Finally, study of large groups of gouty as well as nongouty hyperuricemic persons supports the view that in the majority of such individuals hyperuricemia is not a major independent risk factor for the development of renal insufficiency. In fact, significant renal functional impairment in gout patients is much more likely to be a consequence of disorders known to be strongly associated with (but not consequences of) gout and hyperuricemia, namely hypertension, atherosclerosis, diabetes mellitus, hypertriglyceridemia, obesity, and ethanol abuse. It thus appears that management of patients with hyperuricemia accompanied or unaccompanied by gout should be directed primarily at the amelioration of these significant associated disorders. The decision of whether or how to deal with the hyperuricemia can be approached in a more leisurely fashion and is based on careful consideration of the principles discussed subsequently.

Introduction of drugs to reduce hyperuricemia seems warranted in only a small proportion of persons whose hyperuricemia is asymptomatic or who are likely to be rendered acutely hyperuricemic and hyperuricosuric: (1) men with serum urate concentrations of more than 13 mg per dl and women with serum urate concentrations of more than 10 mg per dl, levels of urate for which there are few substantial data regarding long-term renal risk; (2) patients excreting more than 1100 mg of uric acid in the daily urine, a level of hyperuricosuria associated with a 50 per cent or greater incidence of urolithiasis; and (3) patients with myeloproliferative or lymphoproliferative diseases who are about to undergo chemotherapy or radiation therapy and are thus at risk for acute uric nephropathy, a form of acute renal failure resulting from massive uric acid deposition in the collecting ducts with secondary blockage of renal tubules. When treatment of asymptomatic hyperuricemia is undertaken to avoid consequences of severe hyperuricemia or hyperuricosuria, the principles guiding the choice of hyperuricemic agents are those described later for management of gout. In patients with hyperuricemia, including those not fulfilling the above criteria for hypouricemic drug management, many of the adjunctive measures to be discussed for the treatment of gout are potentially beneficial with little likelihood of untoward reactions. Regardless of the therapeutic decision, thorough patient education and presentation of the treatment options available are critical, since, on the one hand, the risk of a painful clinical event is very real and, on the other, the decision to treat is likely to require a lifelong commitment to compliance.

Management of Gout

The aims of current therapeutic programs in gout are to reduce acute inflammation, to prevent recurrence of gouty arthritis and urolithiasis, to avoid progression of crystal deposition to clinically apparent tophi, and to reverse gouty complications when possible. Prevention of the expression of gout by treatment of asymptomatic hyperuricemia, although usually an attainable goal, is infrequently warranted. Even after one or more clinical manifestations of gout have occurred, a decision regarding long-term management of hyperuricemia must be made in discussion with the patient regarding likely outcome, the need for commitment to lifelong treatment, and the potential hazards of undergoing treatment. Some patients choose to avoid prolonged drug treatment and risk recurrences of arthritis and even of urolithiasis. The wishes of such individuals should be respected and follow-up should be carefully planned, with the physician taking the lead in proposing drug treatment more firmly when convinced of its merit.

It is also important to emphasize the distinctive rationale underlying use of anti-inflammatory and of hypouricemic drugs. Anti-inflammatory agents are used to treat (or in the case of cochicine, to prevent) gouty inflammation; they do not alter the state of hyperuricemia leading to the inflammation. Conversely, uricosuric drugs and allopurinol (Zyloprim) reduce serum urate levels but have no anti-inflammatory properties; their use in acute gouty arthritis is counterproductive.

Acute Gouty Arthritis. The severity of pain and disability associated with acute gouty arthritis usually demands prompt intervention. In general, the earlier treatment is initiated, the more rapid and complete the response to anti-inflammatory agents. The involved joint should be placed at rest; a narcotic analgesic may occasionally be required. Despite the impressive intensity of gouty inflammation, this form of acute arthritis is usually quite promptly and successfully relieved with any of a number of types of anti-inflammatory drugs, including colchicine, the nonsteroidal anti-inflammatory agents, and glucocorticoids.

Orally administered colchicine is usually given in an initial dose of 1.0 to 1.2 mg followed by 0.5 or 0.6 mg hourly until either relief of pain or gastrointestinal symptoms (nausea, vomiting, abdominal pain, or diarrhea). Pain relief and gastrointestinal symptoms often coincide. No more than 8 to 10 doses should be given in the first 24 hours, and 7.0 to 8.0 mg of colchicine should not be exceeded within 72 hours. Intravenous colchicine (1.0 to 2.0 mg in 20 ml of saline, given over 20 min) has the advantage of usually bypassing gastrointestinal side effects. The dose may be repeated in 4 to 6 hours if necessary, but should not exceed 4.0 mg in 24 hours. Care should be taken to avoid extravasation of this extremely sclerotic agent. Colchicine is excreted by the kidney and should be used cautiously and at reduced dose in patients with renal insufficiency.

The nonsteroidal anti-inflammatory drugs (NSAIDs) are the drugs most commonly used in the treatment of acute gouty arthritis. Indomethacin (Indocin), 50 mg, three or four times daily for 2 to 3 days, with subsequent rapid tapering and discontinuation by 1 week, often leads to a prompt response, although headache, agitation, drowsiness, and gastrointestinal intolerance occasionally limit its use. Phenylbutazone (Butazolidin), initially given as a single loading dose of 300 mg, followed by 100 to 200 mg (depending on patient age and severity of attack) every 6 hours for 2 days and tapered over 2 to 3 additional days, has efficacy with occasional side effects of gastrointestinal discomfort and fluid retention, particularly in the elderly. Serious hematologic toxicity, although very uncommon, has limited the acceptance of this drug. Virtually all the newer NSAIDs, including ibuprofen (Motrin), naproxen (Naprosyn), sulindac (Clinoril), and piroxicam (Feldene), have been used successfully in gouty arthritis, reportedly with a lower incidence of gastrointestinal symptoms.

The use of oral glucocorticoids in gout is attended by a variable response and, sometimes, by recurrence of arthritis on discontinuation. Intra-articular steroids after joint fluid aspiration may provide prompt improvement; in postoperative patients requiring parenteral treatment for acute gout, either intra-articular steroid injection or intravenous colchicine may be given.

Improvement in acute gouty arthritis is usually observed within 6 to 12 hours and may be complete within 3 days. In a small proportion of patients, especially those in whom treatment has been delayed, improvement is minimal and resolution slow. When attacks occur regularly after dietary excess, alcohol intake, or other identifiable precipitating events, avoidance of these circumstances by affected patients can reduce the frequency of attacks. In addition, initiation of therapy for recurrent gout with either colchicine or an NSAID at the first premonition or symptom of an impending episode is often successful in aborting full-blown attacks.

Intercritical Gout. Colchicine (0.5 or 0.6 mg, once or twice daily) is an effective agent in the prophylaxis of recurrent attacks of acute gouty arthritis. An unusual propensity of gouty arthritis to occur repetitively in patients early in the course of hyperuricemic therapy with either uricosuric agents or allopurinol is well established. (Such attacks should not, however, prompt discontinuation of the hypouricemic drug, even during treatment for the acute episode.) Colchicine should thus be given prophylactically to all patients receiving hypouricemic agents until after the serum urate concentration has been reduced to a level of 6.0 mg per dl or less for a period of at least 3 to 6 months. Patients still experiencing recurrent attacks and patients with chronic tophaceous gout require more prolonged use of prophylactic colchicine. In patients in whom NSAID treatment is required for chronic joint symptoms or for other reasons, colchicine may usually be omitted since NSAIDs probably exert an adequate prophylactic effect. The identification and abolition of hyperuricemia-provoking environmental influences (e.g., drugs, toxins) and diseases may result in effective prophylaxis through removal of underlying hyperuricemia. The intercritical period is an ideal time to identify such circumstances and to evaluate the need for hypouricemic treatment.

Tophaceous Gout. The body pool of urate is expanded in patients with gout regardless of whether tophi are evident or not. Even at the time of the first acute attack of gouty arthritis, tophaceous deposits too small to be clinically detected are present in most or perhaps all patients. Resolution of tophi, reduction of urate pool size to normal, and removal of the immediate source of further crystallization and clinical events are congruent aims that can be achieved by long-term normalization of serum urate concentration, taking advantage of the availability of two classes of potent hyperuricemic agents—uricosuric drugs and xanthine oxidase inhibitors. Uricosuric drugs increase renal clearance of uric acid; allopurinol, the only xanthine oxidase inhibitor currently available, inhibits urate synthesis. Table 1 presents indications for treatment of gout with hypouricemic agents.

The uricosuric agents commonly used in the United States are probenecid (Benemid), and sulfinpyrazone (Anturane). Both inhibit renal tubular uric acid reabsorption, thus increasing net uric acid excretion. They are the drugs of choice in patients with gout and normal daily uric acid excretion (urinary uric acid < 600 mg daily on a purine-free diet, or < 800 mg daily on a standard diet), a group constituting about 80 per cent of all gout patients. A fluid intake of at least 2 to 3 liters per day is necessary when treatment is begun to avoid urolithiasis during the period of increased uric acid excretion. In addition, prophylactic colchicine should be administered.

The starting dose of probenecid is 0.25 gram twice daily, with a gradual increase over 3 to 4 weeks to 0.5 gram two or three times daily. If serum urate concentration remains more than 6.0 mg per dl, an increase in dose to as much as 2.5 or 3.0 grams daily should be tried. Sulfinpyrazone is started at a dose of 50 mg per day, with a gradual increase to 100 mg three or four times a day. A total dose of up to 800 mg per day may be given to patients requiring further uricosuria.

Gastrointestinal symptoms and skin rash are the most common reactions to uricosuric agents; hepatic necrosis and bone marrow suppression occur rarely. Aspirin and other salicylates are uricosuric at high blood concentrations; however, they should not be used in the treatment of gout because at lower levels salicylates cause uric acid retention by inhibition of tubular urate secretion and salicylates interfere with the action of uricosuric agents. Uricosuric agents are *not* first line drugs in patients with excessive uric acid excre-

TABLE 1. **Indications for Treatment of Gout with Hypouricemic Agents**

Frequent and disabling attacks of gouty arthritis
Tophaceous deposits in soft tissues and/or bone
Chronic gouty joint disease
Gout with renal damage
Recurrent urolithiasis
Severe hyperuricemia (>13 mg/dl in men; >10 mg/dl in women)
Severe uric acid overproduction (urinary uric acid excretion >1100/day)
Prevention of acute uric acid nephropathy in leukemia/lymphoma patients about to receive cytotoxic treatment

tion or with previous histories of urolithiasis or renal insufficiency. These patients, and those in whom uricosuric drugs are ineffective should receive allopurinol. The rate of dissolution of tophi is less with uricosuric drugs than with allopurinol; some physicians consider the presence of tophi an indication for the latter drug.

Allopurinol (Zyloprim) is a hypoxanthine analogue, which undergoes oxidation to oxipurinol, a potent competitive inhibitor of xanthine oxidase, the enzyme catalyzing conversion of hypoxanthine to xanthine and xanthine to uric acid. The result is a diminution in serum and urinary urate concentration. Allopurinol also decreases the rate of purine synthesis de novo. The combination of reduced total purine load presented to the kidney and redistribution of the purines into three compounds (hypoxanthine, xanthine, and uric acid) with independent solubilities reduces the likelihood of stone formation in gout patients. It is advisable to begin treatment with allopurinol at a dose of 100 mg per day and to increase the dose stepwise only after patient tolerance and the need for a higher dose is established. The usual maintenance dose of allopurinol is 300 to 600 mg per day; the drug can be given in a single daily dose. Early in the course of allopurinol treatment, prophylactic colchicine should be administered.

Although uncommon, adverse effects of allopurinol are often severe and occur more often than uricosuric agents. These effects include fever, eosinophilia, dermatitis, elevation of hepatic enzymes, renal failure, headache, diarrhea, and vasculitis. An allopurinol hypersensitivity syndrome consisting of some or all of these features has been described, especially among patients with renal insufficiency or those receiving thiazide diuretics. A high mortality rate (20 to 30 per cent of reported cases) in patients with this syndrome emphasizes the need to restrict use of this agent to patients in whom it is clearly indicated. In patients with renal insufficiency, the dose of allopurinol should be adjusted downward to accommodate the diminished clearance of drug metabolites. In patients receiving allopurinol, the dose of chemotherapeutic agents such as 6-mercaptopurine and azathioprine should be much lower than usual to avoid excessive accumulation of the cytotoxic agent. Xanthine urolithiasis is a rare complication of allopurinol treatment.

Combined treatment with the two classes of hypouricemic agents has occasionally been attempted. The greatest benefit of this combination may be to individuals whose serum urate levels are not adequately controlled with either type of drug alone.

Adjuncts to Management

Maintenance of an adequate level of hydration is an important measure for patients with gout who are at increased risk for urolithiasis. Intake of at least 2 to 3 liters of fluids daily is advisable to maintain urinary uric acid concentrations as minimally supersaturated as possible. It is important to remember that patients treated with uricosuric agents excrete uric acid at a higher rate early in the course of treatment and that both xanthine and oxipurinol are relatively insoluble compounds that may themselves result in stones. Urinary alkalinization can be an extremely useful measure in the treatment of gout patients with uric acid urolithiasis. Such individuals are generally receiving allopurinol as well. Although purine-restricted diets are infrequently advised in long-term management of gout at the present time, specific deletion of one or more purine-rich foods is sometimes advisable when identifiable as provocative agents in acute attacks. Weight reduction can be associated with a reduction in serum urate concentration as a result of a reduced rate of purine synthesis. Weight reduction to or maintenance of lean body mass, with special emphasis on reduced calorie, purine, and protein intake, is a general adjunctive measure especially likely to benefit the gouty population in which obesity, hypertriglyceridemia, and hypertension are highly endemic. Finally, reduction of alcohol consumption represents another approach applicable to the health of the general population that is also especially likely to benefit gouty patients whose hyperuricemia can be potentiated by effects of alcohol on both production and urinary excretion of uric acid.

HYPERLIPOPROTEINEMIA

method of
SCOTT M. GRUNDY, M.D., Ph.D.
University of Texas
Dallas, Texas

Hyperlipoproteinemia signifies an increase in plasma lipoproteins, the carriers of cholesterol and triglycerides. Abnormalities of the plasma lipoproteins are important clinically for several reasons. Most important, an increase in the major cholesterol-carrying lipoproteins seemingly accelerates the development of atherosclerosis. Lipoproteins carrying triglycerides may or may not increase atherogenesis, but when triglyceride levels are very high the result can be acute pancreatitis.

Lipoprotein Metabolism

Chylomicrons are synthesized in the intestinal mucosa and contain mainly dietary triglycerides. They are secreted into intestinal lymph and enter the circulation through the thoracic duct. They then pass into the peripheral circulation where they come in contact with an enzyme, lipoprotein lipase, located on the surface of capillary endothelial cells. Most of the triglycerides undergo lipolysis, and smaller, residual particles, called chylomicron remnants, are released back into circulation and are cleared rapidly by the liver.

The liver likewise secretes a triglyceride-rich lipoprotein named very low density lipoprotein (VLDL). VLDL particles also interact with lipoprotein lipase, and once again, VLDL remnants, or intermediate density lipoproteins (IDL), return to the circulation. IDL contain about equal amounts of cholesterol and triglycerides. IDL particles can have two fates: normally, about half are removed by the liver; the other half are converted to low density lipoproteins (LDL). LDL are the major cholesterol-carrying lipoproteins of plasma. Most plasma LDL are cleared by specific receptors on the surfaces of cells. The liver is the major site of LDL clearance, although other tissues also remove a portion. LDL receptors on liver cells also are responsible for direct removal of IDL from the circulation. A small fraction of LDL is cleared by nonreceptor-mediated processes, presumably by nonspecific pinocytosis.

High density lipoproteins (HDL) belong to another category. The liver and gut secrete precursors of HDL (nascent HDL); nascent HDL are cholesterol-poor and can take up cholesterol from peripheral tissues. HDL thus are important for "reverse cholesterol transport," i.e., transport of cholesterol from peripheral tissues to the liver where it can be excreted. After HDL remove cholesterol from tissues, they transfer this cholesterol to VLDL; in turn, VLDL are catabolized to lipoproteins that are cleared by the liver, namely, IDL and LDL.

The relative atherogenicity of these different lipoproteins is an important issue. The triglyceride-rich chylomicrons seemingly have little atherogenic potential. These large lipoproteins probably are poorly filtered through the arterial intima, and furthermore they carry little cholesterol. VLDL likewise may not be highly atherogenic but are probably more so than chylomicrons. IDL in contrast are moderately atherogenic, and LDL are markedly so. Of all risk factors contributing to atherosclerosis, a high LDL level would seem to be the most important. In contrast, HDL are thought to be antiatherogenic. People with high levels of HDL seem to be protected from coronary heart disease (CHD), while those who have low levels are at increased risk. The mechanism by which HDL protects against atherosclerosis is unknown, but the capacity of HDL to mobilize cholesterol from peripheral tissues likely is involved.

Hypercholesterolemia

Hypercholesterolemia is an elevation of plasma total cholesterol in the presence of normal triglyceride concentrations. A high plasma cholesterol usually is associated with an increase in LDL concentrations. What constitutes an elevated plasma cholesterol is a matter of dispute. One approach to definition of hypercholesterolemia is to use the term to represent any LDL level over the 95th percentile for the general population. For middle-aged Americans, this outer limit of normal corresponds to a total cholesterol value of about 275 mg per dl. An alternate approach is to define hypercholesterolemia according to the relation of plasma cholesterol to risk for CHD. Epidemiologic studies suggest that the desirable cholesterol level is in the range of 150 to 200 mg per dl; populations that have levels in this range have relatively low rates of CHD. Studies indicate that the risk for CHD rises sharply when the cholesterol levels exceed 200 to 225 mg per dl. Above 225 mg per dl, it is no longer reasonable to say that values are desirable or "normal." For this reason, a total cholesterol level in the range of 225 to 275 mg per dl will be called *mild hypercholesterolemia;* levels in the range of 275 to 325 mg per dl will be designated *moderate hypercholesterolemia;* and concentrations over 325 mg per dl will be called *severe hypercholesterolemia.*

Desirable Cholesterol Levels

Cholesterol levels of 150 to 200 mg per dl do not ensure the absence of atherosclerosis. Arterial lesions occur in all populations, even when cholesterol concentrations are low. Nonetheless, the rate of progression of atherosclerosis in people with cholesterol levels of 150 to 200 mg per dl is relatively slow, and most people in this range either avoid clinical manifestations altogether or develop CHD late in life. Still, these cholesterol levels can sustain more rapid atherogenesis in the presence of other risk factors, such as smoking and hypertension. Therefore patients with additional risk factors should not be reassured on the basis of their cholesterol level alone.

An important question is whether people whose cholesterol levels are in the desirable range should be advised to follow a particular dietary regimen. Although some investigators believe not, several arguments can be made for following a diet low in saturated fat and cholesterol, the major dietary factors raising the cholesterol level. One reason for advocating such a diet for all people is the difficulty of obtaining an accurate assessment of a given patient's cholesterol level. A single measurement, or even a series of measurements, do not necessarily reveal a person's average cholesterol level over a long period of time. Even within the so-called "desirable range," those whose cholesterol levels are at the upper end of this range may be at greater risk for CHD than those at the lower end. With regard to plasma cholesterol levels "the lower, the better." Also, the plasma cholesterol concentration may not reveal all the risks for CHD associated with diet. Diets rich in saturated fat and cholesterol may have adverse effects on lipoprotein metabolism and may accelerate atherosclerosis in ways not revealed by fasting cholesterol levels. Several epidemiologic studies are in accord with this concept. Cholesterol concentrations tend to change over time, tending to rise with aging. Consequently, a single value obtained in early adulthood may be misleading because it does not necessarily predict cholesterol levels later in life. For these reasons, a diet low in total fat, saturated fat, and dietary cholesterol can be advocated for all adults. Of course, this is a general recommendation, and in particular patients the physician must make therapeutic decisions and recommendations based on the overall assessment of an individual's needs.

Mild Hypercholesterolemia (Plasma Cholesterol = 225 to 275 Mg per Dl)

The major factor responsible for mild hypercholesterolemia appears to be the diet. Three dietary factors have been implicated: dietary cholesterol, saturated fatty acids, and obesity. The former two raise LDL levels by decreasing LDL clearance from plasma, most likely by decreasing activity of hepatic LDL receptors. Obesity, in contrast, increases LDL concentrations by stimulating the synthesis of the precursor, VLDL. Epidemiologic surveys and metabolic ward investigations indicate that the typical American diet raises the plasma cholesterol by about 50 to 60 mg per dl above that of a diet very low in cholesterol and saturated fat. For many people, this increase is enough to raise the level from the desirable range (150 to 200 mg per dl) into that of mild hypercholesterolemia (225 to 275 mg per dl). Although genetic factors may contribute to mild elevations of plasma cholesterol, dietary factors seem to predominate in the American population.

Mild hypercholesterolemia raises the risk for CHD approximately twofold above that of the desirable range. Therefore an attempt should be made to reduce even mildly elevated levels. In many patients, reduction to the desirable range can be achieved by dietary change and proper use of exercise. The basic goal of diet is to decrease intakes of saturated fat, cholesterol, and total calories. The first step is to restrict caloric intake to obtain desirable weight and to increase exercise to an optimal level; the second step is to alter the composition of the diet. Diet composition can be altered in several ways, including a low fat diet, a diet high in polyunsaturated fatty acids, and a diet rich in monounsaturated fatty acids.

Weight Reduction and Exercise. Some investigators recommend that mild hypercholesterolemia be treated only by weight reduction and maintenance of weight in a desirable range. Such a diet of course should be accompanied by appropriate exercise. Both weight loss and vigorous exercise will lower total cholesterol and LDL levels in many people, and consequently they may be the only treatment required for mild hypercholesterolemia. However, plasma cholesterol levels are not always responsive to exercise and weight loss alone, and unless other changes are made, mildly elevated levels may persist. Nonetheless, it is reasonable to advocate maintenance of desirable weight and exercise as the first step in the control of mild hypercholesterolemia.

Low Fat Diets. The use of a low fat diet for the general public has been advocated by the American Heart Association. This diet consists of a fat intake of 30 per cent of total calories, of which saturated fatty acids, monounsaturated fatty acids, and polyunsaturated fatty acids each make up 10 per cent. Cholesterol intake is recommended at 225 to 300 mg per dl. This diet differs from the typical American diet, which contains approximately 40 per cent of calories as fat (17 per cent saturated, 18 per cent monounsaturated, and 6 per cent polyunsaturated) and about 500 mg per day of cholesterol. The underlying concept of the recommended diet is to lower saturated fatty acids by decreasing total fat intake and by increasing slightly the intake of polyunsaturated fatty acids. The adoption of a low fat diet should lower the plasma cholesterol to the desirable range in many people with mild hypercholesterolemia.

To achieve these changes in diet composition, one must alter the diet mainly in dairy products and meats. As a general rule, meat should not be consumed more than once a day. Turkey, chicken, veal, and fish should be eaten more frequently than beef, pork, or lamb. The latter meats should be restricted to three times a week. When meat and fish are prepared, visible fat and skin should be removed. Organ meats, such as liver and kidney, should be eliminated completely from the diet because of their high cholesterol content.

Skim milk or 2 per cent milk should be substituted for 4 per cent milk, and low fat yogurt and skim milk desserts may be substituted for ice cream. Sherbet also can be used. Cottage cheese containing only 2 per cent fat should be used. Eggs should be limited to three per week, including those used as part of recipes in cooking. Cheese should be selected from those whose fat content is less than 8 per cent. Vegetable oils and soft margarines should be used instead of butter or commercial shortenings.

Diets High in Polyunsaturated Fats. It has been known for many years that polyunsaturated fatty acids will lower plasma cholesterol when substituted for saturated fatty acids. At one time, polyunsaturates were widely recommended. In recent years, however, there has been less enthusiasm for adding large quantities of polyunsaturated fatty acids to the diet. Several factors suggest the need for caution. First, no sizable population has ever consumed large quantities of polyunsaturates for many years with proven safety. Second, in experimental animals, these fats act as cocarcinogens. Third, they produce changes in the fatty acid composition of cellular membrane, and the long-term consequences of these changes are unknown. Thus, most investigators recommend only modest increases in dietary polyunsaturates, not to exceed 10 per cent of total calories.

Diets Rich in Monounsaturated Fatty Acids. The major monounsaturated fatty acid is oleic acid. This fatty acid occurs in large quantities in olive oil, but it is present also in other vegetable oils. Animals also have the capacity to synthesize oleic acid. Large amounts of oleic acid have been consumed in the Mediterranean region for centuries without evidence of harmful effect. In this region, plasma cholesterol levels tend to be low, as do rates of CHD. Monounsaturates also lower LDL concentrations, to about the same extent as those of polyunsaturates. Thus, monounsaturates seem to have all the advantages of polyunsaturates without some of the drawbacks of the latter. Oleic acid, therefore, appears to be the preferred fatty acid to be substituted for saturated fatty acids. Diets rich in monounsaturated fatty acids seem a reasonable alternative to low fat diets, especially for those who cannot tolerate a marked reduction in fat intake.

Moderate Hypercholesterolemia (Plasma Cholesterol = 275 to 325 mg per dl)

Approximately 5 per cent of the adult population has cholesterol levels in this range. The risk for CHD is increased two- to fourfold. Dietary factors (excessive intakes of cholesterol, saturated fatty acids, and total calories) and lack of exercise contribute to moderate hypercholesterolemia in many patients. Genetic factors, however, are important, and unless abnormalities in LDL metabolism are present, plasma cholesterol will not rise to such high levels. The metabolic defect is unknown, but it probably is an abnormality in synthesis of LDL receptors. A metabolic suppression in receptor synthesis seems more likely than a structural defect in the receptor protein, although the latter may be present in some patients. When a definite structural defect in the receptor is present, patients are said to have *familial hypercholesterolemia*. The more general term *genetic hypercholesterolemia* can be applied to the majority of patients with moderate hypercholesterolemia. Some patients with cholesterol levels in the moderately elevated range have overproduction of lipoproteins instead of a clearance defect for LDL, as will be discussed under the section on Hypertriglyceridemia.

In the search for the cause of moderate hypercholesterolemia, two steps are necessary. First, family screening is needed to determine whether the patient has genetic or familial hypercholesterolemia. During screening, other family members who need treatment may be found. Also, secondary causes of elevated cholesterol levels must be ruled out. These include hypothyroidism, nephrotic syndrome, various dysproteinemias, thiazide diuretics, obstructive liver disease, Cushing's disease, and anorexia nervosa.

Management. The first step in the control of moderate hypercholesterolemia is dietary change. A good dietary approach for treatment of hypercholesterolemia has been outlined by the American Heart Association. The recommended regimen is a progressive reduction in intakes of total fat, saturated fat, and cholesterol. The initial phase of dietary change is the eating plan outlined for mild hypercholesterolemia. Once this has been achieved, a further reduction of fat intake to 20 per cent of total calories is advocated. For example, meat consumption other than chicken, veal, and turkey should be decreased to once per week. Fish and vegetable protein should be substituted for pork, beef, and lamb. All milk should be fat free, as should any kind of cottage cheese or cheese. Baking, broiling, and steaming foods should replace frying. Even vegetable oils should be curtailed to reduce total fat intake, and no more than two eggs per week consumed. Many recipes are available for pasta dishes, vegetable dishes, and casseroles in which meat is used as a condiment rather than as the main dish.

In patients with moderate hypercholesterolemia who are especially responsive to dietary change, this regimen will bring cholesterol levels to near the desirable range. However, in many patients drug therapy must be considered. The indications for drug therapy in hypercholesterolemic patients are outlined in Table 1. These indications should be used as a guide and not considered binding. Before starting a patient on drugs, multiple measurements (usually three) are

TABLE 1. **Indications for Drug Therapy in Moderate Hypercholesterolemia**

Persistent moderate hypercholesterolemia on multiple screenings
Premature CHD in patient or family
Presence of other risk factors (e.g., smoking, hypertension)
Failure to respond to dietary therapy (with a fall of total cholesterol to below 250 mg/dl)
Low HDL-cholesterol
Motivation to adhere to drug therapy
Use drugs in men before women, in young to middle-aged men before elderly

needed to confirm persistent hypercholesterolemia and to provide a baseline by which to judge a therapeutic response. Generally, drug treatment is reserved for young to middle-aged adults; for older people, diet therapy alone usually is advocated. In the former, failure to lower total cholesterol below 250 mg per dl by dietary change, either because of poor adherence or metabolic resistance, constitutes a reason to consider drugs. Men should be started on drugs before women. Premature CHD in the patient or family and the presence of other risk factors in the patient favor the use of drugs. Finally, a motivated patient is needed to ensure long-term adherence to drugs.

The potential value of drugs for prevention of CHD was revealed by the recent report of the Lipid Research Clinics Coronary Primary Prevention Trial. In this trial, a large number of patients were treated for 7 years with the bile acid sequestrant cholestyramine or placebo. Those in the treatment group had a significantly lower rate of new onset of CHD than did the placebo controls. Therefore, it has now been demonstrated that cholesterol lowering by bile acid sequestrants will decrease risk for CHD.

The only type of drug that can now be strongly advocated for patients with moderate hypercholesterolemia is the bile acid sequestrant. Two agents of this type are currently available—cholestyramine (Questran) and colestipol (Colestid). Both agents bind bile acids in the intestine and prevent their absorption. Loss of bile acids from the intestine decreases the return of bile acids to the liver and thereby releases the feedback control on conversion of cholesterol to bile acids. As a result, the cholesterol content of liver cells falls, which triggers an increase in synthesis of LDL receptors. The latter causes a fall in LDL levels. At typical doses of 8 to 10 grams twice daily, LDL levels decline by 15 to 25 per cent. Although effective, the sequestrants have certain drawbacks. They are expensive and a nuisance to take. They can lead to a variety of minor gastrointestinal complaints, and they cause varying degrees of constipation. However, prolonged use of sequestrants appears to improve their tolerance.

Severe Hypercholesterolemia (Plasma Cholesterol Greater Than 325 Mg per Dl)

Very high levels of plasma cholesterol frequently are due to familial hypercholesterolemia, although other genetic forms of hypercholesterolemia may be associated with cholesterol levels over 325 mg per dl. Familial hypercholesterolemia is the result of a genetic defect in the molecular structure of the LDL receptor. Most patients have the heterozygosis form, and consequently they have only about 50 per cent of the normal number of receptors. The affected patients commonly have tendon xanthomata, and risk for CHD is increased four- to eightfold. CHD often develops in their 30s or 40s in men and in their 40s or 50s in women. When familial hypercholesterolemia is present, 50 per cent of first degree relatives should have elevated cholesterol levels.

Management. Because of the high risk for CHD in patients with familial hypercholesterolemia, treatment is mandatory. Dietary therapy (i.e., a very low fat diet) should be instituted. Unfortunately, most patients do not show adequate cholesterol lowering with dietary change, and drug therapy must be employed. Frequently, two drugs must be used in combination to obtain an adequate reduction in LDL levels. The first step in drug therapy is to use bile acid sequestrants. These should be pushed to maximum dose: cholestyramine, 24 grams, or colestipol, 30 grams. Some patients cannot tolerate the maximal dose, but they should be urged to take as much as possible. The second step is to employ another drug. The best second agent presently available is nicotinic acid. This drug should be started at low dose (100 mg twice a day) and then increased slowly over a period of several days or weeks as tolerated by the patient. The maximal dose is 5 to 6 grams per day, and a major effort should be made to reach a high dose. Most patients treated with full doses of sequestrants plus nicotinic acid usually have a fall in LDL to near the desirable range. Unfortunately, nicotinic acid has several side effects that limit its usefulness. These include abdominal distress, nausea, vomiting, flushing and itching of skin, hepatic dysfunction, glucose intolerance, and hyperuricemia.

Because of the side effects of nicotinic acid, some patients will require an alternative second drug. Fibric acids (clofibrate and gemfibrozil) can produce incremental cholesterol lowering in some patients. Neomycin, which blocks absorption of cholesterol from the intestine, effectively lowers levels of LDL; unfortunately, this drug has not been used in enough patients to be certain of its safety. Probucol is yet another second step drug. It has been shown to be effective in combination with a sequestrant, but at the same time it decreases HDL as well as LDL, and the HDL/LDL ratio does not improve. Thus, probucol should be reserved for patients who fail to respond to other combinations. Finally, another class of drugs is under study that appears to offer great potential for treatment of familial hypercholesterolemia. Two drugs of this class, compactin and mevinolin, act by inhibiting the biosynthesis of cholesterol. This action causes an increase in LDL receptors and a further reduction in LDL levels. In patients with familial hypercholesterolemia, LDL lowering of 25 to 30 per cent by these drugs alone is typical. They are particularly potent when given in combination with bile acid sequestrants; if they prove to be free of side effects, they may replace nicotinic acid as the second best drug for treatment of severe hypercholesterolemia.

Hypertriglyceridemia

Elevations of plasma triglycerides can occur by one or more of three mechanisms. First, there can be a swelling of VLDL particles by triglyceride secondary to increased synthesis of triglyceride in the liver; in this case the number of VLDL particles produced by the liver is not increased—only the triglyceride content of each particle is increased. Second, the lipolysis of triglycerides in VLDL and chylomicrons can be retarded. And third, the number of VLDL particles secreted by the liver can be increased. It has not been proved that the first two causes of hypertriglyceridemia increase the risk for CHD, but overproduction of lipoproteins almost certainly does.

Overproduction of VLDL can be either primary or secondary. The secondary causes are obesity, diabetes mellitus, and, more rarely, the nephrotic syndrome. The causes of primary lipoprotein overproduction are unknown. The lipoprotein pattern resulting from overproduction of VLDL is variable. If triglyceride synthesis is unusually high, the result will be an increase in VLDL alone [type 4 hyperlipoproteinemia (HLP)]. A concomitant defect in lipolysis causes marked hypertriglyceridemia and fasting chylomicronemia (type 5 HLP). If the patient has an abnormality in clearance of VLDL remnants, the result will be a marked accumulation of these particles (type 3 HLP). Finally, a sluggish clearance of LDL will result in an increased plasma LDL (type 2a) or, if VLDL and LDL both are elevated, type 2b HLP. Some patients with overproduction of VLDL have no defects in processing of lipoproteins, and they will be normolipidemic. However, regardless of the lipoprotein phenotype, there is increased risk of CHD.

TABLE 2. **Indications for Drug Therapy in Hypertriglyceridemia**

For prevention of progressive atherosclerosis
Premature CHD in patient or family
Hypercholesterolemia (elevated LDL) in patients or close relatives
Presence of other risk factors (e.g., smoking, hypertension)
A low HDL-cholesterol
Development of hypercholesterolemia (elevated LDL) on weight loss or treatment with fibric acid derivatives (clofibrate or gemfibrozil)
Absence of secondary causes of hypertriglyceridemia (obesity, diabetes mellitus, or antihypertensive medications)
Presence of type 3 HLP
Use drugs in men before women and in young to middle-aged men before the elderly
For prevention of acute pancreatitis
Severe hypertriglyceridemia (plasma triglycerides >1000 mg/dl)
History of pancreatitis or abdominal pain

Management. Although an elevation of plasma triglycerides alone may not be atherogenic, hypertriglyceridemia is a marker for increased risk in many patients. Approximately 30 per cent of patients with CHD have elevated triglyceride concentrations. The mechanisms for their increased atherosclerosis are not well understood, but they possibly include unusually atherogenic VLDL or LDL, intermittent hyperlipidemia, low HDL, or increased flux of lipoproteins. The aim of therapy is not to lower triglycerides per se but to alter the overall atherogenic process. The first aim is to curtail the overproduction of VLDL; if any concomitant defects in catabolism are present, a second objective is to promote clearance of lipoproteins.

Patients with high plasma triglycerides should be treated first with diet and exercise. Caloric restriction will lower the production of VLDL by the liver. Exercise does the same by diverting excess calories to muscle. Many patients with hypertriglyceridemia respond excellently to these maneuvers. If a patient has diabetes mellitus, glucose levels should be brought to normal; a reduction in triglyceride levels will result. In any patient with hypertriglyceridemia, a diet low in cholesterol and saturated fat can be recommended to produce a maximal reduction in LDL levels. The American Heart Association recommends that most patients with hypertriglyceridemia be treated with a very low fat diet, as advocated for hypercholesterolemia. Nonetheless, some patients with hypertriglyceridemia will respond to a very low fat diet with a further elevation in triglyceride levels; in such patients a diet high in monounsaturated fats is a reasonable alternative.

In some hypertriglyceridemic individuals, drug therapy can be considered. Indications for the use of drugs are listed in Table 2. Drugs can be employed in the attempt to prevent CHD, or to prevent acute pancreatitis in the case of marked hypertriglyceridemia. Patients with primary lipoprotein overproduction are at increased risk for CHD, and many cannot be controlled adequately with diet. In favor of this diagnosis are (1) the absence of secondary causes of hypertriglyceridemia, (2) concomitant hypercholesterolemia in the patient or first degree relatives (or a low HDL/LDL ratio), (3) premature CHD in the patient or other family members, (4) development of elevated LDL cholesterol levels on treatment with a fibric acid, and (5) presence of type 3 HLP. These factors demand consideration of drug therapy. Also, hypertriglyceridemia in young patients or those with other risk factors suggests the need for drugs. In patients with severe hypertriglyceridemia and chylomicronemia, drug therapy should be tried to reduce the risk of acute pancreatitis.

The best drug for treatment of overproduction hyperlipidemia theoretically is nicotinic acid, an agent that reduces the synthesis of VLDL. Therefore, if drug therapy seems indicated, nicotinic acid should be given a trial. Some patients tolerate it well and respond adequately. Others cannot tolerate it. The latter can be tried on a fibric acid derivative. Gemfibrozil (1.5 grams twice daily) (the manufacturer's directive states that the daily dose should range between 900 and 1500 mg per day) seems to be a particularly potent agent. It too decreases synthesis of VLDL and also promotes lipolysis of VLDL triglycerides. The fibric acids have several potential side effects, including increased risk for gallstones and myalgias. Treatment of hypertriglyceridemia with a fibric acid almost always leads to a rise in LDL levels. If levels become unusually high, a bile acid sequestrant should be added as a second drug.

Patients with marked chylomicronemia (type 5 HLP), who are at high risk for pancreatitis, sometimes will respond to drug therapy. Both nicotinic acid and a fibric acid can be tried, either as single agents or in combination. An adequate response commonly occurs, but if it does not the patient must be maintained on a very low fat diet.

Low HDL-Cholesterol

Low concentrations of HDL-cholesterol (HDL-C) are another risk factor for CHD. This is particularly true in countries such as the United States where LDL levels tend to be relatively high. In American men, HDL levels normally range between 35 and 50 mg per dl; in Caucasian women the levels are higher, between 50 and 65 mg per dl. The higher concentrations in Caucasian women may be one factor protecting them from premature CHD. If it is assumed that an HDL-C of 50 mg per dl is desirable in men, the following gives the increasing ratio of CHD risk with progressively lower levels: 50 (1.0), 45 (1.2), 40 (1.4), 35 (1.7), 30 (2.1) and 25 (2.6). In other words, a young to middle-aged adult man with an HDL-C of 25 mg per dl has 2.6 times the risk for CHD as one with an HDL-C of 50 mg per dl.

There are multiple causes of low HDL-C: obesity, sedentary life-style, smoking, hypertriglyceridemia, androgenic hormones, genetic factors, and some antihypertensive drugs such as thiazides and propranolol. Certain diets and drugs that lower LDL levels also reduce HDL. This response has been reported for polyunsaturated fatty acids, low-fat diets, low-cholesterol diets, and probucol. Whether concomitant lowering of LDL and HDL without change in LDL/HDL ratios favorably or adversely affects the risk for CHD is unknown.

Management. Although the mechanisms by which low HDL levels enhance the risk for CHD are unknown, it is reasonable to attempt to raise the HDL in patients with low concentrations. Several measures can be recommended: caloric restriction to achieve desirable weight, increased exercise, stopping smoking, treatment of hypertriglyceridemia, and, when possible, curtailment of drugs that reduce HDL concentrations. Also, when choosing a drug for treatment of hyperlipidemia, those that raise HDL (sequestrants, nicotinic acid, gemfibrozil) would be preferred to those lowering HDL (probucol).

OBESITY

method of
ALBERT J. STUNKARD, M.D.,
and THOMAS A. WADDEN, Ph.D.
University of Pennsylvania
Philadelphia, Pennsylvania

Obesity is characterized by an excessive accumulation of fat in the body. For women, this is defined as a body fat content greater than 35 per cent, with 30 per cent the corresponding figure for men. Because of the difficulty in estimating body fat, however, obesity is usually defined in terms of body weight rather than fat. Both men and women are generally considered obese if their weight is 20 per cent greater than that indicated by standard height-weight tables, such as provided by the Metropolitan Life Insurance Company (Table 1). By this criterion, 23 per cent of men and 30 per cent of women may be judged obese. The comparable estimate for children is about 10 per cent.

Obesity is unevenly distributed in the population. It is more common among women than men and is six times more common in women of low socioeconomic status than in those with higher incomes. In addition, there is a steady increase in the prevalence of obesity from childhood to age 50 years, with a two- to threefold increase between the ages of 20 and 64 years.

Etiology

In one sense the cause of obesity is quite simple: Fat accumulates when more calories are consumed than are expended by the organism. In another sense, the answer eludes us, hidden among the multiple determinants of the regulation of body weight. Two very important determinants (over which neither practitioner nor patient has much control) are genetic and developmental. Studies of twins have suggested that obesity is highly heritable. Whether or not it is heritable, it is certainly familial: 80 per cent of the offspring of two obese parents are obese, compared with 40 per cent of the offspring of one obese parent, and only 10 per cent of the offspring of lean parents.

TABLE 1. **Ideal Weight by Height**

Height (Ft/In)	Weight (25–59 yr) Men	Women
4 10		100–131
4 11		101–134
5 0		103–137
5 1	123–145	105–140
5 2	125–148	108–144
5 3	127–151	111–148
5 4	129–155	114–152
5 5	131–159	117–156
5 6	133–163	120–160
5 7	135–167	123–164
5 8	137–171	126–167
5 9	139–175	129–170
5 10	141–179	132–173
5 11	144–183	135–176
6 0	147–187	
6 1	150–192	
6 2	153–197	
6 3	157–202	
6 4		

Values in this table are for height without shoes and weight without clothes.

(From 1983 Metropolitan Height and Weight Tables. Stat Bull Metrop Life Ins Co *64*:2, 1984.)

A person can be obese as a result of an increased number of fat cells (hyperplastic obesity), an increase in the size of the fat cells (hypertrophic obesity), or both. Hyperplasia is particularly likely in persons who became obese in childhood or adolescence. Whereas the size of fat cells can decrease as well as increase at any time in life, the number of fat cells cannot decrease. When obese people lose weight, it is solely by a decrease in the size of their fat cells. Consequently, in order to achieve ideal body weight, persons with hyperplastic obesity must reduce the lipid content of their individual fat cells to an abnormally low level. This problem helps explain the difficulty that these persons experience in reducing to a normal body weight and their proclivity to regain the weight they have lost.

Regulation of Body Weight

Weight is regulated in experimental animals of normal weight. Obese animals also maintain a remarkably constant weight even in the face of environmental challenges. Their obesity appears attributable to an elevation in the set point about which body weight is regulated, rather than to a failure in regulation.

Humans of normal weight also regulate their body weight with considerable accuracy. But lifetime weight histories of obese persons suggest that they do not; they usually show no level about which their body weight is regulated. Obese people may well have the capacity to regulate their body weight, but the set point about which their weight should be regulated is higher than that approved by society. As a result, they go on diets and reduce their weight below what is biologically normal for them. The consequence is a person who is at the same time statistically obese and biologically underweight, or starved. The theory that obese persons may be biologically underweight is suggested by two facts. First, dieters share psychologic characteristics that distinguish them from nondieters. These characteristics, which include chronic hunger, preoccupation with food, and feelings of depression and irritability, may derive from a body weight that is below set point. Second, a mechanism for elevating a set point has been established by the demonstration of an elevated number of fat cells in some obese persons.

A Classification of Obesity

The classification presented in Table 2 incorporates recent findings concerning adipose tissue morphology and suggests appropriate treatments. The classification, originally proposed by John Garrow and revised by one of us (AJS), is a simple threefold one of mild, moderate, and severe obesity, characterized by body weights that are, respectively, 20 to 40 per cent, 41 to 100 per cent, and more than 100 per cent overweight. Table 2 shows that the percentage of obese women falling into these three categories is 90.5, 9, and 0.5 per cent, respectively. Note that these are percentages of the female obese population, not of the total population. Data for men are similar.

TREATMENT

Mild Obesity

Dietary. Dietary treatment is based on a balanced diet of 1000 to 1200 kcal for women and 1500 kcal for men. Consistent with the dietary goals recommended by the United States Senate Select Committee on Nutrition and Human Needs, the diet should derive about 12 per cent of calories from protein, no more than 30 per cent of calories from fat, and the bulk of the remaining calories from complex carbohydrates. Reduction of fat from the current 42 per cent of calories to 30 per cent is particularly important. In addition to reducing low density lipoprotein cholesterol, reduction in fat intake may cause body weight to be regulated at a lower level, as is the case in laboratory animals.

Persons unable to achieve a satisfactory weight loss on the recommended energy intake should not decrease their caloric intake further. It is virtually impossible to meet all the Recommended Daily Allowances for vitamins and minerals on less than 1000 kcal a day. In addition, the deprivation produced by drastic caloric restriction often leads to binge eating and other undesired behavior patterns. Such persons should increase their physical activity rather than reduce their caloric intake.

Moreover, there is a growing belief that for mildly overweight persons the whole idea of dieting is unwise. *Going on* a diet implies *going off* it and the resumption of old eating habits. For this reason the most effective diet may not be a diet at all but rather a gradual change in eating patterns and a shift to calorically dilute foods (fruits, vegetables, and cereals) that the patient

TABLE 2. **Classification of Obesity (Female Obese Population)**

Type	Mild	Moderate	Severe
Overweight (%)	20–40	41–100	>100
Prevalence (%)	90.5	9.0	0.5
Pathology	hypertrophic	hypertrophic hyperplastic	hypertrophic hyperplastic
Complications	uncertain	conditional	severe
Treatment	behavior therapy (lay)	diet and behavior therapy (medical)	surgical

(From Stunkard AJ: The current status of treatment for obesity in adults, *in* Stunkard AJ, Stellar E (eds): Eating and Its Disorders. New York, Raven Press, 1984.)

can continue to eat indefinitely. This plan probably gives the best chance of maintaining a weight loss, and it is an eminently safe one.

Behavior Modification. Formal instruction in behavior modification may help patients achieve the life style change just described. The behavioral treatment of obesity considers in great detail the *behavior* to be changed, its *antecedents,* and its *consequences*. The primary behavior to be changed is eating, and a number of exercises are designed to slow the rate of eating and allow physiologic mechanisms of satiety to exert their effect.

Even greater attention is paid to modifying the antecedents of eating behavior. Efforts extend from the control of relatively remote antecedents such as shopping for food to more proximate ones such as the ready availability of high calorie food. Patients are taught to remove from their environment such stimuli that might elicit eating, to plan strategies to control eating when such stimuli are present, and to avoid television and reading materials that might distract their attention from their efforts at stimulus control. A third element is the reinforcement of desired changes in behavior. Patients (and their family members) are taught to reward proper eating behaviors and to extinguish undesired ones.

Behavioral treatment includes four other major components:

(1) Self-monitoring of food intake and eating behaviors is perhaps the cornerstone of behavioral treatment. Patients record daily the types and quantities of foods consumed and their caloric value, the frequency with which they display appropriate eating behaviors, and the circumstances surrounding inappropriate eating. Careful record-keeping makes it possible to determine which aspects of diet and behavior need to be modified, to develop programs to modify them, to monitor the effectiveness of these programs, and to use this information to make necessary corrections.

(2) Increased physical activity is important for all patients, but particularly for those who cannot achieve a sufficient energy deficit by diet alone. Patients are taught to increase their life style activity by walking rather than riding and using stairs rather than elevators and escalators. Life style activity is preferable to programmed activity, traditionally referred to as exercise, because it is associated with better long-term adherence.

(3) Nutrition education plays an important role in helping patients make sensible food choices. It is designed to implement the dietary recommendations.

(4) Modification of the self-disparaging attitudes which afflict dieters is an important component of treatment. Patients are taught to identify self-punitive thoughts such as, "I'm a failure. I have absolutely no self-control," and to replace them with more positive, coping statements such as, "I'm upset that I've overeaten, but if I stop now I'll still be ahead for the day." One method of attitude modification is to have patients record their self-disparaging comments on one side of a piece of paper and then write down a more rational coping response on the other side.

Treatment Implementation

Behavior modification is easy to specify and therefore to learn. Many of the key elements are available in easy-to-use treatment manuals (such as that of Kelly D. Brownell, Ph.D., University of Pennsylvania, Department of Psychiatry, Philadelphia, PA 19104 or Richard B. Stuart's Act Thin, Stay Thin, published by Jove Press, 1983). Although few physicians themselves conduct behavioral programs, more and more of them are hiring nutritionists and nurses to conduct weight control groups within their practices. By far the greatest number of obese persons, however, are treated under the auspices of lay-led groups. Prominent among them are Take Off Pounds Sensibly (TOPS) and Overeaters Anonymous (OA), the two largest nonprofit organizations, and Weight Watchers, the largest commercial group, which has a strong behavioral component.

TOPS, founded in 1948, was the first self-help group for obesity, and it now enrolls more than 300,000 persons. The key elements of TOPS are weekly meetings that provide group support, weekly weigh-ins that are a high point of the meeting, and policy supervision from the national headquarters. The membership of TOPS is almost exclusively female, middle-aged, and of lower middle class socioeconomic status; the average member is 60 per cent overweight.

Overeaters Anonymous, though also a nonprofit organization, differs greatly from TOPS. OA was derived directly from Alcoholics Anonymous and follows the procedures of its parent organization in great detail. Thus, there is both pressure for self-revelation and strong social support. Persons who find such a program congenial often obtain substantial benefit for their emotional problems, as well as for their weight.

Commercial weight loss organizations appeal to much the same clientele as do the nonprofit ones, and with somewhat greater success; Weight Watchers opens its doors to approximately 1 million people a week. Weight Watchers has added three important elements to the programs pioneered by the nonprofit groups—behavior modification, inspirational lecturers drawn from successful members, and a carefully designed nutritional program. Weight Watchers is available to persons with even a casual interest in weight reduction and at a cost of only $6 a week.

Treatment Effectiveness

When conducted by professionals, behavior modification programs produce an average weight loss of 0.45 kg (1 lb) a week for up to 6 months. Longer treatment may produce losses even greater than 12 kg. The effectiveness of behavior modification in self-help and commercial programs, however, is difficult to evaluate because of the very high drop-out rates associated with this form of treatment. Attrition as great as 70 per cent has been reported for both TOPS and Weight Watchers. Despite these problems, the low cost and ready availability of lay-led groups make them an important resource for the control of mild obesity. Very large numbers of persons can be reached by these programs and their very low costs result in favorable cost/effectiveness ratios. Physicians can often be of greatest help to patients by encouraging them to enroll in a lay-led program and then enquiring at subsequent office visits about the patients' participation in the program.

Moderate Obesity

Persons 41 to 100 per cent overweight, who have failed to lose weight using conventional approaches, require more aggressive treatment. Very-low-calorie diets and pharmacotherapy are two options, neither of which is entirely satisfactory.

Very-Low-Calorie Diets. These diets provide 300 to 600 kcal per day, with approximately 70 grams of protein and optional small amounts of carbohydrate. The diets are available in the form of an egg- or milk-based formula protein (mixed with water) or as fish, fowl, and lean meat. Both types of diets must be supplemented by a multipurpose vitamin, 30 to 50 mEq of potassium, and small amounts of calcium and sodium. Both diets produce dramatic weight losses, averaging 20 kg in 12 weeks, with even larger losses for longer treatment.

Current very-low-calorie diets (in contrast to the liquid protein diets of 1976–1977) appear to be safe when limited to periods of 3 to 4 months under careful medical supervision. This supervision includes proper selection of patients to eliminate those with a history of cardiovascular, hepatic, or renal disease, type I diabetes, psychosis, or cancer. After an initial physical examination and electrocardiogram, patients must be monitored at least every other week for abnormalities in electrolytes, uric acid, liver function, and blood pressure (hypotension). An electrocardiogram is recommended after every 10 to 15 kg weight loss.

For ease and thoroughness of administration, we recommend referral of appropriate patients to hospitals or clinics specializing in the use of very-low-calorie diets. In addition, we encourage patients to find a program that includes training in behavior modification, for without it they will regain during the ensuing year approximately two thirds of the weight lost (as we discovered in a recent clinical trial). Patients who receive instruction in behavior modification in addition to the very-low-calorie diet achieve a better long-term outcome.

Pharmacotherapy. This is always mentioned among treatments for obesity and had been viewed, until recently, as the cornerstone of medical treatment. A major obstacle to pharmacologic treatment was exerted, however, by the directives of the Drug Enforcement Administration restricting the use of the amphetamines, the most widely used appetite suppressant medication.

Weight regain following pharmacologic treatment is just as serious a problem as it is with very-low-calorie diets. A recent study found that patients treated by fenfluramine (Pondimin) for 6 months lost 14.5 kg but regained more than half of the lost weight in the year following treatment. Efforts to improve maintenance of weight loss with the help of behavioral techniques proved of no avail.

The regaining of weight following treatment

with appetite suppressant medication has been explained by the theory that this medication acts primarily by lowering a body weight set point and only secondarily by suppressing appetite. The implications of this theory are radical: use appetite suppressant medication on a chronic basis or not at all. For if medication lowers a body weight set point, discontinuing medication, with the return of the set point to its previous level, subjects patients to powerful biologic pressures to regain the weight that they have lost.

Severe Obesity

During the past 10 years, surgery has become the treatment of choice for that small percentage of persons who suffer from severe obesity. The first operation to be widely accepted was the jejunoileal bypass, designed to bypass most of the absorptive surface of the bowel and thereby limit the absorption of nutrients. Although it produced large weight losses that were well maintained, complications of the operation, including chronic diarrhea and liver damage, were so serious and unremitting that the jejunoileal bypass is no longer performed. It has been replaced by gastric restriction surgery.

Gastric Restriction. Gastric restriction procedures are designed to reduce the volume of the stomach to as little as 50 ml and the passageway from this restricted stomach to no more than 1.2 cm in diameter. These procedures include the older gastric bypass and the increasingly popular vertical banded gastroplasty. Food intake is greatly reduced, leading to 1 year weight losses of 30 to 55 kg, or about 50 per cent of excess weight. Weight losses tend to be well maintained at 2 years' follow-up, although patients can defeat the purpose of the operation by consuming calorically dense liquid meals or by stretching the stomach's capacity by repeated overeating.

The most common complication of the operation is vomiting, which initially occurs on an average of three times a week but may be a more serious problem in some patients. Health benefits are substantial and include marked alleviation of hypertension, diabetes, hyperlipidemia, arthritis of the weight-bearing joints and, in fact, all the complications attributable to severe obesity. Furthermore, the social functioning of most patients is markedly improved.

Criteria for Electing Surgery. The following points should be addressed in considering surgical treatment:

(1) Patients must be at least 100 per cent overweight and have attempted to lose weight by conventional means.

(2) Patients should be referred to a surgeon who specializes in the operation. The operative mortality of such surgeons is less than 0.5 per cent, and morbidity is correspondingly low.

(3) Behavioral and dietary counseling should be available following surgery to help patients cope with psychologic problems and select a proper diet.

PELLAGRA

method of
JOHN E. CANHAM, M.D.
Alameda, California

Pellagra represents a lack of dietary niacin (nicotinic acid). Niacin, ubiquitous in nature, is generally associated with plant or animal proteins. Humans also synthesize niacin from the amino acid tryptophan, with approximately 60 mg of tryptophan being converted to 1 mg of niacin. Hence, an adequate intake of the vitamin or of a good biologic value protein should protect against pellagra. Unfortunately, a diet deficient in the vitamin but with adequate tryptophan intake may not be adequate if there is an imbalance of the protein's amino acids. Pellagra occurs primarily in population groups in which corn is the main energy source, but is seen in India where sorghum is the staple.

While the tryptophan content of corn is low, that of sorghum and millet is better, but because of the high levels of leucine in these latter cereals, an imbalance appears to be created that alters the enzymatic activities of the metabolic pathway of tryptophan, resulting in decreased production of nicotinamide nucleotide. Though corn's content of tryptophan is low, the niacin content is sufficient to prevent pellagra if it were available. Unfortunately, the niacin in corn and in several other cereals is in a bound form (niacytin) and is unavailable for absorption. In Central America and Mexico, the pretreating of corn prior to cooking with lime water frees the niacin for absorption. Pellagra is rare in these high corn consumption areas. Hence, the dietary pathogenesis of pellagra involves many factors which frequently lead to mixed deficiencies.

Niacin or one of its derivatives is required by all living cells. It is an essential component of two coenzymes: nicotinamide adenine dinucleotide (NAD^+) and nicotinamide adenine dinucleotide phosphate ($NADP^+$), which are employed in the functions of over 250 dehydrogenases. Besides their function in tissue respiration, they are active in lipid, amino acid, and protein metabolism. With performance of such essential functions in all organs and in all cells, it is understandable that a deficiency could have multiple manifestations. Unfortunately, not one measurable biochemical parameter is specific and diagnostic of niacin deficiency.

The practicing physician must have a sufficient level of suspicion whenever a patient is encountered who has a malfunction of one or more of the commonly involved organ systems. It must be remembered that the occurrence of pellagra in the USA today, due solely to dietary deficiencies in otherwise normal humans, is most rare. The identification of niacin as a component of NAD^+ and $NADP^+$ in 1935, the demonstration in 1937 that niacin cured the canine equivalent of pellagra (black tongue), and the subsequent flour enrichment program begun in the early days of World War II provided the knowledge and an approach to eliminate the widespread epidemics of pellagra seen in the southeastern states and parts of the midwest in the first 4 decades of this century. Today pellagra usually occurs as a complication of alcoholism, food faddism, combined dietary deficiencies arising from drug addiction, or the isolation and neglect of the elderly who are unable to care for themselves. It also occurs as a complication of chronic diseases of the gastrointestinal tract, such as Crohn's disease, gastrointestinal neoplasia, and severe malabsorption. The pellagra syndrome has been reported in patients with carcinoid syndrome due to conversion of the majority of ingested tryptophan to 5-hydroxytryptamine with markedly decreased conversion to niacin; with Hartnup's disease—a familial aminoaciduria with multiple manifestations, including impaired absorption and metabolism of tryptophan; and as a consequence of antituberculosis therapy with isoniazid or pyrazinamide.

Active treatment is based on the severity of the disease's manifestations. While all organ systems may be involved, those demonstrating the most signs and symptoms are the skin, the gastrointestinal tract, and the nervous system. The dermatitis classically begins as a bilateral redness usually affecting the backs of hands, forearms, backs of feet, front and sides of neck (Casal's necklace), and those dermal areas exposed to pressure or chronic irritation. The lesions over the pressure points and the exposed surfaces of the body become thickened, hyperkeratotic, and hyperpigmented. Secondary infection may develop. The entire gastrointestinal tract may be involved from cheilosis and fissuring of the lips to inflammation of the anal mucosa. The tongue is most characteristic—with redness, atrophy of the epithelium, hypertrophy of the fungiform papillae with associated pain and discomfort sufficient to limit eating and, sometimes, talking. The involvement of the rest of the gastrointestinal tract is variable; diarrhea and abdominal discomfort are the principal symptoms. Malabsorption may or may not be present. Similarly, the signs of nervous system involvement are quite variable, ranging from depression, fear, and confusion to hallucinations and disorientation. In general, most pellagrins are anorexic, complain of weakness and tiredness, and appear chronically ill. It is wise to remember that pellagra may be present without dermatologic manifestations, particularly in hospitalized patients or individuals with limited outdoor exposure.

Treatment

While therapy with a diet well balanced with high biologic value protein, high in niacin and the other B-complex vitamins, plus supplemented nicotinamide, is ideal, the patient's glossitis, stomatitis, and malabsorption may make that approach difficult. If that be the case, bed rest is essential and is best coupled with the intravenous administration of niacinamide, 50 to 100 mg, two to three times per day. Peripheral parenteral nutrition may be desirable as a means of providing complete mixtures of the other vitamins and a balanced amino acid preparation containing tryptophan. While parenteral nutrition should not be vigorous, it can help alleviate the problem of malabsorption and correct the associated vitamin deficiencies generally found. Oversupply, intravenously, of fluids and glucose in these semistarved individuals can produce an acute refeeding syndrome. The response of the gastrointestinal tract and the nervous system is usually rapid. As soon as is feasible, the patient should be started on a balanced diet—a soft or semiliquid diet may be necessary at first, then proceed to a balanced diet in keeping with the patient's needs and acceptability. As soon as practical, oral nicotinamide, 100 to 150 mg twice a day, should be substituted for the intravenous vitamin. A therapeutic multiple vitamin tablet should be given twice a day.

The goal of therapy is to correct all dietary inadequacies and provide a balanced diet sufficient in protein (1 gram per kg per day) and calories (30 to 35 calories per kg per day) to correct the protein-calorie and vitamin deficiencies that generally accompany pellagra.

During treatment, remember that nicotinic acid (niacin) orally or parenterally can produce distressing vasomotor responses owing to the release of histamine. Nicotinamide is definitely the agent of choice.

Prevention

If the pellagra is due to underlying disease, corrective action is imperative if at all possible. Before returning the patients to their own resources, re-education to ensure an adequate intake of niacin and a good biologic value protein is essential. The assistance of a dietitian may be invaluable in finding foods that are acceptable to the patient from both an economic and organoleptic standpoint.

RICKETS AND OSTEOMALACIA

method of
MICHAEL P. WHYTE, M.D.
Washington University
St. Louis, Missouri

Rickets is the term used to describe the clinical consequences of a generalized failure of skeletal matrix to mineralize in infants and children. *Osteomalacia* refers to the bone disorder that results from the same problem in adults. Neither definition denotes a specific disease—each is a generic term that describes a similar clinical outcome from a variety of pathogenetic mechanisms that disrupt the orderly deposition of mineral into bone matrix. Indeed, the same pathologic processes can cause either rickets or osteomalacia, depending simply on the patient's age. Medical therapy must be designed to correct or to circumvent the specific derangement in mineral homeostasis and, except for dosage, will be the same regardless of the patient's age and whether the clinical diagnosis is therefore rickets or osteomalacia. Nevertheless, it is important to distinguish and understand the differences between rickets and osteomalacia, since the physical and radiographic presentation and the outcome of effective medical therapy differ in each condition.

In rickets, all three processes of skeletal development are adversely affected:

1. Growth—in which cartilage cells in the epiphyses ("growth plates") normally proliferate and then undergo degeneration and calcification (endochondral bone formation), thereby enabling bone to lengthen.
2. Modeling—in which osseous tissue is deposited and removed at the outer and inner surfaces, respectively, of a bone to shape its contour and determine the thickness of its cortex (subperiosteal bone formation and endosteal bone resorption).
3. Remodeling—the process by which cortical (compact) and trabecular (spongy) bone are resorbed and then reformed in accordance with the structural and metabolic needs of the body.

In osteomalacia, only the process of bone remodeling is affected since epiphyses are fused and skeletal growth and modeling have largely ceased; hence, the generalized defect in bone mineralization is usually less apparent clinically than when it occurs before puberty. Rickets is associated with short stature (epiphyseal defects) and deformity of the extremities (modeling defects), whereas both rickets and osteomalacia involve defective bone remodeling that can result in generalized osteopenia or occasionally in osteosclerosis.

Vitamin D Metabolism

During the past two decades, a great deal has been learned about the metabolism and physiologic role of vitamin D (Table 1). Despite fortification of dairy products with vitamin D_2 or D_3 in the United States (400 IU per quart of milk), the majority of antirachitic activity in healthy Americans has been found to come from the cutaneous synthesis of vitamin D_3. 7-Dehydrocholesterol in the skin is converted first to "previtamin D" by ultraviolet light and then to cholecalciferol, which, in turn, is transported by a high affinity binding protein to liver and muscle tissue for storage. Cholecalciferol should therefore no longer be regarded as a vitamin, since its principal source is endogenous. Furthermore, both vitamins D_2 and D_3 undergo a series of bioactivation steps—first in the liver to form the 25-hydroxymetabolite [25(OH)D], and then in the kidney to form 1,25-dihydroxyvitamin D [1,25$(OH)_2$D]—before they act on a variety of target tissues. Vitamins D_2 and D_3 appear equally susceptible to these hydroxylation steps, and their metabolites seem equipotent in regulating mineral metabolism; 1,25$(OH)_2$D is the most potent form of vitamin D as judged by its ability to increase gastrointestinal absorption of calcium. Rightfully, the vitamin D "complex" is now regarded as a group of steroid hormones rather than as a vitamin, since cholecalciferol is metabolized and then acts at sites other than its place of synthesis. Current nomenclature for vitamin D and its metabolites emphasizes the hormonal nature of these compounds (Table 1).

General Guidelines for Therapy

Effective medical therapy can be expected to correct defects in the three processes of skeletal development in rickets and restore bone remodeling in osteomalacia. Since endochondral bone formation is defective in rickets, radiographic changes such as widening of the growth plates and metaphyseal irregularity are helpful in diagnosis and follow-up of therapy (however, they should not be confused with similar radiographic defects that occur in a variety of skeletal dysplasias). Pseudofractures (Looser's zones) are a hallmark of rickets or osteomalacia, although this finding is uncommon. Other radiographic findings are less helpful. Coarsening of trabecular bone is observed in only some patients with osteomalacia. Osteopenia often cannot be distinguished from other causes (e.g., osteoporosis).

Although the patient's history, physical examination, and radiographic and biochemical studies are usually all that is necessary to diagnose and treat most forms of rickets or osteomalacia, the clinician should be aware that defective bone mineralization can be documented and followed with greatest confidence by histomorphometric study of serial specimens of bone tissue that are not decalcified prior to histologic examination. An appropriate specimen can be obtained easily under local anesthetic by trephine biopsy of the iliac crest. However, the patient should receive two 3-day courses of oxytetracycline (Terramycin) or demeclocycline (Declomycin) (about 10 mg per

TABLE 1. **Nomenclature of Vitamin D (Calciferol) and Its Metabolites***

Chemical	Vitamin	Abbreviation
Ergocalciferol	Vitamin D_2	D_2
Cholecalciferol	Vitamin D_3	D_3
25-Hydroxyergocalciferol	25-Hydroxyvitamin D_2	$25(OH)D_2$
25-Hydroxycholecalciferol	25-Hydroxyvitamin D_3	$25(OH)D_3$
1,25-Dihydroxyergocalciferol	1,25-Dihydroxyvitamin D_2	$1,25(OH)_2D_2$
1,25-Dihydroxycholecalciferol	1,25-Dihydroxyvitamin D_3	$1,25(OH)_2D_3$

*Throughout the text, the abbreviations vitamin D, 25(OH)D, and $1,25(OH)_2D$ are used to indicate either the D_2 or D_3 compound or a mixture of each.

kg per day in divided doses)—separated by 2 weeks—before biopsy. (The final dose of the tetracycline preparation should be administered 3 to 4 days before biopsy). In rickets or osteomalacia, when properly stained undecalcified sections of bone are obtained following administration of two courses of tetracycline: (1) routine light microscopy will reveal increased quantities of osteoid covering trabecular bone surfaces, and (2) fluorescence microscopy will fail to demonstrate two discrete tetracycline labels at the osteoid/mineralized bone interface. These two histologic findings (osteoidosis and failure to deposit discrete tetracycline labels) reflect the essence of the pathogenesis of all forms of rickets or osteomalacia, i.e., that osteoblasts have been successful in depositing bone matrix (osteoid), yet there has been failure of the osteoid to mineralize.

Although examination of a bone specimen following administration of tetracycline is the definitive method by which to establish and quantitate defective bone mineralization, it is my opinion that bone biopsy is not mandatory in the routine clinical management of most patients with rickets or osteomalacia. In rickets, clinical history, physical examination, radiographic studies of growth plates (specifically posteroanterior views of the wrists and the anteroposterior views of the knees), and serial biochemical studies are sufficient for diagnosis and follow-up therapy. In osteomalacia, unless there are pseudofractures that can be followed radiographically, symptoms and biochemical studies will be the major parameters to follow. Bone densitometry, if available, is also useful.

Effective therapy for rickets will be associated with normalization of endochondral bone formation (a process that can be observed readily by serial radiographic studies of the growth plates of the wrists and knees) and with correction of abnormal biochemical values. The biochemical parameters that are most useful to follow in either rickets or osteomalacia include circulating calcium and inorganic phosphate concentrations and alkaline phosphatase activity. In most forms of rickets or osteomalacia, urinary excretion of calcium (corrected for creatinine) in 24-hour collections is also a critical parameter by which to judge efficacy of therapy (as well as to monitor for vitamin D toxicity). In rickets, correction of short stature and skeletal deformity are important goals of treatment; therefore, careful physical examination provides significant parameters that can be used to monitor therapy. If, however, there is suspicion that healing of rickets or osteomalacia is not complete, histologic inspection of nondecalcified sections of iliac crest (following two oral courses of tetracycline) is indicated.

Most forms of rickets and osteomalacia can be treated with great success. However, a correct diagnosis is essential not only for a favorable clinical outcome, but to avoid intoxication with vitamin D or its metabolites. Ideally, there will be attention to and correction of the primary pathologic process. Often, however, this will not be possible, and pharmacologic doses of vitamin D (or one of its biologically active metabolites) will be necessary together with mineral supplementation. Currently, four different forms of vitamin D are available in the United States (Table 2). These include vitamin D_2, $25(OH)D_3$, $1,25(OH)_2D_3$, and dihydrotachysterol (DHT). The U.S. Food and Drug Administration (FDA) has thus far approved $25(OH)D_3$ (Calderol) and $1,25(OH)_2D_3$ (Rocaltrol) for use in the treatment of renal osteodystrophy. DHT (Hytakerol) is a synthetic analogue of $1,25(OH)_2D$. DHT and $1,25(OH)_2D_3$ are approved by the FDA for treatment of hypoparathyroidism. FDA approved uses for the metabolites of vitamin D are likely to increase in the future.

The pathogenetic mechanisms for rickets and osteomalacia are fairly numerous. The correct therapeutic regimen (which may involve a choice of vitamin D, or one of its metabolites, in a very great range of therapeutic doses) will depend upon a correct diagnosis and understanding of the mechanism for any underlying aberration in vitamin D stores or metabolism. The appropriate dose and route of administration of vitamin D_2, or some of the more recently available vitamin D metabolites [$25(OH)D_3$ and $1,25(OH)_2D_3$], will depend upon successfully identifying and then correcting or circumventing the precise defect in mineral metabolism. Significant consequences (hypercalcemia, hypercalciuria, nephrocalcinosis,

TABLE 2. **Pharmaceutical Preparations of Vitamin D (and Active Metabolites)**

	Ergocalciferol	Dihydrotachysterol	Calcifediol	Calcitriol
Abbreviation	D_2	DHT	$25(OH)D_3$	$1,25(OH)_2D_3$
Trade Name	Calciferol Drisdol	Hytakerol DHT	Calderol	Rocaltrol
Dosage form	a. Capsules: 1.25 mg b. Liquid: 200 μg/ml c. Intramuscular injection: 12.5 mg/ml in sesame oil	a. Tablets: 0.125, 0.200, and 0.400 mg b. Liquid: 0.250 mg/ml	Capsules: 20 and 50 μg	Capsules: 0.25 and 0.50 μg
Time to reach maximum biologic effects	4–10 weeks	2–4 weeks	4–20 weeks	½–1 week
Persistence of biologic effect after cessation	6–30 weeks	2–8 weeks	4–12 weeks	½–1 week

and renal failure) can result from improper diagnosis and therapy.

The clinician should recognize that the active metabolites of vitamin D have the theoretical advantage of circumventing a defect in vitamin D metabolism. Furthermore, each metabolite has a more rapid onset of action and shorter biologic half-life than the parent sterol. However, they are also more expensive. Also be aware that several preparations are available for calcium and inorganic phosphate supplementation in the treatment of rickets and osteomalacia (Tables 3 and 4, respectively). Oral calcium supplements that are composed of carbonate salt are less expensive (for equal amounts of elemental calcium) than other preparations (gluconate). Although liquid preparations for inorganic phosphate supplementation are least expensive, I have been pleased with the patient acceptability and tolerance of K-Phos-Neutral tablets, which seem to cause less diarrhea.

Although measurement of circulating vitamin D_2 and D_3 levels would seem to provide the most direct biochemical way to assess vitamin D status before treatment, assays for the parent sterols are not readily available. Measurement of the circulating 25-hydroxyvitamin D [25(OH)D] concentration is currently the best way to evaluate vitamin D stores; these assays measure $25(OH)D_2$ and $25(OH)D_3$ together. Accurate assays for circulating 25(OH)D and $1,25(OH)_2D$ levels are now readily available in commercial laboratories.

Appropriate follow-up visits are necessary for all treatable forms of rickets or osteomalacia, but the interval between visits will depend upon the specific diagnosis and type of therapy. Once therapy has been successful in correcting rickets or osteomalacia, it is important to realize that resolution of the "hungry bone syndrome" has occurred and that urinary calcium excretion may abruptly increase as the skeleton no longer acts as a sump for mineral deposition. Normalization of previously abnormal biochemical studies, however, should herald this event. When this observation occurs, readjustment of vitamin D and mineral supplementation therapy is likely to be necessary. Therefore, careful monitoring of urinary calcium excretion is important. Unless there is renal failure, hypercalciuria will generally precede hypercalcemia. Thus, 24 hour urine collections that are assayed for calcium and creatinine (creatinine to assess the reliability of the collection) are especially important in patient follow-up. Increases in urinary calcium from subnormal levels will also provide evidence of therapeutic efficacy, since hypocalciuria is present in many untreated forms of rickets or osteomalacia.

With a correct diagnosis and proper choice of therapy, the astute clinician will often be rewarded with a patient for whom he or she has

TABLE 3. **Calcium Supplements (Oral) for Treatment of Rickets and Osteomalacia**

Preparation	Per Cent Elemental Calcium	Dosage Form	Amount That Contains 1 Gram of Elemental Calcium
Calcium carbonate	40	Suspension	12.5 ml
		Tablets: 420 mg	6 tablets
		650 mg	4 tablets
Calcium lactate	13	Tablets: 325 mg	24 tablets
		650 mg	12 tablets
Calcium gluconate	9	Tablets: 650 mg	17 tablets
		1000 mg	11 tablets
Calcium glubionate	7	Syrup	43.5 ml

TABLE 4. **Phosphate Supplements (Oral) for Treatment of Rickets and Osteomalacia**

Preparation (Trade Name)	Amount Containing 1 Gram Phosphorus
Neutra-Phos	4 capsules*
Neutra-Phos-K	4 capsules*
K-Phos Neutral	4 tablets
K-Phos Original	9 tablets
Fleet's Phospho-Soda	6.7 ml

*Each capsule is reconstituted with 75 ml of water, fruit juice, or cola. A powder concentrate is also available.

been able to eliminate bone pain and muscle weakness, to restore growth, and to prevent fracture and deformity. Therapeutic regimens for specific types of rickets or osteomalacia are outlined in the following sections.

Therapeutic Regimens for Specific Forms of Rickets or Osteomalacia

Vitamin D Deficiency Rickets and Osteomalacia

PRIMARY ("NUTRITIONAL") VITAMIN D DEFICIENCY. Primary deficiency of vitamin D_3 is an unusual but unfortunately persistent cause of both rickets and osteomalacia. Most vitamin D activity comes from cutaneous synthesis of vitamin D_3. In healthy individuals, the minimum daily requirement of vitamin D necessary to prevent this disorder is just 10 micrograms (400 IU) for children and 2.5 micrograms (100 IU) for adults. "Nutritional" rickets or osteomalacia is actually a socioeconomic disease that is due to lack of sunshine when consumption of dairy products fortified with vitamin D has been insufficient to prevent the disorder. Therefore, primary deficiency of vitamin D is generally found in individuals who, because of economic, social, or cultural factors, do not receive sufficient exposure to sunlight (5 to 20 minutes several times weekly) for adequate cutaneous synthesis of vitamin D_3 and whose diets do not contain sufficient foodstuffs fortified with vitamin D. Institutionalized patients, the poor, the elderly, food faddists, and some religious groups (because of diet and dress) are most likely to be affected. Infants who are breast-fed generally receive sufficient antirachitic sterol; however, babies who are bottle-fed with nonfortified milk are likely to become vitamin D–deficient. Measurement of circulating 25(OH)D is useful when a diagnosis of vitamin D deficiency is not readily achieved by routine medical history, physical examination, and biochemical and radiographic studies. Blood levels less than about 6 ng per ml (normal: 10 to 50) are considered diagnostic of vitamin D deficiency.

Although education of the patient (or parents) and the reversal of the etiologic socioeconomic factors would be the most satisfying way to treat and prevent vitamin D–deficient rickets or osteomalacia, this may be difficult to achieve. Pharmacologic therapy is rapid, inexpensive, and effective and is therefore usually indicated. For children who are too young to swallow even small capsules, a liquid preparation of vitamin D_2 is available (see Table 2). They should receive 4000 IU of vitamin D_2 (100 micrograms) daily for several months. With successful therapy, detectable biochemical and radiographic improvement can often be documented in as early as 7 to 10 days. However, a follow-up visit for radiographic and biochemical studies after 2 months of therapy is appropriate. Once there has been healing, as demonstrated by radiographic and biochemical studies, patients can then receive the recommended daily allowance (RDA) of 400 IU per day in their food, either by consuming adequate amounts of fortified foods (dairy products) or by supplementation with pediatric multivitamin preparations that contain the RDA for vitamin D. For children who can take capsules, one 50,000 IU capsule (1.25 mg) of vitamin D_2 orally once *weekly* for three or four doses is an inexpensive, simple, and effective regimen prior to RDA maintenance doses.

For patients with especially severe disease, such as those with hypocalcemia, it is helpful to administer a single "loading dose" of vitamin D_2 (to replete body stores rapidly) and also to supplement calcium intake. I use a single oral dose of about 5000 IU (125 micrograms) of vitamin D_2 per kg of body weight. For a 70 kg adult with severe vitamin D deficiency osteomalacia, this is about 350,000 IU (seven 50,000 IU capsules). Although this single loading dose of vitamin D_2 is massive compared with the RDA (and helps illustrate the body's large storage capacity for vitamin D), it is quick, effective, and safe. When there is symptomatic hypocalcemia, intravenous administration of calcium for several days (20 mg of elemental calcium per kg of body weight *per day* slowly in divided doses) together with a more long-term course of oral calcium supplementation (1 to 2 grams of elemental calcium daily) is advisable. Serum calcium levels should be determined several times daily if calcium is administered intravenously. For individuals who are not intolerant to milk, three to four 8 ounce glasses per day will supply both calcium and inorganic phosphate to mineralize the skeleton. Failure of patients to show biochemical and radiographic improvement, with persistently low 25(OH)D levels after 1 month of therapy, may reflect malabsorption or failure of the patient to comply with therapy. If rickets persists despite documentation of normal circulating 25(OH)D levels, one of the vitamin D–dependent or resistant syndromes (to be discussed) should be considered.

Secondary Vitamin D Deficiency. Despite adequate sunlight exposure and a diet fortified with vitamin D, some patients develop deficiency of vitamin D from a variety of gastrointestinal, pancreatic, or heptobiliary disorders. The mechanism for vitamin D deficiency and deranged mineral metabolism is often complex. Vitamin D and its principal metabolite 25(OH)D are fat-soluble sterols that undergo enterohepatic circulation. Bile salts are necessary for their absorption; hence, hepatobiliary disease or short bowel syndrome may result in steatorrhea and both malabsorption of dietary vitamin D and depletion of endogenous vitamin D_2 and D_3 stores. Here again, occasional assay of circulating 25(OH)D levels [25(OH)D_2 and 25(OH)D_3] may be helpful to document vitamin D deficiency and then monitor therapy. In some instances, however, the underlying skeletal disease in adults will be osteoporosis rather than osteomalacia. In these cases, iliac crest biopsy is useful. It should be noted that vitamin D deficiency and defective skeletal mineralization may result from "subclinical" malabsorption. Furthermore, malabsorption may lead to hypomagnesemia, which, in turn, causes hypocalcemia from impaired parathyroid hormone secretion or action. Circulating magnesium levels should therefore be assayed in patients with skeletal disease due to malabsorption. Hypomagnesemia can be corrected with oral or intramuscular magnesium supplementation.

Although the pathogenesis of this type of rickets or osteomalacia is often complex and involves malabsorption of antirachitic sterols, therapy is generally straightforward and should lead to gratifying results. Since patients with rickets or osteomalacia resulting from these disorders are a heterogeneous group, adequate therapy will require an individualized approach and follow-up. *Pharmacologic* doses of ergocalciferol (vitamin D_2) given orally often prove effective and are relatively inexpensive. Vitamin D_2 is readily converted to 25(OH)D_2 even when there is parenchymal liver disease.

As with severe primary vitamin D deficiency, a single oral "loading" dose of vitamin D_2 of about 125 micrograms (5000 IU) per kg of body weight and intravenous calcium supplementation (20 mg of elemental calcium per kg of body weight *per day* slowly in divided doses) are indicated when there is symptomatic hypocalcemia. Following the "loading" dose of vitamin D_2, patients with secondary vitamin D deficiency will continue to require pharmacologic therapy. It is also important to recognize that patients may need changes in their regimen as rickets or osteomalacia heals and as underlying gastrointestinal or hepatobiliary disease evolves or responds to therapy. Vitamin D_2, 50,000 IU (1.25 mg), orally three times a week, is a reasonable starting dose for milder disease. Again, it must be emphasized that therapy for any disorder with pharmacologic doses of vitamin D_2 requires periodic follow-up. Assay of circulating 25(OH)D levels about 1 month after therapy begins (and continuing about every 6 months thereafter) can be used to assure that oral absorption of vitamin D_2 has been, and remains, successful. Circulating 25(OH)D levels should be maintained in the mid-normal to upper range of normal. Assay of calcium and creatinine excretion in 24 hour urine collections before and periodically during therapy should (1) reveal correction of hypocalciuria, (2) help to assess when skeletal mineralization is complete, and (3) help to guard against vitamin D_2 toxicity (which will often present as hypercalciuria).

Although oral supplementation with vitamin D_2 is usually successful in this group of disorders, if a patient's vitamin D status is not corrected, intramuscular injection of vitamin D_2 should be considered. (In 1979, in the United States, the potency of the two commercially available preparations for intramuscular administration of vitamin D_2 was questioned. Currently, only one product is manufactured (see Table 2); the potency is reported to be 500,000 IU (12.5 mg) of vitamin D_2 per 1 ml of sesame oil.) Vitamin D_2, a fat-soluble sterol, is dissolved in sesame oil during the preparation of this pharmaceutical; therefore, antirachitic activity has delayed bioavailability. Increased circulating 25(OH)D levels will not be observed for several weeks following a single injection of this preparation, but vitamin D_2 release will persist for several months after one dose. A single intramuscular injection of about 500,000 IU (one ml) every few months should provide effective and continuous vitamin D_2 supplementation.

Anticonvulsant Rickets and Osteomalacia

A high incidence of rickets and osteomalacia has been reported for institutionalized subjects receiving anticonvulsant medication. This observation led to extensive studies of the effects of anticonvulsant drugs on mineral homeostasis. Although it was subsequently found that defective bone mineralization could be attributed to primary deficiency of vitamin D in many of these patients, it is now clear that some subjects who receive anticonvulsants (primarily phenytoin) metabolize vitamin D abnormally and may become vitamin D–deficient. Therefore, patients who receive significant doses of phenytoin or phenobarbital should also receive 50,000 IU of vitamin D_2 orally once weekly with periodic assay of levels of circulating 25(OH)D and urinary calcium and creatinine in 24 hour collections if initial values are low.

Vitamin D–Dependent Rickets

Vitamin D–dependent rickets (VDDR) includes autosomal recessive or sporadic disorders that mimic vitamin D deficiency rickets clinically, biochemically, and radiographically. Although the precise metabolic defects remain unknown, abnormalities in the synthesis or action of the active metabolites of vitamin D [25(OH)D and $1,25(OH)_2D$], in the absence of gastrointestinal or renal disease, represent fundamental abnormalities. They are referred to as vitamin D "dependent" because *physiologic* doses of vitamin D_2 fail to generate a good clinical response; however *pharmacologic* doses of vitamin D_2 have been reported to overcome the basic defect in some patients, whereas others respond to physiologic or pharmacologic doses of the biologically active vitamin D metabolites.

VDDR-TYPE I. VDDR-Type I is characterized by normal circulating 25(OH)D levels, but subnormal $1,25(OH)_2D$ concentrations. A fundamental defect appears to be insufficient formation of $1,25(OH)_2D$ at normal circulating substrate [25(OH)D] levels. This defect, at the level of renal 25(OH)D,1α-hydroxylase, can be overcome by pharmacologic doses of vitamin D_2 (20,000 to 60,000 IU per day), which increase circulating 25(OH)D levels. Since there is no defect in the liver's ability to convert vitamin D_2 to $25(OH)D_2$, administration of vitamin D_2—rather than $25(OH)D_3$—is less expensive yet appropriate therapy. Understandably, pharmacologic doses of 25(OH)D or physiologic amounts of $1,25(OH)_2D_3$ are also effective but are more expensive than vitamin D_2 supplementation. The observation that *physiologic* doses of $1,25(OH)_2D_3$ (0.25 to 2.0 μg per day) will correct VDDR-Type I illustrates that the defect is at the renal 25(OH)D,1α-hydroxylase level. Even though use of $25(OH)D_3$ or $1,25(OH)_2D_3$ to treat VDDR-Type I is an expensive approach to therapy, it has advantages. The circulating and physiologic half-lives of these metabolites of vitamin D_3 are much shorter than those of vitamin D_2. Excessive dosing will therefore respond rapidly to modification. Most patients, however, can be managed with vitamin D_2, but periodic follow-up is essential.

VDDR-TYPE II. VDDR-Type II is also a rare autosomal recessive or sporadic disorder. Alopecia is an interesting clinical finding in some patients. In this disorder, even though circulating 25(OH)D levels are unremarkable, $1,25(OH)_2D$ levels are normal or increased. A variety of receptor or postreceptor defects for the action of $1,25(OH)_2D$ account for this form of rickets. Whereas most patients respond to very high doses of $1,25(OH)_2D_3$ (10 to 40 micrograms per day), some show clinical, radiographic, and biochemical improvement with high doses of vitamin D_2 or $25(OH)D_3$. One patient who failed to respond to $1,25(OH)_2D_3$ showed improvement while receiving an experimental preparation of $24,25(OH)_2D_3$.

Hypophosphatemic Rickets and Osteomalacia

The pathogenesis of most, but not all, forms of rickets or osteomalacia includes an aberration in mineral metabolism such that calcium and inorganic phosphate (Pi) levels in extracellular fluid are insufficient to permit normal skeletal mineralization. In the disorders already discussed, deficiency in the action or perhaps the tissue levels of the physiologically active forms of vitamin D resulted in hypocalcemia, secondary hyperparathyroidism, and hypophosphatemia from the phosphaturic action of parathyroid hormone. In these disorders, hypocalcemia and hypophosphatemia act in concert to lower the circulating "calcium-phosphate product" in blood, and subsequently there is defective mineralization of newly synthesized osteoid. There are, however, a group of disorders in which renal Pi wasting and hypophosphatemia (without significant changes in circulating calcium levels) can be regarded as a major pathogenetic defect. The expression "hypophosphatemic rickets" or "osteomalacia" is the term used for this group of metabolic bone diseases. Although the approach to therapy is therefore often similar, it must be recognized that this is, again, a *generic* term that emphasizes the pathogenesis of the skeletal disease. Therapy for each entity in this group of disorders is discussed next.

SEX-LINKED HYPOPHOSPHATEMIC RICKETS (SLHR). This is the most common form of rickets in the United States. It is inherited as an X-linked dominant trait in which hemizygous males are generally more severely affected biochemically and clinically than heterozygous females. Although the precise genetic defect is unknown, renal Pi wasting with subsequent hypophosphatemia is considered the major abnormality that must be addressed therapeutically. However, an important associated defect includes failure to generate increased circulating $1,25(OH)_2D$ concentrations in response to hypophosphatemia. Furthermore, there is malabsorption of calcium from the gastrointestinal tract as an associated, but unexplained, problem.

Demonstration that these patients may show some clinical improvement following high doses of vitamin D_2 therapy alone prompted the term "vitamin D–resistant rickets" (VDRR) in the 1930s. As noted earlier, many forms of rickets have now been identified that can be considered vitamin D–resistant. VDRR, therefore, like hypophosphatemic rickets or osteomalacia, should be regarded as a generic term and should not represent a final diagnosis.

SLHR, when treated in the past with very high doses of vitamin D_2 (e.g., 100,000 IU daily), occasionally healed. However, there were a considerable number of disadvantages to this therapy. Prolonged hypercalcemia, hypercalciuria, nephrocalcinosis, and renal failure were not uncommon. Often, these problems occurred when patients were not followed closely for vitamin D toxicity. The long storage half-life of vitamin D_2 and unexplained periodic fluctuations in circulating calcium levels accounted for the hypercalcemia, which could persist for months after withdrawal of vitamin D_2 supplementation in these cases. An additional disadvantage of "high dose" vitamin D_2 therapy was that it had to be discontinued months in advance of osteotomy to avoid hypercalciuria (induced by immobilization) during the prolonged postoperative course of that era.

When the defect of renal Pi wasting was subsequently addressed, an improved clinical, biochemical, and radiographic response was noted. Augmentation of circulating Pi levels was achieved by frequent oral supplementation (2 to 3 grams of phosphorus, as inorganic phosphate, daily). Pi was given frequently throughout the day (with a dose at bedtime to increase nocturnal Pi levels). Radiographic evidence of healing, increasing growth rate, and histologic improvement were observed in many patients. Lower doses of vitamin D_2 (50,000 IU orally two or three times weekly) were continued to facilitate calcium absorption from the gastrointestinal tract in order to minimize any permissive effect of circulating parathyroid hormone on phosphaturia.

Current clinical trials, however, suggest that pharmacologic doses of $1,25(OH)_2D_3$ (calcitriol) are most efficacious in promoting gastrointestinal absorption of both calcium and Pi in SLHR. When used carefully in conjunction with frequent oral Pi supplementation in compliant patients, $1,25(OH)_2D_3$ has been reported to correct skeletal growth, modeling, and remodeling defects. Indeed, this combination of $1,25(OH)_2D_3$ and Pi supplementation is now considered "state-of-the-art" therapy for SLHR.

$1,25(OH)_2D_3$ and Pi supplementation therapy should begin at an early age in children with SLHR to avoid deformities. However, since significant deformities of the legs do not occur in SLHR until a child stands, therapy might begin at this time. If the child has bowing or knock-knee deformity, orthopedic consultation should be sought since bracing may be important. Monitoring therapy will be difficult until reliable urine collections can be obtained. Unfortunately, only 0.25 and 0.50 microgram capsules of $1,25(OH)_2D_3$ (Rocaltrol) are commercially available at this time (see Table 2); there is no liquid preparation. For young children who are unable to swallow these small capsules, they may be dissolved in applesauce. A therapeutic (pharmacologic) dose of approximately 50 ng (0.050 microgram) per kg of body weight once daily should be achieved after a 2 to 3 month period by gradually increasing the dose. During this time, Pi supplementation should also be introduced (see Table 4). The ideal regimen includes Pi supplements given five to six times daily (with a dose before bedtime) to attempt to correct the hypophosphatemia. The dose of Pi supplementation achieved is, unfortunately, often less than optimal (2 grams per day as phosphorus for an adult) because of its common adverse effect, i.e., gastrointestinal upset, especially diarrhea. If this adverse effect occurs, Pi should be stopped for a few days, then resumed at a lesser (but maximum) amount that can be tolerated without symptoms. Some children develop "tolerance" to the gastrointestinal upset, and the dose can be increased after about 1 month of therapy. In my experience, K-Phos Neutral (see Table 4) is tolerated best by patients. Periodic increments in $1,25(OH)_2D_3$ and Pi supplementation should be anticipated as the child grows and gains weight. Careful biochemical assessment is also necessary for this regimen since $1,25(OH)_2D_3$ is especially potent in increasing calcium absorption from the gastrointestinal tract. As in the era of high dose vitamin D_2 treatment for SLHR, potential adverse effects of therapy include hypercalcemia, hypercalciuria, and so on. Even though these are potential complications with pharmacologic doses of $1,25(OH)_2D_3$, an advantage of $1,25(OH)_2D_3$ therapy is that the short circulating and biologic half-life of this metabolite permits rapid resolution (several days) should hypercalcemia or hypercalciuria occur (see Table 2).

It is important to recognize that hypercalciuria, not hypercalcemia, should be screened for as evidence of early $1,25(OH)_2D_3$ toxicity in patients with SLHR but with otherwise normal renal function. Calcium and creatinine should be assayed in 24-hour urine collections. Initially, these collections should be obtained monthly and then perhaps every other month. Hypercalciuria ($>$ 4 mg of urinary calcium per kg of body weight *or* $>$ 300 mg of urinary calcium per gram of urinary creatinine) may occur suddenly once skeletal mineralization has been successful. A lower dose of $1,25(OH)_2D_3$ will be necessary, but will remain therapeutic at that time. When *hypo*calciuria persists after several months of full dose $1,25(OH)_2D_3$ and Pi therapy, increased milk consumption or $CaCO_3$ supplementation can be used to bring urinary calcium levels into the normal range. The creatinine clearance of patients who receive this regimen should be monitored yearly. Abrupt decreases in high dose Pi supplementation therapy should be avoided, since urinary calcium levels may rapidly rise (Pi binds calcium in the gastrointestinal tract).

Physicians who treat SLHR must not be lulled into thinking that closure of the epiphyses at puberty indicates that therapy has cured their patients and can be discontinued. The metabolic defect of SLHR persists throughout life. Some patients may require therapy during adulthood to prevent skeletal deformity. Furthermore, the approach of the orthopedic surgeon to bowing deformity of the legs in SLHR often is to perform osteotomies only after epiphyses have closed, so as to minimize the possibility of postoperative deformity. Therefore, $1,25(OH)_2D_3$ and Pi therapy may be especially important at this time. With modern techniques, if patients are weight bearing within a few days of surgery, $1,25(OH)_2D_3$ therapy need not be discontinued. However, if immobilization is to be longer, discontinuation of $1,25(OH)_2D_3$ may be necessary until weight bearing resumes (to avoid immobilization hypercalciuria). Similarly, if a child is bedridden for more than a few days for any reason (e.g., fracture), $1,25(OH)_2D_3$ therapy should be temporarily stopped. The efficacy and benefits of long-term $1,25(OH)_2D_3$ and Pi supplementation for adult SLHR require further investigation.

ONCOGENIC RICKETS AND OSTEOMALACIA. This is a rare sporadic disorder that is due to a variety of usually benign mesenchymal neoplasms, especially hemangiopericytoma, nonossifying fibroma, and various bone tumors. These neoplasms appear to elaborate a factor or factors that cause phosphaturia and inhibit renal $25(OH)D,1\alpha$-hydroxylase activity. Impaired hydroxylation of 25(OH)D by the kidney to $1,25(OH)_2D$ (with subnormal circulating $1,25(OH)_2D$ levels) leads to malabsorption of calcium, mild hypocalcemia, and hypocalciuria. The predominant abnormality, however, is significant hypophosphatemia, which is especially important in lowering the circulating calcium-phosphate product. When possible, definitive diagnosis and treatment are achieved by resection of the neoplasm. Therefore, thorough diagnostic evaluation to exclude this disorder is important in sporadic cases of hypophosphatemic rickets or osteomalacia. When resection of a tumor is not possible, Pi supplementation and $1,25(OH)_2D_3$ therapy, often with pharmacologic doses of $1,25(OH)_2D_3$, will be necessary.

ANTACID-INDUCED OSTEOMALACIA Excessive use of phosphate-binding antacids (magnesium and aluminum hydroxides) can result in profound hypophosphatemia and hypophosphaturia and can therefore cause defective bone mineralization. Patients may actually hyperabsorb dietary calcium and become hypercalciuric since their hypophosphatemia acts physiologically to stimulate renal $25(OH)D,1\alpha$-hydroxylase activity, thereby increasing blood $1,25(OH)_2D$ levels. Despite the effects on calcium homeostasis, hypophosphatemia predominates and results in defective bone mineralization.

Since elimination, change, or reduction in the amount or type of antacid should rapidly correct the hypophosphatemia, Pi supplementation and vitamin D therapy will not be necessary. Although dietary phosphorus intake is usually quite variable, it is generally sufficient to allow for proper skeletal remineralization soon after excessive doses of antacid are eliminated. Depending on severity, it may take several months to observe normalization of increased circulating alkaline phosphatase activity as excessive osteoid is mineralized.

SPORADIC HYPOPHOSPHATEMIC RICKETS OR OSTEOMALACIA. Antacid-induced hypophosphatemia, Fanconi's syndrome, oncogenic osteomalacia, and hyperparathyroidism must be excluded prior to making this diagnosis. Some of these patients will represent new mutations for sex-linked hypophosphatemic rickets (SLHR). Therapy with $1,25(OH)_2D_3$ and Pi supplementation (as for patients with SLHR) appears to be most effective.

FANCONI'S SYNDROME. Renal Pi wasting is a frequent complication of proximal renal tubular dysfunction in Fanconi's syndrome. Therapy with $1,25(OH)_2D_3$ and Pi (see section on SLHR) is appropriate in Fanconi's syndrome associated with rickets or osteomalacia. However, urinary calcium levels must be monitored carefully, since hypercalciuria is more likely than in SLHR.

Metabolic Acidosis

Hyperchloremic metabolic acidosis from renal disease occasionally causes rickets or osteomalacia. The pathogenetic mechanisms are complex, but the skeletal disease responds well to vitamin D_2 supplementation and alkali therapy (divided doses of 10 to 15 grams of sodium bicarbonate daily). Alkali therapy to correct the acidosis is important and should be continued after pharmacologic doses of vitamin D_2 help to correct the mineralization defect. Vitamin D_2, about 1.25 mg (50,000 IU) three times a week, is indicated until healing occurs. However, urinary calcium and creatinine must be monitored frequently, since acidosis per se can cause hypercalciuria. Finally, calcium and potassium supplementation may be necessary at the onset of alkali therapy to guard against tetany and hypokalemia.

Renal Failure

In uremia, the most frequent form of skeletal disease (osteitis fibrosa) results from concomitant secondary hyperparathyroidism (in which bone remodeling is rapid). The reader should look elsewhere for details concerning medical therapy for this disorder. However, in some patients with uremia, skeletal disease is characterized by a mineralization defect. Several mechanisms have been documented:

1. *Aluminum intoxication:* Uremic patients who use aluminum-containing antacids to bind dietary phosphate (to prevent secondary hyperparathyroidism) may absorb and deposit excessive amounts of aluminum in bone. This aluminum inhibits skeletal mineralization. Therapy generally consists of altering the antacid regimen. In some cases, deferoxamine (Desferal) has been reported to be a useful chelating agent for aluminum.

2. *Hypophosphatemia*: Overzealous use of phosphate-bindng antacids in uremic patients can produce hypophosphatemia, which, in turn, can cause hypophosphatemic rickets or osteomalacia.

3. *Parathyroid insufficiency*: Devastating osteomalacia has been reported in some uremic patients who have undergone complete or "excessive" parathyroidectomy for treatment of secondary or tertiary hyperparathyroidism. Parathyroid hormone appears to be necessary for bone apposition in uremia. Pharmacologic doses of vitamin D (or its metabolites) and calcium supplementation have been used to treat this disorder, but with little success.

Calcium-Deficient Rickets

Rarely, profound deficiency of dietary calcium intake will result in rickets or osteomalacia. Some untreated cases of hypoparathyroidism or pseudohypoparathyroidism may present with rickets or osteomalacia. In these patients, hypocalcemia is so profound that it causes defective bone mineralization although there is concomitant hyperphosphatemia. Normalization of circulating calcium levels will readily reverse this disorder.

Rickets and Osteomalacia Due to Inhibitors of Bone Mineralization

Rickets or osteomalacia can occur from excessive ingestion of a few inhibitors of bone mineralization:

1. *Aluminum*: Rare case reports suggest that defective bone mineralization can occur in otherwise healthy individuals when high concentrations of aluminum are leached into food from cookware. More frequently, patients with uremia who ingest excessive quantities of aluminum-containing antacids may develop this problem (see earlier section on Renal Failure).

2. *Fluoride*: Pharmacologic doses of sodium fluoride given for prolonged periods of time (most likely in attempted therapy for osteoporosis) may result in osteomalacia. Defective bone mineralization will respond to discontinuation of the fluoride therapy.

3. *Disodium etidronate*: This is a diphosphonate compound used to treat patients with Paget's bone disease and to prevent heterotopic calcification in individuals who undergo hip replacement surgery. Excessive or prolonged therapy with this compound will lead to rickets or osteomalacia as a direct result of its pharmacologic actions to inhibit bone mineralization.

Miscellaneous Disorders

A variety of rare inherited or sporadic conditions present with rickets or osteomalacia even though circulating concentrations of calcium and Pi are normal or even increased. There is no specific medical therapy for these disorders. A correct diagnosis at the outset is important because therapeutic "trials" of vitamin D (or its metabolites) or calcium supplementation may lead to hypercalcemia and hypercalciuria.

Hypophosphatasia is an inherited inborn error of metabolism characterized biochemically by subnormal circulating alkaline phosphatase activity. Defective skeletal mineralization appears to be a direct result of deficient alkaline phosphatase activity in osseous tissue. *Fibrogenesis imperfecta ossium,* a disorder reported in a few sporadic cases, appears to be due to defective skeletal mineralization from a primary defect in the skeletal matrix. *Axial osteomalacia* is characterized radiographically by coarsening of the trabeculae of the axial skeleton. Osteomalacia appears to be due to a primary defect in the osteoblast.

SCURVY

method of
ALAN COHEN, M.D.
Children's Hospital of Philadelphia
Philadelphia, Pennsylvania

Diagnostic Considerations

Scurvy occurs so rarely in the United States and other major industrialized nations that the recognition of this disorder can be considered part of the treatment. Disturbances of the integument, vasculature, bones, joints, and nervous system give rise to clinical findings that are nondistinctive when considered individually but which, in the aggregate, form a singular pattern (Table 1). In young children, irritability, bone tenderness and swelling, and lassitude dominate the clinical picture.

Lind recognized the link between nutritional deficiency and scurvy more than 200 years ago, and awareness of this relationship is no less important today in identifying the susceptible patient. Scurvy occurs in elderly or impoverished individuals who lack sufficient interest or money to eat fresh fruits and vegetables or the numerous canned or frozen foods that are rich in vitamin C (Tables 2 and 3). Infantile scurvy has vir-

TABLE 1. **Clinical Manifestations of Scurvy**

Integument hyperkeratosis perifollicular congestion poor wound healing friable gums	Vasculature easy bruising pinpoint hemorrhage
Bones and Joints fracture subperiosteal hemorrhage scorbutic rosary (children) bone tenderness hemarthrosis loose teeth	Central Nervous System lassitude emotional changes irritability

tually disappeared with the addition of vitamin C to cow's milk formula. Occasional cases of scurvy still occur in exclusively breast-fed infants of mothers with severe vitamin C deficiency.

Iron overload may cause scurvy in patients with normal dietary vitamin C by accelerating the conversion of ascorbic acid to oxalic acid. Other disorders such as hyperthyroidism, infection, thermal burns, and cigarette smoking may increase the requirement for vitamin C without causing frank scurvy.

Low levels of vitamin C in plasma or leukocytes support the diagnosis of scurvy although the correspondence between clinical findings and laboratory measurements is often imprecise. Plasma levels of less than 0.25 mg per dl and leukocyte levels of less than 10 to 15 micrograms per 10^8 WBC usually indicate deficient stores of vitamin C.

Treatment

Administration of vitamin C, 200 to 500 mg daily in single or divided doses, rapidly improves the sense of well-being and reverses the clinical manifestations in patients with nutritional scurvy. Most patients can be treated with oral vitamin C using either ascorbic acid tablets or orange juice. Each ounce of fresh or frozen orange juice contains approximately 15 mg of vitamin C. Intravenous preparations of vitamin C are available for patients who cannot be treated orally. Skin and bone lesions begin to heal after 2 to 3 days of therapy, although complete resolution may require several weeks. Oral or parenteral supplementation with vitamin C should continue until a normal diet has been restored.

The usual therapeutic doses of vitamin C are potentially toxic to iron-overloaded patients. When scurvy occurs in patients with hemochromatosis, the use of low doses of vitamin C (50 to 100 mg daily) with concomitant iron chelation therapy may reduce the risk of treatment.

TABLE 2. **Vitamin C Content in Single Portions of Common Foods**

Broccoli	140 mg
Brussels sprouts	135 mg
Orange juice	124 mg
Orange	113 mg
Cantaloupe	90 mg
Strawberries	88 mg
Cauliflower	69 mg
Spinach	50 mg
Boiled potato	36 mg
Lima beans	29 mg
Asparagus	25 mg
French fried potato	16 mg

TABLE 3. **Differences in Vitamin C Content of Spinach According to Method of Preservation or Preparation**

Type of Spinach	*Wt of 1 Cup (Grams)*	*Vitamin C Content of 1 Cup (Mg)*
raw	55	28
cooked, fresh	180	50
canned	205	29
frozen, chopped	205	39
frozen, whole leaf	190	53

Prevention

The recommended daily allowance of vitamin C to maintain normal stores is shown in Table 4. Normal individuals with well-balanced diets rarely require supplemental vitamin C. Breast milk from vitamin C–replete mothers contains 50 to 60 mg of vitamin C per liter, and infant formulas have been supplemented to achieve similar levels.

Recent studies have refuted earlier claims that high doses of vitamin C prevent the common cold and prolong the survival of patients with advanced cancer. While conventional doses of vitamin C are safe and nontoxic (except in the presence of iron overload), chronic ingestion of doses in excess of 2 to 3 grams has been associated with hemolysis in patients with G6PD deficiency and

TABLE 4. **Recommended Daily Allowance of Vitamin C**

Age (Yr)	*Vitamin C (Mg per Day)*
0–1	35
1–10	45
11–14 (male)	50
11–14 (female)	60
15–51+	60

During pregnancy, add 20 mg per day.
During lactation, add 40 mg per day.

also with the formation of renal stones. Some infants born to mothers receiving large doses of vitamin C develop scurvy when given normal amounts of the vitamin, presumably caused by a temporary metabolic maladaptation. These concerns about toxicity argue cogently for rigorous analysis of the benefits of high doses of vitamin C before such therapy is promoted in the medical or lay press.

VITAMIN K DEFICIENCY

method of
C. THOMAS KISKER, M.D.
University of Iowa
Iowa City, Iowa

Vitamin K is not a single compound but rather a series of compounds, which have in common a naphthoquinone nucleus. Vitamin K_1, a fat-soluble naphthoquinone, is present in many foods and is particularly abundant in leafy vegetables like spinach and cabbage, cauliflower, and broccoli. Vitamin K_2, also fat-soluble, is synthesized by certain bacteria found in the distal large intestine. Because both these naturally occurring vitamin Ks are fat-soluble, effective absorption depends on the presence of bile salts and normal fat absorption. Menadione, vitamin K_3, is a synthetic vitamin K derivative. Water-soluble salts of menadione can be directly absorbed from the intestine but must, however, be converted to an active form by the liver.

The daily requirement for vitamin K in adults may be as little as 0.03 microgram per kg; an infant requires 0.15 to 0.25 microgram per kg per day. Thus, the recommended 100 micrograms of vitamin K per day in the diet is more than sufficient to satisfy the daily requirement. There is little storage of vitamin K in the body, and breast milk contains only 1.5 micrograms per dl. Without supplementation, therefore, the newborn breast-fed infant is at high risk for developing vitamin K deficiency.

Deficiency States (Table 1)

In the absence of vitamin K, core zymogens are synthesized, but the lack of gamma carboxylation prevents their activation in the coagulation cascade. Patients with vitamin K deficiency, therefore, develop a bleeding diathesis. Excessive hemorrhage may follow local trauma or may occur spontaneously in severe deficiency states. Easy bruising, bleeding from puncture wounds or surgical incisions, epistaxis, gastrointestinal bleeding, hematuria, and even intracranial hemorrhage may occur.

Deficiency states occur in a number of clinical settings. Though rare in adults, dietary deficiency may occur in infants who are exclusively breastfed. Older children and adults who are severely anorectic as a result of chemotherapy or major surgery may also develop a deficiency state. Since the dietary forms of vitamin K are fat-soluble, any disorder that impairs absorption of fat, including a reduction of bile salt excretion, may lead to vitamin K deficiency. Patients with chronic diarrhea, cystic fibrosis, sprue, ulcerative colitis, regional enteritis, or obstructive jaundice from any cause are candidates for the development of vitamin K deficiency. The use of broad-spectrum antibiotics often contributes to the development of vitamin K deficiency by reducing intestinal bacteria and secondarily the bacterial synthesis of vitamin K. In these clinical settings, prevention of vitamin K deficiency with supplementation is indicated.

Prevention (Table 2)

Neonates

The lowest concentrations of the vitamin K–dependent coagulation factors are reached on the second or third day of postnatal life. Though this reduction is not necessarily the result of vitamin K deficiency, the gradual increase in the vitamin K–dependent proteins that occurs following the

TABLE 1. **Vitamin K Deficiency Treatment**

Patient	Preparation	Dose	Route
Infant			
Mild deficiency	K_1 AquaMEPHYTON	1 mg × 1	IM
Severe deficiency	K_1 AquaMEPHYTON	1 mg × 1	IV
Severe deficiency with life-threatening bleed	K_1 AquaMEPHYTON Fresh frozen plasma	1 mg × 1 15 ml/kg	IV IV
Older Child and Adult			
Mild deficiency	K_1 AquaMEPHYTON	2.5–10 mg	IM
Severe deficiency	K_1 AquaMEPHYTON	2.5–10 mg	IV
Severe deficiency with life-threatening bleed	K_1 AquaMEPHYTON Factor IX concentrate (Konyne, Proplex)	2.5–10 mg 50 units/kg	IV IV

TABLE 2. **Vitamin K Prophylaxis**

Patient	Preparation	Dose	Route
Infant			
≥2000 grams	K_1 AquaMEPHYTON	1 mg × 1	IM
<2000 grams	K_1 AquaMEPHYTON	0.5 mg × 1	IM
Older Child and Adult			
No restricted intake	K_1 Mephyton	2.5–5 mg daily	PO
Restricted oral intake	K_1 AquaMEPHYTON	2.5–5 mg weekly	IM

initial decrease will be aborted if the infant is vitamin K–deficient. There is little storage reserve of vitamin K in the infant. The infant diet, particularly breast milk, contains little vitamin K, and the infant has inadequate intestinal bacterial flora for synthesis of the vitamin. Thus, significant vitamin K deficiency may occur if additional vitamin K is not provided. One mg of vitamin K_1 (AquaMEPHYTON) should be given intramuscularly to all full-term neonates at birth. For infants weighing less than 2000 grams, 0.5 mg of vitamin K intramuscularly is sufficient. Vitamin K_3 (menadione) or its derivative in high doses is to be avoided in newborn infants, for it may produce hemolytic anemia with subsequent hyperbilirubinemia, particularly in premature infants. The very ill—particularly hypoxic—newborn infant may not respond to vitamin K because of immaturity of the liver and impairment of synthesis of the vitamin K–dependent proteins.

Older Children and Adults

Vitamin K deficiency in the older child or adult may be the result of inadequate intake of vitamin K, decreased production by organisms in the gastrointestinal tract, failure of absorption, or interference with the normal function of vitamin K as a result of administration of a vitamin K antagonist, such as a warfarin-type drug. Regardless of the cause, correction of vitamin K deficiency in the older child or adult is most rapidly achieved by the intramuscular or intravenous administration of 2.5 to 10 mg of vitamin K_1. Following administration, a significant improvement in the prothrombin time will be apparent within 2 to 4 hours, and complete correction is usual within 48 to 72 hours. Care should be exercised in intravenous administration of vitamin K. The rate of administration should not exceed 1 mg per minute, with careful observation for signs and symptoms of anaphylaxis.

When bleeding is severe or life-threatening, immediate correction of the clotting factor deficiencies may be indicated. This can be achieved by the administration of prothrombin complex concentrates (Konyne, Proplex). At present, administration of these concentrates is associated with a risk for the development of hepatitis and aquired immunodeficiency disease (AIDS). Heat treatment of the product is thought to alleviate the risk of AIDS as the AIDS-associated HTLV III virus is very sensitive to heat treatment. However, the concentrates also contain variable amounts of clot-promoting activity, which can cause thrombosis in the recipient. Although these risks may be reduced with future preparations, currently the concentrates are contraindicated in patients with liver disease and in those with prior thrombotic tendencies. When not contraindicated, the intravenous administration of the concentrate at a dose of 50 units of factor IX per kg of body weight will immediately correct the clotting factor deficiencies and provide adequate hemostasis until permanent correction following vitamin K administration has occurred.

Fresh frozen plasma, 15 ml per kg of body weight given intravenously, will also partially correct the bleeding defect in vitamin K deficiency. Plasma transfusion, however, requires additional time, does not achieve full correction of clotting factor activity, and may result in fluid overload. Fresh frozen plasma transfusion, nonetheless, may be a helpful adjunct to vitamin K administration in patients with severe vitamin K deficiency in whom the prothrombin complex concentrates are contraindicated.

OSTEOPOROSIS

method of
ROBERT S. WEINSTEIN, M.D.
Medical College of Georgia
Augusta, Georgia

Osteoporosis is an age-related disorder characterized by a reduction in bone mass below that normally expected for the sex and race of an individual. Bone that remains has a normal ratio of mineral to organic bone matrix. Osteoporosis, therefore, is a condition in which the amount of bone in the skeleton is diminished but the quality of the bone is unchanged. The reduced bone mass leads to mechanical failure and fracture. These fractures occur most commonly in the eighth to twelfth thoracic and the first three lumbar vertebrae, in the proximal femur, in the distal radius, and occasionally in the ribs. Fractures above the sixth thoracic vertebrae are rarely due to osteoporosis and suggest metastatic disease. Women sustain fractures more frequently than men and whites more frequently than blacks. Black individuals with vertebral fractures blacks. Black individuals with vertebral fractures should be considered to have a secondary cause of bone loss. Secondary causes are also suggested whenever blood and urine determinations reveal abnormal calcium or phosphorus concentrations. In the United States, about 1.3 million fractures each year are attributable to osteoporosis, with an estimated annual cost of 3.8 billion dollars.

Bone remodeling is a tightly interlocked regulatory system, and any agent that inhibits bone resorption (e.g., calcium, estrogens, calcitonin) will later reduce the rate of bone formation. If bone remodeling slows, skeletal losses will be attenuated, but the delay in replacement of old or damaged bone may nonetheless lead to skeletal failure.

A few proposed treatments of osteoporosis induce a redistribution of skeletal assets. Administration of a synthetic fragment of human parathyroid hormone or long-term exposure to sodium fluoride may increase the mass of trabecular or cancellous bone at the expense of increased porosity and thinning of the compact cortical bone. Such treatment may reduce the risk of vertebral fractures but lead to fractures at sites composed primarily of cortical bone, such as the proximal femur. Because the consequences and clinical benefits of drug interference with bone remodeling remain unclear, treatment of osteoporosis should begin with general measures.

Treatment

General Therapeutic Strategies. After diagnosis is made based on histologic examination of undecalcified bone and after secondary causes of bone loss have either been excluded or treated, the patient with osteoporosis should be educated and rehabilitated. The physician must avoid pressures to prescribe drugs for osteoporotic fractures before employing more general measures that may otherwise lack emphasis or be neglected.

Patient Education. Patients with documented osteoporosis should be aware that since 10 to 15 million people in the United States have osteoporosis, the problem is not unique. Reassurance that some spontaneous improvement in back pain is likely is usually appreciated. Patients should be instructed on the importance of preventive measures such as avoidance of lifting heavy weights, of stooping or bending to lift objects, and of sports with a risk of trauma or a fall (horseback riding, basketball, volleyball). Loose rugs and stairs without sturdy bannisters should be repaired or else avoided. The use of a cane can provide better balance and reduce the possibility of a fall in wet or slippery weather. Trauma to the spine may be decreased with the use of rubber heels. High heels increase the chance of a fall and must be avoided. Patients should be made aware of the need to remain ambulatory to avoid the further bone loss that occurs with immobilization and should be encouraged to participate in formal exercise and dance programs. Patients should be informed about the lack of value of drug therapy in established osteoporosis and that withdrawal of drugs that impair balance (e.g., barbiturates) or increase bone loss (e.g., glucocorticoids, ethanol) may be far more efficacious.

Physical Therapy and Rehabilitation. Most patients with osteoporosis are asymptomatic. Back pain, when present, is of two types. A new vertebral fracture may be accompanied by the sudden onset of sharp, severe pain, aggravated by motion and located directly over a vertebral process. Muscle spasm is often present but generalized skeletal tenderness and nerve root compression are usually absent. This pain can be diminished by 2 to 3 weeks of bed rest on a hard mattress, with plywood placed between the box springs and mattress to improve spinal support and with a sheepskin covering over the mattress to provide soft contact with the spine. The patient should lie on the back with a thin pillow under the head and a pillow of regular thickness under the knees to avoid undue strain on the spine. Some patients feel better if they lie on their side rather than on their back. A small pillow should then be used to fill the hollow of the flank. In this position, it helps to have the hips and knees somewhat bent and to place a small pillow between the knees. Acetaminophen with 30 mg of codeine should be taken every 6 hours if necessary. A laxative may be necessary. Propoxyphene (Darvon) may substitute for the codeine. Careful use of a heating pad or lamp and gentle massage are often helpful. If pain persists after a 2 to 3 week trial of bedrest, a back support may be necessary to enable ambulation.

Chronic dull back pain is more commonly observed and results from paravertebral muscle spasm without spinous process tenderness. Progressive dorsal kyphosis from vertebral compression fractures leads to forward bending of the torso and prominent horizontal abdominal skin folds. Moreover, this stooped-over posture may decrease the pulmonary vital capacity and result in complaints of easy fatigability and difficulty in breathing. Opiates should be avoided with these long-term problems, but acetaminophen, propoxyphene, and massage are useful to relieve pain and muscle spasm. Optimal treatment requires measures to improve posture, increase muscle tone, and loosen stiffened joints. An excellent back extension exercise can be done in a sitting position: inhale deeply and slowly squeeze the shoulder blades together, exhale and relax. In patients with severe osteoporosis, exercises can be done in a supine position: bring both knees to the chest, hold for a count of five, then return to starting position. Another exercise to strengthen both lumbar and abdominal muscles is to lie supine with one knee brought to the chest, raise the opposite foot 6 inches off the floor while keeping the knee straight, lower the leg slowly to the floor and then repeat with the other leg. Lumbar flexion exercises should be avoided. Each exercise should be done 5 times each day at first, gradually advancing to 20 repetitions as strength increases.

Calcium Therapy. The rationale for the use of oral calcium supplementation in osteoporosis is based on the decline in the ability of the intestine to adapt to a low calcium intake with age and the evidence for low calcium intake in older women. All age-related changes, however, correlate to some degree with loss of bone mass and may not be causal effects. Decreased intestinal calcium absorption may compensate for the reduction in bone formation rate which is characteristic of senescent osteoblasts and may not be an indication for increased calcium intake. On the other hand, patients with lactase deficiency or those with a lifelong avoidance of dairy products appear to be at increased risk for osteoporosis. Although there is some evidence that calcium supplements may reduce the rate of bone loss and the incidence of fractures, the finding is not universal and double-blind controlled studies have not been done. If increased intestinal absorption of calcium is maintained on calcium supplements, the additional calcium absorbed may simply be wasted in the urine. Despite these reservations, calcium therapy is widely used and seems to be safe if hypercalciuria is avoided. Serum calcium determinations are also important since some older women may become hypercalcemic on the calcium supplement. Calcium should not be given to patients with a history of kidney stones.

The current practice is to increase the calcium intake to 1000 to 1500 mg per day. An 8 oz glass (240 ml) of skim milk contains 275 to 300 mg of calcium, but few older people can tolerate enough milk for it to be an adequate supplement. Supplementation with calcium tablets is usually necessary with attention to their elemental calcium content rather than the total weight of the calcium salt. Calcium supplements made from bone meal or mineral clay (dolomite, montmorillonite) may be contaminated with lead and other toxic metals and should be avoided. Calcium carbonate, which is 40 per cent elemental calcium, is inexpensive, generally well tolerated, well absorbed even with achlorhydria, and available as a tablet or suspension. Some patients, however, complain of constipation and may prefer calcium gluconate, which is only 9 per cent elemental calcium and more expensive. Calcium supplements may interfere with other oral medications (e.g., tetracyclines, phenothiazines, iron, levodopa) and should not be taken within 1 to 2 hours of any other drugs.

Estrogen Therapy. The rationale underlying estrogen replacement therapy in osteoporosis is based on the evidence that estrogens can prevent the rapid bone loss that occurs after oophorectomy and retard bone loss after a natural menopause. This prevention requires administration of estrogens within 3 to 6 years after menopause, and the effect may not be sustained because of the tight coupling of bone formation with bone resorption. Estrogen therapy appears to reduce bone turnover without altering the balance between bone resorption and formation, so that the rate of bone loss will decrease after several years of treatment but bone formation will remain less than bone resorption, albeit at a lower level of remodeling. Several studies, however, have suggested a protective effect of estrogen therapy on osteoporotic fractures. In contrast to these findings, convincing evidence that estrogens restore lost bone or reduce fracture rates in patients with established osteoporosis is absent. Furthermore, the rate of bone loss may accelerate when estrogen treatment is discontinued, necessitating lifelong therapy.

The risks of such treatment include an increased incidence of endometrial carcinoma and gallbladder disease. Cyclic therapy with the addition of a progestogen, 1 mg per day of norethindrone (Norlutin) or 10 mg per day of medroxyprogesterone (Provera) during the last 7 to 10 days of the cycle, seems to protect against endometrial cancer but may increase the risk of hypertension, coronary artery disease, fluid retention, and thromboembolic phenomena. Until these risks are more clearly defined, estrogen replacement therapy should be reserved for prevention of osteoporosis in women with a premature or surgical menopause. Dosages for this purpose require at least 0.625 to 1.25 mg per day of conjugated equine estrogen (Premarin), 25 micrograms per day of ethinyl estradiol (Estinyl), or 1 mg per day of 17β-estradiol (Estrace). Therapy should be cyclic and begin on the eighth calendar day of each month.

Vaginal bleeding, whether breakthrough or withdrawal, requires prompt endometrial sampling. Routine endometrial sampling should be considered at yearly intervals. Contraindications include past or present thrombophlebitis, cholestatic jaundice, and estrogen-dependent neoplasia. Relative contraindications are migraine headaches, anticonvulsant drug therapy, and pre-existing problems with salt and water retention.

Other Agents. Over 40 other agents and regimens have been used in osteoporosis but their number attests to their lack of efficacy. Sodium fluoride, an investigational agent, may cause side effects in more than one third of subjects who receive the 40 to 65 mg per day necessary to stimulate bone formation. The plantar fasciitis, arthralgias, epigastric pain, and nausea caused by sodium fluoride treatment are often worse than the underlying osteoporosis.

PAGET'S DISEASE OF BONE

method of
ETHEL S. SIRIS, M.D.,
and ROBERT E. CANFIELD, M.D.
Columbia University
New York, New York

Paget's disease of bone is a localized disorder of the skeleton, characterized by increased rates of bone remodeling in affected sites. The process is believed to begin with a defect in osteoclasts, which are thought to be formed by the fusion of hematopoietic stem cells that take up residence in bone. In Paget's disease the osteoclasts appear to be more prone to fusion with each other, leading to larger than normal cell size, increased numbers of nuclei, and greatly increased rates of bone resorption in involved skeletal sites. Although lytic areas are sometimes noted, new bone formation is also increased, but the high rate of turnover leads to poor control of new bone architecture with an attendant increase in bone size, increased risk of fractures, bowing of weight-bearing limbs, joint pain due to structural changes, and occasional nerve or spinal cord compression. Although the symptoms arising from these changes in bone may produce disability, the majority of patients have minimal if any symptoms and may not require treatment.

No cure exists for this disorder, but considerable histologic and symptomatic evidence suggests that therapy aimed at slowing the rate of osteoclast-mediated bone resorption may produce improvement.

Guidelines for Treatment

The assessment of a patient for treatment includes several factors. Radiographic evidence of involvement at a particular site usually leads to the diagnosis, and a bone scan is the simplest means of assessing whether other skeletal sites are involved as well. The serum alkaline phosphatase level is almost always elevated in patients with active disease and roughly correlates with the extent of skeletal involvement. Elevated urinary total hydroxyproline excretion is viewed as a reflection of collagen degradation in bone but is not widely available as a diagnostic test.

No simple rule assists in making the decision to treat this disorder. The goals of therapy should be either the relief of current symptoms or the prevention of future complications. Symptoms of bone or joint pain in a site of pagetic involvement are the best indication to initiate therapy. Evidence of nerve compression is also an indication, except that no evidence indicates that the treatment reverses eighth nerve compression leading to hearing loss. Spinal cord compression, although rare, is a strong cause for commencing treatment, and surgical decompression also may be indicated.

Although no long-term controlled trials prove that treatment prevents future complications, the restoration of more normal histologic architecture of bone coincident with treatment suggests that this may occur. Accordingly, when Paget's disease occurs close to a joint such as the hip or knee, or in a weight-bearing bone such as the femur or tibia, we are inclined to recommend treatment. Vertebral involvement is a matter of concern, and widespread cranial involvement may lead to increased skull size or to basilar invagination, other factors that lead us to initiate therapy. If disease is localized to a region of the skeleton where there are no symptoms and future complications are unlikely to occur (e.g., the pelvic ilia), no treatment is indicated. The age of the patient is a consideration. A young person may be more apt to progress, whereas treatment to prevent progression in patients aged 70 or 80 years who are discovered to have this disorder is less compelling. Widespread skeletal involvement has been associated with increased cardiac output, but this is usually not a therapeutic issue.

We have found that an investment of time in carefully explaining what is known about the generally benign course of this disease is a source of considerable relief to patients, who are usually quite uninformed about the natural history of the disorder. It is also important to assess symptoms in light of their causes. For example, the symptom of pain in the thigh radiating to the knee in a patient known to have Paget's disease may represent one or more of several causes: pagetic change in the femur itself; degenerative change, with or without pagetic causation, in the lumbar spine; or joint narrowing at the hip, either as a result of Paget's disease of the pelvis or femur or both, or as a primary osteoarthritis without pagetic involvement. Therapy directed at the pagetic process will vary with respect to effectiveness depending on the cause of the symptoms.

Two drugs that decrease osteoclast function have had widespread use over the past decade in treatment. One is etidronate disodium and the other is the synthetic peptide salmon calcitonin. Neither drug cures the disease; each agent at recommended doses usually produces an approximate 50 per cent reduction in biochemical parameters; treatment with either has been shown to relieve certain symptoms.

Calcitonin

Calcitonin is a 32 amino acid polypeptide hormone secreted by the parafollicular cells of the thyroid in mammals and by the ultimobranchial body of birds and fish. The hormone secreted by salmon has been characterized, and synthetic salmon calcitonin is currently approved by the FDA for use in Paget's disease. This form of calcitonin is sold in the United States as Calcimar. It differs moderately in structure from the human hormone by virtue of several amino acid substitutions, and in some patients neutralizing antibodies may develop over time, causing a loss of efficacy.

We generally initiate therapy at a dose of 100 Medical Research Council (MRC) units per day. Salmon calcitonin is prepared as a solution in a vial containing 400 MRC units in 2 ml. Thus, the patient self-injects a 0.5 ml dose subcutaneously each day. Most patients alternate sites in both anterior thighs. Except for the needle insertion, the injection of this fluid is quite painless; occasionally some local redness may occur at the site shortly after injection, but this appears to diminish when the needle is regularly inserted at a 90 degree angle into the skin.

The great majority of patients will improve within 6 months in those symptoms capable of responding to therapy: decreases in heat over affected bone usually occur, headache (often described as a "bandlike tightening") will diminish, aching in the back or the long bones will be reduced, nerve compression syndromes (such as sciatica) are often reduced. However, a bowed extremity will remain bowed and hearing loss is unlikely to reverse, though as mentioned earlier it is conceivable—though unproved—that these problems may progress less rapidly; and severely deformed joints may continue to cause pain and disability without any change. Benefit may be apparent within 2 weeks after initiating therapy, or it may take 2 to 3 months. We generally recommend the 100 MRC units per day dose for a 6 month period and then we reassess the patient, evaluating symptomatic response and reduction in serum alkaline phosphatase levels and in urinary hydroxyproline excretion, if the latter test is available. As noted, we usually see a 50 per cent fall in these indices of bone turnover. If a desirable response has occurred, it is usually possible to decrease the dose of calcitonin to either 50 or 100 MRC units every other day after the first 4 to 6 months of treatment with maintenance of benefit thereafter. Depending on the severity of the pagetic problem, it may be necessary to continue the agent at the lowest effective dose indefinitely. In a patient with mild or monostotic disease, such as tibial involvement alone, who has a complete symptomatic remission and whose blood chemistry values fall to near normal, it may be possible to stop the agent after 6 to 9 months. In such a situation we advise re-evaluating the patient's symptoms and serum alkaline phosphatase level every 6 months thereafter. Some patients have had continuing benefit for 1 to 2 years after stopping calcitonin. With evidence of renewed activity, the agent should be reinitiated. Skin testing is advised prior to starting (or restarting) this agent, although serious allergic reactions are virtually unknown.

The main drawbacks to salmon calcitonin are the need for parenteral administration and its relatively high cost. Most patients will continue to self-inject the agent if they are having a symptomatic response, but many dislike the procedure.

Adverse effects from salmon calcitonin are relatively few and are in the category of annoying rather than serious. About 10 per cent of patients may experience some nausea within the hour following the injection, a symptom that can be ameliorated by taking the medication at bedtime, and one that often ceases to occur with time. Even fewer patients experience cutaneous flushing for up to an hour after injection, a phenomenon that appears to cause no serious sequelae but which can be very unpleasant and may lead to the patient's discontinuation of the drug.

Etidronate Disodium (EHDP)

Etidronate disodium is a pyrophosphate analogue and a member of a class of compounds called diphosphonates. Diphosphonates are bone-seeking agents and are the substances to which radionuclide materials are often linked for bone scanning. Like calcitonin, diphosphonates inhibit bone resorption, presumably through inhibitory effects on pagetic osteoclasts. Etidronate is the only diphosphonate approved in the United States for use in Paget's disease and is the disodium salt of ethane-1-hydroxy-1,1-diphosphonic acid, EHDP, marketed as Didronel.

In most instances, the indications for EHDP treatment are identical to those for calcitonin, and the beneficial effects of the two agents are very similar. As with calcitonin, EHDP use at recommended doses is typically associated with a 50 per cent or greater decrease in both serum alkaline phosphatase levels and urinary hydroxyproline excretion. Both agents are associated with improvements on bone biopsy, and both will provide symptomatic benefit in a majority of patients in whom benefit seems likely to result from inhibition of the pagetic process. The advantages of EHDP are its lower cost and the oral route of administration as a once-a-day medication.

The recommended dose of EHDP is 5 mg per kg per day for 6 months, after which the agent should be discontinued for at least the next 6 months. EHDP comes in both 200 and 400 mg tablets, and the 5 mg per kg dose is 400 mg per day in an average-sized patient. The drug should be taken either 2 hours before or after a meal. The dosing schedule of alternating 6 months of treatment with 6 months of no therapy is the result of information obtained from the early clinical trials with EHDP. It appears that on the average maximum efficacy is achieved after a 6 month course of treatment with the agent, and most patients will sustain the benefit for 6 months without additional treatment. This particular diphosphonate inhibits not only bone resorption—the presumed reason it is helpful in Paget's disease—but at high doses it also inhibits mineralization of newly forming bone. However, at the recommended dose of 5 mg per kg per day for no longer than 6 months per course of treatment, this problem should not occur.

Many patients with relatively mild disease (e.g., only 1 to 2 sites of involvement and serum alkaline phosphatase values in the range of two to four times normal) will respond to a single 6 month course with symptomatic relief and near normalization of the alkaline phosphatase value. At the end of the ensuing 6 month drug-free interval, patients often continue to experience symptomatic improvement and maintenance of the decreased alkaline phosphatase level. We evaluate these patients every 6 months to reassess their clinical and biochemical status, and we reinstitute EHDP at the 5 mg per kg per day dose for a second 6 month course if and when increased pagetic activity returns. Following each 6 month treatment period we observe them for at least 6 months off therapy, as before, with further treatment courses as needed.

Patients with more extensive and active disease may continue to demonstrate significant persistence of activity despite a 50 per cent lowering of the alkaline phosphatase level in response to 6 months of EHDP (e.g., the patient whose alkaline phosphatase decreases from 1600 to 750 units per level), and such patients are generally cycled with EHDP for 6 of every 12 months. On this regimen we have observed the maintenance of lowered blood chemistry values and generally improved symptoms for up to 10 years in some of our patients; others, however, appear to have less benefit from later cycles of therapy.

For most patients, either salmon calcitonin or EHDP provides adequate treatment. If the chosen drug is unsatisfactory, we will switch to the other for a trial or may give them together (each in accordance with the guidelines described) when the disorder is very severe. Our first choice in most cases is EHDP, primarily because of the ease of administration and lower cost, which greatly enhance patient compliance. In certain circumstances, however, calcitonin may be preferred, such as when a severely pagetic individual is immobilized, as after a fracture, and hypercalciuria or hypercalcemia are potential problems; as a therapy to decrease activity over the 3 to 4 months prior to elective surgery on an area of pagetic bone, when a decrease in vascularity is desirable; and as therapy of Paget's disease in the 6 to 12 months following a fracture through pagetic bone. There is also some controversy regarding the use of EHDP in patients who have areas of advancing lytic disease (the so-called "blade of grass") in a weight-bearing extremity; some specialists in this field employ salmon calcitonin preferentially in that setting as well.

Mithramycin

Mithramycin is a cytotoxic antibiotic and a potent osteoclast inhibitor, approved by the FDA for the treatment of hypercalcemia due to cancer. It has been used experimentally in Paget's disease with considerable success in decreasing elevated blood and urine chemistry values and improving symptoms. However, it is a toxic compound, commonly producing nausea, vomiting, and liver enzyme elevations and less often renal dysfunction and low platelet counts at recommended doses, and must be administered intravenously. We reserve its use for very special cases, such as certain patients with progressive spinal cord or nerve compression, in whom rapidly effective medical therapy is desirable either as a preliminary to surgery or, when possible, as an alternative. In essence, this drug has a limited role in treatment of Paget's disease and should be used only when deemed necessary by those who have had considerable experience with this disorder.

Newer Therapies

Currently, clinical trials are being conducted with synthetic human calcitonin. Preliminary results indicate that the parenteral use of this agent is also associated with relief of symptoms and decreases in the biochemical indices of Paget's disease. Unlike salmon calcitonin, the human preparation would not be expected to be associated with the formation of neutralizing antibodies that occurs in some patients. Thus, the human form of calcitonin may be particularly useful in patients whose Paget's disease has become refractory to salmon calcitonin over time. Still an investigational drug, it seems likely that human calcitonin will become commercially available in the future.

Additionally, several new diphosphonates are currently undergoing early phases of investigation. It is possible that some of the members of this class of compounds with more potent osteoclast-inhibiting properties and less active inhibition of mineralization may emerge as new oral therapies for Paget's disease over the next several years.

Analgesics and Nonsteroidal Anti-Inflammatory Drugs

It is important to emphasize the value of analgesics and the NSAID class of agents in patients with Paget's disease. Whether or not specific antipagetic therapy with salmon calcitonin or EHDP is employed, aches and pains often respond to aspirin or acetaminophen. Since this disease occurs in older patients, the coexistence of osteoarthritis is very common and distinguishing between the source of symptoms is sometimes not possible. Moreover, one of the commonest symptoms of Paget's disease that we see is pain related to arthritic change in the spine, hip, ankle, or knee secondary to the presence of pagetic bone. Often impressive relief of symptoms results from the conventional use of naproxen, piroxicam, ibuprofen, or others in this group, for variable lengths of time, as tolerated.

Surgery

Quite wisely, most orthopedic and neurosurgeons are very cautious about performing surgery on pagetic bone, as the surgical manipulation of this very vascular bone may lead to significant loss of blood and the decreased strength of the bone may make working with it quite difficult.

At our institution we have had very good success with hip replacement surgery in patients with severe and refractory pain or joint dysfunction due to pagetic bone in the pelvis, femur, or both. The main goal of surgery has been pain relief and improvement in the quality of the patient's function. In experienced surgical hands, these patients can do quite well.

Surgical decompression of neural structures (due to spinal cord encroachment by pagetic bone or basilar invagination of the skull) is sometimes necessary as a medical emergency and should be undertaken only by highly skilled and experienced neurosurgeons. In most instances, large doses of dexamethasone (up to 16 mg per day in divided doses) are utilized acutely prior to surgery.

PARENTERAL NUTRITION IN ADULTS

method of
EDWARD J. QUEBBEMAN, M.D., Ph.D.
Medical College of Wisconsin
Milwaukee, Wisconsin

Prolonged starvation may accompany severe illness and hospitalization and may cause impaired wound healing, depressed immunologic status, and even death. The ability to provide needed nutrients by the intravenous route represents a major advance in medical care; nutrients can be provided safely and simply to almost any patient in the hospital and at home when required.

The metabolic goals of total parenteral nutrition (TPN) are to provide nutrient materials to correct or prevent protein-calorie malnutrition and to provide protein and energy substrates during periods of stress and thereby prevent excessive breakdown of body protein. Unrealistic goals of TPN therapy are to correct pre-existing malnutrition rapidly or to force patients to heal more quickly by using large quantities of nutrient solutions. Attempts to do this have resulted in metabolic stress and complications such as increased metabolic rate, increased catecholamine output, and excessive deposition of fat in the liver. Malnutrition is easier to prevent than to correct, especially in severely ill and injured patients, and therefore TPN should be used early in a patient's hospital course.

Indications

Since TPN is expensive and is associated with several potential risks, it is important to identify the patients who may benefit from this therapy and not use it indiscriminately. Two indications with proven efficacy are the short gut syndrome and gastrointestinal fistulas. These problems may be caused by Crohn's disease, trauma, or surgical complications, among others.

Additional patients may benefit from TPN if they cannot eat or be fed by enteral means for longer than 7 to 10 days, especially if they are at high risk to develop complications. Patients who actually develop complications (e.g., sepsis, abscess, bowel obstruction, or gastric atony) should begin TPN as soon as the complication is identified. Patients with severe malnutrition prior to a major surgical procedure may require TPN for several weeks before the operation can be safely performed, but a few days of TPN in routine preoperative patients have not been shown to be of benefit.

Several laboratory and anthropomorphic measurements have been proposed to identify patients at high risk for developing complications and for documenting progress on a nutritional therapy program. These measurements need to be correlated with the patient's nutritional and medical history but should probably not be used alone to justify beginning TPN. Specifically, serum albumin concentration is decreased by many processes besides malnutrition, including excess of sodium and water in the patient's extracellular fluid and loss of capillary integrity.

Procedure

Ideally, a patient should be started on TPN with the assistance of a designated team, who can provide the necessary consultation expertise and assist with the technical aspects. This team may consist of various specialists but is often a coalition of physicians, nurses, dietitians, and pharmacists who have an interest in TPN, have standardized procedures, and communicate well with each other.

TPN is begun after inserting a central venous catheter. This access route is necessary because of the high osmolarity of the nutrient solutions; peripheral veins would be rapidly thrombosed. A catheter made of a silicone material is preferred over polyvinyl chloride or Teflon because it is the least thrombogenic material available and probably claims the smallest incidence of infection. The subclavian vein is an ideal access route since the catheter can be easily secured to the flat surface of the chest wall without hindering movement. The person performing the subclavian puncture should be thoroughly familiar with the technique and be able to do it safely. Sterility must be maintained; often a surgeon places these catheters in the operating room. Following placement, a chest radiograph should be obtained to determine catheter position and search for possible complications.

Possible complications include pneumothorax, hemothorax, laceration of the subclavian or carotid artery, damage to the thoracic duct, shearing of the catheter with catheter embolus, air embolus, and myocardial irritation or perforation. In skilled hands, the incidence of these problems should be very small.

The catheter entry site should be dressed once a week, using aseptic technique and a totally occlusive membranous covering (Tegaderm or Op-site). This dressing must prevent movement of the catheter at the entry site and prevent ingress of environmental pathogens.

The nutrient solution is prescribed after first determining the patient's requirements. Calories are calculated from one of several formulas based on patient size and sex. I use the following formulas, which are based on body surface area (BSA):

$$\text{Male REE} = 789 \times \text{BSA} + 137$$
$$\text{Female REE} = 544 \times \text{BSA} + 414$$

These approximate the resting energy expenditure (REE in kcal per day) of the patient, and I provide an additional 20 per cent to provide for physical activity and stress. Other clinicians believe that additional calories need to be prescribed for severe degrees of stress, but this is probably unnecessary except for large surface area burns. The calories should be provided as both glucose and lipid since this will decrease the total glucose load and help prevent hyperglycemia and essential fatty acid deficiency.

Protein is provided almost exclusively as crystalline amino acids in amounts varying between 1 and 2 grams per kg of body weight per day. This amount needs to be decreased for patients with renal or hepatic failure. The exact amount necessary can be determined after TPN has begun by calculating nitrogen balance. If nitrogen balance is negative, more protein may be required.

Solutions high in essential amino acids are available for use in renal failure, but their efficacy over standard amino acid formulations has not been proved. Solutions high in branch chain amino acids are used for hepatic failure and stress; their place and importance in the practice of parenteral nutrition is uncertain but under active investigation.

In addition to calories and protein, all other substances necessary for complete nutrition must be added to the mixture. This includes electrolytes, trace elements, and vitamins. Electrolytes are administered in amounts necessary to meet daily requirements and to replace abnormal losses, which may be due to fistulas, diarrhea, or nasogastric suction. Routine daily needs for electrolytes are sodium chloride—70 mEq, potassium phosphate—60 mEq, magnesium sulfate—10 mEq, and calcium gluconate—10 mEq. These should be decreased in patients with renal failure or increased in patients with severe stress or trauma, or if much higher doses of calories and protein are provided. Trace elements should be provided in adequate amounts from the beginning of TPN even though symptomatic deficiency syndromes may take several weeks to develop. I supply zinc—4 mg, copper—1 mg, manganese—0.5 mg, and chromium—10 micrograms each day, and iodine and iron are frequently added.

Vitamins are required, but the recommended doses range widely. Several vitamin preparations are available from commercial vendors, formulated to exceed known requirements of the water-soluble vitamins and to avoid excess of the fat-soluble vitamins. Vitamin K is generally given as an intramuscular injection once a week.

Monitoring and Complications

Patients receiving TPN need to be observed closely to avoid the many possible complications of this technique and also to be certain that the therapy is adequate and benefiting the patient.

Body weight, fluid intake and output, serum sodium, and osmolality are measured to avoid fluid excess or dehydration. Serum glucose is observed to avoid persistent hyperglycemia, which may cause fat deposition in the liver, and urine analysis is performed to avoid glycosuria, which can lead to nonketotic hyperosmolar coma. Serum potassium is the electrolyte value that is most often abnormal (both increased and decreased), especially during transitions from starved to fed state or following severe stress and trauma. Serum proteins such as albumin and transferrin are often measured to evaluate the visceral protein compartment of the patient. Urine should be collected for 24 hours once a week and urine urea nitrogen measured. Total nitrogen output is then calculated by adding a value of 3 to 4 grams to account for nonurea nitrogen losses. This value is then used to calculate nitrogen balance (total intake minus output) and can be used to adjust the protein intake.

Liver function tests (SGOT, alkaline phosphatase, and bilirubin) should be monitored weekly to detect the development of fatty liver or cholestasis. These abnormalities can be decreased by avoiding excess calorie loads and by preventing persistent hyperglycemia (glucose greater than 180 mg per dl).

One of the most dangerous complications of TPN is sepsis, which may develop from infection of the catheter or contamination of the fluid. Since most solutions are mixed under a laminar flow hood by expert personnel in the pharmacy, primary solution contamination is very uncommon.

Catheter sepsis can be decreased by proper attention to dressing techniques and by avoiding hub contamination when the connecting tubing is changed. If catheter sepsis is suspected, blood should be obtained from the catheter and from peripheral vein sites and cultured for bacteria and fungi. In addition, a careful search should be made for another source of infection (pneumonia, wound abscess). Catheter sepsis is confirmed if the catheter tip and the blood culture grow the same organism, if the fever regresses when the line is removed, and if no other site of infection is identified.

Another complication related to the catheter is central vein thrombosis. This may be overt, as seen with a superior vena cava syndrome, or as subtle as a mild discomfort in the neck. Severely symptomatic patients who require continued use of the catheter may benefit from systemic fibrinolytic therapy; less symptomatic patients may have the catheter removed and prophylaxis of further thrombosis or embolism begun with heparin.

Other complications of TPN that were common in the past, such as fluid overload or essential fatty acid deficiency, are decreasing since fewer total calories are being prescribed and fat is substituted for some of the glucose.

Although complications can still occur, TPN is administered safely to most patients to prevent malnutrition and supply metabolic substrates while other medical therapies are used to treat the underlying disease process.

PARENTERAL FLUID THERAPY FOR INFANTS AND CHILDREN

method of
FRANK G. BOINEAU, M.D.,
and JOHN E. LEWY, M.D.
Tulane University
New Orleans, Louisiana

Replacement of body fluid losses by intravenous therapy is required when an infant or child is unable to meet these needs by oral intake. Parenteral—that is, intravenous—fluid must be given to (1) meet the daily normal losses of water and electrolytes (maintenance), (2) replace deficits that develop before therapy is initiated, and (3) replace abnormal continuing losses that occur during intravenous therapy.

Maintenance Fluid Needs

Maintenance fluid therapy is required to replace physiologic losses of both water and electrolytes. These needs occur because of water losses from the skin and pulmonary system, from the kidneys for excretion of the solute load, and, in infants, from the water contained within the stool. Normally, electrolyte losses occur primarily from the kidney and consist principally of sodium, potassium, chloride, and organic anions.

Skin and pulmonary water losses are best related to calories metabolized. Caloric expenditure depends on body size, expressed in weight. Thus, in this discussion of parenteral fluid therapy, replacement of water and electrolyte needs will be expressed in terms of body weight in kilograms (kg).

Insensible water losses (IWL) is the term given to losses through the skin and pulmonary system. Such losses are proportional to body weight, which is related to age. About two thirds of IWL in infants comes from the skin and one third from the pulmonary system. The usual maintenance fluid losses are shown in Table 1.

Insensible water loss is affected by several factors, including humidity, clothing, body temperature, rate and depth of respiration, and ambient temperature. Insensible water loss in the neonate is especially critical, for the rate is high and affected by therapies that are unique to the neonate. Factors that influence IWL in the neonate include gestational age, phototherapy, and body-warming devices.

TABLE 1. **Components of Maintenance Water Needs in Different Age Groups**

Component	0–6 Months	0.5–5 Years	5–10 Years	Adolescents
	Ml/Kg Body Weight/Day			
Insensible	40	30	20	10
Urinary	60	60	50	40
Fecal	20	10	—	—
Total	120	100	70	50

Table 2 shows the usual IWL for neonates in an Isolette with a relative humidity of 35 per cent and skin temperature controlled at 36.5 C. Radiant body warmers and phototherapy both increase skin water loss of neonates from 80 to 200 per cent. Thus allowances for this increased need should be made when IWL water replacement needs are calculated.

Fever will also increase insensible water loss by 7 ml per kg per day for each degree of temperature above 37.2 C (99 F). This increased fluid need is based on constant temperature elevation and needs to be calculated based on the average temperature elevation.

Urinary water loss is a function of the amount of solute to be excreted and the concentration of the urine. The amount of solute to be excreted is determined by the diet and the metabolic state of the patient. The premature neonate can concentrate the urine to about 400 mOs per liter; the full-term infant, to 800 mOs per liter; and the child, to 1200 mOs per liter. When giving water to replace urinary losses, it is preferable to assume a urinary osmolality of 300 mOs per liter, thus avoiding a burden for the kidney and supplying additional water if the actual solute load is greater than estimated.

The solute load is reduced by giving carbohydrate in the intravenous fluids to prevent cell catabolism and ketosis. Three grams of dextrose per kg of body weight will usually provide sufficient carbohydrate. The solute load of infants and children receiving parenteral fluid containing 5 per cent dextrose averages 20 mOs per kg per day. An average estimate for urine excretion is 50 to 66 ml per kg per day if the urine osmolality ranges from 300 to 400 mOs per liter.

Urine water loss changes if the osmolar load or renal concentrating ability changes. Conditions that produce a large renal osmolar load, such as hyperglycemia, increase obligatory urine water excretion. Thus allowances have to be made and additional water given to replace losses. Conditions that interfere with the urinary concentrating ability require additional parenteral water to replace losses. Shock, surgery, certain diseases, and drugs increase the level of antidiuretic hormone. The urine concentration may be greater than appropriate, leading to abnormal water retention and hyponatremia.

The best guide to the amount of fluid needed to replace urinary losses in the infant and child with renal dysfunction or unusual osmolar loads is the record of the urinary output and its osmolality or specific gravity. Obviously, the anuric infant would be rapidly and markedly overloaded with fluids if "maintenance" urinary replacement were continued after anuria or severe oliguria had been confirmed. Thus, as with IWL, average urinary loss is only an estimate and each patient must be considered individually. When precise replacement of urine loss is necessary, the volume of urine should be measured and replaced volume for volume. Thus under- or overhydration can be avoided. This method is especially helpful when renal dysfunction is present. Weight is the best guide to the adequacy of fluid therapy.

Stool water losses range from 10 to 20 ml per kg per day in infants and toddlers. Stool water loss in older children is very small and can be ignored (see Table 1).

Electrolyte Maintenance

Urine is the major source of electrolyte loss in the healthy child. There is essentially no loss from the lungs. Approximately 0.5 mEq of sodium and potassium per kg of body weight are lost through the skin every 24 hours.

Urinary losses of sodium average 2 to 3 mEq per kg per day and potassium, 1 to 2 mEq per kg per day. Urinary anions are usually chloride and organic anions. Stool losses of electrolytes are minimal in the absence of diarrhea. Supplying a total of 3 mEq per kg per day of sodium, 2 mEq per kg per day of potassium, and 5 mEq per kg per day of chloride usually provides sufficient electrolytes.

An example will serve to illustrate the calculation of daily maintenance of water and electrolyte needs in healthy children. A healthy 6 kg, 7 month old infant requires intravenous fluids for 24 hours. Renal function is normal and he is afebrile. Insensible water loss would be 30 ml per kg per day; urinary loss, 60 ml per kg per day; and stool loss, 10 ml per kg per day. Total daily water needs are (100 ml per kg per day × 6 kg)

TABLE 2. **Insensible Water Loss Needs in Premature Infants***

Birth (grams)	Water Loss (ml/kg BW/day)
1000	64
1001–1250	96
1251–1500	38
1501–1750	22
1751–2000	17

*All infants inside incubator with skin temperature controlled at 36.5 C and humidity controlled at 35 per cent.

= 600 ml per day. Daily sodium needs are 3 mEq per kg or 18 mEq; potassium, 2 mEq per kg or 12 mEq; and chloride, 5 mEq per kg or 30 mEq. These water and electrolyte needs could be provided as 600 ml of 0.2 per cent saline in 5 per cent dextrose and water to which 12 mEq of KCl is added and administered at a rate of 25 ml per hour. Automated intravenous infusion instruments provide a convenient, accurate, and safe method of giving the fluid.

Ongoing Losses

Ongoing losses should be directly measured and replaced. If the normal 7 month old infant described in the preceding example had had abdominal surgery and required a nasogastric tube, nasogastric drainage would be replaced volume for volume. If, for example, 300 ml (0.3 liter) of gastric drainage were collected over 12 hours and it contained a sodium concentration of 75 mEq per liter and a potassium concentration of 15 mEq per liter, the data shown in Table 3 would apply. The usual sodium concentration in gastric fluid is 75 mEq per liter; potassium, 15 mEq per liter; and chloride, 90 mEq per liter.

Deficit Therapy

Deficit fluid therapy is intended to replace losses of body fluids that occurred prior to institution of parenteral fluids. The most common cause of body fluid and electrolyte deficit is gastrointestinal fluid loss from vomiting or diarrhea. Other, less common causes of deficits include disorders of urinary concentrating ability, such as diabetes insipidus or hydronephrosis; osmotic diuresis in diabetes mellitus; excessive losses through skin during vigorous exercise or in patients with cystic fibrosis; and disturbed thirst mechanisms. This discussion will concentrate on replacement of deficits caused by excessive gastrointestinal losses since these are the most common in infants and children. The principles of repair of excessive gastrointestinal losses can be applied to repair of other deficits as well.

TABLE 3. **12 Hour Fluid and Electrolyte Needs for Case Described in Text**

	Water	Na	K	Cl	HCO_3
	ml	*mEq*			
Maintenance	300	9	6	15	—
Replacement	300	22.5	4.5	27	—
Total	600	31.5	10.5	42	—

Fluid prescription
200 ml normal saline,
400 ml 5% dextrose in water,
add 10 mEq KCl,
infuse at 50 ml per hr for 12 hr

The resultant composition of the extracellular fluid depends on the net balance of losses (gastrointestinal) and gains (oral intake) during the evolution of volume and electrolyte depletion. To plan for effective repair of the fluid loss, estimates of both water and electrolyte deficits must be made.

Estimation of water deficit is the first step in planning therapy. The most accurate method of determining the degree of water deficit is to measure weight loss. If a recent weight is not known, less direct methods are required to estimate water deficit. One of these is the use of the child's present height. From earlier examinations, one may know the proportionality between the height and weight of the patient. A well weight can then be calculated by matching the height on a standard growth chart. The difference between the well and sick weight roughly approximates the water deficit.

Obviously, such an estimate must be moderated by clinical judgment. Clinical estimation of the degree of dehydration is very subjective. Signs of dehydration, such as dry mucous membranes, sunken fontanelles, sunken and soft eyeballs, cold and dry skin, decreased skin turgor, and hypotension may not reflect precisely the degree of dehydration. In hypertonic dehydration, for example, the skin turgor may be good and lead one to underestimate the severity of dehydration. In infants, clinical signs of dehydration are usually not present when a less than 50 ml per kg (5 per cent) weight loss has occurred. Vascular instability frequently is present when dehydration exceeds 15 per cent.

Estimation of electrolyte deficit follows an estimation of water loss. The principles are outlined in Table 4. Total body water is the product of the body weight before the illness began times the percentage of body weight that is water. Subtraction of weight loss reveals body water on admission. This figure allows calculation of body solute content present when the subject is well and on admission when sick. The difference reveals the

TABLE 4. **Principles of Estimation of Electrolyte Deficits**

1. Estimated well body weight (kg) × per cent total body water = total body water (L) when well
2. Total body water (L) × normal plasma osmolality (mOs/L) = total body osmols (mOs) when well
3. Deficit water (L) = acute weight loss (kg)
4. Total well body water (L) − deficit water (L) = total sick body water × measured or calculated osmolality on admission (mOs/L) = total sick body osmols (mOs)
5. Solute deficit = step 2 − step 4
6. Cation (or anion) deficit = solute deficit (mOs) ÷ 2
7. Sodium deficit (mEq) = cation deficit − estimated potassium deficit (mEq)
8. Chloride deficit (mEq) = anion deficit − buffer-base deficit

solute deficit, which is divided equally into cations and anions. Sodium and potassium are the principal cations lost. Anion loss is either chloride or buffer anion (HCO_3^-, or organic anion). The buffer-base concentration in the initial blood sample is calculated from pH and tCO_2 or pCO_2 by use of nomograms. This initial buffer-base concentration is subtracted from normal buffer-base concentration to obtain buffer anion deficit, and this difference is multiplied by the body weight and the estimated distribution space for buffer base, which is 0.3.

It is obvious that these calculations require data (serum Na, K, tCO_2, Cl, and blood pH and pCO_2). The initial intravenous fluid in most cases should be half-strength (0.45 per cent) saline in 5 per cent dextrose and water. When laboratory data are available, calculation of electrolyte deficits can proceed and the fluid composition can be changed. Usually, the fluid is given at a rate to correct one half of the water loss in the first 12 hours plus maintenance fluid in 12 hours. When signs of circulatory compromise occur, plasmanate, lactated Ringer's solution, or normal saline should be used. A volume of 10 to 20 ml per kg can be given over 30 to 60 minutes, to expand acutely extracellular fluid volume and plasma volume. If peripheral perfusion is then adequate, the intravenous fluid can be changed to the rehydration solution calculated from the guidelines.

Isotonic volume depletion defines a state in which the net loss of water and sodium is proportional to their usual ratio in the body, resulting in a serum sodium concentration of 130 to 150 mEq per liter. Fluid losses occur from both the extracellular and intracellular compartments. A second example illustrates the repair of isotonic dehydration. Assume that our previously normal 6.0 kg, 7 month old infant develops diarrhea for several days. Oral intake consists of dilute juices. Admission weight is 5.4 kg, and there are signs of moderate dehydration. The blood pressure is 90/60 mm Hg and temperature is 37 C. The electrolyte measurements resulted in a Na level of 132 mEq per liter; K, 4.0 mEq per liter; Cl, 86 mEq per liter; tCO_2, 9 mM per liter; and pH, 7.10. Total fluid deficit is calculated as the total weight loss, since greater than 90 per cent of diarrheal stool is water. Thus, 6.0 kg (well weight) minus 5.4 kg (sick weight) equals total water deficit (600 ml). Total electrolyte losses can be estimated from the weight loss and the serum solute concentration (Table 4).

Solute concentration is best estimated by measuring the osmolality of the serum. If osmolality measurement is not readily available, it can be approximated by measuring the serum sodium and potassium in mEq per liter. If we add the Na + K concentration plus 5 mEq for calcium, magnesium, and trace ions, we will know the total number of milliequivalents of cation per liter. Multiplying this number by 2 approximates the osmolality, since there are an equal number of anionic milliequivalents to balance the cationic milliequivalents. Strictly speaking, the osmolality of total ions is slightly less than twice the total cations, since there is not complete ionization in serum. However, two times the cations does not take into consideration the osmolality of glucose, urea, and other nonionized solutes, and the two inaccuracies tend to balance out. In the normal infant with a serum Na of 135 mEq per liter and a serum K of 5 mEq per liter, estimated osmolality is ($135 + 5 + 5 = 145 \times 2 = 290$ mOsm per liter). This would be the osmolar concentration throughout the body fluids, since water freely moves between compartments to maintain osmotic equilibrium.

The solution concentration (osmolality) multiplied by the volume of total body water equals the total body solute content. Total body water in a 6 kg infant is approximately 70 per cent of weight (6 kg $\times$ 0.7 = 4.2 liters). Therefore, total body solute when well = 290 mOsm per liter $\times$ 4.2 liter = 1218 mOsm.

When the child became ill, the total body weight was reduced by 0.6 kg. Since this is all water, the total body water when ill is reduced by the full amount and equals 4.2 liters − 0.6 liter = 3.6 liters. Solute concentration for this patient when ill is 132 (Na) + 4 (K) + 5 (estimate for Ca, Mg, and so on) = $141 \times 2 = 282$ mOsm per liter; 282 mOsm per liter (solute concentration) $\times$ 3.6 liters (total body water when ill) = 1015 mOsm. Total solute deficit is the difference between the total content well and ill (1218 − 1015 = 203 mOsm). Half this figure is the total cation deficit: 101 mEq, cation.

Note that the total body water is used for this calculation, since rapid water shifts will change intracellular solute concentration to maintain osmotic equilibrium, as our infusion changes principally extracellular solute concentration. The total cation deficit must now be divided into sodium and potassium deficit. Serum potassium levels give little indication of total body potassium losses. However, water deficit and known composition of "average" diarrheal stools allows one to make a rough estimate of the stool contribution to potassium deficit.

Thus, in this infant, a weight loss of roughly 0.6 kg equals 600 ml of net stool. Diarrheal stool contains an average of 44 mEq per liter of K; thus the potassium deficit is 0.6 liter $\times$ 44 mEq per liter = 26 mEq. This is admittedly an underestimate of usual potassium deficit, but, as with all aspects of fluid therapy, it is generally safer to underestimate than to overestimate needs. Total cation deficit (101 mEq) − 26 mEq of K = 71 mEq Na deficit.

The amount of this Na deficit needed to replace buffer-base losses may now be calculated. Using the measured pH value of 7.1, the CO_2 content of 9.0 mEq per liter, and the Singer and Hastings nomogram found in many handbooks, buffer base is calculated to be 23 mEq per liter. Normal buffer base in infancy is approximately 40 mEq per liter, and so buffer base deficit is 17 mEq per liter. The volume of distribution of infused buffer base = 0.3 × (body weight sick + water deficit) = (5.4 + 0.6) × (0.3) = 1.8 liters. Total buffer-base deficit is thus 17 mEq per liter × 1.8 liters = 31 mEq.

The total sodium deficit of 76 mEq can thus be partitioned into 31 mEq of buffer base and the remainder into 45 mEq of Na given as NaCl. Total deficit may be summarized as: 600 ml water; 45 mEq sodium (as NaCl); 31 mEq sodium (as $NaHCO_3$) and 26 mEq potassium. In treating iso- or hypotonic dehydration, one half the fluid and electrolyte deficit should be replaced in the first 12 hours and one fourth in each of the second and third 12 hours. Buffer-base deficit is replaced more rapidly, with one half replacement in the first 12 hours and the remainder in the second 12 hours.

The initial 12 hour fluid repair can now be constructed for this 6 kg child with 10 per cent dehydration. Maintenance fluids should be included in this prescription and will be one half those calculated for 24 hours. Fluid and electrolyte quantities are listed in Table 5. Note that no potassium should be added to the fluids until urinary output and absence of hyperkalemia are assured, and then potassium concentrations should not exceed 40 mEq per liter. Sodium bicarbonate ($NaHCO_3$) is suggested to replace buffer-base deficits. Sodium bicarbonate is available as a 1 mEq per ml solution.

A fluid order may now be written for the first 12 hour bottle, consisting of 200 ml of 0.9 per cent saline plus 400 ml of 5 per cent dextrose and water solution to which 16 mEq of $NaHCO_3$ and 19 mEq of KCl are added. If potassium cannot be added to the bottle at the outset (patient has not urinated), it is imperative that when the potassium is added the amount added does not exceed the maximum concentration of 40 mEq per liter. Thus, if the patient does not urinate for 6 hours and one half the fluid has been infused, the amount of potassium added must be scaled down so that it remains within the permissible range.

The second 12 hour fluid repair can then proceed with intravenous fluid. Before the second 12 hour bottle is started, the child should be reexamined and the fluids adjusted as needed. A weight gain of 300 grams should be expected with correction of one half the sodium and water deficit. The second 12 hour bottle will then contain fluid and electrolytes in the amounts listed in Table 5. A fluid order could thus be written for 135 ml of 0.9 per cent saline plus 315 ml of 5 per cent dextrose and water, to which would be added 15 mEq of $NaHCO_3$ plus 12 mEq of KCl.

The third 12 hour period of fluid repair is identical to the second except that the $NaHCO_3$ is omitted, unless the infant's clinical condition or electrolyte measurements suggest the need for alteration.

Hypotonic dehydration represents the state in which net loss of sodium is proportionately greater than that of water, resulting in a serum sodium of less than 130 mEq per liter. The same logic is used in calculating fluids for repair of hypotonic dehydration as in isotonic dehydration. If hypotonicity is severe (Na $<$ 120 mEq per liter) and associated with seizures, hypertonic (3 per cent) NaCl should be given initially to raise the sodium level to about 125 mEq per liter. In the previous example, if the serum sodium was 118 mEq per liter, then 7 mEq per liter × 4.2 liters (total body water must be used because of water shifts as described earlier) = 29 mEq of sodium is needed to return the serum sodium to 125 mEq per L. Three per cent saline (0.513 molar) contains 0.5 mEq of Na per ml. Infusion of 58 ml would thus raise the serum sodium concentration by 7 mEq per liter.

If hypotonicity is associated with the infant's having received an excess of sodium-free solution and there is thus dilutional hyponatremia without dehydration, hypertonic saline should be given to bring the serum sodium to a relatively safe concentration, approximately 125 mEq per liter; fluid restriction should then be employed to bring both the volume and tonicity of the body fluids back into equilibrium.

Hypertonic dehydration is a state of volume contraction in which net balance of water and sodium losses is out of proportion, with water loss proportionately greater, resulting in hypernatremia. Hypernatremia is defined as a serum sodium of more than 150 mEq per liter. The extracellular compartment is contracted, as is the intracellular compartment. However, extracellular contraction is lessened by osmotically generated water movement from intracellular to extracellular compartments, caused by hypernatremia.

Children with this disorder require particular care, for too rapid a reduction in serum osmolality will lead to intracellular movement of water and cell swelling. Rapid swelling of brain cells may lead to increased intracranial pressure, seizures, circulatory compromise, or vascular thromboses. There is usually a significant volume and solute

TABLE 5. **Repair of Fluid Deficit for Case Described in Text**

	Water *(ml)*	Sodium Chloride *(mEq)*	Sodium Bicarbonate *(mEq)*	Potassium Chloride *(mEq)*
Initial 12 Hour Period				
Maintenance	300	9	—	6
Replacement	300	22	16	13
Total	600	31	16	19
Second 12 Hour Period				
Maintenance	300	9	—	6
Replacement	150	11	15	6
Total	450	20	15	12

deficit initially in patients with hypertonic dehydration. Plasma-volume expansion is often needed with Ringer's lactate or normal saline. After stabilization of plasma volume, repair should proceed slowly. It is important to avoid using an intravenous solution with less than 30 mEq per liter of sodium for repair of dehydration. Potassium can be added once voiding has started and the serum potassium is less than 5 mEq per liter. The "well" serum osmolality is calculated at 300 mOs per liter to reduce the risk of overestimating solute deficit. The serum sodium should not fall by more than approximately 0.5 mEq per hour. Thus, for a serum Na of 170 mEq per liter, the return of Na to normal in 36 hours is reasonable. When it is above 170 mEq per liter, 72 hours is preferable to achieve complete electrolyte correction. However, fluid restoration should proceed over 36 hours.

These principles for the repair of deficits can also be applied to other fluid disorders. Nephrogenic or central diabetes insipidus may result in the loss of hypotonic fluid, which results in hypertonic dehydration. Body water deficit is estimated from the acute weight loss. Solute deficit can also be estimated from net loss of body osmols. Most of the cationic solute deficit is sodium and very little is potassium. Thus all the cationic solute deficit in the first 24 hours is replaced by sodium. After the patient is voiding, renal function is determined to be stable, and hyperkalemia is not present, potassium can be added to the fluids. Anionic solute is replaced with bicarbonate if metabolic acidosis is present. The amount of bicarbonate is determined using the guidelines. The remainder of the anionic solute is replaced with chloride. The serum sodium should fall slowly by 0.5 mEq per hour. Replacement of water deficits should proceed slowly along the guidelines for hypertonic dehydration. If hypotension or reduced peripheral perfusion is present, lactated Ringer's solution, 10 to 20 ml per kg over 30 to 60 minutes, should be given initially, and continued repair of dehydration should proceed as outlined.

Completion of Rehydration Therapy

Frequent observation of the patient is needed following initiation of therapy. Changes in body weight are the best guide to restoration of fluids. Body weight should be measured every 12 hours, and it should increase to reflect rehydration. Blood electrolytes, pH, CO_2, and creatinine should be measured in at least 12 hours. Subsequent measurements of these parameters depend on the degree of dehydration and electrolyte imbalance.

Section 8

The Endocrine System

ACROMEGALY

method of
PETER J. SNYDER, M.D.
University of Pennsylvania
Philadelphia, Pennsylvania

DIAGNOSIS

The diagnosis of acromegaly is first suspected on the basis of growth during adult life: increased shoe and glove size, and coarsening of facial features, as seen through comparison with old photographs. The diagnosis must be confirmed by demonstrating excessive secretion of growth hormone (GH). The diagnosis is confirmed when a supranormal basal serum GH concentration does not suppress to less than 2 ng per ml following an oral glucose load. If this test yields equivocal results, confirmation of the diagnosis may be obtained by demonstrating a GH response to either thyrotropin-releasing hormone or gonadotropin-releasing hormone or by demonstrating a supranormal serum concentration of somatomedin C, the hormone produced by the liver in response to GH and the hormone that directly causes bone growth. As in the case of other pituitary adenomas, diagnostic evaluation should also include tests of basal thyroid and gonadal function and of ACTH reserve, as well as determination of the mass effect of the adenoma by CT scan and visual field and acuity testing. If radiotherapy is planned, hormonal deficiencies can be replaced concomitant with the radiation. If surgery is planned, the patient must be made euthyroid prior to surgery. Perioperative neurosurgical glucocorticoid regimens are sufficient to cover cortisol deficiency.

Treatment

Rationale. In addition to accelerating osteoarthritis and death from cardiovascular disease, acromegaly may also cause damage from an enlarging pituitary gland. This damage can include neurologic problems, including headache, impaired vision, cerebrospinal fluid (CSF) rhinorrhea (which predisposes to meningitis), and deficiency of any pituitary hormone. Because of these potential effects of acromegaly, treatment is desirable, unless a patient's life expectancy is thought to be short for another reason.

When the cause of excessive GH secretion is growth hormone–releasing hormone (GHRH) secretion from a pancreatic or pulmonary tumor, the treatment is excision of the tumor, if possible. The subsequent discussion assumes the more usual situation, a pituitary or hypothalamic cause. Several methods of treatment decrease GH secretion, but none do so completely and reliably, and each has potential side effects (Table 1).

Radiation Therapy

Supervoltage radiation can be directed at the pituitary from a cobalt source or a linear accelerator. Approximately 4500 rad are administered over 4 to 5 weeks. Other forms of radiotherapy, such as heavy particle radiation and implantation of radioactive yttrium into the pituitary, have been used in the past, but the high incidence

TABLE 1. **Treatment of Acromegaly**

Treatment	Indications	Side Effects
Supervoltage radiation	Moderate GH elevation No, or minimal, neurologic effects	Transient loss of hair, smell, and taste Hypopituitarism
Trans-sphenoidal surgery	Marked GH elevation Visual field impairment Severe clinical effects of GH excess	Neurologic deficits, including vision and oculomotor function Hypopituitarism
Transcranial surgery	Residual suprasellar pituitary tissue producing neurologic deficits after trans-sphenoidal surgery	Neurologic deficits
Bromocriptine (Parlodel)	Adjuvant treatment following radiation therapy	Nausea, hypotension

of side effects makes their current use unwarranted.

The serum GH concentration decreases reliably following supervoltage radiation therapy, but the decrease is slow, approximately 50 per cent every 2 years following treatment, and the GH does not always return to normal. As the serum GH concentration decreases, so does the serum somatomedin C concentration and the clinical manifestations that result from the growth of soft tissues, including acral enlargement. Radiation therapy also may decrease the mass effects of the pituitary enlargement, ameliorating headaches and defects in vision.

The side effects of radiation therapy are similar to those due to radiation of other pituitary lesions. Effects that occur during treatment may include nausea, lassitude, and transient loss of smell, taste, and scalp hair. A rare effect during the first year after treatment is loss of vision due to optic neuritis. Between 1 and 10 years following treatment a deficiency can occur of any pituitary hormone that had been secreted normally before treatment.

Surgery

Surgical excision of the pituitary tissue hypersecreting growth hormone should be attempted first by the trans-sphenoidal approach by a neurosurgeon experienced in this technique. The trans-sphenoidal approach is generally associated with less morbidity than is the transcranial approach. The transcranial approach may be necessary, however, when a large amount of adenomatous pituitary tissue remains in a suprasellar position following trans-sphenoidal surgery and is producing neurologic impairment.

The two major advantages of trans-sphenoidal surgery are that the serum growth hormone concentration is usually substantially reduced and that the reduction occurs immediately. The reduction, however, is usually not entirely to normal.

The side effects of trans-sphenoidal surgery are both neurologic and hormonal. Neurologic side effects may include damage to the optic nerves, causing blindness; damage to the oculomotor nerves, causing diplopia; CSF rhinorrhea, which predisposes to meningitis; and hemorrhage. Hormonal side effects may include deficits of any pituitary hormones that had been secreted normally before surgery, including ACTH, TSH, and LH, and of vasopressin. Deficiency of the latter, which produces diabetes insipidus, is often transient but may be permanent. Another potential side effect, peculiar to this approach, is chronic sinusitis. Neurologic side effects are more common from transcranial than from trans-sphenoidal surgery.

Pharmacologic Therapy

Several ergot derivatives that are dopamine agonists have been used successfully to decrease the serum GH in acromegaly. Bromocriptine (Parlodel) is the only one of these drugs now available by prescription in the United States (this use is not listed by the manufacturer), although pergolide, which is more potent, is available on an investigational, compassionate use basis. The inhibitory effect of dopamine agonists in acromegaly is ironic, because in normal humans dopamine agonists stimulate GH secretion.

Although bromocriptine frequently decreases serum GH in acromegaly, it is not nearly so effective in this condition as it is in prolactin (PRL)-secreting adenomas. Rarely, in fact, does bromocriptine reduce the serum GH to normal. Bromocriptine also does not usually produce the dramatic reductions in adenoma size in acromegaly as it does in PRL-secreting adenomas. The best results of bromocriptine in reducing the serum GH are in acromegalics whose adenomas are hypersecreting PRL as well as GH. To minimize side effects, the initial dose of bromocriptine is 1.25 mg at bedtime for one week, then 1.25 mg twice a day for a week, then gradually increasing two or three times a day doses. A total daily dose of 10 to 40 mg is usually required to lower the serum GH concentration.

The side effects of bromocriptine and other dopamine agonists include nausea, hypotension, and nasal stuffiness. These effects can be minimized by the regimen just described but may still occur at the higher doses. No long-term side effects are yet known. Although many women, especially those with PRL-secreting adenomas, have become pregnant while taking bromocriptine and congenital abnormalities have not been greater than expected, bromocriptine is generally discontinued after conception is known.

Choice of Therapy

Either radiation therapy or surgery is preferable to bromocriptine for initial therapy, because it is more effective. If the clinical situation is not urgent and if the serum GH concentration is only moderately elevated, e.g., <40 ng/ml, radiation therapy may be the better initial choice, because of its lesser morbidity. If, however, severe clinical manifestations of GH excess, such as cardiomyopathy, severe osteoarthritis, or even marked facial disfigurement, are already present, or if significant extrasellar extension of the adenoma has already occurred, surgery may be the better initial choice, because it reduces the mass of adenoma tissue and lowers the GH more rapidly.

If the initial therapy is radiation, bromocriptine could be considered for interim treatment while waiting for the full effect of radiation to occur. If the initial therapy is surgery, the need for subsequent treatment depends on the results of the surgery. If the serum GH and somatomedin C levels 4 to 6 weeks after surgery are normal, no further treatment is necessary at that time. If those two measurements are elevated, radiation therapy should be given to prevent regrowth of the remaining adenomatous tissue and even cause a further decrease in GH. Following radiotherapy, bromocriptine might be added as a third treatment modality, especially if the adenoma appears to be an aggressive one.

Evaluation of Therapy

Evaluation of therapy involves determining whether the desired effects have occurred and whether any undesired effects have occurred. Although the principal desired effect is remission of the clinical manifestations of GH excess, clinical remission lags behind the fall in GH, so biochemical assessment must be made. This assessment should include measurement of the serum GH basally and after an oral glucose load and measurement of the serum somatomedin C. Measurements after surgery should be made in 4 to 6 weeks and then every 6 to 12 months; after radiation therapy, measurements should be made every 6 to 12 months. If any mass effects of pituitary enlargement were prominent before treatment, these should be re-evaluated, e.g., by CT scan and visual fields and acuity, at the same intervals.

Four to six weeks after surgery hormonal assessment should be made for possible deficits in the anterior pituitary control of adrenal, thyroid and gonadal function and of vasopressin secretion. The same hormonal deficits of anterior pituitary function, but not of vasopressin, can occur after radiation therapy, but usually not for a year or more, so assessment should be made annually after radiation.

ADRENOCORTICAL INSUFFICIENCY

method of
EMMANUEL L. BRAVO, M.D.
Case Western Reserve University
Cleveland, Ohio

A patient with known adrenal insufficiency should at all times carry a card or tag stating this condition, the need to inject 100 mg of cortisol if the person is severely injured or found unresponsive, the name and telephone number of the patient's physician, and the nearest of kin who should be notified. When traveling in areas where medical care may not be available immediately, the patient should be provided with a needle, syringe, and a water-soluble derivative of cortisol that can be administered parenterally if the patient is unable to take oral medications. The emergency pack of lyophilized hydrocortisone sodium succinate (Solu-Cortef) is recommended for this purpose since it does not require refrigeration. Patients should be advised to increase steroid dosage during exposure to any stressful situation. With any mild upper respiratory tract infection the regular daily dose should be doubled until the infection clears. Immediate medical attention should be considered for any severe infection or gastrointestinal disturbances associated with vomiting or diarrhea.

Treatment

Acute Adrenal Insufficiency

Hypotension, hyperkalemia, and hypoglycemia pose the most immediate dangers. If the diagnosis appears likely, 100 mg of hydrocortisone sodium succinate (Solu-Cortef) should be given immediately as an intravenous bolus injection. From the same puncture site blood should be collected for the measurement of blood sugar, serum electrolytes, BUN, and serum creatinine levels. An electrocardiogram should also be obtained to determine the urgency for reducing the serum potassium level should it be elevated. If no veins are immediately accessible, hydrocortisone sodium succinate may also be given intramuscularly. This should be followed by the rapid administration (over 4 to 6 hours) of another 100 mg of hydrocortisone sodium succinate in 1000 ml of 5 per cent dextrose in 0.9 per cent sodium chloride solution. Continued administration of 3 to 4 liters of isotonic sodium chloride solution with 300 to 400 mg of hydrocortisone sodium succinate is often sufficient to correct the fluid and electrolyte disturbance and stabilize cardiovascular function. In the typical patient with acute adrenal insufficiency the foregoing measures will have dramatic effects within the first 24 hours. The amount of fluid replacement will depend entirely on the degree of dehydration and cardiovascular stability at the time the diagnosis is made and the presence of other diseases (e.g., myocardial disease, chronic renal insufficiency) that could lead to pulmonary edema or hypertension from fluid overload.

Precipitating factors should be identified quickly and treated accordingly. Control of initiating events is usually followed by a dramatic response to therapy, and the patient can then be placed on oral fluids and medications. Steroid dosage can then be tapered but should be initiated only if the patient has been afebrile for at least 24 hours and is eating normally, and if orthostatic hypotension is no longer present. A convenient approach is to give at each succeeding day one half the total daily dose of cortisol of the preceding day until a maintenance dose is reached (usually from 30 to 40 mg of cortisol per day in adults, and 20 mg per M^2 of body surface area per day in children). At this stage, therapy with sodium-retaining steroid should be started and not before then. The usual daily dose is 0.1 to 0.2 mg of fludrocortisone acetate (Florinef).

Chronic Adrenal Insufficiency

Primary Adrenal Insufficiency (Mineralocorticoid, Glucocorticoid and Androgen Deficiency). Replacement therapy for these patients consists of administration of cortisol, a glucocorticoid, and fludrocortisone acetate (Florinef), a mineralocorticoid. The usual dose of cortisol is 30 to 40 mg per day, with two thirds taken on rising in the morning and one third taken in late afternoon. Florinef, in doses of 0.1 to 0.2 mg per day, is taken by mouth with instructions to the patient to liberalize salt intake. Steroid dosage is generally monitored on an empiric basis within these general ranges. Anorexia, weight loss, and increasing fatigue usually mean too little cortisol. Too much cortisol, however, leads to increased appetite, weight gain, euphoria, and insomnia and may be associated with any of the signs and symptoms characteristic of Cushing's syndrome. The effect of fludrocortisone acetate should be monitored by watching the patient for peripheral edema, weight gain, hypokalemia, and hypertension.

Secondary Adrenal Insufficiency (ACTH Deficiency). Adrenal insufficiency secondary to lack of ACTH differs from primary adrenal disease in that mineralocorticoid function is usually intact, since aldosterone production is primarily under control of the renin-angiotensin system. These patients are less likely to develop serious fluid and electrolyte disturbances and do not require fludrocortisone acetate. However, one must keep in mind that patients with cortisol deficiency from whatever cause have some difficulty excreting free water and may present with hyponatremia.

Congenital Adrenal Hyperplasia (Deficiency of Adrenocortical Enzymes Required for Steroidogenesis). Treatment will depend on which enzyme is lacking. All patients with congenital adrenal hyperplasia resulting from a deficiency of 17α-hydroxylase, 21-hydroxylase, or 11β-hydroxylase require substitution therapy with cortisol or a suitable congener. The usual oral dose of cortisol is about 0.6 mg per kg daily in four divided doses, the last one being given as late as possible to maintain overnight suppression of ACTH release. Patients with 21-hydroxylase deficiency will require, in addition, fludrocortisone acetate; the usual dose is 0.05 to 0.2 mg per day. Therapy is guided by gain in weight and height, by urinary 17-ketosteroids (in 21-hydroxylase and 11β-hydroxylase deficiency), and by blood pressure.

Selective Aldosterone Deficiency Syndromes. Selective aldosterone deficiency is an aspect of congenital adrenal hyperplasia due to 18-hydroxylase deficiency. Selective hypoaldosteronism may supervene after removal of an aldosterone-producing adenoma and the syndrome of hyporeninemic hypoaldosteronism may be more common than previously suspected. The clinical hallmark of selective hypoaldosteronism is hyperkalemic hyperchloremic metabolic acidosis, which may or may not be associated with dehydration and hypotension; the latter signs are highly dependent on the patients' salt and water intake. Restricting sodium intake aggravates the various clinical manifestation, especially the hyperkalemia.

The standard treatment includes correction of acidosis, liberalization of sodium intake, and judicious use of fludrocortisone acetate as required to enhance renal secretion of potassium and replete fluid volume without producing hypertension or congestive heart failure. Correction of acidosis is readily accomplished with oral administration of Shohl's solution (contains 140 grams of citric acid and 98 grams of hydrated crystalline salt of sodium citrate per liter of water). The dose must be found empirically and small doses used initially so as not to overtreat.

Special Problems

Surgery in Patients with Chronic Adrenal Insufficiency. Patients undergoing surgical procedures with general anesthesia require adequate preparation and intravenous use of corticosteroids. On the evening of surgery, 100 mg of hydrocortisone sodium succinate (Solu-Cortef) is given intramuscularly. At 6 A.M. of the morning of surgery, an intravenous infusion consisting of 1000 ml of 0.9 per cent sodium chloride with 100 mg of Solu-Cortef is started and administered at a rate of 200 ml per hour throughout the surgical procedure. A similar solution infused at 100 ml per hour should be maintained in the postoperative phase until the patient is fully awake and able to resume taking corticosteroids by mouth. On the first postoperative day, one half the total dose of cortisol administered on the day of operation is given. The dosage is then halved each succeeding day until the preoperative maintenance dosage is attained.

Pregnancy in a Patient with Primary Adrenocortical Insufficiency. Therapy consists of the usual management. If the nausea and vomiting in the first trimester interfere with the oral intake of cortisol, it may be necessary to administer the steroid intramuscularly. In the last trimester, steroid therapy may often be discontinued since the placenta produces cortisol and aldosterone or closely related compounds in significant amounts. The management of delivery is similar to that for the patient coming to surgery. Within 10 days postpartum, the usual maintenance doses of cortisol and fludrocortisone acetate should be reinstituted.

CUSHING'S SYNDROME

method of
GEORGE P. CHROUSOS, M.D.,
and D. LYNN LORIAUX, M.D., Ph.D.
National Institutes of Health
Bethesda, Maryland

Cushing's syndrome results from prolonged exposure to high levels of glucocorticoid hormones. The cause can be exogenous, due to administration of glucocorticoids or ACTH, or endogenous, due to the increased secretion of cortisol or ACTH.

ACTH-dependent Cushing's syndrome, which accounts for about 85 per cent of endogenous cases, is caused by pituitary ACTH secretion in 80 per cent of cases and ectopic ACTH secretion in 20 per cent. Pituitary ACTH secretion is called Cushing's disease. Although the majority of cases of ACTH-dependent Cushing's syndrome can be diagnosed on the basis of clinical and laboratory criteria, occasionally the differential diagnosis is difficult.

ACTH-independent Cushing's syndrome is usually the result of a benign cortisol-secreting adrenal adenoma or an adrenocortical carcinoma. Carcinomas synthesize and secrete cortisol inefficiently. Thus, they are usually large and frequently palpable by the time signs and symptoms appear. A rare form of Cushing's syndrome, micronodular adrenal disease, is caused by multiple, small, bilateral, autonomous, cortisol-secreting adenomas. It is mainly a disorder of children and adolescents.

Depressed or alcoholic patients often have mild hypercortisolism. The hypercortisolism disappears with the resolution of depression or the discontinuation of alcohol. This condition is referred to as a "pseudo-Cushing's state."

DIAGNOSTIC EVALUATION

The first step is to establish hypercortisolism. Urinary free cortisol is the best single laboratory test for this purpose. There are virtually no false-negative results and, with the exception of patients with depression and alcoholism, there are few false-positives. Urinary 17-hydroxysteroid excretion corrected for the urinary creatinine excretion is also useful. Isolated plasma cortisol determinations are of limited value since the normal range is great and patients with hypercortisolism are often in the normal range. Serial measurements, however, can be of assistance since a high 24 hour mean total plasma cortisol with loss of circadian variation suggests the diagnosis of Cushing's syndrome.

Only when hypercortisolism has been established should testing be undertaken directed toward clarifying the differential diagnosis. The tests are of two types, those that examine the integrity of the feedback axis and radiographic techniques used mainly to examine the size and shape of the adrenal glands.

The first category includes the dexamethasone suppression test and the metyrapone test. The dexamethasone suppression test, as described by Liddle (low dose, 0.5 mg orally every 6 hours for 2 days; high dose, 2 mg orally every 6 hours for 2 days), is the standard procedure for differentiating Cushing's disease from the ectopic ACTH syndrome. About 90 per cent of patients with Cushing's disease demonstrate a decrease of urinary 17-hydroxysteroid excretion to values less than 50 per cent of the baseline values. Less than 10 per cent of patients with the ectopic ACTH syndrome respond in this manner.

Metyrapone, 250 mg orally every 6 hours for 2 days, is also useful in this regard. Eighty per cent of patients with Cushing's disease respond with an approximate doubling of their urinary 17-hydroxysteroid excretion. Most patients with the ectopic ACTH syndrome fail to respond in this manner.

The radiologic procedures include computed tomography scanning of the pituitary gland (which has a poor yield in revealing the presence of ACTH-secreting pituitary adenomas, 10 to 20 per cent), and a CAT scan or ultrasound imaging of the adrenal glands. Most cancers are large when patients present with Cushing's syndrome, and hence are easily detectable with these tests. Adenomas are usually smaller (less than 5 cm in diameter), but the majority can be demonstrated with these techniques.

The iodocholesterol scan is useful in differentiating carcinomas from adenomas or ACTH-dependent macronodules. Carcinomas fail to image with this technique whereas adenomas and ACTH-dependent nodules concentrate iodocholesterol and, hence, image.

Promising new tests include corticotropin-releasing factor administration and petrosal sinus sampling. Inferior petrosal sinus catheterization is useful only if ACTH can be reliably measured. Blood is drawn simultaneously from both petrosal sinuses and a peripheral vein. The utility of the test is enhanced if corticotropin-releasing factor is administered during the procedure. A plasma ACTH concentration gradient (petrosal sinus/peripheral vein ACTH greater than or equal to 1.6) verifies a pituitary source of ACTH. Lateralization of ACTH secretion aids in the preoperative localization of the lesion.

If the evaluation supports a diagnosis of ectopic ACTH secretion, the tumor must be found. Approximately 50 per cent of these tumors are within the thorax (oat cell carcinomas, bronchial carcinoids, thymomas), and chest radiographs, lung tomograms, and thoracic CT scans will usually localize the lesion. Other ACTH-secreting tumors are found in the pancreas (islet cell tumors), the thyroid (medullary carcinoma), and the adrenal medulla (pheochromocytoma).

The differential diagnosis between mild Cushing's disease and the hypercortisolism of depression can be a problem. The natural history of the two conditions is different. Depression is usually a self-limited condition, and resolution of the clinical picture of hypercortisolism is associated with improvement in the degree of depression. Patients with Cushing's syndrome, on the other hand, slowly progress and the deteriorating clinical status makes the diagnosis clear.

When the results of the evaluation for Cushing's syndrome are inconclusive, the periodic hypersecretion of cortisol should be suspected. Long-term monitoring (1 to 2 months) with weekly urine collections for the measurement of free cortisol will usually clarify this situation.

Rarely, factitious Cushing's syndrome is encountered. These subjects usually have Cushing's syndrome with low levels of urinary free cortisol excretion because synthetic glucocorticoids, such as prednisone, prednisolone, or dexamethasone, are the most frequently abused agents. Specific plasma or urine assays for these steroids are usually necessary to confirm the diagnosis.

Treatment

Therapy is indicated in all patients with clinical signs and laboratory confirmation of Cushing's syndrome. The treatment of choice depends upon the specific cause of the hypercortisolism. Optimal treatment is the correction of hypercortisolism without permanent dependence on hormone replacement.

Cushing's Disease

Most cases of Cushing's syndrome are caused by small ACTH-secreting pituitary adenomas. These are usually benign, are small (90 per cent are less than 10 mm in diameter), and cause no sellar enlargement. The rare cases of corticotroph cell hyperplasia may represent the hypothalamic hypersecretion of corticotropin-releasing factor. This, however, has not been proved.

Several therapeutic modalities are available for the treatment of these tumors: trans-sphenoidal adenomectomy, pituitary radiation with concomitant therapy with the adrenolytic agent *o,p'*-DDD (mitotane), therapy with *o,p'*-DDD or steroidogenic enzyme inhibitors (aminoglutethimide, metyrapone, trilostane), and bilateral adrenalectomy.

Trans-sphenoidal adenomectomy is the treatment of choice. Successful surgery leads to cure of hypercortisolism with no need for permanent glucocorticoid replacement. Permanent anterior or posterior pituitary hormone deficiencies are rare. Transient diabetes insipidus may occur during the early weeks following surgery. Permanent diabetes insipidus and cerebrospinal fluid rhinorrhea are uncommon complications. The success rate of this operation exceeds 70 per cent in some centers. A small percentage of patients, however, suffer recurrences. Treatment failures are most common in patients with large pituitary tumors. The mortality rate is approximately 1 per cent, less than that of bilateral adrenalectomy.

Pituitary x-radiation, 4500 to 5000 rad given in 180 to 200 rad fractions over a period of 6 weeks, leads to an improvement in 40 to 50 per cent of adult patients and about 80 per cent of children. Biochemical and clinical amelioration is delayed by several months, however, and can be hastened by the addition of mitotane, which is given in four divided doses ranging from 1 to 4 grams per day.

Combined pituitary radiation and mitotane improves the success rate of either modality given alone and is a reasonable alternative treatment following failure of trans-sphenoidal surgery or as the first line of treatment in patients judged unsuitable for surgery. Pituitary radiation leads to progressive anterior hypopituitarism, including growth hormone deficiency, hypothyroidism, and hypogonadism in 30 to 40 per cent of patients.

Mitotane (Lysodren) can cause nausea, vomiting, diarrhea, skin reactions, and neurologic manifestations, primarily lethargy, somnolence, dizziness, and muscle weakness. The drug may affect the zona glomerulosa, leading to hypoaldosteronism that requires replacement with oral fludrocortisone (Florinef), 50 to 200 micrograms per day. The urinary free cortisol excretion should be monitored and the dose of mitotane titrated to maintain urinary free cortisol excretion in the normal range. If adrenal insufficiency is suspected, oral dexamethasone should be added. Since mitotane induces liver mono-oxygenases (P450 enzymes) which metabolize steroids and other drugs, an adequate dose of fluorocortisone or dexamethasone may be higher than expected. The effects of radiation on pituitary ACTH secretion becomes more prominent with time. Thus, the need for mitotane therapy decreases, and the drug can often be discontinued.

Therapy with mitotane alone can be successful in 30 to 40 per cent of patients. Addition of aminoglutethimide (Cytadren), up to 1 gram a day orally in four divided doses, or metyrapone (Metopirone), up to 1 gram a day in four divided doses, can improve the success rate. To our knowledge, long-term studies comparing combinations of adrenolytic-steroidogenic enzyme inhibitor therapies have not been reported. Aminoglutethimide, metyrapone, or trilostane have inhibiting effects on different steroidogenic enzymes. They also have different side effects. Theoretically, combinations should lead to increased therapeutic effectiveness with decreased individual drug doses and, therefore, fewer side effects. The experience with these three agents given alone has shown that, despite some initial beneficial effect, the pituitary-adrenal axis tends to break through therapy.

Aminoglutethimide has gastrointestinal (anorexia, nausea, vomiting) and neurologic (lethargy, sedation, blurred vision) side effects and can cause hypothyroidism in 5 per cent of the patients. A skin rash is frequently observed during the first 10 days of therapy, which usually subsides despite continuation of treatment. Similar side effects have been observed with trilostane, until recently an investigational drug. Metyrapone causes hypertension and hypokalemic alkalosis, a result of blockade of 11-hydroxylase and accumulation of 11-deoxycorticosterone. It also produces gastrointestinal irritation and allergic rash.

Bilateral adrenalectomy, when performed properly, leads to cure of hypercortisolism. The individual is then committed to lifelong daily cortisol replacement. Uncommonly, incomplete removal of the glands can lead to recurrence when adrenal remnants hypertrophy. Operative mortality is approximately 4 per cent. Following bilateral adrenalectomy, ten to 15 per cent of patients with Cushing's disease develop Nelson's syndrome—large pituitary macroadenomas secreting great amounts of ACTH, resulting in skin hyperpigmentation. These adenomas may be locally invasive and extend above the diaphragma sellae, causing visual field defects. Rarely, they can metastasize locally in the brain. Some respond to radiation therapy. Trans-sphenoidal surgery is also an option.

The Ectopic ACTH Syndrome

If the tumor is totally excised, hypercortisolism will be cured. Tumors secreting ACTH are often disseminated at the time of diagnosis, however, and other therapeutic options must be employed. Therapy, other than primary tumor excision, is directed toward the adrenal glands. The use of mitotane and steroidogenic enzyme inhibitors, as described, are the first line of defense. Bilateral adrenalectomy is an alternative approach.

Adrenocortical Tumors

Benign cortisol-secreting adenomas should be treated by excision. Micronodular adrenal disease should be treated by bilateral adrenalectomy. Adrenal carcinomas initially should be treated surgically. Maximal debulking of the tumor should be attempted. Medical therapy includes mitotane at doses higher (up to 16 grams per day) than those used in Cushing's disease or the ectopic ACTH syndrome. About one third of the tumors respond with regression in size. About two thirds of the patients respond to therapy with decreases of urinary 17-hydroxysteroids and 17-ketosteroids. Before initiation of therapy, a tumor mass should be defined, which can be followed objectively by radiologic procedures (usually CAT scan) for monitoring therapeutic efficacy.

In treating adrenal carcinomas, mitotane is used not only to correct the hypercortisolism but also as an adrenocytolytic agent. Occasionally, for the correction of hypercortisolism, steroid synthesis inhibitors are also required. Patients taking mitotane may develop hypoaldosteronism or hypocortisolism and fludrocortisone or dexamethasone should be added as needed.

Postoperative Steroid Replacement

Since a successful trans-sphenoidal operation in Cushing's disease, or removal of an autonomous adrenal adenoma, leads to a period of adrenal insufficiency, glucocorticoids must be replaced. This abnormality of the hypothalamic-pituitary-adrenal axis can last as long as 1 year. Intraoperatively and during the first 2 postoperative days, 100 mg per M^2 per day of hydrocortisone or its equivalent are given intravenously. Oral replacement doses of hydrocortisone, 12 to 15 mg per M^2 per day, are then initiated. Patients who are cured often complain of weakness and lack of energy at these doses, a sign of successful surgery. This regimen is maintained for 1 month and then tapered. Tapering starts by doubling the daily dose and giving it every other day for 2 months. At that time the patient is tested with a short ACTH stimulation test (Cortrosyn, 250 micrograms intravenously, with cortisol measured at 60 min). If the response to this test is normal (plasma cortisol above 20 micrograms per dl) an attempt to discontinue hydrocortisone is made. If the test is not normal, the therapy is continued for another 2 months and the test repeated.

The majority of patients can discontinue glucocorticoid replacement by the tenth postoperative month. During this period patients should be given extra glucocorticoids during stress: minor stress (febrile illness) by doubling the daily dose of hydrocortisone and major stress (trauma, surgery) by giving ten times the replacement dose. All patients should wear medical badges indicating that they are receiving glucocorticoid replacement.

Exogenous Cushing's Syndrome

This is most commonly seen in patients with renal, autoimmune, hematologic, and neoplastic conditions that require chronic pharmacologic glucocorticoid therapy. The symptoms and signs are those of Cushing's syndrome, including hypothalamic pituitary-adrenal-axis suppression and growth stunting in children. These signs and symptoms can be diminished by administering the glucocorticoids in an alternate day pattern. Every effort should be made to minimize the period during which steroids are given daily. Once the disease process has been controlled, the daily dose should be doubled and administered on alternate days. Many glucocorticoid-responsive diseases are now successfully controlled in this manner.

DIABETES INSIPIDUS

method of
JOHN P. FITZGIBBONS, M.D.
Tufts University
Springfield, Massachusetts

Central (or neurogenic) diabetes insipidus results most commonly from head trauma or surgical hypophysectomy. Primary or metastatic tumors to the brain and an idiopathic form of the disease are the next most likely causes. Less common etiologies include vascular abnormalities, infections, granulomatous diseases, histiocytosis, and an inherited form of this disorder. There can be either complete absence of the hormone vasopressin, or a partial defect associated with some ability to concentrate the urine with dehydration.

Nephrogenic diabetes insipidus is most commonly an acquired defect seen in a large number of kidney disorders. Chronic renal failure itself, whatever its etiology, is frequently associated with a relative resistance to vasopressin when the glomerular filtration rate is less than 60 ml per min. Disorders reported to be associated with nephrogenic diabetes insipidus include medullary cystic disease, polycystic kidney disease, chronic interstitial nephritis, sarcoidosis, obstructive uropathy, amyloidosis, pyelonephritis, radiation nephritis, Sjögren's syndrome, sickle cell disease, and light chain nephropathy. There is also a congenital form of nephrogenic diabetes insipidus, which is an inherited defect expressed as a more severe disease in affected males.

Abnormal urine-concentrating ability can also be caused by electrolyte disturbances (hypokalemia and hypercalcemia) and by a number of different drugs. In the evaluation of any patient with polyuria, it is important to rule out any of these disorders, since the appropriate treatment in these circumstances would be to correct either the electrolyte disturbance or withdrawal of the drug, if possible. Among drugs associated with concentrating disorders, the most common ones are lithium carbonate (Lithobid), amphotericin-B, demeclocycline (Declomycin), gentamicin (Garamycin), and methoxyflurane (Penthrane).

In the evaluation of patients with polyuria, it may be difficult to differentiate among partial central diabetes insipidus, nephrogenic diabetes insipidus, and primary polydipsia. Before starting therapy it is important to exclude primary polydipsia as the cause of the polyuria, since any intervention that decreases free water clearance could have potentially catastrophic results in patients with this disorder if they persist in taking in large amounts of fluid.

Hormonal Therapy

Desmopressin acetate (DDAVP), which is a synthetic analogue of vasopressin, is the most commonly used agent in the treatment of central diabetes insipidus. It has the advantage of being administered intranasally, is relatively long acting, and has fewer vasopressor and intestinal smooth muscle effects. The drug comes in 2.5 ml vials with a concentration of desmopressin acetate of 0.1 mg per ml. The agent is administered via a plastic nasal tube with graduations to allow adjustments of the dose delivered. The usual dose is 0.2 ml twice daily, but the amount and frequency of the dose must be adjusted on an individual basis.

Vasopressin tannate in oil (Pitressin Tannate in oil) has the advantage of a longer period of action so that treatment is required only once every 1 to 3 days. Pitressin Tannate in oil must be given as a deep intramuscular injection and does cause contraction of blood vessels and the smooth muscles of the gastrointestinal tract. Sterile abscesses at the site of the injection are a recognized complication. It is important to instruct the patient to warm and vigorously shake the ampule since the pitressin tends to precipitate and must be resuspended. Ampules are 1.0 ml in size containing 5 pressor units per ml. The dose varies between 0.3 and 1.0 ml, with the dosing interval identified by the onset of polyuria.

Lysine vasopressin (Diapid nasal spray) is a synthetic analogue of vasopressin. It has the advantages of being stable and has less vasopressor activity. Its duration of action is between 3 and 8 hours. One spray into the nostril with the container held upright and the patient in a vertical position will dispense approximately 2 pressor units of lysine vasopressin. The usual dose is 1 to 2 sprays four times per day. If this is not effective in controlling the polyuria, the dosage interval should be decreased before the number of sprays is increased. Because of variable absorption from the mucosa, the dose can be quite variable. Many patients use this spray at bedtime to prevent nocturia. Lysine vasopressin comes in an 8 ml nasal spray bottle with a concentration of 50 pressor units per ml.

Aqueous vasopressin (Pitressin) is a synthetic form of 8-arginine vasopressin. It can be given subcutaneously; intramuscularly; or intranasally on cotton pledgets, as a nasal spray, or by dropper. Pitressin causes contraction of the smooth muscles of the gastrointestinal tract and the vascular bed. When given as an injection, the usual dose is 0.25 to 0.5 ml every 3 to 4 hours as necessary to control polyuria. Pitressin is used in the acute treatment of central diabetes insipidus, but because of its short duration of action it is not useful for chronic treatment. When used intranasally, the dose response is highly variable and is adjusted according to the patient's polyuria and thirst. Aqueous vasopressin comes in 0.5 and 1.0 ml ampules containing 20 pressor units per ml.

Nonhormonal Therapy

Chlorpropamide (Diabinese) is useful in the treatment of partial central diabetes insipidus (this use is not listed by the manufacturer). Since its action to decrease urine volume and increase urine osmolarity depends on the presence of some vasopressin, this drug has no effect in complete central diabetes insipidus. In nephrogenic diabetes insipidus, chlorpropamide is usually of no value in improving the intrarenal concentrating defect. The usual dose is 250 mg once or twice daily, although up to 750 mg per day may be used. The effect is not immediate, and it may take several weeks for the maximal response to be achieved. The major side effects of this drug are the potential for hypoglycemia and a disulfiram-like reaction with the concomitant use of alcohol. Chlorpropamide comes in 100 mg and 250 mg tablets.

Thiazide Diuretics

Since nephrogenic diabetes insipidus does not respond to hormonal therapy, thiazide diuretics are the treatment of choice in this condition. Thiazides induce mild salt depletion, which causes an increase in salt and water reabsorption in the more proximal portions of the nephron. Less fluid reaches more distal sites and thus total volume output diminishes. For this form of therapy to be effective the patient must be instructed in and follow a low salt diet. The major complication of diuretic therapy is orthostatic hypotension secondary to excessive salt loss. Thiazides can also be used as an adjunct to hormonal therapy in the treatment of central diabetes insipidus, although such supplemental therapy is rarely necessary. Hydrochlorothiazide (HydroDIURIL) is the thiazide most frequently used. The dose is 50 to 100 mg per day. Hydrochlorothiazide comes in 25, 50, and 100 mg tablets.

Other Therapies

Carbamazepine (Tegretol) and clofibrate (Atromid-S) have both been recommended in the past because of their ability to stimulate vasopressin release. However, because of the toxicity of these drugs and the availability of other forms of therapy they are no longer recommended for the treatment of diabetes insipidus.

Nonsteroidal anti-inflammatory drugs have also been recommended because of their ability to decrease urine output. It has been proposed that this effect results from the action of many of these drugs to decrease intrarenal prostaglandin production. Since prostaglandins interfere with vasopressin's effect on the tubule, prostaglandin inhibition would sensitize the nephron to vasopressin. However, prostaglandin inhibition can also cause a decrease in glomerular filtration rate, especially in the presence of intrinsic renal disease. Since abnormal renal function is common in the conditions causing nephrogenic diabetes insipidus, nonsteroidal anti-inflammatory drugs are not recommended as treatment for this disorder.

NONTOXIC GOITER

method of
LAURA K. BACHRACH, M.D.,
and GERARD N. BURROW, M.D.
University of Toronto
Toronto, Ontario

Goiter is defined as enlargement of the thyroid gland to at least twice the normal size—that is, 40 to 50 grams in North America. Nontoxic goiter is benign thyroid enlargement, which may be diffuse or nodular with solitary or multiple nodules. Nontoxic goiters can be further classified as endemic, sporadic, or compensatory types, the latter occurring after subtotal thyroidectomy. Hashimoto's thyroiditis may also result in nontoxic thyroid enlargement.

Worldwide, iodine deficiency causes the most common type of nontoxic goiter, endemic goiter, which by definition affects more than 10 per cent of the population of an area. In developed areas, where dietary iodine is plentiful, sporadic and compensatory goiters are far more common.

DIAGNOSTIC CONSIDERATIONS

The evaluation of the patient with goiter should establish whether the patient is euthyroid, whether thyroid nodules exist, and whether autoimmune thyroiditis is the cause. Measurement of serum thyroxine (T_4), resin T_3 uptake, and thyroid-stimulating hormone (TSH) will determine functional thyroid status. High positive titers of thyroid antibodies are diagnostic of Hashimoto's thyroiditis. The presence of a nodular goiter, which can be confirmed by thyroid ultrasound or radioisotopic scan, raises the question of malignancy. Further diagnostic studies such as fine needle biopsy are warranted for all solitary nodules. Finally, if the patient complains of local pressure symptoms such as dysphagia, cough, or hoarseness, x-ray studies of the trachea and peak inspiratory and expiratory flow studies will establish whether the goiter is causing upper airway obstruction.

Treatment

Thyroid hormone treatment should be considered for all nontoxic goiters. The rationale for such therapy is suppression of TSH-induced thyroid growth. We believe such treatment serves not only to reduce goiter size but also to prevent nodule formation, which appears to occur as a sequela of prolonged growth stimulation. Even though there is no evidence that multinodular goiter is associated with an increased risk of thyroid malignancy, "lumps" in the thyroid are likely to cause patient and physician concern and may led to unnecessary surgery. Since thyroid hormone therapy is inexpensive and relatively nontoxic, treatment is warranted even for small goiters. In elderly patients, particularly those with nodular goiters that may function autonomously, the physician may consider observation without treatment. This approach is appropriate especially if the patient has risk factors that make T_4 treatment more hazardous, such as cardiovascular disease.

The drug of choice for goiter therapy is L-thyroxine (T_4) since triiodothyronine (T_3) administration causes unphysiologic elevations of serum T_3 concentration. A T_4 dose of 100 to 150 micrograms daily is usually sufficient to achieve TSH suppression. Larger doses may cause clinical or biochemical hyperthyroidism. A blunted TSH response to administered thyrotropin-releasing hormone (TRH) is proof that the T_4 dose is adequate, but this test is not required routinely for nontoxic goiter. Treatment should be monitored with measurement of thyroid hormone concentrations; the serum T_4 concentration may be slightly elevated, but the serum T_3 concentration should be within the normal range. An elevated serum T_3 concentration may indicate autonomously functioning thyroid nodules, which can be confirmed by radioisotopic scan.

Medical treatment successfully reduces the size of the majority of diffuse and multinodular goiters. As many as 33 per cent of nontoxic goiters will resolve completely with T_4 therapy while an additional 33 to 50 per cent show a moderate reduction in size. Goiter regression is more likely to occur with a longer period of medical treatment, and we recommend a minimum of 6 to 12 months of T_4 therapy before declaring that a goiter has failed to respond. If medical treatment results in no reduction in goiter size, the patient may be noncompliant or the dose of T_4 too low to suppress TSH secretion. These possibilities can be excluded with a TRH test. Treatment failures may also be due to fibrosis of the thyroid, and long-standing goiters are less likely to resolve. Persistent goiters also may be explained by the presence of growth stimulators other than TSH. At present, no laboratory assays are routinely available to detect such growth factors and their role in the pathogenesis of goiter remains speculative. Therefore, we recommend continued T_4 treatment even for the goiter that fails to regress, in an effort to prevent further enlargement.

Surgical treatment of nontoxic goiter is rarely indicated. Subtotal thyroidectomy is reserved for large goiters causing upper airway obstruction that fail to respond to T_4 suppression. Postoperatively, these patients require complete T_4 replacement to prevent goiter recurrence.

HYPER- AND HYPOPARATHYROIDISM

method of
DANIEL D. BIKLE, M.D., Ph.D.
University of California, San Francisco
San Francisco, California

Hyperparathyroidism

DIAGNOSTIC CONSIDERATIONS

Hyperparathyroidism is defined operationally by an elevated serum parathyroid hormone (PTH) level. This can be caused by excess secretion of the hormone by an abnormal parathyroid gland (or glands) which fails to respond appropriately to the usually elevated serum calcium level or because of appropriately increased secretion by normal parathyroid tissue responding to a low serum calcium level. Most patients with elevated serum calcium and PTH levels have primary hyperparathyroidism. This disease originates in abnormal parathyroid tissue and can be cured by surgical removal of this tissue. Eighty per cent of the patients with primary hyperparathyroidism have a single hyperfunctioning gland (adenoma), 15 per cent have generalized hyperplasia, and the remainder have two or more adenomas.

When hyperparathyroidism results from a normal response of the parathyroid glands to a hypocalcemic stimulus, the condition is called secondary hyperparathyroidism. Chronic renal failure, vitamin D deficiency, malabsorption, and pregnancy may all result in secondary hyperparathyroidism. Secondary hyperparathyroidism is best treated by reversing the conditions leading to the hypocalcemia. If the hypocalcemic stimulus is prolonged, as in chronic renal failure, the parathyroid glands may become partially or completely refractory to serum calcium levels. When this occurs, a condition similar to primary hyperparathyroidism—elevated serum calcium and PTH levels—results. This condition is sometimes referred to as tertiary hyperparathyroidism. If severe, subtotal parathyroidectomy may be required.

Although most patients with elevated PTH levels can be categorized as having primary or secondary hyperparathyroidism, on the basis of a concomitant serum calcium level, a few special circumstances need to be recognized. A number of solid tumors elaborate a substance that results in hypercalcemia; some radioimmunoassays for PTH detect this substance, which results in an inappropriately elevated PTH value in the face of hypercalcemia. Treatment of such a patient for primary hyperparathyroidism would be an error. Another situation concerns the syndrome of familial hypocalciuric hypercalcemia. Such patients have lifelong hypercalcemia that is untreatable except by total parathyroidectomy—an unnecessary and unjustifiable operation for this benign disorder. These patients may have inappropriately elevated serum PTH levels in some radioimmunoassays. Documentation of a long history of hypercalcemia without any of its complications, the finding of hypocalciuria, and the observation of hypercalcemia in other family members will help make this diagnosis. Lithium therapy can induce a clinical picture similar to that of familial hypocalciuric hypercalcemia in that serum calcium and PTH levels are elevated and urine calcium levels are reduced. Since there is little evidence that such patients develop complications attributable to the hypercalcemia or hyperparathyroidism, attempts to treat the hyperparathyroidism should be limited to discontinuation of the lithium.

Primary Hyperparathyroidism

Surgical Candidates. Surgical removal of the abnormal gland(s) or subtotal parathyroidectomy (removal of 3½ glands) for general hyperplasia by an experienced surgeon remains the treatment of choice for primary hyperparathyroidism. The therapeutic decision, therefore, is not which treatment but who to treat. With the advent of routine serum calcium determinations, more and more patients are being seen with "asymptomatic" hyperparathyroidism. Because of the nonspecific nature of many of the symptoms (malaise, constipation, fatigability, difficulty in concentration), truly asymptomatic hyperparathyroidism is difficult to verify. However, patients who are symptomatic and have a definite diagnosis of primary hyperparathyroidism should be treated when evidence of any of the following conditions exists: progressive nephrocalcinosis or nephrolithiasis, decreasing renal function, bone disease (including generalized osteopenia), gastrointestinal complications (peptic ulcer, pancreatitis), and difficulty in long-term follow-up. Patients with serum calcium levels below 11 mg per dl who do not have any of these complications may not need treatment if long-term follow-up is adequate. We know little about the natural course of the disease in such patients, but data suggest that the course may be benign for a significant number.

Medical Therapy. Medical treatment of primary hyperparathyroidism has not been effective, though several aproaches have been tried. In vitro data indicate that calcium, catecholamines, and histamine all regulate PTH secretion. Accordingly, beta blockers, such as propranolol, and H_2 antagonists, such as cimetidine, have been used to treat primary and secondary hyperparathyroidism. However, despite encouraging initial reports, these drugs are generally ineffective in the treatment of primary hyperparathyroidism. Phosphate therapy can reduce serum calcium levels and may ameliorate the increased bone resorption in patients with hyperparathyroidism, but this therapy raises PTH levels and may cause ectopic calcification. Therefore, this therapy is not recommended.

Secondary Hyperparathyroidism

Surgical Candidates. Subtotal parathyroidectomy may be necessary when secondary hyperparathyroidism has progressed to cause hypercalcemia in the setting of chronic renal failure, especially when accompanied by pruritus, avascular necrosis of the fingers and toes, ectopic calcification, or progressive bone disease. Following a kidney transplant, hypercalcemia and hyperparathyroidism may develop and threaten the function of the transplanted kidney. However, subtotal parathyroidectomy is not always necessary in these patients because the hyperparathyroidism usually resolves, even after as long as 1 year. Accordingly, watchful waiting is preferred to surgery in such patients if the hyperparathyroidism is resolving and is creating no other medical complications. Subtotal parathyroidectomy is not indicated for patients with chronic renal failure and hypercalcemia who have developed the syndrome of low turnover osteomalacia. These patients clinically have symptoms of bone pain, weakness, and fractures. Their PTH levels are low compared with those of other renal failure patients but are still above normal. The mildly elevated PTH value in conjunction with hypercalcemia gives such patients a biochemical profile similar to that of primary hyperparathyroidism. However, subtotal parathyroidectomy may aggravate, not ameliorate, the symptoms of bone pain and weakness.

SURGICAL CONSIDERATIONS AND LOCALIZATION STUDIES. The operation for primary hyperparathyroidism is successful in over 90 per cent of cases. Failures occur when the surgeon fails to find all the glands (four is the usual number, but five or more glands are quite common), which are located nearly anywhere in the neck or mediastinum. In the absence of a family history of hyperparathyroidism or in the absence of polyendocrine disease, removal of only the abnormal gland(s) is generally sufficient in patients with adenomas; subtotal parathyroidectomy (the removal of 3½ glands) is required when all glands are hyperplastic. The removal of all parathyroid tissue with autotransplantation into the forearm is a new procedure still under investigation.

Localization procedures to identify the position of the abnormal gland before surgery include high resolution ultrasonography, computed tomography, selective arteriography (usually combined with selective venous sampling for PTH levels), and ^{75}Se-selenomethionine or thallium scanning (usually combined with ^{99m}technetium thyroid scans). These procedures are probably not needed at the outset since the initial operation is usually successful without them. Localizing techniques may be more valuable if the first operation fails to correct the hyperparathyroidism, although even under these circumstances an overlooked or ectopic gland can usually be found by an experienced surgeon without use of these techniques.

Acute Hypercalcemic Crisis

Occasionally a patient with hyperparathyroidism presents in hypercalcemic crisis with symptoms of mental confusion or coma. Emergency measures begin with large volumes of intravenous saline (500 to 1000 ml per hour). When the patient is rehydrated, sufficient furosemide (40 to 120 mg every 2 hours) is given to ensure a steady diuresis. It is important to correct the dehydration that usually accompanies hypercalcemia before attempting a diuresis. Careful monitoring of input and output and attention to signs of congestive heart failure are required. These measures may reduce the serum calcium levels sufficiently so that parathyroidectomy can be performed safely. If saline diuresis is not successful in reducing serum calcium levels, calcitonin (50 to 200 IU intramuscularly every 6 hours) may be given. Although this therapy often has only a partial and transient effect on serum calcium, it is relatively safe. Mithramycin given intravenously over several hours in 25 microgram per kg doses is more effective than calcitonin in reducing serum calcium within 24 hours, but repeated doses can lead to thrombocytopenia, renal disease, or liver disease. Intravenous phosphate also effectively reduces serum calcium, but the danger of ectopic calcification or hypocalcemia is great, so this form of therapy is not recommended. Glucocorticoids and nonsteroidal anti-inflammatory agents do not effectively treat hypercalcemia resulting from hyperparathyroidism.

Hypoparathyroidism

Hypoparathyroidism results when the secretion of parathyroid hormone is deficient (surgical or idiopathic hypoparathyroidism), the hormone secreted is defective (pseudoidiopathic hypoparathyroidism, a rare disorder), or the target tissues fail to respond to the hormone (pseudohypoparathyroidism and its normocalcemic variant, pseudopseudohypoparathyroidism). Patients with pseudohypoparathyroidism can be subdivided into two groups: those who fail to respond to a PTH infusion with increased renal excretion of cyclic AMP (type I), and those who have a normal cyclic AMP response but an abnormal phosphaturic response to PTH infusion (type II). Pseudohypoparathyroid patients may also show an abnormal skeletal response to PTH, or have an N protein (GTP binding protein) deficiency. Hypomagnesemia, seen in alcoholic patients after a binge or in patients with severe malabsorption, can result in transient hypoparathyroidism that is readily corrected by magnesium supplementation.

The biochemical hallmarks of hypoparathyroidism are hypocalcemia and hyperphosphatemia. In surgical or idiopathic hypoparathyroidism the PTH level is low (although most radioimmunoassays for PTH cannot distinguish low from normal PTH levels). In pseudohypoparathyroidism the PTH level is normal, or may even be elevated. When the phenotypic features of pseudohypoparathyroidism are not present, hypoparathyroidism can be distinguished from pseudohypoparathyroidism by measuring the renal response (cyclic AMP or phosphate excretion or both) to PTH infusion. Regardless of the cause, hypoparathyroidism is treated by correcting the hypocalcemia and hyperphosphatemia that accompany it.

Treatment

Hypocalcemia. The acute treatment of hypocalcemia in a patient with tetany or seizures is the slow infusion of 5 to 20 ml of 10 per cent calcium gluconate. Rapid infusion may provoke cardiac arrhythmias. The chronic treatment of hypocalcemia requires 1 to 2 grams of an oral calcium supplement, generally given in divided doses in the form of calcium carbonate. This inexpensive and readily available formulation of calcium delivers 200 mg of elemental calcium for each 500 mg tablet. If this treatment does not restore the serum calcium level to normal, vitamin D or its potent metabolite 1,25-dihydroxyvitamin D (calcitriol) or its analogue dihydrotachysterol (DHT), should also be given. Vitamin D is the cheapest of the vitamin D preparations to use. It is administered in doses ranging from 25,000 units two or three times a week to 100,000 units or more daily. The principal disadvantage of vitamin D therapy is that many patients unpredictably develop hypercalcemia when given these large doses; because of the long biologic half-life of vitamin D, these patients remain hypercalcemic for weeks or months. Calcitriol is given in daily or twice daily doses of 0.25 to 1 microgram. This relatively expensive metabolite of vitamin D has an advantage over vitamin D in that patients who develop hypercalcemia with its use can be treated quickly (within days) by reducing the dose. DHT is used in doses of 0.2 to 1 mg per day. Its biologic half-life is longer than that of calcitriol but shorter than that of vitamin D.

Thiazide diuretics (not including loop diuretics such as furosemide) aid in the treatment of hypoparathyroidism by reducing the hypercalciuria and thus increasing the serum calcium level. Furosemide increases calcium excretion and should not be used in patients with hypoparathyroidism.

Hyperphosphatemia. Phosphate binders such as an aluminum hydroxide suspension or tablets can be given (300 to 600 mg with meals) to reduce the serum phosphate level and secondarily raise the serum calcium level. Patients also receiving vitamin D therapy benefit from this approach because aluminum hydroxide reduces or prevents the hyperphosphatemia that can develop with vitamin D therapy alone.

HYPOPITUITARISM

method of
RAYMOND V. RANDALL, M.D.
Mayo Clinic
Rochester, Minnesota

The term *hypopituitarism* implies failure of both the anterior pituitary lobe and neurohypothalamic portion ("posterior lobe") of the pituitary, but by common usage the term designates anterior pituitary failure. Hypopituitarism is associated with a deficiency or decreased reserve of one or more of the hormones of the anterior pituitary, namely growth hormone, prolactin, thyroid-stimulating hormone (TSH, thyrotropin), adrenocorticotropic hormone (ACTH, adrenocorticotropin), follicle-stimulating hormone (FSH), and luteinizing hormone (LH). FSH and LH are both gonadotropins and usually fail simultaneously; hence one often speaks of gonadotropin failure rather than FSH failure and LH failure, unless there is deficiency of one and not the other.

Treatment

The treatment of patients with hypopituitarism has two objectives. The first is identification and correction of the underlying cause of the failure, if a remedial condition can be found. The second objective of treatment is correction of the hormonal insufficiency. It is important to realize that in most instances hypopituitarism is secondary to an underlying cause, and idiopathic hypopituitarism is practically unheard of in adults although it does occasionally occur in preadolescent children. Therefore, if a careful search fails to reveal an underlying cause, the patient should be followed carefully since months or years may elapse before signs of the underlying lesion responsible for the hypopituitarism become evident. The new 5th generation computed tomographic scanners are helpful in identifying lesions which heretofore escaped detection on initial search. Whether magnetic resonance imaging (MRI, also known as NMR scanning) will be even more useful as newer generations of this type of equipment become available is as yet unknown.

Hypopituitarism may be partial or involve all the hormones produced by the anterior lobe. With progressive hypopituitarism, as from the growth of a pituitary adenoma or suprasellar lesion such as a craniopharyngioma, the usual sequence of failure is loss of production of growth hormone, gonadotropins, TSH, and finally ACTH. The sequence of failure does not always take place as mentioned here—occasionally the adrenal cortices fail before the gonads, or the thyroid before the gonads, and so on. Where prolactin fits into this scheme is unknown, but it is important to be aware that what seems to be loss of gonadal function from an intrasellar or suprasellar tumor may actually be secondary to hyperprolactinemia.

What role, if any, prolactin plays in the development of the signs and symptoms of hypopituitarism is unclear, and at present we know of no reason why replacement with prolactin is necessary for successful treatment of hypopituitarism. Likewise, the administration of growth hormone is not necessary for the treatment of adults with hypopituitarism, and its lack seems to have no significant clinical indications. However, impaired linear growth (dwarfism) is a major finding associated with decreased secretion of growth hormone in persons who have not reached adult stature.

Theoretically the administration of the tropic hormones would be the ideal treatment for TSH, ACTH, and gonadotropin insufficiency. Although these hormones are available, they are not suited for administration over long periods of time because of their expense, the need for parenteral administration, and their short biologic half-life. The use of hormones similar to those made by the target glands, namely the thyroid, adrenal cortices, and gonads, gives satisfactory results, except that fertility is not restored.

Growth Hormone Replacement

It is essential to give growth hormone to children who have not reached normal adult stature and whose epiphyses of the long bones are still open and capable of growth. Unfortunately, growth hormone from animals other than humans is not effective in humans. A limited supply of human growth hormone is available through the National Pituitary Agency and from commercial sources. The material is expensive and must be given parenterally. It should not be used in patients who do not have well-documented growth hormone insufficiency and whose long bone epiphyses have already closed. The usual treatment is to give 2.0 IU of growth hormone intramuscularly three times a week with a minimum of 48 hours between injections. If the rate of growth is not in excess of 2.5 cm every 6 months the dose can be doubled. Treatment is discontinued when the patient reaches a satisfactory adult height; if the patient ceases to respond with further, adequate linear growth; or if the epiphyses of the long bones close. Adrenal replacement, when indicated, must be given with caution not only to children receiving treatment with growth hormone but also to any growing child, because excessive amounts of glucocorticoids retard or stop linear growth even though adequate amounts of exogenous or endogenous growth hormone are available. The daily dose of hydrocortisone, or an equivalent amount of an associated glucocorticoid, should not exceed a total daily dose of 10 to 15 mg of hydrocortisone per M^2 of body surface. Similar precaution must be observed when giving gonadal replacement, and this will be reviewed later.

Many patients treated with growth hormone develop antibodies to growth hormone, but this usually does not cause failure to respond to the material. Growth hormone has diabetogenic actions; particular care must be given when treating patients with diabetes mellitus or with a family history of this condition.

Thyroid Hormone Replacement

Thyroid hormonal deficiency is treated by giving 0.15 mg of sodium levothyroxine in a single oral dose each day. An occasional patient will require a larger or a smaller dose; measuring the level of serum thyroxine and the response of the patient provide guides to the appropriate dose. Estrogenic materials increase thyroxine-binding globulin and androgens tend to reduce it, thus altering the level of *total* thyroxine in the blood. Hence, measurement of thyroxine-binding globulin or serum free thyroxine is helpful in determining the proper dose of levothyroxine when sex steroids are given.

The serum total triiodothyronine (T_3) level will be in the normal range when adequate amounts of levothyroxine are given as replacement, because there is extrathyroidal conversion of thyroxine to T_3 by peripheral monodeiodination. Most children with thyroid insufficiency require the same replacement dose of thyroxine as adults require. Again, guides to the appropriate dose are measuring the amount of circulating thyroxine in the blood and the response of the patient.

In coronary artery disease, in older persons, or with other contraindications to starting the treatment of thyroid deficiency with the usual daily replacement dose of 0.15 mg per day, it is prudent to begin with a single daily dose of 0.05 or even 0.025 mg per day and gradually increase the dose over a number of weeks or months until a satisfactory daily dose is reached.

The status of adrenal function should be determined before starting thyroid replacement, because full doses of thyroid replacement can precipitate an adrenal crisis in a person with adrenal insufficiency. This does not happen if adrenal replacement begins at the same time treatment with levothyroxine is started. It is not necessary to give glucocorticoids several days or weeks prior to starting thyroidal replacement—they can be started simultaneously.

Triiodothyronine is not a good choice for treating thyroidal deficiency in patients with hypopituitarism, because it must be given in several doses throughout each 24 hour period and the levels of triiodothyronine in the blood fluctuate widely between doses.

Adrenal Replacement

Adrenal replacement is provided by the administration of one of the glucocorticoids, such as hydrocortisone (or hydrocortisone acetate), cortisone acetate, or prednisone. Since hydrocortisone is relatively inexpensive and since it is the major naturally occurring human glucocorticoid I usually use it. However, if cost is a significant factor then prednisone is used.

The usual total daily dose of hydrocortisone is 25 to 30 mg orally, 15 or 20 mg in the morning with breakfast and 10 mg in the late afternoon or with supper. Some patients who take their last dose of glucocorticoid at bedtime may be bothered by insomnia. If cortisone acetate is used, I usually start with a total of 30 mg per day in divided doses, as with hydrocortisone. Occasionally, a patient will need 25 mg of cortisone acetate in the morning and 12.5 mg in the late afternoon or with supper. I give 2.5 mg of prednisone twice daily at the times just mentioned, or in some patients in whom this is not adequate, 5.0 mg of prednisone in the morning and 2.5 mg in the late afternoon or with supper. One should use caution with total doses of 37.5 or 50 mg of hydrocortisone or cortisone acetate per day or 10 mg of prednisone per day, as advocated by some, because patients taking these larger doses, particularly small women, run the risk of developing osteoporosis. An occasional person develops glucocorticoid psychosis with these doses.

In hypopituitarism, the adrenal cortex produces adequate amounts of aldosterone; consequently, it is not necessary to give an electrolyte-retaining hormone. However, we have seen in rare instances a patient with hypopituitarism from a hypothalamic lesion who has been unable to retain adequate amounts of serum sodium and chloride unless given an electrolyte-retaining hormone (mineralocorticoid), such as 0.1 mg of fludrocortisone (Florinef) orally each morning in addition to hydrocortisone, cortisone acetate, or prednisone. An occasional person such as a farmer or steel worker, who is exposed to more than average amounts of heat, may lose enough sodium under these circumstances so that the administration of fludrocortisone is necessary. Such patients must be monitored carefully during the first weeks of treatment with fludrocortisone to guard against excessive retention of sodium, and if such takes place, the daily dose should be reduced to 0.05 mg daily or even every other day.

Patients taking a glucocorticoid are advised to triple each dose of glucocorticoid in the event of a minor febrile illness and to notify their physician at once. They are also given a supply of a parenteral glucocorticoid preparation to keep on hand and use in the event of vomiting or a sudden, severe stressful illness until medical help is available. A convenient form is a prepackaged disposable needle and syringe containing a 1.0 ml solution of 4.0 mg of dexamethasone sodium phosphate (Decadron). Patients are asked to keep two such syringes on hand and inject one in a medical emergency. If medical help cannot be obtained a second dose is taken 6 to 8 hours after the first dose. We teach members of the family as well as the patient how to administer the material. Each package has an expiration date, and the material should be replaced when outdated.

In the event of severe physical stress, such as operation, trauma, or severe illness, patients with hypopituitarism should be given adrenal support in the form of large parenteral doses of hydrocortisone or one of the related steroids. In a hospital setting we usually give 40 mg of prednisolone phosphate sodium (Hydeltrasol) intramuscularly every 6 to 8 hours. The material can also be given intravenously in a dose of 40 mg by constant drip over a 6 to 8 hour period, following an initial intravenous dose of 40 mg over 3 to 5 minutes. It is important to remember that large doses of hydrocortisone or cortisone acetate have significant mineralocorticoid action (sodium retention), and hence caution must be used in the simultaneous administration of intravenous fluids containing sodium.

Gonadal Replacement

Males can be given androgens by the intramuscular, oral, or buccal routes. The intramuscular preparations are more effective and do not carry the risk of cholestatic jaundice that occasionally occurs with the use of oral or buccal preparations. I prefer to use testosterone enanthate in sesame oil (Delatestryl) or testosterone cypionate in cottonseed oil (Depo-Testosterone) in doses of 200 mg intramuscularly every 3 weeks. Testosterone enanthate in sesame oil comes prepackaged, 200 mg in a disposable 1.0 ml syringe with a needle. Some patients occasionally may need 200 mg every 2 weeks whereas other patients may go a month between injections. A member of the family or the patient is usually instructed to administer this material intramuscularly into the buttocks or large anterior thigh muscles. If the patient prefers to use an oral preparation, fluoxymesterone (Halotestin, Ora-Testryl, Ultandren) can be given in a single oral dose of 10 to 20 mg per day. Methyltestosterone (Metandren, Neo-Hombreol-M, Oreton-Methyl) can be given orally in doses of 20 to 60 mg per day or buccally in doses of 15 to 30 mg per day. The oral and buccal preparations of methyltestosterone are more effective when given in 2 or 3 doses per day.

Preferably, androgens are not started in adolescent males as long as the epiphyses of the long bones are open and the patient has not reached an acceptable adult height. Under such circumstances the epiphyses close later than normal, and the rate of growth will be less than average if there is a deficiency of growth hormone or if growth hormone has not been started until after the patient has had a period of delayed growth. These patients are often caught in an emotional turmoil between a desire for greater height and a desire for sexual maturation at a time when their peers are maturing. If treatment with androgens is elected under these circumstances, 75 to 100 mg of testosterone enanthate or cypionate is given intramuscularly once a month until the epiphyses have closed, and then the dose is increased to 200 mg every 3 weeks.

Side effects of androgen therapy include acne and occasionally gynecomastia. As the patient gets older, balding will take place if the patient has an inherited tendency to become bald. Prostatic hypertrophy may develop in older patients since androgen therapy is continued throughout the life of the individual. Patients should be warned about possible side effects, and in older patients the prostate should be checked annually, or more often if indicated, for possible malignant change. In older patients the dose can be decreased from 200 mg of the intramuscular preparation every 3 weeks to once every 4 weeks.

Females of menstrual age can be given adequate replacement by the oral route, and intramuscular preparations are not necessary although they are often prescribed. Estrogenic materials are given cyclically for the first 21 days of each month or daily for the first 3 of every 4 weeks. A progestational agent is added from day 12 through day 21 of each cycle. A convenient way of giving these materials is to use one of the oral contraceptive pills containing both an estrogenic agent and a progestational agent. If the physician prefers to use separate preparations of each, conjugated estrogens (Premarin, Mesest, SK-Estrogens) are given orally in a single daily dose of 0.625 or 1.25 mg for the first 21 days of each month or daily for the first 3 of every 4 weeks. Ethinyl estradiol (Estinyl, Lynoral), 0.01 or 0.02 mg orally each day, can be given on the same schedule. Progestational preparations such as medroxyprogesterone acetate (Provera) are given in a single oral dose at a rate of 10 mg daily starting on day 12 and ending on day 21 of each cycle of estrogenic preparation.

The precautions for giving androgens to growing adolescent men should also be observed when treating adolescent women with estrogens and progesterone. The patient should also be alerted to the possibility of developing thrombophlebitis, hypertension, and other side effects ascribed to estrogens and birth control pills. However, my impression (not proved statistically) is that patients with hypopituitarism who are given these compounds rarely have these side effects. I believe that women should be given these hormones until 50 to 55 years of age unless there is some contraindication. Patients of either sex are prone to develop osteoporosis if they are deficient in sex steroids during early adulthood and middle age.

Some female patients, especially those who develop pituitary insufficiency in their adolescent or preadolescent years, will have poor development of sexual hair and poor libido despite receiving adequate replacement therapy with estrogenic and progestational agents. In an attempt to correct this, the physician can prescribe cautiously small doses of adrogens, such as 2 mg of fluoxymesterol (Halotestin) orally every 1 to 2 days for 6 to 9 months. The patient must be monitored closely because these small doses can cause hyperandrogenism in some women, and the same precaution about possible cholestatic jaundice applies to women as to men. Patients who have a good libidinous response to androgens usually want to continue the treatment indefinitely, which may ultimately lead to undesirable androgen effects such as acne, hirsutism, clitoral enlargement, and deepening of the voice.

What appears to be gonadal insufficiency from the destructive effects of an expanding pituitary tumor or other process in that area may actually be secondary to hyperprolactinemia, and reducing the level of prolactin (as discussed in the next article, on Hyperprolactinemia) will restore gonadal function if that is the cause.

Fertility can often be restored in a patient with hypogonadism by the use of gonadotropins. This complex treatment requires close monitoring and cannot be discussed adequately in the space provided here.

Medical Information Tag

Patients with hypopituitarism should wear a medical information necklace or bracelet inscribed with the information that they have a pituitary problem and should be given adrenocorticosteroids in a medical emergency. The bracelet or necklace should also be inscribed with other pertinent information, such as drug allergies or other illnesses. In my opinion the most satisfactory tag is either the Medic Alert bracelet or necklace available from Medic Alert Foundation International, P. O. Box 1009, Turlock, CA 95381-1009. Application forms are obtained by writing to this nonprofit foundation or calling 1-800/344-3226 (in California, 1-209/668-3333).

HYPERPROLACTINEMIA

method of
RAYMOND V. RANDALL, M.D.
Mayo Clinic
Rochester, Minnesota

Hyperprolactinemia is the presence of excessive amounts of prolactin in the blood; it can be without effect or associated with the manifestations shown in Table 1. The exact effects depend upon the levels of prolactin in the blood, the individual sensitivity of the patient to these levels, and the age of the patient when hyperprolactinemia begins. In addition, the patient may have symptoms related to an underlying condition associated with or causing hyperprolactinemia.

The treatment of hyperprolactinemia consists of not only treating the hyperprolactinemia but attempting to identify and correct the underlying associated condition. In some instances, correcting the underlying condition will terminate the hyperprolactinemia. Examples are the removal of a prolactin-producing pituitary adenoma, correction of hypothyroidism, and stopping a medication.

Diagnostic Considerations

The most frequent causes of hyperprolactinemia are medications, physiologic states, hypothyroidism, and

TABLE 1. **Endrocine Manifestations of Hyperprolactinemia**

Women
Galactorrhea
Regular menses
Ovulatory
Anovulatory
Irregular menses
Ovulatory
Anovulatory
Amenorrhea
Secondary
Primary
without delayed puberty
with delayed puberty
Menorrhagia (rare)
Men
Galactorrhea, usually with gynecomastia
Spermatogenesis
Normal
Decreased (oligospermia)
Absent (azoospermia)
Hypotestosteronemia
Delayed puberty
Both Sexes
Refractoriness to exogenous sex steroids

pituitary adenomas. The first three should be easy to identify. A pituitary adenoma is relatively easy to identify if it is 5 mm or greater in diameter, but it can be elusive when only 2 to 3 mm in diameter. Fortunately, these smaller adenomas can usually be demonstrated by the new 5th generation computed tomographic scanners with scans taken in the coronal and axial planes during the infusion of contrast medium.

The finding of a pituitary adenoma in the presence of hyperprolactinemia does not necessarily mean that the adenoma is secreting prolactin. Large pituitary adenomas, particularly those that expand the sella and protrude above the diaphragm, can cause hyperprolactinemia by preventing prolactin-inhibiting factor, which is secreted by the hypothalamus, from reaching the normal prolactin-producing cells of the anterior pituitary. Released from the influences of inhibiting factor, these normal prolactin-producing cells secrete excessive amounts of prolactin. Likewise, the demonstration of an enlarged sella on plain roentgenograms of the skull does not establish a diagnosis of pituitary adenoma, much less one producing excessive amounts of prolactin. An empty sella cannot be differentiated from a pituitary adenoma on plain roentgenograms of the skull, and some empty sellas are associated with hyperprolactinemia.

Treatment

No single plan of treatment is appropriate for all circumstances under which hyperprolactinemia occurs. This is because of the multiple causes, varying objectives of treatment, and diverse opinions about the optimal treatment for prolactin-producing pituitary adenomas (Table 2).

TABLE 2. **Treatment of Hyperprolactinemia**

Hyperprolactinemia not associated with prolactin-producing pituitary adenomas*
Hyperprolactinemia associated with prolactin-producing pituitary adenomas*
Diffuse and invasive adenomas
Fertility not a consideration
Fertility a consideration
Microadenomas
Fertility not a consideration
Fertility a consideration
Other considerations

*Adenomas classified as microadenomas, ≦10 mm in diameter; diffuse adenomas, >10 mm in diameter, not invasive; invasive adenomas, adenomas of any size invading dura or dura and bone.

Hyperprolactinemia Not Associated with Prolactin-Producing Pituitary Adenomas

Correction of an underlying condition associated with hyperprolactinemia leads to cessation of hyperprolactinemia and, within a few weeks or so, reversal of the findings. There are exceptions, however, and in some patients who are treated for hypothyroidism abatement of hyperprolactinemia may not occur for a number of weeks after the serum thyroxine and TSH levels have become normal. Hyperprolactinemia associated with the use of certain drugs may not disappear until a number of weeks after administration of the drug has ceased. When it is desirable to terminate hyperprolactinemia, as in lactation following pregnancy or situations in which the underlying cause cannot be treated rapidly or successfully, or when it is not possible to change medications, as in a patient taking antipsychotic medications, medical treatment for hyperprolactinemia is usually successful. In some instances it may not be necessary or practical, for reasons of cost, to treat the hyperprolactinemia. For example, mild hyperprolactinemia that occurs from the administration of certain drugs can be ignored if it is causing minimal symptoms, such as slight galactorrhea. However, the physician should be aware that hyperprolactinemia over long periods of time can lead to decreased production of sex steroids and osteoporosis.

Dopaminergic drugs have been used successfully in treating hyperprolactinemia for over a decade. The ones commonly used are bromocriptine (Parlodel), lisuride, and pergolide. Bromocriptine has been available in the United States for only the past several years. While it has been approved by the FDA for the treatment of physiologic lactation and galactorrhea not associated with a pituitary adenoma, it has not been approved for treating pituitary adenomas associated with hyperprolactinemia.

Bromocriptine is usually effective in oral doses

of 2.5 to 10 mg per day in the treatment of most instances of hyperprolactinemia, including that associated with prolactin-producing pituitary adenomas. As with other medications, the physician using bromocriptine should be familiar with the side effects associated with the use of this medication. The most common ones are transient nausea and transient postural lightheadedness, both of which usually disappear after 5 to 7 days of treatment. Serious side effects such as drug rash or hallucinations occur in rare instances.

Bromocriptine is taken orally. It should be given during meals and, when given at bedtime, with food. When we plan to use bromocriptine for longer than 7 to 10 days, we usually have the patient take 1.25 mg (one half of a 2.5 mg tablet) of bromocriptine with food, at bedtime, rather than starting with 2.5 mg once or twice a day, which will cause nausea in about 50 per cent of patients. After 5 to 7 days, if the patient is having no symptoms from the medication we increase the dose by prescribing another 1.25 mg each morning during breakfast. After another 5 to 7 days the bedtime dose is increased to 2.5 mg a day, and after another 5 to 7 days the morning dose is increased to 2.5 mg, with the patient then taking 2.5 mg twice a day. When the patient has been taking 2.5 mg twice a day for a minimum of 7 to 10 days, we measure the serum prolactin to see whether there has been an adequate response. If the prolactin values are still above normal, the dose is increased in successive steps of 1.25 mg each every 5 to 7 days until the patient is taking 2.5 mg at breakfast and 5.0 mg at bedtime. If a larger dose is indicated, a third dose is given during lunch and increased stepwise to 2.5 mg. The level of serum prolactin is checked as the dose is increased, with the goal being to suppress prolactin values to within normal limits with the smallest daily dose possible. This is important when it is planned to continue treatment over long periods, because currently a 2.5 tablet of bromocriptine costs $0.70 to $0.75 in the United States. Fortunately, total doses of 10 mg or less each day will suffice to control hyperprolactinemia in almost all instances except for some prolactin-producing pituitary adenomas for which total daily doses of 20 to 30 mg may be required. The usual dose to stop postpartum lactation is 2.5 mg orally twice a day for 7 to 10 days.

Hyperprolactinemia Associated with Prolactin-Producing Pituitary Adenomas

The treatment of hyperprolactinemia associated with prolactin-producing pituitary adenomas (also known as prolactinomas) is controversial because there is no single way of successfully treating all such tumors. Medical treatment such as bromocriptine will control the hyperprolactinemia in about 80 to 85 per cent of cases and, when effective, decreases the level of prolactin within a few hours after an optimal therapeutic dose is reached. Although bromocriptine and related dopaminergic drugs may reduce the size of a prolactinoma, often dramatically, they do not eradicate the tumor. If bromocriptine is stopped, the tumor re-expands within a few days, and the serum prolactin returns to its previous levels and may even rise above pretreatment levels before returning to pretreatment levels.

Conventional radiation with high voltage x-rays, cobalt-60, or linear accelerator will reduce the levels of prolactin in an estimated 70 to 80 per cent of instances but may take months or 8 to 10 years or longer to be effective. There is no way of predicting which adenomas will respond to radiation.

Successful trans-sphenoidal microsurgery will return the prolactin levels to normal within a matter of hours after the tumor has been removed. Surgical treatment is successful in 33 to 74 per cent of patients with prolactinomas of all sizes, including microadenomas (noninvasive adenomas with a diameter of 10 mm or less), diffuse adenomas (tumors larger than 10 mm in diameter but confined within the dura even though there may be suprasellar extension), and invasive adenomas (adenomas of any size that invade the dura or dura and bone). The best surgical results, with up to a 91 per cent success rate, have been in patients with a microadenoma and preoperative prolactin values of 200 ng per ml or less. Unfortunately, operative results are less beneficial in men with prolactinomas, with successful results being reported in only about 25 per cent. These poor results are not unexpected because when men come for treatment, they usually have large, often invasive tumors and only rarely is a microadenoma present.

The lack of one single method of successful treatment in dealing with prolactinomas means that combinations of treatment using operation, chemotherapy, and radiation are often employed. The exact combination depends upon the treatments available at the time and those available in the past. For example, dopaminergic agents have been in use in Europe for over a decade and are often preferred to operation. On the other hand, these medications have not been available for as long in Canada, and for even less time in the United States. This, plus the application of image intensification, the operating microscope, and the concept of selective resection of a pituitary adenoma to trans-sphenoidal surgical techniques by Dr. Jules Hardy of Montreal, has led to widespread adoption of the trans-sphenoidal procedure in Canada and especially the United States. Hence, the plans of treatment we use at our institution are based, in part, on our extensive experience with trans-sphenoidal procedures and are subject to debate, particularly in regard to microadenomas.

In general, our plan of treatment for an individual patient with a prolactinoma depends upon whether that patient is in the reproductive portion of life and whether pregnancies are desired now or in the future. Another determining factor is whether the prolactinoma is a microadenoma, a diffuse adenoma, or an invasive adenoma. Other factors must be considered as well. The smaller the pituitary adenoma the better the chance of surgically removing the tumor totally and without disrupting the function of the anterior pituitary. Although there is no evidence that the use of bromocriptine by either women or men has deleterious effects upon offspring or patient, experience is limited to just over a decade of use and possible long-term side effects cannot be accurately predicted, as was the case with diethylstilbestrol.

Diffuse and Invasive Adenomas

Fertility Not a Consideration. For both men and women with large prolactinomas in whom pregnancy is not a consideration, our usual plan is to attempt by trans-sphenoidal operation to remove or reduce the size of the tumor. If the prolactin values do not return to normal following surgery, we give a course of radiation therapy. Radiation therapy in patients who have not previously received it consists of a total of 4000 to 4500 rad in doses of 180 to 200 rad with a linear accelerator using 360 degrees' rotation.

While awaiting the effects of radiation therapy, which may take from months to 8 to 10 years or more, we attempt to reduce the prolactin levels by giving bromocriptine in the doses mentioned earlier. The bromocriptine is discontinued once a year and the serum prolactin measured just prior to stopping bromocriptine and every 2 weeks thereafter. If the prolactin values rise after stopping the bromocriptine, bromocriptine is again given in the same doses as before and continued for another year. If the prolactin values rise only 10 to 20 ng per ml above normal, we restart the bromocriptine and stop it 6 months later, again observing the behavior of the prolactin values. When the prolactin values remain within normal limits after stopping bromocriptine, the patient should be followed with prolactin determinations every 2 to 3 weeks for a minimum of 3 to 4 months, because some patients will have a late rise in prolactin values. We also continue to measure prolactin values every 6 months for an indefinite period if the values did not rise within the first several months of stopping bromocriptine.

Some patients will never have an adequate response to radiation therapy, and they should continue bromocriptine indefinitely. As mentioned, bromocriptine not only suppresses the prolactin values but also decreases the size of prolactinomas and keeps the tumor cells suppressed as long as the medication is continued. We have never seen a prolactinoma that escaped the suppressive effects of bromocriptine while the patient was using the medication as prescribed, with the exception of one patient who had a metastatic prolactin-producing pituitary carcinoma.

Fertility a Consideration. Women in this category are usually treated with radiation and bromocriptine. There is about a 30 per cent chance that a woman with a diffuse or large invasive prolactinoma will develop pressure symptoms, such as headache and visual field defects, during pregnancy if she is treated only with bromocriptine and not in conjunction with radiation. The bromocriptine is stopped as soon as pregnancy is suspected or if 5 days beyond the expected date of menses elapse and the patient has not been protected against conception. Radiation therapy prior to restoring fertility with bromocriptine almost always prevents the development of pressure symptoms during pregnancy.

If a patient has anterior pituitary failure in addition to hyperprolactinemia when first seen, the chance of restoring fertility with bromocriptine is small, particularly in the presence of a large prolactinoma. The usual plan is trans-sphenoidal operation plus radiation therapy and bromocriptine if the prolactin levels do not fall to normal following the operation. However, before proceeding with the operation, a trial of bromocriptine for a few months is reasonable to see whether there is a return of menses and ovulation (determined by basal body temperatures). If there is a favorable response to bromocriptine, then radiation therapy along with continuation of bromocriptine is warranted. We would not attempt this if the patient has visual field defects or extension of the pituitary adenoma beyond the confines of the sella, particularly in a superior or lateral direction.

Men with diffuse or invasive prolactinomas without extensive spread beyond the sella who wish restoration of fertility can be treated with bromocriptine alone, if there is a satisfactory response to treatment, until the desired number of their partner's pregnancies has taken place. They can then be treated by trans-sphenoidal operation, with the bromocriptine being stopped at the time of operation. Radiation therapy is given postoperatively if the prolactin levels fail to fall to normal.

Microadenoma

Pregnancy Not a Consideration. In both men and women with microadenomas, we attempt to remove the tumor by trans-sphenoidal operation. If the operation is not successful, we use radiation therapy and bromocriptine, as described. Other physicians believe that bromocriptine is the treatment of choice in this situation. We do not use bromocriptine initially or solely because it is not definitive treatment; rather it is a holding measure that must be continued indefinitely and is expensive.

Fertility a Consideration. In rare instances when a microadenoma is found in a man, we prescribe bromocriptine until the desired number of the partner's pregnancies and then advise trans-sphenoidal operation. The operation is followed by radiation therapy and bromocriptine, if it did not restore prolactin levels to normal. The length of treatment with bromocriptine depends upon the outcome of radiation therapy, as discussed earlier.

Controversy attends the treatment of women who have a microprolactinoma and desire fertility. The main drawback to trans-sphenoidal operation is the possibility that anterior pituitary failure may occur during removal of the adenoma. The chances of this are small, but it does occur rarely. The problem with using bromocriptine alone is that it is stopped as soon as pregnancy occurs, and these tumors may grow during pregnancy. Fortunately, chances of a microadenoma enlarging enough to cause problems during pregnancy are small.

We usually advise surgical removal, particularly if the microadenoma is 8 to 10 mm in size. However, if a patient prefers to try bromocriptine after an unbiased discussion of the pros and cons of medical versus surgical treatment, we give bromocriptine. Patients are followed carefully in case they develop symptoms of an expanding pituitary adenoma. We also do perimetry testing of the visual fields at the 5th and 8th months of pregnancy or if visual symptoms develop. Approximately 3 months after delivery, we perform a CT scan of the pituitary area with axial and coronal views during the infusion of contrast medium, and at the same time test thyroid and adrenal function. If the patient plans additional pregnancies and she is not nursing, we restart bromocriptine. Before a second pregnancy is attempted, we again do CT scanning of the pituitary and measure thyroid and adrenal function. When the patient has had the desired number of pregnancies, or should there be evidence that the tumor grew significantly during the preceding pregnancy, we advise trans-sphenoidal pituitary operation as definitive treatment.

Other Considerations

In deciding to use bromocriptine as initial treatment for a prolactinoma, one should be as certain as possible that the patient will comply with treatment and not discontinue medication without medical advice. There is ample evidence that large prolactinomas that regress with the use of bromocriptine will expand in a matter of days after bromocriptine is discontinued. Because of the continuing expense of using bromocriptine over long periods, particularly when doses of 20 mg or so each day are necessary to suppress the tumor, patients may request definitive therapy in the hopes that the medication can be discontinued. When treating with bromocriptine, we measure prolactin values two or three times every year to determine whether the tumor remains suppressed, although we have yet to see a benign adenoma escape from the suppressive effects of bromocriptine.

Some evidence suggests that the chances of successful operation upon a patient with a microadenoma are less if the patient has been treated previously with bromocriptine for more than 1 year. This possibility has not been satisfactorily resolved one way or another, but if true would reinforce the advisability of early operation on patients who have a microadenoma.

About 20 per cent of patients with a prolactinoma do not respond satisfactorily to treatment with bromocriptine. Hence, when bromocriptine is chosen as initial therapy, a change in treatment is indicated if there is not a significant fall in prolactin values after the maximal advisable dose of 20 to 30 mg a day has been tried for several weeks.

As mentioned earlier, some patients with a pituitary adenoma that is not secreting prolactin may have hyperprolactinemia, and the prolactin values return to normal with bromocriptine treatment. No conclusive evidence at present suggests that bromocriptine will alter the course of these pituitary adenomas associated with hyperprolactinemia but which are not secreting prolactin—that is, pseudoprolactinomas. Two guidelines are helpful. Generally, pseudoprolactinomas are large tumors, not microadenomas, and the prolactin levels are almost always less than 250 ng per ml. On the other hand, the prolactin values associated with prolactinomas are usually directly proportional to their size. Large prolactinomas occasionally may be associated with prolactin values under 200 ng, but usually the values are 300 ng or more and at times measure in the thousands.

Large tumors that are thought to be prolactinomas must be monitored carefully when one elects to give only bromocriptine as initial treatment. If CT scanning fails to show regression in the size of the tumor after prolactin values have been suppressed for a month or so, one is either dealing with a prolactinoma resistant to treatment or a pseudoprolactinoma, and a change in treatment is indicated.

At present no single treatment is satisfactory in the management of all prolactin-producing pituitary adenomas. The best chances for complete eradication and preservation of pituitary function come with early diagnosis, a small tumor, and trans-sphenoidal operation. However, with the various forms of treatment available the vast majority of prolactinomas, regardless of size or invasiveness, can be managed satisfactorily.

HYPERTHYROIDISM

method of
LEONARD WARTOFSKY, M.D., Col, MC, USA
Walter Reed Army Medical Center
Washington, D.C.

Hyperthyroidism (or thyrotoxicosis) is a syndrome caused by supraphysiologic circulating blood and tissue levels of the thyroid hormones thyroxine or triiodothyronine or both. Toxic diffuse goiter (Graves' disease) is the most prevalent cause, but hyperthyroidism due to hyperfunctioning nodules (single or multiple) of the thyroid gland is also quite common. Appropriate thyroid function tests are required to confirm the clinical diagnosis prior to initiation of treatment since the diverse forms of the syndrome may require different therapeutic approaches. For example, a 24 hour radioiodine uptake (RAIU) will differentiate causes of hyperthyroidism with high uptake (diffuse and nodular toxic goiter) from those with low uptake (thyroiditis and factitial ingestion of thyroid hormone). Obviously, a course of antithyroid drug therapy or surgical or radioiodine ablation of the thyroid gland would all be inappropriate therapies for the latter cause of hyperthyroidism.

Graves' Disease

Today the treatment of thyrotoxicosis in Graves' disease is concerned primarily with producing a reduction in the hypersecretion of the thyroid hormones. This may be effected by two general methods. The first constitutes ablative procedures such as the use of radioiodine (^{131}I) or surgical thyroidectomy. The effects of ablative procedures are relatively predictable, and either permanent remission or permanent hypothyroidism necessitating replacement thyroid medication can be expected. The second type of therapy involves the use of chemotherapeutic agents that inhibit or block various steps in thyroid hormonal synthesis or release. In 1986, agents such as perchlorate, thiocyanate, and iodine are rarely used in the routine management of hyperthyroidism, whereas the so-called antithyroid drugs of the thionamide type are now the mainstay of medical therapy. In the United States, the only generally prescribed drugs of this class are propylthiouracil (PTU) and methimazole (Tapazole).

Use of Antithyroid Drugs

In general, antithyroid drugs act to block intrathyroidal new hormone synthesis and do not affect continuing secretion of preformed thyroidal hormone stores or the ongoing metabolic effects of increased thyroid hormone levels in the systemic circulation and peripheral tissues. As a consequence, it may take weeks to months of antithyroid drug therapy for the thyrotoxic patient to achieve a euthyroid state, similar to the delayed effect of radioiodine treatment. With the latter, the delay is due to the time required for the destruction of dividing thyroid follicular cells. With the antithyroid agents, the duration of the delay in improvement depends in large part upon the magnitude of the intrathyroidal hormone pool (colloid stores) and its rate of discharge. Once the pool is reduced, clinical improvement should follow rapidly, provided the dose is adequate to ensure blockade of new hormone synthesis. We employ a beta blocker such as propranolol (discussed later) for relief of symptoms during this initial treatment interval. Once serum thyroid hormone levels are comfortably within the normal range, the propranolol is discontinued.

The decision about which antithyroid drug to choose is often quite arbitrary. On a weight basis, methimazole (Tapazole) is approximately 10 to 12 times more potent than PTU. Often the decision to use one of these agents may be based on a demonstrated toxic reaction to the other drug. The most commonly encountered side effects are rash or pruritus, which occur in 5 to 7 per cent of patients, whereas the more worrisome toxic reaction of agranulocytosis occurs in 0.2 to 0.3 per cent of patients. The latter usually occurs within the first few months of treatment. We do not routinely monitor white blood cell counts to detect this rare complication, but patients should be advised to come in for a complete blood count with differential count should they note any fever or sore throat. Virtually all patients recover from

---

The opinions or assertions contained herein are the private views of the author and are not to be construed as official or reflecting the views of the Department of the Army or the Department of Defense.

the agranulocytosis, especially when it is detected early.

One theoretic advantage to the selection of PTU over methimazole is that PTU has a peripheral effect, inhibiting the conversion of thyroxine to triiodothyronine, in addition to its effects on new hormone synthesis. Since most of the metabolic effects of thyroid hormone derive from T_3 rather than T_4, the patient thus may attain more rapid clinical improvement with PTU when given in comparable dose. It is customary to start either drug in a larger initial dose in order to more rapidly achieve an effect. Since the frequency and severity of toxic reactions appear to be related to dosage, the initial dose usually should not be greater than 30 to 60 mg per day of methimazole, or 400 to 800 mg per day of PTU. Because of their relatively short half-life (especially while the patient is still hypermetabolic), it is advisable to administer the drugs in a divided dose, e.g., every 8 hours.

Once the serum T_4 level declines into the normal range, the dose is tapered, dropping toward the maintenance dose required to ensure that T_4 levels neither fall into the hypothyroid range nor begin to rise again into the hyperthyroid range. Thus, there is usually a trial and error adjustment period of a few months to establish the correct maintenance dose, which averages 10 to 30 mg per day for methimazole, or 150 to 450 mg per day for PTU. In practice, this is done by seeing the patient every 2 to 3 weeks for the first few months, then once monthly thereafter for both clinical assessment and serum T_4 determination. The dose that maintains euthyroidism is then continued for approximately an additional 9 to 18 months. Enlargement of the thyroid gland during treatment may indicate either worsening thyrotoxicosis related to increased circulating thyroid-stimulating immunoglobulins, or it could signify antithyroid overdosage with the increasing gland size due to drug-induced hypothyroidism. In the latter case, the goiter is due to thyroid stimulation from increased pituitary release of thyrotropin (TSH), and the differential diagnosis may be resolved by obtaining a serum TSH determination. On the other hand, decreasing goiter size during therapy is a good sign of impending remission of Graves' disease.

With this management, permanent remission of the thyrotoxicosis of Graves' disease may be seen in 20 to 40 per cent of patients. The remainder of patients will relapse at some time after discontinuation of antithyroid drugs and will then become candidates for either ablative radioiodine treatment or surgical thyroidectomy, to be discussed later. Generally, patients who fail one well-managed course of antithyroid drugs are less likely to have a successful outcome with an additional course of treatment. Antithyroid drugs also may be effectively employed as adjuncts to other therapy, e.g., temporarily to achieve euthyroidism in anticipation of either ^{131}I or surgical management.

Selection of Patients for Antithyroid Therapy

While the antithyroid drugs are worth trying under many circumstances, many thyrotoxic patients are more appropriate candidates for ablative therapy. To enhance the possibility of a remission of antithyroid drugs, we rely on certain characteristics that more regularly correlate with a predictably favorable outcome. These characteristics include a small goiter (less than 50 grams), disease of short duration (less than 6 months), absence of prior history of failure with antithyroid medications, and a low dosage requirement for antithyroid maintenance once initial control of the disease is established. In such patients, we make every effort to attempt a full therapeutic trial of antithyroid treatment before abandoning this therapy.

Danger of Iodine as Sole Therapy for Hyperthyroidism

Iodine may act to ameliorate hyperthyroidism by two major mechanisms. First, this substance will inhibit synthesis of T_4 and T_3 (Wolff-Chaikoff effect), and second, iodine will rapidly inhibit proteolysis of colloid and the release of T_4 and T_3 into the blood. The Wolff-Chaikoff effect is only transient, and in the absence of concomitant antithyroid blockade of organification, T_4 and T_3 synthesis will proceed. Therefore, since the administered iodine is only serving to block discharge of hormone into the blood, the result is a progressive enrichment of hormonal stores in the gland. The ultimate and dreaded consequence of this may be "escape" from the iodine block on release (which can occur after 3 to 8 weeks of therapy) and an abrupt aggravation of the thyrotoxicosis with possible "thyroid storm" due to the large hormone stores.

To make matters worse, the clinician is unable to use iodine for treatment at this point and must rely on other forms of chemotherapy that are generally slower in their onset of action. Thus, iodine is most safely used only with a concomitant antithyroid drug blockade that would not permit iodine enrichment of glandular stores but rather would tend to deplete pre-existing stores of hormone. Given the possibility of an iodine-induced worsening of the disease, combined iodine-antithyroid therapy is best administered in consultation with an endocrinologist and only for very specific indications, such as thyroid storm, preparation of patients for surgery, and in elderly thyrotoxic patients with thyrocardiac disease.

Role of Beta-Adrenergic Blockade in Therapy

The apparently increased activity of the sympathetic nervous system in hyperthyroidism led to the use of adrenergic blocking agents in this disorder when these drugs first became available. Propranolol, a specific beta-adrenergic blocking agent, has proved so effective that it has supplanted the use of reserpine and guanethidine. Patients may be made to feel significantly better with as little as 10 mg three times daily, although very severely thyrotoxic patients may require as much as 80 mg every 6 hours. This drug will ameliorate tremor, palpitations, sweating, hyperreflexia, tachycardia, and other arrhythmias and will decrease nervousness and promote a feeling of general well-being. Propranolol is effective within hours of use, and we have found it to be an invaluable adjunct to therapy, especially while awaiting the attainment of euthyroidism following initiation of antithyroid drug treatment or the administration of radioiodine. We do not recommend the use of propranolol as the sole preparation for surgery, as has been recently proposed; we believe this to be a course of management that may be required in a rare emergency situation but otherwise appears imprudent. In practice, propranolol is usually started simultaneously with antithyroid drug therapy or is given to patients programmed to receive radioactive iodine treatment. In either case, there is no need to continue the beta blockade after the patient attains normal iodothyronine blood levels and clinical euthyroidism.

Use of Radioiodine Therapy in Young Adults and Children

Radioiodine represents both effective and cost-effective therapy for adult patients with hyperthyroidism. Moreover, several medical centers are now evaluating the efficacy of ^{131}I therapy for pediatric patients with thyrotoxicosis. Although preliminary results could be considered satisfactory, there is reason to condemn this practice on theoretic grounds. Radioiodine therapy has been in use for approximately 35 years with increasing frequency, so the majority of patients have been treated within the past 20 years. It has been established from recent experience based upon other radiation treatment models that tumors such as undifferentiated carcinoma and sarcoma may arise in x-ray–treated areas 20 or even 30 years after the initial therapy is administered. Thus the possibility is raised of subsequent harm from therapeutic doses of ^{131}I. In patients from 40 to 70 years of age, a "guarantee" of 30 years without late complications appears acceptable, but to treat a 12 year old child with the meager foreknowledge of complications only to age 40 to 45 years seems needlessly cavalier.

From the unfortunate experience in areas exposed to radioactive fallout, such as Japan and the Marshall Islands, we have learned that the child's thyroid is unusually susceptible to radiation in comparison with the adult or mature thyroid gland, which is undergoing less frequent mitoses. We have also become increasingly aware of the dangers of radiation to the area of the head and neck in childhood in predisposing to later thyroid malignancies. It may take another 15 to 20 years before adequate follow-up on young persons treated with ^{131}I will be sufficient to fully evaluate and possibly justify such management. Until then, radioiodine therapy should not be routinely used in these patients.

Use of Antithyroid Drugs in Conjunction with Thyroid Hormone

Physicians who advocate administering some form of thyroid hormone along with full blocking doses of antithyroid compounds maintain that this type of management will tend to avoid the ups and downs of too much or too little antithyroid drug and thus keep the patient in a steady state of euthyroidism. However, the patient is then taking two drugs instead of one, requiring a greater dose of antithyroid than would ordinarily be required without supplemental thyroid hormone. There is also a potentially greater incidence of drug reactions, difficulty in the interpretation of thyroid function tests, and greater difficulty assessing when and if a spontaneous remission has occurred.

We prefer to keep patients on maintenance doses of an antithyroid drug only, in the smallest doses compatible with good control. The patient is seen at monthly intervals, and the dose is increased or decreased in accordance with both the clinical response and the serum T_4 and T_3 levels. In this way, a patient may be gradually tapered down to very small doses of drug and ultimately weaned completely. A triiodothyronine suppression test (with a radioactive iodine uptake performed before and after 10 days' treatment with 75 to 100 micrograms of T_3 per day) may then be performed to assess whether remission has occurred. We have used combined thyroid-antithyroid therapy only in patients with severe progressive ophthalmopathy, since it has been empirically stated that stability of thyroid control may be desirable to possibly avoid exacerbation of the eye problems. More recently, we have favored radioablation of the thyroid gland, followed by early thyroid replacement, as an alternative means of ensuring rapid control and stability in such patients.

Recent data have lent theoretic support to the concept of combined therapy, based on studies indicating that the antithyroid drugs may have immunosuppressive effects distinct from their effects on thyroid hormone synthesis. Better remission rates were seen with higher than with lower antithyroid doses, presumably because the higher doses were more effectively blocking production of the abnormal thyroid stimulator of Graves' disease. Thyroid hormone supplements need to be given with the higher antithyroid drug doses to avoid hypothyroidism. Additional studies need to be performed to confirm this interesting work before this approach can be recommended.

Thyroid Storm

Thyrotoxic storm or crisis is a relatively rare but life-threatening syndrome characterized by exaggerated manifestations of hyperthyroidism. Prior to the availability of pharmacologic agents to inhibit thyroid hormone synthesis and release, storm often was seen in the immediate postoperative setting after thyroidectomy. Presumably, this was the result of augmented hormonal release secondary to surgical manipulation compounded by other effects of the surgical stress. Probably the most commonly associated precipitating event today is infection.

The therapy of thyroid crisis may be considered in terms of four components and the relative importance of each for survival will vary in a given patient. In view of the serious implications of thyroid storm, no one component of this therapeutic approach should be overlooked:

Therapy Directed Against the Thyroid Gland. The antithyroid drugs propylthiouracil (PTU) and methimazole (Tapazole) are given to block new hormone synthesis. PTU should be started in a dose of 1200 to 1500 mg daily given as 200 to 250 mg every 4 hours. Methimazole in a daily dose of 120 mg should suffice (given as 20 mg every 4 hours), but PTU has the additional advantage of inhibiting conversion of T_4 to T_3, a property not shared by methimazole. As a consequence, a more rapid amelioration of symptoms is possible with PTU. Nevertheless, the major effect of both drugs is on new hormone synthesis, with no reduction demonstrable in thyroidal release of preformed glandular stores of hormone. Consequently, separate treatment must be administered to inhibit proteolysis of colloid and release of T_4 and T_3 into the blood. For this purpose, either stable iodine or lithium carbonate may be employed. There is considerably more experience with the use of iodines, which may be given orally as either Lugol's solution or saturated solution of potassium iodide (8 drops every 6 hours) or by intravenous drip as sodium iodide (0.5 to 1 gram every 12 hours), which is generally available as a sterile preparation.

An extremely important aspect of this combined therapeutic approach to the thyroid is to remember to administer the thiourea compound prior to initiation of iodine therapy. Use of iodine alone is to be rigorously avoided since the absence of concomitant antithyroid drug blockade of new hormone synthesis will allow enrichment of hormone stores within the gland, thereby generating the potential for further exaggeration of thyrotoxicosis by virtue of a massive release of hormone.

Other agents that may be employed in this manner are the radiographic contrast dyes ipodate (Oragrafin) and iopanoate (Telepaque). These drugs act to decrease hepatic uptake of T_4 and the per cent of free T_4 in plasma, and their use can be associated with remarkable clinical improvement. Ipodate may be administered as 3 grams orally on a daily basis and should be used (like Lugol's iodine) only with simultaneous antithyroid blockade with PTU or methimazole to avoid the tremendous enrichment of glandular iodine stores that would occur otherwise.

In those occasional patients who may be allergic to iodine, lithium carbonate may be used as an alternative agent to inhibit hormonal release. Lithium should be administered initially as 300 mg every 6 hours with subsequent adjustment of dosage as necessary to maintain serum lithium levels at approximately 1.0 mEq/liter.

Therapy Directed Against Systemic Decompensation. Fever should be treated promptly with antipyretics, preferably acetaminophen rather than salicylates since the latter might theoretically temporarily worsen the clinical situation because of an increase in free hormone resulting from inhibition of binding and displacement of T_4 from binding sites. External cooling with alcohol sponging, ice packs, or a hypothermia blanket also may be employed. Fluid losses due to the hyperpyrexia and diaphoresis, as well as to vomiting or diarrhea when present, must be vigorously replaced to avoid vascular collapse. Care and judicious replacement of fluids is required in the elderly patient with congestive heart failure or other potential cardiac compromise. Intravenous fluids containing 10 per cent dextrose in addition to electrolytes will serve to aid restoration of depleted hepatic glycogen stores. Hypercalcemia, if present, will usually be reversed by hydration, and vitamin supplements may be added to the intravenous fluids to replace probable coexistent deficiency.

Congestive failure when present may be treated with digitalis and diuretics, although somewhat greater than usual doses may be required for initial digitalization as well as maintenance in the patient with severe hyperthyroidism. Antiarrhythmia therapy for specific arrhythmias also may be indicated, as well as pressor therapy in the event of hypotension not readily reversed by adequate hydration. Large doses of glucocorticoids have been given on empiric grounds for several decades on the basis of a theoretic relative adrenal insufficiency. This indication notwithstanding, the more recently demonstrated ability of steroids such as dexamethasone or hydrocortisone to inhibit T_4 to T_3 conversion is additional justification for their use. An initial dose of 300 mg of hydrocortisone followed by 100 mg every 8 hours during the acute phase of this syndrome should be adequate.

Therapy Directed Against Ongoing Effects of Thyroid Hormone in the Periphery. As mentioned, some workers have attempted to reduce the burden of excessive circulating concentrations of the thyroid hormones by either peritoneal dialysis or plasmapheresis. Hemoperfusion through a resin bed which removes T_4 and T_3 has been demonstrated to be effective experimentally but has not been reported as yet under clinical circumstances. Perhaps because of the difficulty attending these procedures, most physicians tend to rely on more traditional measures although such aggressive management should be considered in a severe case. The use of beta-adrenergic receptor blockade to ameliorate the manifestations of thyroid hormone excess evolved from the earlier demonstration that agents such as reserpine and guanethidine could blunt the apparently enhanced sympathetic activity seen in thyrotoxic patients. Propranolol is the agent most commonly employed today, at least in the United States. The usual oral dosage of 20 to 40 mg every 6 hours may have to be increased to 60 to 120 mg every 6 hours in thyroid crisis. Indeed, due to the more rapid metabolism of the drug in severe hyperthyroidism, even larger oral doses, or preferably intravenous doses, must be given. A plasma propranolol level in excess of 50 ng/ml may have to be maintained to establish clinical response. When employed intravenously, an initial dose of 0.5 to 1.0 mg should be given cautiously while the patient's cardiac rhythm is continuously monitored. Subsequent doses of 2 to 3 mg may be given by intravenous infusion over 10 to 15 minutes every several hours while awaiting for orally administered drug to take effect. While it has been assumed for many years that the primary role of propranolol was to attenuate the effects of catecholamines, it has become apparent in recent years that this drug will also inhibit the conversion of T_4 to T_3, albeit incompletely, and may serve to ameliorate the thyrotoxicosis to some degree on this basis.

Therapy Directed Against the Precipitating Illness. Although the therapies outlined in the three preceding sections may be clearly life-saving, a careful search and early treatment of the underlying illness that may have precipitated the thyroid crisis is also important. Those patients with enhanced thyroidal secretion due to withdrawal of thiourea therapy or to administration of iodine, iodinated contrast dyes, or ^{131}I require some special concern. The need for continuing effective blockage of hormonal biosynthesis and release beyond the period of immediate improvement must be recognized, since premature withdrawal of treatment could result in a recurrent exacerbation of thyrotoxicosis. Once treatment with antithyroid drugs is instituted, measures such as diuresis or dialysis designed to deplete iodine in the patient with iodine-induced thyrotoxicosis are no longer necessary. Those patients with thyroid storm related to hypoglycemia, ketoacidosis, pulmonary thromboembolism, or stroke require the same vigorous management ordinarily indicated for each respective specific event. It is obviously important to be alert to the fact that these conditions may underlie thyroid crisis, particularly in the obtunded or psychotic patient since the dramatic manifestations of severe thyrotoxicosis may overshadow the clinical presentation of these disorders.

Therapy of Thyrotoxicosis Complicating Pregnancy

In my view, the best management consists of using the smallest quantity of antithyroid drugs required to control the clinical thyrotoxicosis and to bring the serum T_4 concentration down to the normal range *for pregnancy*. This is emphasized since it must be remembered that increased estrogens (as in pregnancy) increase serum T_4 levels, and the normal serum T_4 in pregnancy may be as high as 11 to 15 micrograms per dl, depending upon the T_4 assay system employed. The patient is seen in intervals of 2 or 3 weeks, and the antithyroid dose is tapered as rapidly as possible, consistent with the guidelines mentioned previously. For unknown reasons, many patients undergo spontaneous remission of their hyperthyroidism during pregnancy, and the antithyroid drug may be totally discontinued if such is detected. Had such a patient been treated with a combined thyroid-antithyroid program, however, the remission would not have been recognized, and the fetus would have been unnecessarily endangered.

Toxic Nodular Goiter

Multinodular Toxic Goiter

By and large, patients with toxic multinodular goiter tend to be over 35 years of age, thus more eligible for ^{131}I treatment than for surgery. In either case, we do not think it wise to treat extremely toxic patients with radioiodine or by surgical thyroidectomy without first rendering them euthyroid. Therein lies the role for the antithyroid agents in toxic nodular disease—to prepare patients for ablative therapy. The rationale for such preparation is based on the potential danger (albeit small) that radioiodine may cause a radiation thyroiditis, with resultant release of hormonal stores and aggravation of an already marginal clinical state; similarly, a thyroid crisis or "storm" may occur in the intra- or postoperative period of the patient who had not been properly prepared. By first treating these patients with antithyroid drugs for 4 to 8 weeks, one can render them euthyroid prior to either of these definitive therapies, as well as deplete the store of hormone in their thyroid glands and thus obviate the possibility of thyroid crisis. When radioiodine is the choice for therapy, it is given according to the approximate formula:

$$\frac{160\ \mu\text{C/gram estimated thyroid weight} \times \text{No. grams estimated thyroid weight}}{\text{24 hr radioiodine uptake}}$$

This calculation results in a total dose that ranges between 12 and 30 millicuries, representing a dose of 4 to 15 millicuries to the thyroid. These doses are higher than those used in patients with comparably sized goiters from Graves' disease because of the relatively greater radioresistance of the multinodular goiter.

Solitary "Hot" Nodules

Solitary autonomous thyroid adenomas most often exist in euthyroid individuals and require only observation to ensure that hyperthyroidism is not evolving or that growth of the nodule may not be signaling an associated carcinoma. The latter is exceedingly rare. The hyperthyroid patient with a "hot" nodule is a candidate for either surgery or ^{131}I therapy, depending upon age, clinical state, and other factors. Generally, we refer those hyperthyroid patients under age 25 years to surgery, and the procedure recommended is a unilateral thyroid lobectomy. Patients over age 50 years are treated with ^{131}I, and therapy is individualized for those patients falling between these age ranges. One should not make the mistake of treating the euthyroid patient who has a hot nodule with thyroid medication under the erroneous impression that the nodule is somehow being suppressed. The autonomous nodule is, by definition, nonsuppressible. Hence, administered thyroid hormone will only add to that being produced by the nodule itself, and the result may be the development of hyperthyroidism.

The thiourea compounds act by inducing a block in the synthesis of the thyroid hormones, which restores serum T_4 and T_3 levels to normal. During the antithyroid therapy of Graves' disease it is hoped that a remission might occur. However, the solitary autonomous nodule or the toxic multinodular goiter (Plummer's disease) with associated thyrotoxicosis will not spontaneously remit, as will Graves' disease. Hence, a remission cannot be expected, except in the rare event of infarction of toxic nodules.

HYPOTHYROIDISM

method of
WILLIAM L. GREEN, M.D.
State University of New York
Brooklyn, New York

A deficiency of circulating thyroid hormones can be the result of intrinsic thyroid disease (primary hypothyroidism) or secondary to deficient secretion of thyroid-stimulating hormone (TSH) by the pituitary. TSH deficiency can be due either to a diseased pituitary (secondary hypothyroidism) or to a decline in secretion of the hypothalamic TSH-releasing hormone called TRH (tertiary hypothyroidism). Primary hypothyroidism is almost invariably associated with elevated levels of TSH in plasma, and the radioimmunoassay for TSH has become an important diagnostic test. Secondary and tertiary forms of hypothyroidism usually occur as part of a more generalized deficit in hypothalamic-pituitary function, and are more fully discussed elsewhere.

Hypothyroidism in the Juvenile and Adult

Hypothyroidism can be acquired in several ways: (1) spontaneous (nongoitrous) hypothyroidism with insidious onset of symptoms, probably secondary to autoimmune destruction of the gland or "atrophic thyroiditis"; (2) Hashimoto's thyroiditis, also thought to be an autoimmune disease, in which euthyroid goiter is the most common presentation, but which often is accompanied by varying degrees of thyroid hypofunction; or (3) post-thyroidectomy or post-^{131}I treatment for hyperthyroidism or thyroid cancer. Less commonly, goiter and hypothyroidism may be induced by therapy with amiodarone, iodide, or lithium salts; when this occurs, the patient usually has an underlying thyroid abnormality, such as Hashimoto's thyroiditis or ^{131}I-treated Graves' disease.

Congenital Hypothyroidism (Cretinism)

When hypothyroidism is present in utero and becomes evident soon after birth, it is usually due to either maldevelopment of the thyroid, including aplasia and failure to descend from the foramen cecum, or genetic errors in thyroid hormone synthesis. In the latter case, goiter typically appears, although it may not be present at birth. Unless promptly treated, congenital hypothyroidism may cause permanent damage to the developing brain. Screening tests for hypothyroidism should be done routinely in neonates to permit early detection and treatment.

Low Thyroid Hormone Levels in Seriously Ill Patients

The increased use of thyroid function tests as screening procedures has revealed that many seriously ill patients have low plasma levels of T_4 and T_3, suggesting a thyroid deficiency state. With more detailed testing and follow-up, it has been proved that most such patients do not have thyroid disease, and that the low hormone levels are an adaptation to illness. Therefore thyroid hormone therapy is not indicated unless there are definite hypothyroid symptoms accompanied by a high TSH level.

Choice of Drugs for Treatment

The naturally occurring thyroid hormones are L-thyroxine (T_4) and L-triiodothyronine (T_3), which are normally produced in the body in a molar ratio of about 2:1 but, because of T_3's much greater metabolic clearance rate, are present in plasma in a ratio of about 50:1. T_3 is more potent than T_4 and thus mediates most of the thyroid hormone effect in the body, despite its relatively low blood level. A large proportion, perhaps three fourths, of the circulating T_3 is derived from peripheral deiodination of T_4. Levels of both hormones show little diurnal fluctuation, since T_4 itself has a long-life, about 7 days, and provides a large precursor pool from which T_3, with the much shorter half-life of about 1 day, is formed at a steady rate. The treatment that most closely mimics this physiologic state is administration of synthetic T_4, levothyroxine (Synthroid, Levothroid). During long-term treatment with 0.1 to 0.2 mg of T_4 daily, the usual replacement dose, most hypothyroid subjects become euthyroid and have normal circulating levels of both T_3 and T_4; therefore synthetic T_4 is the agent of choice to treat hypothyroidism.

Clinical hypothyroidism can also be reversed by treatment with desiccated thyroid U.S.P. and thyroglobulin (Proloid), which are produced from animal thyroids. Because of their T_3 content, they cause fluctuations in plasma T_3, with peak levels soon after ingestion that may rise well above the normal range. Despite this theoretic disadvantage, desiccated thyroid has proved to be an effective treatment over several decades, has the advantages of wide availability and low cost, and is an acceptable second choice; the adult replacement dose is 96 to 160 mg (1½ to 2½ grains) daily. Occasional batches of inactive desiccated thyroid have been found; this should not occur if a biologically standardized preparation, such as that provided by Armour, is employed. Other available drugs include liothyronine (Cytomel), a synthetic T_3, and liotrix (Euthroid, Thyrolar), a combination of synthetic T_4 and T_3. At present there are no clear advantages to liothyronine or liotrix that would justify their greater cost.

Regimen for Beginning Treatment

In younger patients with mild hypothyroidism and no evidence of heart disease, treatment can be started immediately with a full replacement dose. When heart disease is present, which is quite common in older patients with spontaneous hypothyroidism, sudden initiation of full replacement has led to cardiovascular catastrophes. Therefore the usual practice is to start therapy with small doses, e.g., 0.05 mg of T_4 per day, increasing the dose to 0.1 mg daily after 2 to 4 weeks; if no adverse effects result, the dose can be increased to 0.15 mg 4 weeks later. In patients with concurrent symptomatic heart disease, an initial dose of 0.025 mg may be advised. Particular caution is merited if desiccated thyroid is employed, because relatively small doses may produce transient elevations in the T_3 level. A few patients may have worsening angina and be unable to tolerate full replacement. However, with appropriate caution, treatment of myxedematous patients who have heart disease may produce more benefit than harm; for example, improvement of pre-existing angina pectoris is not uncommon when a euthyroid status is restored.

In hypothyroid infants, the initial dose of levothyroxine is about 0.05 mg daily, increasing to about half of full adult doses during the second year and to full adult replacement dose by the age of 10 years.

Determining Adequacy of Therapy

In adults, clinical criteria usually suffice to determine whether treatment is optimal; overdosage produces thyrotoxic symptoms, especially nervousness and palpitations. The best laboratory test to detect insufficient dosage is the TSH level, which should be normalized by an adequate dose of thyroid hormone. To test for overtreatment, measurements of T_4 and T_3 are useful. For reasons that are not well understood, when some hypothyroid patients become clinically euthyroid on standard doses of T_4 they have high T_4 levels whereas the T_3 concentration is low normal. In such cases, the T_3 level is the better guide, and dosage should not be reduced.

In children, progression in height, weight, and indices of skeletal maturation provides additional criteria for adequate treatment.

Conditions That Alter Hormone Requirements

There is a rough correlation between optimal T_4 replacement dose and body weight, and replacement needs decline somewhat with age. However, once a suitable dose has been determined it may remain the same for many years. Although the hormones are only partially absorbed from the intestinal tract (T_4 absorption, 40 to 70 per cent; T_3, 70 to 90 per cent), variations in absorption and serious malabsorption have occurred infrequently. One well-documented problem, however, is created by soybean formulas in infancy; they prevent absorption of T_4 and can frustrate the therapy of cretinism. A similar problem is created by cholestyramine and colestipol, two cholesterol-lowering agents that can bind T_4 and T_3 in the intestine and prevent their absorption.

Conditions Associated with Hypothyroidism

Numerous associations with autoimmune thyroiditis have been reported, including pernicious anemia, type 1 diabetes mellitus, premature menopause, Addison's disease, hypoparathyroidism, and vitiligo. In most instances, these associations are based on finding organ-specific antibodies rather than clinical disease. For example, many more patients with hypothyroidism have antibodies to gastric parietal cells than have significant megaloblastic anemia. It has not been our practice to test patients for these associated conditions, unless clinical observation gives some evidence of their presence.

In postsurgical hypothyroidism, parathyroid damage is sufficiently common that questioning about symptoms of tetany and serum calcium determinations are routinely advised.

Myxedema Coma

An occasional patient with profound myxedema will lapse into a coma caused by the thyroid hormone deficiency, which can be reversed only by vigorous thyroid hormone treatment. This usually occurs in elderly subjects with spontaneous myxedema, but it can be a feature of any type of hypothyroidism. Our approach to management follows:

1. Obtain adequate blood samples to allow later confirmation of diagnosis (T_4, TSH, cortisol).

2. Give a loading dose of levothyroxine intravenously, usually 0.3 to 0.5 mg, and follow this with 0.05 to 0.1 mg intravenously daily, adjusting the dose downward at any evidence of untoward cardiovascular effects. On switching to oral maintenance, the daily dose should be increased to compensate for the partial absorption of levothyroxine. Although liothyronine is said to act more rapidly, these large doses of levothyroxine have a fairly prompt effect and provide a smooth rise in T_4 and T_3 levels toward normal rather than the very high T_3 levels produced by large doses of T_3.

3. Give replacement doses of cortisol appropriate to the stress of the disease, e.g., 200 mg of hydrocortisone sodium succinate (Solu-Cortef) intravenously on the first day, tapering the dose over 4 to 7 days as the patient improves. This may prevent adrenal crisis in the occasional patient who has panhypopituitarism presenting as myxedema coma and will prevent manifestations of the functional adrenal cortical impairment which sometimes occurs in hypothyroidism.

4. Give appropriate ventilatory assistance; in some cases CO_2 narcosis is a major feature of the myxedematous state, and measures that lower the PCO_2 value may reverse the coma.

5. Look for complicating infection and treat it promptly; pneumonia is particularly common in patients with myxedema coma.

6. Provide adequate oxygenation. Since hypoxia may be a factor in coma, the cautious use of oxygen and correction of anemia, if present, by transfusion of packed red cells are recommended. Vasopressor agents, however, should be avoided, because they may synergize with thyroid hormones to produce dysrhythmias.

THYROID CANCER

method of
MELVIN A. BLOCK, M.D.
University of California, San Diego
La Jolla, California

The definitive treatment for thyroid carcinoma requires surgery. Radioactive iodine remains an important therapeutic adjunct, especially for well-differentiated thyroid carcinoma.

Basic Principles in Treatment. Although thyroid carcinoma is relatively rare and, in general, has a good outlook, the high frequency of thyroid nodules, which always introduces the possibility of carcinoma, and the obligation to effect a high rate of cure make the subject important. Thyroid carcinoma can be classified for clinical purposes on the basis of pathologic varieties as follows:

I. Well-differentiated.
   A. Papillary—approximately 70 per cent.
   B. Follicular—approximately 20 per cent.
II. Medullary—approximately 7 per cent.
III. Anaplastic—approximately 3 per cent.

Critical factors used in determining the extent of operation are:

1. Clinical evidence of extent of carcinoma in the neck, presence or absence of distant metastases.
2. The pathologic variety of carcinoma.
3. Miscellaneous:
   a. Age—prognosis worse over 40 years for well-differentiated carcinomas, justifying more aggressive treatment.
   b. History of previous external radioactive therapy—increases likelihood of multicentricity.
   c. Size of primary neoplasm and its locally invasive characteristics.

Lobectomy is considered by most surgeons to be the basic operative procedure for a carcinoma located in one lobe of the thyroid. The extent of operation will vary on the basis of the factors just noted and will be briefly outlined. Needle biopsy preoperatively is of significant value in directing management, including operation, for thyroid carcinoma.

Extent of Thyroidectomy

For papillary thyroid carcinoma evidenced only by a unilateral nodule less than 1.5 cm in diameter, the risk of later difficulty following thyroid lobectomy is so low as to make this the accepted operation. For larger lesions, for cases with evidence of multicentricity, for patients who have had external radiation therapy previously, for patients with regional lymph node or distant metastases, a total or near-total thyroidectomy is justified. Judgment is required to match extent of operation to the demonstrated need and also avoid undue morbidity.

The treatment of follicular carcinomas varies primarily on the basis of the pathologic variety. Low-grade, well-encapsulated, follicular thyroid carcinomas, without evidence of distant metastases, are managed satisfactorily by thyroid lobectomy. Angioinvasive follicular carcinomas are best treated by total thyroidectomy to ensure removal of multiple foci and permit effective use of radioactive iodine, frequently indicated. Hürthle cell carcinomas justify total or near-total thyroidectomy.

Medullary thyroid carcinomas are considered in two categories: the hereditary variety as part of the multiple endocrine neoplasia (MEN) 2a syndrome in which the carcinoma is always bilateral, and the sporadic variety which is unilateral. In general, total thyroidectomy is performed since it is not always possible to be certain of the variety without thyroidectomy.

Anaplastic thyroid carcinoma rarely is operable; management usually is restricted to biopsy for confirmation of diagnosis and radiation or chemotherapy, which rarely provides significant palliation.

Primary lymphomas of the thyroid gland are rare. These and small cell anaplastic thyroid carcinoma respond to external radiation therapy with an overall 5 year survival rate of approximately 50 per cent.

Extent of Cervical Lymph Node Removal

The likelihood of metastases to cervical lymph nodes varies with the histologic variety of thyroid carcinoma but can occur with any of the categories. The surgeon attempts removal of suspicious lymph nodes adjacent to the thyroid gland during the operative procedure on the thyroid gland.

For well-differentiated thyroid carcinomas, lymphadenopathy as clinical evidence of lymph node metastases is a reliable determinant of the need for lateral cervical lymph node removal. A modified radical cervical lymph node dissection provides the best long-term results in patients requiring this. A delay of lymph node dissection until clinical lymphadenopathy denotes metastases does not appear to significantly impair prognosis. Biopsy of a midjugular lymph node to check for the presence or absence of metastases can also be used as a determinant for performing modified lateral cervical lymph node dissection. Local invasion of metastases outside of cervical lymph nodes, especially in older patients, justifies a radical rather than a modified radical thyroidectomy.

For medullary thyroid carcinoma manifested by a palpable thyroid nodule, ipsilateral cervical lymph node dissection is indicated because of the frequent presence of microscopic metastases and the seriousness of the disease. For patients with occult hereditary medullary thyroid carcinoma recognized only by screening for elevated levels of serum calcitonin, biopsy of midjugular lymph nodes to check for evidence of microscopic metastases can govern the need for lateral cervical lymph node dissection.

On occasion, especially with well-differentiated thyroid carcinomas, extended cervical procedures are justified by which segments of invaded trachea or esophagus or both are removed.

In all operative procedures on the thyroid, efforts to preserve parathyroid and recurrent laryngeal nerve function are emphasized.

Postoperative Management

Administration of thyroid hormone is usually advised to provide for replacement needs after total or near-total thyroidectomy and to suppress thyroid-stimulating hormone (TSH) stimulation of residual, well-differentiated thyroid carcinoma. The dose should be such as to suppress serum TSH to low levels. The initiation of this treatment varies with policies for timing of postoperative neck and total body scans, and for radioactive iodine uptake. Continued administration of thyroid hormone indefinitely is emphasized.

Postoperative scanning for evidence of residual well-differentiated thyroid carcinoma in the neck or distant metastases is justified whenever the possibility for such metastases exists and, in general, is performed for patients treated by total or near-total thyroidectomy. In the interpretation of postoperative scans, it is important to avoid designating residual normal thyroid tissues erroneously as metastases. The dose of radioactive iodine will vary with the evident amount and function of remaining carcinoma.

For medullary thyroid carcinoma, periodic determination of serum calcitonin levels provides an assessment of residual or recurrent disease. However, patients have been found to have elevated but stable serum calcitonin levels for many years without clinical evidence of persistent or recurrent disease.

Periodic re-examination of the neck, chest radiograph, and scans are performed on the basis of the initial extent of disease.

Thyroid carcinoma not controlled by surgery or, in the case of well-differentiated thyroid carcinoma, by radioactive iodine and thyroid hormone therapy, rarely responds significantly to currently available chemotherapeutic agents. Papillary carcinoma does respond to external radiation therapy, and this can be used when localized disease is not amenable to operation. In such cases, external radiation therapy is palliative for varying periods of time.

Medullary thyroid carcinoma, or a variation of this pathologic type not treatable by operation has been reported to occasionally respond, at least to varying degrees of palliation, to thyroid hormone therapy or external radiation therapy even though the origin from parafollicular thyroid cells would not logically explain this.

PHEOCHROMOCYTOMA

method of
LEWIS LANDSBERG, M.D.
Harvard Medical School
Boston, Massachusetts

Pheochromocytoma is a catecholamine-secreting tumor that arises, in most cases, from the chromaffin cells of the adrenal medulla. Those tumors that arise from extra-adrenal chromaffin cells are commonly located about the sympathetic ganglia; they are called extra-adrenal pheochromocytomas or paragangliomas. The clinical manifestations of pheochromocytoma are usually the consequence of excessive and unrestrained catecholamine release from the tumor with the consequent intensive stimulation of adrenergic receptors.

Pheochromocytoma is a rare disease, occurring in less than 0.1 per cent of unselected hypertensive patients. The rarity of pheochromocytoma should not belie its importance: correctly diagnosed and properly treated, pheochromocytoma is almost always curable; if it is misdiagnosed or improperly treated, it is often fatal. Autopsy series, moreover, demonstrate that well over 50 per cent of pheochromocytomas are found unexpectedly at postmortem examination; in many of these the tumor appears to have contributed to the fatal outcome. It seems likely, therefore, that many potentially curable patients are not discovered during life. It has been estimated that over 30,000 cases are at present unrecognized in the United States. Furthermore, since pheochromocytoma occasionally occurs in familial form in association with other endocrine tumors, the diagnosis of pheochromocytoma may alert the physician to the presence of other potentially lethal tumors in the patient or in members of his family. If diagnosed early, these other tumors may be cured.

DIAGNOSTIC CONSIDERATIONS

The characteristic manifestations of pheochromocytoma are hypertension, paroxysmal attacks or crises, and signs and symptoms of increased metabolic rate. The disease is most common in early to mid-adult life and uncommon over the age of 65 years. Some series show a slight female predominance. The majority of patients with pheochromocytoma (approximately 60 per cent) have sustained hypertension. Characteristically, however, the hypertension is labile, and spontaneous fluctuations in blood pressure are common. Distinct crises or paroxysms occur in about half the patients with sustained hypertension. The hypertension is truly paroxysmal in about 25 per cent of patients with pheochromocytoma; in this group an elevated blood pressure can be demonstrated only during attacks. In most patients with paroxysmal hypertension the paroxysms occur frequently, and it is usually possible for the physician to witness an attack over the course of 1 or 2 days. In some patients, however, the attacks are sporadic and may occur at intervals as long as weeks or months. The hypertension in patients with pheochromocytoma is often severe, and occasionally it is malignant. Characteristically the blood pressure does not respond to treatment with drugs that are effective in essential hypertension. The physician should also keep in mind that on rare occasions the initial manifestation of pheochromocytoma may be unexplained hypotension or shock in association with surgery or trauma.

Preoperative Medical Management

The definitive treatment of pheochromocytoma is surgical removal of the tumor. Prior to surgery, however, it is essential that the manifestations of excessive adrenergic stimulation be reversed by treatment with adrenergic blocking agents. Three agents are generally used for this purpose.

Phentolamine (Regitine) produces a short-acting, competitive alpha-receptor blockade. As an intravenous bolus it is useful in controlling hypertensive crises or paroxysms in patients with pheochromocytoma. Phenoxybenzamine (Dibenzyline) produces a long-lasting, stable, noncompetitive alpha-receptor blockade; oral administration of this agent is particularly suitable in preparation for surgery as well as for long-term control of blood pressure and paroxysms. Propranolol (Inderal) is the usual beta-blocking agent employed; it is effective orally and intravenously in patients with pheochromocytoma. It diminishes the heart rate and is useful in the treatment of catecholamine-induced cardiac arrhythmias.

Treatment of Hypertensive Crisis or Paroxysm. Phentolamine is administered intravenously in the treatment of a severe hypertensive episode in a patient with a known or suspected pheochromocytoma. After a stable intravenous infusion is established, a test dose of 0.5 mg is given as a bolus; if there is no response, the remainder of a 5.0 mg ampule may be administered intravenously. The blood pressure should be recorded frequently (every 30 seconds). The response to phentolamine is maximal 2 or 3 minutes after the bolus and lasts 10 to 15 minutes. Norepinephrine (Levophed) or phenylephrine (Neo-Synephrine) should be on hand in case a severe hypotensive reaction ensues. If the response to phentolamine is satisfactory, the dose may be repeated as necessary to control the blood pressure.

The Induction of Stable Alpha-Adrenergic Blockade. An adequate course of alpha-adrenergic blockade is the cornerstone of successful surgical treatment of pheochromocytoma and should always be instituted prior to surgery and prior to invasive localization procedures. The patient should be placed on phenoxybenzamine as soon as the diagnosis of pheochromocytoma is established. Adjustment of the phenoxybenzamine dosage should be performed in the hospital. The blood pressure and pulse should be checked with the patient supine and upright several times each day. The usual initial dose is 10 mg every 12 hours. Because of the long duration of action of phenoxybenzamine (the biologic effect persists for more than 24 hours), the therapeutic effects are cumulative and the optimal dose must be achieved gradually. Increments of 10 or 20 mg may be added every few days until the blood pressure is controlled and the paroxysms disappear. A transient postural fall in blood pressure is common as the dose of phenoxybenzamine is increased; this does not necessarily mean that an adequate dose has been achieved, especially if the supine blood pressure remains high. As the plasma volume expands, postural signs tend to diminish. Most patients require between 40 and 80 mg of phenoxybenzamine per day, although some patients require considerably more. It is satisfactory to administer one half of the daily dose every 12 hours. Intravenous phentolamine can be given as needed for paroxysms that occur while treatment with phenoxybenzamine is being initiated.

In patients without sustained hypertension, adjustment of the dose of phenoxybenzamine is more difficult. In these patients, phenoxybenzamine should be titrated to the point at which all paroxysms cease; when persistent postural signs and symptoms develop, the dose should be stabilized or slightly diminished. The appearance of nasal stuffiness or diarrhea indicates a high degree of adrenergic blockade, but it is not necessary or desirable to push alpha-adrenergic blockade until these symptoms appear.

Prazosin (Minipress), the selective alpha-1 receptor antagonist, has had a limited trial in the management of patients with pheochromocytoma. Doses in the range of 1.5 to 2.5 mg every 6 hours provide effective blood pressure control. No advantages of prazosin over phenoxybenzamine have been noted, however, and the shorter duration of action of prazosin may be a significant disadvantage in preoperative preparation when prolonged stable blockade is desirable. In hypertensive patients in whom the diagnosis of pheochromocytoma is considered but not established, prazosin is a reasonable drug to incorporate into the antihypertensive regimen during the period of investigation.

Alpha-adrenergic blockade should be continued for about 2 weeks prior to surgery. During this time a liberal salt diet will allow the expansion of the plasma volume and will permit recovery from the effects of excessive adrenergic stimulation that dominated the pretreatment period. Phenoxybenzamine can be continued through the morning of surgery.

Beta-Receptor Blockade. Beta-receptor blocking drugs have an important, albeit secondary, role in the treatment of pheochromocytoma. Propranolol will be required in most patients with pheochromocytoma, but it should be administered only after alpha-adrenergic blockade is undertaken, since the administration of beta-adrenergic blocking agents alone may cause a paradoxic increase in blood pressure because of unopposed alpha-receptor stimulation. During the development of alpha-adrenergic blockade small doses of propranolol should be administered when a clinically significant tachycardia develops. Patients with pheochromocytoma are sensitive to beta-adrenergic blockade, and the usual starting dose of propranolol is 10 mg three to four times a day. The dose is titrated upward to control the pulse rate. Only rarely will more than 60 to 80 mg of propranolol be needed per day. Propranolol may also be useful in controlling ventricular ectopic beats and supraventricular arrhythmias, particularly those associated with the administration of anesthetic agents. Intravenous boluses of propranolol in doses of 0.5 to 2.0 mg may be used for this purpose. If congestive heart failure has been present or is suspected, propranolol must be used cautiously. Other beta-blocking agents are presumably effective as well, but experience with other agents in the setting of pheochromocytoma is not extensive.

Inhibition of Catecholamine Biosynthesis. In doses ranging from 0.3 to 4.0 grams per day, alpha-methyl-paratyrosine (Demser) inhibits catecholamine production by 50 to 80 per cent. There is no clear need for this agent in the usual case of pheochromocytoma, but, when catecholamine production is markedly increased by a very large tumor, it may be of use along with phenoxybenzamine in preoperative preparation. The major use of alpha-methyl-paratyrosine is in the long-term treatment of unoperable patients, such as those with malignant pheochromocytoma.

Adverse Drug Interactions. The clinical course of pheochromocytoma may be complicated by drugs or diagnostic agents that affect catecholamine metabolism. Severe and even fatal crises have been induced by opiates, histamine, ACTH, saralasin, and glucagon. These drugs appear to induce a paroxysm by releasing catecholamines directly from the tumor. The potent opiate agonist fentanyl (Sublimaze) has been implicated in precipitation of crises during anesthesia induction in patients with unsuspected pheochromocytoma undergoing incidental surgery. Radiographic contrast media, when administered intra-arterially, also release catecholamines; arteriography, therefore, may induce a severe paroxysm if performed in patients with pheochromocytoma before the administration of adrenergic blocking agents. Intravenous pyelography, however, can be safely performed. In addition, patients with pheochromocytoma accumulate increased amounts of catecholamines in the sympathetic nerve endings, since neuronal uptake is a major inactivating mechanism for circulating catecholamines. Indirect-acting sympathomimetic amines, including intravenously administered alpha-methyldopa, may be associated with an unpredictable increase in blood pressure by releasing catecholamines from the augmented stores within nerve endings. Proprietary cold remedies, which contain sympathomimetic amines as decongestants, are frequent offenders and may worsen the hypertension and increase the symptoms in pheochromocytoma patients. A third type of adverse interaction involves drugs that block the neuronal uptake of catecholamines, such as guanethidine or tricyclic antidepressants; these agents inhibit a major inactivating process and thus enhance the physiologic effects of circulating catecholamines. All these drugs should be specifically avoided in patients with known or suspected pheochromocytoma, and all medications should be considered carefully and administered cautiously in this group of patients.

Operative Considerations

The removal of a pheochromocytoma is a technically demanding operation and should not be undertaken lightly. Surgery should be performed in centers that have experience in dealing with this disease. Successful surgery requires adequate preoperative preparation with phenoxybenzamine. A 2 week course of alpha-adrenergic blockade will allow restoration of the plasma volume and recovery from the adverse effects of vasoconstriction and hypertension. As noted earlier, phenoxybenzamine should be administered until and including the morning of surgery.

Although opinion differs with regard to the relative merits of various preanesthetic medications and muscle relaxants, short-acting barbiturates and scopolamine along with succinylcholine are generally successful. A combination of anesthetic agents made up of thiopental, nitrous oxide, narcotics, and enflurane is usually employed. (Narcotics can be safely administered in the well blocked patient.) All the halogenated hydrocarbon anesthetics (including enflurane) sensitize the heart to the arrhythmogenic properties of catecholamines; since these arrhythmias are effectively antagonized by beta-adrenergic blockade, it is, therefore, customary to continue beta-adrenergic blocking agents up to the time of surgery and to administer propranolol during the operative procedure itself if cardiac arrhythmias develop.

Careful observation of the patient during the operation is of critical importance, and continuous monitoring of arterial pressure (via intra-arterial catheter), central venous pressure, and the electrocardiogram should be carried out. An accurate assessment of blood loss should be recorded from the outset and saline, albumin, or blood should be administered to replace losses as they occur. Intraoperative hypotension responds better to volume replacement than to the administration of vasoconstrictors; the central venous pressure is helpful in estimating the need for volume replacement. If heart failure has been present, or if cardiac reserve is significantly impaired, pulmonary capillary wedge pressure should be monitored as well.

Hypertension and cardiac arrhythmias occur most frequently during induction of anesthesia, intubation, and manipulation of the tumor. Hypertension can usually be controlled adequately by the intravenous administration of phentolamine in 1 to 5 mg boluses as needed. Large amounts are sometimes required. Nitroprusside is also effective in controlling hypertension in patients with pheochromocytoma; infusion of nitroprusside may be used in addition to phentolamine to lower the blood pressure during the operation, particularly during manipulation of the tumor. Sinus tachycardia or ventricular ectopy will usually respond promptly to the intravenous administration of 0.5 to 2.0 mg of propranolol. Lidocaine may also be used in the treatment of ventricular irritability. In the rare event that a vasopressor is required, norepinephrine or phenylephrine should be used; indirect-acting sympathomimetic amines that release norepinephrine from the nerve endings have an unpredictable response in patients with pheochromocytoma.

The surgical procedure itself depends upon the preoperative localization of the tumor. In the unusual circumstance in which localization has not been accomplished prior to surgery, complete exploration of both suprarenal areas, the sympathetic ganglia around the abdominal aorta, and the paravertebral areas must be undertaken. When preoperative studies have localized the site of the tumor to one adrenal gland, the exploration can be limited to the adrenal containing the tumor. Most surgeons prefer a thoracoabdominal approach to the flank on the involved side under these circumstances. The pheochromocytoma should be removed with the capsule intact, including surrounding connective tissue and fat; each tumor should be handled as a potentially malignant lesion and the entire adrenal gland should be removed, since it is impossible to remove the tumor and spare the underlying normal adrenal tissue. Malignant disease cannot be predicted with confidence on the basis of the histologic appearance of the tumor; metastatic deposits and microvascular invasion are the only reliable indications. The blood pressure should fall after the tumor is removed. Infusions of albumin or blood will usually control hypotension that occurs after resection of the tumor. If both adrenals are removed, hydrocortisone should be administered; the dose and route of administration are similar to those employed in patients undergoing bilateral adrenalectomy for any reason.

In the immediate postoperative period, hypertension may recur; this usually reflects fluid shifts and autonomic instability and does not necessarily indicate residual pheochromocytoma. Persistent hypertension may indicate residual pheochromocytoma or an intraoperative complication, such as damage to a renal artery. Postoperative hypotension may reflect volume depletion, persistent adrenergic blockade, or hemorrhage at the operative site, but the possibility of adrenocortical insufficiency should be considered, particularly if both adrenal glands have been explored.

Postoperative Management

One to two weeks after operation urinary catecholamines or catecholamine metabolites should be measured to confirm that all functioning pheochromocytoma has been removed. It is wise to repeat these analyses 6 months to 1 year after operation as further confirmation that no functioning pheochromocytoma remains. In those patients in whom operative removal of the tumor is impossible either because of malignancy or because of an intercurrent illness that prevents surgery, long-term medical management is necessary. This will usually involve the chronic administration of adrenergic blocking agents and, as described earlier, alpha-methyl-tyrosine. At the present time there are no generally available ways of destroying unresectable tumor by external radiotherapy or chemotherapy, although the use of ^{131}I-metaiodobenzylguanidine (MIBG) in high dose has been employed experimentally to radiate the tumor.

Familial Pheochromocytoma

A careful evaluation of the possibility of familial pheochromocytoma should be made in each patient, especially if bilateral tumors are present. If the history suggests the familial occurrence of pheochromocytoma, or one of the associated familial diseases (medullary carcinoma of the thyroid, hyperparathyroidism, mucosal neuromas, von Recklinghausen's neurofibromatosis, and von Hipple–Lindau retinal cerebellar hemangioblastomatosis), screening of the patient's family for pheochromocytoma is indicated. This evaluation should include urinary catecholamines with specific measurement of urinary epinephrine. All members of a kindred with familial pheochromocytoma (except those with von Recklinghausen's or von Hipple–Lindau disease) should also be screened for medullary carcinoma of the thyroid, since early diagnosis of this lesion may result in the cure of what is otherwise a progressive and usually lethal tumor.

Pheochromocytoma in Pregnancy

Management of pheochromocytoma during pregnancy is a considerable challenge. Spontaneous labor and delivery in unprepared patients must be avoided. Once the diagnosis is established, adrenergic blocking agents sould be prescribed (as described earlier). In early to mid-pregnancy, the tumor should be removed after suitable preoperative preparation. The pregnancy need not be terminated prior to or during the surgery, but the risk of spontaneous abortion is high. In late pregnancy, if the fetus is of sufficient maturity, cesarean section followed by tumor resection may be undertaken. The safety of adrenergic blockade during pregnancy has not been established, but in several cases these agents have been used without untoward effects, and no alternative is available.

Prognosis

In experienced hands surgical mortality is less than 3 per cent. In the usual case of benign pheochromocytoma, the 5 year survival rate after surgery is over 95 per cent and the recurrence rate is less than 10 per cent. After the removal of benign pheochromocytoma, the survival rate approaches the age-adjusted norm. The hypertension is completely cured in approximately 75 per cent of patients. In the remaining 25 per cent hypertension remains or recurs but is usually well controlled on a standard antihypertensive regimen. In this group, underlying essential hypertension or irreversible vascular damage secondary to pheochromocytoma may contribute to the persistent high blood pressure. In malignant pheochromocytoma, the 5 year survival rate is less than 50 per cent.

THYROIDITIS

method of
THOMAS F. NIKOLAI, M.D.
Marshfield Clinic
Marshfield, Wisconsin

Acute Thyroiditis (Bacterial, Suppurative)

Although common many years ago, acute thyroiditis is now quite rare. It is usually caused by *Staphylococcus aureus,* beta-hemolytic streptococcus, *Streptococcus pneumoniae,* and *Escherichia coli.* Often what appears to be a suppurative infection of the thyroid is actually infection in the adjacent structures. The onset of the disease is characterized by difficulty in swallowing, severe neck pain often radiating to the ear area, and a localized, tender, hot mass, which progresses in several days to abscess formation and involvement of adjacent structures and septicemia unless the course is interrupted by antibiotic therapy. Culture of needle aspirate or abscess fluid will help direct antibiotic therapy. *Treatment* should be started early and consists of high dose, wide spectrum antibiotic therapy such as nafcillin (Nafcil, Unipen), orally or intravenously, and incision and drainage when abscess appears.

Riedel's Thyroiditis

The cause of Riedel's thyroiditis is unknown. It is extremely rare and may be associated with mediastinal or retroperitoneal fibrosis. A sclerosing fibrosis involves the thyroid and adjacent structures, leading to a stony hard thyroid and obstruction and compression of local structures, such as the trachea, esophagus, and recurrent laryngeal nerves. A needle or open surgical biopsy specimen is necessary to make the diagnosis. *Treatment* consists of surgical decompression of the involved adjacent structures. Corticosteroid and thyroxine therapy do not appear helpful, although thyroxine therapy may be necessary if hypothyroidism develops.

Subacute (deQuervain's, Giant Cell, or Granulomatous) Thyroiditis

This disease appears to be caused by a viral infection of the thyroid gland or an immunologic reaction in the thyroid secondary to a viral infection. It often follows an upper respiratory infection, with a tendency to seasonal or geographic aggregation. Multiple viruses (measles, mumps, Coxsackie B) have been implicated through noting a marked rise in viral antibody titers during the course of the disease. Rarely has the virus been actually cultured. Onset occurs within a few weeks after the upper respiratory infection and is heralded by malaise, headache, fever, neck pain radiating to the ear areas, and exquisite tenderness localized to one or both lobes of a slightly enlarged thyroid. In severe cases, extensive follicular disruption releases excessive amounts of preformed thyroid hormone into the serum, causing typical signs and symptoms of thyrotoxicosis. Laboratory tests show a mild anemia in about 50 per cent of the patients and a high erythrocyte sedimentation rate—greater than 50 mm per hour—in most cases. Patients with thyrotoxicosis have elevated serum levels of T_4, T_3 uptake, and T_3 but a depressed radioactive iodine uptake. Patients often thought to have mild forms of subacute thyroiditis because of mild thyroid tenderness almost always are found to have chronic lymphocytic thyroiditis on needle biopsy examination.

Treatment consists of aspirin, 650 to 975 mg

four times a day for 2 to 3 weeks, or another nonsteroidal anti-inflammatory agent in mild to moderate cases. In more severe or prolonged cases, corticosteroid therapy gives prompt, dramatic improvement, so much so that the prompt response can be used as the diagnostic test. A 3 to 4 week course of prednisone is given, starting with 40 to 60 mg per day with gradual reduction by 10 mg every 5 to 7 days. Up to 10 per cent of patients will have an exacerbation of their disease even after 3 to 4 weeks' therapy and may require another course of treatment. Propranolol, 80 to 160 mg daily in divided doses, gives relief of thyrotoxic symptoms.

About 50 per cent of the patients who are thyrotoxic go through a transient hypothyroid phase that lasts about 1 to 2 months while the damaged thyroid regenerates. They may require L-thyroxine therapy, 100 to 150 micrograms daily, during this time. Permanent hypothyroidism or any form of thyroid disease after a bout of subacute thyroiditis is rare.

Chronic Lymphocytic Thyroiditis (Hashimoto's Disease, Autoimmune Thyroiditis, Struma Lymphomatosa)

Chronic lymphocytic thyroiditis is a common disease, and it appears to be gradually increasing in frequency since World War II. Women are affected four to ten times more often than men. There appears to be a strong family hereditary tendency, often involving whole families and often associated with Graves' disease. Circulating autoantibodies to thyroglobin and microsomal thyroid fractions are often present in medium and high titers. The disease presents most often as an asymptomatic euthyroid goiter (occasionally slightly tender) or as primary hypothyroidism. The thyroid gland is characteristically diffusely enlarged, firm, rubber-like, and bosselated. The thyroid tests are variable, reflecting the clinical thyroid state present ranging from normal to frank hypothyroidism with a low serum T_4 and very high serum thyroid-stimulating hormone (TSH).

Diagnosis is made clinically on the basis of the firm, diffusely enlarged, or slightly nodular thyroid. The finding of high titers of serum thyroid microsomal antibodies is confirmatory. Needle biopsy of the thyroid should be done to establish the disease with certainty.

Treatment consists of lifelong thyroid suppression or replacement with L-thyroxine in a dose ranging from 75 to 150 micrograms daily, enough to keep the serum T_4 in the mid or upper range of normal and the serum TSH suppressed in the low range of normal. Therapy usually results in a dramatic reduction in thyroid size to normal or near-normal within 2 to 4 months and in relief of all symptoms. It should be started at one-half therapeutic levels for 2 to 4 weeks in patients who are healthy and under age 50 years. In those over the age of 50 years or who have cardiopulmonary disease, caution is advised and initial therapy begun at 25 micrograms daily. Triiodothyronine (Cytomel) therapy can be used for suppression therapy, starting with 12.5 micrograms two to three times daily and observing the fall in the serum T_4 that occurs with it. The full dose of triiodothyronine is 25 micrograms three or four times daily. Maximum suppression of the thyroid will decrease the serum T_4 to 2 to 3 micrograms per cent. Failure of the thyroid to decrease in size with therapy is unusual and should alert one to the possibility of other disease, such as thyroid malignancy. Desiccated thyroid thyroglobulin (Proloid) and balanced T_4 and T_3 preparations (Euthroid, Thyrolar) should not be used as the contents of T_3 and T_4 vary, and high levels of serum T_3 are present for 6 to 8 hours every day from these drugs. Corticosteroid therapy usually results in a rapid decrease in thyroid size, but the goiter generally recurs after it is stopped.

Surgery is rarely indicated except to make a diagnosis in questionable cases in which there are enlarged or suspicious nodules or when there are obstructive symptoms and signs. Surgery should be approached with caution by an experienced surgeon, as it has been my experience that the incidence of vocal cord paralysis increases especially when inexperienced surgeons are concerned about possible malignancy in these firm, fibrotic glands and attempt near-total excision.

Silent Thyroiditis (Lymphocytic Thyroiditis with Spontaneously Resolving Hyperthyroidism, Painless Thyroiditis, Postpartum Thyroiditis)

Silent thyroiditis appears to be an early or a variant form of chronic lymphocytic thyroiditis. It usually presents as a transient form of thyrotoxicosis lasting 2 to 4 months with a painless, normal-sized or slightly enlarged gland. The initial impression after finding thyrotoxicosis in these patients is that they have Graves' disease until a suppressed radioactive iodine uptake is found. Thyroid biopsy needs to be done to confirm the diagnosis in questionable cases. This disease was first described in the mid-1970s and has been shown to have an increased incidence since that time. It comprises between 5 and 20 per cent of all cases of hyperthyroidism in recent reports. About 10 per cent of the cases occur in the immediate postpartum period when it is very common, affecting 5 to 10 per cent of women. This variant has been labeled postpartum thyroiditis and appears to be related to a resurge in the immune system that occurs after the generalized immunosuppression of pregnancy. Postpartum thyroiditis may present initially as transient or permanent hypothyroidism.

The *treatment* of silent thyroiditis depends on recognition. Failure to distinguish it from Graves' hyperthyroidism has resulted in inappropriate treatment with radioactive iodine, surgery, and thionamides. The severity of the hyperthyroidism ranges from mild to severe. In most cases, no therapy or only sedatives, tranquilizers, and beta-adrenergic blockers are all that is needed to give symptomatic relief. Patients need to be advised of the transient (1 to 3 months) nature of the disease. In more severe cases, corticosteroid therapy is quite effective and causes rapid reduction in thyroid size and decrease of thyroid function tests to normal within 7 to 10 days. Prednisone is given for 3 to 4 weeks, with an initial dose of 40 to 60 mg daily and gradual reduction by 10 mg every 4 to 6 days. On recovery, about 50 per cent of the patients develop a transient hypothyroidism lasting 4 to 6 weeks. This may require L-thyroxine therapy, 75 to 150 micrograms daily for 6 to 8 weeks. About 10 per cent of the affected patients develop persistent hypothyroidism and probably require lifelong thyroid replacement therapy. Long-term follow-up reveals that 10 to 20 per cent of patients have recurrent episodes of silent thyroiditis 1 to 5 years apart, with up to five episodes reported in one patient. Approximately 50 per cent of the patients go on to chronic thyroid disease, which includes chronic euthyroid goiter, hypothyroidism, and decreased thyroid reserve. All affected patients need to be followed indefinitely.

Section 9

The Urogenital Tract

BACTERIAL INFECTIONS OF THE URINARY TRACT—MALE

method of
KEITH N. VAN ARSDALEN, M.D.
University of Pennsylvania
Philadelphia, Pennsylvania

Male bacterial infections of the urinary tract occur in all age groups and may involve all parts of this system. With the exception of the first 3 months of life, these infections are much less common in males than in females. The lower incidence, however, becomes less dramatic in the elderly when infections in males increase significantly, presumably associated with the development of prostatic disease. It has been estimated that less than 1 per cent of men between the ages of 50 and 59 years have bacteriuria, with the incidence rising to 3 to 4 per cent after the age of 70 years. Bacteriuria may be three to four times this figure in hospitalized elderly men.

The ascending route is the most common pathway for bacteria entering the urinary tract, although hematogenous infection may also occur. An antibacterial factor isolated from prostatic secretions may normally prevent the retrograde ascent of bacteria. In the absence of instrumentation, the factors that are important in overwhelming the natural defense mechanisms of the urinary tract are generally unclear. The pathogenic organisms are usually various serotypes of *Escherichia coli* and, less commonly, other gram-negative rods, including *Klebsiella, Proteus, Enterobacter,* and *Pseudomonas.* Gram-positive organisms such as *Enterococcus* and *Staphylococcus* are occasionally involved. The common sexually transmitted organisms include *Neisseria gonorrhoeae, Chlamydia trachomatis,* and *Ureaplasma urealyticum.*

Urethritis

Urethritis is generally subdivided into gonococcal and nongonococcal. Both forms may be associated with dysuria, itching, and a urethral discharge. However, symptoms may be unreliable for diagnosis as one fourth of men with gonorrhea and two thirds of men with nongonococcal urethritis (NGU) may not complain of the discharge. Gonococcal urethritis is associated with the gram-negative diplococcus *N. gonorrhoeae.* Nongonococcal urethritis is diagnosed by demonstrating urethritis in the absence of gonorrhea. NGU is now approximately twice as common as gonococcal urethritis. *C. trachomatis* is thought to be the most common etiologic organism, followed by *U. urealyticum.* These organisms may coexist with *N. gonorrhoeae* and may account for the development of postgonococcal urethritis. The treatment of NGU consists of tetracycline, 500 mg orally four times daily for 7 days, or doxycycline (Vibramycin), 100 mg orally twice daily for 7 days. Alternatively, erythromycin, 500 mg orally four times daily for 7 days, may also be given. The patient's sexual partner or partners should also be evaluated and treated, and follow-up cultures on both patient and partner should be obtained.

The standard treatment of gonococcal urethritis in men has been aqueous procaine penicillin G, 4.8 million units intramuscularly, with 1.0 gram of probenecid orally. Alternatively, amoxicillin, 3.0 grams, or ampicillin, 3.5 grams orallly with 1 gram of probenecid orally, may be used. Each of these single dose regimens insures compliance with approximately 95 per cent effectiveness of therapy. The major disadvantage of the aqueous procaine penicillin regimen is the possible procaine reaction. Also, neither of these regimens is effective against coexisting chlamydial infections. Treatment with tetracycline, 500 mg orally four times daily for 7 days, is now recognized as effective against *N. gonorrhoeae* while simultaneously being effective against *C. trachomatis.* Compliance with this longer regimen, however, is essential to assure adequate treatment and to prevent the development of tetracycline-resistant strains of *N. gonorrhoeae.* Lastly, mention should be made of treatment of urethritis due to penicillinase-producing *N. gonorrhoeae.* These organisms account for persistent *N. gonorrhoeae* infections after the aforementioned regimens. Recommended treatment includes spectinomycin (Trobicin), 2.0 grams intramuscularly, or cefoxitin (Mefoxin), 2.0 grams intramuscularly plus 1 gram of probenecid orally.

Epididymo-Orchitis

Acute epididymitis generally develops secondary to spread of infection to this area from a primary site in the urethra, prostate, or bladder. Secondary involvement of the testicle in association with acute epididymitis is relatively common. In sexually active males under 35 years of age, the most common infecting organisms are those producing urethritis, that is, *N. gonorrhoeae* and *C. trachomatis,* as noted. Although these organisms may also infect older men, the most common organisms in the latter group are the gram-negative rods that are responsible for cystitis and prostatis.

Treatment of epididymo-orchitis in men with infections suspected to be secondary to sexually transmitted organisms is initiated with tetracycline, 500 mg orally four times daily for at least 10 days. Amoxicillin, 500 mg orally four times daily, may be used in place of tetracycline for gonococcal epididymitis. Erythromycin, 500 mg orally four times daily, may be used if nongonococcal epididymitis is noted. Supportive measures include bedrest and scrotal elevation. Once again, the sexual partner or partners should be treated. Further evaluation of the genitourinary tract is usually unrewarding as underlying pathology is rare.

The treatment of epididymo-orchitis secondary to bacteriuria begins initially with the administration of broad-spectrum antibiotics. A cephalosporin is often used and may be administered orally or intravenously, depending upon the clinical setting. A fever above 101 F, an elevated white blood cell count, or advancing age usually warrants admission to the hospital and intravenous therapy. The results of the urine culture and sensitivity studies determine subsequent therapy. Bedrest and scrotal elevation are again important supportive measures. The genitourinary tract should be evaluated for underlying pathology. An intravenous urogram may be made as soon as the patient is stable, but endoscopy should be delayed 4 to 6 weeks after therapy if possible.

Prostatitis Syndromes

See the article on Prostatitis later in this section, page 553.

Cystitis and Pyelonephritis

Cystitis and pyelonephritis are seen most commonly as ascending infections of the genitourinary tract, particularly the prostate. In this regard, the most common offending pathogens are the gram-negative rods although infections caused by gram-positive organisms such as enterococci and occasionally staphylococci may also be noted. Therapy for acute pyelonephritis is generally started with gentamicin, 3 to 5 mg per kg per day in three divided intravenous doses, plus ampicillin, 1 gram intravenously every 6 hours. Depending upon the culture results and the antibiotic sensitivities, a change may be made to oral therapy after the patient has become afebrile. Medication should be continued for at least 10 to 14 days. Acute cystitis without evidence of upper urinary tract infection may initially be treated with oral antibiotics. If there is a known history of chronic bacterial prostatitis, trimethoprim-sulfamethoxazole double strength (Bactrim DS, Septra DS) twice daily or carbenicillin indanyl sodium (Geocillin), two tablets four times daily, may be started. Alternatively, nitrofurantoin (Macrodantin), 50 to 100 mg four times daily or the oral cephalosporins (Keflex, Velosef), 250 to 500 mg four times daily, may also be used until results of the urine culture and sensitivity testing are available. A complete urologic investigation is warranted in cases of pyelonephritis and cystitis to identify associated genitourinary abnormalities. Complete lower urinary tract localization studies are also recommended because of the association of these infections with the presence or persistence of bacteria within the prostate.

BACTERIAL INFECTIONS OF THE URINARY TRACT—FEMALE

method of
ABDOLLAH IRAVANI, M.D.
University of Florida
Gainesville, Florida

Urinary tract infections (UTIs) are highly prevalent in women of child-bearing age. It is estimated that 6 to 8 per cent of young women develop UTIs each year, compared with only 2 to 3 per cent of female infants and prepubertal girls. Bacteria responsible for these infections originate from the normal constituents of fecal flora that colonize the periurethral mucosa. Because of a variety of host factors, bacteria ascend the urethra and invade the urinary tract. The most common urinary pathogens in women are *Escherichia coli* and *Staphylococcus saprophyticus*. The other organisms, in order of decreasing incidence, are strains of *Proteus, Klebsiella*, and *Enterobacter* species. Infection may be limited to the lower tract (cystitis) or also involve the upper tract (pyelonephritis). Over 95 per cent of young women with UTIs have simple uncomplicated infections with normal urinary tracts, but the recurrence rate is high. Urinary tract infections carry a great risk when they are complicated by underlying abnormalities of the urinary tract such as calculi, obstruction, pregnancy, or systemic diseases such as diabetes mellitus, lupus erythematosus, and sickle cell disorder.

Diagnosis

The diagnosis of urinary tract infection is confirmed when $\geq 10^5$ colony-forming units of one bacterium per milliliter of urine are present in a clean-catch, midstream specimen. Bacteria seen in a microscopic examination of an unspun clean-catch, midstream urine specimen suggest bacteriuria but do not confirm the diagnosis. Pyuria (WBC > five per high-power field) is noted in 50 to 60 per cent of women with UTI. However, pyuria may occur without bacterial infection or may be due to contamination of urine with vaginal secretions. Therefore, documentation cannot be based on the presence of pyuria.

Management

Selection of Antimicrobial Agents

Most antimicrobial agents that reach a high urinary concentration in active form usually produce a rapid, effective therapeutic response. Besides a drug's effectiveness, other selection criteria should be (1) little or no adverse effects on major organ systems, (2) minimal emergence of bacterial resistance, (3) low incidence of *Candida* vaginitis, (4) low cost, and (5) convenient administration. The following antimicrobial agents meet most of these requirements.

Duration of antimicrobial treatment may range from a single dose to short-term (3 to 10 days) or long-term (more than 10 days) courses, depending on the site and severity of the infection and the presence of underlying urologic abnormalities.

Sulfonamides. Sulfonamides are synthetic bacteriostatic agents. Of the urinary pathogens, 75 to 85 per cent are susceptible to these agents. Commonly used oral sulfonamides are sulfisoxazole (Gantrisin), 0.5 to 1 gram every 6 hours, or sulfamethoxazole (Gantanol), 0.5 to 1 gram every 12 hours. Sulfamethoxazole has a slower renal excretion rate than sulfisoxazole; however, both drugs are highly soluble. Sulfonamides are low in cost. Common side effects are headaches, rashes, and nausea.

Trimethoprim. Trimethoprim is a synthetic bacteriostatic agent. It blocks a step in microbial folate metabolism that immediately follows the reaction inhibited by sulfonamide. Trimethoprim (Proloprim, Trimpex), 100 mg twice daily or 200 mg once daily, is an effective oral agent against more than 95 per cent of urinary pathogens. Since trimethoprim is secreted in high concentrations in the vagina, it is suitable for use in prophylaxis of recurrent UTIs. Trimethoprim is tolerated well by over 95 per cent of patients. The common adverse reactions encountered are maculopapular rash and nausea.

Trimethoprim/Sulfamethoxazole. Because of the synergistic antibacterial action of trimethoprim and sulfonamides, a fixed combination of trimethoprim, 80 mg, and sulfamethoxazole, 400 mg (Bactrim, Septra), (or double-strength tablets) is available. This combination is effective against more than 95 per cent of urinary pathogens. Adverse reactions commonly noted with this combination are the same as those known to occur with sulfonamides and trimethoprim when used separately. Leukopenia has been reported with the use of this combination. *Candida* vaginitis, a common side effect of antimicrobial treatment, develops less often after use of sulfonamides, trimethoprim, or trimethoprim/sulfamethoxazole.

Aminopenicillins. Among the aminopenicillins are ampicillin (250 to 500 mg every 6 hours), amoxicillin (250 to 500 mg every 8 hours) and bacampicillin (400 mg every 12 hours). These agents have similar activity against the common urinary pathogens and enterococci. Bacampicillin is not active against bacteria in vitro but is converted to ampicillin in the intestinal wall. Amoxicillin and bacampicillin are preferable to ampicillin because doses are less frequent and patient tolerance is higher. Amoxicillin has been the aminopenicillin of first choice. More than 20 per cent of urinary pathogens of non-nosocomial UTIs are resistant to these agents. The most common mechanism of bacterial resistance is inactivation of penicillins by beta-lactamases. A fixed combination of amoxicillin (250 mg) and the beta-lactamase inhibitor clavulanic acid (125 mg) has now become available (Augmentin). This combination is effective against most bacteria resistant to amoxicillin. A reasonable approach for therapy is to initiate treatment with amoxicillin–clavulanic acid until the results of bacterial susceptibility testing become available. Aminopenicillins must, of course, be avoided in patients with histories of allergy to penicillins. Common adverse reactions include diarrhea and rashes. *Candida* vaginitis is a common side effect, occurring in 10 to 16 per cent of patients treated with aminopenicillins.

Nitrofurantoin. Nitrofurantoin is active against most gram-negative bacteria and enterococci. *Proteus* and *Pseudomonas* species are usually resistant to this agent. Because nitrofurantoin is absorbed in the small intestine, it does not promote the emergence of resistant bacteria in the fecal flora. Nitrofurantoin macromolecules (Furadantin, Macrodantin), at oral doses of 50 to 100 mg every 6 hours, should be taken after meals to prevent nausea and vomiting. *Candida* vaginitis is an unusual complication of this agent.

Nalidixic Acid. Nalidixic acid (NegGram) has a wide spectrum of antibacterial activity against gram-negative organisms except *Pseudomonas* species. *Staphylococcus saprophyticus* is resistant to this drug. The presence of *S. saprophyticus* should be ruled out by microscopic examination of the urine before nalidixic acid is prescribed. The dose is administered as 1 gram every 6 hours orally. Common side effects include visual disturbances, photosensitivities, and dizziness. *Candida* vaginitis occurs rarely following treatment with nalidixic acid.

Cephalosporins. Cephalosporins have antibacterial activities similar to those of aminopenicillins. Oral cephalexin (Keflex) or cefaclor (Ceclor), 250 to 500 mg every 8 hours, is used in treatment of UTI. Adverse reactions are rare. Cross-reactivity to cephalosporin is present in 20 per cent of patients with a history of anaphylactic reactions to penicillins. *Candida* vaginitis develops in 6 to 14 per cent of women treated with these agents.

Simple Uncomplicated Infections

Simple uncomplicated infections are differentiated from complicated infections by their response to treatment. In patients with uncomplicated infections, symptoms are usually relieved and urine becomes sterile within 2 days of therapy. Persistence of symptoms and bacteriuria may be due to a variety of conditions, such as bacterial resistance, urinary calculi, or obstructive uropathy. On the other hand, resolution of symptoms alone is not a reliable indicator of therapeutic success and elimination of the urinary pathogen; therefore, it is suggested that urine cultures be repeated at 1 week and 1 month after therapy.

Duration of antibiotic treatment of UTI is a controversial issue. The history of the individual patient must be considered, with attention to whether she has had single episodes with long disease-free intervals or frequent repeated infections, or whether systemic symptoms are present such as fever, vomiting, and dehydration. Patients with simple lower tract infections are usually afebrile and respond favorably to a short course of therapy. In fact, a single dose of any of the aforementioned antimicrobial agents has been shown to be effective in these patients. However, a better alternative to single dose treatment is 3 to 5 days of therapy. Antimicrobial therapy should be started with the finding of microscopic bacteriuria on urinalysis rather than be delayed for the results of urine culture and susceptibility testing.

Acute Pyelonephritis

Acute pyelonephritis is a bacterial infection of the renal parenchyma. It is distinct and more serious than lower tract infections. The symptoms may vary from flank pain, fever, chills, vomiting, and dysuria to no symptoms at all. Depending on the severity of the clinical findings and general condition of the patient, antimicrobial agents may be administered orally or parenterally for 10 to 14 days. Ampicillin, 1 gram every 6 hours, trimethoprim/sulfamethoxazole (Bactrim, Septra), 160/800 mg every 12 hours, or cefazolin sodium (Ancef, Kefzol) or cefamandole nafate (Mandol), 1 gram every 6 hours, may be given intravenously for 3 to 5 days or until the patient can tolerate an oral antimicrobial agent. Therapy with an oral antimicrobial agent should be continued for a total of 10 to 14 days, according to the bacterial susceptibility testing results.

An intravenous pyelogram or a sonogram of the urinary tract is suggested within 1 month after therapy.

Recurrent Urinary Tract Infections

Recurrent UTIs are a major problem in women. Thirty to 40 per cent of women with an episode of UTI develop another within 3 months, and 75 to 80 per cent within 2 years after therapy. Recurrent UTIs are costly and inconvenient and interfere with all aspects of daily life. Over 80 per cent of recurrences are reinfections caused by fecal bacteria that have colonized the vagina and periurethral area and migrate into the urinary bladder or to the level of the kidneys.

Each episode of recurrence is treated with an appropriate antibacterial agent for 3 to 10 days. Personal hygienic precautions alone are not effective in preventing recurrent infections, whereas long-term, low dose antimicrobial therapy has been proved effective. Prophylactic therapy is indicated when recurrences occur at frequent, closely spaced intervals. After the active infection is cleared, a low dose of an antimicrobial agent is prescribed to be taken at bedtime for 3 to 9 months. The antimicrobial agents commonly used for prophylaxis include trimethoprim, 100 mg; trimethoprim/sulfamethoxazole 80/400 mg; nitrofurantoin, 100 mg; cinoxacin, 250 mg; and cephalexin, 250 mg. A complete blood cell count (CBC) and liver profile tests (transaminase enzymes) are indicated every 3 months to evaluate the safety of the drug being used. Sulfonamides and aminopenicillins cause rapid emergence of bacterial resistance in fecal flora and are not recommended for prophylactic therapy.

An intravenous pyelogram or a renal sonogram is suggested for patients with more than four recurrences in a 12 month period.

Asymptomatic Urinary Tract Infections

Asymptomatic UTIs may occur in either anatomically normal or abnormal urinary tracts. Treatment of these infections is controversial. Asymptomatic UTIs, detected on a medical screening, are usually treated with a short course of an antimicrobial agent, after which the patient is observed for recurrent infections. Asymptomatic UTIs are of greater significance, and treatment is essential in patients with ureteral reflux, obstructive uropathies, or primary parenchymal renal disease or during pregnancy.

Urinary Tract Infections in Pregnancy

Urinary tract infections can be a serious problem in pregnancy. Pregnant women are more susceptible to UTIs than are nonpregnant women, due largely to hormonal and physiologic changes. During pregnancy, hydroureter and vesicoureteral reflux may develop and facilitate pyelonephritis and renal scarring. The incidence of symptomatic UTI in pregnant women is reported as high as 15 per cent, whereas the incidence of asymptomatic UTI is 4 to 6 per cent (similar to that of nonpregnant women). Acute pyelonephritis is a common sequela of untreated asymptomatic bacteriuria. Recommended antimicrobial agents include aminopenicillins, cephalosporins, nitrofurantoin, and sulfonamides. A 7 to 10 day course of therapy usually eradicates the infection. Sulfonamides should not be used during the third trimester since they may cause kernicterus in the neonate. Periodic screening for asymptomatic bacteriuria is recommended during pregnancy.

Complicated Urinary Tract Infections

The incidence of complicated infections is less than 5 per cent in young women with UTIs. *Pseudomonas* species, enterococci and Enterobacteriaceae other than *E. coli* commonly cause these infections. Urinary pathogens are usually resistant to most antimicrobial agents. Management of complicated infections may require both antimicrobial therapy and surgical intervention. Consequent renal damage and scarring depend on the nature and degree of the obstruction and the time lapse between onset of infection and establishment of antimicrobial therapy and adequate drainage. Bacteriuria may often persist or repeated relapses occur at short intervals, in spite of long-term antimicrobial therapy.

BACTERIAL INFECTIONS OF THE URINARY TRACT—FEMALE CHILDREN

method of
STUART B. BAUER, M.D.
Harvard Medical School
Boston, Massachusetts

Urinary tract infection (UTI) is the second most common infection of childhood, after upper respiratory infection. Girls seem to be afflicted 50 times more frequently than boys. About 1 in 20 girls will have a urinary tract infection during their school years. After one infection, there is an 80 per cent chance a girl will have another one within a year.

DIAGNOSTIC CONSIDERATIONS

The most important aspect of UTI is proper diagnosis. Symptoms are often not suggestive of a UTI. In infants, fever, anorexia, vomiting, diarrhea, central nervous system signs, anemia, and failure to thrive are common. Older girls may have dysuria, frequency, and incontinence, making one more suspicious of the diagnosis. Fever and other systemic symptoms do not signify that the infection is predominantly upper urinary tract. Conversely, an infection confined to the bladder may not produce only lower urinary tract symptoms.

Appropriately collected specimens are paramount in making the diagnosis. A midstream sample of a clean voided specimen in a toilet-trained girl who has thoroughly cleaned herself off and spread her labia is the only way to obtain an accurate sample of urine. Girls who have not been toilet-trained should be catheterized for a urine sample. Suprapubic taps may be utilized in neonates and infant girls, who are difficult to catheterize. Bag specimens are considered invalid (unless the culture is negative) because they are invariably contaminated within 20 minutes of being applied to the perineum. Once a properly collected specimen is obtained, it should be cultured, not just examined microscopically. Fifty per cent of specimens exhibiting pyuria or bacteriuria will not be infected, whereas half of infected specimens will not show any pyuria or bacteriuria. The diagnosis of UTI is made when the cultured specimen grows out 100,000 colonies per ml of a single organism. It is interesting that the validity of one positive culture is only 80 per cent, whereas three specimens approach 95 per cent. Therefore, I like to obtain at least two properly collected samples in a girl suspected of having a UTI.

My reasons for being so specific in diagnosing a UTI in girls are because of the far-reaching implications of this diagnosis. I advise that all girls under the age of 2 years with one documented UTI undergo radiographic evaluation of the urinary tract. Any girl over the age of 2 years who has a UTI from an organism other than *Escherichia coli* should also undergo radiographic studies, for it is likely that her first UTI was either missed or not clinically evident. Because *Escherichia coli* is such a protean organism, I tend not to order radiographic studies until a girl has two such infections. However, any girl who has constitutional symptoms suggesting an upper urinary tract infection, an infection that fails to clear with an adequate course of antibiotics, or a repeated infection with the same or another organism within a short period of time should have a radiographic investigation of the urinary tract.

Treatment

Once the diagnosis of a UTI is made, the treatment will depend on the organism and its sensitivities and the type and extent of symptoms. Most uncomplicated UTIs can be treated with 7 to 14 days of sulfisoxazole (Gantrisin), trimethoprim-sulfamethoxazole (Bactrim), nitrofuradantoin macrocrystals (Macrodantin), or amoxicillin. The dosage schedule for each is as follows: Gantrisin, 50 mg per kg per day; Bactrim, 1 teaspoon per 10 kg twice daily; Macrodantin, 5 to 7 mg per kg per day; amoxicillin, 50 mg per kg per day, usually in three divided doses. Urinary infections involving organisms other than *E. coli* require more potent antibiotics, such as cephalexin (Keflex) or cefaclor (Ceclor); their dosage is 25 mg per kg per day in three or four divided doses. Organisms resistant to most oral antibiotics, such as *Pseudomonas*, generally require intravenous administration of antibiotics for 7 days, usually necessitating hospitalization for that period of time.

When a girl has constitutional symptoms of highly elevated temperature, malaise, nausea, and vomiting resulting in a toxic or dehydrated state, hospitalization may be necessary even though the organism is sensitive to an orally administered antibiotic. Intravenous administration of the appropriate drug for 24 to 48 hours should result in the rapid disappearance of symptoms. The child can then be switched to oral antibiotics and discharged from the hospital.

CHILDHOOD ENURESIS

method of
GEORGE W. KAPLAN, M.D.
Children's Hospital
San Diego, California

Enuresis may be defined as the involuntary loss of urine after an age at which a child should be toilet trained. This discussion will center on pure nocturnal enuresis; however, children with nocturnal enuresis often have daytime frequency as well. Children with both day and night wetting are a slightly different problem; in this latter group organic lesions are most likely to be found. Obstructive and neurologic problems are quite rare in children with nocturnal enuresis only.

One issue of concern is the timing of intervention. Most reserchers agree that as many as 10 per cent of normal children are enuretic to age 5 years; my feeling is that therapy for any large segment of the population such as this is inappropriate. I prefer to delay active intervention until children are 7 or 8 years of age, at which time they themselves are becoming concerned about the problem and are more interested in and cooperative with therapy.

Treatment

Multiple modalities have been employed in the management of enuresis. In evaluating the results of any intervention, there is an approximate 40 per cent placebo effect. Hence, almost any intervention is likely to be successful in a sizable minority of cases. The modality that has consistently proved most successful has been conditioning therapy. This method involves the use of a buzzer and pad system. When there is a wetting event, an electrical circuit is completed so that an alarm will sound. In some series, the success rate with such devices has been as high as 90 per cent; in my own experience it has not been quite that successful. This system is most effective when the child and the parents are motivated. Because many of the enuretic children are deep sleepers, I find it helpful to have an adult sleep in the room with the child during the early stages of therapy so that the child can be awakened when the buzzer sounds. The relapse rate is relatively high (about 50 per cent) after successful therapy, but the buzzer can be reintroduced if there is recidivism, and a high degree of success can be achieved the second time as well.

Certain medications are also effective. These include imipramine (Tofranil), anticholinergics, and DDAVP (vasopressin). In general, the anticholinergics have not been terribly helpful in the management of primary nocturnal enuresis, but a double blind study of oxybutynin (Ditropan) has shown some efficacy. The medication is administered in two doses: 5 mg late in the afternoon and a second 5 mg dose at bedtime. If such therapy is successful, it must be continued for several months to reinforce the behavior of voiding only when awake. (The safety and efficacy of imipramine and oxybutynin in children under 6 years of age have not been established.)

Perhaps the mainstay of therapy in the United States has been the drug imipramine (Tofranil). Multiple double-blind cross-over studies have shown its superiority to placebo. The drug is usually administered as a single night-time dose of 25 mg. If success is not attained within a few weeks, the dose can be increased to 50 or even to 75 mg. The dose should never exceed 1 mg per kg per dose. The major problem of imipramine is its toxicity—an overdose can be fatal. Younger children often will emulate their older siblings and may ingest their sibling's medications. For this reason, it is of paramount importance that imipramine be kept under lock and key and administered only by a responsible adult.

A newer medication that has recently become available is DDAVP (vasopressin) which is administered as a nasal spray (20 micrograms per dose). Early studies indicate that this medication is good for episodic use such as at camp or on vacations. Its mode of action is presumably by producing an antidiuresis. However, long-term use has not proved unusually beneficial when compared with placebo.

Traditional psychiatric approaches have not proved efficacious for primary nocturnal enuresis. They are occasionally beneficial when identifiable anxieties and conflicts are present, but these constitute a definite minority of cases. Elimination diets have been proposed by those who feel that enuresis may be a manifestation of food allergy, but controlled studies have failed to support their efficacy. Fluid restriction and waking the child at intervals for voiding have not proved to be particularly effective. Fluid restriction is sometimes viewed by the child as punitive and for that reason is best omitted in my opinion.

Bladder control training has been used by some as an adjunct to therapy, based on the observation that enuretic children have a reduced functional bladder capacity. The goal of this type of therapy is to increase the bladder capacity during the day and thereby increase the nocturnal capacity and eliminate the wetting events. Although I have no objection to its use, I have not observed that this is a particularly effective form of therapy and do not routinely recommend it.

URINARY INCONTINENCE

method of
EDWARD J. McGUIRE, M.D.
University of Michigan
Ann Arbor, Michigan

Incontinence may be due to abnormalities of urethral or bladder function. Bladder abnormalities include poor reservoir function manifested by decreased compliance or an increase in pressure with increasing volume. These abnormalities are relatively subtle and often poorly diagnosed and poorly managed. Abnormalities of the control of bladder reflex activity are probably the most common reason for incontinence, although the etiology of this kind of abnormality is multiple. In addition, "paradoxic" or overflow incontinence results from lack of reflex bladder contractility.

TREATMENT

Bladder-Related Incontinence

Disorders of Compliance. An abnormal increase in intravesical pressure with filling, indicating loss of bladder reservoir function, occurs after radical pelvic surgery, in cases of peripheral neuropathy, in patients with myelodysplasia, and in sacral cord or sacral root injuries or disease. These disorders are frequently associated with lack of reflex bladder contractility, but the major abnormality is a loss of low pressure volume accommodation. The increased pressure volume relationship has a direct hydraulic effect on ureteral delivery of urine to the bladder and induces leakage across a fixed continence mechanism at low to moderate vesical volumes. The intent of treatment is to periodically empty the bladder and preserve and protect low pressure storage of urine. This can usually be accomplished by intermittent catheterization and anticholinergic drugs. If vesical pressures cannot be kept below 35 cm of H_2O at the volumes obtained at the time of intermittent catheterization, some method to improve reservoir function is essential to preserve upper tract function. This can be by augmentation cystoplasty using bowel tissue or by reducing the outlet resistance and lowering the pressure at which leakage occurs (with the acceptance of more incontinence). Increasing urethral resistance to improve continence is directly prejudicial to upper tract function if vesical compliance (volume tolerance at pressures under 35 cm of H_2O) is inadequate.

Disorders of the Control of Reflex Vesical Activity. These disorders may be associated with spinal cord injury or disease and multiple sclerosis, in which case control of reflex bladder activity is poor or absent and both the storage and voiding phases of bladder activity are disordered. Approximately 70 per cent of the patients can be managed by anticholinergic medication and intermittent catheterization. Because the major effect of such lesions in men is related to upper tract changes related to high bladder pressure, sphincter obviation procedures and condom catheter drainage are frequently used—these sacrifice continence. In women, bladder pressures are lower and continence is of major importance. Interruption of reflex pathways at the trigone, or sacral root, or cord levels or partial cystectomy and augmentation cystoplasty can be used to achieve good vesical storage function, with intermittent catheterization used for periodic bladder emptying. Quadriplegic women are a special problem; provision for a continent stoma to allow self-catheterization permits avoidance of treatment by Foley catheter drainage or ileal loop diversion; both methods have a dismal long-term outlook.

Treatment of male spinal-injured patients by ileal loop diversion, cutaneous ureterostomy, suprapubic tube, or Foley catheter drainage is associated with equally dismal long-term complications.

"Idiopathic" Detrusor Contractile Incontinence. Poor control of reflex vesical activity without high pressure bladder dysfunction is a fairly common problem that is frequently encountered in the elderly, those with cerebrovascular disease or lesions of the basal ganglia, adult men and women without neurologic disease, and children. The urodynamic finding is basically a sudden bladder contraction that occurs without its owner's permission.

Warning of detrusor events is poor, and reflex contractility is provoked by volume. Treatment is directed at delay of the reflex bladder response with anticholinergic agents such as oxybutynin chloride (Ditropan), 5 mg three times daily, propantheline bromide (Pro-Banthine), 15 to 30 mg three times daily, dicyclomine (Bentyl), 20 mg four times daily, or imipramine (Tofranil), 10 to 25 mg three times daily or 50 mg at bedtime. These should be coupled with a regular program of timed voiding, which tends to short-circuit the uninhibited response of the bladder to filling. Urodynamically, no qualitative differences distinguish hyperactive bladder activity in one group from that in another. Poor response to one agent often can be circumvented by using two agents that act differently—e.g., imipramine, 10 mg three times daily, and oxybutynin, 5 mg three times daily.

Obstructive Uropathy. Poor control of reflex vesical activity is also associated with obstructive uropathy—most comonly, benign prostatic hyperplasia. Residual urine or symptoms suggesting obstruction—for example, hesitancy or a slow stream—should prompt investigation and initially contraindicate anticholinergic therapy.

Stress Incontinence

Stress incontinence related to poor urethral support in women, associated with visible urethral hypermobility, responds most predictably to surgical repair. Alternative methods include tampon use to achieve urethral support, and temporary treatment with drugs with alpha-stimulating properties (e.g., phenylpropanolamine, 25 mg three times daily, or imipramine (Tofranil), 25 mg three times daily). These agents are not FDA approved for this usage and have somewhat limited value.

Weakness of urethral sphincter function in elderly women, not associated with urethral hypermobility with an increase in intra-abdominal pressure, responds reasonably well to intravaginal Premarin (on third of an applicator at night and imipramine, 10 mg three times daily). Men with very mild postprostatectomy incontinence *may* respond to alpha-stimulating agents, but this does not happen often.

When internal sphincter function is absent in patients with myelodysplasia and following radical prostatectomy, and occasionally following radical surgery for uterine or rectal malignant disease, medication is of no benefit, and usually complicated surgical procedures are required for relief.

EPIDIDYMITIS

method of
GERALD H. JORDAN, M.D.
Eastern Virginia Medical School
Norfolk, Virginia

Epididymitis is an inflammatory condition involving the convoluted tubule that is interposed between the rete testis/ductuli efferentes and the vas deferens. The condition can affect any age group but most commonly is seen in the sexually active male in his 20s or 30s. Classically, it presents with an insidious or semiacute onset of unilateral scrotal pain and swelling. Early in the course of the inflammation, the affected epididymis is indurated and tender, either focally or diffusely. As the inflammation progresses, the entire testicle and overlying tissues of the hemiscrotum can become swollen, tender, and indurated. This diffuse inflammation, which is often referred to as epididymo-orchitis, is often accompanied by a secondary hydrocele. When the inflammation has progressed to the diffuse stage, the diagnosis is often obscure, and the differential diagnoses of testicular tumor, torsion of the spermatic cord/testicular appendage, or scrotal abscess must be entertained.

Treatment

Antibiotics. For the young, sexually active male who is afebrile, tetracycline, 500 mg orally every 6 hours, is the antibiotic of choice. Recent literature has recommended higher doses of tetracycline; however, these higher doses often cause nausea and compliance is poor. Other effective alternatives include doxycycline, minocyline, or erythromycin in standard doses for age. In the young patient or older male, more aggressive therapy is usually warranted, as these patients frequently appear toxic with fever and leukocytosis. In these patients a parenteral cephalosporin such as cefazolin, 500 mg intravenously every 8 hours, should be given either singly or in combination with an aminoglycoside, such as gentamicin or tobramycin in standard doses following a loading dose. When using aminoglycosides, appropriate hydration along with the monitoring of serum drug levels and serum creatinine is necessary.

Immobilization. Diminished activity seems to be

as important in the treatment of epididymitis as does antibiotic therapy. The use of scrotal support with sedentary activity until the patient's hemiscrotum is no longer tender will expedite the resolution of inflammation in less severe cases. In more severe cases, strict bed rest is necessary with the patient flat or slightly in the Trendelenburg position until his scrotum is nontender. A simple scrotal support in the more severe cases often causes discomfort, and the use of a Bellevue bridge type support (tape from thigh to thigh such that the scrotum is supported on the platform created) is suggested. The patient will appreciate the shaving of the area of the thighs to be taped when the time comes to discontinue the bridge.

Topical and Oral Anti-Inflammatory Measures. Application of an ice pack to the affected hemiscrotum during the first 24 to 48 hours of immobilization often greatly diminishes the patient's discomfort. The use of oral anti-inflammatory agents is controversial. In my experience, the use of these agents is effective in reducing the morbid period only in relatively localized or segmental cases. I have found no benefit to their use in the more severe cases. Indomethacin (Indocin), 25 mg orally every 8 hours, or ibuprofen (Motrin), 400 mg every 6 hours, are useful. Motrin also has mild analgesic properties, which makes it my choice. I have stopped using phenylbutazone (Butazolidin) or oxyphenbutazone (Tandearil) because of concern about side effects. If anti-inflammatory drugs are going to be effective, it appears that their effect is maximal during the first days of therapy, and I seldom prescribe these medications for longer than 4 to 5 days. All these agents cause gastrointestinal irritation and should not be used in any patient with a known or suspected history of peptic ulcer disease. In other patients, symptoms of dyspepsia can be alleviated by the use of antacids.

Analgesia. Immediate pain relief can be obtained by infiltrating the spermatic cord as it crosses the pubic tubercle with 5 to 8 ml of a 50/50 mixture of 1 per cent lidocaine (Xylocaine) and 0.5 per cent bupivacaine (Marcaine). This "cord block" can be invaluable during the examination and makes the application of supports and the early immobilization period much more comfortable. Cord block should be used only by those practitioners familiar with the anatomy of the spermatic cord and experienced in the technique. Thereafter, agents such as Tylenol with codeine or oxycodone with acetaminophen (Tylox, Percocet) usually suffice to keep the patient comfortable. Should torsion, as opposed to epididymitis, be found following cord block, manual detorsion is often facilitated because of the block. However, these patients must be watched very closely as acute retorsion can occur which might not be accompanied by recurrence of pain.

Surgery. The dictum of "explore if in doubt" applies to all cases of acute scrotal pain and swelling. Early urologic consultation in these cases is mandatory. An epididymitis that is explored will often improve symptomatically immediately following exploration for reasons that cannot be explained. A testicle that is the victim of a torsion of the spermatic cord will infarct unless the torsion is reduced. The generally accepted time frame from onset of symptoms to loss of the testicle is 6 to 8 hours. Spermatogenic function can be lost after approximately 3 to 4 hours. A radionuclide scan is very accurate in distinguishing epididymitis from torsion. Exploration, however, should not be delayed for a scan if the diagnosis of torsion is strongly suspected.

The older male with epididymitis warrants a word of special caution. The older male often does not respond to the more conservative measures already described. Early epididymectomy, or more likely epididymo-orchiectomy, must be performed to preclude the complications of scrotal abscess or sepsis. In any case complicated by abscess or fistula formation, incision and drainage should be performed. Occasionally the testis and epididymis will undergo necrosis and epididymo-orchiectomy may be necessary.

In some patients, epididymitis becomes a chronic relapsing process associated with episodic or constant orchialgia. Epididymectomy may be required to relieve the chronic infection and pain in these cases.

GLOMERULAR DISORDERS

method of
MICHAEL P. MADAIO, M.D.
Tufts University
Boston, Massachusetts

Patients with glomerular disorders usually present symptoms that can be grouped into one of two major clinical syndromes: acute glomerulonephritis (hematuria, proteinuria, and red blood cell casts) or the nephrotic syndrome (greater than 3.5 grams of urinary protein per square meter of body surface area, per day). The accompanying signs and symptoms associated with these syndromes may vary considerably, depending on the underlying disease process and its severity. Occasionally patients with glomerular disease visit the physician for the first time with signs and symptoms of uremia and irreversible renal failure. In this situation, no therapy is effective in reversing the underlying disease process and restoring glomerular function.

Acute Glomerulonephritis

Poststreptococcal Glomerulonephritis

This form of glomerulonephritis usually occurs following either a cutaneous or a pharyngeal infection, with a relatively limited number of serotypes of beta-hemolytic streptococci. When these nephritogenic strains spread quickly through a community, glomerulonephritis may occur in epidemic form. Treatment of the infection with antibiotics will not prevent the nephritis; however, it will diminish the antibody response to the extracellular products of streptococci, commonly used to diagnose recent infection. The serum level of the third component of complement is usually depressed at initial presentation, and then it returns to normal after 6 to 8 weeks. Persistent hypocomplementemia, therefore, suggests an alternate diagnosis.

For children, the clinical signs and symptoms of glomerulonephritis are usually self-limited, with spontaneous resolution the rule within weeks of onset. In adults the course is more variable; however, the development of progressive renal insufficiency is unusual. Thus, conservative management aimed at control of symptoms is usually sufficient therapy for both adults and children. Occasionally a patient will present with crescentic glomerulonephritis and rapidly progressive renal failure. Anecdotal success in managing these patients has been reported using various combinations of steroids, cyclophosphamide, and antiplatelet and antithrombotic agents. Spontaneous recovery has been reported as well, and therefore it is difficult to determine whether there is any benefit to these therapies. Since the outcome with crescentic glomerulonephritis is less favorable, in selected adults I favor the administration of methylprednisolone, 15 to 30 mg per kg intravenously over several hours on 3 successive days. This is followed by 60 mg of oral prednisone per day for 4 weeks, and then tapering of the prednisone over the next 4 weeks.

Membranoproliferative Glomerulonephritis

This is a primary renal disease of unknown etiology that affects both children and adults. Clinically patients may present with acute glomerulonephritis, nephrotic syndrome, or both simultaneously. Most patients have a chronic, progressive course; approximately 50 per cent require dialysis after 10 years. Occasionally spontaneous remissions may occur. The patients can be divided on the basis of morphologic patterns seen on kidney biopsy specimens. Type I is characterized by prominent C3 deposits localized along the glomerular capillary wall and in the mesangium, with IgG and IgM present in similar locations. Electron-dense deposits are located diffusely in subendothelial and mesangial locations. In type II membranoproliferative glomerulonephritis, there are C3 deposits in the peripheral capillary wall and the mesangium, but immunoglobulins are conspicuously absent. The glomerular basement membrane is diffusely thickened with electron-dense deposits, hence the term "dense deposit disease."

The majority of patients have type I disease. In this form, dipyridamole (Persantine), 225 mg, and aspirin, 975 mg, given daily in three divided oral doses, have been shown to preserve renal function and delay the development of end-stage renal disease (this use of dipyridamole and aspirin is not listed in the manufacturer's directive). Prolonged use of this regimen continues to provide benefit. Patients with type II disease have a worse prognosis than those with type I. Although there are no controlled trials of patients with type II disease, I recommend treating these patients with the regimen already outlined. At this time, however, this therapy should be regarded as experimental.

A number of other therapeutic regimens have been reported to have a favorable effect in patients with MPGN, including daily oral doses of prednisone and prednisone in combination with cyclophosphamide, dipyridamole, and warfarin. In randomized controlled trials, however, these therapies have not been observed to have a clear-cut benefit on the preservation of renal function.

Infectious Endocarditis, Shunt Nephritis

Glomerulonephritis may be associated with subacute bacterial endocarditis, infected ventriculoatrial shunts, or viceral abscesses. In each situation the primary therapy should be directed at eradicating the infection as rapidly as possible. The glomerulonephritis usually resolves with appropriate antibiotic or surgical treatment of the underlying process.

Occasionally patients develop diffuse crescentic glomerulonephritis with rapidly progressive renal failure. In these individuals the risk of high dose intravenous or oral steroid therapy must be weighed against the detrimental and potentially life-threatening effect that such therapy might have on the course of the underlying infection. If the infection has not been adequately treated, I would not administer high dose steroids. If acute crescentic glomerulonephritis with progressive renal failure persists after the underlying process has been eradicated, I would consider treating the patient with intravenous methylprednisolone 15 to 30 mg per kg given over several hours on 3 successive days, followed by a short course (4 weeks) of oral prednisone (60 mg per day). I would not initiate this therapy unless I was certain that the infection was eradicated. Since this approach has not been subjected to controlled trials, it should be considered experimental.

Cryoglobulinemia

Cryoglobulinemia may be associated with a variety of diseases, including myeloma, autoimmune disorders, infections, lymphoproliferative disorders, and liver disease, or may be idiopathic. The cryoglobulins can be entirely monoclonal (type I), mixed with a monoclonal component (type II), or of a mixed polyclonal variety (type III). Essential mixed cryoglobulinemia is a term used to describe patients with mixed-type cryoglobulins (type II or III) in the serum, who have no apparent systemic disease. Glomerulonephritis is commonly associated with cryoglobulins of the mixed variety, and it is often accompanied by purpura, hepatosplenomegaly, arthralgias, and Raynaud's phenomenon. The electron microscopic appearance of the kidney is often characteristic, with microstructural deposits typical of cryoglobulins located in glomeruli.

The patients should avoid exposure to cold. Therapy in symptomatic patients should be directed at the underlying condition associated with the cryoglobulinemia. For nonresponders and patients with essential mixed cryoglobulinemia, combined therapy with plasmapheresis (beginning with 3 four-liter exchanges weekly), oral doses of prednisone (60 mg daily), and cyclophosphamide (Cytoxan) (1.5 to 3.0 mg per kg daily) is effective in lowering the serum cryoglobulin concentration, often with improvement in renal and other severe systemic manifestations. (This use of cyclophosphamide is not listed by the manufacturer.) Dramatic responses to this treatment, including recovery from acute renal failure and remission in proteinuria, have been reported. Controlled clinical trials, however, have not yet been performed. Following treatment, the serum cryoglobulin concentration should be monitored closely. As the level declines, the frequency of plasma exchange can be decreased. If the levels remain low after cessation of plasmapheresis, the prednisone can be tapered slowly. After prolonged remission, the cyclophosphamide can be discontinued. Penicillamine has been utilized to dissociate cryoglobulins and reduce the cryoprecipitate in these patients; however, this therapy is of little clinical benefit.

Systemic Lupus Erythematosus

Although all patients with active lupus have some form of renal involvement, severe glomerulonephritis requiring treatment occurs only in the minority. In practice, when there is no evidence of clinical renal disease, the physician can assume the patient does not have severe glomerulonephritis, and therapy should be directed at controlling the extrarenal manifestations. When considering therapy, however, it is useful to classify patients according to the microscopic appearance of the kidney.

Minimal and Mesangial Lupus Nephritis. Minimal lupus nephritis is characterized by scant mesangial immune deposits and an otherwise normal microscopic appearance of the kidney. With mesangial nephritis there are more mesangial deposits, and this is associated with mild mesangial expansion and proliferation. Typically patients with these forms of nephritis have normal renal function and minimal proteinuria. The goal of the therapeutic regimen is to control the extrarenal manifestations of lupus. No specific therapy is required for this form of glomerular disease. If the serum creatinine level increases or heavy proteinuria occurs, the clinician should suspect the development of a more severe form of disease.

Focal and Diffuse Proliferative Lupus Nephritis. Focal lupus nephritis is characterized by focal and segmental glomerular lesions that are often associated with necrosis and intracapillary fibrin thrombi. Focal crescents may be observed. Typically, immune deposits are extensive, involving the mesangium and the glomerular capillary wall. Diffuse proliferative lupus nephritis involves almost all glomeruli and is characterized by extensive glomerular hypercellularity, necrosis, capillary wall thickening, and fibrinoid changes. Extensive crescent formation is common. Abundant immune deposits are located in mesangial, subendothelial and even subepithelial regions. Patients with these more severe forms of disease typically have heavy proteinuria, an active urine sediment, and reduced glomerular filtration rate.

High oral doses of prednisone (60 to 80 mg daily) constitute the initial treatment of choice for most patients with either severe focal or diffuse proliferative lupus nephritis. This should be continued for 1 to 2 months and then tapered. For patients with rapidly progressive renal failure (usually associated with crescentic nephritis), I recommend initiating therapy with intravenous methylprednisolone, 15 to 30 mg per kg on three successive days, followed by high dose oral prednisone treatment. An attempt should then be made to get the patient on the lowest dose of prednisone required to control extrarenal disease. It may be possible to switch selected patients to alternate-day steroid therapy. There is no proved benefit in adding either cyclophosphamide or azathioprine to the initial therapeutic regimen in acute lupus nephritis. However, the addition of these agents to the chronic regimen as the prednisone is tapered is associated with preservation of renal function and a reduction in the number of clinical renal flares. After the prednisone is tapered below 30 mg per day, I recommend adding cyclophosphamide (Cytoxan), either 1.0 to 3.0 mg per kg daily in oral form, or 0.5 to 1.0 gram per square meter of body surface intravenously as a single dose, every 3 months. Azathioprine (Imuran), 1.0 to 2.0 mg per kg orally, may be substituted for cyclophosphamide. (This use is not listed by the manufacturer.)

Note that deterioration in renal function is not always due to active renal disease. Extensive scarring, including glomerular sclerosis and interstitial fibrosis, can irreversibly and progressively reduce the glomerular filtration rate. In this situation, the risk of continued immunosuppressive therapy is much greater than any potential benefit. Therapy should be directed at controlling extrarenal disease.

Membranous Lupus Nephritis. Like idiopathic membranous nephropathy, this form of lupus is characterized by diffuse capillary wall thickening with immune deposits located in the subepithelial space. In addition, mild mesangial changes with mesangial immune deposits are also present. Heavy proteinuria is common. The clinical course is more indolent than in the proliferative forms of nephritis. Although there are no controlled therapeutic trials in this form of lupus nephritis, I recommend treating patients with prednisone, 120 mg orally every other day for 8 weeks. Over the next 4 weeks the prednisone is tapered. Higher doses of prednisone may be necessary to control extrarenal lupus.

Necrotizing Vasculitis

Glomerulonephritis may complicate polyarteritis nodosa, hypersensitivity vasculitis, or Wegener's granulomatosis. In polyarteritis nodosa (medium-sized vessel vasculitis), the initial therapy should consist of 60 to 80 mg of prednisone daily for 4 to 6 weeks. The dose can then be slowly tapered provided disease activity is quiescent. If clinical manifestations do not subside, or should they recur, cyclophosphamide should be administered in oral dosages of 1 to 2 mg per kg daily (this use is not listed in the manufacturer's directive). Most patients with hypersensitivity vasculitis (small vessel vasculitis) respond to high dose steroid treatment alone; however, those with an overlap syndrome (mixed small and medium vessel vasculitis) may also require cyclophosphamide.

The combination of oral doses of cyclophosphamide (Cytoxan), 1 to 2 mg per kg per day, with prednisone, 40 to 60 mg per day, is the initial therapy of choice in Wegener's granulomatosis. After 1 year of therapy the cyclophosphamide can be discontinued. Although no controlled clinical trials using this regimen have been performed, dramatic results have been observed, including many long-term remissions.

Idiopathic Rapidly Progressive Glomerulonephritis

Rapidly progressive glomerulonephritis (RPGN) is a term used to describe patients with fulminant glomerulonephritis associated with progressive renal insufficiency that develops over weeks to months. Morphologically, all patients have extensive glomerular crescent formation. If untreated, the likelihood of developing end-stage renal disease is predictable. Early diagnosis and treatment are therefore essential. Any disease that causes acute glomerulonephritis can also result in crescentic glomerulonephritis. (The more common disorders are referred to in the text.) The location of glomerular immunoglobulin deposition by immunofluorescence of the kidney biopsy specimen is helpful in both delineating the underlying process and planning effective therapy. Approximately one fifth of patients will have circulating antiglomerular basement membrane antibodies and linear deposits of IgG along the glomerular basement membrane unassociated with the pulmonary hemorrhage that characterizes Goodpasture's syndrome. Another 40 per cent will have granular immune deposits within the glomerular capillaries; most of these cases are associated with a systemic disease. The remaining 40 per cent are idiopathic with no glomerular immune deposits.

The initial therapy of antiglomerular basement membrane antibody–mediated disease should include plasmapheresis combined with oral prednisone, 60 mg, and cyclophosphamide, 1.5 to 3 mg per kg daily. Azathioprine given orally in doses of 1.5 to 3 mg per day may be substituted for cyclophosphamide. Plasmapheresis consisting of 4 liter exchanges should be performed daily for the first two to five exchanges. The frequency of plasma exchange should then be gradually reduced over 2 to 4 weeks, depending on the serum antiglomerular basement membrane antibody level and the clinical response. After 2 to 3 months, the cyclophosphamide or azathioprine can be discontinued, and the prednisone should be slowly tapered. The serum antibody level should be followed closely. The likelihood of a beneficial therapeutic response is greatest in nonoliguric patients with an initial serum creatinine level of less than 8 mg per dl. For patients with prolonged oliguria or renal failure, a more conservative approach with dialysis and transplantation is indicated (see also Goodpasture's syndrome). Plasma exchange therapy without simultaneous immunosuppression should not be used because it may lead to clinical relapse from an increase in circulating antibody level.

The initial treatment of patients with RPGN associated with granular immune deposits consists of intravenous doses of methylprednisolone, 15 to 30 mg per kg, given over several hours on 3 to 5 successive days. This therapy seems to be most effective in nonoliguric patients who are treated early in the course of their disease. Beneficial responses, however, also have been reported in oliguric patients on dialysis. This initial therapy should be followed by oral prednisone, 60 to 80 mg daily, for 1 to 2 months. The prednisone can then be gradually tapered. Although large controlled clinical trials have not yet been performed, most experts agree that therapy with this dose of oral steroids alone is insufficient. Anecdotal success has been observed in patients treated with the combination of oral steroids and either cyclophosphamide or azathioprine; however, controlled trials in proliferative glomerulonephritis have not demonstrated a benefit from these regimens. For patients who fail to respond to intravenous methylprednisolone, combination therapy including plasmapheresis, prednisone, and cyclophosphamide (as described earlier for antiglomerular basement antibody–mediated disease) has been associated with dramatic improvements in renal function. Recovery has been observed in patients requiring dialysis for over 10 days. It is emphasized that the use of combined therapy in patients with renal failure is associated with significant mortality from life-threatening infections. Therefore, it may be more appropriate to treat selected patients conservatively with dialysis, including those not likely to respond to therapy, those at high risk of infection, and those likely to tolerate systemic infections poorly.

Intravenous methylprednisolone therapy appears to be most effective in patients with RPGN associated with no glomerular immune deposits. I recommend that this initial treatment be followed by oral prednisone, 60 mg daily, for 4 to 6 weeks. There is little evidence that combination therapy with plasmapheresis is beneficial in this group of patients. Although anecdotal success has been reported using anticoagulants (heparin, warfarin) and antithrombotics (dipyridamole) in combination with prednisone and cyclophosphamide, the high risk of life-threatening complications, including bleeding or sepsis or both, outweigh any potential benefit.

Goodpasture's Syndrome

Goodpasture's syndrome is characterized by pulmonary hemorrhage, acute glomerulonephritis, and the production of antibodies to glomerular basement membrane. The therapeutic approach depends on the severity of the clinical manifestations. For patients with severe pulmonary hemorrhage, intravenous methylprednisolone, 15 to 30 mg per kg given daily over several hours, may be life-saving. Oral doses of prednisone, 1 mg per kg per day, should follow. If the glomerulonephritis is mild and the antiglomerular basement membrane antibody levels are low, this therapy may be sufficient. For patients with more severe glomerulonephritis, plasmapheresis (4 liter exchanges) should be initiated to remove circulating antiglomerular basement membrane antibodies. At the same time, oral cyclophosphamide (1.5 to 3.0 mg per kg per day) should also be added to suppress the production of pathogenic antibodies. Azathioprine, 1.5 to 3.0 mg per kg per day, may be substituted for the cyclophosphamide. (This use of cyclophosphamide and azathioprine is not listed by the manufacturers.) After daily plasmapheresis for 2 to 5 days, alternate-day therapy should be continued for several weeks. The clinical response and antiglomerular basement membrane antibody level should be monitored closely and used to decide on the need for additional plasma exchange therapy. Pulmonary hemorrhage that does not respond to high dose steroid therapy usually responds to this regimen. Although nonoliguric patients with a serum creatinine level of less than 8 mg per dl are most likely to benefit from this therapeutic approach, some patients regain renal function after initiation of dialysis. If a prompt improvement in renal function does not occur, however, a more conservative approach with dialysis and transplantation should be utilized. To minimize the risk of recurrence of this disease in the transplanted kidney, patients should have low or undetectable serum antibody levels for 3 to 6 months after immunosuppressive therapy has been discontinued.

Henoch-Schönlein Purpura

Henoch-Schönlein purpura is characterized by a leukocytoclastic vasculitis involving skin, the gastrointestinal tract, and glomeruli. Typically there are IgA deposits in the kidney and skin. The glomerulonephritis can vary in severity from very mild to quite severe. In most cases, this is a self-limited disorder that does not lead to end-stage renal disease; only a small percentage of patients develop a relapsing course with progressive renal failure. Occasionally patients may present with crescentic glomerulonephritis. Treatment of the renal disease is not generally effective; however, a short course of oral steroids may abbreviate the abdominal symptomatology.

IgA Nephropathy

Approximately 20 to 25 per cent of patients with IgA nephropathy will develop end-stage renal disease over a period of 5 to 20 years. A number of therapies have been tried in these patients, including prednisone alone and prednisone in combination with cytotoxic agents. Unfortunately, no treatment is of proved benefit. Oral phenytoin has been shown to decrease levels of circulating IgA, but this was not associated with preservation of renal function. Recently enthusiasm was high for the long-term administration of tetracycline; however, this treatment has not been shown to be of benefit in preventing the development of end-stage renal disease. At present, I do not recommend specific treatment for patients with IgA nephropathy.

Nephrotic Syndrome

In children, the overwhelming majority of patients will have idiopathic nephrotic syndrome, whereas in adults approximately one third of patients will have an associated systemic disease, drug, or toxin. The most common systemic diseases include diabetes, amyloid, systemic lupus, and neoplasms. Diabetic nephropathy is almost always accompanied by other manifestations of microangiopathy, including retinopathy and neuropathy. There is no known specific therapy for the renal disease; however, rigorous blood glucose and blood pressure control can delay the development of end-stage renal failure. Amyloidosis may be primary or associated with a variety of systemic diseases. If an underlying disease can be identified, it should be treated if possible. Unfortunately, there is no specific therapy of proven benefit for amyloidosis. Anecdotal success has been reported using melphalan and prednisone, given in 3 day cycles each month for 1 year; however, this therapy should be considered experimental. In patients with familial Mediterranean fever, colchicine will diminish the frequency of attacks and prevent the development of amyloidosis.

Many neoplasms have been associated with the nephrotic syndrome. If the neoplasm can be effectively treated, the nephrotic syndrome often remits. It is also worth emphasizing that a multitude of drugs have been associated with the nephrotic syndrome, including nonsteroidal anti-inflammatory agents, captopril, gold, and penicillamine. The nephrotic syndrome usually abates when the offending agent is discontinued.

Minimal Change Disease

This disease accounts for over 90 per cent of children with the nephrotic syndrome and for from 10 to 15 per cent of idiopathic nephrotic syndrome in adults. When treating patients with this disorder, it is essential to remember that preservation of renal function is the rule, whether or not treatment is administered. Thus, the indications for treatment are primarily symptomatic. There is almost universal agreement that initially all children should be treated. The risk of additional therapy, however, should always be balanced against the complications of the nephrotic syndrome in the individual patient. Older patients with minimal symptoms or other complicating diseases may be managed more effectively by conservative measures alone, including salt restriction and diuretics.

For the initial bout of nephrotic syndrome in children, I recommend oral prednisone, 60 mg per square meter of body surface area (maximum dose, 80 mg) given as a single daily dose for 4 weeks, then on an alternate-day basis for an additional 4 weeks (60 mg every other day). As soon as the nephrotic syndrome completely remits (urine protein excretion less than 200 mg per day), switch to alternate-day steroid therapy. If the dose of prednisone at the time of remission is 60 mg per day, I recommend switching to 120 mg of prednisone every other day. The prednisone should then be slowly tapered over the remainder of the 8 week treatment period. Alternate-day treatment can also be used as the initial therapy; however, the time required to induce remission is somewhat longer than that with daily treatment. In adults, especially those with less severe symptoms, I prefer this latter regimen.

This approach effects a remission in over 90 per cent of the patients. Approximately 60 per cent of these patients, however, subsequently relapse. In patients who relapse infrequently (one to two relapses per year or less), a repetition of the initial therapy is usually effective. Those patients who achieve a complete remission but then frequently relapse many weeks after discontinuation of prednisone may benefit from the addition of either daily oral cyclophosphamide (Cytoxan), 2 mg per kg, or chlorambucil (Leukeran), 0.15 mg per kg, given daily with prednisone for 2 months (this use is not listed by the manufacturers). These combinations have been shown to induce more sustained remissions. Patients who relapse as the prednisone dose is being tapered or immediately after the prednisone is discontinued are considered to be steroid-dependent. Although these patients can sometimes be maintained in remission on a low dose of steroids, side effects, including growth retardation, may complicate the situation. The benefit of cyclophosphamide or chlorambucil in inducing a lasting remission in this group is less well established than in frequently relapsing patients who are not steroid-dependent; however, slightly higher doses of oral chlorambucil (0.15 to 0.3 mg per kg per day) for 5 to 15 weeks have been shown to decrease the relapse rate in this group as well. Higher doses of chlorambucil (greater than 0.3 mg per kg per day) provide no additional benefit, and the risk of adverse effects is greatly increased. Both of these alkylating agents should be used with great caution, especially in young children who are at high risk from viral diseases. The white blood cell count, hematocrit, and platelet count should be measured weekly, and if signs of bone marrow toxicity develop the dose of the alkylating agent should be immediately reduced or discontinued. To avoid gonadal dysfunction, the total cumulative dose of chlorambucil should be kept under 7 mg per kg, and the total dose of cyclophosphamide should be less than 300 mg per kg. Although hemorrhagic cystitis is unusual at this dose of cyclophosphamide, the urinalysis should be monitored carefully for hematuria. These agents have also been associated with the late development of malignancies, including leukemia and lymphoma.

Given the risk of severe side effects with the use of alkylating agents and the natural history of this disease, the majority of patients should not be treated with these drugs. These agents should be reserved for frequently relapsing patients who are debilitated from both the consequences of the nephrotic syndrome and the long-term side effects of steroid therapy.

Focal and Segmental Glomerulosclerosis

The majority of patients with nephrotic syndrome secondary to this disorder develop progressive renal failure, hypertension, and end-stage renal disease. Approximately 50 to 60 per cent of patients require dialysis after 5 years. Patients who achieve a partial remission (less than 2 grams of urine protein per day) have a better prognosis than those with persistent heavy proteinuria. Although the results of controlled clinical trials have been inconclusive thus far, some patients have a remission in proteinuria associated with steroid therapy. Steroid-responsive patients also appear to have a clinical course characterized by less rapid deterioration in renal function. For this reason, if there are no contraindications to steroid therapy and renal function is well preserved (creatinine less than 2 mg per dl), I recommend 120 mg of oral prednisone on alternate days until a complete remission occurs or for a maximum of 8 weeks. The prednisone should then be tapered over the next 4 weeks.

There is no proved benefit to this therapy. However, in otherwise healthy patients the risk of side effects from short-term alternate-day prednisone therapy is very low, and the potential benefit is great. If there are contraindications to steroid therapy, more conservative management with salt restriction and diuretics is indicated. There is no evidence that alkylating agents are of benefit in preserving renal function in this disease. Rare patients, however, with a frequently relapsing, steroid-dependent nephrotic syndrome with severe steroid side effects, may have a prolonged remission in proteinuria when either cyclophosphamide, 2 mg per kg per day, or chlorambucil, 0.15 to 0.30 mg per kg per day, is administered with prednisone for 8 to 10 weeks. This treatment should be reserved for patients with both steroid-responsive disease and severe detrimental effects from the nephrotic syndrome and steroid treatment.

Membranous Nephropathy

This disorder accounts for over 50 per cent of patients with adult idiopathic nephrotic syndrome. The initial treatment of patients should include 120 mg of oral prednisone on alternate days until a complete remission occurs (less than 200 mg of urine protein per day) or for a maximum of 8 weeks. The prednisone should then be tapered over the next 4 weeks. Relapses in proteinuria should be re-treated with a similar course of prednisone. This regimen, when administered to patients with a relatively normal glomerular filtration rate, has been shown to preserve renal function and prevent the development of end-stage renal disease. This benefit is achieved whether or not the patient has a remission in proteinuria; however, the likelihood of remission is higher in patients treated with prednisone. Spontaneous remissions in untreated patients may also occur but they do so less frequently and later in the course of disease. Combination therapy, consisting of 1 gram of intravenous methylprednisolone for 3 consecutive days, followed by alternating monthly cycles of oral prednisone, 0.5 mg per kg per day, and then chlorambucil, 0.2 mg per kg per day, for a total of 6 months is also beneficial for preserving renal function (this use is not listed in the manufacturer's directive). In addition, this therapy may be more effective than alternate-day steroids alone in inducing and sustaining complete remissions in proteinuria. In patients with a diminished glomerular filtration rate (serum creatinine greater than 2 mg per dl), the beneficial effects of steroid therapy are not documented. However, since the risk of short-term, alternate-day steroid therapy in otherwise healthy adults is low, I recommend using this form of treatment. If there are contraindications to steroid therapy, more conservative management with salt restriction and diuretics alone is indicated.

Renal vein thrombosis appears to occur more frequently in patients with the nephrotic syndrome due to membranous nephropathy. Venography should not be performed routinely in these patients, but it is indicated when there is either (1) evidence of pulmonary emboli or (2) edema that cannot be explained on the basis of hypoalbuminemia. Occasionally renal vein thrombosis will lead to deterioration in renal function. Patients with documented thromboembolic events during an episode of nephrotic syndrome should receive anticoagulation with coumadin during relapses.

General Management of Glomerular Diseases

In addition to specific treatment of the underlying disorder, management of patients with glomerular diseases also includes therapy directed at relief of symptoms, correction of deficiencies resulting from urinary losses, and preservation of renal function.

Edema. Edema may occur in patients with glomerular disease for a variety of reasons. (1) Hypoalbuminemia resulting from heavy proteinuria reduces plasma oncotic pressure, leading to a redistribution of Starling forces in the peripheral capillary. As a result, fluid moves from the intravascular space into the interstitial space. In turn, decreased intravascular volume leads to increased reabsorption of sodium chloride and water by the kidney. Since plasma oncotic pressure remains decreased, most of the retained salt and water moves into and accumulates in the interstitial space. (2) Avid sodium chloride reabsorption may accompany glomerular disorders in the absence of hypoalbuminemia. (3) A decrease in the glomerular filtration rate may limit urinary sodium chloride and water excretion. The latter two mechanisms are usually associated with intravascular volume expansion. In an individual patient, multiple mechanisms may operate.

Patients with minimal edema do not need to be treated. Moderate salt restriction (2 gram sodium diet) may be sufficient in others to control edema. For symptomatic or more severe edema, diuretics should be added. If the glomerular filtration rate exceeds 50 ml per minute, hydrochlorthiazide may be effective. The more potent loop diuretics furosemide or ethacrynic acid can be substituted when hydrochlorthiazide is ineffective or the glomerular filtration rate is more severely reduced. The dose of diuretics should be sufficient to induce a diuresis, and this varies from patient to patient. When using hydrochlorthiazide, begin with 25 mg and double the dose until the desired effect is achieved or to a maximum of 100 mg per day (the initial dose of furosemide is 20 mg and of ethacrynic acid, 25 mg). For patients with moderate edema, increase the dose every few days. In hospitalized patients with more severe edema, the dose can be doubled every 6 to 12 hours. Patients requiring chronic therapy can take diuretics once or twice daily.

It is emphasized that the dose of diuretic should be adequate to induce a diuresis; giving half of an effective dose twice daily is often ineffective. Intravascular volume depletion may limit the effectiveness of diuretics and may be associated with either orthostatic or even frank hypotension. In addition, severe intravascular volume depletion may further reduce the glomerular filtration rate. Thus, the physician must balance the risks of edema against the risks of hypotension and reduced glomerular filtration rate. It should be realized that it is not possible to rid every patient of edema completely. The addition of spironolactone, amiloride or triamterene may be useful when the patients become potassium-depleted; however, these agents should be used with caution when the glomerular filtration rate is diminished.

Hypertension. Hypertension associated with glomerular disorders may be secondary to either volume expansion or excess systemic vasoconstriction. Both factors may be operative in an individual patient. Sustained hypertension will accelerate the progressive and irreversible loss of renal function, whatever the underlying disorder. Therefore, when hypertension is documented it should be treated promptly. Clinically evident volume expansion should be treated with diuretics. For patients who do not appear to have volume expansion, diuretics should also be the initial therapy. Hydrochlorthiazide, administered twice daily, can be utilized for patients with an adequate glomerular filtration rate. Furosemide (Lasix) or ethacrynic acid (Edecrin) should be given to patients with a glomerular filtration rate below 50 ml per minute. The dose of diuretic should be sufficient to induce a diuresis but not reduce glomerular filtration rate or lead to severe volume depletion. If the patient remains hypertensive despite diuresis, therapy should be increased in the usual stepwise manner. I prefer adding a beta-blocker like propranolol (Inderal), 40 mg twice daily, and increasing the dose gradually until either the blood pressure is controlled, the total dose is 160 to 320 mg per day, or side effects occur. If hypertension is still not adequately controlled, I then add hydralazine (Apresoline), beginning with 25 mg twice daily. The dose can be increased to 200 mg per day if necessary. For resistant hypertension, minoxidil (Loniten) may be substituted for hydralazine, or a calcium channel blocker such as nifedipine (Procardia) can be added.

A few words of caution about the use of specific antihypertensive medications in patients with glomerular disease. (1) Acute interstitial nephritis may complicate sulfonamide diuretic use and lead to deterioration in renal function that is more rapid than expected from the underlying glomerular disease. In this situation, ethacrynic acid can be substituted. (2) The beta blockers nadolol and atenolol are excreted primarily by the kidney. If the glomerular filtration rate is diminished, they should be used with extreme caution and in reduced dosage. (3) The dose of angiotensin-converting enzyme inhibitor, captopril (Capoten), should be reduced in patients with impaired renal function. Captopril has been associated with the development of membranous nephropathy in a small number of patients. In addition it has also been associated with neutropenia, especially in patients with systemic lupus erythematosus. (4) The active metabolites of methyldopa may accumulate in patients with severe renal failure, and the dose should be reduced to avoid side effects.

Nutritional Therapy

In patients with heavy proteinuria, hypoalbuminemia and hypogammaglobulinemia can occur. If protein losses are profound and sustained, malnutrition may develop. Patients with the nephrotic syndrome, therefore, should be advised to eat a diet that contains enough protein of high biologic value to maintain normal nitrogen balance. If urine protein losses are severe, associated zinc, iron, copper, and vitamin D losses may be helped by replacement therapy. Hyperimmune gammaglobulin may be beneficial in patients with severe hypogammaglobulinemia and recurrent infections.

The optimal dietary intake for patients with renal insufficiency remains to be established. Clinical evidence suggests that moderate dietary protein restriction may retard the progression of renal disease in patients with a reduction in glomerular filtration rate. The safety and efficacy of this diet in patients with either heavy proteinuria, insulin-dependent diabetes, or active systemic disease are not well known, and it may be potentially harmful. This dietary regimen should not be used in growing children. Given these reservations, at the present time I advise selected patients that this diet has potential benefit. Initial therapy includes a diet containing 0.6 to 0.7 gm per kg of protein and dietary counseling. It is possible that these diets may be deficient in vitamins, minerals, and trace elements; therefore, the patients should be followed closely. Particular attention should be devoted to maintenance of body weight, serum albumin concentration, and serum transferrin level. For the first 3 to 6 months, patients are frequently dissatisfied with the diet. Repeated dietary adjustments by the nutritionist, with reinforcement by the physician, are needed to assure continued dietary compliance.

PYELONEPHRITIS

method of
DANIEL B. CRAIG, M.D.
Dwight David Eisenhower Army Medical Center
Fort Gordon, Georgia

Pyelonephritis is inflammation of the renal parenchyma associated with bacterial infection. Acute pyelonephritis is usually the result of infection ascending from the lower urinary tract, except for infants in whom hematogenous infection is more common. Chronic pyelonephritis results from repeated episodes of urinary tract infection and is almost always associated with anatomic abnormalities of the urinary tract. Many other tubulointerstitial diseases of the kidney may result in identical pathologic changes and clinical presentations, but they are rarely associated with recurrent infections.

Acute Pyelonephritis

Acute pyelonephritis is often difficult to distinguish from infection of the lower urinary tract. Fever greater than 38.3 C (101 F), white blood cell casts, and flank pain are generally present; however, none of these is diagnostic of upper tract infection. Recent evidence indicates that the response to a single dose of antibiotics may help differentiate pyelonephritis from lower tract infection in otherwise healthy young women. However, no similar data exist for men, pregnant women, or patients with structural abnormalities of the urinary tract.

Management

In general, patients who appear toxic, have structural abnormalities of the urinary tract, or are unable to take oral antibiotics should be admitted to the hospital and treated with intravenous antibiotics. Selected nontoxic patients may be treated as outpatients with oral antibiotics and close observation. Initial evaluation of the patient with pyelonephritis includes complete blood count with differential, urinalysis, serum creatinine, BUN, and electrolytes along with cultures of blood and urine. Empiric selection of antibiotics should be guided by a Gram stain of uncentrifuged urine and the clinical setting. The presence of gram-positive cocci on the Gram stain usually indicates enterococcal infection, for which ampicillin is the drug of choice. In the severely ill patient, gentamicin may be added for synergy.

The opinions or assertions contained herein are the private views of the author and are not to be construed as official or as reflecting the views of the Department of the Army or the Department of Defense.

The majority of patients, however, have infections caused by gram-negative bacilli, and those with a hospital-acquired infection require treatment with an aminoglycoside. The choice of aminoglycoside should be based upon the sensitivity patterns in that particular hospital. Patients who are hospitalized with community-acquired pyelonephritis caused by gram-negative organisms can be treated equally well with an aminoglycoside or intravenous trimethoprim-sulfamethoxazole. For outpatient therapy, trimethoprim-sulfamethoxazole offers the broadest spectrum of activity, with ampicillin or oral cephalosporins being alternatives for the patient who is allergic to sulfa.

After 48 hours of appropriate antibiotic therapy, most patients will be afebrile, will be improved clinically, and will have a sterile urine. Failure to become afebrile during this time suggests obstruction or perinephric abscess requiring surgical drainage, and an ultrasound examination is indicated. A normal ultrasound result does not eliminate the possibility of acute obstruction without dilation of the collecting system; if clinical suspicion remains high, an intravenous pyelogram or other radiologic procedure may be indicated. When the patient has been afebrile for 24 hours and is able to take oral medications, oral antibiotic therapy may be started based upon the sensitivity of the infecting organism. The total duration of therapy should be 14 days.

Follow-Up

Seven to ten days after the completion of therapy, culture of the urine should be done. Recovery of the same organism indicates relapse and the need for an additional 4 to 6 weeks of therapy. Women with a documented relapse and all men with urinary tract infections require an intravenous pyelogram to exclude correctable structural abnormalities of the urinary tract.

Chronic Pyelonephritis

Chronic pyelonephritis is usually detected during evaluation of renal insufficiency, hypertension, or an abnormal sediment. The criteria required for the diagnosis are tubulointerstitial disease, recurrent bacterial infections and evidence of pelvocalyceal inflammation, fibrosis, and deformity on radiographic evaluation. Almost invariably this is associated with anatomic anomalies, obstruction, or vesicoureteral reflux.

Management

The primary goal of treatment is to prevent further renal damage due to infection. This requires sterilization of the urine with antibiotics and surgical correction of the structural abnormality. Most authorities recommend a 6 to 12 week course of antibiotics based upon the sensitivity of the infecting organism, and some would continue suppressive therapy for up to 2 years. Antibiotics commonly chosen for suppression include trimethoprim-sulfamethoxazole (Bactrim, Septra), trimethoprim alone (Proloprim, Trimpex), and methenamine mandelate (Mandelamine).

When the structural abnormalities cannot be corrected, it is usually impossible to maintain a sterile urine even with chronic suppression. The most reasonable management of a patient who has failed to achieve a sterile urine is to treat symptomatic infections only and to limit treatment to 10 to 14 days. Each patient should also be routinely evaluated for complications of chronic pyelonephritis, including renal tubular acidosis, salt wasting, hypertension, and nephrolithiasis. When diagnosed, each of these will require specific therapy.

TRAUMA TO THE GENITOURINARY TRACT

method of
ALEXANDER S. CASS, M.B.B.S.
University of Minnesota
St. Paul, Minnesota

In the multiply injured patient the management of life-threatening injuries takes precedence over urologic injury, so the diagnosis of genitourinary trauma is usually delayed. A method of immediate diagnosis by radiologic evaluation and immediate surgical management can optimize the restoration of function and continuity of the urinary tract.

Immediate Evaluation

Following external trauma the indications for immediate radiologic evaluation of the urinary tract are hematuria (gross, microscopic), perirenal hematoma found during laparotomy for intra-abdominal injury, fractures of the transverse processes of the lumbar vertebrae, fall from a height, and pain, tenderness, or mass in the side of the abdomen or flank.

In the adult, a retrograde cystogram with 400 ml of radiopaque dye is performed. After the anteroposterior film is taken the bladder is emptied of the dye and washed out with normal saline, then another anteroposterior film is taken as the washout film. Following this an intravenous pyelogram with a large dose of dye (100 ml in an adult) is performed with 5, 10, and 20 minute exposures made. When the intravenous pyelogram (IVP) findings show extravasation, incomplete filling, or delayed visualization, a computed tomography (CT) scan is performed. If the IVP shows nonfunction, a renal arteriogram is made.

When blood is found at the external urinary meatus,

retrograde urethrography with radiopaque dye is performed before any instrumentation of the urethra is attempted. This will determine the integrity of the urethra for insertion of a catheter, which could convert a partial rupture into a complete rupture of the urethra.

Renal Injuries

Renal Contusions

Contusions include bruises or minor tears of the renal tissue with an intact renal capsule. Renal contusions comprise 92 per cent of renal injuries (74 per cent of renal injuries found during laparotomy for intra-abdominal injury). The IVP is usually normal. The subcapsular hematoma is limited in extent. Conservative treatment is indicated, which consists of bed rest, monitoring vital signs (blood pressure, pulse, hemoglobin, hematocrit), and examining each voided urine specimen for the degree of hematuria. When the gross hematuria has cleared, the patient is mobilized. Renal contusions almost always settle to normal unless there is a pre-existing renal lesion such as hydronephrosis, cyst, or tumor.

Renal Lacerations

Lacerations are parenchymal disruptions with damage to the renal capsule with or without calyceal disruption. Renal lacerations comprise 5 per cent of renal injuries (16 per cent of renal injuries found during laparotomy for intra-abdominal injury). The IVP shows extravasation of dye. The perirenal hematoma with renal laceration can be large and can fill the perirenal space and expand Gerota's fascia, which acts as a tampon. The management of renal lacerations is controversial. Some state that renal lacerations almost characteristically self-heal, whereas others state that surgical management is needed. Conservative management consists of bed rest, monitoring of the vital signs, and recording the degree of hematuria in the voided specimens. If the patient becomes clinically unstable or septic or has persistent or recurrent gross hematuria requiring transfusion, then surgical exploration is indicated.

Immediate surgical management involves an anterior approach with incision of the peritoneum in the lateral colic gutter. The colon and its mesentery are reflected medially to expose the area of the renal artery and renal vein. Dissection is carried out through the retroperitoneal tissues to isolate the renal vein and then the renal artery lying behind it. Vascular clamps are applied to give preliminary vascular control, then Gerota's fascia is opened with evacuation of the perirenal clot. With preliminary vascular control, deliberate surgical repair of the laceration is performed with either renorrhaphy or partial nephrectomy, depending on the extent of renal laceration found. When all ischemic or macerated tissue is debrided, the collecting system, if open, is closed with a continuous suture. If a partial nephrectomy is performed, the renal surface is left open and the kidney replaced in Georta's fascia. Retroperitoneal drains are placed in position.

Renal Rupture

Rupture consists of fragmentation or shattering of the kidney. Renal ruptures comprise 1 per cent of renal injuries (4 per cent of renal injuries found during a laparotomy for intra-abdominal injury). A large expanding perirenal hematoma accompanies renal rupture, and the patient becomes clinically unstable from the continued bleeding. The IVP shows extravasation of dye or little function. Renal exploration, with preliminary pedicle control with vascular clamps and nephrectomy, is the treatment of choice.

Renal Pedicle Injury

Renal pedicle injuries include tearing or occlusion of the renal vein or artery, its main branches, or polar arteries. Renal pedicle injuries comprise 2 per cent of renal injuries (6 per cent of renal injuries found during laparotomy for intra-abdominal injury). The IVP shows nonfunction with renal artery occlusion. With blunt trauma the most common renal pedicle injury is thrombosis of the renal artery secondary to intimal tear with intact outer and medial layers of the renal artery. There is bruising surrounding the renal artery but no perirenal hematoma present with renal artery thrombosis. A large perirenal hematoma is present with disruption or rupture of the renal artery or renal vein or any of their branches.

With immediate radiologic evaluation, renal pedicle injuries can be diagnosed early. Thrombosis or disruption of the renal artery or vein should be repaired within 12 hours of the injury if renal blood flow is to be restored to achieve a viable kidney. If renal artery thrombosis is limited in extent, then excision with end-to-end anastomosis of the renal artery is performed. If thrombosis is more extensive, a bypass graft from the aorta to the distal renal artery, using a saphenous vein graft, is done. Laceration or rupture of the renal vein is repaired by direct suture.

Renal Pelvic Rupture

Rupture of the renal pelvis involves extravasation of urine into the perirenal space and along the psoas muscle. The IVP shows a normally functioning kidney and calyceal system with extravasation of dye. Renal pelvic rupture is rare and is often misdiagnosed as a small renal laceration. The patient develops high fever and increasing abdominal pain and tenderness as the extravasation of urine continues into the retroperitoneal space. A retrograde pyelogram should be performed as soon as possible to make the diagnosis. The rupture should be repaired by continuous or interrupted sutures with adequate drainage. A double J stent or a nephrostomy with a ureteral catheter should be used if there is any question of the viability of the repair or in the presence of surrounding infected tissues.

Ureteral Injuries

These are the rarest of all genitourinary injuries from external trauma. With blunt trauma there is rupture at or just below the ureteropelvic junction due to hyperextension of the spine with the lower end of the ureter fixed at the trigone of the bladder. With penetrating injuries there can be contusion and partial or complete rupture of the ureter. Gunshot wounds can cause contusion of the ureter when the path of the bullet is beside the ureter; shock waves damage the vessels in the ureteral wall, resulting in bleeding or thrombosis. Upon surgical exploration the path of the bullet is traced beside the ureter, and the ureteral wall appears intact or shows slight bruising. If thrombosis of the vessels in the ureteral wall occurs, then delayed necrosis with a urinary fistula will result.

Direct laceration or rupture of the ureter found upon exploration of penetrating injuries to the abdomen should be repaired at the time of initial laparotomy. The ureteral wall must be debrided until completely viable tissue is obtained. End-to-end anastomosis with continuous or interrupted sutures is performed provided no tension results. If the gap in the ureter is too long for a tension-free anastomosis, then mobilization and descent of the kidney should be done to provide extra length when the injury is in the upper half of the ureter. If the injury is in the lower half of the ureter, the gap can be bridged by reimplantation of the ureter in the bladder, and upward mobilization of the bladder with a psoas hitch or a Boari bladder flap. A double J stent should be used if there is any doubt about the anastomosis.

Bladder Injuries

The bladder is an intra-abdominal organ in a child but is situated deep in the bony pelvis in the adult; it is thus protected from all but severe injuries to the trunk. Bladder injuries are the second most common injury to the genitourinary tract after renal injury and are usually associated with a fracture of the pelvis. An exception is intraperitoneal rupture of the bladder, which occurs with a sudden deceleration injury when the bladder is full, resulting in a large rent in the dome of the bladder.

Bladder Contusion

Bladder contusion is bruising of the bladder wall with hematuria. The cystogram shows an intact bladder outline. With a fractured pelvis there is often a large hematoma inside the bony pelvis, causing displacement of the bladder either superiorly or laterally. Management is conservative as the bruise of the bladder wall resolves, leaving an intact bladder wall.

Intraperitoneal Rupture of the Bladder

The cystogram will show intraperitoneal extravasation of dye along both paracolic gutters and between the coils of intestine. Exploration of the abdominal cavity and repair of the large rupture in the dome of the bladder are required. The bladder wall is debrided and a two layer closure performed—the first layer with the mucosa and the second layer with the seromuscular layer of the bladder. A urethral and a suprapubic catheter are placed in position and a drain placed in the prevesical space. With accompanying pelvic fracture the drain is removed as soon as possible in the posterative period.

Extraperitoneal Rupture of the Bladder

A retrograde cystogram will show extravasation along the lateral wall of the pelvis and behind the bladder. The washout film is most helpful when the extravasation is predominantly behind the bladder and obscured by dye in the full bladder film of the cystogram. Until recently exploration was done, with repair of the extraperitoneal rupture. However, with a single extraperitoneal rupture and small extravasation, urethral catheter drainage alone has been used successfully. The catheter remains indwelling for 10 to 14 days, and the cystogram is repeated to verify that the rupture has healed, at which time the urethral catheter is removed.

Urethral Injuries

Injuries may occur to the posterior (prostatomebranous) urethra or to the anterior (bulbous and penile) urethra. Posterior urethral injuries are usually associated with fracture of the pelvis whereas anterior urethral injuries are the result of direct blows (fall-astride injuries, straddle injury, kick).

Urethral Contusion

The retrograde urethrogram is normal but there is blood at the external urinary meatus. The contusion heals upon conservative management, with or without an indwelling urethral catheter.

Partial Urethral Rupture

The retrograde urethrogram will show a limited extravasation of dye at the site of injury, with dye passing up into the bladder. Partial ruptures are managed by an indwelling urethral catheter alone or with a suprapubic cystostomy. After 14 days a small feeding tube is placed into the external urinary meatus beside the indwelling catheter and dye is injected as a retrograde urethrogram around the catheter. When the partial rupture has healed, there will be no extravasation and the indwelling urethral catheter can be removed.

Complete Urethral Rupture

The retrograde urethrogram will show a large extravasation of dye at the site of injury with no dye passing up into the bladder.

This should be surgically repaired in the anterior urethra by debridement of the ruptured ends and end-to-end anastomosis. Suprapubic catheter drainage is used to divert the urinary stream, and a small urethral stent is used to splint the anastomosis.

When there is complete disruption of the posterior urethra, controversy exists about using primary alignment of the ruptured urethra with suprapubic cystostomy or suprapubic cystostomy alone with delayed urethral reconstruction in 4 to 6 months. With primary alignment, the bladder is opened and the urethra realigned using the railroad technique with two sounds and a Foley catheter pulled into the bladder. Traction is applied on the catheter at a 45 degree angle to the bed in the postoperative phase to pull down the bladder and prostate and thus maintain realignment of the urethra. After 14 days, a retrograde urethrogram is performed with a feeding tube along-side the urethral catheter to see whether the rupture has healed. If extravasation is present, the urethral catheter is left and the retrograde urethrogram repeated 7 days later. When no extravasation is seen on the retrograde urethrogram the indwelling urethral catheter is removed. With management by suprapubic cystostomy alone, the area of the rupture and the prevesical tissues are left intact. The pelvic hematoma absorbs, and the bladder and prostate settle down toward the perineal membrane, with a resulting stricture of the urethra. At 4 to 6 months a delayed reconstruction of the urethra is performed at the site of the stricture.

The main advantage claimed for management by suprapubic cystostomy alone is the decreased impotence rate, although recent studies with long-term follow-up have shown that the impotence rate is approximately the same with both methods of management. The other long-term complications of urethral stricture and incontinence are similar with both methods of management.

Injuries to the Genitalia

Testicle

The mobility of the testis, cremaster muscle contraction, and the tough capsule of the testis (tunica albuginea) are responsible for its infrequent injury in the patient multiply injured from a traffic accident. A direct blow with impingement of the testis against the symphysis pubis results in a testicular injury. The testicular injury is either contusion or a testicular rupture. In both cases the tunic vaginalis sac is filled with blood (hematocele) resulting in a large, swollen, tender, blue scrotal mass. Early exploration with evacuation of blood clots in the tunica vaginalis and repair of the testicular rupture, if present, result in a shorter hospital stay, a greatly reduced period of disability, and a faster return to normal activity compared with patients managed conservatively. Conservative management is complicated by secondary infection of the hematocele or the injured testis, and the pressure effect of the tense hematocele can result in subsequent atrophy of the testis after the hematocele resolves.

Penis

Self-inflicted injuries of the penis include vacuum cleaner injuries and blade injuries. Vacuum cleaner injuries cause extensive injury to the glans penis as well as some loss of the urethra, requiring debridement of devitalized tissue and reshaping or reconstruction of the injured glans penis and urethra. Blade injuries to the penis can range from superficial lacerations of the prepuce or the glans penis to complete or partial amputation of the penis. Amputation of the penis is managed by replantation or local reshaping measures involving closure of the open corpora and meatoplasty. Primary anastomosis (replantation) is preferable if the distal segment is available, in good condition and ischemia time is less than 18 hours.

Traumatic rupture of the corpus cavernosa of the penis or fracture of the penis occurs when the erect penis impacts forcibly on a hard object (sexual partner's pubis or the floor) receives a direct blow or is subjected to abnormal bending. A cracking sound is heard followed by penile pain, immediate detumescence and rapid swelling, and discoloration and distortion of the penis. The management is immediate surgical evacuation of the blood clot and repair of the tear in the tunica albuginea of the corpus cavernosum.

Loss of penile skin by avulsion injury or burns is managed by split skin grafts after the denuded penis is clean and noninfected. The avulsed skin should not be reapplied for it invariably becomes necrotic and infected and must be subsequently removed. With loss of scrotal skin the testicle should be housed in the remaining scrotal skin even though the reconstruction places it under considerable tension. Usually within a few months the scrotum will have returned to nearly normal size.

Zipper injury to the penis consists of entrapment of the foreskin by the zipper fastener of the trousers. Extraction by manipulation of the zipper is usually prolonged and painful, and it is preferable to use bone-cutting pliers to cut the median bar or diamond of the zipper, which will result in the entire zipper falling apart with release of the entrapped foreskin.

The penile tourniquet syndrome due to a constricting agent such as hair, penile ring, steel washer, or metallic nut presents early with pain and swelling of the glans penis. The constricting agent should be removed or cut.

BENIGN PROSTATIC HYPERTROPHY

method of
FRANK HINMAN, JR., M.D.
University of California
San Francisco, California

Prostatic hypertrophy, a disease of middle and later years, progresses slowly with time, although the symptoms show ups and downs. The chance of a 50 year old man requiring prostatectomy before age 60 is 1.5 per cent; this rises to 7 per cent in the next decade. Today a man probably has one chance in four of requiring a prostatectomy in his lifetime.

Hormonal Factors

Androgens are needed to allow the initiation of BPH, but they seem to have little influence once the growth begins. Hormonal manipulation or castration does not measurably influence the disease, although the effects of such therapy are difficult to quantify. Nonsteroidal agents, such as those that reduce cholesterol, also have not proved useful clinically. At the present time, no agent is available to shrink the prostate effectively.

Neurophysiologic Treatment

The internal bladder sphincter and the prostatic capsule contract during α-adrenergic stimulation. Since BPH fills the capsule and bladder neck, an increase in adrenergic activity will promote obstruction; thus, administration of an α-blocker may partially relieve obstruction. Phenoxybenzamine hydrochloride (Dibenzyline), 10 mg at bedtime, may carry a patient through an obstructive episode. Conversely, medications for coryza that contain ephedrine will increase obstruction. Acute urinary retention from overstimulation of the adrenergic receptors may in some cases be relieved by a more rapidly acting agent, such as Regitine, 10 mg given slowly intravenously with monitoring. Trying to stimulate the detrusor with parasympathetic agents such as bethanechol (Urecholine) will fail.

Response to Obstruction

Obstructed voiding is detected urodynamically by simultaneously measuring urinary flow rate and bladder pressure, but only 65 per cent of patients can be diagnosed by these techniques. Normally a balance exists between the work of the detrusor and the resistance of the outlet. With prostatic hypertrophy, the detrusor works harder but tires more easily as the outlet resistance rises. The net result is a stream that starts slowly as the resistant outlet opens, runs slowly, and finishes indeterminately with dribbling and residual urine as the bladder fatigues. At first the detrusor can cope, but eventually residual urine increases and urinary retention supervenes.

DIAGNOSTIC STEPS

For an orderly work-up:

1. Observe the flow rate (time the void with a stopwatch).
2. Perform urinalysis to detect infection.
3. Check for bladder distention by palpation.
4. Examine the prostate rectally to judge size (which will affect the type of operation selected) and detect malignancy. Remember, size is not related to obstruction; large glands are not necessarily obstructive.
5. Estimate residual urine by sonography, phenolsulfonphthalein (PSP) test, or catheterization. Serial determinations over the years are helpful in the decision for operation.
6. Determine renal function by serum creatinine test.
7. Excretory urography is probably not indicated in the patient without other stigmata.
8. Instrumentation (panendoscopy) can be done at the time of operation.
9. Urodynamic studies are reserved for atypical cases or postoperative problems.

Treatment

Conservative Management. If the patient doesn't feel his daily life is disturbed and he is not suffering renal damage, he will be managed conservatively. He is re-examined every 6 months to detect incipient damage (and to pick up incidental carcinoma). To carry a patient through an obstructive crisis, alpha-blocking agents might be used.

Intermittent self-catheterization is an alternative for a few diehards. It is simple and safe, but operation is preferable for most cases.

Indications for Operation. *Mandatory indications* are overflow incontinence and persistent total obstruction. Recurrent infection, vesical calculi, and severe bleeding are also strong indications for surgery.

Optimal indications are more flexible. If frequency interferes with daytime activities and nocturia disturbs sleep, surgery may be worthwhile, especially if the obstructive symptoms of a slow stream (less than 10 ml per sec) and dribbling are present also. Residual urine volumes over 60 ml probably warrant correction.

Patient Counseling. *Impotence* occurs in 16 to 30 per cent of patients. The expected *retrograde ejaculation* may be psychologically upsetting. *Incontinence* is a rare complication.

Operative Treatment

The surgical objective is to remove all the adenoma and leave the true prostate (surgical capsule) behind.

Transurethral prostatic resection (TUR) is the method of choice except for glands so large they would be technically difficult to remove this way. A sheath in the urethra carries a fiberoptic light, a lens, a movable loop activated to cut by an electrosurgical unit, and a tube for water flow. Drawing the loop through the tissue under vision allows progressive resection down to the distinctive tissues of the surgical capsule. Hemostasis is provided through the same loop. All the pieces are evacuated from the bladder at the end of the operation, when a catheter is placed to remain 2 days. Total hospitalization is 4 days or less.

Spinal anesthesia is preferred. Water is satisfactory for irrigation since the syndrome following extravasation from the capsule is from hypervolemia and hyponatremia, not from hemolysis. It is treated by diuretics and an intravenous infusion of sodium to restore the serum level to normal. The operative mortality rate is less than 0.4 per cent.

Suprapubic or retropubic prostatectomy is limited to large glands that could not be removed transurethrally in the safe period of 1 hour. In these operations the bladder is opened transabdominally and the adenoma is shelled out with the fingers. Sutures of the prostatic arteries secure hemostasis, which may be reinforced with compression from a balloon catheter.

The results of operation are usually good. Urethral strictures occur in 6 per cent, a result of urethral manipulation by the resectoscope. The obstructive symptoms resolve if the operation has been done adequately and the irritative ones generally clear.

BPH is a common disease that may disable the patient and damage his urinary tract. Since operation carries a low incidence of morbidity and mortality, at present it is the treatment of choice for those men who have sufficient functional impairment to warrant it.

PROSTATITIS

method of
LINDA M. DAIRIKI SHORTLIFFE, M.D.
Stanford University
Stanford, California

Diagnosis

To make the diagnosis of prostatitis, the prostatic fluid must be examined microscopically. In true prostatitis (inflammation of the prostate), the prostatic fluid must be inflamed and show more than 10 white blood cells per high power (× 400) microscopic field. If clinical symptoms of voiding disturbance, ejaculatory pain, perineal aching, low back pain, and prostatic tenderness to palpation alone are relied upon for diagnosis, many of the patients will be found not to have prostatic inflammation. Once a patient is found to have prostatic inflammation, it must be determined whether he has the bacterial or nonbacterial variety.

Acute Bacterial Prostatitis

Patients with acute bacterial prostatitis usually have a sudden onset of malaise, low back and perineal pain, chills, fever, and obstructive and irritative voiding symptoms, such as dysuria, urinary frequency, and intermittent urine stream. The prostate may feel nodular or normal, but the patient has severe pain when the prostate is palpated. Gram-negative bacteria can usually be cultured from the patient's prostatic fluid, but because of prostatic pain and the risk of prostatic massage disseminating bacteria from an acutely infected prostate into the systemic circulation, acute bacterial prostatitis is probably one condition in which prostatic massage to obtain fluid should not be done. Most of the time acute bacterial prostatitis is accompanied by bacteriuria, so the bacterial pathogen may be cultured from the voided urine specimen. These infections usually involve the Enterobacteriaceae—*Escherichia coli, Enterobacter, Serratia, Klebsiella,* and *Pseudomonas* species—or less commonly enterococcus.

Since some of these men are severely ill, they may need to be hospitalized for treatment with parenteral antimicrobial agents, such as an aminoglycoside *and* ampicillin or a cephalosporin (gentamicin [Garamycin] or tobramycin [Nebcin], 1 to 1.5 mg per kg of body weight every 8 hours, *plus* ampicillin or cefazolin [Ancef], 1 gram every 6 hours intravenously). When the patient has improved and the organism and its antimicrobial sensitivities have been identified, treatment with an oral agent such as trimethoprim-sulfamethoxazole (Bactrim, Septra), 160 mg/800 mg twice a day, or carbenicillin indanyl sodium (Geocillin), 764 mg four times a day, can be started and continued at full dosage for 3 to 4 weeks to prevent the development of chronic bacterial prostatitis. Urinary retention that may occur because of bladder outlet obstruction from the inflamed and swollen prostate is probably best treated with a temporary percutaneous suprapubic drainage catheter. A urethral catheter may increase prostatic irritation. The prostate should be re-examined several months after the infection to ensure that any nodules that were present at the time of the acute infection have disappeared.

Chronic Bacterial Prostatitis

Men with chronic bacterial prostatitis have a variety of complaints, such as intermittent bladder irritative symptoms, perineal aching, and low back pain, but some are almost asymptomatic. The most common characteristic of these patients is a history of recurring urinary infections. Since bacteria that are hidden in the prostate are the nidus for the infections, routine courses of antimicrobial agents only temporarily clear the bladder of infection until prostatic bacteria reinfect the bladder.

The therapy for chronic bacterial prostatitis is often frustrating. Few antimicrobial agents have been shown to diffuse into the prostate and prostatic fluid in concentrations adequate to cure infection by the responsible gram-negative bacteria; these bacteria are usually the same organisms that cause acute bacterial prostatitis. In addition, infected prostatic calculi may cause persistence of bacterial infection. Two drugs that can be given orally and have been used to cure chronic bacterial prostatitis when the bacteria are sensitive are trimethoprim-sulfamethoxazole (Bactrim, Septra), 160 mg/800 mg twice a day, and carbenicillin indanyl sodium (Geocillin), 764 mg four times a day. Once started, these drugs should be continued for at least a month and possibly as long as 3 months. If the patient continues to have chronic bacterial prostatitis after this treatment, as about 50 per cent of patients will, parenteral aminoglycoside therapy may be given to try to cure a few more patients if the organism is sensitive. Intravenous or intramuscular tobramycin (Nebcin) or gentamicin (Garamycin), 1.0 to 1.5 mg per kg every 8 hours, netilmicin (Netromycin), 150 mg every 12 hours, or amikacin (Amikin), 500 mg every 12 hours for 7 to 10 days, can be given while serum creatinines are measured every other day to ensure that nephrotoxicity has not occurred.

In some men radical transurethral resection of the prostate may be curative, but in most the bacteria tend to be located in areas of the prostate not routinely removed in this operation. Often the potential complications of radical transurethral resection of the prostate, such as retrograde ejaculation or incontinence, and the suboptimal success rate make this option unacceptable to patients. In those men in whom treatment fails, daily low dose antimicrobial therapy with a drug to which the organism is sensitive, such as nitrofurantoin (Furadantin, Macrodantin), 100 mg per day, cinoxacin (Cinobac), 250 mg per day, trimethoprim-sulfamethoxazole (Bactrim, Septra), 40 mg/200 mg a day, or cephalexin (Keflex), 250 mg a day, will prevent relapsing bladder infections and render the patient asymptomatic by sterilizing the urine daily and suppressing bacteriuria.

Even though zinc levels from the prostatic fluid of patients with bacterial prostatitis are lower than those from normal men, there is no convincing evidence that oral zinc administration improves or cures bacterial or nonbacterial prostatitis.

Nonbacterial Prostatitis

The patients with nonbacterial prostatitis usually have complaints similar to those of patients with bacterial prostatitis but without documented prostatic infection or episodes of bacterial cystitis. The prostatic examination is usually normal to palpation, but the prostatic fluid shows greater than 10 white blood cells per high power (× 400) microscopic field. The urine is normal by microscopic examination. Although *Ureaplasma, Chlamydia, Haemophilus influenzae,* and even anaerobic organisms have been implicated as causes of nonbacterial prostatitis, none of these agents have been proved to be responsible for the majority of cases.

Since *Chlamydia* and *Ureaplasma* must be cultured using techniques rarely available in most bacteriology laboratories, a therapeutic trial with doxycycline (Vibramycin), 100 mg twice a day, or erythromycin, 500 mg four times a day for a few weeks, may be reasonable. If, however, no improvement is seen, treatment should be stopped and no further antimicrobial agents used. Occasionally a patient will gain symptomatic relief with anti-inflammatory agents such as indomethacin (Indocin) or ibuprofen (Motrin). It is important that the patient be counseled that he has prostatic inflammation, but that his symptoms are unrelated to prostatic cancer or venereal disease.

Prostatodynia

This term has been used to describe patients with prostatic complaints similar to those just described, but who have no evidence of prostatic inflammation upon microscopic examination of the prostatic fluid. The reason for the symptoms is not understood, but various findings such as perineal muscle spasm during voiding and psychologic disturbance have been associated with it. Before this diagnosis is made, however, patients with persistent frequency, voiding discomfort, and suprapubic pain may need evaluation to eliminate a diagnosis of bladder tumor, carcinoma in situ, or interstitial cystitis. Since no definite causes for these symptoms have been identified, no single therapy is effective. Some patients experience symptomatic relief with short trials of prazosin hydrochloride (Minipress), 1 mg three times a day (although this is not a use described by the manufacturer), or diazepam (Valium), 5 mg once or twice a day. Although their symptoms may improve, these men should be warned that the symptoms may recur or persist, but that no serious prostatic disease has been discovered.

ACUTE RENAL FAILURE

method of
ROBERT A. GUTMAN, M.D.
Duke University
Durham, North Carolina

Sudden loss of glomerular filtration function and decrease of urine flow complicates serious medical and surgical disease as frequently as 1 in 500 hospitalized patients. Even more common is a less sudden but still ominous reduction of glomerular filtration rate without a concomitant reduction of urine flow. Acute renal failure (ARF), may also appear without apparent preexisting disease or in the complete absence of earlier illness. Many causes of ARF are recognized, and several may simultaneously contribute to a clinical reduction of renal function. Do not be lulled into the facile diagnosis of "acute tubular necrosis" (ATN) without considering the other possibilities.

DIAGNOSTIC CONSIDERATIONS

Assessment of plasma volume depletion: There is no reliable laboratory assessment of the volume of extracellular fluid (ECF). Bedside evaluation requires a reasonable appreciation of the patient's previous health. For example, poor skin turgor, traditionally regarded as useful in judging hydration, is not useful in the evaluation of a previously ill older person, though it is in a previously well youngster. A careful search for edema not only around the ankles, shins, and sacrum but especially around the thighs (the most dependent area in a bedridden patient) is important because edema and appreciable ECF depletion seldom coexist. If the external jugular vein of the completely recumbent patient can be seen when the vein is occluded at the thoracic inlet but falls flat when the examining hand is lifted, the ECF may be depleted. Assessment of both pulse and blood pressure before and after standing may indicate fluid depletion. Sitting is usually insufficient provocation of an orthostatic change of these parameters. However, advanced age, longstanding diabetes, or antihypertensive therapy may impair autonomic adjustment to the erect position and convey falsely the impression of ECF depletion.

Urinalysis may be useful if it is not done perfunctorily. Formed elements may indicate both the nature and chronicity of the renal problem. Renal tubular cells and casts of these cells support the diagnosis of acute tubular necrosis. A heavy burden of oxalate crystals in the urine, occasionally seen in small numbers in normal urine, suggests ethylene glycol exposure. A large number of uric acid crystals in the urine of a patient who has undergone induction therapy for cancer suggests acute uric acid nephropathy. Occasionally acute glomerulonephritis may present as ARF. The presence of a large number of red or white cells and casts containing these cells helps clarify the situation. Very broad and waxy casts indicate a substantial degree of pre-existing chronic renal disease. Eosinophiluria strongly suggests the possibility of acute interstitial nephritis; eosinophils are most reliably found by a Wright's stain of urine sediment prepared by the cytospin technique.

Renal ultrasound in the hands of skilled imaging experts is very nearly as reliable as the much more invasive use of retrograde ureteral catheterization and for that reason has nearly completely replaced it for seeking signs of obstruction above the urinary bladder. Moreover, evaluation of kidney size and the echogenicity of the renal parenchyma gives reliable clues about the presence of pre-existing chronic disease in which echoes are usually present.

FENa is the nephrologist's jargon for *fractional excretion of filtered sodium.* It is an easy, noninvasive test of tubular function. Its purpose is to differentiate functional oliguria, which occurs when ECF depletion, sepsis, or hepatic or cardiac disease reduces renal blood flow, from the more serious renal damage usually termed acute tubular necrosis. The putative difference between the two conditions is that in the functional disturbance, the GFR is relatively well preserved and the oliguria is the consequence of avid tubular resorption of sodium and water, whereas in the latter case the oliguria is largely the consequence of marked reduction of GFR and accompanying failure of tubular resorption. Several measurements of tubular function have been advocated to allow this assessment, including the ratio of urinary creatinine to serum creatinine (UCr/SCr), a crude measure of tubular water resorption, and the urinary sodium to serum sodium ratio

(UNa/SNa), which is a function of tubular sodium resorption. Experience has shown that the most reliable distinction is given by assessment of the fraction of filtered sodium that is excreted. The calculation for this is $FENa\% = (UNa \times SCr/SNa \times UCr) \times 100$. Determining urinary osmolality has been a popular method of making the same judgment. It is not as reliable unless the ratio of urinary to measured plasma osmolality is over 1.5, and then it is less sensitive. Urine specific gravity is very unreliable because the density of urine is not a direct consequence of tubular function.

The relative merits of measuring *serum creatinine* and *blood urea nitrogen* levels for the assessment of the loss of the GFR require understanding, especially when the rate of production of urea is likely to change. Inasmuch as the rate of creatinine production seldom changes, its concentration is more closely linked to the level of filtration function. On the other hand, the BUN level may change as a consequence of either changing GFR, increasing catabolism, gastrointestinal bleeding, or glucocorticosteroid usage. For the same reasons, the ratio of BUN to creatinine, which has been touted as a very robust method for recognizing prerenal azotemia, may not be reliable in patients whose BUN is elevated for these other reasons.

Treatment

Reversible Causes

The most common reversible cause of ARF is obstruction. Relief of bladder obstruction must be prompt and may be as simple as the placement of a urethral catheter. However, in the event of a severely obstructed urethra, suprapubic catheterization may be necessary. Similarly, if urinary obstruction is higher, either retrograde or antegrade renal pelvic catheterization is required early. If arterial occlusion is suspected after a renal scan, consideration must be given to surgical or even angioplastic treatment of the obstruction. There are reports of return of useful renal function even when many weeks elapsed between the obstruction and the repair.

Recognition of functional renal insufficiency or so-called "prerenal azotemia" may lead to prompt improvement of renal function and urine flow by repletion of ECF or partial correction of severe heart failure. The physician must guard against overenthusiastic replacement of fluid in this and other causes of renal failure, remembering that more than 3 liters of ECF depletion is uncommon and more than 5 is usually incompatible with life.

Drug-induced renal toxicity is becoming the most common cause of ARF and has several mechanisms. The aminoglycosides cause direct damage to renal tubular cells when excess concentrations in the blood and filtrate are resorbed by tubular epithelial cells that are unable to handle the burden. Other antibiotics, including members of the penicillin and cephalosporin groups, may cause acute interstitial nephritis, which occasionally can be recognized by the presence of eosinophiluria. Nonsteroidal anti-inflammatory agents (NSAIDs) cause renal failure by at least two mechanisms. The best known is related to their pharmacologic effect; since they do interfere with prostaglandin synthesis, they impair the normal defensive medullary vasodilatation that is taking place in the renal circulation of most patients under stress. Thus they may impair the GFR even if the patient had been taking the NSAID without ill effect before requiring hospitalization for a new problem. 11NSAIDs may also cause acute interstitial nephritis.

Radiologic contrast–induced renal failure occurs in 5 to 35 per cent of certain high risk groups, including those with pre-existing renal insufficiency, diabetes mellitus, and multiple myeloma. Captopril, the angiotensin-converting enzyme inhibitor being used for the treatment of hypertension and heart failure, seems to cause a sudden decline in GFR, especially in patients with bilateral renal artery stenosis or a single kidney. This drug can also cause interstitial nephritis and proteinuria.

Although acute glomerulonephritis is not always a reversible process, its early diagnosis can lead to successful therapy. Treatment with glucocorticosteroids, cytotoxic agents, and plasmapheresis all have their role and clearly are more likely to be effective if started soon. Malignant hypertension can cause severe and partially reversible loss of GFR. Even though the serum creatinine level often rises further after control of blood pressure is effected, the antihypertensive program should continue. Only in this way may healing and then improvement of function take place.

Principles of Management

1. *Attempt to establish diuresis*. Diuretic therapy has become widely used in the hope that it will induce a diuresis and hasten the patient's recovery. Indeed, there is some evidence from animal research that the effort has a scientific basis, and most nephrologists are willing to try giving a potent diuretic, usually furosemide (Lasix) or ethacrynic acid (Edecrin), to an oliguric patient with ARF. Many experienced physicians believe they have seen a diuresis effected and adverse consequences are rare. However this approach has never been proved rigorously to be effective. The usual dose of Lasix is approximately 240 mg intravenously over 10 to 20 minutes. This may be repeated several times but should not become part of the daily regimen unless the patient is clearly benefiting.

2. *Control fluid and electrolyte disturbances.* There are four distinguishable potential areas of disturbance of body fluid and electrolytes. The first two of these should be considered together because they are often confused. Clinically detectable losses of ECF, discussed earlier and often called "dehydration," are the consequence of the net loss of isotonic fluid. This means that the losses do not change the serum sodium concentration because large amounts of both sodium and water losses have occurred. This may be thought of conveniently as "saline depletion," and replacement is done properly with an isotonic fluid such as normal saline, lactated Ringer's solution, or even blood or plasma. Once replacement has been accomplished—usually this can be done rapidly—it may be dangerous to continue. Rarely, an edematous person benefits from further isotonic fluid, unless red blood cells are needed. Once the patient is considered euvolemic, ECF may be maintained best by daily estimates of sodium balance and body weight.

For example, if the patient is experiencing a 2 liter per day loss of gastrointestinal fluid, he or she is losing approximately 200 mEq per day of sodium, which needs to be replaced to maintain ECF; this can be given in any concentration suitable for electrolyte "free water" losses. Free water losses, by contrast, raise serum and whole body (including cellular water) effective osmolality. The increased effective osmolality is usually best reflected by the serum sodium concentration unless the patient is hyperglycemic, hyperlipidemic, or (rarely) hyperproteinemic.

In summary, there is a fundamental difference between isotonic fluid and free water disturbance with regard to their causes, recognition, treatment, and consequences. Moreover, it is not uncommon for a patient to have an excess of the one and a deficit of the other. For example, an edematous patient with hypernatremia needs water (usually given as 5 per cent dextrose in water), but sodium, even quarter normal saline, should be avoided if possible.

Acid-base problems are a third area of potential disturbance. Most ARF patients tend to be acidotic and may benefit from the administration of sodium bicarbonate. The serum bicarbonate concentration does not need to be made normal, but the physician should take advantage of any opportunity to partially correct the acidosis of an ECF-depleted patient by giving a substantial amount of the necessary isotonic sodium solution as bicarbonate rather than as chloride. Generally, if the serum bicarbonate is under 12 mEq per liter, the acidosis should be treated; if the patient cannot tolerate further sodium administration, dialysis may be needed. Most authorities recommend that bicarbonate deficits be repaired over at least a 72 hour period. A very rough guide to the bicarbonate deficit can be reached by assuming that the body deficit is equal to twice the total ECF deficit; in turn, this is equal to the difference between the present and normal concentration multiplied by the estimated volume of ECF. Alkalosis may occur in ARF patients despite the loss of hydrogen ion excretory function. This may be the consequence of previous vomiting, excessive use of bicarbonate, or prolonged earlier use of diuretics. In any case, it is usually not treated unless the bicarbonate concentration is over 35 mEq per liter.

Finally, disturbance of body potassium must be addressed in most ARF patients. Serum potassium is a useful first approximation of the body's need for the mineral when the effects of acid-base disturbance, if any, are taken into consideration. While potassium excess is more common in ARF, not only because of the loss of excretory function but because of the loss of cellular integrity, deficits are seen regularly. Potassium deficit can and occasionally should be repaired with due regard for the potential for later excess. Potassium excess is perhaps the most important treatable hazard in the management of the early phase of ARF.

Frequent measurement of the serum potassium may be important, but most physicians feel that close monitoring of the electrocardiogram is essential because it does reflect the severity of the hyperkalemia even if its changes do not correlate closely with the measured potassium values. There is a crude relationship; peaked T waves will appear first in the evolution of hyperkalemia, usually at about 6.3 mEq per liter; then loss of P waves (if the patient was in normal sinus rhythm) and a shortened Q-T interval; finally, widening of the QRS complex; and lastly the development of a sinus wave and a chaotic tracing with ineffective heart pumping. If this last feature is encountered, intravenous calcium gluconate (at least 4 and preferably 12 mEq) may be lifesaving.

For less severe manifestations of hyperkalemia, intravenous sodium bicarbonate, 50 mEq over 2 to 5 minutes will result in temporary intracellular transfer of potassium; this may be especially useful in patients who are acidemic or hyponatremic. The effect is transitory, and hypertonic sodium bicarbonate should not be used repeatedly because of the danger of ECF excess or hypernatremia.

The other method of achieving a temporary resolution of hyperkalemia is to administer intravenous regular insulin and sugar simultaneously. This therapy facilitates the cotransport of potassium with glucose into the cells, especially the liver, in the process of glycogen manufacture and storage. As much as 200 mEq of potassium capacity may be created this way, but again the effect is only transient and does not remove the potential excess. One formulation is to add 10 units of insulin to 200 ml of 5 per cent dextrose in water to be administered over 30 minutes.

True losses of potassium can be accomplished by only one of three ways: recovery of renal function, the effective use of dialysis, or the use of sodium polystyrene sulfonate resin (Kayexalate). Kayexalate may be given either orally or per rectum. In the presence of functioning bowel, I prefer to give it orally as long as an osmotic agent such as sorbital is given first to prevent the resin from binding the bowels. Generally, the resin is also mixed in sorbitol, by adding 25 grams per 100 ml of 20 per cent sorbitol. Five to 10 grams orally every half to one hour or 25 to 50 grams as a retention enema are useful. With an adequately functioning bowel, dialysis will rarely be necessary for the control of hyperkalemia per se. Nevertheless, customary practice holds that, if possible, dialysis should be applied rather than continue to remove potassium with resin alone. There is good reason for this practice. Most patients with a potassium excess are hypercatabolic and are probably developing an appreciable degree of uremia. In addition, the Kayexalate adds to the patients' ECF because it exchanges sodium for potassium.

3. *Indications for dialysis: uremia versus azotemia.* In the modern era, no reason exists for the patient with acute renal failure to wait for dialysis until one of the classic urgent needs is manifest. This is not to say that hyperkalemia, acidemia, and ECF excess are not indications: rather they are late indications, especially if they occur together. On the other hand, the mere presence of oliguria and azotemia, even a BUN of greater than 100 mg per dl, does not require that dialytic therapy be instituted. The application of this therapy, like other invasive treatments, requires bedside judgment and a reasonable appraisal of the alternative possibilities. As an example, a patient who is oliguric and showing signs of early *uremia* (lethargy, nausea, neuromuscular irritability) may well need dialysis much more than the clinically stable patient with a greater degree of *azotemia* (BUN) whose renal function and urine flow rate shows signs of impending improvement.

The principal purpose of dialysis treatment for acute renal failure is to return the patient to the degree of health he or she would have had without the oliguria—that is, to provide short-term maintenance dialysis while renal function is given time to improve. Consequently, one of the modern indications for dialysis therapy is to provide a means to allow adequate nutritional therapy to be applied. Without regularly scheduled dialysis treatments, feeding—especially by the parenteral route—will result in fluid overload. Finally, we must acknowledge that we see patients dying with, rather than of, uremia whose prognosis is hopeless. For them, dialysis therapy should be replaced by common sense and the good judgment to allow a peaceful passing.

4. *Choice of dialysis modality.* In many cases, either hemodialysis or peritoneal dialysis can be used with equal overall value and equal risks. The local nephrology group will pick the modality most suitable to their program and resources in these cases. Hemodialysis is preferred when extremely rapid fluid or potassium removal is desired or when correction of acidosis must be done promptly. Peritoneal dialysis is preferred for the unstable patient or the patient with technically difficult vascular access. Contraindications exist for both modalities, including recent abdominal surgery or ileus in the case of peritoneal dialysis and extreme hypotension in hemodialysis.

CHRONIC RENAL FAILURE

method of
JAMES F. WINCHESTER, M.D., FRCP
Georgetown University
Washington, D.C.

Enormous variation in individual tolerance to uremia occurs, and many so affected remain asymptomatic until 80 per cent of nephrons are destroyed, i.e., a glomerular filtration rate (GFR) below 20 ml per min. Ultimately, nephron loss is so great that dialysis and transplantation are required to sustain life. This usually occurs, however, near a glomerular filtration rate (usually measured by endogenous creatinine clearance) of 5 ml per min. Individual variations may be so great that many patients can tolerate uremia down to glomerular filtration rates of 2 ml per min with conservative management, whereas others require dialysis at higher glomerular filtration rates. Modern approaches favor dialysis well before severe uremic symptoms occur.

Symptoms and Signs

Symptoms and signs of chronic renal failure differ remarkably from patient to patient, depending to a great extent on the rapidity with which renal failure ensues. The classic symptoms of fatigue, effects of anemia, effects of hypertension, and symptoms of renal bone disease are still commonly seen. However, it is rare today to see severe acidosis (with Kussmaul respiration), uremic frost, and pericarditis if the patient has been adequately managed. The goal is to prevent the development of any severe uremic symptoms, with early institution of substitution therapy. The subtle signs of impending uremia include changes in mental capacity and changes in taste and smell (particularly a metallic taste).

Symptoms and signs of renal disease are thought to be due to retention of end products of protein metabolism, such as urea and creatinine and its derivatives (methylguanidine, guanidinosuccinic acid); to electrolyte and mineral disturbances; to retention of so-called middle molecules; and to failure of the endocrine activity of normal renal tissue. The last leads to anemia (loss of erythropoietin) and bone disease. No single molecular compound is likely to cause the state of uremia, and it is generally accepted that the uremic state is multifactorial in origin.

Management (of Phases I and II)

Management of end-stage renal disease (ESRD) is divided into three main phases (Table 1), depending upon the degree of reduction in glomerular filtration rate. Phase I (GFR > 20 ml/min) consists of correction of reversible factors and conservative therapy (measures other than dialysis and transplantation); phase II (GFR 20 to 5 ml/min) consists of conservative therapy with dietary management; and phase III (GFR < 5 ml) consists mainly of dialysis and transplantation. In phases I and II, conservative management may retard or halt progression of renal disease and provide symptomatic therapy. Every measure is taken to fully exclude any reversible factor at any phase.

Progression of renal disease in an individual can be estimated by the reciprocal of serum creatinine ($1/S_{Cr}$) versus time plotted semilogarithmically, to give a rate of fall in GFR. For most

TABLE 1. **Plan for the Management of Chronic Renal Failure**

Phase I (GFR >20 ml/min)
Correction of the following reversible factors:
Treatable renal diseases (e.g., systemic lupus erythematosus, polyarteritis nodosa)
Hypertension
Sodium/water balance
Electrolyte/acid-base balance
Cessation of analgesic drugs; avoidance of nonsteroidal anti-inflammatory drugs and other drugs affecting renal function
Systemic or renal infection
Cardiac failure
Exclude obstruction
Phase II (GFR 5–20 ml/min)
Correction of reversible factors as above
Introduction of dietary protein restriction ± essential amino acids/alpha-ketoacids
Introduction of vitamin D analogues and phosphate binders
Creation of vascular access or implantation of peritoneal dialysis catheter
Phase III (GFR ≤ 5 ml/min)
Dialysis or transplantation
Continue vitamin D and phosphate binders
Control of blood pressure

patients, the progression to ESRD is relentless, although there are several diseases amenable to therapy. Treatable renal diseases may include collagen vascular diseases, particularly systemic lupus erythematosus and polyarteritis nodosa, and other diseases such as Goodpasture's syndrome, rapidly progressive glomerulonephritis (nonoliguric), membranous glomerulonephritis, analgesic nephropathy and possibly diabetes mellitus, and secondary amyloidosis.

Even progressive diseases may be amenable to treatment by correcting factors that adversely influence their course. The most important of these contributory factors is hypertension, which potentiates glomerular injury both in glomerulonephritis and in diabetes mellitus. In patients with primary or secondary hypertension, renal damage may progress to the point at which dialysis is required. Even in these cases, there are many reports of patients who have recovered GFR sufficient to discontinue dialysis after control of hypertension. Further reduction of GFR with antihypertensive drugs may occur, but the benefits of lowering blood pressure to normal limits outweigh the risks of temporary reduction in GFR. Even in phase II chronic renal failure, any reduction in GFR is usually followed by improvement. Modern drugs such as minoxidil (Loniten), diazoxide (Hyperstat), captopril (Capoten), and enalapril slow progression of renal disease, such that nephrectomy is rarely necessary to control hypertension. Greater success is achieved if drugs with different modes of action are chosen, since injudicious use of two drugs of the same class (e.g., vasodilators) increases side effects without appreciably controlling blood pressure.

Analgesic nephropathy due to phenacetin may have caused ESRD, but analgesics such as aspirin and other nonsteroidal anti-inflammatory agents (NSAID) have been shown to reduce GFR whether or not accompanying interstitial nephritis or papillary necrosis develops. Nonsteroidal anti-inflammatory agents reduce renal prostaglandin production, limit renal blood flow, and result in further reduction of GFR in the renal-impaired patient. A careful drug history is mandatory in patients in whom the etiology of renal disease is not clear, since NSAID cessation can stabilize or improve renal function. Iodine containing radiology dyes and anticancer drugs such as *cis*-platinum may also lower GFR in the renal-impaired subject.

Cardiac failure from relative volume expansion and anemia is common in ESRD patients. Cardiac failure is frequently of the high-output type, but it may also be due to impaired left ventricular function (observed in over one third of patients). Pericardial effusion is frequent.

Any possible obstruction of the renal tract

should be ruled out so that the obstruction can be relieved early. It is important that the classification of a patient's disease as "end-stage" should be made only after obstruction has been ruled out.

Renal Adaptive Mechanisms

Adaptive mechanisms occur in diseased and failing kidneys that preserve natriuresis and sodium balance, even to very low GFR (2 ml per min). When the GFR is below 25 ml per min, acute changes in sodium intake may not result in homeostasis, since the patient is unable to excrete more than 150 to 200 mEq of sodium per day, accompanied by some extracellular fluid volume expansion. In contrast, obligatory sodium excretion of 25 mEq per day occurs, and abrupt reduction of sodium intake is not accompanied by reduced sodium excretion, as in normal subjects. Rather, sodium continues to be excreted at a rate two to three times over the intake. This is true for most renal diseases, whether glomerular or tubular and, if high, may give rise to "salt-losing nephropathy." This is commonly associated with chronic pyelonephritis, polycystic renal disease, and nephrolithiasis. It is therefore clear that routine restriction of dietary sodium is to be avoided in renal patients. In those with evidence of total body sodium excess (congestive heart failure, edema, and hypertension) reduction in dietary sodium should be made. If negative sodium balance precipitated by fever, gastrointestinal bleeding, vomiting, diuretics, or dietary sodium restriction occurs in those with obligatory sodium loss, they may become volume contracted, thereby decreasing renal blood flow and GFR. Such events may occur in previously stable patients and may precipitate the need for dialysis.

As renal function declines, excretion of isosmotic urine, i.e., isosthenuria (osmolality of urine equal to that of plasma) results. Isosthenuria is present regardless of the intake of water, because patients are unable to concentrate or dilute the urine maximally. The patient may become volume contracted with fluid restriction but rapidly fluid overloaded with excessive fluid intake. Since the rate of urine formation during chronic renal failure is relatively constant day and night, nocturia is an early feature of chronic renal disease. At very low filtration rates, fluid intake should be monitored and maintained around 2 liters per day.

Potassium, like sodium, is excreted at a greater rate per nephron owing to decreased fractional reabsorption but, unlike sodium, is added to urine via distal tubular secretion. Consequently, potassium balance is better maintained in chronic renal failure than is sodium balance. In addition, the colon secretes potassium and shows an adaptive increase in fecal potassium secretion in renal failure. It follows that potassium intake should not be restricted until the late stages of ESRD unless other circumstances exist, e.g., intercurrent illnesses, metabolic acidosis, and volume contraction. Constipation should be avoided, since the contribution of the colon to potassium secretion is impaired. Potassium-sparing diuretics (amiloride, spironolactone, and triamterene) can upset the adaptive balance and thus should be avoided.

As renal failure progresses, the kidneys cannot excrete an acid load, which leads to metabolic acidosis. The immediate factor responsible is decreased ammonium excretion, which is associated with an excessive anion gap. The retained acid moieties are largely buffered in bone, which eventually contributes to renal osteodystrophy. Treatment of the acidosis must be weighed against the risk of sodium overload (from sodium bicarbonate), and therefore serum bicarbonate concentrations should be maintained at about 20 mEq per liter. Volume contraction may produce hyperchloremic alkalosis, and excessive use of phosphate binders (aluminum hydroxide) may restrict the availability of urinary phosphate (the major buffer for acidity). Systemic infections or local renal infections may contribute to the acidosis, while volume contraction from vomiting or diarrhea may further reduce GFR. Such conditions should be rapidly treated. Correction of reversible factors is equally important in phase II disease as in phase I, and every potential reversible component should be sought and dealt with.

Diets

Dietary protein restriction has long been known to ameliorate symptoms of chronic renal failure. Recent evidence strongly suggests that low dietary intake of high biologic value proteins, providing 0.5 to 0.6 gram protein per kg per day, may retard renal deterioration (by reducing renal hyperfiltration) and delay dialytic therapy. Dietary phosphate restriction and calcium supplementation may also slow the progression of renal failure. In addition, a low-protein diet produces a rise in plasma bicarbonate that lasts for many years if the diet is maintained. Such dietary manipulation has opened up new possibilities for managing ESRD. Results of a multicenter study on the effect of protein restriction on the progress of glomerular filtration are eagerly awaited.

Dietary protein restriction has been used for at least 30 years in the management of chronic renal failure, being introduced to manage patients before hemodialysis became available. The Giordano-Giovanetti diet used 18 grams of protein (largely pasta and eggs) and supplementation of

0.5 gram methionine in order to reverse negative nitrogen balance. Since this low-nitrogen diet was abundant in essential amino acids, depletion of tissue amino acids and proteins was prevented, and nitrogen was conserved. The diet reduced serum urea nitrogen, uric acid, and inorganic phosphate, while hemoglobin and hematocrit stabilized or rose, and anorexia, nausea, vomiting, hiccuping, itching, and drowsiness became less frequent. Although most of these studies were encouraging, many patients had no prolongation of renal function and died suddenly with acidosis. Other investigators found that negative nitrogen balance ensued with time. Approximately 0.6 gram of high biologic value protein per kg per day was required to achieve neutral or positive nitrogen balance. Accordingly, the usual ESRD diet consists of 40 to 60 grams of high biologic value protein, 60 mEq of sodium, and 60 mEq of potassium, along with 1000 to 1500 ml of fluid derived from food or from fluid intake.

Recently, semisynthetic diets containing very low quantities of protein but supplemented with essential amino acids or alpha-ketoacids (which generate essential amino acids) have been introduced. By using 20 grams of essential amino acids with 20 grams of high-quality protein, nitrogen balance may become neutral or positive, compared with isonitrogenous diets containing protein as a sole source of nitrogen. Alpha-ketoacids and alpha-hydroxyacid analogues of essential amino acids provide pure amino acids without increasing the nitrogen load. Adding ketoacid analogues of phenylalanine, valine, and tryptophan allows a faster adaptation to the low nitrogen intake than does the nonketoacid diet. Moreover, renal function can be stabilized or increased using this regimen, although it is unclear whether this is due to the ketoacids, the low serum phosphate levels, or the low calcium phosphorus product.

Although compliance with restricted-protein diets is variable, careful counseling will achieve a high rate of success. In highly compliant patients, substantial delay in the introduction of substitution therapy may be achieved.

When dialysis is necessary, dietary protein restriction may be relaxed to 80 grams of protein, 60 mEq of sodium, and 60 mEq of potassium. In nephrotic syndrome or in patients receiving peritoneal dialysis, renal or peritoneal protein losses must be supplemented by additional dietary protein. In addition to protein, it is recommended that renal diets contain at least 2000 calories per day to prevent nitrogen catabolism.

Unfortunately, supplementary diets produce a rise in cholesterol and triglycerides, which increases the risks from hyperlipidemia.

Phosphate Binders and Vitamin D Analogues

Renal osteodystrophy includes osteitis fibrosa cystica (and other features of hyperparathyroidism), osteomalacia, osteoporosis, and osteosclerosis. Renal bone disease creates deformation, resorption, fractures, and retardation of growth. The etiology of renal osteodystrophy is multifactorial, but the basic common defects are vitamin D resistance, vitamin D deficiency (osteomalacia), and secondary hyperparathyroidism. Vitamin D_3 (cholecalciferol) from animal sources and vitamin D_2 (ergocalciferol) from plants are the two major vitamin D parent compounds. Vitamin D_3 is hydroxylated in the liver, followed by conversion in the kidney to the biologically active 1,25-dihydroxy–vitamin D_3. The failing kidney exhibits impaired 1,25 dihydroxy–vitamin D_3 (calcitriol) production. Hypocalcemia, calcium deficiency, and hypophosphatemia augment calcitriol formation. Calcitriol, in turn, is transported by its carrier protein, enhances gastrointestinal absorption of calcium and phosphorus, and acts on bone in the presence of parathyroid hormone to mobilize calcium and stimulate mineralization of osteoid tissue. Clinical features of vitamin D deficiency are proximal myopathy (calcitriol facilitates protein synthesis in muscle) and impaired mineralization of osteoid. In addition, there is low intestinal absorption of calcium and phosphate in the absence of vitamin D, which leads to hypocalcemia and produces hyperparathyroidism, a renal phosphate leak, and subsequent hypophosphatemia.

Parathyroid hormone (PTH) production is stimulated by lowered blood calcium, and small changes in plasma calcium (7.5 mg per dl to 10.5 mg per dl) can influence secretion. PTH biotransformation occurs in the liver and kidney, with release of carboxy-terminal (C-terminal) fragments that are biologically inactive. The active amino terminal (N-terminal) fragment has a rapid half-life of 4 to 5 minutes and is removed by the kidneys, whereas the N-terminal fragments are metabolized in the skeleton. Consequently, C-terminal PTH is high in the absence of renal conversion of vitamin D_3, and converts mesenchymal cells to osteoclasts (which increase bone resorption) as well as activating osteoblasts. The overall effect of PTH in bone is to increase bone resorption and formation and increase bone turnover.

Since renal disease begins early in phase II chronic renal failure, the aim is to reduce plasma phosphate and elevate serum calcium. Since hyperphosphatemia usually occurs when the GFR falls below 25 ml per min, modest dietary phosphate restriction combined with aluminum hydroxide gels to adsorb excessive dietary phosphate should be introduced. In addition, low plasma levels of vitamin D_3 are almost invariable as renal failure advances. However, therapy may potentiate renal bone disease, since aluminum may deposit in bone and cause defects in mineralization. Pruritus, common in advanced renal failure, may be due to a high ionized calcium or high calcium phosphorus product and is associated with hyperparathyroidism. In children, growth retardation and delayed epiphyseal ossification result from vitamin D resistance and other unidentified factors. In advanced bone disease, fractures of the axial skeleton, including ribs, vertebrae, hips, and long bones, are common. Rarely, calcium deposits around joints of elbows, hands, and shoulders (x-ray diffraction reveals hydroxyapatite crystals). These patients respond to anti-inflammatory agents as well as parathyroidectomy.

The recommended measures for prevention of renal bone disease are as follows: Dietary calcium should be 1 gram per day and the calcium-phosphorus product should be maintained at around 40 to 50, since a higher calcium-phosphorus product is associated with vascular calcification and pruritus. Serum calcium should be maintained at around 9 to 11 mg per dl, and serum phosphate should be controlled with aluminum hydroxide gels. Although the exact role of magnesium in renal bone disease is unclear, persistent hypermagnesemia is undesirable. One-25-dihydroxy vitamin D_3 or 1,alpha-hydroxy D_3 promotes calcium absorption and mineralization of bone and should be employed. Hypercalcemia may fall more rapidly when 1,25-dihydroxy vitamin D_3 is used. Parathyroidectomy for secondary hyperparathyroidism (formerly termed tertiary hyperparathyroidism) may be necessary in patients who do not respond to the vitamin D sterols, or those in whom vitamin D sterols produce complications. Since total removal of parathyroid glands may contribute to osteomalacia, subtotal parathyroidectomy with preservation of the parathyroid tissue in liquid nitrogen (for subsequent implantation, should this be necessary) is recommended. Parathyroidectomy is most often required in phase III uremia.

Angioaccess

In a patient with slowly declining renal function, a time is reached when vascular access for subsequent hemodialysis should be created. The Cimino-Brescia fistula introduced in the 1960s has been the preferred method of angioaccess for hemodialysis. Since 4 to 6 weeks of "maturity" for arterialization of the venous portion of the forearm fistula is required, the experienced nephrologist will anticipate this well in advance of the institution of hemodialysis. If the patient presents with a GFR less than 5 ml per min, other access methods are available, e.g., the Scribner shunt, subclavian venous lines, and femoral venous lines. Arteriovenous fistula formation may be unsuccessful, e.g., in the diabetic patient with chronic renal disease or in the elderly female or failed vascular access patient; placement of a synthetic graft in the form of Dacron or Goretex vessels between artery and vein in the subcutaneous tissue of the forearm or upper arm may be necessary. In the patient who selects peritoneal dialysis (PD), a peritoneal catheter should be inserted surgically, by trocar, or by peritoneoscope.

In this phase it is equally important to exclude reversible renal factors, continue dietary protein restriction, and control phosphate. Vitamin D analogues should be continued. In phase III chronic renal failure, the principal therapeutic intervention is dialysis or transplantation.

Management of Phase III

Dialysis is the term for transfer of a solute across a semipermeable membrane. Hemodialysis entails the passage of anticoagulated (heparinized or citrated) blood, obtained via vascular access, through synthetic membranes in the form of flat plates, hollow fibers, or coil dialyzers. On the side of the membrane opposite the blood is dialysate (rinsing fluid) containing sodium, magnesium, calcium, glucose, chloride, acetate, and bicarbonate. The last two compounds serve to buffer any hydrogen ion excess. Clinically important uremic toxins not included in the dialysis fluid (urea, creatinine, uric acid, phosphate, and hydrogen ion, sodium, potassium, and water) are removed. Since volume expansion exists in ESRD, water and sodium removal is a necessary part of dialytic management.

During a single 5-hour dialysis, usually performed three times a week on alternate days in the outpatient setting or at home, serum urea nitrogen, creatinine, and phosphate will fall 40 to 50 per cent. Ultrafiltration through the membranes removes 2 to 4 liters of water each session. Patients may experience symptoms from shifts in osmolality, serum sodium, and fluid balance, with hypotension and other unphysiologic responses. Unphysiologic response to dialysis is more common in elderly, diabetic, and other debilitated patients but is uncommon in the majority. Many patients now select peritoneal dialysis for their management. Intermittent PD has largely been replaced with long-dwell PD. Long-dwell PD (continuous ambulatory peritoneal dialysis, or CAPD, and continuous cycling peritoneal dialysis, or CCPD) employ the peritoneal membrane for solute transfer. Intermittent peritoneal dialysis uses hourly cycling of peritoneal dialysis fluid into and out of the peritoneal cavity. CAPD consists of four exchanges (approximately every 6 hours) of 2 to 3 liters of sterile dialysis fluid in adults (less in children). CCPD uses 3-hour dwell times at night, with machine-controlled instillation and removal of peritoneal dialysate every 2 to 3 hours during sleep. Both CAPD and CCPD are employed daily, in contrast to intermittent PD, in which a total treatment of 40 hours per wk is divided into two or three sessions. CAPD has grown rapidly since its introduction in the late 1970s; at the time of writing, 20,000 patients are receiving long-dwell peritoneal dialysis throughout the world (with half in the United States). The total quantity of solute removed often exceeds that attained with hemodialysis, certain molecules, such as "middle molecules," being more efficiently removed with CAPD than with intermittent hemodialysis. Long-dwell peritoneal dialysis achieves stable serum chemistries and abolishes the large fluid and electrolyte shifts that occur with hemodialysis. Consequently, hypertension is more easily controlled in these patients, and improved nutrition and a rise in hematocrit occur. The most serious disadvantage of peritoneal dialysis is peritonitis, which develops in more than one half of patients within the first year. Peritonitis accounts for approximately 27 per cent of all causes for discontinuing CAPD and is responsible for frequent hospitalization. Although solute removal through the peritoneum does not diminish with time, there are isolated reports of membrane failure due to thickening of its mesothelial surface. Sclerosing encapsulating peritonitis has rarely been reported, but its etiology is uncertain and does not relate to frequency of peritonitis. Current evidence points to the type of dialysate involved, possible plastic particles in the dialysate, or the antiseptics used.

Alternatives to Standard Dialysis. Sorbents (activated charcoal along with urease, zirconium phosphate, and hydrated zirconium oxide) in a canister are used widely for the regeneration of dialysate to reduce the total volume of dialysate in a single hemodialysis session. Urea is split by urease into ammonium, which is adsorbed on activated charcoal. Zirconium phosphate exchanges ammonium, calcium, magnesium, and potassium for hydrogen and sodium ions. Hydrated zirconium oxide also exchanges phosphate for acetate. Activated carbon adsorbs creatinine, uric acid, phosphate, and other organic compounds. Regeneration of dialysis fluid is a convenient form of reducing dialysate volume; it also increases the portability of such dialysis equipment and reduces the need for expensive plumbing in the home dialysis setting. Bicarbonate dialysis may correct acidosis more readily than acetate dialysis and may be associated with better control of blood pressure in the dialysis session. In addition, slow continuous ultrafiltration and hemodiafiltration are techniques that use more porous membranes to effect solute and water removal. The former is a useful approach for continuous removal of fluid in the postoperative management of fluid control in a renal-impaired patient.

Dialysis Survival. As might be expected, age and other medical conditions complicating renal failure significantly influence survival in patients undergoing dialysis or transplant therapy. In Europe and the United States, many patients are still alive after 10 years of hemodialysis. All studies show that a greater survival occurs in the home hemodialysis patient. In contrast to in-center dialysis, home dialysis patients are selected because of improved medical status and compliance. The majority of deaths in ESRD are due to cardiovascular complications—myocardial infarction and cerebrovascular accidents. The second most common cause of death is sepsis, most likely introduced via arteriovenous needles. Another factor contributing to the frequency of sepsis is that ESRD patients are immunocompromised. Mortality rates do not appear to differ significantly between hemodialysis and CAPD when age corrections are made, but "dropout" from CAPD is a significant problem. This is predominantly related to peritonitis.

Transplantation

As mentioned, transplantation offers an alternative therapy. Living related donor transplantation and cadaveric transplantation are accepted therapies, with greatly reduced mortality and a high rate of success compared with 20 years ago. Immunosuppressive therapy, in the form of azathioprine, prednisolone, and antilymphocytic serum, is used in the majority of patients. In patients with a history of previous rejection or presensitization, the new immunosuppressive agent cyclosporine offers a real benefit in creating tolerance to the renal allograft. Major complications of transplant are sepsis from immunosuppression and cardiovascular disease (from the second year on). The previous relative unpredictability of successful outcome is now much improved with DR matching and/or demonstration of mixed lymphocyte culture unreactivity. Although cyclosporine represents a major advance in immunosuppression, it is associated with nephrotoxicity and T cell–dependent tumor induction (lymphoma and Kaposi's sarcoma), both of which are dose-dependent. It is likely that with further experience and other analogues of cyclosporine such complications will be minimized.

Although the patient never achieves complete

normality on hemodialysis or peritoneal dialysis (since at best a state of mild uremia is induced), a better quality of life may be obtained with transplantation. However, the adverse effects of a transplant must be weighed against the benefits. Furthermore, metabolic abnormalities that are present on dialysis are not completely corrected after transplantation (e.g., atherosclerosis, hypertension, hyperlipidemia, and renal osteodystrophy). It must be stressed that the patient is free to choose any type of therapy, none of which are mutually exclusive, depending on their medical suitability.

Drug Handling In Uremia

It is known that in patients with renal impairment the incidence of drug side effects is higher than in patients with normal renal function. This is due to the fact that many drugs that are cleared by normal renal tissue accumulate in the presence of reduced renal function. The physician therefore should use reduced dosage of such drugs or lengthen the period between successive doses of the particular drug, as well as monitor blood levels of drugs that may produce serious side effects (e.g., aminoglycosides and digoxin). Among those drugs that should be administered in accordance with these rules are aminoglycosides, digoxin, cephalosporins, sulfamethoxazole-trimethoprim, cimetidine, and vancomycin. Drugs that should not be administered are tetracycline (antianabolic and produces a rise in SUN) and nitrofurantoin (produces pulmonary fibrosis and does not achieve therapeutic levels in the urine).

GENITOURINARY TUBERCULOSIS

method of
JAMES G. GOW, M.D.
Lourdes Private Hospital
Liverpool, England

The diagnosis of genitourinary tuberculosis should be established by culture prior to instituting therapy, unless there is overwhelming clinical evidence in favor of the disease. Tuberculosis is now largely under control in the Western world but still poses problems in underdeveloped countries, where case finding and adequate follow-up examinations are often impossible to organize.

Therapeutic Plan

In the past, prolonged triple drug therapy has been the standard treatment, but this is now no longer necessary. Because of the efficiency of the new drugs rifampin, isoniazid, and pyrazinamide, short courses of treatment have now become standard practice, and for genitourinary disease, the course should last no longer than 4 months. This can even be reduced to 3 months in cases which are not severe, or when tuberculous epididymitis is the only presenting symptom.

General Management

It is no longer necessary to treat patients in the hospital. Patients should be encouraged to carry on their normal work, unless bladder symptoms are severe, and take the drugs as outpatients. They should be examined weekly to ensure that no toxic signs are developing. They should take a nourishing diet, but the addition of vitamins is not required.

All contacts, especially close family members, should be screened by tuberculin skin tests and chest radiographs. Adult converters should have skin testing and chest films every 3 to 6 months, to exclude the development of pulmonary tuberculosis.

Chemotherapy

The most effective drug therapy is the administration of isoniazid, together with rifampin and pyrazinamide. The course can be restricted to 4 months, because in renal lesions fewer organisms are present than in the pulmonary disease, all the drugs penetrate cavities, there is a high concentration of the drugs in the urine, and there is a bactericidal concentration of the drugs in renal, ureteral, and bladder tissues.

The first intensive chemotherapy, which lasts 2 months, consists of rifampin (Rifadin, Rimactane), 450 mg per day; isoniazid, 300 mg per day, and pyrazinamide, 25 mg per kg per day. All these drugs are taken together and are best given last thing at night, possibly in milk, as this helps reduce gastric intolerance. After 2 months, rifampin, 900 mg, and isoniazid, 600 mg, are continued three times a week for a further 2 months and then discontinued, making a total course of 4 months. If there is intensive disease, particularly with severe bladder symptoms, streptomycin, 1 gram daily, can be added for the initial 2 months of intensive treatment. In my experience using this regimen, (130 patients over a period of 10 years), no organisms have been isolated from urine after 2 months of intensive chemotherapy.

There is no place for the use of ethambutol in this initial first-line treatment. Ethambutol is a bacteriostatic drug, whereas the other four mentioned are bactericidal; not only is it less effective, but it is also more toxic and considerably more expensive. Ethambutol should only be used if there is resistance to one or more of the primary drugs, but this is rare in genitourinary tuberculosis, especially in developing countries where in nearly every case the organisms are sensitive to the three primary agents.

In underdeveloped countries, it might be possible to consider giving the drugs three times a week from the start of treatment, because there is accumulating evidence that this regime is just as effective as daily treatment, and less expensive. However, if this regime is used, total compliance is essential, otherwise resistant strains will rapidly develop.

The initial 3 to 4 weeks of treatment are the most important. The population of *Mycobacterium tuberculosis* will be reduced 1000-fold during the first 3 or 4 weeks of treatment, but only if there is absolute adherence to the course of treatment, so compliance is a most important factor in treating this disease.

Surgical Treatment

Now that short course chemotherapy is the standard method of treatment, it is important to reappraise the use of surgery. There are two surgical approaches: the removal of diseased tissue and reconstructive surgery. Removal of diseased tissue consists of nephrectomy, partial nephrectomy, and epididymectomy. All these have a place in the modern management of genitourinary tuberculosis. Nephrectomy, partial nephrectomy, and epididymectomy should be carried out when the organs are grossly diseased, are unlikely to recover function, and would always remain a source of problems if left in situ. This will enable the high concentration of circulating chemotherapeutic agents to destroy any small foci that are present anywhere in the body.

Reconstructive Surgery

This consists of reimplantation of the ureter or augmentation cystoplasty. Reimplantation of the ureter is nearly always carried out at the ureterovesical junction, where a stricture is present in about 9 per cent of cases. Sometimes it is due to edema caused by an acute infection; therefore, in the initial stages, steroids are not necessary. The intensive chemotherapy is closely monitored by a weekly intravenous urogram, one film being taken at 25 minutes; only if there is no improvement after 3 or 4 weeks should steroids be used. If after steroids have been added to the routine chemotherapeutic regime for 2 weeks and there is still no improvement, reimplantation of the ureter should be carried out.

The ureter is reimplanted into a normal area of bladder using a reflux-preventing technique, which means a tunnel of at least 5 cm in length. If the stricture of the ureter is long, then a Boari bladder flap should be used, adopting the same reflux-preventing technique. Rarely, strictures occur at the pelviureteral junction, and these can be repaired either by a Culp or an Anderson Hynes technique. The kidney pelvis should always be drained and irrigated with a mixture of 1 per cent isoniazid and 5 per cent rifampin. This helps control any residual infection in the pelvicalyceal system.

Augmentation Cystoplasty

This is performed for intolerable frequency, which means half-hourly voiding during the day and night, together with a small capacity bladder—less than 100 ml—in which the mucous membrane has been destroyed and replaced by intermural fibrosis. Such a bladder will never recover, and therefore augmentation enteroplasty should be performed, using either colon or cecum, according to the usual practice of the surgeon. Before surgery, urinary flow studies should be carried out to exclude outflow obstruction. In this way the bladder capacity can be increased and the frequency improved. If there is reflux or a stricture of the lower end of the ureters, using the cecum is the best technique because the ureters can be reimplanted into the ileum and then the cecum attached to the fundus of the bladder. The anastomosis of the ureters to the ileum should always be performed before the cecum is attached to the bladder, otherwise the technical difficulties may be considerable.

Follow-Up Studies

With the present regimen, patients need not be followed up for more than a year in an uncomplicated case. Intravenous urograms, if indicated, are carried out at 6 months and 1 year, and the urine is tested for *M. tuberculosis* by three or possibly five consecutive early morning specimens of urine on each attendance. If the intravenous urogram is satisfactory and the urine sterile after 1 year, then the patient can be discharged but told to report back if urinary symptoms recur.

If, however, calcification is found, patients are treated like any other patient with renal stones. Annual radiographs are done to ensure that the calcification is not increasing, because I have seen many cases in which there is insidious, slow, symptomless enlargement of the calcification, which so damages renal parenchyma that eventually the kidney is completely destroyed. It may be necessary to follow cases of calcification for more than 10 years.

MALIGNANT TUMORS OF THE UROGENITAL TRACT

method of
HARRY W. HERR, M.D.
Memorial Sloan-Kettering Cancer Center
New York, New York

Urologic neoplasms constitute approximately 25 per cent of male and 4 per cent of female cancers in the United States. Most malignant tumors of the genitourinary system occur in the latter decades of life. With increased life expectancy, a larger proportion of the population is exposed to the risks of urologic cancer–related morbidity and mortality, and in the future these neoplasms will assume greater medical importance.

Adrenocortical Carcinoma

This rare neoplasm arises from the adrenal cortex. Between 50 and 80 per cent of these tumors retain endocrine function, usually resulting in Cushing's syndrome due to excessive production of glucocorticoids, or virilization due to excessive production of androgens. Less commonly, feminization due to estrogen secretion by the tumor or hypertension and hypokalemic alkalosis due to aldosterone production may be the main clinical feature.

The preferred treatment for adrenal carcinoma is complete excision. A subcostal, flank, or thoracoabdominal incision is used, depending on the size and location of the tumor. Since resectability influences survival, aggressive surgical therapy is indicated in patients with locally advanced disease. This includes regional lymphadenectomy, adjacent nephrectomy and tumor thrombectomy, including resection of a portion of the inferior vena cava, if involved. The overall 5-year survival for stage I (tumor less than 5 cm) is 80 per cent; for stage II (greater than 5 cm with neither local invasion nor metastases), 50 per cent; for stage III (nodal metastases or local invasion), 11 per cent; and for stage IV (distant metastases), 0 to 5 per cent.

The role of radiotherapy is unclear. The insecticide op'DDD (mitotane) (Lysodren) is the only chemotherapeutic agent active against adrenocortical carcinoma. However, its effects are palliative and generally of short duration, and the drug often produces severe gastrointestinal side effects and depression. Its mechanism of action is unknown. The usual dose is 3.0 to 5.0 grams daily orally, increased in 2.0 gram increments every few days until a total daily dose of 20 grams is reached (this dosage exceeds manufacturer's recommendation). Urinary steroid excretion can be measured at regular intervals and combined with radiographic parameters of response in patients with steroid-producing cancers. Amino-glutethimide and metapyrone used to achieve medical adrenalectomy may be helpful to counteract the steroid effect produced by functioning tumors. Patients must maintain surveillance after surgery for many years. They are followed at 3-month intervals with chest x-ray and liver function tests, and, if the latter is elevated, periodic steroid excretion tests. A rising steroid excretion will often indicate recurrence of the tumor before there is palpable or radiologic evidence of disease.

Renal Cell Carcinoma

Perifascial (radical) nephrectomy is the preferred treatment for patients without clinically detectable metastatic disease. An ipsilateral hilar lymphadenectomy is performed to further stage the tumor but has little therapeutic value. I prefer an extrapleural, extraperitoneal flank approach through the bed of the tenth or eleventh rib. On occasion, a midline transperitoneal or thoracoabdominal incision is required, especially to facilitate removal of a tumor thrombus from within the lumen of the inferior vena cava (10 per cent).

The 5-year survival for patients with tumor localized to the kidney or perirenal fat ranges from 50 to 80 per cent. If disease involves contiguous organs or metastases to regional lymph nodes, the 5-year survival is 20 per cent. The median survival of untreated patients with metastatic disease ranges from 8 to 11 months, although an occasional patient with limited, asymptomatic bone or pulmonary metastases may survive for many years. Patients who present with a solitary metastasis (less than 5 per cent), or who develop a solitary metastatic deposit after nephrectomy, should have this tumor excised, if possible. Five-year survival in this clinical setting is 35 per cent. Radical nephrectomy is not indicated for patients with multiple metastases, except if life-threatening renal hemorrhage or pain is present. These sequelae from a large renal tumor can often be alleviated by angioinfarction. Overall, the prognosis for patients with renal cell carcinoma has not changed substantially over the past 20 years.

Patients with small (2 cm or less) primary tumors involving a solitary kidney or an ectopic kidney (and selected patients with a normal contralateral kidney) undergo partial nephrectomy. Local control and survival achieved with conservative renal parenchyma–sparing surgery are similar to results after total nephrectomy.

Radiation therapy does not have an adjunctive therapeutic role pre- or postoperatively. It may palliate some patients with bone metastases. In metastatic renal cancer, chemotherapy has been unrewarding, but immunotherapy with interferon has shown modestly encouraging results. About 20 per cent of patients have partial remissions or stabilization of disease. High-dose medroxyprogesterone acetate (Depo-Provera) is ineffective and may produce undesirable side effects.

After nephrectomy, patients are followed every 3 months for 3 years, every 6 months for 2 years, and annually thereafter. At each visit, a chest x-ray, urinalysis, hemoglobin value, and serum liver and kidney function test are obtained. A CT scan of the remaining kidney is obtained yearly.

Wilms' Tumor

This tumor occurs in children or young adults. Most are detected before the age of 6 years. Treatment has been defined largely by the collaborative efforts of the National Wilm's Tumor Study.

Patients with clinically localized disease undergo transperitoneal nephrectomy. The contralateral normal kidney should be examined for bilateral disease. Surgical removal of all local disease is performed. Patients with bilateral Wilms' tumor (5 per cent) undergo radical nephrectomy for the larger lesion and partial nephrectomy for the smaller tumor in order to avoid dialysis and renal transplantation. Patients in whom primary surgical extirpation is deemed hazardous because of local extension into vital areas (e.g., the root of the mesentery, duodenum, pancreas), or extensive involvement of the inferior vena cava, are treated initially with chemotherapy, with or without supplemental radiation therapy. This usually facilitates complete and safe removal of the primary tumor at a later date.

Chemotherapy (actinomycin D and vincristine, with or without doxorubicin) is given for 15 months to all patients with local-regional Wilms' tumor after nephrectomy. Radiation therapy (2000 rad) is added to control soft tissue extension of tumor or incompletely excised tumor, or after surgical spillage of tumor, but is not needed if disease is confined to the kidney. Durable survival for most patients with Wilms' tumor exceeds 80 per cent. Patients with unfavorable (sarcomatous) pathology or stage IV (metastatic) disease present a major challenge, since most of these children are not treated successfully.

Retroperitoneal Tumors

This category of neoplasms comprises a wide variety of rare tumors that can originate from any retroperitoneal tissue or organ, i.e., the adrenal gland, kidney, or ureter. Approximately 85 per cent of primary retroperitoneal tumors are malignant. Excluding renal cell carcinoma, the most common retroperitoneal neoplasm is lymphoma. Presenting as vague abdominal or nonspecific back pain, lymphoma may occur primarily within the kidney or retroperitoneum, or may be a further manifestation of systemic disease. Surgical excision is the treatment of choice in the former case, whereas in the latter, treatment for systemic lymphoma is required (combination of chemotherapy and radiotherapy).

Sarcomas are the the second most common retroperitoneal tumor. Complete surgical resection should be attempted and generally can be accomplished. Postoperative radiation therapy (5000+ rad) may reduce the incidence of local recurrence. Adjuvant doxorubicin (Adriamycin) may improve subsequent survival and produces up to 30 per cent objective response rates in patients with metastatic disease. Prognosis is poor for patients with high-grade sarcomas or metastatic disease. Patients are followed at 3-month intervals with chest x-ray and serum liver function tests. A periodic abdominal CT scan is performed. Local recurrences are common; the lesion should be surgically excised if metastases are not detected concomitantly.

Neuroblastoma

This neoplasm is one of the more common pediatric solid tumors. It may arise from the adrenal gland or sympathetic ganglia in the retroperitoneum or pelvis. The peak incidence occurs at 2 years of age. Elevated serum and urinary catecholamine levels and an abdominal radiogram showing stippled calcifications are helpful in diagnosis. The staging system utilized is:

- Stage I—tumor confined to the organ of origin.
- Stage II—presence of regional spread that does not cross the midline.
- Stage III—tumors extending across the midline.
- Stage IV—distant metastases.
- Stage IV-S—patients with small primary tumor and metastases limited to the liver, skin, or bone marrow without radiographic evidence of bone metastases.

Complete surgical excision is the initial goal of treatment. Unfortunately, complete resection may be hazardous or impossible because of involvement of adjacent vital structures or soft tissues. Resection of contiguous viscera in an attempt to remove all tumor has not improved survival. Many surgeons feel, however, that debulking of as much tumor as possible should be attempted, although this may result in brisk bleeding. The benefit of resecting the primary tumor in the face of metastases has not been established.

Combination chemotherapy (vincristine, cyclophosphamide, nitrogen mustard, doxorubicin, and the maturating agent papaverine) is necessary and is often combined with radiation therapy for inoperable or gross residual disease after surgery. Despite the advent of multimodal therapy and the improved response rates, dismal survival rates have remained essentially unchanged.

Urothelial Tumors

Renal Pelvic Carcinoma. Carcinoma of the renal pelvis accounts for only 7 per cent of all renal neoplasms. The peak incidence occurs in the sixth and seventh decades. Hematuria is the most common symptom. There is a male to female preponderance of three to one. Diagnosis is established with excretory urography, positive cytology for malignant transitional cells, and biopsy obtained indirectly by retrograde brushing of the tumor or directly by ureteroscopy.

Staging of urothelial tumors at all sites is similar:

Stage 0—neoplasms confined to the mucosa.
Stage A—lesions that have invaded the submucosa.
Stage B—tumors that have infiltrated the muscle layer.
Stage C—lesions that have infiltrated through the urothelium to involve adjacent fat or kidney.
Stage D—neoplasms with regional or systemic metastases.

A radical nephrectomy and complete ureterectomy with excision of a bladder cuff are performed. The rationale for this approach includes (1) The low incidence of low-grade, low-stage lesions that can be treated conservatively (most are invasive and multifocal); (2) the high incidence of recurrence (up to 30 per cent) in a retained ureteral stump; (3) the low incidence of synchronous (2 per cent) or asynchronous (5 per cent) tumors; and (4) the high incidence of renal (30 per cent) or perinephric fat invasion.

The role of lymphadenectomy and postoperative radiation therapy is unclear. Selected patients with small papillary tumors within the renal pelvis or ureter, and patients with solitary kidneys, may be treated with conservative ureteroscopic resection and fulguration combined with topical chemotherapy or immunotherapy. Conservative approaches to favorable tumors probably will parallel results achieved with more aggressive surgery.

The prognosis in this malignant tumor is influenced by both the stage and the grade of the tumor. The overall 5-year prognosis ranges from 70 per cent for stage I and some stage II tumors to less than 20 per cent for stage III lesions. Because 30 per cent of these patients subsequently develop bladder cancer, they are followed cystoscopically every 3 months for 3 years, every 6 months for 2 years, and annually thereafter. Urinalysis, urine cytology, and chest x-ray are performed at each visit. Excretory urography is carried out annually.

Carcinoma of the Ureter. These tumors are less frequent than tumors of the renal pelvis, but they are also transitional cell carcinomas. The peak incidence occurs in the sixth and seventh decades and is associated with a male predominance of two to one. There is a predilection for these tumors to arise in the distal one third of the ureter (75 per cent), and approximately 10 per cent of patients will have concomitant bladder tumors. Hematuria is the most common presenting symptom. Detection is similar to that employed for renal pelvic tumors. The staging system for this neoplasm is based on the degree of ureteral wall penetration and is similar to that for carcinoma of the renal pelvis.

Patients with proximal ureteral tumors are treated with radical nephroureterectomy, since these tumors tend to be multifocal in origin and locally invasive when first discovered. On the other hand, distal ureteral tumors tend to be low-grade and not invasive. Therefore, these lesions can be managed either conservatively with ureteroscopic resection and fulguration, or, if this proves inadequate, with distal ureterectomy with reimplantation of normal proximal ureter into the bladder. The prognosis of patients with primary carcinoma of the ureter is influenced by the stage and grade of the neoplasm. Overall, 5-year survival for proximal ureteral tumors is 50 per cent; for distal ureteral tumors, it is 70 to 80 per cent. Patients with this malignancy are followed exactly as those with carcinoma of the renal pelvis.

Carcinoma of the Urinary Bladder. This is a common neoplasm. There are approximately 36,000 new cases of bladder cancer diagnosed annually in the United States. It is estimated that 12,000 patients die every year with this disease. Etiologic causes include aromatic amine exposure and schistosomiasis. There is an increased incidence of bladder cancer in patients occupied as textile workers, leather tanners, dye workers, and rubber and cable workers as well as those in the petrochemical industry. Phenacetin and saccharine (artificial sweeteners) have also been incriminated as cocarcinogens. Bladder cancer is highly associated with cigarette smoking. The peak incidence is in the sixth and seventh decades, but the disease may occur at any age beyond puberty. There is a male predominance of three to one. Hematuria is the leading symptom, but pain and frequency of voiding are present in many patients. The diagnosis and staging are established by cystoendoscopy and biopsy. Most patients present with disease localized to the bladder.

Patients with superficial (stage 0, A) papillary tumors are managed by transurethral resection and fulguration (TUR). This generally requires anesthesia but in some instances can be accomplished as an outpatient procedure. Superficial bladder tumors represent 75 per cent of all urothelial tumors. TUR of existing and recurrent tumors (occurs in 30 to 80 per cent of cases) produces an 80 to 90 per cent 5-year survival rate. Patients who present with four or more tumors, a history of multiple recurrent tumors at frequent cystoscopic evaluations, symptomatic irritative voiding symptoms associated with papillary tumor, or diffuse high-grade flat carcinoma in situ should receive topical intravesical therapy as an adjunct to TUR. I prefer intravesical BCG (this use of BCG not listed by manufacturer) (Pasteur strain) given as 120 mg in 50 ml saline (retained for 2 hours) once a week for 6 consecutive weeks. The rationale for this regimen is that patients who present with the foregoing criteria have up to a 30 per cent incidence of developing subsequent invasive bladder cancer, and intravesical BCG seems to prevent progression (and delay cystectomy) of local disease in up to 70 per cent. Intravesical chemotherapy using mitomycin C (40 mg weekly for 8 weeks) or doxorubicin (Adriamycin) (40 to 80 mg for 6 weeks) may also be useful. Thiotepa (30 or 60 mg in 30 or 60 ml saline once a week for 6 weeks) is effective for some patients with recurrent low-grade papillary tumors but is not as effective in patients with more extensive tumors. Patients who manifest recurrent bladder tumors or prostate involvement after intravesical therapy should be considered for radical cystectomy. Conservatively treated patients are followed with cystoendoscopy and urine cystology every 3 months for 3 years, every 6 months for 2 years, and annually thereafter.

Infiltrating bladder cancers are treated with radiation therapy, radical cystectomy, or a combination of both methods. Most stage B and stage C tumors, and some stage A lesions, require an aggressive approach. I favor preoperative pelvic irradiation (2000 rad in 5 days) followed by bilateral pelvic lymph node dissection, radical cystectomy, and ileal conduit urinary diversion. Male patients with tumors that involve the bladder neck or prostatic urethra or both, undergo concomitant total urethrectomy. Radiation therapy is employed for medically poor-risk patients or those who refuse surgery. Dose level required is 6000+ rad, side effects are often significant, and, most importantly, radiation therapy does not prevent new tumor formation within the bladder. However, salvage cystectomy may be performed safely in selected patients whose tumors fail to respond to therapeutic radiation. Some patients (5 per cent) with limited stage B lesions may be managed by transurethral resection. Partial (segmental) cystectomy is indicated only in patients who fulfill the following criteria: (1) tumors inaccessible to transurethral resection; (2) solitary lesion with well-defined margins without any other mucosal abnormalities; (3) no prior history of malignant urothelial disease in the bladder; and (4) location of the tumor permitting a 2 cm surgical margin.

The prognosis in patients with superficial invasive disease (stages A, B_1) ranges from 60 to 80 per cent 5-year survival, whereas patients with deep muscle-infiltrating tumors (Stages B_2, C) have a 30 to 50 per cent survival. Until recently, prognosis for patients with pelvic nodal or systemic disease was extremely poor (5 to 10 per cent). Combination chemotherapy has improved the prognosis of patients with locally advanced or metastatic urothelial tumors arising in all sites. At present, I am using the M-VAC protocol. This employs the most active single agents that have demonstrated objective responses in patients with metastatic bladder cancer. M-VAC (monthly cycles of methotrexate, 30 mg/m^2, followed 24 hours later by vinblastine, 3 mg/m^2, Adriamycin, 30 mg/m^2, and cisplatin, 70 mg/m^2, with vinblastine and methotrexate repeated on days 15 and 22) produces significant tumor regression in 71 per cent of patients and, more importantly, produces complete remissions of all metastatic disease in 40 per cent. The M-VAC regimen is toxic and requires hospitalization and careful supervision during therapy. Responses have been detected both within the bladder and at distant sites. M-VAC is also employed with radiation therapy (rather than cystectomy alone) in selected patients with operable infiltrating cancers, preoperatively in patients with inoperable locally advanced bladder cancers, and as an adjunct postoperatively in patients with positive pelvic lymph node metastases. It is hoped such an aggressive multimodal approach will ultimately preserve the bladder with complete control of disease in some patients, permit removal of nonresectable tumors in others, and improve the dismal 5 to 10 per cent 5-year survival rates of patients with regional or disseminated disease.

Female Urethral Carcinoma. Fewer than 1000 cases of this uncommon neoplasm have been reported. The most common presenting symptom is urethral bleeding (not hematuria). Urethral carcinoma is the only genitourinary malignancy more common in women than in men. Squamous cell carcinoma is the most common histologic type, followed by adenocarcinoma and then transitional cell carcinoma. Urethral carcinoma may arise in a urethral diverticulum, but this is rare.

There is no predilection for location of these tumors along the female urethra. They often infiltrate the muscle of the adjacent vagina and mucosa as well as other adjacent structures such as bladder, labia, and clitoris. Metastasis to inguinal lymph nodes alone may occur in up to 25 per cent initially or subsequently.

Treatment recommendations and prognosis are determined by the stage and location of the tumor. For treatment purposes, tumors are classified as involving the distal urethra (one third) only or proximal (entire) urethra. Distal urethral tumors may be managed with local excision (or in some cases, distal urethrectomy), which results in 5-year survival rates of 50 to 70 per cent. Tumors involving the proximal urethra tend to be larger and invasive; they have a poor prognosis despite the extent of surgical excision. Patients with small (2 cm or less), mobile tumors are treated by local excision plus interstitial radiation therapy using iridium-192 or iodine-125, and supplemental external radiation therapy, to achieve a total tumor dose of 5000 to 7000 rad. Larger proximal tumors require more aggressive treatment. I favor preoperative irradiation followed by anterior exenteration and urinary diversion. A prophylactic groin dissection is not performed because limited experience suggests that inguinal lymphadenectomy for nonpalpable nodes does not improve overall survival. Moreover, the inguinal regions can be regularly assessed for metastases, and ilioinguinal dissection is associated with high morbidity, e.g., lower extremity edema.

Local radiotherapy combined with radiation sensitizers (e.g., misonidazole), M-VAC, and radiation therapy, followed by limited surgical resection and M-VAC for regional or systemic metastases, is now undergoing evaluation. Of note, M-VAC combination chemotherapy is effective in patients with squamous or transitional cell carcinoma but is not effective for adenocarcinoma. Despite such innovative approaches, prognosis remains poor, with 5-year survival rates of approximately 50, 35, 25, and 10 per cent reported for stages A, B, C, and D, respectively.

Male Urethral Carcinoma. Only 400 cases of this rare neoplasm have been reported. Urethral pain, discharge, and a narrowed urinary stream are common presenting symptoms. The disease is often associated with a prior history of urethral stricture or venereal disease. Most are squamous cell carcinoma or adenocarcinoma. The most frequent location is the bulbomembranous urethra, although tumors may arise from any portion of the male urethra from the bladder neck to the meatus. Clinical staging is as follows:

Stage 0—tumors confined to mucosa.
Stage A—tumors that have not invaded beyond the submucosa.
Stage B—neoplasms invading into but not beyond the corpus spongiosum or prostate (extremely difficult to determine clinically).
Stage C—direct extension into tissues beyond the corpus spongiosum.
Stage D1—regional metastases involving inguinal or pelvic nodes, or both.
Stage D2—distant metastases.

For treatment and prognostic considerations, male urethral cancers are divided into anterior or posterior lesions. Treatment is predicated on the stage and location of the tumor in the urethra. Superficial tumors (stages 0 and A), regardless of location, may be adequately treated by transurethral resection. Regular follow-up cystoscopic examination every 3 months is recommended for these patients. Stage B or C lesions of the anterior urethra are best managed by partial penectomy to obtain at least a 2 to 3 cm disease-free urethral margin. Bulky, invasive posterior carcinomas are treated aggressively with preoperative irradiation (anterior, posterior, and perineal ports with 2000 rad in 1 week) followed by total excision of the penis, prostate, bladder, inferior aspects of the symphysis pubis and pubic rami, and bilateral pelvic lymph node dissection. Total emasculation may be required if the tumor involves the scrotum and its contents. Radical exenterative surgery produces 5-year survivals of not more than 40 per cent, but it is justified because most patients (60 per cent) develop and die from local recurrences after less radical surgical procedures or radiation therapy used alone. Since the value of surgery in patients with positive pelvic inguinal nodes is not well established, surgery is generally not indicated. Combination chemotherapy may improve the outlook for such patients.

In general, the prognosis for anterior urethral lesions is good (60 to 70 per cent), whereas that for posterior urethral cancers remains poor (20 per cent). As with female urethral cancer, patients are followed at 3-month intervals for 3 years, every 6 months for 2 years, and annually thereafter with careful pelvic examination, chest x-ray, and serum liver function tests.

Prostate Cancer

This neoplasm is the second most common cancer in males and is the third most common cause of male cancer deaths. Adenocarcinoma of the prostate is detected in approximately 70,000 males annually and results in over 22,000 deaths every year. Most affected males are over 50 years of age; the peak incidence occurs at age 70. Clinically silent prostate cancer is estimated to be four times more common than the clinical incidence. Prostatic cancer tends to be a slow-growing tumor, but the disease may progress rapidly in some individuals. Since the rate and the pattern of prostatic tumor growth are unpredictable in an individual patient, categorical treatment recommendations for any given stage of prostatic cancer remain uncertain. There is no more controversial topic concerned with cancer in general than the treatment of early prostatic cancer.

Treatment is generally based upon the clinical stage of disease:

Stage A—(incidentally discovered carcinoma); generally detected after prostatic surgery performed to relieve urinary obstruction from clinically benign prostatic enlargement (BPH).

Stage B—a nodule confined to the capsule of the prostate on digital rectal examination.

Stage C—locally advanced carcinoma invading prostatic capsule or seminal vesicles.

Stage D—pelvic nodal or systemic metastases, most commonly detected in bone.

Stages A, B, and C are potentially curable. Unfortunately, only 20 to 30 per cent of patients present with localized disease. The majority have detectable metastatic disease when first seen, and palliative therapy is all that can be offered. For localized disease, options of therapy include observation only (70 to 75 years and older), radical prostatectomy (either retropubic or perineal approach), megavoltage external radiation therapy, interstitial irradiation using I-125 seeds or gold-198 grains, or a combination of modalities. With disease confined to the prostate gland, the 5-, 10-, and 15-year survival data with external beam irradiation, radical excision, or interstitial irradiation are 80 per cent, 50 per cent, and 30 per cent, respectively. The treatment selected depends on the age of the patient, concurrent medical illnesses, and consideration of side effects of treatment, especially consequences of bladder, bowel, and sexual function after therapy. Radical excision and I-125 implantation are preferred for small and well-defined prostatic carcinomas, whereas stage C lesions are preferably treated with megavoltage radiation therapy (6000+ rad in 6 to 8 weeks). Prognosis regarding disease progression depends on volume of tumor within the prostate; stage, grade, and presence or absence of pelvic nodal metastases; and responsiveness of the tumor to irradiation.

Patients with stage D disease usually receive some form of hormonal therapy. This includes orchiectomy, diethylstilbestrol (DES) at a dose of 1 to 3 mg daily, and/or antiandrogen (flutamide) 750 mg per day orally or one of the newer LHRH analogues (Leuprolide) given as a daily subcutaneous injection or intranasal spray. Patients with asymptomatic local or systemic disease are observed until they become symptomatic (bone pain, urinary obstruction, weakness, fatigue, and so forth). They are not treated, because of (1) the side effects that may occur (psychologic, sexual impotence, fluid retention, aggravation of preexisting cardiovascular disease, phlebitis, gynecomastia) and (2) lack of evidence that early versus late initiation of endocrine therapy significantly affects survival or quality of life. I treat symptomatic patients with either orchiectomy or DES. The patient is begun on 1 mg per day and evaluated for relief of pain. Adequacy of dose required to suppress androgens is monitored by serial plasma testosterone determinations along with serum acid phosphatase. DES is increased to 3 mg per day if bone pain or obstructive urinary symptoms are not improved after 1 month, or if the patient subsequently relapses after responding to the lower dose. Orchiectomy is preferred in patients with a history of cardiovascular disease, since daily drug doses of 3 to 5 mg or greater are associated with myocardial infarction, angina, and stroke. Antiandrogen therapy offers some advantages with regard to side effects of treatment, but these drugs are not yet approved for general use. Approximately 70 to 80 per cent of patients will respond to hormonal therapy for 1 to 2 years. Unfortunately, most patients relapse with progressive disease. Local or spot radiation therapy is useful to palliate symptomatic bone metastases. Analgesics combined with steroids also give short-term relief. Further attempts at alternative hormonal methods of control are ineffective. Patients with obstructive urinary symptoms due to locally advanced prostatic carcinoma are generally treated with hormonal therapy; on occasion, however, a transurethral resection of the prostate (TURP) may be necessary to restore adequate voiding and obviate the need for an indwelling catheter, and in the patient who is still sexually active. Cytotoxic chemotherapy has been tried in a large number of patients with hormone-refractory metastatic carcinoma of the prostate gland. Unfortunately, chemotherapy trials have failed to demonstrate convincing evidence of significant objective regressions or meaningful survival advantages for such patients. Moreover, palliation of symptoms and maintenance of acceptable levels of quality of life have been realized by only a few patients. Therapeutic use of cytotoxic nonhormonal chemotherapy in patients with metastatic prostatic cancer, or its use as an adjunct in patients who are found to have positive pelvic lymph node metastases, is not recommended.

All patients with localized or advanced disease are followed at least three times a year with careful digital rectal examination of the prostate combined with periodic acid and alkaline phosphatase determination, and serum kidney and liver function test as well as an IVP or renal ultrasound and bone scan yearly.

Sarcoma of the Prostate and Bladder. The most common type is rhabdomyosarcoma, which occurs in children, adolescents, and young adults. Compared with rhabdomyosarcoma in other sites, genitourinary sarcomas have a more favorable prognosis, owing to (1) low incidence of regional (20 per cent) or systemic (10 per cent) spread at presentation; (2) propensity to reach massive size before interfering significantly with adjacent organ function; (3) established sensitivity to chemotherapy and radiotherapy; and (4) a favorable (embryonal) histologic type.

Pelvic rhabdomyosarcoma usually arises in the bladder or prostate but may originate in the retrovesical soft tissues, and in females from the uterus, cervix, vagina, or urethra. Wide local excision of the tumor is performed initially if this can be accomplished without removing pelvic organs. VAC (vincristine, actinomycin D, and cyclophosphamide) chemotherapy is administered thereafter for 18 to 24 months. Three-year disease-free survival is 80 per cent. Similar survival rates can be achieved with centrally located pelvic sarcomas involving bladder and prostate, but this requires a pelvic exenteration, diversion of the urinary stream and possibly the fecal stream, and postoperative pelvic radiotherapy and chemotherapy. Because of the morbidity and functional sacrifices imposed by such initial surgical therapy, patients are now treated first with pulse VAC chemotherapy and radiotherapy (PCR). Appropriate (perhaps limited) surgery is reserved for nonresponding patients. This PCR approach has yielded a 70 per cent durable survival with preservation of bladder and bowel functions in 40 per cent of patients. Similar results have been achieved in rhabdomyosarcoma in adults.

Other types of pelvic sarcomas (e.g., leiomyosarcoma, fibrosarcoma) in adults have a much poorer prognosis. Despite the combination of aggressive radical surgery, chemotherapy, and radiotherapy, 5-year survival rates are less than 20 per cent, unless such tumors are small (less than 2 cm) and involve an area of the bladder amenable to segmental cystectomy. Patients with favorable tumors are generally cured of their disease with complete excision.

Malignant Intrascrotal Tumors (Excluding Testis)

These are relatively uncommon neoplasms arising from the epididymis, spermatic cord, or scrotum wall. Approximately one half are malignant, whereas the other half represent benign lipoma of the spermatic cord. The most common presenting symptom is an intrascrotal or inguinal mass.

Treatment depends on the site of origin. Most common are sarcomas arising from the spermatic cord. The treatment is radical orchiectomy, removing the testicle and entire spermatic cord to the level of the internal inguinal ring. Tissue surrounding the cord to the aponeurosis of the external oblique muscle is included, as is a hemiscrotectomy. Wide local excision alone yields 60 to 80 per cent 5-year survival. Similarly, wide local excision of scrotal tumors is performed; pelvic lymph node dissection and radical ilioinguinal groin dissection are also included in patients with histologically proved inguinal metastases.

The most common of these tumors in children is rhabdomyosarcoma of the spermatic cord. This tumor has an excellent prognosis when treated by radical (inguinal) orchiectomy followed by bilateral retroperitoneal lymph node dissection (40 to 60 per cent of such patients will have retroperitoneal nodal metastases). Chemotherapy (VAC) is given for 18 months postoperatively. Para-aortic radiotherapy is also given at a dose of 3000 to 4000 rad to patients with positive retroperitoneal nodes. Five-year survival in patients with negative nodes is over 80 per cent; it is 60 per cent in those with positive nodes. Patients who present with systemic disease or bone marrow involvement have a less than 5 per cent 3-year survival despite treatment.

Testis Cancer

This neoplasm affects males between 15 and 39 years and is the most common cause of cancer deaths in this age group. The incidence rate in the last decade has risen from 2.2 to over 6 per 100,000 males, but is rare in blacks. Testicular cancer occurs two to eight times more frequently in the cryptorchid testis. Orchiopexy is not protective in decreasing this incidence of malignancy. The most common presenting symptom of testicular cancer is an enlarging, relatively asymptomatic hard scrotal mass, although trauma to the testis may alert the patient to the presence of a testicular tumor.

Any patient who presents with an intrascrotal mass suspected of being a neoplasm should undergo an inguinal orchiectomy. Scrotal biopsy or orchiectomy may spill the tumor, contaminate scrotal structures, alter lymphatic pathways of spread, and significantly complicate management. Furthermore, a delay in diagnosis of more than 3 months may result in more therapy and a worse prognosis.

For therapeutic purposes, germ cell neoplasms of the testis are classified as seminoma or nonseminomatous tumors. Both types are staged as follows:

Stage I—tumors confined to the testis.
Stage II—retroperitoneal metastases.
Stage III—distant metastases (usually in lung), often with concomitant retroperitoneal disease.

After radical orchiectomy, stage I and stage II seminoma are treated by para-aortic and ipsilateral inguinal and pelvic radiation therapy (3000 rad in 3 weeks). Prophylactic mediastinal or supraclavicular radiation is not needed. Bulky retroperitoneal or systemic disease is treated with combination chemotherapy. Current drug combinations include vinblastine, actinomycin D, bleomycin, and cisplatin (VAB-6 or PVB regimen). Survival for stages I and II seminoma treated with radiotherapy is 96 per cent and 80 per cent respectively; for stage III seminoma treated with chemotherapy, survival is 70 per cent. Patients for whom conventional therapy for seminoma is not successful (or those with an elevated alpha-fetoprotein level) are treated as for nonseminomatous tumor.

My current therapeutic plan of management for nonseminomatous testicular cancer is the following:

Patients with clinical stage I (normal serum tumor markers, abdominopelvic CT scan, ipsilateral pedal lymphangiogram, and chest x-ray) are offered the option of observation only at monthly intervals for 2 years versus retroperitoneal lymph node dissection. This procedure is associated with a 50 per cent incidence of infertility due to ejaculatory dysfunction. Patients who elect surveillance have a 20 per cent chance of relapse, but my present experience suggests they may be "salvaged" by appropriate chemotherapy or surgery, or both. Limited (nonbulky or less than a 5 cm mass) stage II patients are treated with retroperitoneal lymph node dissection followed by adjuvant chemotherapy (two cycles) with VAB-6 or PVB. Patients are followed at monthly intervals for 2 years. Patients with bulky retroperitoneal disease (mass greater than 5 cm) or disseminated metastases are treated with chemotherapy for three cycles (3 months). Retroperitoneal lymph node dissection or thoracotomy, or both, are undertaken if there is evidence of a "tumor" mass following chemotherapy. Pelvic lymphadenectomy is performed on patients who have had prior inguinal surgery or scrotal violation, or in whom there is involvement of the epididymis or the spermatic cord. The overall survival of patients with stages I and II nonseminomatous tumors is greater than 90 per cent; it is 70 per cent for patients with stage III. The application of multimodal therapy to testicular cancer represents one of the few success stories of solid tumor therapy and is often used as a model for treatment strategies directed to other tumor types. Such success can be attributed to a favorable patient population and improved effective combination chemotherapy regimens and staging modalities of disease, most notably the availability of specific serum tumor markers. As a result, we now have the luxury of considering optimal therapy for all patients, i.e., treatment of those who truly need it and omission of therapy in those who do not. Such approaches have maintained high survival rates and at the same time reduced the therapeutic burden for many patients.

Yolk sac (infantile embryonal carcinoma) is a neoplasm of the testes that occurs in children. This tumor is associated with a low incidence of retroperitoneal metastases. It also produces high levels of alpha-fetoprotein (AFP) in the serum, which may be used as a marker to monitor the course of disease. Although some recommend retroperitoneal lymph node dissection, my policy is to perform inguinal orchiectomy and follow the patient at monthly intervals with AFP levels and chest x-ray. Chemotherapy is indicated at first sign of relapse. Cure rate with a conservative approach is 90 per cent.

Carcinoma of the Penis

Carcinoma of the penis represents less than 1 per cent of all male malignancies. The peak incidence is in the sixth and seventh decades, but the lesion has been seen in patients younger than 40 years of age. Neonatal circumcision is a well-established prophylaxis that almost entirely eliminates the occurrence of penile cancer. In the noncircumcised male, general hygiene and degree of phimosis may play a role in the development of this malignancy. The most common symptom is the presence of a visible lesion associated with purulent penile discharge. Approximately 80 per cent of the lesions are located on either the glans penis or the prepuce, and most are locally infiltrating. About half the patients will have inguinal nodal metastases, but systemic metastases are a late manifestation of disease.

Therapy is dependent on the location of the neoplasm as well as the clinical stage. Patients with disease located on the prepuce may be candidates for a circumcision only. With involvement of the glans or distal one third of the penile shaft, partial penectomy is the treatment of choice. In general, a 2 cm margin for the proximal extent of the cancer is desirable and allows upright voiding and adequate sexual function. More extensive tumors may require total penectomy and creation of a perineal urethrostomy. For selected noninvasive (in situ) tumors limited to the glans penis, external or interstitial irradiation may be an acceptable treatment alternative.

After control of the primary tumor, the groins are examined 6 weeks later. Evidence of adenopathy at this time necessitates biopsy and will reveal metastatic tumor in 50 per cent of cases. Since disseminated disease is rare, bilateral pelvic and ilioinguinal groin dissection is performed and results in 50 to 70 per cent 5-year survival. If, at 6 weeks, careful palpation of the inguinal lesions reveals no adenopathy, the patient is carefully observed. Lymphadenectomy is not recommended prophylacticly because of (1) the high incidence of inflammatory adenopathy at presentation; (2) uncompromised survivorship following delayed lymphadenectomy; and (3) the high incidence of associated operative morbidity, i.e., lower extremity edema.

Patients with inoperable and fixed inguinal nodes may be treated palliatively with either radiation or chemotherapy (cisplatin or methotrexate). Metastatic disease is treated with systemic chemotherapy using one or both of these agents.

Patients are followed every 3 months for 3 years, every 6 months for 2 additional years, and annually thereafter. Careful examination of the genitalia and inguinal regions and chest x-ray are performed at each visit.

URETHRAL STRICTURE

method of
JOHN F. REDMAN, M.D.
University of Arkansas
Little Rock, Arkansas

A practical approach to the management of urethral strictures is to consider treatment based on the location of the stricture within the urethra. It should be assumed for this discussion that the stricture is mature and well delineated. Strictures associated with acute tissue reaction at times require treatment prior to maturation of the scar; however, a period of diversion to allow the reaction to subside is preferable.

Management

Transurethral Methods

Urethral Dilatation. Urethral dilatation is a euphemistic term. In general, the so-called dilatation of a stricture actually involves fracture of the circular cicatrix, which as a result produces multiple tears that in time heal by increased fibrosis. Forcible urethral dilatation usually is a short-lived management of a urethral stricture. In forcible dilatation, a small caliber instrument is passed through the stricture, carrying behind it a portion of the instrument or instruments of a higher caliber. Van Buren sounds may be utilized for the denser strictures. A filiform may be passed thorugh the stricture, followed by a Phillips follower that has been screwed to the proximal end of the filiform. Le Forte sounds have also been employed. These are modifications of the Van Buren sound, with a threaded male tip that will screw into the proximal end of a filiform. In particularly dense strictures the so-called soft dilation technique is at times employed: a small follower or a small catheter is left in place for a period of 24 to 36 hours. Upon removal, a catheter of large diameter can be immediately placed through the stricture as softening of the stricture occurs. This process may be repeated over several days until the desired urethral caliber is achieved.

Blind Internal Urethrotomy. Urethral strictures may be incised by the Otis urethrotome. The body of the instrument allows it to be stretched by means of a proximally located wheel, which places the urethra on stretch. A knife blade that remains hidden in the distal end of the shaft can then be drawn through the urethral stricture, producing a clean cut. The disadvantage of the instrument is that although the knob is calibrated for selection of a specific urethral diameter, the stretch of the urethra may produce far deeper cuts than one would desire. Also, normal urethral mucosa is unnecessarily incised.

Visual Urethrotomy. A most useful recent addition to the tools for management of urethral strictures is the visual urethrotome. A blunt-ended sheath is placed into the urethra. Using a Foroblique lens system and a working element, a knife blade can be introduced into the stricture, and under visualization the stricture can be incised until a normal urethral caliber is achieved. The advantage is that the procedure is done under direct visualization so that only abnormal tissue is incised. A catheter may be put in place for several days to several weeks following incision of the stricture. A further advantage is that the procedure can be done using only topical anesthesia in most cases. Reports of the long-term efficacy of this procedure vary. Even though it requires repetition, it is preferred by some patients as an alternative to an open operative procedure.

Open Operative Techniques

One-Stage Procedures

Excision of Stricture Followed by Urethrourethrostomy. With short anterior urethral strictures, the urethral stricture may be totally excised. The ends of the urethra are spatulated and then reapproximated over a splinting catheter.

Patch Graft Urethroplasty. In selected anterior urethral strictures, the stricture may be incised, carrying the incision a centimeter at least proximally and distally into normal urethra. A free patch graft may then be sewn into the defect over a splinting catheter. An ideal skin to use for a patch graft is the inner leaf of the prepuce. If this skin is not available, penile skin is often taken from the dorsal aspect of the prepuce just proximal to the corona, with the lines of the incision perpendicular to the long axis of the penis.

Free Skin Graft. Free skin grafts may be used, utilizing either a full-thickness skin graft taken from the prepuce or penile skin. The skin is tubed and anastomosed to the proximal and distal remaining urethral segments. Free full-thickness skin grafts taken from other sites, such as the inner aspect of the upper arm, tend in the long run to restricture.

Staged Open Operative Procedures

A frequently utilized technique is to first externalize the stricture by incising through the stricture and then anastomosing the skin to the urethral mucosa itself. After a period of externalization, usually 6 months, the urethra can be reconstructed over a catheter, incorporating the now adjacent skin into the repair. Several techniques are available to bring the skin to the urethra. This is particularly true for bulbous urethral strictures.

Regional Management

Meatal Stenosis. Meatal stenosis is managed by urethral dilatation or by proximal incision of the meatus. A technique often employed to maintain a good urinary stream without splattering is to perform an advancing V flap, described by Horton and Devine, in which V flap of glandular epithelium with its base placed distally is elevated. The urethra is then incised dorsally until the normal caliber is reached, and the tip of the V flap is sewn into the apex of the incised urethra.

Anterior Urethral Strictures

Pendulous Urethral Strictures. These may be managed by urethral dilatation, blind or visual urethrotomy, excision with urethrourethrotomy, patch graft urethroplasty or skin graft, or staged urethroplasty. Bulbous urethral strictures may be handled in all of the aforementioned ways. Staged procedures require good preplanning for the incision. My preference is to swing a perineally based flap, with the tip of the flap being based on the scrotum or just adjacent to the scrotum, as described by Blandy. Flaps of this nature may be moblized deep into the bulbous urethra.

Membranous Urethral Strictures. Membranous urethral strictures may be managed by all the previously described techniques. A urethrourethrostomy, particularly when the defect is rather long, may be accomplished through a perineal incision or may be approached anteriorly through a transpubic incision, often combined with a perineal incision. In these cases the urethra is freed in the perineum and from its attachments to the corpora cavernosa. The prostatic urethra is incised on its anterior aspect, and a spatulated anastomosis is accomplished.

RENAL CALCULI

method of
JOHN R. BURNS, M.D.
University of Birmingham
Birmingham, Alabama

Urolithiasis is a medical problem throughout the world. Bladder calculi are most common in underdeveloped countries and renal calculi in industrialized countries. It has been estimated that 12 per cent of people in the United States will eventually form urinary calculi.

Urolithiasis is a chronic disease. Eighty per cent of patients will have a recurrent stone within 20 years. Long-term follow-up of urinary stone formers is necessary to assess both the effectiveness of treatment and patient compliance. Proper management of a recurrent stone-former involves a long-term commitment by both patient and physician.

In the United States, sterile calcium (calium oxalate and calcium phosphate) calculi account for approximately 80 per cent of urinary calculi. Other commonly encountered calculi are struvite (magnesium ammonium phosphate, infected phosphate), uric acid, and cystine. While the management of the different calculi varies in many respects, the need for adequate hydration and for modification of dietary habits is common to stones of all types.

Diagnostic Considerations

All patients with recurrent stone disease merit full investigation. Patients with cystine, uric acid, and infected phosphate calculi should be evaluated completely. The extent of evaluation of a patient with an initial episode of sterile calcium lithiasis depends on age, sex, and race. Children require complete investigation. Because "idiopathic" stone disease is uncommon in blacks, the etiology should be determined. For a white adult with a first sterile calcium stone, laboratory evaluation consisting of stone analysis, SMA 18 or its equivalent, and determination of urinary acidification is adequate.

On the initial visit to our stone clinic, a patient is instructed to bring a 24 hour urine collection and a diet record. The diet record includes the amounts of all foods, liquids, and medications consumed each day over a 1 week period. The patient is also instructed to record the pH, measured with nitrazine paper, of the first two specimens of voided urine each day. Any stone previously passed is sent to a specialized laboratory for analysis.

General Therapy

Regardless of stone type, increasing the fluid intake is the most effective method of preventing stone recurrence. Rather than prescribing consumption of a fixed amount of fluid (such as 1 gal per day), it is more effective to focus on urine output. A daily output of 3 to 4 liters is ideal. Patients should also be instructed to distribute their fluid intake throughout the day. Risk is maximal in the 2 to 3 hours after a meal and during sleep, so it is necessary to stay well hydrated during these periods. Fluid intake during the evening is sufficient if a patient is required to awaken once to urinate during sleeping hours.

Before any specific antistone therapy begins, the number and size of pre-existing calculi are estimated. Plain films of the abdomen or renal tomograms are obtained to serve as a baseline for judging the effects of therapy. Without them, it is impossible to distinguish the passage of pre-existing calculi from the passage of new stones. Follow-up plain films can then be obtained at 6 month intervals. For patients with a high degree of metabolic stone activity, more frequent radiographs may be required.

Most large studies dealing with treatment for stone disease have demonstrated a placebo effect of 50 per cent or greater. The placebo effect probably occurs as a result of changes in diet and hydration. Patients are instructed as to proper diet on the basis of stone analysis, and the beneficial effects of hydration are stressed.

Cystine Calculi. Patients should submit a 24 hour urine collection for quantitative cystine analysis. Urine of all consanguineous relatives should be screened for cystine with a sodium nitroprusside test. The patient's dietary protein should be limited to less than 56 grams per day.

The mainstay of therapy in these patients is hydration. Urine output must be spaced evenly through the day. Urinary alkalinization is usually required to increase cystine solubility. Alkali should be administered to keep urinary pH above 7.5. Sodium bicarbonate tablets, 40 grains orally every 6 hours is the usual starting dose. Patients are instructed to use nitrazine pH paper and to titrate their dose of alkali by monitoring urinary pH. Patients unable to tolerate a large sodium load can take Polycitra, 15 ml four times daily.

In patients with markedly increased cystine excretion (>1 gram per day), D-penicillamine (250 to 500 mg four times daily) is often necessary. The usefulness of penicillamine is often limited, however, by its toxicity. Common adverse effects include rashes, arthralgia, fever, and proteinuria. Penicillamine should be used only when attempting to dissolve pre-existing calculi or in patients unresponsive to hydration and alkali therapy.

Uric Acid Calculi. Serum calcium should be determined, to rule out hyperparathyroidism, because uric acid stone disease and calcium stone disease may coexist. Initial therapy for uric acid stone formers includes limitation of protein to 56 grams per day and an increase in fluid intake. Sufficient alkali is administered to achieve a constant urinary pH of 6.7 to 7.0. Either sodium bicarbonate or Polycitra is taken at 6 hour intervals.

If the above measures are inadequate to control stone growth or to cause stone dissolution, allopurinol can be added in a single daily dose of 300 mg. Dissolution of pure uric acid calculi occurs rapidly if the aforementioned measures are followed.

Infected Phosphate Calculi. Infected phosphate calculi are composed of a mixture of struvite ($MgNH_4PO_4 \cdot 6H_2O$) and carbonate apatite [$Ca_{10}(PO_4)_6CO_3$]. These calculi can form only after the introduction of a urease-positive bacterial urinary infection, most often with *Proteus*. Patients with neurogenic bladder or foreign bodies in contact with the urinary stream are at high risk for this type of calculi.

The initial management of infected phosphate calculi should be surgical, since infection cannot be adequately controlled until the kidney is free of stones. Surgery is preceded by at least 24 hours of appropriate parenteral antibiotics. Postoperative antibiotics (parenteral followed by oral) should be given for at least 2 to 3 weeks.

Before surgery, serum calcium should be measured. Many menopausal women with infected phosphate calculi have hyperparathyroidism as an underlying disease, and infection is superimposed on metabolic calculi. If hyperparathyroidism is documented, it should be corrected before surgical removal of the calculi.

If retained stone fragments are found postoperatively, irrigation of the kidney with either Renacidin or Urologic G solution is started. Irrigations are continued until the fragments are no longer detected by radiography.

Urinary phosphorus excretion should be maintained below 450 mg per day either by diet or by aluminum gel antacids (Amphogel, 45 ml four times daily, or Basaljel, 30 mg four times daily). Patients should also avoid magnesium-containing medications such as milk of magnesia, Maalox, and Mylanta.

If the above measures are unsuccessful, administration of acetohydroxamic acid should be considered. Acetohydroxamic acid inhibits the action of bacterial urease. Dosage is based on weight and renal function.

Sterile Calcium Calculi. Possible metabolic causes of calcium urolithiasis should first be eliminated. Primary hyperparathyroidism, renal tubular acidosis, and medullary sponge kidney disease account for over 90 per cent of metabolic sterile calcium calculi. Primary hyperparathyroidism can usually be excluded with a fasting serum calcium determination. If the calcium concentration is greater than 10.2 mg per dl, a parathyroid hormone (iPTH) level should be checked.

Renal tubular acidosis accounts for less than 1 per cent of stone formers in most series. Treatment consists of administration of absorbable alkali, with 100 to 150 mEq per day of cation taken in four equally divided doses. Either sodium bicarbonate, potassium bicarbonate, or Polycitra can be used. The dose is titrated until the systemic acidosis is corrected and until urinary citrate excretion has been maximized.

Patients with medullary sponge kidney disease are managed with hydration, dietary modification, and control of infection. Hydrochlorothiazide (50 mg every 12 hours) can be added if these measures fail.

After excluding metabolic causes of calcium urolithiasis, one is left with a large group of "idiopathic stone formers." Through outpatient metabolic evaluation, this group of patients can be subdivided into various categories, including absorptive hypercalciuria, renal leak hypercalciuria, hyperuricosuric calcium oxalate urolithiasis, and enteric hyperoxaluria. For patients with a high rate of stone recurrence, such an evaluation is worthwhile.

For a recurrent sterile calcium stone former with low urinary output and a highly lithogenic diet, medication is initially withheld. The patient is given a several month trial period in which to adhere to a low calcium–low oxalate diet and increase fluid intake. A 24 hour urine collection is obtained after 2 to 3 months. Urine volume and the concentrations of offending stone salts (calcium, oxalate, and uric acid) are measured. If these characteristics do not show improvement, medical therapy is started.

Medical Therapy

Thiazides. Hydrochlorothiazide is effective in treatment for sterile calcium stones. It is most effective in patients with hypercalciuria ($>$ 250 mg per 24 hours). It is, however, also effective in patients with normal urinary calcium and should be considered in any sterile calcium stone former who does not respond to diet modification and increased hydration. Hydrochlorothiazide acts primarily by decreasing urinary calcium. The mean reduction is 150 mg per day. The decrease in urinary calcium is maximal within 1 to 2 weeks. Urinary oxalate may also decrease after long-term administration.

The major adverse effects of thiazides are hypokalemia, hyperglycemia, and hyperuricemia. Potassium supplements are required in approximately 50 per cent of patients. Administration of potassium will prevent the common adverse effects of lassitude, dizziness, and muscle weakness. Development of hyperuricemia in thiazide therapy can be managed either with the administration of allopurinol (300 mg once a day) or by changing to an alternative antistone therapy. In the rare patient who develops diabetes mellitus as a consequence of therapy, thiazides should be discontinued and phosphate therapy instituted. Side effects of thiazide therapy occur in 30 to 35 per cent of patients, usually early in the course of treatment. To reduce the incidence of side effects, patients should be started at 25 mg per day, with increases in the dosage weekly by 25 mg per day until the maintenance dosage of 50 mg twice a day is reached.

Thiazide preparations other than hydrochlorothiazide have been shown to be effective in preventing sterile calcium stones. Bendroflumethiazide (2.5 mg twice daily) and trichlormethiazide (2 mg twice daily) appear to be as effective as hydrochlorothiazide. (This use of these agents is not listed in the manufacturers' directives).

Phosphates. Treatment with orthophosphates increases the urinary excretion of pyrophosphate, a known inhibitor of calcium phosphate and calcium oxalate crystallization. Urinary calcium also decreases; the effect is most pronounced in patients with hypercalciuria.

Orthophosphates are available as acidic, neutral, and alkaline preparations. Therapy in most patients should be started with a neutral preparation. Alkaline phosphates, although possibly more effective than neutral phosphates, contain large amounts of sodium, which may aggravate hypertension or fluid retention. The minimal effective dose for men is 1500 mg or more of phosphorus given in divided doses at 8 hour intervals. A slightly smaller dose, 1250 mg, may be effective in women. If stone disease is not adequately controlled, the dose is gradually increased. A daily dose of 2250 mg of phosphorus may be required.

The major side effect of orthophosphate therapy is diarrhea. This usually occurs early in the course of therapy and may gradually subside. Diarrhea occurs to some extent in all patients and can be minimized by taking the medication after meals rather than before. Patients may also tolerate orthophosphates better if they are started at a lower dose and then gradually increased to therapeutic amounts. Patients with ulcer disease, irritable colon, or pre-existing chronic diarrhea usually will not tolerate orthophosphate therapy. Orthophosphates should be used with caution in patients with recurrent urinary tract infections.

Magnesium. Magnesium deficiency is not common in sterile calcium stone formers. However, many stone formers have low urinary magnesium in relation to calcium. In normal persons, the average molar calcium-to-magnesium (Ca/Mg) ratio is 1.98. In calcium oxalate stone formers, the average ratio rises to 2.76.

Patients with sterile calcium stones and hypercalciuria should first be treated with thiazides. If the molar calcium-to-magnesium ratio remains greater than 2, then magnesium supplements may be worthwhile. Patients are started on one milk of magnesia tablet every 8 hours; 24 hour urine collections are periodically analyzed for calcium and magnesium, and the dosage is titrated to achieve a Ca/Mg ratio of 2 or less.

Allopurinol. The use of allopurinol (300 mg once daily) in the treatment of sterile calcium calculi is controversial. Some series show that in calcium oxalate stone formers with hyperuricosuria, allopurinol markedly reduces the incidence of stone recurrence. The rationale for this beneficial effect is unclear.

In most calcium oxalate stone formers, hyperuricosuria is caused by excessive purine ingestion. A reduction in animal protein intake to 6 to 8 ounces per day will usually reduce uric acid excretion to an acceptable level. Because of the potential adverse effects of allopurinol, it is reserved for patients who form mixed calcium oxalate–uric acid calculi and cannot be controlled by dietary or other conservative measures.

Sodium Cellulose Phosphate. Sodium cellulose phosphate is an ion-exchange resin that combines with calcium in the intestinal lumen, thereby reducing calcium absorption. Gastrointestinal magnesium absorption is also diminished. The usual dosage is 2.5 to 5 grams with each meal or 10 to 15 grams per day. It is important that it be taken with meals for maximal benefit.

Magnesium supplements must be given to avoid any decrease in urinary magnesium excretion. Milk of magnesia tablets (1 tablet twice a day) should be given separately from sodium cellulose phosphate. Patients must also be on a low oxalate diet, because binding of dietary oxalate with intestinal calcium is limited during therapy.

Side effects of sodium cellulose phosphate include dyspepsia, diarrhea, and mild intestinal discomfort. A major consideration in its use is cost. For the average patient on 15 grams per day, the daily cost would exceed $4.00. Thiazides and orthophosphates have been shown to be effective in both absorptive and renal hypercalciuria, so sodium cellulose phosphate would not be considered an ideal first-choice drug. In the occasional patient with absorptive hypercalciuria who cannot tolerate or is otherwise unsuited to thiazides or phosphates, sodium cellulose phosphate would be the drug of choice.

Section 10

Sexually Transmitted Diseases

CHANCROID

method of
TED ROSEN, M.D.
Baylor College of Medicine
Houston, Texas

Chancroid is a sexually transmitted disease which, on clinical grounds, may mimic such diverse disorders as primary syphilis, herpes progenitalis, and granuloma inguinale. Although chancroid is generally considered uncommon in the United States, the recent development of an enriched, selective culture media has led to the recognition of epidemics in California, Georgia, and Canada. Thus, it is likely that the number of verified cases will be higher in the future.

The ability to grow *Haemophilus ducreyi* readily in the laboratory has enabled in vitro antibiotic sensitivities to be determined. Considerable variation occurs in antibiotic susceptibility patterns for organisms recovered from different endemic, epidemic, or sporadic geographic locations. Nonetheless, plasmid-mediated resistance to antibiotics previously considered "standard" therapy for chancroid has become widespread. As a consequence, the treatment regimens suggested in most textbooks have been rendered obsolete.

Treatment

Local washing with soap and water will facilitate removal of crusts and exudates. No ointments or creams should be applied.

Erythromycin, 500 mg orally four times daily for 10 days or until there has been complete resolution of both cutaneous erosions and lymphadenopathy, is the current therapy of choice.

Trimethoprim 160 mg/sulfamethoxazole, 800 mg (Bactrim-DS, Septra-DS), given twice daily for 14 days, has proved to be an effective alternative. Single dose trimethoprim/sulfamethoxazole (640 mg and 3200 mg, respectively) is also efficacious and may be the proper treatment when patient compliance is questionable. Streptomycin, 1.0 gram intramuscularly daily for 6 days, often is effective. As resistance to both of the former drugs of choice, tetracycline and sulfisoxazole, has become common, neither agent is currently recommended as a single therapy. However, the combination of tetracycline, 500 mg, and sulfisoxazole, 1.0 gram, both given orally four times daily, may be effective therapy for patients intolerant of the preferred drugs.

Small series of patients have been successfully treated with minocycline, cephalothin, and amoxicillin. However, data on these antibiotics are too scant to support their use in chancroid unless exceptional circumstances warrant it.

Both erythromycin and tetracycline mask syphilis; trimethoprim/sulfamethoxazole is ineffective against syphilis and does not invalidate tests for lues.

When present, fluctant lymph nodes should be aspirated with an 18 gauge needle. Incision may be performed if needed for adequate drainage.

Concurrent sexually transmitted disease should be suspected and actively sought in all cases of chancroid. Coinfection, particularly with herpes simplex, may be a reason for slow response to adequate antibiotic treatment.

GONORRHEA

method of
MARGARET L. SIMPSON, M.D.
Minneapolis, Minnesota

Although the annual incidence of reported cases of gonococcal infections in the United States has been decreasing, the increasing presence of strains of *Neisseria gonorrhoeae* resistant to penicillin has generated changes in the recommended therapeutic regimens. Another change in the last decade has been rise of the need to inquire about a person's sexual preference in order to appropriately assess for acquisition of a sexually transmitted disease.

UNCOMPLICATED GONORRHEA

Treatment regimens for cervicitis and urethritis:

1. Ampicillin, 3.5 grams (or amoxicillin, 3.0 grams) by mouth, with 1 gram of probenecid by mouth.
2. Tetracycline, 500 mg by mouth four times daily for 7 days or doxycycline (Vibramycin), 100 mg by mouth twice daily for 7 days.
3. Procaine penicillin G, 4.8 million units intramuscularly, with 1 gram of probenecid orally.
4. Spectinomycin (Trobicin), 2 grams intramuscularly.

Treatment regimens for proctitis:

1. Procaine penicillin G, 4.8 million units intramuscularly with 1 gram of probenecid.
2. Spectinomycin (Trobicin), 2 grams intramuscularly.
3. Tetracycline, 500 mg by mouth four times daily for 7 days.

Treatment regimens for pharyngitis:

1. Procaine penicillin G, 4.8 million units intramuscularly, with 1 gram of probenecid by mouth.
2. Tetracycline, 500 mg by mouth four times daily for 7 days.
3. Trimethoprim/sulfamethoxazole (80 mg/400 mg) (Bactrim, Septra), 9 tablets by mouth daily for 5 days. (Use of this agent for this purpose is not listed in the manufacturer's directive.)

Uncomplicated gonorrhea refers to gonococcal infections that remain localized to the site(s) of initial inoculation without causing disabling symptoms and resolve without sequelae if appropriately treated.

The majority of cases of urethral infections are symptomatic; however, cervical, rectal, and pharyngeal infections are frequently asymptomatic. All urethral, cervical, and rectal infections should be appropriately treated with the delineated regimens, whether symptomatic or asymptomatic. The appropriate site should always be cultured in patients with pharyngeal or anal sexual contact, to ascertain whether infection is present.

For urethritis and cervicitis the oral ampicillin (amoxicillin) and probenecid regimen has proved to be almost as efficacious as intramuscular penicillin. To alleviate the problem of the intramuscular injection and the possibility of procaine reactions, this oral regimen might be preferred over intramuscular penicillin in an outpatient facility. Spectinomycin is an excellent alternative for urethral, cervical, and rectal infection but is not effective in the treatment of pharyngeal infections. Tetracycline is inexpensive, but compliance with its administration may be difficult since the dose timing must avoid meals and dairy products. Gastrointestinal intolerance is also a problem with this medication. These problems with tetracycline are not as great as those with an analogue, doxycycline. However, doxycycline is much costlier. A major advantage of the tetracyclines is that they will concurrently eradicate genital infections caused by *Chlamydia trachomatis* and *Ureaplasma urealyticum* (etiologies of postgonococcal urethritis, nongonococcal urethritis, mucopurulent cervicitis, and proctitis). Many advocate administering single dose ampicillin/probenecid followed by a 1 week course of tetracycline, to heterosexual men and women with *Neisseria gonorrhoeae* infections. This provides coverage for the possibility of a coinfection with *Chlamydia trachomatis,* which may occur in up to 40 per cent of heterosexual men and women with gonococcal infections.

Symptomatic proctitis from *Neisseria gonorrhoeae* may occur in men and women with rectal sexual contact. Asymptomatic anorectal infections may occur in women with cervical gonococcal infection, and eradication of infection at this site needs to be documented by a rectal culture after therapy. Asymptomatic infections of the rectum should be treated. Procaine penicillin with probenecid is the best regimen for anorectal infection. Spectinomycin is an excellent alternative, and tetracycline can be used but is associated with more failures. For prolonged symptoms, a single dose treatment may be followed by ampicillin (amoxicillin), 500 mg by mouth four times daily for 7 to 10 days. A thorough examination should be performed, looking for tears, abscesses, or other problems. Presently there is debate over the need to treat asymptomatic pharyngeal gonorrhea, and the majority of infections are asymptomatic. Infections are probably not very transmissable from this site; however, persistent infection at this site may lead to disseminated gonococcal infection. Efficacious regimens for infection at this site include procaine penicillin with probenecid or a 7 day course of tetracycline. An alternative regimen is trimethoprim/sulfamethoxazole—9 single strength tablets by mouth daily for 5 days (use of this agent is not listed in the manufacturer's directive). Local symptoms should be treated with saline gargles and analgesia.

The penicillin regimens and the tetracycline regimen are thought to eradicate incubating syphilis. People being treated with spectinomycin should be followed more closely, as this agent does not treat incubating syphilis.

Infections With Penicillin-Resistant Strains

During the last five years there has been a dramatic increase in the number of infections caused by penicillin-resistant strains of *Neisseria gonorrhoeae* in the United States. The majority of these strains are resistant to penicillin because of the presence of penicillinase; they have also frequently demonstrated increased resistance to other antibiotics, including tetracycline. Treatment failures with the penicillin regimens (when reinfection has been ruled out) should be recultured and the organism tested for penicillinase production, as well as having antibiotic sensitivities performed. These tests are usually available through state health departments and also through the Centers for Disease Control, Atlanta, Georgia. Patients with a history of sexual contact in Africa or Asia should be treated initially for penicillin-resistant *Neisseria gonorrhoeae.*

Treatment regimens for penicillin-resistant *Neisseria gonorrhoeae* infections include the following:

1. Spectinomycin (Trobicin), 2 grams intramuscularly.
2. Cefoxitin (Mefoxin), 2 grams intramuscularly accompanied by 1 gram of probenecid orally.
3. Cefotaxime (Claforan), 1 gram intramuscularly.

All three regimens are effective for uncomplicated genital infections. Spectinomycin is known to be effective with anorectal infections, and cefoxitin and cefotaxime are probably efficacious at this site. For pharyngeal infection with penicillin-resistant strains of *Neisseria gonorrhoeae,* trimethoprim/sulfamethoxazole, 9 single strength tablets by mouth daily for 5 days is the therapy of choice. (This use not listed in the manufacturer's directive).

COMPLICATED GONOCOCCAL DISEASE

Pelvic Inflammatory Disease

In the United States, *Neisseria gonorrhoeae* is isolated from the cervix in 40 to 50 per cent of women with pelvic inflammatory disease (PID). Other etiologic organisms to consider when salpingitis is diagnosed include *Chlamydia trachomatis,* aerobic and anaerobic bacteria, *Mycoplasma hominis,* and *Ureaplasma urealyticum.* Presumptive therapy initially may need to be broad-spectrum to cover the organisms included in the differential diagnosis.

Women who should be hospitalized for salpingitis are those with severe peritonitis (temperature greater than 38 C, severe nausea, rebound tenderness on examination), a suspected pelvic abscess, failure to respond to antibiotics given as an outpatient, or an unclear diagnosis of salpingitis. Some people feel that all women with the diagnosis of pelvic inflammatory disease should be hospitalized.

For gonococcal PID, outpatient regimens include the following:

1. Ampicillin, 3.5 grams (or amoxicillin, 3.0 grams) by mouth with 1 gram of probenecid orally *or*
2. Procaine penicillin G, 4.8 million units intramuscularly with a gram of probenecid orally.

followed by

1. Ampicillin (or amoxicillin), 500 mg orally four times daily for 10 days *or*
2. Tetracycline, 500 mg four times daily (or doxycycline [Vibramycin], 100 mg twice daily) by mouth for 10 days.

For women allergic to penicillin, the tetracycline (or doxycycline) regimen may be used. Tetracycline derivatives cannot be used in pregnant women.

Regimens for women hospitalized with gonococcal PID include:

1. Penicillin G, 3 to 4 millions units intravenously every 4 hours.
2. Doxycycline (Vibramycin), 100 mg intravenously twice daily.
3. Cefoxitin (Mefoxin), 1 to 2 grams intravenously every 4 hours.

The intravenous regimen should be continued for 48 hours after defervescence or marked improvement in symptoms. One of the oral regimens should then be used to complete a 10 day course of therapy.

For PID caused by penicillin-resistant *Neisseria gonorrhoeae* strains, the cefoxitin regimen or spectinomycin, 2 grams intramuscularly twice daily, may be used.

Women in whom a pelvic abscess is suspected need broad coverage for aerobic and anaerobic bacteria.

To provide coverage of *Chlamydia trachomatis* in the treatment of PID some physicians are strong proponents of a tetracycline (or doxycycline) regimen. However, tetracyclines cannot be used in pregnant women.

Epididymitis

In sexually active young men, the most common causes of epididymitis are infections with *Neisseria gonorrhoeae* or *Chlamydia trachomatis.* In older men, coliform bacteria or *Pseudomonas aeruginosa* accounts for the majority of cases. For gonococcal urethritis with epididymitis, one of the following regimens should be used:

1. Procaine penicillin, 4.8 million units intramuscularly with 1 gram of probenecid, orally *or*
2. Ampicillin, 3.5 grams by mouth (or amoxicillin, 3.0 grams) with a 1 gram of probenecid by mouth.

followed by

1. Ampicillin (amoxicillin), 500 mg orally four times a day for 10 days *or*
2. Tetracycline, 500 mg orally four times a day (doxcycline [Vibramycin], 100 mg twice daily) for 10 days.

The tetracycline (doxycycline) regimen will also cover *Chlamydia trachomatis* and should be used in sexually active young men in whom *Neisseria gonorrhoeae* is not isolated.

With penicillin-resistant *Neisseria gonorrhoeae* as the etiology, intravenous cefoxitin or trimethoprim/sulfamethoxazole may be used for treatment.

Disseminated Gonococcal Infections (Arthritis-Dermatitis Syndrome)

Mild cases may be managed on an outpatient basis with careful follow-up. Regimens for the ambulatory patient include the following:

1. Procaine penicillin G, 4.8 million units intramuscularly with 1 gram of probenecid orally *or*
2. Ampicillin, 3.5 grams (amoxicillin, 3 grams) orally with 1 gram of probenecid orally.

followed by

1. Ampicillin (amoxicillin), 500 mg orally four times a day for 7 days.
2. Tetracycline, 500 mg orally four times a day for 7 days.
3. Erythromycin, 500 mg orally four times a day for 7 days.

The tetracycline regimen is the alternative regimen in the penicillin-allergic patient but cannot be used in pregnant women. Erythromycin may be used during pregnancy.

Patients who have frank septic arthritis, are somewhat toxic and febrile, or have severe tenosynovitis probably should be hospitalized and started on parenteral antibiotics. Initial therapeutic regimens include:

1. Aqueous crystalline penicillin G, 10 million units intravenously per day in 4 to 6 divided doses.
2. Spectinomycin (Trobicin), 2 grams intramuscularly two times a day (not listed in manufacturer's directive).
3. Cefoxitin (Mefoxin), 1 gram intravenously four to six times a day.

The parenteral antibiotics can be changed to one of the oral regimens when definite improvement in the condition has occurred. A total of at least 7 days of antibiotics should be administered. Parenteral antibiotics are usually needed for a longer period of time with septic arthritis. Repeated aspiration may be needed initially in a patient with septic arthritis, in addition to joint immobilization. Intra-articular antibiotics do not need to be administered.

For penicillin-resistant disseminated infections, cefoxitin or spectinomycin (not listed in the manufacturer's directive) may be used. Trimethoprim/sulfamethoxazole (not listed in the manufacturer's directive), 9 single strength tablets orally per day may be used as an alternative.

Pregnancy

Any of the penicillin or ampicillin type of antibiotics are safe in pregnancy and may be used to treat gonococcal infections. In the pregnant patient who is penicillin-allergic, cefoxitin, cefotaxime, or spectinomycin may be used, although the safety of these drugs in pregnancy has not been thoroughly proved. Erythromycin may be used to treat the possibility of coinfection with *Chlamydia trachomatis* since tetracycline administration is contraindicated during pregnancy.

Infants and Children

Because an infant born to a mother with gonorrheal infection is at high risk for infection, the infant should be treated with aqueous crystalline penicillin. A dose of 50,000 units for full-term infants or 20,000 units for low birth weight infants should be administered intravenously or intramuscularly. This is not adequate treatment for clinical gonococcal disease.

Ophthalmia Neonatorum

The prevention of ophthalmia neonatorum has been accomplished by the use of 1 per cent silver nitrate. More recently the use of 0.5 per cent erythromycin or 1 per cent tetracycline has been increasing. The antibiotic eye drops cause less chemical conjunctivitis and may provide some coverage for *Chlamydia trachomatis* also.

The treatment of ophthalmia neonatorum is with aggressive systemic therapy. Aqueous crystalline penicillin G, 50,000 units per kg per day parenterally should be given in two divided doses for 7 days. Topical therapy should include irrigation with saline or buffered ophthalmic solutions immediately and then hourly until the discharge is eliminated. Untreated ophthalmia neonatorum is very contagious and may rapidly lead to blindness.

Infections with penicillin-resistant organisms

should be treated with cefotaxime or gentamicin in appropriate neonatal doses.

Uncomplicated Genitourinary Infection, Proctitis, and Pharyngitis

For children weighing 45 kg (100 lbs) or greater, the adult doses of the antibiotic regimens can be used. The therapy for vulvovaginitis and urethritis includes:

1. Amoxicillin, 50 mg per kg orally, plus probenecid, 25 mg per kg (maximum 1 gram) orally, *or*
2. Procaine penicillin G, 100,000 units per kg intramuscularly with probenecid, 25 mg per kg (maximum 1 gram) orally.

The second regimen should be used for pharyngeal and rectal infections.

Disseminated Complicated Infections

Children not very ill may be treated on an outpatient basis. Children weighing more than 45 kg (100 lbs) should receive the adult doses of antibiotics.

Hospitalized children should receive aqueous crystalline penicillin, 75,000 to 100,000 units per kg divided into 2 to 4 doses for 7 to 10 days. Alternative regimens for penicillin-allergic children include spectinomycin, and cefoxitin or cefotaxime in appropriate doses.

Any child diagnosed with a gonococcal infection should be actively investigated for sexual abuse.

PREVENTION, EPIDEMIOLOGY, AND FOLLOW-UP

The use of condoms, the diaphragm, a cervical cap, or spermicidal agents may reduce the transmission of genital infection. Urinating, washing, or douching after intercourse are not believed to be beneficial. Although the prophylactic administration of antibiotics immediately before or soon after sexual exposure reduces the risk of infection, this is not recommended.

Patients who have had sexual contact within the last 30 days with a person documented as having a gonococcal infection should be treated after cultures are obtained without waiting for the results. Male contacts of women with gonococcal pelvic inflammatory disease (PID) frequently have asymptomatic gonococcal urethritis. Treatment of male contacts of patients with PID may be extended to sexual contact within 90 days.

Test-of-cure cultures should be obtained 3 to 7 days after the course of treatment has been completed. All known infected sites should be recultured. In women with documented endocervical infection, anorectal cultures should also be obtained at the follow-up visit.

GRANULOMA INGUINALE

method of
MAX R. TAYLOR, M.D.
University of Mississippi
Tupelo, Mississippi

Granuloma inguinale is caused by *Calymmatobacterium granulomatis,* a bipolar staining bacillus found within histiocytes, using Giemsa or Wright's stain on crush preparations of the lesion. The organism does not grow predictably on routine media and in vitro susceptibility data are lacking. Controlled, comparative clinical trials of antimicrobials are also not available. Initial therapy should be tetracycline hydrochloride, 500 mg orally four times daily for a minimum of 3 weeks or until the lesion heals. Duration of therapy generally depends on the size of the lesion and may take 4 to 6 weeks. If no response occurs after 2 weeks, resistance to tetracycline is possible, or another diagnosis should be considered.

Successful alternative regimens are the double strength tablet of trimethoprim-sulfamethoxazole taken orally twice a day or erythromycin, 500 mg, taken orally four times daily. Chloramphenicol, gentamicin, and streptomycin, although more toxic, are efficacious alternatives that are reserved for resistant cases. Relapses occur occasionally and prolonged observation after therapy is recommended, because the pathogenesis of the disease is poorly understood. Coexistent sexually transmitted diseases should be sought in patients and contacts.

LYMPHOGRANULOMA VENEREUM

method of
MAX R. TAYLOR, M.D.
University of Mississippi
Tupelo, Mississippi

Lymphogranuloma venereum is caused by serotypes L–1, L–2, and L–3 of *Chlamydia trachomatis*. The primary lesion is usually inapparent and is followed by invasion of lymphatics and constitutional symptoms. The primary lesion and secondary phase, which usually presents as tender or suppurative lymphadenopathy, are treated with tetracycline hydrochloride, 500 mg orally four times daily for 3 to 6 weeks. Needle aspiration of fluctuant nodes is preferred over incision or spontaneous drainage, which may result in a chronic draining sinus. Untreated, the secondary phase leads to a tertiary phase of chronic sinuses, fistulas, strictures, and lymphedema. These chronic sequelae usually require combined antimicrobial and surgical therapy. Response to therapy is indicated more by reduction in size and fluctuance of lymph nodes and closure of sinus tracts and fistulas than by falling serologic titers.

Chlamydia grow in tissue culture; therefore, standard antimicrobial susceptibilities are not available. Erythromycin, 500 mg orally four times daily, or sulfisoxazole, 1.0 gm orally twice a day, are also used, if tetracycline is not tolerated or fails. Chloramphenicol, 500 mg four times daily, and other tetracycline derivatives have also been useful. Coexistent sexually transmitted diseases should be sought in patients and contacts.

SYPHILIS

method of
MICHAEL F. REIN, M.D.
University of Virginia
Charlottesville, Virginia

There is no evidence that the spirochete of syphilis has become resistant to penicillin or other antibiotics. Virulent *Treponema pallidum* is killed at the maximum rate by concentrations of penicillin G as low as 0.1 μg per ml. Penicillin G remains the treatment of choice for all forms and stages of syphilis in patients who are not allergic to the drug. Clinical and laboratory data support the value of relatively long duration therapy for the successful treatment of syphilis. The single dose regimens used for treating gonorrhea cannot be assumed to cure established syphilis.

Contacts to Infectious Syphilis

One third to one half of the sexual partners of patients with primary or secondary syphilis will contract the infection. Clinical and serologic evidence of infection may develop as late as 90 days after exposure (although it usually becomes manifest in about 21 days). Patients exposed during the previous 90 days should be treated as if they had early syphilis, since the probability of infection is high. Treating the patient prior to the appearance of a syphilitic lesion will prevent spread of infection to other sexual partners. Adequate treatment given before a patient's nontreponemal serologic test becomes reactive will prevent the development of seroreactivity.

Early Syphilis

For therapeutic purposes, early syphilis is defined as primary or secondary syphilis or latent syphilis of less than 1 year's duration. The diagnosis can be made on clinical grounds or by a nonreactive serologic test within the past year.

The regimen of choice because of its efficacy and convenience is benzathine penicillin G, 2.4 million units total by intramuscular injection, half the total dose being administered in each buttock.

Patients allergic to penicillin may be treated with tetracycline hydrochloride, 500 mg four times daily by mouth for 15 days. Patients should be cautioned to take the drug on an empty stomach (60 minutes before or 2 hours after eating) and not with milk or antacids.

Penicillin-allergic patients for whom tetracycline is also contraindicated (late pregnancy, hypersensitivity, gastrointestinal intolerance) may be treated with erythromycin, 500 mg four times daily by mouth for 15 days. The drug should be administered as the enteric-coated base, stearate or ethylsuccinate. Erythromycin estolate has no obvious therapeutic advantage and has been associated with hepatic enzyme elevations.

More than half the patients treated for early syphilis will experience a Jarisch-Herxheimer reaction. Usually beginning within 6 hours of treatment, the reaction consists of fever, transient exacerbation of skin lesions or adenopathy, occasional arthralgias, and, rarely, transient hypotension. The reaction is usually mild and abates in less than 24 hours. It can be managed with aspirin and reassurance.

Latent, Cardiovascular, and Late Benign Syphilis

It is generally thought that syphilis of longer duration requires therapy of longer duration. This may be because more spirochetes are present, they are reproducing more slowly, or they may be residing in microenvironments relatively protected from antibiotics. There is little to suggest that antibiotics reverse the pathology of cardiovascular syphilis.

From the standpoint of efficacy and convenience, the regimen of choice is benathine penicillin G, 7.2 million units total: 2.4 million units by intramuscular injection divided into two doses and administered at the same session. This treatment is administered weekly for three visits.

No published clinical data adequately document the efficacy of drugs other than penicillin for syphilis of more than 1 year's duration. Thus, a history of penicillin allergy should be carefully documented before alternatives to penicillin are used. In this setting, skin testing for immediate hypersensitivity to penicillin may be particularly useful. Patients allergic to penicillin may be treated with tetracycline hydrochloride, 500 mg four times daily by mouth for 30 days. The drug should be taken on an empty stomach, either 60 minutes before or 2 hours after eating, and should not be taken with milk or antacids. Penicillin-allergic patients who cannot take tetracycline may be treated with erythromycin, 500 mg four times daily by mouth for 30 days. The drug should be administered as the enteric-coated base, stearate, or ethylsuccinate.

Neurologically asymptomatic patients with syphilis of undetermined duration should have an examination of the cerebrospinal fluid (CSF) to rule out asymptomatic neurosyphilis. Considerable doubt exists as to whether any of the aforementioned regimens is effective in the treatment of neurosyphilis.

Symptomatic or Asymptomatic Neurosyphilis

Optimal therapy for syphilis of the central nervous system is controversial. Published data on the efficacy of benzathine penicillin G are limited. Many patients treated with benzathine penicillin G have undetectable penicillin levels in CSF, and there are anecdotal reports of patients failing to respond to benzathine penicillin G who apparently responded to subsequent treatment with higher dose regimens.

The treatment of choice for patients with documented neurosyphilis is crystalline penicillin G (potassium or sodium), 20 million units intravenously per 24 hours by continuous infusion or in divided doses every 3 to 4 hours for 15 days. Although there are no supporting clinical data, some experts recommend following this with benzathine penicillin G, 2.4 million units intramuscularly weekly for 3 weeks.

Alternatively, one might administer procaine penicillin G, 2.4 million units intramuscularly daily for 15 days along with probenecid, 500 mg by mouth four times daily. This, too, might be followed by the benzathine penicillin G regimen described in the preceding paragraph.

The United States Public Health Service also recommends benzathine penicillin G, 2.4 million units by intramuscular injection weekly for 3 successive visits.

The treatment of neurosyphilis with drugs other than penicillin is empiric. Penicillin allergy should be well documented before alternative therapies are employed. Patients whose allergy does not involve anaphylaxis might be treated with cefotaxime (Claforan), 2 grams intravenously every 4 hours for 15 days. If the patient has had an anaphylactic reaction to penicillin, neurosyphilis on theoretic grounds might be treated with chloramphenicol (Chloromycetin), 500 mg orally four times daily for 30 days. Hematologic parameters should be followed weekly. Chloramphenicol penetrates well into the central nervous system. Alternatively, one might consider the administration of erythromycin (stearate, ethylsuccinate, or enteric-coated base) or tetracycline in the same doses.

Syphilis in Pregnancy

The pregnant woman should be treated with a penicillin regimen appropriate to her stage of syphilis. Such regimens are highly effective in preventing the stigmata of congenital syphilis in the baby.

Because the efficacy of nonpenicillin drugs in preventing congenital syphilis is not adequately established, documentation of penicillin allergy in pregnant women is important. The penicillin-allergic pregnant woman should be treated with erythromycin in doses appropriate to her stage of syphilis.

Pregnant women who have been treated for syphilis should have monthly quantitative nontreponemal serologic tests for the remainder of the current pregnancy. Women showing a fourfold rise in titer should be retreated. After delivery, follow-up is the same as for nonpregnant patients.

Congenital Syphilis

Infants with congenital syphilis should have an examination of the CSF before treatment to serve as a baseline. All infants, however, should receive a regimen effective against neurosyphilis. They should be treated with aqueous crystalline penicillin G, 50,000 units per kg intramuscularly or intravenously daily in two divided doses for a minimum of 10 days. Alternatively, one may administer procaine penicillin G, 50,000 units per kg intramuscularly daily for a minimum of 10 days.

Immediate hypersensitivity to penicillin is not a problem in neonates. Babies born to mothers whose gestational syphilis was treated with a drug other than penicillin should be given penicillin at birth as if they had congenital syphilis.

Older children with congenital syphilis should be treated with similar regimens, but the total dose of penicillin need never exceed that administered to adults. Children under the age of 8 years who are allergic to penicillin should be treated with erythromycin, 30 to 50 mg per kg per day in four oral divided doses for 2 weeks. Older penicillin-allergic children may be treated with erythromycin or tetracycline.

The Jarisch-Herxheimer reaction may be observed in the treatment of congenital syphilis.

Follow-Up

Adequate therapy for all stages of syphilis is suggested by a fourfold drop in titer of a quantitative nontreponemal test (VDRL, RPR, ART) for syphilis. Patients treated for syphilis should return for nontreponemal serologic tests every 3 months until a fourfold drop in titer is observed. Thereafter, patients should return for serologic testing every 3 to 6 months until the quantitative nontreponemal test has become nonreactive or the titer has remained stable for 6 months. Documentation of the patient's lowest post-treatment titer is important to detect relapse or reinfection. After a patient has demonstrated a fourfold drop in the titer of a nontreponemal test for syphilis, a subsequent fourfold rise is highly suggestive of relapse or reinfection. The same nontreponemal test must be used in following a patient's course. Titers obtained with the RPR (rapid plasma reagin) test and the ART (automated reagin test) are frequently two to eight times higher than those obtained with the VDRL (Venereal Disease Research Laboratory) test, and interchanging results from different tests may prove confusing.

After adequate treatment for primary syphilis, most patients manifest a fourfold drop in the nontreponemal titer in 3 months, three fourths of patients will have a nonreactive VDRL test result within 1 year, and 97 per cent will be seronegative within 2 years. After treatment for secondary syphilis, 42 per cent of patients will have a nonreactive VDRL test result within 1 year, and three fourths will be seronegative within 2 years. Patients having untreated syphilis for more than 2 years are unlikely to become nonreactive with the nontreponemal tests but should still show a fourfold drop in titer within 12 months of completing therapy. The FTA-ABS (fluorescent treponemal antibody absorption) test or the MHA-TP (microhemagglutination test for *Treponema pallidum*) generally remains reactive even after adequate therapy. A persistently reactive treponemal test is not, therefore, an indication for retreatment.

The efficacy of drugs other than high dose penicillin for the treatment of asymptomatic neurosyphilis is uncertain. CSF should be examined two years after completing therapy for syphilis if

—The patient was treated with a nonpenicillin regimen.

—The patient had syphilis of greater than 1 year's or unknown duration and CSF was not examined at the time of therapy.

—*Possibly*, in all cases of syphilis treated with benzathine penicillin G. Spirochetes invade the central nervous system in many patients with early syphilis. If these organisms are not eradicated by regimens that kill extrameningeal spirochetes, apparently cured patients may later develop symptomatic neurosyphilis. Recent preliminary data suggest that this may rarely occur in patients whose early syphilis was treated with benzathine penicillin G.

Patients treated for neurosyphilis should have a re-examination of CSF every 3 months until an adequate response is demonstrated. After adequate treatment, 60 to 80 per cent of patients no longer show CSF pleocytosis within 3 months. CSF protein levels return to normal within 6 months, and the VDRL titer in CSF generally shows a fourfold drop within 6 months. Patients treated for neurosyphilis should be followed for several years.

Section 11

Diseases of Allergy

ANAPHYLAXIS AND SERUM SICKNESS

method of
JAMES EASTON, M.D.
University of California, Los Angeles
Los Angeles, California

ANAPHYLAXIS

Anaphylaxis is an immunologic reaction resulting from re-exposure to an antigenic substance, previous exposure to this substance or to an antigenically cross-reactive substance having caused the production of IgE antibodies, which became fixed on the surfaces of basophils and tissue mast cells. Upon re-exposure, interaction of antigen with these antibodies results in the secretion of many chemical mediators from the cells, of which histamine appears to be of primary importance in anaphylaxis. These mediators, in turn, act on the vasculature, airway smooth muscle, and mucous glands, causing the pathophysiologic changes and clinical manifestations. Anaphylactoid reactions are clinically indistinguishable from anaphylaxis but are the result of nonimmunologic mechanisms. Agents responsible for this type of reaction are thought to have a direct (IgE antibody not involved) effect on basophils and mast cells, causing mediator release. In this situation previous exposure to the etiologic factor is unnecessary.

The number of causative agents implicated in anaphylaxis or anaphylactoid reactions is exhaustive; apparently any drug can be responsible. Agents most frequently involved are listed in Table 1. Recently an unusual symptom complex of urticaria, angioedema and anaphylaxis induced by strenuous physical exercise has been described.

Clinical manifestations and their rapidity of onset and severity vary considerably from individual to individual. Usually they begin within minutes of exposure to the etiologic agent but may be more delayed, particularly with ingested agents. In general the more rapid the onset, the more severe the overall course. Major signs and symptoms are shown in Table 2. Cutaneous manifestations are the most common whereas respiratory and cardiovascular involvement are the most serious.

TABLE 1. **Common Etiologic Agents**

Anaphylaxis
Antibiotics
penicillins
cephalosporins
sulfa and trimethoprim-sulfa
clindamycin
Other drugs and therapeutic agents
allergy extracts
heterologous antisera
insulin
chymotrypsin and chymopapain
ACTH
egg protein–containing vaccines
Foods
fish
shellfish
eggs
nuts
legumes
Anaphylactoid Reactions
Aspirin and nonsteroidal anti-inflammatory agents
Iodinated radiographic contrast media

TABLE 2. **Major Manifestations of Anaphylaxis and Anaphylactoid Reactions**

Cutaneous
pruritus
flushing
urticaria
angioedema
Respiratory
hoarse voice and stridor
wheeze
cough
dyspnea
cyanosis
Cardiovascular
rapid weak pulse
hypotension
arrhythmias

Treatment

Prevention is the most important aspect of the management of anaphylaxis and anaphylactoid reactions. A history suggesting even mild symptoms associated with these reactions is an integral part of any medical record, and avoidance of the etiologic agent and immunologically cross-reacting substance, such as cephalosporins in penicillin-sensitive patients, is essential whenever possible. Skin tests to detect the presence of IgE antibodies can be performed for a limited number of drugs such as penicillin, horse serum, insulin, chymopapain, and some vaccines, and are helpful when the history is equivocal and no alternative therapeutic agent is acceptable. Skin testing is of *no* value in anaphylactoid reactions. Testing should be performed or supervised by someone familiar with the technique, interpretation of results, and possible hazards. A negative skin test significantly reduces but does not completely eliminate the possibility of anaphylaxis.

When a patient is felt to be at risk for anaphylaxis and no alternative agent is satisfactory for use, "desensitization" may be attempted and is usually successful. This is most frequently done in individuals sensitive to penicillin or horse serum. Specific protocols are beyond the scope of this discussion but can be found in standard allergy texts and in the package inserts of most antisera. Desensitization should be supervised by a physician knowledgeable with the procedure and performed where emergency equipment and drugs are immediately available.

Anaphylactoid reactions to iodinated radiographic contrast media can be significantly modified and in many instances prevented in patients who have had a previous reaction and in whom repeat studies are essential. Prednisone, 50 mg orally, is given at 6 hour intervals for three doses, with the last dose given 1 hour before the procedure. Diphenhydramine (Benadryl), 50 mg intravenously or intramuscularly, and ephedrine, 25 mg orally, are given at the same time as the last dose of prednisone.

Persons with known anaphylaxis or anaphylactoid reactions should wear Medic-Alert bracelets obtainable from Medic-Alert Foundation, Turlock, CA 95380. Patients with reactions to Hymenoptera stings or to food which they may accidentally ingest in some "hidden" form and the occasional patient for whom no etiologic agent can be established should carry a preloaded epinephrine-containing syringe for self-administration, having been properly instructed in its use.

Anaphylaxis and anaphylactoid reactions are true medical emergencies, and the prompt institution of appropriate therapy is essential (Table 3). Since these reactions may be rapidly progressive, it is important that therapy be started even with minimal manifestations. All physicians must have well in mind a basic plan of treatment, as well as having emergency equipment and drugs immediately available. A list of basic supplies is found in Table 4. If the etiologic factor is an insect sting or medication given subcutaneously or intramuscularly, further systemic absorption can be minimized by the application of a tourniquet proximal to the injection site, remembering to loosen it periodically. Aqueous epinephrine 1:1,000 is the primary therapeutic agent and is given in doses of 0.3 to 0.5 ml by deep subcutaneous or intramuscular injection. This dose may be repeated at intervals of 15 to 20 minutes if necessary, based on frequent monitoring of pulse and blood pressure. In the most profound reactions a 1:10,000 concentration may be given intravenously. In all but very mild reactions an intravenous site should be established promptly. Hypotension occurs as the result of loss of adequate circulating blood volume and is managed by rapid infusion of physiologic saline solution sufficient to maintain a reasonably normal blood pressure. Additional management of hypotension, if necessary, can be accomplished

TABLE 3. **Outline of Treatment of Anaphylaxis and Anaphylactoid Reactions**

Primary Therapy
1. Apply tourniquet above injection site if appropriate
2. Aqueous epinephrine 1:1,000, 0.3 to 0.5 ml, repeated every 15 to 20 minutes if necessary
3. Establish intravenous site
4. Administer oxygen
5. Monitor pulse and blood pressure frequently
6. Physiologic saline solution intravenously for hypotension

Secondary Therapy
1. Diphenhydramine (Benadryl), 25 to 50 mg intravenously
2. Aminophylline, 5 mg/kg diluted in 50 ml of physiologic saline, administered intravenously over 10 to 15 minutes for bronchospasm; repeat every 4 to 6 hours as indicated
3. Hydrocortisone (Solu-Cortef), 500 to 1000 mg, or methylprednisolone (Solu-Medrol), 125 to 250 mg intravenously every 4 to 6 hours
4. Metaraminol (Aramine), 0.3 to 0.4 mg/kg in 500 ml of intravenous fluid for additional control of hypotension

TABLE 4. **Basic Equipment for Treatment of Anaphylaxis**

Aqueous epinephrine 1:1,000
Diphenhydramine (Benadryl) for injection
Oxygen
Tourniquets
Syringes, needles, and tubing for subcutaneous and intravenous use
Physiologic saline for intravenous infusion
Sphygmomanometer
Metaraminol (Aramine)

by the use of metaraminol bitartrate (Aramine), 0.3 to 0.4 mg per kg in 500 ml of physiologic saline with adjustment of the rate of administration based on frequent blood pressure monitoring.

Airway obstruction, either as the result of upper airway edema or bronchospasm in lower airways with asthma-like symptoms, usually responds to epinephrine administration. Intravenous aminophylline, 5 mg per kg diluted in 50 ml of physiologic saline given over 15 to 20 minutes, may be used for additional control of bronchospasm. Hypoxemia exists in the face of even mild airway obstruction, and supplementary oxygen should be administered.

Recent reports indicate that anaphylaxis may be more severe in individuals taking beta-adrenergic blocking agents, and much more aggressive therapy is required.

Corticosteroids and antihistamines are secondary therapeutic agents to be given only after the previously discussed measures have been implemented. Hydrocortisone sodium succinate (Solu-Cortef), 500 to 1000 mg, or methylprednisolone sodium succinate (Solu-Medrol), 125 to 250 mg, is given intravenously at 4 to 6 hour intervals, and diphenhydramine (Benadryl), up to 50 mg intravenously or intramuscularly, can be administered every 4 hours.

Mild recurrences of symptoms are common for 24 to 48 hours following remission of the acute stage. Slow-release epinephrine suspension (Susphrine), 0.15 to 0.2 ml subcutaneously, and diphenhydramine (Benadryl), 50 mg orally every 4 to 6 hours, should be used for control.

Important aspects of overall management are discussions with the patient regarding the etiologic agent (if known) and cross-reacting substances, follow-up investigations if indicated, the possibility of future reactions, and the availability of effective desensitization injections in the case of insect sting anaphylaxis.

SERUM SICKNESS

Serum sickness is a more slowly evolving immunologic reaction presumed to be mediated by immune complexes of IgG and antigen. In its classic form, clinical manifestations begin 7 to 12 days after initial exposure to the antigen, but if a previous exposure has resulted in development of appropriate antibodies it may begin within hours of re-exposure (accelerated serum sickness). Therapeutic agents, particularly antibiotics, are the most common causes.

Common clinical manifestations include urticaria, angioedema, arthralgias, and frequently low grade fever. Vasculitis and immune complex nephritis occur rarely. Laboratory tests are not often helpful. A mild to moderate leukocytosis is often present, whereas eosinophilia may or may not be present. Depressed levels of total hemolytic complement (CH_{50}) or the complement components C_3 and C_4 are helpful if present, as is a positive test for circulating immune complexes. One must remember, however, that laboratory abnormalities may reflect the underlying disease state for which a therapeutic agent was given initially.

Treatment. Discontinuance of the etiologic agent, if determined, is the most important aspect of management. Symptoms frequently last several days and occasionally as long as 2 to 3 weeks after discontinuance, but recovery is generally complete. Antihistamines such as hydroxazine (Atarax, Vistaril), 20 mg three to four times daily, are helpful for the urticaria and pruritus, and aspirin is useful for arthralgia. In more severe cases corticosteroids may be required for control. Prednisone orally in doses of 1 to 2 mg per kg per day (maximum, 60 mg) in three divided doses for 5 to 7 days, followed by relatively rapid tapering of the dose over an additional 4 to 6 days, is generally used. In the occasional prolonged severe case, prednisone may be continued, using the smallest amount necessary for control of symptoms, as a single morning dose on alternate days.

ASTHMA IN THE ADOLESCENT AND ADULT

method of
W. JAMES METZGER, M.D.
East Carolina University
Greenville, North Carolina

Asthma is a syndrome of reversible obstructive airways characterized by hyperresponsiveness to a variety of stimuli. It is usually associated with excessive production of mucus, mucosal inflammation and edema, and eosinophilia of blood, airways, tissue, and sputum. The degree of reversibility is said to be essentially complete. Traditionally, asthma has been classified as being extrinsic (allergic), intrinsic (idiopathic or infectious), mixed, or aspirin-sensitive. These designations imply pathogenesis.

Perhaps it is more useful to consider precipitating factors or "triggers" for asthma, which exacerbate already hyperresponsive airways to constrict, become edematous, and produce excessive mucus (Fig. 1). Asthma affects thousands of adults and adolescents each year, causing time lost from work or school, multiple hospitalizations and emergency room visits, and several thousand deaths. Occupationally induced or precipitated asthma has become increasingly important as new technology brings new exposures to irritants and sensitizers. Exercise, in this era of physical fitness, limits possibilities for some asthmatics. For these reasons it is important to understand what constitutes asthma, how it can be prevented or treated, and the prognosis for each individual.

CUMULATIVE THERAPY FOR ASTHMA

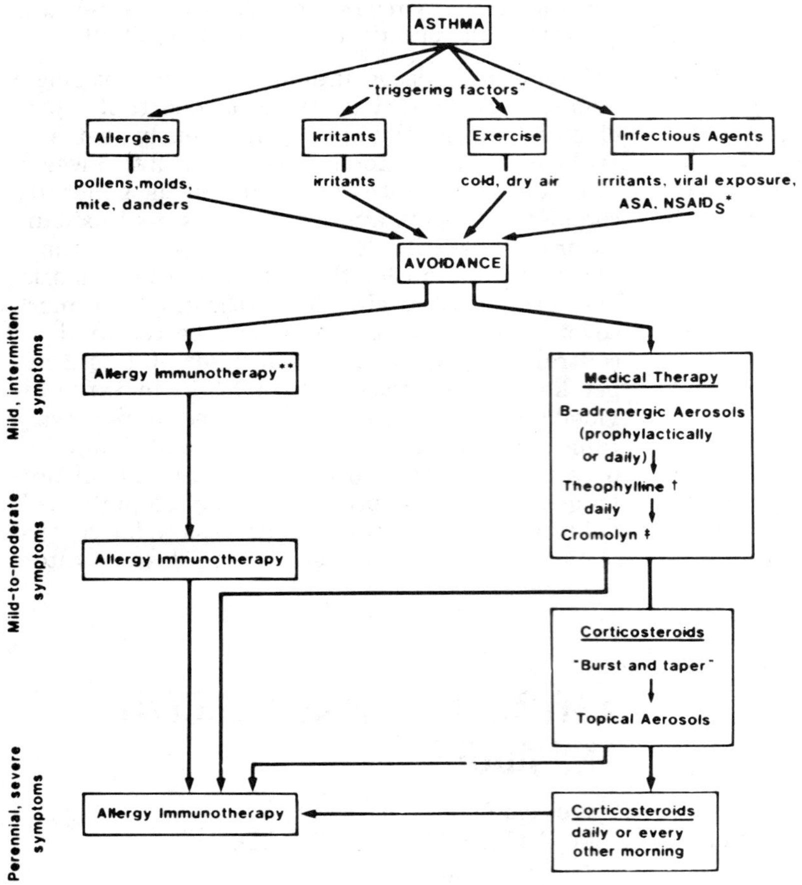

* NSAIDS nonsteroidal anti inflammatory drugs.

** Immunotherapy may be used alone, in addition to avoidance, or in conjunction with other medical therapy.

† Sustained release preparations promote compliance, reduce side effects, and facilitate monitoring.

‡ Cromolyn may be used before theophyline and may be useful for exercise induced asthma or intermittent exposure, such as animal danders.

Figure 1. An algorithm showing the cumulative method for developing a therapeutic regimen for symptomatic asthma.

Bronchoprovocation

Bronchoprovocation with histamine or methacholine "triggers" asthma and differentiates asthmatics from normal subjects based upon the degree of hyperresponsiveness. Those with allergic rhinitis or intermittent asthma fall between these two groups. Aerosol challenge with these chemicals causes bronchospasm followed by spontaneous reversal and is limited to an immediate response. Allergen bronchoprovocation produces an immediate (early) asthmatic response and, in some individuals, also a late asthmatic response. These *dual* responses usually resolve by 24 hours but may persist for several days. The late response has been associated with *increased* airways hyperresponsiveness, and the severity of the late response is related to the degree and duration of the increased responsiveness. Thus, the late asthmatic response is said to "induce" hyperresponsiveness of the airways.

The late asthmatic response is an inflammatory response with cellular inflammation of the airways. Eosinophils, neutrophils, and lymphocytes are all increased in bronchial lavage specimens following allergen bronchoprovocation. This inflammation may account for defects of both immune regulation and neural overactivity.

Asthma is airway obstruction in both central and peripheral airways that results in an early decrease in maximal flow rates (FEV_1, FEF 25 to 75 per cent, or peak flow) followed by an increase in lung volumes (RV or residual volume and TLC or total lung capacity). These changes are often dramatic but with proper treatment are equally dramatically reversible. TLC may increase as much as several liters and apparently be retained as "trapped air," upon which the asthmatic must breathe in short shallow breaths. This "breathing with a lung already full of air" results in rapid tiring and eventual respiratory failure. Blood gases are helpful to alert the physician to this process. Normally, a mild asthmatic will hyperventilate to maintain reasonable oxygenation. As muscles fatigue, however, the asthmatic will begin to retain CO_2, and the Pco_2 will return toward normal, while the Po_2 remains low. When this occurs, the patient is beginning to experience respiratory failure and requires close observation. It is not a sign of improvement.

It is often helpful to categorize patients by the severity of their asthma. Several methods can be used, but it usually suffices to divide them into mild, moderate, and severe, recognizing also the "asthma variants." These can be thought of as stages of progression, but frequently an individual remains in one or the other of these categories for most of his life. Those with *mild* asthma have occasional asthmatic episodes, perhaps associated with exercise or animal dander exposure. Their FEV_1 may be slightly reduced (<30 per cent) and easily reversed. Those with *moderate* asthma may have chronic symptoms either throughout the year or during several seasons and require medications to maintain near-normal function. Their FEV_1 is usually reduced less than 50 per cent but is reversible. *Severe* asthmatics are those with chronic debilitating symptoms requiring regular medication, often corticosteroids. Their life style is markedly altered, and they frequent emergency rooms and clinics if inadequately treated.

Status asthmaticus is severe asthma that is unresponsive to the usual medical therapy. It may require hospitalization and close observation. "Asthma variant" is hyperresponsive airways or asthma that may present as a cough, exertional dyspnea, a "tight or congested chest," or nighttime wheezing as a result of late responses or a relative deficiency in corticosteroids during the early morning hours. Sometimes the asthma variant may precede the onset of chronic asthma or remain after a recent upper respiratory infection. A methacholine or histamine challenge is usually positive when the patient presents with one of these variants of asthma.

Evaluation of the Patient

A thorough history and physical examination of the patient are the cornerstones of good management. This history should emphasize environmental exposure to seasonal allergens; occupational exposure (in detail); pets in the home; smoking or exposure to smokers; exposure to irritants such as smog, fumes, dust, and so forth; the use of aspirin or nonsteroidal anti-inflammatory drugs; previous use of steroids for asthma; and frequent ingestion of yellow dyes or metabisulfites. The physical examination should emphasize the head, neck, and chest examination but not to the exclusion of the other organ systems. The throat should be examined for posterior lymphoid hyperplasia, suggesting postnasal discharge; sinuses should be palpated; and the nasal passages should be examined for polyps. The thyroid should be examined for enlargement, as hyperthyroidism is occasionally associated with worsening asthma or increased airways hyperresponsiveness. Examination of the chest often reveals clues to the presence of other illness, while listening during a forced expiratory maneuver may bring out quiet wheezing. Pulmonary functions are useful to document progression during therapy and the extent of recovery.

A chest x-ray is often helpful to consider the complications of asthma and to rule out other chest diseases and search for infiltrates, but it is of little value in treating the initial episode. Sinus films may be useful in some; a high incidence of sinusitis (50 per cent) and nasal polyps (20 per cent) is found with chronic idiopathic asthma (nonallergic). If the allergic asthmatic is experiencing an exacerbation of his symptoms or is exposed to a moldy environment, an intradermal skin test for *Aspergillus*, total serum IgE, and serum precipitins for *Aspergillus* (IgG antibody) are helpful to suggest allergic bronchopulmonary aspergillosis (ABPA). A lung infiltrate and marked eosinophilia may be found, and central bronchiectasis can be confirmed by tomography or a CT scan. An early diagnosis of ABPA is important, as inappropriate treatment may lead to irreversible lung pathology.

Treatment

Patient education is essential for maximal benefit from any treatment program; much care and time must be invested in this enterprise. Symptom diary scorecards on which to record daily medications and symptoms may be helpful in evaluating patients requiring oral steroids or receiving allergy injection therapy. One must use specific criteria, such as number of days in hospital, number of emergency room visits, epinephrine injections, or days lost from school or work, to quantitate year-to-year progress. A distinction should be drawn, for example, when evaluating the response to allergy immunotherapy, between allergen-induced (such as seasonal) symptoms and a flare-up due to nonspecific inciters or inducers of asthma, such as exercise or viral infections; otherwise immunotherapy may appear to have been ineffective.

The cumulative use of therapeutic medications is a convenient method of designing a treatment regimen based upon the categories of asthma severity (see algorithm in Figure 1).

Avoidance

Avoidance of both allergens and nonspecific irritants is central to any treatment regimen. House dust mite control, for example, has now been shown to reduce airway reactivity. Without attention to avoidance, immunotherapy is often ineffective. If animals cannot be placed outside the home, they should at least be kept out of bedrooms. Occupational exposure can be avoided with improved ventilation, filters, or masks. Avoiding sidestream smoke, irritants such as household cleaning solutions, cold air, and air pollution may be as helpful to the asthmatic as protection against pollens. In those with nonallergic asthma and sinusitis or nasal polyps, aspirin and nonsteroidals should be restricted unless they are essential for the treatment of other diseases.

Medications

Medications for treating asthma are numerous and for the most part safe. They may be given intermittently or regularly but are most helpful when given prophylactically.

Beta-Adrenergic Agonists. Beta-adrenergic agonists are widely prescribed, convenient, and very effective for treating asthma. As pressurized inhalers, they are quick-acting and give moderately prolonged relief if the asthma is mild. One of the physician's most important roles is to educate the patient as to the proper use of inhalers. Two principles must be emphasized: first, sequential dosing, and second, timing the inhalation with a slow, deep breath to deposit the medication in the airways instead of the throat. For maximal benefit, the first inhalation should be followed in 10 to 15 minutes by a second inhalation. This can increase the efficiency of the drug up to 50 per cent. The inhalation should begin at FRC (functional residual capacity) and proceed with a slow, deep breath while the canister is activated. Breath-holding for 10 seconds also improves deposition of the drug. Since many patients cannot time this adequately, an extender such as Aerochamber (Monaghan Medical Corp., Plattsburgh, N.Y.) or Breathancer (Geigy, Ardsley, N.Y.) has been helpful in allowing relaxed inhalation of the aerosolized powder. For some, a home nebulizer may provide more adequate treatment. Short-acting beta-agonists are sufficient for mild or intermittent asthma, but the more specific beta-stimulants, such as metaproterenol and albuterol, may last up to 4 hours or more and can be used on a regular basis (two puffs every 4 to 6 hours) for better control. These are also the most effective medications for exercise-induced asthma when used prophylactically or during exercise.

Oral beta-agonists are less effective than aerosols and associated with tremor, palpitation, and "jitteriness." They may be useful in those who cannot use aerosols or who are unable to use theophylline.

Theophylline has gained great favor in this country in spite of its side effects and risk for serious complications. It is a good bronchodilator but is not as potent as inhaled bronchodilators. The distinct advantage of theophylline is the availability of long-acting preparations such as Theo-Dur or Slo-bid, which, if given at a dose of approximately 6 mg per kg every 12 hours, will maintain a fairly constant blood level. This blood level can be measured any time during that 12 hours to confirm that it is in the desired 10 to 20 μg per ml range. Levels less than 5 μg per ml have little clinical benefit, and those over 20 μg per ml can be hazardous. The principal advantage of the long-acting preparations for adults is to insure compliance and to protect the individual during the nighttime hours, when it is inconvenient to take medication and when pulmonary function is at its worst. Normally, only one theophylline level 5 days after beginning a twice-daily dosage of between 200 to 400 mg of Theo-Dur is sufficient to establish a therapeutic level. Drugs such as cimetidine or erythromycin may increase the blood level beyond the therapeutic range, causing toxicity in a previously stabilized patient.

Corticosteroids. Although most asthmatics will respond to intermittent or daily beta-adrenergic aerosols, or to the combination of beta-agonists plus daily theophylline, some patients need corticosteroids to initially "clear" their asthma or to treat a flare and correct the presumable inflammation of asthma. Corticosteroids have gained a bad reputation, and not undeservedly, but when bronchodilators are ineffective, it is detrimental to withhold the proper use of corticosteroids. Oral corticosteroids may be used in one of several ways: For the severe asthmatic, a daily morning dose or an every-other-morning dose may be needed; for those with recurrent viral infections that lead to asthma, a "burst and taper" regimen of 7 to 10 days is usually sufficient. The goal with all steroid therapy is to give enough to suppress and control the asthma, and then to reduce the dose as quickly as possible while maintaining the improvement. It is important to initially give a large enough dosage to suppress the asthma before moving too quickly to smaller doses in an attempt to limit side effects. Usually, 40 to 60 mg of prednisone in divided doses for 1 to 2 weeks is sufficient to clear most asthma flares, while more prolonged dosing may be needed to induce a remission or control asthma that has been present for a longer time. Usually, the initial dose given to clear the asthma can be tapered 5 mg every 3 to 4 days. Corticosteroids help reestablish apparent beta-adrenergic sensitivity and may be especially helpful in hospitalized patients who were previously refractory to beta-agonists.

Topically effective corticosteroids, such as beclomethasone dipropionate, can be rapidly degraded to biologically inactive metabolites with one pass through the liver. In the usual starting dose of two puffs orally every 6 hours, there are no significant side effects. These are able to control the symptoms of a majority of asthmatics (75 per cent), but one usually needs to begin with a short course of oral prednisone to "clear" the patient, followed by inhaled beclomethasone. Most asthmatics will also need oral prednisone for occasional flares or postviral wheezing, even while taking inhaled steroids with good control. Although oral candidiasis may result from the use of beclomethasone, it can be prevented by rinsing the mouth after each use and by the use of an extender. Unnecessary antibiotics or prednisone may predispose to this complication. If candidiasis does occur, it can be controlled with antifungal agents. The sudden switch to inhaled topical steroids from long-term oral steroids has resulted in adrenal insufficiency in some, and caution should be used to slowly taper oral steroids in this situation.

In spite of these remarkable advances, a few severely steroid-dependent asthmatics may be controlled only with daily doses of oral prednisone, often more than 10 mg per day. Although every effort should be made to taper and eliminate prednisone, continually trying to do this will often lead to using more prednisone than needed and to poor control. Patience is essential to long-term follow-up. The usual side effects are weight gain, fluid retention, increased appetite, hypertension, cataracts, glaucoma, and, occasionally, a mild increase in diabetes. The worst complication is osteoporosis, especially in postmenopausal females. Various regimens have been recommended without full agreement, but certainly mobility must be emphasized. Calcium supplements and replacement estrogens have been suggested for the most severe situations.

Cromolyn Sodium. Although cromolyn has found great popularity in Europe, it has never gained similar status here, perhaps because of its cost. It is useful, however, for prophylaxis in exercise-induced asthma and specific occupational or animal-induced exposures. It has essentially no toxicity. Normally, it controls allergen-induced asthma very well, but it has been relatively ineffective for other types of adult asthma. The newer nebulized form may find more usefulness, but it is cumbersome and therefore limits patient compliance. Cromolyn should probably receive a trial for at least 6 weeks in severe asthmatics who require corticosteroids. It may help reverse airway reactivity.

Anticholinergic Antagonists. Atropine and other anticholinergic drugs are effective bronchodilators but appear to work in a small subpopulation only. A new anticholinergic agent, ipratroprium bromide (Sch-1000), is clinically effective as an aerosol and essentially nontoxic but is not yet available in the United States. It may be helpful for cough or to prevent exercise-induced wheezing.

Alpha-Adrenergic Antagonists. Some asthmatics have been shown to have alpha-adrenergic hyperresponsiveness. Thus, alpha-adrenergic blockers have been tried with some success experimentally, especially for exercise-induced asthma. These agents have potentially serious side effects, such as hypotension, and are not recommended for routine use.

Other Treatment Modalities

Immunotherapy. Immunotherapy has been used for many years to treat allergic asthma. Clinical studies have generally supported the efficacy of immunotherapy for allergen-induced asthma. Since asthma is multifactorial, however, it has been difficult to provide definitive studies. These are currently being done. There is some evidence to suggest that high-dose immunotherapy may reverse airway reactivity and modify late responses. Therefore, in the appropriately chosen patient, it can be a very effective tool.

Antibiotics. Most infections encountered by adult asthmatic patients are virally induced and not bacterial. Therefore, antibiotics are not routinely recommended in spite of what appears to be purulent sputum. The yellow or green look to the sputum in asthmatics is generally due to eosinophils and other inflammatory cells. Triacetyloleandomycin (Troleandomycin, Tao), a macrolide antibiotic, is effective in conjunction with methylprednisolone, but not with prednisone, to treat severe steroid-dependent asthma. The incidence of hepatic dysfunction is high with this drug. Although not currently an approved method of therapy for asthma, it has been used by some in dire situations to preserve the patient from severe steroid side effects.

Antihistamines are generally ineffective for clinical asthma. Their sedative and drying effect on the mucosal membranes is not a contraindication for their use in those who have concomitant rhinitis. This principle is frequently misunderstood.

Establishing a Treatment Regimen

In asthma, as with other allergic diseases, education and prevention are the two most important goals. Once the patient understands what asthma is, and what the usual precipitating factors are, avoidance can be undertaken with more enthusiasm.

Treatment with medication is accomplished in a "cumulative" fashion, as demonstrated in Figure 1. Beta-adrenergic aerosols may be used prophylactically, as in exercise asthma or animal exposures, and for mild intermittent asthma. For moderate asthma, they may be used on a regular basis. If wheezing is occurring two to three times per week, theophylline may be used as a long-acting preparation to maintain bronchodilatation around the clock. Theophylline supplemented with intermittent or regular use of beta-adrenergic aerosols is sufficent to control most asthmatics. If mild-to-moderate asthma is precipitated by allergens, allergy immunotherapy may be used alone or in conjunction with the above-named medications. Cromolyn sodium should also be considered, either alone or in conjunction with other medications. If all of these are insufficient, corticosteroids, either as a "burst-and-taper" or as a daily dosage, may be needed. This may be followed by inhaled beclomethasone or flunisolide. If a major portion of severe asthma is precipitated by allergen(s), immunotherapy may be helpful. All of these measures may be necessary in the most severely afflicted patients.

In-Hospital and Emergency Therapy

Many patients present to the office or the emergency room with an exacerbation of their asthma. Predicting whether or not hospitalization is necessary can be lifesaving. Most patients respond to medical intervention, corticosteroids, and a change in their previous regimen. Treated inadequately, many return several times before hospitalization is considered necessary. *This can be avoided by treating the patient vigorously during the first visit.*

Several recent studies have tried to establish guidelines for assessing status asthmaticus and predicting the need for hospitalization. The "Fischil Index" was developed to predict relapse and the need for hospitalization. The usefulness of this index was not confirmed by recent studies. Such decisions, therefore, remain essentially dependent upon clinical judgment.

An assessment of blood gases is not helpful in mild-to-moderate asthma, but will indicate a downward trend toward respiratory failure by a rise in P_{CO_2}. The precipitating factor(s) for the acute exacerbation should be sought because they may modify the approach to treatment. Patients with sudden and intermittent exposures to allergens (e.g., seasonal or immunotherapy), animal danders, or occupational inhalants (e.g., toluene diisocyanate, laboratory animals, wood dust) usually respond well to therapy and do not require admission. Those who have had recent viral infections or exacerbations that have lasted for several days to weeks, or who have needed previous treatment with steroids, will more often need extreme treatment and perhaps admission.

The initial emergency room treatment of asthma should include (1) epinephrine 0.3 ml at 1:1000 solution subcutaneously, repeated twice more at 20-minute intervals if necessary; (2) aminophylline 0.5 mg per kg per hour intravenously, preceded if necessary by a loading dose; and (3) corticosteroids, either prednisone 60 to 80 mg orally followed by 10 to 15 mg four times a day or hydrocortisone 2 mg per kg followed by 0.5 mg per kg per hour intravenously. Oxygen should be administered at 2 to 4 liters per minute, and adequate fluids should be given to mobilize secretions. Metaproterenol sulfate 5 per cent by nebulizer (25 mg in 2.5 ml saline) every 2 to 4 hours, or terbutaline 0.25 mg subcutaneously, may be used until the patient's condition begins to clear.

There may be some cardiovascular risks to the combination of high-dose theophylline therapy and inhaled sympathomimetics, and patients should be monitored closely. Positive-pressure therapy (IPPB) is not indicated for the treatment of asthma because of the attendant risks of pneumothorax and pneumomediastinum.

Prognosis for Asthma

In general, the prognosis for asthma is very good. Asthma tends to "wax and wane," and therefore good times follow the bad. Asthma is not caused by psychologic problems, although anxiety and stress may trigger asthma. Asthma does not inflict permanent damage on the airways but is primarily a reversible disease. With many effective medications for asthma, it is unusual that a patient cannot be treated to the point of suitable function within his life style. The exceptions might be those who are in highly competitive athletics or involved in certain sports such as soccer or basketball, or those who are steroid dependent. We now know that dust control in the home can improve airways reactivity and that immunotherapy may also do the same. Therefore, the prognosis for most asthmatics is bright.

ASTHMA IN CHILDHOOD

method of
THOMAS F. SMITH, M.D.
Emory University
Atlanta, Georgia

Asthma is a chronic disease characterized by airway hyperreactivity to a variety of stimuli, which results in obstruction to airflow. Asthma is an extremely variable disease, and treatment regimens must be individualized. Children with simple asthma have completely reversible airflow obstruction. Other diagnoses should be sought in children in whom complete resolution of airflow obstruction cannot be documented by objective measurement or examination. Allergy plays a significant role in causing or triggering asthma in children more often than it does in adults; however, not all children with asthma have allergies, and many other stimuli besides allergens will trigger an allergic child's asthma.

Although the basic cellular defect in asthma has not yet been identified, much is known about its pathogenesis, and an effective treatment program should be possible for each child with asthma. Errors in the management of childhood asthma include failure to recognize reversible airflow obstruction, underestimation of lung function abnormality, tolerance of ongoing airflow obstruction, and undertreatment either in level or in duration of therapy. Reasonable goals of therapy for the majority of children should include complete control of symptoms, normal pulmonary function, and full activity.

The therapeutic options for an asthmatic child include (1) avoidance of avoidable triggers of symptoms, (2) pharmacotherapy for symptoms from unavoidable triggers, and (3) immunotherapy in some situations. These should be presented in an ongoing program of education and support for the parents and the child.

Treatment

Avoidance

Stimuli that are definite or probable triggers of asthma should be avoided through environmental control measures. For example, house dust mites are a common allergen; exposure to mites can be reduced by frequent cleaning; by covering mattresses, springs, pillows, and upholstered furniture in plastic; by removing rugs; and by decreasing humidity in the home. Animals should be prohibited indoors, since animal dander is a common allergen and also adds to the particulate load in a house. Tobacco smoke is a very common nonallergic trigger for asthma, and smoking indoors also should be prohibited. Other irritants, including smoke from wood stoves, aerosol sprays, or strong odors such as certain perfumes, provoke symptoms in some children and should be avoided. Food allergy is not a common problem in asthmatic children, and restrictive diets usually are not warranted. Avoidance of aspirin is suggested because of the frequency with which aspirin triggers asthma.

Pharmacotherapy

Pharmacologic management is the foundation of therapy for most children with asthma. Asthma medicines are most useful when instituted before symptoms appear, and the level of therapy should be advanced quickly if symptoms persist or increase. Asthma medicines fall into four major categories.

Theophylline. Oral theophylline is the most commonly used drug for maintenance therapy of asthma in the United States. Theophylline pharmacokinetics have been well studied, and serum theophylline levels usually are readily available to guide treatment. Although a serum level of 10 to 20 μg per ml is considered optimal for treating asthma, many children will have complete resolution of symptoms at levels below 10 μg per ml, whereas others will experience adverse effects at levels below 20 μg per ml. Therapy in children aged 1 to 9 years usually is started at 20 mg per kg per day divided into equal doses according to the preparation used. This dose is increased until there is good clinical response or until adverse effects occur. Children younger than 1 year or older than 9 years usually are slower metabolizers of the drug and thus require lower dosage. Measuring serum levels is useful when noncompliance is suspected, when there are persistent symptoms in spite of high dose, or when adverse effects are encountered. In addition, measuring levels at intervals in children doing well will predict dosage changes necessitated by changes in metabolism and the child's growth.

Adverse effects of theophylline administration include local gastric irritation and CNS symptoms such as headache, nausea, vomiting, and behavior changes. The last is a significant problem in many children and may affect school performance. In some children, tolerance will develop to this adverse effect; in others, it can be avoided by prescribing a decreased dose. However, there are children for whom theophylline is not a therapeutic option. In children especially, theophylline metabolism varies over time and may change because of intercedent factors such as concomitant medicine use and viral respiratory infection. For example, erythromycin usually prolongs serum theophylline half-life, and it is prudent to decrease theophylline dose when erythromycin is prescribed. Headache, nausea, or vomiting in the context of presumed viral infection must be assumed to be a side effect of theophylline unless a nontoxic serum theophylline level is documented. Theophylline relaxes smooth muscle nonspecifically and may cause or increase gastroesophageal reflux and constipation. Pulmonary function can be maintained and side effects reduced by administering a decreased dose of theophylline in conjunction with a beta-agonist (discussed below) because of synergy between these bronchodilators.

There are many preparations available for use in children. Products containing xanthines that are converted to theophylline, such as oxtriphylline (Brondecon, Choledyl), or theophylline salts, such as aminophylline (Phyllocontin, Somophyllin), must be prescribed in terms of their anhydrous theophylline equivalent. Other xanthines such as diphylline (Lufyllin, Dilor) are not metabolized into theophylline, have a very short serum half-life, and should not be used. Products containing alcohol, dyes, and combinations of drugs should be avoided. Liquid preparations (Aquaphyllin, Slo-Phyllin, Somophyllin, Theolair) are available for infants and small children. In general they are unpalatable; they also must be given every 6 hours around the clock to most children.

Sustained-release preparations (Slo-bid, Theo-bid, Theo-Dur, Theolair) permit maintenance of effective blood levels when taken in equally divided and spaced doses two or three times each day. Children unable to swallow pills may be given slow-release granules from capsules (e.g., Slo-bid) mixed with food. These preparations are well accepted by both patients and parents and improve compliance. They are not useful for intermittent therapy because of the delay in achieving an effective blood level when first taken. There also is variation in absorption of these products that is produced by meals. Young children with nausea or vomiting from gastroenteritis should be given rectal theophylline solutions only after a nontoxic serum theophylline level has been demonstrated. Rectal suppositories are contraindicated because of erratic absorption.

Beta-Adrenergic Agonists. Beta agonists act rapidly and are useful for intermittent therapy and for acute bronchospasm; they also are effective in prophylaxis of symptoms. They are especially useful in preventing exercise-induced asthma. By inhalation, beta agonists offer the most beneficial effect with the least adverse effect. Adverse effects of beta agonists include tachycardia (beta-1) and tremor (beta-2). Tremor usually will disappear over time as skeletal muscle receptors become tolerant. In general, patient education will prevent abuse of metered dose inhalers, and currently used formulations are safer than those associated with increased mortality in the past. Maximum delivery into the lung occurs when the drug is inhaled slowly, through open airways, to a full inspiration. Efficacy of inhalation can be increased for some children by the use of spacing devices (Aerochamber, Brethancer, InspirEase, Inhal-Aide). Delivery of aerosols is most effective after nebulization using a portable air compressor unit (Maximyst, Pulmonaide) and mouthpiece.

Currently available adrenergic agonists, such as metaproterenol, terbutaline, and albuterol, offer beta-2 selectivity and long duration of action; they have largely replaced products such as isoproterenol (Isuprel) and isoetharine (Bronkosol) for the ambulatory management of asthma. Metaproterenol (Alupent) is available as a liquid preparation for children. Metaproterenol (Alupent), terbutaline (Brethine, Bricanyl, Brethaire), and albuterol (Proventil, Ventolin) are available as tablets and in metered dose inhalers. Metaproterenol (Alupent) also is available as a solution for use in nebulizers; terbutaline for injection (Brethine Ampuls) has been used this way as well. Not all of these medicines are recommended for children below a given age or by the route listed; use of them other than as approved or recommended should be made with discretion and with the consent of patients or parents.

Cromolyn. Cromolyn (Intal) is a topically active prophylactic agent that is particularly useful in the treatment of children with allergen-triggered or exercise-induced asthma. It may serve as a first-line drug; however, it alone will not reverse bronchospasm, and other treatment modalities should be used when airflow obstruction is present. It requires open airways and some operator skill to deposit cromolyn into the lung. Cromolyn alone may induce coughing or bronchospasm in some patients; this usually can be avoided by pretreatment with an inhaled beta agonist. Cromolyn is available as a dry powder for use with the Spinhaler delivery device and as a solution for nebulization. The usual starting dosage for children 2 years of age and older is 20 mg (one capsule or ampule) four times a day. The frequency of administration often can be decreased after the child's symptoms have stabilized.

Corticosteroids. Corticosteroid administration is mandatory when a child experiences bronchospasm incompletely responsive to bronchodilators alone. Thus, corticosteroids are given in high dose for a short course for an acute exacerbation of asthma, such as occurs with viral respiratory infection. In this situation, prednisone 1 mg per kg given twice a day (or an equivalent dose of another corticosteroid) is added to the bronchodilator regimen for 3 to 5 days. Early institution of prednisone improves its effectiveness. Short courses of high-dose steroid given no more often than once every 2 weeks will not induce significant adrenal suppression and may be stopped without tapering.

In children who have chronic symptoms or frequent, acute, severe exacerbations of asthma not controlled by bronchodilators and cromolyn, maintenance therapy with corticosteroids should be started. Initially, oral therapy with a rapidly metabolized corticosteroid (prednisone, methylprednisolone) is used to normalize lung function. For example, prednisone 2 mg per kg per day is given daily for 5 to 7 days, followed by 2 mg per kg every other day in the morning. Prednisone dosage then may be reduced in small increments every 2 weeks until the lowest alternate-day dosage providing symptom control is determined.

Corticosteroids by oral inhalation provide an alternative to every-other-day dosage. Beclomethasone (Beclovent, Vanceril), flunisolide (AeroBid), and triamcinolone (Azmacort) are administered using a metered dose inhaler two to four times each day, according to the product used. Inhaled corticosteroids usually permit reduction in oral dosage for children experiencing adverse effects from long-term, high-dose therapy. At usual doses, alternate-day prednisone and inhaled corticosteroids are both effective and safe. In most children, prednisone is preferable because of its ease of administration and lower cost.

Oral inhalation of steroids requires open airways and some skill. It should not be used in younger children, who cannot inhale it effectively, or in children with increasing airflow obstruction. Corticosteroids given orally or parenterally are mandatory for children with status asthmaticus or with adrenal suppression in times of stress.

Other Drugs. Atropine sulfate by inhalation (0.05 to 0.10 mg per kg) and other anticholinergic agents have been shown to decrease bronchospasm in many patients with asthma. These drugs presumably block vagally mediated bronchoconstriction. Atropine is not approved for use by inhalation, and a clinical trial with this agent should be preceded by an adequate course of more conventional therapy. Antihistamines do not adversely affect asthma and may be used for coexisting allergic disease. The efficacy of expectorants is controversial. Guaifenesin has not yet been shown to have any effect on lower respiratory tract fluids. Iodides have many side effects and are not recommended unless there is clear-cut evidence of reproducible benefit. Acetylcysteine (Mucomyst) causes bronchospasm and is contraindicated for asthmatics. Antibiotics should not be used routinely for exacerbations of asthma; they should be reserved for patients who have objective evidence of bacterial infection or immunologic abnormality.

Immunotherapy

Immunotherapy (hyposensitization) can reduce airway hyperreactivity in patients with allergen-triggered asthma. Successful therapy depends on identifying a candidate who has symptomatic hypersensitivity to a relevant allergen, and then administering an adequate dose of the purified allergen. Lack of standardization of allergen extracts makes the latter difficult. Immunotherapy generally is reserved for truly allergic patients whose symptoms have not been well controlled on a reasonable trial of avoidance and pharmacotherapy or who experience adverse effects from medicines necessary to provide symptom relief.

Treatment of Acute Asthma

Acute exacerbations of asthma are best managed in advance, by maintaining normal lung function, by recognizing early clinical signs or symptoms that warn of an oncoming exacerbation, and by promptly increasing the level of pharmacotherapy when these early signs appear.

Initial evaluation of a child with acute asthma should include a concise history and physical examination, with particular attention to degree of respiratory difficulty (respiratory rate, work of breathing, airflow on auscultation of the chest, and fatigue). A history of prolonged symptoms, frequent hospitalizations, or respiratory failure should warn of a child who needs more cautious and aggressive treatment. Spirometry should be obtained on all children old enough to perform a forced expiratory maneuver. Arterial blood gases should be obtained and oxygen by mask started in moderately and severely ill children. It is important that supplemental oxygen be added before giving beta agonists, since they may decrease Pa_{O_2} in children who are bronchodilator-unresponsive. Beta agonists may be given subcutaneously (e.g., aqueous epinephrine 1:1000, 0.01 ml per kg up to 0.3 ml) or by inhalation after nebulization (e.g., isoproterenol 0.25 to 0.50 ml, isoetharine 0.25 to 0.50 ml, or metaproterenol 0.1 to 0.5 ml). These may be repeated once or twice at 20-minute intervals if blood pressure and heart rate are not unduly elevated.

IPPB should never be used to treat asthma. An optimal serum theophylline level should be assured. Patients not taking theophylline should receive a loading dose of 6 to 7 mg per kg. Oral therapy is usually acceptable, with intravenous administration being reserved for more severely ill patients. In all cases, serum theophylline levels should be measured to adjust dosage. Corticosteroids should be given early to children whose symptoms do not respond rapidly and completely to bronchodilator therapy and to children at risk for increasing symptoms or respiratory failure.

Admission to hospital for further management should be considered for children who fail to respond to these therapies; who have acidosis, significant hypoxemia, or normal to elevated P_{CO_2}; who have a history of prolonged symptoms or respiratory failure; or in whom appropriate care at home cannot be assured. Prolonged efforts to clear symptoms in the emergency room are not worthwhile. Children whose symptoms resolve in response to emergency room treatment should be discharged on a drug regimen increased from that used before, since the previous level of therapy was inadequate to prevent the acute exacerbation. Medicines added with an acute exacerbation should be continued long enough to permit lung healing, which is beyond the time when overt symptoms of asthma have resolved.

In-patient therapy of acute asthma is an extension of that detailed above. Its goal should be to provide maximum therapy to decrease the likelihood of respiratory failure and decrease time in hospital. Oxygen should be continued to maintain Pa_{O_2} above 70 torr. An optimal serum theophylline level should be maintained and assured by repeated measurement. One should continue beta agonists orally and by inhalation at the doses listed above while monitoring heart rate and blood pressure. Corticosteroids are given at increased dosage, e.g., methylprednisolone 1 mg per kg every 4 to 6 hours or an equivalent dose of hydrocortisone may be used. Respiratory failure (Pa_{O_2} < 40 torr or < 75 torr on maximal oxygen, or rising Pa_{CO_2}) necessitates intubation and assisted ventilation; it should be considered imminent in any child with faint or absent breath sounds, increasing fatigue, or altered sensorium regardless of arterial blood gas values. Intravenous isoproterenol has been used at some centers to treat impending respiratory failure, but this mode of therapy is associated with significant risk, including myocardial infarction. Sedatives are contraindicated, since they may depress respiratory effort.

Prognosis

Asthma remains a chronic, incurable disease, but the outlook for children with asthma is generally good. Children with onset of asthma after age 2 years usually will have an eventual spontaneous amelioration of their disease, although those under age 2 years may have more severe and more prolonged symptoms. With appropriate support, education, and management, morbidity from asthma in children should be minimal and mortality should be eliminated.

ALLERGIC RHINITIS CAUSED BY INHALANT FACTORS

method of
DAVID I. BERNSTEIN, M.D.,
and I. LEONARD BERNSTEIN, M.D.
University of Cincinnati
Cincinnati, Ohio

Allergic rhinitis is defined as nasal mucosal inflammation resulting from local release of vasoactive mediators from IgE-sensitized mast cells. Symptoms are often easily recognized and include rhinorrhea, nasal stenosis, prominent ocular lacrimation, and itching. Palatal itching and symptoms due to eustachian tube obstruction are common associated complaints. Secondary acute or chronic sinusitis may result from persistent inflammatory obstruction of the ostial openings of the sinus cavities. Symptoms may occur acutely following brief exposure to inhalant aeroallergens such as pollen and animal proteins or may become chronic when propagated by continuous exposure to multiple aeroallergens to which the patient has become sensitized. Allergic rhinitis may follow a predictable seasonal pollination pattern, as with short ragweed, which occurs from mid-August to early October, or become a perennial problem in which clear seasonal exacerbations are not easily recognized. Table 1 lists common seasonal and nonseasonal aeroallergens that are the most frequent causes of acute or chronic allergic rhinitis, as well as other less frequently encountered environmental and occupational allergens. A thorough knowledge of the pollinating seasons endemic to a particular region is absolutely necessary for arriving at an accurate diagnosis of seasonal allergic rhinitis (Table 1).

DIAGNOSIS

Diagnosis of seasonal allergic rhinitis patients is rarely difficult. However, a continuous history of perennial nasal obstruction and rhinorrhea without prominent ocular itching or seasonal exacerbations may necessitate an extensive evaluation to distinguish allergic from nonallergic etiologies. Infectious rhinitis may be suspected when thick purulent nasal discharge containing copious amounts of neutrophils is detected, in contrast to classic allergic rhinitis in which copious amounts of clear nasal secretions containing eosinophils are often found. However, the presence of nasal eosinophils observed on a Wright stain of a nasal smear is often nonspecific and may be found in patients with nonallergic rhinitis or nasal polyposis. Nasal polyps, which usually occur independently of allergic factors, can easily be identified by a thorough examination with a nasal speculum and should be considered in any patient presenting with chronic rhinorrhea and nasal congestion. Asthma and aspirin sensitivity are found in a significant number of such patients. Chronic nasal obstructive symptoms can also be related to chronic use or abuse of medications (rhinitis medicamentosa), such as topical sympathomimetic agents (phenylephrine [e.g., Neo-Synephrine]), estrogens (e.g., contraceptives), and antihypertensive agents (e.g., reserpine, guanethidine).

Hypertrophic (hyperplastic) nonallergic rhinitis, an uncommon disorder, can be recognized when swollen edematous nasal turbinates fail to shrink in response to topical vasoconstrictors. Perennial nasal symptoms that occur independently of allergenic stimuli most often are due to vasomotor rhinitis. This common condition is characterized by lacrimation, rhinorrhea, and nasal congestion that is provoked by temperature, humidity, and positional changes as well as environmental irritants. This condition may be due to an intrinsic vasomotor instability resulting in exaggerated changes of the vascular bed in the nasal mucosa in response to physical stimuli.

Following a thorough environmental and allergic history, diagnostic skin testing with a battery of common inhalant aeroallergens may be indicated. Skin tests are usually initiated with the less sensitive puncture or prick method and, if negative, are followed by the intradermal method. A positive wheal and flare response to a particular aeroallergen that correlates well with a clinical history of exposure is indicative of clinical sensitivity. In general, the correlation between clinical sensitivity and skin tests is better for the prick test than the intradermal method. An elevated serum total IgE in a patient may be useful for further defining atopic status. However, we discourage the routine use of serum-specific IgE measurements, such as the radioallergosorbent test (RAST), because of their relative higher cost and reduced sensitivity in comparison with skin tests.

TABLE 1. **Allergens That Induce Allergic Rhinitis**

Allergens	Sources of Exposure
Pollens (major sources from trees, grasses, and ragweed)	outdoors—seasonal
Mold (Fungi Imperfecti, *Basidiomycetes, Oomycetes, Zygomycetes,* etc.)	outdoors—ubiquitous indoors—damp basement, barns, contaminated air conditioners, humidifiers, indoor plants
House dust (*D. pteronyssinus, D. farinae* mite species, insect casts and particulates, fungi, algae, animal and human proteins)	bedding, carpeting, drapes, upholstered furniture, aquaria
Feathers	bedding, comforters
Animal-derived allergens (cat, dog, horse, rodent, and avian species are most common)	home and workplace (laboratory animal workers)
Nonhouse dust, arthropod–derived allergens	
Arachnids	grain handlers (grain mites)
Crustaceans—shrimp, *Daphnia*	food-related industries
Hexapods (insects)	seasonal endemic exposure (mayflies), household exposure (cockroaches), workplace exposure to larval emanations (i.e., beetles, moths)
Other plant-derived proteins	
Enzymes (subtilisins, papain, etc.)	household detergents, food and enzyme manufacturing sites
Kapok	pillows, mattresses, sleeping bags
Pyrethrum (Compositae family)	insecticides (cross-reactive with ragweed)
Miscellaneous—castor and coffee bean dust, wood dusts (western red cedar, *Quillaja* bark)	occupational—transport, food, lumber industries
Small molecular weight chemicals (phthalyl and trimellityl anhydrides, diisocyanates, penicillin, sulfonechloramide, etc.)	chemical industries, consumer do-it-yourself kits

Treatment

Effective treatment of allergic rhinitis encompasses avoidance and pharmacologic and immunologic modalities.

Avoidance

Rational therapy of seasonal or perennial allergic rhinitis is predicated on accurate identification of relevant environmental allergens. If possible, specific avoidance measures are considered as the initial treatment strategy. Such recommendations should be tailored to the socioeconomic and emotional conditions of individual patients. For example, when removal of a family pet is perceived as unacceptable for emotional reasons, the recommendation can be tempered by suggesting that pets can be housed in heated shelters in garages or any area of the house that is not connected to the heating ventilation system. When possible, attempts should be made to control and reduce indoor housedust allergen exposure in dust-sensitive patients. The use of snug plastic encasings on the pillow and mattress may be helpful. Because ambient mite concentrations in homes correlate highly with the presence of high pile carpeting, replacement of such floor covering may be an effective measure. Installation of central electrostatic filters may effectively reduce indoor airborne dust particulates. Occasionally, use of a surgical face mask during housecleaning may effectively reduce symptoms.

Recommendations for reduction of indoor mold exposure should be given to mold-sensitive patients, especially when excessively damp or mildewed areas are identifiable. A dehumidifier placed in a damp or leaky basement may help control mold growth. Special attention should be given to identification of possible contamination of humidifiers or air conditioning units as these provide excellent culture media for growth of indoor allergenic molds. Aerated aquaria are potential sources of exposure to allergenic molds or algae. If extreme mold contamination is present, fumigation of a room with formalin for 24 hours can be attempted, although this measure is only temporarily effective. When severe mold-sensitive patients, who often have coexistent asthma, fail to respond to intensive environmental manipulation or medical and immunologic modalities, relocation to a new living environment may be indicated. Although complete avoidance of pollen allergen is impossible, central air conditioning may effectively reduce daytime and nocturnal seasonal symptoms during the pollinating season.

In most cases of allergic rhinitis, even the

strictest avoidance measures are inadequate, necessitating pharmacologic or immunologic treatment or both.

Pharmacologic Treatment

The pharmacologic treatment of allergic rhinitis is often successful because of the wide spectrum of oral antihistamines-decongestants, intranasal cromolyn sodium, and topical corticosteroids. Systemic oral or parenteral corticosteroids are not indicated for routine treatment of acute or chronic allergic rhinitis because of their unfavorable risk/benefit ratio. Long-term use of topical vasoconstrictors should be avoided because of their potential to cause rebound symptoms and rhinitis medicamentosa. Selection of particular agents should depend on overall symptom severity and chronicity. For example, patients with longstanding allergen-induced nasal mucosal edema and inflammation may be less responsive to oral antihistamines and topical cromolyn sodium, necessitating the initial use of a topical corticosteroid agent such as beclomethasone (Beconase, Vancenase) or flunisolide (Nasalide).

A schematic approach for rational drug therapy of allergic rhinitis is presented in Table 2. Oral antihistamines alone or combined with pseudoephedrine and phenylpropanolamine decongestants are the drugs of first choice, and many of these agents are available as timed-release preparations. The latter symptomatic agents should not be administered to patients with pre-existing hypertension, coronary artery disease, or arrhythmias because these agents may exacerbate these conditions.

H_1 antagonists are classified according to the chemical group attached to the ethylamine chain into six major groups (ethanolamine, ethylenediamine, alkylamine, piperazine, phenothiazine, piperidine). Commonly used drugs representing each of these classes with recommended dosages are listed in Table 3. There is wide interpatient variability among different antihistamines with regard to efficacy and associated side effects. Many good antihistamine-decongestant preparations are now available over the counter (e.g., Disophrol, Actifed, and Dimetapp) and many patients will have been self-medicated prior to consulting physicians. Thus, a poor response to a prescribed antihistamine in such a patient would not be unexpected. However, on occasion, a patient who is unresponsive to a particular H_1 antagonist may improve following a trial of an antihistamine from a different class. Patient intolerance to soporific and anticholinergic side effects (dry mouth, urinary retention) may also be remedied by switching to an alternate agent from a different class. The mechanism of action of antihistamines is through competitive inhibition of H_1 cellular histamine receptors. Azatadine (Optimine, Trinalin) is an antihistamine that has the additional property of in vitro inhibition of basophilic histamine release.

Intranasal topical 4 per cent disodium cromoglycate (Nasocrom) is also effective as a prophylactic agent because of its ability to inhibit significant release of primary and secondary mediators from submucosal mast cells. It is most effective when used prophylactically and initiated, for example, just prior to the pollination season or before exposure to a known allergen. The mechanisms of action of cromolyn on tissue mast cells may be related to blockade of calcium transport across the mast cell membrane, resulting in inhibition of release of primary and secondary mediators. Because of its putative inhibitory effects on mediator release, we frequently find azatadine (manufacturer warns not intended for use in children under 12 years of age) in combination with nasal cromolyn for treatment of moderate or severe rhinitis symptoms most effective.

The availability of nasal topical corticosteroids

TABLE 2. **Strategy for Pharmacologic Treatment of Allergic Rhinitis**

Clinical Presentation	Treatment
(1) Seasonal or episodic allergic rhinitis due to a common inhalant allergen (i.e., pollen, animal dander)	Intranasal cromolyn H_1 antihistamine 0.5 hour before and every 6 hours as needed
(2) Perennial allergic rhinoconjunctivitis (i.e., mold and dust sensitivity) in the absence of nasal obstruction	Begin with H_1 antihistamines **If no response:** Add intranasal cromolyn sodium and substitute with another class of antihistamine **If no response:** Intranasal flunisolide or beclomethasone
(3) Perennial allergic rhinitis with chronic nasal mucosal inflammation and obstruction	Use antibiotics as needed for secondary sinusitis. Initiate intranasal corticosteroids for 2 wks and H_1 antihistamines **With good response:** Gradually taper intranasal steroids. Continue H_1 antihistamines or intranasal cromolyn sodium for maintenance

TABLE 3. **Classes and Dosages of Oral Antihistamines**

Class	Example	Recommended Adult Dosage	Recommended Pediatric Dose
I. Ethanolamine	Diphenhydramine HCl (Benadryl)	25–50 mg qid	5 mg/kg/24 hr
II. Ethylenediamine	Tripelennamine* (Pyribenzamine)	25–50 mg qid	5 mg/kg/24 hr*
III. Alkylamine	Chlorpheniramine maleate (Chlortrimeton)	4 mg qid	2–4 mg tid
IV. Piperazine	Hydroxyzine HCl (Atarax, Vistaril)	10, 25 or 50 mg qid	50 mg/24 hr/divided doses
V. Phenothiazine	Promethazine HCl (Phenergan)	12.5 mg qid	6.25–12.5 mg tid
VI. Piperidine	Azatadine (Optimine)	1–2 mg bid or tid	Not recommended under age 12 years
	Cyproheptadine HCl (Periactin)	4 mg tid	0.25 mg/kg/24 hr

*Manufacturer states: Do not use tripelennamine in children.

has greatly enhanced the treatment of allergic rhinitis. Aerosolized dexamethasone (Decadron Turbinaire) was the first such drug introduced and was shown to be effective at the recommended dose of 2 puffs four times daily or a total dose of 0.7 mg. This medication may be effective for short periods of treatment. However, long-term use of dexamethasone should be avoided because significant systemic absorption and adrenal suppression may occur at recommended dose levels. In recent years, topical beclomethasone and flunisolide have replaced dexamethasone as preferred agents for treatment of allergic rhinitis symptoms that are nonresponsive to cromolyn or antihistamines. Intranasal beclomethasone (Vancenase and Beconase) is recommended at an initial dose of 2 sprays (50 micrograms) four times daily. The dose frequency may then be tapered, after an initial clinical effect has been observed, to a maintenance dose of 2 sprays once or twice daily. Beclomethasone is rapidly metabolized to beclomethasone 17-mono-proprionate, which has minimal adrenal suppressive effects. The local anti-inflammatory effects account for the efficacy of both beclomethasone and flunisolide for allergic rhinitis. Sneezing and rhinorrhea may occur after administration secondary to the irritant effects of the Freon aerosol vehicle. Flunisolide may be better tolerated for this reason because it is delivered in a polyethylene glycol solution via a spray device. At the recommended dosage of flunisolide (Nasalide)—2 sprays (25 micrograms each) delivered three to four times daily—adrenal suppression does not occur. Nausea and bad taste are infrequent side effects. No evidence of atrophic nasal mucosal changes or nasal septal perforation has been found with long-term administration of intranasal beclomethasone or flunisolide.

Immunotherapy

Allergen immunotherapy or hyposensitization should be considered in patients with moderate to severe symptoms who fail adequate trials of topical and systemic pharmacotherapy. Numerous studies have demonstrated overall efficacy of immunotherapy for pollen- and nonpollen-induced allergic rhinitis. However, specific indications, as well as the cost:benefit ratio, must be considered as this treatment involves a considerable financial and time investment. We recommend immunotherapy most often to patients with perennial symptoms. This treatment is also generally indicated for individuals who have seasonal rhinitis during two or more of the pollinating seasons and are nonresponsive or intolerant to the effects of antihistamines and topical medications. Immunotherapy is strongly indicated for patients who have developed coexistent extrinsic asthma in which a beneficial response could result in long-term reduction of asthma-related morbidity. Rarely, immunotherapy may be indicated for patients who have single seasonal symptoms that are severe enough to result in temporary functional impairment and days lost from work.

Prior to initiating immunotherapy, it is absolutely essential to confirm clinical sensitivity, as determined by history with prick or intradermal skin tests to relevant aeroallergens. Only those allergens that are determined to be clinically significant based on the history should be included in the starting allergen extract mixture. For example, a patient living in the Midwest with a history of allergic rhinitis during August and September who exhibits cutaneous reactivity to many other tree, grass, mold, and dust allergens should be treated only with ragweed. In most allergy clinics, preparation of mixtures of multiple allergens for patients sensitive to such things as pollens, mold, dust, and weeds has been found to be the most expedient method without sacrificing treatment efficacy. Standard immunotherapy dose schedules are shown in Table 4.

Considerable variation with regard to the standard beginning concentration of the extract mixture (usually 10^{-6} to 10^{-4} dilutions) may be found among different practitioners. However, there is general consensus that significant improvement in symptoms is achieved in most pa-

TABLE 4. **Hyposensitization Schedules**

	Series I (twice a wk)		**Series II (twice a wk)**		**Series III (every wk)**		**Series IV (every 2 wk)**		**Series V (every 3–4 wk)**	
	*Wt by Vol**	*PNU*†	*Wt by Vol*	*PNU*	*Wt by Vol*	*PNU*	*Wt by Vol*	*PNU*	*Wt by Vol*	*PNU*
POLLENS	1:100,000	5/ml	1:10,000	50/ml	1:1000	500/ml	1:100	5000/ml	1:33	15,000
Initial dose (ml):	0.10	0.5	0.10	5	0.10	50	0.05	250	0.03	450
Increase by (ml):	0.15–0.20		0.10–0.15		0.10		0.05		0.03	
Final dose (ml):	0.80	4.0	0.80	40	0.90	450	0.90	4500	0.50	7500‡
	Wt by Vol	*PNU*	*Wt by Vol*	*PNU*	*Wt by Vol*	*PNU*	*Wt by Vol*	*PNU*	*Wt by Vol*	*PNU*
MOLDS	1:100,000	5/ml	1:10,000	50/ml	1:1000	500/ml	1:100	5000/ml	1:50	10,000
Initial dose (ml):	0.10	0.5	0.10	5	0.10	50	0.05	250	0.03	300
Increase by (ml):	0.15–0.20		0.10–0.15		0.10		0.05		0.03	
Final dose (ml):	0.80	4.0	0.80	40	0.90	450	0.90	4500	0.50	5000‡
	Wt by Vol	*PNU*	*Wt by Vol*	*PNU*	*Wt by Vol*	*PNU*	*Wt by Vol*	*PNU*		
HOUSE DUST	1:100,000	5/ml	1:10,000	50/ml	1:1000	500/ml	1:100	5000/ml		
Initial dose (ml):	0.10	0.5	0.10	5	0.10	50	.05	250		
Increase by (ml):	0.15–0.20		0.10–0.15		0.10		.05			
Final dose (ml):	0.80	4.0	0.80	40	0.80	450	.50	2500‡		

*Wt by Vol: grams of allergen per volume of extracting fluid. Thus a 3% (1:33) extract means that 3 grams of allergen have been extracted in 100 ml of extracting solution.

†PNU: Approximate number of protein-nitrogen units contained in corresponding Wt by Vol solution.

‡Maintenance dose.

tients only after higher maintenance doses of allergen concentrations ($> 10^{-2}$ dilution) are reached. Optimal results in our clinic have been obtained when an endpoint maintenance dose (1:30 for pollens and 1:50 for mold allergens) is achieved. In house dust therapy, commerical extracts that have been fortified with mite allergen are preferred. Most patients exhibit objective clinical responses to immunotherapy within the first year of allergen injections and can work up to maintenance injection intervals of 3 to 4 weeks. Because some patients have a delayed response, an initial trial of at least 3 years is encouraged. When a good to excellent response is observed, cessation of immunotherapy is considered after 3 to 5 years. However, approximately 40 per cent of such patients may experience a recurrence of symptoms.

In mold-sensitive patients, it is essential that indigenous allergenic fungal species be used in preparation of the extract mixture. Immunotherapy for animal protein allergens (e.g., cat and dog) should not be routinely recommended for control of sensitivity to house pets. This form of therapy may be justified for patients whose livelihood (e.g., veterinarians, laboratory animal workers) depends on frequent exposure to animals. Patients undergoing this therapy should be informed of the known increased risk of immediate systemic reactions following injections and the potential unknown risks of long-term parenteral immunization with heterologous animal proteins.

Postulated mechanisms responsible for the overall efficacy of immunotherapy include (1) the formation of IgG "blocking" antibodies; (2) the induction of T cell–dependent immune tolerance associated with in vitro identification of specific T suppressor cells in treated patients; (3) the formation of antigen-specific anti-idiotypic antibodies that regulate specific IgE production downward; and (4) the induction of B cell tolerance leading to decreased IgE production.

The major adverse effects of allergen immunotherapy are local or systemic immediate allergic reactions occurring within 15 minutes after an allergen injection. Thus we recommend that patients be observed for at least 20 minutes following each allergen injection. Because life-threatening anaphylaxis is a possible but rare occurrence, epinephrine (1:1000) must be readily available. In the event of systemic allergic reactions, 0.3 ml of epinephrine (1:1000) should be administered subcutaneously. An additional 0.2 ml may be given at the site of an allergen injection to vasoconstrict and minimize systemic absorption of antigen. Benadryl, 50 to 100 mg orally or intramuscularly, should be given, although this drug should not be considered as the drug of first choice for the treatment of anaphylaxis. Intravenous hydrocortisone sodium succinate (200 mg of Solucortef) should be administered immediately and prednisone orally four times daily is also recommended for 2 days after a systemic reaction to modify any late clinical responses (e.g., urticaria, angioedema, and bronchospasm), which are common following severe IgE-mediated reactions.

When intensive pharmacotherapeutic and immunologic modalities are insufficient in a patient, the physician must periodically re-evaluate other contributing factors. Nonallergic diseases such as coexistent vasomotor rhinitis or chronic sinusitis may hinder response to treatment. Daily irritant exposure at work or home (e.g., sulfur dioxide, cigarette smoke) may cause toxic or irritant inflammatory reactions in the nasal mucosa. Acquisition of a new house pet after the initial allergic evaluation can account for a recent onset of symptoms in a previously stable patient. Interventions such as stricter avoidance measures and antibiotic treatment for acute or chronic sinusitis may be necessary to enhance overall response of the patient.

Surgery is rarely indicated or effective as a primary treatment for allergic rhinitis. Nasal polypectomy or sphenoidethmoidectomy may be necessary in patients with severe coexistent chronic sinusitis in whom intensive medical treatment has failed. However, polypectomy should not be performed as an alternative to medical treatment since the polyps recur in the majority of patients.

ALLERGIC REACTIONS TO DRUGS

method of
JOHN A. ANDERSON, M.D.
University of Michigan
Detroit, Michigan

Adverse reactions to drugs or *drug sensitivity* represents unintended and undesirable effects following the usual or appropriate use of specific agents in the diagnosis, treatment, or prevention of disease. These reactions may be further broadly classified on the basis of the involvement of immune mechanisms. *Allergic reactions to drugs* refer to those adverse reactions that involve immune mechanisms. *Drug intolerance* is a term that represents all other reactions—both those that are clearly based on nonimmune mechanisms and others in which the cause is unknown. Drug intolerance includes reactions because of *drug overdose, drug side effects, secondary drug effects, drug interactions, drug-induced teratogenicity, maternal-fetal/maternal-child toxic drug transfers,* as well as *drug idiosyncrasy.*

Most of the adverse reactions to drugs fall into the food intolerance or nonimmune category. Allergic reactions to drugs (immunologic reactions) account for 25 per cent or less of all adverse reactions. Truly allergic reactions (Types I, II, III, and IV) probably only represent 6 to 10 per cent of the total (Table 1). Since some drug reactions are suspected of involving immune mechanisms (but are not proved allergic) and other reactions resemble allergic reaction, two other classifications are used: *possible drug allergy* and *pseudoallergic drug reaction.* The most important and potentially most serious allergic drug reaction is *anaphylaxis,* which is discussed in a separate article.

TABLE 1. **Allergic and Allergic-Like Reactions to Drugs**

DRUG ALLERGY (immunologic adverse reactions)	
Type I:	*IgE-mediated hypersensitivity* (e.g., penicillin, chymopapain and insulin anaphylaxis)
Type II:	*Cytotoxic antibodies or antitissue antibodies* (e.g., quinidine thrombocytopenia, penicillin hemolytic anemia)
Type III:	*Arthus, immune complex antigen-antibody and complement-mediated reactions* (e.g., serum sickness from any drug, procaine amide lupus-like reaction, pituitary snuff allergic alveolitis)
Type IV:	*Cell-mediated hypersensitivity* (e.g., neomycin and paraben contact dermatitis)
POSSIBLE DRUG ALLERGY (suspected reactions involving immune mechanisms)	
Many drug-associated skin reactions (e.g., erythema, erythema multiforme, maculopapular rash, fixed drug reaction)	
Drug fever	
Eosinophilic pneumonitis	
Drug-induced cholestasis and hepatitis	
Interstitial nephritis	
Lymhadenopathy	
PSEUDOALLERGIC DRUG REACTION (pseudohypersensitivity, drug idiosyncrasy)	
Anaphylactoid (anaphylaxis-like) reaction (e.g., radiocontrast media)	
Salicylate intolerance (in some cases due to modification of mediator production or release)	
Febrile mucocutaneous syndrome (erythema multiforme, Stevens-Johnson syndrome, toxic epidermal necrolysis, or Lyell's syndrome) (e.g., associated with penicillin, sulfonamides, barbiturates, or hydantoin)	
Jarisch-Herxheimer reactions	
Ampicillin rash	

Assessment of Patients with a History of Prior Adverse Reaction to Drug

The circumstances concerning a prior history of an adverse reaction to a drug should be carefully scrutinized by the physician to distinguish allergic (and allergic-like) reactions from nonallergic or drug intolerance reactions, as well as from reactions that are only coincidentally related to drug exposure. The term allergy is often misused by the patient to indicate any perceived abnormal or unexpected event which the patient relates to the exposure to a medication. Often the true circumstances are misinterpreted by the patient. Also, even though a reaction from a drug exposure did occur, the character of the reaction can be explained as a recognizably minor side effect of the drug and not that of a significant, possibly life-threatening adverse reaction. It may be important to clarify this situation so that usual medications are *not* excluded from potential use simply because of the perception of "an allergic reaction."

If a reasonable likelihood of an allergic or an allergic-like reaction to a drug-of-choice exists, then alternative approaches to management should be considered. The issue of cross-reactivity should be in the physician's mind when choosing alternative medications. Examples include the following cross-reactivities: (1) all beta-lactam antibiotics (penicillin, semisynthetic penicillin, and, to some degree, cephalosporin), (2) cross-reactivity of the *p*-aminophenyl group of local anesthetics, such as procaine, tetracaine, and benzocaine (but the lack of cross-reactivity of lidocaine or carbocaine), (3) possible cross-reactivity of aspirin with other nonsteroidal analgesics and anti-inflammatory agents, i.e., Motrin (but not sodium salicylate and acetaminophen), (4) cross-reactivity of sulfonamide with sulfonyl urea and oral hypoglycemic agents, diuretics related to sulfa (e.g., thiazide) hydrate inhibitors, and disulfiram, and (5) cross-reactivities of ethylenediamine with promethazine, antozoline, and aminophylline.

TABLE 2. **Penicillin Skin Testing***

Skin Test Type	*Drug Conc*	*Test Vol*
Major Determinant:		
Penicilloyl-Polylysine (PPL)†		
1. Prick or scratch	skin test strength	1 drop
2. Intradermal	skin test strength	0.02 ml
Minor Determinant:		
Penicillin G‡		
1. Prick or scratch	10,000 μ/ml	1 drop
2. Intradermal	(100 μ/ml optional)	0.02 ml
	(1000 μ/ml optional)	0.02 ml
	10,000 μ/ml	0.02 ml

*Prick skin tests first read at 10 minutes and, if positive, no further tests are necessary. If negative, intradermal tests are then performed.

†Kremers Urban Co.—supplied in skin test strength.

‡Freshly prepared in buffered saline.

Immunologic Assessment of Allergic Drug Reactions

Practical office and laboratory assessment of allergic drug reaction is limited to the measurement of IgE drug allergen-specific antibodies for Type I hypersensitivity by either direct immediate-reacting allergy skin testing or the in vitro measurement of serum IgE antibodies. These studies can be used to help confirm the presence of the following drug reactions: penicillin, insulin and protamine, animal serum, chicken egg and egg-containing vaccine, semisynthetic penicillin, cephalosporin, chymopapain, and possibly local anesthetics.

Patients who have a history of a prior adverse reaction involving penicillin should not be given penicillin (or semisynthetic penicillin) without investigation. Alternative treatments should be considered. (A small percentage of truly penicillin-allergic patients may also react to cephalosporin antibiotics, so these drugs should not be considered as alternative antibiotics without prior patient investigation.)

Immediate-reacting IgE skin testing, which measures IgE antibodies to penicillin and penicillin metabolites, is an indicator of the patient's probable response to the next dose of penicillin. Table 2 demonstrates the skin test procedure for freshly prepared penicillin G (as a measure of minor allergen determinant) and penicilloyl-polylysine, Pre-Pen (as a measure of major allergen determinant). These skin tests are preferably administered and interpreted by physicians familiar with this type of evaluation. The reliability of testing for the major determinant using PPL alone is about 75 per cent. The addition of the minor determinant, as represented by penicillin G, will single out most (but not all) additional allergic individuals. Most investigators have shown that testing in this fashion to penicillin G and PPL also reliably identifies most of the patients sensitive to the semisynthetic penicillins—because of cross-reactivity. In selective patients, however, specific semisynthetic penicillin (as well as cephalosporin) skin testing is possible and may be of value. The exact risk of cephalosporin sensitivity in patients known to be allergic to penicillin is not known but is probably smaller than originally reported. In vitro assays of penicillin-specific IgE antibodies (RAST/ELISA) are possible but are not as helpful as screening techniques, as are the penicillin skin-testing methods.

Diabetic patients who develop either local or systemic (unusual) reactions to insulin or protamine can be studied using both prick/intradermal allergy skin testing and in vitro IgE allergen-specific measurements (RAST/ELISA). Studies of this type should be performed by allergists and diabetologists. Since human insulin (HI) has been introduced, approximately 50 per cent of the patients shown to be allergic to either beef or pork animal insulins have been found to be safely converted to HI—even without skin testing—especially in the case of local reactions.

Egg sensitivity can result in urticarial reactions or systemic anaphylaxis in allergic persons receiving vaccine containing trace amounts of chicken egg protein allergen. Vaccines with this potential include influenza, yellow fever, rubeola (measles), mumps, and typhus. Patients who cannot safely eat chicken eggs can be skin-tested using prick/intradermal allergy skin testing techniques with both chicken egg and with 1:10 and 1:100 weight/volume strength of the vaccine to identify sensitivity.

Patients with back problems who are to undergo chemonucleolysis may be at risk for sensitivity to chymopapain. The risk is increased in patients who are atopic as well as in patients who have had a prior exposure to papain. Prick (but not intradermal skin testing, since chymopapain is an enzyme) as well as in vitro RAST/ELISA allergen-specific IgE measurements can be helpful to identify some (but not all) patients who are at risk for anaphylaxis to chymopapain (overall risk is approximately 1 per cent).

True allergic reactions to local anesthetics probably make up less than 1 per cent of all adverse local anesthetic reactions (such as to procaine or benzocaine). Allergy skin-testing for suspected sensitivities, as well as to other *prospectively safe* and generally noncross-reactive local anesthetics, such as lidocaine and carbocaine, may be performed to confirm or rule out sensitivity. In most cases, these tests are followed by the serial and subcutaneous injection of a local anesthetic which has been shown to be negative on prick/ID skin testing. Volumes of local anesthetic of 0.1, 1:100 w/v; 0.1, 1:10 w/v; and 0.1 undiluted local anesthetics are followed by 0.5 and 1.0 ml of undiluted local anesthetic successively at 20 to 30 minute intervals while the patient is under controlled conditions.

In most cases of adverse drug reaction, in vivo or in vitro tests are not available to confirm adequately the suspicion of an adverse reaction. In these cases, *direct challenge* under controlled conditions is the only method available to obtain proof of sensitivity. In a few drug sensitivities, procedures such as outlined in the situation with local anesthetics have been worked out to standardize challenge techniques. Examples also include a graded IV challenge for radiocontrast media reactions and for inhalation challenge with sulfur dioxide for patients possibly sensitive to the sulfite contained in inhalation medication.

TABLE 3. **Penicillin Desensitization**

Dose	Units	Route	Dose	Units	Route
ORAL ROUTE—					
Dose injected at 15 minute intervals					
1	100	oral	10	50,000	oral
2	200	oral	11	100,000	oral
3	400	oral	12	200,000	oral
4	800	oral	13	400,000	oral
5	1600	oral	14	200,000	subcutaneous
6	3200	oral	15	400,000	subcutaneous
7	6400	oral	16	800,000	subcutaneous
8	12,800	oral	17	1 million	intramuscular
9	25,000	oral	18	full therapeutic dose (IV)	

Dose	IV Units	Dose	IV Units
INTRAVENOUS ROUTE—			
Dose injected at 15 minute intervals			
1	10	10	5000
2	20	11	10,000
3	40	12	20,000
4	80	13	40,000
5	160	14	80,000
6	320	15	160,000
7	640	16	320,000
8	1280	17	640,000
9	2500	18	1,250,000

Desensitization and Premedication for the Patient Proved to Be or Suspected of Being Sensitive to Drugs

Desensitization, or the cautious administration of progressively larger doses of drug allergen, has been successfully applied to the management of the following drug sensitivities: penicillin, insulin, heterologous antiserums, egg-containing vaccines, and aspirin.

If penicillin must be administered to patients who are known to be anaphylactically sensitive to penicillin or semisynthetic penicillin, desensitization may be performed under controlled conditions. This procedure is best done by physicians familiar with the management of penicillin allergy. Table 3 gives examples of formats for the oral desensitization procedure (which is reported to be the safest route of administration) and the intravenous route of desensitization (which has the advantage of more control). With both these methods, any anaphylactic symptoms and signs that emerge can be controlled, allowing the patient to receive the necessary drug therapy.

In patients with a history of immediate hypersensitivity reaction to animal-derived insulin, the substitution of human insulin alone is often possible. If desensitization with any form of either animal-derived or human insulin is used, it is first desirable to do immediate-reacting prick and intradermal skin tests using serial tenfold dilution of U-100 regular insulin. In this fashion, the physician is able to identify the *least* reactive insulin type at the highest concentration of insulin that does not cause an immediate intradermal wheal and flare response. Insulin at this dose in units is then administered subcutaneously in a volume of 0.05 ml. Continued administration of the insulin by the subcutaneous route is done with progressively doubling doses (in units—not volume) at 30 minute intervals until therapeutic doses are achieved.

Desensitization for either heterologous antiserum (e.g., vaccine prepared in horses) or egg-containing vaccine may require individual formats depending upon the degree of the reactivity. One program would require 10 plus doses progressively administered at 15 minute intervals, from 0.1 ml of 1:1000 w/v strength serum or vaccine administered intradermally and progressing as follows: 0.2 ml, 1:1000 intradermally; 0.1 ml, 0.5 ml, 1.0 ml, 1:1000 subcutaneously; 0.2 ml, 0.5 ml, 1.0 ml, 1:100 subcutaneously; and 0.2 ml, 0.5 ml, 1.0 ml, 1:10 subcutaneously. At this point, the equivalent of 0.17 ml of undiluted serum/vaccine will have been administered. Subsequent administrations can be given by the subcutaneous and intramuscular route in graded doses to reach the desired total dose (e.g., vaccine total desired dose = 0.5 ml will require two additional doses of 0.13 and 0.2 ml undiluted subcutaneously).

The treatment of choice in aspirin-sensitive patients is almost always avoidance. If there is a compelling indication for the use of a nonsteroidal anti-inflammatory agent, however, or if aspirin-sensitive asthma is difficult to control by any other means, aspirin desensitization by trained personnel *may* be attempted under strictly controlled conditions. If the patient has asthma, desensitization should not be attempted if severe impairment of pulmonary function exists, since a further drop in pulmonary function can be anticipated during the desensitization process. Investigators have used a desensitization schedule that involves the oral administration of progressive doses of aspirin at 3 hour intervals with doses of 10 mg, 20 mg, 40 mg, 80 mg, 160 mg, 320 mg, and 650 mg. If the schedule is interrupted at night, it may be resumed the following morning beginning with the last or the next to the last tolerated dose. As in any other desensitization procedure, adverse effects that occur during the procedure must be treated vigorously (and the pulmonary function return to baseline) before progressing to the next dose on the desensitization schedule. The aspirin desensitization procedure continues until the full dose of aspirin is achieved. Usually other nonsteroidal drugs are tolerated at this point. In the aspirin-sensitive asthmatic patient, the state of "desensitization" is maintained only for a few days—however, if this is used in treatment, additional doses of aspirin should be given daily. (Once several days have elapsed without ASA, another dose of aspirin may cause a life-threatening attack of asthma.)

Occasionally patients are encountered who are at risk for developing anaphylaxis or anaphylactoid reactions unexpectedly. In a few of these patients, medications may be a factor. In these patients, as in patients sensitive to stinging insects or to foods, it is advisable to instruct the patient to carry Adrenalin for self-administration, either in a preloaded syringe or in a spring-loaded device (Ana-Kit or Epi-Pen/Epi-Pen Jr.).

Patients who have experienced an anaphylactoid reaction to radiocontrast media (RCM) are at increased risk of reaction upon re-exposure to this diagnostic agent. Additional possible risk factors include an age of 50 or more years, preexisting cardiac disease, acute renal failure, atopy, asthma, or serious debilitating illness. Alternative diagnostic procedures should be used in patients at risk for a radiocontrast medium reaction, whenever possible. If radiocontrast media must be used again, however, then it is usually preferable to use prophylactic medication.

TABLE 4. **Radiocontrast Media (RCM) Prophylactic Medication Program for Patients at Increased Risk**

Drug	Dose	Instructions
Diphenhydramine (Benadryl)	50 mg	Give PO 1 hr before or IV 5 min before RCM administration
Cimetidine (Tagamet)	300 mg	Give PO 1 hr before
	or	
Ranitidine (Zantac)	150 mg	Give IV 5 min before (cimetidine) RCM
Prednisone	50 mg	Give PO q 6 hr for 4 doses beginning 18 hr before RCM administration—*in severe risk situations*
Ephedrine sulfate	25 mg	Give PO 1 hr before RCM
Anhydrous theophylline	200 mg	Give PO 1 hr before RCM (or equivalent dose of aminophylline IV 5 min before RCM) when patient has a history of bronchospasm

Table 4 outlines the various drugs recommended for such prophylactic management. Diphenhydramine (Benadryl) should be given to all such patients. Cimetidine or ranitidine H_2 antihistamines may be considered, but their value is debatable. Patients who are at increased risk, especially those with a history of prior life-threatening systemic anaphylaxis or those with serious debilitating illness, should be started on prednisone (or its equivalent) 18 hours before RCM administration. Recently ephedrine sulfate has been recommended to reduce further the risk of reaction on subsequent RCM exposure. Theophylline also has been recommended as an additional therapy, especially in patients who are known to be asthmatic or who have developed bronchospasm with a prior exposure to RCM. Note, however, that in spite of all these prophylactic medications, including corticosteroids, patients with a prior history of severe reaction to RCM may be at risk at the rate of 50 per cent for another reaction upon subsequent RCM exposure. Knowing this fact, all staff in attendance should be prepared to treat a systemic anaphylactoid reaction, including bradycardiac shock.

INSECT STING ALLERGY

method of

MARTIN D. VALENTINE, M.D.

The Johns Hopkins University
Baltimore, Maryland

The normal local response to an insect sting consists of transient redness and swelling, usually with itching and occasionally with pain, all of these confined to the area of the sting and usually gone within 24 hours. This response is due to the vasoactive and pain-producing amines and polypeptides found in the venoms. By contrast, generalized allergic reactions to stings of the Hymenoptera (honeybees, yellowjackets, hornets, wasps, and fire ants) are due to prior sensitization to one or more of the protein constituents of the venoms. The allergens of importance in the common Hymenoptera venoms are seen in Table 1.

Allergic reactions to stings are generally classified by reaction pattern as well as severity within reaction type. Fewer than 50 deaths annually are reported in the United States from insect sting reactions; the unreported number must be many times this figure. Surveys of various populations suggest that between 0.5 and 5 per cent of the population has had a systemic reaction to a sting; the prevalence of the sensitized state probably approaches 20 per cent, the likelihood of having a positive skin test being greater if a recent sting has occurred. Although over 90 per cent of patients who report systemic reactions to stings have positive skin tests to one or more of the available venoms (honeybee; yellowjacket; yellow hornet; baldfaced hornet; *Polistes* sp.), the positive skin tests without a prior history of a systemic reaction do not predict what risk may exist for that individual for a future reaction.

In adults who have not been immunized with venom, the risk of future systemic reactions when one has already occurred is between 50 and 60 per cent. Immunotherapy with the appropriate Hymenoptera venoms reduces the risk of future systemic reactions to 3 per cent or less. In children up to age 16 years whose systemic reactions have been confined to the skin (e.g., generalized urticaria), the risk of future reactions appears smaller (10 per cent); if such a patient does have a reaction to another sting, the reaction is generally no worse in severity than the previous one.

TABLE 1. **Allergens of Hymenopteran Venoms**

Honeybee
Phospholipase A_2
Hyaluronidase
Acid phosphatase
Melittin
*Vespid**
Antigen 5
Phospholipase A_1
Hyaluronidase
Acid phosphatase

*"Vespid": Yellow jackets, hornets, and wasps.

Treatment Criteria

To be considered a candidate for venom immunotherapy, an adult must have had at least one prior systemic reaction to a sting and have evidence of a positive skin test to venom. "Prick" or "scratch" test techniques reduce the risk of systemic allergic reactions to skin testing and are used before intracutaneous tests in patients whose prior histories include severe or near-fatal reactions. In patients whose prior histories are less severe, the starting intracutaneous test concentration of venom that has generally proved safe is 0.01 microgram per ml. Venoms are tested individually to a maximum concentration of 1.0 microgram per ml (higher concentrations than these may be somewhat irritating to normal skin and produce nonspecific positive reactions). Alternatively, a serum sample may be assayed for IgE antibodies to venoms. Such assays should be performed only by a laboratory with an established reputation and broad experience in in vitro testing. Up to 20 per cent of individuals with positive histories and positive skin tests may have a negative "RAST" test due to insufficient serum antibody to be detectable in such an assay. These are regarded as false-negatives.

Treatment

Immunotherapy with venoms is recommended for any adult with a history of a systemic sting reaction and positive skin tests. With the exception of children whose reactions have been limited to the skin, the same criteria apply in childhood. Each venom that produces a distinct positive skin test at 1 microgram or less is included in the patient's treatment. A sample treatment regimen is shown in Table 2. Injections are given at weekly intervals until 100 micrograms of each relevant venom can be administered in a single dose without undue local or systemic reaction. After this level is reached, doses are repeated at increasing intervals until a 4 week interval is attained. This interval is used for the next 6 months, at which point the interval is usually extended to 6 weeks. The progress of immunotherapy may be checked by obtaining IgG

TABLE 2. **Venom Immunotherapy Schedule**

Day	Dose (μg)
1	0.1, 1.0, 3.0*
8	10
15	20
22	40
29	60
36	80
42	100

*On Day 1, the three doses are given at approximately 30 minute intervals, provided no untoward reaction develops. Systemic reactions to injections are rarely severe, but physicians administering any allergenic extract should be prepared to treat acute allergic reactions from immunotherapy. The suggested progression of doses should be modified if systemic reactions occur.

antibody levels for the respective immunizing venoms. If IgG levels lower than 3 micrograms per ml are found after the 100 microgram venom dose is attained, consideration is given to increasing the immunizing dose to 150 or 200 micrograms of each venom, which usually results in an improvement in the IgG response. It is not known how long venom immunotherapy may need to be maintained. Presumably this may be as long as skin tests to venom remain positive. This question is under study.

Sting Avoidance

Ordinary insect repellents do not appear to prevent stings from Hymenoptera. Nesting areas should be avoided and patients are counseled to avoid eating outdoors and to avoid going barefoot. Unimmunized patients with prior sting reactions should carry an emergency kit such as the Ana-Kit (Hollister Laboratories, Spokane, Washington) or the Epi-Pen (Center Laboratories, Port Washington, New York). The Epi-Pen is an automatic self injector, which some people find easier to use than the Ana-Kit. The advantage of the Ana-Kit is that it provides the option of a second 0.3 mg dose of epinephrine if needed after the first dose is delivered. The advantage of the Epi-Pen is that it is designed to provide an automatic injection when appropriately applied: a second advantage is the availability of a "junior" size designed to deliver 0.15 mg of epinephrine rather than the 0.3 mg in the regular version. Antihistamines such as chlorpheniramine or diphenhydramine may be quite helpful in reducing pruritus locally and systemically, but these drugs will not help greatly in more severe anaphylactic reactions. Whether corticosteroids are of benefit is moot since even when administered parenterally they take several hours to begin working and are clearly not a first choice drug for a severe reaction.

Large Local Reactions

Some patients experience redness, pain, swelling, and itching contiguous with the skin site but peaking at 24 to 72 hours after the sting and involving an area of greater than several centimeters. An example of such a reaction would be swelling of an entire distal extremity when a person was stung on a toe or finger. Some care must be taken to distinguish this from local cellulitis. Large local reactions to stings can generally be treated with antihistamines and aspirin or acetaminophen; some believe that oral corticosteroids for several days hasten resolution of large local reactions. Approximately 90 per cent of patients with large local reactions also have positive skin tests, and about 5 per cent may eventually have a systemic reaction to a sting. This progression rate to systemic reactions is generally not considered high enough to warrant prescribing immunotherapy for all patients with large local reactions.

Section 12

Diseases of the Skin

ACNE VULGARIS AND ROSACEA

method of
ALAN R. SHALITA, M.D.
State University of New York
Brooklyn, New York

Acne Vulgaris

Acne vulgaris is the most common skin disease. It affects approximately 80 per cent of the teenage population and, contrary to popular belief, may persist well into the third and fourth decades of life. Acne is a disease of the pilosebaceous follicle with a multifactorial cause. The pathogenesis includes an androgen-dependent increase in sebum production, proliferation of the follicular microflora (principally *Propionibacterium acnes*), and alterations in follicular keratinization. This results in the clinical lesions of acne—namely, open comedones (blackheads), closed comedones (whiteheads), papules, pustules, and nodulocystic lesions. Current therapy is directed toward suppression of these lesions by affecting one or more of the pathogenic factors. Treatment is remarkably effective in most patients.

Topical Therapy

Many patients may be successfully treated with topical therapy alone. For comedonal and mild inflammatory acne, therapy is initiated with tretinoin (Retin-A) cream, 0.05 per cent, or 0.01 per cent tretinoin gel applied daily. The patient should be advised that an initial erythema and exfoliation may occur, that an exacerbation of inflammatory lesions is possible during the first month of therapy, and that an increased sensitivity to sunburn is likely. For the latter condition it is advisable to limit sun exposure and to recommend a suitable (SPF 15) sunscreen.

Patients who demonstrate little or no response and who have exhibited little or no erythema or desquamation may be placed on higher concentrations of the drug, either the 0.1 per cent cream or 0.025 per cent gel. A few patients may require the 0.05 per cent liquid, the most irritating form of the drug, before achieving a satisfactory therapeutic response. Significant therapeutic improvement does not usually occur before 4 to 6 weeks, and 12 weeks are usually required for optimal therapeutic benefit. Topical tretinoin appears to exert its effect on the keratinizing epithelium of the follicle.

For the more inflammatory forms of acne, the addition of a benzoyl peroxide gel (Desquam-X, Persa-Gel, PanOxyl) is frequently beneficial. Benzoyl peroxide is a potent antibacterial agent that significantly reduces the intrafollicular population of *P. acnes*. Therapy is usually initiated with the 5 per cent gel applied daily, although some patients may achieve a satisfactory response to the 2.5 per cent concentration. Refractory cases and patients with considerable involvement of the back and chest may require the 10 per cent concentration. Although little erythema usually occurs, there may be considerable desquamation. In addition, a small percentage of the population may exhibit contact allergy to benzoyl peroxide.

Our preferred method of topical treatment is the sequential use of topical tretinoin and benzoyl peroxide, one applied in the morning and the other at night. The effects of the two drugs appear to be additive. Some patients, however, will not tolerate the "dryness" produced by this regimen. One may then try therapy with each drug on alternate days. Eventually, most patients will accommodate to these local side effects and will be able to use both drugs on the same day.

Topical antibiotic solutions, such as those containing erythromycin (T-Stat, Staticin, ATS, Ery-Derm) and clindamycin (Cleocin-T), are useful alternatives to benzoyl peroxide in the treatment of inflammatory acne. They offer the advantage of being essentially nonsensitizing but may result in the overgrowth of resistant organisms. Erythromycin solution, 1.5 to 2.0 per cent, and clindamycin solution, 1.0 per cent, appear to be equal in therapeutic value. They may be used in conjunction with topical tretinoin, as described for benzoyl peroxide. Recent investigations suggest that combining benzoyl peroxide and a topical antibiotic produces better results than when either agent is used alone. A stabilized formulation of erythromycin, 3 per cent, and benzoyl peroxide, 5 per cent (Benzamycin), has recently become available and may be used in the sequential regimen with tretinoin. For those patients easily irritated by hydroalcoholic gels or solutions, meclocycline cream (Meclan) or erythromycin ointment (Akne-mycin) may be used satisfactorily.

Preparations containing various combinations of sulfur, resorcin, and salicylic acid, particularly in tinted lotions and creams, may be useful when used judiciously. They accelerate the resolution of inflammatory lesions while providing cover. In addition, cleansers containing salicylic acid may be useful, particularly in patients who do not tolerate topical tretinoin. Salicylic acid has mild comedolytic properties.

Systemic Therapy

Broad-spectrum antibiotics remain valuable tools in the treatment of inflammatory acne. They are generally reserved for patients with inflammatory acne and have achieved a remarkable record of safety in long-term use. Therapy is usually initiated with 500 to 1000 mg of tetracycline hydrochloride or erythromycin. The dose is decreased at appropriate intervals according to the therapeutic response. Minocycline (Minocin), 50 mg daily to four times daily is useful in those patients who appear to be refractory to the aforementioned agents. An alternative is larger doses of tetracycline, up to 3000 mg daily.

Recent evidence suggests that many women with inflammatory acne may have elevated androgens, either of adrenal or ovarian origin. In these patients, treatment with oral contraceptives, low dose dexamethasone, or a combination of the two may be quite beneficial.

Patients with severe, recalcitrant, nodulocystic acne who have failed to respond to the treatment regimens outlined may achieve remarkable improvement with isotretinoin (Accutane). Isotretinoin is administered in a dose of 1 mg per kg daily. Patients with severe involvement of the back and chest may require as much as 2 mg per kg daily. The course of treatment is from 4 to 5 months, and improvement is variable during this time period. Some patients may not achieve maximum improvement until they have completed the course of treatment. Relapses are rare and remissions lasting as long as 6 years have been reported. In any case, it is advisable to wait at least 3 to 4 months before retreating the refractory patient.

Isotretinoin therapy is accompanied by numerous side effects. Most noteworthy is the fact that the drug is teratogenic in humans. Women of child-bearing age, therefore, should have pregnancy tests before initiation of therapy, practice strict contraception during treatment, and be constantly reminded of the teratogenic effects of the drug. It appears safe for conception to occur 1 month after discontinuing treatment. The drug is not mutagenic and has no effect on the ability to conceive and no apparent effects on spermatozoa. Most additional side effects relate to the fact that the drug causes a pronounced reduction in sebum production. Thus there is dryness of the skin, marked chapping of the lips, and cheilitis; dryness of the mucosa, which can lead to epistaxis and conjunctivitis; and some pruritus. All of these can be alleviated by the use of emollients. Although a variety of laboratory abnormalities may occur, the most significant is triglyceride elevation. For this reason it is recommended that baseline fasting triglycerides be obtained before treatment and every 2 weeks thereafter until a plateau has been reached. Dietary modification, prohibition of alcohol, and dose reduction will usually reduce these triglyceride elevations. If not, it is recommended that patients whose triglyceride levels rise above 750 mg per dl discontinue the drug. Bone pain, muscle aches, headache, and fatigue have been reported with some frequency. Most are relieved with simple analgesics. Pseudotumor cerebri has also been reported and appears to occur with increased frequency in patients taking isotretinoin and a tetracycline concomitantly. Therefore, the use of these two drugs together appears contraindicated. Finally, there are rare reports of decreased night vision and bony exostoses of the cervical vertebrae. The latter appear to be asymptomatic. Given this side effect profile, it is evident that the drug should be limited to the most severe forms of the disease or to those patients who have proved to be totally refractory to conventional forms of acne treatment.

Systemic glucocorticoids are rarely required in the management of acne except as noted in the low dose treatment of women with increased androgen secretion. Larger doses (30 to 40 mg daily) may be used for brief periods of time in patients who develop flares of their disease during the course of isotretinoin treatment. Local injections of glucocorticoids such as triamcinolone acetonide (2.5 mg to 5.0 mg per ml) are useful for the treatment of individual nodulocystic lesions and for the exuberant granulation tissue that may develop during treatment with isotretinoin. The use of a 1 ml syringe with a 30 gauge needle provides excellent control of the amount of material injected. No more than 0.5 mg should be injected in any one site. Triamcinolone hexacetamide, 5 mg per ml, is longer lasting but may produce more atrophy and should be limited to lesions of the chest and back. It is also useful for the treatment of hypertrophic scars.

The physical removal of comedones with a comedo extractor is frequently beneficial. Incision and drainage of inflammatory lesions rarely accomplishes more than intralesional steroids.

Rosacea

Rosacea is a not uncommon disease of the skin that usually occurs from the fourth decade of life onward. It may be preceded by seborrheic dermatitis and appears to be more common in fair-skinned individuals of Celtic background. It is characterized by facial erythema, particularly of the perinasal area. More pronounced involvement may include the glabella, perioral areas, and the chin. As the disease progresses, telangiectasia, papules and pustules, and granulomatous tissue may form. The disease appears to be aggravated by all factors that increase blood flow to the head and neck, such as strenuous exercise, hot foods, increased temperature, hypertension, alcohol ingestion, and emotional stress.

Therapy

Most patients with rosacea will respond to combined therapy with oral tetracycline and topical anti-inflammatory measures. Tetracycline therapy is initiated at 1000 mg daily and reduced at monthly intervals to a maintenance dose of 250 mg daily. Many patients will achieve enough of a response to discontinue tetracycline for varying periods of time, but most will relapse at one time or another. Topical therapy should consist of the judicial use of hydrocortisone alone or in combination with 3 per cent precipitated sulfur or 10 per cent sodium sulfacetamide. Fluorinated steroid preparations are contraindicated since they will produce rebound telangiectasia. Even hydrocortisone (1 to 2.5 per cent) should be limited to twice daily applications for brief periods of time to control the symptoms. Topical antibiotic therapy is occasionally beneficial, but many patients with rosacea do not tolerate the hydroalcoholic vehicles. For these patients erythromycin ointment (Akne-mycin) or meclocycline cream (Meclan) may be tried, although neither has been subjected to rigorous clinical evaluation for this purpose.

Isotretinoin has been reported to be particularly effective in patients with the more severe papulopustular and granulomatous forms of the disease. Reports conflict as to whether or not this drug has any effect on the telangiectasia. A dose of 0.5 mg per kg has been reported to be effective for this disease.

Telangiectasia may be treated by gentle electrodesiccation using an epilating needle with the lowest current available. Exuberant tissue such as that found in rhinophyma may be removed by electrosurgery, dermabrasion, or laser treatment.

Some patients with rosacea may develop ophthalmologic complications. Blepharitis is common and frequently is accompanied by conjunctivitis. Keratitis is less common but left untreated may result in visual impairment. All respond to oral tetracycline therapy. The addition of sodium sulfacetamide ophthalmic ointment is frequently of added benefit. Refractory patients should be referred to an ophthalmologist.

DISEASES OF THE HAIR

method of
NORMAN ORENTREICH, M.D.,
New York University
and DAVID S. ORENTREICH, M.D.
Mount Sinai School of Medicine
New York, New York

Alopecia can result from pathologic processes that involve either the living hair matrix and dermal papilla or the dead keratinized hair shaft. When only the hair shaft is involved, the hair loss is temporary and due to breakage; the follicle continues to produce hair without interruption.

In anagen defluvium, matrix arrest interrupts hair growth, usually with hair shaft breakage; the follicles remain in anagen. Shedding begins 1 to 2 weeks after the insult. Anagen defluvium may be induced by cytostatic agents, thallium, x-rays, and alopecia areata. When the insult is removed, the hair matrix resumes hair production. Alopecia secondary to chemotherapy can be ameliorated or prevented by applying a tourniquet to or cooling the scalp during administration of the antineoplastic agent, but there is a risk of preventing treatment of subclinical scalp metastases.

In a telogen defluvium, anagen hair follicles are prematurely thrown into telogen; excessive shedding of club hairs (telogen) occurs approximately 3 months later when anagen resumes. Telogen defluvium occurs after childbirth, high fever, hemorrhage, starvation, accidental or surgical trauma, and administration of certain drugs (megadoses of vitamin A, heparin, coumarin, triparanol, carbamazepine, lithium, indomethacin, allopurinol, gentamicin, propranolol, levodopa, Dilantin, carbimazole, and thiouracil).

When either the entire follicle or the dermal papilla is destroyed, loss of that hair is permanent (cicatricial alopecia).

Physiologic Shedding

Resting and growing hairs are randomly distributed throughout the scalp; approximately 10 to 15 per cent are in telogen and the rest are in anagen. With approximately 100,000 hairs on the scalp, there is a random shedding of 50 to 150 hairs a day. Normal shedding is seasonally increased in the fall and decreased in the spring in the north temperate zone. If not performed daily, shampooing is accompanied by increased shedding because it harvests several days accumulation of telogen hairs.

Congenital Alopecia

Congenital alopecia can be diffuse, complete, or patchy. It may occur with other congenital ectodermal anomalies (e.g., teeth and nails). A biopsy proves the absence of hair follicles; focal congenital alopecia is correctable by punch autografts.

Endocrinopathy-Associated Alopecias

The following endocrinopathies can produce alopecia: hyperpituitarism; hypopituitarism; hyperthyroidism; hypothyroidism; hypoparathyroidism; hypocorticoidism; diffuse adrenocortical hyperplasia; benign and malignant androgenic adrenocortical tumors; benign and malignant androgenic ovarian tumors; polycystic ovaries; and diabetes. These conditions may be helped by appropriate endocrinologic medical therapy or surgery, but hair regrowth may not occur for many months.

Relative hyperandrogenic states that can trigger androgen-dependent alopecia in genetically predisposed individuals are puberty, menopause, the postpartum period, after relatively estrogenic contraceptive therapy, and during relatively androgenic oral contraceptive therapy.

Androgenetic Alopecia

Androgenetic alopecia (AGA), or androchronogenetic alopecia, is the most common type of hair loss in both sexes. It occurs only in scalp follicles with the genetic potential to be inhibited by androgens over time. Male pattern baldness is its common name.

For both men and women, the androgenic dermatoses include AGA, oily skin, and acne. Women may also exhibit varying degrees of hirsutism: darker, longer, coarser hair of the chin, upper lip, sideburns, body, arms, and legs; a masculinized pubic hair distribution, including midline hairs from the pubis to umbilicus; and periareolar breast hair. Menstrual irregularity may accompany skin symptoms.

AGA is controlled by a single, dominant, sex-limited, autosomal gene and may be influenced by polygenic modifying factors affecting expressivity of the trait. Hormonal and aging influences are operative at the genome level; no expression of baldness occurs in the absence of circulating androgens. The genetic potential is expressed if the appropriate androgen enters the target cells of the hair papilla and/or matrix, binds with a specific cytosol receptor protein, and is translocated to the nucleus, where it interacts with the cell's genetic material.

Medical Treatment

Medical treatment of AGA is directed toward the androgenic component, because treatment cannot be effectively directed against the chronogenetic components. Because of the inherent lag time in hair growth response, no clinically noticeable therapeutic effect can be expected in less than 3 to 6 months. Frequent shampooing (preferably daily) removes scalp sebum, a source of dihydrotestosterone (DHT).

Surgical or medical castration arrests but does not reverse the balding process. Any reduction of androgen levels sufficient to stop hair loss also produces gynecomastia and a decrease in libido and potency. (Theoretically, reduction of only plasma DHT levels would be free of these undesired effects.)

Scalp skin contains the 5-alpha-reductase enzyme that converts testosterone to DHT; reducing local production of DHT is possible by increasing the scalp level of progesterone, a competitor for the 5-alpha-reductase enzyme. In the presence of progesterone, 5-alpha-reductase makes less DHT and more dihydroprogesterone (DHP); DHP in turn competes against residual DHT for the cytosol nuclear binding protein, further reducing the amount of DHT making gene contact. Since progesterone only partially inhibits DHT production and since DHP incompletely inhibits cytosol nuclear binding of residual DHT, local progesterone at best can ameliorate AGA; it cannot arrest AGA. Treatment lapses result in the resumption of DHT production from testosterone.

Topical progesterone is usually administered as a 1 to 4 per cent tincture in males. It may be combined with 1 per cent spironolactone, an inhibitor of nuclear DHT uptake.

Topical minoxidil (Loniten) is used for the treatment of AGA in both men and women. Minoxidil is an antihypertensive, peripheral vasodilator that presumably works by increasing the blood supply to the scalp; by raising skin temperature, the rate of hair growth is increased. Treated hairs show elongation, thickening, and enhanced pigmentation. Topical minoxidil, in concentrations of 2 to 3 per cent, is effective in approximately 20 per cent of patients. Upon cessation of therapy the hypertrichosis abates. (This use of minoxidil is not listed by the manufacturer.)

Topical therapy is the same for men and women with one notable exception; menstrual irregularity from excess percutaneous absorption of progesterone can occur if more than 2 ml of a 2 per cent solution (40 mg) is applied daily.

Plasma hyperandrogenism is not rare in women with multiple androgenic dermatoses. Estrogen therapy, or surgery when indicated, reduces ovarian hyperandrogenism. Adrenal androgens can contribute significantly to androgenization of women, especially in the second and third decades of life when dehydroepiandrosterone and its sulfate (DHEAS) are at their highest levels. Excessive adrenal production of androgens (as measured by serum DHEAS) can be effectively and safely reduced by as little as 2.5 mg of prednisone taken orally at bedtime; there is no significant change in cortisol levels or adrenal reserve capacity. Eliminating exogenous androgens that may precipitate or aggravate AGA is beneficial. Exogenous sources are androgenic drugs; androgenic birth control pills; and foods such as wheat germ oil, peanut oil, and brewer's yeast that contain testosterone and/or DHT.

Testosterone and DHT circulate in the blood mostly bound to plasma proteins, especially sex hormone–binding globulin (SHBG); however, only the free hormone can enter a cell. Deficient liver production of SHBG results in higher levels of free testosterone and DHT. Estrogens and thyroids stimulate liver production of SHBG and thereby reduce free plasma androgen levels.

Estrogens in the form of birth control pills that contain nonandrogenic progestins may be prescribed after gynecologic consultation. L-triiodothyronine (Cytomel, 37.5 to 75 micrograms orally in the morning) or other thyroid agents can be administered to euthyroid women in good health; relative contraindications are hypertension, arteriosclerotic heart disease, tachycardia, cardiac arrhythmia, and tremulousness. (This use of Cytomel is not listed by the manufacturer.)

Cyproterone acetate, a remarkably effective systemic antiandrogen in the treatment of all androgenic dermatoses, is not available in the United States.

Cimetidine, a histamine H_2 antagonist, has been reported to be effective in hirsutism. Although there are no publications on its effects in alopecia, informal clinical use indicates some benefit.

Surgical Treatment

Sites of advanced AGA can be effectively and permanently corrected with full thickness, hair-bearing punch autografts obtained from the AGA-resistant occiput. In their new location, transplanted follicles continue to produce hair at the same rate and of the same texture and color as they did in the occipital scalp. When indicated, bald scalp reduction can reduce the area requiring hair transplants.

Neoplastic Alopecia

Benign and malignant neoplasms can produce hair loss by pressure, displacement, replacement, or systemic influences. Internal pressure, typically from a cyst, may cause a localized alopecia. Permanent alopecic areas that remain after treatment of the neoplasm may be corrected with hair-bearing scalp transplants.

Acquired Traumatic Alopecia

Acute Traction. Plucking, combing, or brushing may break the hair shaft but does not disrupt continuity of growth; evulsing growing scalp hair from follicles induces telogen and a temporary (3 month) cessation of growth.

Chronic Traction. Tight "pony tails," "corn rowing" braids, curlers, hair pins, bobby pins, styling combs, and barrettes can cause alopecia. Alopecia is temporary if the traction is not prolonged, but permanent follicular destruction by avascular necrosis can result from prolonged traction.

Avulsion. The forcible tearing away of scalp tissue may, if untreated, cause not only loss of the hair-bearing skin but also injury to the underlying skull. If the avulsed area is small, then immediate replacement of the avulsed skin may "take," with partial or complete regrowth of hair. Prompt microvascular anastomosis of an entire avulsed scalp can prevent avascular scalp necrosis and permanent alopecia. Laceration may cause alopecia at the site of injury that can be permanent if there is scarring. Punch autografts are a suitable therapy for acquired traumatic alopecia and scars of the scalp.

Friction. Occupational or sporting gear can cause hair shaft breakage close to the scalp. Hair breakage is commonly seen on an infant's head in the area of frictional contact with the mattress or crib. This condition invariably improves after removal of the eliciting cause. Lichen simplex chronicus (neurodermatitis) can produce a self-inflicted frictional alopecia.

Edema. Prolonged general anesthesia, especially in the Trendelenburg position, may cause a temporary alopecia in the area of dependent edema.

Electrical Burns. Electrical burns that destroy the hair follicles produce permanent hair loss; superficial burns result only in temporary alopecia.

Thermal Trauma. Extreme heat or cold can cause permanent hair loss if there is deep necrosis with hair follicle destruction.

Chemical Contactants. Industrial or cosmetic chemical contactants usually produce only partial or complete disintegration of the hair shaft, resulting in hair breakage and temporary alopecia. Severe primary irritant reactions that destroy hair follicles produce permanent alopecia. Allergic eczematous contact dermatitis does not produce permanent alopecia.

Ionizing Radiation. Temporary alopecia can be

caused by ionizing radiation when only the epithelial elements are affected; in 3 to 5 weeks hair loss is complete, but regrowth may be seen in as early as 10 weeks. When radiation destroys the dermal papilla (more than 1,500 rads of a single dose of superficial x-rays with a half value layer of 0.9 mm Al or more), alopecia is permanent, invariably associated with radiodermatitis and an increased predisposition to skin cancers; there is no safe permanent epilating dose.

Infections

Localized Infection. Superficial infection seldom causes alopecia; deeper involvement can disrupt the follicular matrix and cause hair breakage or induce telogen, causing temporary alopecia. Follicular destruction can be caused by viruses (herpes simplex, varicella zoster, and variola) and bacteria (tuberculosis, leprosy, and pyogenic organisms). Most fungal infections involve the hair shaft and produce only breakage, although kerion celsi and favus can cause follicular destruction unless prompt treatment is instituted.

Systemic Infection. The high fever associated with systemic infection frequently causes transient telogen defluvium. The shedding is frequently associated with a Beau line—a transverse depression in the nail plate developed at the peak of illness. A corresponding narrowing in the hair shaft is called the Pohl-Pinkus mark.

Patchy, "moth-eaten" telogen defluvium is a typical sign of secondary syphilis; antibiotic therapy cures both conditions.

Neurologic and Psychiatric Alopecia

There is insufficient evidence to establish direct neurogenic or psychiatric effects on follicular function.

Trichotillomania

This subconscious or conscious pulling out, twisting, or breaking off of one's own hair from the scalp, eyebrows, or occasionally eyelashes is not uncommon and is frequently misdiagnosed as alopecia areata. The removed hair may be discarded or hidden; if ingested it occasionally results in a trichobezoar. To confirm the diagnosis with the "trichotillo test," firmly attach an occlusive substance or suture a bandage to an affected area; hair growth will be evident after removing the patch 4 to 8 weeks later. Psychiatric referral is recommended if the test is positive, especially if the patient continues to deny or cannot stop the compulsive, neurotic behavior. Chronic trichotillomania may produce permanent alopecia; for every 100 hairs plucked, 1 dermal papilla will be extirpated.

Nutritional and Metabolic Alopecia

Caloric deprivation must be severe (kwashiorkor, sprue, and celiac disease) to produce hair loss. Increased shedding sometimes occurs after marked weight loss for obesity. Anemia, diabetes, hyper- and hypovitaminosis, and zinc deficiency may be associated with alopecia.

Dermatologic Alopecias

Alopecia Areata. Alopecia areata is a group of alopecias probably with an autoimmunologic etiology. It may take many forms—areata, concentric, guttate, diffuse localized, diffuse generalized, ophiastic, totalis, or universalis. The hair loss is usually sudden and asymptomatic except for mild erythema and occasional premonitory paresthesia. Pathognomonic "exclamation point" hairs are present in the early, active phase. Fine grid-like pitting of the nails occurs in about 20 per cent of the patients, and dermatoglyphics may show an increased number of arches. Although single patches frequently regrow spontaneously within a few months, the course is unpredictable (including the rare extension to totalis or universalis) and recurrences are common. Alopecia areata is associated with various autoantibodies and with such autoimmune diseases as thyroiditis, vitiligo, Addison's disease, pernicious anemia, hyperparathyroidism, diabetes mellitus, myasthenia gravis, and rheumatoid arthritis.

Treatment

Hair growth in response to injection of anti-inflammatory corticosteroids into an alopecic site is both diagnostic and therapeutic. Usually only the most severe active phases of this disorder, or those where there has already been inflammatory destruction of the hair papilla, do not respond to this treatment. Under- or overdosage of injected corticoid may also account for therapeutic failure. The corticoid of choice is short-acting triamcinolone acetonide (Kenalog) at 5 mg per ml; the long-acting, less soluble triamcinolone hexacetonide (Aristospan) at 5 mg per ml may be substituted for some or all of the acetonide to provide a prolonged cutaneous depot. Injection of approximately 0.05 to 0.1 ml, at 1 to 2 cm intervals, usually produces good regrowth within 4 to 6 weeks and little, if any, temporary atrophy. Previously injected sites that are actively growing hair do not need reinjection. Total dosage depends upon the severity of the condition, but even the most severe involvement can usually be treated with 50 mg or less per month.

Since triamcinolone acetonide may have a progestational effect, especially above 20 mg, treatment can be given within a few days before or during menstruation to reduce menstrual irregularities. Topical spray cryogens (ethyl chloride,

Cryoesthesia, or Freon) usually produce sufficient anesthesia; block anesthesia of a scalp wedge can be achieved with lidocaine injections to the scalp perimeter through which innervation passes. Hair regrown from treatment is usually of the original texture and color but occasionally is darker or curlier; spontaneously regrown hair may be hypopigmented. Pigmented hair is sometimes more susceptible to loss during recurrences; occasionally all pigmented hair is lost, creating apparent overnight graying, which is really partial and selective alopecia areata.

Oral anti-inflammatory corticosteroids have been given alone or in conjunction with intralesional injections for extensive alopecia areata or alopecia totalis and alopecia universalis but are best avoided, since a safe and therapeutic regimen is rarely achieved. Furthermore, in cases with a good response to therapy, hair loss often develops after therapy is discontinued.

Jet injector techniques are wasteful. Tattooing and iontophoresis of corticoids usually fail to produce adequate regrowth. High potency topical steroids, occasionally with occlusion, sometimes produce good regrowth and are frequently used to treat children.

Topical sensitizers are thought to produce an immunologic reaction, blocking the lymphocytes that mediate the hair loss in alopecia areata. Immunotherapy with contact allergens such as dinitrochlorobenzene (DNCB), diphenylcyclopropenone, and squaric acid dibutyl ester is partially successful. Unlike DNCB, diphenylcyclopropenone is not mutagenic in the Ames assay. Sensitization is first achieved in a localized 1 cm area; subsequently, the areas of alopecia are painted with a very dilute solution of the allergen.

Oral and topical 8-methoxypsoralen photochemotherapy is occasionally successful and probably works through an immune mechanism.

Isoprinosine, a synthetic immunomodulator, has been used for alopecia areata and alopecia universalis and produced some clinical response, disappearance or decrease in autoantibodies, and enhancement of T lymphocyte function.

Topical irritants, such as phenol or anthralin, are usually ineffective. Our trials with 1 to 5 per cent topical minoxidil have been disappointing; others have reported somewhat better results.

Cicatricial Alopecias. Other than those already mentioned, cicatricial alopecias occur in a number of atrophic cutaneous diseases, e.g., pseudopelade, lupus erythematosus, lichen planus, and scleroderma. Intralesional steroids administered as for alopecia areata are usually effective in the active phase. Hair-bearing normal scalp may be transplanted into clinically inactive alopecic sites.

Pseudofolliculitis Barbae

Pseudofolliculitis barbae (PFB) is a chronic recurrent disease usually of the beard area caused by ingrown hairs after shaving. The incidence ranges from 45 to 80 per cent in black men who shave frequently. The higher prevalence in blacks is accounted for by their tightly curled hairs that grow at a more acute angle than those of other races. Curiously, shaving the moustache area rarely causes PFB. When present in whites, PFB is usually mild. Other hairy areas (e.g., axilla and legs) that are closely and/or repeatedly shaved can be affected as well. Women who shave, pluck, or wax hairy areas may develop PFB. The disease can mimic acne, but comedones and cysts do not occur unless acne exists concomitantly.

The ingrown hairs of PFB act as foreign bodies and cause erythematous firm papules and pustules that are pruritic and tender. The inflammatory lesions of PFB either are sterile or contain normal skin flora. Additional trauma and secondary bacterial infection may result from excoriation and superficial nicks from shaving. The inflammatory reaction and clinical manifestations resolve spontaneously once the distal ends of the embedded hairs are released or removed. The chronic sequelae of PFB are fine, linear, depressed, occasionally criss crossed scars, alopecia, hypertrophic or keloidal scarring, and postinflammatory hyper- and hypopigmentation.

Management

Management of an acute eruption begins with the physician or nurse removing the distal penetrating ends of ingrown hairs with a number 11 blade and splinter forceps. Tetracycline or erythromycin, 250 mg 2 to 4 times a day, treats secondary infection and reduces inflammation. Hot compresses and anti-inflammatory/antibiotic topical preparations are salutary. Shaving is counterproductive in the acute phase of the disease. Painful inflammatory papules respond rapidly to intralesional injection of 0.05 to 0.1 ml of triamcinolone acetonide 2.5 mg per ml.

Long-term management is best accomplished by abstinence from shaving for an indefinite period. This approach is both curative and preventive, for as the hairs lengthen, spring-like forces operate to withdraw the offending penetrating hairs from their "pseudofollicles," allowing the violated inflamed tissues to heal. Moreover, because the hairs have lengthened, they are, for the most part, not rigid enough to repenetrate the skin. This salutary result can be achieved with a beard having a length of approximately 10 mm, which takes most men about a month to grow. Unfortunately, a beard is not acceptable to all patients with PFB because of personal preference, societal expectations, or occupational prohibitions.

Chemical depilatories (Magic Shave, Nair, Surgex) may be superior to other methods of temporary depilation. Depilatories dissolve beard hairs, leaving a rounded tip that makes it difficult for the curved hair to re-enter the skin. However, they are time-consuming, irritating, and foul smelling. Electrolysis is time-consuming and expensive and may be complicated by keloid development and postinflammatory hyperpigmentation.

Electric razors are not a satisfactory means of controlling PFB. However, electric clippers (trimmers) with a triple "O" head are useful and leave about 1 mm of beard protruding from the skin. The user must be willing to accept a visible stubble. When combined with twice daily facial epidermabrasion accomplished with a polyester fiber web skin-cleansing sponge (Buf-Puf), this regimen proves effective in most patients with PFB. The Buf-Puf tugs at hair loops to help dislodge ingrown hairs and prevent hair tips from penetrating the skin. Patients may also liberate incarcerated hair tips by lifting with a splinter tweezers. Plucking is discouraged, since it traumatizes the skin and leads to transfollicular penetration if the plucked hair breaks within the follicle.

A disposable, foil-guarded shaver (PFB Shaving System) is available from the American Safety Razor Company, Staunton, Virginia. This razor has a single blade covered by a serrated foil guard that prevents too close a shave while not leaving a visible stubble. Shaving is best performed by using short strokes in the direction of hair growth while avoiding pulling the skin taut.

Postinflammatory hyperpigmentation may respond to topical hydroquinone (2 to 4 per cent), mild chemical peel (e.g., 20 per cent trichloroacetic acid), or cryotherapy. Hypertrophic or keloidal scarring is treated with intralesional triamcinolone acetonide, 2.5 to 10 mg per ml (in aliquots of 0.1 ml per cubic centimeter of scar). Depressed scars are amenable to silicone/collagen augmentation. Ice pick scars respond to punch autografting. Dermabrasion is useful for sharp-edged scarring and has been used therapeutically by us for recalcitrant PFB. Besides removing trapped hairs, epithelialized tunnels, and labyrinths, dermabrasion alters the collagen architecture surrounding pilosebaceous openings and may reduce the tendency for hairs to ingrow.

SKIN CANCER

method of
RICHARD G. BENNETT, M.D.
University of California
Los Angeles, California

Skin cancer is the most common form of cancer, with a high prevalence in populations composed of fair-complexioned individuals who have poor tanning ability. It is estimated that approximately 500,000 new cases of skin cancer occur annually in the United States; however, because the majority of these cancers are small and easily cured, valid statistics are difficult to obtain.

The three major types of skin cancers are basal cell carcinoma, squamous cell carcinoma, and melanoma. In addition, several rarer types of skin cancer include locally invasive malignancies, such as dermatofibrosarcoma protuberans, as well as more aggressive skin cancers, such as angiosarcoma, which has a great potential for metastasis.

Many physicians view skin cancers like basal cell carcinoma or squamous cell cancers on sun-exposed areas as "nonmalignant" because of their extremely low metastatic potential and slow growth rates. However, these malignancies, if ignored or improperly treated, will eventually invade and destroy surrounding tissue, leading to cosmetic as well as functional problems. Some patients with many skin cancers may become discouraged and psychologically depressed. Such patients need to have their skin cancers dealt with in a systemic manner.

Diagnosis

Any lesion suspected of being a skin cancer should be biopsied adequately. A biopsy serves several purposes: it definitely establishes a diagnosis that allows the physician to decide intelligently the most appropriate form of therapy. Second, the patient and physician will know the precise diagnosis. Patients appreciate the effort made to establish a diagnosis. Third, a biopsy serves as a permanent record that may be useful for future review should further treatment become necessary.

Basal Cell Carcinoma

Basal cell carcinoma (BCC) usually arises on sun-exposed skin as a small papule which over time enlarges to form a pearly, translucent surface. With additional growth, a nodule ensues which may be ulcerative ("rodent" ulcer). Such large lesions frequently have telangiectasia, a rolled, raised border, and a depressed center.

Factors in Selection of Treatment Modalities

The treatment of basal cell carcinoma is based on four variables: location, size, histology, and previous treatment. Other factors to consider include the age and disability of the patient, the desires of the patient and family, and various psychosocial problems.

Location. Basal cell carcinomas that occur in certain locations are known to be more prone to recurrence with all modalities of therapy. These locations include the inner canthus of the eye, the nasolabial crease, the ear (especially the postauricular sulcus and external auditory canal), the nasal septum, and the scalp. For unknown reasons, lesions located in these areas tend to spread insidiously and deeply.

Size. Lesions greater than 2 cm on the trunk or extremities and greater than 1 cm on the head and neck are more prone to recurrence because of deeper tumor extensions. Therefore, prior to therapy all lesions should be measured to determine whether they fit into one of these high risk categories.

Histology. Not all basal cell carcinomas are histologically similar; some varieties tend to be more infiltrative (morphea or adenoid basal cell carcinomas) whereas other types tend to be less aggressive (superficial or nodular basal cell carcinomas). The clinical borders of morpheaform basal cell carcinomas in particular are indistinct, and these lesions are quite prone to recurrence.

Previous Treatment. Previous treatment failure of a basal cell carcinoma foretells the likelihood of success or failure of subsequent treatment, for the basal cell carcinoma that recurs subsequent to previous therapy is more difficult to eradicate. Tumor becomes trapped in or beneath scar tissue from previous treatments and is difficult to detect.

Treatment

Figure 1 provides an algorithm for treatment. Each of the six treatment modalities to be discussed has advantages and disadvantages as well as different rates of cure associated with different tumors based on the variables of location, size, histology, and previous treatment as just discussed.

Curettage and Electrodesiccation. This method utilizes a special instrument, the dermal curette, to literally scrape away the basal cell carcinoma from the surrounding skin. Its success is based upon the curette's ability to separate tumorous tissue from surrounding normal stroma. In addition, an electrosurgical apparatus is used to stop bleeding and to destroy additional tissue as a margin of safety. It is currently recommended that this method of curettage followed by electrodesiccation be done sequentially three times. Three times may not be necessary, though, on small superficial lesions, particularly if on the trunk and extremities—areas known to be less prone to treatment failure.

Cryosurgery. This form of therapy destroys tumor cells by freezing. Used appropriately, it requires careful monitoring of the depth and adequate freezing of the tumor to be effective. Less than adequate freezing of the tumor leads to treatment failure. Cryosurgery should not be used on large or recurrent tumors unless palliation is the goal.

Radiotherapy. This method requires special equipment and training and is best given by those experienced in its use. Properly given for skin cancer, radiation doses must be fractionated into at least 15 treatments. It may be inconvenient for patients or their families to complete a full course of therapy. However, radiotherapy avoids

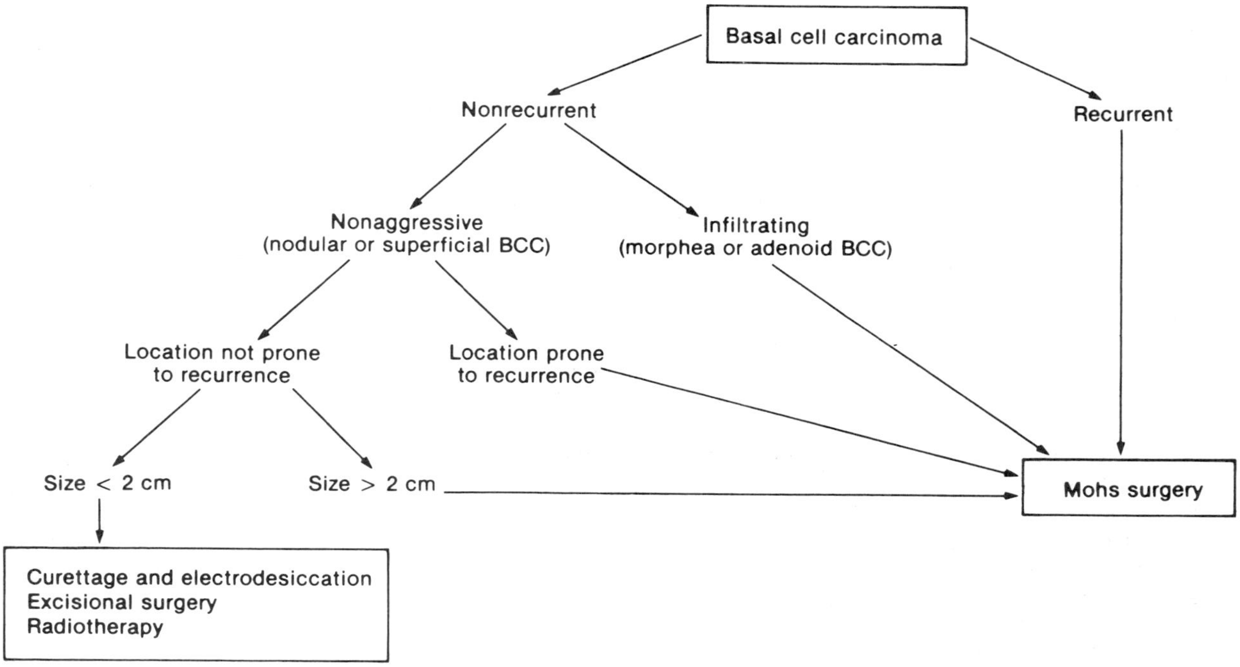

Figure 1. Algorithm for treatment of basal cell carcinoma.

surgery for those at high risk and is useful for palliation if this is the goal.

Excisional Surgery. After curettage and electrodesiccation, the most commonly used form of therapy for basal cell carcinomas is excisional surgery. Usually this may be done with only local anesthesia in an outpatient setting. Once excised, the surgical wound may be immediately closed, either with a simple closure or if necessary more complex procedures such as skin grafts or flaps. The excellent cosmetic results of excisional surgery and the high likelihood of cure make this an excellent treatment method.

Topical Chemotherapy. 5-Fluorouracil is occasionally useful for "superficial" basal cell carcinomas, particularly on the trunk and extremities. It cannot be overemphasized that superficial basal cell carcinomas are a clinicopathologic entity that must be substantiated both by the clinical appearance of a scaly macular lesion as well as by a typical histologic appearance. Treatment with 5-fluorouracil is twice a day for at least 4 to 6 weeks for malignancies, and treatment should be carefully monitored by the physician. 5-Fluorouracil provides an excellent cosmetic result and may be quite useful for palliation. It should not be used routinely on nodular or morphea basal cell carcinomas.

Mohs Surgery. A specialized form of excisional surgery developed by Dr. Frederic Mohs combines a special (tangential) method for removal of tissue with special methods for dyeing, mapping, and histologic processing of removed tissue. Because of its unique precision in localization of tumor, Mohs surgery affords the highest possible cure rates. Therefore it is most useful when the previously discussed types of therapy have already been used or when tumors are more likely to recur. It will preserve as much normal tissue as possible. Mohs surgery is properly performed only when the same physician who performs the surgery also serves as the pathologist to prepare and interpret the histologic specimens.

Variants of Basal Cell Carcinoma

A rare autosomal dominant syndrome, *basal cell nevus syndrome,* is characterized by multiple basal cell carcinomas that begin at an early age (around puberty) and are associated with palmar and plantar pits and bony abnormalities. Although many of the basal cell carcinomas developing in such patients are superficial, some may become aggressive and therefore should be treated with the same respect as basal cell carcinomas arising de novo.

Basal cell carcinoma associated with radiodermatitis is a distinct entity. Here prior radiotherapy, usually 25 to 30 years previously and given for therapeutic reasons, results in the development of malignancies, commonly basal and squamous cell carcinomas. It is important to realize that many such lesions may develop *separately* in a radiation field and should be treated individually. Such lesions may be just as aggressive as lesions appearing in nonradiation-damaged skin.

Squamous Cell Carcinoma

Squamous cell carcinomas represent another common form of skin cancer. These lesions arise de novo, associated with actinic keratoses or in association with Bowen's disease. Squamous cell carcinoma arising on the sun-damaged surfaces of the body has little likelihood of metastasizing. However, when it occurs on the mucous membranes, such as the lower lip, or in old scars that have resulted from burns, trauma, or inflammatory processes, the possibility of metastases is reported to be anywhere from 6 to 14 per cent.

Treatment

Like other forms of skin cancer, the variables of size, location, histology, and previous therapy all influence which treatment method is chosen. The histologic features of the lesion are perhaps of more importance in determining the potential for recurrence and metastases. Lesions that are poorly differentiated have a higher likelihood for metastases whereas well-differentiated lesions tend to be only locally invasive.

Variants of Squamous Cell Carcinoma

A few special common types of SCC deserve special comment because of their peculiar growth patterns that influence therapy.

Bowen's disease is an intraepidermal squamous cell carcinoma. This type of tumor tends to extend down hair follicles, therefore superficial forms of therapy (C & E or 5-fluorouracil) may result in treatment failure. Patients with Bowen's disease on nonsun-exposed surfaces should be searched for additional lesions. Some patients with many Bowen's disease lesions and keratoses of the palms and soles have previously been exposed to arsenic, either medically or occupationally. Such patients may be at higher risk for the development of internal malignancies, particularly of the female genital tract, gastrointestinal tract, or bladder. Such patients should be carefully evaluated and followed.

Keratoacanthoma is probably a variant of squamous cell carcinoma, which grows rapidly, enlarges, and then involutes within a few months. It is a clinicopathologic diagnosis that requires both a typical clinical as well as pathologic appearance. It is essential to realize that the behavior of a keratoacanthoma will determine its malignant potential. It should be treated or removed and should not be expected to resolve on its own. Cases have been recorded of "keratoacanthomas" that have progressed to metastasizing squamous cell carcinomas. Any recurrent keratoacanthoma should be viewed as probably of great malignant potential and definitively treated.

Basosquamous cell carcinomas are probably squamous cell carcinomas with features of basal cell carcinomas. They behave like squamous cell carcinoma and may metastasize, therefore these lesions should be treated aggressively.

Malignant Melanoma

Perhaps the most deadly form of skin cancer, malignant melanoma is being reported with increasing frequency. Whether this reflects a true increased incidence or increased detection is unknown. The features typical of melanomas are a pigmented lesion with an *irregular border, irregular pigmentation* (usually brown or black), and *irregular surface.* All three features are usually present.

The treatment of melanomas is detemined by the biopsy and the clinical presence or absence of palpable nodes. Lesions should be classified histologically by both Clark's levels of invasion *and* Breslow's depth of invasion. Lesions measuring 0.76 mm or more in thickness are more likely to metastasize. Such lesions should be treated with wide excision, and the possibility of node dissection should be entertained. Wide excisions may be anywhere from 3 to 5 cm and include underlying subcutaneous tissue to muscle fascia. From a practical point of view this may not be feasible—for instance, on the face. Here special monitoring of the pathologic margins should be done. Mohs surgery should be considered for locally recurrent melanomas or those occurring in areas where preservation of normal tissue is of great importance.

Melanomas have both a vertical downward as well as a horizontal growth phase. Where the horizontal growth phase is predominant, the lesion is referred to as a *superficial spreading melanoma.* If the vertical growth phase predominates, a nodule is the prime lesion and the melanoma is thus a *nodular melanoma.* On the face, a special type of melanoma may arise in which the malignant cells are mainly confined to the epidermis as irregular melanocytes but with some invasion of these cells into the dermis. This is known as a *lentigo maligna melanoma.* When the tumor cells are simply confined to the epidermis, the tumor is known as a *lentigo maligna.*

Two exceptions to the above classification systems are acral lentiginous melanomas and pedunculated melanomas. These two unusual variants are usually more aggressive than they appear, as judged by the grading systems worked out by Clark and Breslow.

Treatment

Treatment of melanomas is primarily surgical. For lesions of a greater thickness than 0.76 mm, referral should be made to physicians specializing in the care of such patients. Lesions less than 0.76 mm thick may be treated primarily by simple excisions. If maximum preservation of normal tissue is desirable, Mohs surgery should be considered.

Dysplastic Nevus Syndrome. A syndrome consisting of atypical-appearing moles ending in melanomas in patients with first degree relatives with melanomas has been recently described. A family history of melanoma is essential to be included in this syndrome, although such a history may be difficult to obtain with certainty. However, atypical-appearing moles on patients with strong family histories of melanoma should be viewed cautiously and biopsied if suspicous in appearance. One should, however, not be overly aggressive in biopsying lesions unless truly suspicious. Photodocumentation with careful follow-up is also recommended for patients in this category for whom multiple biopsies are untenable.

Rare Forms of Skin Cancer

Rarer forms of skin cancer may require specialized forms of treatment, and such malignancies present unique problems in management.

Dermatofibrosarcoma protuberans is a low grade sarcoma arising from the fibrous tissue of the skin. Treatment is excision. Recurrences are common with standard excisional approaches because this tumor extends much farther than can be appreciated by either inspection or palpation alone. Mohs surgery affords the highest likelihood of cure.

Extramammary Paget's disease is a tumor that usually occurs in the groin, perineum, or perirectal areas. Histologically, one sees invasion of the epidermis by a glandular neoplasm usually arising in nearby tissue. The glandular carcinoma is most often apocrine in origin although underlying rectal glands may also be the cause. Treatment consists of excision, with careful histologic monitoring of the surgical margins to confirm total extirpation as well as to detect the source of the underlying neoplasm.

Angiosarcoma is an extremely aggressive malignancy arising from the vascular structures within the skin. Such lesions are notorious for a high metastatic potential. They should be treated aggressively with surgery.

Kaposi's sarcoma is a low grade malignancy of the vascular tissues, usually occurring in the lower legs as purple nodules in the elderly. There it may persist for many years, growing insidiously. Impairment of the lymphatic drainage may occur, with marked lymph stasis. Treatment is either local excision or radiotherapy. Localized thermal treatment may be useful combined with radiotherapy. Low dose vinca alkaloids have been reported to be successful in treating refractory cases.

A newly recognized variant of Kaposi's sarcoma occurs with the acquired immune deficiency syndrome (AIDS). Here the vascular lesions occur at a relatively young age (between 20 and 40 years) and may appear as vascular macules. This type of Kaposi's sarcoma may be quite lethal, progressing to death within a short period of time.

Mycosis fungoides is an unusual type of T cell lymphoma, which may be confined totally to the skin but frequently involves several organ systems. Its treatment involves topical nitrogen mustard, radiotherapy, and systemic chemotherapy. Treatment is ideally given by those with experience in its management.

Additional Comments

Careful Follow-Up. Careful follow-up visits are an essential part of the treatment plan for all skin cancer patients. We have found that follow-up visits scheduled at 1, 3, and 6 months and 1 year and then yearly after treatment are ideal. For more aggressive lesions, such as undifferentiated squamous cell carcinoma, follow-up visits should be more frequent—every 3 months for the first year and every 6 months thereafter.

There are two main reasons for follow-up visits. First, it is desirable to detect evidence of recurrent skin cancer as soon as possible so that retreatment will have a higher likelihood of cure. Second, patients with skin cancer are likely to develop other separate skin cancers in the future. Early detection will lead to early treatment.

Palliation. Under some circumstances, for instance when the patient is quite elderly and in poor medical condition, the treatment aim may be to make the patient more comfortable rather than to subject him or her to extraordinary measures to effect a cure. Any of the nonsurgical methods of therapy should be considered, including cryosurgery, radiotherapy, or topical 5-fluorouracil. However, both the patient and family should have a clear understanding that these forms of therapy are being used for palliation only.

Assessment of Surgical Margins. In reality, only a relatively small sampling of the cut surgical margins are actually examined routinely by the pathologist. Statements to the effect that the margins are "clear," "close," or "uninvolved" should be interpreted as the *margins that are examined* are "clear," "close," or "uninvolved." Most of the margins will not be examined routinely.

Prophylactic Measures. Patients with skin cancer developing on sun-exposed skin should be counseled to use moderation with respect to future sun exposure and if possible to utilize regularly a sunscreen of strength appropriate to their potential for sunburning.

Tumor Conference. For patients with difficult-to-manage lesions, interdisciplinary tumor conferences are available for consultation at most medical centers and many smaller hospitals and should be used, when needed, for advice in management.

Research. Newer forms of therapy currently being investigated for the treatment of skin cancers include synthetic retinoids and vitamin A. Although promising results have been documented with these substances, the side effects of long-term usage, which would be necessary, clearly outweigh some of the advantages. Newer topical approaches for skin cancer include the use of DNCB (dinitrochlorobenzene) for multiple lesions where other forms of therapy would produce multiple unsightly scars.

PAPULOSQUAMOUS ERUPTIONS

method of
THOMAS F. ANDERSON, M.D.,
and JOHN J. VOORHEES, M.D.
University of Michigan
Ann Arbor, Michigan

The papulosquamous eruptions are a group of skin conditions of diverse etiology that have in common the presentation of well-marginated macules, patches, papules, and plaques, often exhibiting a characteristic scale. Grouped together because of their superficial epidermal involvement, similar presentation, and overlapping treatment regimens, papulosquamous disorders include seborrheic dermatitis (and other chronic eczematous dermatoses such as lichen simplex chronicus or nummular eczema); pityriasis rosea (and chronic parapsoriasis); lichen planus; and psoriasis. These scaly inflammatory conditions can usually be differentiated from each other by their clinical presentation and characteristic scaling pattern. However, they must first be distinguished from other scaly disorders.

SEBORRHEIC DERMATITIS

Seborrheic dermatitis is a chronic, recurrent papulosquamous eruption characteristically localized in the sites of greatest concentration of sebaceous glands. The most common presentation is erythematous patches or plaques often surmounted by a greasy yellow scale distributed to the scalp, eyebrows, and periauricular or presternal regions. Less frequently, it occurs in the intertriginous, or fold, areas, such as the axilla and inframammary, perianal, and periumbilical regions. When it occurs on the chest or back it often takes an annular or circinate pattern and may be difficult to distinguish from nummular eczema. Often pruritic, chronic scratching may lead to lichenification, resulting in thickened patches indistinguishable from those of lichen simplex chronicus. Extension to a more generalized papulosquamous eruption and even erythroderma occurs commonly in infantile seborrheic dermatitis and rarely in adults.

Severe seborrheic dermatitis may often be precipitated by hospitalization for a serious illness in another organ system. This is especially true with disorders of the central nervous system, such as stroke, Parkinson's disease, and seizure disorders. Overtreatment, superimposed contact dermatitis, or secondary infection may also aggravate seborrheic dermatitis. Sunlight and the chronic use of fluorinated topical corticosteroids may also accentuate seborrheic dermatitis.

Occasionally, severe seborrheic dermatitis may be found on a continuum with psoriasis, prompting the term sebopsoriasis for a condition that appears to be psoriasis found in a seborrheic distribution. Seborrheic dermatitis can usually be distinguished from psoriasis by its distribution, lack of nail involvement or Koebner phenomena, typical histologic pattern on biopsy, and usual prompt response to treatment. The etiology of seborrheic dermatitis is unknown. However, it has been hypothesized that it may be an inflammatory hypersensitivity response to an overgrowth of sebotropic cutaneous flora. Thus, many antiseborrheic shampoos have been formulated with agents that are bacteriostatic and fungistatic. These keratolytic shampoos also inhibit epidermal proliferation and remove excessive oil.

Treatment

Seborrheic dermatitis is a chronic, recurrent condition, and the expectation of control rather than cure must be stressed to the patient. Mild seborrheic dermatitis of the scalp may often be controlled by increasing the frequency of shampooing and by using over the counter "medicated" antidandruff shampoos such as Selsun Blue selenium sulfide, Head and Shoulders, Danex, Sebulon, Zincon, or one of a variety of tar shampoos (e.g., T-Gel, Vanseb-T, Sebutone, Zetar, and DHS tar). The "resistance" that commonly occurs with continued use of these shampoos may be avoided by rotating different shampoos every 1 to 2 weeks. Severe oiliness or scaling may be improved by the use of keratolytic and drying shampoos such as Sebulex, Metasep, or Meted.

More severe inflammation and pruritus in the scalp may be ameliorated with the application of hydrocortisone solutions, such as Texacort scalp lotion, Aeroseb-Dex, and Barseb Thera-Spray. More resistant cases may be improved with the use of fluorinated corticosteroid solutions such as fluocinolone acetonide 0.01 per cent (Synalar or Fluonid solution), betamethasone valerate 0.1 per cent (Valisone solution), or Kenalog (triamcinolone) spray. A few drops or a small spray of these agents following shampooing and as needed for pruritus is often initially necessary in the management of seborrheic dermatitis or during severe flare-up. Lastly, patients should be warned to avoid oily or greasy hair dressings and conditioners. Alternatives include Drest, Sebucare, and Ionil rinse.

Inflammatory seborrheic dermatitis in the eyebrows, around the ears, or in the intertriginous folds can usually be managed with 1 per cent hydrocortisone cream or lotion. Occasional resistant cases may require 2 to 2½ per cent hydrocortisone cream or lotion or Tridesilon cream or ointment. Patients should be warned not to use fluorinated corticosteroids in these locations.

When seborrheic dermatitis becomes more generalized on the trunk, moderate strength fluorinated corticosteroids, such as 0.025 per cent triamcinolone acetonide (Kenalog or Aristocort) or fluocinolone acetonide (Synalar or Synemol cream), may be used once or twice daily for 1 or 2 weeks and then tapered to 1 per cent hydrocortisone. Occasionally in adults a short course of systemic prednisone, 30 mg daily for 4 days, reduced to 20 mg daily for 4 days and then to 10 mg daily for 4 days, may be helpful in addition to topical therapy. Rarely, resistant seborrheic dermatitis may require the addition of a tar cream lotion or bath oil (Zetar, Polytar, Balnetar, or T-derm oil) or topical sodium sulfacetamide lotion (Sebizon lotion).

PITYRIASIS ROSEA

Pityriasis rosea is a common papulosquamous eruption most often seen in young adults. Although often thought to be due to a virus, the etiology is unknown. Typically, the usual presentation begins with a single (occasionally multiple) papulosquamous annular plaque approximately 2 to 5 cm in diameter. Most often this plaque is easily confused with a ringworm infection. However, examination of the scales under a microscope will reveal no fungal elements. This so-called herald patch often (but not necessarily) precedes a more generalized papulosquamous eruption from 2 days to 2 months. This generalized eruption tends to appear in crops with primary involvement on the upper third of the trunk and extremities and only rarely involves the face, scalp, or genitalia.

Typically, pityriasis rosea is characterized by round or oval patches or plaques surmounted by fine scale, which tends to peel peripherally. The long axis of the oval lesions tends to follow parallel lines of cleavage. Patients may present with an asymptomatic eruption or may complain of varying degrees of pruritus. Generally, pityriasis rosea is self-limited and lasts only 2 to 8 weeks; rarely, it may last longer. However, if the eruption persists longer than 3 months, a biopsy should be performed to rule out the possibility of a more longstanding form of parapsoriasis, such as pityriasis lichenoides chronica. Any atypical presentation must be differentiated from guttate psoriasis, a lichenoid drug eruption, and, most importantly, secondary syphilis. It has been recommended that a serologic test for syphilis be obtained on any patient who does not present with the classic picture of pityriasis rosea or certainly if he presents with lesions on the palms and soles, fever, malaise, adenopathy, or a history consistent with a previous primary chancre.

Treatment

Treatment of pityriasis rosea is primarily symptomatic. Often, no treatment is necessary once patients are reassured about the self-limited nature of this condition. Mild pruritus can be treated with emollients or systemic antihistamines at bedtime. More severe pruritus can be treated with topical corticosteroids, tar preparations, and occasionally a short-tapering systemic burst of corticosteroids (such as 30 mg per day for 4 days, 20 mg per day for 4 days, 10 mg per day for 4 days). If the patient is extremely symptomatic and systemic corticosteroids are contraindicated, a short course of ultraviolet light therapy, either natural or artificial, is often helpful in combination with emollients or tar preparations. Most patients will respond following one to eight minimally erythemogenic ultraviolet light exposures spread over 1 to 3 weeks.

Chronic parapsoriasis may respond to emollients or 1 per cent hydrocortisone but often requires chronic ultraviolet light therapy, psoralen photochemotherapy (PUVA), or, rarely, low dose methotrexate therapy. Patients with chronic parapsoriasis must be followed carefully, and biopsies should be performed periodically on any suspicious lesions to rule out the development of a cutaneous T cell lymphoma.

LICHEN PLANUS

Distinctive among the papulosquamous eruptions, lichen planus is characterized by the develpment of angular flat-topped violaceous papules covered by a faint gray white network of lines (Wickham's striae) over the surface. This extremely pruritic eruption tends to involve the flexural regions, particularly the volar aspect of the wrists, forearms, and trunk, equally in men and women between the ages of 20 and 50. In 50 per cent of patients, mucous membranes will be involved, with a white net-like reticulated patch, which uncommonly may become erosive or leukoplakic. Fingernails may be involved with longitudinal ridging or thinning of the nail plate. Follicular involvement of the scalp may rarely result in small patches of atrophic alopecia. Lichen planus may vary in presentation from the typical acute pruritic polygonal papules to more chronic hypertrophic lesions, especially on the lower legs. Rarely, lichen planus may present with atrophic or vesicular lesions.

The etiology of lichen planus is unknown. However, local trauma may aggravate the condition (Koebner phenomenon), resulting in typical lesions of lichen planus occurring in a linear scratch mark. Acute generalized lichen planus tends to be self-limited, with clearing in 2 months to 2 years. More chronic forms, erosive mucous membrane lesions, and nail and scalp involvement tend to last for many years. When lichen planus involvement in the skin does resolve, residual hyperpigmentation may last for many months. Care must be taken to differentiate true lichen planus from lichenoid drug reactions or the other papulosquamous eruptions. A skin biopsy in difficult cases is generally diagnostic.

Treatment

With acute generalized lichen planus, the patient should be warned to avoid trauma to the skin or activities that worsen pruritus (such as the use of harsh soaps, hot water, or strenuous exercise). Often an antipruritic lotion such as menthol 0.3 to 0.5 per cent with or without phenol 0.5 to 1 per cent lotion (e.g., Sarna lotion) applied three times daily or as needed may be helpful. One per cent hydrocortisone or more potent topical steroid preparations may occasionally offer some relief as well. Antihistamines, such as diphenhydramine (Benadryl), 25 to 50 mg, or hydroxyzine (Atarax), 10 to 25 mg, at bedtime may be helpful in preventing nocturnal pruritus. Severe acute generalized lichen planus often requires a 2 to 4 week tapering course of systemic corticosteroids. If there are no contraindications a typical dosage would be 40 to 60 mg for 4 to 6 days, gradually tapered to an alternate day schedule and finally off. Although lichen planus typically relapses after withdrawal of corticosteroids, it is occasionally easier to treat or is milder.

If it does not respond to these treatments and the symptoms are disabling, patients may respond to a course of tar and ultraviolet light therapy (Goeckerman therapy) or psoralen photochemotherapy (PUVA) (see treatment of psoriasis).

Localized chronic lichen planus often requires more potent fluorinated corticosteroids, such as fluocinamide (Lidex) 0.05 per cent or desoximetasone (Topicort) 0.25 per cent, applied after a cool tap water compress one to three times daily. Alternatively, triamcinolone or hydrocortisone may be applied under an occlusive plastic covering (e.g., Saran Wrap) or in the form of a steroid-impregnated tape, such as flurandrenolide tape (Cordran Tape), for 4 to 8 hour periods. Patients must be followed carefully and treatment discontinued if any evidence of inflammatory folliculitis or unwanted atrophy occurs. In addition, intralesional corticosteroid therapy may be beneficial. Using a 1 mm Luer-Lok tuberculin syringe mounted with a 26 to 30 gauge, ½ inch needle, one can inject triamcinolone acetonide (Kenalog-10), 10 mg per ml, diluted with equal parts 1 per cent lidocaine, in amounts up to 1 to 2 ml depending on the size of the hypertrophic lesion. The injection should be intradermal and, if no signs of atrophy occur, may be repeated every 4 to 6 weeks if necessary.

Mucous membrane lichen planus often responds to triamcinolone acetonide in a special base (Kenalog in Orabase) designed to adhere to mucous membrane surfaces. The mucous membrane must be dried prior to application of this product. Intralesional corticosteroid therapy as described previously is also helpful. Pain in erosive lichen planus may be partially alleviated by using diphenhydramine elixir (Benadryl) as a mouth gargle for 1 to 3 minutes three times daily. This should not be swallowed unless sedative or antihistaminic effects are desired. Experimental treatments using topical corticosteroid gels and retinoic acid formulations may be useful in the future. Any indurated or thickened white area in or around erosive lichen planus should be biopsied to rule out carcinomatous transformation. Lichen planus of the nails may respond to psoralen photochemotherapy or monthly intralesional corticosteroid injections in the proximal nail fold.

PSORIASIS

Psoriasis is the most chronic papulosquamous eruption and potentially the most debilitating. The most common form, psoriasis vulgaris, is characterized by erythematous scaling plaques that often begin in the scalp, genitalia, or extensor areas of the body (elbows, knees, sacrum). It varies in extent from one elbow or knee to generalized involvement. Typically, psoriatic plaques are covered with thick adherent or flaking, micaceous silvery white to yellow scale, which typically produces pinpoint bleeding when it is removed traumatically (Auspitz sign). Thirty per cent of patients with psoriasis report new lesions form exactly in the site of skin trauma (Koebner phenomenon). Thirty to 80 per cent of psoriasis patients also have nail involvement characterized by onycholysis (separation of the nail bed from the nail plate), pitting (indentations of the nail plate), and subungal hyperkeratosis and discoloration. Approximately 6 to 7 per cent of psoriasis patients also suffer from an inflammatory, asymmetric, seronegative destructive arthritis, often affecting the joints of the fingers, toes, or vertebral spine.

Other variants of psoriasis include exanthematic, pustular, and erythrodermic forms. Acute guttate psoriasis is characterized by generalized erythematous papules in a young person, occurring in crops following an upper respiratory tract infection (often streptococcal). Localized pustular psoriasis of the palms and soles characterized by painful sterile pustules can be disabling. The most severe, life-threatening forms of generalized pustular psoriasis and exfoliative or erythrodermic psoriasis often present with fever, leukocytosis, and severe debilitation. Like the other papulosquamous eruptions, the etiology of psoriasis is unknown. However, it appears to be a genetic misregulation of proliferation, differentiation, and inflammation in the skin, resulting in excessive epidermal proliferation and dermal inflammation.

Treatment

The treatments for psoriasis involving the scalp, genitalia, or extensor skin are all different and must be individually designed. The practical limitations of each therapy, including the costs, constraints of the therapeutic setting, requirements for patient travel, time off work, and compliance, must be considered along with the patient's physical or emotional state, sophistication, and expectations. In general, patients with psoriasis can be classified into three major groups based on extent of disease and disability: mild, moderate, and severe. Treatment regimens can be grouped into preventive measures, suppressive therapy, and aggressive programs.

Preventive Treatment

Patients should be warned to avoid drugs known to exacerbate or worsen psoriasis if at all possible. Lithium and beta-blockers such as propranolol and, less commonly, nonsteroidal anti-inflammatory agents such as indomethacin have been reported to worsen or precipitate psoriasis. Early treatment of streptococcal and upper respiratory tract infections should also be encouraged. Patients should be warned to avoid activities that tend to damage or irritate the skin. In particular, they should be encouraged to use mild soaps, tepid water for washing, and bland moisturizers and emollients, such as Vaseline Petroleum Jelly, Eucerin, Lubriderm, and mineral oil. Mild psoriatic plaques may stabilize and even regress with continued use of moisturizing, occlusive emollients.

Keratolytic Therapy

In addition to emollients, plastic occlusive dressings (such as Saran Wrap, plastic gloves, or total body vinyl suits) have been shown to be useful in the treatment of hyperkeratotic psoriasis. Occlusive dressings are generally used only intermittently for 2 to 4 hour periods or, at most, overnight to prevent maceration or folliculitis. Chemical keratolytic agents, such as urea 20 to 40 per cent or salicylic acid 2 to 6 per cent, are useful in helping to remove excessive hyperkeratosis of the palms and soles or recalcitrant scale from psoriatic plaques elsewhere on the body.

Propylene glycol solutions in a concentration by volume of 40 to 60 per cent in water are particularly useful in removing thick scale when used under moist plastic occlusion. A combination of 6 per cent salicylic acid in a 60 per cent glycol gel (Keralyt) can be applied to thickened areas such as the palms and soles, followed by the application of damp cotton gloves or stockings. Large plastic gloves, booties, or Saran Wrap sheets are then taped down, forming a watertight but not constricting seal. After a 3 to 4 hour period during the day or overnight, this plastic dressing is removed and excess keratin atraumatically scraped away with a washcloth, a polyester fiber sponge (Buf-Puf), or an abrasive tool such as a pumice stone. An occlusive moisturizing ointment is then applied to avoid excessive drying of the skin, which may result in the formation of painful fissures. If a painful fissure or superficial erosion occurs, the area must be protected with an emollient or zinc oxide paste prior to any further treatment. Urea in a 20 to 40 per cent concentration in hydrophilic petrolatum can be used as an alternative to Keralyt in this procedure.

Corticosteroids

Topical glucocorticosteroids are one of the most commonly prescribed treatments for psoriasis. Although expensive, they are anti-inflammatory, antimitotic, and nonstaining and may only need to be applied once a day to once a week. Ointments are generally more effective than creams in treating thick hyperkeratotic psoriasis. Hairy areas are best treated with creams or lotions, and solutions, gels, and sprays are the easiest preparations to apply to the scalp or pubic area. Corticosteroid solutions (e.g., Synalar or Fluorobate) are helpful in treating psoriasis of the ear canal and fingernails.

A high potency corticosteroid such as fluocinanide 0.05 per cent (Lidex), desoxymetasone 0.25 per cent (Topicort), or betamethasone diproprionate 0.05 per cent (Diprosone) may be used initially for a short period of time to bring about fast resolution of the inflammation in psoriasis. The frequency of application and potency of these products are gradually tapered to hydrocortisone or even moisturizing emollients to prevent adverse cutaneous side effects such as atrophy, telangiectasia, and acneiform eruptions. Continued use of topical corticosteroids in psoriasis is often associated with loss of effectiveness and occasionally with a rebound phenomenon resulting in a more severe form of psoriasis or one that is difficult to treat. Considering their expense, side effects, and loss of effectiveness over time, topical corticosteroids are best used for short periods (less than 3 weeks) and never as the sole therapy for psoriasis.

Systemic corticosteroids are generally not recommended for the treatment of psoriasis, as there have been case reports of severe generalized pustular psoriasis following the withdrawal of systemic corticosteroid treatment. However, intralesional corticosteroids can be an invaluable treatment adjunct with a minimum of side effects. One quarter to 1 milligram (0.1 to 0.4 ml) of triamcinolone acetonide injected from a concentration of 2.5 to 10.0 mg per ml (Kenalog) may result in a prolonged resolution of the psoriatic papule or plaque, lasting weeks to months. Adverse reactions following intralesional corticosteroids include the development of sterile abscess or cellulitis, pain, atrophy, hyper- and hypopigmentation, and telangiectasia. Care must be taken to avoid reinjection at the same site for 4 to 6 weeks.

Tar Products

A wide variety of crude or refined coal tar products are available. Side effects of tar therapy include folliculitis, photosensitivity, and allergic hypersensitivity, in addition to their staining properties and unpleasant odor. Crude coal tar in a 1 to 5 per cent concentration may be incorporated in Aquaphor, washable petrolatum, or a zinc oxide paste to treat large, thick psoriatic plaques. These agents should not be applied to intertriginous or hairy areas or under moist plastic occlusion to avoid primary irritation and folliculitis. A less irritating alcohol extract of tar, liquor carbonis detergens (LCD), is commonly used in a 10 per cent concentration in hydrophilic creams, lotions, or bath oils for generalized acute guttate psoriasis. Other tar extracts formulated in creams or gels such as Fototar, Estar, or psoriGel have recently been developed as less messy alternatives for scalp and general treatment. A wide variety of tar-based shampoos and bath and body oils is available without prescription. Generally, tar products are applied once or twice daily for a minimum of 2 hours or overnight. After the tar agent is washed off a moisturizing ointment or cream is then applied to the skin.

Anthralin Products

Anthralin is a synthetic trihydroxyanthracene compound that is useful for treating thick, recalcitrant plaques of psoriasis. Unfortunately, it is a potent cutaneous irritant and more likely to stain the skin and clothing than tar. It must not be used in acute inflammatory psoriasis or on flexural areas or the face. Accidental contact with the eyes may produce severe chemical conjunctivitis.

Anthralin is generally compounded in a 0.1 to 2.0 per cent concentration in a stiff zinc oxide paste, to which 0.2 to 4.0 per cent salicylic acid has been added as a stabilizing agent. Commercially available anthralin preparations include 0.1 to 1.0 per cent concentration in a cream or ointment base (Drithocreme or Lasan). Patients are treated with the lowest concentration initially, gradually increasing the strength every few days until either the desired response or irritation occurs. Unlike tar, which is usually applied on psoriasis as well as normal skin, anthralin must be carefully applied only to the psoriatic plaques. To prevent irritation and the spread of psoriasis to the surrounding skin, the plaques are often ringed with a protective coat of petrolatum or plain zinc oxide paste. Anthralin-covered plaques may often be dusted with talc or covered with tube gauze or stockinette bandages for 4 to 12 hour periods. Bath oil or mineral oil with an added emulsifying agent (such as 5 per cent sodium lauryl sulfate) is then used to remove the paste prior to the next application. Staining and irritation may be lessened by applying lower concentrations or using anthralin for short periods of time (under one half hour). As psoriasis responds to anthralin, lesser concentrations or shorter application periods must be utilized to prevent irritation. The concomitant use of a low potency corticosteroid such as 1.0 per cent hydrocortisone may blunt this irritant effect.

Ultraviolet Light Therapy

Sunlight and artificially produced midrange "erythemogenic" ultraviolet radiation (UVB) are also effective treatments for psoriasis. There is often an added and possibly synergistic effect when combined with anthralin or tar products, but, at minimum, ultraviolet light therapy must be combined with emollients and moisturizers. Titrated exposures of increasing doses of ultraviolet light can be delivered to the skin through a template with a series of small openings. In this manner, the dose of ultraviolet light necessary to produce a minimum degree of erythema (the minimum erythema dose) can be determined. Starting at a dose just below that necessary to produce erythema, daily treatments are delivered gradually, increasing the exposure time by approximately 10 to 50 per cent until minimum erythema is maintained approximately 6 to 24 hours after phototherapy. Twenty to 40 exposures are generally necessary to obtain the best results. The end point of treatment is the gradual desquamation and thinning of individual psoriatic plaques in association with a diminution of erythema within the psoriatic plaque. If the capillary refill time after compression of the treated psoriatic plaque approximates that of the surrounding uninvolved skin, ultraviolet light phototherapy may be discontinued or reduced to maintenance therapy frequency of once or twice a week.

Adverse reactions to ultraviolet light phototherapy include acute sunburn-like responses, which can usually be prevented by careful monitoring of dosage and reduction of therapy when desquamation of the uninvolved skin takes place. The face, breasts, axillae, popliteal fossae, and genitalia are areas that tend to sunburn more easily, and they may require a double layer of cloth shielding or a UVB sunscreening agent during all or part of the phototherapy exposures. Psoriasis can be worsened by too much ultraviolet light, and leg edema is a common side effect as well. Acute painful exposure keratitis and chronic cataract formation can be prevented by wearing ultraviolet light opaque sunglasses or goggles with each exposure.

Chronic side effects of phototherapy include pruritus, xerosis, premature aging, freckling, and hyperpigmentation. Experimental evidence suggests that ultraviolet light with or without coal tar produces a cutaneous immunosuppression and is carcinogenic. However, experience suggests that the incidence of cancer in psoriatic patients treated with phototherapy or tar is not significantly greater than that in the general population.

Aggressive Phototherapy Protocols

Hospitalization

For moderately severe to severe psoriatic patients who are undergoing an acute, generalized eruptive flare of psoriasis, those who are suffering with greater than 20 per cent of body surface area involvement, and those who are disabled by their disease, hospitalization for a combination of all the previously described treatments is the treatment of choice. Since its introduction in the 1920's by the Mayo Clinic dermatologist William Goeckerman, this treatment regimen has proven cost effective over time. Patients undergoing this aggressive treatment regimen often experience prolonged remissions lasting months to years after one hospitalization. Initially, patients are treated with corticosteroids and moist occlusive dressings and/or soothing baths. Once acute inflammation has been lessened, tar ointments, bath products, and shampoos are added to the regimen in addition to once or twice daily ultraviolet light treatments. Intralesional corticosteroids, anthralin, and extra ultraviolet light phototherapy are added for recalcitrant plaques to speed their resolution.

Scalp psoriasis is treated with topical corticosteroid gels or solutions such as Valisone, Synalar, or Fluobate. This is followed by the application of a thick coat of Baker's P & S scalp oil if there is a lot of hyperkeratotic scale. The scalp is then dressed with a moist gauze turban, which is then covered with a plastic Saran Wrap occlusive dressing or shower cap. This occlusive dressing remains in place for 4 hours or overnight, after which the scalp is shampooed with a tar shampoo such as T-gel, Zetar, or 10 per cent LCD in a mild shampoo base. After shampooing, the topical corticosteroid is then reapplied to the scalp without occlusion. The occlusive therapy is continued for 3 or 4 days, after which it is tapered gradually to daily treatment with a tar shampoo followed by a weak topical steroid solution or gel such as hydrocortisone. Recalcitrant scalp disease is occasionally treated with an anthralin or tar pomade gel applied 10 to 30 minutes prior to shampooing.

Nail psoriasis is treated with a combination of surgical management, keratolytic therapy with 20 to 40 per cent urea under occlusion, and topical corticosteroid solution or 5-fluorouracil (Efudex) applied daily without occlusion. Intralesional corticosteroids are a painful but often effective treatment in select patients. Intertriginous fissuring often responds to a mixture of 1.0 per cent hydrocortisone with 25,000 units/ml of nystatin in Cetaphil or Wise's shake lotion.

Patients are treated in the hospital until virtually all the psoriasis is flat and showing evidence of slow capillary refill. In general, the less psoriasis at discharge, the longer the clinical remission. A typical psoriasis hospitalization may last from 3 to 6 weeks. Any residual psoriasis at the time of discharge is treated with outpatient tars, anthralin, or ultraviolet light therapy. Scalp, nail, or intertriginous psoriasis is treated as previously described.

If psoriasis patients develop painful chemical irritation from anthralin and tar or a sunburn response from ultraviolet light, a moderate strength corticosteroid, such as triamcinolone (Kenalog, Aristocort) is sometimes used for one or two applications to help decrease inflammation and avoid a Koebner response. Pruritus following phototherapy treatments or tar therapy may be treated with an antihistamine such as hydroxyzine (Atarax), 10 to 25 mg every 6 to 8 hours, and topical counterirritants such as 0.5 per cent menthol with or without 1.0 per cent phenol in Cetaphil lotion. Staining of the skin from anthralin can be removed by using a few daily applications of a keratolytic such as Keralyt.

Systemic Therapy

The rare patients who respond poorly to this modified Goeckerman regimen, who require multiple hospitalizations (with only partial improvement), and who continue to be disabled by their disease are candidates for psoralen photochemotherapy (PUVA) or systemic antimetabolite therapy. Psoralen photochemotherapy is administered as described by the guidelines published in the Journal of the American Academy of Dermatology *1*:106, 1979. Psoralen is administered in a dose of 0.6 mg per kg of methoxsalen twice weekly 2 hours prior to graduated exposures to long wave ultraviolet light type A. Alternatively, methotrexate, 15 to 30 mg, can be given orally or intramuscularly as a single dose on a weekly basis following the guidelines published in the Journal of the American Academy of Dermatology *6*:145, 1982. Methotrexate has an added advantage in that it seems to help in the treatment of psoriatic arthritis. Unfortunately, as PUVA therapy is associated with an increased risk of cutaneous carcinoma and methotrexate is associated with a cumulative dose-dependent hepatotoxicity, patients on these regimens must be followed carefully by physicians experienced in their use. Fortunately, the vast majority of patients with psoriasis respond to topical suppressive programs and only the minority require hospitalization or systemic therapy. Pustular forms of psoriasis are extremely difficult to treat. However, new synthetic retinoid agents are being developed that appear to be effective in both pustular and erythrodermic psoriasis. Psoriatic arthritis treatment is similar to the treatment of rheumatoid arthritis coupling nonsteroidal anti-inflammatory drugs, intra-articular corticosteroid injections, orthodic devices, and occasionally orthopedic surgery. Severe cases may require methotrexate.

EXFOLIATIVE ERYTHRODERMA

All of the papulosquamous eruptions may on occasion result in a generalized exfoliative erythroderma. In addition to psoriasis, lichen planus, and seborrheic dermatitis, a widespread eczematous dermatitis, such as atopic dermatitis or contact dermatitis, may result in this generalized reaction. In addition, the entire skin may become red and desquamate with infections with yeast or fungi or as a toxic reaction to bacterial infection. Rare dermatoses such as pityriasis rubra pilaris or pemphigus foliaceous must also be considered. Drug eruptions and malignancies such as T cell lymphomas, leukemia, myeloma, and visceral carcinoma may also manifest with this generalized eruption.

Treatment

When a patient presents with this picture, biopsy is needed. Because of excess water loss and hypermetabolism of the skin, fluid intake and output must be monitored to prevent dehydration, and electrolyte and protein balance must be maintained by oral or intravenous supplementation. Patients must be monitored for bacterial infection and kept in a warm environment to prevent excessive heat loss. Tepid baths containing an emollient (Aveeno oilated) or bath oils such as Domol, Alpha Keri, or Lubath and occasionally coal tar products given 3 or 4 times a day followed by a lubricating moisturizer such as Aquaphor or Petrolatum may be helpful prior to the institution of specific therapy based on the results of the skin biopsy. In addition, topical application of steroids (0.025 to 1.0 per cent hydrocortisone and 0.1 per cent triamcinolone in a lotion or cream) following moist compresses of Burow's solution (1 tablet or packet of Domeboro's or Bluboro's per quart of cool water) may be helpful. Alternatively, corticosteroids may be applied under moist occlusive dressings for short periods. Patients who are treated with corticosteroids must be monitored very carefully, as extensive and rapid vasoconstriction of the skin secondary to corticosteroid use may result in volume overload in a patient prone to congestive heart failure. Rarely an erythroderma may be chronic and idiopathic, requiring systemic corticosteroids or antimetabolites for a variable length of time.

SCLERODERMA
(Systemic Sclerosis)

method of
ROBERT C. SIEGEL, M.D.
University of California, San Francisco
San Francisco, California

Systemic sclerosis (scleroderma) is a chronic disease of unknown cause with therapy that must be considered largely palliative rather than curative. Proper management of the patient with systemic sclerosis continues to challenge the patience and resourcefulness of the concerned physician.

Diagnosis of the type of systemic sclerosis requires exclusion of both localized forms and the two systemic masqueraders, mixed connective tissue disease and fasciitis with eosinophilia. Localized forms include linear scleroderma and morphea. Morphea may be either localized in plaques or generalized. Evolution of the localized forms into systemic sclerosis is extremely rare to nonexistent. However, some patients with linear scleroderma may have mild systemic complaints such as fatigue, weakness, and arthralgias. Serologic tests such as antinuclear antibodies may be positive in younger patients with linear scleroderma. The principal problem associated with linear scleroderma is atrophy of the underlying structures. Tissues down to bone in an extremity or into the brain in the case of facial hemiatrophy may be atrophic and scarred. Patients with involvement of the head should be tested neurologically to define the extent of the lesion.

Treatment of localized forms is limited. Morphea frequently resolves spontaneously but may clear more rapidly with local corticosteroid injections. Phenytoin (Dilantin) may be effective in decreasing the disfigurement of linear scleroderma. It promotes increased connective tissue synthesis in the areas of linear scleroderma so that there is less apparent atrophy. (This use is not listed by the manufacturer.)

Mixed connective tissue disease (MCTD) has characteristics of several rheumatic diseases. It has features of systemic sclerosis, with Raynaud's phenomenon, cutaneous induration, esophageal motility disorder, and pulmonary hypertension. As in systemic lupus erythematosus, there is high serologic reactivity, polyserositis, and arthritis. The muscle inflammation present may initially suggest polymyositis. MCTD is distinguished by high titer, speckled antinuclear antibodies that are digestible with ribonuclease. Treatment with high dose prednisone often results in remission or improvement.

Fasciitis with eosinophilia was first described in 1975. There is often a characteristic history of rapid onset of cutaneous induration after exercise that had been unusually strenuous for the affected person. There is marked proximal extremity and truncal involvement without Raynaud's or sclerodermatous digital changes. There may be peripheral eosinophilia as high as 30 per cent in some patients. Diagnosis is made by biopsy en bloc from indurated skin through the fascia to underlying muscle. The fascia may be 60 times the normal thickness, with eosinophil and mononuclear cell infiltration. Although the cutaneous induration frequently responds to high dose corticosteroids, the natural history is uncertain. Late hematologic sequelae, such as aplastic anemia and Hodgkin's disease, have been described recently.

The two principal subtypes of systemic sclerosis are the acrosclerotic, or inflammatory, form and the diffuse form. The acrosclerotic form comprises the majority of cases. Patients have a high frequency of Raynaud's phenomenon, which may precede other symptoms by 1 to 2 years. There is a three to one female predominance, with early digital sclerosis and slowly progressive visceral involvement. The 10 year survival is over 50 per cent. Certain patients with this subtype may develop the CREST syndrome: *C*alcinosis, *R*aynaud's, *E*sophageal motility disorder, *S*clerodactyly, and *T*elangiectasia. Since calcinosis usually doesn't occur until 7 to 10 years of disease, this finding implies a more benign course and better prognosis. The patients may be recognizable as a subgroup early in their disease by the presence of anticentromere antibody, but more data are required at present before this test can be considered to be an absolute indicator of a benign course. Some investigators have classified all patients with the acrosclerotic inflammatory disease as having CREST syndrome. This may lead to confusion since they recognize CREST and diffuse systemic sclerosis only as subtypes. Many patients in their CREST group are described as "incomplete CREST" patients. Patients with the CREST syndrome generally have little visceral impairment. However, they may develop fulminant pulmonary hypertension as a late complication more than 20 years after disease onset.

Diffuse systemic sclerosis is a more aggressive disease. There is less frequency of Raynaud's phenomenon and equal male to female incidence. There is early truncal induration and visceral involvement. The 5 year survival is approximately 50 per cent. Severe and early renal, pulmonary, or cardiac involvement causes the lowered life expectancy. Recognition of these different subtypes and prognoses is obviously important in weighing the relative risks and benefits of various therapeutic agents for each patient.

General Treatment

A number of general measures are beneficial for all patients with systemic sclerosis. These include avoidance of cold and smoking, continued physical therapy, proper skin care, and education. Regardless of the type of disease, cold temperatures precipitate both cutaneous and visceral arterial spasm, which causes decreased nutritional blood flow and disease progression. Patients should wear gloves and hats, use multilayer clothing, and try to keep the ambient temperature in their homes high enough to prevent Raynaud's phenomenon. They should also try to stay 5 to 10 per cent above their ideal weight to benefit from the insulating effect of fat. Patients should avoid cigarette smoking because it may precipitate local digital vasospasm by local absorption of nicotine as well as accelerate pulmonary complications.

Physical therapy is often neglected in the long-term treatment program because of expense and poor insurance coverage. This is unfortunate since physical therapy frequently can make the difference between function and disability. Aggressive physical therapy can contribute significantly to maintaining joint range of motion and preventing contractures. Newer dynamic splinting techniques and progressive casting frequently can restore lost range of motion and improve function. Without a continued program to preserve or regain function, the effects of various pharmacologic agents on joint mobility will be less than potentially achievable.

Prospective care to prevent skin drying, fissures, and ulceration is essential. The first step is avoidance of cold. Emollient skin creams containing lanolin or aloe vera should be used several times a day. If fissures or ulcers begin to develop, they should be promptly treated with topical antibiotics and rest of the affected part. If they continue to progress, then systemic agents to promote nutritional blood flow are indicated. These drugs are used for treatment of ulcers, which are usually on the fingers or hands as a consequence of Raynaud's. Healing occurs as the ratio of nutritional blood flow and tissue to be nourished is shifted by either increased blood flow or loss of tissue by atrophy. Chronic ulcers or areas of pressure may develop subcutaneous calcinosis for which there is no effective preventive therapy. Treatment consists of control of infection and surgical excision where necessary.

Patients will often experience depression and frustration at the lack of effective therapy and the frequent experience of hearing about an effective new agent that is then discarded after careful testing. Most patients can expect many years with little impairment, but they will be haunted by anecdotes of severely afflicted patients. They should be encouraged to learn about their disease and should be given an estimate of their prognosis, which is often much better than they expect. The Scleroderma Foundation, P.O. Box 724, Watsonville, California 95076, is a valuable source of information. Patients who are not actively denying their disease often will benefit from the activities and information sponsored by the Foundation. There are now chapters in most major cities.

Systemic Treatment

Symptoms related to Raynaud's phenomenon are usually the first ones to require drug therapy. Since nutritional blood flow reduction by the arteriolar vasospasm of Raynaud's occurs in internal organs such as the heart, kidneys, and lungs, as well as the skin, the presence of Raynaud's may imply that potential visceral damage is occurring. Raynaud's phenomenon should be treated if there is interference with normal daily activities or if digital ulcers refractory to conservative therapy are present. A wide variety of agents is available, but their efficiency will be limited by the extent to which the arteriolar supply to the affected part has been obliterated by the disease. Nitroglycerin applied topically may be helpful for refractory ulcers by promoting cutaneous vasodilation. For short-term systemic treatment, the calcium channel blocker nifedipine (Procardia), which is also a peripheral vasodilator, is often effective. It often becomes less effective after 1 to 2 months of continuous use. Other useful drugs are the alpha blockers, phenoxybenzamine (Dibenzyline) and tolazoline; arteriolar dilators, such as methyldopa (Aldomet) and prazosin (Minipress); and the beta-agonist terbutaline (Bricanyl). The selective type II serotonin antagonist ketanserine is reported effective in short-term investigational studies. Other promising investigational agents are prostacycline infusions to inhibit thromboxane-induced vasospasm and dazoxiben, which inhibits thromboxane synthesis. Captopril (Capoten), the angiotensin-converting enzyme inhibitor useful for hypertensive crisis, also may promote healing of digital ulcers. Fibrinolytic agents (discussed subsequently) like stanozolol (Winstrol) may also be helpful.

Treatment with drugs to try to slow disease progression rather than for a specific problem, such as digital ulcers, requires careful weighing of the risk to benefit ratio. Patients with CREST syndrome or mild acrosclerosis and anticentromere activity should not be treated with a disease-modifying agent unless a specific organ problem exists, such as early edematous disease, myositis, pulmonary hypertension, congestive heart failure, or hypertension. Early edematous disease or myositis may respond to low dose corticosteroids. Other problems will be discussed later.

Patients with diffuse systemic sclerosis or rapidly progressive acrosclerosis are candidates for treatment with disease-modifying agents. The principal drug in this category is D-penicillamine (D-Pen, Cuprimine), which is best given early in the disease, before significant functional impairment occurs. Preliminary evidence indicates that early treatment may delay or prevent visceral complications. Patients treated with D-penicillamine should have baseline pulmonary, renal, and cardiac evaluations as well as careful documentation of cutaneous involvement and joint motion. The "go low—go slow" approach is preferable to minimize side effects. Dosage should be slowly increased over 3 to 4 months from 125 to 250 mg initially to 750 mg a day. Potential renal or hematologic toxicity with leukopenia or thrombocytopenia should be monitored monthly. The decision to treat should imply a commitment to continue for several years, since improvement may be slow and a portion of the benefit may be in the delay of late complications.

Drugs affecting the coagulation system are currently under active investigation as disease-modifying agents. Patients with active systemic sclerosis have an activated clotting system with impaired fibrinolysis. This is shown by a shortened fibrinogen half-life, increased circulating platelet aggregates, and prolonged euglobulin clot lysis time. Stanozolol (Winstrol) affects both laboratory improvement in fibrinolysis and clinical improvement in Raynaud's and cutaneous induration. Antiplatelet adhesive drugs such as dipyridamole (Persantin) are also in the early stages of investigation, and improvement in laboratory parameters have been shown. Plasmapheresis with high dose prednisone and cyclophosphamide (Cytoxan) has been used with best effects on muscle strength, Raynaud's, and digital ulcers. However, the potential side effects of these medications severely limit its applicability. Lymphoplasmapheresis without other medication may be just as effective but this procedure is investigational and clearly should be restricted to the most severely afflicted patients in whom other therapies have failed.

Specific Organ Systems

Fulminant renal failure is the most dreaded complication of systemic sclerosis but is now often treatable. Rapid skin tightening, schistocytes, and recent onset of hypertension may be clues that this is imminent. Hypertension should be treated early with conventional agents. Since depletion of intravascular volume is a potential risk factor for renal failure, potent diuretics should be avoided. Aggressive treatment with conventional antihypertensive agents like minoxidil (Loniten) or captopril (Capoten) has shown that renal failure is reversible. Recovery of sufficient renal function to allow termination of dialysis can be expected in over 50 per cent of cases although restoration of normal renal function is rare. Anticoagulation with coumarin (Coumadin) or heparin may be useful.

Gastrointestinal problems are frequent. Many patients will have asymptomatic gastroesophageal reflux. If motility testing or cine esophagram confirms this, patients require chronic antacid therapy to prevent esophagitis and stricture. Occasionally metoclopramide (Reglan) will raise lower esophageal sphincter pressure sufficiently to prevent reflux. Otherwise, the selective H_2 antagonists ranitidine (Zantac) or cimetidine (Tagamet) or conventional antacids should be used. The latter may also relieve constipation due to decreased intestinal motility. Decreased motility may also cause malabsorption as a consequence of bacterial overgrowth and bile salt deconjugation. Recognition may require specific testing since bowel habits may not change significantly. Treatment with tetracycline or ampicillin is usually effective.

Pulmonary hypertension and pulmonary fibrosis are frequent late sequelae. CREST syndrome patients are at increased risk for late fulminant pulmonary hypertension. Pulmonary function testing may show considerable variation with time in assessment of therapeutic agents and is difficult. Penicillamine (Cuprimine) may be useful in early fibrosis. Hydralazine (Apresoline) or prazosin (Minipress) may reduce pulmonary artery pressures, but evaluation requires right heart catheterization because the response is not predictable and sudden death has been reported. Nifedipine (Procardia) may also reduce pulmonary artery pressures.

Much of the current therapy of systemic sclerosis has resulted from the use of agents originally developed for other diseases. Prognosis is clearly improving, and most patients can look forward to many years of productivity and less disability than previously.

DERMATOMYOSITIS

method of
W. P. DANIEL SU, M.D.,
and FRANK C. POWELL, M.R.C.P.I.
Mayo Clinic
Rochester, Minnesota

Dermatomyositis is an inflammatory disease of skin, skeletal muscle, and sometimes blood vessels. Polymyositis occurs in patients who have muscle involvement without skin lesions. Some of these patients may later present skin findings and be diagnosed as having dermatomyositis at that time. Rarely patients may have only cutaneous findings without myositis. In general, cutaneous and muscular manifestations occur concomitantly or within a few months of each other in patients with dermatomyositis. Systemic symptoms are common and may be the early findings.

Diagnosis

Five major criteria are recognized for the diagnosis of dermatomyositis: (1) weakness and pain of proximal muscles, (2) cutaneous findings, including poikiloderma, periorbital edema and erythema, Guttron's sign, calcinosis cutis, and atrophic plaques over elbows and knees, (3) suggestive electromyographic findings, (4) necrosis of type 1 and type 2 muscle fibers on biopsy, and (5) elevation of muscle enzymes. The suggestive electromyographic findings are short, small, polyphasic motor units, fibrillations, positive sharp waves and insertional irritability; and bizarre high frequency repetitive discharges. Creatinine kinase, aspartate transaminase (AST, previously SGOT), and lactate dehydrogenase are elevated in active myositis. To determine the clinical status of dermatomyositis as a guide to monitoring therapeutic dosage, the gross muscle power, changes of skin lesions, and results of muscle enzymes should all be considered.

In adults, dermatomyositis may occur on its own or in association with other collagen vascular diseases such as scleroderma, lupus erythematosus, rheumatoid arthritis, and so on. In patients over 45 years old, a sudden and severe onset of dermatomyositis should be investigated for possible associated malignancy, particularly tumors of the ovary and stomach, although this occurs in only a minority of patients. Two types of juvenile dermatomyositis are seen. The Banker type is characterized by a rapid course, vascular changes, lack of response to steroid medications, and poor prognosis. Calcinosis cutis is rare. In contrast, the Brunsting type has a slower course of inflammatory myositis without vascular or visceral changes, and calcinosis cutis is often extensive. Patients usually respond well to systemic steroids and, thus, the prognosis is better in the Brunsting type of juvenile dermatomyositis.

TREATMENT

The major therapeutic measures in the management of dermatomyositis are listed in Table 1.

General Measures and Skin Care. Hospitalization with bed rest is necessary in the initial stages to stabilize advancing inflammatory disease. A negative nitrogen balance may be caused by inflammatory myositis; therefore, high protein, high energy diet supplements are needed, and a daily calorie count should be kept. A minimum of 2500 calories per day is necessary. Total parenteral nutrition may rarely be required, for example, in childhood dermatomyositis (Banker type) with visceral lesions. In addition to expert dietary supervision, gentle physical therapy should be started early. In this situation, a delicate balance must be achieved between exhausting the patient with active muscle disease and allowing muscle contractures and disuse atrophy to develop. An experienced physical therapist must supervise treatment.

Dermatologic care includes advice regarding sun protection, as many of the cutaneous features may be precipitated or exacerbated by ultraviolet

TABLE 1. **Treatment of Dermatomyositis**

General Measures
High protein diet
Physical therapy
Bed rest at acute stage
Antibiotics for secondary infection
Surgical excision of calcinosis cutis at sites of pain and pressure
Topical Treatment
Topical lubricating cream or emollient regularly
Topical steroids usually of little benefit
Systemic Medications
Systemic steroids—treatment of choice
Methotrexate or azathioprine (with steroid-sparing effect) in more severe cases
Cyclophosphamide, chlorambucil, and 6-mercaptopurine may be helpful, but data are insufficient
Antimalarials
Plasmapheresis

light. Topical lubricating creams applied twice daily help to improve general skin condition. Topical steroid creams are usually of little benefit in the management of the cutaneous lesions.

Antibiotics may be used to treat infection about sites of cutaneous calcinosis. However, these deposits need to be surgically excised if they cause ulceration or physical disability. The benefit of aluminum hydroxide or low calcium diets to prevent the development of cutaneous calcification is questionable.

Corticosteroids. Although spontaneous remissions may occur in up to 30 per cent of patients, treatment with systemic medications is usually required. Oral prednisone is the mainstay of treatment and should be used in full therapeutic levels, since low dose therapy can be associated with significant side effects without controlling the disease. Initial doses in adults range from 40 to 100 mg per day, which may need to be given in divided dosages. In children, the initial dose should be approximately 1.5 to 2.5 mg per kg per day. Control of the disease is indicated by regression of inflammatory skin lesions, reduction of muscle enzyme level, and improvement in muscle power. Even as clinical improvement is manifested, 40 to 60 mg of prednisone daily should be given for at least three months; then the level of steroid dosage can be gradually reduced by 10 mg every 3 to 4 weeks until a maintenance level of between 10 and 30 mg per day is reached; then tapering becomes more gradual. Although the response rate varies from weeks to months, treatment is usually required for many months and often for a total treatment period of up to two years. For long term maintenance, alternate day steroid therapy may be preferable to daily treatment. If relapse of the disease occurs, the dose of prednisone needs to be increased by 10 to 20 mg per day until clinical improvement again is evident, after which tapering is carried out at a more gradual pace. This approach should control the great majority of cases. Patient progress is monitored by regular evaluations of muscle enzyme levels and sedimentation rate in addition to clinical parameters. Occasionally, difficulty in distinguishing a steroid-induced myopathy from relapse of myositis may necessitate rebiopsy of muscle. Rarely, high dose intravenous pulse steroid therapy has been used, but serious biochemical alterations may occur with this form of therapy and it is not recommended except as a last resort. Because long-term use of steroids is usually required, patients must be monitored closely for side effects of treatment, such as osteoporosis, diabetes, Cushing's syndrome, hypertension, and gastrointestinal bleeding.

Other forms of immunosuppressive therapy are generally used in conjunction with oral prednisone to enable more rapid reduction in the dose of steroids or to achieve more complete control of the disease.

Methotrexate. Methotrexate has been used with varying success in the management of both childhood and adult dermatomyositis (use not listed in manufacturer's directive). Both oral and intravenous routes have been employed, usually given as a single weekly dose of 10 to 25 mg orally or 10 to 20 mg intravenously. With control of the disease, the methotrexate treatment can be reduced by spacing the therapy to every 2 weeks, every 3 weeks, and then once per month, or by reducing the dosage level. The potential hepatotoxicity of this drug must be remembered, and it should not be used in patients with impaired liver function, alcoholism, severe renal disease, or blood dyscrasias. The earliest manifestations of methotrexate toxicity are oral ulcerations and leukopenia. Close supervision of therapy is required with frequent checks of hepatic, renal, and hematologic function. With long term therapy, liver biopsy with histologic evaluation of the degree of fibrosis should probably be carried out before treatment and then repeated every 1 to 2 years. Liver function testing alone is inadequate to detect the hepatotoxicity of methotrexate. Improvement in cases treated with methotrexate is usually noted in 2 to 3 months, and significant steroid-sparing can be achieved.

Azathioprine. This agent may be used at a dosage of 1 to 3 mg per kg per day (use not listed in manufacturer's directive). The dose level may be adjusted upwards until mild leukopenia supervenes. Two to 3 months of treatment may be required before benefit is observed, and this medication is generally used in conjunction with oral prednisone to achieve steroid-sparing. As control of the disease is achieved, the prednisone dose is gradually tapered. Side effects are primarily hematologic (leukopenia, anemia, thrombocytopenia, hemorrhage), but GI upset, alopecia, arthralgia, jaundice, higher incidence of infections, and drug eruptions may occur. The complete blood count should be checked two or three times per week during initiation of therapy and while high dose levels are being used, and at least weekly or biweekly during maintenance therapy.

Other Immunosuppressive Agents. Cyclophosphamide, chlorambucil, and 6-mercaptopurine have also been used in the management of dermatomyositis. Clinical experience with the use of these agents in this disease is limited, and no clear guidelines exist for their administration. Encouraging results have been reported, however, with short-term cyclophosphamide therapy.

Antimalarials. Antimalarials have been shown to be helpful in treating dermatomyositis with primarily cutaneous changes. The usual dosage is hydroxychloroquine (Plaquenil), 200 mg twice daily for 1 week, then 200 mg once daily. When the skin lesions show a definite improvement, the dosage can be decreased to 200 mg once every other day and gradually tapered. Before the patient is placed on hydroxychloroquine, ophthalmologic examination should be done as a baseline and should be repeated every 3 to 6 months to rule out any ocular toxicity while the patient is on therapy. Quinacrine hydrochloride (Atabrine), 100 mg per day, can be used alone or added to hydroxychloroquine in more severe cases. Quinacrine rarely causes ocular side effects but commonly induces yellowish discoloration of the skin. (This use of Plaquenil and Atabrine is not listed by the makers.)

Plasmapheresis. Plasmapheresis has recently been reported to be of benefit in some patients with dermatomyositis who have had inadequate clinical response to prednisone or immunosuppressive agents. Some of these patients could subsequently be maintained in remission with prednisone alone following plasmapheresis and cytotoxic therapy. This procedure may prove to be a useful therapeutic modality in patients resistant to more established methods of therapy. Plasmapheresis may be carried out weekly for up to 10 weeks, and then at gradually lengthening intervals as response dictates. Between 10 and 30 exchanges are usually required.

LUPUS ERYTHEMATOSUS

method of
DENNY L. TUFFANELLI, M.D.
University of California, San Francisco
San Francisco, California

Discoid Lupus Erythematosus

In discoid or chronic cutaneous lupus erythematosus (LE), the manifestations are primarily cutaneous. Discoid lupus is a part of the systemic lupus erythematosus (SLE) spectrum, and patients should be regarded as having potential for developing SLE. Cutaneous lesions in patients who have discoid lupus lesions as part of their SLE are managed in the same manner as those seen in pure discoid LE. Discoid LE may be minimal or extensive and may be a major or minor cosmetic problem. The individual lesions may subside or may progress with scarring and disfigurement. Therapy should be individualized, because different patients respond in different manners to the cosmetic problem.

A complete general and medical examination is indicated. All patients with discoid LE are concerned about the possibility of developing SLE. The appropriate tests to evaluate this possibility are CBC, urinalysis, and measurement of sedimentation rate, antinuclear antibody, anti-DNA, total hemolytic complement, CH50, and C3. If the patient has Raynaud's phenomenon an extractable nuclear antigen (ENA) test is done. Skin biopsy for routine histologic and immunopathologic evaluation is done if the diagnosis is in question.

Treatment

Following laboratory tests, an extensive discussion with the patient concerning prognosis and therapy is held. The patient with completely negative laboratory test results should be informed that the problem is primarily cosmetic and that the possibility of the development of systemic lupus erythematosus is unlikely. If the major problem is cosmetic, make-up, wigs, and sun exposure are discussed with the patient. Some patients are more sun sensitive than others, so the patient is advised to avoid sun bathing and other forms of long sun exposure. With reasonable precautions, an ordinary life style can be followed. The patient should wear a hat and sunscreens when there is significant sun exposure. Testing for photosensitivity is occasionally helpful. Sunlight phobia should be avoided. The patient is also advised that plaques of discoid lupus occur in traumatized area—the Koebner reaction. Picking, excoriating, and injury to the skin in the forms of burns should be avoided.

Local Therapy. Numerous sunscreens are available. They are labeled with their sun protection factors (SPF), which range from 2 to 19. Patients with cutaneous LE should use sunscreens within the 15 to 19 range on all exposed areas. Sunscreens are available with alcohol or moisturizing bases. The patient should experiment with sunscreens until a cosmetically satisfactory one is found.

Topical Therapy. Topical corticosteroids are the most common form of therapy for cutaneous LE. They are particularly beneficial for erythematous plaques. Chronic scarred lesions obviously will not respond. Medium or high concentration topical corticosteroids can be utilized, but high potency topical corticosteroids should be used with caution if needed for long periods on the lips and face. One should watch for the side effects of facial telangiectasia and cutaneous atrophy. Plastic film occlusion with low or medium strength topical corticosteroids is occasionally worthwhile. Tape impregnated with steroid (Cordran tape) is useful. Intralesional corticosteroids are useful in more chronic refractory lesions. About 0.1 ml of triamcinolone 2.5 mg per ml is injected with a number 27 needle into 1 cm square areas. This is particularly useful for lesions on the lips and refractory lesions of the hand and face. The possibility that the injected area may develop subcutaneous atrophy or hypopigmentation should be discussed with the patient.

Surgical excision and grafting are rarely indicated because of the possibility of Koebner's reaction.

Systemic Therapy. If the lesions are not controlled with topical or intralesional therapy, antimalarial drugs can be considered. Risks and benefits should be discussed at length with the patient. Antimalarials may lead to the clearing of old lesions and prevent the appearance of new lesions. Three different antimalarials, chloroquine diphosphate (Aralen), hydroxychloroquine sulfate (Plaquenil), and quinacrine (Atabrine), are used. Each has advantages and disadvantages. Hydroxychloroquine, 200 to 400 mg daily, is the safest. If there is no response after 3 to 6 months, chloroquine 250 mg daily may be utilized. If there is no response to this routine, quinacrine, 100 mg a day, can be added to the chloroquine. The patient should be cautioned that quinacrine causes a yellowish discoloration of the skin. Retinal toxicity can occur, and ophthalmologic examinations should be performed before and during therapy. Side effects of the antimalarials include gastrointestinal disturbances, myopathy, hyper- and hypopigmentation of the skin, hair, and nails, pruritus, and erythema multiforme. Hematologic side effects, including leukopenia, anemia, and aplastic anemia, are more common with quinacrine. Ocular changes include a reversible keratopathy, irreversible retinopathy, and cycloplegia. (This use of Atabrine and Chloroquine is not listed by the makers.)

Other Measures. Low dosage corticosteroids, cytotoxic agents, and dapsone will occasionally benefit extensive cutaneous lesions that are unresponsive to the preceding measures. However, they should be used only in special circumstances by those with experience in their usage.

Systemic Lupus Erythematosus

Systemic lupus erythematosus (SLE) is a multisystem disease of unknown etiology. Treatment depends on the systems involved and the severity of symptoms. Most patients with SLE can be well controlled.

General Management

An assessment of the extent of disease includes a complete examination and extensive laboratory tests. All studies utilized in the work-up of a patient with chronic cutaneous LE are employed in working up the patient with SLE. In addition, a complete general work-up including studies of renal function should be obtained. Serologic abnormalities such as C3 values and levels of anti-DNA antibodies often give a good indication of disease activity.

Patient Education. SLE is a chronic disease, and patient education is of major importance. Patients should be referred to the several lupus foundations, whose membership consists of persons with the disease and which are dedicated to patient education. In addition, a discussion of prognosis, therapy, and preventive measures is useful. Continuing patient education is a major aim of the follow-up office visit.

Most commonly, affected patients are young women with very active life styles. They should be cautioned against pushing daily activities too far. Infections may lead to a flare of SLE. Since patients with SLE do not handle bacterial infection well, these infections should be treated rapidly and adequately. Blood cultures should be obtained in patients on steroid therapy with significant infections and chest x-ray films in patients with persistent cough.

The same precautions with regard to sunlight in discoid lupus erythematosus (DLE) apply to SLE. Patients with a history of toxicity following extensive sun exposure should be particularly careful and should use sunscreens.

Pregnancy must be discussed extensively with each patient, since there is the possibility of a flare during pregnancy or the immediate postpartum period. There is no contraindication to pregnancy in most patients with SLE, but the risks, adverse effects of medications, and effect of LE on the fetus must be discussed.

Oral contraceptives and estrogen therapy may be deleterious. Other forms of contraception should be utilized if at all possible. Drugs known to induce LE, such as procainamide and hydralazine, should be avoided. The effect of environmental chemicals is not well known, but various insecticides and hair dyes have been implicated.

Systemic Therapy

For many patients with SLE, salicylates alone are useful. The dose varies from 4 to 8 grams or 60 to 120 grains of aspirin or its equivalent daily given with milk. The dosage can be increased until there is significant clinical improvement or side effects occur. The precise role in SLE of other nonsteroidal anti-inflammatory drugs has not been adequately ascertained. Until more information is available, I continue to use aspirin.

Antimalarials. Patients with photosensitivity, arthralgias, or cutaneous lesions appear to respond particularly well to antimalarial therapy. These agents can also be used in some patients to aid in the reduction of steroid dosage. The usage, cautions, and side effects of antimalarials are listed under Discoid Lupus Erythematosus.

Systemic Corticosteroids. Adrenal corticosteroid compounds, the mainstay of therapy of active SLE, suppress the inflammatory reaction. In some patients with mild chronic forms of the disease, rest, salicylates, and possibly antimalarials are frequently helpful. If this approach does not control the disease, corticosteroids are utilized in a dosage of approximately 15 mg a day. However, in a severely ill, febrile, toxic patient, a larger initial dose (40 to 80 mg) of prednisone is given daily. This dose can be increased until control is achieved. Other indications for corticosteroids include thrombocytopenia, hemolytic anemia, significant nephropathy, pericarditis, and CNS involvement. Once the disease is controlled, the dosage is diminished as rapidly as possible. My approach is to reduce the dose by 5 to 10 mg increments weekly until a level of 15 mg daily is reached. At this point the dose may be reduced by 1 or 2 mg every few weeks. Alternate day steroid doses are rarely effective in managing systemic lupus erythematosus, with the possible exception of renal manifestations. Side effects of steroids, which are proportional to the dosage given, include cushingoid appearance, ecchymoses, atrophic fragile skin, hirsutism, acne, tuberculosis, glycosuria, osteoporosis, mycosis, muscle weakness, peptic ulcer, and aseptic bone necrosis. Following a patient on steroids requires frequent urinalysis and determinations of blood pressure, weight, blood cell counts, and chemical profiles. In stressful situations, such as following operation or infection, the dose of steroids should be significantly increased.

Immunosuppressives. Currently, there is some interest in the use of immunosuppressives and antimetabolites, particularly in the therapy of lupus nephropathy. In the treatment of patients with active lupus glomerulonephritis, it is unclear whether a combination of adrenocorticoids and cytotoxic drugs is more effective than adrenocorticoids alone; this is the situation in which immunosuppressives are most commonly used. In addition, patients with other forms of LE in whom steroid side effects or steroid failure is a problem are candidates for immunosuppressive therapy. Immunosuppressive agents are still experimental and should be used only by experienced investigators. They have both immunosuppressive and anti-inflammatory effects. Antimetabolites such as 6-mercaptopurine and azathioprine, alkylating agents such as cyclophosphamide and nitrogen mustard, and folic acid antagonists such as methotrexate have been used. The drugs predispose to viral, bacterial, and fungal infections. Other risks include bone marrow depression, the development of lymphoproliferative disorders, teratogenic effects, and chromosomal abnormalities.

When the nephritis of SLE has progressed to end stage renal failure, medical management is ineffective in improving renal function. Such patients generally have been denied acceptance into chronic renal dialysis programs. Hemodialysis, bilateral nephrectomy, and renal transplantation have been utilized in a few patients.

CUTANEOUS VASCULITIS

method of
JOSEPH L. JORIZZO, M.D.
University of Texas
Galveston, Texas

"Vasculitis" has become a much abused "wastebasket" diagnosis. Physicians attribute many signs or symptoms that are otherwise unidentified to this process, much as they did in earlier years to the diagnosis "viral infection." The gross pathologic characteristics of systemic vasculitides—at least as they present cutaneously—can be determined from careful examination of the skin. Categorization into small vessel vasculitis or large vessel vasculitis is often easily done clinically and can be confirmed histologically by the microscopic detection of leukocytoclastic vasculitis.

Small Vessel Vasculitis

A preferred synonym for small vessel leukocytoclastic vasculitis is necrotizing venulitis. Other synonyms and subgroups of necrotizing venulitis include hypersensitivity angiitis, Henoch-Schönlein purpura, urticarial vasculitis, essential mixed cryoglobulinemia, erythema elevatum diutinum, and hypergammaglobulinemic purpura of Waldenström. These small vessel vasculitides may affect the skin without apparent systemic illness, although they should be considered systemic diseases. The typical cutaneous lesions consist of palpable purpura on the lower extremities.

The evidence to support a circulating immune complex–mediated vasculitis pathogenesis for necrotizing venulitis is compelling. Each patient should be evaluated carefully for involvement of internal organs. An etiologic agent is discovered in only about half of patients, although a search could encompass infection (streptococcal, *Mycobacterium tuberculosis,* hepatitis B); drugs (aspirin, penicillin, phenothiazines, sulfonamides, iodides); chemicals (insecticides); foreign proteins (serum sickness, allergy testing); autoimmune disease (systemic lupus erythematosus, rheumatoid arthritis, ulcerative colitis); and underlying malignant tumors (Hodgkin's disease and others).

Diagnosis of large vessel vasculitis in the skin is made by the detection of digital necrosis or necrosis of wedges of tissue, in a manner consistent with occlusion from vasculitis of small or medium-sized muscular arteries. Histologic confirmation requires incisional biopsy of deep tissue. The microscopic appearance of the specimen will be of leukocytoclastic or granulomatous vasculitis of the small or medium-sized muscular arteries that supply the affected necrotic skin. Synonyms and subgroups of large vessel vasculitis include polyarteritis nodosa; Wegener's granulomatosis (also of small vessels); allergic granulomatous angiitis of Churg and Strauss; giant cell arteritis; and the large vessel vasculitis seen in systemic lupus erythematosus, rheumatoid arthritis, and other collagen vascular diseases. A thorough evaluation for internal involvement and etiology, similar to that done for small vessel vasculitis, is warranted for all patients.

Treatment

General Measures

The mildest types of small vessel vasculitis might require no treatment. Close monitoring for internal organ involvement and a search for etiologic precipitants, however, is always warranted. A simple maneuver—discontinuing a medication, for example, or treating underlying infection, paraproteinemia, or an autoimmune disorder—might result in prompt improvement in the vasculitis. Bedrest or support stockings might help heal the lesions that occur on the skin of ordinarily dependent structures. Potent topical corticosteroids may result in more rapid clearing of cutaneous lesions, but prolonged use can induce cutaneous atrophy. Patients with small vessel vasculitis who have significant involvement of internal organs, and all patients with more serious large vessel vasculitis, require systemic therapy.

Corticosteroids

Systemic corticosteroids are still the treatment to use for severe vasculitic syndromes, particularly for those with a rapidly progressing course or with renal, neurologic, or cardiopulmonary involvement, or for syndromes in which the patient suffers from severe serum sickness–like manifestations—fever and arthralgias and so on. There is not convincing experimental evidence to prove the efficacy of this therapy. Because of the potential of high dose systemic corticosteroid therapy to induce adverse reactions, physicians need to be well informed about the risks and care of complications.

If systemic corticosteroid treatment is strongly indicated, however, therapy should be begun at 1 mg per kg per day, in a single oral dose in the morning (prednisone, 60 to 80 mg per day). Split-dose therapy carries a proportional increase in clinical response and in side effects, so no advantage is achieved over the higher, single dose regimen. Alternate-day therapy is effective in diseases such as dermatomyositis or bullous pemphigoid but seems to be ineffective for diseases that are mediated (presumably) by circulating immune complexes, such as systemic vasculitis. Systemic daily corticosteroid therapy should be tapered usually to zero over a several week to month period while all affected organ systems are monitored closely by clinical and laboratory examinations.

"Pulse" therapy, with massive doses of methyl prednisolone (given as 1 gram per day, intravenously, for 3 to 5 days) has been used in patients with life-threatening large vessel vasculitis, in an attempt to gain rapid control of the disease process. Long-term, oral, traditional dose therapy is required for maintenance after pulse therapy. The patient must be monitored in hospital for cardiac arrythmias and sudden electrolyte shifts that may accompany pulse therapy.

Azathioprine (Imuran)

Patients who require massive doses of prednisone may benefit from the addition of azathioprine to the regimen, as a single oral dose of 100 to 200 mg per day (use not listed by the makers). The benefits of adding azathioprine may not be apparent for as long as 4 to 6 weeks. Close monitoring for the possibility of hematologic toxicity is required. Long-term risks of combined immunosuppressive and corticosteroid therapy may include reduced immune surveillance with increased likelihood of internal malignancy.

Cyclophosphamide (Cytoxan)

Patients with life-threatening vasculitis, especially those with polyarteritis nodosa, Wegener's granulomatosis, and severe rheumatoid vasculitis, may best be treated with cyclophosphamide with or without prednisone (use not listed by the makers). The dosage schedules and monitoring are similar to those for azathioprine; beneficial effects will be apparent at about the same time, and side effects are similar, with the added significant toxicity for cyclophosphamide of hemorrhagic cystitis. Careful attention to adequate hydration is required to help prevent hemorrhagic cystitis.

Plasmapheresis

Plasma exchange can be an adjunct to therapy of severe diseases that are characterized by circulating immunoreactants, such as vasculitis. A number of exchanges are required, and they must be performed in a hospital setting. This therapy can protect the patient through a severe flare of disease, although systemic therapy, as reviewed earlier, will be required for long-term management.

Other Systemic Therapies

A number of agents have been used—reported primarily in an anecdotal fashion—to treat patients with small vessel vasculitis that is difficult to manage but is not severe enough to require therapy with systemic corticosteroids or immunosuppressive agents.

Antihistamines, for one, have been advocated because local histamine release in tissue might trigger deposition of circulating immune complexes. They have seldom been effective in treating vasculitis.

Nonsteroidal anti-inflammatory drugs have been used to treat vasculitis because the products of arachidonic acid metabolism may play a role in inducing vasculitis, and because platelet aggregation is inhibited by these agents. They may be more useful for their anti-inflammatory effects in patients with joint involvement than for their effects on cutaneous systemic vasculitis.

Antimalarial agents such as hydroxychloroquine (Plaquenil) have been used in the treatment of various forms of vasculitis, and they are generally safe if the patient is closely monitored for signs of ocular, hematologic, and hepatic toxicity. The results with them, however, are not generally beneficial.

Diaminodiphenyl sulfone (dapsone) has been reported to be effective treatment for various forms of small-vessel vasculitis, particularly in erythema elevatum diutinum. Oral doses of 100 to 200 mg per day may be used, but hematologic monitoring must be extremely careful. The mechanism of action may be related to inhibitory effects on neutrophils.

Colchicine in oral doses of 0.6 mg two to three times daily may be of some benefit in treating mild cases of small vessel vasculitis that affect skin and joints. The mechanism of action may lie in inhibition of neutrophil migration. Side effects, such as diarrhea or nausea, respond to lowering of the dosage. Hematologic status, especially for neutropenia, must be monitored closely.

NAIL DISEASES

method of
ORVILLE J. STONE, M.D.
Pacifica Hospital
Huntington Beach, California

Nail problems have a reputation for being difficult to treat. This, at least to a degree, is deserved. Diverse diseases can produce similar defects, making diagnosis difficult. The slow growth of nails also makes it difficult to get quick results and it is difficult to get penetration of medication into the nail area. Fingernails grow about 0.1 mm to 0.15 mm per day, and toenails grow at about one half that rate. Fingernails, therefore, require 4 to 6 months to regrow and toenails double that time. In judging the rate of healing to be expected, ask the patient about the usual growth rate of his or her nails. Nails are of great cosmetic importance to many patients.

Reaction to Cosmetic Procedures

This is the most common nail problem in my practice. The reactions occur most commonly to acrylic nails, glues for split or broken nails, or penetrating nail hardeners. The substances applied have irritated the nail bed and produced separation or hyperkeratosis. In patients doing a lot of wet work, secondary yeast or bacterial infection can move into the pocket under the nail. The great majority of these lesions will heal without consequence. If the pocket is not infected and there is no debris, I use fluocinonide acetonide gel (Lidex gel). If it is wet and has secondary bacterial infection, I use topical clindamycin, 1 per cent solution (Cleocin T). If considerable hyperkeratosis is present in the subungual area, I use 6 per cent salicylic acid in a gel base (Keralyt gel). These treatments can be combined.

It is safe to continue to use nail polish to cover the defects until regrowth occurs, but one should not use penetrating nail hardeners or glues. About 90 per cent of patients can continue the use of acrylic nails. The color changes under the nail are due to saprophytic bacteria or fungi that are not causing the problem. However, patients insist on calling this fungus of the nail. Cutting back the nail speeds results, but this is so unpopular I suggest it only for emergencies.

Fungal Infections

Fungal infections of the nail bed and subungual area are very common, particularly in persons who have had chronic fungal infections of the feet and hands. It is extremely important to prove the diagnosis, because long-duration therapy is required. I discuss seriously with the patient the degree of compliance that is necessary to treat fingernails for 5 months or toenails for a year. Topical treatment offers very little benefit, and the best treatment is microsized griseofulvin (Grisactin), 500 mg twice a day with meals. Treatment is continued for 3 to 4 weeks after a clinical and laboratory cure. I occasionally avulse part of the nail to speed healing, but I do this in less than 10 per cent of patients. There are several chemical methods of debriding nails but they are very irritative and one should study them in detail before using. I commonly use 6 per cent salicylic acid gel (Keralyt gel) under occlusion for treating hyperkeratotic aspects of nail problems, but I seldom use more aggressive substances to eat away nails. I currently favor Grisactin for fungus of the nail but ketoconazole (Nizoral), 200 mg daily, is also effective. I feel obligated to follow use of this latter drug more closely.

Bacterial Infections

Green Nails. Green nails result from secondary growth of *Pseudomonas aeruginosa* in pockets of wetness. This responds best to keeping the area dry and using drying antibiotics such as alcohol drops of topical 1 per cent clindamycin (Cleocin T).

Acute Pyodermas. Acute pyodermas are treated

like acute infections at other sites except more aggressively since there is a greater tendency to rapid spread. The tissue in the area is also tight, so pyodermas tend to be more painful. The acute infections tend to be streptococcal so I usually use erythromycin, 250 mg four times a day. If there is considerable pain, consider that there may be a pocket of pus under the nail, which should be drained.

Chronic Paronychia. This disorder is chronic swelling and retraction of the posterior nail fold. It occurs in people who frequently have their hands in water. Acute flares occur under the posterior nail fold, and pus drains from the area. The best treatment is to keep the area dry, spray it three or four times a day with triamcinolone acetonide spray (Kenalog Spray) using a scalp-adaptor that has been cut short, and follow each spraying with clotrimazole or miconazole. Many clinicians recommend culturing these lesions. I have done extensive cultures and although multiple organisms were found in each lesion, *Candida albicans* is the basic cause of the problem.

Traumatic Lesions. If a hemorrhage forms under the nail, the pressure should be relieved by a nail drill or a hot paper clip. In the hot paper clip technique, the paper clip is heated in an open flame and then applied to the nail over the hematoma. The nail is easily penetrated and the blood pours out, relieving the pressure. If a splinter is under the nail, I may try to remove it directly, but if removal appears difficult, I do a digital block first. A bright light under the fingertip makes it easier to locate a foreign body.

Ingrown Nails. This varies from a mild to a severe problem. In the milder forms, a piece of cotton can be placed under the lateral edge of the nail; this is gradually moved daily proximally until the nail has been lifted out of the soft tissue. The cotton also acts as a pad to decrease discomfort. In the more severe or persistent forms, I do a digital block, excise the granulation tissue, and cauterize the base. I destroy the nail matrix only for special reasons—for example, where the nail is extremely curved.

Tumors. Benign tumors around the nail are most likely to be warts. The edge of the wart showing around the nail is only part of the wart, which almost always extends under the nail and makes the failure rate of removal very high. I usually use a digital block, cut away the nail over the wart, and thoroughly curette the wart. It tends to bleed vigorously and requires postoperative pain medication.

Mucocele (Mucinous Cyst). These are common and have a strong tendency to recur. I surround the lesion with 0.2 ml of triamcinolone suspension (10 mg per ml) and then inject 0.1 ml directly into the lesion.

Pyogenic Granulomas. These vascular growths are excised under local anesthesia and the base cauterized. The specimen should be sent for histopathologic examination.

Cancer or Melanoma. These lesions should be referred directly to surgeons who do a lot of hand surgery. Biopsy of the nail matrix usually causes scarring. If the lesion is away from the matrix, a diagnostic biopsy can be performed, and then appropriate therapy initiated.

Nail Disorders

Onycholysis. This is a common disorder in women, especially those with thyroid or hormone disorders. It tends to resolve slowly but has a strong tendency to recur over years. In some patients it comes and goes. I treat it the same as separation of the nail described earlier under Reaction to Cosmetic Procedures. An old standard therapy used by many is 4 per cent thymol in chloroform. (Note: The latter preparation has not been approved for use by the Food and Drug Administration.)

Psoriasis. This is a common and frustrating problem. Intralesional steroids are the best approach, but it is certainly uncomfortable treatment. If the lesions are in the superficial nail, I inject triamcinolone acetonide suspension (10 mg per ml) into the posterior nail fold. If the lesions are under the nail, I do a digital block and inject a small amount (0.1 ml) of the same material into the involved area. If there is marked hyperkeratosis, I use 6 per cent salicylic acid (Keralyt gel) under occlusion overnight.

KELOIDS

method of
LOUIS A. BROWN, JR., M.D.
Bala Cynwyd, Pennsylvania

Keloids are cutaneous lesions composed of excessive collagenous tissue and clinically characterized by a nodular appearance. They arise in genetically predisposed patients and when arising in scars, usually exceed the initial dimensions of the inciting trauma. Other features include a predilection for sites of increased skin tension, such as the presternal and deltoid regions, as well as areas of increased mobility such as the neck. The ear is another common site of occurrence.

Diagnosis

Making the diagnosis is not usually a problem; however, it is useful to distinguish a keloid from the more therapeutically amenable hypertrophic scar. The hypertrophic scar may arise in any individual in whom the normal wound healing process is interfered with due to repeated or excessive trauma, persistent foreign particles, or infection. As for keloids, the most distressing feature, both for the patient and the physician, is the recalcitrance to therapy.

Treatment

The mainstays of treatment include intralesional corticosteroid injection, surgical excision, pressure dressings, radiotherapy, and most recently laser surgery. A multitude of other methods has been tried with varying degrees of success, including use of immunosuppressive agents like methotrexate, thiotepa, and nitrogen mustard, or agents affecting collagen metabolism, such as asiaticoside, β-amino proprionitrile (BAPN) fumarate, colchicine, and retinoic acid. Still other modalities have been found to be efficacious by serendipity, such as topically applied zinc and ultrasound treatment.

Regardless of the modality chosen, both the physician and the patient must understand that follow-up management of at least 2 years' duration after any definitive procedure is necessary to reduce and control recurrences.

Corticosteroids

Recommendations for corticosteroid administration include use of triamcinolone acetonide in a concentration of 40 mg per ml to be injected with a 25 gauge needle initially into the surface of the lesion. The surface of the lesion can be frozen with ethyl chloride or liquid nitrogen and the injection made upon thawing. The use of a Luer-Lok type of syringe can enhance drug delivery. On subsequent visits, at monthly intervals, when the lesion has softened the injection can be made into its base with blanching as the desired result. Care should be made to avoid injecting or freezing surrounding normal-appearing skin. Should hypopigmentation arise in the surrounding skin, the patient should understand that it will resolve over a period of 6 to 12 months. The response to steroid injections is unpredictable. In some cases lesional growth is arrested within a period of months, whereas in others growth may continue despite more than 2 years of routine injections. The indications for use of corticosteroid intralesional injections include a symptomatic lesion, a relatively small lesion (i.e., $<$5 cm in diameter), or as an adjuvant to surgical excision. Side effects to be anticipated include atrophy and hypopigmentation.

Surgery

When surgically excising keloids, the clinician should be careful to use atraumatic sterile technique. For closure, use inert suture material such as silk or prolene. A minimum of one corticosteroid injection should be administered at least 1 month prior to the surgery. Postoperative follow-up should extend to a minimum of 2 years, with more frequent visits in the immediate postoperative period. Postoperative intralesional injection into the surgical scar site should be performed 3 to 4 weeks following excision and also at the first glimpse of recurrence. Another important adjunct is the use of pressure dressings postoperatively. Elastic dressings can be customized for various parts of the body and, if possible, should be left in place for a 2-year period to optimize the result. For postoperative earlobe management, plastic molds or earring clasps should be used. Despite these measures patient and physician should be prepared for the possibility of recurrence.

Radiotherapy

Radiotherapy can be used in keloid management either alone or in conjunction with surgery. Prevention of the reported complication of thyroid cancer due to radiotherapy is enhanced with lead shielding. In addition, eye and gonadal regions should be protected. Total doses of 1500 to 3000 rad may be used in divided doses. A typical regime, used in conjunction with surgery, can include preoperative irradiation 14 to 21 days prior to surgery, with 150 to 200 rad to the depth of the lesion. Factors used are 96 KV—2.7 mm of AL with HVL adequate to 3.3 mm of AL. Intraoperatively, radiation with 150 to 200 rad using factors of 85 KV—5 MA and 0.8 mm of AL may be employed. Postoperative irradiation may include a dosage of 300 rad using factors of 100 KV and 4 MA with 1.0 mm of aluminum.

Laser

Use of the carbon dioxide laser beam is recommended. This is invisible to the human eye and has a wavelength of 10.6 μm in the infrared spectrum. This "light scalpel" to excise keloids minimizes damage to adjacent soft tissue, thereby eliminating the possible stimulation of excessive collagen production. Additionally, hemostasis is obtained while excising, owing to scaling of vessels less than 0.5 mm in diameter, which in turn greatly facilitates visualization during surgery, thereby eliminating unnecessary trauma. Typical CO_2 settings include a spot size of 2.0 mm, power 20 watts, power density 500 watts/cm^2, and use of the continuous node. In addition, postoperative injection of the base of the lesion with corticosteroids is recommended.

The postlaser course of treated lesions is characterized by epithelialization over a 10 day to 2 week period and clinical healing by 1 month. If no additional measures are used besides laser extirpation, the keloid is likely to recur within 4 months postoperatively. Thus, measures discussed earlier for surgical management of keloids should be employed.

VERRUCA VULGARIS (WARTS)

method of
DUANE C. WHITAKER, M.D.
University of Iowa
Iowa City, Iowa

Common warts, plantar warts, condyloma acuminatum (genital warts), and flat warts are all caused by the human papilloma virus (HPV). Warts are presumed to be contracted from direct human contact through a break in the skin barrier. Although a high percentage of warts will spontaneously resolve in healthy individuals, many patients request treatment because of the physical appearance of warts or the pain caused by them (particularly in plantar and periungual lesions). Warts are also of concern because of their transmissibility and potential oncogenicity. The infectious nature of warts presents a public health problem among groups living in close contact, and HPV is tumorogenic in animals and humans. This has clinical importance in the immune-suppressed host and probably in patients with extensive and prolonged genital warts. These patients appear to be at a higher risk to develop frank carcinoma at or adjacent to wart-infected tissues. Such patients can present severe management problems, which warrant discussion beyond the scope of this article. Thus in this group of patients as well as in healthy individuals there are good reasons why most warts should be treated.

Treatment

The most important factors to be considered when deciding which type of treatment to use for a given wart are the anatomic location, type, and number of lesions as well as patient characteristics such as age, other medical conditions, and previous treatment failures. Cryotherapy, keratolytic agents (salicylic acid compounds), trichloroacetic acid (TCA), electrodesiccation, curettage, retinoic acid, 5-fluorouracil (5-FU), intralesional bleomycin, and carbon dioxide laser are frequently used therapeutic modalities. A solution of podophyllin resin can be useful in treating condyloma acuminatum but generally is not helpful in other types of warts. Cantharidin (Cantharone) continues to be used by some physicians; however, I find limited use for it. Superficial x-ray has long been used for treatment of resistant plantar warts; with availability of the carbon dioxide laser there is probably no longer any role for this, particularly in younger patients.

Common Warts

Therapy for ordinary warts is usually based on wart size, number, body location, and the ability of the patient to cooperate with therapy. Many warts are successfully treated with a single application of liquid nitrogen cryotherapy. However, if there are many lesions or previous therapy has failed, then multiple treatments can be anticipated. Manipulation and trauma of warts are a frequent cause of "recurrence" or development of new lesions. While cryotherapy is easily applied without anesthesia in the adult, this is not as easy in children, and stronger consideration should be given to a painless therapy such as repeated application of a keratolytic agent. The method of application of liquid nitrogen is with a cotton-tipped applicator until the wart is frozen white. Thicker warts may require several freeze-thaw cycles and repeat therapy at 3 to 4 week intervals. The freeze should be sufficient to destroy the wart but not so deep as to cause a dermal slough or to injure the underlying structures. Superficial structures requiring particular care are the digital nerves on fingers and the ulnar nerve at the elbow. If the physician has any concerns about lesions on these sites, it is sometimes best to infiltrate the lesions with a small amount of local anesthesia and then treat the warts with electrodesiccation and curettage, although this carries a greater chance of scarring. The use of electrodesiccation and curettage is particularly advantageous when there is a small number of warts since there is less chance that seeding of the virus to other sites has already occurred. Periungual warts are harder to eradicate because the wart may extend under the nail and into the nail bed or matrix so that the whole wart is inaccessible to therapy. Intralesional bleomycin, diluted 1 unit per 1 ml of saline, injected in a very small quantity (0.1 or 0.2 ml) into the lession has been used for this and other recalcitrant warts. This use is not directed by the product manufacturer and can cause local skin sloughing. It is not known if there are any long-term effects. The CO_2 laser is also effective for periungual warts.

Plantar Warts

The mainstay of therapy is the continuous application of keratolytic agents to loosen the verrucous tissue, which can then be carefully debrided. This avoids any invasive disruption of the dermis such as would be caused by cryotherapy, electrodesiccation or excision of plantar warts. The use of 40 per cent salicylic acid plaster, 40 per cent salicylic acid ointment, salicylic acid and lactic acid (Duofilm) coupled with proper occlusive dressing, paring, and debridement can result in painless elimination of plantar warts. Surgical excision is notoriously unsuccessful and should be avoided. However, judicious use of cryotherapy, either alone or combined with other agents, can be used for small plantar warts. While CO_2 laser is most effective for plantar warts, it is generally reserved for those unresponsive to conventional therapy.

In general, the most effective treatment is that which requires the least effort on the part of the patient. If warts can be eliminated in one or several office visits with therapy applied by the clinician, then success approaches 99 per cent. However, when applications by the patient are required on a regular basis, the success rate falls off dramatically. If home treatment is required, patient education and a clear explanation of the treatment plan are essential.

Flat Warts

Flat warts are both smaller and flatter than common warts, and they frequently appear in fairly large numbers. They are usually elevated in their vertical dimension no more than 3 mm and usually are 5 mm or less in diameter. Frequently patients are not aware of them until many lesions are present, and therefore they are often spread by trauma such as shaving. They are best visualized with indirect lighting. Because of their multiple numbers and small size, special care is required to destroy them without causing scarring or hyper- or hypopigmentation. This is especially problematic since they are so frequently seen on the face or neck. Treatment with topically applied retinoic acid cream or gel is usually preferred initially. This is started with the lowest concentration and is usually applied once or twice daily just to obtain slight erythema. The duration of treatment is variable but usually extends over several weeks. A second choice is a low concentration of 5-fluorouracil cream, but this is recommended only if the clinician has experience with 5-FU therapy. When these are ineffective, then cryotherapy, trichloroacetic acid, or light electrodesiccation with a very low epilating current may be used with extreme care. Flat warts are often refractory to therapy and usually require multiple treatments.

Condyloma Acuminatum

Genital warts are classified as a sexually transmitted disease. It is unknown whether there can be a prolonged incubation period between exposure to the virus and clinical appearance of the warts (months to years) and whether warts of the genitals can be contracted in ways other than direct skin to skin contact. Therefore genital warts in any pediatric patient warrant thorough medical and social investigation.

Retrograde spread of genital warts into the anal canal and urethra is likely in men and women who have extensive condylomata clustered about either orifice. The vaginal mucosa and cervix should be examined in patients with condylomata. Either of these can be a source of seeding and skin recurrence. Patients with genital warts often are more disturbed about their lesions than other patients with verruca. This may relate to concern about how they contracted the disease, to whom they may have exposed the warts, and how this affects their sexual activity and self-image. A sexual history should be obtained and all sexual partners examined. Patients should abstain from sexual activity while being treated. If this is not likely, then the male partner should use a condom. These patients are at risk for having additional sexually transmitted diseases.

Podophyllin has long been the standard treatment for genital warts. A 20 to 30 per cent solution of podophyllin in tincture of benzoin, either with or without salicylic acid, is used. Sitz baths or cleaning of the area 2 to 4 hours after treatment is usually recommended. When in doubt this should be done; however, the meticulous application of podophyllin to only the wart tissue and not treating large areas at one time obviates the need for such cleansing. Podophyllin should not be used in pregnant women and nursing mothers and should never be given to patients for self-application. While podophyllin treatment can be effective in the treatment of condylomata, many patients do not respond. Therefore other treatments such as cryotherapy, electrodesiccation, and curettage or electrosurgery may be necessary.

Perhaps the most effective therapy is carbon dioxide laser. Patients who have had multiple treatment failures for condyloma acuminatum can often be cured with one or several CO_2 laser sessions. Because of the oncogenic potential of HPV, female patients with extensive condylomata should have regular Pap smears regardless of age. This is even more important in patients who are immune suppressed. In my experience few patients with genital warts are cured with one session by any of the methods outlined, therefore a plan for regular treatment and follow-up should be established at the outset.

NEVI AND MALIGNANT MELANOMAS

method of
JUNE K. ROBINSON, M.D.
Northwestern University
Chicago, Illinois

clinician because of the need to identify premalignant or malignant processes. Acquired nevi are classified according to the position of the melanocytes in the skin: *junctional,* nests of melanocytes lie at the epidermal-dermal junction; *intradermal,* in the dermis; and *compound,* at both the epidermal-dermal junction and in the dermis. There are also two special and somewhat controversial variants of nevi that bear special recognition of their role as precursors to melanoma: congenital nevi and dysplastic nevi. Identification and appropriate management of such precursors could significantly reduce the incidence and mortality from melanoma. The reported incidence of melanoma is 6 to 10 cases per 100,000 persons per year. Early detection is the key to increased chances of survival following surgical resection.

Dysplastic Nevus

Dysplastic nevi, distinctive lesions both clinically and histologically, are both markers and precursors for familial melanoma. Morphologically, dysplastic nevi have both macular and papular components and have borders that usually are irregular and frequently are ill-defined (Table 1). Many features resemble those of melanoma. Histopathologic features include (1) basilar melanocytic hyperplasia with elongation of rete ridges, (2) cytologic atypia with enlarged hyperchromatic nuclei, (3) melanocytes, spindle-shaped and arranged horizontally, or epithelioid, aggregating in nests of variable size and fusing with adjacent rete ridges to produce bridging, (4) lamellar or concentric dermal fibroplasia, and (5) patchy dermal infiltrate of lymphocytes.

Dysplastic nevi, which can be found in 2 to 8 per cent of the population, have been associated with a 10 per cent risk of developing malignant melanoma. The lifetime risk for developing melanoma in the general population is 1 per cent. The dysplastic nevus syndrome (the presence of dysplastic nevi in two or more family members, and a family history of melanoma) can be associated with a 100 per cent lifetime risk of melanoma and may have an autosomal dominant transmission.

Patients having dysplastic nevi are a heterogeneous group composed of those with a family history of melanoma, without a family history of melanoma, and with or without a family history of dysplastic nevi. The relative risk of developing melanoma varies with these other factors and so does the management of the individual. Patients having dysplastic nevi but no family history of melanoma or dysplastic nevi require less frequent examination of the entire skin than those with a family history of familial melanoma or dysplastic nevi. The diagnosis should be confirmed by excisional biopsy and accurate recording of the lesions by photography, with a numbering system and measurement of the lesions. Those with dysplastic nevi and a family history of melanoma should be examined every 3 to 6 months by a physician. Any lesion that is suspected to be early melanoma should be excised. This decision will be influenced by variation in color, size of the lesion relative to the patient's other nevi, or progression based upon previous observation. Scalp lesions should be removed because they are

TABLE 1. **Differentiation Among Common Acquired Nevi, Dysplastic Nevi, and Malignant Melanoma**

	Common Acquired Nevus	Dysplastic Nevus	Malignant Melanoma
Size	Less than 5 mm	5–12 mm	Greater than 6 mm
Appearance	Initially macular, then papular	Both macular and papular components in each lesion (pebbled)	Macular and papular components
Borders	Sharp, even	Irregular, fades out	Notching indistinct
Color	Evenly pigmented tan, brown	Variegated tan to dark brown on a pink background	Hues of tan, brown, black, gray-blue, red, often with white areas of regression
Skin Markings	Present	Slightly altered	Absent
Location	Sun-exposed areas; scalp, breasts, buttocks rarely involved	Truncal, including sun-protected areas; may occur on scalp, breast, buttocks	Primarily sun-exposed sites
Number	20–40	100	—
Age	Appear in childhood, stop at age 30 years, involute at 40 years	Appear in adolescence, continued after age 35 years	

hard to locate and observe. An effort should be made to examine all first-degree relatives and educate them. It would be prudent for them to avoid excessive sun exposure and to use sun screens. Patients may perform self-examinations each month. Women with dysplastic nevus syndrome should avoid oral contraceptives. Pregnancy should be carefully considered, as it may precipitate changes that lead to the development of new melanomas. Pregnant women with dysplastic nevus syndrome should be carefully examined monthly by a physician. Suspicious lesions must undergo biopsy as they appear, which may mean removal of 2 to 3 nevi every month during the pregnancy.

Congenital Nevi

Melanoma may develop in congenital nevi, especially when the lesion is larger than 20 cm. Congenital nevi are found in less than 1 per cent of all neonates, but most are less than 1.5 cm in diameter. There is no accurate indication of the association between small lesions (less than 1.5 cm in diameter) and melanoma risk. The lifetime risk of melanoma in patients with large congenital nevi (greater than 20 cm) has been estimated to be 5 to 20 per cent. Patients with small lesions should be followed periodically for changes and the lesions measured and photographed. Patients and relatives should perform periodic examinations.

The larger lesions (greater than 20 cm) should be surgically excised before puberty. The management of such patients must be individualized to accommodate factors such as technical difficulty and cosmetic and functional consequences. A changing lesion should be handled by an excisional biopsy in toto whenever it is feasible. Biopsy under local anesthesia would remove a small nevus.

It is not certain whether dermabrasion of congenital nevi in the first few months of life can remove a sufficient number of nevus cells prior to their migration into the deep dermis to lower the risk of subsequent melanoma.

Indicators for Removal of Acquired Nevi

It must be emphasized that in young people nevi may appear rapidly, and a history of growth is not necessarily a danger signal. Some darkening of nevi can be expected during pregnancy. Any mole which changes in size, shape, or color, ulcerates or bleeds, itches or causes pain or demonstrates "run off" of pigment into adjacent skin at the border, or has variation in pigmentation should be removed for diagnostic purposes. The lesion should be excised in toto, extending into the adipose tissue and with a narrow margin (2 to 3 mm) of uninvolved skin. In this situation the clinical suspicion of a melanoma necessitates removal in a way that allows the best pathologic examination of the area of deepest penetration of the atypical cells. If the lesion is too large to remove totally, the most suspicious area should be selected for incisional biopsy and include subcutaneous tissue.

Nevi that are subject to chronic trauma should be removed to eliminate the inconvenience and discomfort that they cause. Patients often find raised, dome-shaped moles unsightly. When there is no suspicion of melanoma, these may be removed by a shave biopsy. When deciding whether to perform a fusiform excisional biopsy or a shave removal, it is better to choose the excisional method in a number of benign processes than to run the risk of doing a shave biopsy in a melanoma, which prohibits the ability to level that lesion. The level of the melanoma determines the proper surgical approach. When the risk of melanoma is small and the area is cosmetically difficult to achieve a good result in (tip of nose), the shave procedure can obtain a nice cosmetic result and sufficient material for histologic evaluation.

PREMALIGNANT LESIONS

method of
GEORGE A. FARBER, M.D.
Tulane University
New Orleans, Louisiana

For small lesions, excisional biopsy is the preferred method of both evaluation and therapy. For larger lesions, single or multiple punch biopsies serve well to delineate the nature and stage of the precancerous lesion. Dysplastic microscopic changes indicate definitive excision or destruction.

Problems in management occur when a patient presents with multiple premalignant lesions. In these instances, clinical evaluation for the purpose of selecting the more clinically advanced lesions for diagnostic biopsy may be helpful in planning the overall therapy.

The available forms of therapy for the precancerous lesions include scalpel surgery, electrodesiccation surgery, cryosurgery, chemical exfoliation or chemosurgery, laser surgery, and variations or combinations of these approaches. In all probability, within the foreseeable future, immunologic approaches to therapy of premalignant conditions will be developed to increase the armamentarium available to the practitioner.

Primary Lesions

Actinic Keratosis. This condition is the most common of the premalignant conditions. The actinic keratoses vary in appearance according to their stage, duration, and anatomical location. The lesions tend to occur on sun-exposed areas, although they may occur anywhere on the body, which is sometimes a paradox. The lesions may be single, few and scattered, or multiple and everywhere on the sun-exposed areas. Often, the anatomic location determines the method of treatment.

The most conservative treatment consists of topical 5-fluorouracil (5-FU) for 2 to 3 weeks followed by 2 to 3 weeks of a palliative medication, such as topical corticosteroid cream. For lesions of the face and scalp, particularly in balding individuals, 5-FU treatment is sufficient. On the extremities and upper torso, a 3 to 4 week course of 5-FU medication is usually required. Midway through therapy, the actinic lesions will become erythematous, even to the point of producing pain, tenderness, and considerable discomfort. It is important that the patient be adequately prepared in advance. Otherwise, serious complaints and loss of confidence develop, and compliance decreases as the redness and tenderness increase.

At the completion of the recommended schedule, a moderate to strong topical corticosteroid cream, such as triamcinolone or betamethasone valerate, is applied three times daily for 2 to 3 weeks, until satisfactory resolution occurs.

In purely premalignant lesions, 5-FU treatment is very rewarding and eliminates 85 to 95 per cent of the visible actinic lesions. However, malignant lesions or suspected deep malignant lesions should not be treated with this regimen. Whenever there is a question as to the depth or degree of metaplasia, biopsy or excision should be performed.

After treatment with 5-fluorouracil, recurrent lesions should be treated with excisional surgery and careful evaluation of the pathologic specimen.

This topical treatment may be repeated at intervals of 3 to 5 years, depending on the patient's response and compliance.

The surgical approaches to actinic keratoses include simple excision and repair, shave excision, and either electrodesiccation or light dermabrasion using refrigerant anesthesia. In some cases cryosurgery is quite useful. There is an advantage to surgical procedures that provide pathologic specimens.

With the shave excision technique, multiple procedures can be done at each visit. The best results are obtained on the face, forehead, and scalp; on the neck and trunk, shave excision tends to leave visible scars for considerable periods. The patient should be so advised preoperatively.

Malignancies develop in the basal areas of the epidermis, and the changes can spread peripherally throughout the epidermis, but when they penetrate the basement membrane, their significance alters considerably, and the dermal component is not premalignant. Hence the value of pathologic evaluation.

It is not uncommon to see almost the entire lower lip involved with actinic damage or keratoses; a more definitive procedure such as vermilionectomy may be indicated. The nose may be the site of multiple actinic keratoses. Multiple procedures, if the lesions are individually identified, may be accomplished, using any of the modalities indicated. If the actinic lesions are a continuum, special treatment may be indicated, such as dermabrasion or chemo-exfoliation (chemical peel).

When actinic lesions involve most of the face and forehead, two special surgical procedures are effective: the full face dermabrasion, and the full face phenolic chemical peel or exfoliation. Both procedures are more definitive and much more effective than topical 5-fluorouracil. Most patients, regardless of age, appear to tolerate the procedures well. In addition to removal of the premalignant lesions, there is marked rejuvenation of the skin, resulting in excellent cosmetic improvement.

Another approach, if the patient can tolerate the procedure and is properly instructed, is multiple sessions of cryosurgery using liquid nitrogen. The healing time and the residual scars may be less preferential than with other procedures.

In all cases, supportive instruction of the patient, avoidance of additional sun exposure, and adequate use of emollients to maintain the hydration of the skin are important.

Leukoplakia. This term means "white plaques" and generally refers to such plaques in the vermilion areas of the lip and mucocutaneous areas of the oral, anal, and genital regions. Not all leukoplakia is premalignant.

When leukoplakia occurs in a sun-exposed area, it is more likely to be premalignant and multiple selected biopsies are in order. When the biopsy site is to be sutured, silk suture is preferred to the monofilament material for postoperative comfort.

When lesions occur within the oral cavity but have a reddish hue, they may be known as erythroleukoplakia. They have a much higher rate of degeneration to malignancy. Such lesions should be excised in toto.

Once a definitive diagnosis is established and the pathologic changes are considered premalignant, for a lesion on the lower lip and occasionally on the upper lip, a vermilionectomy is the simplest and best procedure, if most of the lip is involved. If the disease is localized, a wedge resection is preferred.

Leukoplakia on the genital or anal area requires special consideration. It is absolutely imperative to rule out malignant degeneration before any surgical or medical treatment is initiated. Multiple selected biopsy sites may be utilized to establish the diagnosis.

When leukoplakia occurs on the vulva or perianal area, there is no satisfactory and reliable medical treatment. Therefore, planned excisional therapy, if location and size of the lesions are amenable, is the preferred method. Consideration of anatomic function and structure is part of the surgical planning. Often, the leukoplakic areas are small in relation to overall pathologic areas, and hence specific excisions may be accomplished. When surgery is not to be considered, nonsteroidal topical medications, particularly emollients, may be useful.

Lentigo Maligna. Lentigo maligna, sometimes referred to as the melanotic freckle of Hutchinson, is most probably a form of actinic keratosis. The freckles tend to occur on sun-exposed areas, primarily on the face and most often on the malar or lateral cheek areas. They begin as small brownish macules (flat) and, in time, usually years, enlarge peripherally and may obtain silver dollar size or larger.

The significance of these lesions is primarily in regard to malignant degeneration. There is obviously a pigmentary alteration, and one of the potential malignant degeneration forms is that of malignant melanoma. When such lesions develop basement membrane level lateral extension, they are considered superficial. Once the dysplastic or malignant changes penetrate the basement membrane, they should be considered melanomas and treated as such.

Focal areas of increased pigmentation, papule or nodule development, or variegate color changes should be sampled for biopsy to determine whether they are malignant or premalignant.

In the premalignant state, treatment is similar to that of actinic keratosis. In view of the pathologic changes, surface excision by shave technique, electrodestruction, dermabrasion, phenol peel, or strong (50 per cent) trichloracetic acid is simple, rapid and effective. Small lesions respond well to superficial cryosurgery. Treatment techniques that provide a pathologic specimen are preferred.

Bowen's Disease. This condition is actually a malignancy in situ. The lesions are quite similar to actinic keratosis in appearance. In general, if the lesions occur on nonsun-exposed areas, they may be a sign of internal malignancy. Hence, such patients deserve a clinical workup for occult malignancy, most particularly of the GI tract and pulmonary system. If the lesions occur on a sun-exposed area, they are statistically less likely to be a sign of internal malignancy. Nevertheless, reports over the years have raised significant questions as to whether or not Bowen's disease is a precursor or indicator of internal malignancy.

Essentially all Bowen's disease lesions are slow-growing and small. The average size at presentation for clinical evaluation is about 0.5 inch in diameter. They tend to be annular or circular, flat, slightly scaly, and slightly pinkish or erythematous. The extremities are the most common site.

The preferred method of treatment is complete excision. If there is a question in diagnosis, a punch biopsy in the center of the lesion should suffice. Since most lesions are less than 1 inch in diameter, simple excision and closure are usually adequate and definitive.

After specific diagnosis, cryosurgery may be effective. Mohs' chemosurgery is an optional though unnecessary approach. The effectiveness of 5-fluorouracil therapy is indefinite although its use has been reported.

Erythroplasia of Queyrat. This is a unique disease occurring on the glans penis or foreskin. It is equivalent to Bowen's disease occurring elsewhere. Because of the glabrous type of skin, with the epidermis and dermis much thinner than that of the extremities, the possibility of development into squamous cell carcinoma, with the threat of metastasis, is more likely.

Diagnosis is the key to treatment. A punch biopsy is invaluable before definitive surgery. When the lesion is clinically definable, surgical excision with adequate margins is an effective cure. On uncircumcised males, circumcision is advised.

For extensive lesions of erythroplasia of Queyrat, particularly when considerable foreskin is involved on an uncircumcised male, Mohs' chemosurgery may be the treatment of choice.

Keratoacanthoma. The natural history of keratoacanthoma is rapid development of a craterform lesion with a central keratin plug. There is a tendency for these lesions to resolve spontaneously, over a period varying from 6 months to many years. The significance of these lesions, despite their rapid onset, is their histologic similarity to squamous cell carcinoma.

A punch biopsy of keratoacanthoma lesions may be very misleading. The microscopic appearance of portions of lesions may so resemble squamous cell carcinoma that the pathologist cannot make a definitive diagnosis under the light microscope. Therefore, unless the lesion is excessively large, complete excision is the preferred method of treatment.

There have been many reports of wide excision and consequential disfigurement or deformity when such lesions are clinically misdiagnosed preoperatively. A wedge biopsy on selected lesions may be a preferred method of diagnosis prior to complete excision. The wedge biopsy should contain a portion of the center and should extend peripherally to apparently normal skin.

In cases of multiple keratoacanthomas, selected lesions may be excised, and after several lesions have been evaluated to rule out squamous cell carcinoma, those remaining may be treated through several options. These include cryosurgery, intralesional 5-fluorouracil at full strength, intralesional corticosteroids (triamcinolone), and electrodestruction and curettage.

Multiple keratoacanthomas of the eruptive type, which can number in the dozens or more, may be candidates for systemic therapy with methotrexate or other antineoplastic agents such as bleomycin. Intralesional injection of bleomycin may be another approach. There is reported use of oral methotrexate in combination with topical bleomycin (Blenoxane).

Arsenical Keratoses. Arsenical keratoses are raised keratotic lesions that tend to involve epidermis and the outer keratin layers and may occur on the palms, soles, or anywhere on the body cutaneum. There is no distinct microscopic feature.

Usually the source of arsenic is unknown to the patient. It may have been ingested or inhaled. In certain types of mining and smelting, particularly of copper, gold, and bauxite, the smeltery will perfuse the air with arsenic fumes for several miles around. For years, arsenic was contained in pesticides and other farm products, and over many years, well water became contaminated with detectable levels of arsenic. Persons using such water were subject to development of arsenical keratoses. Tobacco products may contain detectable levels of arsenic. Certain famous brand name cigars and pipe tobaccos have been measured by reliable laboratories and found to contain from 15 to 29 ppm of arsenic.

Palmar and plantar arsenical keratoses rarely develop into malignancy but lesions on other areas of the skin or mucous membrane margins are likely to become malignant. Hence, treatment for arsenical keratoses should be equivalent to that for actinic keratosis except when they occur on the palmar and plantar surfaces.

Palmar and plantar arsenical keratoses can be treated by simple curettage, electrosurgery, cryotherapy, or use of keratolytic topical agents.

Tar Keratoses. This unusual condition is seen in persons with a long history of exposure to coal, pitch, tar, or their byproducts. Treatment may be simple, using electrodestruction, cryosurgery, or shave excision and light dermabrasion. Preventive measures include avoidance of the exposure to tar, pitch, soot, crude paraffin, asphalt, and related byproducts. Sun screens are helpful to decrease photoactivation of tar products. Occupational changes may be most practical.

Paget's Disease. Lesions are irregularly shaped, have scaling and erythema, and are typically found around the nipple or areola. Typical locations for extramammary Paget's disease include the genital, axillary, and perianal areas. This condition is a form of carcinoma in situ. It may relate to an underlying ductal or apocrine carcinoma when it occurs on the mammary area. The cutaneous aspect may only be a small focus of the entire process. Therefore, aggressive diagnosis and surgical intervention are advisable.

Cutaneous Horn. These lesions may be small or very large and may be fast- or slow-growing. There is often squamous cell carcinoma at the base. Therefore, treatment consists of excision, including a reasonable margin of apparently normal tissue at the base. Surgical methods that do not provide a surgical specimen for pathologic evaluation are not recommended. Large lesions may be sampled at several points along the base before definitive surgery is planned. Small lesions are best treated by total excision.

Giant Condyloma Acuminatum of Buschke-Lowenstein. The initial lesions resemble condylomata but have a tendency to progress to carcinoma. Multiple specimens may be required for histologic examination before true carcinoma can be diagnosed. When diagnosis is in doubt, surgical excision is the wisest choice of therapy. Fortunately, this condition is rare.

Oral Florid Papillomatosis. These lesions resemble leukoplakia of the oral mucosa and are usually found on the lower lips. The tendency to malignant degeneration is much less than that of actinic keratoses. Therefore, after biopsy to establish diagnosis, conservative treatment such as special topical or intralesional steroids may merit a trial. Vermilionectomy may be definitive. Pipe smoking, chewing tobacco, and snuff are possible causative agents.

Epithelioma Cuniculatum. This unusual condition involves the inner digital and plantar surfaces. Lesions may be quite large and hence difficult to cure because the most satisfactory treatment is complete surgical excision. Other acceptable modes of therapy for small lesions detected early include electrodestruction using curettage and electrodesiccation, cryotherapy, and radiation therapy.

Secondary Lesions

Congenital Nevocellular Nevus. There are two types of pigmented lesions, the giant hairy pigmented nevus (bathing trunk nevus) and the smaller, nonhairy congenital pigmented nevus. The latter may be single or multiple and tends to develop during the first 2 decades of life. The giant hairy pigmented nevus may be small or huge. The huge lesions, in themselves, are not amenable to simple therapy. There are reports of malignant melanomas developing in 2 to 15 per cent of the lesions. In large lesions there is some merit for dermabrasion at early age and, in amenable lesions, for excision and full-thickness skin grafting. In any giant hairy pigmented nevus, unusually heavily pigmented areas, or thicker areas within the lesion should be sampled for pathologic evaluation.

The more common and smaller pigmented nonhairy congenital nevi are usually quite amenable to excisional therapy. The incidence of malignant degeneration varies from 2 to 25 or 30 per cent but is most likely closer to 3 per cent. At least one suspected congenital nevus should be excised and evaluated histopathologically. If more than one lesion shows dysplastic changes, methodical excision of all visible lesions should be planned. Malignant degeneration is more likely to occur once dysplasia has been detected. For the congenital nevocellular pigmented nevus, such procedures as dermabrasion, cryosurgery, chemical exfoliation, and electrodestruction are not recommended.

In regard to the giant bathing suit black hairy nevus in otherwise healthy infants, there is considerable merit in accomplishing dermabrasion procedures early. Such procedures usually will remove most of the pigment cells through the depths of the papillary dermis before the natural phenomenon of abtropfung, or dropping down of cells to the mid and lower dermis, occurs. Whether this is a definitive procedure to prevent malignant degeneration is questionable. However, there is some probability that degeneration will occur and great probability that the cosmetic and psychologic effects offer the patient considerable benefit.

Organoid Nevus (Nevus Sebaceus of Jadassohn). These lesions tend to develop later in life in the hairy scalp areas. Malignant degeneration is generally slow and usually appears in adulthood. Surgical removal should occur early, particularly when lesions are smaller.

Small lesions are usually amenable to simple excisional surgery. In larger lesions, relaxing galeotomies and considerable undermining may be required to effect primary closure or advancement or pedicle full-thickness grafting.

The pathologic nature of these lesions implies involvement of the appendages to mid and deep dermis; hence, superficial curettage and electrodestruction, cryosurgery, and chemo-exfoliation (peel) are not indicated. Mohs' chemosurgery may be the preferred treatment once a malignant lesion has been detected.

Chronic Conditions. These may predispose to malignant degeneration, though usually long-term. Suspicious change in any lesion should undergo biopsy and the appropriate definitive surgery chosen, depending on the size and site. These conditions include but are not limited to radiodermatitis, thermal and chemical burns, lupus erythematosus, long-standing cutaneous ulcers particularly of the feet and ankles, chronic irritation from ill-fitting appliances or dentures or exogenous means such as pipe-smoking, chronic cheilitis, lichen sclerosus et atrophicus, lichen planus, and lupus vulgaris. The presenting signs and symptoms of malignant development may be obscure, and it is incumbent upon the patient and the physician to recognize and evaluate any changes appearing in such areas.

Hereditary Conditions

The genodermatoses in this category (xeroderma pigmentosum, basal cell nevus syndrome, dysplastic nevus syndrome with B-K mole, neurofibromatosis, pachyonychia congenita, dyskeratosis congenita, and epidermodysplasia verruciformis) have a known tendency to malignant degeneration. We do not have as yet the means to prevent the malignant degeneration, so careful monitoring is necessary for early detection and surgical intervention. Those conditions activated by ultraviolet light require supportive care and avoidance of ultraviolet light exposure.

The basal cell nevus syndrome can manifest as several lesions or a multitude. Once a patient has allowed the lesions to go untreated for years and has developed myriads of lesions, treatment is limited. However, if the condition is detected early, regular "maintenance therapy" with semiannual excision of lesions as they manifest, makes it possible to "keep up" with malignant degenerations. The same principle applies to dysplastic nevus syndrome, wherein visible lesions are excised as early as possible in the hope that specific malignant degeneration will be preempted by prompt surgical intervention.

Sarcomatous degeneration of neurofibromas is unusual. However, rapid growth, pigmentary changes, and ulceration, even of the small lesions, may be a sign of malignant degeneration. The only hope is early and adequate excision. Unfortunately, neurofibromatosis can develop in areas where it is not detectable clinically until considerable malignant changes have occurred.

Miscellaneous Conditions

Parapsoriasis. The en plaques type of parapsoriasis tends to develop quite similarly to psoriasis and has a tendency to develop in irregular asymmetric patterns, with bizarre shapes and forms of dry scaly patches on the skin, principally the trunk. The typical end stage of this somewhat unusual condition is mycosis fungoides.

Treatment is nonsurgical, other than biopsy for diagnosis. Included in the forms of therapy are topical corticosteroids, ultraviolet light therapy, anticancer drugs such as methotrexate, systemic corticosteroids, and careful monitoring during the premalignant stage. Once the disease is established as malignant, there is no specific cure.

Cowden's Disease. This rare and unusual complex cutaneous disorder is characterized by multiple hamartomas and by co-existence of multiple ectodermal, mesodermal, and endodermal neoplasias that tend to develop after the third decade. Abnormalities may occur in any or all of the internal organs or glands, most notably the breast. Fibrocystic disease may be an early manifestation, followed by carcinoma. Neural tumors are known to develop and result in mental and neurologic changes. The disease is named after its originally presenting patient. Multiple diagnostic regimens are required, with surgical therapy directed toward individual lesions and organ systems. There is no known medical therapy for this rare, unusual, and slowly devastating disease.

Bowenoid Papulosis. This relatively new condition occurs on the cutaneum and mucous membrane tissues of the anogenital area. Lesions are small and usually multiple and generally involve the shaft and glans of the penis but may also involve the foreskin. Although the etiology is not specifically defined, bowenoid papulosis is believed to be caused by the human papillomavirus, perhaps Type 16. Although the micropathology is fairly distinctive, there is sufficient similarity to condyloma acuminatum to consider bowenoid papulosis a variant. There has been recent concern in the literature that this disorder is a precursor to invasive carcinoma.

Bowenoid papulosis usually is not responsive to podophyllin therapy but is amenable to electrodestruction, which is the preferred method of treatment. In cases in which large clusters of such lesions exist on the foreskin, it may be amenable to circumcision as a form of surgical removal.

Cryosurgery is not recommended, because it is usually unacceptable to the patient and its definitive therapeutic effectiveness may be questionable in such instances. Notwithstanding, it is a potential alternative treatment to electrodestruction.

Condyloma Acuminatum. These lesions are believed due to the human papillomavirus, probably Type 16, and may be precancerous. See discussion in Verruca Vulgaris earlier in this section.

Calcifying Epithelioma of Malherbe. This rare condition is usually not diagnosed preoperatively. The lesions may develop in late childhood through late adulthood and manifest as an apparent epidermal inclusion cyst, often on the scalp. Lesions have been seen on legs, scalp, trunk, and upper extremities. Simple excision is usually adequate. The true nature of this disorder remains unknown.

Dermatofibroma. This lesion occurs in male and female adults, although it may appear in the second decade. Etiology is unknown. The lesion manifests as a firm nodule attached to the skin and often has either an external scaly appearance or a flat, shiny appearance, depending on anatomic location. There is a very low potential for malignant degeneration. However, it is an open question whether or not these lesions degenerate into a form of sarcoma, known as dermatofibrosarcoma protuberans, or develop superficial basal cell epitheliomas above and around them or coincidentally in association with basal cell epithelioma. The lesion itself may be a form of sclerosing hemangioma. In any case, it is abnormal and amenable to simple excision. Simple excision is the treatment of choice.

Seborrheic Keratosis. These lesions are also known as senile warts or barnacles and present as unsightly waxy or pigmented scaly lesions on the surface of the skin. They tend to be superficial with a minor potential for malignant degeneration. Basal cell epitheliomas and occasionally squamous cell carcinomas develop in or around the base, either coincidentally or as a form of malignant degeneration per se. Some forms of seborrheic keratoses tend to develop fine strands of basophilic cells, which migrate into the papillary and mid dermis. These may be labeled fibroepitheliomas and may have a tendency to develop into basal cell epitheliomas. Most lesions are extremely superficial and can be simply shaved off the surface of the skin, with fine electrocautery or superficial dermabrasion to complete the therapy. Whenever the lesion is inflamed, irritated, or otherwise abnormal clinically, it should be excised, and the entire specimen submitted for microscopic evaluation. Some lesions may be confused with basal cell epitheliomas or keratotic squamous cell carcinomas.

BACTERIAL DISEASES OF THE SKIN

method of
LAURA LAYDEN, M.D.,
and SAMUEL E. WILSON, M.D.
Harbor–UCLA Medical Center
Torrance, California

The skin has the largest surface area, approximately 2 M^2, of any organ of the body. The normal flora are constituted predominantly of Micrococcaceae (including *Staphylococcus*), *Corynebacterium acnes*, and aerobic diphtheroids, which act as a defense against bacterial infection by providing a mechanical barrier and producing free fatty acids from skin lipids. The common bacterial inflammations occur when a break in the skin becomes infected by *Staphylococcus aureus* and streptococci (primarily group A beta-hemolytic streptococci). Streptococcal infections have a spreading erythematous character with necrosis, lymphadenopathy, and lymphangitis and often involve the lower extremities. Staphylococcal infections are characterized by bullae or pustules of the hair follicles or exocrine sweat glands, often on the face. The severity of these infections can range from benign cutaneous lesions or lesions reflecting systemic disease to rapidly progressing destructive infections as seen with necrotizing cellulitis.

Hidradenitis Suppurativa

A disease of the apocrine sweat glands first described by Velpeau in 1839, hidradenitis suppurativa is a chronic infection characterized by painful abscesses, fistulas, and scarring. It is typically found in the axilla, groin, perineum, and perirectal area but occasionally involves the antecubital fossa, popliteal fossa, and periumbilical area. These apocrine sweat glands consist of a straight excretory duct that empties into the hair follicle, as well as a coiled secretory duct. Hidradenitis suppurativa probably begins with ductal obstruction caused by inspissation of keratinous secretions in the gland, progressing to rupture of the gland into the dermis. This sets up a cascade of bacterial infection, draining sinuses, fibrosis, and scarring. Predisposing factors are thought to include poor hygiene, tight-fitting clothing, diabetes, and acne. In the acute setting, incision and drainage is appropriate therapy. Bacterial cultures show various organisms but commonly include *Proteus* species, *Staphylococcus epidermidis,* and *Staphylococcus aureus.* Doxycycline, 200 mg by mouth initially then 100 mg twice a day, may be used in the acute setting. In the chronic setting, tetracycline, 250 to 500 mg, is given by mouth four times a day for 10 days, followed by a dose of 500 mg daily for an additional 2 weeks.

When local incision and drainage, heat, and antibiotics fail to control chronic hidradenitis, definitive treatment consists of excision of all the apocrine glands, along with the overlying skin. Various methods besides wide local excision have been employed, including application of isotretinoin (Accutane), topical antibiotic lotions (clindamycin), and radiation, all of which are inferior to complete removal of the disease. After complete excision of the area the defect can be managed by primary closure, delayed healing by secondary intention, split thickness skin graft initially or later, Silastic foam dressings, or rotation flaps. Each case should be individualized according to the site of the defect as well as patient compliance. Axillary defects are unsuitable for immediate grafting because of vascularity and heavy bacterial contamination of the subcutaneous fat. Although immobilization of the arm along with a painful donor site is a disadvantage of split thickness skin grafts to the axilla, centers have reported good outcomes with the procedure. Silastic foam dressings allowing open granulation have been employed in Wales with success but have the disadvantage of a longer healing time. The disease may recur even after wide excision.

Erysipelas and Cellulitis

Erysipelas and cellulitis are both examples of a true pyodermatitis, secondary to a break in the skin. Erysipelas is a superficial dermal infection and cellulitis involves the deep dermal layer. Both these infections are caused by group A beta-hemolytic streptococcus. *Erysipelas,* also known as St. Anthony's fire, is an acute but rare and benign condition since the advent of antibiotics. It is characterized by a tender, erythematous area with sharp margins, bullae, and vesicle formation. Just as in cellulitis, there may be fever and regional adenopathy. The face is the most frequently involved site in erysipelas but the lower limbs are more commonly involved when tinea pedis and diabetes mellitus are present.

Cellulitis, in contrast, has less distinct margins and is serpiginous, tender, and erythematous, occurring most frequently on the lower extremities. Predisposing factors are tinea pedis, contact dermatitis, stasis dermatitis, and skin ulcers. Fever, malaise, adenopathy, and lymphangitis may be present. Central necrosis and suppuration may occur at a later stage. Streptococcal cellulitis may progress to a necrotizing infection that is difficult to distinguish from erysipelas because bleb formation is seen after proteolytic enzymes are released. Streptococcal cellulitis spreads rapidly, with intense pain, erythema, and purplish skin color changes as well as the bleb formation. Fevers up to 102 F, tachycardia, and generalized toxemia may also be present. Intense swelling can lead to operative intervention; incision and drainage may be necessary to decompress nerves or relieve muscle ischemia.

Bed rest with hospitalization may be required for the diabetic, immunocompromised, or toxic patient, as well as the noncompliant patient. The affected extremity should be elevated to promote lymphatic outflow, and warm, moist compresses applied. Wound cultures can seldom be obtained. Appropriate antibiotic coverage in the hospitalized patient is penicillin G, 2 million units intravenously every 4 hours, and oxacillin, 1 gram every 6 hours. For the less severely ill patient use oral penicillin VK, 250 to 500 mg every 6 hours or, for penicillin-allergic patients, erythromycin, 250 mg per mouth every 6 hours. These dosages should be continued for 5 to 10 days, depending on clinical response. Failure of the inflammation to subside after 48 to 72 hours of antibiotic therapy suggests that an abscess has developed, and incision and drainage are indicated.

Streptococcal gangrene, progressive bacterial synergistic gangrene, or Meleney's ulcer are all names given to an infection described by Meleney that can occur at postoperative wound sites, including abdominal wounds. It appears a few days to a few weeks postoperatively as an erythematous, tender area juxtaposed to the wound. The area progresses to a gangrenous wound with purple margins, bullae, and spreading boundaries.

Organisms responsible for this entity include *Peptostreptococcus,* usually isolated from the gangrenous margins, and *Staphylococcus aureus* or Enterobacteriaceae, which are cultured from the central portion. Treatment includes debridement of gangrenous skin as well as drainage of surrounding tissues. Penicillin, 2 million units every 4 hours, and an aminoglycoside (e.g., gentamicin 1.5 mg per kg every 8 hours) should be employed regardless of whether operative intervention is required.

Fornier's gangrene is a necrotizing cellulitis and fasciitis of the genitals, scrotum, perineum, penis, or abdominal wall. It occurs as a sequela of local trauma, perirectal or perianal infection, paraphimosis, and operations involving these areas. Gram stain shows gram-positive and gram-negative organisms and can be used to differentiate Fornier's gangrene from streptococcal, clostridial, or phycomycotic infections. The commonly cultured organisms are Enterobacteriaceae, enterococci, anaerobic streptococci, and *Bacteroides.*

Treatment includes radical debridement of devitalized structures, with wounds kept open by packing for drainage. Antibiotic therapy should be directed at aerobic and anaerobic organisms; blood cultures are often positive with this infection. Ampicillin, 1 gram every 6 hours, clindamycin (Cleocin), 900 mg every 8 hours, and gentamicin, 1.5 mg per kg every 8 hours, are the first choice unless blood cultures mandate otherwise. The natural proclivity of this disease is toward a high morbidity and mortality rate. Patients with an underlying disease, such as renal failure or diabetes mellitus, have the highest risk.

Impetigo

Impetigo can be defined as bullous or nonbullous. Bullous impetigo will be discussed in the next section. Nonbullus impetigo is caused by the beta-hemolytic streptococcus, although staphylococcus is frequently isolated on culture. It is highly contagious in infants but less so among children and adults. The hallmark lesion of impetigo is a honey-colored crust which occurs after the erythematous macule becomes a vescicle. Lymphadenopathy and fever may accompany the disease.

Treatment consists of thorough cleansing of the area with antibacterial soap and removal of the crust. Warm compresses and washings with topical Neosporin cream three times a day are advantageous. If impetigo is severe, associated with fever, malaise, or lymphadenopathy, or located on the face, intravenous penicillin for 5 to 7 days is recommended. Intravenous penicillin, 50,000 to 250,000 units per kg per day in children over 3 months of age and 2 million units every 4 hours in adults for 5 to 7 days, is recommended. Although intravenous antibiotics may decrease the contagiousness of the disease, it remains contagious until all lesions are healed. For less severe infections, penicillin, 25,000 to 50,000 units per kg per day, should be given to children and 250 to 500 mg every 6 hours by mouth to adults. Penicillin-allergic patients can be treated with erythromycin, 500 mg orally every 6 hours. Complications include glomerulonephritis, which may follow a persistent course of impetigo when the major pathogens are the nephrogenic strains of streptococci.

Staphylococcal Scalded Skin Syndrome and Bullous Impetigo

Staphylococcal scalded skin syndrome affects neonates and young children and is produced by certain strains of *Staphylococcus aureus,* particularly bacteriophage group 2, which produces an epidermolytic exotoxin. This exotoxin causes loss of the stratum corneum and stratum granulosum, but the lower epidermis is preserved. The disease originates from a focus of infection and is a fairly common cause of exfoliative dermatitis in neonates and young children. Clinically, the findings are tender skin areas with erythema and a positive Nikolsky's sign (slippage of the superficial layer of the epithelium on gentle pressure) on both involved and uninvolved skin. Fever may be present. The skin lesions commonly affect the neck, groin, and axilla, but spare the palms, soles, and mucous membranes. Bullae form and rapidly rupture. Healing occurs promptly, usually after 2 to 5 days, with a very low mortality rate. Scalded skin syndrome can be treated with local care and antibiotics. A beta-lactamase–resistant antibiotic such as oxacillin (Prostaphlin), 1 gram intravenously every 6 hours, or nafcillin (Nafcil), 500 mg intravenously every 4 hours, should be used. In penicillin-allergic patients, vancomycin (Vancocin), 500 mg every 6 hours, a first generation cephalosporin, or clindamycin (Cleocin), 900 mg every 8 hours (possibly in conjunction with an aminoglycoside), are indicated. Less severe infections can be treated with dicloxacillin (Dynapen), 250 mg, cephalexin (Keflex), 250 mg, or erythromycin (E-Mycin), 500 mg. All are taken every 6 hours. *Staphylococcus* does not grow from cultures of blister fluid.

Prevention can be accomplished by careful attention to the skin and minor wounds, incision and drainage when necessary, and antibiotics by mouth (dicloxacillin or erythromycin in doses listed previously). Dicloxacillin will produce blood levels nearly comparable to those resulting from intravenous antibiotics.

Bullous impetigo is a more localized form of disease caused by the same exotoxin. Again bullae are formed by the exfoliate toxin, producing an epidermal separation. After the bulla ruptures, the underlying skin is found to be red, resembling a second degree burn. Subsequently a brown crust forms. Bullous impetigo is commonly seen in infants and young children; due to the contagiousness of the disease, isolation is imperative. Cultures from these bullae do grow *Staphylococcus aureus*. Antibiotic therapy is the same as for staphylococcal scalded skin syndrome.

Toxic Epidermal Necrolysis

Toxic epidermal necrolysis, or Lyell's disease, is a reaction secondary to drugs such as sulfonamides, barbiturates, and hydantoins. It is exceedingly important to differentiate this severe manifestation of erythematous tissue from scalded skin syndrome; toxic epidermal necrolysis usually affects adults, involves mucous membranes, and is characterized by large, flaccid blisters on an erythematous base. These lesions may be found anywhere on the body. A positive Nikolsky sign occurs over skin bordering on the blisters. Toxic epidermal necrolysis, in contrast to scalded skin syndrome, includes necrosis of the entire epidermis, including the basal layer, with dermal-epidermal separation. Treatment is aimed at correcting dehydration from fluid loss. High dose systemic corticosteroids are recommended. There is a 25 to 50 per cent mortality rate even with appropriate and aggressive treatment.

Differentiation between toxic epidermal necrolysis and toxic shock syndrome is also important as both can present a diffuse erythema. Early clinical manifestations in toxic shock syndrome include fever greater than 102 F and erythema but no vesicular lesions, as seen with toxic epidermal necrolysis. Skin biopsies can help distinguish between the two, with frozen section or hematoxylin and eosin stains showing interface dermatitis in toxic epidermal necrolysis, compared with a superficial perivascular dermatitis in toxic shock syndrome.

Folliculitis, Furuncles, and Carbuncles

Superficial folliculitis, or Boeckhart's impetigo, is a perifollicular form of impetigo. Found on the scalp and extremities, superficial folliculitis is characterized by a pustule pierced by hair, surrounded by erythema. These pustules result from plugging of the hair follicles with grease or epithelial debris, complicated by proliferation of resident staphylococci, which can be confirmed by Gram stain and cultures. Contributing factors include chronic friction, poor personal hygiene, plastic occlusive dressings, and tar-containing medications applied to hairy skin.

Treatment includes an antibacterial soap such as hexachlorophene (Phisohex) and a topical antibiotic such as Neosporin. Intravenous oxacillin, 1 gram every 6 hours, or a cephalosporin active against penicillinase-resistant *Staphylococcus* is needed for widespread and chronic folliculitis. Penicillin-allergic patients can be treated with clindamycin (Cleocin), 900 mg every 8 hours, or erythromycin (Erythrocin), 15 to 20 mg per kg per day. Prophylaxis includes improved personal hygiene, avoidance of above-mentioned risk factors, and a regular use of hexachlorophene or chlorhexidine gluconate soap.

Furuncles are the deep variety of folliculitis almost exclusively caused by *Staphylococcus aureus,* presenting as perifollicular erythema with surrounding edema. Furuncles are usually found on the face, neck, buttocks, thigh, perineum, breast, and axilla. After several days, the lesions become fluctuant with a beige head and can rupture spontaneously.

Carbuncles are multiloculated abscesses resulting from two or more infected hair follicles. These occur more often in the thick-skinned areas, such as the nuchal area, and are less likely to drain spontaneously and therefore spread subcutaneously.

Treatment for both furunculosis and carbunculosis includes warm compresses three or more times a day. In lesions that do not spontaneously drain, incision and drainage are necessary, using topical ethyl chloride spray. Complications include bacteremia, and rarely osteomyelitis and cavernous sinus thrombosis. Antibiotic coverage may prevent seeding of adjacent follicles and is indicated for individual lesions in important areas or for recurrent or extensive disease. Dicloxacillin, 250 mg orally every 6 hours, cefaclor (Ceclor), 250 mg every 8 hours, and cephalexin (Keflex), 250 mg every 6 hours, are all useful; penicillin-allergic patients can be treated with erythromycin (E-Mycin), 500 mg every 6 hours. Parenteral antibiotics are used for patients with evidence of systemic toxicity, and in these instances, nafcillin (Nafcil), 500 mg every 4 hours, oxacillin (Prostaphlin), 1 gram every 6 hours, cefazolin (Kefzol), 1 gram every 6 hours, kanamycin (Kantrex), 15 mg per kg per day (given in two doses per day and not to exceed 1.5 grams per day), or gentamicin (Garamycin), 1.5 mg per kg every 8 hours, is recommended. Recurrent disease is usually attributable to penicillin-resistant *Staphylococcus,* found in the nares or perineum. Regular use of topical Neosporin cream in these areas will help reduce the staphylococcal population and prevent recurrence in susceptible patients.

HERPES SIMPLEX AND HERPES ZOSTER

method of
RICHARD D. ANDERSEN, M.D.,
and WARREN W. PIETTE, M.D.
University of Iowa
Iowa City, Iowa

HERPES SIMPLEX

The Virus

Herpes simplex virus (HSV) is a member of the herpesvirus family, which also includes varicella-zoster virus, cytomegalovirus, and Epstein-Barr virus. HSV infections occur throughout the world and throughout the year. From 60 to 100 per cent of the human race, depending on geography and age, demonstrate antibodies to type 1 HSV in their blood. A considerably smaller segment of the human population, perhaps 10 to 20 per cent, demonstrate serologic evidence of encounters with type 2 HSV. Because of the association of type 2 HSV with genital infection, the latter figures are more heavily influenced not only by age but also by sexual activity. Most but not all oral HSV infections are caused by type 1 HSV. Similarly, most but not all genital HSV infections are caused by type 2 HSV.

The interaction of HSV with the human immune system is notably complex. Most importantly, the virus is capable of reactivation on numerous occasions following primary infection. Reactivation occurs despite the presence of circulating antibodies against HSV and is made possible by the ability of the virus to persist in a latent state in certain sensory ganglia near the site of reactivation. Whereas many individuals experience frequent oral or genital lesions caused by HSV, an equally large proportion of the population demonstrates no clinical symptoms with latent HSV in neural ganglia or with colonization of the oropharynx and female genital tract.

Clinical Manifestations. Herpetic gingivostomatitis typically appears as ulcerative, painful lesions of both gums and the oral mucous membranes. It is thought to represent a primary encounter with the virus and is more commonly seen in infants and toddlers than in older children and adults. The systemic manifestations include fever and malaise, which, along with the lesions, often persist for up to 2 weeks. Most gingivostomatitis is caused by type 1 HSV, though type 2 virus may be present with or without a history of oral-genital sexual activity. The severity of the accompanying dysphagia, particularly in infants and toddlers, is occasionally great enough to compromise nutrition and hydration and warrant hospitalization.

Herpes labialis is probably the most common manifestation of HSV infection, typically recurring in a large proportion of the population. The lesion is typically a localized vesicle or cluster of vesicles on an erythematous base, occurring at the junction of mucous membrane and epidermis on or near the lips. The colloquial terms used to describe such lesions (cold sores, fever blisters) reflect the long-recognized association of recurrences with intercurrent viral illness and fever, as well as with stress, menstruation, and other minor physiologic disruptions. Recurrent herpes labialis tends to produce few or no systemic signs, in contrast to primary gingivostomatitis. Most episodes are brief and self-limited, lasting less than 1 week. The duration and severity of each recurrence may vary considerably, even within the same individual, but tend to lessen with time. As with gingivostomatitis, most but not all herpes labialis is caused by type 1 HSV.

Genital HSV infections parallel oral HSV infections in that primary genital HSV is usually more severe and more prolonged. The duration of primary infections may be 1 to 2 weeks. Genital herpetic infection begins as erythematous plaques, which subsequently develop vesicles and erosions on epidermal surfaces and erosions alone on mucous membrane surfaces. Periurethral erosions are often associated with dysuria. Primary infection is often associated with fever, malaise, lymphadenopathy, and other systemic manifestations.

Most but not all primary genital herpes is caused by type 2 HSV. It appears that primary infections with type 2 HSV are more likely to be followed by recurrent lesions than primary genital infections with type 1 HSV, and episodes due to either type tend to become less frequent over time. In a small percentage of women, asymptomatic colonization of the uterine cervix may be present. The frequency of this finding varies considerably with geography and sexual behavior.

Other forms of direct inoculation and reactivation of herpetic infection include those that occur in traumatized skin, such as with burns, abrasions, and minor cuts. Such direct inoculation may occur during contact sports like wrestling and has been termed herpes gladiatorum. Herpetic whitlow is HSV infection of fingertips, most typically occurring in dental and medical personnel, contracted during patient examination.

Neonatal herpes simplex infections represent a less common but more serious part of the disease spectrum caused by HSV. The apparently increasing frequency, the life-threatening potential, and the neurologic and cutaneous sequelae of neonatal HSV infection have brought increased attention to this entity. Most HSV infection in the neonate can be categorized into three general patterns. Some newborns, usually during the first week of life, experience widely disseminated infection of internal viscera, often in the absence of neural or cutaneous disease. Mortality is highest in this group, perhaps due both to the rapidity of dissemination and to the difficulty of diagnosis in the absence of vesicles. A second subset of neonates will experience disease limited to skin, eyes, and mucous membranes, presenting in the first several weeks of life. These neonates appear to have a good prognosis for survival but have a disturbing frequency of occult, unrecognized central nervous system involvement. A third subset of neonates will experience localized, overt central nervous system disease. They tend to be seen beyond the first week of life but within the first month, and brain involvement may be diffuse or focal. In all these instances, natal acquisition of HSV appears to be more common than a postnatal or in utero acquisition. Roughly three fourths of neonatal HSV infections are caused by type 2. Probably because of obstetric strategies with overt maternal HSV disease, most neonates with HSV infection are now born to parents with no history of such infection. In most instances this presumably reflects asymptomatic maternal genital colonization. Thus, neonatal HSV must be considered in various clinical settings, particularly in the presence of unexplained fever and even in the absence of parental history of HSV infection.

HSV infections in the immunocompromised host are of two kinds. Most commonly, gingivostomatitis or orofacial lesions occur and persist well beyond the usual duration of these conditions in the normal host. Immunocompromised or debilitated patients may also develop small, discrete, grouped ulceration in the sacral, perianal, or perineal regions. Such patients are often bedridden with chronic neurologic or oncologic conditions, may require frequent physical therapy and nursing assistance, and may pose an unsuspected source of occupational hazard. Rarely, HSV may produce disseminated multisystem disease, usually in the severely immunocompromised patient, and is thought to be associated with primary infection. Extensive visceral involvement implies a poor outcome, though antiviral therapy has improved the likelihood of survival.

HSV ocular infection may occur in two settings. First, keratitis or keratoconjunctivitis due to HSV may occur in the neonate, the normal child, and the adult. In this situation, dendritic ulcerative changes are seen in the cornea, usually with accompanying pain. Reactivation of the lesions may occur and in some patients become a serious problem. Ocular disease with HSV may also be manifested by the appearance of chorioretinitis in association with disseminated disease of the neonate or immunocompromised host.

Patients with atopic dermatitis, ichthyosis, Darier's disease, pemphigus, and other cutaneous diseases may develop a potentially serious complication of HSV infection termed eczema herpeticum. After an incubation period of approximately 10 days, crops of vesicles develop and may become widely distributed. These vesicles usually become pustular, may be hemorrhagic, and may be associated with significant cutaneous edema. New crops of vesicles may continue to appear, and the patient may develop high fever, regional adenopathy, and systemic symptoms. Death rarely may result from visceral involvement. This same clinical syndrome has also occurred in association with the same types of cutaneous disorders following exposure to vaccinia virus (eczema vaccinatum). This is rare but continues to occur, now almost exclusively in family members of inoculated military personnel. The Tzanck preparation of lesions due to vaccinia is negative, however. The term Kaposi's varicelliform eruption has been used for both eczema herpeticum and eczema vaccinatum.

Diagnosis. Most minor mucocutaneous manifestations of HSV infection do not come to medical attention. When a physician does encounter herpes labialis, for example, diagnosis is made by visual inspection alone, and further diagnostic measures are neither necessary nor indicated. In an increasing number of HSV infections, however, precise viral diagnosis is desirable, particularly with the availability of effective antiviral therapy.

Definitive diagnosis of HSV infection is made by tissue culture, performed in diagnostic virology laboratories, utilizing a variety of human and non-human cell lines to grow the virus. The increasing number of such laboratories and the ability of HSV to survive transport to such laboratories in appropriate viral transport media have made culture diagnosis practical in most circumstances. Within 48 to 72 hours, most clinical specimens containing HSV will produce characteristic cytopathic changes in the cell sheet, permitting presumptive diagnosis. In serious HSV infections, such as neonatal herpes, disseminated herpes, and herpes encephalitis, reliable tissue culture of appropriate specimens is mandatory and daily inspection of the culture is essential.

More rapid diagnostic techniques may permit a presumptive diagnosis, which may be critical in instituting early antiviral therapy in serious HSV disease. Historically, the most useful approach to rapid presumptive diagnosis of HSV has been the use of cell scrapings from skin vesicles or oral ulcers. Using the Tzanck smear with Wright or Giemsa stains may demonstrate the typical multinucleated giant cells. This finding is specific to HSV and varicella-zoster virus but does not distinguish between them. Because of the potential false-positive and false-negative interpretation of these smears, their use must never be regarded as a substitute for tissue culture in serious HSV infection. In experienced hands, however, cytologic diagnosis may be a valuable aid in therapeutic decision making.

Currently, other rapid diagnostic techniques are emerging, using antigen-detection in clinical specimens by such techniques as enzyme immunoassays or immunofluorescence assays. Until recently, antibodies to type 1 or 2 HSV have been sufficiently cross-reactive such that type-specific diagnosis has not been possible. Promising developments with highly type-specific monoclonal antibodies may circumvent these difficulties. These techniques may also provide a valuable exclusionary test for varicella-zoster virus, which may be of particular value in the immunocompromised host.

The special circumstances of HSV encephalitis (discussed elsewhere) and herpes keratitis may necessitate other special diagnostic procedures. In the former, brain biopsy has provided definitive diagnosis, which has not been possible using more indirect methods such as cerebrospinal fluid examination.

Treatment

For many years, a multitude of topical and oral treatments has been in use for oral and genital HSV infections. Very few, however, were subjected to rigorous clinical study, and their efficacy remains unproved. In the 1970s, nucleoside analogues with clear-cut activity against HSV were described. One in particular, vidarabine (adenine arabinoside, Ara-A) was shown to be efficacious in parenteral treatment of serious HSV infections, such as neonatal HSV, herpes encephalitis, and HSV in the compromised host. With these conditions, it became the standard of comparison for later antiviral agents.

In the 1980s, vidarabine has been largely superseded by acyclovir (acycloguanosine, Zovirax), though comparative study of the two drugs in neonatal HSV is still in progress. Acyclovir, with a unique mechanism utilizing a virus-specific enzyme, has been shown efficacious in a variety of HSV infections. Further, its availability in intravenous, topical, and oral formulations allows varying approaches according to the nature and severity of HSV infection.

Intravenous acyclovir has been shown to be efficacious in primary genital HSV and HSV in the compromised host. Both clinical symptoms and virus shedding are significantly shortened. In two comparative trials, acyclovir also has been shown to be superior to vidarabine in HSV encephalitis (beyond the neonatal period) and is currently the drug of choice in proven HSV encephalitis.

Studies of topical acyclovir ointment in a variety of less severe HSV conditions have consistently shown reduction of viral shedding and variable attenuation of clinical symptoms. The use of topical therapy would appear most appropriate in minor cutaneous infection early in the course of lesions, especially in the compromised host. Many have voiced concern that use of this agent for minor lesions in the normal host will cultivate resistant strains and generally be initiated after viral replication has largely ceased.

Recently, oral acyclovir has been approved for use in the United States. It may be of particular value in reducing symptoms in the compromised host with HSV infections whose systemic signs do not warrant hospitalization. It has also been shown to be of value in short-term prophylaxis of recurrent genital HSV. The optimal use of oral acyclovir for extended prophylaxis and in patient-initiated treatment is a subject of continuing debate and intense public interest. The potential and proved benefits must be weighed against cost considerations and the problem of drug-resistant strains.

Neonatal HSV infection, even if restricted to skin and mucous membranes, should be treated for 10 days with intravenous antiviral therapy. Presumptive diagnosis of HSV, e.g., with the Tzanck test, is sufficient for initiating parenteral therapy while definitive tissue culture diagnosis is pending. It is not as yet clear whether higher dose vidarabine (30 mg per kg per day) or acyclovir (30 mg per kg per day) will prove to be more efficacious or less toxic. Optimally, neonates with this condition should be treated under the existing two-drug protocol at major centers until this question is resolved.

HERPES ZOSTER

The Virus

The clinical phenomenon of zoster, colloquially known as shingles, was long recognized to have features similar to those of herpetic disease and has thus been known as herpes zoster. Within the last century, the causative agent, varicella-zoster virus, was identified and distinguished from herpes simplex virus. Whereas varicella (chicken pox, discussed elsewhere) generally represents a primary encounter with the virus, zoster is a localized reactivation of the same virus. Varicella-zoster virus, like herpes simplex virus, is a member of the herpesvirus family. Like all herpesviruses, it is a large, enveloped DNA virus, with capacity for latency and complex interaction with the host immune system.

Clinical Manifestations. Zoster typically begins as an erythematous plaque or plaques in a dermatomal distribution. These plaques then usually develop vesicles, which may evolve into umbilicated pustules. The virus reactivates from a sensory ganglion, but the viremia, fever, and high degree of contagion associated with chicken pox do not generally occur. Age and immunologic status are critical determinants of the occurrence and character of zoster. Zoster in the normal host tends to be a disease of the elderly. Individuals experiencing primary varicella in the neonatal period or early infancy appear to be at increased risk of zoster in childhood or early adulthood. Timing of antecedent varicella is less a factor in the overtly immunocompromised patient, in whom the degree of depressed immunity is the overriding factor. Dissemination to internal viscera appears to occur almost exclusively in the compromised host. Ocular involvement in herpes zoster is a serious complication and should prompt immediate ophthalmologic referral. It should be suspected with a trigeminal distribution and presumed with nasociliary branch involvement evidenced by lesions on the nasal tip. Similarly, involvement of the external ear or tympanic membrane may be associated with facial palsy and loss of taste (Ramsey-Hunt syndrome), and also tinnitus, vertigo, or deafness. Postherpetic neuralgia, the painful and sometimes prolonged dermatomal sequel to zoster, tends to occur more frequently in older patients, affecting up to one third of zoster patients above age 55 years.

Diagnosis. The diagnosis of zoster is usually not difficult, given the distinctive distribution and vesicular nature of the rash. Some diagnostic confusion may arise if the eruption fails to vesiculate, if the patient has no history of prior chicken pox, or if the dermatomal distribution is not immediately apparent. In the presence of vesicles, a Tzanck smear of the lesions generally will support the diagnosis by demonstration of multinucleated giant cells. This histologic finding does not differentiate herpes simplex infection or primary varicella from zoster; this is important because herpes simplex infection occasionally occurs in a zosteriform distribution. Tissue culture of early vesicles provides definitive diagnosis, but the slower viral growth and lower sensitivity of the technique make it less useful than for herpes simplex virus. In the usual instance in which disseminated cutaneous zoster must be differentiated from primary varicella, demonstration of virus-specific antibody in serum at onset supports a diagnosis of zoster. Finally, rapid diagnostic tests are emerging that enable detection of virus-specific antigen in vesicle scrapings or tissue; in certain situations (to be discussed), these tests will allow institution of therapy earlier in the course of illness.

Treatment

The treatment of zoster has been controversial for many years. Until very recently, therapy has been directed toward modification of symptoms, often through modification of host response. The emergence of antiviral agents, particularly acyclovir (acycloguanosine, Zovirax), allows for direct interference with the virus replication. Since not all manifestations are due solely to viral replication, especially postherpetic neuralgia, treatment options are still not ideal.

In the usual zoster episode, wet-to-dry dressings provide both some pain relief through evaporative cooling and vital, gentle debridement, important in preventing secondary infection. Additional pain relief is afforded by acetaminophen, aspirin, or codeine. The frequency and severity of postherpetic neuralgia does appear to be roughly predictable by the magnitude of pain before and during the acute episode. Systemic corticosteroids may be of value in reducing the incidence of postherpetic neuralgia if given within 5 days of onset of zoster. Because older patients are most at risk for this complication, corticosteroid use has greatest value in the otherwise healthy elderly patient seen with early zoster. Controversy continues whether the probable benefit in this instance is outweighed by the possible risk of promoting dissemination. Diphenylhydantoin, carbamazepine, and cimetidine, as well as other agents, are of possible value in chronic postherpetic neuralgia, but patients with refractory, severe pain may well benefit from a combination of therapeutic approaches available through specialized pain clinics.

Treatment of zoster with antiviral agents has only recently become possible. Acyclovir represents the optimal currently available agent, and it is now approved for use in topical, intravenous, and oral forms. The decision to treat, as well as the route of administration, may be influenced by host status, duration and distribution of vesicles, and presence or absence of other systemic symptoms. With recent availability of oral acyclovir, it may become unnecessary to hospitalize certain patients to achieve acceptable efficacy. As in the treatment of herpes simplex, the efficacy of acyclovir is most readily demonstrable with more severe zoster and more severe compromise of host defense.

Indications for systemic acyclovir are clearest in immunocompromised patients with evidence of dissemination of zoster to internal viscera. In addition, intravenous acyclovir appears efficacious in preventing progressive cutaneous and visceral dissemination in immunocompromised patients. Finally, patients with cutaneous dissemination (many lesions outside primary or contiguous dermatomes) will experience more rapid viral clearance with intravenous acyclovir.

In the normal host, intravenous acyclovir has been shown to reduce pain during acute zoster and to accelerate the rate of healing. Limited information has emerged with respect to oral acyclovir and zoster. The comparative efficacy of intravenous and oral acyclovir in this setting and others is under investigation.

PARASITIC DISEASES

method of
LAWRENCE CHARLES PARISH, M.D.,
Thomas Jefferson University
and JOSEPH A. WITKOWSKI, M.D.
University of Pennsylvania
Philadelphia, Pennsylvania

Scabies

Scabies, once called the 7 year itch, is a pruritic disease caused by *Sarcoptes scabiei*. The fertilized adult female subsists and deposits eggs just under the stratum corneum to create the burrows that are diagnostic. These burrows appear as short, zigzag disruptions of the horny layer and are most often found on the sides of the fingers, wrists, elbows, and penis. Small noninflammatory vesicles, erythematous urticarial papules, excoriations, eczematous patches, and pyoderma are seen in association with the burrows but are also found on the anterior axillary folds, the breasts of women, the belt line, the lower part of the buttocks, and the scrotum. Occasionally reddish brown nodules are seen on the elbows, anterior axillary folds, and the male genitalia. Lesions are more widespread in children and include the face, neck, and feet. In the mentally retarded, the physically debilitated, and the immunologically incompetent, thick scaly patches on the hands and feet, nail dystrophy, and generalized erythema may be seen.

The diagnosis of scabies can frequently be made clinically based on the morphology, distribution, presence of contact cases, nocturnal pruritus, and therapeutic response. Some clinicians prefer to make the diagnosis only if a positive scraping is obtained, using potassium hydroxide or mineral oil, that demonstrates the mite or its products. Since scratching may remove the mite, the best place to scrape is an area that is not excoriated.

Specific Therapy. The treatment of scabies is remarkably simple. One per cent lindane lotion or cream (Kwell) is applied from the neck to the toes. Although some evidence suggests that 6 hours of application is sufficient, 12 hours provides adequate insurance that the mite will be killed. Care should be given to apply the medication under finger nails so that all mites are destroyed. At the end of 12 hours, a bath may be taken to wash off the insecticide. Reapplication is usually unnecessary, and there is no known lindane resistance by the scabies mite.

Itching will be reduced by 50 per cent within 24 hours. This pruritus represents an immunologic reaction to the products of the scabies mite. Topical steroid creams, colloid baths, and systemic antihistamines may be necessary to relieve pruritus and signs of inflammation over the next several days. The patient who continues to itch may have underlying atopic dermatitis or neurodermatitis, but reinfestation should also be considered. This is why bed partners and other members of the household should be treated at the same time. Because household pets such as dogs and cats are not afflicted by *Sarcoptes scabiei humanus,* they need not be treated. In fact, lindane is lethal to cats because they lick their skin. Although clothing, towels, and bed linens should be laundered on the day of treatment, there is no need to fumigate the living quarters. Because we think the merits of lindane lotion outweigh any alleged neurotoxicity, we are not concerned about application of lindane to infants and pregnant women, provided it is used correctly. Only the amount necessary for treatment should be prescribed, and prescriptions should not be renewable. The alternative treatments are far less effective. These include the use of crotamiton 10 per cent (Eurax), applied daily for 3 days, or 6 per cent precipitated sulfur in hydrophilic petrolatum applied for up to 6 days. The latter can often cause contact dermatitis.

Pediculosis

Of the enormous numbers of the Anoplura family, only three lice afflict humans. These include the head louse, the body louse, and the pubic louse. Although each has its own domain, it sometimes can be found in other areas of the body.

Pediculosis Capitis

The head louse *Phthirus capitis* afflicts white children and infrequently adolescents. Black children almost never develop pediculosis capitis for unknown reasons. The louse, which measures 1.0 to 1.5 mm, can be seen on gross inspection on the hair. More often nits or eggs are found. These are whitish oval bodies that are firmly attached to the hair shaft. Since ova are laid on the hair shaft near the scalp surface, the duration of the infection can be judged by the distance of the nit from the skin. Although adult lice die within several days when away from humans, nits may remain viable for as long as 30 days.

The head louse is easily transmitted by contact so that many children in a family or classroom can be afflicted, usually in the fall and winter. For unknown reasons, the epidemics of pediculosis capitis die down in the spring. Generally, pediculosis capitis proves to be merely a nuisance. No disease is carried by the head louse. Only rarely does the intense itching of the scalp result in secondary pyodermas and cervical lymphadenopathy.

Treatment. Lindane 1 per cent shampoo (Kwell) is applied undiluted to the dry scalp for 4 minutes. This is then wet with warm water, worked into a lather, and rinsed off. Contact with the eyes and mouth should be avoided. Although some clinicians prefer to repeat this in 7 days, we believe the momentum is lost that way and prefer to repeat treatment the following day. To the best of our knowledge, there is no evidence that head lice are resistant to lindane.

The nits turn gray and may take several weeks to fall off the hairs. Their removal can be hastened by the use of a stiff fine-toothed comb.

Alternative treatments include pyrethrin shampoos, such as RID, applied to the scalp for 10 minutes and then washed off. A second application should be made a day later.

Treatment should be carried out among all children in a household. When pediculosis capitis has reached epidemic proportions, it is necessary for all children in a classroom, including contacts in after school activities, to be treated.

Although the nits that fall off a child's head may remain viable, it is generally unnecessary to fumigate the living quarters. It is advisable to wash all clothing the child has been wearing and to dry clean all hats and coats.

Pediculosis Corporis

This terribly itchy disorder, characterized by parallel scratch marks on the shoulders, trunk, and buttocks and by secondary infection, is caused by *Phthirus corporis*. This louse is slightly larger than the head louse. It does not live on the body but rather in the seams of clothing, where it deposits its eggs. It attacks the body, biting the skin for its blood meal. The bites can be seen as small urticarial papules. Postinflammatory pigmentation is a common clinical feature.

Treatment. Treatment consists of washing the clothes and bed linens in hot water or placing them in a sealed plastic bag for 30 days. Clothes not washable should be dry cleaned. Because the louse does not live on the body, it is unnecessary to apply an insecticide to the skin. Nevertheless, many clinicians and especially nursing staffs in hospitals and extended care institutions prefer to treat the patient with Kwell shampoo applied to the entire body for 4 minutes.

The pruritus that may remain for several days can be treated with topical corticosteroids, colloid baths, and systemic antihistamines. If there is marked secondary infection, it is most often due to *Staphylococcus aureus* or *beta-hemolytic streptococci*. Tegopen, 500 mg four times a day, or erythromycin, 250 mg four times a day, can be employed. Although the body louse is known to carry epidemic typhus and relapsing fever in other parts of the world, this has not been found in the United States. Lindane resistance of body lice has not been demonstrated in the United States.

Pediculosis Pubis

This intensely itching disease is caused by *Phthirus pubis,* called the crab louse because it resembles this crustacean. Its usual site of predilection is the pubic area but it can also attack the eyelids and eyebrows (pediculosis ciliaris) and any other hairy part of the body. Contact dermatitis in response to self-prescribed medications is a common complication. Grayish-blue macules called maculae ceruleae are occasionally seen.

Treatment. Lindane shampoo should be applied to the entire body for 4 minutes on two successive days. Bed linen and clothing should be washed in a washing machine or dry cleaned.

Treatment of contacts is necessary to prevent reinfestation and continual spread of this parasite.

If itching remains after the second day, hydrocortisone 1 per cent (Hytone) cream may be applied three times a day. The eyelashes are most effectively treated by 1 per cent yellow oxide of mercury ointment applied three times a day for 1 week. The nits may be manually extracted from the lashes either by the physician or by the patient.

Creeping Eruption

This is most often caused by the cat and dog hookworm larva *(Ancylostoma braziliense)*. *Ancylostoma canium* and *Ancylostoma duodenali* are less common etiologic agents in the United States. A pruritic erythematous papule develops at the site of penetration of the larva. After several days the larva migrates, producing the characteristic erythematous serpiginous linear lesions. Excoriations and secondary bacterial infections often result from the intense pruritus.

The infestation is most common in warm, sandy, coastal areas after periods of rainy weather. The infective larvae develop in the soil from eggs deposited in the feces of cats and dogs. Infections occur while people are walking barefooted on the beaches, playing in sand boxes, or working in crawl spaces.

Treatment. Thiabendazole suspension (Mintezol) applied three times daily will result in clearing in 7 to 14 days. Generally itching is decreased by the end of 3 days.

Alternative methods include the use of ethylchloride spray or dry ice. To be effective, the affected area must be sufficiently frozen to cause sloughing of the epidermis and the larva. In recalcitrant cases, oral thiabendazole in a dosage of 10 mg per pound (25 mg per kg) body weight twice daily for 2 to 4 days is usually effective. It is available as a suspension of 500 mg per 5 ml and 500 mg chewable tablets. The secondary infection that would usually be caused by *S. aureus, beta-hemolytic streptococci,* can best be treated with Tegopen, 500 mg four times per day, or erythromycin, 250 mg four times per day, for 10 days.

Prevention

It is obvious that walking barefoot in contaminated areas, particularly in the tropics or subtropics, leads to the disease and thus should be avoided. Where the disease is endemic in dogs or cats, they should be kept away from beaches and sand boxes in which they may choose to defecate. Deworming the animals will also stem an epidemic.

FUNGAL DISEASES

method of
EDGAR B. SMITH, M.D.
University of Texas
Galveston, Texas

The most common fungus infections of the skin are dermatophytosis, tinea versicolor, and candidiasis. These conditions can be mimicked by a variety of other dermatoses. The resulting treatment of nonfungal conditions with antifungal medications is a common cause of treatment failure. Mycologic confirmation of clinically suspected superficial fungus infection should always be obtained before antifungal therapy is begun. The identification of fungal hyphae on microscopic examination of scales from the suspected lesion in a potassium hydroxide preparation is the quickest and most useful means of obtaining this confirmation. Culturing of material on mycologic media, such as Sabouraud, Mycosel, or DTM, is essential when it is desirable to accurately identify the causative organism. However, some organisms, such as *Pityrosporum orbiculare,* do not grow on the usual media for fungi, and others grow slowly. The potassium hydroxide preparation can be done when the patient is seen initially and is a most valuable guide to choosing appropriate therapy. Wood's light examination was once a useful confirmatory test in some dermatophyte infections of the scalp. However, *Trichophyton tonsurans* is now the predominant organism causing scalp infections in the United States, and this organism does not produce fluorescence. Wood's light examination is of no use in identifying fungus infections of the nonhairy skin.

Antifungal Agents
(Table 1)

Topical Preparations

1. Whitfield's ointment (salicylic acid 3 per cent and benzoic acid 6 per cent): An inexpensive preparation useful in treating chronic scaling dermatophytosis of the feet and hands.

2. Castellani's paint (carbol fuchsin, phenol, and resorcinol in acetone-alcohol): A colored solution useful in treating macerated interdigital dermatophyte infections of the feet.

3. Gentian violet solution, 1 per cent: An effective but messy topical agent for the treatment of oral candidiasis and candidal intertrigo.

4. Undecylenic acid (Desenex: ointment, powder, and spray): An older agent effective in dermatophyte infections. The main component of most over-the-counter preparations.

5. Tolnaftate (Tinactin, Aftate: 1 per cent cream, lotion, or powder): Useful in treating dermatophyte infections. Routine daily use of powder is effective in preventing recurrences.

6. Nystatin (Mycostatin, Nilstat: cream or ointment, 100,000 units per gram; vaginal tablets, 100,000 units; oral suspension, 100,000 units per ml; oral tablets, 500,000 units): A polyene antibiotic effective against *Candida albicans* infections. Tablets are useful in reducing the yeast flora of the gastrointestial tract, but systemic absorption is negligible.

7. Amphotericin B (Fungizone: 3 per cent cream, lotion, and ointment): A polyene antibiotic useful in treating candidiasis.

8. Haloprogin (Halotex: 1 per cent cream and lotion): An iodinated trichlorophenol compound effective against yeast infections and dermatophytosis, the first of the newer broad-spectrum agents introduced in the United States.

9. Thymol (3 per cent in absolute alcohol): An effective drug agent for use in candidal paronychia and onycholysis with secondary candidal infection.

10. Aluminum chloride hexahydrate (Drysol 20 per cent; Xerac AC 6.25 per cent in anhydrous alcohol): These preparations are effective antiperspirants and are useful in treating hyperhidrosis, which predisposes to fungal infections of the feet.

11. Miconazole (Monistat-Derm, Micatin: 2 per cent cream or lotion, Monistat 7 vaginal cream)

12. Clotrimazole (Lotrimin, Mycelex: 1 per cent cream or lotion; Gyne-Lotrimin: 1 per cent vaginal tablets or cream; Mycelex troche: 10 mg)

13. Econazole (Spectazole: 1 per cent cream)

Numbers 11, 12, and 13 are imidazole compounds, which are broad-spectrum agents effective in dermatophytoses, candidiasis, and tinea versicolor. They are comparable in effectiveness. However, the econazole preparation is free of parabens and propylene glycol and can be used in patients with sensitivity to these preservatives.

14. Ciclopirox olamine (Loprox: 1 per cent cream): A pyridone-ethanolamine salt that has

TABLE 1. **Therapy for Superficial Fungal Infections**

	Topical Therapy		Oral Therapy		
	Preparation	*Duration*	*Preparation*	*Daily Dose*	*Duration*
Tinea capitis	No	—	Griseofulvin	5 mg/lb	1–2 months
Tinea corporis	Only if localized	2–4 weeks	Griseofulvin	500–1000 mg	1 month
Tinea cruris	Imidazoles Haloprogin Ciclopirox	2–4 weeks	Griseofulvin	500–1000 mg	1 month
Tinea pedis—toewebs	Imidazoles Ciclopirox	2–4 weeks	No	—	—
Tinea pedis—planter	Imidazoles Ciclopirox Whitfield's	6 weeks	Griseofulvin	1000 mg	2–3 months
Tinea manuum	Imidazoles Ciclopirox Whitfield's	Chronically	Griseofulvin	500–1000 mg	2 months
Tinea unguium	Ciclopirox	6–12 months	Griseofulvin	1000–1500 mg*	6–12 months
Candidiasis	Imidazoles Haloprogin Ciclopirox	1–2 weeks	No	—	—
Chronic mucocutaneous candidiasis	No	—	Ketoconazole	100–400 mg	5 days
Tinea versicolor	Selenium sulfide	Daily for 1 week	Ketoconazole	400 mg	Single dose

*1500 mg may exceed manufacturer's recommended dose.

the same broad spectrum as haloprogin and the imidazoles. This agent appears to penetrate nails better than other topical agents.

15. Selenium sulfide (Selsun, Exsel: 2½ per cent suspension): Originally developed as an antidandruff shampoo, this agent is very useful in the treatment of tinea versicolor. It also has an effect on spores of the dermatophytes causing scalp infections. Regular shampooing will reduce the spread of infectious organisms and is a useful adjunct in the management of dermatophytoses of the scalp.

16. Clotrimazole-betamethasone dipropionate (Lotrisone cream): A combination imidazole-corticosteroid preparation that produces more rapid responses in inflammatory fungal infections.

Topical agents are very effective in the management of localized infections. In general, they should be applied sparingly to the infected skin and to a 1- to 2-inch area of the surrounding normal-appearing skin.

Systemic Agents

1. Griseofulvin (Grifulvin V, Fulvicin-U/F, Grisactin: 250 mg and 500 mg tablets; suspension 125 mg per 5 ml): Griseofulvin is an effective oral agent against dermatophytes but has no effect on the causative agents of candidiasis or tinea versicolor. In recent years some relatively resistant strains of dermatophytes have appeared, resulting in refractory infections. Griseofulvin is best given after meals. Its common side effect is headache. Nausea, urticarial reactions, phototoxicity, and exacerbation of porphyria cutanea tarda may occur. Griseofulvin induces hepatic microsomal enzymes and decreases the effect of warfarin and related anticoagulants, necessitating increased anticoagulant dosage. Discontinuation of griseofulvin in patients who have been also taking anticoagulants may result in bleeding if the anticoagulant dosage is not decreased. Phenobarbital may interfere with the absorption of griseofulvin and its effectiveness as an antifungal agent.

2. Ketoconazole (Nizoral tablets, 200 mg): An oral imidazole with broad-spectrum activity against dermatophytes, *Candida,* and *Pityrosporon* species as well as many of the deep fungi. Ketoconazole is given as a single daily dose, usually 200 mg, and is well tolerated. It is best taken with meals. Ketoconazole requires acid for absorption and should not be given with antacids or cimetidine and other H_2 antihistamines. Ketoconazole is the most effective drug for chronic mucocutaneous candidiases. It is effective in the management of extensive or severe cases of dermatophytoses unresponsive to griseofulvin. It is useful in candidal paronychia and extensive or unresponsive tinea versicolor. The drug rarely causes an idiosyncratic hepatitis (approximately

1 in 10,000 persons), and at least one fatality has occurred as the result of liver damage. Ketoconazole can also interfere with testosterone and cortisone synthesis and there have been reported cases of decreased libido, impotence, and gynecomastia.

Dermatophyte Infections

Scalp and Beard

Fungus infections of the scalp and beard area are caused by organisms in the *Microsporum* and *Trichophyton* groups that invade hairs. This leads to broken hairs and alopecia as well as varying degrees of inflammation in the adjacent epidermis and dermis. Hairs from suspected lesions should be selected for potassium hydroxide preparations and cultures.

These infections rarely respond to topical therapy, and orally administered griseofulvin is the treatment of choice. We use the microcrystalline form of griseofulvin in the following dosages: for very small children, 125 mg of griseofulvin suspension daily; for children from 30 to 50 pounds, 250 mg daily; for children over 50 pounds, 500 mg daily; for adults, 1 gram daily. The total daily dosage is divided into two equal doses and is best given after meals. Griseofulvin should be continued for approximately 2 weeks after the infection is clinically clear and laboratory examinations are negative. In most cases, the usual course of therapy is 6 to 8 weeks. Concomitant use of shampoos every 2 to 3 days with selenium sulfate, 2½ per cent suspension, may reduce dissemination of organisms. Siblings and pets should be examined and treated, if infected, to prevent reinfection of the patient. With modern therapy, it is not necessary for children to remain home from school.

Occasionally, a severely inflammatory fungus infection of the scalp, or kerion, is seen. This represents an immunologic response to the fungi in hair follicles. Mild cases will respond to the use of topical steroids. In very severe cases, short (1 to 2 week) courses of systemic steroids are useful in suppressing the inflammatory reaction and reducing the risk of scarring and permanent hair loss.

Nonhairy Skin

These infections can be caused by many *Microsporum* and *Trichophyton* species and *Epidermophyton floccosum* and may result in classic ringworm. Most infections can be successfully managed topically with haloprogin, ciclopirox, or one of the imidazole preparations. The medication should be continued for about 1 week after the lesions are cleared. The usual duration of treatment is 2 to 4 weeks. Oral griseofulvin, microcrystalline form 500 mg twice daily for 1 month, is indicated in patients with extensive cutaneous involvement, with lesions at hard-to-reach sites, and with chronic or recurring infections. Recalcitrant infections can be treated with ketoconazole, 200 mg daily, for 1 month.

Dermatophytosis of the inguinal folds, or tinea cruris, is a common variant that occurs frequently in young athletically active patients and is frequently associated with dermatophyte infections of the feet. Patients should be advised to reduce sweating and chafing in the groin area by avoiding tight or highly occlusive synthetic material underclothing. The treatment is otherwise the same as that for other dermatophyte infections of the glabrous skin.

Feet

There are two main variants of foot infection with dermatophytes. The most common involves the toe webs and the instep of the sole, is most frequently due to *Trichophyton mentagrophytes,* and responds more readily to therapy. Most infections of this type can be successfully treated with haloprogin, ciclopirox, or an imidazole applied twice daily for about 4 weeks. This type of infection is often complicated by secondary bacterial infection, usually with *Streptococcus* or *Staphylococcus*. If pustules or purulent exudate are present, cultures should be taken and the patient started on a program of bed rest, elevation of feet with compresses or soaks with warm tap water for 15 to 20 minutes three times daily, and systemic antibiotics. After bacterial infection resolves, appropriate antifungal treatment should be initiated.

The dry, scaly diffuse type of infection of the soles is usually due to *Trichophyton rubrum* and tends to be chronic. However, most infections will respond at least temporarily to topical treatment with imidazoles or ciclopirox. Treatment should be continued for 5 to 6 weeks. Refractory infections of this type are treated with a combination of a topical medication and orally administered griseofulvin or ketoconazole. Relapses are quite common even with such combined therapy. The patient should be advised to keep the feet cool and dry and to wear cotton socks rather than the more occlusive nylon or other synthetic fabrics. Wearing of sandals or perforated shoes is also helpful. Prophylactic use of tolnaftate powder will reduce the frequency of recurrences.

Hands

Dermatophytosis of the hands is usually unilateral and clinically resembles the dry, scaly, diffuse type of infection of the feet with which it is frequently associated. These chronic infections of the palmar skin usually require combination therapy with imidazoles or ciclopirox and oral griseofulvin or ketoconazole.

Nails

Infections of the hands and feet are frequently accompanied by infection of the nails. In general, nail infections do not respond well to topical therapy. Ciclopirox appears to penetrate nails better and will occasionally produce cures if used persistently until the infected nail grows out. Infections of the fingernails that do not respond to ciclopirox can usually be treated successfully with griseofulvin 500 mg twice daily. Therapy should be continued until the nail appears completely normal; this usually requires 4 to 6 months. Toenail infections will occasionally respond to ciclopirox and/or griseofulvin, but cure rates are quite low even with very prolonged therapy. I often discourage patients from treating toenail infections unless the resulting thickness of the nail plate produces pain and mechanical problems with footwear. In these relatively rare cases, the nail is avulsed and the patient is placed on oral griseofulvin for 6 to 8 months as a new nail is growing out.

Tinea Versicolor

Tinea versicolor, caused by *Pityrosporum orbiculare,* is quite common in areas of warm temperatures and high humidity. It is characterized by asymptomatic, scaling patches on the upper trunk and neck that vary from slightly red to brown and white. Since a few organisms can be found on the normal skin of most persons, this condition can be considered the result of overgrowth of this yeast in more susceptible persons. Tinea versicolor responds well to a variety of topical antifungal agents, but relapses are common with all. Since infections are often extensive, I consider selenium sulfide (Selsun), 2.5 per cent suspension, to be the treatment of choice. Following the bath or shower, the suspension is applied as a lather to all of the skin of the neck and upper trunk, allowed to dry for 10 to 15 minutes, and then washed off well with a washcloth. This treatment is repeated each day for 1 week. This treatment will usually eradicate active infection characterized by the presence of scaling, but hypopigmented spots may remain for several months. For very susceptible patients who have frequent relapses, I recommend repeating the above regimen once or twice monthly as a form of maintenance therapy. The newer antifungal agents, such as haloprogin, the imidazoles, and ciclopirox, are quite effective in tinea versicolor, but the expense of these agents limits their usefulness to those with relatively small areas of involvement. Patients with severe refractory infections may be treated effectively with ketoconozole 400 mg in a single dose or 200 mg daily for 2 weeks.

Candidiasis

Cutaneous candidiasis, caused by the yeast *Candida albicans,* occurs frequently in young, active persons who work or play in hot, humid environments. It most frequently involves intertriginous areas such as the groin, perineum, axillae, and inframammary areas. Older patients who are obese or who have diabetes mellitus are also predisposed to infections with this organism. Acute infections are quite inflammatory and should be treated with moist compresses of cool tap water for 10 to 15 minutes three times daily. After the compresses are removed the skin should be allowed to dry, and a broad-spectrum antifungal agent, such as an imidazole or ciclopirox, or nystatin lotion should be applied. Concomitant application of a topical steroid with the anticandidal agent will suppress the inflammation and hasten resolution. I do not recommend use of commercially available nystatin-steroid combinations containing ethylenediamine or parabens because of their potential sensitizing properties. The compresses can be discontinued when weeping and erosions have resolved, but the medications should be continued until the eruption has completely cleared. This usually occurs within 1 to 2 weeks. The patient should be instructed to keep the involved area cool and dry. Loose cotton underclothing is useful in achieving this goal.

Candida albicans can also cause chronic infections of the nail folds (paronychia) and separation of the nail plate from the nail bed. These infections most frequently occur in persons whose work involves continuous wetting of the hands. The patient must be instructed to keep his hands out of water as much as possible. Paronychial infections are treated with applications of an anticandidal agent four times daily. Nystatin cream (Mycostatin) or one of the newer agents such as clotrimazole (Lotrimin), 1 per cent solution; miconazole (MicaTin), 2 per cent lotion; or haloprogin (Halotex), 1 per cent cream are all quite effective. Response is slow, and treatment must be continued for 2 or 3 months. When onycholysis and infection of the nail bed are present, the overlying nail plate should be trimmed back as far as possible; then thymol, 4 per cent, in ethanol, is applied thoroughly under the nail three times daily until the nail grows out in a normal fashion. Refractory infections are best treated with ketoconazole, 200 mg daily, for 1 month.

DISEASES OF THE MOUTH

method of
HENRY W. RANDLE, M.D.
Scott and White Clinic
Temple, Texas

Oral mucous membranes are specialized, thin membranes that lack a thick, horny layer (except on the dorsum of the tongue and hard palate), making them susceptible to physical and chemical injuries. They may be the site of allergic, infectious, metabolic, nutritional, or systemic disorders or may present with congenital anomalies or benign or malignant tumors.

Most oral malignancies are related to life style and environmental factors, including chronic irritation from excessive use of alcohol and tobacco (including smokeless), dental and denture irritations, poor oral hygiene, solar radiation (carcinoma of the lower lip), syphilis, and iron deficiency (Plummer-Vinson syndrome).

GENERAL MEASURES

For optimal treatment of oral disease, poor dental hygiene must be corrected. Control of periodontal disease is the starting point for providing good oral hygiene. The physician must insist that plaques, calculus, periodontitis, caries, ill-fitting dental appliances, and malocclusion be treated by the dentist. The patient must have an adequate intake of oral fluoride and must regularly cleanse with a toothbrush and fluoride toothpaste, dental floss, and perhaps an irrigating instrument such as a WaterPik.

Bad breath or bad taste may reflect oral sepsis or excessive dryness. Adequate hydration must be maintained with frequent mouthwashes immediately before and after meals and several times during the day. A mild alkaline mouthwash such as a solution of cetylpyridinium chloride, phosphate buffers, and alcohol (Cepacol) diluted 1:4 with water may be a useful preparation. A very soothing, inexpensive solution is made by dissolving ½ teaspoonful of sodium bicarbonate in an 8 ounce glass of warm water. One ounce of this preparation held in the mouth may be preferable to the frequently used diluted hydrogen peroxide (1 teaspoonful per 8 ounce glass of water), saline (1 teaspoonful of table salt to 8 ounces of lukewarm water), or commercial preparations, which are frequently irritating to an already inflamed mouth.

Topical anesthesia is sometimes necessary to relieve discomfort and pain before eating. Swishing ½ teaspoonful of viscous lidocaine (Xylocaine) per 2 teaspoonsful of water around in the mouth for 2 to 3 minutes is effective. An alternative would be equal parts of Kaopectate and elixir of diphenhydramine hydrochloride (Benadryl) as a mouthwash prior to eating. Swallowing this preparation will give an additive sedative effect in anxious patients. Dyclonine solution (Dyclone) applied topically will anesthetize the tissue. When anesthesia is used, the patient must be cautioned against traumatizing the oral tissues during eating.

For inflammatory and ulcerative diseases, the diet should be limited to cool bland soups, milkshakes, and ice cream. Hard, hot, acid, sharp, irritating foods should be avoided, as should tobacco. These measures often provide dramatic relief of oral disease. In addition, any associated systemic disorder should be identified and managed or treatment may fail.

LESIONS OF THE LIPS

A variety of lip lesions that require medical attention may occur at or shortly after birth.

Cleft Lip and Cleft Palate. Craniofacial deformities, cleft lip and cleft palate being the most common, may vary from a small depression to extensive, deforming, and mutilating abnormalities that involve the nostrils, hard and soft palates, tongue, and mandible. There may be associated anomalies of other organ systems. Extensive anomalies require long-term management and rehabilitation by specialized teams of pediatricians, plastic surgeons, oral surgeons, pedodontists, dentists, speech therapists, and counselors specializing in long-term management of these defects. Specially designed nipple and palatal obturators are important for feeding and for prevention of nasal aspiration and ear infection. Cleft lip repair is usually undertaken at about 4 weeks of age, but palatal surgery is deferred until later, when speech is beginning to develop.

Vascular Lesions. Capillary and cavernous hemangiomas may involve the lips as well as other oral structures. Most lesions involute spontaneously over several years and do not require treatment. Management is supportive and requires careful evaluation and frequent re-examination. Residual scarring may require some reconstructive surgery; this is generally done at approximately 5 years of age for capillary hemangiomas and at puberty for cavernous hemangiomas. Covermark makeup by Lydia O'Leary will effectively conceal small lesions. Rapid growth of such lesions, especially when vital functions or organs are compromised, requires intervention. Hemangiomas regress with steroid therapy, which should be administered and monitored by a specialist. Radiation therapy, if utilized, must be of such quality and quantity that the teeth buds and bone centers are not harmed. Surgical intervention, cryosurgery with liquid nitrogen probes, and laser surgery are alternative therapies.

Lymphangiomas are rare tumors of the lips and tongue and may require radical surgical intervention. Venous ectasias (lakes) are common among the elderly. No treatment is required, but they may be destroyed by laser, electrodesiccation, or cryoprobes (avoiding the vermilion border) for cosmetic reasons.

Small telangiectasias occur on the lips in patients with scleroderma and hereditary hemorrhagic telangiectasis (Osler-Weber-Rendu disease). If these disorders are suspected, a general examination should be performed.

Cheilitis. Redness and alternating areas of dryness, flaking, and vesiculation are common to most forms of cheilitis. Physical trauma resulting from wind, sunlight, cold, lip licking, tics, and desiccation will cause desquamation. White petrolatum (Vaseline) is helpful for mild to moderate cheilitis. For more severe inflammation, the application of a corticosteroid such as 0.1 per cent triamcinolone acetonide ointment (Aristocort, Kenalog) is usually effective.

Further occurrences may be prevented by application of zinc oxide paste, photoprotective lip balm such as PreSun Lip Protection, or petrolatum. The dry and desquamating lips of severely ill patients should be kept greased with petrolatum.

CONTACT CHEILITIS. Contact cheilitis affects women more often than men, and the vesiculation often extends to the adjacent skin. This is usually caused by lipstick (perfume, dyes, or the base), lip salves, and food. Elimination of the offending agent and the use of topical steroids are helpful.

ANGULAR CHEILITIS. This condition is usually due to a low grade intertrigo from drooling (such as occurs with ill-fitting dentures) with or without candidiasis. Local treatment with an ointment containing nystatin, neomycin sulfate, gramicidin, and triamcinolone acetonide (Mycolog Ointment) (because the cream contains sensitizers) and drying measures (to prevent macerations) are helpful. The buccal mucosa should be examined to be certain there is no additional evidence of candidiasis.

ACTINIC CHEILITIS. Actinic cheilitis is a premalignant lesion seen predominantly on the vermilion of the lower lip in men who have spent considerable time outdoors. The lesions most likely to be dysplastic or neoplastic are those with heavy keratinization, erosion, ulceration, and erythema. Lips with any of these changes should be biopsied for histopathologic examination to exclude malignancy.

For mild actinic cheilitis, cryotherapy with liquid nitrogen and the spray technique with a thaw time of 60 to 90 seconds is rapid and effective and gives a good cosmetic result. Thin lesions can be removed by applying dichloracetic acid until the lesion turns dead white. An alternative would be topical application of 5-fluorouracil (Efudex), 5 per cent cream applied to the vermilion two times each day for about 3 weeks or until erosion of the affected area is produced. This method is effective but may be exceedingly painful. Electrosurgery is more likely to produce excessive scarring. All persons with actinic cheilitis should protect the lips with a photoprotective lip balm (PreSun Lip Protection) and have periodic examinations for possible development of squamous cell carcinomas. For severe actinic cheilitis, surgical excision of the full thickness affected vermilion should be performed. This may be completed by primary closure of the wound by advancement of the labial mucosa.

Squamous cell carcinomas of the lip (usually lower) are treated surgically by wedge excision and primary reconstruction, occasionally combined with an upper or complete neck dissection, depending on the staging and histologic differentiation of the tumor. Radiotherapy may be used as primary treatment.

CHEILITIS GLANDULARIS APOSTEMATOSA. This uncommon entity is the result of inflammation and irritation of the mucous glands along the exposed surface of the lower lip and is manifested by numerous pinhead-sized openings of the ducts of the mucous gland and enlargement of the lips. Cleansing of the lips with tap water upon arising is usually sufficient to remove accumulated debris. Protection of these tissues from the sun and wind with a photoprotective lip balm (PreSun Lip Protection) applied during the day does much to allay symptoms. The disease tends to be self-limited and disappears spontaneously after a number of years. In severe cases, plastic surgery of the lower lip may be helpful.

FACTITIAL CHEILITIS. Continual licking or biting should be suspected in obsessive neurotic patients who present with nonhealing lesions.

Cheilitis may occur in scarlet fever, hereditary polymorphic light eruption, Kawasaki's syndrome (mucocutaneous lymph node syndrome), erythema multiforme, glucagonoma syndrome, and, less commonly, discoid lupus erythematosus. It is also present in nearly all patients receiving isotretinoin (Accutane).

WHITE LESIONS OF THE MOUTH

All white hyperkeratotic lesions of the mouth should be studied by biopsy unless an infection (thrush) or other obvious cause is recognized. The lesions should be classified histopathologically as benign, dysplastic, or malignant, and the patient should be treated and followed appropriately.

The diagnosis of leukokeratosis should be reserved

for white lesions that show no dyskeratosis on histopathologic examination. These lesions are benign white plaques usually caused by trauma such as cheek biting, irritation of tobacco, sharp margins of carious teeth, ill-fitting dental appliances, or "aspirin burns." Correction of dental abnormalities, good oral hygiene, and avoidance of tobacco are frequently followed by considerable improvement. The chronic cheek chewer is helped by a mouth guard appliance worn at night to prevent chewing while sleeping.

Leukoplakia and Carcinomas

Leukoplakia is a descriptive term meaning "white patch" but usually implies a premalignant condition. Biopsy reveals cellular dysplasia, and this lesion shows a tendency toward malignant transformation into squamous cell carcinoma. Many lesions show marked clearing within 6 weeks after irritating factors are removed. Resistant plaques may be destroyed by cryosurgery. Frequent re-evaluations are important. Any change, especially induration, ulceration, or the development of erythroplasia-like areas, is an indication for additional biopsies. Because leukoplakic lesions of the tongue and floor of the mouth show the greatest potential for malignant transformation, they should be excised promptly.

Early detection of malignancy is important since the survival rate is 70 per cent before lymph node involvement, contrasted with 30 per cent 5 year survival of patients who have nodal disease. Other potential precancers or cancers of the oral cavity that require consideration of biopsy include hyperkeratotic, papillomatous, verrucous lesions; chronic ulcers that do not heal within 2 to 3 weeks; lesions that do not resolve after potential injury is eliminated; tissue enlargement that cannot be attributed to trauma or bacteria; pigmented lesions; cysts; and painful or enlarging bony lesions.

Treatment

Over 95 per cent of intraoral cancers are squamous cell carcinomas. They are treated by two major modalities: surgical excision and radiation therapy, either singly or in combination. These carcinomas grow locally, with invasion spreading along lymphatic channels to regional nodes. Treatment decisions are based on prognosis as predicted by the staging classification "TNM" (Tumor-Node-Metastasis). Side effects of treatment must be considered for each individual patient. Radiation therapy results in xerostomia and stomatitis and is adversely affected when there is bone or muscle involvement. Surgery requires highly skilled surgeons and may result in significant cosmetic and functional disfigurement requiring skilled prosthodontists. Therefore, treatment must be individualized to give the greatest chance of cure with the least morbidity and alteration of function.

In general, smaller tumors are excised, since this may be easiest for the patient. Radiation is reserved for small, posteriorly situated, ill-defined inaccessible tumors and those on the soft, movable mucosa. Medium-sized tumors may be treated surgically if there is a good prosthodontist available or by radiation therapy, which will minimize deformity. Larger cancers probably benefit by combined surgery and radiation. Extensive disease with bone, muscle, and cervical node metastasis has a poor prognosis and is treated by a combination of surgical excision, neck dissection, and radiation. If the lesions are obviously incurable, palliation with radiation, cryosurgery, chemotherapy, and laser excision is achieved with the aim to decrease the size of bulky tumors, relieve pain, facilitate deglutition, and improve respiration. Squamous cell carcinomas of the oral cavity are usually chemoresponsive, although responses are of short duration. Methotrexate is the standard single agent treatment. In most cases, these adjunctive measures are not considered curative for intraoral cancers.

Rehabilitation is enhanced by the use of a prosthesis designed by a maxillofacial prosthodontist. A speech pathologist may assist in speech recovery and swallowing, two of the most important postoperative concerns. If extensive deformities occur, psychological assistance may be required during the first 2 years after surgery, emphasizing the importance of a multidisciplinary approach to oral cancer treatment.

Smoker's Keratosis of the Palate (Leukokeratosis Nicotine Palati)

Enlargement of palatal mucous glands and dilation of their ducts produce papules with a central red spot on a grayish white, wrinkled palatal mucosa. These occur predominantly on the hard palate in pipe smokers. Cessation of smoking leads to gradual resolution of the problem. Another form of papillary hyperplasia of the palate is due to dentures. These papillae may be removed by light curettage with a sharp curette.

Lichen Planus

Lichen planus may resemble leukoplakia with painful erosions and ulcerations, particularly on the buccal mucosa and tongue. To exclude malignancy, a biopsy for histopathologic examination may be helpful. The hyperkeratotic lesions are most likely to remit, whereas atrophic, ulcerative, and bullous lesions seem to persist. Drug-induced lichenoid reactions (gold, thiazide diuretics, antimalarials, and, rarely, phenothiazine, methyldopa, and penicillamine) should be excluded and usually clear when the drug is discontinued.

Treatment

Good oral hygiene, as stressed earlier, should be strongly encouraged for all persons with oral lichen planus. Although there is no cure, several treatments may be satisfactory in relieving symptoms. Only symptomatic lesions need to be treated. When the lesions are painful, a topical steroid in the form of 0.05 per cent fluocinonide (Lidex gel), applied five to six times each day preceded by a mouthwash, may alleviate the discomfort in 7 to 10 days. In severe, localized lesions, intralesional injections of triamcinolone acetonide (5 mg per ml), 0.1 ml per square centimeter of tissue, may be used.

Griseofulvin in doses of 250 mg of the ultramicrosize (Grisactin Ultra, Gris-PEG) two times daily for 6 to 12 weeks is effective in about 50 per cent of cases. (This use of griseofulvin is not listed in the manufacturer's official directive.)

In severe disabling disease, short courses of corticosteroids may be administered orally in a prednisone equivalence of 60 mg each day for 7 days, followed by 30 mg each day for 7 days, and then discontinued. There have been reports of the development of squamous cell carcinoma in longstanding lichen planus, so those persons with chronic disease should be periodically re-examined.

Candidiasis (Thrush)

White plaques may be localized or may involve the intraoral tissues diffusely. They may extend into the esophagus or may affect the corners of the lips, producing maceration and fissures (perleche). To confirm the diagnosis, plaques are removed by scraping and the material is examined microscopically in 10 per cent potassium hydroxide.

Treatment

Dilute hydrogen peroxide mouth rinses will soothe the oral discomfort. Holding 1 teaspoonful of nystatin solution in the mouth for 2 minutes before swallowing, sucking on 1 tablet (500,000 units) of nystatin (Mycostatin) three times daily, or dissolving a lozenge of clotrimazole (Mycelex troche) in the mouth five times each day for 14 days may be used. Lesions in infants and young children may be carefully removed by a cotton applicator dipped into a nystatin suspension (Mycostatin Oral Suspension or Nilstat Oral Suspension). Anticandidal creams such as clotrimazole (Lotrimin, Mycelex), miconazole nitrate (Monistat-Derm), or haloprogin (Halotex) applied under the dentures and at the corners of the mouth (perleche) will be effective. Ketoconazole (Nizoral) in a single daily dose of 200 mg orally for 1 to 2 weeks will clear most cases of oral candidiasis. Ketoconazole is the treatment of choice for the severe disorder but must be given for 6 to 12 months or longer.

Candidiasis is an opportunistic infection and may occur in immunosuppressed patients or may be superimposed on other oral diseases. Failure to improve within 2 weeks or frequent recurrences indicate the need for a general examination of the patient's health.

Fordyce's spots are sebaceous glands that appear clinically as 1 to 3 mm whitish papules on the lips and buccal mucosa. These are asymptomatic and require no treatment except to reassure the patient that the process is neither malignant nor premalignant.

There are several uncommon disorders that may produce white lesions in the mouth. Darier's disease causes whitish "cobblestone" papules on the buccal or palatal mucosa. The lesions in this autosomal dominantly inherited disorder are benign and do not require treatment. Another autosomal dominant disorder is the white sponge nevus. If this benign disorder is suspected, a biopsy should be taken, and the histopathologic examination will reveal thickened mucosa with characteristic features. The lesions are asymptomatic and do not undergo malignant degeneration; therefore, no treatment is indicated. An appreciation of this disorder is important so that it can be differentiated from other white lesions of the oral cavity. Two other rare inherited syndromes are pachyonychia congenita and dyskeratosis congenita. These rare disorders consist of opaque white or grayish white plaques on the dorsum of the tongue or the buccal mucosa along with associated cutaneous features. Oral lesions may become malignant and should be removed surgically if they become irritated, ulcerated, or thickened.

EROSIVE, ULCERATIVE, AND VESICULOBULLOUS LESIONS

A variety of inflammatory diseases may produce vesicles, bullae, erosions, and ulcers in the oral mucosa. Vesicles and bullae are quite friable and are easily eroded in the mouth, producing erosions and ulcers. Diagnosis frequently must be confirmed by histopathologic and/or immunopathologic examination. Tissue situated adjacent to the primary lesion (perilesional tissue) should be studied by biopsy, since this specimen is more likely to provide diagnostic material than is lesional tissue.

Aphthous Stomatitis

This common disorder of multiple, shallow, recurrent, painful ulcerations may be of three types: (1) minor aphthous ulcers, which recur in crops of one to five lesions and are less than 1 cm in diameter each and usually affect the lips, buccal mucosa, mucobuccal and mucolabial sulci, and tongue; (2) major aphthous ulcers, which are greater than 1 cm in diameter, begin as solitary nodules, and subsequently destroy deeper tissue, resulting in scarring that affects the movable oral mucosa and posterior mucosal surfaces; and (3) herpetiform ulcers, which are recurrent, multiple, shallow, pinpoint lesions 1 to 2 mm in diameter that may affect any part of the mucosa. The cause for any of the three types is not known, although autoimmune mechanisms are suspected.

Nutritional deficiencies of vitamin B_{12}, folate, and iron may be present, and persons with these deficiencies may respond to replacement therapy. For most patients, however, treatment for these lesions represents a challenge to both the physician and the patient, and it is therefore necessary to be optimistic and to have a variety of approaches available.

Treatment

Look for correctable causes such as nutritional deficiencies. If there are none, try to reduce any oral trauma. Local cleansing, good oral hygiene, avoidance of irritants, and pain relief measures as discussed previously are fundamental. Patients should avoid sharp-surfaced foods such as peanuts, popcorn, potato chips, and tacos. They should use a soft-bristled toothbrush and brush the teeth carefully, avoiding banging the toothbrush into the buccal mucosa. Efforts should be made to reduce dental trauma by correcting dentures or sharp-edged teeth, and the patient should avoid talking while chewing. During flare-ups of the condition, certain foods such as spices, citrus fruits, and acidic foods that aggravate the lesions should be eliminated from the diet. Specific foods such as chocolate, nuts, and strong cheeses should also be avoided if these are recognized as precipitating bouts of aphthous stomatitis.

If a few lesions are present, 0.1 per cent triamcinolone acetonide in emollient dental paste (Kenalog in Orabase), applied by gently pressing against the mucosa with the fingertip two times each day, is the first choice of treatment and is effective for many patients. Fluocinonide (Lidex Gel) is an alternative.

Escharotics, such as silver nitrate or negatol (Negatan), may be applied in the physician's office to very early lesions and may decrease pain. These agents should not be used for late lesions, however, as they will only increase the amount of tissue necrosis.

Tetracycline in a variety of preparations may be used effectively for aphthous stomatitis. Herpetiform-type ulcers often respond to systemic administration of 10 ml (2 teaspoonsful) of the tetracycline oral suspension (Achromycin V Oral Suspension) swished in the mouth for 1 to 2 minutes four times each day and then swallowed. A 2 week course of this syrup may be repeated as necessary to control recurrences. An elixir made of tetracycline syrup (60 ml), diphenhydramine (60 ml Benadryl Elixir), and fluocinolone acetonide solution (20 ml Synalar) may be used as a mouthwash, 1 teaspoonful three times each day.

A short course of systemic corticosteroids in a prednisone equivalence of 60 mg orally for 7 days followed by 30 mg orally for 7 days, is indicated for patients with continuous or major types of aphthous stomatitis.

Behçet's Syndrome

Behçet described the classic trisymptom complex of recurrent oral ulcers, ocular inflammation, and genital ulcerations. These may be accompanied by a variety of other systemic manifestations. When neurologic deficits are present, the mortality rate is high; therefore, these patients require a general examination and frequent follow-up visits.

Treatment

Colchicine, 0.6 mg two times each day as suppressive therapy, or systemic corticosteroids may be tried and are helpful for individual episodes but do not alter the natural course of the disease. Severe complications have been managed with cytotoxic drugs such as azathioprine, cyclophosphamide, and chlorambucil. (This use of these agents is not listed in the manufacturers' directives.)

Herpes Simplex

Prevention of eliciting factors such as fever, sunburn, windburn, and trauma by photoprotective lip balms (PreSun Lip Protection) should be stressed. Aspirin may be used to reduce fever and inflammation.

Topical zinc sulfate solution (2 per cent) or witch hazel may diminish symptoms. The amino acid lysine (Enisyl) in doses of 1 gram daily may be tried as suppressive therapy for patients with frequent recurrences of herpes simplex. It should be used in conjunction with a diet low in arginine with the avoidance of peas, cereals, peanuts, cashews, beer, colas, chocolates, and gelatin. (This use of Enisyl is not listed in the manufacturer's official directive.)

Acyclovir (Zovirax) (ointment capsules or intravenous infusion) is indicated for herpes simplex infections in immunocompromised patients and in primary herpetic gingivostomatitis.

Erythema Multiforme

Many allergic stimuli have been implicated in precipitating these shallow, painful lip and oral ulcerations. If possible, these agents should be identified and eliminated. For patients with recurrent erythema multiforme due to herpes simplex infections, measures to prevent these infections should be used (see Herpes Simplex). Acyclovir ointment (5 per cent) or capsules (200 mg) every 4 hours for 5 days should be used for recurrent herpes simplex infections as soon as they are noted.

For mild cheilitis, fluocinonide gel 0.05 per cent (Lidex Gel) is applied three to four times daily. Alternatives are white petrolatum (Vaseline) or bacitracin ointment. For painful mucosal erosions, frequent mouthwashes with Cepacol diluted 1:4 with water several times daily are recommended. A soothing mixture of 1:1 Kaopectate plus diphenhydramine elixir (Benadryl) or viscous lidocaine diluted 1:4 with water may alleviate pain if held in the mouth for 2 to 3 minutes. If there is any evidence of secondary infection, erythromycin, 1 gram per day, can be given for several days. Severe lesions are managed with systemic corticosteroids in prednisone equivalence of 60 mg daily until the disease is controlled, at which point drug dosage is slowly reduced over a period of 3 weeks.

Pemphigus and Pemphigoid

Oral lesions (blisters or ulcers) may be the precipitating manifestation in patients who have pemphigus vulgaris. They may also occur in bullous and cicatricial pemphigoid (benign mucous membrane pemphigoid). For histopathologic and direct immunofluorescent studies, biopsies should be taken of any persistent, erosive, ulcerative, or bullous lesions. An early diagnosis will facilitate early treatment and may prevent extensive lesions.

Treatment

Treatment of pemphigus vulgaris and bullous pemphigoid is discussed elsewhere in this text. Cicatricial pemphigoid is a chronic condition but may respond to dapsone in doses of 50 to 150 mg per day. (This use of dapsone is not listed in the manufacturer's official directive.) Acute episodes may respond to short courses of prednisone, 60 mg per day tapered over 3 weeks. Cyclophosphamide (Cytoxan) is reserved for severe cases refractory to the medicines previously listed. Patients with this condition should be followed by an ophthalmologist, since blindness may result.

Other Causes

There are a variety of other causes of oral ulcerations. Mucositis and ulceration constitute significant problems in patients receiving chemotherapy. Soothing mouthwashes and supportive care as discussed previously should be used in these patients. Systemic infections such as blastomycosis, histoplasmosis, cryptococcosis, tuberculosis, syphilis, leprosy, and other chronic infections may present as chronic ulcerative lesions of the mouth. Actinomycosis may form multiple sinus tracts in the skin adjacent to the mouth. Gonorrhea of the oral mucosa presents with a fiery red appearance and scattered white pseudomembranes. Leishmaniasis may cause red, granulating, capillary configurations with ulceration and fibrosis of the mucosa. Treatment is as indicated elsewhere in the text for the specific type of infections. Hand, foot, and mouth diseases caused by the Coxsackie virus may have small red vesicles or ulcers in the oral mucosa that last from 1 to 6 days without specific therapy.

Leukokeratotic, atrophic, inflammatory, erythematous, ulcerative, and hemorrhagic plaques may be seen in both systemic lupus erythematosus and discoid lupus erythematosus, primarily on the buccal and palatal mucosa. Histologic examination and direct immunofluorescent methods will confirm the diagnosis.

Treatment

Symptomatic local therapy as for lichen planus, especially the application of the topical steroid 0.05 per cent fluocinonide (Lidex Gel) five to six times each day, is soothing, but ultimate resolution of lesions depends on systemic control of the lupus erythematosus. Hydroxychloroquine (Plaquenil), 200 mg twice daily, is effective for severe oral involvement. Severe mucosal ulcers may be a component of other multisystem diseases, such as the hypereosinophilic syndrome, neutropenia, ulcerative colitis, or regional enteritis, so virtually any nonhealing mouth ulcer should prompt a general examination.

GINGIVAL AND PERIODONTAL MEMBRANES

Gingival Hyperplasia. Localized enlargement of the gums may be evidence of a periodontal abscess, malignancy, or a hyperplastic growth caused by local irritating factors. Plaque and calculus deposits and faulty dental restorations should be corrected.

Generalized enlargement of the gums may be seen in various inherited conditions as well as in some patients who take phenytoin (Dilantin). Careful dental prophylaxis should begin as soon as phenytoin is started because occurrence of the hyperplasia does not justify cessation of drug therapy. The condition can be managed by removing excessive gingival tissues surgically. Afterward, the construction of a positive pressure mouthguard may reduce the regrowth of tissue.

Diffuse gingival enlargement may also occur with leukemic infiltrates. Hemorrhage is the complicating factor, and surgery is contraindicated in these patients. Gentle cleansing of the teeth with a WaterPik may be helpful in reducing irritation from dental deposits. If hemorrhage occurs, topical hemostatic agents such as Gelfoam may be applied.

Huge granular magenta gingiva and interdental papillae with diffuse petechial markings are characteristic of Wegener's granulomatosis.

Epulides. Epulides are localized "lumps on the gums" and may be of a giant cell or fibrous type.

Or they may be a pyogenic granuloma that results from irritation or inflammatory change on the gingival margin. To exclude malignant processes, histopathologic examination should be carried out.

Removal of the irritant may suffice for treatment. However, a more rapid result is obtained by surgical removal of the hyperplastic and fibrotic tissue.

Gingivitis and Periodontitis. Patients with these common inflammatory reactions involving the supporting structures of the teeth should be promptly referred to the dentist for removal of plaques and calculus to prevent infection of the gingiva and tooth surface.

Acute Necrotizing, Ulcerative Gingivitis (Vincent's Disease, Trenchmouth). This acute bacterial (fusospirochetal) infection is usually localized in the marginal gingival tissue presenting as painful, punched-out erosions in debilitated patients with pre-existing gingival disease. Oral penicillin V, 250 mg four times each day for 4 or 5 days, is the antibiotic of choice. Erythromycin and tetracycline are alternatives. As discussed previously, mouth rinses with warm, dilute hydrogen peroxide should be used for the first few days, and necrotic tissue should be removed by gently swabbing with a cotton swab moistened with hydrogen peroxide. After the acute phase, the patient's dentist should correct any periodontal disease. Smoking is an aggravating factor.

Chronic Desquamative Gingivitis. The cause of this diffuse erythema of the marginal and attached gingiva with desquamation and occasional vesicle formation is obscure. It may be a manifestation of various disorders, such as bullous pemphigoid, cicatricial pemphigoid, or pemphigus vulgaris. A biopsy should be performed to establish an accurate diagnosis with subsequent appropriate systemic disease treatment. If there is no evidence of a systemic problem, then topical medication is often helpful. Regular lavage with soothing washes such as those previously discussed may reduce inflammation, as will the frequent application of a topical steroid such as fluocinonide (Lidex Gel 0.05 per cent) to a dry field. This should be gently massaged into the inflamed area with the fingertips.

Pericoronitis. An inflammatory reaction may develop around erupting third molars (wisdom teeth). These may become infected, and antibiotic treatment is necessary. Removal of the offending tooth or teeth is necessary for relief.

Eruption Cysts. The redness and swelling of the mucosa that may accompany the eruption of teeth may be treated by making an incision in the overlying tissue. Topical anesthetic ointments may be necessary to relieve discomfort in children. Aspirin may also be used for its analgesic effect.

Dental Sinus. A dental sinus may develop from an apical abscess and present near the infected tooth intraorally or in the skin, most commonly on the face below the inferior border on the mandible or in the lateral part of the neck. These findings should prompt consideration of roentgenographic investigation of the dental arches. Treatment involves extraction of the infected tooth and excision of the sinus tract if it fails to heal. Successful root canal procedures often lead to spontaneous resolution of the sinus and its manifestations on the skin.

LESIONS PECULIAR TO THE TONGUE

Geographic Tongue (Glossitis Areata Migrans, Benign Migratory Plaque, Wandering Rash of the Tongue, and Pityriasis Linguae). The cause of this rapid shedding and growing of the papillae on the tongue is not known, although it is occasionally seen in patients with psoriasis or Reiter's disease. The patient may be reassured that this is a harmless, recurrent, self-limited condition that usually requires no therapy. For patients who have associated symptoms of burning and discomfort or who are concerned about the appearance, topical tretinoin 0.05 per cent (Retin A Solution) applied with a cotton swab two times daily for several days may be used, but it is painful. (This use of Retin A is not listed in the manufacturer's official directive.) Soothing measures, such as the use of topical anesthetics and avoidance of excessively hot or spicy food, are recommended.

Scrotal Tongue. This fissuring of the tongue is a congenital anomaly that usually occurs as an isolated finding; however, it is important to consider since it is an occasional occurrence in Down's, Sjögren's, and Melkersson-Rosenthal syndromes. No treatment is required, but local hygienic measures should be encouraged, since these deep, narrow fissures may act as a site of irritation and infection.

Black Hairy Tongue. Elongation and hyperplasia of the filiform papillae of the tongue, discolored brown or black by pigment-producing oral flora, may occur after treatment with antibiotics.

In most instances, brushing the tongue with a soft-bristled toothbrush and hydrogen peroxide solution is satisfactory. Resistant cases may be treated with local anesthesia with viscous lidocaine (Xylocaine), the elongated papillae carefully snipped away with sharp scissors, and the area painted with 15 per cent trichloroacetic acid. Several treatments are usually required. Antibiotics, smoking, chewing tobacco, and all oral irritants should be avoided.

Smooth Tongue. The absence or atrophy of the filiform papillae of the anterior two thirds of the tongue is commonly seen in many nutritional deficiency states such as Plummer-Vinson syndrome, pellagra, and pernicious anemia and the malabsorption state of sprue and celiac disease. Treatment of the underlying process is indicated.

Infection with *Candida* may also lead to atrophy of the filiform papillae. Treatment for this is discussed in the section on white lesions of the mouth.

Macroglossia. A variety of conditions may lead to an enlarged tongue. Tumors, infectious processes, metabolic processes (especially amyloidosis), and conditions such as angioneurotic edema, superior vena cava syndrome, and sarcoidosis should be suspected.

Median Rhomboid Glossitis. A depressed area on the dorsum of the tongue that is red and sharply demarcated from the adjacent white pink papillary surface may be of developmental origin or may represent a response to chronic infection by *Candida*. These lesions respond poorly to topical treatment, but oral ketoconazole may be tried if *Candida* is present. If the lesion does not have the typical appearance sufficient for diagnosis, a biopsy may be done to exclude carcinoma. If chronic irritation becomes a problem, surgical excision of the rhomboid lesion may be performed.

OTHER PAINFUL LESIONS OF THE MOUTH

Sore mouth may be an idiopathic condition or may be caused by ill-fitting dentures, drug reaction, irritant or allergic reaction, nutritional deficiency, or a psychoneurotic state. A specific diagnosis is often difficult, but an investigation should be carried out to exclude organic causes.

Glossodynia. The condition of a painful, burning tongue is usually idiopathic and occurs almost exclusively in middle-aged and elderly women with a normal-appearing tongue. It is generally attributed to a psychoneurotic condition. However, the disease is not limited to this population.

A diagnostic investigation should consider organic causes such as diabetes mellitus; pernicious anemia; deficiencies of folic acid, zinc, and iron; xerostomia; denture sore mouth; candidiasis; stomatitis medicamentosa; trigeminal neuralgia; vascular thrombosis; and hypoestrogenism. These "secondary" glossodynias frequently have an associated abnormal morphology of the tongue or symptoms such as loss or perversion of the sense of taste. If no organic cause is found, then the patient should be reassured that the problem is not malignant or serious. If this is not acceptable, amitryptyline hydrochloride (Elavil) may be used. Good dental hygiene and adequate nutrition should be maintained. Occasionally, psychiatric consultation is indicated.

Contact Stomatitis. The mucous membranes are less susceptible to irritant and allergic sensitization than is the skin. Removal of the offending agent is ideal, but frequently it is difficult to identify. A wide variety of contactants must be suspected with the hope that careful history and clinical examination will identify the source of the problem. Routine patch testing is occasionally helpful.

Elimination of potential irritants such as aspirin, strong mouthwashes, hot, spicy, and citrus foods, commercial dentifrices, chewing gum, candy, and lozenges is necessary. Cheilitis may be treated with cool tap water compresses and the application of a topical fluorinated steroid (such as Lidex Gel 0.05 per cent) and protective ointments. Gargling with 5 ml of diphenhydramine (Benadryl Elixir) may give symptomatic relief.

The condition of atypical gingivostomatitis, which presents with fire engine red gingiva, is frequently caused by gum chewing. Elimination of gum chewing will frequently result in resolution of this problem.

Denture Sore Mouth. This condition is most common in postmenopausal women and is attributed to bone loss in the jaw, which alters the fit of dentures. It is frequently compounded by *Candida* infections. Removal of the dentures every night and application of an anticandidal cream such as haloprogen (Halotex 1 per cent) to the oral mucosa and denture itself is often helpful. Construction of a new denture may be necessary.

Drugs are frequently associated with alterations in the mucosa and may cause sore mouth. Gingival hyperplasia may occur in patients using phenytoin (Dilantin); mouth ulcers may result from cytotoxic drugs; antibiotics can cause a black hairy tongue or overgrowth of *Candida*; gold or penicillamine therapy may produce a lichen planus–like stomatitis under the tongue; local burns may be produced by aspirin; and a variety of drugs may cause xerostomia.

Oral Burns. Mild thermal, electrical, and chemical burns of the lips, tongue, and palate are usually minor and heal uneventfully in 1 week. Use of one of the local anesthetic preparations previously discussed will relieve pain and promote healing.

Xerostomia. Dryness of the mouth is a sign of impaired salivary gland function and may be temporary or permanent. Transient causes include emotional stress, drugs such as anticholinergic compounds and antihistamines, excessive mouth breathing, and sialolithiasis. There is atrophy of the salivary gland with age and following radiation therapy to the head and neck. These changes are irreversible. If none of these are apparent or if keratoconjunctivitis sicca is present, then a general evaluation should be performed to look for systemic disorders such as Sjögren's syndrome, scleroderma, rheumatoid arthritis, diabetes mellitus, lupus erythematosus, sarcoidosis, paraproteinemias, and malignancies.

Treatment of xerostomia is difficult. If the cause is a drug, it may not be practical to withdraw the patient from the medication. If the problem is salivary gland atrophy, then there is no effective way to increase saliva production, although chewing sugarless gum may stimulate saliva flow. Symptomatic relief may be obtained by frequent sips of water or a saliva substitute (XeroLube, Scherer Laboratories).

Dental caries often occurs rapidly in patients with xerostomia; therefore, good oral hygiene, prompt referral to a dentist, and intermittent fluoride treatments are necessary.

OTHER BENIGN TUMORS

Melanocytic Nevi. Pigmented nevi of all types may be seen in the mucosa, including lentigos and blue, junctional, compound, and dermal nevi. Excision to exclude the possibility of melanoma is appropriate treatment.

Occasionally, bluish brown macules located on the posterior gingiva and adjacent buccal mucosa (amalgam tattoos), which represent the submucosal inclusion of amalgam particles inoculated traumatically, may be mistaken for melanocytic nevi. These metallic particles may be identified by softer tissue x-ray films, and no treatment is indicated.

Oral Pigmentation. Other oral pigmentary problems of systemic importance include those resulting from heavy metal exposure (bismuth and mercury cause black lines at the gingival margin, and lead and silver leave a diffuse grayish color on the gingiva), ingestion of antimalarial agents or phenothiazine, Addison's disease, hemochromatosis, neurofibromatosis, and Peutz-Jeghers syndrome. If there is any evidence of these disorders, the patient should undergo a general evaluation. Physiologic, asymptomatic pigmentation is common in the oral mucosa of black patients.

Mucocele. Mucous cysts are most commonly located on the lower lip and represent the reaction of oral mucous glands to obstruction of the duct carrying the mucoid secretion to the mucosal surface. They may be produced by trauma or infection. Because these usually lack a true cyst wall, excision may result in the development of further cystic lesions, since healing may obliterate other ducts in the area that were severed in the surgical procedure.

An alternative form of therapy is cryosurgery with a liquid nitrogen probe, although this may require more than one treatment. Persistent lesions may be incised and the enlarged glandular tissue carefully teased and squeezed out through the opening. The base should not be desiccated, since this may promote recurrence.

Fibromas and Papillomas. These pedunculated, fibrous, and benign epithelial neoplasms may occur anywhere in the mucosa and may be removed by simple excision.

Warts. Verruca vulgaris and condyloma acuminata may occur on the vermilion border or the oral mucosa. Simple excision may be carried out and histologic studies performed if there is any possibility of verrucous carcinoma. Light electrodesiccation and curettage under local anesthesia are usually successful. Local application of 20 per cent podophyllin in tincture of benzoin to a few lesions weekly or cryosurgery with a liquid nitrogen probe may give excellent results. Areas of treatment should not be sutured, since this may deposit the virus along the suture tract and result in additional lesions.

It should be remembered that these are intraepithelial growths and that deep, destructive measures are not warranted. Multiple verrucae on the lips and oral mucosa should raise the suspicion of Cowden's syndrome.

Torus Palatinus and Mandibularis. These are benign, simple bony growths on the hard palate or lingual surface of the mandible. Surgical removal may be performed when a prosthetic appliance is necessary.

OTHER MALIGNANT TUMORS

The majority of oral cancers are squamous cell carcinomas (over 95 per cent). Most others are adenocarcinomas arising from minor salivary glands. Definitive treatment is surgical. These are radioresponsive but probably not radiocurable. Melanomas are rare and usually advanced when diagnosed and are treated by radical excision. Other unusual primary oral tumors include lymphoma, fibrosarcoma, rhabdomyosarcoma, liposarcoma, neurofibrosarcoma, angiosarcoma, and Kaposi's sarcoma. Basal cell carcinoma may occasionally involve the mucosa of the lip as an extension from the skin surface. Mucosal basal cell carcinoma is probably an extraosseous ameloblastoma. Therapy is dependent upon the histologic differentiation, location, and size of tumor. One per cent of oral malignancies are metastatic from the breast, lungs, kidney, thyroid, prostate, and, occasionally, other sites. Most occur in the mandible and are usually asymptomatic. Current therapeutic modalities are insufficient, and the prognosis of these patients is generally poor.

STASIS AND OTHER SKIN ULCERS

method of
HENRY H. ROENIGK, JR., M.D.
Northwestern University
Chicago, Illinois

Ulceration of the lower extremities is a common medical problem, which may be caused by a wide variety of processes. In many cases systemic disease is present in the patient with a leg ulcer and can affect the ability of the ulcer to heal. Table 1 lists many of the disorders that may cause or complicate a leg ulcer.

TABLE 1. **Classification of Leg Ulcers**

Vascular Disorders	Metabolic Disorders
Arterial	Diabetic ulcer
Thromboangiitis obliterans	Necrobiosis lipoidica diabeticorum
Arteriosclerosis obliterans	Pyoderma gangrenosum
Livedo reticularis	Gaucher's disease
Hypertension	Gout
Chronic pernio (chilblains)	Porphyria cutanea tarda
Venous (chronic venous insufficiency)	Tumors
Lymphatic (elephantiasis nostras, lymphedema)	Basal cell carcinoma
Vasculitis	Squamous cell carcinoma
Atrophie blanche	Kaposi's hemorrhagic sarcoma
Allergic vasculitis	Lymphoma
Lupus erythematosus	Lymphosarcoma
Necrotizing angiitis	Mycosis fungoides
Periarteritis nodosa	Malignant melanoma
Rheumatoid arthritis	Miscellaneous
Degos' disease	Drugs
Hematologic Disorders	Halogens
Sickle cell anemia	Ergot
Spherocytic anemia	Methotrexate
Thalassemia	Chemical burns
Polycythemia vera	Trophic injury
Leukemia	Thermal injury
Dysproteinemia	Lichen planus
Infections	Weber-Christian disease
Fungal	Acrodermatitis chronica atrophicans
Blastomycosis	Insect bite
Coccidioidomycosis	Radiation
Histoplasmosis	Frostbite
Sporotrichosis	Factitial (self-induced injury)
Maduromycosis	
Syphilis	
Bacterial infections	
Tuberculosis	
Erythema induration	
Lupus vulgaris	
Papulonecrotic tuberculid	

Vascular Disorders

Arteriosclerosis Obliterans. See Peripheral Arterial Disease, Section 4.

Venous Insufficiency. Ulcerations usually occur in the region of the ankle near the internal malleolus and may develop spontaneously or secondary to trauma. Aseptic cellulitis may develop in surrounding skin. The base of the ulcer is usually moist, with extensive granulation tissue, and is often secondarily infected. The ulcers may be painful but, in contrast to ulcers caused by arteriosclerosis obliterans, are often relieved by rest and elevations of the extremity.

Hypertension. Chronic ischemic ulcers of the lower extremities may develop in patients who have had essential hypertension of long duration. Women in their fifth or sixth decades are most commonly affected, although ulcers occur in men. The ulcer usually starts as a painful, reddish-blue plaque over the lateral malleolus. The plaque ulcerates and is surrounded by a cyanotic or purpuric halo. The ulcer usually has little granulation tissue and is very painful. Control of essential hypertension is vital in the treatment of these ulcers.

Vasculitis

Cutaneous lesions of vasculitis vary from erythematous macules, purpura, hemorrhagic vesicles, urticarial lesions, nodular and eventually necrotic lesions, and ulcerations. The skin is easily accessible for biopsy, and this often will confirm the diagnosis of vasculitis. The histopathologic changes seen in skin biopsy specimens reveal swelling and degeneration of the endothelial cells of the blood vessels, thickening of the vessel walls, and a fibrinoid degeneration of the perivascular tissue. A severe inflammatory infiltrate composed of mostly polymorphic neutophils and eosinophils with some lymphyocytes is often seen. The most common finding in acute vasculitis of the skin is leukocytoclasis or nuclear dust. This classic feature of vasculitis is the result of fragmentation of nuclear material from surrounding inflammatory cells. Other laboratory studies that may help confirm a more generalized type of vasculitis include blood hemoglobin, leukocyte count, erythrocyte sedimentation rate, antinuclear factor, renal function studies, hepatitis B antigen, cryoglobulins, and rheumatoid factor.

Treatment. The treatment of vasculitic ulcerations of the lower extremities involves treatment of the systemic disease producing the vasculitis. This may include administering antibiotics for an underlying infection, stopping a course of medications (hypersensitivity reaction), or administering a systemic steroid, as in systemic lupus erythematosus. Stronger immunosuppressive agents, such as cyclophosphamide or azathioprine, are sometimes needed to control the vasculitis.

Hematologic Disorders

Various types of hematologic disorders will result in ulceration of the lower extremities. Sickle cell anemia, a genetically transmitted abnormality that results in an abnormal hemoglobin molecule in homozygous persons, is found almost entirely in the black race. The cutaneous manifestations of sickle cell anemia are indolent ulcers or scars on the lower parts of the legs, which develop in about 75 per cent of older children or adults with the disease. The ulcers, which have sharply defined edges, are usually single but may be multiple and bilateral. There is no distinctive feature of this ulcer, but in a young black patient with no other obvious cause of the ulcer, sickle cell anemia and the sickling phenomenon can be demonstrated in a moist, sealed, coverslip preparation.

Hereditary spherocytosis may produce ulceration of the lower extremities. Chronic ulcers of the leg in the region of the malleoli are reported to occur in 6 per cent of patients. The ulcers are usually several centimeters in diameter and are surrounded by an area of hyperpigmentation. Increased fragility of erythrocytes in hypotonic saline solution has been recognized as a characteristic feature of hereditary spherocytosis.

Other hematologic disorders that rarely produce leg ulcers are listed in Table 1.

Infectious Diseases

Deep Fungal Infections. These are produced as two distinct types. The rarer form, the chancriform syndrome, is an example of primary cutaneous inoculation. This form of the disease most commonly follows trauma to the skin, with an introduction of the pathogenic organisms into the tissue. An area of erythema and induration develops at the site of inoculation. In 1 to 2 weeks, a chancre appears with subsequent lymphangitis and lymphedema of the involved limb.

The common forms of the deep fungal infections are those associated with systemic involvement. The appearance of the lesion is usually a papular, pustular nodule that enlarges peripherally to form an elevated, ulcerated, verrucous granuloma. The greatest activity of infection occurs at the periphery, which is clearly demarcated from normal skin.

The deep fungal infections that most commonly produce a lower extremity ulceration are listed in Table 1.

Syphilis. Syphilitic gumma, a late form of syphilis, develops as a deep subcutaneous fixed nodule or plaque that may be singular or multiple. Clinically, it appears as a firm, well-defined, painless, indolent nodule or plaque. The lesions often ulcerate or extrude a thick, sanguineous secretion. The ulcers are clearly demarcated, deep, and have a purulent base. The ulcer heals from the base and leaves a contracted scar.

Bacteria-Infected Ulcers. Peripheral vascular ulcers of the leg often become secondarily infected and produce an increased inflammation of the ulcer and surrounding tissue. The clinical signs are erythema, edema, and purulent exudate or a heavy eschar with pronounced peripheral inflammation. These ulcers respond to local antiseptic agents and topical or systemic antibiotics, depending on the degree of inflammation and the size of the ulcer. Appropriate cultures and antibody sensitivity tests are indicated.

Tuberculosis. Lupus vulgaris of the lower extremities appears as a well-demarcated, reddish-brown patch or patches containing small papules. The papules show a yellowish-brown color when the glass slide is pressed against them in diascopic examination. These yellow lesions gradually become atrophic and show multiple areas of ulceration; occasionally the borders develop a verrucal growth. Squamous cell carcinomas can occur in these chronic lesions. A biopsy shows a typical tubercle with moderate caseation in the upper dermis. Acid-fast stains reveal the presence of small numbers of tubercle bacilli.

Metabolic Disorders

Necrobiosis Lipoidica Diabeticorum. Plaquelike lesions that occur over the anterior surface of the leg and are reddish-yellow with a smooth glistening surface and numerous telangiectasias are often a clue to underlying diabetes mellitus. Necrobiosis lipoidica diabeticorum (NLD) presents these distinctive clinical features, which can be confirmed by skin biopsy.

Occasionally, as a result of minor trauma, the lesions of NLD will become ulcerated. Treatment with topical antibiotics and Unna boot often results in re-epithelialization of the lesions. When the ulceration is extensive, split-thickness skin grafting may be necessary.

Pyoderma Gangrenosum. Acute necrotizing ulcerations of the lower extremity that have a rolled vegetating border are suggestive of pyoderma gangrenosum. The skin lesions usually begin as erythematous papulonodules that enlarge rapidly into plaques up to 12 or more cm in diameter. The active border is deeply violaceous, and the central portion is necrotic and ulcerated. A halo of erythema surrounds the lesion. Lesions of pyoderma gangrenosum are often extremely painful and, although they usually occur on the lower part of the leg, they may occur anywhere on the skin.

Although pyoderma gangrenosum at one time was considered pathognomonic of an underlying chronic ulcerative colitis, today other conditions such as regional enteritis, myelogenous leukemia, empyema, and rheumatoid arthritis may be associated with it. Therapy is directed primarily at the underlying systemic disorder. When the chronic ulcerative colitis is active, treatment with salicylazosulfapyridine, adrenocorticotropic hormone, or corticosteroids usually results in prompt healing of the ulcerations.

Tumors

Frequently the presenting signs of benign and malignant tumors (see Table 1) are ulcerations of the lower extremities. In each case, the diagnostic skin biopsy is essential to the correct diagnosis and thus early appropriate treatment.

Decubitus Ulcer

These areas of tissue necrosis and erythema develop in skin and subcutaneous tissue over areas of bony prominences. They are usually the result of ischemia of tissue from external pressure, friction, or prolonged lying in bed with fecal or urinary material left on skin as an irritant. These areas of necrosis are then susceptible to infection, causing more tissue damage.

The most common locations for decubitus ulcers are the sacrum, greater trochanters, ischial tuberosities, knees, tibial crest, malleoli, heels, iliac spines, spinous processes, and elbows.

The quality of nursing care of the patient's general health, nutrition, and ability to ambulate are important factors in the development of decubitus ulcers.

Poor nutrition, associated with anemia, hypoproteinemia, and vitamin deficiency, as well as motor paralysis accompanied by muscle atrophy, superficial sensory loss with absence of awareness of pain or pressure, reduction of fatty tissue between the skin and underlying bone, and disturbed vasomotor function are conditions that greatly predispose the patient to the formation of decubitus ulcers. Also at great risk are bedridden obese or mentally disturbed patients who fail to change their body positions frequently or refuse to cooperate with the nursing care.

The treatment of decubitus ulcers is similar to the treatment of all other ulcers. It is necessary, however, to pay more attention to the nursing care, nutrition, and physical therapy of the patients.

Miscellaneous Disorders

Among the large group of miscellaneous causes of leg ulcers, probably the most fascinating are factitial or self-induced ulcerations. They are not confined to the lower extremity but are found in areas easily accessible to the patient. Bizarre ulcers are produced by chemicals, cigarettes, syringes, and other devices used by psychotic patients. A feature that may serve as a clinical clue is the presence of square or angulated borders of the ulcer.

Management of Leg Ulcers

The goal of treatment of all leg ulcers is to stimulate good granulation tissue and restore epithelial regrowth. General measures include clearing the surrounding skin (stasis eczema) with use of compresses, topical corticosteroids, and, occasionally, topical antibiotics. Bed rest and reduction of edema speed healing. In ulcers caused by arteriosclerosis obliterans, bed rest is helpful, but the head of the bed should be elevated.

Local treatment of the ulcer is important in clearing the infection and in stimulating granulation tissue that can accept either an entire skin graft or epithelial regrowth from the borders of the ulcer.

Topical enzymes and antibiotics are often used to debride leg ulcers. Another excellent method of local debridement is to apply topical viscous lidocaine (Xylocaine) and use a small sharp curette to remove the moist eschar that adheres to the granulation tissue and inhibits re-epithelialization of the ulcer. Occasionally a forceps and small scissors can be used to cut away thicker eschar that cannot be removed by the curette.

Benzoyl Peroxide. This potent oxidizing agent, widely used in treating acne vulgaris, has been reported to give an excellent result in promoting granulation tissue in ulcers.

A piece of terry cloth cut in the exact shape of the ulcer is moistened with normal saline solution, impregnated with 20 per cent benzoyl peroxide lotion (investigational, but 10 per cent lotion may be substituted), and applied to the ulcer. The normal skin margins of the ulcer are protected with petrolatum, and the padded ulcer is then occluded with plastic wrap. The dressings are changed every 8 to 12 hours. Excessive granulation tissue at epithelial borders may be cauterized with 10 per cent silver nitrate solution. Benzoyl peroxide probably acts by providing bactericidal action, stimulating granulation tissue, and producing hyperbaric oxygen and debridement.

Initially there is some local pain and irritation, but soon the infection starts to clear and the rolled borders of the leg ulcer will flatten and begin good re-epithelialization. Excessive granulation tissue at epithelial borders may be cauterized with 10 per cent silver nitrate solution.

Dextran Polymer Beads. The treatment of leg ulcers with Debrisan consists of applying to the ulcer a thick layer of a three-dimensional network of porous dextran polymer beads 0.1 to 0.3 mm in diameter. The beads are highly hydrophilic and absorb fluid until saturated, swelling in the process. When placed on the discharging ulcer surface, the beads promptly absorb the exudate, bacteria, and tissue degradation residues from the ulcer surface. The dextran polymer beads are pharmacologically inert, and their action is entirely physical. By absorbing the protein-rich fluids from the ulcer surface, they prevent crust formation, greatly reduce the bacterial load on the ulcer surface, and remove inflammatory mediators and toxins produced by bacteria, allowing more vigorous cell metabolism in the ulcer base. They can cause excessive drying of granulation tissue and, therefore, are generally stopped after infection is cleared and healthy granulation tissue begins to appear.

Unna Boot. The Unna paste boot is a flesh-colored roll bandage impregnated with a uniformly spread paste of zinc oxide, calamine, glycerine, and a gelatin. Before the boot is applied, the leg is cleansed with lukewarm water or mineral oil to remove debris and any previous medication. Gentian violet is applied directly to the ulcer. A fluocinolone acetonide ointment or a topical antibiotic is then applied to the surrounding skin if there is stasis dermatitis. The Unna boot is applied from the foot to an area just below the popliteal space. The foot should be kept at a right angle to minimize chafing.

The bandage is placed around the foot, then directly obliquely over the heel and up the calf in much the same manner as an elastic bandage is applied. It should be applied in a "pressure gradient manner," with the greatest pressure at the ankle and lower third of the leg. A double layer of Tubegauze is placed over the Unna boot and secured at the upper and lower limits with tape. The Unna boot is changed weekly or more often if there is excessive drainage through the boot or if the boot becomes loose due to reduction of edema.

The Unna boot is ideal for stasis ulcers and stasis eczema, but it also can be used with a variety of other ulcers since it helps remove edema and protects the ulcer from external trauma. The patient may be ambulatory while wearing the Unna boot.

New Wound Dressings. In the past few years new dressings have been developed which do more than just cover the wound and keep it clean. These occlusive or semiocclusive dressings vary in the degree of debridement, cleansing, and wound granulation that speed the healing process. It is well accepted that epithelial migration occurs more readily in a moist environment such as that created by occlusive dressings. Some examples are Op-Site, Tegaderm (polyurethane), Bioclusive, Vigilon (polyethylene oxdihydrogel with polyethylene film backing, thicker hydrogel films on both sides, and gel in the middle), and DuoDerm (hydrocolloid material surrounded by an inert, hydrophobic polymer that is adhesive).

Most of these dressings, except DuoDerm and Vigilon, will transport water, and all except DuoDerm will transport oxygen. They all absorb bacteria, except Vigilon, and only DuoDerm is not transparent. All except Vigilon are self-adhesive to the skin. There is excessive accumulation of fluid under some of these dressings, especially Op-Site. There can be exacerbation of infection and cellulitis if these dressings are used on an infected leg ulcer. They are best used when all infection is cleared and there is good granulation tissue and re-epithelialization is sought. They are also useful in conjunction with skin grafts.

The final goal in the treatment of all leg ulcers is to provide adequate skin coverage of the ulcer. Conservative methods may stimulate granulation tissue, with regrowth of epithelial tissue from the borders of the healing ulcer, but healing by this method is not always satisfactory, since the epithelium may be fragile and ulceration can recur.

Surgical Treatment

The underlying etiologic factors—such as venous or arterial insufficiency and hypertension—must be determined because, in general, skin grafting will not take well if the arterial blood supply is poor.

It is not necessary to keep the patient in bed for many weeks to achieve good healing of a leg ulcer by secondary intention or re-epithelialization from the edges of the ulcer. Once there is good granulation tissue, a skin graft can be considered to speed up the recovery time for the patient.

Excision of Ulcer and Grafting. Ulcers that have poor granulation tissue, necrotic or fibrotic tissue at the borders, and no signs of epithelial ingrowth can be completely excised. If a split-thickness skin graft, usually taken from the thigh or buttocks, is placed on this area, it will take readily, and fibrosis of the recipient site does not occur because of the immediate coverage. Skin grafts over such areas are soft and supple.

Rotational Flaps and Pedicles. When bone and periosteum have been damaged by superimposed infection or areas of little subcutaneous support (anterior tibial surface), split-thickness skin grafts will not take, and full-thickness skin and subcutaneous tissue with a vascularized pedicle must be provided. Small advancement flaps to poorly healing ulcers, especially over the anterior tibia, are good examples of the use of this procedure.

Pinch Grafts. Small pinch grafts (4 mm) taken from the thigh can be used to cover a good granulation base of an ulcer that is not infected. This will cause the ulcer to heal more rapidly and stimulate re-epithelialization even in the areas where the pinch grafts do not take completely.

The donor site is properly cleansed and the skin is marked with gentian violet. The areas are anesthetized with 1 per cent Xylocaine. A 25 gauge needle is used to tent up the skin and then a No. 15 scalpel blade or a sterilized single-edge razor blade is used to cut off a 4 to 5 mm split-thickness graft. There should be some dermis but no fat on the grafts. These grafts are then placed in a Petri dish with sterile saline. The recipient site is properly prepared, and a curette is used to stimulate bleeding. The pinch grafts are laid onto the granulation base. The ulcer is sprayed with Skin Prep, a spray adhesive dressing, and a topical antibiotic, a Telfa dressing or Op-Site, and a pressure bandage are applied. The dressing is left in place for at least 4 days unless there are signs of infection or pain in the area of the grafting. Op-Site has the advantage of being clear and thus allowing observation of the wound for signs of infection daily without actually disturbing the grafts. If excessive purulent discharge is seen, the dressing should be changed. The donor sites can be sutured closed or just left to heal by secondary intention. After the dressing is removed from the grafted area, careful postoperative care is needed, since the grafts usually are not secure for several more days. Careful cleansing with 70 per cent alcohol and allowing the area to remain open will help improve the postoperative results from pinch grafts.

ATOPIC DERMATITIS

method of
JOHN W. P. TOOLE, M.D.
University of Manitoba
Winnipeg, Manitoba

Atopic dermatitis is characterized by early age of onset, chronicity, and pruritus. This combination produces frustration in patients and their parents.

Once the diagnosis is made, a thorough discussion of the natural history of the disease and the goals and limitations of therapy should be undertaken. The majority of patients experience improvement or resolution of their disease by adolescence, and this should be pointed out. One should explain that the goal of therapy is to relieve the symptoms of the disease and prevent secondary infection. Finally patients must realize that the therapy is effective only when used, is expensive, and is not a cure. Patients and their parents who understand the goals of therapy and the limitations are likely to be more compliant.

The skin of patients with atopic dermatitis is particularly susceptible to irritants. Patients should be advised to avoid or minimize exposure to solvents, wool, nylon, harsh detergents, fabric softeners, and highly scented cosmetic products and soaps. Choice of hobbies and future occupations might be discussed in this regard as well.

Treatment

The majority of patients with atopic dermatitis have dry skin, which aggravates their dermatitis. Most patients will improve when the hydration of the skin improves. Frequent bathing is helpful in this regard. It is important to define bathing specifically. I advise patients to soak in a tub of tepid water with one-quarter cup of oilated Aveeno powder and no soap for 20 minutes daily. Immediately following the bath I suggest a general application of Dermabase and white petrolatum, mixed in equal parts, applied to moist skin. Frequent showers and short soapy baths should be avoided.

The role of diet in atopic dermatitis is controversial. The majority of patients show little or no clinical response to dietary restriction. When parents notice a repeated and consistent flare in the dermatitis on ingestion of a specific food, it is reasonable to eliminate the food. Restrictive diets formulated on an empirical basis are not justified.

The skin of patients with atopic dermatitis is particularly susceptible to colonization by virus. Exposure to herpes simplex and vaccinia virus should be avoided.

Specific therapy of the eczema itself involves the efficient use of topical steroids. Most patients will require repeated applications over a number of years; hence it is important that these products be used efficiently to minimize side effects.

I prefer to initiate therapy with less potent steroids, such as hydrocortisone 1.0 per cent cream applied to the involved skin three times daily. Treatment of facial and flexural skin should be limited to hydrocortisone 1.0 per cent.

In situations in which the eczema fails to respond to 1.0 per cent hydrocortisone, I favor the use of betamethasone valerate cream (Valisone). This product is available in strengths ranging from 0.1 per cent to 0.01 per cent. Intermediate strengths can be dispensed by dilution with a cream base. The weakest effective strength should be used. I find it most effective to have the creams applied three times daily to affected skin for several days, then tapered off completely when the eczema is in remission.

Patients, particularly children, requiring large amounts of cream for prolonged periods should be checked regularly for striae, cataracts, and the stigmata of Cushing's syndrome.

In the acute exudative stages of the disease, cool compresses of aluminum sulfate (Domeboro) aqueous solution 1:40 to the affected skin three times daily will be of more value than the topical steroids.

Antihistamines are of value in relieving pruritus and producing sedation. I prescribe hydroxyzine (Atarax) tablets or suspension at bedtime when sleep is being disrupted by pruritus.

Secondary bacterial infections are common in atopic dermatitis. These infections are best treated systemically. After swabs for culture I prescribe erythromycin (Erythrocin) for a 7-day course.

On follow-up visits it is important to adjust the amount and potency of topical steroids, alter any changes in habit or environment that may be aggravating the dermatitis, and treat secondary infection.

THE ERYTHEMAS

method of
ROBERT G. CARNEY, Jr., M.D.
Decatur, Illinois

The erythemas are a group of dermatoses that are diverse in their frequency, characteristics, and age of onset but seem to have the common denominators of causing pink to red eruptions and representing hypersensitivity reactions to a variety of agents.

Erythema Multiforme

This is the most common of the erythemas. It may occur at any age, although children are frequently afflicted with the more severe forms. The reaction occurs about three times more commonly in boys.

The eruption of erythema multiforme may involve erythematous macules, urticarial plaques, and even nodules. The classic lesion is a centrifugally enlarging "target" or "iris" lesion, often involving more than one concentric ring. More severe forms show central vesicle or bulla formation, often with hemorrhage.

Erythema multiforme may affect both skin and mucous membranes. The oral and other mucosae are usually severely affected in the major form, commonly called the Stevens-Johnson syndrome. In this form, bullous erythema multiforme can cause permanent damage or even death.

The reaction pattern of erythema multiforme may be induced by a wide variety of agents. The most common are herpes simplex virus and mycoplasma infections, especially "primary atypical pneumonia." Other infections, malignancies, pregnancy, collagen vascular diseases, sarcoidosis, and many drugs can induce erythema multiforme, although in perhaps half of patients the cause cannot be found.

Treatment. Mild eruptions should be treated symptomatically. Cool compresses, calamine lotion, and other soothing preparations are helpful. Antihistamines are often useful in mild to moderate forms of erythema multiforme. Feel free to change antihistamine daily until one is found that stops pruritus without causing drowsiness or hyperactivity.

More severe reactions with mucous membrane involvement may require parenteral fluids and medications if the patient is unable to eat or drink. Mucous membranes can be moisturized with antibiotic ointment to prevent dryness and soreness and, of course, secondary infection. This is particularly important in the eyes, since blindness has been known to occur.

The use of systemic steroids, such as intravenous hydrocortisone 100 mg every 8 hours or oral prednisone 60 to 80 mg daily in divided doses, is helpful in giving symptomatic relief but may not alter the course of the disease. Doses, which occasionally must be higher, can usually be reduced over 2 to 4 weeks. Oral or parenteral antibiotics should be used if there is evidence of bacterial intervention.

When recurrences of bullous erythema multiforme are caused by repeated episodes of herpes simplex, Zovirax ointment or capsules have been advocated. This may not reduce recurrences of herpes simplex enough to stop erythema multiforme reactions, but it is probably not harmful, if the usual treatment schedule is followed.

Erythema Nodosum

Erythema nodosum is a second fairly common immunologic reaction pattern to a rather varied group of inducing agents. The most frequent causes are streptococcal infections, sarcoidosis, tuberculosis, viral and fungal infections, and drugs, notably sulfonamides and oral contraceptives. Erythema nodosum is perhaps six times more common in women.

The eruption of erythema nodosum occurs mainly on the anterior shins with occasional spread to the thighs and forearms. The lesions are tender, dusky erythematous nodules involving both skin and subcutaneous tissues. The clinical diagnosis is usually not difficult.

Treatment. Erythema nodosum is generally a self-limiting reaction, lasting 3 to 6 weeks. Thus bed rest and mild analgesics are normally all that are required. Discovery and treatment of the cause of the condition are important to help prevent recurrences. Moreover, infectious causes must be eliminated if systemic corticosteroid therapy is being considered in a severe case. Start prednisone at 40 to 60 mg daily in divided doses, then taper over about 2 weeks.

Fixed Erythemas

The fixed erythemas include several reactions whose appearance is similar to that of erythema multiforme. However, the lesions often last much longer, sometimes weeks to months, and grow into larger rings and other polycyclic shapes. The most common, erythema annulare centrifugum, has a list of causes very similar to that of erythema multiforme, with the notable addition of carcinomata and blood dyscrasias. Erythema chronicum migrans is usually a solitary, tick bite–induced reaction. The causative agent is often a rickettsial infection and has recently been associated with the spirochetal "Lyme arthritis." Erythema marginatum often accompanies rheumatic fever or juvenile rheumatoid arthritis. The lesions have a distinctive narrow active border. The eruption usually lasts from several hours to days but may recur.

Treatment. Erythema annulare centrifugum and erythema marginatum usually are asymptomatic and require no treatment. When erythema chronicum migrans is diagnosed, it is important to discover the causative agent, since treatment with tetracycline or penicillin is rapidly curative.

BULLOUS DISEASES

method of
RONALD P. RAPINI, M.D.,
and ROBERT E. JORDON, M.D.
University of Texas
Houston, Texas

This section discusses three of the bullous diseases: dermatitis herpetiformis, pemphigus, and pemphigoid. Dermatitis herpetiformis (DH) has a peak incidence in the third to fourth decade. Pemphigus most commonly presents in the fourth to fifth decade, and pemphigoid usually affects individuals in the sixth to eighth decade. Dermatitis herpetiformis usually presents as grouped ("herpetiform"), very pruritic papules and vesicles on the sacral area, shoulders, scalp, and extensor surfaces of the extremities. Patients usually have a mild, asymptomatic gluten-sensitive enteropathy.

Pemphigus is divided into two major types, each with a variant. Pemphigus vulgaris produces flaccid vesicles or bullae that result in crusted, weeping, or denuded areas of skin. Mucous membrane involvement is extremely common. A rare variant, pemphigus vegetans, produces vegetating lesions, especially on the lips or in intertriginous areas. Pemphigus foliaceus represents a more superficial, less severe disease. Erosions and eczematous patches are usually more prevalent than vesicles or bullae. Pemphigus erythematosus is a variant of pemphigus foliaceus that shows clinical features suggesting lupus erythematosus.

The pemphigoid group of diseases includes bullous pemphigoid, cicatricial pemphigoid ("benign" mucous membrane pemphigoid), localized scarring pemphigoid (Brunsting-Perry), and pemphigoid gestationis ("herpes" gestationis). In bullous pemphigoid, tense bullae are generally much larger than those of pemphigus or DH.

Pemphigus, pemphigoid, and DH all appear to be immunologically mediated. Routine histopathology often shows changes characteristic of each disorder. However, the clinical and routine histopathologic changes may overlap between these disorders, and other skin diseases may enter the differential diagnosis. Therefore, direct immunofluorescence of skin biopsy specimens should be used to confirm the diagnosis for each of these three disorders. In addition, indirect immunofluorescence of serum may be useful in pemphigus and bullous pemphigoid.

Treatment

Routine topical care for any eroded, weeping, or blistering skin disorder involves the use of wet compresses for 30 minutes four times daily. Such compresses have a soothing effect on the skin and remove crusts and debris that may harbor bacteria. The important ingredient of all compresses is water, with additives varying with the personal preference of the physician. The favorite seems to be aluminum acetate (Domeboro, Bluboro). Some physicians use topical antibiotics, such as a combination of polymyxin and bacitracin (Polysporin ointment), or topical steroids following the compresses. Patients with ocular lesions should be followed by an ophthalmologist to help prevent scarring and possible blindness.

For those patients with severely denuded areas, a powdered bed (cornstarch) may afford considerable relief of discomfort. Patients with oral or esophageal involvement of their blistering disorder may experience problems with adequate food or fluid intake. A soft diet and viscous lidocaine (Xylocaine) before meals may be helpful.

Systemic corticosteroids are the mainstay of treatment for pemphigus and pemphigoid. Pemphigus vulgaris can be life-threatening, and patients are often hospitalized and treated with initial doses of prednisone ranging from 100 to 200 mg per day. The dose is increased until suppression of new blister formation occurs. Some patients may require up to 500 mg per day. In difficult cases, intravenous corticotropin (ACTH), 40 to 80 units daily, will help control new blistering. Some physicians monitor pemphigus antibody titers along with the clinical response to therapy, but such titers do not always correlate with disease activity in every patient. In general, pemphigus antibody titers correlate with disease activity, whereas pemphigoid titers do not. Once control of the disease is attained, the steroid dose can usually be decreased somewhat rapidly to 40 to 60 mg per day. Further tapering must be gradual, by no more than 5 to 10 mg per week. Eventually, alternate-day treatment should be achieved.

Pemphigoid and less severe forms of pemphigus often respond to lower daily initial doses of prednisone (60 to 100 mg). In patients with mild or localized disease, the benefits of therapy must be weighed against the well-known systemic side effects of corticosteroids. The physician should constantly watch for signs of opportunistic infection, a leading cause of death in these patients, particularly those with severe forms of pemphigus vulgaris. Occasional patients with mild disease can be managed with topical steroids or intralesional triamcinolone acetonide, 3 to 5 mg per ml. Oral lesions may be treated with topical triamcinolone acetonide in emollient dental cream (Kenalog in Orabase).

Immunosuppressive therapy is often used for long-term treatment of patients with pemphigus or pemphigoid. Immunosuppresive drugs are not effective for the acute phases of these diseases. They are usually not started until the prednisone dose has been tapered to 40 to 60 mg. These drugs seem to facilitate a reduction in the corticosteroid dose, but it is important to remember that it takes 3 to 4 weeks for them to exert an effect. For some patients, it may be possible to eventually stop corticosteroid therapy altogether while maintaining immunosuppressive therapy. This is an advantage, since the side effects of immunosuppressives are usually less of a problem than those experienced on long-term, high-dose corticosteroid therapy.

The most widely used immunosuppressive agent today is azathioprine (Imuran—use not listed in maker's directives). Doses of 50 to 150 mg daily are used. Side effects include hematopoietic depression, hepatotoxicity, and an increased long-term risk for development of malignancy.

Less frequently, methotrexate or cyclophosphamide (Cytoxan) has been used. Methotrexate is started at 25 to 30 mg once weekly. This is given intramuscularly or orally in one dose or is divided into three doses given every 12 hours over a 36-hour period. At this low dosage, the main side effect is hepatotoxicity. Many physicians obtain pretreatment and annual liver biopsies. Initial doses of cyclophosphamide are 100 to 200 mg daily, which is tapered to 100 mg daily after about 3 weeks. Because side effects are more prevalent than with azathioprine or methotrexate, cyclophosphamide is usually reserved for more refractory patients.

Gold therapy has been used for pemphigus vulgaris, with or without corticosteriods. As with immunosuppressive drugs, gold injections may allow a decrease in the required doses of corticosteroids. Treatment is begun with a test dose of 10 mg of gold sodium thiomalate (Myochrysine—use not listed in maker's directive) or gold thioglucose (Solganal) intramuscularly. Gold thioglucose is preferable because it rarely causes the nitritoid reaction (an anaphylaxis-like reaction) soon after injection. One week later, 25 mg is given, followed by subsequent weekly doses of 50 mg. A complete blood count (CBC) with platelet count and urinalysis is obtained prior to each dose to check for proteinuria, hematuria, leukopenia, thrombocytopenia, or eosinophilia. Once clinical improvement or a drop in serum pemphigus antibody titer is noted, maintenance doses of 50 mg intramusclarly every 2 to 4 weeks may be given.

Plasmapheresis, especially in combination with prednisone and azathioprine, has sometimes been helpful in the treatment of patients with pemphigus vulgaris that was previously refractory to therapy.

Dapsone (diaminodiphenylsulfone, DDS, Avlosulfon) is the drug of choice for the treatment of DH. Most patients note a dramatic clearing of lesions and improvement of pruritus within 3 days. Such a rapid response used to be used as a diagnostic criterion, but it is now known that certain other dermatologic conditions may also respond to this drug. If the drug is discontinued, signs and symptoms of DH return rapidly. The usual starting dose is 100 mg daily. Occasional patients may require 200 mg or more, but higher doses usually result in bothersome side effects. Some patients respond to maintenance doses as low as 50 mg weekly.

Since dapsone and other sulfones are potent oxidizers, the most common side effect is anemia resulting from hemolysis. This is present to some degree in all patients taking the drug and does not usually indicate that the drug needs to be stopped. Most patients initially develop a reduction of their hemoglobin by 2 grams per dl, but this is usually largely corrected as treatment is continued. Methemoglobinemia and cyanosis are frequent. Patients with pulmonary or cardiovascular diseases should be treated cautiously with this drug. Other side effects include agranulocytosis (rare, but sometimes fatal), infectious mononucleosis–like syndrome, skin eruptions, cholestatic jaundice, and polyneuropathy (occurs after years of treatment). Pretreatment laboratory tests should include glucose-6-phosphate dehydrogenase (G6PD) level, since patients deficient in this enzyme may experience severe hemolysis. It is reasonable to follow a CBC weekly for the first month of treatment, and then monthly. A multisystem chemical profile should be obtained every 3 months. Dapsone has occasionally been used successfully in certain forms of pemphigoid.

Sulfapyridine may be used as a substitute for dapsone for those patients who cannot tolerate dapsone's side effects. Sulfapyridine is less effective than dapsone but does not cause hemolysis as frequently. Other side effects are similar to those of dapsone. Sulfapyridine may precipitate in the kidney because of its poor water solubility. Renal function should be monitored, and patients should continue a high fluid intake. The drug is supplied in 500 mg tablets. Patients are usually started at 500 mg twice to four times daily, which is increased until a response is noted (rarely up to 6 grams daily). The average maintenance dose is 1.5 grams daily. Because of side effects, attempts should be made to use the smallest effective dose.

A gluten-free diet is valuable in the treatment of DH. Apart from its beneficial effect on the skin lesions, it is the only treatment that is effective for the gastrointestinal symptoms, which fortunately are mild to absent in most patients with DH. Only a *strict* gluten-free diet is effective, and the diet must be followed for 6 to 12 months before the dose of dapsone can be reduced. Some patients may be able to stop dapsone altogether after 2 to 3 years of the diet; however, even minute amounts of gluten in the diet will produce new skin lesions. Because the teratogenic effect of dapsone is unknown, a gluten-free diet is the treatment of choice for pregnant females.

Patients must be extremely motivated and intelligent to follow this difficult diet. The advice of a well-trained dietician is important. Several companies specialize in supplying gluten-free foods. Special gluten-free recipes are available from such support groups as the Gluten Intolerance Group of North America, P. O. Box 23053, Seattle, Washington 98102, or the New England Chapter of the National Celiac Sprue Society, 5 Jeffrey Road, Wayland, Massachusetts 01778.

CONTACT DERMATITIS

method of
WILLIAM L. EPSTEIN, M.D.
University of California
San Francisco, California

Contact dermatitis is a common skin condition. It has several modes of presentation, which taken together constitute approximately 10 per cent of a clinical dermatologist's practice.

Acute Contact Dermatitis

When the cause is an irritant, the clinical diagnosis usually is self-evident. Although this sort of injury can occur in the home or during recreational activity, it is more common as an occupational hazard. In work places such as caustic plants and biochemisty laboratories, where this poses a significant potential, emergency showers are available to quickly wash off the offending chemical and minimize the degree of injury. Office treatment of this dermatitis is simply supportive. One should make certain no residual chemical is left, and the damaged area is treated with cool soaks. Depending upon the extent of injury, the patient may be advised to rest at home for a day or two until the area begins to heal. The use of nonsteroidal anti-inflammatory drugs, sedatives, and analgesics may be indicated in patients with extensive chemical burns, but there is no benefit from the use of systemic or topical corticosteroids. Fortunately, these lesions tend to heal quickly, and the problem is rapidly resolved.

Allergic contact dermatitis is a diffent matter. This is a form of cell-mediated immunity and as such has a delayed onset (2 to 7 days after exposure) and presents as erythema, edema, vesiculation, intense pruritus, and, in extreme cases, bullae. Except for poison oak–poison ivy dermatitis, most patients are unaware of the cause, at least during the initial bout.

In mild to moderate cases seen 2 to 4 days after onset of the eruption, therapy should be conservative, with the prospect of self-healing in 7 to 10 days. Treatment includes cool soaks of water or Burow's solution (1:40), tepid baths (starch and soda, Aveeno), and shake lotions (calamine lotion without additives). Topical antihistamines in the acute phase may induce contact sensitization. Systemically, aspirin in large doses (0.6 gram [10 grains] every 3 to 4 hours) or antihistamines in sedative doses may reduce pruritus. A hypnotic at bedtime (chloral hydrate, 0.5 to 2.0 grams [7½ to 30 grains]) is required occasionally. If edema becomes noticeable, as often happens when the dermatitis occurs on the face or genitalia, I use systemic corticosteroids (see further on). In the healing stages, when the skin is dry and scaly, pruritus is best controlled by use of topical corticosteroids.

Acute contact dermatitis from plants in a very sensitive person should be considered a dermatologic emergency, requiring timely and aggressive therapy. In this situation, the dermatitis begins within hours of exposure to the plant and is associated with erythema and marked tissue edema. Definitive therapy requires the use of large doses of systemic corticosteroids. I have had best results with ACTH-gel, 80 units given intramuscularly as soon as the patient is seen, followed by a second injection 8 to 10 hours later. If the disease effervesces in 2 or 3 days, a second injection of 80 units of ACTH-gel is given. A modified regime calls for 20 tablets of the physician's favored corticosteroid (most dermatologists choose prednisone). My choice is dexamethasone 0.75 mg, 4 tablets given five times during the day. This is repeated on two consecutive days and then abruptly stopped. Again, the patient is seen 2 days later and, if necessary, given 20 more tablets to ingest. Usualy this is sufficient to result in healing. An alternative favored by many is to give 80 mg of prednisone for the first few days and then reduce the dose over a period of 2 to 3 weeks, with alternate-day therapy at the end.

During the first few days of severe acute allergic contact dermatitis it is best to have the patient rest at home. Hospitalization is not indicated because of the possibility of secondary infection and expense. Besides, Diagnosis-Related Groups (DRG's) do not include this sort of patient.

Chronic Contact Dermatitis

Chronic contact dermatitis presents an entirely different problem, and different strategies are needed. The main approach is the judicious use of topical corticosteroids. When the disease affects areas such as the face, the hands, and the folds, one must be careful not to use fluorinated steroids for prolonged periods. Corticosteroid gels are not recommended because of the possibility of systemic effects from absorbed drug. I frequently use triamcinolone acetonide alone or with occlusion at bedtime for a few weeks, switching as healing begins to the less potent corticosteroids, such as hydrocortisone or desonide.

Systemic antihistamines also are indicated but are not nearly as effective antipruritics as Atarax and the tricyclic antidepressants, which can be given in small doses throughout the day or as a large single dose at bedtime, according to tolerance.

An important consideration is the use of emollients, and these should be tailored to the acceptance of the patient. Some prefer greasy preparations such as ointments or oils, whereas others like a cream base. One should not be too rigid in prescribing these preparations. It is more important that the patient feel comfortable and obtain subjective relief from whatever topical agent is used. Sometimes, with chronic contact dermatitis, particularly on the hands and feet, the involved areas become markedly thickened and hyperkeratotic. This calls for keratolytic agents, such as Keralyt Gel and urea, and propitious use of tars. However, these formulations may produce additional irritation and aggravate the situation. Another common occurrence is the appearance of deep, painful fissures. Our preferred treatment is the use of Castellani's paint with or without added phenol.

Alternative therapy includes the use of grenz rays for chronic hand eczema. Oral psoralen plus long wavelength ultraviolet light therapy (PUVA) is another therapy of merit, especially for localized dermatitis on the hands and feet. This is a nonspecific treatment for chronic dermatitis.

Prophylaxis

Another strategy, in addition to avoiding contact, is immunologic prophylaxis. Although specific desensitization can be accomplished in experimental animals, this has not proved practical for use in man. Nevertheless, a severe bout of poison ivy dermatitis is recognized clinically to produce a state of temporary desensitization in some patients, and the phenomenon is well recognized in certain industries where workers who are repeatedly exposed to potent sensitizing chemicals can achieve a state of nonreactivity called "hardening." On the other hand, there have been many proposals over the years to induce hyposensitization to poison oak or ivy by systemically administering increasing doses of the allergenic chemical. A reliable active oleoresin is supplied by Hollister-Stier Laboratories (107 S. Division Street, Spokane, Washington 99202). The standard desensitization set contains 15 ml each of 1:100, 1:50, and 1:25 dilutions of oleoresin in corn oil (a total of 1050 mg of allergen). Instruction sheets are enclosed. The important point is to increase the dose of allergen in a stepwise fashion as rapidly as the patient's tolerance allows. Onset of itching means that the increment is too great. When this happens, the dose is reduced by 1 to 3 drops; after pruritus subsides, it is increased again. Other untoward reactions, such as dermatitis, urticaria, or dyshidrosis, may occur if the cardinal symptom of pruritus is ignored or not recognized. This preparation occasionally causes pruritus ani; dividing the dose tends to reduce this complication. The total dose for hyposensitization varies between 2000 and 3000 mg. (After the first set is completed, 1:25 dilutions should be used in doses of 1 to 1.5 ml daily.) Once hyposensitization therapy is completed and the drug is stopped, sensitivity tends to return within 2 to 3 months, so that many patients are required to remain on a maintenance dose year round. According to tolerance, this can be 1 to 2 ml of 1:25 dilution two to three times a week.

SKIN DISEASES OF PREGNANCY

method of
KIM B. YANCEY, M.D.
Uniformed Services University of the Health Sciences
Bethesda, Maryland

Herpes Gestationis

Herpes gestationis (HG) is a rare, nonviral, subepidermal blistering disease of pregnancy and the puerperium. HG may begin during any trimester of pregnancy or present shortly after delivery. Lesions are usually distributed over the abdomen (frequently in the periumbilical region) and the extremities; mucous membrane lesions are rare. Lesions in HG can be quite polymorphous and may include urticarial papules and plaques, vesiculopapules, and frank blisters. Lesions are almost always very pruritic. Severe exacerbations of HG frequently occur after delivery (within 24 to 48 hours), and patients should be carefully evaluated at this time even if their disease was previously controlled by treatment or was inactive. HG tends to recur in subsequent pregnancies, may flare briefly with resumption of menses after delivery, and may recur if patients use oral contraceptives. Occasionally, infants born of affected mothers also demonstrate cutaneous lesions; however, these lesions are usually transient and last no more than the first few weeks of life. Several investigators feel that HG is associated with an increased risk of fetal morbidity and mortality.

Direct immunofluorescence microscopy on normal, perilesional skin from patients with herpes gestationis reveals the immunologic hallmark of this disorder—linear deposits of C3 along the cutaneous basement membrane zone. Biopsies from 30 to 40 per cent of these patients also demonstrate linear deposits of IgG at this location; it is hypothesized that an avid complement-fixing IgG antibody is responsible for C3 deposits in both patients and their offspring. The cause of autoantibody formation in this disease is unknown, but its relationship to pregnancy suggests that it is hormonally modulated. In HG it is advisable to obtain skin for demonstration of immunoreactants bound in situ (specifically, linear deposits of C3 at the cutaneous basement membrane zone), rather than to rely on routine indirect immunofluorescence techniques for demonstration of a circulating autoantibody.

Treatment

The goal of therapy is to prevent the development of new lesions, relieve the intense pruritus associated with this disorder, and care for any erosions at sites of blister formation. Specific theraputic measures depend on the character, extent, and severity of the patient's eruption. Most patients with HG require treatment with moderate doses of daily systemic corticosteroids. Twenty of 40 mg of prednisone daily usually provides substantial clinical and symptomatic relief within several days; occasionally, divided doses of prednisone (i.e., every 12 hours) may hasten initial improvement. When the eruption and symptoms have been controlled, prednisone should be tapered approximately 5 mg every 1 to 2 weeks until only an occasional lesion develops or symptoms recur. If a post-partum exacerbation of HG occurs, patients should be restarted on 20 to 40 mg prednisone daily; patients unable to tolerate oral medications can be treated with an equivalent amount of daily hydrocortisone intravenously. Rarely, post-partum exacerbations of HG are quite severe and may require treatment with high doses of systemic corticosteroids. Exacerbations associated with resumption of menses are usually mild and normally can be managed by a small dose of daily prednisone (e.g., 20 mg) or vigorous use of a topical corticosteroid cream alone. In mild cases of HG, vigorous use of potent topical corticosteroids such as fluocinonide 0.05 percent (Lidex) or triamcinolone acetonide 0.5 per cent (Aristocort) four to six times each day may control the eruption and obviate the need for treatment with systemic medications. As with systemic therapy, topical corticosteroids in HG should be gradually tapered to the lowest effective dose. Weeping, moist skin lesions can be dried with open wet dressings of saline or tap water used for 10- to 15-minute intervals three to four times each day. Erosions should be carefully inspected for sites of secondary infection.

Pruritic Urticarial Papules and Plaques of Pregnancy

Pruritic urticarial papules and plaques of pregnancy (PUPPP) is a distinctive pruritic eruption that usually presents during the third trimester in primigravidas. The clinical manifestations of PUPPP almost always first appear on the abdomen and begin within periumbilical striae distensae in approximately 50 per cent of cases. Additional common sites of involvement include the buttocks, thighs, legs, and upper inner arms; facial lesions are very rare. Lesions consist of small erythematous urticarial papules, which often coalesce to form plaques covering a significant portion of the body surface area. Urticarial lesions are frequently rimmed by faint pallor. Although pruritus in this disorder is extreme and often interferes with sleep, patients rarely demonstrate excoriations. PUPPP usually promptly responds to treatment or resolves with delivery. Experience to date suggests that PUPPP does not flare after delivery, recur with subsequent pregnancies, or develop if patients are later exposed to oral contraceptives. Preliminary data also suggest that PUPPP is not associated with an increased risk of fetal morbidity or mortality. The cause of this relatively common eruption of pregnancy is unknown. Since no specific diagnostic test is available, the diagnosis of PUPPP is based on the characteristic clinical presentation of this disorder.

Treatment

Frequent applications (i.e., four to six times daily) of potent topical corticosteroids usually provide symptomatic relief and halt lesion formation. Agents frequently employed for initial therapy include fluocinonide 0.05 per cent (Lidex) or triamcinolone acetonide 0.1 percent (Aristocort or Kenalog). Less potent topical corticosteroids and less frequent treatment schedules should be employed once the eruption is controlled; therapy should be continued until the disorder resolves and then slowly tapered. In selected severe cases not completely controlled by topical therapy, a brief tapering course of systemic corticosteroids may be required. In those cases, 20 to 40 mg of daily prednisone usually promptly controls the eruption and associated pruritus; systemic corticosteroids can be rapidly tapered by 5 mg at 2- to 3-day intervals, especially when combined with vigorous topical therapy. Experience has demonstrated that oral antihistamines are less effective therapeutic agents than is vigorous use of topical corticosteroids alone.

PRURITUS ANI AND VULVAE

method of
JAMES E. RASMUSSEN, M.D.
University of Michigan
Ann Arbor, Michigan

Both renal and imaginary diseases can produce excruciating pruritus of the anus and vulvae. Although there are many possible causes, most patients who itch in these locations have one of three diseases: intertrigo, psoriasis/seborrheic dermatitis, or lichen simplex chronicus. Other potential causes of pruritus are insects (pediculosis), parasites (pinworms), fungal diseases (tinea cruris, candida), allergic contact dermatitis (particularly from the "caine" group of topical antibiotics as well as perfumes), warts, lichen sclerosis et atrophicus, and rarely carcinomas.

Mild, intermittent pruritus in the genital or anal region is normal in many individuals and only needs treatment when it interferes with the patient's life.

General Therapy

Considerable effort should be focused on attempts to reduce friction, sweating, and bacterial overgrowth. Obese patients should be encouraged to lose weight, and all patients should be encouraged to wear loose-fitting undergarments made with cotton. Tight-fitting slacks and pantyhose should not be worn if at all possible. Absorptive powders (Zeasorb, baby powder) will reduce friction and absorb sweat.

Bacterial and fungal colonization is common in most patients with pruritus ani. Reducing the sweating will help this problem, but attention also should be paid to the use of antibacterial soaps (provided scrubbing isn't carried out vigorously enough to injure the tissue) and the use of broad-spectrum antibacterials such as miconazole (but not the sensitizing neomycin). Bacterial contamination from the stool may be reduced by oiling the perimeter of the anus with mineral oil or petrolatum jelly. This and the use of soft toilet tissues will reduce bacterial implantation and trauma. Mild astringents such as witch hazel (Tuck's) are often helpful.

Finally, all attempts should be made to reduce possible causes of inflammation such as perfumed or rough toilet tissue and local sensitizers (benzocaine, neomycin). Chronic vaginal discharge should be investigated and treated when appropriate.

Specific Treatment

The treatment of patients with pediculosis, fungi, pinworms, and candidiasis is given in other sections of this text. The treatment of intertrigo and intertriginous psoriasis will be discussed here.

Intertriginous psoriasis is most difficult to treat. Medications that are effective in other areas of the body, such as high potency steroids, anthralin, and ultraviolet light, are often too irritating or produce far too many side effects to be used for longer periods of time in the groin or perianal areas. I usually begin therapy with 1 per cent hydrocortisone cream alternating with either nystatin or miconazole. If there is no success with this regimen I will then switch to a short course of a more potent topical steroid (1 week of Lidex or Topicort), but I never use intermediate/high potency steroids for long periods of time. They are well known to produce atrophy, ulcers, and striae. Low concentrations of tar (Fototar or Ichthyol) are often effective in more resistant cases.

Lichen simplex chronicus is also a difficult entity to treat since the patient gets particular pleasure from the itch/scratch cycle. Mild topical steroids should be tried first along with the use of nonsensitizing topical anesthetics (Pramosone). This is frequently ineffective, and I am forced to resort to either a short course of a more potent topical steroid or the use of intralesional corticosteroids. In my opinion, intralesional corticosteroids are much more effective since they do not require patient compliance. I use triamcinolone acetonide, 2.5 to 5.0 mg per ml, infiltrated superficially throughout the lichenified areas. If this fails and the patches are small, then cryotherapy is very effective, but can produce substantial blistering. Patients with prolonged and intractable lichen simplex of the anus and vulvae may have an underlying phobia regarding cancer, venereal disease, or sexual function. Often a frank discussion of this will bring underlying problems into view.

Finally, when all else fails I use 1–2–3 ointment, which is a soothing, mild astringent composed of one part Burow's solution, two parts Aquaphor, and three parts Lassar's paste. Other good old-time anti-itch medicines are Schamberg's lotion (menthol, 0.5 grams; phenol, 1.0 grams; zinc oxide, 2.0 grams; calcium hydroxide, 40 ml; and peanut oil, qs ad 100 ml) and Weiss' shake lotion (Burow's solution, 9 mg; zinc oxide, 18 grams; talc, 18 grams; glycerin, 14.4 mg; slaked lime, 139 mg; and water, qs ad 100 ml).

URTICARIA AND ANGIOEDEMA

method of
LARRY E. MILLIKAN, M.D., FACP
Tulane University
New Orleans, Louisiana

Urticaria presents as localized edema in the skin, usually involving the upper dermis. In contrast, angioedema usually has deeper involvement throughout the epidermis, and it often manifests in areas of low tissue pressure around the eyes and lips but can also be seen in other parts of the body, including the extremities and genitalia. Urticarial lesions are transient, usually have minimal associated erythema, and are usually pruritic. There is sometimes confusion with urticarial vasculitis, which usually is much more erythematous with lesions often persistent in excess of 18 hours. Traditionally, urticaria is classified as acute or chronic—the former occurring for less than 6 weeks and the latter for more than 6 weeks.

Urticaria is a symptom complex, not a primary disease, and the etiology is often elusive. The physician's primary role may often be that of symptomatic therapy only.

The best chance for detecting underlying etiology is found in acute urticaria. Here the reaction is of short duration and the patient's memory of possible causes may provide the answer.

It is always important in unclear cases to have the patient keep a careful record of exposure to possible urticariogens. Stress to the patient the significance of the syndrome and its potential problems for airway compromise. The first order of business on the initial visit, therefore, is to institute appropriate medication to minimize the possibility for catastrophic events and begin an initial review of possible underlying causes so that ultimately therapy can be effective. Certain key areas are important in the initial review, including foods, drugs, any other ingestants, infection—apparent or inapparent, physical causes, infestations, and certain underlying systemic diseases. Acute urticaria rarely is precipitated by such things as collagen vascular disease and cancer, but these have been reported; therefore this must be borne in mind, for one cannot predict which patient with acute urticaria will persist to the chronic stage because of serious underlying disease.

In acute urticaria, therapy is begun immediately while a complete, intensive search is made for underlying etiology. Chronic urticaria usually is recurrent and episodic and in most cases is assumed to be due to the same source. It is possible that repetitive episodes of acute urticaria over a period of time could be confused with chronic urticaria, which further may render determination of the underlying etiology difficult.

Treatment

Acute urticaria of a limited nature usually is responsive to oral medications. The antihistamines are preferred. Of these, the most useful are hydroxyzine and cyproheptadine. In each, dosage often must be pushed to the maximum to achieve optimal results.

Hydroxyzine (Atarax, Durrax) generally requires 25 mg twice daily and 25 to 50 mg at bedtime. The dose for cyproheptadine (Periactin) is 4 mg three times daily and 8 mg at bedtime. This can be pushed to the maximum recommended dose of 40 mg per day. In severe or widespread urticaria, or in most cases with possible airway embarrassment, parenteral medications are often necessary immediately. Intravenous antihistamines can be dramatically beneficial. Diphenhydramine (Benadryl), 50 mg intravenously, often will stop progression of the urticaria immediately and clear it rapidly. If this is unsuccessful, beta-agonists are appropriate, including epinephrine, 0.3 to 0.5 ml of the 1:1000 preparation intramuscularly. Sometimes sustained-release preparations of antihistamine, with or without beta-agonist decongestants, may also be useful (Dimetane, Dimetapp, Drixoral). These usually require higher dosage. With severe cases, maintenance of beta-agonists such as pseudoephedrine (50 mg two or three times daily) or a slow taper of steroids (1 mg per kg for 2 days in divided doses four times a day, decreasing to 0.75 mg per kg for 3 days and then 0.5 mg per kg for 3 days) may be necessary. Usually one can withdraw the medication at that time without difficulty. If the source of the acute urticaria has not been determined, a careful follow-up is necessary after withdrawing all medications. While the patient is on a tapering dose of corticosteroids, one of the aforementioned antihistamines should be maintained and continued for 10 to 14 days after discontinuing the steroid.

Chronic urticaria provides additional challenges in therapy and extensive problems in the orderly search for underlying etiology, which is discovered in less than 30 per cent of patients. Therefore, the primary role of the physician in chronic urticaria may be to supply symptomatic treatment. Therapy initially is the same as for acute urticaria and is begun immediately.

My initial approach to discovery of the etiology of chronic urticaria is an extensive review of drugs. Of particular interest are aspirin, salicylates, and nonsteroidal anti-inflammatory agents because of their effect on prostaglandin metabolism. Antibiotics are also high on the list, and penicillin has been an important culprit. A careful review of the patient's use of over-the-counter medications and a subsequent diary of all medicaments and other ingestants is an essential first step.

Occult infection is also high on the list of common causes of chronic urticaria. In the literature, sinus, dental, and urinary tract infections are particularly important causes.

Foods also can be a major cause. More often than not, food additives, food colorings, and other possible agents rather than the foods themselves are the problem. Special elimination diets can be found readily in most textbooks. On the first visit it is important to begin a diary of foods ingested to get an idea of the possibilities. Some of the food dyes, especially tartrazine, have been considered significant in the past. Tartrazine relates to the previously mentioned aspirin and prostaglandin metabolism.

Certainly, one of the most essential accomplishments of the first visit for a patient with a long history of urticaria is review of the patient's understanding of the process and appropriate education. This will provide the patient with greater insight and enhanced ability to avoid future urticariogens.

Drug treatment of chronic urticaria involves the same principles as those for acute urticaria. In general, these patients are less responsive to therapy and a more involved approach to achieve symptomatic relief is necessary. Patients with chronic urticaria are often good candidates for the use of prolonged-release forms of antihistamine, since there can be serious compliance problems when a combination of several different drugs is attempted. Long-acting antihistamines such as dibrompheniramine maleate (Dimetane Extentabs) allow simplicity in dosing and assure greater patient compliance.

Other traditional first choices for the antihistamines are hydroxyzine and cyproheptadine in the same dosages as previously mentioned. Chlor-Trimeton is an additional antihistamine that may be of use (4 mg three or four times daily). Each of these three drugs belongs to a different class of antihistamines structurally and therefore each may have some potential added benefit in regard to differing side effects, effectiveness, and potential for additive effect. When a second antihistamine is added, care is always taken to make sure that this drug is not of the same pharmacologic group in order to at least potentially enhance the possibility of more beneficial response. Sustained-release preparations may be useful to enhance patient compliance. Patients who do not respond well to antihistamines alone are candidates for beta-agonists and pseudoephedrine. Terbutaline (2.5 mg three times a day) is one of the newer $beta_2$-adrenergic stimulators that has shown some promise.

Recent evidence has also suggested the efficacy of an ataractic, doxepin (Sinequan), which has a potent H_1 and H_2 blocking effect. Data are thus far insufficient to convince me that doxepin should be a routine therapeutic modality rather than being reserved for complicated, difficult, and unresponsive cases.

Only patients who have flares of their chronic urticaria associated with severe symptoms or who may have potential airway involvement are candidates for steroids. When steroids are needed, aggressive therapy is begun immediately. When the acute flare that has destabilized the patient is controlled, steroids are tapered rapidly. Beginning with prednisone, 1 mg per kg per day at 8 A.M. for 4 days is given, tapering to 0.5 mg per kg per day at 8 A.M. for 4 days, then 0.25 mg per kg for 4 days. This will usually get the patient over the acute flare and allow restabilization of the condition. Some patients, however, may require a more prolonged course of steroids. This is undertaken only after extensive manipulation of H_1 and H_2 antihistamines and beta-agonists. A small percentage of patients require steroids over a long period of time.

An additional approach to therapy has been the use of systemic antibiotics. This, on occasion, has proved efficacious and presumably is associated with therapeutic correction of an occult infection. In many instances, a broad-spectrum antibiotic over a short course may be far less expensive than the extensive work-up to determine the underlying occult infection.

It is also important to be aware of the potential problem of physical urticarias. These may be subtle, and the patient may be unaware of their potential. The most common ones to consider are cholinergic, cold, pressure, and solar.

Cholinergic Urticaria

Cholinergic urticaria is related to abnormalities in the cholinergic sweating system and classically presents with grouped hives of 3 to 5 millimeters (pencil eraser size). Patients generally have urticaria precipitated by sweating, either from exercise, heat, or on an emotional basis. This may be a particular problem to the patient. A careful history of precipitating factors is often all that is necessary to sustain the diagnosis.

One characteristic of cholinergic urticaria is its predictable response to hydroxyzine (Atarax, Durrax). The dosage may vary from 10 to 50 mg four times daily to control symptoms. I have seen patients with a long history of urticaria who became symptom-free for the first time in many years upon the institution of hydroxyzine. Not all patients respond to hydroxyzine. Some require an additional H_1 blocker such as cyproheptadine (Periactin) and possibly even the addition of an H_2 blocker such as cimetidine (Tagamet) or ranitidine. There has been interest in some of the ataractics that have H_1 and H_2 activity, such as doxepin (Sinequan). This can be tried cautiously in patients who fail to respond to the aforementioned treatment.

Cold Urticaria

The diagnosis of cold urticaria is usually obvious. A very rare familial variant of this syndrome has a slightly different presentation. The classic finding of localized urticaria in the area of cold exposure makes the diagnosis self-evident.

The first step in cold urticaria is education of the patient to avoid unnecessary further cold exposure. This is not entirely possible, therefore systemic therapy is usually required. The first line of therapy in cold urticaria is the use of cyproheptadine (Periactin) at a dose of 4 mg four to six times a day. This generally has to be pushed to 40 mg a day, which is the maximum recommended dosage. Periodic rechallenge of the patient with an ice cube will allow indirect evidence of success of therapy. When the patient is well controlled, the ice cube test will result only in an erythematous flare and minimal to no urtication. A certain percentage of patients will not respond to cyproheptadine alone. In these patients, hydroxyzine is also added. Usually the cyproheptadine dose remains the same and gradually the hydroxyzine (Atarax) dose is increased from 10 mg four times a day to a maximum dose of 50 to 75 mg four times a day as the patient tolerates. In my experience, the most common mistake is the use of inadequate dosages of the medication, resulting in therapeutic failure.

Since the majority of patients have cold urticaria unrelated to any known cause, therapy is continued with maximal intensity during the periods that the patient faces cold stress, withdrawn during the warmer months, and initiated in anticipation of the patient's return to cold exposure.

Pressure Urticaria

Pressure urticaria can present as an immediate or a delayed phenomenon. Simple dermographism is considered a minor manifestation of pressure urticaria. In these patients, careful review of history, signs, and symptoms is usually sufficient to establish the diagnosis. The diagnosis is easy, but the treatment is difficult. Most of the patients are initially tried on the usual antihistamines and almost invariably fail to respond. Most ultimately require steroids. As with cold urticaria, many of these patients will ultimately outlive their urticaria and the etiology is never discovered.

Solar Urticaria

Solar urticaria may be easily diagnosed in most instances. The characteristic distribution is classic. Solar urticaria is perhaps the most complicated of all the urticarias and has several subcategories related to a transferable serum factor and in some cases different portions of the ultraviolet spectrum as the causative agent. Diagnosis must be confirmed, after ruling out photosensitivity due to underlying disease or drugs. Certain sunscreens are sometimes effective, depending on the portion of the spectrum wherein the sensitivity lies. Beta-carotene is also useful in some patients. The porphyrias can sometimes present as apparent solar urticaria.

Urticarial Vasculitis

In the last 5 years, urticarial vasculitis has received increasing interest. The lesions persist far longer than those of simple chronic or acute urticaria and are often more erythematous. Collagen vascular disease has been found in many of these patients. Treatment differs little from that for chronic urticaria, but the underlying disease primarily requires treatment.

Angioedema

A very rare syndrome is that of hereditary angioedema, or Quincke's edema. It is associated with hereditary deficiency of the protein C-1 esterase inhibitor. This substance is either absent in these patients or is functionally absent, which requires a functional assay for the enzyme to be detected. There are clinical differences so that urticaria and urticarial vasculitis are rarely confused with angioedema. Abdominal pain is one of the most common premonitory signs and symptoms. The urticaria is of the deeper tissues, and the possibility of airway obstruction is greatest in this syndrome.

Many of these patients are hospitalized at the onset of an attack so that a tracheostomy can be provided immediately if airway obstruction occurs. Fresh-frozen plasma has also been beneficial.

Danazol (Danocrine), 200 mg daily then tapering to 200 mg every other day, has been found uniquely to stimulate production of the missing protein. Stanazolol (Winstrol), 2.5 to 10 mg daily, has also been successful in angioedema. Careful regulation of these drugs can allow the patient to live a nearly normal life.

PIGMENTARY DISORDERS

method of
JOSIANE S. LEDERMAN, M.D.,
and ARTHUR J. SOBER, M.D.
Harvard Medical School
Boston, Massachusetts

Melasma

Melasma is an acquired macular hypermelanosis of sun-exposed areas primarily of the face and neck. It develops progressively to usually become symmetric and uniformly light or dark brown. It is by far more frequent in women than in men. Melasma has both genetic and hormonal causes and has been associated with pregnancy, oral contraceptives, and phenytoin. When an offending agent is present, cessation of the agent is needed as part of the therapy.

Solar exposure exacerbates melasma, and its avoidance is fundamental for successful management. Transparent sunscreens are of limited value. An opaque sunscreen absorbing both ultraviolet and visible light must be applied every morning in all seasons during and after therapy such as RV Paque, Reflecta, or Covermark, which also evens out the complexion. Fair to good bleaching is obtained with hydroquinone cream 2 per cent (Esoterica, Eldoquin) with or without retinoic acid cream 0.05 to 0.1 per cent. Good results are obtained with an alcoholic solution of 2 per cent hydroquinone and 0.05 or 0.1 per cent retinoic acid or with Melanex, which is a 3 per cent hydroquinone solution. Prior to use on the face, the hydroquinone should be applied for several days to a small site on the arm to test for hypersensitivity. The hydroquinone formulation must be applied sparingly twice daily for at least 3 months and limited to the hyperpigmented areas. If irritation occurs, the treatment must be stopped because of the risk of postinflammatory hyperpigmentation. Hydrocortisone cream 1 to 2.5 per cent can be applied to the irritated areas.

We do not recommend the use of monobenzyl ether of hydroquinone (MBEHQ) for melasma, since it can cause an irreversible confetti-like depigmentation, both at the site of application and at distant sites.

Postinflammatory Hyperpigmentation

This is the most commonly encountered pigmentary disorder, especially in dark skinned caucasians, blacks, and orientals. It may follow any inflammatory condition (e.g., lichen planus, eczema, chronic stasis dermatitis). Most often the pigmentation fades slowly with time. There is no known effective treatment.

Lentigines

Lentigines are discrete, hyperpigmented macules of varying size. They are most often sporadic, occurring in middle-aged patients on the light-exposed areas of the face, forearms, and backs of the hands. When more diffuse, they can be part of a familial syndrome: LEOPARD syndrome (generalized lentiginosis, electrocardiographic abnormalities, ocular hypertelorism, pulmonary stenosis, abnormalities of genitalia, retardation of growth, deafness), Peutz-Jeghers syndrome (periorificial lentigines, intestinal polyposis) or centrofacial lentiginosis (butterfly pattern of lentigines, neuropsychiatric disorders).

No treatment is as yet satisfactory. Temporary lightening can be obtained with long and regular applications of hydroquinone cream 2 to 5 per cent for the generalized lentigines, or with a single light freeze with liquid nitrogen for solar lentigines. Sun avoidance and use of sunscreens may limit the development of new lesions.

Vitiligo

Vitiligo is an idiopathic acquired amelanosis of the skin affecting at least 1 per cent of the population. It has been associated with autoimmune and endocrine disorders such as pernicious anemia, adrenocortical insufficiency, alopecia areata, hyperthyroidism, and diabetes mellitus. The depigmentation can also result from exogenous exposure to phenols, thiols, and quinones.

Therapy of vitiligo is long and tedious, often requiring more than 1 year. Anticipated results also depend on the site of involvement. Facial repigmentation is more successful than that of extremities. When the disease is limited or of little cosmetic concern to the patient, appropriate measures include reassurance about the lack of seriousness of vitiligo itself, with no therapy undertaken, or simple measures such as application of a camouflage make-up product that approximates the normal skin color (Covermark) or with quick tanning agents (Vitadye, Dyoderma).

At present repigmentation of the vitiliginous areas is best achieved with administration of psoralens and exposure to ultraviolet A radiation (320 to 400 nm). Topical photochemotherapy is recommended when the patient has only a few small lesions (less than 20 per cent of cutaneous involvement). A 1 per cent solution of 8-methoxypsoralen (8-MOP) diluted with 50 per cent propylene glycol and 50 per cent ethanol to a final concentration of 0.1 per cent is painted with a cotton-tipped swab strictly to the vitiliginous patches 1 hour before exposure for 3 to 10 minutes to noon sunlight or alternatively to an artificial UVA source starting at 0.5 to 2.0 J per cm^2, the dose depending on skin type. The treated area should then be washed well with soap and water to remove the nonbound psoralen.

In children under 12 years of age, topical therapy given two or three times a week on alternate days often gives satisfactory results. Topical corticosteroids (hydrocortisone 1 per cent) may be used simultaneously for 6 to 8 weeks for small macules.

Treatment of large lesions requires ingestion of 0.4 to 0.6 mg per kg of trimethylpsoralen, or 8-MOP, taken 2 hours before light exposure and three times a week on alternate days. The light source is either natural sunlight or artificial UVA. The combination of psoralen and UVA therapy is termed PUVA. The PUVA dose depends on skin type. For natural sunlight the initial exposure of 15 minutes is gradually increased by five minute intervals to a maximum of 1 hour depending on response (mild erythema). When the maximum time has been reached, the dose of psoralen may be increased to the maximum of 0.7 mg per kg, accompanied by a decrease in exposure time to 30 minutes. Exposure time can then be gradually increased again to 1 hour as tolerated. The therapeutic goal is to obtain a mild erythema 24 to 36 hours after each exposure. Overexposure must be avoided as burning may enhance the vitiliginous process. Significant repigmentation is usually apparent after 3 to 4 months of therapy. One hundred treatments of PUVA may be needed for a maximum response. If no evidence of repigmentation is seen after 15 to 20 treatments, oral PUVA is considered a failure.

Prior to initiating oral therapy, an antinuclear antibody test and an eye examination must be done. Annual follow-up eye examinations are recommended. Contraindications to treatment with oral psoralen include pregnancy, less than 12 years of age, pre-existing photosensitive dermatoses, ingestion of phototoxic drugs, previous history of skin cancer, and cataract.

Photoprotection consisting of applications of a broad-spectrum sunscreen containing benzophenones, especially on amelanotic areas, will prevent sunburn. Sunscreens are numbered according to the sun protection factor (SPF), with the higher number giving more protection. Patients with vitiligo should use a sunscreen with an SPF of 15 or higher (Presun 15, Total Eclipse 15, Sundown 15). Special sunglasses that block UVA light should be worn indoors and outdoors for the first 24 hours after ingestion of the psoralen and outdoors for the second 24 hours.

For extensive vitiligo (more than 50 per cent), depigmentation of the remaining melanized skin can be undertaken by the application of 20 per cent of monobenzyl ether of hydroquinone (Benoquin) twice daily. Complete and irreversible depigmentation is obtained after 1 year of continuous therapy. Patients must constantly use highly protective sunscreens to avoid sunburns, as the tanning ability has been completely destroyed. This therapeutic option is usually reserved for patients over age 40 years; after failure of an adequate trial of PUVA; for nonlactating, nonpregnant women; and for individuals wishing to have a uniform color. The social implications of the color change must be completely understood by racially pigmented patients.

OCCUPATIONAL DERMATOSES

method of
JAMES S. TAYLOR, M.D.
Cleveland Clinic Foundation
Cleveland, Ohio

Occupational skin disorders still account for almost half of all reported work illnesses, despite the fact that they are almost fully preventable. No industry, whatever its size, scope, or location, is immune to their occurrence. Occupational skin diseases are produced from old chemicals in processes both old and new, new chemicals in new processes, and a wide variety of biologic and physiologic agents. The major categories of work-related skin disorders are contact dermatitis (allergic, irritant, and photosensitivity), acne and follicular eruptions, and pigmentary abnormalities.

Contact Dermatitis

In this category are most occupational dermatoses. They may be caused by some of the hundreds of thousands of chemicals used in industry. About 80 per cent of contact dermatitis is produced by irritants, 20 per cent from allergic sensitization, and a small percentage, often overlooked, from photosensitivity. Most affected are the hands, but any part of the body may be involved.

Acute Contact Dermatitis. 1. Avoid contact with the offending agent. This may require several days away from work or temporary transfer to another job.

2. Avoid contact with potential aggravating factors such as excessive soap and water, alcohol, thimerosal, and sensitizers such as topically applied antihistamines, antibiotics (neomycin or nitrofurazone), and anesthetics ("caine" preparations). Other contributing factors to be avoided are heat, friction, and radiant energy.

3. Apply cool wet compresses to weeping and blistered areas for 15 minutes two to three times daily. Isotonic saline solution may be used. With commercial preparations of Burow's solution (Bluboro powder or Domeboro powder or tablets), 1 packet or tablet per 500 ml (pint) of water makes approximately a 1:40 dilution. Make certain the mixture is completely dissolved before application. A soft cloth such as Kerlix gauze, an old, clean thin white handkerchief, or a towel is immersed in the solution. The cloth is wrung slightly and applied to the affected area of the skin. When the cloth begins to dry, remove it completely and resoak in the solution before reapplying. Do not pour the solution directly on the dressing; a fresh solution should be prepared before each treatment.

As an alternative the patient may soak the affected part, such as a hand or a foot, directly in the solution for the same period of time.

For generalized involvement hospitalization may be necessary. Compresses may be applied to all affected areas of the body, and in some cases baths such as with Aveeno colloidal oatmeal may be preferable.

Treatment should be continued for no more than a few days (usually 3 to 4) to avoid excessive drying of the skin.

4. Immediately following the compresses, soaks, or baths, apply a topical corticosteroid spray (triamcinolone [Kenalog] spray or betamethasone [Valisone] aerosol). A 2 or 3 second spray to each affected area is sufficient. One of the many topical corticosteroid creams such as betamethasone valerate (Valisone), triamcinolone (Kenalog), or fluocinolone acetonide (Synalar) may be used when the acute dermatitis is not extensively vesicular. Avoid ointments in the acute stages.

5. Do not apply fluorinated topical corticosteroids to the face for more than 2 weeks; prolonged use may produce severe sternoid rosacea.

6. Oral antihistamines such as cyproheptadine (Periactin), hydroxyzine (Atarax), or diphenhydramine (Benadryl) help relieve itching. It is imperative that workers be warned not to drive or operate dangerous machinery while taking antihistamines.

7. Systemic use of corticosteroids is indicated in patients with severe, localized dermatitis, such as a vesiculobullous eruption of the hands or feet, or with severe, generalized dermatitis. An injection of triamcinolone acetonide suspension (Kenalog-40 injection) may be given, or oral corticosteroids such as prednisone (Deltasone), 30 to 60 mg daily in two or three divided doses, is begun initially and tapered over 10 to 30 days.

Subacute and Chronic Contact Dermatitis. 1. Avoidances as outlined in (1) (2) and (5) above. 2. Do not compress or soak. 3. Use a topical corticosteroid cream or ointment two to three times daily and continue treatment for 2 to 3 weeks after the skin appears normal. 4. Oral antihistamines as in (6) above. 5. I wish to emphasize that frequently recurring cases of acute contact dermatitis should be considered "chronic," and frequent use (more than once every 3 months) of short courses of systemic corticosteroids should be avoided. In these patients a tireless search for precipitating and aggravating factors is necessary.

Secondarily Infected Contact Dermatitis. In my experience this is infrequent. A low grade bacterial infection such as from a coagulase-positive *Staphylococcus* may occur. In these patients compresses or soaks with povidone-iodine (Betadine solution) are helpful. Bacterial cultures should be made, and antibiotic therapy such as erythromycin stearate (Erythrocin), 250 mg three to four times daily for 10 days, is initiated. As infection resolves, topical corticosteroid therapy may be reinstituted. Acute cellulitis with accompanying chills, fever, and lymphangitis may require more aggressive and closely supervised antibiotic therapy; hospitalization may be necessary.

Ancillary Measures

Resources to Identify Causative Agent(s). It is imperative that the causative agent(s) be identified in every patient. Unless this is done, treatment may be doomed to failure and the patient will experience recurrences of the dermatosis. A careful work history should be obtained to determine in detail all the patient's industrial contacts. Inquiry into exposures from second jobs, hobbies, and household contacts is essential. In this regard I have found it most helpful to consult standard texts on occupational and contact dermatitis. In addition, two other resources are helpful:

1. Division of Technical Services, National Institute for Occupational Safety and Health, United States Public Health Service, 4676 Columbia Parkway, Cincinnati, Ohio, 45226.

2. The patient's employer (with the consent of the patient), such as the plant manager, industrial research department, or the plant physician, nurse, safety officer, industrial hygienist, or personnel manager.

Together these resources may provide lists of chemicals contacted in various occupations, information on cutaneous and systemic toxicity of chemicals, suggested patch-testing concentrations, and information on sources of products and processes that contain a particular chemical. The latter is extremely important, because a worker may be exposed to the same chemical at home and at work (e.g., rubber, metal, chromates, dyes, plastic resins) or in several sources at work.

Diagnostic Patch-Testing. Patch-testing, when properly performed and correctly interpreted, is unquestionably of great value in identifying the causative agent(s) of allergic contact dermatitis. Initial testing is usually done with the most frequent contact allergens (nickel, chromates, rubber, medicaments, preservatives, dyes, and resins). Other materials, found at home or work, may also have to be tested *in appropriate concentrations* to distinguish occupational and nonoccupational factors. Patch-testing should be employed only by physicians highly experienced with this technique. Pre-employment patch-testing generally should be avoided. The same recommendations and precautions apply to photopatch-testing, which is used to diagnose photoallergic contact dermatitis.

Preventive Measures. It is impossible to separate treatment from prevention. Personal measures such as wearing protective clothing may be required when they can be used safely. Barrier or protective creams should be used only as a last resort and should never be applied to inflamed skin. Environmental control such as good housekeeping, engineering controls, and removal of physical and chemical hazards is also important.

Fiberglass Dermatitis

This special form of pruritic papular, eczematous, and occasionally purpuric dermatitis is produced by mechanical irritation from glass fibers. Body folds and areas of tight-fitting clothing are common sites of involvement. Hardening usually occurs after several weeks of exposure.

Treatment. 1. Limitation of further exposure to fiberglass by environmental control. 2. Wearing of loose-fitting clothing which is changed daily. 3. Frequent skin cleansing. 4. Topical corticosteroid creams (see Contact Dermatitis above). 5.

Lightly apply a thin coating of talcum powder. 6. Workers with dermographism or urticaria should not work with fiberglass.

Oil Acne

Most cutting fluids used today are synthetic or semisynthetic and most frequently produce contact eczema. Treatment of these patients should follow measures described previously for contact dermatitis. However, exposure to insoluble, straight cutting fluids may produce folliculitis ("oil boils") in areas uncommon for acne vulgaris, usually the extremities.

Treatment. 1. Avoidance of contact with oils and grease. 2. Daily changes of work clothing. 3. Frequent cleansing of the skin with soap and water. 4. The worker should avoid cleansing the skin with fabric waste, which is intended only for cleaning machines and tools. 5. Local acne medications (benzoyl peroxide 5 per cent gel [PanOxyl 5]) or retinoic acid cream 0.05 to 0.1 per cent (Retin A).

Chloracne

This extremely refractory form of industrial acne is produced by exposure to various polyhalogenated aromatic compounds, such as naphthalenes, biphenyls, dibenzofurans, and phenol and aniline herbicide intermediates.

Treatment. 1. Absolute avoidance of chemical exposure through a totally enclosed manufacturing process. 2. Appraisal of possible systemic toxicity, including liver, kidney, neurologic, and porphyrin studies. 3. Work clothing should be laundered at work. 4. Double locker rooms (clean and dirty) with adequate shower facilities. 5. Protective creams should not be used. 6. Optimal control is obtained by preventing formation of the toxic chloracnegenic chemical by changing the synthetic process.

Pigmentation Disorders

Staining. A number of chemicals stain the skin by direct external contact. The stain usually responds to attempts at cleansing, avoidance of chemical exposure, and the passage of time.

Hyperpigmentation. Exposure to tar, pitch, and chemicals such as psoralens in combination with ultraviolet light may produce increased pigmentation of the skin. Protective clothing and sunscreens may be helpful. Hydroquinone (Eldopaque Forte), applied twice daily, may help reduce the pigmentation.

Hypopigmentation. Exposure to paratertiary butyl phenol or catechol, or paratertiary amyl phenol (germicidal disinfectants, oils, plastics, paints, or resins) and certain chemicals may produce occupational leukoderma. Treatment involves avoiding chemical exposure and using stains for the skin (Vitadye, Dy-O-Derm). Photochemotherapy with oral psoralen (methoxsalen [Oxsoralen]) and black ultraviolet light (PUVA) may occasionally be effective in this form of leukoderma.

Other Occupational Dermatoses

Microbial infections (sporotrichosis), granulomatous reactions (foreign bodies), ulcerations (chrome), neoplasms, (tar, pitch), and repeated mechanical trauma (calluses, blisters) may occasionally occur. The spectrum of these and other occupational dermatoses is wide, and therapy depends upon cause. The hallmarks for the successful treatment of occupational dermatoses are identifying the causative agent(s), early therapy, and prevention of further chemical exposure.

SUNBURN AND PHOTOSENSITIVITY

method of
DAVID R. BICKERS, M.D.
Case Western Reserve University
Cleveland, Ohio

Sunlight consists of a broad spectrum of radiant energy from very short, highly energetic x-rays to very long radiowaves. However, only a small fraction of solar radiation is of importance in terms of sunburn and photosensitivity disease. This component is known as the photobiologic action spectrum and consists of the ultraviolet (UV) and visible wavelengths. The UV has been arbitrarily divided into three major components: the UVA (320 to 400 nm), the UVB (290 to 320 nm), and the UVC (200 to 290 nm). Since the UVC is completely absorbed by the stratospheric ozone and does not reach the earth's surface, only the UVA, UVB, and visible (400 to 700 nm) wavelengths are major factors in producing sunburn and photosensitivity disease.

It is important to recall that the sun's capacity to produce a biologic effect in the skin requires that its energy must first be absorbed. This absorption process is a chemical reaction, caused by the presence within the skin of a variety of chemical substances or *chromophores* capable of absorbing radiant energy. Examples are DNA, RNA, proteins such as melanin and keratin, and constituent amino acids.

The action spectrum for a specific photobiologic effect consists of those wavelengths of solar energy that can be shown to produce the response, whereas the absorption spectrum of a chromophore consists of those wavelengths of energy that it can absorb. To produce a photobiologic effect, energy must be absorbed by a chromophore that exhibits an absorption spectrum within the action spectrum for the effect. *Whereas the action spectrum and absorption spectrum need not be identical, they must overlap at some point.*

Sunburn

Sunburn erythema results either from direct damage to the vascular endothelium in the dermis or from the diffusion of vasoactive mediators from irradiated epidermis to the dermal vasculature. There is also some evidence that mast cells may release proinflammatory substances when injured by UV radiation.

A search for inflammatory mediators in suction blisters obtained from UVB-irradiated human skin has revealed elevated histamine levels immediately after radiation, which returned to normal at 24 hours. Prostaglandin E_2 (PGE_2) increases to approximately 150 per cent of control levels after 24 hours and then diminishes. Prostaglandins are known to evoke redness and pain in human skin after intradermal injection and are present in elevated amounts in suction blisters after UV irradiation of the skin.

By far the most effective treatment of acute sunburn is prevention. Protection of the skin with light-opaque clothing and minimizing exposure between 10 A.M. and 3 P.M. when the intensity of solar UVB is greatest largely will prevent severe reactions, even in individuals highly susceptible to sunburn. A wide variety of chemical and physical sunscreens is available commercially; these are effective if used regularly and reapplied frequently prior to and during sun exposure. A qualitative indicator of sunscreen efficacy is known as the *S*un *P*rotective *F*actor (SPF). Simply stated, SPF is a ratio of the dose of sunlight required to produce visible erythema of the skin to which the sunscreen has been applied, to that dose that evokes erythema without sunscreen. Thus an SPF of 10 indicates that an individual could remain outdoors exposed to sunlight ten times longer than if sunscreen were not applied and achieve the same degree of redness. Unfortunately, the SPF numbers used by some sunscreen manufacturers have been derived under artificially controlled temperature and humidity conditions and do not account for the inevitable loss of efficacy that occurs as a result of exercise, sweating, and swimming.

TABLE 1. **Photoallergenic Drugs and Chemicals**

Halogenated Salicylanilides	*Sulfonamides*
tetrachlorosalicylanilide	
tribromosalicylanilide	*Sunscreens*
dibromosalicylanilide	PABA esters
trichlorocarbanilide	digalloyltrioleate
bithionol	
	Whiteners
Antifungal Agents	stilbenes
Multifungin	
Fenticlor	*Fragrances*
Jadit	musk ambrette
	methylcoumarin
Phenothiazines	
chlorpromazine	*Nonsteroidal anti-inflammatory agents*
promethazine	piroxicam

Once an acute sunburn has developed, the only forms of management currently available are symptomatic. Cool, topical soaks using moist compresses of tap water or Burow's solution 1:40 may reduce discomfort. Topical corticosteroids are of little benefit. Systemically administered nonsteroidal anti-inflammatory agents (NSAIDs), which can inhibit the cyclo-oxygenase pathway of arachidonic acid metabolism and thereby reduce prostaglandin production, may be helpful if administered within the first several hours after exposure. Systemic corticosteroids in doses of 1 to 1.5 mg per kg can be employed and probably shorten the course of the severe discomfort that accompanies very severe sunburn.

More prolonged exposure may lead to blister formation and epidermal sloughing. In rare cases, it may be desirable to transfer such patients to a burn center where experienced personnel can manage any complications.

Photosensitivity Dermatitis

The capacity of environmental chemicals to produce cutaneous photosensitivity dermatitis is now well recognized. The two major types are photoallergic and phototoxic. Regardless of the type, the cutaneous manifestations of photosensitivity dermatitis include changes involving primarily the face, neck, ears, dorsa of the hands, rims of the ears, and "V" of the neck. There is usually a sharp line of demarcation between sun-exposed skin and body areas covered by clothing.

Photoallergic Dermatitis. A large number of compounds are thought to be capable of producing photoallergic dermatitis; some are listed in Table 1. A number of cases have been reported of individuals who have used cosmetic products containing the halogenated salicylanilides or the

TABLE 2. **Phototoxic Drugs and Chemicals**

Dyes	*Furocoumarins*
anthraquinone	psoralen
eosin	8-methoxypsoralen
methylene blue	4,5,8-trimethylpsoralen
rose bengal	
	Drugs
Coal tar derivatives	nalidixic acid
acridine	phenothiazines
anthracene	sulfonamides
phenanthrene	tetracyclines
pyridine	thiazides

fragrance musk ambrette. Most recently the nonsteroidal anti-inflammatory drug piroxicam (Feldene) has also been shown to cause acute photosensitivity.

The pathogenesis of photoallergic dermatitis has puzzled investigators for many years. The diagnostic technique of photopatch-testing in which suspected photosensitizing chemicals are applied to normal-appearing skin of affected individuals and subsequently irradiated with UVA in an effort to reproduce a localized eczematous lesion has shown that both the photosensitizing chemical and UVA radiation are required to elicit an abnormal response. This led to the hypothesis that certain photosensitizers such as the halogenated salicylanilides, which are low molecular weight compounds, may function as haptens and after absorption of light become bound to a carrier protein, thereby creating a "photoantigen" that can evoke the photoallergic response.

In addition to having photoallergic dermatitis, many of these individuals may also be contact-allergic to composite plant oleo resins, certain fragrances, and lichens, and this contact-allergic sensitivity is often an aggravating facator.

Phototoxic Dermatitis. Chemically induced photosensitivity reactions in the skin can also be produced by a nonimmunologic process in which the photosensitizing chemical is excited by light and can damage cutaneous tissue directly. This form of reaction is known as phototoxicity; some of the agents that can produce it are listed in Table 2.

The management of photosensitivity disease, whether photoallergic or phototoxic, centers on the identification and elimination of the offending photosensitizing chemical and the reduction of sun exposure. The identity of the photosensitizer often can be obtained by a careful history and confirmed by the technique of photopatch-testing. Once the chemical has been eliminated and sun exposure minimized, the majority of patients will notice slow but steady improvement of their dermatologic disease. Rarely, the condition may persist for months or years. Severe flares of the disease can be managed with moist compresses and topical corticosteroids. Systemic corticosteroids may be necessary in selected cases. Unfortunately, sunscreens have proved relatively ineffective in this regard.

Section 13

The Nervous System

BRAIN ABSCESS

method of
JOEL N. ABRAMOVITZ, M.D.
Tufts University
Boston, Massachusetts

Bacterial infection of the brain begins as cerebritis, a diffuse infection analogous to cellulitis in other tissues. As the center of the infected area becomes necrotic, it is properly called an abscess. Ultimately, a gliotic capsule surrounds the abscess. The brain responds to the inflammatory mass with surrounding edema, increasing the apparent mass effect, causing neurologic deficits, and subjecting the patient to the dangers of increased intracranial pressure.

The goals of therapy are to make a bacteriologic diagnosis in order to achieve sterilization, and to relieve symptoms of intracranial mass.

Antibiotic Therapy

When the diagnosis is made during the stage of cerebritis, or at any time prior to firm encapsulation, antibiotic therapy is often successful without operation. Drugs useful in the treatment of brain abscess are listed in Table 1. Nonsurgical treatment may be considered (a) when the causative organism is known, as in the setting of a systemic infection or when one of multiple abscesses has been aspirated, and (b) when the neurologic deficits due to the intracranial mass are mild and not life-threatening.

Repeated CT scans must be employed to monitor the success of treatment. Systemic parameters such as fever, leukocyte count, and sedimentation rate cannot be used as they are often normal in brain abscess. While careful serial neurologic examination is important, it cannot solely be relied upon to rule out progression of an abscess.

Antibiotics are used in conjunction with surgical treatment. In the acutely ill patient, antibiotics should be started immediately following the surgical procedure at which specimens are obtained and prior to bacteriologic identification. The likely source of the infecting organism may be used to guide the choice of antibiotics until culture and sensitivity data are available (Table 2).

Prior to obtaining specimens, the bacteriology laboratory should be alerted so that the specimen may be properly processed for the wide variety of possible organisms, including anaerobes and fungi.

TABLE 1. **Antibiotics Useful in Treatment of Brain Abscess**

Drug	Organism	Dose
Penicillin G	Streptococci: some anaerobes	2 million units IV q 2–4 hr
Oxacillin	Staphylococci	2 grams IV q 4 hr
Chloramphenicol	Gram-negative bacilli *Bacteroides*	1 gram IV q 6 hr
Metronidazole	Anaerobes	7.5 mg/kg IV q 6 hr

TABLE 2. **Organisms Likely to Cause Brain Abscess, by Site of Origin**

Setting	Organism
Scalp or skull wound	Staphylococci
Basilar fracture with CSF leak	Staphylococci Pneumococci Anaerobes
Otitis, sinusitis	Same Anaerobic streptococci
Dental procedures or infections	Anaerobes Anaerobic streptococci
Cyanotic heart disease	Staphylococci Streptococci Gram-negative bacilli
Endocarditis	Same
Immunosuppressed states	*Actinomyces* *Nocardia, Aspergillus*
Idiopathic	Staphylococci Streptococci Anaerobes Gram-negative bacilli

Indications for Surgical Treatment

In most cases, operation will be required to make a bacteriologic diagnosis. If abscesses are multiple, only one need be sampled.

Operation is mandatory when neurologic deficits are severe or progressive, and particularly when signs of brain stem compression (herniation) are present. This is particularly urgent when the abscess is in the posterior fossa. Abscess drainage is by far the most rapid and effective method of reduction of intracranial pressure in the setting of a severe deficit.

When the abscess abuts the ventricular wall, the patient is at risk for rupture of the abscess. Drainage is indicated to prevent this possibility, which would lead to disseminated meningeal infection. Operation is also indicated when serial computed tomography (CT) scans show progression of an abscess under antibiotic treatment.

Surgical Methods

Prior to operation, accurate localization of the lesion is essential. This can almost always be accomplished by CT scan.

Steroids are useful adjuncts for reduction of edema caused by the operative procedure. Dexamethasone (Decadron), 4 to 10 mg intravenously every 4 hours, is adequate as an initial dose. Since prolonged use is not anticipated, any immunosuppressive effects may be ignored. Anticonvulsants such as phenytoin (Dilantin), 100 mg intravenously or orally every 8 hours, or phenobarbital, 30 to 60 mg intravenously every 6 to 8 hours, should be used. Blood levels of anticonvulsants should be used to guide selection of the ultimate dose. Antibiotics should be begun as stated. The regimen will be modified when culture results are available.

Most abscesses can be drained via needle puncture performed freehand through a burr hole. This may be done under local anesthesia, an advantage in seriously ill patients. Needle drainage may be repeated thereafter as necessary using the same burr hole. While a single drainage is often adequate, the possibility that several may be required should be anticipated. When the abscess is located in a deep or neurologically sensitive site, CT-guided stereotactic equipment may be used to perform the drainage.

If the abscess is large or multiloculated, craniotomy with abscess drainage under direct vision may be performed. Open technique will permit loculations to be broken down and the abscess cavity to be irrigated with Ringer's lactate or an antibiotic solution such as bacitracin (1000 units per ml). A drainage catheter may be left in the cavity and brought out through a separate stab incision. A closed-suction system like the Jackson-Pratt drain is ideal for this purpose. Significant drainage does not usually continue beyond 48 hours from operation, and the catheter may then be removed. Risks of associated superinfection are therefore slight.

Craniotomies should be performed, if possible, through an osteoplastic (vascularized) bone flap. This will minimize the risk of osteomyelitis from the inevitable contamination of the flap. Such a flap may be conserved, eliminating the need for a cranioplasty at a later date. Even when a free bone flap must be used, osteomyelitis is not likely, and an attempt to retain the flap is justified.

Abscess drainage may usually be accomplished through a small craniotomy. An exception is the case in which the abscess is secondary to a traumatic cerebrospinal fluid leak through a fracture of the anterior fossa floor. In this case, a full frontal flap is needed to repair the leak at the same time the abscess is drained.

A rare, highly mature abscess with a firm capsule occasionally may be excised in toto without rupture. This should not be attempted unless obviously and easily feasible since it is not necessary for treatment and does not eliminate the need for antibiotic therapy. Excision of an abscess or of a postabscess scar occasionally may benefit the patient who has seizures that have resisted ordinary treatment.

Postoperative Care. CT scans must be performed to confirm that drainage has achieved its goal and that progressive resolution of the abscess is taking place. In the past, radiologic contrast materials have been instilled into the abscess cavity, permitting observation of the size and location of the cavity with plain radiographs. This procedure is now primarily of historic interest.

Antibiotics should be continued for 6 to 8 weeks following drainage. They may be then discontinued, even though there will usually be residual abnormality on the enhanced CT scan. Such an abnormality should be re-examined by CT about a month after the antibiotics are stopped, to rule out re-emergence of the abscess.

Steroids may be tapered rapidly as the patient's neurologic condition improves. They will not usually be required for more than a week following drainage. Persistent neurologic symptoms at this point may require repeated drainage of a residual abscess.

Anticonvulsants should be continued until the abscess has definitely resolved. At that point, they may be stopped if the patient has been free of seizures. The patient must be aware that seizures may recur and that long-term anticonvulsants may be required.

ALZHEIMER'S DISEASE

method of
ROBERT J. JOYNT, M.D.
University of Rochester
Rochester, New York

Alzheimer's disease was described in 1907 but has attracted widespread attention of the lay public and medical profession only in the last decade. It is now recognized as one of our major health care problems. The disease is a progressive deterioration of the brain resulting in memory loss, cognitive deficits, and altered behavior. The prevalence of the disease is not clearly established and estimates vary from 10 to 15 per cent of the population over age 65. The major brunt of the disease is in the eighth and ninth decades, and this is the segment of the population increasing most rapidly in number. With advances in medical care, the survival rate of patients with dementia has been increasing. So the increase in the size of the at risk population and in survival makes the search for solutions a high priority.

Alzheimer's disease is one of the many causes for dementia so that two admonitions are pertinent. One is that dementia is a symptom and there are many causes, and, two, that some of these causes are treatable. This places a great burden on the diagnostician, as the specter of a failing mind in a healthy body has immense implications for the patient, family, and society.

Treatment

Alzheimer's disease has as yet no specific treatment, but many things can be accomplished in care for both the patient and the family. Once a diagnosis is established, there should be active consultation set up between the family and someone knowledgeable in the disease. This is important not only for the care of the patient but for the support of the family.

The personal physician should monitor the patient's general health closely. Patients with dementia often do fairly well if otherwise healthy, but mild congestive failure, anemia, urinary tract infection, and so on will often make them much worse as their "brain reserves" are low.

Life should remain as uncomplicated as possible, and major changes in living patterns should be avoided. Patients with mild dementia can often do very well in a familiar home setting. Often a patient can be maintained outside a nursing home or supervised facility with minimal supervision or intermittent assistance. The apathy that is a hallmark of dementia necessitates a simple and largely unvarying routine.

Many patients can be successfully cared for at their home or a family member's home if their sleep pattern coincides with that of the family. In general, sedation does not work very well, although medication such as chloral hydrate, 0.5 to 1.0 gram, may be tried. Generally, the most common cause of nighttime wandering is the frequent naps taken during the day. If the patient is kept active (e.g., walking or visiting a day care program) this will often eliminate the problem.

Medications should be kept to a minimum, as these patients often are very sensitive to medications. At the same time, there are obvious indications for medication for specific medical problems. Also, it should be recognized that early in the disease depression may be present so that an antidepressant, such as amitriptyline, 25 to 100 mg per day, may be useful and if given at night may promote sleep. Rarely, patients may be combative and a psychotropic such as haloperidol, 2 to 4 mg per day, may be useful.

A major component of the care is the concern for the family. This is an extremely trying time for spouses, children, and friends. All that was human and endearing in a person is disintegrating. Major stresses in the family appear as guilt, accusations, and shifting and denial of responsibilities. In many instances, the best in human nature comes out and the loving care of a spouse or child is remarkable. Therefore, efforts should be made for support and respite. There are major support groups throughout the country, and these should be identified for the family. Respite during the day or for more extended periods of time is provided by many different groups and agencies. Relief of the constant burden of care for a few hours or days will be of great benefit.

Research has been very active in this area. The most significant finding has been the identification of a cholinergic deficit in the brains of patients dying with Alzheimer's disease. The original hope was similar to that of a few years ago when Parkinson's disease responded to dopamine precursors to correct a basal ganglion dopamine depletion. Therefore, precursors of acetylcholine, such as lecithin and choline, and drugs to increase the action of acetylcholine, such as physostigmine, have been tried. There is no convincing evidence that any of these are beneficial. Similarly, there is no evidence that cerebral vasodilators work in this disorder. Various modes of therapy are being developed and tried. If any of these therapies are tried, and in some instances the families insist, it must be clearly explained that the efficacy has not been established.

INTRACEREBRAL HEMORRHAGE (Nontraumatic)

method of
LOUIS R. CAPLAN, M.D.,
and L. DANA DEWITT, M.D.
New England Medical Center,
Tufts University
Boston, Massachusetts

Intracerebral hemorrhage (ICH) is a major cause of morbidity and death and accounts for approximately 10 per cent of all strokes. Although many hemorrhage syndromes are identifiable by their clinical presentations, the management of ICH has been revolutionized by the advent of computed axial tomography (CT). CT accurately documents the size and location of the hematoma, the presence and extent of mass effect, the presence of hydrocephalus, and the presence of spontaneous dissection of the hematoma into the ventricular system and subarachnoid space.

Selection of treatment for the individual patient with ICH depends on six key factors: (1) etiology of ICH, (2) locale of the lesion, (3) lesion size, (4) lesion age, that is, time since onset, (5) presence of significantly increased intracranial pressure (ICP), and (6) clinical course while under observation, that is, is there improvement, stabilization, or worsening of neurologic signs or level of consciousness. The available medical and surgical treatment modalities are outlined in Table 1.

TABLE 1. **Treatment of Intracerebral Hemorrhage**

Medical
Control of hypertension
trimethaphan camsylate (Arfonad)
0.5 to 1 mg per min intravenously by drip
nitroprusside sodium
15 to 200 micrograms per min intravenously by drip
hydralazine hydrochloride (Apresoline)
50 to 100 mg twice daily orally
Reversal of bleeding diathesis
fresh frozen plasma
antihemophilic factor
phytonadione (vit. K, aquaMEPHYTON) 20 to 40 mg intravenously
platelet transfusion
fresh blood transfusion
"Medical" decompression for increased intracranial pressure
intubation and mechanical hyperventilation
dexamethasone (Decadron) 4 mg every 6 hours
mannitol 0.5 to 1 gram per kg every 4 hours intravenously
glycerol 1 to 1.5 ounces orally every 6 hours
furosemide (Lasix) 40 mg (4 mg per min) intravenously
Surgical
Drainage of hematoma
Ventricular drainage or shunt
Removal of bleeding AVM or tumor
Repair of aneurysm

Treatment Related to Specific Etiologies

Hypertension

Hypertension is the most common cause of spontaneous ICH. Bleeding is usually from deep penetrating arteries of the circle of Willis, especially lenticulostriate, thalamostriate, and thalamoperforating branches and similar penetrating branches from the vertebrobasilar arterial system. Hypertension-induced pathologic changes in these arteries include fibrinoid necrosis and microaneurysm formation, changes that predispose to bleeding. Hypertensive hemorrhages have a definite predilection for certain regions and are distributed approximately as follows: putamen, 40 per cent; lobar, 22 per cent; thalamus, 15 per cent; pons, 8 per cent; cerebellum, 8 per cent; caudate, 7 per cent.

Control of arterial hypertension is important in stemming the bleeding and in preventing subsequent episodes of ICH. If the blood pressure is extremely high, we begin a drip of trimethaphan camsylate (Arfonad) using an intravenous drip delivering 0.5 to 1 mg per min of the drug while titrating blood pressure. Alternatively, nitroprusside sodium can be given by intravenous drip in a dosage of 15 to 200 micrograms per min, again titrating the arterial pressure. We attempt to reduce the systolic blood pressure to 120 to 150 mm Hg and the diastolic pressure to 80 to 90 mm Hg. Hydralazine hydrochloride (Apresoline), 50 to 100 mg orally twice daily, is then frequently used to maintain the lower blood pressure levels. We carefully monitor the blood pressure for abrupt hypotension, which can occur with these agents. In large hemorrhages, the increased ICP causes a secondary rise in blood pressure, which is needed to maintain a sufficient arterial to venous gradient to ensure adequate cerebral perfusion. In such patients excessive reduction of blood pressure can lead to hypoperfusion of the brain and clinical deterioration. Neurologic signs and level of alertness should be monitored carefully as the blood pressure is lowered. If the patient worsens, we allow the blood pressure to rise to see if the findings are sensitive to changes in arterial pressure and perfusion.

Bleeding Diathesis

Oral anticoagulant use has become an important iatrogenic cause of ICH. Oral anticoagulant hemorrhages progress more slowly and are more commonly lobar and cerebellar than hypertensive ICH. Mortality is high. Reversal of hypoprothrombinemia should be immediate using phytonadione (vitamin K), 20 to 40 mg intravenously. Hemorrhage due to hemophilia or deficiency of other coagulant factors can be treated with infusion of fresh frozen plasma or antihemophilic factor. Thrombocytopenia-related ICH is treated by platelet transfusion or infusion of fresh blood.

Drugs

Cocaine, phencyclidine (PCP), amphetamines, and phenylpropanolamine have effects on catecholamine metabolism and release and can cause sudden blood pressure elevations and ICH. Amphetamines and the intravenous use of drugs prepared for oral use, such as methyl phenidate (Ritalin), pentazocine (Talwin), and tripelennamine (Pyribenzamine), can cause a cerebral vasculitis and ICH. Arteriography may show focal narrowing and beading of small intracranial surface arteries in such patients. Medical control of increased ICP is usually sufficient to allow survival. Cessation of drug abuse is essential.

Bleeding Lesions (Arteriovenous Malformations, Aneurysms, Tumors)

Arteriovenous malformations (AVM) and aneurysms pose a slightly different problem to those already considered, that of potentially serious rebleeding. Tumors require treatment unrelated to the propensity for bleeding. The identification of these lesions by CT or angiography is essential for optimal treatments. AVMs should be suspected in young patients with superficial hemorrhages in the absence of hypertension, drugs, or trauma. Preceding headache, seizures, and abnormal cranial calcifications are clues to the presence of these lesions. Often an enhanced CT will show abnormal vessels. Aneurysms can cause meningocerebral hemorrhages; hematomas are usually contiguous to the brain base, and associated subarachnoid bleeding is seen on CT. Tumors are also often identifiable on CT. The presence of prior neurologic signs and a known primary tumor, such as bronchogenic carcinoma, melanoma, or choriocarcinoma should raise a suspicion of this etiology. If hematomas require surgical drainage, it would be optimal to repair the AVM or aneurysm and remove the tumor at the same time.

Amyloid Angiopathy

Cerebral amyloid angiopathy is becoming an increasingly frequent cause of ICH. These lesions are prevalent in older patients and affect primarily the cerebral lobes. They do not begin in the basal ganglia, thalamus, pons, or cerebellum, loci with infrequent vascular amyloid. The friable blood vessels predispose these patients to bleeding or oozing after surgery. Suspicion of cerebral amyloid angiopathy should deter surgery unless the situation is life-threatening.

Locale and Age of the Hematoma as Treatment Determinants

Some ICH locations lend themselves more readily to surgical drainage. Lobar hemorrhages are relatively close to the brain surface and can usually be drained through a cortical incision. Putaminal hemorrhages can be drained through an incision into the lateral ganglionic lesion through the insula. Cerebellar hemorrhage, though often deep, can usually be readily drained through a posterior fossa surgical approach. Well localized round or oval hematomas are easier to drain than lesions that are slit-like or that extend longitudinally along white matter fiber tracts. Thalamic and brain stem hemorrhages, especially those in the pons, are relatively inaccessible to drainage and are usually considered nonsurgical lesions. Although surgical damage to cerebral, cerebellar, or basal ganglionic structures near hematomas can usually be tolerated, damage to the thalamus or pons is more likely to cause severe disability or death. Surprisingly, after extensive surgical decompression of the cerebellum with removal of the large hematoma, there may be little lasting clinical deficit except lack of agility on navigating turns. Caudate hemorrhages usually drain themselves spontaneously and early into the adjacent lateral ventricles and rarely if ever require surgical drainage. Thalamic hemorrhages sometimes cause obstruction of the ventricular system that can be managed by ventricular drainage.

Soft or nearly liquid blood is much easier to drain than firm clot. Early in the course of the ICH, during the first 24 hours, blood is still semiliquid and can usually be removed by suction through a small incision. After 24 hours blood solidifies and a wider incision is needed to extricate the clot. Much later (5 to 10 days) the clot is again more liquified, although by this time the clinical condition has stabilized and drainage is seldom indicated.

Size, Presence of Increased Intracranial Pressure, and Clinical Course of the Lesion

Death from ICH is usually due to the consequences of increased intracranial pressure. The addition of extra mass in the form of hematoma, surrounding edema, or dilated ventricles increases intracranial pressure. Pressure increases maximally in the region of the hematoma and can cause shifts or herniation of tissues through dural compartments and fatal brain stem compression. Increased ICP also compromises cerebral blood flow. The skull and dura mater are effective fortresses that protect the brain from external injury; these structures also act as a prison when intracranial pressure rises internally. Atrophy, common in the elderly, can provide reserve room for local volume expansion not available in healthy, young patients. Medical and surgical control of serious increased intracranial pressure can be life-saving.

On the other hand, there is no evidence that reduction of slight increase in ICP or drainage of small hematomas that do not threaten life will reduce long-term morbidity in patients with ICH. Hematomas gradually resolve and leave slit-like scars that disconnect cortical regions. Drainage of these lesions also leaves a scar unlikely to be smaller than the natural one.

Medical decompression or surgical drainage is unnecessary in small lesions that are less than 2 cm in diameter. Small hematomas heal spontaneously, and, when not located in vital regions such as the thalamus and brain stem, recovery is usually good. Treatment of small lesions is limited to control of blood pressure and other etiologic factors previously discussed that could cause recurrence or later extension of the lesion. Massive hemorrhages usually increase ICP rapidly and cause fatal, irreversible brain stem cerebral damage even before the physician can treat the patient. Treatment of these massive lesions is seldom if ever effective. Survival when it occurs is usually vegetative. The most important patients to treat are those with moderate sized or large, well localized hematomas greater than 3 cm in diameter who develop signs of increased intracranial pressure but are still awake on arrival at the hospital.

Most studies correlate mortality and increased ICP with the size of the lesion. Lobar, cerebellar, and putaminal lesions over 3 cm in diameter have a much higher incidence of increased ICP and death than smaller lesions. ICP can be monitored by clinical signs or CT changes or by direct pressure measurements requiring a surgically placed intracranial monitor. It has not been our practice to advise placement of intracranial pressure monitors unless the clinical situation is unusual or a surgical procedure is going to be performed and the monitor can be incidentally placed at the same time.

Careful monitoring of the patient's neurologic signs and state of alertness is critical if the physician is to quickly respond to the need for decompressive intervention. Nothing can substitute for frequent and careful examination by a physician experienced in central nervous system disease. As intracranial pressure begins to rise, the patient usually complains of headache and often vomits. In posterior fossa ICH, the neck becomes stiff. Further rises in intracranial pressure cause a progressive decline in the level of consciousness. Lethargy is followed by agitation and delirium and finally stupor and coma as pressure rises to critical levels. In putaminal or ganglionic ICH, an increase in the effective size of the lesion due to continued bleeding or edema causes fixed conjugate deviation of the eyes to the side of the hematoma. Compression of the contralateral hemisphere and brain stem causes an ipsilateral extensor plantar reflex and later bilateral conjugate gaze palsy and third cranial nerve dysfunction in the form of an ipsilateral fixed or dilated pupil. When these signs develop while the patient is under observation, in our experience, the hematoma invariably proves fatal unless decompression measures are quickly instituted. Papilledema is not a very helpful sign since it is often absent. Worsening neurologic signs and a decreasing level of alertness are ominous prognostic signs and warrant urgent intervention.

CT findings also can document the development of significant pressure. Compression of the ipsilateral lateral ventricle, dilatation of the contralateral lateral ventricle because of compression of the foramen of Monro, symmetric hydrocephalus, shift of the midline, and compression of the rostral brain stem cisterns are helpful signs to note. Deviation of the proximal cisternal segment of the anterior choroidal or posterior cerebral arteries and shift of the anterior cerebral artery to the opposite side are also helpful angiographic signs of herniation. When a monitor is in place, elevation of the ICP above 20 torr (mm Hg) is worrisome. Pupillary dilatation often occurs if ICP exceeds 28 torr.

We administer phenytoin sodium (Dilantin), 500 mg intravenously, if seizures occur and continue this drug orally in doses of 100 mg three times a day. We do not prophylactically use anticonvulsants. Higher doses of phenytoin or other anticonvulsants are used if seizures are not controlled.

Method of Managing Patients with Increased Intracranial Pressure Due to ICH

We perform CT scanning immediately in patients suspected of having an ICH. Repeat CTs are ordered if the patient worsens in order to monitor changes in the effective size of the lesion and ventricular system and to detect important pressure shifts. Lumbar puncture is not indicated in the evaluation of patients with known ICH. In smaller lesions that do not communicate with the ventricles or subarachnoid space, taps are invariably clear, and in large hematomas puncture increases the chances of herniation while yielding little useful additional data. If the clinical syndrome and CT findings are those of a typical hypertension hemorrhage in the basal ganglia, caudate, thalamus, pons, or cerebellum, we do not perform angiography. If the hemorrhage is in an atypical location for hypertensive ICH or the patient is young and nonhypertensive, we pursue angiography to exclude an AVM, aneurysm, vasculitis, or tumor, since the presence of any of these lesions would affect treatment. We routinely order coagulation parameters, such as prothrombin time, partial thromboplastin time, bleeding time, and platelet count. If the patient is not fully alert, arterial blood gases are drawn to detect hypoventilation.

We try to nurse the patient in the upright posture when possible to help reduce ICP. Intubation with forced mechanical hyperventilation is the most effective and rapid means of reducing ICP and takes effect in less than 1 minute. We use hyperventilation when deterioration is rapid and urgent measures are needed. Mannitol is infused in doses of 0.5 to 1 gram per kg every 4 to 6 hours or 0.25 gram per kg every 2 to 3 hours. Dexamethasone (Decadron) is given in doses of 4 mg every 6 hours. Although some advocate "megadose" levels of steroids we are not persuaded that they are more effective and feel they probably do increase the risk of steroid therapy. Steroids do not work immediately. If the situation is not urgent, glycerol in doses of 1 to 1.5 ounces can be given orally or in nasogastric tubing every 4 to 6 hours. Glycerol is often effective in controlling increased intracranial pressure and can be effective and tolerated for longer periods than mannitol. Diuretics and fluid restriction are helpful if increased intracranial pressure is slight.

Osmotic agents can cause rapid but usually temporary increases in intravascular volume. The patient should be monitored carefully for congestive heart failure or pulmonary edema. Hyponatremia can be caused by the diuretic or osmotic agents or inappropriate antidiuretic hormone release so that electrolytes and urinary output should be closely watched. These "medical" decompressive measures may suffice to pull the patient through the critical first 24 to 72 hours and may obviate the need for surgery. They are also adjuncts to surgical treatment and probably reduce the mortality associated with operations in patients with increased ICP.

If the patient does not improve and become more alert after the previously described treatment or if he deteriorates, surgical drainage should be considered. We would like to re-emphasize the crucial role of monitoring the patient's progress in the therapeutic decision. In lesions of the cerebral hemisphere and basal ganglia, the physician should carefully consider the likely nature of the residual disability before deciding on drainage. A large putaminal hemorrhage that destroys the internal capsule and undercuts the speech cortex will leave a right-handed person aphasic and hemiplegic. Occipital, parietal, frontal, anterior temporal, right posterior temporal, and right putaminal lesions are less likely to cause deficits as severe. Age, prior morbidity, general health, available support systems, and a host of other factors also help predict how well the patient will adapt to his deficit. His stated wishes concerning disability are also important. When uncertain, we give the patient the benefit of the doubt and urge surgical drainage of accessible cerebral and ganglionic ICH in life-threatening circumstances when there is a reasonable chance of a good outcome. Cerebellar hematomas are a special circumstance for two reasons: (1) sudden change in the lesion can compress the caudal brain stem and lead to respiratory arrest without warning, and (2) removal of cerebellar lesions usually leaves little serious disability. If the cerebellar hematoma is larger than 3 cm in diameter we advise surgical decompression in most circumstances. In thalamic hemorrhage, although direct surgical drainage is seldom useful, ventricular drainage can be life-saving if obstructive hydrocephalus develops.

FOCAL ISCHEMIC CEREBROVASCULAR DISEASE

method of
ANTHONY J. FURLAN, M.D.,
and JOHN R. LITTLE, M.D.
Cleveland Clinic Foundation
Cleveland, Ohio

The term "focal ischemic cerebrovascular disease" applies to a spectrum of diagnoses ranging from the asymptomatic carotid bruit to completed brain infarction. The primary treatment goal in such patients is to prevent or minimize the risk of neurologic dysfunction due to brain ischemia. The majority of focal cerebrovascular ischemic problems are related to atherosclerosis (artery-to-artery embolism, atherothrombosis, arteriolar lipohyalinosis) or embolism from the heart.

Asymptomatic Carotid Bruits

There are many causes of neck bruits other than stenosis of the carotid arteries. Localized bruits high in the neck near the jaw angle, especially if there is a diastolic component, are best correlated with underlying internal carotid artery stenosis; about 4 per cent of the population over age 65 harbors such an asymptomatic bruit.

Epidemiologic studies have shown that patients with asymptomatic carotid bruits have an increased risk of stroke, *but* this applies to all kinds of stroke in all vascular territories. Hence, asymptomatic carotid bruits are best viewed as markers of atherosclerotic disease.

Treatment

There is no randomly controlled evidence that repairing an isolated asymptomatic internal carotid artery stenosis, regardless of severity, significantly alters long-term stroke risk. Since the risk of stroke in patients with asymptomatic bruits is about 2 per cent per year, in patients over age 70 asymptomatic carotid bruits should *not* be investigated with noninvasive tests (NIT) or intravenous digital subtraction angiography (IV-DSA). In younger patients who are in good general medical condition, asymptomatic carotid bruits are often screened for high grade (greater than 90 per cent) internal carotid artery stenosis with either NIT or IV-DSA. Patients with stenosis greater than 90 per cent can then undergo endarterectomy if there is access to a surgeon with operative morbidity and mortality rates less than 2 per cent. Patients with lesser degrees of stenosis patients over age 70 are managed medically through risk factor modification, education about transient ischemic attacks, and aspirin, 5 to 10 grains daily. Serial NIT or IV-DSA is done in selected cases at 6 to 12 month intervals.

Transient Ischemic Attacks

A transient ischemic attack (TIA) is a temporary, *focal* episode of neurologic dysfunction of vascular origin, typically lasting less than 5 minutes but occasionally as long as 24 hours. TIAs are classified as carotid or vertebrobasilar depending on the vascular territory of the ischemia. The risk of stroke after TIA depends on a number of variables, including the cause of the attack and the presence of other stroke risk factors. Among all patients with TIA who do not die of a cause other than stroke, about 33 per cent have a stroke within 5 years of the first attack. Of these, more than 20 per cent have their stroke within 1 month and 50 per cent within 1 year of the initial attack. After the first 6 months following the onset of TIA, the incidence of stroke is about 6 per cent per year, which is approximately six times the expected rate for a matched normal population.

Treatment

When TIAs are due to atherosclerotic disease of the internal carotid system, a decision must be made as to whether the patient is a candidate for cerebrovascular surgery or medical therapy. Extracranial/intracranial (EC/IC) bypass surgery is reserved for patients with symptomatic occlusion of the internal carotid artery or inaccessible severe stenosis of the intracranial internal carotid artery or middle cerebral artery. Carotid endarterectomy has yielded the best results in patients with typical hemispheric carotid TIA or amaurosis fugax who have demonstrable atherosclerosis in the extracranial internal carotid artery on the same side as the symptoms. Stenosis usually must exceed 50 per cent for a patient to qualify for surgery, but endarterectomy is performed occasionally in patients with deep, irregular ulcerations and milder stenosis.

In the best surgical hands, the risk of endarterectomy is between 1 and 7 per cent, depending on a number of variables, primarily the medical and neurologic condition of the patient. In some hospitals, the combined morbidity and mortality rate for carotid endarterectomy may be as high as 21 per cent. Thus, in addition to the patient's symptoms, the surgeon's skill and the patient's condition are critical factors in determining the efficacy of endarterectomy.

Patients with vertebrobasilar TIA are usually managed medically. Vertebral artery surgery or EC/IC bypass surgery of the posterior circulation is done in selected cases. The benefit of carotid endarterectomy for most patients with nonlocalizing symptoms or vertebrobasilar TIA has not been established.

Antiplatelet therapy is the preferred form of medical treatment for most patients with TIA, either as the sole treatment or following cerebrovascular surgery. Warfarin is preferred in patients with cardiac conditions such as atrial fibrillation or rheumatic heart disease and in patients with severe inaccessible stenosis of a major vessel such as the basilar artery. Sometimes warfarin is employed for 2 or 3 months after the onset of TIA and then the patient is switched to antiplatelet therapy. In practice, however, most physicians begin with antiplatelet therapy and switch to warfarin if this fails.

The only antiplatelet agent that has been shown to decrease the frequency of TIA and reduce the risk of stroke is aspirin. Aspirin and many nonsteroidal anti-inflammatory drugs interfere with platelet aggregation by blocking the enzyme cyclooxygenase, an important rate-limiting enzyme in the arachidonic acid cascade. As a result, the formation of thromboxane (a potent platelet aggregant and vasoconstrictor) as well as prostacyclin (an antiaggregant and vasodilator) is inhibited.

In clinical trials, aspirin dosages between 1,000 and 1,500 mg per day have been used. Considerable in vitro evidence indicates that much lower dosages (i.e., less than 300 mg per day) inhibit platelet cyclooxygenase, the major site of thromboxane formation, while sparing prostacyclin production, which occurs in blood vessel endothelium. This is a theoretical advantage in patients with cerebral ischemia. However, prescription of so-called minidose (30 mg) aspirin in patients with TIA is premature. The protective action of aspirin may involve pathways other than the arachidonic acid cascade. Also, on the basis of clinical trials many physicians prescribe 300 mg four times daily or 600 mg twice daily. Others advise 300 mg twice daily. If patients experience gastrointestinal side effects lower aspirin doses, coated aspirin, or aspirin combined with antacid can be considered.

The other available antiplatelet agent is dipyridamole (Persantine—this use not listed by maker). The usual dosage is 50 mg 3 times a day or 75 mg twice a day, combined with aspirin. Dipyridamole is an adjunct treatment in patients with TIA; the only evidence that dipyridamole lowers stroke risk is in patients with prosthetic heart valves who are also receiving warfarin. The mechanism by which dipyridamole prevents platelet aggregation is different from that of aspirin. Dipyridamole elevates platelet cAMP levels by blocking the enzyme phosphodiesterase; this interferes with platelet calcium release and aggregation.

Antiplatelet drugs that selectively block thromboxane synthesis or interfere with platelet function while permitting prostacyclin synthesis are under investigation.

Progressing Stroke (Stroke in Evolution)

If a patient is seen within 24 hours of the sudden onset of a focal neurologic deficit and that deficit has not yet resolved, it is uncertain whether the event is a TIA, a stroke that may still progress, or a completed infarct. In this situation the physician must decide whether to institute immediate medical or surgical therapy in an attempt to prevent neurologic deterioration.

Treatment

Although emergency angiography and endarterectomy are sometimes employed in these patients, surgery carries a high risk and is of uncertain benefit in reversing the ischemic process, especially when there has been any lapse of time since the onset. Some of these patients will improve spontaneously. Often, however, the question arises as to the efficacy and timing of acute anticoagulant therapy with heparin in an attempt to prevent progressive thrombosis or recurrent embolization. Unfortunately, a decision regarding therapy in evolving stroke often must be made despite the lack of precise information regarding the etiology of the stroke or the mechanism of progression.

Patients with severe deficits or decrease in level of consciousness should not be placed on heparin. In patients with milder deficits, acute heparin therapy can be employed if no contraindications exist (severe hypertension or active peptic ulcer disease) and if intracranial hemorrhage has been excluded by performing a nonenhanced CT scan.

The optimal dose of heparin to prevent arterial thrombus formation and to minimize the risk of brain hemorrhage in patients with acute cerebral ischemia has not been well studied. In cerebrovascular patients, in whom the risk of intracranial hemorrhage may be high, it would seem safest to employ the lowest possible antithrombotic dose. Bolus injections should be avoided, and heparin should be administered by constant pump infusion. Dosage is usually monitored with the activated partial thromboplastin time, which can be supplemented with various heparin assay systems in high risk patients. Most patients will require 300 to 400 units of heparin per kg per 24 hours either to keep the activated partial thromboplastin time between 1½ and 2 times control or to maintain a blood heparin level between 0.2 and 0.5 units per ml.

In patients with evolving stroke in a carotid distribution, heparin therapy is continued for about 72 hours or until the neurologic picture stabilizes. The patient may then undergo angiography, may be switched to aspirin or warfarin, or may be provided with supportive care depending upon the final neurologic outcome. In patients with progressing brain stem infarction, heparin therapy may have to be continued for up to 2 weeks, at which point the patient is usually placed on either antiplatelet therapy or long-term warfarin.

Although many stroke victims have a prior history of hypertension, blood pressure may be acutely and transiently elevated following an infarction. Unless the elevation is extreme, a period of bed rest is often sufficient to lower the blood pressure to its prestroke level. Cerebral blood flow autoregulation is often impaired in an area of infarction, and some acute stroke victims are passively dependent upon mean arterial pressure to maintain cerebral blood flow. Also, patients with chronic hypertension and atherosclerotic vessels require higher than usual mean arterial pressures to maintain cerebral blood flow. Hence, precipitous drops of the blood pressure into the normotensive range should be avoided in hypertensive patients with acute evolving stroke. If lowering of the blood pressure is necessary, a graduated decrease into the low or medium hypertensive range is best achieved by using a sodium nitroprusside drip. Mean arterial blood pressure should be maintained at or slightly above premorbid levels, as any reduction in pressure could have a deleterious effect on perfusion in the ischemic zone.

We sometimes use the rheologic agent low molecular weight (LMW) dextran when heparin is contraindicated. A 500 ml loading dose is administered over 2 to 4 hours followed by 500 ml every 12 hours over a 48 to 72 hour period. Patients receiving LMW dextran should be closely monitored for signs of renal or cardiac failure, and excessive hemodilution (i.e., hematocrit less than 30 per cent) should be avoided.

Cerebral edema can lead to increased intracranial pressure, herniation, and death after acute brain infarction. There is no effective treatment for infarct-associated edema. Dexamethasone does not prevent or ameliorate infarct-associated edema and may raise blood glucose levels. Elevated blood glucose during the preischemic period has a deleterious effect in ischemia, possibly by elevating brain lactic acid levels. Attempts to control infarct-associated edema can be made with infusions of Lasix and mannitol.

Traditional forms of therapy for evolving stroke will probably soon be supplanted by new treatment modalities based on a better understanding of the pathophysiology of acute focal brain ischemia. The use of high dose barbiturates in treating acute focal cerebral ischemia appears promising, but treatment must be initiated before or at the onset of the ischemic event. Consequently, the potential clinical applications of this form of therapy are very limited. Other areas currently being explored include opiate antagonists (e.g., naloxone); free radical scavengers; modification of prostaglandin metabolism (e.g., prostacyclin, thromboxane, leukotrienes); and calcium entry blockers.

Reversible Ischemic Neurologic Deficit

Treatment

The timing of angiography and possible endarterectomy following a small completed brain infarction or a so-called reversible ischemic neurologic deficit (RIND) poses a special management problem. If the patient has no or minimal neurologic deficit and an enhanced CT scan done more than 48 hours after onset is normal, angiography and, if necessary, endarterectomy can be performed during the immediate post-stroke period. If there is an infarct on CT it is safest to defer angiography and possible cerebrovascular surgery for 4 to 6 weeks. If angiography is to be postponed the patient is usually discharged on antiplatelet therapy.

Cardiogenic Embolic Infarction

Treatment

The risk of recurrent embolism must be weighed against the risk of brain hemorrhage in deciding on the timing and use of anticoagulant therapy after acute nonseptic embolic brain infarction. Early recurrent brain embolism occurs in 10 to 13 per cent of patients with embolic stroke from a variety of cardiac sources. Aggregate data from recent studies suggest that early heparin therapy can reduce the rate of early recurrent brain embolism by as much as 67 per cent. Less than 5 per cent of nonseptic embolic infarcts will be hemorrhagic on CT performed within 48 hours of onset. As many as 22 per cent of large embolic infarcts will undergo spontaneous hemorrhagic transformation within 8 days of onset. The Cerebral Embolism Study Group estimates that about 5 per cent of unselected embolic stroke patients who are immediately anticoagulated will experience worsening associated with brain hemorrhage. In one third of such patients with large embolic strokes, the prevalence may reach 20 per cent, which exceeds the risk of early recurrent embolism. The Study Group recommends immediate anticoagulation of small and moderate sized nonseptic embolic infarcts, regardless of embolic source, if a CT performed after 24 hours from stroke onset does not show hemorrhage. In patients with large infarcts who are at special risk for spontaneous, late onset hemorrhagic transformation, a delay of at least 7 days before initiating anticoagulation seems prudent. Bolus doses of heparin, excessive anticoagulation, and elevated blood pressure should be avoided. In patients who are receiving anticoagulants at the time of stroke onset, the Study Group recommends continuing anticoagulation in patients with submassive infarcts who do not show hemorrhage on CT and in whom blood pressure is well controlled.

Anticoagulation should still be considered contraindicated in patients with infectious endocarditis and septic embolism. However, in patients with prosthetic valve endocarditis who are receiving warfarin, anticoagulation may be continued in the absence of systemic or brain embolism. Anticoagulation should also be considered in patients with multiple embolic events, but in this situation it is safest to first perform cerebral angiography to exclude a mycotic aneurysm.

There is ample evidence that long-term anticoagulation decreases the risk of embolism in patients with mechanical prosthetic valves. The addition of dipyridamole or other antiplatelet agents probably affords additional protection but may increase the risk of hemorrhagic complications. Antiplatelet agents are ineffective in preventing embolism when used alone in patients with prosthetic valves. Long-term anticoagulation is also an accepted form of therapy in patients with rheumatic mitral stenosis and atrial fibrillation. In patients with acute myocardial infarction, anticoagulation is sometimes used for a 6 month period to allow organization of mural thrombus in patients who have embolized. Long-term anticoagulation is also recommended for patients with chronic atrial fibrillation who have suffered any embolic event. Patients with mitral valve prolapse who have embolized are usually first treated with antiplatelet agents and then anticoagulation should this fail. The role of long-term antiplatelet therapy in patients with cardiac embolic sources has been incompletely studied. Prophylactic antiplatelet therapy should be considered in patients with chronic atrial fibrillation or other cardiac conditions that carry a significant stroke risk but in whom the dangers of long-term anticoagulation do not seem justified.

REHABILITATION OF THE PATIENT WITH HEMIPLEGIA

method of
JEROME S. TOBIS, M.D.
University of California
Irvine, California

Hemiplegia as the result of cerebrovascular disease is a major health problem in our nation. It is the third most common cause of death. It is estimated to have a prevalence of over 2,000,000. In England, according to one report, one fifth of all hospital beds are occupied by stroke victims 65 years of age and older. The incidence is estimated to be about 2 per 1,000 for the population at large. However, the majority of strokes occur in older individuals, so that 75 per cent occur in persons 65 years and older. The incidence rate for men slightly exceeds that for women. Residual loss of function as the result of hemiplegia is a major rehabilitation and social problem, for it results in disability in at least 50 per cent of the survivors.

Management

Immediately following the acute stroke episode, the physician should assure an adequate airway if the patient is comatose. The cardiopulmonary status must be evaluated. A significant number of strokes have associated cardiac episodes such as myocardial infarction. The diagnosis must be established for the stroke, ruling out tumor, subdural hematoma, and subarachnoid hemorrhage secondary to arteriovenous malformation or aneurysm. Such diagnoses warrant definitive procedures that will not be reviewed in this presentation.

Bladder Function

Attention should be given to fluid intake and urinary output. An indwelling catheter should be discontinued if any voluntary control is present. A condom collecting system may be substituted. Intermittent catheterization in facilitating continence retraining is preferable to an indwelling catheter. Frequent opportunities for voluntary voiding should be provided. It should be remembered that incontinence may be due to the patient's inability to communicate his needs. Prolonged use of an indwelling catheter perpetuates incontinence as well as urinary tract infections.

Positioning in Bed

The paretic lower extremity should be maintained in a neutral position with the hip and knee straight. The use of sandbags or pillows to prevent external rotation of the hip may be used. A pillow under the knee should be avoided. The foot should be maintained at 90 degrees by the use of a footboard, a foot support, or a shoe.

The paretic upper extremity tends to be adducted and internally rotated at the shoulder, flexed and pronated at the elbow, and flexed at the wrist and fingers. To reduce the risk of contracture, the shoulder should be maintained in slight abduction with the use of a pillow in the axilla. A pillow might also be placed under the elbow to raise the forearm above the level of the heart and thereby avoid dependency edema, which is so common in the paretic hand. Later, the use of an elastic glove may reduce this phenomenon. The presence of the edema transudate, which is rich in proteinaceous fluid, may contribute to fibroblast activity with consequent fibrosis and contracture. The wrist should be maintained in a neutral position. If this is difficult to achieve a splint for wrist and hand may be applied for optimal positioning.

If there is significant loss of sensation on the paretic limbs, special care may be needed to prevent decubitus ulcers from forming over the bony prominences such as the heel, the greater trochanter, and the sacrum.

Early Rehabilitation Activities

Passive range of motion of all paretic joints should be carried out by a nurse or therapist or a family member instructed in carrying out these procedures cautiously. In addition to preventing contractures, this activity may be valuable for the kinesthetic experience.

Active movement of the nonparetic limbs may be started as soon as there is no progression of the neurologic deficits. By the second day, if the condition is stabilized, the patient may sit up in bed. By the third day, standing with assistance may be attempted. In the presence of an intracerebral hemorrhage more conservative time constraints may have to be followed.

Ambulation

By the nature of hemiplegia, the paralysis or weakness of the involved extremities tends to cause us to focus upon the motor system. However, whether the patient will have a functional lower extremity in order to walk more often depends on the severity of the sensory loss. Ninety per cent of those stroke victims whose disability is limited to a motor loss will be able to walk effectively with or without additional support such as a brace (ankle foot orthosis) and/or a cane. However, a high percentage of those with severe sensory loss (especially proprioception) will not achieve functional ambulation, that is, more than learning to transfer from bed to wheelchair or chair or standing transfers for toileting.

Ambulation training should be seen as part of a graduated activity program. It may start with regaining sitting balance on the side of the bed, then in a chair, and then standing in parallel bars with assistance. If there is a drop foot present, the application of an Ace bandage around a shoe and ankle may temporarily brace the foot until an ankle foot orthosis is obtained. Instability at the knee may be aided by Ace bandaging or a posterior knee splint. If the patient ultimately requires a full length leg brace there is little likelihood that the patient will be a functional walker. However, knee bracing early may be a temporary measure that may be discarded as the patient regains skill of balance and alternation of gait. Occasionally, elevation of the shoe of the uninvolved side with a ½ inch shoe lift may permit more easy clearance for the swing-through phase of the paretic limb.

Gait training is usually provided by a physical therapist utilizing tilt table, parallel bars, a therapeutic gymnasium, and the assistance of various devices such as a walker, quadripod cane, J-shaped cane, and appropriate bracing as indicated. Such resources are usually available in the hospital setting. However, in a home setting substitutions can be devised, such as two rows of parallel chairs for the parallel bars.

Falls are not infrequent in hemiplegics, with 5 per cent experiencing hip fractures. The goal of gait training is safe, functional walking. If this is not feasible, a wheelchair with foot rests that can be lifted should be prescribed to permit the patient to use his unimpaired leg to propel the chair.

Upper Extremity Function

In the presence of subluxation of the shoulder associated with shoulder pain, I recommend the use of a sling. Such a complaint is most often found in the presence of a nonfunctional arm and hand. In addition to reducing the subluxation and the pain, the sling provides partial elevation of the hand to reduce the risk of edema of dependency. In addition, it may prevent involuntary arm movements that interfere with body and arm function of the unimpaired extremity.

Occasionally in the presence of exquisite touch and friction tenderness associated with edema and vasomotor changes, a diagnosis of a shoulder-hand syndrome should be entertained. The use of oral steroids and stellate ganglion nerve blocks may be indicated.

The objective for the patient with a nonfunctional arm and hand is to learn to perform two-handed activities unimanually. This entails learning to carry out all self-care activities of feeding, dressing, bathing, and toileting with the uninvolved arm. The occupational therapist is well qualified to help the patient to relearn such skills. Special equipment such as supports for the tub, shower, and toilet and self-help devices such as adapted utensils and elastic shoe laces may be obtained from medical supply companies.

Perceptual and Other Disturbances

The lesion that results in hemiplegia is rarely limited in its damage to the motor system. Loss or diminution of the sensory modalities of proprioception, touch, and temperature has been mentioned. Hemianopia when present may interfere with the visual field and the ability to read the printed page completely. Disturbances in verticality and the imperception of the true upright may interfere with balance and stability of gait. The phenomenon of constructional apraxia, which is the inability to accurately perceive spatial relationships (as in geometric designs), may interfere in self-care activities and ambulation. Any of these deficits exposes the patient to increased risk of accident. A retraining program should take these factors into account once they are recognized after evaluation.

Psychologic Factors

Aphasia

Aphasia is one of the most disabling consequences that may result from a stroke. It has been estimated to affect 40 per cent of those who suffer strokes initially. A significant number of this group improve within 6 months of the acute episode. Global or total aphasia is associated with severe dysfunction in all language modalities and has a poor prognosis for recovery.

Speech therapy should be provided by a qualified therapist. However, communication skills can be improved by all care providers, including family members and friends, who have an ongoing relationship with the patient. Guidance for such activities should be the responsibility of the speech pathologist. Often communication needs may be partially met by the use of gestures. One admonition to all who are in contact with the patient is to avoid any conversation that would not be expressed if the patient had full comprehension.

Dementia

Disruption of cortical function, as occurs in stroke, may lead to disturbances in cognition, memory, and judgment. Bilateral lesions or multi-infarct episodes are more prone to lead to these behavioral changes. The severity of the dementia will also depend upon the extent of the cerebral lesions as well as their locations.

Early after the stroke, the patient may be obtunded; after several days there may be greater lucidity and improved orientation. Gross evaluation of these cognitive functions can be determined by the physician with traditional testing. The Double Simultaneous Stimulation Test and the Imperseverance Test of Benton are shortcut tests to quickly estimate the severity of the cognitive losses. If a more detailed evaluation is indicated, a qualified neuropsychologist should be consulted.

Depression

Reactive depression following catastrophic illness such as a stroke is appropriate. In fact, I am concerned about those patients who do not experience a mourning period for their loss. Such depression may, however, produce a change in behavior that may appear as dementia, a phenomenon that might be called pseudodementia. The patient may appear apathetic and laconic, may be poorly motivated with poor appetite, and may have a sleep disorder. For persistent depression psychotherapy and the use of antidepressant drugs may be helpful.

Expectations

It is apparent from what has been discussed that the severity of impairment that will ultimately result depends on the losses suffered. The individual with a totally nonfunctional hand is more disabled than one with minimal use of finger flexion and extension and thumb opposition. However, there is little correlation between the severity of disability and the reaction to it. One may see the severely impaired hemiplegic more accepting of his or her disability than the one with mild residual loss. It is as if the mildly impaired feels obliged to compete with the able-bodied norm, whereas the severely damaged can no longer compete and does not try.

In this regard a mild impairment may have profound consequences. Minimal loss of finger dexterity in a professional violinist may be a catastrophic disability. A banker who becomes a wheelchair-bound hemiplegic without intellectual deficits may be minimally disabled.

Social Support Systems

Family Counseling

Stroke is a family illness. Its consequences are as profound on the care givers as on the patient. Much of the prognosis for successful rehabilitation depends on the quality of the support system available. A caring spouse and other family members may make the difference between a severely disabled hemiplegic being capable of residing in the community or needing long-term institutional care. Often, I have seen patients 6 months to 1 year after they are discharged from a rehabilitation center continue to improve when placed in a sympathetic, well structured, stimulating environment. Persistent incontinence of bladder and bowel may resolve, and communication in the aphasic may continue to improve.

The primary care physician should be aware of these very important considerations for successful home placement. Physical modifications of the home should be evaluated. The advice of an occupational therapist or visiting nurse may be very helpful. This may include changing steps to a ramp, moving a bed from the second floor to a ground floor, or widening the doorway of a bathroom to permit access.

The family physician may be called upon to provide many aspects of family counseling.

Day Care Centers

Many communities have day care facilities for the physically disabled, including hemiplegics, where therapeutic services may be received on an outpatient basis. These may be an extension of free-standing rehabilitation centers, outpatient services of hospitals, or independently established facilities. Many hemiplegics may derive benefit from such therapies after discharge from hospital. Speech, physical, and/or occupational therapies may be prescribed for selected indications, such as continuing improvement in motor skills, easing persistent pain, or increasing limited range of motion due to contracture.

Home Care

With the expanding therapeutic services available today, many of the resources of the hospital or rehabilitation center may be brought into the home. With judicious use of these services, the patient's functional capacity may continue to improve slowly. In the familiar well structured home setting the patient may perform at a higher level than might be achieved in the hospital environment.

Stroke Club

Many communities in this country and abroad have organized community recreation facilities for the stroke victim. These may be found in community centers. They provide social contact for the isolated, home-bound stroke victim. Such programs provide a respite for the family care givers. They may also have support groups that provide counseling for family members.

Other Considerations

Stroke involves more than one side of the body. Studies done on hemiplegic gait show that there are abnormalities of the motor pattern of the "unimpaired" lower extremity. Studies of the "uninvolved" upper extremity show that there are prolonged latencies and reduced performance in psychomotor skills. Family members should be aware of these limitations that may impair performance below their expectations.

In this regard, the use of the terms "good" arm and "good" leg should be avoided. It tends to imply a "bad" arm and leg, with the tendency to avoid using those extremities to their maximum capacity.

Rehabilitation Is a Learning Process

The patient who is involved in a rehabilitation program must be capable of learning new techniques or relearning old ones in order to improve his functional capacity. Further, he must be able to retain what he has learned the day before. This is a critical consideration in determining how ambitious the therapeutic program may be. During the acute phase after the ictus, much of what is done involves the patient passively (e.g., range of motion exercises). Later the patient must be an active participant for successful functional gains beyond the limited biologic recovery that occurs early.

Nutrition

Inanition may result from numerous factors in the stroke victim. It may be the result of a pseudobulbar palsy due to bilateral cerebral lesions or a bulbar palsy involving the brain stem. Aspiration of food, especially liquids, may result. Training by those skilled in this problem, such as an occupational or speech therapist, may be very helpful.

Malnutrition may also result from poor-fitting dentures. It is a frequent observation that prestroke dentures fit poorly after the stroke. This may be the result of atrophy of the alveolar ridge or the musculocutaneous tissues of the buccal cavity. An edentulous mouth or poor-fitting dentures lead to a soft diet high in carbohydrates. This in turn may contribute to obesity. Hemiplegics tend to be more sedentary than they were prior to their stroke and therefore should reduce their caloric intake to avoid obesity. The obese patient has greater difficulty in walking.

Immobilization

The patient who is kept immobilized and bedridden is vulnerable to venous thrombosis, hypostatic pneumonia, and decubitus ulcers. Frequent turning of the bedridden patient from side to side is advisable. Passive range of motion of the extremities may reduce the risk of phlebothrombosis, decubitus in the absence of sensation of an extremity, and contracture.

Spasticity

This phenomenon is a frequent concomitant of the motor paralysis. Spasticity and gravity are the two factors that contribute to contracture. Spasticity often may prevent weak voluntary movement in the paretic hand from being recognized and utilized. When spasticity is severe and a major obstacle to function, such as ambulation, it may be treated with a spasmolytic agent such as diazepam (Valium), dantrolene sodium (Dantrium), or baclofen (Lioresal). None of these drugs should be prescribed casually, since their side effects may be deleterious. Valium leads to somnolence, habituation, and possibly depression. The others are potentially hepatotoxic.

Occasionally, spasticity may be beneficial and may provide stability for weight bearing on an unstable knee joint due to a weak quadriceps muscle.

On rare occasions, the use of a phenol block to selected muscles may provide a more optimal muscle balance for a spastic limb and thereby increase functional capacity in the lower or upper extremity. If successful, such blocks may be repeated after several months.

Sexual Counseling

For too long the hemiplegic has been presumed to have lost all sexuality. This may be partly due to the fear instilled in the patient or the spouse that sexual activity may induce another stroke. Other factors may include the pain that may be caused by positioning for the sex act itself.

Sexual activity, including caressing, might be perceived as a form of communication and caring. As such, sexual activity and interest should be discussed with the patient and spouse. When interest is displayed, the physician may provide suggestions for facilitating the sex act. For example, the able-bodied partner, male or female, may take the more active role or the hemiplegic might assume the supine position.

Return to Work

Since stroke victims are usually elderly, the likelihood of them being employed prior to the stroke is not great. However, in one recent study, it was found that those who returned to work 1 year after the stroke tended to be younger patients under 55 years. The physician's or nurse's subjective opinion of the patient's degree of disability at the time of admission was a strong predictor of the probability of return to work. The likelihood of a patient who held a professional or managerial position prior to the stroke being able to return to work is at least five times as great for blue collar workers and almost as high for farmers.

EPILEPSY IN ADOLESCENTS AND ADULTS

method of
RICHARD W. FINCHAM, M.D.
University of Iowa
Iowa City, Iowa

The various epilepsies affect about 1 per cent of the general population. Pharmacologic agents provide the basis of therapy. Lifetime treatment is required for many. Potential problems with drug toxicity and undesired pharmacologic effects, as well as therapeutic effectiveness, are concerns for the physician who cares for these individuals.

Three questions must be addressed before treatment is undertaken: (1) are the spells epileptic?; (2) what kind of spells are present?; (3) what is their cause? Affirmation of the first question requires that a number of issues be discussed with the patient by the doctor and as many other persons (nurse, social worker, psychologist, vocational rehabilitation worker, cleric, family, support groups such as may be organized through the Epilepsy Foundation of America) as the patient will have need for in understanding, accepting, and living with the diagnosis of epilepsy. The effectiveness of drug therapy will be greatly enhanced if the patient and family understand what epilepsy is, how it is to be treated, and that vocational and emotional support are available.

Although a single seizure does not fulfill the requirement for recurrent attacks that indicate a diagnosis of epilepsy, you may sometimes feel that an initial single seizure is a first episode in what will become a recurrent disorder (the patient has a history or physical findings of cerebral injury or abnormality, the EEG shows generalized spike wave or other clear epileptiform change, or there is a strong family history, e.g., a sibling with epilepsy) and choose to begin treatment. The patient should know that epilepsy is not a disease but a symptom of disturbed brain function in which, for diverse and often unknown reasons, large groups of neurons discharge paroxysmally and without control to produce varying kinds of seizures in accordance with the location and spread of abnormal neuronal discharge. The patient will need assurance that epilepsy, if properly treated, does not bring about a progressive deterioration and dementia (unless it is associated with an untreatable and progressive neurologic disease of some kind).

Patients with epilepsy need to know about routine precautions that should be followed when consciousness and motor control are impaired. They must understand and follow the interdiction against motor vehicle operation for as long as required by law; limit swimming to pools with the company of a knowledgeable companion (if at all); not take baths in locked rooms, and then only when someone is available for help should a seizure occur; and limit other activities in keeping with their seizure control. Vocational placement may pose an immediate and significant problem. Encouragement will be needed in an early and persistent fashion from the patient's family as well as a variety of professional workers.

If the patient is a woman in her child-bearing years she must be made aware that drugs required to control her seizures may cause fetal malformations and that the precise risk for specific drugs and anomalies is not clearly established. None of the presently available antiepileptic drugs have been shown to be free of possible teratogenic effects. Children from treated pregnancies have malformations about two times more often than those from untreated pregnancies, but studies have not established whether the difference is due to medication alone. If the patient's seizures require medication for control, she must either take medications with the knowledge that drug therapy provides a possible basis for fetal malformations or not take the medications and suffer the consequences of uncontrolled seizures. The possible teratogenic effects of medications are ordinarily far less risky than uncontrolled epilepsy.

Management of the patient during a seizure should be discussed with the patient and family. Objects should not be thrust into the mouth of a patient experiencing a tonic-clonic seizure to pry the teeth apart, since injury to teeth, tongue, and oral mucosa may ensue. No effort should be made to stop the muscle contractions. The patient should be protected from injury during the spell, and the witness should stand by until consciousness is clearly regained to see if the person wishes or needs postictal assistance.

Patients must know that drug therapy is not curative but a way of providing freedom from epileptic attacks and that therapeutic effectiveness depends on careful compliance with planned treatment and achievement of adequate serum concentrations of medication to control the seizures. They need to know about potential toxicity or undesired effects of medication to help guard against such untoward effects. Careful follow-up evaluations are particularly important in caring for patients with epilepsy.

What Kind of Seizures are Present?

An individual may experience more than one kind of seizure. It is important to identify the type of seizures for diagnostic confirmation and choice of therapy. A brief outline of a classification recently provided by the International League Against Epilepsy for these purposes is given in Table 1. Special efforts have been and are currently being made in the testing of new drugs to identify specific antiepileptic agents for specific types of seizures.

TABLE 1. **Classification of Epileptic Seizures***

I. Partial (focal, local) Seizures
  A. Simple partial seizures (consciousness not impaired)
    1. With motor signs.
    2. With somatosensory or special sensory symptoms (simple hallucinations, e.g., tingling, light flashes, buzzing).
    3. With autonomic symptoms or signs (including epigastric sensation, pallor, sweating, flushing, piloerection, and pupillary dilatation).
    4. With psychic symptoms (disturbances of higher cerebral functions).
  B. Complex partial seizures (with impairment of consciousness)
    1. Simple partial onset followed by impairment of consciousness.
      a. With simple partial features (A1–A4) followed by impaired consciousness.
      b. With automatisms.
    2. With impairment of consciousness at onset.
      a. With impairment of consciousness only.
      b. With automatisms.
  C. Partial seizures evolving to secondarily generalized seizures (this may be generalized tonic-clonic, tonic, or clonic).

II. Generalized Seizures (convulsive or nonconvulsive)
  A. 1. Absence seizures.
      a. Impairment of consciousness only.
      b. With mild clonic components.
      c. With atonic components.
      d. With tonic components.
      e. With automatisms.
      f. With autonomic component.
      Note: b. through f. may occur alone or in combination.
    2. Atypical absence.
      a. Changes in tone that are more pronounced than A1.
      b. Onset and/or cessation that is not abrupt.
  B. Myoclonic seizures.
  C. Clonic seizures.
  D. Tonic seizures.
  E. Tonic-clonic seizures.
  F. Atonic seizures (astatic).
  (B–F: combinations are possible)

III. Unclassified Epileptic Seizures

IV. Addendum
  A. Fortuitous attacks: come unexpectedly and without apparent provocation.
  B. Cyclic attacks: come at more or less regular intervals (e.g., in relation to menses or sleep-waking cycle).
  C. Provoked attacks.
    a. Nonsensory factors: fatigue, alcohol, emotion, etc.
    b. Sensory factors: "reflex epilepsy."

*From International League Against Epilepsy.

What Causes the Seizures?

A specific etiology must always be sought, although one is not always found. Antiepileptic drug therapy is not the primary therapeutic modality for metabolic etiologies such as the hypoglycemia associated with an insulinoma or marked hyponatremia. On the other hand, drug therapy for seizures related to tumor or trauma is often required indefinitely even after successful surgical treatment of the primary condition.

TREATMENT OF EPILEPSY

Some Pharmacokinetic Considerations

Accurate measurement of antiepileptic drug concentrations in serum permits a rational approach to drug therapy previously unobtainable. These measurements permit insights into absorption, distribution through the body, metabolism, and excretion of drugs that are helpful in many clinical decisions.

The patient must realize that drug therapy is designed to prevent the recurrence of seizures and that the effectiveness of the medication depends on an adequate serum concentration of drug, which, in turn, depends on compliance with the dosage regimen outlined. Each drug has a therapeutic range in the serum that provides most patients with seizure control without toxicity. Although these ranges give helpful limits for planning dosage schedules, some individuals may have seizures that will be fully controlled with less than a "therapeutic" concentration. Others may not attain control with maximal concentrations. If no evidence of toxicity is present, cautious increments somewhat beyond the upper limits of "therapeutic" levels may be considered for these patients with attentive watchfulness for signs or symptoms of toxicity if the seizures are controlled. Seizure control may be attained with a single drug, but a careful follow-up evaluation is always required. The upper limit of the "therapeutic" range should not be greatly exceeded.

The timing of the serum sampling in relation to drug ingestion is of importance, particularly in drugs with short half-lives (time for serum level to decrease by 50 per cent). A trough plasma level is useful in identifying the lowest blood level of drug in a 24 hour period. This is drawn at the end of the longest dose interval, usually just before the first morning dose. Samples are most often taken after the drug is in steady state (when the tissue distribution of the drug is in equilibrium with the plasma and when absorption is equal to metabolism and excretion) and are most useful on a comparative basis when the sampling times are the same for each analysis.

The final action of antiepileptic drugs takes place within the brain. Free or unbound (to serum proteins) drugs are able to penetrate the blood brain barrier and exert their action at appropriate receptors. The standard laboratory reports of antiepileptic drug concentrations include both free and bound drug concentrations. Different anticonvulsants bind with different affinities to serum proteins (Table 2). This information is important to consider for those drugs that are highly bound. When serum proteins are not available (hypoproteinemia), are saturated with other drugs (polypharmacy), or are altered by various pathologic states (such as in renal or hepatic disease), increased amounts of free antiepileptic drug may complicate the interpretation of the usual plasma measures of these drugs (bound plus free). Free levels of the drug in question must be measured to identify toxic states and plan appropriate dosage adjustments.

How to Begin Antiepileptic Therapy

The objective is full control of the patient's seizures without drug toxicity. We have noted the usefulness of pharmacokinetic principles in this undertaking. A brief outline of an approach to induction of therapy follows.

Control with a single drug represents the ideal. The choice of medication is determined by type of seizure and other considerations such as potential toxicity. The drug therapy is begun after baseline hemogram and blood chemistry series have been found to be in an acceptable range. Steady state serum concentrations are checked at an appropriate time, and if this value and associated blood count and chemical parameters are in an acceptable range and the patient's seizures are under control without any signs or symptoms of drug toxicity, then the ideal of seizure control with monotherapy has been attained.

Should the seizures persist after the full serum level of antiepileptic concentration has been reached, the patient should be given the option of adding a second drug and bringing this into "therapeutic" range. The goal of monotherapy can then be continued with a gradual phasing out of the initial drug. The patient needs to understand that seizures may break through as these manipulations are made, and a physician must be available to guide alterations in therapy as the initial adjustments take place. A third, and rarely a fourth, drug may need a trial in this way in patients with refractory seizures. The goal of monotherapy may not be attainable in perhaps 15 per cent of patients, and a combination of antiepileptic drugs may be required to attain the best possible control. Here, careful attention must be given to possible drug interactions and added toxicity.

Summary of Specific Drugs

The antiepileptic drugs reviewed here are often effective, and untoward effects do not often occur. Undesirable effects include idiosyncratic (rare and unpredictable) reactions, toxicity related to excessive serum concentrations of drug, and toxic reactions without excessive serum concentrations (side effects). Since at least two thirds of the patients require lifelong therapy, attention to potential untoward effects is important for both patient and physician. Idiopathic reactions such as skin rash and thrombocytopenia require prompt discontinuation of the causative drug therapy (another value of monotherapy).

Phenobarbital

Type of Seizure. May be tried in adults for all types except absence seizures.

Pharmacokinetics. Most absorption takes place slowly over 6 to 18 hours in the small intestine (intramuscular injection provides relatively rapid and complete absorption), with an equal distribution taking place throughout the body (about 50 per cent is bound to serum proteins). Biotransformation takes place in the liver.

Usual Adult Dose. 2 to 3 mg per kg (the possibility of toxicity exists and must be carefully watched for whenever the dose is greater than 200 mg per day). Prolonged half-life supports giving a single dose (although a twice daily schedule may be preferred by patients). Attainment of steady state requires 2 to 3 weeks.

TABLE 2. **Binding Affinity of Anticonvulsants**

Drug	Protein Binding (%)	Therapeutic Range (mcg/ml)	Serum Half-Life (hours)	Steady State (days)
phenobarbital	50	15–30	50–120	14–21
phenytoin	90	10–20	3–50 22 (mean)	5–7
primidone	20–25	6–15	6–15	2–3
ethosuximide	0	40–100	30–60	4–8
carbamazepine	75–80	4–12	5–26	4–6
clonazepam	47	0.02–0.07	19–46	4–6
valproic acid	90	50–100	7–10	2–3

Toxicity

DOSE-RELATED. Sedation and slowed mentation; ataxia.

IDIOPATHIC. Dermatitis; agranulocytosis; aplastic anemia; hepatitis.

Side Effects (with Prolonged Usage). Folate deficiency with or without microcytic anemia; vitamin D deficiency with or without hypocalcemia and osteomalacia; vitamin K–dependent bleeding problems are possible in the newborns of mothers using phenobarbital.

Drug Interactions. Valproic acid commonly elevates serum phenobarbital concentration when it has been added to phenobarbital therapy. Folic acid and dicumarol may lower concentrations, whereas chloramphenicol may elevate concentrations of phenobarbital in the plasma.

Phenobarbital may lower plasma drug concentrations of dexamethasone, digitoxin, clonazepam, and chloramphenicol.

Disease States. The risk of phenobarbital intoxication must be monitored carefully in renal and hepatic disease.

Phenytoin (Dilantin)

Type of Seizure. May be used in adults for all types except absence.

Pharmacokinetics. Nearly complete absorption takes place in the small intestine. Suspensions must be thoroughly shaken before ingestion to obtain proper dosage. Phenytoin should not be given intramuscularly, since this route does not provide effective absorption. Generic phenytoin and Dilantin Kapseals vary in bioavailability, and serum levels must be monitored if a change is made in the patient's medication. Phenytoin is bound to serum protein (90 per cent) with the free fraction (10 per cent) rapidly entering the brain, liver, muscle, and other tissues, where it binds to proteins and phospholipids.

Biotransformation is accomplished in the liver.

Usual Adult Dose. 4 to 5 mg per kg. A single daily dose may be effective for some patients, whereas others do better with two or three separate daily doses. The half-life varies greatly from individual to individual, and serum concentrations must be followed carefully. The establishment of stable plasma and brain levels follows saturation of body binding and storage sites so that steady state can require 4 to 5 weeks instead of the usually expected 5 to 7 days. Drug withdrawals can be accomplished in four equal reductions spaced at 4 day intervals. The medication is available in 30 and 100 mg capsules and 50 mg tablets. A syrup for oral usage and a parenteral form are also available.

Toxicity

LOCAL. Gastric distress with early treatment can often be alleviated by taking medication with meals.

DOSE-RELATED. Cerebellar signs (ataxia, limb movement, dysarthria, nystagmus); encephalopathy; changes in mental state ranging from dysphoria and mild confusion to coma; choreiform movements; increased seizure frequency.

IDIOSYNCRATIC. Dermatitis (usually morbilliform and appearing within the first 2 weeks of therapy); agranulocytosis, thrombocytopenia, and aplastic anemia; lymphoma-like syndrome (usually appears within 4 weeks of starting therapy and may be associated with skin rash and other signs of systemic disease). Phenytoin has rarely been associated with malignant lymphoma in those individuals not having previously experienced an antecedent pseudolymphoma; hepatitis; thyroiditis; systemic lupus erythematosus; hyperglycemia.

Side Effects. Hirsutism (in an estimated 5 per cent of patients); gingival hyperplasia (can be minimized with careful dental hygiene and avoidance of high serum concentrations); accelerated scar formation, thickening of subcutaneous tissues of face and scalp; Dupuytren's contractures; enhanced problems with acne; folic acid, vitamin K, and vitamin deficiency problems as noted in the discussion of phenobarbital are possible with the chronic use of phenytoin; low levels of immunoglobulin A; peripheral neuropathy (usually without clinical manifestations).

Drug Interactions. Disulfiram, isoniazid, and chloramphenicol may elevate serum phenytoin concentrations. On occasion, the concurrent use of valproic acid and phenytoin may lead to competition for binding sites on serum proteins such that phenytoin will be significantly displaced from these binding sites. Measure of standard antiepileptic drug concentrations may show a "therapeutic" level (10 to 20 mcg per ml) and yet the patient may manifest signs of phenytoin intoxication that are explicable only when free serum phenytoin concentrations are determined and found to be in excess of the usual upper norm of slightly more than 2 mcg per ml. Carbamazepine, clonazepam, and, variably, phenobarbital may cause decrements in serum concentrations.

Carbamazepine biotransformation is enhanced by concurrent treatment with phenytoin such that increased doses of carbamazepine may be required to maintain desired serum concentrations of carbamazepine. Phenytoin has also been observed to enhance the amount of derived phenobarbital in the presence of dual therapy with primidone and phenytoin. Ineffectiveness of contraceptive pills with phenytoin therapy has been described in some epileptic patients.

Disease States. Phenytoin intoxication is not likely in renal disease, but relatively high concentrations of free or unbound drug are present and may need to be specifically determined at times. There is some risk of phenytoin intoxication in hepatic dysfunction.

Primidone (Mysoline)

Type of Seizure. May be tried on all types of adult seizures except absence epilepsy.

Pharmacokinetics. Primidone is rapidly absorbed from the gastrointestinal tract. Tissue distribution has not been thoroughly investigated. Binding to serum proteins may take place at about 20 per cent of its total serum concentration. Biotransformation of primidone leads to the formation of two metabolites, phenobarbital and phenylethylmalonamide (PEMA). Each has antiepileptic activity along with primidone per se. The rate of conversion to phenobarbital is enhanced by concurrent use of inducing drugs such as phenytoin. When primidone is given as a singular drug, the derived phenobarbital concentration may be less than the serum concentration of primidone. Concurrent use of inducing drugs will often provide serum concentrations of primidone that are one third those of the metabolically derived phenobarbital. Concurrent use of primidone and phenobarbital should be avoided to prevent phenobarbital toxicity (this is further enhanced if a third drug with metabolic induction qualities is employed).

Usual Adult Dose. Special care is needed with the induction of this therapy, particularly in patients who are starting drug treatment for the first time. Previous treatment with phenobarbital (which should be discontinued if primidone is to be used) allows for a smooth introduction of this drug. The patient should take the initial dose prior to bedtime, and no more than 125 mg (50 mg tablets are available for induction and it is often best to begin with a dose of this size) should be given. The patients need to be forewarned about side effects such as unusual drowsiness, possible dizziness and nausea, and unsteadiness, which will usually disappear with continuing use of small initial doses. A night's rest will allow most of these problems to be gone by the next day and eventually allow employment of a full program of therapy (rarely more than 250 mg four times daily). Hallucinatory states have rarely been observed at the time of induction. Some individuals seem unable to tolerate this drug, but most will pass through the initial phase of difficulty and tolerate the medication well thereafter. Dosage adjustments are made with the goal of attaining serum concentrations at not greater than 15 mcg per ml (2 hours after ingestion). Drug withdrawal is done gradually with four reductions at 1 week intervals. Fifty and 250 mg tablets and a suspension are available.

Toxic Reactions

DOSE-RELATED. Sedation; ataxia.

IDIOSYNCRATIC. Dermatitis; leukopenia and thrombocytopenia; agranulocytosis and aplastic anemia; lymphadenopathy; hepatitis; lupus erythematosus; personality change.

Side Effects. Prolonged therapy may be associated with folate, vitamin D, and vitamin K deficiency, as previously noted with phenobarbital and phenytoin.

Drug Interactions. Enhanced conversion of primidone to its metabolite phenobarbital in the presence of concurrent treatment with phenytoin has been emphasized. Carbamazepine may cause a similar effect. Isoniazid has been observed to inhibit the metabolism of primidone in one patient, causing elevation of primidone concentration and half-life with lessened concentrations of phenobarbital and PEMA.

Disease States. The risk of primidone toxicity is enhanced in instances of renal disease; its effect on hepatic disease is less clear.

Carbamazepine (Tegretol)

Type of Seizure. Partial and tonic-clonic seizures.

Pharmacokinetics. Absorption from the alimentary tract is followed by a fairly equal distribution in the body with 75 to 80 per cent binding to serum proteins. Hepatic biotransformation to epoxide and a variety of other metabolites—some with antiepileptic properties—is followed by renal excretion, only 1 per cent of which is unmetabolized carbamazepine.

Usual Adult Dose. Treatment is initiated at 100 or 200 mg twice daily and gradually increased to 200 mg three or four times daily in the ensuing 2 weeks. Adult dosage exceeding 1200 mg per day is not routinely recommended. Great variability is seen from patient to patient in relation to dose and serum concentration. Decreasing serum concentration can occur with increasing oral doses in the presence of concurrent antiepileptic drugs (another reason to pursue monotherapy whenever possible). Careful monitoring of the serum concentration is important to determine optimal dosage for each patient. A fasting morning sample for a trough level is preferable to a random sample, although it may be important to time samples to coincide with clinical toxicity or impaired control of seizures. Drug withdrawal should be gradually managed over several weeks. Two hundred mg tablets are available along with 100 mg chewable tablets.

Toxicity

LOCAL. Gastric irritability (usually managed by taking the drug after meals).

DOSE-RELATED. Diplopia or blurred vision; dizziness, drowsiness; ataxia; headache; tremor, dystonia, chorea; depression, irritability; psychosis; convulsions; water retention (inappropriate ADH-like syndrome); congestive heart failure; cardiac arrhythmias.

IDIOSYNCRATIC. Anemia, agranulocytosis, leukopenia, thrombocytopenia; hypersensitivity syndrome (dermatitis, eosinophilia, lymphadenopathy, splenomegaly); cholestatic and hepatocellular jaundice.

Drug Interactions. Carbamazepine tends to decrease the plasma-to-dose ratio of other concurrently given antiepileptic drugs, and, conversely, carbamazepine level-to-dose ratio is decreased by other antiepileptic drugs used concomitantly.

Propoxyphene, triacetyloleandomycin, and erythromycin should not be given with carbamazepine, as they will probably lead to intoxication by inhibiting carbamazepine metabolism.

Disease States. Carbamazepine may precipitate or enhance congestive heart failure. Its use should be avoided in this setting or where major arrhythmias are a concern. Plasma levels and potential toxicity need to be closely watched if the drug is necessarily used in instances of renal or hepatic disease.

Ethosuximide (Zarontin)

Type of Seizure. Absence and some myoclonic seizures.

Pharmacokinetics. This drug is readily and almost completely absorbed in the alimentary tract followed by rapid and uniform distribution to body tissues except body fat, which contains a lesser concentration. There is little or no binding to serum proteins. It is transformed in the liver to either a ketone or an alcohol metabolite, which is then excreted with or without glucuronide conjugation.

Usual Adult Dose. 15 to 30 mg per kg in 3 to 4 doses per day. Drug withdrawal should be done with four equal reductions at 1 week intervals. Medication is available as a syrup or a 250 mg capsule.

Toxicity

LOCAL. Gastric irritation, anorexia, nausea, vomiting.

DOSE-RELATED. Drowsiness, dizziness, headache.

IDIOSYNCRATIC. Psychosis; interference with cognitive function; skin rashes; lupus erythematosus; dyskinesia, akathisia, bradykinesia, and parkinsonian changes; pancytopenia, agranulocytosis, and aplastic anemia.

Drug Interactions. An increase in serum phenytoin concentration is possible. Enzyme induction does not appear to be a common problem. Drug interactions are uncommon.

Disease States. Renal and hepatic disorders do not appear to pose major problems for enhanced toxicity of ethosuximide.

Clonazepam (Clonopin)

Type of Seizure. Atypical absence (Lennox-Gastaut syndrome), absence seizures refractory to previous drug therapy, and sometimes atonic and myoclonic attacks.

Pharmacokinetics. Clonazepam appears to be well absorbed by the alimentary tract with subsequent rapid distribution due to its solubility. It is 47 per cent protein bound. Extensive biotransformations take place, and less than 0.5 per cent is recovered from the urine as clonazepam.

Usual Adult Dose. 1.0 mg per day in three doses initially. An increase of 1 mg per day may be made at 3 to 4 day intervals until seizure control is attained or a maximum dose of 20 mg per day is reached. A clear correlation between plasma clonazepam levels and seizure control has not been achieved. The drug should be withdrawn very slowly to avoid withdrawal convulsions. Tablet sizes include 0.5, 1.0, and 2.0 mg.

Toxicity

DOSE-RELATED. Drowsiness; ataxia; behavioral change (irritability, depression, psychosis); dysarthria; diplopia.

IDIOSYNCRATIC. Skin rash; hair loss; anemia, leukopenia, and thrombocytopenia.

Drug Interactions. Concurrent use of amphetamines and methylphenidate may cause central nervous system depression and respiratory irregularities. Depressant effects may also be enhanced by alcohol, antianxiety and antipsychotic drugs, antidepressants, and other antiepileptic drugs. Concurrent use of valproic acid has, in some individuals, been associated with the development of absence status.

Disease States. Renal disease is unlikely to affect the elimination of clonazepam, but liver disease may require decreased dosage and lengthening of dose intervals for this drug.

Valproic Acid (Depakene)

Type of Seizure. Simple and complex absence seizures occurring singly or in combination with generalized seizures. In the latter setting this drug holds the unique prospect of controlling both absence and tonic-clonic seizures with monotherapy.

Pharmacokinetics. Valproic acid is rapidly and completely absorbed after oral administration, with a slight delay in absorption if taken after meals. It is then rapidly and evenly distributed throughout body tissues with binding to serum proteins at 90 per cent. Primary metabolism is by hepatic hydroxylation and conjugation with glucuronide. Valproate also appears in the bowel and undergoes enterohepatic circulation. Beta and omega oxidation may also take place. Excretion as glucuronide in the urine follows with minor amounts lost in feces and expired air.

Usual Adult Dose. Therapy is started at 15 mg per kg and gradually increased by 5 to 10 mg per kg every week until therapeutic success is achieved, a maximum dose of 60 mg per kg is reached, or the serum concentration exceeds 100 mcg per ml. Valproic acid (Depakene) is available in 250 and 500 mg tablets and as a syrup. It is also available as enteric-coated divalproex sodium, a stable coordinate compound (Depakote), which is available in 125, 250, and 500 mg tablets. The absorption of this enteric-coated compound is delayed by about 1 hour with a peak concentration reached in 3 to 4 hours.

Toxicity

LOCAL. Anorexia, nausea, and indigestion are common early gastrointestinal symptoms that rarely include vomiting and diarrhea. These symptoms are significantly improved with the enteric-coated preparation.

DOSE-RELATED. Elevated serum transaminases (usually transient but could be harbinger of serious hepatic disease); tremor.

IDIOSYNCRATIC. Thrombocytopenia; pancreatitis; hyperammonemia; hepatic necrosis; stupor and coma; hair loss; "worsened behaviors"; depression.

Side Effects. Weight gain.

Drug Interactions. Valproic acid slows hepatic hydroxylation and elimination of other concurrently used antiepileptic drugs and causes their serum concentrations to rise. Phenobarbital has been shown to be so affected. Careful monitoring of antiepileptic drug concentrations is imperative in this setting.

The strong affinity for serum protein binding sites can result in competitive displacement of phenytoin from these binding sites and bring about phenytoin intoxication with "therapeutic" serum concentrations. This state can be confirmed only when free levels of phenytoin are determined and found to be elevated.

Although valproic acid does not induce its own metabolism or that of other drugs, other drugs induce hepatic enzymes and enhance the metabolism and clearance of valproic acid. Once again, the careful monitoring of plasma concentrations—sometimes free as well as total concentrations—will help guide therapy in these situations.

Disease States. The use of valproic acid is probably best avoided in the presence of liver disease.

Withdrawal of Antiepileptic Therapy

The question about when it is appropriate to discontinue antiepileptic medication is not easily answered. Two situations have a relatively bright prognosis. Rolandic epilepsy, an autosomal dominant disorder that is usually remittent by the age of 20, responds quite well to antiepileptic drugs during its active phase between the ages of five and nine. The interictal electroencephalogram shows spike and slow wave activity over the rolandic area. The seizures characteristically involve the face and cause arrested speech, although appendicular and tonic-clonic seizures are also a part of this type of epilepsy. Full control of such seizures for several years, along with a normal electroencephalogram and, very importantly, the approach of the expected remission time for this seizure, is an important factor in planning discontinuation of drug therapy. Patients with only simple absence seizures and a family history of similar problems known to be outgrown by perhaps the late teens are also individuals who may look forward to eventual discontinuation of drug therapy.

The decisions are more difficult for most other types of seizures. Persistent epileptiform electroencephalographic abnormalities or neurologic abnormalities do not bode well for discontinuation of drug therapy. Full control of seizures for 4 to 5 years and a normal electroencephalogram may warrant consideration of a trial phaseout of antiepileptic drug therapy but not without cautioning the patient that recurrent seizures are possible.

TREATMENT OF STATUS EPILEPTICUS

Status epilepticus occurs "whenever a seizure persists for a sufficient length of time or is repeated frequently enough that recovery between attacks does not occur." Three categories of status may be considered: convulsive, nonconvulsive, and continuous partial seizures (epilepsia partialis continua). Prompt efforts at control of all types is important, but urgent control of tonic-clonic and probably partial complex status (a very rare type of status) is of crucial importance to prevent significant residual neurologic deficit or death.

Identification of the type of status epilepticus proceeds with consideration of the causative factors (inadequate concentrations of antiepileptic drugs, cerebral tumor, trauma, infarction, infection, or various toxic metabolic derangements), as the appropriate drug is chosen to control the specific types of status. Careful observation of respiratory, cardiovascular (electrocardiographic monitoring), and renal fucntioning is appropriate. Electroencephalographic monitoring is desirable.

Tonic-Clonic Status

This form of status is a medical emergency. The more rapidly it is brought under control, the less the risk of serious sequelae or death.

1. Protect the patient from injury, establish a patent airway, and be prepared to support respiration as the patient is observed to confirm the diagnosis of tonic-clonic status. Check arterial blood gases and pH. Establish intravenous routes for blood samples (anticonvulsant levels, complete blood count, blood chemistry and electrolyte series) and give 50 ml of 50 per cent glucose (if hyperglycemic state is not likely) and a bolus of B vitamins.
2. Begin intravenous diazepam at 2 mg per min until 20 mg have been given. Intravenous phenytoin should be started concurrently at 50 mg per min to complete a total dose of 18 mg per kg (with slowing of infusion if hypotension evolves).
3. In the presence of persistent seizures following the completion of the phenytoin infusion, phenobarbital may be given intravenously, no faster than 100 mg per min up to a total loading dose of 20 mg per kg. Respiratory support may be needed at this point.
4. General anesthesia with halothane and neuromuscular blockade may be required if the status continues despite all the previous treatments.

Absence status usually responds quickly to antiabsence drugs or intravenous diazepam. The concerns of fatality or serious sequelae seen with tonic-clonic status are not present in absence status. Similarly, epilepsia partialis continua, which may also be refractory to drug therapy, does not appear to carry the grave risks of uncontrolled tonic-clonic status.

Follow-Up Evaluation

Epilepsy, which tends to appear early in life and persists for long periods, if not a lifetime, requires special attention and follow-up appraisals. Effective management depends on effective communication between patient and physician. Besides conveying a genuine concern for the patient's well-being, the physician must consider these issues in follow-up evaluations: (1) how are the seizures responding to treatment; (2) is drug toxicity present; (3) are the patient's life adjustments in need of support; (4) is there evidence of progressive neurologic disease (a previously unsuspected tumor or degenerative process); (5) are adjustments in drug therapy needed; (6) should a new antiepileptic drug be tried?

EPILEPSY IN INFANTS AND CHILDREN

method of
F. E. DREIFUSS, M.B., FRCP
University of Virginia
Charlottesville, Virginia

Epilepsy refers to spontaneously recurring seizures that are the result of abnormal electrochemical discharge of neurons which, if sufficiently synchronized, causes interruption of normal motor, sensory, or cognitive brain function. Individual seizures are expressed according to the origin, rapidity, and direction of spread of the electrical discharges. In childhood more than half of the cases are of unknown etiology, and these frequently have a genetic predisposition.

Classification of Seizures and the Epilepsies

Because the epilepsies are etiologically diverse and because the development of antiepileptic drugs has tended more toward specific drugs for specific types of seizures, classification of the convulsive disorders has assumed an importance transcending taxonomy. Once a diagnosis of epilepsy has been made, the type of seizures and the syndrome to which the seizures belong must be established. This determination will lead to the formulation of a prognosis on which the therapeutic process may be predicated.

The classification of epileptic seizures is shown in Table 1 of the preceding article, on page 706. From a practical point of view, it is important to distinguish seizures that are primarily generalized and those that are secondarily generalized because of the different responses to medication and the different medication recommendations. It is also important to distinguish between absence seizures and complex partial seizures, which may be indistinguishable at first glance. The use of inappropriate medications should always be avoided.

Classification of Epilepsy Syndromes

Epileptic syndromes are concatenations of symptoms including seizure type, etiology, precipitating factors, age of onset, severity and chronicity, diurnal and circadian cycling, family history, and prognosis. Childhood epilepsy syndromes may be classified according to age. Thus one may recognize neonatal seizure syndromes, infantile spasms, the syndrome of febrile convulsions, the Lennox-Gastaut syndrome, pyknoleptic petit mal, benign juvenile partial seizures, juvenile epileptic myoclonus, epilepsia partialis continua, and the reflex epilepsies as well as etiologically identifiable diseases such as lipidoses, progressive myoclonic epilepsy, and other storage diseases presenting with seizures. It is important to realize that most of these syndromes consist of two main syndromic subgroups, primary or idiopathic epilepsy and secondary, lesional, or symptomatic epilepsy. The primary epilepsies are unassociated with underlying pathology. There is frequently a positive family history, the child is usually normal up to the time of the development of the seizures, which are often self-limited and responsive to medication. Symptomatic epilepsies are frequently associated with neurologic abnormalities and abnormal neurologic development. The seizures are frequently more difficult to control and often persist despite treatment. These subdivisions may be applied to nearly all the childhood seizure syndromes including neonatal convulsions, infantile spasms, febrile seizures, astatic myoclonic seizures, and absence seizures of the petit mal syndromes.

Management

Appropriate treatment includes the reversal of metabolic disorders, the removal of surgically remediable diseases such as tumor or abscess, the treatment of inflammatory lesions, and the elimination of toxins. In most instances, epilepsy will continue to have to be treated symptomatically, and the mainstay of therapy is anticonvulsant medication. Occasionally a decision not to treat may be made, such as in appearance of the first febrile seizure or instances where recurrence is unlikely. The decision not to treat may be reached by weighing the statistical chance of seizure recurrence against the potential deleterious consequences of long-term therapy.

The choice of a specific drug will be determined by its potential efficacy and its relative freedom from side effects. Whichever drug is used, the patient and family must be educated about the importance of compliance, the need for therapeutic blood level determinations, and the recognition of both dose-related and idiosyncratic side effects. Drugs should be gradually introduced to lessen the incidence of side effects. Monotherapy should be the therapeutic aim, but substitution of another drug may be mandated by failure of the first drug. The first drug is then slowly withdrawn as the second drug is introduced. Occasionally more than one drug may be necessary but if polytherapy is used, knowledge of potential drug interactions is essential.

Management of Specific Seizure Type

Neonatal Seizures

Neonatal seizures frequently have an identifiable etiology. Many are the result of prematurity or birth trauma, including intracranial hemorrhage, infection, and metabolic disorders such as hypoglycemia or hypocalcemia. Cerebral malformations, metabolic diseases, and drug withdrawal may underlie neonatal seizures. Occasionally the seizures may be benign, self-limited, and familial. Rapid diagnosis and immediate removal of underlying remediable causes are essential. Hypoglycemia is treated with intravenous 25 per cent glucose, 2 to 4 ml per kg, and blood glucose is then monitored continuously. Hypocalcemia is managed with intravenous 5 per cent calcium gluconate, 200 mg per kg, while monitoring the fetal heart rate. Hypomagnesemia is treated with 0.2 ml per kg 50 per cent magnesium sulfate intramuscularly. Because pyridoxine deficiency may cause continuing seizures, pyridoxine, 50 mg, can be given intravenously during electroencephalography, although this is a relatively rare cause of neonatal convulsions.

Specific anticonvulsant treatment is undertaken while awaiting definitive therapy or if the cause cannot be ascertained or seizures persist. In the neonate the drug of choice is phenobarbital, which may be given intravenously in two divided doses to a total of 20 mg per kg. Subsequent oral phenobarbital therapy may be used to maintain satisfactory blood levels. If phenobarbital does not control neonatal convulsions, phenytoin (Dilantin) may be used but must be given intravenously very slowly because of the danger of cardiac arrhythmia. Up to 20 mg per kg may be administered at 1 mg per kg per minute. Oral phenytoin therapy results in unpredictable blood levels in the neonate. Phenobarbital is maintained at 3 mg per kg per day and phenytoin at 6 mg per kg per day while obtaining frequent blood levels. Duration of therapy depends on the underlying etiology and EEG findings. If the cause can be identified, treatment may be necessary for only a few weeks. In the case of an ongoing process, impaired development, or persistent EEG abnormality, long-term therapy may be needed.

Infantile Spasms

Infantile spasms are an early childhood epilepsy syndrome characterized by myoclonic flexion or extension spasms that are usually bilateral. They often occur in clusters and are often associated with an EEG pattern of hypsarrhythmia, although the actual EEG pattern during spasms may be electrodecremental. In the idiopathic variety neurologic development is normal until the onset of the condition during the first year, usually around four months of age. Symptomatic infantile spasms frequently begin in the postnatal period and are usually associated with severe brain disease, anoxia, congenital malformations, or metabolic abnormalities such as nonketotic hyperglycinemia. Infantile spasms due to tuberous sclerosis behave more like the idiopathic variety. The treatment of choice is intramuscular ACTH, and it is generally believed that early treatment is associated with better prognosis than delayed therapy. The dosage is 30 to 40 units of ACTH gel daily for 4 to 6 weeks. If ACTH is not successful, benzodiazepines, particularly nitrazepam (Mogadon) (not yet approved for use in the United States) or clonazepam (Clonopin), 0.05 to 0.2 mg per kg, may be used. Sodium valproate (Depakene), 30 to 60 mg per kg, may also be effective. Side effects from ACTH include hypertension, cushingoid changes, and interference with immunity. Elective immunizations should not be given during this time. Side effects from benzodiazepines include hypotonia and increased respiratory secretions. If valproate is used, liver function should be carefully monitored.

There is no consensus regarding long-term therapy. Relapse after discontinuation of ACTH therapy is less common in the idiopathic than the symptomatic group. Reinstitution of ACTH therapy is usually unsuccessful. Some authorities recommend long-term corticosteroid therapy, but I prefer valproate. In the symptomatic group, other seizure types such as the Lennox-Gastaut syndrome frequently emerge and have to be treated on their own merits.

Febrile Seizures

This is a common disorder, occurring in approximately 50 per 1000 children between the ages of 3 months and 5 years, and in each case intracranial infection or other known causes must be excluded.

Idiopathic or benign febrile seizures are not associated with a major risk of subsequent epilepsy but if frequently recurrent should be treated. Major risk factors that predispose to recurrence or to the development of nonfebrile seizures include a family history of epilepsy, an abnormal neurologic development prior to the onset of febrile seizures, prolonged seizures (longer than 15 minutes), an element of focality, and a series of seizures. Those children at increased risk (two or more risk factors) should receive long-term prophylaxis. The drug of choice continues to be phenobarbital with the aim of reaching blood levels between 15 and 25 micrograms per ml until a two year seizure-free interval has been attained. Because of the side effects of hyperactivity and possible interference with cognitive development, some prefer to use valproate prophylaxis, but the danger of hepatotoxicity detracts from the attractiveness of this alternative. In Europe, the availability of rectal diazepam offers the choice of intermittent therapy during fever episodes and is gaining increasing popularity.

Lennox-Gastaut Syndrome

Lennox-Gastaut syndrome is characterized by astatic myoclonic seizures, atypical absence, and frequently localization-related seizures. In most cases this is a very severe disorder attended by developmental delay and mental retardation as well as extreme intractability to most medication regimens. A relatively benign form of astatic myoclonic epilepsy may respond to valproate therapy, and this is the drug of first choice. In these cases the interictal EEG usually has a relatively normal background.

In the severe form the interictal EEG background is usually very slow. The multiple spike and wave pattern is usually that of a slow spike and wave, and here valproate is not as successful. Akinetic drop attacks are quite resistant, and several anticonvulsant drugs are frequently given in combination, including benzodiazepines and a major anticonvulsant such as carbamazepine (Tegretol). (The safety and efficacy of carbamazepine in children under the age of six years have not been established.) As a last resort, a 3:1 ketogenic diet may be tried. In this diet three fourths of the caloric intake is derived from fat. When a ketogenic diet is used, anticonvulsant drugs should not be dispensed in a carbohydrate vehicle such as sweetened syrups.

Petit Mal Syndrome

Petit mal syndrome is characterized by recurrent absence seizures consisting of sudden onset, interruption of ongoing activities, a blank stare, and, frequently, a brief upward rotation of the eyes. In addition, there may be mild clonic components, changes in postural tone, automatisms, or autonomic components. The ictal EEG usually consists of regular and symmetric three cycle per second spike and wave complexes. In "atypical absence" there may also be astatic myoclonic components. Absence may occur in the form of status or "spike wave stupor," which is characterized by continuing absence activity for hours or even days with stuporous, confused, or dazed behavior. The treatment of choice in absence is ethosuximide (Zarontin) monotherapy, 10 to 30 mg per kg, with an effective blood level of 40 to 100 micrograms per ml. The principal side effects include gastrointestinal disturbance, hiccups, drowsiness, and headache. Idiosyncratic side effects include erythema multiforme, blood dyscrasia, and systemic lupus erythematosus. The next drug of choice is valproate, which is equally effective and is ranked second only because of the potential seriousness of idiosyncratic hepatic side effects. It is given in a dose of 30 to 60 mg per kg with an expected trough blood level of 50 to 100 micrograms per ml. In the case of myoclonic absence a combination of ethosuximide and valproate may be more successful than either drug alone.

In the treatment of petit mal, sedative anticonvulsants should be avoided as these potentiate absence seizures. If generalized tonic-clonic seizures emerge, valproate becomes the drug of choice for the treatment of both conditions. Clonazepam is effective in the treatment of absence in a dose of 0.05 to 0.2 mg per kg and a therapeutic blood level range between 13 and 72 nanograms per ml, but the side effects reduce its popularity, as does the emergence of tolerance.

The treatment of choice for absence status is the intravenous use of diazepam followed by ethosuximide or valproate.

Treatment of petit mal may be discontinued after a two year seizure-free interval. The pyknoleptic petit mal syndrome has a good prognosis for spontaneous resolution in adolescence.

Rolandic Epilepsy

This benign form of partial seizure associated with a centrotemporal spike EEG abnormality and a stereotyped characteristic focal childhood attack responds well to most anticonvulsant drugs. Carbamazepine or valproate is the drug of choice. Some pediatric epileptologists recommend no treatment for this usually self-limited condition. Because the prognosis is never certain and because of the anxiety induced by the attacks, my practice is to administer carbamazepine, aiming for a therapeutic blood level range of 8 to 12 micrograms per ml.

Juvenile Myoclonic Epilepsy

This condition occurs in childhood and adolescence and is characterized by frequent myoclonic jerks, usually occurring in the mornings, interspersed with generalized tonic-clonic seizures. Sleep deprivation is a common precipitating factor, and these patients are frequently photically sensitive. Sleep deprivation and strobe lights should therefore be avoided. The drug of choice is valproate. Despite the efficacy of treatment, discontinuation of medication after a period of time usually judged to be appropriate frequently leads to recurrence of seizures, and therapy should therefore be long-term.

Reflex Epilepsies

Reflex epilepsies include those with seizure regularly induced by external stimuli such as flashing lights, certain noises, or certain proprioceptive stimuli or by reading or listening to music. The majority of these reflex epilepsies respond well to valproate monotherapy. Clonazepam and carbamazepine are also effective.

Epilepsies Characterized by Partial Seizures

The drugs of choice for partial seizures, both simple and complex, include carbamazepine (Tegretol), phenytoin (Dilantin), phenobarbital, and primidone (Mysoline). Until recently, carbamazepine was used adjunctively but it is evident that it is effective as monotherapy in most forms of partial seizures, particularly those of the complex variety. Serious side effects are infrequent, and carbamazepine is a relatively benign drug in children in relation to central nervous system toxicity. The side effects of primidone are sufficiently troublesome to reduce its popularity in children. Phenytoin continues to be a popular

TABLE 1. **Drugs of Choice in the Management of Seizure Types**

NEONATAL SEIZURES	
A. Benign familial	No therapy
B. Others	phenobarbital (Luminal)
INFANTILE SPASMS	
A. Primary generalized	ACTH
B. Symptomatic	nitrazepam valproate (Depakene)
FEBRILE SEIZURES	
A. Primary benign	No treatment or phenobarbital or valproate
B. Symptomatic	phenobarbital or valproate
ABSENCE SEIZURES	
A. Primary petit mal	ethosuximide (Zarontin) or valproate (Depakene, Depakote)
B. Symptomatic	ethosuximide plus valproate
C. Myoclonic	ethosuximide plus valproate
ASTATIC-MYOCLONIC SEIZURES	
A. Generalized	valproate
B. Lennox-Gastaut	valproate ± clonazepam (Clonopin) carbamazepine (Tegretol)
BENIGN ROLANDIC SEIZURES (primary partial epilepsy of childhood)	carbamazepine or valproate or no treatment
JUVENILE MYOCLONIC SEIZURES	valproate
REFLEX EPILEPSIES	valproate or benzodiazepines or carbamazepine
PARTIAL SEIZURES	
A. Limbic	carbamazepine plus/or phenytoin (Dilantin) plus/or valproate
B. Extralimbic	carbamazepine plus/or phenytoin plus/or primidone (Mysoline)
GENERALIZED TONIC-CLONIC SEIZURES	
A. Primary	valproate or carbamazepine or phenytoin
B. Secondary	carbamazepine or phenytoin

drug in the treatment of most forms of seizures, including partial seizures, but is becoming less popular than carbamazepine because of the prevalence of side effects during long-term therapy. It has the advantage of requiring only once daily administration, which improves compliance. Moreover it is relatively inexpensive, which is an important economic consideration. In the case of carbamazepine, blood counts should be performed periodically. Transient leukopenia is common, but persistent leukopenia should lead to reduction or discontinuation of this drug.

Epilepsies Characterized by Generalized Tonic-Clonic Seizures

The drugs used in the treatment of partial seizures are also generally employed in the management of generalized tonic-clonic seizures, but the order in which the drugs are used may depend upon the setting in which the seizures occur. In concomitant absence seizures, valproic acid (Depakene, Depakote) is the treatment of choice, as one is dealing with primary generalized epilepsy. Under other circumstances, carbamazepine, phenytoin, or phenobarbital might be preferred, particularly if there is evidence that one is dealing with secondarily generalized seizures. When seizures are secondarily generalized, when there is evidence of other neurologic dysfunction such as intellectual impairment or the presence of abnormal neurologic signs, and when other seizure types are also present, the prognosis becomes less favorable. It is here that control with a single drug is less predictable, as is the prognosis for cessation of seizures with maturation. Here, more than one drug may have to be given, leading to the potential complications inherent in drug interactions.

Status Epilepticus

Status epilepticus is defined as recurrent seizures without intervening recovery. The term is usually used after 30 minutes of seizure activity. Status epilepticus represents a medical emergency because of the threat to life and to continued integrity of brain function posed by anoxia, hypoglycemia, increasing acidosis, and, of course, the disorders leading to the status epilepticus in the first place. A treatment plan must include maintenance of vital functions including airway, oxygen, and blood pressure. An intravenous line should be placed to provide blood for glucose, electrolyte, and anticonvulsant levels and to provide access to glucose and anticonvulsant drugs. Glucose is administered as 50 per cent dextrose in water, 1 gram per kg to children. Pharmacologic management consists of the administration of a benzodiazepine and/or phenytoin or phenobarbital intravenously. A benzodiazepine, either diazepam (Valium) or lorazepam (Ativan), is the drug of choice in a previously untreated patient, followed by a longer-acting drug such as phenytoin. In a patient previously treated with phenobarbital, diazepam may cause respiratory and cardiovascular depression, and phenytoin or more phenobarbital might be preferred. In the case of diazepam, this is given to children 0.25 to 0.4 mg per kg over 2 minutes with a maximum injection of 5 to 10 mg. This may be repeated once. In the case of lorazepam, experience with children is limited and the recommended dose is 0.05 to 0.2 mg per kg. Both benzodiazepines are followed by a longer-acting drug. Phenytoin is delivered at 20 mg per kg intravenously at a rate of 1 to 2 mg per kg per minute. Alternatively, phenobarbital may be administered as 5 to 10 mg per kg at 30 mg per minute, and this may be repeated to a maximum of 25 mg per kg. All intravenous anticonvulsants may cause apnea and hypotension, and the patient should be carefully monitored in an intensive care unit. If seizures are not controlled by these medications, general anesthesia may have to be used. In children, continuing seizures despite adequate intravenous therapy are usually the result of severe brain disease.

Partial status, or epilepsia partialis continua, may be treated similarly but constitutes considerably less of an emergency. It does, however, usually represent the expression of a severe focal underlying lesion, and management should be directed toward the underlying cause and the realization that unduly vigorous anticonvulsant drug treatment may further jeopardize the patient. Epilepsia partialis continua in a child is usually a progressive intractable condition of poor prognosis that ultimately leads to severe neurologic impairment including hemiparesis.

General Considerations in the Management of Children with Epilepsy

Children should be guarded against developing psychosocial consequences of epilepsy by giving attention to those factors that influence a person's coping style. These include factors inherent in the epilepsy, such as age of onset, site of lesion, and the nature and dose of medication employed, as well as the child's underlying personality, family support, and innate mechanisms for coping with stress. Coping factors should not be further interfered with by trying to shield the child from competition and exploratory activities that are necessary for the attainment of independence and confidence. Restrictions should be confined to threatening situations such as the operation of a motor vehicle, solo bathing, and contact sports in which head injury is a frequent and predictable consequence. However, most ath-

TABLE 2. **Drug Therapy in the Management of Seizures**

Drug	Dosage: *Starting*	Dosage: *Maintenance*	Blood Level	Side Effects	Precautions
carbamazepine (Tegretol)	Child: 5 mg/kg/day	10–25 mg/kg/day	5–12 μg/ml	*Dose-related:* Diplopia, drowsiness, vertigo, headache, diarrhea, inappropriate ADH, leukopenia *Idiosyncratic:* Aplastic anemia, hepatotoxicity, arrhythmia	Blood counts and SGOT monthly for 6 mo, then every 4 mo
clonazepam (Clonopin)	0.05 mg/kg/day	0.2 mg/kg/day	13–72 ng/ml	*Dose-related:* Drowsiness, hypotonia, increased secretions, behavior problems, tolerance	Begin with small dose. Extreme caution on withdrawal
ethosuximide (Zarontin)	20–25 mg/kg/day	20–25 mg/kg/day	40–100 μg/ml	*Dose-related:* Drowsiness, headache, hiccup, nausea *Idiosyncratic:* Aplastic anemia, erythema multiforme, Stevens-Johnson syndrome, SLE	Blood counts monthly. Report skin, joint, or mucous membrane symptoms, sore throats
phenytoin (Dilantin)	Child: 4–8 mg/kg/day	4–8 mg/kg/day max. 300 mg	10–20 μg/ml	*Dose-related:* Dizziness, ataxia, diplopia, athetosis, gingival hyperplasia, hirsutism, coarse facies, folate deficiency, vit. D deficiency, cerebellar dysfunction *Idiosyncratic:* Skin rashes, erythema multiforme, SLE, pseudolymphoma, teratogenicity	Annual blood counts. Oral hygiene. Avoid in pregnancy if possible. Warn of possible effect on birth control meds
primidone (Mysoline)	Child 1–2 mg/kg/day	10–25 mg/kg/day		*Dose-related:* Sedation, vertigo, behavior disturbances *Idiosyncratic:* Skin rashes, fever	Begin with very small dose. Avoid in school age children if possible
phenobarbital (Luminal)	Neonate: 10–20 mg/kg/day Child: 3–4 mg/kg/day In Status Epilepticus Child: 20 mg/kg IV	3–4 mg/kg/day 5 mg/kg/day	10–30 μg/ml	*Dose-related:* Sedation, hyperactivity, irritability *Idiosyncratic:* Skin rash, exfoliative dermatitis, fever	
valproate (Depakene, Depakote)	Child: 15 mg/kg/day	up to 60 mg/kg/day	50–120 μg/ml trough level	*Dose-related:* Drowsiness, GI disturbances, alopecia, weight gain, tremor, SGOT elevation *Idiosyncratic:* Leukopenia, thrombocytopenia, hepatitis, pancreatitis, teratogenicity	CBC, platelets, SGOT and SGPT every 2 weeks for 2 mo then every mo for 1 year

Adapted from Dreifuss FE: *In* Porter R (ed): BIMR Neurology. Vol. 5, Epilepsies. London, Butterworth's.

letic activities can be engaged in, and supervised swimming is not usually contraindicated. Treatment participation by social workers, educational consultants, and vocational counselors may add to the quality of life and directly influence the degree of seizure control.

HEADACHE

method of
JOHN EDMEADS, M.D.
University of Toronto
Toronto, Ontario

Headache is one of mankind's most common afflictions. It has many causes. Expanding intracranial lesions, such as a neoplasm or a hematoma, produce progressively worsening *traction headaches*. Irritation of pain-sensitive structures by blood or pus in the meninges causes cataclysmic *inflammatory headaches*. Periodic dilatation of cranial blood vessels causes the paroxysmal *vascular headaches* of migraine and cluster headache. Physical and emotional stress, sometimes through sustained contraction of scalp and neck muscles but more often through unknown mechanisms, produces chronic recurrent *tension headaches*.

Traction and inflammatory headaches are very uncommon, accounting for only a small fraction of all patients with headaches. Vascular headaches are quite common, affecting 10 to 15 per cent of the population. Tension headaches are endemic; it is an exceptional person who has never had a tension headache, and many people have them frequently.

The first step in the management of any patient with headache is a detailed history and a thorough physical examination. Not only will this provide a diagnosis, which will lead to definitive treatment of patients with traction and inflammatory headaches, but in the much larger group of patients with vascular and tension headaches it will demonstrate that the physician is taking their symptoms seriously, an important consideration for patients who have been told too often that their headaches are "functional" or "imaginary."

CLUSTER HEADACHE

This severe and dramatic headache is believed to arise from recurrent paroxysmal distention and inflammation of the internal carotid artery, probably produced in turn by abnormal influences from the hypothalamus and other neural centers. The patients are nearly always male. They experience one or more headaches (usually up to five) every day for several weeks and then may have months or years without headaches until the next recurrence. The syndrome derives its name from the tendency of the headaches to cluster in time. Rarely remission may fail to occur; these patients have "chronic cluster headaches."

Each headache last 30 to 120 minutes. It involves one eye and the adjacent cheek, temple, and forehead. It is associated with redness and watering of the affected eye, sometimes drooping of the eyelid, and stuffing or running of the ipsilateral nostril.

Treatment

Treatment of the acute attack is often unrewarding; the headache, although intense, is usually brief enough that it has begun to settle spontaneously by the time oral analgesics and ergotamine have been absorbed from the gastrointestinal tract. Rectal absorption of ergotamine is quicker, but the compulsion for these people to pace with the headache makes it difficult for them to retain suppositories. Sublingual ergotamine may be quickly absorbed but often not quickly enough to be of significant help. Three things may work: (1) inhalation of 100 per cent oxygen by mask, at a rate of 7 liters per minute, may shorten the attack by about 50 per cent in 50 per cent of patients; (2) inhaled ergotamine (Ergotamine Medihaler), in a dose of one puff (0.36 mg) every 5 minutes to a maximum of five puffs per day, may shorten the attack; (3) placing a nifedipine (Procardia, Adalat, 10 mg) capsule that has been punctured with a pin under the tongue may allow sufficient sublingual absorption to shorten the headache (note: nifedipine and ergotamine should not be used together).

Prevention of cluster headaches is definitely preferable. Methysergide (Sansert) is the traditional therapy; 1 tablet (2 mg) is given three or four times daily, preferably with food or milk to avert gastric irritation. Long-term side effects are not usually a problem, since a cluster rarely lasts for more than 3 to 4 months. The methysergide is given for the expected length of the cluster (but never for more than 5 months) and is then slowly withdrawn.

Lithium carbonate, 1 tablet (300 mg) two to four times daily, is useful when methysergide is either ineffective or contraindicated by coexistent disease. It is customary to obtain weekly serum lithium levels during treatment to ensure that toxicity is not developing. Fine tremor of the outstretched fingers may occur even at subtoxic levels and if bothersome to the patient can be controlled by propranolol (Inderal), 40 mg two or three times daily. Although currently considered the drug of choice for chronic cluster headaches, lithium is also effective in "ordinary" cluster headache.

Prednisone may be helpful if methysergide and lithium are ineffective. An initial dose of 80 mg per day for the first 3 days is used to break the cluster, and then the dose is reduced slowly to the smallest amount that will keep the patient comfortable. It is discontinued when it is determined that the cluster has run its course. Note that there is an increased incidence of peptic ulcer in patients with cluster headache and that this is a contraindication to the use of prednisone in some individuals.

The most recent treatment to be introduced for cluster headache is calcium channel blockers. What appears from investigational studies to be the most appropriate agent for headache, nimodipine, is not yet on the market. Nifedipine, 20 mg three times daily; verapamil, 80 mg three times daily; or diltiazem, 60 mg three times daily, does not have the same specificity as nimodipine but has been reported beneficial for some patients with "ordinary" and chronic cluster headaches.

Ergotamine tartrate, 1 to 2 mg orally two or three times daily, has been used on a short-term basis for the treatment of nonchronic cluster headache.

When all of these treatments used singly have failed, various combinations may be tried, including lithium and ergotamine, prednisone and methysergide, and methysergide and lithium.

Chronic paroxysmal hemicrania is a rare variant of cluster headache characterized by its occurrence in women, by very frequent (up to 20 per day) brief attacks, and by its unique responsiveness to indomethacin (Indocin), 50 mg three or four times daily. Other forms of cluster headache do not respond to indomethacin or any other nonsteroidal anti-inflammatory drug.

When medication fails, surgery may be considered for the patient with chronic cluster headache. Procedures available include radiofrequency lesions of V1 and V2; instillation of glycerol into Meckel's cave around the trigeminal ganglion; and section of the greater superficial petrosal nerve, the nervus intermedius, or the sphenopalatine ganglion. Surgery confers only inconsistent benefit but can be worthwhile in desperate cases.

MIGRAINE

Migraine is a group of constitutional disorders characterized by paroxysmal disturbances of cephalic neurovascular function and presenting predominantly as episodic headaches associated with autonomic, visual, somatosensory, and/or psychologic symptoms of variable prominence. When the neurologic aspects of the attack are clear-cut and prominent and precede the headache (as in the fortification figures of the visual aura), the attack is said to be a "classic migraine." When the neurologic accompaniments are less marked and consist mainly of autonomic disturbances such as nausea, vomiting, chilliness, and so on, the attack is described as "common migraine." As the name implies, common migraine is much more frequent than classic migraine; only about one migraine sufferer in eight has attacks of classic migraine.

It is believed that in the migraine sufferer genetically vulnerable cranial blood vessels, when subjected to attack by internal and external environmental factors (such as the neurochemical changes of stress, the hormonal concomitants of the menstrual cycle, chemical components in food, and so on), react by painful vasodilatation, producing headache. Mediating this reaction are thought to be neural and humoral factors.

Treatment

Educating the patient about what migraine is, how it occurs, and what may trigger it is the first step in therapy. Sometimes it is appropriate to emphasize the relationship between life style and headache and to advocate the elimination of stress and the cultivation of equanimity. Where a specific trigger can be identified with confidence, it should be eliminated; examples are skipping meals, sleeping in, alcohol ingestion, and oral contraceptive medication. In common migraine it may be worthwhile to suggest a trial of discontinuation of oral contraceptive medication, since this may aggravate the migraine in some individuals. In classic migraine it is much more important to discontinue oral contraceptives because of the alleged relationship between these medications and the production of permanent neurologic sequelae following attacks of classic migraine.

Recently there has been emphasis on the role of food allergy in the production of migraine, but this appears to have been overdone. Only about 10 per cent of the migrainous population have identifiable food triggers, such as chocolate, old cheese, red wine, and food additives such as monosodium glutamate and sodium nitrite. Putting a migraine patient on a diet may help in ways unrelated to elimination of food triggers; for example, the general regulation of life style that frequently attends adhering to a diet is often beneficial to the patient with a migraine.

Treatment of the Acute Attack of Migraine

When attacks of migraine are no more frequent than two to four times a month it is more reasonable to treat them as they occur rather than to attempt to prevent them with daily prophylactic medication (see hereafter). Treatment of the acute attack may involve analgesics, antinauseants, sedatives, or ergotamine in various combinations.

Many people have learned that over the counter analgesics, such as acetylsalicylic acid or acetaminophen, taken in a dose of 650 mg very early in the attack will abort the attack when a much larger dose taken later will not. Some people absorb oral medication poorly during a migraine attack because of the gastric stasis that may accompany the headache; in this situation effervescent acetylsalicylic acid may be much better absorbed and thus more effective. Another strategy is to administer a stimulant of gastric contraction, such as metoclopramide (Reglan), in a dose of 1 tablet (10 mg) 10 minutes prior to taking the analgesic. Stronger analgesics, such as compounds of acetylsalicylic acid or acetaminophen with codeine or oxycodone (Percodan or Percocet), may be tried in patients who in previous attacks have not responded to the more innocuous acetylsalicylic acid or acetaminophen alone, but a physician prescribing these potentially addictive drugs must accept the responsibility for monitoring the intake carefully and ensuring that dependence does not occur. This precaution is especially important in compounds of barbiturate, codeine, caffeine, and acetylsalicylic acid (for example, Fiorinal-C½); this can be quite effective for the treatment of occasional headaches but has the potential of producing habituation if taken more frequently than 2 days out of every week.

A few patients derive more benefit from taking a nonsteroidal anti-inflammatory drug, such as naproxen (Naprosyn) or ibuprofen (Motrin), than they do from acetylsalicylic acid or acetaminophen; these medications are more likely to cause gastrointestinal upset, however.

Midrin is a compound of acetaminophen, dichloralphenazone (a mild sedative), and isometheptene mucate (a mild vasoconstrictor). This can be helpful taken in a dose of 2 capsules at the onset of an attack followed by 1 capsule every half hour as needed, to a maximum of 5 capsules per day.

Antinauseants such as dimenhydrinate (Dramamine, Gravol) or chlorpromazine (Thorazine) may be added to the previously mentioned combinations, using the oral, rectal, or parenteral route.

Ergotamine is the traditional drug of first choice for aborting an acute attack of migraine, but there are problems in its use. First, it must be taken very early in the course of an attack if it is to work, and many people have trouble comprehending this even after being told repeatedly. Second, through its action on the vomiting center in the brain, it can worsen the nausea and vomiting of an attack (some manufacturers offset this by adding an antiemetic, e.g., Cafergot-PB,

TABLE 1. **Ergotamine Preparations**

Format	Dosage
Oral: Cafergot, Cafergot PB, Wigraine, Ergodryl, Gravergol	2 tablets at onset; 1 every 1/2 hour as needed to maximum of 5 for any one attack
Sublingual: Ergomar, Ergostat, Wigrettes	1 tablet at onset; repeat once in 1 hour if needed
Inhaled: Ergotamine Medihaler	1 puff at onset; repeat every 5 minutes as needed to maximum of 5 puffs per day
Rectal: Cafergot PB, Wigraine	1/2 to 1 suppository at onset; repeat once in 1 hour if needed
Intramuscular: dihydroergotamine (DHE-45)	1 ml at onset; repeat once in 1 hour if needed

Ergodryl, Gravergol). Third, some forms of the oral tablet may be slowly and incompletely absorbed (uncoated are best), correct use of the sublingual and inhaled forms requires careful instruction of the patient, rectal suppositories are spurned by many patients as unesthetic and inconvenient, and injected dihydroergotamine (DHE-45) poses logistic problems. Many people feel it easier to treat their attacks with analgesics.

Nevertheless, in a dose and format carefully chosen by the physician and carefully followed by the patient, ergotamine can be very effective. Table 1 gives specific recommendations. Ergotamine is contraindicated in patients with vascular disease (hypertension, atherosclerosis, Buerger's disease, Raynaud's disease), liver and kidney disease, infection, and pregnancy. The recommended maximum dosages should not be exceeded to avoid producing either toxicity (vomiting, muscle cramps, vasospastic changes) or habituation. It is prudent to advise the patient not to take ergotamine more than 1 day in 3; if consumption exceeds this, a migraine prophylactic regimen should be instituted (see hereafter).

Whether ergotamine or analgesics or both are taken in an attempt to abort the attack, *rest* is a very important part of the treatment. Patients should learn to accept that, in many instances, migraine is a symptom of overload and, therefore, that medication should be followed by at least a few hours rest and, preferably, sleep. Physical adjuncts include a quiet darkened room, elevation of the head slightly above horizontal, and application of cold to the head (a 3M Cold Comfort Pack is ideal).

Some patients may be trained to use biofeedback techniques to limit the extent of a migraine attack, providing that the onset is not too sudden; some others gain benefit from self-hypnosis. In general, however, the backbone of abortive treatment is analgesics and/or ergotamine, coupled with rest and adjunctive measures.

Prophylactic Treatment of Migraine

Migraine prophylactic medication is indicated when the frequency of attacks exceeds three or four per month. It may also be used when headaches occur on a predictable schedule; for example, headaches occurring within the few days preceding menstruation (menstrual migraine) may sometimes by prevented by starting a prophylactic medication 1 week after ovulation each month and continuing until menstrual flow ceases. A wide variety of agents are available.

Beta-blockers are the most widely used migraine prophylactics. Propranolol (Inderal) is the best known, but other beta-blockers, including nadolol (Corgard), timolol (Blocadren), atenolol (Tenormin), metoprolol (Lopressor), and perhaps pindolol (Visken), may also be useful. The potency of these drugs as beta-blockers does not seem to be the major determinant of their antimigraine effect; the exact way in which they exert this effect is obscure. Beta-blockers are contraindicated in allergic asthma, insulin-dependent diabetes, heart failure, and heart block.

Propranolol is started in a dose of 20 mg twice daily and increased by 20 mg every day until improvement is achieved, bradycardia and/or hypotension occur, or the dosage reaches 320 mg per day. Most people respond well to about 160 mg per day; some need more.

Cyproheptadine (Periactin) is useful for the prophylaxis of migraine in children; it seems not to be as effective in adults. It is believed to exert its antimigraine effect through its antiserotoninergic and antihistaminic properties. The usual dose is 2 to 4 mg three times daily.

Pizotifen (Sandomigran) is available in Canada but not in the United States. It is a more powerful antiserotoninergic and antihistaminic than cyproheptadine and is effective in adults. Like cyproheptadine it can cause appetite stimulation and drowsiness. These side effects can be minimized by giving the daily dose (3 to 6 mg) all at once at bedtime. Also, like cyproheptadine, it is contraindicated in glaucoma, prostatic hypertrophy, and pyloric stenosis.

Amitriptyline (Elavil) is becoming increasingly popular. It seems to work not primarily on the basis of its antidepressant effect but rather because of its action on serotonin dynamics. Other antidepressants, such as doxepin (Sinequan), protriptyline (Vivactil), and imipramine (Tofranil), also have antimigraine effects. Amitriptyline may be given in one dose at bedtime, beginning with 10 to 25 mg and increasing slowly to 100 to 150 mg. Weight gain and drowsiness are common side effects of amitriptyline, especially at the higher dosage.

Calcium channel blockers are being increasingly used as migraine prophylactic agents. Verapamil (Isoptin), 80 mg three times daily; nifedipine (Procardia), 20 mg three times daily; and diltiazem (Cardizem), 60 mg three times daily may be helpful (this use not listed by the makers). There is not yet enough experience to choose between them. We have learned that the calcium channel blockers may take up to 1 month to begin to exert their antimigraine effects and that in some patients they are more helpful for the migraine prodrome than for the headaches.

These medications are reasonably effective in preventing migraine in most patients and are unlikely to produce serious side effects. Patients not responding to them can be moved up to methysergide (Sansert) or phenelzine (Nardil). Both these drugs are quite effective; both have the potential of producing serious side effects. (This use of phenelzine not listed by maker.)

Methysergide (Sansert), in a dose of 1 tablet (2 mg) three to four times daily, can bring about significant improvement within a few days. It should be given with food to minimize gastrointestinal upset and should not be given too close to bedtime to prevent bad dreams. Under no circumstances should methysergide be given for more than 4 or 5 months without discontinuing it for at least 4 weeks in order to minimize the chances of dangerous long-term side effects such as retroperitoneal, pleuropulmonary, and cardiac fibrosis.

Phenelzine (Nardil) is a monoamine oxidase inhibitor that can be helpful in some patients resistant to all other medications. How it exerts its antimigraine effect is not known. The usual dose is 15 mg three or four times daily. Patients taking Nardil must receive careful instructions about avoiding certain foods (those containing tyramine) and certain drugs, particularly over the counter medications with sympathomimetic properties, such as "cold tablets," "diet pills," and nasal sprays.

A number of other medications have been used for the prophylaxis of migraine. In general they are not useful for most patients, but in occasional migraine sufferers they may work better than anything else and therefore are worth trying in resistant cases.

Lithium carbonate is not as uniformly useful in migraine as it is in cluster headache but has helped some people with migraine whose attacks tend to cluster in time. The dose for migraine is the same as that used for cluster headache. *Clonidine (Catapres)*, popular in Europe as a migraine prophylactic medication, has been disappointing to most North American clinicians. The usual dose is 0.05 to 0.2 mg twice daily. (This use of lithium and clonidine is not listed by the makers.) *Nonsteroidal anti-inflammatory drugs* have proved more useful for the prevention of exercise-induced migraine than for "garden variety migraine" but may be helpful in the latter condition. Indomethacin is the representative drug, with the usual dose between 25 and 50 mg three times daily. These medications tend to produce GI distress; some clinicians find it useful to give over the counter antacids (Gelusil, Maalox) with each dose. *Platelet-disaggregating agents* like dipyridamole (Persantine) are occasionally helpful in preventing migraine in people with well-marked auras. The usual dose is 25 to 50 mg three times daily. *Bellergal Spacetabs*, a compound of phenobarbital, belladonna alkaloids, and ergotamine, is helpful in a small percentage of people with migraine and is worth trying, especially since its side effects are so uncommon.

Treatment of Status Migrainosus

When an attack of migraine persists for at least 36 hours, with the patient remaining in severe distress due to pain, vomiting, dehydration, and apprehension, "status migrainosus" is said to exist. Since these patients are frequently dehydrated because of vomiting and because of nausea with little oral intake of fluids, an intravenous line should be set up with normal saline. Nausea and apprehension may be settled by small doses of intravenous chlorpromazine (10 to 25 mg), taking care to keep the patient flat in case hypotension occurs. Not infrequently it is found that the chlorpromazine (and the rest and reassurance inherent in being under close medical care) is sufficient to relieve the pain, but if there is still significant headache 4 hours after the chlorpromazine, then intravenous corticosteroids can be given as either Solu-Cortef 250 mg or Solu-Medrol 40 to 80 mg. In general, narcotic analgesics are less helpful in "breaking" status migrainosus than the combination of rest, hydration, intravenous chlorpromazine, and possibly intravenous corticosteroids.

TENSION HEADACHES (MUSCLE CONTRACTION HEADACHES)

The classic view that these intermittent (or sometimes constant) dull, diffuse, nonthrobbing headaches are due to sustained muscle contraction is not as generally accepted as it had once been since it has been demonstrated that many patients with these headaches have no EMG evidence of muscular overactivity. We must now accept that we simply do not know the pathophysiologic substrate of these headaches. There is a general feeling that they are, through unknown mechanisms, often the somatic manifestations of fatigue, stress, or depression. Most of us have these headaches from time to time, and a few have them nearly all the time.

There is a minority view that these headaches may be caused by cervical spondylosis, temporomandibular arthritis, and a number of other conditions that also occupy the head and neck, but most feel that these are incidental. Improvement of headaches following treatment directed to the neck, the jaw joints, and other structures may well be on the basis of either placebo response or shared efficacy (for example, nonsteroidal anti-inflammatory drugs prescribed for cervical spondylosis may help tension headaches simply by virtue of their general analgesic effect).

Treatment

Treatment of occasional tension headaches is seldom a problem. Most patients are aware of the relationship between these occasional headaches and specific stressful situations and know to remove themselves from that situation as soon as possible. They also know of the general effectiveness of over the counter analgesics for these occasional headaches.

However, an increasing frequency of tension headaches is often accompanied by a decreasing insight into the relationship to stress. With this failure to recognize that life style is a major cause of the symptom comes increasingly frequent resort to analgesics, sometimes containing codeine and/or barbiturate, and the risk of dependency and habituation. For patients in this situation, education is the first treatment. When the environment or the patient's reaction to it is the major stress generator, then to this educational and insight-developing therapy may be added, very carefully, anxiolytic medications such as diazepam or chlordiazepoxide. As noted, resorting to medication too readily may become a problem with these patients and may come to include these anxiolytic medications, so very close and careful supervision is mandatory. In patients with depression, tricyclic agents such as amitriptyline or doxepin are indicated.

In these patients with frequent but not constant tension headaches, all medications, including analgesics, anxiolytics, and antidepressants, should be viewed as short-term measures. Definitive therapy over the long term includes psychotherapy (which may be in a short informal format) and, for motivated patients who have developed insight, biofeedback training. Biofeedback can be extremely useful in teaching the patient, through relaxation, to cope with his symptoms without recourse to medication.

Physical therapies such as massage, heat, and so on may be helpful in the short term but are seldom of long-term value because they tend to emphasize the passive approach to headache therapy ("here I am, fix me up") rather than teaching the patient to take responsibility for his headaches and their treatment.

Patients with absolutely constant tension headaches are, unfortunately, not at all uncommon. Sometimes, overlain onto these chronic constant tension headaches are intermittent attacks of common migraine (so-called mixed headaches). These patients can be daunting to any physician. They are characterized, usually, by complete lack of insight into the social and psychologic factors that are probably determining their headaches, by a completely passive approach that places all responsibility for their treatment on someone else, and often by habituation to analgesics (sometimes including narcotics) and ergotamine.

These patients have almost always seen a number of practitioners, have proven resistant to migraine prophylactic medication used alone and antidepressant medication used alone, and have often manifested side effects (sometimes bizarre) to these agents. They often report that biofeedback has failed to help, as have hypnotherapy, reflexology, and numerous other modalities. Some of them have gone, usually at the insistence of a physician, to a psychiatrist. Not infrequently they have emerged with a psychiatric opinion of "no psychiatric disease"; this can occur because these people are very well defended and because many conventional schools of psychiatric thought do not view persistent nonorganic symptoms and consequent personal and interpersonal disruption as necessarily representing a psychiatric disorder.

A combined therapeutic approach is highly desirable, and chances of success are enhanced in an inpatient environment. Gradual reduction of analgesic medication and ergotamine is accomplished under "cover" of chlorpromazine or another phenothiazine. While this is being done, educational and psychotherapeutic maneuvers are carried out; often, a group format is used in addition to a one on one approach. Antidepressant medication (usually a tricyclic, but in resistant cases a monoamine oxidase inhibitor) can be added, and, where the migrainous component is significant, a migraine prophylactic medication such as propranolol is helpful. Coping techniques, to be used with the advent of individual attacks, are taught; these include relaxation therapy, biofeedback training, and/or self-hypnosis.

Using this combined approach, many people with chronic daily tension headaches are able to achieve striking reduction in symptoms without dependence on medication. Follow-up after discharge is essential, because, left to their own devices, many patients relapse.

EPISODIC VERTIGO

method of
THOMAS BRANDT, M.D.
University of Munich
Munich, West Germany

Vertigo is not a clinical unity but a multisensory syndrome which is induced by either physiologic stimulation or pathologic dysfunction. It is characterized by a combination of phenomena involving perceptual, oculomotor, postural, and vegetative manifestations: vertigo, nystagmus, ataxia, and nausea. Management includes pharmacologic and physical therapy as well as surgery and psychotherapy. Persuaded by the pharmaceutical industry, physicians tend to overestimate the benefit of antivertiginous drugs. These have only three clear indications for symptomatic relief of nausea and vertigo: in acute peripheral vestibulopathy, in acute brain stem lesions near the vestibular nuclei, and for prevention of motion sickness.

Peripheral Labyrinthine Vertigo Syndromes

Acute Unilateral Peripheral Vestibulopathy

The chief symptom of the acute (idiopathic) labyrinthine lesion (also known as vestibular neuronitis) is severe rotational vertigo associated with spontaneous nystagmus, postural imbalance, and nausea. Normal vestibular end-organs generate a tonic resting firing frequency equal from the two sides that is transmitted to the vestibular nuclei via vestibular nerves. Pathologic processes involving an end-organ alter its firing frequency, thereby creating a tone imbalance. The imbalance causes most of the manifestations of the vertigo syndrome. The symptoms abate when the tone is re-equalized by either peripheral restitution or central compensation.

During the first 3 to 5 days when nausea is prominent, vestibular sedatives can be administered for symptomatic relief, such as the antihistamine dimenhydrinate (Dramamine), 50 mg every 6 hours parenterally, or the anticholinergic scopolamine (Transderm-Scōp), 2.5 cm^2 every 72 hours transdermally or 0.6 mg parenterally. The major side effect is general sedation. The transdermal application of scopolamine hydrobromide avoids some of the side effects of the conventional dosage forms. Alternative choices include the antihistamines promethazine hydrochloride (Phenergan), 50 mg, cyclizine (Marezine), 50 mg, meclizine (Bonine), 25 mg, flunarizine (Sibelium), 10 mg, or cinnarizine (Stugeron), 15 mg, as well as the phenothiazines prochlorperazine (Compazine), 5 mg, thiethylperazine (Torecan), 10 mg, buclizine (Bucladin-S), 50 mg, or diphenhydramine (Benadryl), 50 mg. (Flunarizine and cinnarizine are not available in the United States.)

The capacity to antagonize acetylcholine by competitive inhibition is the only known similarity among the drugs to counter labyrinthine vertigo and motion sickness. The most probable sites of primary action are the synapses of vestibular nuclei that exhibit a reduced discharge and diminished neuronal action to body rotation.

These drugs should not be given longer than nausea lasts because they prolong the time course of central compensation. Further management is physical therapy, using the Cawthorne-Cooksey exercises modified according to current knowledge of vestibular physiology (Table 1). Vestibular exercises consist mainly of eye, head, and body movements designed to provoke a sensory mismatch; they enhance compensation by facilitating central recalibration, although the symptoms initially are uncomfortable.

Central vestibular compensation for labyrinthine lesions requires reorganization of commissural brain stem connections between the vestibular nuclei and probably involves the cholinergic system. Pharmacologic and metabolic studies in animals suggest that alcohol, phenobarbital, chlorpromazine, diazepam, and ACTH-antagonists retard compensation; caffeine, amphetamine, and ACTH accelerate compensation; cholinomimetics, cholinesterase inhibitors, adrenergic agents, GABA agonists, and alcohol may (re)produce decompensation.

Benign Paroxysmal Positional Vertigo (BPPV)

In benign paroxysmal positional vertigo, attacks of rotational vertigo and concomitant positional nystagmus are precipitated by head extension as well as with lateral head tilt toward the affected ear. The natural history for BPPV is spontaneous recovery in weeks or months, but in some patients the condition persists for years. The histologically proved explanation of cupulolithiasis led us to construct a most effective form of mechanical therapy for these patients in order to promote the loosening and ultimate dispersion of the degenerated otolithic material from the cupula (Fig. 1).

Therapeutic protocol: Patients are seated, with their eyes closed, and tilted laterally with the lateral aspects of their occiputs resting on the bed to ensure proper plane-specific stimulation of the posterior semicircular canal. They remain in this position until the evoked vertigo subsides or for at least 30 seconds, and then sit up for another 30 seconds before assuming the opposite head-down position for another 30 seconds. The sequence of positioning is repeated about five times at each session. The maneuvers are carried out by the patients themselves every 3 hours while awake and are terminated after 2 consecutive vertigo-free days.

Certainly such a regimen should be undertaken over 2 to 4 weeks in all patients with unremitting BPPV in whom a surgical procedure is contemplated. In the rare patients refractive to prolonged physical therapy, surgical transection of

TABLE 1. **Physical Therapy for Acute, Unilateral Labyrinthine Lesions**

Clinical Stage	Physical Exercise	Strategy
I. Approximately days 1–3 Nausea Spontaneous nystagmus with fixation	No exercise; bed rest Head immobilization	Prevent falls Avoid active head accelerations leading to "cross-coupled" effects
	Eyes closed	Avoid visual-vestibular mismatch
II. Approximately days 3–5 No spontaneous nausea Incomplete suppression of spontaneous nystagmus by fixation straight ahead	Exercise in bed (supine and sitting) 1. Fixation straight ahead; voluntary saccades and eccentric gaze-holding (10, 20, and 40° horizontal/vertical); reading exercise	Visual control of stabilization of gaze in space by suppressing spontaneous nystagmus through voluntary fixation impulse (retinal slip)
	Smooth pursuit (finger movements or pendulum ± 20–40°, 20–60°/sec)	Visually guided control of target fixation
	Active head oscillations with fixation of a stationary target at 1 meter distance (0.5–2 Hz; ± 20–30°; yaw pitch $>$ roll)	Provoke vestibular stimuli for recalibration of VOR under visual control of retinal slip of the viewed target
	2. First balance exercise—free sit and stance and guided gait (eyes open, eyes closed)	Circulatory training, prophylaxis of thrombosis
Approximately days 5–7 Suppression of spontaneous nystagmus with fixation straight ahead, but continued gaze nystagmus in the direction of fast phase, and spontaneous nystagmus with Frenzel's glasses	1. Static stabilization: Four point stance; Stance on one knee and one foot Upright stance (eyes open/eyes closed; head upright/head extension)	Recalibrate visuovestibulospinal reflexes for postural control and eye-head coordination at free body movements
	2. Dynamic stabilization: Smooth pursuit and head oscillation exercises at free stance as described in preceding section Exercises with rope, ball, and club under fixation (eye and head) of the instrument (sitting/standing/walking)	
IV. Approximately weeks 2–3 No spontaneous vertigo Weak spontaneous nystagmus with Frenzel's glasses	Complex balance exercise, successive increase in difficulty, above the demands for postural control under daily life conditions	Expose the subjectively "recovered patient" increasingly to unstable body positions in order to facilitate rearrangement and recruitment of control capacities

the posterior ampullary nerve via a middle ear approach can be considered. This operation provides relief of vertigo; it is, however, not easy to locate the particular semicircular canal nerve surgically, and sensorineural hearing loss is a possible complication. Drug therapy with antimotion sickness medications has not proved particularly efficacious.

As distinct from BPPV, positional exacerbation of intractable vestibular vertigo (associated with auditory signs and symptoms) has been described as a consequence of eighth cranial nerve compression by blood vessels, with therapeutic benefit from microvascular decompression at the cerebellopontine angle.

Menière's Disease

Because management of Menière's syndrome due to endolymphatic hydrops is discussed elsewhere, only three aspects of therapy are mentioned here. (1) Nowadays, less than 5 per cent of patients ultimately require surgical treatment, such as middle fossa vestibular nerve section or labyrinthectomy, since the success of regular "endolymphatic sac shunt operations" has been shown to be a placebo effect. (2) The histamine derivative betahistine hydrochloride, 8 mg three times daily, has been advocated as the drug of first choice. Encouraging reports, however, have not been proved in prospective double blind studies. (3) Intratympanic treatment with ototoxic antibiotics such as gentamicin sulfate, 8 to 24 mg instilled daily via a plastic tube inserted behind the anulus by the transmeatal approach, is obviously able to selectively damage the secretory epithelium (and thereby to improve endolymphatic hydrops) before significantly affecting vestibular and cochlear function. Instillations (up to 10 days), therefore, should be stopped when daily audiograms or a check of spontaneous nys-

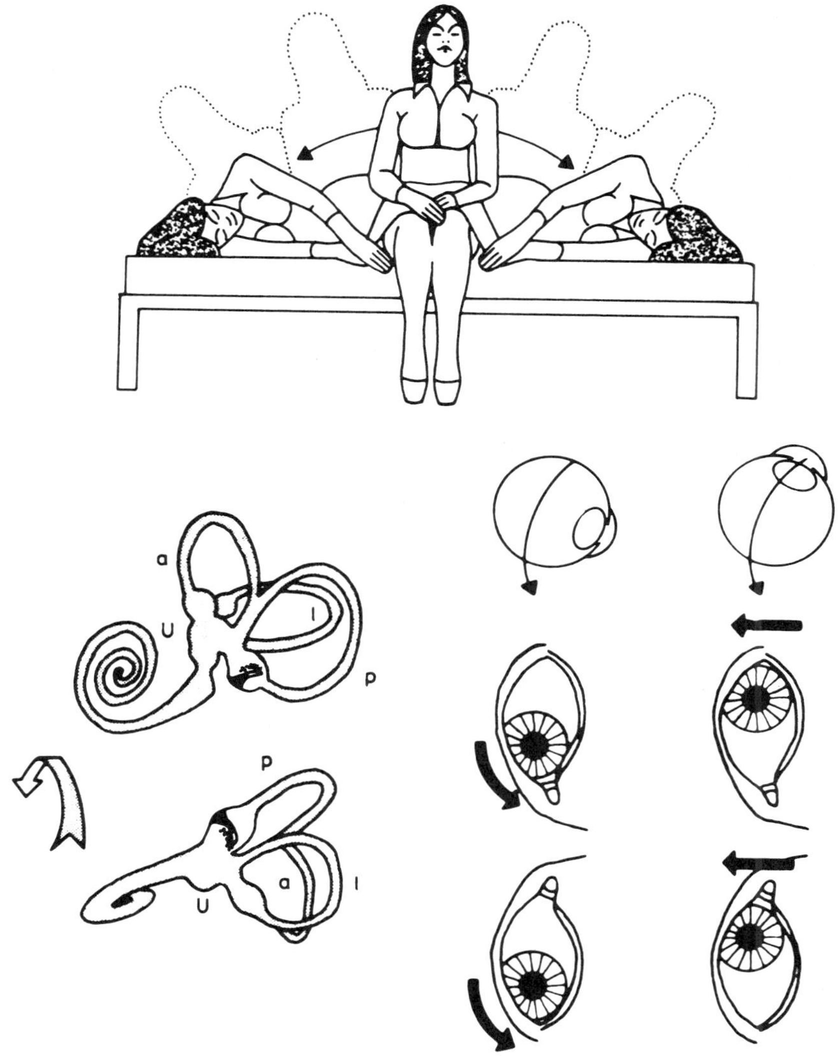

Figure 1. Sequence of repetitive positionings in patients with benign paroxysmal positional vertigo in seated position, with eyes closed (top) (physical therapy after Brandt and Daroff, 1980). Corresponding location of the right labyrinth is depicted at bottom, with the concomitant nystagmus precipitated by the critical position of the head. The nystagmus is horizontal-rotary, with the fast phases beating toward the undermost ear; the nystagmus beats upward (toward the forehead) when the gaze is directed toward the uppermost ear.

(U—utricle; a, p, l—anterior, posterior, lateral semicircular canal.)

tagmus by use of Frenzel's glasses indicates end-organ dysfunction.

Vestibular Drop Attacks (Tumarkin's Otolithic Crisis)

Rarely, in late stages of endolymphatic hydrops, vestibular drop attacks may occur when sudden changes in endolymphatic fluid pressure cause inadequate end-organ stimulation with a reflex-like vestibulospinal loss of postural tone. Pharmacologically, administration of fentanyl and droperidol (Innovar) has been tried with questionable success. Surgical treatment may be the latest thinking and is most effective. It consists of either ipsilateral labyrinthectomy or selective section of vestibular nerve in order to preserve serviceable hearing of the affected ear.

Perilymphatic Fistula

Perilymphatic fistulas may lead to episodic vertigo and sensorineural hearing loss owing to a pathologic elasticity of the bony labyrinth, usually at the round or oval window. Despite some typical clinical fistula tests, a definite diagnosis can be made only by exploratory tympanotomy.

In the acute case medical management is universally recommended since most often these fistulas heal spontaneously and the result of surgical interventions are not encouraging. Medical care consists of absolute bed rest with head elevation for 5 to 10 days; avoidance of straining, sneezing, or coughing; and use of stool softeners. With persistent symptoms over 3 to 4 weeks, exploratory tympanotomy is indicated under local anesthesia, with the Valsalva maneuver or gentle palpation of the footplate to make the leak apparent. For patching the fistula, perichondrial graft from the tragus is superior to fat.

Miscellaneous Central Vestibular Vertigo Syndromes

Basilar Insufficiency and Basilar Artery Migraine

Transient attacks of vertigo of central origin are the commonest early symptom of basilar insufficiency because of the steep pressure gradient from the aorta to the terminal pontine arteries. These are long, tenuous, circumferential arteries and therefore provide a most vulnerable blood supply for the vestibular nuclei. Whereas basilar insufficiency is a disease of the elderly, sudden attacks of basilar artery migraine occur predominantly in adolescent girls (see Headache). The benign paroxysmal vertigo of childhood with onset within the first 4 years of age is probably related to migraine. The sudden attacks of vertigo last seconds to minutes and do not require drug therapy. The natural history is spontaneous relief within months or years.

Vestibular Epilepsy

Vestibular seizures ("vertiginous epilepsy") are secondary to focal discharges from either the temporal lobe or the parietal association cortex receiving vestibular projection from the thalamus. Also absences (petit mal) may be experienced as episodic vertigo by the patient. For treatment, see the Epilepsy article.

Downbeat Nystagmus Vertigo Syndrome

Postural instability, oscillopsia, and downbeat nystagmus in the primary or lateral position of gaze is a well-defined clinical sign, almost specific for a structural lesion of the paramedian cranial cervical junction near the vestibular nuclei. About 30 per cent of the cases are due to Arnold-Chiari malformation. That downbeat nystagmus usually is a permanent syndrome may be due to the site of the lesion between the vestibular nuclei when the vestibular commissure is affected, a structure necessary for central compensation of a tone imbalance. A surgical suboccipital decompression because of the compression of the herniating cerebellum against the caudal brain stem may gradually improve part of the distressing symptoms. Clonazepam has been described to partially suppress nystagmus and associated oscillopsia. Rarely, when the nystagmus is inhibited by convergence, improvement of visual acuity can be achieved simply by use of "base out prisms." Physical balance training improves postural instability significantly.

Upbeat nystagmus caused by intra-axial brain stem lesions of either the tegmentum of the pontomesencephalic or the pontomedullary junction may be associated with severe vertigo, ataxia, and nausea particularly at first; depending on the etiology, the natural history mostly shows a gradual improvement or disappearance as opposed to downbeat nystagmus.

Ocular Tilt Reaction. This is a rare, paroxysmal oculocephalic synkinesis consisting of skew deviation and torsion of the eyes with lateral head tilt, due to rostral tegmental brain stem lesions. Carbamazepine or baclofen have been used with some benefit to control these paroxysms.

In general, physical therapy is most important for all central vestibular vertigo forms such as Wallenberg's syndrome. The differential effects of balance training on postural sway in normal subjects clearly show that the process of sensorimotor arrangement with subsequent postural stability is related to the degree of the initial instability. The greater the initial risk of falling, the greater the per cent reduction in sway amplitudes by training. Consequently, this should stimulate the clinician to make it a strategy in ataxia therapy to expose the patient increasingly to unstable body positions to facilitate recruitment of control capacities. Stance and gait aids will alleviate only transiently patients' balance problems, but when used continuously they will worsen the symptoms because the multiloop control rapidly adapts to the additional feedback and support that they provide. In patients with peripheral or central vestibular ataxia, the amount of rapid improvement by training within the first session frequently makes it possible to predict the long-term benefit of physical therapy.

Physiologic Stimulation Vertigo

Vertigo may be induced by physiologic stimulation or pathologic dysfunction of any of the stablizing sensory systems: vestibular, visual, and somatosensory. The functional ranges of the individual systems overlap, enabling them to compensate partially for each other's deficiencies. The intensity of vertigo is a function of the magnitude of the mismatch and is increased if the intact sensory systems are eliminated, such as with eye closure during pathologic vestibular vertigo.

Motion Sickness. This is induced during passive locomotion in vehicles and is generated either by unfamiliar accelerations to which a person has therefore not adapted, or by an intersensory mismatch involving conflicting vestibular and visual stimuli.

Physical prevention of motion sickness involves vestibular training to promote central habituation, as well as head fixation and head position during stimulation to avoid cross-coupling effects (Table 2). Motion sickness is significantly reduced when ample peripheral vision of the stationary

TABLE 2. **Physical Prevention of Motion Sickness**

Strategy	Mechanisms
Chronic	
Vestibular training Repetitive exposure to stimuli during active head movements	Acceleration-specific central habituation
Simulator training	Using the benefit of positive visual-vestibular habituation transfer
Acute	
Head fixation	Avoidance of additional acceleration and cross coupling—e.g., Coriolis effects
Head position (relative to g-vector) ship: supine; car: supine, head in driving direction; helicopter: sitting	Using the benefit of the natural habituation for head-z-axis accelerations
Counterbalance of vehicle-induced body motions	
Visual control of vehicle motion if not possible: eyes closed	Avoidance of visual-vestibular mismatch

surroundings is provided during vehicle accelerations. Conversely, the symptoms are heightened in closed ship cabins or while reading and, to a lesser extent, while simply sitting in the back seat of a moving vehicle. This creates a visual vestibular conflict, with the vestibular signals of acceleration being contradicted by visual information of a seemingly stationary environment.

Antimotion sickness drugs, such as the belladonna alkaloid scopolamine, 0.6 mg, and the antihistamine dimenhydrinate (Dramamine), 50 to 100 mg, are effective in preventing both vestibular and optokinetic motion sickness. In cases of exceptionally strong motion sickness, combinations of either D-amphetamine sulfate and L-scopolamine hydrobromide or promethazine with D-amphetamine provide far better protection than any single drug without increasing distressing side effects.

Physiologic Height Vertigo. Height vertigo, a visually induced syndrome, commonly experienced atop high structures, is manifested by a subjective instability of posture and locomotion, coupled with a fear of falling and vegetative symptoms, which spontaneously remit after termination of the inducing stimulus. Physiologic postural instability under height vertigo conditions is secondary to a geometrically explainable, visually induced postural imbalance, when the distance between the observer and the nearest stationary contrasts in the environment becomes critically large.

Susceptible subjects should avoid the free upright stance in critical situations at high altitudes. This is done intuitively by grasping for stationary framework or leaning against a wall for support. When looking down, one should obtain stationary cues from nearby contrasts in the peripheral visual field. Staring at moving objects such as clouds increases the danger of falling because additional postural destabilization through linear vection may be induced. One should avoid long exposure times, because height vertigo usually takes several seconds to develop. Looking through binoculars is very dangerous because it restricts the visual field and introduces the unusual and therefore unadapted-to magnification factor. Body and head position should be adjusted to the gravitational vector because vision will receive a relatively greater sensorial weight (which is undesirable) if the otoliths are displaced beyond their optimal working range by extreme head tilt. It may also be true on the basis of other observations that the feet should be firmly planted on an "earth horizontal" surface.

Psychosomatic Phobic Vertigo

Acrophobia, Agoraphobia. Panic attacks in phobic vertigo syndromes such as acrophobia and agoraphobia require a neurotic personality as well as the eliciting stimulus situation, which is often uncomfortable even for healthy subjects. Although the dissociation between the objective and subjective risk of falling is typically realized by acrophobic patients, they cannot overcome their avoidance behavior.

Psychotherapy is dominated by behavioral approaches that can be classified as either systematic or in vivo desensitization procedures. Systematic desensitization is based on the construction of a graduated hierarchy of anxiety-provoking visual scenes, which, after a training phase in muscle relaxation, are subsequently visualized by the patient while in a relaxed state. Although therapist or self-directed (tape-recorded) desensitization has been widely used, in vivo desensitization is more effective in the treatment of phobia.

In vivo desensitization techniques aim to reduce avoidance behavior or anxiety by increasing contact with real life rather than the patient imaging provoking stimuli. Successive approximation to the feared situation is supported by instructions and reinforcement. Contact desensitization stresses the advantage of joint participation and physical contact with the therapist model (participant modeling). Flooding, an alternative technique, also uses exposure to real phobic stimuli but without a graduated approach. It is based on getting the patient into the feared situation and maintaining the exposure for prolonged periods of time.

Drugs used for symptomatic relief from panic attacks in phobic patients are either tranquilizers or antidepressants like imipramine. The long-term course of untreated anxiety neurosis, however, indicates that during a 5 year interval most children and 50 per cent of adults have either recovered from their phobias or substantially improved.

MENIERE'S DISEASE

method of
I. KAUFMAN ARENBERG, M.D.
Porter Memorial Hospital
Denver, Colorado

Meniere's disease, or endolymphatic hydrops, is a common disorder of the inner ear characterized by episodic vertigo, fluctuating hearing loss, tinnitus, and pressure or fullness of the ear afflicting between 2.4 and 7 million Americans. The most widely accepted definition of Meniere's disease was given in 1972 by the American Academy of Otolaryngology: "A disorder of the membranous inner ear characterized by deafness, vertigo, usually tinnitus and has as its pathophysiologic correlate distension of the endolymphatic system." Classic Meniere's disease is a fluctuating or progressive, nonfluctuating sensorineural hearing loss with episodic vertigo and tinnitus. Other forms include cochlear Meniere's disease in which there is no vertigo and vestibular Meniere's disease in which no sensorineural hearing loss occurs.

All types of Meniere's disease are caused by excess fluid in the inner ear under pressure (hydrops), which can produce any or all of the inner ear symptoms: episodic vertigo, dysequilibrium, hearing loss, tinnitus, pressure, and associated disability. The mechanism of endolymphatic hydrops is thought to be a malfunction of the endolymphatic sac, which is the resorptive mechanism within the inner ear. This can be caused by fibrosis or other factors that affect its resorptive capabilities and cause backup of endolymph within the endolymphatic system, producing the endolymphatic hydrops or endolymphatic hypertension. This is a situation analogous to glaucoma, in which an excess of fluid under pressure in a closed fluid system results in a reversible sensory system deficit.

Treatment

Most patients with Meniere's disease get better. Sixty to 80 per cent respond to conservative treatment by a variety of medical, dietary, and allergic regimens. The two primary therapeutic concerns that remain are patients who continue to experience acute attacks, and those 20 to 40 per cent who do not get better. It is important to realize that many patients with Meniere's disease who seem to get better are merely experiencing fewer disabling attacks of vertigo. Although the vertigo is gone, the acute attacks are exchanged for some form of chronic, often disabling, dysequilibrium. Vestibular tests show that these patients continue to lose balance and auditory function. However, their vertigo is dissipated. This is not considered successful management, particularly when over 50 per cent will develop bilateral involvement during a 5 to 10 year period of follow-up.

Management Goals

The most obvious goal of treatment is to control or even eliminate vertigo. However, the long-term improvement or stabilization of sensorineural hearing loss can be more important. Vertigo, one way or another, can be controlled. However, once the hearing deficit loses its reversible component, chances for improved hearing and speech discrimination are lost. The best treatment plan is to address not only the short-term symptomatic relief of vertigo, but also attempt to preserve or improve both auditory and vestibular system function for the long term. The "good ear" should be checked periodically. Unless this is done symptoms continue to be attributed to the bad ear until it becomes very obvious that the good ear is also affected. The rate of bilateral involvement is much greater than previously thought.

Acute Attacks

Some attacks of vertigo occur without warning. Others occur with a prodrome of increased aural fullness and pressure on one side with ipsilateral tinnitus. An attack of vertigo then ensues with a concomitant or sequential loss of auditory sensitivity. An irritative nystagmus can usually be documented. The patient is often nauseated, with occasional vomiting, and has significant exacerbations of dysequilibrium and vertigo with positional changes.

The management of the acute episodes of vertigo varies with the severity as well as the frequency of attacks. The patient should be put at bed rest and rehydrated with intravenous fluids. For the control of most severe attacks, droperidol (Inapsine) intravenously can be given if the patient is monitored carefully in the hospital. Or, 0.5 to 1.0 ml can be given intramuscularly every 6 hours along with 0.4 to 0.6 mg of atropine subcutaneously or intramuscularly. This requires appropriate observation for about 1 hour but can be repeated every 4 to 6 hours in a 24 hour period on an outpatient basis. It is unusual for a second dose to be required. Another approach is diazepam (Valium), 5 mg intravenously slowly titrated up to 20 mg. This can be given over a 4 to 8 hour period, with an initial dose of atropine as above, and possibly one second dose. If there is significant nausea and vomiting, a 10 mg Compazine suppository can be given. Intravenous fluids also may be necessary to adequately rehydrate the patient. In the mild attack, one injection of atropine with 5 mg of diazepam can be given intramuscularly. This can be followed with oral diazepam, 5 mg four times a day. With general rest and stress reduction, this may be sufficient to bring the vertigo under control.

Long-Term Management

Before embarking on and getting locked into a long-term treatment plan, confirmation of the definitive diagnosis is most important. Medical treatment should be tried for all patients prior to any surgical intervention. It is imperative, therefore, to reassure the patient that one way or another the vertigo most likely can be controlled. The importance of patient compliance with the medical treatment should be emphasized.

Medical Management

(1) Low salt diet. No added salt, no salt in cooking, and avoid foods high in sodium content, such as pork, bacon, and preserved foods. It need not be a no salt diet.

(2) Diuretics. Hydrochlorothiazide (HydroDIURIL), 25 to 50 mg each morning with orange juice or other potassium-rich food. The potassium should be monitored as indicated clinically. This is an attempt to reduce systemic extracellular fluid volume and secondarily to reduce intralabyrinthine fluid and, it is hoped, reduce endolymphatic pressure.

(3) Diazepam (Valium), 2 mg (low dose) four times a day, but not prn. This is done to establish an even, nonfluctuating blood level of diazepam. This is the most effective oral vestibular suppressant, and the muscle relaxant and stress reduction properties of Valium are often greatly appreciated by these patients. It is also helpful in breaking the cycle of periodic recurrences. It is usually not necessary to use this drug for more than 3 months. I have found this more effective than meclizine (Antivert), 12.5 to 25 mg three times a day.

(4) Zinc sulfate, 25 to 50 mg daily, may be clinically useful although there are no current studies to support the use of this or lipoflavonoids or any other vitamin-mineral supplement. However, patients are encouraged to make sure that they receive an adequate supply of the routine vitamins and minerals each day.

(5) Cawthorne positional exercises. This is a very effective general vestibular exercise program that reduces vestibular dysfunction if compliance is good.

(6) Avoid CATS: *C*affeine, *A*lcohol, *T*obacco, *S*tress. A good general aerobic exercise program is also often helpful.

(7) Reassurance. "Something can be done!" If metabolic, endocrinologic, or allergic disorders are identified, they must be appropriately treated and then the Meniere's disease process reassessed.

Medical Treatment Failure

Medical treatment failure is defined as recurrence of symptoms despite adequate patient compliance. If compliance is "good," a 3 month trial is considered sufficient. If compliance is only fair, a 6 month trial may be necessary. However, if after the 3 month trial, patient compliance is nil, it is unlikely that further medical treatment will be helpful. It is important to watch for patients who are "better," i.e., attacks of vertigo are fewer and less severe, but who are still experiencing chronic imbalance, dysequilibrium, and possibly progressive sensorineural hearing loss. The degree of work and social disability should also be critically assessed in evaluating medical treatment failure. Determine whether vertigo or sensorineural hearing loss is the primary basis for surgical intervention, and remember to consider the status of the patient's other ear.

Conservative Surgical Treatments

It is apparent from the number of procedures listed in Table 1 that there is no unanimity about

TABLE 1. **Conservative Surgical Treatments**

Distal Endolymphatic System Surgery:

A. *Endolymphatic system surgery without implant*
   - Endolymphatic sac decompression and drainage procedure (Portmann)
   - Simple endolymphatic sac decompression (Shambaugh)

B. *Endolymphatic system surgery with implant from endolymphatic sac and duct; drainage into the mastoid*
   - Silastic sheeting and endolymphatic sac enhancement (Paparella)
   - Capillary tube (Morrison and Austin)
   - Pressure-sensitive unidirectional valve implant (Arenberg)

C. *Endolymphatic system surgery with implant from the endolymphatic sac; drainage to the subarachnoid space*
   - Subarachnoid shunt (House)
   - Angled subarachnoid shunt (Brackmann)

Proximal Endolymphatic System Surgery:

D. *Endolymphatic system surgery involving stapes foot plate*
   - Sacculotomy (Fick)
   - Tack procedure (Cody)
   - Sacculocentesis (Shea)

E. *Endolymphatic system surgery involving the round window*
   - Cochleostomy (Morrison)
   - Cochleosacculotomy (Schuknecht)
   - Otic-periotic shunt (House-Pulec)
   - Intracochlear shunt (Shea)

the best conservative surgical approach. In general, vertigo can be eliminated in 70 to 90 per cent of the patients who failed medical treatment. About 70 to 80 per cent will have stabilized or improved hearing better than the worst at the preoperative hearing level.

Destructive Procedures

Destructive procedures should be considered only if more conservative procedures have failed. The procedures available are vestibular nerve section, which can usually preserve existing hearing, or labyrinthectomy, which will eliminate both auditory and vestibular function.

Destructive Procedures That Attempt to Preserve Hearing. Selective sections of the vestibular division of the 8th cranial nerve can be performed to alleviate the attacks of vertigo. If the hearing is approximately 50 decibels or better with 60 per cent discrimination, one should always try to preserve existing hearing. These operations eliminate vertigo in over 95 per cent of cases. The most likely cause of failure is early bilateral disease. There are two major variations of the surgical technique: (1) middle cranial fossa vestibular nerve section (House, Glasscock, Fisch, and Garcia-Ibanez), and (2) retrolabyrinthine vestibular nerve section (Silverstein and Brackmann).

It is possible in specially selected patients to combine the best of the destructive procedures (retrolabyrinthine vestibular nerve section), which will eliminate vertigo from the operated ear, with a valve implant, which has a good chance to improve or stabilize the hearing and improve or eliminate the pressure and the tinnitus by treating the hydrops directly.

Destructive Procedures That Destroy Hearing. If the hearing is not worth preserving (i.e., there is a greater than 50 decibel loss and less than 50 per cent discrimination), a complete labyrinthinectomy will most likely eliminate both the vertigo and the residual hearing. This can be done either transcanal, oval window (Cawthorne); transcanal connecting the oval window and round window (Schuknecht); or translabyrinthine labyrinthinectomy (House, Glasscock).

VIRAL MENINGITIS/ENCEPHALITIS

method of
STANLEY PERLMAN, M.D., PH.D.,
and WILLIAM BELL, M.D.
The University of Iowa
Iowa City, Iowa

Viral infections of the central nervous system include a number of different conditions with varying clinical manifestations and ranges of severity. Viral invasion of the cerebrospinal fluid (CSF) or brain can occur in any age group including the fetus (rubella, cytomegalovirus) and the newborn infant (herpes simplex, enteroviruses). In most instances, viral encephalitis is an acute illness, but chronic forms (subacute sclerosing panencephalitis, progressive multifocal leukoencephalopathy, Creutzfeldt-Jakob disease) also occur, especially in the immunosuppressed patient.

ASEPTIC MENINGITIS

Aseptic meningitis is a common illness characterized by signs of meningeal irritation, a cellular response in CSF in the absence of bacterial or fungal pathogens, and a benign course in the majority of cases. Nonviral causes include the introduction of chemotherapeutic or other chemical agents into the subarachnoid space, the presence of cystic or solid mass lesions adjacent to the subarachnoid space, or as a complication of a variety of disorders such as systemic lupus erythematosus, Sjögren's syndrome, and the mucocutaneous lymph node syndrome. Infectious but nonviral causes of aseptic meningitis include the *Leptospira* sp. and *Mycoplasma pneumoniae.* Mollaret's meningitis is a type of aseptic meningitis noted for its transient and benign attacks lasting 1 to 4 days but followed by periodic recurrences over the course of years. Large endothelial-like cells are often described in the CSF on the first day of each recurrence. The cause of Mollaret's meningitis is not known.

Numerous viruses can provoke aseptic meningitis, but most cases result from a small number of common viruses. The enteroviruses, including many serotypes of the echoviruses and the Coxsackie group B viruses, are the most common.

VIRAL ENCEPHALITIS

In patients with viral encephalitis, fever and signs of increased intracranial pressure are often present in conjunction with encephalitic features such as confusion, disorientation, lethargy, coma, seizures, long tract signs, and cranial nerve signs. Focal signs may evolve in patients with encephalitis caused by many different viruses but are especially common with acute encephalitis caused by herpes simplex type I. Meningeal signs may or may not be present in these patients.

The arboviruses cause seasonal encephalitis corresponding to the summer and fall activity of the mosquito vectors. St. Louis encephalitis affects persons of all ages, with morbidity and mortality being greatest in the very young and the elderly. The illness can occur over a large portion of the country but has its highest incidence in the Midwest and South. California virus encephalitis has a decided predilection in children, with peak age of involvement being four to eight years of age. California encephalitis can be seen in many parts of the country but is most prevalent in the upper midwestern states. Western equine encephalitis also occurs widely but most frequently west of the Mississippi River. Eastern equine encephalitis is confined geographically to regions along the East coast and to certain southern states. It is not a common cause of human encephalitis but is associated with high morbidity and mortality.

The enteroviruses usually cause aseptic meningitis but can cause a mild acute encephalitis, although disease may be severe, especially in the newborn infant. Infection with influenza, parainfluenza, and adenoviruses may result in either an acute encephalitis or an acute encephalopathy in the form of Reye's syndrome. Adenovirus encephalitis can be a complication of immunosuppression, as are varicella and herpes zoster encephalitis. Acute measles encephalitis is now quite infrequent subsequent to the control of measles with vaccine, and rabies encephalitis is even more rare but with an almost uniformly fatal outcome.

Herpes simplex type I virus is the most common cause of sporadic, severe encephalitis in this country. Herpes simplex encephalitis is usually preceded by 1 to 3 days of generalized symptoms such as fever, malaise, anorexia, headache, and pharyngitis. These early symptoms are then followed by confusion, decline in responsiveness, and the development of signs of focal cerebral dysfunction due to involvement of the orbitofrontal or medial temporal lobe in most instances. Localized brain involvement can usually be documented by EEG, computed tomography, or isotope brain scans, but early in the course of the illness these studies may be normal. Absolute diagnosis of herpes simplex encephalitis usually depends on brain biopsy, which is most desirable in the early stages of the illness before the patient becomes comatose.

Herpes simplex encephalitis in the newborn infant is most often caused by type II virus, the so-called genital strain. Encephalitis is usually a component of disseminated disease in the neonate with pulmonary, hepatic, or cutaneous-mucosal involvement. Less often, neonatal herpes simplex encephalitis occurs in isolated fashion. Diagnosis of the newborn illness again depends on either isolation of the virus in tissue culture or demonstration of viral antigen in infected tissues or skin lesions when present.

Treatment

Treatment of viral meningoencephalitis includes both general supportive therapy and specific antiviral treatment in the case of herpes simplex and zoster encephalitis. Most cases of viral aseptic meningitis are transient illnesses followed by recovery and require only symptomatic treatment. The primary reason for hospitalization in most instances is to exclude other possible disorders, including bacterial meningitis and other nonviral causes of an acute meningeal syndrome. Colchicine has been used in some instances of Mollaret's relapsing aseptic meningitis but with variable results. Certain cases of postviral perivenous demyelinating encephalomyelitis and acute hemorrhagic leukoencephalitis respond favorably to corticosteroid treatment.

General Supportive Therapy

This includes measures used in the treatment of patients with any severe illness as well as modalities appropriate for neurologic disease. An adequate airway must be maintained, and cardiovascular support, including the use of vasopressors, must be provided as required. The patient must be well hydrated, although this should be done carefully in the patient with neurologic disease, since these patients often develop inappropriately elevated levels of antidiuretic hormone (ADH). Fluid status should be monitored by frequent measurement of serum and urine electrolytes and osmolality.

Careful monitoring of neurologic function, including level of consciousness, should be performed, and appropriate therapy for the cerebral effects of viral meningoencephalitis should be administered. Seizures in patients with encephalitis may result from many causes, including hyponatremia (secondary to inappropriate levels of ADH), hypoxia, toxic encephalopathy resulting from widespread tissue injury, and inflammatory vasculitis. Seizures cause an increase in the metabolic requirements of the brain, particularly in the presence of fever, and should be vigorously treated. Correctable causes, such as hyponatremia, should be treated appropriately. Anticonvulsant medications should be administered for seizures of other etiologies. Phenobarbital should be administered intravenously with a loading dose of 10 to 15 mg per kg (up to 300 mg), with a total dose of 20 to 25 mg per kg over the first 12 hours (up to 1 gram). Maintenance dosage is 60 to 200 mg per day. If seizures are not controlled or if they recur in the presence of adequate levels of phenobarbital, phenytoin (Dilantin) should be administered at a loading dose of 10 to 15 mg per kg administered intravenously at a rate no faster than 50 mg per min. Additional phenytoin up to a total of 18 mg per kg may be administered initially. Maintenance dosage is 300 to 600 mg per day in adults and 5 to 8 mg per kg per day in children. If seizures are not controlled by either phenobarbital or phenytoin, intravenous diazepam at a dosage of 10 to 15 mg or 50 per cent paraldehyde administered rectally (0.3 ml per kg, max 10 ml) may be required. Respirations should be carefully monitored during diazepam therapy. If seizures are not controlled by any of these measures, paralysis with artificial ventilation may be required for control.

Increased intracranial pressure (ICP), a frequent complication of vital meningoencephalitis, results from either exposure to the toxic byproducts of tissue destruction or inflammatory vasculitis. Severe increased ICP, as determined by rapid deterioration in clinical status, elevated opening pressure measured by lumbar puncture, or findings on CT scan (e.g., collapse of lateral ventricles, loss of sulci), should be aggressively managed. Appropriate therapy includes (1) hyperventilation to maintain PCO_2 at 20 to 25 mm Hg. This may be achieved only by intubation and artificial ventilation; (2) fluid restriction with administration of intravenous mannitol (0.25 to 0.5 gram per kg) every 4 to 6 hours for 1 to 2 days to achieve a serum osmolality of 300 to 320 mosm per liter. After this time, mannitol may lose its effectiveness; (3) placement of an intracranial pressure monitor, which allows more exact determination and regulation of intracranial pressure; (4) initiation of pentobarbital coma, with a loading dose of 5 to 6 mg per kg with hourly doses of 1 to 3 mg per kg. This therapy should be used only when all other measures have failed. Corticosteroids are often used to treat increased intracranial pressure, but no data exist to show they change outcome, and they may enhance viral replication by depressing host immunologic function. If the decision is made to start corticosteroid therapy, dexamethasone should be administered with a loading bolus of 10 mg followed by 5 mg every 6 hours.

Specific Treatment

Specific treatment of herpes simplex encephalitis is now available. Adenine arabinoside (ara-A, vidarabine, Vira-A) has been shown to decrease the morbidity and mortality associated with herpes simplex encephalitis and is the only drug presently approved by the FDA to treat this disease. The diagnosis of herpes simplex encephalitis usually requires a brain biopsy, and the severity of the illness may necessitate transfer to a referral center equipped to handle the complications of this disease. Once the diagnosis is established, ara-A in a dose of 15 mg per kg given in a single 12 hour infusion each day for 10 days should be initiated. Ara-A is believed to inhibit viral DNA polymerase, although it may affect host cell DNA synthesis as well. Ara-A is not highly soluble in aqueous solutions and must be administered at a concentration no greater than 700 mg per liter. Dosage should be reduced in the presence of renal disease. Side effects include gastrointestinal complaints, neurologic dysfunction, particularly tremors, and rarely bone marrow suppression.

Acyclovir (Zovirax), an acyclic nucleoside analogue of guanosine, has shown great promise in the treatment of herpes virus infections, including encephalitis, but is not yet licensed for this purpose. Acyclovir is selectively phosphorylated by viral deoxynucleoside kinase and is also a selective inhibitor of viral DNA polymerase. Acyclovir is useful in clinical settings for infections caused by herpes simplex virus, varicella-zoster virus, and Epstein-Barr virus but is not effective in cytomegaloviral infections. Host cell function is not affected by acyclovir, and, as a result, acyclovir has a high therapeutic index. Acyclovir is administered at 250 to 500 mg per square meter every 8 hours, with dosage reduction in the presence of renal disease. Side effects are rare and include occasional renal dysfunction with a reversible rise in serum creatinine level and a transient elevation in liver transaminases. Central nervous system dysfunction, including delirium and tremors, has been reported but its relationship to drug administration has not been fully established.

REYE'S SYNDROME

method of
JOEL A. THOMPSON, M.D.
Primary Children's Medical Center
Salt Lake City, Utah

In 1963 Reye and coworkers described a disease entity termed "encephalopathy and fatty degeneration of the viscera." By 1974 the reported incidence of this disease was 2 cases per 100,000 children 18 years and younger, with a mortality rate of approximately 40 per cent.

Since 1981 the incidence of Reye's syndrome has dropped substantially and the mortality rate at institutions skilled at diagnosis and treatment has dropped to 10 per cent. This may reflect decreased salicylate use secondary to heightened public awareness of its contraindication in children with chichenpox or influenza-like illness.

DIAGNOSIS

Early recognition and immediate therapy are critical to reduction of morbidity and mortality from Reye's syndrome. The diagnosis should be strongly suspected in any child with an antecedent viral infection, particularly varicella or influenza, who appears to be recovering and then develops unexplained pernicious vomiting followed by deterioration in level of consciousness over a period of minutes to hours. The diagnosis is supported by laboratory studies that, at a minimum, show a threefold elevation of SGOT or SGPT. Most children will also demonstrate hyperammonemia, hypophosphatemia, and prolongation of the prothrombin and partial thromboplastin times.

PHYSIOLOGIC BASIS FOR THERAPY

Reye's syndrome is presumably a temporary viral-induced disturbance in the function of most mitochondria-borne enzymes resulting in a complex disturbance of carbohydrate, lipid, and protein metabolism. Accumulation of ammonia, free fatty acids, and lactic acids as well as other metabolic by products results in a progressive encephalopathy. Hypoglycemia, diminished production of high energy phosphate compounds, and a deficiency in clotting factors are also noted. Preventive therapy is specifically and empirically aimed at preventing catabolism of carbohydrates, proteins, and lipids, which results in the accumulation of toxic products. Glucose is the mainstay of metabolic therapy. Hyperglycemia reduces gluconeogenesis and lipolysis and, respectively, reduces generation of ammonia and free fatty acids. Hyperglycemia may also promote sufficient brain levels of glucose.

Therapeutic Approach

Assessment of Severity

A staging system is utilized to evaluate disease severity (Table 1) and determine the intensity of therapeutic support (Table 2).

Therapeutic Components

Supportive Care (All Stages)

Unpredictable rapid progression of Reye's syndrome makes admission to a hospital with pediatric intensive care and neurosurgical capabilities advisable. Careful attention should be given to the physical protection of the delirious patient, but sedation is not recommended because it may impair assessment of level of consciousness. Vital signs and neurologic status should be assessed at frequent intervals by individuals capable of determining their significance.

Metabolic Management (All Stages)

Meticulous metabolic management dictates hourly serum glucose determinations. Serum electrolytes, SGOT, ammonia, phosphate, and osmolarity should be obtained at 4 hour intervals. After the first 24 hours, frequency of laboratory studies may be decreased.

GLUCOSE. The serum glucose is maintained at 200 to 300 mg per dl for at least 24 hours. A central venous line is usually necessary to allow continuous infusion of hypertonic solutions. An initial bolus of 50 per cent glucose at 1 ml per kg intravenously should be given on diagnosis, and, if the hourly serum glucose is less than 200 mg per dl, a bolus of 25 per cent glucose at 1 ml per kg intravenously should be given with coincident upward adjustment in the strength of the hypertonic glucose maintenance solution.

FLUID AND ELECTROLYTE THERAPY. Most patients with Reye's syndrome are dehydrated and hyperosmolar. Fluid therapy is aimed at maintenance of sufficient vascular volume to avoid shock and ensure adequate urine output (1 ml per kg per hour). It is important to give fluids that will not precipitously drop serum osmolarity and induce cerebral edema. Most patients can be maintained with fluid volumes of two thirds to full maintenance if serum osmolarities are carefully monitored along with intake and output. Proper fluid management usually necessitates use of a urinary catheter, nasogastric tube, central venous line, and arterial line, particularly in patients in stage III or deeper.

HYPERAMMONEMIA. This is most effectively managed by maintaining a high serum glucose and preventing catabolic production of ammonia. Neomycin enemas (25 to 50 mg per kg per dose) and lactulose may be helpful, but hemodialysis and exchange transfusions are rarely indicated.

HYPOPHOSPHATEMIA. This may be corrected by giving potassium phosphate instead of potassium chloride in the maintenance intravenous solution and titrating this against the serum phosphate. Avoid high serum phosphate levels.

CLOTTING ABNORMALITIES. Prolonged prothrombin and partial thromboplastin times indicate clotting abnormalities, which are treated with vitamin K (AquaMEPHYTON), 1 mg intravenously or 5 mg intramuscularly. Fresh frozen plasma, 10 ml per kg, may be necessary in patients with actual hemorrhage. On rare occasions, thrombocytopenia occurs and may require treatment with platelet transfusions.

Intracranial Pressure (Stages III–V)

Patients in stage III or deeper may have increased intracranial pressure, which requires careful monitoring to prevent transtentorial herniation and cerebral ischemia.

Intracranial pressure is monitored utilizing a subarachnoid bolt or intraventricular catheter. Pressures greater than 20 mm Hg for longer than 5 minutes or a cerebral perfusion pressure (mean arterial pressure minus intracranial pressure) of

TABLE 1. **Staging Reye's Syndrome**

	I	II	III	IV	V
Level of consciousness	Lethargy; follows verbal commands	Combative/stupor; verbalizes inappropriately	Coma	Coma	Coma
Posture	Normal	Normal	Decorticate	Decerebrate	Flaccid
Response to pain	Purposeful	Purposeful/nonpurposeful	Decorticate	Decerebrate	None
Pupillary reaction	Brisk	Sluggish	Sluggish	Sluggish	None
Oculocephalic reflex (doll's eyes)	Normal	Conjugate deviation	Conjugate deviation	Inconsistent or absent	None

TABLE 2. **Summary of Therapy for Reye's Syndrome**

Stages I and II	Hospitalization; intravenous fluids; meticulous management of glucose, fluid, and electrolyte balance
Stages III, IV, and V	Intensive care support; mechanical ventilation; continuous monitoring of intracranial pressure; treatment of increased intracranial pressure with osmotic agents or barbiturate coma

less than 40 mm Hg dictates therapy for increased intracranial pressure.

METHODS OF PRESSURE CONTROL

Head inclination by 30 degrees improves venous return from the brain. Be careful not to turn the head, thus compressing the jugular venous system.

Hyperventilation reduces the pCO_2 and causes cerebral vasoconstriction, which reduces cerebral blood volume. This is best accomplished by paralyzing the patient with pancuronium bromide (Pavulon), 0.1 mg per kg, and utilizing a mechanical ventilator. A pCO_2 of 22 to 25 mm Hg is optimal.

Increasing the pO_2 to 100 to 125 mm Hg will also cause cerebral vasoconstriction and lower the intracranial pressure but is not as effective as reducing pCO_2. Avoid a high pO_2, which may cause pulmonary oxygen toxicity.

Osmotherapy with mannitol is effective in decreasing intracranial pressure, assuming that renal function is intact. Mannitol (20 per cent solution) may be given by intravenous push at a dosage of 0.5 to 1.0 gram per kg every 4 hours as long as the osmolarity does not exceed 330 mOsm per liter and the patient is not hypotensive. Intracranial pressure is very responsive to serum osmolarity, and it is important not to increase volumes of maintenance fluid following a dose of mannitol unless the patient is in shock, since this will drop osmolarity and increase intracranial pressure.

Barbiturate coma reduces intracranial pressure by causing cerebral vasoconstriction. It may also be of benefit by reducing cerebral metabolic rate. We have not found barbiturates to be more effective than the previously listed methods for controlling intracranial pressure, although they may have an infrequent role in control of refractory pressure. Barbiturates do fix and dilate the pupils, removing all major parameters for assessment of neurologic function. They can cause cardiac arrhythmia and hypotension.

If barbiturates are used, a loading dose of pentobarbital, 3 to 6 mg per kg, is given followed by a maintenance dosage of 1 to 3 mg per kg. Optimal therapeutic effect is attained by maintaining a burst of suppression pattern on continuous EEG monitoring with a suppression phase of no longer than 20 to 30 seconds. Serum pentobarbital levels should not exceed 5.0 micrograms per ml.

COMPLICATIONS OF REYE'S SYNDROME

Autonomic collapse, manifested by a sudden drop of blood pressure and loss of cerebral autoregulation, is usually fatal and may occur either early in the course of the illness or later as the patient begins to awaken. This is to be distinguished from hypotension resulting from barbiturate coma or volume contraction from osmotherapy. Although volume expanders such as Plasmanate at 10 ml per kg and vasopressors may help remedy the problem, they are often ineffective.

Uncontrollable increased intracranial pressure is an infrequent but usually fatal complication, commonly reflecting severe underlying cerebral injury.

Hemorrhage is an infrequent complication and usually involves the gastrointestinal tract. Blood loss in the gastrointestinal tract may also aggravate hyperammonemia.

Hypoglycemia is more common in children under five years of age and usually occurs early in the course of the illness, resulting in additional encephalopathy, which often proves fatal.

Seizures are an indication of hypoglycemia if they occur early in the course of the illness and may occur later as a preterminal event reflecting severe encephalopathy. Correction of hypoglycemia and therapy with phenytoin (Dilantin) in a loading dose of 15 mg per kg may be indicated.

Pancreatitis and renal failure are very rare occurrences with Reye's syndrome and are treated symptomatically.

Prognosis

The mortality rate in children who do not progress beyond stage III is often no greater than 10 per cent. Failure to recognize hypoglycemia, late diagnosis (stages IV and V), and inadequate therapy increase the mortality substantially. Presentation with a serum ammonia of greater than 400 mg per dl suggests a poor outcome.

MULTIPLE SCLEROSIS

method of
KENNETH P. JOHNSON, M.D.
University of Maryland
Baltimore, Maryland

Multiple sclerosis (MS) is a complex, episodic, and progressive disease of the central nervous system

(CNS) that generally appears in young adult life and then produces increasing neurologic damage and disability throughout life. It is more common in Caucasians and in women and currently, at least in the U.S., has an average duration of over 30 years after diagnosis. The care of patients with MS requires much more than simply the administration of various drugs. Rather, it implies long-term medical, neurologic, and psychologic support of patients with a highly unpredictable disease that has increasing disability.

A PHILOSOPHY FOR LONG-TERM CARE OF MULTIPLE SCLEROSIS

The successful practitioner must be willing to enter into a long-term and often frustrating role as a support person for the MS patient and his family. This, in reality, implies an informal contract to undertake psychologic, sociologic, and neurologic care that changes as various facets of the disease appear. A willingness to undertake an intensive educational process of the patient and his family when the diagnosis of MS is first determined is essential. New MS patients have a right to know the diagnosis when it has been clearly established. They are generally young adults who have major life decisions to make, and they must know the diagnosis and its implications.

Once the diagnosis has been established (this can be done with certainty in over 90 per cent of early cases), the majority of patients will enter various stages of increasing dependency. This process may extend over several years or even decades. Patients often must change employment and finally terminate gainful activities. Need for aids in ambulation is common. They must often rely on others to undertake the responsibilities of family life, such as active involvement in child rearing. Later, some patients become wheelchair bound or bedridden.

Treatment of the Acute MS Attack

MS often appears in acute episodes of new neurologic disease, especially during the early years. In general, young patients have episodic disease or attacks with some remission, whereas patients beyond the age of 40 or 45 are more likely to have a progressive course. Acute attacks may be superimposed on the progressive disease and may occur even beyond the age of 50 or 60. Relatively good scientific evidence exists that treatment of the acute MS attack with intravenous, high dose ACTH reduces the duration of the episode. ACTH is usually given in a dose of 60 units per day for 10 or 12 days by a slow intravenous infusion in the hospital. ACTH gel may also be given intramuscularly in a dose of 80 to 120 units per day for 12 to 15 days to treat major new attacks. Some evidence of therapeutic benefit may be noticeable within 5 to 7 days; however, improvement may be delayed for as long as 30 days after the course of therapy is complete. ACTH, either intravenously or intramuscularly, has a variety of complications with which the physician should be familiar. These include fluid retention with electrolyte abnormalities, osteoporosis and aseptic necrosis of long bones, peptic ulcer, hypertension, menstrual abnormalities, and posterior subcapsular cataracts.

An alternative to ACTH therapy is the use of oral prednisone or other adrenocorticosteroids. Prednisone is given in a single morning dose of 60 to 80 mg for 10 to 12 days with a tapering dose over the next 3 weeks. The adverse side effects previously listed for ACTH may also be seen with steroid therapy. A rare but frightening complication of either steroid or ACTH therapy is an acute psychosis that is reversible when the dose is lowered and the medication terminated.

Treatment of Chronic, Progressive MS

Many chronic MS patients have a slow increase in disability measured over months or years. In such patients, no specific therapy is available or recommended, although the numerous complications listed hereafter frequently require therapeutic intervention. Some patients show relatively rapid progression; over a matter of months or 1 or 2 years they develop major, irreversible neurologic disability. In these progressive patients, an attempt should be made to reduce the tempo of increasing disability. The most common medication used during this phase of disease is oral prednisone, given in a single morning dose on alternate days. The dose can be as high as 200 mg, although the disease can often be controlled with alternate day doses of 100 mg or less. Once stabilization is evident, it is necessary to reduce the dose and terminate therapy. Often the dose is reduced in small steps of 5 or 10 mg at 1 or 2 week intervals. The risk of complications of steroid therapy listed previously is much greater with chronic therapy, even on an alternate day basis. Thus reduction of dosage should be a constant goal. Most patients complain of urinary frequency on the day of medication.

Over the last two decades, MS treatment centers have attempted to control the progressive course with various immunosuppressive drugs. The most widely used of these is azathioprine (Imuran), which must be given chronically, for it seldom has much effect in less than 6 to 12 weeks. Several experimental studies of azathioprine are now underway. The current available data suggest that azathioprine is not a useful drug for chronic, progressive MS. In addition, there is a recent disconcerting report from France of a significant increase in carcinoma in MS patients treated for prolonged periods with azathioprine.

Another potent immunosuppressant recently employed in MS is cyclophosphamide (Cytoxan) (this use not listed by maker), administered in a short-term, high dose intravenous course often with concurrent ACTH. The recommended dose is 400 to 500 mg given daily in a slow intravenous infusion until the peripheral white blood count drops to 3500, at which time the medication is stopped. Generally the leukopenia continues for 3 to 4 days, at times getting to extremely low levels, at which point it is prudent to maintain the patient on a reverse isolation procedure to reduce infection exposure. Patients commonly develop nausea, vomiting, and significant body hair loss during cyclophosphamide therapy; however, these changes are reversible once the drug course is completed. Cyclophosphamide may induce an acute hemorrhagic cystitis and, possibly, late carcinoma of the bladder; therefore, when treating MS, large amounts of fluids are given and the urine is checked daily for hematuria. Persistent microscopic hematuria should signal termination of therapy. It is important to note that cyclophosphamide therapy will probably not reverse MS neurologic abnormalities but will simply stabilize the process. Thus, the true benefit of therapy can only be determined after the condition has been stabilized for 6 to 12 months following therapy.

Treatment of Complications of MS

Spasticity is a major finding in MS, especially when the disease afflicts the spinal cord. Of several medications available, the most effective is baclofen (Lioresal), 15 to 80 mg per day in divided oral doses. Approximately 80 per cent of MS patients with spasticity benefit from baclofen; however, the required dose varies widely for different patients. Baclofen is especially useful for control of nocturnal spasms. In approximately 20 per cent a limp, weakened sensation precludes use. Other medications of possible value for MS spasticity are diazepam (Valium), which produces an unfortunate drowsiness or psychic detachment, and dantrolene sodium NA (Dantrium), which has been associated with severe hepatic toxicity.

Physical and Occupational Therapy

There is no good evidence that physical or occupational therapy alters, in any way, the fundamental course of MS. Nevertheless, these activities play an important role in the care of the patient. Most major new attacks, especially those affecting the motor system, are followed by significant neurologic improvement. Therefore, during recovery from periods of transient disability, physiotherapy can contribute a good deal, especially in maintaining muscle, joint, and pulmonary function until neurologic recovery is evident.

During the chronic, progressive stages of disease, various exercise programs are of real value. Even though a fixed neurologic deficit is in place, active or passive exercises will help maintain peripheral vascular and joint function. Such exercise programs prevent disabling contractures and give the patient and the family a sense of participating actively in maintaining the best condition possible. In most instances, such exercise programs can be taught during one or two sessions, and repeated visits to the physiotherapy department are unnecessary.

Occupational therapy has an important role during the various transitional phases of increased dependency in MS. Home assessments may be of value to provide suggestions for increased efficiency for wheelchair living, for instance.

Vocational rehabilitation is also an important aspect of MS care. Many patients are skilled yet unemployable because of concern, often unfounded, on the part of employers. Community education campaigns in which the physician can participate may alter the attitudes of employers to permit increased opportunity for employment of MS patients.

Ambulation aids are essential to maintain optimum mobility and independence. Most patients require increasing aids in a progressive fashion from a cane to canadian crutches to a walker and finally to a wheelchair. The transition from full ambulation to a wheelchair is a serious neurologic and psychologic one that should be delayed as long as possible. When a wheelchair existence is necessary, patients should be taught the proper methods of transfer by competent professionals. Family and other care givers are frequently required. A variety of wheelchair designs are available. One of the most useful for patients who have adequate vision and hand control is the Amigo electric chair (or other similar machines). These chairs are much more maneuverable, especially in public places, than the standard wheelchair. Importantly, they do not display the same degree of invalidism that a standard wheelchair does, thus the public impression of and reaction to the wheelchair-bound patient are quite different and much more positive. Lightweight travel wheelchairs may allow patients to be transported to social events and other public places. Continued social contact is highly important in maintaining the morale and psychologic health of patients with chronic MS.

Urinary Problems

The spinal cord is a major site of MS lesions, which frequently produce abnormalities of urinary tract function. Urgency, frequency, nocturia, incontinence, and an increased susceptibility to urinary tract infections are commonplace complaints. Most or all of these conditions can be attributed to a spastic bladder produced by lack of inhibitory control by higher nervous system centers. Adequate care of urinary complications requires a careful urinary history, measurement of residual urine volume following voiding, and, often, formal urodynamic studies.

Once the various combinations of incontinence, or "failure to store" urine, and retention, or "failure to empty the bladder," are identified, a series of stepwise control measures can be initiated. In many patients, anticholinergic medications will achieve control. Propantheline bromide (Pro-Banthine), 30 to 90 mg per day in divided doses, is most often used. In some cases, the addition of imipramine (Tofranil), 75 to 150 mg per day in either divided doses or one bedtime dose, is helpful both for its effect on bladder control and as an antidepressant.

Recurrent bladder infections can at times be prevented by chronic acidification of the urine by ascorbic acid, 4 grams orally each day. Cranberry or citric juices may also be of benefit. Once the urine is acidic, use of nitrofurantoin (Macrodantin), 200 to 400 mg per day in divided oral doses with food, may also maintain sterile urine.

Residual urine may be a problem in some patients regardless of the medications used; intermittent self-catheterization throughout the day is then indicated. The patient or other care givers must be carefully taught the technique. Clean, washed catheters can often be used repeatedly at 4 to 6 hour intervals. An effort should be made to keep the bladder residual below 400 ml at the time of catheterization. Unfortunately, some patients with quadriplegia or severe ataxia must be given indwelling catheters, which should be changed monthly or more often as needed. A high fluid intake will aid in preventing serious urinary tract infections. Whenever signs of active infections appear, such as chills, fever, and flank pain, appropriate antibiotics must be given, usually parenterally. After a urine and blood culture is obtained, a broad spectrum aminoglycoside or cephalosporin should be administered until appropriate culture and sensitivity data are obtained.

Impotence in the male is a frequent MS complication. It is generally due to neurologic dysfunction secondary to spinal cord lesions. In some cases, however, psychologic depression clearly plays a role. The preservation of spontaneous nocturnal erections, pudendal nerve–evoked response testing, and other urogenital diagnostic procedures may allow the differentiation between organic and psychologic impotence. In the case of psychologic impotence, therapy and counselling may be of benefit, whereas impotence caused by organic neurologic dysfunction can at times benefit from one of a variety of penile implants.

A final clinical note concerns the abrupt increase in nocturnal spasms and degree of spasticity in the legs. This may be due to new spinal cord damage but also frequently results from a cryptic bladder infection, which increases sensory input into the damaged spinal cord. Identification and treatment of the infection frequently relieve the distressing motor symptoms.

Depression

Reactive depressions are frequent in MS, especially during periods of increasing dependency. The standard antidepressive medications are frequently valuable in combating depression if used conservatively for periods of 1 to 3 months. Rarely is it necessary to maintain long-term antidepressive therapy in MS, especially when other attempts are made to improve the patient's environment.

Pain

MS is said to be a relatively painless disease; however, most patients do experience a variety of pain syndromes periodically. Often the pain can be traced to low back stresses due to muscle imbalances or to peripheral nerve entrapments in the extremities. A variety of pain syndromes intrinsic to the MS process are also recognized, however. The most characteristic of these is trigeminal neuralgia, which, if it appears in a younger adult, should always suggest the possibility of MS. However, many patients complain of other neuritic-type pain syndromes, often citing a burning or boring numbness in one extremity or in a series of contiguous dermatomes. The pain is generally unnatural, unrelenting, and poorly localized. Terms such as "gnawing," "boring," or "burning" are frequently used. Such sensory syndromes rarely respond to the usual mild analgesics. Because of the chronic nature of MS, it is generally unwise to use narcotics. Pain relief is frequently accomplished by use of anticonvulsants such as carbamazepine (Tegretol), 200 to 1200 mg per day in divided doses. The well known concern about bone marrow depression with carbamazepine must be recognized. Phenytoin (Dilantin), 300 to 500 mg per day in divided oral doses, is also effective at times in relieving MS-produced neuritic pain.

Current Trials of Experimental Therapy in MS

The clear determination that MS is an immunopathic condition has led to a large number of clinical trials of new therapies to modulate or inhibit the immune response. Ongoing trials of immunosuppressants such as azathioprine, cyclophosphamide, and cyclosporin are being watched with interest. Copolymer 1, a synthetically produced fragment of myelin basic protein, and myelin basic protein itself have been used to induce immunologic tolerance. Several immune modulators, some produced by recombinant DNA technology such as alpha, beta, and gamma interferon, are also undergoing clinical trial. Procedures such as plasmapheresis and hyperbaric oxygen therapy are also being tested. None of these treatments have been convincingly shown to be of major therapeutic value throughout the wide range of MS patients. Possibly some of these treatments will be of value during specific stages in MS but are useless or even hazardous in other stages. Continued testing of these and other new forms of therapy in well designed clinical trials will hopefully provide improved forms of rational therapy within the next few years.

MYASTHENIA GRAVIS

method of
DAVID GROB, M.D.
State University of New York
Brooklyn, New York

Diagnostic Considerations

In 95 per cent of patients with generalized myasthenia gravis and in 60 per cent of patients with localized ocular disease, there is an elevated serum level of antibodies to acetylcholine receptor protein of skeletal muscle. These antibodies react with the receptor protein and decrease and alter the sensitivity of this protein to acetylcholine. This is presumably the basis for the weakness, although the level of antibodies correlates poorly with the severity and clinical course of the disease, except in individual patients over a long period of time. The reduced sensitivity to acetylcholine of the altered receptor protein can be partly overcome by the administration of an anticholinesterase compound, which, by inhibiting muscle cholinesterase, delays the hydrolysis of acetylcholine and thereby partly compensates for the reduced sensitivity. This response serves as the basis for clinical diagnosis and symptomatic management of the disease. Occasionally, the improvement produced by an anticholinesterase compound may be difficult to distinguish from that produced by a placebo. In such patients, diagnosis is aided by determination of the serum level of acetylcholine receptor antibody, which is not elevated in patients with other diseases. Exceptions include some patients with thymoma and a few with other autoimmune diseases, such as systemic lupus erythematosus (which may be associated with or precede myasthenia gravis), and some relatives of patients with myasthenia gravis.

Symptomatic management of the disease relies on anticholinesterase drugs and, when necessary, mechanical assistance of ventilation, removal of secretions, and nasogastric feeding. Management by altering immunologic mechanisms is provided by corticosteroids, immunosuppressant agents, plasmapheresis, and thymectomy.

Anticholinesterase Drugs

The day-to-day management of myasthenia gravis relies mainly on anticholinesterase drugs, which are administered for the amelioration of weakness. The most useful of these are pyridostigmine (Mestinon), neostigmine (Prostigmin), and to a lesser extent ambenonium (Mytelase). Another and shorter-acting anticholinesterase compound, edrophonium (Tensilon), is useful in diagnosis and in evaluation of adequacy of doses of the longer-acting compounds, but is too short acting for use in management. The maximum strength obtained after optimal doses of any of these compounds is approximately the same. The compounds differ mainly in their duration of action (ambenonium > pyridostigmine > neostigmine > edrophonium) and in the severity of their parasympathomimetic side effects (neostigmine > ambenonium > pyridostigmine > edrophonium). The administration of graded doses of any of these compounds results in an increase in strength in muscles affected by the disease, but the maximal strength obtained is usually below normal, and may be far below normal. Most patients become less responsive to all anticholinesterase medication after prolonged administration, particularly of large doses. Responsiveness cannot be restored by changing from one anticholinesterase compound to another, but may be restored by reducing the dose or by a drug-free period, with assisted ventilation if needed.

Before regulation of a patient on anticholinesterase medication is attempted, the diagnosis should be established and the maximal strength determined by the response to an injection of edrophonium (10 mg intravenously) or neostigmine (1.5 mg intramuscularly), administered when the patient has been off all anticholinesterase medication for at least 8 hours. The effect of intravenous edrophonium is manifest within 30 seconds and lasts 5 to 10 minutes, whereas that of intramuscular neostigmine begins in 20 minutes and lasts 3 hours. Atropine (0.6 mg intramuscularly) should be given half an hour prior to neostigmine to prevent parasympathomimetic side effects, and prior to edrophonium in older patients to prevent bradycardia and hypotension. Strength should be evaluated before and after administration of a test dose of an anticholinesterase compound by measuring the width of the palpebral fissures before and after 1 minute of sustained upward gaze, range of ocular movement, grip strength, vital capacity, and ability to elevate the neck and extremities and to cough, swallow, and talk. Any change after atropine serves as a placebo response. Regulation of anticholinesterase medication is then initiated by the administration of a dose below that necessary to produce maximal strength, and the dose is gradually increased until the same degree of maximal improvement has occurred as after the test parenteral dose. Further increase in dose seldom results in further increase in strength, and excessive dosage is likely to produce generalized weakness, the so-called cholinergic crisis.

If the patient is able to swallow, pyridostigmine is the drug of choice, in an initial oral dose of 60 to 90 mg every 3 to 4 hours when awake. In patients with predominantly peripheral weakness who have not been satisfactorily regulated on pyridostigmine, ambenonium may be tried in an initial oral dose of 5 mg every 4 hours when awake. In patients with mild myasthenia, neostigmine may be employed instead, in an initial dose of 15 mg every 3 hours when awake. Pyridostigmine and ambenonium produce the same peak strength as neostigmine, but their longer duration of action results in more even strength, better endurance, and greater residual effect during the night and on awakening and generally permits the patient to omit medication during sleeping hours. These drugs also produce fewer gastrointestinal symptoms than neostigmine, although higher doses are more likely to cause headache. Pyridostigmine is somewhat less likely to produce weakness after an overdose than is ambenonium and is therefore usually the oral drug of choice. In patients who have difficulty chewing or swallowing, anticholinesterase medication may be administered 30 minutes before meals. In those who are troubled by muscarinic side effects of the medication, oral administration with milk or food delays absorption and reduces these side effects. When the patient is unable to swallow, intramuscular neostigmine (0.5 to 1 mg every 2 to 3 hours) generally produces the most satisfactory regulation, because adjustment in dose and effect of drug can be made more rapidly than in the case of other anticholinesterase compounds and overdose more easily avoided.

Pyridostigmine (Mestinon). This drug is the most satisfactory for the regulation of myasthenic patients who are able to swallow. It is available in quarter-scored 60 mg tablets and in a syrup containing 12 mg per ml. The syrup is particularly useful in children and in patients being fed through a nasogastric tube. Pyridostigmine is less likely to cause muscarinic side effects than neostigmine, but may, particularly when administered in large doses and on an empty stomach, produce gastric distress, abdominal cramps, diarrhea, and occasionally headache. Most patients who are regulated on pyridostigmine do not require atropine, but this may be administered when necessary to relieve abdominal cramps or diarrhea. Pyridostigmine is administered every 3 to 4 hours while the patient is awake, beginning with a dose of 60 to 90 mg and increasing the dose by 15 mg increments at intervals of 48 hours or more until there is no further improvement in strength. Except for those who are severely ill, most myasthenic patients do not require anticholinesterase medication while they are asleep. If the patient is very weak on awakening, a long-acting preparation, Timespan pyridostigmine (Timespan Mestinon), can be administered at bedtime in scored tablets containing 180 mg of pyridostigmine, of which one third is released for immediate effect and two thirds more slowly. This preparation has a duration of action 2 to 2.5 times that of regular pyridostigmine. It is seldom advisable to use the Timespan preparation during the day, because release of the drug is less predictable than that of regular pyridostigmine.

Pyridostigmine is also available for parenteral administration in a solution containing 5 mg per ml. Whether given intravenously or intramuscularly, 2 mg is equivalent to one 60 mg tablet of regular pyridostigmine. Parenteral pyridostigmine is less likely to produce excessive salivation and bronchial secretion than parenteral neostigmine and is occasionally useful in patients who are troubled by excessive secretion. However, since pyridostigmine is longer acting than neostigmine, cumulation and overdose are more likely to occur, so that neostigmine is generally preferred in patients who require parenteral anticholinesterase medication.

Neostigmine (Prostigmin). Some patients, especially those with mild myasthenia, can be satisfactorily regulated with neostigmine bromide, administered initially in a dose of 15 mg (1 tablet) orally every 3 or 4 hours when awake and increased by increments of one fourth to one half tablet at intervals of 1 or more days until there is no further improvement in strength. Some patients with severe myasthenia obtain slightly more strength when a small dose of neostigmine (15 mg) is administered orally 1 hour after each dose of pyridostigmine or ambenonium. However, the greatest use of neostigmine is its parenteral administration in the management of patients who are unable to swallow and in newborn infants with myasthenia. The intramuscular dose of neostigmine methylsulfate is 0.5 mg every 2 to 3 hours, which may be increased by increments of 0.1 or 0.2 mg at intervals of 3 or more hours until there is no further improvement in strength. Muscarinic side effects are more pronounced after neostigmine than after pyridostigmine or ambenonium and may include increased salivation and bronchial secretion, sweating, diarrhea, abdominal cramps, and occasionally bradycardia and hypotension. These may be relieved by 0.6 mg of atropine intramuscularly or intravenously.

Ambenonium (Mytelase). This drug is slightly longer acting than pyridostigmine and sometimes has a slightly greater effect on the peripheral musculature. It is occasionally more useful than pyridostigmine in patients who have predominantly peripheral weakness and who are not satisfactorily regulated on pyridostigmine. The initial oral dose is 5 to 7.5 mg (½ to ¾ tablet) every 4 hours when awake, with increments of 2.5 mg at intervals of 48 hours or more until there is no further improvement in strength. The side effects of ambenonium are less than those of neostigmine, but are somewhat more pronounced than those of pyridostigmine and may include abdominal cramps, diarrhea, and headache.

Edrophonium (Tensilon). This drug is used in establishing the diagnosis of myasthenia gravis and in assessing the adequacy of the dose of anticholinesterase medication. It has rapid onset and short duration of action. The test dose of 10 mg (1 ml) is administered intravenously 8 or more hours after any prior anticholinesterase medication. Since some patients, and some muscles, respond better to less than the full test dose, this is injected in increments of one third at 30 second intervals and muscle strength is evaluated after each increment. When the patient is on anticholinesterase medication, edrophonium is useful in assessing the adequacy of dose and for this purpose is administered intravenously in a single dose of 2 mg (0.2 ml) 1 hour after the last dose of anticholinesterase medication. A transient increase in strength, beginning in 30 seconds and lasting 3 to 5 minutes, indicates that the dose of anticholinesterase medication can be increased if necessary. A transient decrease in strength, sometimes accompanied by fasciculations, lacrimation, salivation, sweating, cramps, or nausea, indicates that the dose of anticholinesterase medication should not be increased and that it should probably be decreased. If none of these changes occurs, it can generally be assumed that the patient is at or near his or her optimal dosage level, although occasionally patients who are overdosed may exhibit no further change. Muscarinic side effects produced by edrophonium may include bradycardia and hypotension, especially in older patients. These muscarinic side effects can be prevented or relieved by the intravenous or intramuscular administration of 0.6 mg of atropine.

Regulation of Dose

Measurements of strength are carried out daily, and the dose of anticholinesterase medication is increased by increments of one fourth the initial dose until no further increase in strength occurs. The time between doses may be decreased by 0.5 to 1 hour if this proves to be necessary to maintain strength. Since the duration of action of pyridostigmine and ambenonium is longer, adjustments in dose of these drugs should be made at intervals of 1 to 2 days, as an increase in dose at shorter intervals may result in cumulation of drug and consequent overdose. The dose of neostigmine may be adjusted at shorter intervals, and when parenteral neostigmine is employed, the dose may be adjusted several times a day if necessary.

Whenever augmentation in dose of any anticholinesterase drug results in no further increase in strength, the dose should be reduced to the previous level, in order to administer the least amount of drug necessary to produce a maximal level of strength. Unfortunately, the manifestations of drug overdose, such as difficulty in holding up the head and in chewing and swallowing, are similar to the symptoms of myasthenia gravis, and it may be difficult to decide what adjustment to make in dose. The problem is further complicated by the fact that various muscle groups may have different drug requirements, so the level of drug at which overdose occurs may vary with different muscles. The muscles of the neck and of chewing and swallowing often show manifestations of overdose first, occasionally after as little as 120 mg of pyridostigmine or 10 mg of ambenonium every 4 hours. The muscles of the shoulder girdle and upper extremities may be affected next. The pelvic girdle and extraocular muscles are usually most resistant to the effects of excessive drug and may be unaltered or even improved in strength when the other muscles have become weaker owing to overdose. The muscles of the legs are also often at good strength at this time, although they may fasciculate and in this manner warn of excessive drug administration. Careful attention to the time of onset of weakness may aid in the differentiation between overdose and underdose of (or resistance to) anticholinesterase medication. Onset of weakness 1 hour after drug administration is suggestive of overdose, and onset 3 or more hours after administration is suggestive of underdose or resistance. Muscarinic signs and symptoms indicate overdose, but may be absent, especially if the patient has received atropine. Observation of the effect on muscle strength of 2 mg of edrophonium intravenously is helpful in assessing whether the patient is overdosed, underdosed, or resistant to anticholinesterase medication.

Use of Atropine to Control Side Effects

Atropine sulfate (0.6 mg) may be administered orally, intramuscularly, or intravenously as needed to suppress or prevent the muscarine-like effects of anticholinesterase compounds, such as excessive salivation, bronchial secretion, sweating, nausea, vomiting, abdominal cramps, diarrhea, bradycardia, and rarely hypotension. Myasthenic patients, particularly those receiving anticholinesterase compounds, generally have a higher threshold for the development of these effects than do nonmyasthenic subjects. During the initial period of drug regulation, atropine is best administered only as needed to ameliorate these side effects, so that the occurrence of cumulation and overdose of an anticholinesterase compound may be more easily detected. A sudden increase in side effects alerts the physician to the more serious effects of overdose on neuromuscular transmission, including weakness, frequently accompanied by muscle fasciculations, "tightness," and cramps. After satisfactory regulation has been attained, atropine is usually not required, but may be administered if needed to prevent side effects, usually in a dose of 0.3 to 0.6 mg orally or intramuscularly every 6 to 8 hours. However, overatropinization should be avoided, as this may produce inspissation of bronchial secretions, atelectasis, and increased pulmonary infection, as well as tachycardia, flushing, urinary retention, and disorientation.

Exacerbation of Myasthenia Gravis

This is characterized by increased weakness, often with dysphagia, weakness of cough, obstruction of the upper airway, and respiratory weakness. Exacerbation may result from upper respiratory tract infection, other infectious illness, emotional tension, or inadequate or excessive anticholinesterase medication. During severe exacerbation, the patient becomes less responsive to anticholinesterase medication, presumably because more receptors have become insensitive or desensitized to acetylcholine. It is this insensitive state that constitutes the main problem in management of the disease and often leads to the administration of large doses of anticholinesterase medication and confusion as to whether the patient is overdosed (in "cholinergic crisis") or underdosed (in "myasthenic crisis"). Many patients who are thought to be overdosed are in an insensitive state, and administration of large doses of anticholinesterase compound often renders the patient more insensitive as a result of agonist-induced desensitization.

Exacerbation is managed by carefully adjusting the dose of anticholinesterase medication, with the help of the edrophonium test, in order to administer the smallest dose that will have an optimal effect on swallowing, cough, and respiration. Mechanical measures are employed when needed to maintain respiration and remove secretions. Corticosteroids are administered, and if the patient does not improve, plasmapheresis is used as well.

Adequate hydration should be maintained and infection treated with an appropriate antibiotic. When dysphagia or respiratory weakness is severe, oral medication should be discontinued and the patient managed with intramuscular neostigmine. If respiration is being supported mechanically, the dose of neostigmine should be reduced to the smallest dose necessary to sustain respiration in case of failure of mechanical support. There may be some advantage to discontinuing all anticholinesterase medication for 48 to 72 hours, which may restore the responsiveness of the receptors to acetylcholine, but this should be done only if there is adequate observation of the patient.

Maintenance of Airway and Artificial Respiration

Severe dysphagia and weakness of pharyngeal and tongue muscles may result in upper airway obstruction and choking spells. If there is airway obstruction or if respiratory movements are severely impaired, an endotracheal catheter should be inserted and mechanical respiration instituted. The endotracheal tube should not be left in place more than 2 to 3 weeks because it produces edema of the larynx, which may result in airway obstruction when the tube is removed. Since many myasthenic patients continue to have severe dysphagia after withdrawal of the tube, it may be necessary to perform a tracheostomy under local procaine anesthesia while the tube is still in place, if it cannot be removed. The tracheostomy tube is changed weekly to allow a tract to form, and the inner tube is cleaned or replaced daily. A short tube should be employed to prevent pressure on the tracheal wall. Suction should be carried out at frequent intervals, with 1 to 2 ml of saline instilled every few hours. The inspired air or piggy-backed oxygen should be humidified. The head should be turned from side to side to allow the catheter to be inserted into each bronchus. The cuff of the endotracheal tube or tracheostomy should be deflated for at least 5 minutes of every hour to prevent pressure necrosis of the trachea. Mechanical respiration can be maintained with humidified air, unless the arterial Po_2 falls below 60 mm Hg, in which case oxygen can be piggy-backed for short periods of time. Pure oxygen should be avoided, as it causes destruction of cilia, drying, and atelectasis. Signs of anoxia may include elevation of pulse and blood pressure, sweating, confusion, and arrhythmia. When these signs occur, intensive tracheal suctioning should be carried out. A pressure-cycled respirator usually suffices, as lung compliance is usually good. However, if inspissated secretions or chronic lung disease causes decreased compliance, a volume-cycled respirator may be more effective. The lungs should be hyperinflated periodically with an Ambu bag to prevent atelectasis, and back slapping and postural drainage should be employed.

Adequate fluid intake should be maintained to prevent dehydration and inspissation of mucus in the bronchioles. Atropine should be employed only if absolutely necessary to diminish excessive secretions, and then used in small doses to avoid overatropinization. Electrolyte balance should be maintained by intravenous administration of sodium chloride and potassium chloride daily. If the patient is unable to swallow by the third day, a nasogastric tube should be inserted and feeding begun to maintain an adequate nutritional state and for the administration of pyridostigmine if desired. Antacid and cimetidine (Tagamet) or ranitidine (Zantac) should be administered to prevent peptic ulceration induced by anticholinesterase compounds, anoxia, stress, or steroid administration. Although the value of prophylactic administration of antibiotics to patients on respirators has been questioned, it is probably helpful to administer penicillin or cephalothin parenterally, because the dysphagia and impairment of cough and respiration that precede institution of artificial respiration predispose to atelectasis and pneumonia. The tracheostomy can be utilized as long as dysphagia persists or recurs, for years if necessary. The overlying skin may be allowed to close whenever the patient's condition permits, but the sinus tract of the tracheostomy persists and can be utilized again if necessary.

If facilities for intubation and mechanical respiration are not immediately available, artificial respiration can be instituted by mouth-to-nose or mouth-to-mouth means. During this procedure the hand is placed at the angles of the patient's mandible, which is pulled up and forward, and the head is tilted back as far as possible, in order to prevent the base of the tongue from blocking the airway. Breathing can also be maintained by an Ambu bag, which is rhythmically deflated with one hand while the other hand applies a face mask and supports the mandible. The occurrence of atelectasis necessitates bronchial suction, which can usually be carried out through a catheter passed into the trachea and bronchi, with the help of proper positioning of the patient. Bronchoscopic suction is occasionally required.

Management of Overdose of an Anticholinesterase Compound. Discontinuation of anticholinesterase medication, with assisted respiration if needed, will result in the gradual return of responsiveness to medication, as indicated by periodic testing of the response to 1 or 2 mg of edrophonium intravenously. Although seldom required, return of strength and drug response can be accelerated by the intravenous administration of 500 mg of pyridine 2-aldoxime methiodide (2-PAM, Protopam) at 10-minute intervals until strength improves. The oxime reverses the inhibition of cholinesterase enzymes by anticholinesterase compounds. Since overtreatment may convert cholinergic weakness to myasthenic weakness, strength should be evaluated after each injection and no more than 2 grams administered, except for the treatment of organophosphate poisoning.

Other Forms of Treatment

Corticosteroids. In patients with generalized myasthenia gravis who are responding poorly to anticholinesterase compounds, the next step in management is use of corticosteroids or thymectomy. If the patient is extremely weak, the risk of thymectomy can be reduced if the procedure is performed after improvement in strength has been brought about by corticosteroids, supplemented by plasmapheresis if necessary.

Corticosteroids in adequate doses usually produce an initial exacerbation of weakness in patients with generalized myasthenia, so that treatment should be begun in the hospital. High doses of hormone are more likely to produce exacerbation, but also bring about more rapid improvement. If the patient is severely ill, treatment should be initiated in an intensive care unit with 60 mg of methylprednisolone intramuscularly or 100 mg of prednisone or 12 mg of dexamethasone orally, in divided doses, or 100 units of corticotropin gel intramuscularly, daily for 10 days. Exacerbation of weakness may occur during the first week and may require intubation and assisted respiration. Improvement usually begins during the second or third week. If it does not, repeat courses of high doses of hormone should be reinstituted within 1 to 2 weeks until improvement begins, after which the dose may be gradually reduced, aiming at maintenance with smaller doses of oral prednisone (35 mg) or dexamethasone (4 mg) every other day. If exacerbation of the disease recurs, higher doses of steroid should be reinstituted, if necessary daily. If weakness is more pronounced on the "off days," small doses of steroid may be administered on these days. In patients who are less severely ill, steroid can be initiated in smaller doses (25 mg of prednisone or 3 mg of dexamethasone orally daily) and the dose gradually increased in an effort to achieve improvement with less marked initial exacerbation. However, the resulting improvement is slower in onset and usually less pronounced than following larger doses.

During hormone administration, the patient should be given antacid and cimetidine or ranitidine and supplementary potassium chloride (2 grams orally three times a day after meals in a dilute solution). Since prolonged use of corticosteroids or corticotropin may cause peptic ulcer, osteoporosis, aseptic necrosis of the femoral heads, cataracts, and increased susceptibility to infection, this should be limited to patients with disabling myasthenia, and the hormone should be reduced in dose and discontinued when possible.

Nonsteroidal Immunosuppressant Drugs. Azathioprine (Imuran), 150 to 200 mg (2 to 3 mg per kg) daily by mouth, has been widely used in myasthenia gravis patients in Europe, but this use is not yet listed in the manufacturer's instructions. Onset of improvement is slower than following corticosteroids, usually occurring after 2 to 12 months of administration, and becoming maximum in 4 to 24 months. Complications include leukopenia, thrombocytopenia, nausea, and vomiting, which are dose and duration related and are reversible. The white blood count should be monitored, although leukopenia may develop suddenly and be indicated by infection. Cyclophosphamide (Cytoxan) is similar in dose, complications, and effect, but may also cause alopecia and hemorrhagic cystitis. The risk of acquired malignancy in patients treated with either drug for long periods is not known, nor is the potential for genetic damage if given to women of childbearing age. In view of these hazards, these drugs should be limited to patients with severe, generalized myasthenia gravis who have failed to respond to steroids and thymectomy, or as an adjunct to steroids in patients who require excessive amounts of hormone or added immunosuppression following plasmapheresis.

Plasmapheresis. A series of exchanges of plasma for an equal volume of saline and albumin (usually 2 liters three times a week) usually results in temporary improvement, attributable to removal of circulating antireceptor antibody, although this is not well correlated with the level of antibody. Improvement usually starts after the first to fourth exchange, becomes maximal after the first to fourteenth exchange, and lasts a few weeks (or longer if supplemented by steroids, azathioprine, or thymectomy). It is not clear to what extent plasmapheresis adds to these other measures, but the short-term improvement produced by plasma exchange is useful in patients in myasthenic crisis, in those unresponsive to other measures, and to improve respiration and swallowing prior to thymectomy.

Thymectomy. Although the natural course of the disease is usually one of gradual improvement after the first 1 to 3 years and no prospective trial of thymectomy has been performed, most patients who have had removal of a hyperplastic thymus do appear to improve more than matched controls (20 per cent during the first year and 50 per cent within 5 years). Some, but not all, investigators report the best results in younger patients, in those with disease of recent onset, in females, and in patients after removal of all detectable thymic tissue by splitting the sternum and examining not only the anterior mediastinum but also the lower cervical and pleural regions. Others recommend transcervical thymectomy because of lower morbidity, with splitting the sternum and further exploration reserved for patients who do not improve within a few years. Either procedure will remove small, unsuspected thymomas or prevent their later development. Since either procedure has a mortality of 1 or 2 per cent and since thymoma is rare in patients with localized ocular myasthenia gravis, thymectomy is recommended only in patients with generalized disease. Some investigators do not recommend thymectomy in patients with mild disease who are able to carry out normal activity on anticholinesterase medication and small doses of steroids, in patients over age 60 years who have no thymus visible on computed tomography (CT), and in children under age 10, even though there is as yet no evidence of untoward effect on the immunologic system. For several days after thymectomy, anticholinesterase medication may produce more parasympathomimetic effects and fasciculations. Therefore, these drugs should be reduced or discontinued at this time and respiration supported mechanically if necessary. Radiation of the thymus is not of proven value and is contraindicated in children, because thyroid carcinoma may develop later in life.

Adjuvant Drugs. Approximately one third of myasthenic patients experience a slight increase in strength after the oral administration of ephedrine sulfate (25 mg orally three times a day) as an adjuvant to anticholinesterase medication, and a smaller number have a similar response to potassium chloride (2 grams orally three times a day after meals, in a dilute solution). Ephedrine should not be given after 4 P.M., as it may cause wakefulness. An occasional patient may improve when calcium gluconate (1 gram orally four times a day), theophylline, spironolactone, or triamterene is added to anticholinesterase medication. If there is no significant improvement after 1 to 2 weeks of trial of any of these drugs, they should be discontinued. Certain drugs may increase neuromuscular block and should be avoided. These include streptomycin, colistin, colistimethate, neomycin, kanamycin, vancomycin, novobiocin, polymyxin B, D-tubocurarine, succinylcholine, quinine, quinidine, procainamide, beta blockers, calcium channel blockers, and magnesium sulfate. Morphine should not be used. Sedatives are best avoided or prescribed in half the usual dose.

Ocular Myasthenia Gravis

In 16 per cent of patients, myasthenia gravis is limited to the extraocular muscles and orbicularis oculi. Ptosis is usually, although not always, relieved by anticholinesterase medication, whereas diplopia responds less satisfactorily. Lid crutches attached to eyeglasses may be more effective in relieving ptosis, and alternately patching one eye may be more helpful in relieving diplopia than anticholinesterase medication. A short trial of a corticosteroid may also be helpful, but large doses should not be administered over prolonged periods because of side effects.

Associated Clinical Problems

Thymoma. Fifteen per cent of patients with myasthenia gravis, mainly those over the age of 40 years and with generalized disease, have a thymoma; 60 per cent a hyperplastic thymus containing germinal centers; and 25 per cent a thymus that is normal, or, in the elderly, normally involuted or undetectable. Ninety per cent of thymomas are asymptomatic and are detected on routine lateral x-ray film or CT scan as a density in the anterior mediastinum. The tumor should be promptly removed, since 75 per cent are fully encapsulated at operation and can be entirely removed, while the remainder have already invaded adjacent structures and are not fully resectable. Only 3 per cent have metastasis to regional lymph nodes and 1 per cent have more distant metastases, regardless of the "malignant" appearance of cells in the tumor. While local invasion may be slowed by irradiation, it is usually fatal within 5 years.

Thirty per cent of patients with thymoma have myasthenia gravis, and a few develop the disease even after total thymomectomy. Twenty per cent have or develop nonthymic cancer, and 5 per cent have or develop one of the other diseases of autoimmunity, especially red cell or bone marrow aplasia. The associated disease usually determines the prognosis. Myasthenia gravis in patients with thymoma tends to be more severe and to have double the mortality of myasthenia in patients without thymoma. Removal of thymoma, even in toto, does not usually affect the course of myasthenia gravis or of other associated disease.

Other Associated Diseases. Diseases that are associated with myasthenia gravis more frequently than chance would predict include hyperthyroidism, hypothyroidism, thyroiditis, rheumatoid arthritis, lupus erythematosus, polymyositis, and pemphigus. The most frequent association is with hyperthyroidism, which occurs in 3 per cent of myasthenic patients. These patients should therefore have an assessment of thyroid function every few years. One per cent of thyrotoxic patients have or develop myasthenia gravis, which should be suspected when there is ptosis, weakness of the orbicularis oculi, or complete limitation of extraocular movement, and confirmed by the response to an anticholinesterase drug. In patients with both diseases, hyperthyroidism should be treated in the usual manner, but it is advisable to avoid induction of severe hypothyroidism. Corticosteroids may be administered to patients with disabling myasthenia gravis and have been reported to induce remission of associated hyperthyroidism.

Surgical Procedures. Oversedation with pre- or postoperative medication should be avoided, and the patient should be carefully observed for exacerbation of the disease and change in requirement for anticholinesterase medication. During the operative procedure, maintenance doses of intramuscular neostigmine can be administered if the patient is not being ventilated, but are not needed while the patient is being ventilated. D-Tubocurarine and succinylcholine should be avoided. Local, regional, or spinal anesthesia may be employed if feasible. If general anesthesia is needed, sodium pentothal, nitrous oxide, cyclopropane, or halothane (Fluothane) may be employed. Postoperatively, intramuscular neostigmine is administered as needed, and careful attention is paid to adequacy of the airway and of respiration. Meperidine (Demerol) may be administered for relief of pain.

Pregnancy. This may have no effect on myasthenia gravis or may result in improvement or exacerbation (especially after delivery) in approximately equal numbers of patients. There is no medical indication for termination of pregnancy or cessation of needed corticosteroids. Cesarean section is not necessary unless there are obstetrical indications unrelated to myasthenia. If the mother is taking anticholinesterase medication, breast feeding is contraindicated, because the medication may be transferred through breast milk. Children born of myasthenic mothers are normal except for 10 per cent who have neonatal myasthenia, which is manifested by weakness at birth, lasting 1 to 6 weeks, and followed by complete recovery if the infant survives the transient weakness. If the infant has difficulty breathing, the bronchial tree must be aspirated thoroughly and artificial respiration started, with endotracheal intubation if necessary. Neostigmine methylsulfate, 0.03 mg per kg, is administered intramuscularly every 2 to 3 hours. If muscarine-like side effects develop, atropine sulfate, 0.01 mg per kg, may be administered every 4 to 8 hours as needed, but overatropinization should be avoided. The dose of neostigmine may be adjusted after observing the response to edrophonium, 0.04 mg per kg intravenously, or twice this amount intramuscularly, administered 1 hour after the last dose of neostigmine. As the infant improves, the requirement for anticholinesterase medication will decrease, and the dose should be reduced and the drug discontinued when possible.

Myasthenia gravis rarely develops in children of nonmyasthenic mothers at birth and seldom occurs before the age of 1 year. Infants born of nonmyasthenic mothers who have respiratory difficulty at birth are infinitely more likely to be suffering from cerebral anoxia, brain damage, airway obstruction, pulmonary disease, or the effect of sedative or hypnotic drugs administered to the mother than from myasthenia gravis.

TRIGEMINAL NEURALGIA

method of
JACK WILBERGER, M.D.,
and JOSEPH C. MAROON, M.D.
University of Pittsburgh
Pittsburgh, Pennsylvania

Trigeminal neuralgia, or tic douloureux, is a relatively common disorder that can cause excruciating facial pain. The disorder usually develops in middle age and is more common in women than men. Initially, it is often misdiagnosed as pain due to dental problems, and many patients will have one or more tooth extractions without relief before the correct diagnosis is established. Tic douloureux is characteristic in that the patient has severe, brief episodes of lancinating pain, often described as electric shock–like or lightening in character, that is restricted to the trigeminal nerve distribution, more commonly in the lower part of the face (V2 and V3 distributions). First division trigeminal neuralgia is relatively uncommon, occurring in less than 15 per cent of patients with the disorder. Pain attacks can last a few seconds to an hour. They may be sporadic or may occur more than 100 times per day. Frequently, the patient will have a trigger zone and the lightest touch initiates the pain. Cold water, tooth brushing, or eating may precipitate an attack, and patients have been known to lose weight because of this. Tic douloureux is a chronic unremitting pain that can virtually always be totally relieved by either medicinal or surgical intervention.

The etiology of trigeminal neuralgia is variable and at times obscure. Approximately 1 to 3 per cent of affected patients will have a tumor in the posterior fossa causing trigeminal nerve compression and subsequent pain in the trigeminal distribution mimicking trigeminal neuralgia. Approximately 5 per cent of patients with multiple sclerosis will have associated trigeminal neuralgia because of plaque deposition in the trigeminal nerve. Arteriovenous malformations and aneurysms have also been reported to cause trigeminal neuralgia. The leading pathophysiologic theory of the etiology of trigeminal neuralgia is that proposed by Jannetta. This theory presupposes that normal atherosclerotically elongated or otherwise tortuous vertebrobasilar vessels impinge on the trigeminal nerve, usually at the root nerve entry zone into the brain stem. Such vascular compression distortion is thought to be responsible for the abnormal neural functioning associated with trigeminal neuralgia.

Medical Management

Narcotic analgesics have not proven to be of particular value in the long-term treatment of trigeminal neuralgia, but other drugs may be quite useful. The primary drugs in use today for the treatment of tic douloureux include phenytoin (Dilantin) (use not listed by maker), carbamazepine (Tegretol), and baclofen (Lioresal). Approximately 80 to 90 per cent of patients suffering from tic douloureux can be expected to achieve satisfactory pain relief with medicinal therapy.

In spite of its potential side effects, we initiate therapy with carbamazepine, which is successful in controlling tic pain in greater than 80 per cent of patients. The dose of the drug must be titrated to the patient's tolerance and should be gradually increased over a 7 to 10 day period. Initial doses should be in the range of 200 to 400 mg per day. If this dose is tolerated well, then dose increases of 100 mg a day can be instituted until either pain control is achieved or toxicity develops. With doses in excess of 800 mg per day, toxicity and side effects are quite high and the likelihood of achieving pain relief with higher doses is small.

The most common side effects leading to intolerance of carbamazepine are gastrointestinal complaints, such as nausea, vomiting, and abdominal cramping. The most serious side effects are the potential for bone marrow suppression leading to leukopenia, thrombocytopenia, and, on rare occasions, aplastic anemia. For this reason, patients on carbamazepine require careful monitoring of complete blood count with differential and platelet count. We recommend following these parameters on a monthly basis for the first 4 months of treatment and 2 to 3 times a year thereafter. The rarely reported complications of carbamazepine use include ataxia and incoordination, mental obtundation, liver function abnormalities, and rises in BUN and creatinine.

Phenytoin is the second drug of choice in the treatment of trigeminal neuralgia. It is effective in controlling the tic pain in approximately 30 per cent of patients. An initial dose of 300 to 400 mg per day can be given. It is not necessary to give a loading dose of phenytoin, as it has been shown that plasma serum levels of phenytoin do not correlate well with the therapeutic pain response. The more common side effects of phenytoin administration include gum hyperplasia, rashes, and gastrointestinal upset. Toxic levels of the drug may be associated with incoordination, nystagmus, and dysarthria. Bone marrow suppression has also been reported from the use of phenytoin.

If phenytoin or carbamazepine is unsuccessful alone in controlling the patient's trigeminal neuralgia, they may be used in combination with some effectiveness in a small number of patients.

Baclofen, a drug that is primarily used for spasticity, has recently been found to be useful in patients suffering from trigeminal neuralgia. Although baclofen experimentally has been shown to significantly decrease spontaneous aberrant trigeminal nerve discharges, its use clinically has not been as successful. Only 5 to 10 per cent of patients will benefit from this drug. In some instances, patients with atypical facial pain will respond better to baclofen than those with typical trigeminal neuralgia. The usual dose of baclofen is from 20 to 80 mg per day. The initial dose, 20 to 30 mg a day, can be gradually increased over 7 to 10 days unless side effects develop or pain relief is achieved.

Surgical Management

A multitude of surgical procedures have been devised to relieve the pain of trigeminal neuralgia in the 15 to 20 per cent of patients who are not relieved by a pharmacotherapy trial. Peripheral nerve avulsions are popular, easy to accomplish, and of low risk, but they always lead to undesirable facial anesthesia and rarely give pain relief from trigeminal neuralgia for more than 1 year. The same is true of alcohol blocks of the gasserian ganglion. Both procedures must be repeated frequently, requiring multiple visits or hospitalizations. The most frequent patient complaints following these procedures are loss of facial sensation, which in some is more undesirable than the previous facial pain. Currently, the most popular and successful surgical procedures for the treatment of trigeminal neuralgia are radiofrequency percutaneous gasserian ganglion lesioning, microvascular decompression of the fifth cranial nerve, and percutaneous glycerol trigeminal rhizotomy.

Percutaneous Radiofrequency Gasserian Ganglion Lesioning

Percutaneous radiofrequency lesions have proven to be very reliable for the relief of pain of trigeminal neuralgia. This procedure is performed under local anesthesia; a long needle is placed through the cheek into the foramen ovale at the base of the skull under fluoroscopic guidance. Once the trigeminal fibers that are to be lesioned are identified by electrical stimulation, a coagulating current is passed so as to injure the adjacent trigeminal ganglion and roots. The positioning of the needle and the subsequent lesioning can be repeatedly checked by examination of the awake patient.

Percutaneous radiofrequency lesioning has a relatively high recurrence rate—up to 61 per cent in some series—with one procedure. Surgeons experienced in this procedure report a recurrence rate of 20 to 30 per cent. This rate is reduced to less than 5 per cent of patients with persistent facial pain after four or more such procedures. Complications from this procedure are low. The most disturbing complication is first division trigeminal analgesia and subsequent loss of the corneal reflex. For this reason, many surgeons are reluctant to advocate radiofrequency lesioning for first division tic. Many patients complain of the loss of facial sensation that this procedure not infrequently brings.

The most feared complication of radiofrequency lesioning is anesthesia dolorosa. This is a severe deafferentiation pain that occurs as a result of partial destruction of the trigeminal fibers. In such patients, the pain of anesthesia dolorosa is frequently more severe than the original tic pain and is extremely difficult to treat successfully with medications or other surgical procedures.

The major advantage of percutaneous radiofrequency lesioning is that it can be done under local anesthesia, and, thus, elderly patients with significant medical problems can undergo the procedure with minimal risk of associated morbidity.

Microvascular Decompression

The concept of microvascular decompression of the trigeminal nerve for the treatment of trigeminal neuralgia was introduced in 1967 by Jannetta after rediscovery of many previous observations that tic might be caused by mechanical distortion of the trigeminal nerve by associated normal vascular structures in the posterior fossa. Since that time, thousands of such procedures have been performed, with a long-term success rate of approximately 70 to 80 per cent for the relief of the pain of trigeminal neuralgia.

The procedure involves a major intracranial operation under general anesthesia. The trigeminal nerve is approached through a retromastoid craniectomy and identified with the use of the operating microscope. The superior cerebellar artery and anterior inferior cerebellar artery have been found to be the most common vessels causing compression of the trigeminal nerve at its root entry zone into the brain stem. The vessels are manipulated away from the root entry zone, and prosthetic material such as Teflon felt or Ivalon is placed between the vessels and the trigeminal nerve to prevent them from reassuming their previous compressive position.

As this is a major intracranial operation, the procedure is not without possible complications. The incidence of hearing loss and/or facial weakness approaches 5 to 10 per cent in various series. Aseptic meningitis occurs in approximately 25 to 30 per cent of patients. There have been approximately 5 deaths in 1,500 patients secondary to brain stem infarction from vascular manipulation and/or postoperative hypertension. Thus this procedure, while giving good relief of pain on a long-term basis and having little associated incidence of loss of facial sensation, is generally reserved for patients in good medical condition under the age of 65 years.

Percutaneous Glycerol Trigeminal Rhizotomy

The effectiveness of glycerol in the treatment of tic pain was incidentally discovered by Hakenson and his group in Sweden when a stereotactic technique was being developed to study the effect of gamma irradiation of the trigeminal ganglion for tic. Glycerol mixed with tantalum dust was instilled into the trigeminal cistern to serve as a radiographic marker to guide the gamma irradiation. It was observed that many patients had complete relief of their pain subsequent to the glycerol injection and prior to any irradiation. The mechanism by which glycerol abolishes tic pain is not well understood. Glycerol is a highly hypertonic solution and acts as a dehydrating agent. The glycerol may exert some specific neurolytic effect on small myelinated fibers, which are responsible for mediation of the pain associated with trigeminal neuralgia. It has also been postulated that defective nerve fibers, which are responsible for ephaptic, or "cross talk," transmission within the trigeminal ganglion, are particularly sensitive to glycerol. Once this ephaptic transmission is abolished, the tic pain is relieved.

The glycerol injection is performed with the patient awake and under local anesthesia. A small gauge spinal needle is inserted through the cheek and directed fluoroscopically toward the foramen ovale. Once the trigeminal cistern is entered (as evidenced by free flow of cerebrospinal fluid and documented by contrast injection), the glycerol is injected around the trigeminal fibers.

Since its introduction in 1978, several large series have evaluated the results of percutaneous glycerol trigeminal rhizotomy and enumerated potential complications of the treatment. The success rate of complete relief of tic pain with one injection approaches 85 per cent. Pain relief is often not immediate, and up to 50 per cent of the patients will experience episodic tic pains for up to 7 to 10 days following the glycerol injection. The incidence of glycerol injection–associated facial sensory loss is controversial. Up to 35 per cent of patients will experience some mild hypalgesia and hypoesthesia as a result of the injection. No complete loss of facial sensation has been reported, and no occurrences of anesthesia dolorosa have been reported. Complications reported in association with the procedure include aseptic meningitis and ipsilateral herpetic facial eruptions. There have been no reports of cranial nerve or vascular injury from insertion of the needle. It is common during manipulation of the trigeminal nerve to produce bradycardia, which, on occasion, is associated with hypotension. This must be carefully watched in all elderly patients who are undergoing the procedure. This procedure, at least preliminarily, seems to be quite useful, particularly in elderly patients suffering from trigeminal neuralgia, in whom the use of general anesthesia is contraindicated.

OPTIC NEURITIS

method of
JOEL M. WEINSTEIN, M.D.
University of Wisconsin
Madison, Wisconsin

Optic neuritis, inflammation of the optic nerve, may be related to an infectious agent or to an autoimmune or demyelinating disorder or may be idiopathic. In a few patients, an infectious agent such as tuberculosis or syphilis can be identified. In some patients optic neuritis is associated with a relatively well defined autoimmune disorder, e.g., sarcoidosis or systemic lupus erythematosus. In still another group of patients, optic neuritis is seen in the setting of a previously diagnosed demyelinating disorder, usually multiple sclerosis. The majority of patients with optic neuritis, however, have an idiopathic disorder; i.e., no identifiable infectious or autoimmune etiology can be found. This article will deal only with the idiopathic form of optic neuritis. To avoid diagnostic confusion, the term optic neuritis should not be used for other forms of optic neuropathy, e.g., ischemic optic neuropathy, nutritional optic neuropathy, and so on.

Clinical Features

The typical patient with optic neuritis is between 15 and 40 years of age. Women are more frequently affected than men. The onset of blurred vision occurs over hours to days and may be accompanied by mild ocular or periorbital pain. The pain is often accentuated by eye movement. Some patients note "phosphenes," pinpoint flashes of light that are also accentuated by eye movements. Ocular examination reveals a monocular decrease in central acuity in the vast majority of patients. However, about 15 per cent of patients have normal central vision but a demonstrable peripheral visual field defect. The optic disc is usually normal, although about 15 to 25 per cent of patients demonstrate (unilateral) optic disc swelling. The presence of bilateral disc swelling with severe visual loss in a young woman should suggest an autoimmune disorder. The optic disc is not pale at the time of onset. Well established disc pallor should suggest pre-existing disease, e.g., optic nerve compression. An afferent pupil defect (Marcus Gunn pupil) is almost always present, and its absence casts serious doubt on the diagnosis unless visual loss is bilateral. Some patients notice worsening of vision with heat or exercise (Uhthoff's sign), and this disturbing symptom may persist after recovery is otherwise complete.

Approximately 85 per cent of patients recover vision of 20/40 or better within 3 to 6 months. Severe visual loss (hand movements vision or worse) is often associated with poor recovery. Despite recovery of good acuity, many "recovered" patients continue to complain of poor perception of color and low contrast objects. Visual evoked potential testing usually demonstrates residual demyelination in such patients. Over a long period of follow-up, approximately 35 per cent of patients who have had a single episode of optic neuritis without other neurologic deficits will develop clinically apparent multiple sclerosis. The risk is significantly lower for men (11 per cent) and higher for women (45 per cent). The presence of oligoclonal bands in the cerebrospinal fluid is associated with a higher risk for development of multiple sclerosis.

Treatment

It is essential to rule out other causes of optic neuropathy before treating. The disorder most commonly misdiagnosed as optic neuritis is a compressive lesion of the optic nerve, often a parachiasmal tumor or aneurysm. Because corticosteroid treatment may have a temporary beneficial effect on edema caused by such space-occupying lesions, a dramatic response to steroid therapy should prompt reconsideration of the diagnosis of optic neuritis.

Several investigators have conducted controlled prospective trials of oral, parenteral, and periorbital steroid therapy with rather disappointing results. The accumulated evidence suggests that steroid therapy may accelerate recovery but does not improve the final visual outcome. It has been pointed out, however, that the number of patients tested is insufficient to exclude a small subgroup who may derive a significant benefit. Several further clinical trials are under way. Because prolonged therapy seems to have no advantage, we and several other centers use methylprednisone (Solu-Medrol), 250 mg every 6 hours given over 30 minutes for 3 days. Because the efficacy of steroid therapy is in doubt, we reserve treatment for the following situations:

1. Severe involvement, i.e., vision decreased to perception of hand movements or worse.
2. Bilateral visual loss in which other causes of optic neuropathy have been carefully ruled out.
3. Second eye affected by optic neuritis if the first eye had a poor recovery.
4. Persistent pain when all other causes of optic neuropathy have been ruled out.
5. Patients whose vocation requires rapid recovery of binocular vision, e.g., surgeons, bus drivers, and so on.

ACUTE PERIPHERAL FACIAL PARALYSIS
(Bell's Palsy)

method of
CHARLES DIAMOND,
and IVOR FREW
University of Newcastle upon Tyne
Newcastle upon Tyne, England

Bell's palsy accounts for 60 to 80 per cent of all cases of peripheal facial paralysis. Bell's palsy may be defined as an isolated idiopathic acute peripheral facial paralysis unrelated to disease elsewhere in the body. The first step in treatment is diagnosis. It is important not to misdiagnose Bell's palsy in a patient whose facial paralysis is due to other causes, as in Table 1. Herpes zoster oticus and the Melkersson-Rosenthal syndrome are usually treated in a similar fashion to Bell's palsy. Treatment of facial paralysis due to otitis media calls for antibiotic therapy in the acute stage. In chronic otitis media treatment involves antibiotic therapy combined with surgical removal of the disease. In the presence of middle ear sepsis the facial nerve sheath should not be slit in an attempt to decompress the nerve. Tumors of the parotid gland and temporal bone are treated by surgical excision followed by nerve repair if indicated.

Treatment

Reassurance

Patients with Bell's palsy are frightened and disfigured. They frequently fear that the paraly-

TABLE 1. **Differential Diagnosis**

Causes of Acute Peripheral Facial Paralysis	Associated Features
Bell's palsy	Abrupt onset, paralysis usually reaches its maximum development within 48 hours
Herpes zoster oticus (Ramsay Hunt syndrome)	Herpetic vesicles around pinna, neck, mouth, or palate; deafness and vertigo often present
Tumors of temporal bone or parotid gland	Account for 5 per cent of all peripheral facial paralyses; usually a slowly progressive paralysis developing over weeks or months; primary and metastatic tumors cause an abrupt onset of paralysis in minority (approx. 20 per cent) of cases
Acute and chronic otitis media	Conductive deafness; inflamed intact tympanic membrane or perforated tympanic membrane and aural discharge
Melkersson-Rosenthal syndrome	Unilateral facial edema; fissured tongue; history of recurring facial palsy
Traumatic facial paralysis	History of trauma; paralysis usually immediate; occasionally onset delayed 1–7 days after injury

sis is due to a brain tumor or that it is the first stage of a stroke or hemiplegia. They are haunted by the thought that the grotesque facial deformity, the drooling of saliva, and the slurred thick speech will be permanent. They should be reassured in layman's language that the disease is due to a defect in a single nerve and not to brain disease. They need to be encouraged by the hopeful prospects of recovery. The natural history of Bell's palsy provides a sound basis for optimism. In the Copenhagen area of Denmark the spontaneous course of the paralysis was studied in an unselected series of 1,011 patients with Bell's palsy during a 15 year period. No therapy to improve muscle or nerve recovery was administered. All patients with postparalysis sequelae, namely, residual muscle weakness, contracture, and associated movements (synkinesis), were followed up for at least 1 year. The results of the study are summarized in Table 2, which divides the postparalysis sequelae into four grades.

Patients can be reassured that there is an 84 per cent chance of complete or near complete spontaneous recovery and that treatment is aimed at improving this recovery rate.

Treatment of the Paralyzed Face

Protection of the Eye

There is danger of exposure keratitis, conjunctivitis, and corneal ulceration because the patient is unable to close the eyelids and because the lacrimal flow is decreased in some patients with Bell's palsy. Therefore it is crucial to protect the eye. Methylcellulose artificial tears may be used immediately and instilled every 2 or 3 hours during the day. A suitable eye ointment can be applied at night before retiring. Tape may be used to close or support the eyelids, or the eye can be covered with an eye patch. The use of a moisture chamber eye shield is often preferred because it gives very good protection and does not impede vision. In cases in which a quick recovery of facial nerve function is not anticipated a temporary tarsorrhaphy should be considered.

TABLE 2. **The Results of Untreated Bell's Palsy**

Grade	Percentage	Definition
0	71	Normal facial function without contracture or synkinesis
1	13	Slight palsy with barely visible contracture (less than 1 mm) and without synkinesis
2	12	Moderate palsy with clearly visible contracture and synkinesis
3	4	Severe palsy with disfiguring contracture and synkinesis

After Peitersen.

The protection of the eye is the single most important step in the treatment of facial paralysis. It is also the only noncontroversial part of the treatment. All other steps in the management of Bell's palsy continue to be subject to debate and disagreement.

Treatment of the Paralyzed Muscles

Active exercise of the facial muscles by practicing grimacing movements in front of a mirror may well be helpful and is certainly harmless. It can be performed for 5 to 10 minutes three or four times daily. There is some evidence that the simultaneous use of the masseter muscle, by clenching the teeth while grimacing, improves recovery. The masseter muscle is innervated by the trigeminal nerve. It is well known that there are anastomoses between the terminal branches of the facial and trigeminal nerves, although the function of these anastomotic links is not understood. It is believed that some trigeminal fibers may pass through the anastomotic plexus to innervate paralyzed facial muscle fibers.

Electrical stimulation of the paralyzed muscles by weak galvanic current has been carried out enthusiastically in the past. The aim of treatment was to prevent disuse atrophy of the muscles so that they would be in a better condition to receive and react to the nerve impulses when regeneration occurred. Most authorities now agree that this treatment confers no benefit. Some believe that the excessive use of electrical stimulation may promote the development of contractures.

Medical Treatment

Steroid Therapy

The pathologic mechanism of nerve paralysis in Bell's palsy is considered to be edema and congestion of the facial nerve in its rigid bony canal, which results in compression of the nerve fibers. Initially the edema causes a neuropraxia. However, if the edema increases, compression of the nerve fibers causes axonal degeneration. The adrenocorticotrophic hormone (ACTH), prednisolone, and prednisone have been advocated frequently in the treatment of Bell's palsy as a means of reducing edema and compression damage to the nerve. A short course of steroid therapy is a safe form of treatment in patients who are not pregnant, do not suffer from diabetes, and do not have a history of tuberculosis or peptic ulcer. Provided steroid therapy is not contraindicated, it is our practice to treat new cases of Bell's palsy with prednisone for 8 days. On the first day 40 mg of prednisone is given and the dosage is reduced by 5 mg daily until the course is completed. Although some studies have shown that steroids produce no significant benefit, the majority of studies have claimed decreased denervation and improved recovery in patients treated early in the course of the disease.

Vasodilator Therapy

The use of vasodilator drugs is based on the concept that Bell's palsy is due to ischemia of the facial nerve caused by circulatory changes inside the fallopian canal. Nicotinic acid in flushing dosage has been recommended in an attempt to overcome the ischemia. Physicians who believe that the paralysis is due more to edema than ischemia tend to avoid vasodilator therapy in case it increases the congestion inside the nerve sheath.

Mast Cell Degranulation Inhibitors

There is recent evidence to support an immunologic concept of Bell's palsy. This theory attributes the paralysis to an edematous neuropathy of the facial nerve caused by an immediate hypersensitivity reaction. This reaction triggers the degranulation of specific mast cells, which results in an allergic type of edema in the facial nerve. Sodium cromoglycate (cromolyn sodium) has been recommended by certain internationally recognized experts in the United States to inhibit this degranulation. The advocates of this treatment recommend that a 20 mg capsule of cromolyn be used by inhalation every 2 or 3 hours night and day for about 2 weeks. They claim that good results are obtained provided treatment is started within 4 or 5 days of the onset of paralysis. We have no experience with this form of treatment and therefore must suspend judgment until more evidence of its effectiveness is available.

Surgical Treatment

Surgical decompression of the facial nerve is the most controversial of all the remedies used in Bell's palsy. The purpose of surgical decompression is to relieve the congestion and swelling of the nerve in its bony canal before compression edema damages nerve fibers and causes axonal degeneration. In order to be effective the operation should be done as early as possible in the course of the disease. Since 84 per cent of patients can be expected to have a spontaneous good recovery, the problem lies in accurately identifying, during the first 2 weeks of the disease, the small minority of patients who will not recover and might benefit from surgical decompression.

Surgical decompression is not free from risk. It is believed that compression frequently involves that part of the nerve that lies in the internal auditory canal and labyrinthine section of the fallopian canal. Decompression of the nerve in this region requires a middle fossa exploration. The rest of the nerve in the temporal bone can be exposed by a transmastoid operation. Injury to the nerve by surgical instrumentation can add further insult to an already damaged nerve. Injury to the closely related auditory and vestibular system can cause deafness and vertigo. A middle cranial fossa procedure can produce the complications associated with intracranial operations. Decompression of the facial nerve is a major surgical undertaking that demands a very high degree of skill. Supporters of the operation claim that the degree of residual paralysis contracture and synkinesis will be less after operation than it would have been if decompression had not been carried out. There is no way of validating this claim.

For the past two decades the treatment of Bell's palsy by surgical decompression has been abandoned in Great Britain.

In these times when physicians are faced with the problems of litigation and informed consent it is important that patients be made aware that the treatment of Bell's palsy is controversial. It must be emphasized that, at present, there is no scientific proof of the efficacy of any of the medical or surgical treatments.

PARKINSONISM

method of
MARGARET M. MAIER HOEHN, M.D., FRCP(C)
University of Colorado
Denver, Colorado

The parkinsonian syndrome, or parkinsonism, is characterized clinically by the classic triad of tremor, rigidity, and akinesia, accompanied by abnormalities of posture and balance. Neurochemically, there is a deficiency of dopaminergic inhibition of cholinergic neurons in the striatum, although other neurotransmitters and neuromodulators, such as peptides, probably are also involved to a lesser degree.

The term Parkinson's disease is usually reserved for the primary or idiopathic form of parkinsonism first described by James Parkinson in 1817. The most conspicuous and consistent pathologic change is the loss of pigmented neurons in the zona compacta of the sustantia nigra. These neurons synthesize dopamine and store it within their terminals in the striatum. Degeneration of these cells of the nigrostriatal dopamine pathway results in an absolute and measurable deficiency of dopamine in the striatum. The signs and symptoms of Parkinson's disease appear when there has been a loss of approximately 80 per cent of the cells.

Destruction of dopamine-synthesizing cells of the substantia nigra and the syndrome of parkinsonism also occur secondary to known etiologic factors. It was a common sequela of von Economo's encephalitis lethargica, which occurred in epidemic proportions after World War I and sporadically until the early 1930's. Parkinsonism also has been described following other viral encephalitides. MPTP, a chemical inadvertently produced during the synthesis of meperidine, produces specific destruction of cells of the substantia nigra, with resultant severe parkinsonism. Damage to the nigrostriatal dopamine system can occur concomitantly with more diffuse cerebral damage from tumors, trauma, toxins, anoxia, calcification secondary to hypoparathyroidism, and degenerative diseases such as progressive supranuclear palsy, the Shy-Drager syndrome, low pressure hydrocephalus, nigrostriatal degeneration, olivopontocerebellar atrophy, Huntington's disease, and Wilson's disease.

These conditions produce an absolute depletion of dopamine. However, functional dopamine deficiency can result from interference with the storage, release, and reuptake of dopamine and with its access to the dopamine receptor cells of the striatum. Usually this is the result of the actions of drugs such as reserpine, haloperidol, and the phenothiazines, all of which can produce the parkinsonian syndrome.

Effective treatment depends upon accurate diagnosis, differentiation between the primary and secondary forms, and treatment of the cause if possible. When the syndrome is secondary to diffuse cerebral damage, diagnosis may be aided by the presence of neurologic signs in addition to those of parkinsonism. However, especially in patients with mild and early disease, the signs of primary and secondary parkinsonism may be indistinguishable. An exceedingly careful history may provide the only clue. In other patients, final diagnosis must await the development and progression of the disease over time or even postmortem examination. Two additional points may be helpful. Secondary parkinsonism responds less well to treatment; occasionally a poor response provides the first indication that the disease is not idiopathic Parkinson's disease. Second, Parkinson's disease frequently is missed because it is thought to be a disease of the elderly. It should be remembered that, although the mean age at diagnosis is in the 50s, approximately 20 per cent of patients are diagnosed in their 40s and 10 per cent before the age of 40.

TREATMENT

General Approach

It is essential that patients with Parkinson's disease and their families understand the nature of the disease. They must be reassured that, while it is a progressive disease with no known cure, since the development of levodopa, improvement of function and mobility is a reasonable expectation from proper therapy; approximately half of patients have no disability even after 10 years of illness; and life expectancy is approximately equal to that of the unaffected population. Because of this long duration, they must learn to live their lives as normally as possible without undue expectations and with every attempt to counteract the depression and withdrawal that are so common. Patients must be encouraged to remain as active and to do as much for themselves as possible, no matter how long these activities take to perform.

As with any chronic, progressive, and debilitating disease, psychologic support for both the patient and the family is essential. This can be facilitated by the physician's allotting additional time to patients with Parkinson's disease. In addition, they should be encouraged to become members of local support groups and national educational foundations. The sharing of experiences, problems, and their solutions can be very beneficial to both patients and their families. With regard to specific therapy, they must understand the limitations of drug therapy, that it must be individualized, the wide range of effective dosages of drugs, and the variability of both beneficial and adverse effects from patient to patient. They must be aware from the onset of therapy that the physician cannot prescribe a fixed dosage, that a great deal of patience and time are required for the trial and error process of determining the optimal drug regimen for an individual patient, and that their own observations, understanding, and communication to the physician of the effects of the drugs are essential.

They also should understand that combinations of low dosages of several drugs often are more beneficial, with fewer side effects, than larger dosages of a single drug.

Drug Treatment of the Symptoms and Signs of Parkinsonism

Present drug treatment is aimed at re-establishing the normal relationship between dopamine and acetylcholine by decreasing cholinergic and/or increasing dopaminergic activity in the basal ganglia. This is accomplished by three approaches: the enhancement of endogenous dopaminergic activity (usually by inhibition of cholinergic activity), the replenishment of dopamine, and the replacement of dopamine.

Enhancement of Endogenous Dopaminergic Activity

Anticholinergic Agents. Since 1867, when Ordenstein recommended the use of the belladonna alkaloid hyoscyamine, natural and synthetic compounds with anticholinergic properties have been used to treat parkinsonism (Table 1). A deficiency of dopamine or a blockade of dopamine receptors disinhibits the striatal cholinergic interneurons, resulting in overactivity and a marked release of acetylcholine. Anticholinergic agents not only dampen this overactivity but probably also block the reuptake of dopamine by the presynaptic nerve terminals, making more of the neurotransmitter available for stimulation of postsynaptic receptors and inhibition of cholinergic activity. All of the drugs listed in Table 1 are useful, but, in general, the anticholinergics are more potent than the antihistamines; the antiparkinson effects of the latter depend on their anticholinergic properties but may, especially in patients with severe tremor, also be useful for their sedative effects. The most commonly used are trihexyphenidyl HCl (Artane), benztropine mesylate (Cogentin), and diphenhydramine (Benadryl), although the others theoretically are equally effective and, in occasional patients, are more beneficial. Benztropine mesylate and diphenhydramine are useful in severely ill or postoperative patients because they come in a parenteral as well as an oral form. Ethopropazine (Parsidol) is the only phenothiazine that can be given to patients with parkinsonism without the risk of blocking dopamine receptors and exacerbating the disease.

Dosages should be started low, usually with ½ of the smallest tablet two or three times daily, increasing gradually every 5 to 14 days to observe both beneficial and adverse effects at each level. Anticholinergics and antihistamines seldom effect more than 20 per cent improvement.

Because of their parasympathetic blocking action, these drugs produce blurred vision and poor accommodation; dryness of the mouth; urinary hesitancy and retention; constipation; drowsiness; tachycardia and cardiac arrhythmias; sleep disturbance; impairment of memory; confusion; hallucinations; and nightmares. The mental disturbances may be significant: memory impairment interferes with work potential in the younger patients, and toxic psychosis may occur in the elderly. For this reason, I try to avoid the use of anticholinergics, although this is not always possible. It should be remembered that abrupt discontinuance of these drugs can cause life-threatening atropine withdrawal symptoms.

Amantadine HCl. Because of its relatively uniform dosage of 200 to 300 mg daily, the simplicity of administration two to three times daily, and the low incidence of adverse reactions, amantadine (Symmetrel) is one of the most useful of the less potent antiparkinson drugs, used either alone or as an adjunct to levodopa. It probably releases dopamine from neuronal pools, making more available at receptor sites; it also may have a direct action on dopamine receptors in the striatum. It is slightly more potent than the anticholinergic agents, effecting 15 to 25 per cent improvement. Adverse reactions include peripheral edema and livedo reticularis, thought due to abnormal permeability of dermal blood vessels, since total body water and electrolytes are not abnormal. Especially at dosages over 200 mg daily, hyperexcitability, increased tremor, jerkiness, insomnia, and nightmares may occur.

Central Nervous System Stimulants. Amphetamine acts by releasing monoamines from storage sites and/or via a direct action on dopamine receptor cells. Before levodopa, it frequently was used as an ancillary drug, especially in postencephalitic parkinsonism. Both amphetamine and methylphenidate (Ritalin) occasionally also alleviate levodopa-induced somnolence.

Tricyclic Antidepressants. Drugs such as imipramine HCl (Tofranil), amitriptyline HCl (Elavil), and desipramine (Norpramin) are useful because of their anticholinergic properties and because they treat the depression that so frequently accompanies the disease. A dosage of 25 to 150 mg daily can be given in divided doses or as a single bedtime dose. The combination of levodopa, amantadine or an anticholinergic, and a tricyclic antidepressant is a common regimen for parkinsonism. Adverse reactions occur infrequently and are similar to those from other anticholinergic agents.

Monoamine Oxidase Inhibitors. Monoamine oxidase (MAO) inhibitors increase dopamine's effective life by blocking its oxidative deamination. At the present time, deprenyl, an inhibitor of monoamine oxidase type B, is being used exper-

TABLE 1. **Drugs that Enhance Endogenous Dopaminergic Activity**

Drug	How Supplied	Daily Dosage (mg)
Anticholinergics		
trihexyphenidyl HCl (Artane)†	2, 5 mg tabs 5 mg sust rel caps 2 mg/5 ml elixir	6–30
biperiden (Akineton)	2 mg tabs*	2–8
procyclidine HCl (Kemadrin)	2, 5 mg tabs	7.5–25
Antihistamines		
diphenhydramine HCl (Benadryl)†	25, 50 mg caps* 12.5 mg/5 ml elixir	75–150
orphenadrine HCl (Disipal)	50 mg tabs	150–400
Anticholinergic-Antihistamines		
benztropine mesylate (Cogentin)	0.5, 1, 2 mg tabs*	0.5–8
Phenothiazine-Anticholinergic-Antihistamines		
ethopropazine HCl (Parsidol)	10, 50 mg tabs	40–400
Unclassified		
amantadine HCl (Symmetrel)	100 mg caps	100–300
Central Nervous System Stimulants		
amphetamine sulfate (Obetrol)†	2.5, 5, 10 mg tabs 15 mg sust rel caps	5–15
dextroamphetamine (Obetrol, Dexedrine)†	2.5, 5, 10, 15 mg tabs 5, 10, 15 mg caps 5, 10, 15 mg sust rel caps 5 mg/5 ml elixir	5–15
methylphenidate (Ritalin)	5, 10, 20 mg tabs 20 mg sust rel tabs	10–30
Tricyclic Antidepressants		
imipramine (Tofranil, Janimine, Pramine)†	10, 25, 50 mg tabs* 75, 100, 125, 150 mg caps	25–150
amitriptyline HCl (Elavil, Endep)†	10, 25, 50, 75, 100, 150 mg tabs*	25–150
desipramine HCl (Norpramin, Pertofrane)	10, 25, 50, 75, 100, 150 mg tabs	25–150
Monoamine Oxidase Inhibitors		
deprenyl‡	5, 10 mg tabs	30

*Also available for parenteral use.
†Available in generic preparations.
‡Experimental.

imentally at a usual dosage of 5 to 10 mg three times daily. It improves the signs of parkinsonism and smoothes out the fluctuation of response some patients have when on levodopa. When approved, it will be a valuable adjunctive drug. In addition, the recent indications that MAO inhibitors interfere with the development of 1-methyl-4-phenyl-1,2,3,6-tetrahydropyridine (MPTP)-induced parkinsonism make their possible future use exciting. Side effects include hypertension, hypotension, cardiac arrhythmias, confusion, agitation, depression, insomnia, nausea, anorexia, exacerbation of gastrointestinal ulcers, and levodopa-induced dyskinesias.

Replenishment of Dopamine

Parkinsonism has been established as essentially a dopamine deficiency disease, and the severity of the signs is correlated positively with the degree of dopamine deficiency in the basal ganglia. Dopamine itself does not cross the blood-brain barrier and is an ineffective and impractical therapeutic agent. In 1967, George Cotzias demonstrated that the administration of dopamine's precursor, DL-dopa, resulted in marked amelioration of the signs and symptoms of the disease. Approximately one quarter of orally administered levodopa (or L-dopa, an analogue of DL-dopa) enters the brain. The resultant dopamine, synthesized by the brain, is stored in the striatum. Although many of the neurons that synthesize and store dopamine have degenerated in Parkinson's disease, this capacity is not entirely lost, at least in the early stages of the disease. It has been demonstrated that levodopa-treated patients who responded well have, at postmortem, markedly higher striatal dopamine levels than do patients who responded poorly. Impairment of synthesizing and storage ability with progression of the disease may account for the apparent decreasing effectiveness of levodopa after many years of treatment.

During the past 15 years, levodopa has become the treatment of choice for parkinsonism. Although about 20 per cent of patients do not respond in a satisfactory and/or longlasting manner to levodopa, in some patients levodopa may produce up to 80 per cent improvement. The duration of illness at each stage of severity has increased by 3 to 5 years. After 10 years of illness, the proportion of patients disabled (stages IV and V) or dead has decreased from over 80 per cent to approximately 50 per cent. Quality of life has been improved, and the mean age at death has increased by 6 years, from the late 60s to the early 70s. Sixty per cent of patients now are over 75 years old at the time of death, as compared with only about 20 per cent before levodopa. Life expectancy is approximately equal to that of the nonaffected population. Some neurologists delay the use of levodopa as long as possible, depending upon the less potent agents used during the early stages of the disease. This practice is based upon the belief that late problems in the management of parkinsonism are due to prolonged use of levodopa. My practice is to initiate treatment with levodopa during the first year after diagnosis because of the improved quality of life it provides, the fact that there is some evidence to indicate that disability is postponed, and the belief that late problems are due to severity and progression of the disease process rather than to length of treatment with levodopa.

Levodopa is administered in two forms: levodopa alone or, since the mid 1970's, in combination with the peripheral decarboxylase inhibitor carbidopa (Table 2).

Levodopa (Larodopa). When levodopa is used alone, extremely large dosages are required because approximately 75 per cent of it is rapidly decarboxylated to dopamine in the periphery and never reaches its therapeutic target in the brain. Severe side effects, such as anorexia, nausea, and vomiting, occur in almost all patients. The drug must almost always be given with food, which impairs absorption and transport, thus decreasing its effectiveness. Induction must be extremely slow, and it often takes many months to achieve tolerance of side effects and to attain optimal effects. At the beginning, most patients can tolerate 250 mg two or three times daily. The dosage then is increased by 250 or 500 mg every week or so; frequently it is necessary to temporarily decrease the dosage to a previous level when adverse reactions supervene. Average maintenance dosage is 4 or 5 grams daily, with a range from 1 to 10 grams and occasionally more.

Because of the slowness and difficulty of induction of therapy and because some patients never cease being nauseated from the drug, during the past 10 years most patients have been switched from levodopa alone to its combination with a peripheral dopa decarboxylase inhibitor. However, a small percentage of patients still does better on levodopa alone.

Levodopa Combined with a Peripheral Dopa Decarboxylase Inhibitor. In the United States, levodopa has been combined with the decarboxylase inhibitor L-alpha-methyldopahydrazine, or carbidopa, in a preparation known as Sinemet. Outside the United States, another inhibitor, benzerazide, is combined with levodopa and marketed under the trade name Madopar. Carbidopa is a peripheral decarboxylase inhibitor that does not cross the blood-brain barrier; it therefore preferentially inhibits the extracerebral metabolism of levodopa without preventing the synthesis of dopamine from levodopa within the brain. As a result, peripheral adverse reactions are reduced, induction is smoother and more rapid, and the dosage of levodopa can be reduced by approximately 75 per cent.

Between 75 and 150 mg of carbidopa are required to fully inhibit peripheral decarboxylation. Sinemet comes in tablets containing either 10 or 25 mg of carbidopa, combined with 100 or 250 mg of levodopa (10/100, 25/100, and 25/250). Sinemet 25/100 is the preparation of choice in initial treatment, since full peripheral inhibition

TABLE 2. **Drugs That Replenish or Replace Dopamine**

Drug	How Supplied	Daily Dosage
levodopa (Larodopa, Dopar)	100, 250, 500 mg tabs 100, 250, 500 mg caps	1.0–10 grams
carbidopa/levodopa (Sinemet)	10/100, 25/100, 25/250 tabs	300–2000 mg levodopa
bromocriptine (Parlodel)	2.5 mg tabs 5.0 mg caps	2.5–100 mg

of decarboxylation can be attained rapidly while the dosage of levodopa is still low, thus avoiding many adverse reactions. Treatment usually is started with ½ tablet two or three times daily. The dosage can be increased by ½ tablet every 3 or 4 days to 1 tablet three or four times daily. Usually the dosage is maintained at this level for several weeks to determine response. If additional levodopa is required, 6 tablets daily may be taken. The average daily dosage of levodopa is between 600 and 700 mg, but there is wide variability from less than 300 mg to as much as 2,000 mg. If more than 6 tablets of Sinemet 25/100 are required, the dosage of levodopa can be increased by gradually substituting the 25/250 preparation. Dosages of 25/250 should not exceed 8 tablets, since there is only limited experience with dosages of carbidopa over 200 mg daily. If, in the rare patient, additional levodopa is required, it should be added in its uncombined form.

On this regimen, some patients still become nauseated at first. In most it can be avoided by administering Sinemet after meals. The nausea usually subsides with continued treatment, and many patients later can take Sinemet on an empty stomach. This increases its efficacy, since amino acids interfere with the transport of levodopa. Hydroxyzine pamoate (Vistaril), 25 to 50 mg, is a useful antiemetic, since it is a mild anticholinergic and is not a dopamine antagonist.

Other adverse reactions to levodopa include palpitations, malaise, fatigue, severe somnolence, especially after individual doses, a burning sensation of the tongue, bitter taste in the mouth, episodic flushing and sweating, and orthostatic hypotension, dizziness, and syncope. The latter can be treated with increased salt intake, elastic stockings, fludrocortisone (Florinef), 0.1 to 0.2 mg, or ephedrine, 25 mg, two or three times daily. As with all antiparkinson drugs, mental disturbances may occur and include euphoria and hypomania, depression, confusion, insomnia and nightmares, paranoid ideation, and particularly vivid hallucinations. Severe psychotic episodes are best treated by temporarily discontinuing Sinemet until mentation has returned to normal, usually in 12 to 36 hours, and then resuming Sinemet at a lower dosage. Discontinuance for this short a time usually does not cause significant deterioration of the parkinsonism. However, especially in the elderly with severe disease, it may be necessary to compromise between optimal antiparkinson benefits and an entirely clear sensorium; many patients tolerate mild and nonthreatening hallucinations, if they understand the cause, rather than suffer helpless akinesia.

Abnormal involuntary movements (AIMs, dyskinesias) occur in almost all patients treated with levodopa if the dosage is high enough. They may be choreic, athetotic, dystonic, myoclonic, ballistic, or slow with an almost purposive character. They may involve the face and extremities and/or the axial, abdominal, and respiratory muscles. When mild, they frequently are not noticed by the patient and are more disturbing to the family. In approximately 30 per cent of patients they are severe enough to interfere with or prevent function. There are two types of AIMs; they are related to the dosing schedule of Sinemet and must be clearly differentiated. *Peak dose dyskinesias* are thought to be associated with overdosage, high circulating levels of dopamine, and excessive stimulation of striatal receptors. They occur when levodopa is exerting its most beneficial antiparkinson effects. Reduction of levodopa dosage relieves peak dose dyskinesias, but often at the expense of deterioration of parkinsonism. The other types of AIMs have been called *off dose dyskinesia, off period dystonia, diphasic dyskinesia*, or the *dystonia-improvement-dystonia (DID) response*. These movements frequently are dystonic and painful but may have charateristics impossible to distinguish, except for the timing of their occurrence, from those of peak dose dyskinesia. They occur before taking the first dose of levodopa in the morning; after taking a dose but before the beneficial effects appear; and/or after the beneficial effects of a dose have worn off or are wearing off. Often they last only 5 to 30 minutes but occasionally last many hours. They disappear with the full re-emergence of parkinsonian signs and when the parkinsonism is relieved. They are not relieved by decreasing the dosage of Sinemet. Some relief can be obtained by taking doses more frequently and by the addition of other antiparkinson agents, especially the dopamine agonists.

Fluctuations of therapeutic response are the most troublesome problem of chronic levodopa therapy, and, again, there are several types. Subtle *diurnal fluctuations* are common. Usually patients feel best in the morning, worse in the late afternoon, and slightly better again during the evening. Some deteriorate as the day progresses, others improve. Surprisingly, many patients feel very well before the first morning dose despite the long interval since the bedtime dose; this is thought to be due to the storage of endogenous dopamine during rest. With the *wearing off effect* or *end of dose akinesia*, the effects of individual doses of levodopa begin to last for progressively shorter periods and become erratic in time of onset and degree of benefit. Occasionally the *on-off phenomenon* is associated with the wearing off effect; fluctuations are extreme and abrupt, often occurring within seconds. The expression was coined by patients who described it "like a light turning on and off." When fluctuations are completely unpredictable and unrelated to the dosing schedule, it is called *yo-yoing*.

Some fluctuations of response occur in almost all patients; severe and unpredictable fluctuations that interfere with function occur in about 30 per cent of patients but seldom before the third year of treatment. They are much more frequent in patients with a young age at onset of disease: almost 70 per cent of patients whose disease began before the age of 50 develop severe fluctuations; they occur in less than 10 per cent of those whose onset was after the age of 60. Another type of fluctuation is *episodic freezing* or *peak dose freezing*. These are very brief episodes during which the patient is unable to move. They occur almost at random, even when all other aspects of parkinsonism are under control, and often are associated with hypotonia and falling. The cause of fluctuations is unknown; they have been ascribed to changes in the sensitivity of dopamine receptors, decreased ability of presynaptic neurons to store dopamine, and progression of the disease.

Treatment is difficult when the fluctuations are severe. Dividing the total daily dosage of levodopa into multiple small and more frequent doses, as well as eating multiple small meals with decreased dietary protein, may be of some benefit. A "drug holiday" has been advocated and has been moderately successful for a few months in a few patients. One approach is to discontinue levodopa for 1 to 2 weeks and then restart it at a lower dosage; however, this requires hospitalization and may produce severe, rapid, and life-threatening deterioration. I do not recommend it except in patients with the most severe and intractable fluctuations in whom all other methods of treatment have failed, leaving the patient nonfunctional. An alternative approach, which does not require hospitalization, is to stop levodopa for 1 or 2 days each week, either on consecutive or alternate days. The addition of other antiparkinson agents may smooth the response to some extent, especially the longer acting ones. However, by far the best approach to the treatment of fluctuations is the addition of the dopamine agonists.

Replacement of Dopamine

The degree to which levodopa can replenish deficient dopamine levels depends on the number of remaining nigrostriatal neurons that can synthesize and store dopamine. However, nigrostriatal cells are degenerated in patients with parkinsonism, perhaps by 75 to 80 per cent before the signs of the disease appear. In addition, there is a deficiency of aromatic amino acid decarboxylase, which is responsible for the conversion of levodopa to dopamine. Since the early 1970's, there has been a search for agents that would stimulate the striatal dopamine receptors directly, thus bypassing the need for the brain to synthesize dopamine. Apomorphine was the first dopamine agonist discovered, but it is too toxic for chronic use. Piribedil, lergotrile, lisuride, pergolide, mesulergine, ciladopa, and bromocriptine are all ergot alkaloids and effective dopamine receptor stimulants, but only bromocriptine (Parlodel) is available on the market. It has unequivocal antiparkinson effects, either alone or in combination with levodopa. However, it is very expensive, and, at high dosages, as many as 40 per cent of patients have had to discontinue the drug because of adverse reactions.

Treatment should be started with 1.25 mg daily and increased very slowly by 1.25 to 2.5 mg every 1 to 2 weeks. It should be given in divided doses three or four times daily. Approximately one quarter of patients respond at 7.5 mg daily, half at 12.5 mg daily, and two thirds at 20 mg daily. Some patients require much higher dosages, up to 100 mg daily, for optimal results. Bromocriptine is the drug of choice for alleviating the wearing off effect and treating off dose dystonia. It is less effective for the on-off phenomenon and episodic freezing, and it seldom effects significant improvement in those patients who have severe disease and an inadequate response to levodopa.

Adverse effects of bromocriptine are similar to those of levodopa and may be cumulative when the two drugs are given together and the dosage of levodopa is not reduced. However, usually it is possible to reduce the levodopa. Peak dose AIMs usually can be reduced by this approach, while still maintaining the improvement effected by the addition of bromocriptine. Mental disturbances similar to those seen with levodopa are frequent but are less of a problem at the lower dosages. In addition, acute personality and affective disturbances can occur. Vascular constriction, peripheral edema, livedo reticularis, and exacerbation of angina pectoris may require reduction of dosage or discontinuance.

Nonpharmaceutical Treatment

Exercise is essential to maintain mobility and psychologic health. To a large extent, this can be achieved by encouraging normal occupational and social activities and personal independence. Because of the tendency to withdraw that is a part of the disease, many patients require a more formally structured exercise program. This may be done individually or in groups with a professional physiotherapist. In addition, the United Parkinson Foundation (360 West Superior St., Chicago, IL 60610) has published an exercise program specifically designed for patients with

Parkinson's disease; with the physician's approval, it can be followed at home, with other members of the family, or in groups of patients without the supervision of a professional physiotherapist. It should be remembered that patients with Parkinson's disease fatigue easily, and exercise should not be too strenuous and forced.

The *surgical* destruction of a small area of the thalamus was popular before the advent of levodopa. When successful, it decreased tremor and rigidity on the contralateral side but usually did not improve, and occasionally worsened, akinesia. The complications, especially when performed bilaterally, were severe, and it seldom is used today. Transplants of fetal brain and adrenal gland are still in the very early experimental stage. To date, they have been only partially successful in decreasing signs and have not been curative.

PERIPHERAL NEUROPATHIES

method of
PHILIP G. McMANIS, M.D.,
and PHILLIP A. LOW, M.D.
Mayo Clinic
Rochester, Minnesota

A useful way of approaching peripheral neuropathies is to place patients into one of several diagnostic categories based on the distribution of nerves affected, the type of nerve fiber involved, and the time course of the disease (Table 1).

In many instances there is no specific treatment for a particular type of neuropathy. It is important to keep in mind the value of general supportive measures in alleviating symptoms. Range of motion exercises to prevent joint contractures and braces and splints for weakened muscle groups are often invaluable in maintaining mobility. Patients with severe lower extremity weakness often derive considerable benefit from the stability provided by a cane. The importance of protection and care of insensitive feet, particularly in the patient with diabetes, cannot be overemphasized. Patients should be instructed to trim their toenails with great care and to be fastidious about foot hygiene. Any fungal or bacterial infection requires prompt medical attention. The need for well-fitting shoes should also be stressed. In addition, patients should be warned that the lack of sensation makes their feet more susceptible to damage from frostbite in winter, an event with potentially disastrous consequences.

TABLE 1. **Diagnostic Categories of Peripheral Neuropathies**

1. Distal symmetric sensorimotor neuropathy ("glove and stocking")
2. Polyradiculoneuropathy
3. Mononeuritis multiplex
4. Large fiber neuropathy
5. Small fiber neuropathy

Patients with peripheral neuropathy severe enough to confine them to bed are at risk for deep vein thrombosis and respiratory complications. Care should be taken to prevent these complications or to treat them promptly if they arise.

HEREDITARY NEUROPATHIES

Inherited peripheral neuropathies are an important group to recognize. Many undiagnosed neuropathies are eventually found to be familial, and it is important to look for the clues of hereditary neuropathies before undertaking an expensive diagnostic work-up. The presence of pes cavus, clawed toes, and scoliosis together with a youthful age at onset or very longstanding symptoms are strongly suggestive of hereditary neuropathy. If possible, family members should be examined for similar findings, and electromyography may be warranted to attempt to identify subclinical neuropathy in relatives.

Even though there is no specific treatment for the vast majority of hereditary neuropathies, the patients can be given genetic counseling regarding the likelihood of their progeny developing the disorder. They can also be informed about the prospective severity of their disease and counseled about suitable employment. Treatment can be offered to a few patients with inherited neuropathies: some of them have a peculiar predisposition to developing pressure palsies, and measures can be taken to avoid situations likely to produce these and to treat them if they occur. Another group of patients inherit a disorder that is very similar to chronic inflammatory demyelinating polyradiculoneuropathy and have elevated cerebrospinal fluid protein levels. This group obtains considerable benefit from prednisone therapy in the same doses used to treat the acquired form of disease (see hereafter).

ACQUIRED PERIPHERAL NEUROPATHIES

Distal Sensorimotor Neuropathy

Sometimes called "glove and stocking" neuropathy, this is the most commonly encountered form of peripheral neuropathy. Many different conditions produce this pattern of distal muscle wasting and weakness with decreased or absent tendon reflexes and loss of sensation. In general, these are "dying back" or "axonal" neuropathies, but some demyelinating neuropathies present in the same way. This category may cause considerable frustration for the physician because specific therapy is usually not available. In addition the causes often lack distinguishing features to aid in diagnosis. In most cases the treatment is directed toward the underlying disease or involves eliminating the offending drug or toxic agent.

Neuropathies with Predominant Axonal Degeneration

Most distal sensorimotor neuropathies are caused by primary degeneration of axons. At times the same clinical picture can be produced by a demyelinating neuropathy and electromyography may be very helpful in differentiating these groups. In axonal degeneration the amplitude of the evoked motor or sensory response will be low (or absent), whereas conduction velocities will be relatively unaffected. Needle examination of muscles will show changes of acute and/or chronic denervation in distal muscles. In demyelinating neuropathies the main abnormality is a prominent reduction in maximum nerve conduction velocities.

Metabolic and Endocrine Disorders

UREMIA. The neuropathy associated with renal failure follows a pattern typical of distal neuropathies, with distal loss of strength and sensation and decreased reflexes. One notable feature, however, is that sensory symptoms are common; patients frequently complain of unpleasant pulling or drawing sensations in their legs together with burning or tingling discomfort in the feet. Frequent cramps and restless legs may appear during the early development of the neuropathy.

Uremic neuropathy occurs only in end stage renal failure. Treatment of the neuropathy depends on correction of the chronic metabolic abnormalities, but hemodialysis is generally not effective in improving the symptoms and may even fail to prevent progression. On the other hand, renal transplantation is almost always followed by a significant improvement in the neuropathy. This may influence the choice of treatment in patients with severe uremic neuropathy.

DIABETES MELLITUS. In this condition the neuropathy may be predominantly axonal, demyelinating, or angiopathic, but more commonly features of different types of pathologic processes are present in the same patient. Some diabetics will have the picture of mononeuritis multiplex, whereas others will present with predominant involvement of either large or small nerve fibers (see hereafter). However, the most common form of peripheral neuropathy is a mild to moderate distal sensorimotor neuropathy, which is almost invariably present in patients with longstanding noninsulin-dependent diabetes. This is frequently asymptomatic, although patients may admit to mild distal tingling or numbness. Florid autonomic nervous system symptoms are less common with this type of diabetic neuropathy than with the small fiber type of neuropathy.

The aim of treatment is to obtain the best possible control of the blood sugar level. If this cannot be achieved with diet alone or with oral hypoglycemic agents, then insulin therapy may be indicated. However, caution should be exercised when first beginning insulin treatment as some diabetics develop the acute onset of painful tingling and hypersensitivity of their extremities at this time. The cause is uncertain but may be related to the sudden normalization of blood (and nerve) glucose levels. Diabetic nerves have endoneurial hypoxia so that there is an increased dependence on anaerobic glycolysis for energy metabolism. When the substrates for anaerobic glycolysis are suddenly reduced, the nerve is unable to meet its energy requirements and nerve damage results. Thus, a gradual reduction in the elevated blood sugar levels may be preferable to a rapid change.

Experiments are currently under way with sorbinil, an aldose reductase inhibitor that reduces the elevated nerve sorbitol levels. Preliminary results suggest that a small improvement in nerve conduction velocity may occur during treatment with this drug, but the relevance of this observation to the pathogenesis of diabetic neuropathy is quite uncertain. It has also been found that myoinositol is reduced in nerves in experimental diabetes, but an improvement in human diabetic neuropathy has not been demonstrated with myoinositol supplementation. At present neither drug can be recommended as treatment of diabetic neuropathy.

OTHER METABOLIC DISORDERS. A peripheral neuropathy may be seen in acromegaly. In this condition, nerves are edematous and are susceptible to compression. Patients may present with carpal tunnel syndrome or ulnar nerve compression at the elbow. In the absence of focal compressions, the neuropathy is usually mild. A dramatic improvement in symptoms may be seen after hypophysectomy.

Patients with chronic liver disease often have a distal neuropathy. However, there is usually another cause for the nerve disease such as alcoholism, diabetes, or connective tissue disease. Treatment of neuropathy is usually directed toward the cause of the liver disease.

Distal sensorimotor neuropathy may also occur in rare disorders such as porphyria and recurrent hypoglycemia secondary to an insulinoma. Both of these are predominantly motor neuropathies and tend to affect the upper extremities before the lower. Porphyric neuropathy may produce greater weakness in proximal muscles than distal muscles and is characteristically associated with autonomic disturbances, abdominal pain, and psychiatric symptoms. Again, the treatment is that of the underlying disease process.

Drugs and Toxins

Many drugs are known to cause a peripheral neuropathy. The pattern of disease is variable: some agents produce a mild distal sensory neuropathy, whereas others result in a generalized motor neuropathy, sometimes affecting proximal and upper limb muscles more than distal lower limb muscles. It is essential that a careful drug history be taken from any person with neuropathy so that suspect drugs can be removed from the therapeutic regimen.

Most toxic agents produce a typical pattern of neuropathy: symptoms are very symmetric and begin in the feet, with the severity and rate of proximal progression being dose-related. Upper limbs are affected later in the course. Sensory nerves are more affected than motor fibers. The patient complains of distal burning and tingling together with prominent hypersensitivity. Examination reveals impaired sensation. The sensory deficit may be very mild relative to the symptoms in milder cases. Weakness is not a prominent feature early in the course or in mild to moderate toxic neuropathy. Exceptions to this pattern include glue sniffer's neuropathy, which is due to the chronic inhalation of *n*-hexane, and lead neuropathy. Both produce predominantly motor abnormalities. In addition, lead intoxication may result in a mononeuritis multiplex picture and often preferentially affects the upper extremities.

Treatment of these neuropathies is dependent on the identification of the toxin. Recovery generally follows the withdrawal of the causative agent but is slow and frequently incomplete. Specific therapy is available for metal poisoning (arsenic, lead, mercury, thallium); this is best and most safely treated with d-penicillamine. The usual dose is 250 mg four times daily, and therapy should be continued until urinary excretion of the metal returns to the normal range.

Vitamin Deficiencies and Alcohol

ALCOHOLIC NEUROPATHY. Alcoholics frequently develop a sensorimotor neuropathy characterized by distal muscle wasting and weakness with prominent sensory symptoms. Hypersensitivity and burning discomfort in the soles of the feet are frequent complaints, and calf tenderness is often present. Examination reveals distal lower limb weakness with absent ankle jerks and mild to moderate reduction of all sensory modalities. The upper extremities are relatively spared. The skin over the legs is often thin, pigmented, and shiny. Although a direct toxic effect of alcohol on nerve cannot be completely excluded, it is much more likely that the nerve damage is due to nutritional deficiencies, especially a lack of thiamine and other B group vitamins. Alcoholic neuropathy occurs in the setting of grossly abnormal dietary intake, whereas heavy drinkers who maintain a satisfactory diet rarely develop peripheral neuropathy. For these reasons, treatment of the neuropathy consists of a balanced high protein diet with B vitamin supplements. The recommended daily vitamin doses are thiamine 100 mg, pyridoxine 50 mg, niacin 100 mg, riboflavin 10 mg, and panthothenic acid 10 mg. Abstinence from alcohol should be encouraged, as this is likely to lead to an improvement in diet.

VITAMIN B_{12} DEFICIENCY. In contrast to the vitamin deficiency syndromes seen in alcoholics and others, lack of vitamin B_{12} is not caused by reduced dietary intake. In most cases the condition is due to an inability of the gut to absorb the vitamin, resulting from an autoimmune disease that reduces the production or blocks the action of intrinsic factor. This substance is essential for the absorption of vitamin B_{12}. Examination of these patients reveals prominent loss of vibration and joint position sense in the lower limbs. This often results in a sensory ataxia. Because weakness and reflex changes appear later in the course, the presence of neuropathy may be masked by a concurrent myelopathy. Treatment consists of intramuscular injection of B_{12} and must be continued indefinitely. The usual dose is 1000 micrograms five times the first week followed by the same dose once a month.

OTHER B GROUP VITAMIN DEFICIENCIES. Other nutritional neuropathies are rarely due to a single vitamin deficiency. Patients with neuropathy due to poor diet will usually have other evidence of malnourishment, such as loss of fat and muscle bulk. These patients will have clinical signs similar to those seen with alcoholic neuropathy and should be treated in the same way with a balanced diet and supplementary vitamins.

Pellagra is a vitamin deficiency syndrome consisting of diarrhea, dermatitis, and dementia. These symptoms respond to treatment with niacin. On occasion a peripheral neuropathy occurs in conjunction with the classic triad, but it is rarely responsive to niacin supplementation. In these cases the neuropathy will improve with pyridoxine and other B group vitamins. In the United States pellagrins are usually alcoholics, and vitamin supplements should be given in doses similar to those recommended for alcoholic neuropathy except that the niacin dose should be increased to 100 mg three times daily.

Deficiency of three other B group vitamins, thiamine, pantothenic acid, and pyridoxine, is also thought to produce a peripheral neuropathy. As a rule, these are seen only as part of a general nutritional deficiency except for pyridoxine. This substance may be specifically deficient in some patients during treatment with the antituberculous drug isoniazid. This causes a neuropathy characterized by a symmetric numbness and tingling in the feet followed by burning pains and calf tenderness. It has been shown that the neuropathy results from markedly increased excretion of pyridoxine and that it can be prevented by the administration of pyridoxine in a dose of 50 to 100 mg daily.

It is important to note that patients with peripheral neuropathy of unknown cause rarely benefit from the indiscriminate use of vitamins. In particular, large doses of B_6 (pyridoxine) can cause a very severe sensory neuropathy that responds only slowly to withdrawal of the vitamin. Patients taking vitamin supplements should be advised to adhere to recommended dosage regimens.

Neoplasms

Neoplasia is associated with several different neuropathic syndromes, including large fiber sensory neuropathy, acute pandysautonomia, subacute neuropathy resembling the Guillain-Barré syndrome, and other demyelinating neuropathies. However, the most common form is a mild, chronic distal sensorimotor peripheral neuropathy. This can be detected in many cancer patients if specifically sought but does not often cause significant symptoms. This may be partly explained by the fact that it commonly appears during the terminal stages of cancer. Improvement with treatment of the underlying neoplasm has not been documented except in the case of solitary plasmacytomas of bone and osteosclerotic myeloma. Irradiation of these tumors may result in improvement of the neuropathy.

Neuropathies with Predominant Demyelination

Neuropathies with primary demyelination of the peripheral nerves commonly present with the clinical pattern of polyradiculoneuropathy. The prototypes of this pattern are acute and chronic inflammatory demyelinating polyradiculoneuropathy (see hereafter). In these conditions proximal and sometimes trunk and cranial muscles are weak. Less commonly, some patients with a distal sensorimotor neuropathy are found to have primary demyelination or mixed demyelination and axonal degeneration on pathologic examination of the nerves. The clinical symptoms and signs may be indistinguishable from those of distal sensorimotor neuropathies with primary axonal degeneration. However, electromyography may be very helpful as outlined previously, and the cerebrospinal fluid protein is more likely to be elevated in demyelinating neuropathies.

Lead. Although lead is ubiquitous in the environment, lead neuropathy is now a rare disease. This situation has come about because of the awareness of the toxic nature of lead and the institution of effective precautions to minimize lead exposure. Nevertheless, lead neuropathy may still occur in certain groups exposed to high lead concentrations, especially those in lead-working industries. Children with pica may ingest lead-containing paint from old houses, but lead-intoxicated children will usually present with an encephalopathy rather than neuropathy.

The clinical picture is one of a motor neuropathy mainly affecting upper limbs, often in the pattern of a mononeuritis multiplex. Wrist drop is a prominent feature but sensory symptoms are virtually absent. Lead-poisoned children are more likely to have a symmetric distal motor neuropathy. A hypochromic microcytic anemia with basophilic stippling of red blood cells is almost always present.

The optimal method of treatment is controversial, but, as with other metal intoxications, most cases of lead neuropathy can be treated safely and effectively with oral d-penicillamine, 250 mg four times daily.

Acromegaly. In this condition the distal sensorimotor neuropathy is frequently accompanied by entrapment neuropathies, particularly median nerve compression in the carpal tunnel. The nerves are edematous and often palpably enlarged. Hypophysectomy is followed by a rapid and complete recovery from the neuropathy.

Hypothyroidism. Hypothyroid patients may develop a severe demyelinating neuropathy that mainly affects large sensory fibers. Clinically there is distal sensory loss, particularly of proprioception and vibration, whereas loss of strength is minimal. There may be an associated proximal myopathy, and cerebellar degeneration may combine with the proprioceptive loss to produce severe ataxia. Cerebrospinal fluid protein level is usually elevated. Treatment with thyroid hormone replacement leads to a complete resolution of the neuropathy.

Paraproteinemia. Patients with paraproteinemias who develop neuropathy may present with a distal sensorimotor neuropathy or with a polyradiculoneuropathy. Most patients with an abnormal serum protein have a monoclonal gammopathy of uncertain significance (MGUS) and only a minority have myeloma, amyloidosis, or Waldenström's macroglobulinemia. About 10 per cent of MGUS patients develop neuropathy, and it is thought that the paraprotein contains antibodies directed against peripheral nerve myelin in these cases. On the other hand, the neuropathy in patients with myeloma and macroglobulinemia is often associated with amyloid deposits in nerves. The clinical picture in these cases is of a dominantly sensory peripheral neuropathy, unlike primary amyloidosis, which causes a small fiber neuropathy with prominent autonomic dysfunction.

An unusual form of myeloma with osteosclerotic bone lesions has a strong association with neuropathy, either the distal sensorimotor form or a polyradiculoneuropathy. These patients also have a high incidence of endocrine abnormalities such as hirsutism, hypogonadism, gynecomastia, and skin pigmentation. Bony lesions may be solitary or multiple and either sclerotic or mixed lytic and sclerotic.

Treatment of the paraproteinemic neuropathies seen with macroglobulinemia or multiple myeloma is difficult, as there is no therapy available for amyloid infiltration. The treatment of the underlying disorder with prednisone and melphalan or chlorambucil could conceivably help if the paraprotein itself is neurotoxic. On the other hand, the neuropathy of osteosclerotic myeloma often improves with excision or irradiation of the bony lesions. The response is not as good in patients with widespread disease. The treatment of the neuropathy of MGUS is still being evaluated in clinical trials, but prednisone, immunosuppressive agents, and plasma exchange all hold promise. Some groups recommend prednisone in the high doses used to treat chronic inflammatory demyelinating polyradiculoneuropathy (120 mg and 7.5 mg on alternate days, gradually tapering to a low maintenance dose over several months). Others use a combination of prednisone with melphalan or chlorambucil and treat those who fail to respond with plasma exchange. More definite recommendations will have to await the results of these trials.

Other Demyelinating Neuropathies. Diabetes may result in demyelination of peripheral nerves as already discussed. Sarcoidosis can produce a demyelinating distal sensorimotor neuropathy but more commonly presents with the picture of mononeuritis multiplex or polyradiculoneuropathy.

POLYRADICULONEUROPATHY

The next major group of peripheral neuropathies consists of disorders producing the clinical picture of a polyradiculoneuropathy. These may be acute, subacute, or chronic. Although sensory and motor fibers are usually involved together, weakness is much more prominent than sensory complaints. Nerve roots and proximal portions of nerves are frequently affected, resulting in proximal limb, trunk, and cranial nerve involvement. Weakness may be severe and life-threatening. Tendon reflexes are universally hypoactive or absent. Minor abnormalities of sensation can often be detected. Examination of the cerebrospinal fluid usually reveals a high protein level with normal cell counts, and nerve conduction studies show marked slowing of conduction velocities in most cases.

Acute Inflammatory Polyradiculoneuropathy

Often known as Guillain-Barré syndrome, this neuropathy is abrupt in onset and rapidly progressive. There is often a precipitant such as preceding viral infection, vaccination, or bee sting, and the syndrome may be seen in association with diseases such as infectious mononucleosis, viral hepatitis, sarcoidosis, lymphoma, and leukemia. The clinical picture is of a rapidly ascending weakness of all four extremities, which frequently progresses to involve respiratory, facial, and bulbar muscles. Sphincter muscles are invariably spared. Sensory loss is usually mild but in some patients may be the dominant feature of the illness. Autonomic neuropathy may be present and in some cases may be severe and life-threatening with sustained or paroxysmal tachycardia or hypertension.

The most important aspect of treatment for this disorder is early diagnosis and admission to hospital, since mild weakness may progress to respiratory failure within hours. The respiratory function and pulse rate must be closely monitored, and assisted ventilation should begin if the vital capacity falls below 1 liter. Meticulous pulmonary hygiene must be maintained. Physical therapy to prevent contractures should begin early, and great care should be taken to avoid complications of prolonged bed rest such as decubitus ulcers and hypostatic pneumonia. If tachycardia or sustained hypertension develops, propranolol should be given. Paroxysmal fluctuations in blood pressure generally require a combination of alpha and beta blockers.

Recovery often begins 1 to 3 weeks after onset, and in these cases the prognosis for recovery is good. Patients whose illness continues to progress for more than 6 weeks are more likely to have a chronic or relapsing course.

Specific therapy for the Guillain-Barré syndrome remains controversial. The role of corticosteroids and ACTH is now in doubt; recent studies show no benefit from these agents and one trial documented a slower recovery in patients treated with prednisone. Steroids also reduce the patient's resistance to respiratory and urinary infection. More recently the use of plasmapheresis has become popular in the management of this condition. This is based on the proposal that weakness is caused by demyelination and conduction block produced by a circulating antibody. If this is so, plasma exchange should be effective because the antibody would be removed by the procedure. Anecdotal reports have described dramatic responses to plasmapheresis. A large multicenter study of the effectiveness of plasmapheresis in Guillain-Barré syndrome has been claimed to demonstrate a statistically significant benefit. Patients undergoing plasma exchange were shown to improve more rapidly and to have shorter hospital stays. On the other hand, two other controlled clinical trials failed to show an unequivocal benefit. Other problems in the use of this therapy are the expense, the inconvenience to the patient, and the potential for anaphylactic reactions to the products used to replace the serum. Because of these uncertainties, recommendations on the use of plasmapheresis in acute inflammatory polyradiculoneuropathies must be tentative. It is not recommended for the patient with mild or improving neuropathy. For the patient with severe (tetraplegia) or rapidly progressive disease a course of plasma exchange (for example, three times a week for 2 weeks) may be given early.

Chronic Inflammatory Polyradiculoneuropathy

In this disorder the initial rate of progression is slower than that in the Guillain-Barré syndrome. The time to maximum disability is greater than 6 weeks in most cases and may be a year or more in some. There is rarely a history of an antecedent illness or other precipitating factor. Other features differentiating the two disorders include nerve thickening, more prominent sensory symptoms, and a more protracted course, sometimes with spontaneous remissions and relapses, in chronic inflammatory polyradiculoneuropathy. Clinical symptoms and signs are otherwise similar; evidence of a generalized neuropathy with proximal weakness is essential to the diagnosis of both. The cerebrospinal fluid protein is elevated and nerve conduction velocities are slowed in both disorders, although these abnormalities are more common and more marked in the chronic form.

Despite the apparent similarities it is important to distinguish this disorder from the Guillain-Barré syndrome because the response to treatment is different. Recent evidence strongly suggests a definite benefit from prolonged prednisone therapy in the chronic form. For moderate to severe disease, a trial of at least 3 months is indicated. Prednisone is given in doses of 120 mg and 7.5 mg on alternate days initially. If a response occurs, the doses are slowly tapered over 9 months, but if there is no beneficial effect after 2 months the prednisone is reduced more rapidly. For patients with less severe disease the potential benefit must be weighed against the risks of long-term corticosteroid therapy such as infection, cataracts, and elevated blood sugar level. Plasmapheresis has been shown in a double blind sham-controlled clinical trial to be beneficial. It, therefore, should be considered in the management of patients with severe disease unresponsive to conventional treatment.

Before making a diagnosis of chronic inflammatory polyradiculoneuropathy, certain conditions that mimic this condition must be excluded. A similar clinical picture with increased cerebrospinal fluid protein may be seen in diabetes, sarcoidosis, various neoplastic disorders (especially lymphoma and paraproteinemic neuropathies), and some of the hereditary neuropathies. These diseases should be sought by careful clinical examination including testing of relatives and appropriate laboratory tests.

MONONEURITIS MULTIPLEX

This distinctive pattern of peripheral nerve disease is characterized by marked asymmetry of limb involvement and is the result of damage of individual peripheral nerves rather than diffuse disease. The nature and distribution of symptoms are determined by the nerves that are involved.

Mononeuritis Multiplex of Gradual Onset

The commonest cause of a slowly progressive mononeuritis multiplex is entrapment or pressure palsies of multiple nerves. Many of the peripheral nerves are vulnerable at well known sites, such as the median nerve in the carpal tunnel, the ulnar nerve at the elbow, the radial nerve in the upper arm, and the peroneal nerve at the fibula head. When these nerves are chronically compressed, symptoms can be alleviated in most cases by surgery and avoidance of maneuvers known to compress these nerves. However, if damage to axons has been severe, recovery will be slow and incomplete.

Several medical conditions predispose to the development of pressure palsies. In rheumatoid arthritis, bony deformities may result in chronic nerve compression and surgery may be necessary to correct the deformity or move the nerve to a less vulnerable site. Hypothyroidism and acromegaly are associated with multiple focal neuropathies, and correction of the hormonal abnormalities leads to rapid symptomatic relief. Amyloidosis may cause local pressure palsies by infiltrating tight compartments. This is most common in the carpal tunnel. Surgical decompression will relieve the compressive neuropathy but there is currently no effective treatment for amyloidosis. Mononeuritis multiplex is also one of the most common manifestations of sarcoidosis involving the nervous system and is often seen in association with large areas of sensory loss over the trunk. This probably represents involvement of thoracic nerve roots. Nerve lesions in sarcoidosis tend to worsen slowly and then gradually recover, but prednisone therapy is usually warranted as it is believed to abbreviate the course of neuropathy and to prevent new lesions from appearing. The recommended dose is 60 mg daily with gradual tapering to 15 mg daily. This dosage should be maintained for several months and then slowly withdrawn.

Lead neuropathy is currently a rare disorder but typically presents as a mononeuritis multiplex with a predilection for the radial nerves. Treatment is discussed in the section on demyelinating neuropathies.

Mononeuritis Multiplex of Abrupt Onset

When a patient develops a flurry of individual nerve lesions with each one evolving almost overnight, the underlying process is usually a vasculitis. Typically, the onset of paralysis is preceded by severe pain and paresthesias, which are often more distressing than the weakness that follows. The clinical picture is easily recognized but the diagnosis can be confirmed on sural nerve biopsy. Even if this nerve is not involved clinically, the pathologic changes of the underlying angiopathy can almost always be demonstrated. Nerve has low metabolic demands and a richly anastomotic blood supply, so angiopathic changes must be extensive before nerve infarction develops.

Many diseases are known to produce this pattern of disease: polyarteritis nodosa and the Churg-Strauss syndrome, rheumatoid arthritis, systemic lupus erythematosus, Sjögren's syndrome, diabetes, Wegener's granulomatosis, cryoglobulinemia, and cranial arteritis. With the exception of diabetes and cryoglobulinemia, these conditions are treated with high doses of prednisone, 60 to 100 mg daily for 2 weeks, then 100 mg on alternate days. Disease progression sometimes occurs on this schedule, so cyclophosphamide, 2 mg per kg, is often added (this use not listed by maker). A high fluid intake is recommended to avoid hemorrhagic cystitis, and regular checks of the blood count and platelet count, blood sugar level, and blood pressure are essential on this drug regimen. The use of cyclophosphamide may permit a lower corticosteroid dose than would otherwise be necessary, and weaning from steroids can often be started earlier.

The management of diabetic mononeuritis multiplex is essentially the same as for other types of diabetic neuropathy discussed previously. Cryoglobulinemia causes nerve infarction by occluding vessels with proteins that precipitate on exposure to the cold. Essential (idiopathic) cryoglobulinemia is best dealt with by simple avoidance of cold exposure, but cryoglobulins produced in plasma cell dyscrasias as a paraprotein often require more aggressive treatment. This is usually directed toward the cause of the paraprotein, but in some cases plasma exchange can be of great benefit in decreasing the total amount of the cryoglobulin.

LARGE FIBER NEUROPATHY

Some peripheral neuropathies cause selective dysfunction of the largest nerve fibers. This produces an easily recognizable clinical syndrome resulting from the loss of proprioceptive sense that travels in these large fibers. Patients with this disorder have a severe ataxia in darkness or with eyes closed. Examination shows disproportionate loss of vibration and joint position sense with relative preservation of pain, temperature, and touch sensations. The inability to sense the position of the joints may cause pseudoathetosis or "searching" movements of fingers and toes, particularly when attempting to maintain a specified posture.

Neoplastic Sensory Neuropathy

In some patients with carcinoma, a slowly progressive large fiber neuropathy occurs and may antedate the diagnosis of the cancer by up to 3½ years. The associated malignancy is almost always an oat cell carcinoma of the lung, but occasional instances of other primary lung neoplasms or carcinoma of the cecum or esophagus are found. The usual symptoms are peripheral numbness and tingling associated with clumsiness and falls due to the sensory ataxia. Treatment of the neoplasm does not appear to influence the course of this neuropathy.

Drug-Associated Sensory Neuropathy

The chronic abuse of nitrous oxide can produce a large fiber neuropathy with sensory ataxia. This is usually found in medical personnel with ready access to the drug but has also been reported with the inhalation of nitrous oxide from canisters used to prepare whipped cream. Cessation of the abuse is generally followed by improvement but a residual deficit may persist. Large doses of pyridoxine (vitamin B_6) can lead to a severe large fiber sensory neuropathy with slow recovery after stopping the drug. Clioquinol, a drug once commonly used for travelers' diarrhea, is thought to be the cause of a degenerative disorder of spinal cord and optic nerves known as subacute myelo-optic neuropathy. An associated large fiber neuropathy has been described but not clearly documented.

Other Large Fiber Neuropathies

Some of the classic causes of this syndrome have already been discussed in earlier sections. These include hypothyroidism, which is associated with a demyelinating large fiber neuropathy that is exquisitely responsive to replacement therapy, and diabetes mellitus, which can cause selective damage to large sensory fibers as well as other types of peripheral neuropathy. Vitamin B_{12} deficiency produces a large fiber neuropathy, but the peripheral abnormalities are often overshadowed by the presence of myelopathy. The treatment of these disorders is described in the appropriate sections.

SMALL FIBER NEUROPATHY

Patients with this type of neuropathy can sometimes cause diagnostic difficulties because pain and discomfort may be severe in the absence of the usual clinical signs of neuropathy. The main complaints are of intense pricking, tingling, and burning pains in the feet and sometimes in the hands. Symptoms of autonomic nervous system dysfunction are also common and consist of postural dizziness, bloating, diarrhea, and impotence in males. Severe autonomic neuropathy may cause urinary and fecal incontinence. Examination reveals normal distal strength and reflexes, whereas sensory testing shows marked impairment of pain and temperature sensation with preserved joint position and vibration sense. Electromyography is often completely normal in the beginning but may show mild abnormalities with progression.

Diabetes. This form of neuropathy is seen most commonly in insulin-dependent juvenile diabetics. Adult diabetics whose blood sugar level is normalized rapidly with insulin may also develop a neuropathy with prominent positive symptoms that may be associated with a less severe dysautonomia. The prognosis for recovery from the painful symptoms is good with satisfactory control of the blood glucose, but recovery from autonomic neuropathy is unusual.

Amyloidosis. The next largest group of patients with small fiber neuropathy are those with primary amyloidosis. These patients are usually middle aged or elderly males with postural syncope, impotence, and impaired sweating. Examination shows decreased pain and temperature sensation. About 90 per cent have an abnormal protein band on immunoelectrophoresis of serum and urine. There is no treatment available at present for this condition. Amyloidosis secondary to myeloma, macroglobulinemia, or chronic inflammation does not often produce this type of neuropathy.

Other Small Fiber Neuropathies

Occasionally, this syndrome occurs in patients with lung cancer. In these cases the autonomic failure may be severe with complete anhidrosis and marked postural hypotension, and peripheral nerve symptoms may be absent. Treatment of the malignancy has been reported to improve the autonomic function. Rare hereditary neuropathies such as Fabry's disease, Tangier disease, and hereditary sensory neuropathy type 1 can present with dysautonomia and the sensory symptoms. Autonomic function may be prominent in acute inflammatory demyelinating polyradiculoneuropathy.

Treatment of Painful Neuropathies

Pain is a prominent feature in some peripheral neuropathies and can be the most distressing part of the disease. The quality of the pain is usually an intense burning or pricking sensation and is often associated with marked hypersensitivity to light touch. Some patients complain of deep-seated aching and pulling sensations or tightness. Certain neuropathies are more prone to produce these sensations than others: the worst offenders are generally axonal degenerations, particularly alcoholic and uremic neuropathies; metal intoxications; and the small fiber neuropathies of diabetes and Fabry's disease. Pain is often severe in nerve infarction resulting from angiopathy and in the neuropathy produced by some drugs such as gold and vincristine. In addition, some patients with very little clinical evidence of neuropathy complain of prominent positive symptoms but do not have the marked loss of pain and temperature sensation and the dysautonomia that characterize small fiber neuropathies. These patients probably have an idiopathic minimal sensory neuropathy.

Treatment of these symptoms can be challenging, as they often do not respond well to conventional analgesics, and there is a real risk of drug dependence developing. Mild symptoms can be relieved by soaking the extremities in cold tap water (about 15C) for 20 minutes. If this is done late in the evening and combined with 600 to 900 mg of acetylsalicylic acid orally, the patient may be able to sleep undisturbed. When more severe symptoms are present, phenytoin or carbamazepine can be tried in standard anticonvulsant doses. Amitriptyline, 25 mg in the morning and 50 mg at night, sometimes provides very effective relief. This can be augmented with fluphenazine (Prolixin), 1 to 2 mg twice daily except in the elderly, in whom there is a significant risk of inducing dyskinesias. Transcutaneous nerve stimulation is often effective at the outset but the benefit is often transient.

ACUTE HEAD INJURIES IN ADULTS

method of
KAMRAN TABADDOR, M.D.,
and THOMAS KAYE, M.D.
Albert Einstein College of Medicine
Bronx, New York

Head injury is the leading cause of death in young adults under the age of 40. The cause of head injury varies according to the population density and socioeconomic status of the community. Auto accidents resulting in head injury are more prevalent in suburban and rural communities, whereas violence is the predominant cause of injury in urban and inner city populations. The clinical importance of the cause of injury is its association with intracranial pathology. Intracranial hematomas are more often observed in the victims of violence and falls.

Sixty to 70 per cent of the head trauma mortalities occur prior to hospital admission. Death in these patients is directly related to the extensive brain injury, which is usually beyond repair. It therefore appears that the most effective means of reducing trauma-related deaths is prevention. The influence of alcohol has been implicated in over 50 per cent of fatal motor vehicle accidents in the United States. Recent efforts to increase the legal age for purchase of alcoholic beverages and to enforce "drunk driver" laws have already produced promising results in many states.

NEUROLOGIC ASSESSMENT

The temporal course of the patient's level of consciousness is particularly relevant; a history of a lucid interval in an unconscious patient strongly suggests an expanding intracranial hematoma. Direct blows to the head are associated with a higher rate of intracranial hematoma formation, whereas acceleration/deceleration injuries more often result in diffuse axonal damage.

The level of consciousness is the sentinel point in evaluating the extent of injury. Certain terms used to describe the patient's level of consciousness, such as "semicomatose," "stuporous," and "obtunded," have different meanings to different examiners and thus are unclear. This confusion can be avoided by recording the patient's response to various intensities of external stimuli. A practical scale has been developed by Jennett and colleagues to quantify the state of consciousness and response to the specific stimuli. The Glasgow Coma Scale (GCS) consists of three components: eye opening, motor response, and verbal response (Table 1). Scores of less than 8 on this scale are an indication of severe brain injury, scores of 9 to 12 indicate moderate brain injury, and scores above 12 suggest a mild cerebral trauma.

TABLE 1. **Glasgow Coma Scale**

Best Verbal Response:	
None	1
Incomprehensible sounds	2
Inappropriate words	3
Confused	4
Oriented	5
Eyes Open:	
None	1
To pain	2
To speech	3
Spontaneously	4
Best Motor Response:	
None	1
Abnormal extensor	2
Abnormal flexion	3
Withdraws	4
Localizes	5
Obeys	6
Total Coma Scale	____

The GCS scores correlate well with both severity and outcome of injury. The most sensitive component of the scale in predicting outcome in severe injuries is motor response. Verbal response more accurately describes the level of consciousness in mild and moderate categories. However, in some circumstance the GCS scores may not reflect the severity of injury. Associated injuries such as bilateral orbital trauma or cervical spinal cord damage can lower the scores inappropriately. Evaluation of verbal response in an agitated, uncooperative, dysphasic, or intubated patient may not be possible. Also, the scale cannot be applied to preverbal children. Furthermore, since the motor score is recorded from the side with the best response, it fails to reflect unilateral deterioration. This can be avoided by recording the motor response of both sides.

Treatment

Early Care of Head Injury

Head injury constitutes a dynamic process and has a variable course depending on both uncontrollable and controllable factors, which if treated appropriately can alter the outcome. Uncontrollable factors include severity of the initial injury, age, pre-existing medical condition, and the mechanism of injury. Severity of injury is the single most important factor determining the outcome, but the contribution of the other factors cannot be overlooked.

Among controllable factors, hypoxia, ischemia, and delay in diagnosis of an expanding lesion deserve special attention. Since the goal of resuscitation and management in these patients is to prevent secondary brain damage, these factors must receive immediate attention. The ability to talk after head trauma implies that the traumatic force exerted on the cranium was not lethal, and if fatal outcome ensues it must be explained by other intervening factors. In patients known to have talked after head injury but who did not survive, hypoxia and shock were the most common extracranial causes; and misdiagnosis or delay in diagnosis of a surgically treatable lesion was the most common intracranial cause of death. Thus every effort must be made to establish an optimal tissue oxygenation and perfusion followed by prompt diagnosis of intracranial pathology. The following therapeutic guidelines take into account these principles.

Resuscitation on the Scene

A well-designed and executed resuscitative protocol is essential for achieving the best potential recovery. The ABCs of trauma management (airway, breathing, circulation) should be applied to every trauma victim. Once adequate ventilation and circulation are established, the patient should be transported to a trauma care facility for definitive management. Delay in transportation to such facilities may result in increasing morbidity and mortality, especially in the case of expanding intracranial lesions.

Upper respiratory tract obstruction is the most common cause of impaired ventilation in comatose patients following head injury. Obstruction may occur when the tongue falls backward or when the mouth and oropharynx are occluded by hemorrhage from facial injuries. Upper airway obstruction may also occur as a result of aspiration of gastric contents. Thus the mouth and oropharynx should be manually cleared of foreign objects and food fragments. The trachea should be suctioned if there is evidence of aspiration. Patients with a depressed level of consciousness may require tracheal intubation. If rapid and smooth intubation is not possible, an esophageal obturator and a face mask can be used. An esophageal obturator will prevent regurgitation of stomach contents and gastric distention during manual ventilation. This technique also obviates the need for turning the patient to a lateral position during transport.

The next step in emergency care is to ensure adequate cerebral perfusion. Sustained hypotension after head injury in adults frequently points to extracranial sources, but transient hypotension shortly after injury is not an infrequent occurrence. In infants, intracranial hemorrhage, particularly if associated with galeal laceration or subgaleal hemorrhage, can lead to hypovolemia. In adults, intracranial hematomas do not reach a volume sufficient to cause hypovolemic shock. Therefore, sustained hypotension in adults is due to other systemic injuries or to brain stem failure. The latter condition commonly is a terminal event. Concomitant spinal cord injury may cause shock secondary to loss of sympathetic tone. This vasoparalysis results in a sudden increase in the vascular bed and pooling of blood volume into the lower extremities. Elevating the legs above the level of the heart or using MAST trousers is the management of choice for this condition.

Emergency Room Management

The resuscitative principles outlined previously should be followed in the emergency department. The oxygen requirement of an injured brain is higher than that of the normal brain. A borderline hypoxia ordinarily tolerated by a normal brain can result in hypoxic damage in the acutely insulted brain. Endotracheal intubation must be considered if both a patent airway and adequate spontaneous ventilation cannot be maintained. Ventilatory adequacy is determined by arterial blood gases. An arterial oxygen partial pressure (PaO_2) of less than 70 mm Hg or an arterial carbon dioxide tension ($PaCO_2$) of greater than 40 mm Hg is an indication for ventilatory assistance. Intravenous administration of succinylcholine prior to intubation can prevent bucking and struggling, which can lead to increased intracranial pressure. The use of this paralyzing agent is not advisable in patients in whom cervical spine stability has not yet been determined, as any stability provided by muscle spasm will be affected by the paralyzing agents. However, cervical fractures are rare when compared with the frequent occurrence of hypoxia in patients with traumatic coma. Therefore, the need for establishing an airway should take precedence over the concern for potential cervical instability.

Hypoxia secondary to neurogenic pulmonary shunting is a common finding in severe head injury and usually responds to positive end expiratory pressure (PEEP). Although there is some evidence that PEEP may increase intracranial pressure (ICP), reduced thoracic compliance and head elevation may prevent such pressure elevation. Improvement in arterial oxygenation and intracranial compliance outweighs the potential deleterious effects of PEEP. If increased pulmonary shunting is secondary to fluid overload, it can be corrected with a loop diuretic such as furosemide. Osmotic diuretics such as mannitol should be avoided in this situation.

Hypotension after injury usually falls into one of the following categories: hypovolemic, neurogenic, vasogenic, and cardiogenic.

Hypovolemic hypotension is the predominant cause of shock in trauma patients. Any systolic blood pressure of less than 100 mm Hg is commonly accepted as evidence of shock. This phenomenon is often seen in patients with multisystem injury with or without external bleeding, such as closed hip fractures or intra-abdominal organ lacerations.

Shock must be vigorously treated with the administration of intravenous fluids. The best replacement is Ringer's lactate, which is similar to extracellular fluid. Along with rapid infusion of 2 liters of fluid, any external source of bleeding should be brought under control. In the absence of cardiogenic or vasogenic shock, blood transfusion is indicated. Blood transfusion not only improves the circulating volume but also increases the oxygen-carrying capacity of the circulation.

Once the patient is fully resuscitated and all system evaluations are completed, the alignment of the cervical spine must be radiographically established before the patient is positioned for other radiographic assessments. Evaluation of the neck is not complete unless all seven vertebrae and their relation with adjacent vertebrae are visualized. With the advent of CT scanning, the indications for obtaining skull x-ray films are limited to such conditions as penetrating injuries, depressed skull fracture, or evaluation of basal skull fractures. About one third of patients with severe head injury may have a normal CT scan initially. Any unexplained deterioration in neurologic condition, even a few hours after the first scan, is an indication for repeat evaluation by CT scanning. This study not only can demonstrate or rule out operative pathology, it can provide information suggesting increased ICP, such as the presence of a midline shift greater than 5 mm, compressed ventricles, or subarachnoid cisterns.

If CT scan demonstrates a surgically treatable lesion the patient must promptly receive appropriate surgical management. Palliative procedures such as exploratory burr hole or twist drill in the emergency department only delay definitive treatment.

Management of Intracranial Hypertension

Increased ICP is the most common pathophysiologic change observed in severe closed head injuries. It is assumed that ICP elevation is the cause of death in most instances. The deleterious effect of elevated ICP is reduction of cerebral blood perfusion. The pressure by which the brain is perfused is the function of mean systemic arterial blood pressure and mean ICP (PP [perfusion pressure] = mean BP − mean ICP). Traumatized brain may require a higher level of perfusion pressure than normal brain. In general a perfusion pressure of 70 mm Hg is desirable. In order to achieve and maintain this level of cerebral perfusion, the determination of ICP is necessary.

ICP can be monitored in one of the three anatomic locations: epidural, subarachonid, and intraventricular. Epidural and subarachnoid monitoring have a lower risk of significant infectious complications. Also brain cannulation and its potential side effects are avoided. However, the high rate of failure and relative lack of accuracy have led most neurotrauma surgeons to use ventricular monitoring as the preferred method. Furthermore, ventricular cannulation permits withdrawal of fluid, which is a useful adjunct to the management of intracranial hypertension. By using the CT scan for ventricular localization, ventriculostomy can be successfully performed in over 80 per cent of the cases.

The infectious complications of ICP monitoring can be minimized by careful attention to sterility at the time of insertion and avoiding prolonged monitoring beyond 3 days. If a longer period of monitoring is required, a new cannula should be inserted, preferably in the contralateral ventricle.

The optimal level of ICP is considered to be 15 to 20 mm Hg. Although higher levels of ICP in some other conditions, such as pseudotumor cerebri, are well tolerated by the patients, any ICP level above 20 mm Hg in head trauma is potentially harmful. ICP values provide useful information only when used in conjunction with other clinical data.

The present experience with ICP monitoring in patients with head trauma has led to the identification of several factors critical in the management of intracranial hypertension. Elevated ICP in the presence of a unilateral mass lesion is associated with a higher morbidity. As a lesion expands, it produces pressure gradients between compartments of the intracranial space, leading to structural displacement and, ultimately, brain stem compression. Displacement of the midline structures is related to the location of lesions within the cranium. Frontal lobe masses commonly are associated with marked elevation of ICP before they manifest clinical signs of brain stem compression. Monitoring ICP in these patients can provide a margin of safety before tentorial herniation occurs. On the other hand, temporal lobe lesions can result in tentorial herniation before ICP levels become markedly elevated. The safety margin is, therefore, quite narrow, and any elevation of ICP requires medical or surgical treatment.

In patients with basilar skull fractures and cerebrospinal fluid (CSF) leaks, ICP does not accurately reflect the influence of an expanding lesion. As the volume of a mass increases, CSF is forced out of the cranium without a significant rise in ICP. Under these circumstances, a normal ICP should not militate against the surgical treatment of a focal intracerebral mass lesion.

Once all surgical lesions are removed, intracranial hypertension should be managed using appropriate pharmacologic agents. The medical treatment commonly employed to reduce ICP is primarily aimed at reducing cerebral swelling and edema. Recent pathophysiologic studies have led to a clear distinction between "edema" and swelling. Brain swelling is defined as an increase in the cerebral blood volume, whereas brain edema is used to describe an increase in water content of the extravascular spaces. Brain swelling results from vasoparalysis and may last from several hours to several days. This hyperemia often leads to vasogenic edema and an additional rise in ICP. The characteristic CT scan finding in cerebral hyperemia is a slight increase in brain density, which can be enhanced with intravenous contrast infusion. The edema, on the other hand, appears as low density expansion of white matter on CT scan and usually develops after 1 day post-trauma.

Hyperventilation

The influence of hyperventilation on ICP is based on reduction of tissue CO_2 and extracellular alkalosis. Hypocapnia directly affects vascular muscles and causes constriction of cerebral resistance arterioles. This results in the reduction of cerebral blood flow (CBF) and blood volume. An acute reduction of 10 mm Hg in the $Pa{CO_2}$ can produce a 22 per cent reduction in CBF. The effect of hyperventilation on ICP begins in less than 1 minute and usually stabilizes within 5 minutes. If hyperventilation is continued, ICP slowly rises and becomes stable after 3 to 5 hours, usually at a level lower than the original pressure. The cerebral vascular response to hypocapnia is markedly reduced or abolished in the presence of hypoxia. Therefore, the shallow rapid respiration of neurogenic hyperventilation, which is commonly accompanied by hypoxia, is ineffective in lowering ICP. In addition, spontaneous hyperventilation leads to fatigue, increased body metabolism, and hyperthermia, all of which in turn raise the cerebral metabolic demand. Under these circumstances it is best to sedate the patient and mechanically control the respiration.

When rapid temporary reduction of ICP is desired, hypocapnia of 25 mm Hg can be effective. For long-term treatment of ICP, $Pa{CO_2}$ levels of around 30 mm Hg may be as effective as lower levels. It is in the early post-traumatic phase that hyperventilation is expected to be most effective. In patients with compromised CBF, the pressure response might rapidly become adapted to hyperventilation.

Steroid Therapy

The purported beneficial effects of steroids in head injury remain controversial. The brain's reaction to impact injury is complex and, depending on the time course, may consist of various combinations of swelling, vasogenic edema, cytotoxic edema, ischemic reactions, and infarcts. Whereas corticosteroids have been reported to be beneficial in treating vasogenic edema associated with brain tumors, abscesses, and cryogenic lesions, the contribution of this form of edema to traumatic head injury is variable. The other pathologic reactions of the brain to injury appear to be unaffected by corticosteroids. Therefore the effect of steroids could vary in different patients.

Dexamethasone (Decadron) is the most commonly used steroid for treatment of central nervous system disease. This preparation has the minimum mineralocorticoid function and does not result in water retention. The conventional dosage used in head trauma is 16 mg daily in divided doses, but higher doses up to 100 mg per day have been suggested under certain conditions. The side effects of steroid therapy include reduction of immune response to infections, particularly opportunistic and nosocomial infections. Specifically, an increased incidence of gram negative pneumonias has been reported. Steroids can also interfere with wound healing by impeding normal collagen synthesis. The incidence of gastrointestinal hemorrhage may be increased with steroid administration.

Diuretics

Various diuretics have been used to lower ICP. The most frequently used diuretic is mannitol. This agent not only reduces ICP, it improves intracranial compliance and CBF. The mechanism by which this agent affects ICP is based on a rapid rise of serum osmolality, which creates an osmotic gradient between blood and brain compartments, facilitating a shift of water from the brain. Areas most likely to respond are those with normal capillary endothelial permeability. In the presence of vasogenic edema, mannitol may shrink normal areas of the brain that are interspersed with edematous tissues.

After a rapid infusion of mannitol over a period of 15 minutes, serum osmolality reaches peak level within 30 minutes. Diuresis begins within 45 minutes followed by a blood brain osmolality equilibrium 4 to 6 hours later. Once equilibrium has been reached, mannitol no longer lowers ICP; hence continuous infusion becomes rapidly ineffective. The ICP reduction is usually noted within 5 to 10 minutes following mannitol administration. This early response cannot be easily explained by the osmotic effect of this agent. Recent studies suggest a vascular mechanism reducing cerebral blood volume resulting in lowered ICP.

The effect of mannitol on ICP is dependent on the serum osmolality. Mannitol is no longer effective when serum osmolality reaches 320 mOsm per liter. Any further increase in serum osmolality can result in intravascular volume contraction, cerebral depression, and metabolic acidosis. It is important that a state of mild dehydration without hypovolemia be maintained. This condition can be controlled by monitoring central venous pressure. If prolonged administration of mannitol is expected or if the patient's cardiopulmonary condition is unstable, a flow-directed balloon (Swan-Ganz) catheter is more desirable. In patients with impending heart failure, mannitol should be used with extreme caution. A nonosmotic diuretic such as furosemide (Lasix) is the drug of choice in this condition. Also, when further diuresis is needed in the presence of high serum osmolality, furosemide (Lasix) can be used.

With the exception of clinical emergencies, mannitol should not be used without monitoring ICP and serum osmolality. The mannitol dose must be titrated according to the ICP. An initial dose of 0.5 gram per kg body weight rapidly infused may effectively lower the ICP. This dose can be repeated every 4 to 6 hours if needed. If more frequent treatment is needed or if this dose fails to control ICP, higher doses up to 1 gram per kg can be used.

Chronic use of mannitol can induce hemolysis and hemoglobinuria, which can result in renal failure. No specific toxic dose has been established for this complication, but a state of dehydration is a major predisposing factor. This complication is commonly reversible with termination of mannitol therapy.

Acetazolamide (Diamox) is another diuretic that is effective in reducing the CSF production. Because of its vasodilating effect on the cerebral vessels, it is not indicated in head trauma management.

Aggressive Management of ICP

If ICP elevation in comatose patients does not respond to hyperventilation, steroids, anticonvulsants, head elevation, and diuretics, more aggressive management is required. CT scan must be repeated to rule out development of a new lesion that requires surgical treatment. Intravenous morphine sulfate can be used for sedation at a rate of 4 to 10 mg every hour. Spontaneous or provoked reflex posture can contribute to ICP elevation. Pancuronium bromide (Pavulon) is an effective agent in eliminating muscle tone and reducing ICP. The effect is usually apparent within 5 to 10 minutes. The initial dose of 0.1 mg per kg can achieve the best result. Subsequent doses can be titrated to produce complete paralysis. The maintenance dose may vary from 0.02 to 0.1 mg per kg every hour.

When using these pharmacologic agents, neurologic assessment is limited to pupillary light reactivity. Under these circumstances extensive physiologic monitoring, e.g., on line arterial pressure, pulmonary artery pressure, and pulmonary wedge pressure, is necessary. Ventricular pressure monitoring provides an added advantage over other methods of ICP monitoring in allowing intermittent fluid withdrawal. Paralyzed patients are unable to clear their bronchotracheal secretions and require a frequent pulmonary toilet. This effect on pulmonary function may be further compounded by dehydration, resulting in thickening of bronchial secretions.

Mild hypothermia (around 35 C) also has a beneficial effect on ICP.

If the previously mentioned treatment fails to control the ICP, pentobarbital (Nembutal) can be utilized. Although the effect of this agent on ICP is adequately demonstrated, its beneficial effect on outcome remains controversial. Adequate hydration is necessary before pentobarbital is administered. Inadequate hydration may result in cardiovascular decompensation and may precipitate hypotension. A pulmonary wedge pressure of 8 to 10 mm Hg usually suggests adequate hydration.

The initial loading dose of pentobarbital is 10 mg per kg administered intravenously over 10 to 15 minutes. The ICP response is usually observed within 5 minutes. If the ICP is not sufficiently reduced, a similar dose can be given in 30 minutes. The maintenance dose varies from 2 to 5 mg per kg per hour. This regimen usually provides a serum pentobarbital level, which should be determined on a daily basis, of 2 to 4 mg per cent. The success of this treatment protocol is dependent on the availability of a well trained professional staff and a well equipped intensive care unit.

Management of Post-Traumatic Epilepsy in the Emergency Room

Post-traumatic epilepsy has been implicated as one of the avoidable causes of death in head-injured patients. The incidence of early post-traumatic epilepsy rises when the head injury is associated with a depressed skull fracture or laceration of the dura and the brain. In penetrating injuries and gunshot wounds, the incidence of seizures is even higher. Other contributing factors are intracranial hematomas, retained intracerebral foreign bodies, infectious processes, and the location of injury. Seizure activity may not only cause respiratory embarrassment but also increases cerebral blood flow and cerebral blood volume, resulting in elevation of ICP. The risk of complications is markedly higher when seizures become repetitive and progress to status epilepticus. Intravenous phenytoin (Dilantin) is the drug of choice to achieve a sustained anticonvulsant effect. Phenytoin should be infused at a rate of 50 mg per minute for a total dose of 15 mg per kg. This slow rate of infusion is required to avoid cardiovascular complications. With this regimen, an adequate blood level is obtained within several minutes. Intravenous phenobarbital may also be used for this purpose, but in order to achieve a satisfactory anticonvulsant effect in a short time sedative doses are required. This effect is not always desirable and may compromise the value of subsequent neurologic examinations.

HEAD INJURIES IN CHILDREN

method of
RICHARD L. WEINER, M.D.,
and HOWARD M. EISENBERG, M.D.
The University of Texas
Galveston, Texas

Management of head injuries can be complex, requiring attention not only to the central nervous system but to metabolic, respiratory, and cardiac systems as well. Occasionally, a child who seems well in the early period following injury may later abruptly develop signs and symptoms of progressive deterioration of central nervous system function. It is essential, therefore, that patients with significant head injuries be cared for in a setting where a neurosurgeon and an anesthesiologist are available full time along with fully trained nursing personnel experienced in handling these problems in the intensive care unit.

INJURIES TO THE SCALP, SKULL, AND MENINGES

Scalp

Simple lacerations are the most common injury of the scalp. Management includes a careful examination of the injured area, looking particularly for foreign bodies. Irrigation of the wound is important and in some patients debridement of scalp edges and deeper tissues may be necessary. Simple lacerations are generally best closed using a single layer of monofilament suture, but in those rare instances of severe laceration or evulsion, rotational skin flaps and skin grafts may be necessary for repair. Bleeding from the scalp may be profuse and in a small child or infant may cause hypotension.

Skull

Injury to the skull is a common result of head trauma in children. Our policy is to have skull x-ray films made on all patients with a history of head injury, although the most common skull injury, the linear skull fracture, frequently occurs without injury to the central nervous system and requires no specific therapy. It is, however, an indication of severity of impact and therefore it is prudent to hospitalize for observation all children with acute skull fractures. We recognize that the incidence of neurologic deterioration in such patients is quite small.

Particular attention should be paid to fractures that overlie dural venous sinuses or cross the middle meningeal artery, as these are more likely to be associated with intracranial hematoma. The signs of the hematoma may not be present on the initial evaluation. Skull fractures below the tentorium also warrant special consideration. Posterior fossa hematomas that occur as a result of trauma are almost always associated with fracture. Hematomas that develop in the posterior fossa, although rare, can cause precipitous brain stem compression and respiratory arrest.

Basilar Skull Fracture and Cerebrospinal Fluid

Fractures at the base of the skull may extend into the air sinuses. These basal fractures are difficult to visualize without special x-ray films and may not be seen even after careful radiologic studies. Hemotympanum and Battle's sign are the most frequent signs of fracture in the mastoid region.

Treatment

Since basal skull fractures may be complicated by bacterial contamination of the meninges, there is a continuing debate as to whether prophylactic antibiotics should be used in these patients. Our current policy is not to use prophylactic antibiotics in cases of uncomplicated basal skull fracture in an otherwise healthy child.

Basal skull fractures can be associated with a tear in the meninges, resulting in a fistula from the subarachnoid space to the exterior. Cerebrospinal fluid rhinorrhea is frequently caused by a fracture of the cribriform plate, whereas cerebrospinal fluid otorrhea is generally due to fractures of the petrous or mastoid portions of the temporal bone. These associations are, however, not invariable and the pathway of the leak cannot be safely assumed until specific diagnostic tests are done.

When an active cerebrospinal fluid fistula is present without evidence of meningitis, treatment initially consists of positioning the child with the head elevated approximately 45 degrees. Infants can be placed in recliners or infant car seats to maintain the elevated head position. If the leak persists, daily lumbar punctures are done to remove 25 to 50 ml of fluid to further decrease the velocity of CSF drainage. Alternatively, a spinal drain can be used for several days. Lumbar punctures and spinal drainage should be used only if no intracranial masses are present.

Prophylactic antibiotic administration remains controversial in that usage may select out resistant nasal or auricular flora contaminating the meninges. Our preference is to avoid using antibiotics unless clinical infection occurs or spinal drainage is used. For CSF otorrhea, the outer edge of the ear canal and auricle is gently cleansed and a small urine or colostomy bag is applied to cover the ear. This allows quantitation of CSF drainage and prevents further wound contamination.

Operative repair, in general, should be delayed at least 10 days, as 85 to 90 per cent of all traumatic CSF fistulas close spontaneously within this time. A workup of persistent CSF fistula should include tomograms or CT scans of the base of the skull to show the associated fracture. Radionuclide cisternography can aid in demonstrating the pathway of the leak. Metrizamide cisternography with CT scanning using 5 mm cuts along the plane of the base of the skull has been useful in demonstrating CSF leaks in the region of the sphenoid and ethmoid sinuses. The treatment of persistent cerebrospinal fluid post-traumatic fistula after anatomic definition of its pathway is operative repair of the torn meninges.

Depressed Skull Fractures

Fractures that distort the contour of the skull require special consideration. These depressed fractures may be associated with scalp lacerations and are then compound. Operative repair should be considered in all patients with compound depressed skull fractures and in those with noncompound fractures in which the depression is greater than 5 mm or in whom a focal neurologic deficit correlates with the fracture site. CT scans or x-ray films with tangential views are frequently necessary to judge the degree of displacement. At one time it was thought that the skull deformity, if not corrected, would press on the growing brain, resulting in a cortical injury and a seizure focus. This argument for repair of these fractures has not been subjected to serious study, and it is probable that when seizures do develop, they are due to damage to the cortex at the time of injury. Not infrequently bone fragments lacerate the dura and sometimes the cortex. This may occur when there are no signs or symptoms of cerebral injury. We consider repair of these fractures to be good practice so that bone fragments can be removed and the torn dura can be repaired.

An unusual sequela of a linear fracture is the growing fracture or "leptomeningeal cyst." This is seen almost exclusively in children under five years of age, and the majority occur in those two years old or younger. They most frequently occur when the edges of the fracture are acutely separated by 4 mm or more. In young children the dura is firmly attached to the skull at the suture lines and those fractures whose edges are widely separated may cause disruption of the dura. This pathologic situation may lead to the formation of an arachnoid cyst or, more commonly, a cerebral cicatrix, which is associated with erosion of the underlying bone and further separation of the bone edges. In some patients the fracture may expand with surprising rapidity within a few weeks after the injury. The management of a young child with a linear skull fracture whose fracture edges are separated by 4 mm or more should include follow-up x-ray films within 3 months after injury. The condition is usually suspected by finding a subcutaneous mass over the fracture site. Once the condition develops, it is progressive and may cause injury to the underlying brain. Correction of these lesions is done by exposure of the fracture and repair of the dura followed by a cranioplasty.

INJURY TO THE CENTRAL NERVOUS SYSTEM

The large majority of traumatic brain injuries are not severe and a full recovery can be expected. Typically, after a fall or other type of impact, there is momentary or brief loss of consciousness. This is generally followed by a rapid recovery of awareness, although in some patients drowsiness may be prolonged. In these children, protracted severe vomiting frequently occurs. This sometimes is the most alarming symptom. Most of the signs and symptoms usually resolve within 24 hours. In young children it may be impossible to document their brief loss of consciousness. Although these injuries usually resolve spontaneously, they do indicate the severity of the impact. Our practice is to admit any child with a history of loss of consciousness or suspected loss of consciousness to the hospital for at least 24 hours of observation, since a very small percentage of them may later develop signs of central nervous system deterioration owing to delayed mass effect.

Although there is almost always a full recovery after these mild injuries, certain transient sequelae may follow. Not uncommonly, these children develop a postconcussion syndrome characterized by feelings of dizziness, headache, and loss of concentration. The symptoms generally resolve within days or weeks. Children with mild head injuries may have deficits documented by neuropsychologic testing, and, although they are usually not severe, they may affect learning and school behavior for varying periods of time.

A small number of children with head injury will have a persistent loss of consciousness. In some of these patients there may be progression of the injury due to brain compression by an intracranial hematoma or the development of brain swelling. These effects are secondary to the initial brain insult. Distinguishing between primary force and secondary compressive injuries is important. In one, the injury is immediate and is due to forces of impact; in the other, the injury is progressive owing to expanding forces of an intracranial mass and may become evident after variable periods. Both types of injury may coexist in the same patient. The second type of injury, although progressive, can frequently be successfully treated by reducing mass effect (e.g., surgical removal of an expanding hematoma). If it is not treated the compression almost always results in hemorrhagic infarction of the brain stem and either a persistent vegetative state or death.

EVALUATION

In the initial evaluation, information about the level of consciousness from the time of injury should be sought. It is also important to know whether seizures have occurred, since these can alter the neurologic state. A good deal of attention is now being paid to the precise description of impaired consciousness. The Glasgow Coma Scale (GCS) has gained wide acceptance as an accurate means of assessing and communicating the patient's level of consciousness (see Table 1 in preceding article, page 765). This scale grades responses in terms of eye opening, movements, and localization. This information can be quickly and unambiguously transmitted to others involved in the treatment of the head-injured patient, thus allowing for continuity of care during the critical eary assessment period. The best response on each of the three criteria is scored, using a numerical system.

The definition of coma, according to the Glasgow group, is that there is no eye opening, even to painful stimuli, and the patient does not obey commands or speak words. Coma in babies (before development of speech) may be defined as no eye opening and an absence of crying or appropriate withdrawal from painful stimulus. Children and adults whose GCS score is greater than 8 are not considered to be in coma by this definition. This distinction is of predictive importance in that patients with GCS scores greater than 8 account for 70 per cent of all head-injured hospital admissions but less than 5 per cent of the deaths. Conversely, patients with GCS scores less than 8 account for only 30 per cent of admissions but greater than 90 per cent of deaths. The scale can be used to describe the impairment of consciousness observed on the initial evaluation and to document progress or deterioration.

PHYSICAL EXAMINATION

After assessment of consciousness, additional specific neurologic signs should be sought. The neurologic examination should also include a search for abnormal patterns of respiration, abnormal position or movements of the eyes, and abnormal motor response. An acute change in vital signs may indicate neurologic deterioration or the presence of a concomitant systemic injury. Hypotension never occurs as a result of an acute brain injury except as a terminal event of medullary failure. One must always look for a source of acute blood loss to explain a low blood pressure. Occasionally, blood loss from large scalp lacerations, especially in infants and small children, may cause hypovolemic shock. The pattern and depth of respiration should be observed; many of these patients have inefficient ventilation and require prompt intubation and assisted ventilation. The Cushing reflex (hypertension with widened pulse pressure and bradycardia) usually occurs as a consequence of elevated intracranial pressure following dramatic changes in level of consciousness. A unilaterally dilated pupil, provided there is no evidence of direct injury to the eye, indicates the presence of an intracranial mass (hematoma and/or swelling) and that temporal lobe herniation has occurred. Frequent serial evaluation of the patient should be used to determine whether there is a progressive neurologic dysfunction.

Eye movements can be evoked in the comatose patient using the doll's head maneuver or caloric stimulation. The doll's head maneuver entails rapid rotation of the head in the horizontal plane from side to side. A stronger stimulus for eye movement is caloric stimulation, which involves injecting cold water into the external auditory canal. In an unconscious patient the doll's head maneuver causes the eys to move in a direction opposite that of the rotation, whereas cold caloric stimulation causes the eyes to deviate toward the stimulated side. Other eye movements or lack thereof generally indicates an injury to the brain stem more severe than one that causes impairment of consciousness alone. The doll's head maneuver should not be done until one has confirmed that there is not an unstable injury of the cervical spine, and cold water should not be injected into the ear unless the tympanic membrane is known to be intact. Flexion of the arms and extension of the legs, the decorticate posture, and extension of both arms and legs generally indicate severe brain stem injury. The initial evaluation should also include a search for other injuries, particularly those of the cervical spine, chest, abdomen, and extremities. There is a need for great urgency in the treatment of these comatose children, and initial treatment should not be withheld until all phases of this outlined evaluation are completed.

Treatment

Initial Management

Our policy is to insert an endotracheal tube in all comatose patients and to control breathing with a ventilator. The correct and aggressive management of the airway and ventilation is the single most important step in the initial management of these patients. Intravenous catheters are inserted, and, unless the patient is hypotensive, intravenous solutions containing saline are given at a slow rate. A nasogastric tube and Foley catheter are inserted. Venous blood samples are submitted for typing and cross matching in the event that an operation becomes necessary and for a complete blood count, BUN, serum electrolytes, and clotting studies (disseminated intravascular coagulation is associated with brain injury). Other routine diagnostic procedures include x-ray films of the skull, cervical spine, and chest.

In our institution all comatose patients routinely undergo CT scanning (without contrast enhancement). Special attention should be paid to the temporal fossa cuts to look for a temporal lobe contusion and extradural hematoma. Occasionally a subdural hematoma may not be readily apparent on CT scanning because its coefficient of absorption is not sufficiently different from that of the surrounding brain. These hematomas may, however, cause a shift of the midline, and the tissues surrounding the hematoma may be visualized by radiographic enhancement techniques. CT scanning also allows visualization of areas of brain contusion and edema.

Of interest, particularly in children, is a scan showing small ventricles without midline shift and with compression or absence of brain stem cisterns. In young patients this brain swelling may be due to engorgement of the cerebrovascular system rather than cerebral edema. This diffuse hyperemia most likely represents a vasomotor paralysis secondary to the impact injury. This feature of the injury may account for sudden neurologic deterioration when the blood volume is rapidly expanded during treatment of shock.

Specific Treatment

This depends on whether there is a mass effect. Mass effect may be due to a hematoma, which in some patients may enlarge after the initial impact, or to edema or vascular engorgement of the brain, which may also develop later. Most patients with significant hematoma also develop cerebral edema. These conditions cause progressive neurologic deterioration of the patient as a result of either compressive forces that produce cerebral herniation and secondary injury to more remote areas of the brain or impairment of cerebral blood flow, causing infarction. Cerebral blood flow is dependent on cerebral perfusion pressure: the difference between the mean intracranial and mean arterial blood pressures. Maintenance of normal systemic blood pressure is critical. Mass effect is detected by neurologic deterioration, masses, shifts, and herniations seen on CT scans and by measured elevation in intracranial pressure.

Many comatose patients with mass effect do not have a hematoma. These patients are the most difficult to manage. In these patients the mass effect is due, as mentioned previously, to cerebral edema or vascular engorgement. It is our practice to continuously monitor the intracranial pressure in all patients in coma with suspected increased intracranial pressure. This is done by either placing a catheter through the skull into a lateral ventricle or catheterizing the epicortical subarachnoid space using a specially designed bolt-like catheter that is fixed to the skull. The pressure is then continuously monitored using a pressure transducer. Arterial blood pressure in these patients is also monitored and the cerebral perfusion pressure is determined. The electrocardiographic and ventilatory movements are also monitored continuously. A concerted effort is made to bring and keep the intracranial presure below 15 mm Hg (200 mm of water)

If there is any evidence of mass effect as indicated by neurologic deterioration, elevation of intracranial pressure, or findings on CT scanning, hyperventilation is immediately started manually or by using a ventilator. The arterial pCO_2 is lowered to 20 to 30 torr. CO_2 is a potent cerebral vasodilator, and lowering the pCO_2 decreases intracranial volume by constricting the cerebral blood vessels, thereby compensating at least temporarily for mass effect. In addition, patients whose conditions are deteriorating are given an osmotic diuretic (mannitol, 0.25 to 1.5 grams per kg as a bolus repeated every 4 to 6 hours as needed, or Lasix, 0.5 to 1.0 mg per kg intravenous bolus). If a significant hematoma (e.g., $>$ 25 ml or causing shift) is found, an operation is virtually always indicated.

The primary measures to control intracranial pressure are intubation, oxygenation, lowering of arterial pCO_2 by hyperventilation, and administration of mannitol or Lasix. Administration of glucocorticoids (Decadron, Solumedrol) has not been shown to be of benefit in acute head injuries, although their use continues at some neurosurgical centers. In some patients, small volumes of CSF can be removed through the ventricular cannula to abort sharp rises in intracranial pressure (CSF should not, however, be removed by lumbar puncture). Small doses of morphine as well as neuromuscular blockade with Pavulon may be useful in controlling intracranial pressure. The patient is kept normothermic using antipyretics or a cooling blanket if necessary.

Despite these efforts, some patients continue to have high intracranial pressure. Elevated intracranial pressure refractory to these measures may be lowered by giving high doses of barbiturates, 3 to 5 mg per kg of pentobarbital (Nembutal) every hour if necessary. Barbiturate levels are measured frequently. An adequate blood level for control of high intracranial pressure is believed to be in the range of 2.5 to 3.5 mg per 100 ml. These drugs should be administered only in an intensive care unit with pressure monitoring equipment staffed by experienced physicians and nurses, and this regimen should be considered experimental.

Our policy is to give all of our patients with severe head injuries anticonvulsant doses of phenobarbital, 3 to 5 mg per kg per day, or phenytoin (Dilantin), 5 to 8 mg per kg per day. The drugs used to decrease mass effect can cause severe abnormalities of fluid and electrolyte imbalance. In addition, these patients are subjected to abnormalities of fluid and electrolyte balance, such as inappropriate antidiuretic hormone (ADH) secretion. Routine care must then also include a strict record of intake and output and monitoring of serum electrolytes and osmolarity.

Outcome

The clinical literature suggesting neuroplasticity in children with resultant significant improvement in neurologic deficit consists of studies of recovery from focal lesions. There is no impressive evidence that the immature brain confers any advantage in withstanding the effects of diffuse cerebral insult. Actually, several studies have shown that residual neuropsychologic deficits are more profound when diffuse head injury occurs in young children as compared with adults.

Apparent good recovery may be misleading if the patient's progress is measured only in terms of resumption of daily childhood activities and motor function, i.e., ambulation. Marked cognitive impairment may result following a severe closed head injury in children.

Neuropsychologic assessment is of great importance in evaluating the long range implications of deficits detected during the early stage of recovery. Impairments in language, memory, behavior, and intellectual ability should be identified. Baseline and follow-up assessments contribute greatly to parental counseling with regard to resumption of school activities (academic and social), evaluating future vocational opportunities, and dealing with social maladjustment problems. We feel that neuropsychologic assessment is indicated during the recovery phase in all severe and moderate head injuries (initial GCS 9 to 12) and in mild head injuries (GCS 13 to 15) if behavior deficits continue beyond 3 to 4 weeks.

BRAIN TUMORS

method of
NICHOLAS A. VICK, M.D.
Northwestern University/Evanston Hospital
Evanston, Illinois

Primary brain tumors inspire justifiable fear out of proportion to their frequency, which, although not inconsequential, is dwarfed by cancers such as those of lung and breast. Approximately 17,000 new instances of primary brain tumors occur in this country each year. Of them, the majority are malignant and fundamentally incurable by current methods. Although it is true that some lower grade gliomas (well differentiated astrocytomas and oligodendrogliomas) can be definitively resected by a neurosurgeon, these comprise less than 10 per cent of this class of primary brain tumors. Most are the malignant gliomas (glioblastoma multiforme and anaplastic astrocytoma), which are surgically inseparable from the brain tissue in which they arose and remarkably resistant to eradication by radiotherapy and chemotherapy.

The concept of malignant disease in the brain is a peculiar one and is different in important ways from cancer elsewhere. For example, meningiomas, which arise from the dura and which comprise approximately 20 per cent of intracranial tumors, are generally benign histologically and eminently curable by surgery. However, they may occur in a position inside the skull that precludes complete surgical resection. At times, they may be unusually destructive, greatly impairing the quality of life and even proving fatal. Location, therefore, is a critical factor in the concept of malignancy with reference to brain tumors. On the other hand, the matter of metastasis, so important in systemic cancer, is a minor issue. Even the most aggressive primary brain tumor rarely metastasizes to distant sites, although some spread to contiguous structures within the brain or to the spinal cord.

There are important differences in the pattern of tumor type and location between adults and childen. Tumors in children occur primarily in the posterior fossa. Among them are some of the most treatment-resistant tumors (medulloblastoma, brain stem glioma) and some of the most responsive and even curable (cystic astrocytoma of the cerebellum). The presenting symptoms in children are usually quite different from those that occur in adults. In children, ataxia, signs of increased intracranial pressure such as nausea and vomiting, and cranial nerve dysfunction predominate. Adults with brain tumors usually present with symptoms of localized cerebral hemisphere dysfunction such as hemiplegia, aphasia, hemianopia, or convulsions. It is fair to say that any healthy adult who has a first convulsive seizure, even if nonfocal on clinical grounds, must be considered to have a brain tumor until disproven by a CT scan with contrast.

Headaches are distinctly less frequent as a presenting symptom than signs or symptoms of localized cerebral dysfunction. Nevertheless, they occur often enough to warrant the concern that a new, persistent headache engenders in both patients and physicians. It has long been recognized that a CT scan is more accurate than the most skilled neurologist's guess as to the possibility of new, persistent, and progressive headaches being the first symptom of a brain tumor.

Except for meningiomas, which occur considerably more often in women than in men, and glioblastoma multiforme, which tends to predominate in men, there are neither important sex patterns, epidemiologic features, nor proven environmental factors that lead to the occurrence of primary brain tumors. Only in neurofibromatosis of von Recklinghausen, which rarely causes intracerebral tumors but which may be associated with some instances of acoustic neuroma (especially if bilateral), is there a known genetic predisposition.

Metastatic brain tumors are somewhat more common than primary brain tumors and, in general, carry a grave prognosis. Untreated, few patients with brain metastases survive more than 3 to 4 months. Radiotherapy is effective for some and is almost always worth doing in that it often doubles useful lifespan. The best prognosis is achieved by surgical resection, followed by radiotherapy, of solitary metastases in patients with small, localized primaries. The decision to resect a solitary metastasis is always a complicated one. Critical factors include the patient's general condition and the location of the tumor within the brain. Unlike the primary malignant brain tumors, metastases are often remarkably demarcated from adjacent brain and can be resected completely as far as can be seen by the surgeon's eye.

Treatment

Steroids

Once the correct diagnosis is made, which is not often a problem in the CT era, initial treatment in almost all cases, whether in adults or children and whether the tumor is a primary or a metastasis, is corticosteroids. This group of drugs has a remarkable effect in reducing the brain swelling that so often surrounds brain tumors, especially those that have grown rapidly such as the malignant gliomas or metastases.

Dexamethasone (Decadron) is the customary steroid to use, although the reasons are less scientific than habitual. Possibly, its remarkably long half-life may be a factor in its perceived special efficacy in reducing peritumoral edema. In acutely ill patients with consequential neurologic signs, large doses, such as 50 mg, should be given intravenously. This should be followed by doses in the range of 8 to 24 mg twice daily. Dexamethasone is well absorbed by mouth and this is always the preferred route when possible.

The beneficial effect is usually evident within 24 hours; if the signs of neurologic impairment do not remit within 48 hours, it can be concluded with a high degree of confidence that the neurologic impairment is due to destruction by the tumor of the affected brain region and not simply peritumoral edema. This is important to know, since to some extent it predicts the results of surgery. Patients who improve dramatically with dexamethasone usually do better.

Oral dexamethasone is almost always well tolerated if it is given with meals. Because of its very long half-life, a twice daily schedule is more than adequate. It has never been established with any degree of confidence that oral corticosteroids induce gastrointestinal ulceration or bleeding. Although almost all physicians insist that patients who take oral corticosteroids use antacids, there is no real evidence that this is of value. Moreover, there is no role whatsoever for drugs such as cimetidine or ranitidine in brain tumor patients. In fact, more than a few experience confusional states when given these drugs, which, possibly, may be due to their increased access to the brain because of altered, hyperpermeable capillaries within brain tumors and in the surrounding brain.

Although a few adult patients present with such marked signs of intracranial pressure that rapid intravenous infusion of mannitol (1 gram per kg) is required, most do not and dexamethasone suffices in the preoperative period. A higher proportion of children require mannitol and even shunt procedures to control intracranial pressure before definitive surgery can be undertaken. This is because their tumors are so often in the posterior fossa and in or near the ventricular system. The long-term use of mannitol presents a number of problems because of systemic fluid and electrolyte balance. This can, at times, be minimized by using lower doses of mannitol on an intermittent basis instead of the usual high dose given as initial treatment in the emergency period.

Surgery

The ideal treatment of a brain tumor consists of its complete surgical removal without damage of contiguous brain tissue. Although this goal, obviously, cannot always be achieved, it is more likely when there have been accurate preoperative studies. CT scanning with anterior-posterior reconstructions may appear sufficient, but many neurosurgeons feel that cerebral angiography is necessary to provide details of blood supply and precise localization. Magnetic resonance imaging (MRI), as it becomes more generally available, will add considerable information, but it seems that this powerful technique's main value in the field of brain tumors will be with tumors within the ventricular system, in or near the midline, and at the base of the brain. Refinements of technique may minimize the sometimes confusing image that results in instances of primary malignant brain tumors and metastases; at present, most of the images do not permit separation of the tumor itself from the surrounding swollen brain.

The neurosurgeon should be expected to resect all that can be safely resected; small biopsies should be avoided if at all possible. There is no question that patients do better when as much tumor as possible is removed. When considerable tumor bulk remains, radiotherapy and chemotherapy are invariably less effective. Although there are some patients who will be considered inappropriate candidates for surgery, such as the very old or those who have major systemic illnesses, almost all patients can, technically, be at least biopsied and a diagnosis thereby established. In fact, if a patient is to be considered for palliative treatment with radiotherapy, it is almost always wrong to proceed without a tissue diagnosis. Even the most inaccessible-appearing lesions can be safely biopsied by neurosurgeons who are experienced with stereotactic procedures that are linked with CT scanning.

Although the CT appearance of most brain tumors is reasonably characteristic, this radiologic tool does not provide a histologic diagnosis. Radiotherapy is too potent to deliver in error to patients with evolving infarctions, brain abscesses, unusual infections, and focal demyelinating disorders. These conditions will, at times, appear indistinguishable from a brain tumor by CT.

Radiotherapy

After surgery, treatment will vary considerably depending upon the type of tumor found and its anatomic location. Most meningiomas and acoustic neuromas, as histologically benign extra-axial neoplasms, will be "cured." However, it is wise to plan periodic follow-ups of these patients. There is, at times, recurrence, especially if any tumor tissue has been left behind because of inaccessibility or adherence to vital structures such as dural sinuses. Patients with solitary metastases, glioblastoma multiforme, and anaplastic astrocytoma should all have postoperative radiotherapy even when gross total resection has been achieved. There is ample evidence in the literature to indicate that useful lifespan is doubled and recurrence is considerably retarded. Careful fractionation of dosage and avoidance of a total dose greater than approximately 6000 rads are critical in the effort to avoid radionecrosis of normal brain tissue. Primary brain lymphoma usually responds well, at least initially, to much lower doses of radiation, but other malignant brain tumors are undertreated with much less. Dexamethasone can usually be tapered down and off within 2 weeks after surgery. There is no clear evidence that maintenance of low dose dexamethasone during radiotherapy provides any real benefit.

During radiotherapy only a few patients will experience transient symptoms such as nausea and lethargy. Except for hair loss, which is a sensitive matter that should always be fully discussed ahead of time, this mode of treatment is well tolerated. Unfortunately, at doses the brain can tolerate, complete control or cure is extraordinarily rare. Studies are being conducted to determine if a neutron boost to the tumor bed is more effective than photons alone. Interstitial radiation via surgical implantation is also being studied for recurrent tumors and as primary postsurgical treatment. In children, radiotherapy may alter intellectual development. This is a problem of major concern. Radiotherapy to the spine may lead to growth delay, such as is seen with some instances of medulloblastoma where treatment of the entire neuraxis is usually recommended. In adults, there is a disturbing incidence of blunting of immediate memory function and intellectual acuity after radiotherapy. These changes may be subtle and difficult to distinguish from the effects of the tumor itself. There are, of course, instances of radionecrosis of brain, especially in the area of brain adjacent to the tumor, even when radiotherapy has been properly delivered with fractions of less than 200 rads daily and with a total dose not in excess of 6000 rads. It seems likely that external beam radiation has reached its limit in efficacy, given the almost exponential increase in the incidence of radionecrosis when dosages greater than 6000 rads are given.

Control of Seizures

Convulsive seizures are a major problem for many brain tumor patients. Although not all patients present with seizures, almost all are given phenytoin (Dilantin) after surgery because of the relatively high incidence of seizures thereafter. The side effects of phenytoin are usually inconsequential in adults who are managed properly. A clear understanding on the part of the patient as to the nature of potential effects of excessive dosage, such as ataxia, is important. Plasma levels should be kept in the range of 15 to 20 micrograms per ml. The daily need of phenytoin for an adult varies from 200 to 700 mg; most patients are adequately managed with a dosage in the range of 300 to 400 mg daily, but this can be established only with plasma levels. The very long half-life of phenytoin permits the total daily dosage to be given once daily, such as at bedtime.

Carbamazepine (Tegretol) is just as effective as phenytoin and, despite its reputation to the contrary, actually has slightly fewer side effects. There is really no reason why it should not be used more frequently except for its cost and the unwarranted fears of hematologic toxicity. It is easier to adjust to its therapeutic plasma range of 8 to 12 micrograms per ml than phenytoin because of more orderly kinetics, but its shorter half-life demands that it be given in at least three separate daily doses. Phenobarbital, primidone, and clonazepam should be considered adjunctive drugs for those patients who do not achieve complete control of their seizures with phenytoin or carbamazepine. Now and then, patients who are intolerant of or allergic to these two major drugs will need to be managed primarily with one of these alternatives. As is true in the management of seizures of any cause, it is best to work with one drug alone to its maximal potential benefit before prescribing two simultaneously.

Chemotherapy

After radiotherapy, it is reasonable to consider chemotherapy for certain types of brain tumors. There are several promising experimental protocols for medulloblastoma and other childhood tumors. Generally, chemotherapy is not considered for the lower grade gliomas in adults, but most patients with glioblastoma multiforme and anaplastic astrocytoma should be encouraged to participate in experimental treatment protocols. Without chemotherapy, the current median survival of glioblastoma patients is approximately 8 months. Anaplastic astrocytoma, which is differentiated from glioblastoma histopathologically only on the basis of its lacking areas of necrosis, leads to a median survival of approximately 28 months. Obviously, the two must be considered separately, and the blurring of the diagnosis that occurs with the outmoded and simplistic Roman numeral grading scheme should be avoided. It has been amply clear for many years that younger patients do considerably better and, indeed, that age seems to be the most important variable in overall prognosis for adult patients in both groups.

Intravenous nitrosoureas, such as BCNU, are the most commonly used drugs at present for the malignant gliomas. Others are being studied for their efficacy, and there is reason to believe that treatment with multiple drugs, such as has become customary with many systemic cancers, will yield more favorable results. The relative impermeability of brain tumors to drugs in the blood stream remains a major impediment to the use of many of the water-soluble drugs in regular use for systemic cancers. Most chemotherapeutic agents being tried for malignant brain tumors are lipid soluble and can enter normal brain as well as the brain tumor. This poses a considerable problem for intra-arterial chemotherapy. There are a disturbing number of instances where tumors are controlled but the normal brain is injured by intra-arterial BCNU. This appears to be true of dosages that, when given intravenously, do not seem to cause detectable adverse effects on normal brain. It remains to be seen whether lower doses of intra-arterial BCNU and other lipid-soluble drugs will prove to be as efficacious as when given by the intravenous route. In general, it is fair to say that chemotherapy of brain tumors has been both disappointing and difficult, although there is no question that, for unknown reasons, about 10 per cent of patients will respond very well. Immunotherapy trials, being conducted at a few centers, are in their infancy, although there is intensive research in this area.

Follow-up

Perhaps the main advantage for most patients with malignant brain tumors who are referred for postradiation chemotherapy is the increased likelihood of their being involved with a comprehensive care program. Total care of brain tumor patients is complex and demanding. All too often, they slip between the specialties of primary care, neurosurgery, neurology, and oncology. Their problems are just too complicated and have too great an impact upon quality of life issues to be left at loose ends. Even those patients with less aggressive tumors who do well need to be followed at intervals. Their problems can range from seizures to the need for rehabilitative efforts, both physically and psychologically.

Now and then the decision needs to be made about reoperation, not only for recurrent low grade tumors but also for the occasional patient with a glioblastoma, anaplastic astrocytoma, or metastasis who might be best managed with a second operation. Although the risks of reoperation are somewhat higher than those of the primary procedure, well selected patients can, at times, be greatly helped. It is not as difficult as it might seem to suggest reoperation, since modern neurosurgery usually goes so well that patients and families do not look back at the first procedure with dread. Neurosurgical morbidity is almost always slight as compared with intra-abdominal procedures; it is the diagnosis, not the surgery, that causes the anguish.

When malignant brain tumors recur despite radiotherapy and chemotherapy—and they usually do—the human suffering is considerable, the cost high, and the outcome invariably fatal. Sometimes, enormous doses of dexamethasone, up to 50 mg twice daily, will maintain function for a few months, although the price to pay for this is usually unacceptable. Patients become grossly cushingoid in appearance, may suffer pathologic spine fractures, and may have difficulties with steroid-induced diabetes mellitus and myopathy. Steroid-induced hypokalemia, which may not be reflected by the serum potassium, can easily be overlooked, and it is often useful to provide oral potassium supplementation of this predominantly intracellular cation.

The terminal brain tumor patient rarely suffers. His family suffers as they watch progressive neurologic impairment give way to coma from increased intracranial pressure. Sensitive and realistic families and physicians will stop dexamethasone when it becomes clear that there is no hope to maintain quality of life. At this point, it is often worthwhile to increase the dexamethasone dosage significantly for a trial period of 3 days to establish whether there will be benefit. If not, it is then easier to arrive at a definite decision to withdraw the drug completely, since lack of improvement strongly suggests that the impairment and decline are due to the tumor itself and not to edema.

Section 14

The Locomotor System

RHEUMATOID ARTHRITIS

method of
JOHN T. SHARP, M.D.
University of Colorado
Denver, Colorado

Rheumatoid arthritis is a complex disease with many manifestations and a variable course. Successful treatment requires an understanding of the natural history of the disease and a careful analysis of the patient's problems. It is especially important to determine whether the main symptoms are the consequence of active inflammation in the joints, are the result of systemic effects of the illness, or are due to destruction of articular cartilage and bone from long-continued inflammation. Appraisal of the status of the articular system usually can be accomplished by a thorough history and physical examination without resorting to histologic study. Prolonged morning stiffness, easing of stiffness and pain with mild exercise, prominent synovial effusions, an excess of synovial tissue, and tenderness to gentle pressure are features indicating active inflammation. On the other hand, the presence of instability and severe degrees of crepitation represents destruction of cartilage and the supporting tissues that has reached an irreversible stage rather than current inflammation. Additional evidence of joint damage can be obtained by radiologic examination to determine the extent of cartilage destruction and bony erosion. In general, early disease is associated with active inflammation, but in this context, "early" refers to the stage of illness and not to elapsed time from onset, since there is great variability in the rate of progression of disease in different patients. Patients with intermittently active arthritis, namely, patients who have periods with symptoms and signs followed by the complete disappearance of active inflammation, either do not have serious damage to their joints or have minimal, slowly progressive changes. In contrast, those patients in whom inflammation is continually present for many months or years usually develop serious sequelae.

Treatment

The treatment of rheumatoid arthritis should be considered under several broad headings: the general program, physical therapy, occupational therapy, drug therapy, and surgical therapy. The general program includes a regular, normal diet with some adjustment of calories if the patient needs weight reduction or gain. Much has been written in the lay literature about diet and arthritis, and much of it is nonsense. Unfortunately, many arthritis patients are grasping at straws for help and may adopt dietary habits that are potentially dangerous. For this reason, dietary history should be reviewed and the importance of normal nutrition stressed. The patient should get a regular night's sleep; when the disease is particularly active and fatigue is an important symptom, added periods of rest during the day are helpful.

Patient education is essential. Psychologic support is usually provided by the rheumatologist or primary care physician, but specialized help may be required.

Physical therapy is regularly prescribed to maintain muscle strength and a normal range of joint motion insofar as possible. The importance of an active physical therapy program cannot be overstated. General body conditioning is as central to maintaining a sense of well-being in arthritis patients as it is in healthy people. In addition, a full range of motion exercise program for each individual joint will help to preserve joint function. The help of an occupational therapist is enlisted to instruct the patient on methods of protecting inflamed and weakened joint structures, to review activities of daily living, and to suggest devices to improve function, when needed.

Drug Therapy

Many drugs have been advocated for the treatment of rheumatoid arthritis. None is curative, and none is universally effective. Many have serious side effects. In spite of these limitations, appropriate use of available agents will ease the pain of arthritis and improve function, and some may slow the progression of the disease. In this discussion, drug therapy will be considered in terms of analgesics, anti-inflammatory agents, drugs that appear to be relatively specific in reducing the inflammation of rheumatoid arthritis, steroids, and cytotoxic agents.

Use of an appropriate, well-tolerated, *nonsteroidal anti-inflammatory drug (NSAID)* is indicated in all patients with rheumatoid arthritis who have active synovitis. This group of drugs has proliferated in recent years, and a large number are now available. There are seven classes of NSAIDs based on chemical composition (see Table 1). Aspirin is the oldest, best known, and, in the past, most frequently used NSAID. There is no evidence that its effectiveness in rheumatoid arthritis is surpassed by any of the newer agents. Unfortunately, aspirin causes a slight increase in blood loss through the gastrointestinal tract in virtually all patients, and occasionally, serious bleeding occurs. For that reason, enteric-coated or buffered aspirin is preferred.

Patients who have a history of peptic ulcer disease or gastritis or a previous episode of gastrointestinal bleeding are given one of the propionic acid derivatives instead of aspirin. These latter agents appear to be equally effective when used in the recommended doses. Those with a longer half-life are more convenient because administration can be reduced to every 8 or 12 hours. Recommended doses and intervals of administration are shown in Table 1. Although these drugs are no more effective than aspirin, they are effective substitutes in patients in whom aspirin is contraindicated.

The indole derivatives are another class of NSAID represented by three agents: indomethacin (Indocin), sulindac (Clinoril), and tolmetin (Tolectin). These drugs may be used instead of aspirin, but they are no more effective and their gastrointestinal toxicity is similar. Renal side effects may be more frequent.

Piroxicam (Feldene) is the only drug in the oxicam class currently available. This drug has the advantage of having a long half-life, so it can be given once daily. Phenylbutazone is no longer recommended because of serious side effects. Acetaminophen (Tylenol) appears to be less po-

TABLE 1. **Drug Therapy for Rheumatoid Arthritis**

Drug	Total Dose (mg)	Half-Life (hrs)	Recommended Frequency of Administration
*NSAIDS**			
ASA and other salicylates	3000–4000/day	3–30†	every 4–6 hrs
Propionic acid derivatives			
Ibuprofen (Motrin, Rufen)	1200–2400/day	2	″ 3–6 hrs
Naproxen (Naprosyn)	500–1000/day	13	″ 8–12 hrs
Fenoprofen (Nalfon)	1200–3200/day	3	″ 6–8 hrs
Ketoprofen (Orudis)‡	100–200/day	1–4	″ 12 hrs
Indoles			
Indomethacin (Indocin)	50–200/day	2	″ 3–6 hrs
Sulindac (Clinoril	300–400/day	8	″ 12 hrs
Tolmetin (Tolectin)	600–1200/day	1	″ 3–6 hrs
Oxicams			
Piroxicam (Feldene)	10–20/day	>30	″ 24 hrs
Phenylbutazone	Not recommended	>80	″ 24 hrs
Meclofenamate sodium (Meclomen)	200–400/day	2–3	″ 4–6 hrs
Acetaminophen	2000–3000/day	1–3	″ 4–6 hrs
SAARDs§			
Gold (Myochrysine, Solganal)	25/wk	Not relevant to current practice	″ wk
Penicillamine	250–750/day	″	″ 24 hrs
Hydroxychloroquine (Plaquenil)	200/day	″	″ 24 hrs
Methotrexate	7.5–15/wk	″	″ wk
Azathioprine (Imuran)	75–200/day	″	″ 24 hrs
Cyclophosphamide (Cytoxan)‖	75–150/day	″	″ 24 hrs
Chlorambucil (Leukeran)‖	4–8/day	″	″ 24 hrs
Steroids	Recommended for limited situations. Dose and frequency of administration highly variable.		
Experimental Agents			
Total lymphoid irradiation			
Lymphopheresis			
Plasmapheresis			

*NSAIDs = nonsteroidal anti-inflammatory drugs.
† Dose-dependent. Longer half-life associated with higher doses.
‡ Not available in United States at time of writing.
§ SAARDs = Slow-acting antirheumatic drugs, some of which have been demonstrated to be disease-modifying agents.
‖This use is not listed in the manufacturers' directive.

tent than the other drugs, and its long-term use may be associated with renal disease. It has the advantage of being well tolerated in the gastrointestinal tract.

In general, all the drugs in the NSAID class appear to be interchangeable when treating rheumatoid arthritis. However, when satisfactory response is not obtained with a particular drug, a trial of another agent in another class may provide relief. On some occasions, drugs may be combined with added benefit. In general, combinations should include drugs from different classes. Feldene is not combined with aspirin because of the reported increased incidence of gastrointestinal complications.

NSAIDs are well tolerated by most patients, but occasionally serious toxicity occurs. Gastritis, gastrointestinal bleeding, toxic hepatitis, reduced renal blood flow, interstitial nephritis, and renal failure are serious complications that are occasionally seen.

Most of the anti-inflammatory agents are also analgesic. In some instances, an additional analgesic is helpful, but unfortunately, most of the potent analgesics are addictive. Even Darvon and Talwin are habit-forming and, if used to excess, can produce physiologic addiction. For this reason, only occasional use of Darvon is recommended, and the drug is never used on a regular schedule. Talwin has little or no advantage over narcotics.

NSAIDs usually effect a significant decrease in morning stiffness and improve comfort and function. Unfortunately, their effectiveness is limited, and in many patients progressive joint damage occurs if these drugs are used alone. Therefore, if active synovitis continues for 6 to 12 months, a *slow-acting antirheumatic drug* (SAARD) is recommended. This class of drugs includes gold, penicillamine, and chloroquine. Each has been demonstrated in controlled trials to be effective in relieving the symptoms of rheumatoid arthritis. In addition, gold therapy slows the progression of radiologic changes. Effectiveness of these agents is usually not apparent for 2 to 6 months. Their mechanism of action is not known, but all affect lymphocyte function in vitro and thus may alter immune responses.

Gold therapy is routinely given weekly for a period of 20 to 40 weeks, using a dose of 25 mg gold sodium thiomalate or gold sodium thioglucose. During this time, a detailed joint examination defining the extent of active synovitis is performed monthly. If the disease goes into complete remission, the frequency of injections is reduced to every 2 weeks for a period of 4 to 6 months. Then, if the patient remains in remission, the frequency of injections may be reduced to every third or fourth week. If active synovitis recurs in the course of this reduction, weekly injections may be resumed in an attempt to suppress the flare-up. Thereafter, the optimal interval of injections is reassessed. If no benefit is observed after 40 weeks of injections, gold therapy is discontinued. Throughout the duration of weekly injections, the patient is examined by the physician prior to each injection to exclude toxic reactions, the most prominent of which include stomatitis, dermatitis, pruritus, diarrhea, agranulocytosis, thrombocytopenia, and nephritis. Weekly white blood cell counts and differentials, platelet counts, and urinalyses are monitored.

When *penicillamine* is used, therapy is begun with 250 mg daily. At 6- to 8-week intervals the dose may be increased to 500 mg, and then 750 mg, daily if response is not optimal on the lower dose. The patient is examined for skin rash, mouth ulcers, muscle weakness, and respiratory symptoms biweekly until the dose has been stabilized for 3 months, and then monthly thereafter. Initially, blood counts and urinalyses are checked weekly, and frequent monitoring is continued until the dose is stabilized. Later, laboratory tests are done at the same interval as the examination.

Hydroxychloroquine is used in patients who have mild but persistent disease with progression of x-ray changes and who either failed to respond to gold or penicillamine or had toxic reactions that precluded their use. Hydroxychloroquine is given in a dose of 200 mg daily. Although serious ophthalmic toxicity is uncommon with this dose, a complete ophthalmologic checkup must be completed before starting treatment and repeated at 6-month intervals.

Glucocorticoids, when given in large doses, relieve the inflammation of rheumatoid arthritis. Unfortunately, effective steroid doses regularly induce hypercorticism. In many patients these effects are worse than the original disease, and in some the side effects are disastrous. For these reasons, systemic corticosteroid therapy is not recommended.

Immunosuppressive drugs used in the treatment of rheumatoid arthritis include cyclophosphamide (Cytoxan), azathioprine (Imuran), and methotrexate (this use of cyclophosphamide and methotrexate is not listed by the makers). Cyclophosphamide has been associated with an increased incidence of tumors and, therefore, its use is limited to patients with life-threatening episodes of systemic vasculitis associated with rheumatoid arthritis. Imuran is suspected of causing an increased incidence of tumors, although this side effect is not well documented. Its use is not recommended when other agents are available.

Methotrexate has recently been shown in short-term trials to provide significant relief of the pain and discomfort of synovitis in rheumatoid arthritis. Long-term studies have not determined whether the disease progression is altered. Unfortunately, the drug is potentially quite toxic, with serious depression of bone marrow occurring acutely and liver and lung disease occurring with chronic use. Because of its potentially serious toxicity, its use is reserved for patients who have not responded to, or have not tolerated, gold, penicillamine, or hydroxychloroquine. The drug is given once weekly in a dose of 2.5 mg the first week and, if well tolerated, 7.5 mg the second week. This dose is continued for 6 to 8 weeks. Liver function tests are obtained prior to beginning therapy and every 3 months thereafter. A complete blood count is done before treatment and weekly during treatment. If the drug is well tolerated at 7.5 mg weekly, the dose may be gradually increased at monthly intervals if the initial response is not satisfactory, but a total dose of 15 mg per week is rarely exceeded. Patients should be advised not to use alcohol while taking methotrexate. Depression of the leukocyte count requires adjusting the dose downward or discontinuing medication. Significant abnormalities of liver functions require discontinuing the drug or performing a liver biopsy. Unfortunately, the prognostic value of minor changes in the liver biopsy in determining the safety of continued therapy is not clear. Some physicians recommend periodic liver biopsy even if liver function tests remain normal, since progressive fibrosis may occur in spite of normal tests. However, experience is too limited to judge whether regular biopsies are necessary to give the drug safely for prolonged periods.

Surgery

Although most patients have disease in many joints and drug therapy is the preferred mode of preventing progression, in some instances a synovectomy may provide relief of inflammation localized to a single joint. However, the number of joints that are easily accessible to thorough synovectomy, which is required to produce lasting benefit, is somewhat limited. The procedure is frequently successful only in the knees, ankles, elbows, and wrists.

Patients who have disease that has already produced deformities and destruction of cartilage and bone must be analyzed carefully to determine whether inflammation is a continuing process. At this stage, these patients usually have had disease for several years. If, in addition to the permanent damage there are physical signs of active inflammation, they may benefit from drug therapy, particularly if previous therapy was inadequate. If surgical correction of deformities is indicated, it is often wise to delay surgery to permit the suppression of active inflammation by treatment.

In patients who have deformities and radiologic changes, but in whom the inflammation has subsided, the permanent changes in the cartilage, bone, and supporting structures will not be affected by drug therapy, and surgical reconstructive procedures may be the only treatment to consider. Such procedures, at the present time, are generally extensive and often require total joint replacement with a prosthetic device. The most successful of these has been the total hip prosthesis. Somewhat less successful, but remarkably good in properly selected patients, have been the total knee and the shoulder prostheses. Still under study are total joint replacement procedures for ankles, wrists, and elbows. Hand surgery often provides cosmetic benefit, but the functional improvement may be limited.

Other forms of surgical therapy are occasionally useful. Total joint replacement procedures have reduced the necessity of performing arthrodeses in most joints, but fusion is still the mainstay of treatment for the patient with severe cervical subluxation and occasionally may be the appropriate treatment of subtalar subluxation and instability.

Proper analysis of each patient's problems, with application of the appropriate therapeutic regimen, will provide some relief for most, will slow or halt progression of disease during the inflammatory phase in many, and can restore major degrees of functional ability in those with "burned-out" disease.

JUVENILE RHEUMATOID ARTHRITIS

method of
JERRY C. JACOBS, M.D.
Columbia University
New York, New York

The goals of treatment for juvenile rheumatoid arthritis are to (1) control pain, if present; (2) suppress signs and symptoms of inflammation; (3) maintain or improve motion and function; and (4) promote physical, emotional, and intellectual growth. Achievement of these goals will be facilitated by positive functional physician attitudes, and by education of the patient, parents, siblings, and teachers about the nature and management of this disorder. Education need not be the exclusive responsibility of the physician. A considerable amount of educational materials (pamphlets, books, slide/tape packets) suitable for patients, parents, and teachers is available through the Arthritis Foundation locally and nationally.

Regardless of onset pattern, the long-term prognosis for most patients is excellent. Twenty-eight per cent of patients recover completely within 5 years and greater than 75 per cent of patients properly treated have good function after 10 years of disease, even if all signs of active disease have not disappeared. The functional prognosis is poorest for those who have systemic polyarticular onset or rheumatoid factor.

Drug Therapy

Salicylates. Aspirin (ASA), slow release aspirin (Zorprin, Encaprin, Ecotrin capsules), salicylsalicylic acid (Disalcid), or choline salicylate (Arthropan, Trilisate), in doses of 90 mg per kg per day, is safe and usually sufficient. Suppression of synovitis, as well as fever, rash, and generalized toxicity, is best accomplished with constant anti-inflammatory doses of salicylates. These should be given in regular divided doses to achieve a steady-state blood salicylate level of around 25 mg per dl. It will require 7 to 10 days of constant administration to achieve a steady state. Systemically ill patients often require higher doses. Antacids lower serum levels and are unnecessary.

ASA hepatotoxicity, manifest by mild elevation of liver enzymes without other symptoms, is not an indication to discontinue the drug. It occurs usually at full anti-inflammatory doses, with serum salicylate levels in excess of 25 mg per dl. Reduction of the dose is usually sufficient to allow correction of the enzyme elevation. Other toxic effects of aspirin include rare bleeding, and bruising from hypoprothrombinemia. The possible relationship of aspirin therapy to Reye's syndrome remains to be determined. Signs and symptoms of salicylism in children include change in personality (irritability, lability, depression), nausea, vomiting, and hyperpnea. These symptoms require determination of the salicylate level and temporary discontinuation of the drug. Monitoring salicylate and serum transaminase (SGOT and SGPT) levels should minimize the chances of salicylism.

Other Nonsteroidal Anti-Inflammatory Drugs (NSAIDs). At present, only tolmetin sodium (Tolectin) and naproxen (Naprosyn) have been approved for general use by children under 14 years of age. These drugs are as effective as anti-inflammatory doses of ASA in suppressing synovitis. These drugs are useful for children who do not tolerate ASA, or who have hepatotoxicity from aspirin. Occasionally, some children with JRA respond better to tolmetin or naproxen than to salicylates. The dose of tolmetin is 20 to 30 mg per kg per day in four divided doses or 10 to 15 mg per kg of naproxen in two or three divided (8 to 12 hr) doses daily. The most common toxicities include gastrointestinal irritation, headache, rash, and ulcers. Indomethacin (Indocin), 2 mg per kg per day in four divided doses, may also be used in severe cases.

Remission-Inducing Drugs. Salicylates and other nonsteroidal anti-inflammatory drugs suppress inflammation but do not prevent progressive joint damage. However, gold, antimalarials, and D-penicillamine may occasionally induce remission of disease and may sometimes modify the long-term outcome. Because JRA has a generally better prognosis than does adult rheumatoid disease, these drugs are less frequently required. Due to the complexity of these drugs and the probable progressive nature of the disease, it is advisable to seek a consultation before starting.

Antimalarials. Though not listed in the manufacturer's directive, hydroxychloroquine (Plaquenil) is prescribed by rheumatologists for JRA patients who have persistent chronic synovitis despite an adequate conservative program. The effectiveness of this drug has been established in adult rheumatoid disease but is only presumed in JRA. The dosage is 3 to 5 mg per kg per day. It should be added to the previous regimen and not used instead of it. A trial of at least 4 to 6 months is necessary to assess efficacy. Gastrointestinal distress (usually diarrhea), rash, bleaching of hair, and mild photosensitivity represent the major toxic effects. Retinal toxicity is a potential hazard from long-term use and requires special ophthalmologic examinations every 3 months.

Gold Salts. In patients who have failed to get good suppression of synovitis from the previous regimen, one can use gold salts instead of hydroxychloroquine. There is equal effectiveness between gold sodium thiomalate (Myochrysine) and gold thioglucose (Solganal), both of which are administered by deep intramuscular injections weekly. One begins with 0.25 mg per kg for the first two doses and increases to 1 mg per kg thereafter for 20 to 26 weeks. If there is good objective improvement of synovitis, a decrease in the number of joints involved, and a fall in the erythrocyte sedimentation rate (ESR), the injections should be decreased to every 2 weeks and subsequently, if possible, to monthly. Before every injection, the patient should be observed for rash (or pruritus) and stomatitis. A blood count, platelet count, and urinalysis should be obtained prior to commencing the course of gold and before every injection thereafter.

A decrease in hematocrit of 4 per cent or more, a 50 per cent or greater decline in white blood count (WBC) or total neutrophil count (TNC), a WBC of less than 4500 and a TNC of less than 2000, a platelet count of less than 100,000, or eosinophilia over 10 per cent requires withholding the gold injections. Proteinuria of 2+ or more that is confirmed also requires withholding gold. Definite marrow or renal toxicity caused by gold interdicts any retrial of this agent. However, if mild-to-moderate stomatitis or dermatitis occurs, gold can be cautiously reintroduced when the toxic manifestations have fully cleared. Other uncommon gold toxicities include vasomotor reactions, diarrhea, pneumonitis, and corneal chrysiasis. An oral preparation of gold, auranofin (Ridaura), is under clinical investigation for juvenile rheumatoid arthritis. Patients with systemic JRA may be at risk for consumption coagulopathy after the second injection of gold; this is potentially fatal.

D-Penicillamine. Another slow-acting, possibly remission-inducing drug is D-penicillamine (Cuprimine, Depen). (Manufacturer's warning: Effectiveness of D-penicillamine in juvenile rheumatoid arthritis has not been established but is being evaluated in a clinical trial.) Its benefits have been established in adult rheumatoid disease but are still not certain in JRA. It is administered orally at a dose of 2.5 to 5.0 mg per kg per day for 6 to 12 weeks. If well tolerated and benefit is incomplete, the dose is increased to 5.0 to 7.5 mg per kg per day. At subsequent 6 to 12 week intervals, the dose can be progressively increased to a maximum of 10 mg per kg per day. Clinical observation of at least 6 months is necessary to assess benefit. It should never be given simultaneously with gold or hydroxychloroquine. Because major toxicities include marrow suppression (including selective thrombocytopenia) and nephritis with proteinuria, microhematuria, or casts, biweekly blood counts, platelet counts, and urinalyses must be done. Other toxicities include rash, gastrointestinal disturbance, and transient hypogeusia. Patients have been reported to develop a pemphigus-like eruption, myopathy, lupus-like syndrome, and myasthenia gravis. These are reversible by discontinuing the drug.

Corticosteroids. Without doubt, these are the most potent anti-inflammatory agents. However, in addition to the usual problems characterized by Cushing's syndrome, which occurs from prolonged corticosteroid therapy, there is also interference with growth and development in children. While corticosteroids suppress inflammation, they do not prevent progressive joint damage. Therefore, systemic steroid therapy as a supplement to aspirin or other NSAIDs should be reserved for patients who have (1) uncontrolled visceral involvement such as pericarditis or myocarditis; (2) severe systemic disease unresponsive to adequate doses of salicylates; (3) vision-threatening uveitis unresponsive to local therapy; and (4) severe unremitting synovitis threatening to make the child bed- and chairbound. In situations 1 through 3, high dose prednisone (or its equivalent) is used in doses of 0.5 to 2.0 mg per kg per day if alternate morning doses are not sufficient. For severe synovitis, only 5 to 10 mg of prednisone or its equivalent are needed on alternate mornings. Gradual tapering of dosage is necessary during steroid withdrawal to allow adrenal recovery and to avoid rebound flares of disease. Adding corticosteroids lowers salicylate levels; withdrawing steroids raises salicylate levels; monitoring is necessary.

Intra-articular steroids are sometimes effective when used infrequently and selectively for joints out of character with the general level of disease in a given patient. Depot long-acting nonabsorbable suspensions are best. These include hydrocortisone tertiary butyl acetate (Hydeltra T.B.A.), methylprednisolone (Depo-Medrol), triamcinolone acetonide (Kenalog), and triamcinolone hexacetonide (Aristospan). Aristospan is also used for intrapericardial injections for large pericardial effusions when myocarditis does not require systemic steroid therapy.

Cytotoxic Agents. Cytotoxic or immunosuppressive drugs such as cyclophosphamide (Cytoxan), methotrexate, chlorambucil (Leukeran), or azathioprine (Imuran) are experimental in the treatment of JRA. Potentially life-threatening complications from the use of these drugs, as well as the potential long-term risks of infertility and malignancy, relegate their use to a few seriously ill patients.

Physical and Occupational Therapy

Casting is never necessary or advisable. Even painful, inflamed joints can and should be put through daily passive ranges of motion to prevent permanent deformity. Heat, in the form of hot packs, and whirlpool by home tub often will alleviate pain and help with range-of-motion exercise. Night splints may help maintain position.

Physical and occupational therapists experienced in childhood arthritis can teach the patient and parents the basic information about maintaining function by a selective set of range-of-motion, isometric, and muscle-strengthening exercises. These should be done at regular times daily by the patient at home or in school. Bicycle riding and swimming are excellent.

Positive functional attitudes without physician-imposed restrictions are an important part of comprehensive care, along with social services and case management. Negative physician attitudes and unnecessary restrictions and clinic visits add to disability and reduce the quality of life for these children and their families.

Eye Care

Iridocyclitis can be a serious complication in 15 per cent of patients and formerly resulted in total blindness in 2 per cent of all children with JRA. It is more common in girls, and especially those who have relatively early onset of pauciarticular disease and who also have a positive antinuclear antibody (ANA) test. Young children often are asymptomatic until the process is well developed. Early vigorous treatment has a much better prognosis. Regular slit-lamp examinations are advised at 3 month intervals in children with pauciarticular disease and positive ANAs. Those with negative ANA or polyarticular disease should have eye examinations at 6 month intervals.

Surgery

Because of the generally good prognosis of this disease, and with adequate and persistent treatment, surgical intervention is rarely required. Synovectomy has been advocated for large, persistently active joints. Unfortunately, this is not curative, and the synovitis usually recurs. Furthermore, rehabilitation after such surgery is variable. Reconstructive surgery is usually reserved for those with severe, progressive deformity and impairment. While hip or knee resurfacing has been successful in selected patients, joint replacement surgery is generally delayed as long as possible and is limited to patients who cannot be ambulatory or have reasonable quality of life without it. Initial results may be excellent, but later failure is frequent. Reconstruction of mandibular dysplasia in teenagers who wish this cosmetic surgery is usually successful when performed by experienced surgeons. Special surgical techniques have restored vision to some patients with complicated cataracts resulting from uncontrolled uveitis.

ANKYLOSING SPONDYLITIS

method of
JOHN P. GOFTON, M.D.
University of British Columbia
Vancouver, British Columbia

Ankylosing spondylitis (AS) is a disease in which a chronic inflammation of unknown etiology involves the sacroiliac joints in all patients and the spine to a varying extent in most patients. This is the classic form of the condition and is the core problem in all patients.

Aims of Treatment

Good medical treatment of AS is management of the disease. To date no cure is possible.

If a patient is destined to suffer eventually from a rigid spine, it is of crucial importance to insure that fixation takes place in an extended position, thus permitting a full upright posture and a reasonably normal gait. Physical disability in such patients is surprisingly small. The pitiful picture of a stooped, bent man who cannot raise his head to see where he is walking is a relic of the past and should not occur today. Two means assure that a good posture is preserved. The first is adequate control of pain, which, of course, has the added purpose of allowing the patient to live a reasonable life. When pain is controlled a simple program of daily extension exercises will usually preserve spinal configuration in extension.

Control of Pain

The inflammatory process of AS is similar under the microscope to that seen in rheumatoid arthritis but is usually controllable by drugs the effect of which in rheumatoid arthritis is much more modest. On the other hand, aspirin is very much less effective in AS and is seldom useful.

Phenylbutazone (Butazolidin) and oxyphenbutazone (Tandearil) were the first drugs to demonstrate major and usually complete suppression of back pain in AS. They remain effective but unfortunately the rare but potentially fatal side effects of bone marrow suppression cannot be predicted, and these drugs are rightfully reserved now for rare cases where nothing else is effective.

Indomethacin (Indocin) in doses of 75 to 150 mg per day has been shown to be effective in most patients. The 75 mg sustained-release form given at bedtime is often useful. Other nonsteroidal anti-inflammatory drugs (NSAIDs) initially advised for rheumatoid arthritis and osteoarthritis have been extending their indications to include AS. These drugs show puzzling individual differences in effect in different patients, and in the present stage of our knowledge one can do little better than to try one or another and eventually select one which is both effective for pain relief and well tolerated.

Because the inflammatory process and the resultant pain fluctuate, full doses will be needed at times for adequate control whereas at other times patients may be active and pain-free on as little as two or three tablets per week. Because subjective pain is the determining factor, the physician and patient must understand the aim of treatment. To a large extent intelligent patients can adjust their own dosages.

Gold, systemic steroids, chloroquine, and cytotoxic agents are not recommended in AS. X-ray therapy has been shown to confer a significant risk of leukemia in later years and is not recommended.

Prevention of Deformity

A number of recipes are available for an extension exercise program which the patient must be taught to do himself. This brief daily program should be encouraged in the strongest terms. If an experienced physiotherapist is available, the physician can use this service for initial instruction and for follow-up. In simple terms, spinal extension and the strength of the extensor muscles must be preserved. A pain-ridden patient will seek relief by resting in bed in a curled-up position, which results in spinal fixation in a flexed posture. With adequate pain relief from drugs, the patient must understand the importance of continually seeking to hold the back in extension. Persistent pain induces atrophy in muscles whose activity is inhibited by it. With pain relief, extension exercises will preserve the strength of the extensor spinal muscles.

Patients tend to become bored with daily exercises that are preventive in nature and show no immediate postural gains. It is useful to explain that the disease will attempt to take away a fraction of an inch per day of spinal extensibility and that this will accumulate in time to a significant amount. The exercise program is designed to regain this small amount each day. The preventive aspects must be emphasized. Some recommend the persistent adoption of erect postures when standing or sitting, and no doubt this is helpful when patient compliance is good. Frequent follow-up is important in the early stages of the disease so the physician can detect progressive deformity and re-emphasize the need for faithful adherence to exercises. It may be useful to have the patient stand with his or her back to a wall—heels and buttocks against the wall. A patient with a normal spine can bring the upper back to touch the wall. However, if one is losing spinal extensibility, this can be demonstrated on subsequent visits and may be useful to reinforce the recommendations. Detailed descriptions of exercise programs may be found in pamphlets and in texts and occasionally are useful to the physician and patient.

Prevention of deformity is relevant to the early stages of the disease. Unfortunately, when some degree of flexion deformity is aleady present little can be done to regain it. However there is every reason to believe that further deformity can be minimized by persistent attention to spinal exercises.

Other useful procedures for the physician to encourage include the use of a firm mattress and a small pillow to avoid undue flexion when the patient sleeps. Rest periods with the patient lying on the stomach also are useful. Most patients will be able to engage in numerous activities, such as swimming, and often will enjoy sports that encourage spinal mobility. Whether or not this inhibits the development of ultimate ankylosis is unknown.

Counseling

This will be important for any patient with early disease and for many patients at whatever stage the physician is first consulted. It is of first importance to discuss the nature of the disease and its consequences. Many patients will have mild disease and will develop minimal deformity, so an optimistic outlook should be encouraged. Young people may find it difficult to accept their disease and the inevitable limitations it will impose. All the implications may not be taken in at one visit. The supportive physician should accept the inevitable reiteration of facts and treatment aims. An initially rebellious patient usually will come to terms with these in time and will return to the physician whose counsel has been dispassionate, understanding and patient.

Some patients will ask about the risk of AS in their children. Many will have read about HLA B27, and the physician should have an elementary understanding in order to discuss the problem. Most patients with AS possess the B27 antigen. Not all people in the population who have B27 antigen are destined to develop the disease, however. The risk of developing AS in B27-positive people varies from as high as 1 in 5 in some studies to as low as 1 in 15 in others. The child of a B27-positive parent with AS has about one chance in two of inheriting the B27 antigen. At worst, then, this child may have a risk of developing AS in the order of 1 in 10, and at best it may be as low as 1 in 30. It also should be emphasized that over half of all patients with AS will develop only minimal disability. This perspective should encourage the patient to consider having a family, but the final decision will be a personal one.

Females with AS who become pregnant may require cesarean section because of rigidity of pelvic ligaments. Sexual counseling may be important in some patients, paticularly those with hip disease.

Some thought must be given by the patient to choice of occupation. Young people who propose to embark on training or apprenticeship would be wise to choose work that can be done even if the future is destined to produce moderate or severe disability. Thus their disease will not seriously impair their ability to earn a living.

Special Features, Associated Conditions, and Complications

Through the course of the illness, one or more special problems may arise requiring treatment considerations beyond those described for the typical core disease.

Fever and Systemic Illness. Unlike the case in rheumatoid arthritis, this is rarely seen in AS so most patients will lead active lives if their pain is controlled. When systemic illness is present appropriate measures must be taken to minimize physical stress, and reasonable rest may be indicated. However, rest in improper postures should be avoided and every attention paid to maintaining spinal extension.

Iritis. Acute idiopathic iritis is often seen during the course of AS and occasionally precedes musculoskeletal symptoms. This was once thought of as a complication of AS but it is now considered to be an independent risk of B27 positivity. Since most patients with AS are B27-positive, the two conditions will frequently be seen together. Local steroids and mydriatics usually control the self-limiting process, but occasionally patients will develop severe and recurrent disease requiring the help of an ophthalmologist.

Peripheral Joint Disease. This occurs in some patients, usually involving the hips or knees and occasionally other large joints. The small joints of the hands and feet are rarely involved. Inflammatory synovitis in large joints resembles that seen in rheumatoid arthritis. Intra-articular steroids may be useful. Inflammation followed by a bony erosion is also seen at tendon insertions, usually at the calcaneus or at the shoulder. This may produce pain and disability mimicking that seen when active synovitis is present in a joint itself. The injection of steroids into tendon insertions should be cautioned against since the processes of repair may be impaired. Synovitis in the knee joint may be relatively bland whereas hip joint involvement probably always progresses to major destruction.

Cervical Spine Complications. The ligament that holds the odontoid process of C2 against a portion of C1 may deteriorate, producing dangerous laxity at the C1–2 articulation. This condition is more frequently seen in rheumatoid arthritis. Patients with this subluxation are vulnerable to stresses—a whiplash injury in particular—and a cervical supporting collar may be advisable. In rare cases operation may be required. Intubation for anesthesia may be contraindicated by this lesion.

Aortic Insufficiency. The aortic valve is involved by inflammation in about 1 per cent of patients and significant regurgitation may occur. Involvement of connective tissues at the base of the heart may produce a variety of conduction abnormalities, most commonly some form of block.

Chest Problems. Involvement of the costovertebral and costochondral joints may produce chest wall pain. Patients with manubriosternal involvement may develop symptoms mimicking angina. Tenderness over the manubriosternal joint will usually lead to the correct diagnosis and radiographs of this joint may show erosion. Restraint of chest cage movement may be severe but rarely leads to impairment of respiratory function. In rare instances there may be fibrosis of the lung apices.

Trauma to the Ankylosed Spine. The ankylosed spine is especially susceptible to trauma. Sudden back pain following trauma may be due to vertebral fracture. One form of this commonly seen in AS is known as spondylodiscitis, in which a fracture and sometimes collapse of a vertebral end plate occurs. This usually heals in time with rest, but spinal cord damage has occurred. Cauda equina syndrome and other kinds of spinal cord compression are rare and of course deserve appropriate consultations.

Surgery. Hip joint destruction is the commonest indication for surgery in AS and is used to salvage function. Unfortunately, some AS patients develop periarticular calcification, which may compromise the end result of hip replacement.

Age and Sex Differences. It was once thought that AS affected men many times more frequently than women. Recent evidence suggests that the frequency of the disease is about equal for the two sexes but that it appears to be milder in women. Treatment is essentially the same for either sex.

The inflammatory phase of ankylosing spondylitis will usually cease after the age of 40 years although there are exceptions. It is equally unusual for the disease to begin after the age of 40 years. This has some implications for diagnosis and treatment. If a patient has had good pain control in a partially ankylosed spine, and after the age of 40 years has several years free from pain without medication and then develops back pain, it often fails to respond promptly to drugs that had been effective previously. It should not be assumed that such a patient has a flare-up of AS; it may be due to some other cause, possibly spondylodiscitis.

BURSITIS AND CALCIFIC TENDINITIS

method of
MIRIAM COHEN, M.D.,
and MICHAEL H. ELLMAN, M.D.
Michael Reese Hospital and Medical Center
Chicago, Illinois

Bursitis

Bursae are sacs lined with a synovium-like membrane that serve to decrease friction between contiguous musculoskeletal tissues. There may be as many as 70 bursae on each side of the body, most being nameless. Some bursae are anatomically constant and some develop only in response to abnormal stresses (adventitious bursae). Bursal inflammation is a common medical problem, producing both acute and chronic pain.

Bursitis usually develops because of trauma, infection (septic bursitis), or crystal deposition (gout, pseudogout, calcium hydroxyapatite). Bursitis is common in the inflammatory arthritides, such as rheumatoid arthritis. The history and physical examination will usually point to the diagnosis of traumatic bursitis, e.g., the patient who rests his elbows on a desk for 8 hours a day presenting with an olecranon bursitis (draftsman's elbow). Bursitis associated with fever, chills, and a history of an antecedent penetrating injury assuredly is septic bursitis. Calcium hydroxyapatite deposition (calcific bursitis), gout, and, rarely, pseudogout (calcium pyrophosphate dihydrate deposition disease) may also cause acutely painful bursitis and mimic septic bursitis.

Bursae should be aspirated when bursal fluid is present and the diagnosis uncertain. Aspiration is mandatory when infection is suspected. We use aseptic technique with a 20- or 21-gauge needle (18- or 19-gauge if infection is likely) usually without local anesthesia, collecting the fluid in sterile tubes for bacterial culture and heparin-containing tubes. We routinely request white blood cell count and differential as well as Gram stain and bacterial culture if infection is possible. We examine the aspirate microscopically for the presence of crystals. A polarizing light microscope is helpful in this regard. If the bursal fluid is hemorrhagic or serosanguineous, but with less than 200 white blood cells per cu mm, trauma is the probable cause. A white blood cell count greater than 1000 white cells per cu mm is usually due to the presence of crystals or to septic bursitis, although it is common to see frank pus in the latter.

The knee is surrounded by many bursae, including the large suprapatellar bursa that freely communicates with the knee joint. The prepatellar (housemaid's knee) and infrapatellar (clergyman's knee) bursae are common sites of inflammation because they are frequently exposed to trauma. The anserine bursa, located medial and inferior to the knee, is also frequently a source of pain, especially in patients with knee joint osteoarthritis or rheumatoid arthritis. In the latter disease, the bursa may present as a soft tissue mass. The subdeltoid bursa, lateral to the glenohumeral joint and lying beneath the superior portion of the deltoid muscle, is a frequent site of shoulder pain. It is exposed to external trauma but is often involved when shoulder joint and tendon inflammation occur within the shoulder. When there is rupture of the rotator cuff, there is free communication between the shoulder joint and the subdeltoid bursa. The olecranon and trochanteric bursae are frequent sites of inflammation and must be distinguished from elbow and hip arthritis, respectively. Retro- and subcalcaneal bursae are traumatized during running and jogging and are the bane of the long-distance runner.

Tendinitis

Tendons are seldom accorded their due importance as a source of pain and disability. Tendinitis is a common problem, usually resulting from the strain of repetitive motion at insertion sites, especially over bony prominences. Systemic disorders such as sarcoidosis, rheumatoid arthritis, and systemic lupus erythematosus are associated with tendon or tendon sheath involvement. Tenosynovitis (tendon sheath inflammation) is common in gonococcal infection. Calcific tendinitis resulting from an alteration in tendon vascularity is due to calcium hydroxyapatite deposition.

Some common tendons that are involved with inflammation include the tendon insertions of the rotator cuff at the shoulder and the short and long head of the biceps as they insert into the coracoid process and the glenoid fossa, respectively. "Tennis elbow" or lateral epicondylitis is a tendinitis of the wrists and finger extensors, resulting in lateral epicondylar pain. Although frequently associated with tennis playing, it may result from any repetitive pronation-supination activity of the arm. On examination, pain occurs with wrist extension and there is often exquisite local tenderness over the epicondylar area, but elbow joint motion is normal. DeQuervain's tendinitis is common; it involves the abductor pollicis longus and extensor pollicis brevis tendons as they pass over the radial styloid. There is local tenderness at the radial styloid, and a simple test is often pathognomonic for this condition: This is the "Finkelstein test," in which a fist is made with the thumb abducted and clasped within; upon ulnar deviation of the fist there is pain at the styloid and lateral surface of the wrist.

Treatment

Basic Measures

The purpose of treatment is to alleviate pain and maintain function. When repetitive trauma is the etiology, rest and cessation of the offending cause may be adequate treatment. Heat application is often helpful for chronic pain, but for acute tendon and bursal inflammation, cold application may be more salutary. Some forms of tendinitis, particularly tennis elbow and deQuervain's tendinitis, are particularly resistant to therapy, and a simple program of rest, splinting, heat or cold application, and assurance is the basis of treatment. True tennis elbow (actually due to tennis playing) may require re-education in the proper execution of ground strokes.

Drug Management

The nonsteroidal anti-inflammatory medications (NSAIDs) are often helpful in relieving bursa and tendon inflammation. These are excellent anti-inflammatory and analgesic drugs that are reasonably safe for short-term use. They all cause gastrointestinal irritation to some degree and should be administered with food or antacid.

The drugs affect platelets and may cause central nervous system abnormalities such as headache and depression. We like the rapid-onset, short-acting NSAIDs, such as indomethacin and ibuprofen, the former in doses of 50 mg immediately and 25 mg every 4 to 6 hours, slowly decreasing the dose with the pain resolution. Ibuprofen is usually started at 600 to 800 mg immediately and 400 mg every 4 to 6 hours, slowly tapering as the patient improves. Usually a 5 to 10 day course of treatment is necessary. Other NSAIDs may be equally as effective. Aspirin is not as effective as indomethacin in acute bursitis or tendinitis and should not be used in gout. For chronic bursitis and tendinitis, aspirin is helpful. Septic bursitis and septic tenosynovitis require specific, and usually bactericidal, antibiotic therapy. Aspiration of bursal fluid with Gram stain and culture on appropriate media is obligatory prior to treatment.

Local Corticosteroid Use

If infection has been excluded and oral NSAID use contraindicated, not tolerated, or unhelpful, then corticosteroid injection may be tried. For tendinitis, 0.2 to 0.4 ml (4 to 8 mg) of prednisolone tebutate or similar non–water soluble preparation is mixed with 0.8 ml of 1 per cent lidocaine and, using a 25- or 26-gauge needle, is carefully injected into the tendon sheath. As much as 20 mg of a water-insoluble corticosteroid mixed with 4 ml of 1 per cent lidocaine may be used in bursitis. Postinfection flares due to corticosteroid crystal and white blood cell interactions are common but usually resolve with splinting and ice application. Patients should be warned of this possibility. Tendon injections should rarely be repeated; bursal injections may be repeated once or twice during a 12-month period. Surgical excision of bursae or reattachment of tendons may be considered if all other treatment fails.

LYME DISEASE

method of
GREGORY J. KUNDRAT, M.D.,
and STEVEN W. LUGER, M.D.
Old Lyme, Connecticut

Lyme disease is a clinical syndrome of single or multisystem involvement, caused by infection from a tickborne spirochete. The disease may present as a flu-like illness or with a pathognomonic rash and progress to neurologic, cardiac, or arthritic manifestations.

History

In 1975, Lyme disease (initially termed *Lyme arthritis*) was described as a specific entity based on a clustering of cases of arthritis among children in the town of Old Lyme, Connecticut. Subsequent investigation led to the discovery that the disease was transmitted to humans by a tick vector. Further study isolated a spirochete (*Borrelia bergdorferi*) from the *Ixodes dammini* tick, and later from patients with Lyme disease, proving this organism to be the etiologic agent.

Epidemiology

In the years since 1975, three distinct geographic areas have been recognized as endemic for Lyme disease. These include the eastern seaboard from Massachusetts to Virginia, the northern Midwest (Minnesota, Wisconsin), and the far Northwest (California, Oregon, Nevada). Scattered cases have been reported from several other states and from Europe and Australia.

Early Stage Disease

Lyme disease may occur at any age and in either sex. Its peak incidence is in June and July, although cases appear as early as March and as late as November. The best early clinical marker for Lyme disease is erythema chronicum migrans (ECM) occurring in 30 to 40 per cent of patients. The rash is characterized by a central red macule or papule at the site of the tick bite, which then expands centrifugally in a flat annular fashion with partial central clearing and light red outer borders. The size of the ECM lesion ranges from 1 to 24 inches. These lesions may be singular or multiple, even in the presence of a single tick bite and may at times show areas of central necrosis. The rash usually appears within 3 to 32 (median 7) days after the tick bite. An actual history of tick bite is obtained from only 30 per cent of patients with ECM, due mainly to the small size of the *Ixodes* tick (1 mm) and the fact that the bite is painless. The rash is usually nonpruritic and painless but may be warm to the touch. The lesions have appeared everywhere except the palms, soles, or mucous membranes. Untreated, ECM will spontaneously disappear within 1 to 3 weeks; however, recurrences have been reported in as many as 26 per cent of patients 1 to 14 months later.

Another common presentation of Lyme disease is a symptom complex consisting of malaise, fatigue, headache, stiff neck, fever, myalgia, lymphadenopathy, and arthralgia. ECM may or may not be present at this time. Various combinations of these symptoms may appear in a given patient. If they occur in midsummer, Lyme disease should be considered, particularly if the patient has recently traveled to an endemic area.

Late Stage Disease

Later manifestations of Lyme disease involve the nervous system, heart, and joints. There is some evidence that patients carrying the HLA-DR2 alloantigen may be more susceptible to this stage of illness. It is important to note that a patient's *initial* presentation of Lyme disease may be one of the late stage complications with no history of tick bite, ECM, or prodromal illness.

Common neurologic findings include meningoencephalitis, cranial neuropathies (particularly Bell's palsy), and peripheral radiculopathies. These occur in approximately 15 per cent of patients with untreated Lyme disease. The onset of neurologic symptoms ranges from 2 to 11 (median 4) weeks after tick bite. In untreated patients, neurologic abnormalities typically last for months but may resolve within 2 to 3 weeks.

Approximately 8 per cent of untreated patients will develop cardiac abnormalities. Cardiac involvement is usually limited to variable degrees of AV block and/or myopericarditis, but the heart valves have not been affected. The onset of cardiac manifestations ranges from 3 to 21 (median 5) weeks after the tick bite and typically lasts 1 week with a range from 3 days to 6 weeks. Patients presenting with cardiac symptoms (shortness of breath, syncope, palpitations, or chest pain) who have a suspicious clinical or travel history for Lyme disease should have an electrocardiogram.

The most common late manifestation of Lyme disease is the development of arthritis. This is usually a monoarticular or asymmetric oligoarticular variety, involving large joints, primarily the knees. It can be very difficult clinically to differentiate this form of the disease from juvenile rheumatoid arthritis, particularly when it presents as the initial manifestation. As many as 60 per cent of untreated patients may develop arthritis. Onset is usually 2 to 24 (median 6) weeks from the time of the tick bite. Generally, the acute arthritis lasts weeks to months and may recur for several years if untreated. It may also progress to a chronic arthritis (10 per cent of Lyme disease patients with arthritis) with actual destruction of bone and cartilage similar to rheumatoid arthritis.

Laboratory Testing

Laboratory testing can be helpful in confirming the diagnosis of Lyme disease or in arousing the physician's suspicion. The erythrocyte sedimentation rate (ESR) is elevated in a majority of patients, even in the earlier stages. ESR ranges from 21 to 68 have been reported with a median of 35. Complete blood counts and serum chemistries are typically normal. Elevation of total serum IgM occurs in one third of patients during early stages of the disease. C1q binding activity, as a measure of circulating immune complexes, is elevated during the early stages of Lyme disease in almost all patients.

A specific spirochetal antibody test has been developed using both immunofluorescent antibody and enzyme-linked immunosorbent assay techniques. The diagnosis is confirmed if an initially high titre is obtained or if a fourfold rise in titre is demonstrated. Close to a 100 per cent sensitivity rate is present in patients with late manifestations, whereas during the earlier stages of disease, a 50 to 70 per cent sensitivity rate is seen.

Treatment

Early Stage Disease

The drug of choice for adults and children aged 8 years and older is tetracycline, 250 mg four times daily for 10 days, extended to 20 days if symptoms persist. For children younger than 8 years old, one should use penicillin V, 50 mg per kg daily in divided doses, but not less than 1 gram or greater than 2 grams per 24 hours. Again, the recommended duration of treatment is 10 days.

For those adults unable to take tetracycline, penicillin V is recommended, 500 mg four times daily for 10 days. In the penicillin-allergic patient, erythromycin may be used at a dose of 250 mg four times daily; however, because of its somewhat decreased effectiveness, we recommend a 20-day course. Children unable to take penicillin should receive erythromycin, 30 mg per kg per day in divided doses to a maximum of 250 mg four times daily. Again, the course of treatment should be 20 days.

Cephalosporins have not been effective in treating Lyme disease, even if given during the early stage. It is interesting to note that in recent *in vitro* studies, ampicillin has been shown to have a lower MIC to the Lyme disease spirochete than penicillin; however, it has not yet been used in any clinical trials.

To our knowledge, patients treated with tetracycline during early stage disease have not developed late stage symptoms. The same cannot be said, however, for penicillin and erythromycin, even though the early stage symptoms may resolve quickly.

Late Stage Disease

Neurologic System. Patients with late stage neurologic symptoms of Lyme disease (meningitis, cranial nerve palsies, and peripheral radiculopathies) may be treated initially with oral tetracycline, 500 mg four times daily for 20 days. If the patient does not respond or the clinical condition does not permit outpatient therapy, hospitalization for intravenous penicillin therapy has proved to be effective. The dosage is 20 million units daily in divided doses for 10 days.

In our experience, high dose (1 mg per kg) prednisone therapy for cranial nerve palsies has proved to be very effective when given concomitantly with antibiotics, regardless of the length of time symptoms have been present prior to treatment. A tapering dose of this medication over 7 to 14 days is the recommendation.

Cardiac Disease. The patient with cardiac manifestations of Lyme disease (AV block, myopericarditis) should also be treated with antibiotics using the same schedule as for neurologic disease. The addition of prednisone to the treatment regimen has been shown to hasten resolution of heart block within 24 to 48 hours in patients with this finding.

Patients with high-degree AV block or first-degree block with PR intervals greater than or equal to 0.30 should be considered for hospitalization, cardiac monitoring, and possible temporary pacemaker placement.

Arthritis. The initial treatment for the arthritic manifestations is tetracycline, 500 mg four times daily for 20 days. Patients who do not respond may be considered for intravenous or intramuscular penicillin. The intravenous dosage of aqueous penicillin G is 20 million units daily in divided doses for 10 days. Alternatively, benzathine penicillin G may be given at a dose of 2.4 million units intramuscularly weekly for 3 successive weeks. Unfortunately, even with high-dose antibiotic therapy, some patients do not respond and may develop chronic arthritis.

Nonsteroidal anti-inflammatory agents can be helpful in alleviating symptoms when given concomitantly with antibiotics. Steroids given orally or intra-articularly may help in alleviating symptoms but do not alter the course of disease. Surgical intervention (*i.e.*, synovectomy) should only be considered when all other treatments have failed and the patient's clinical course is one of chronic deterioration and disability.

OSTEOARTHRITIS

method of
ARTHUR L. WEAVER, M.D.
University of Nebraska
Lincoln, Nebraska

Osteoarthritis (osteoarthrosis, hypertrophic arthritis, degenerative joint disease) is not one but a group of diseases that may have different pathogeneses. It is the most common of rheumatologic disorders and the major cause of disability and limitation of activity in the elderly population.

Treatment

The principal objectives in the management of patients with osteoarthritis are to reassure the patient, relieve the symptoms of pain and stiffness, preserve function or minimize functional loss, and delay progression of the disease.

Patient Education

Patient education and reassurance are of vital importance to the successful management of all rheumatic diseases. It is important for patients to understand clearly the chronic nature of osteoarthritis and to know that symptoms are generally mild, that pain can usually be managed effectively with available medication, and that the progression of the disease is slow. Patients should be reassured that they do not have an inflammatory arthritis, such as rheumatoid arthritis, and that osteoarthritis rarely causes deformity, crippling, or fatal complications. A useful and helpful educational resource is the booklet entitled *Osteoarthritis* published by and available from the Arthritis Foundation.

In chronic disease, when pain and disability are common, continued surveillance by the physician for associated anxiety and depression is essential. Dietary counseling for the overweight patient is important because excessive weight probably exacerbates progression of the damage in the low back and weight-bearing joints. Other than weight reduction, there is no evidence that dietary manipulation has a role in the treatment of osteoarthritis. Specific advice as to modification of sexual activities may benefit those patients with spinal and lower extremity involvement.

Prolonged and repeated overuse of involved joints is detrimental, and the need for rest and protection of these joints must be emphasized as one of the most effective ways of alleviating the pain and slowing the progression of osteoarthritis. Periods of daily joint rest should be prescribed in accordance with the site and extent of joint involvement. The serious misconception that vigorous exercise is beneficial for an involved joint must be dispelled at the time of initial evaluation. Patients must be advised to modify or avoid stressful activities such as participation in certain sports and recreational activities. For example, upper extremity involvement may necessitate modification of knitting, crocheting, typing, and playing certain musical instruments; weight-bearing joints will benefit from avoidance of jogging, long walks, squatting, kneeling, and stair climbing and descending. Occupational activities must be assessed and, if necessary, modified to prevent disease progression in those patients with significant joint involvement.

Physical and Occupational Therapy

Patients with osteoarthritis should be involved in an exercise program designed to improve general fitness as well as a program of graduated exercise for involved joints. Such a program will enhance their general well-being, help prevent muscle atrophy and osteoporosis, decrease muscle spasm, and help maintain a full range of joint motion. Active rather than passive and isometric rather than isotonic exercises are preferred. Moist heat (moist packs, soaks, hydrotherapy, paraffin baths) has excellent muscle relaxant effects and facilitates an exercise program. Physical and occupational therapists can provide instruction in joint protection, work simplification, energy conservation, postural training, back care, and positions of rest in addition to instruction in exercise programs and methods of heat application. Specific aids such as canes (always used in the hand opposite the affected joint), crutches, splints, walkers, cervical collars, braces, corsets, prescribed shoes and shoe inserts, and assistive devices such as grab bars, hand railings, extended and built-up handles, and elevated chairs and toilet seats can reduce weight-bearing and stress on involved lower extremity joints, reduce pain and stiffness, provide stability, and promote continued independence. Transcutaneous electrical nerve stimulation has proved beneficial in some cases of painful osteoarthritis of the spine.

Nonsteroidal Anti-Inflammatory Drugs (Including Aspirin)

Nonsteroidal anti-inflammatory drugs (NSAIDs), including aspirin, are the foundation of the pharmacologic treatment of osteoarthritis. There is little evidence that these agents alter the course of osteoarthritis, but they often keep the patient functional by relieving pain and inflammation. The choice of an NSAID is a matter of physician preference, but the majority of clinicians initiate therapy with aspirin because of its significantly lower cost. Serum salicylate concentrations in the range of 15 to 25 mg per dl are necessary to obtain an anti-inflammatory effect; 650 to 1300 mg (10 to 20 grains) of aspirin three or four times daily are required to achieve these levels. Tinnitus and hearing loss begin to appear at salicylate levels in excess of 25 mg per dl; in the elderly, hearing loss may develop before tinnitus and simulate confusion.

Aspirin allergy is rare but important to recognize and is characterized by the triad of urticaria, asthma,and nasal polyps. Aspirin inhibits prostaglandin synthesis by blocking cyclo-oxygenase, irreversibly blocks platelet cyclo-oxygenase, and enhances the effects of oral anticoagulants and oral hypoglycemic agents. Gastrointestinal erosions and bleeding occur frequently in patients taking soluble aspirin preparations (ASA, Bufferin, Ascriptin, CAMA) and may be lessened by stressing the importance of taking aspirin with meals or by switching to enteric-coated preparations (Easprin, Ecotrin, Encaprin) or zero-release aspirin (Zorprin). The nonacetylated salicylates include magnesium salicylate (Magan, Mobidin), choline magnesium salicylate (Trilisate), salsalate (Disalcid), and diflunisal (Dolobid). These agents offer advantages of twice daily administration and significantly less gastrointestinal irritation.

The continued search for effective aspirin substitutes with fewer side effects has resulted in the development of several new NSAIDs. These agents as a group are acidic, protein bound, readily absorbed by the gastrointestinal tract, and rapidly metabolized and excreted by the liver and/or kidney. These drugs are divided into several groups based on chemical structures. The indole derivatives are indomethacin: Indocin, 25 to 50 mg three times daily, and Indocin SR, 75 mg once or twice daily; tolmetin (Tolectin), 200 to 400 mg four times daily; and sulindac (Clinoril), 150 to 200 mg two times daily. The propionic acid derivatives include ibuprofen (Motrin, Rufen), 400 to 800 mg four times daily; fenoprofen (Nalfon), 300 to 600 mg four times daily; and naproxen (Naprosyn), 250 to 500 mg two times daily. Phenamic acid is the parent compound of meclofenamate (Meclomen), 50 to 100 mg four times daily, and the available oxicam derivative is piroxicam (Feldene), 10 to 20 mg once daily. Improved patient compliance has been demonstrated with agents administered only once or twice daily.

The philosophy of selecting a given NSAID should include considerations of cost, efficacy, tolerability and safety, flexibility of dosage, range of therapeutically active doses, and frequency of administration. These agents are more expensive and better tolerated than aspirin and demonstrate a cross-sensitivity in aspirin-allergic patients. They are analgesic and anti-inflammatory due to blockage of cyclo-oxygenase; they reversibly block cyclo-oxygenase in platelets and potentiate oral anticoagulants and oral hypoglycemic agents.

All the NSAIDs have comparable side effects. The mechanism of upper gastrointestinal irritation and bleeding is the same mechanism by which these drugs are therapeutic: they inhibit cytoprotective prostaglandin synthesis and their antiplatelet effect contributes to bleeding. The other side effects include skin rash, central nervous system signs and symptoms, hepatitis, hypersensitivity reactions, and nephrotoxic phenomena. Special note should be made of the risk factors associated with nephrotoxic reactions, most of which are related to inhibition of prostaglandins. The risk factors include age over 50 years, hypertension, diabetes, congestive heart failure, and the concomitant use of diuretic agents. An appropriate therapeutic trial for each of these agents should be 4 weeks, and if no response is obtained, several of these agents (preferably in different chemical groupings) should be tried in sequence. It is unknown whether these agents are synergistic or antagonistic with salicylates or with each other.

Analgesics and Muscle Relaxants

Pure analgesics such as acetaminophen, propoxyphene (Darvon, Dolene), and codeine preparations may be useful as adjuncts to the NSAIDs. Muscle relaxants such as cyclobenzapine (Flexeril), methocarbanol (Robaxin), orphenadrine (Norflex), carisoprodol (SOMA), and diazepam (Valium) can be used to reduce muscle spasm adjacent to osteoarthritic joints but must be dispensed cautiously.

Intra-articular Corticosteroids

Systemic corticosteroid therapy clearly has no place in the treatment of osteoarthritis. However, intra-articular corticosteroid therapy can provide quick and sometimes lasting relief when used judiciously in select patients. Such therapy is adjunctive and most effectively used in patients who have one or two persistently painful and inflamed joints or in those patients with associated crystal deposition disease. Using meticulous aseptic technique, such joints should be aspirated and injected with a longer-acting steroid preparation such as triamcinolone hexacetonide (Aristospan) or prednisolone tebutate (Hydeltra-TBA). Patients should be advised to rest the joint for several days after injection, and a given joint should not be injected more often than once every 4 to 6 months. If no benefit occurs following injection, further steroids are best avoided, because repeat injections are unlikely to succeed.

Surgery

Surgical intervention in osteoarthritis is indicated for patients with intractable pain unrelieved by medical measures, significant loss of function, and marked joint instability. Débridement of cartilage and spurs and removal of loose bodies can be accomplished via arthroscopy and arthrotomy. Osteotomy of the knee (if the disease is localized to the medial or lateral compartment) may be an effective temporizing procedure. Total joint arthroplasty is reserved for patients with severe disease of the hip or knee and results in excellent pain relief and near-normal motion in most instances. Total joint replacement should not be used to return the patient to a vigorous physical life style. These operations are not without complications of loosening with prosthetic failure and infection, and the patient should be informed of these possibilities prior to surgery. Arthrodesis is of value in patients whose weight or physical activity is too demanding for total joint replacement and as a salvage procedure for failed total joint replacement.

POLYMYALGIA RHEUMATICA AND TEMPORAL ARTERITIS

method of
M. BASHAR KAHALEH, M.D.
Medical University of South Carolina
Charleston, South Carolina

Polymyalgia rheumatica (PMR), a clinical syndrome of unknown cause, occurs most commonly in individuals older than 50 years of age. It is characterized by aching and stiffness in the shoulder and pelvic girdles. Common constitutional symptoms include low-grade fever, malaise, and weight loss. Mild anemia and marked elevation of Westergren erythrocyte sedimentation rate (WESR) are usually seen. A close association between PMR and temporal arteritis (TA) has been firmly established. The presence of unilateral or bilateral temporal headache, jaw claudication, tenderness or decreased pulsations of the temporal arteries, or visual disturbances in patients with PMR should suggest the presence of TA. Patients with TA may have a symptom complex consistent with PMR in 50 per cent of cases, and about 15 per cent of the patients with PMR have positive temporal artery biopsy findings in the absence of symptoms of TA. With this degree of overlap, it is difficult to make a clinical distinction between these two disease processes.

Treatment

Patients with PMR will respond dramatically to low doses of oral glucocorticosteroids (5 to 15 mg of prednisone per day). This dose of prednisone is associated with almost complete resolution of musculoskeletal symptoms and fall in WESR. After several weeks, the dosage of glucocorticoids can be decreased slowly by 1 to 2 mg per day at weekly intervals to the lowest daily dose needed to control symptoms. PMR may not always be a self-limited disease that runs its course within 2 years. Long-term studies indicate that the course is often prolonged and unpredictable; up to 50 per cent of patients are still on steroids after 24 months of treatment. Most patients have no evidence of complications and are comfortable on a prednisone dosage sufficiently low to prevent cumulative toxicity. Trial and error is the only way to tell when prednisone can be discontinued.

Once the diagnosis of TA is established, glucocorticoid treatment should be instituted. In patients with strong clinical suspicion of TA, particularly in those with visual disturbances, therapy should be started immediately because of the known efficacy of steroids in preventing blindness and other vascular complications. Glucocorticoids should not be used as a "therapeutic trial"; as soon as possible, a firm diagnosis should be established by temporal artery biopsy. Most patients with TA will respond rapidly to treatment. Within days, systemic symptoms and localized vascular manifestations begin to resolve. The optimal dose may vary from patient to patient. Because irreversible damage from a vascular occlusion can occur, the usual practice is to give large initial doses (40 to 60 mg) of prednisone orally in divided daily doses for 1 month before beginning a gradual taper. The dose is then gradually reduced by a maximum of 10 per cent of the total daily dose each 1 or 2 weeks over 6 months to a daily maintenance dose of 5 to 7.5 mg. The steroid dose is tapered according to the patient's symptoms rather than the sedimentation rate. Recent studies have cast doubt on the use of WESR as an entirely reliable diagnostic and therapeutic aid in PMR/TA. A small percentage of patients with TA do not respond as readily to corticosteroids. Such patients are indistinguishable from responsive patients by pretreatment symptoms or histopathologic findings. Once symptoms resolve and laboratory tests return to normal, patients with TA should be managed as patients with pure PMR.

With rapid diagnosis and appropriate treatment prior to a life-threatening ischemic event, the prognosis is excellent and the patient may anticipate a normal life expectancy. In general, visual impairments are not reversible, although functional vision may rarely be restored.

In a minority of patients, glucocorticoids may not be effective or may be associated with a high degree of toxicity. Cyclophosphamide, azathioprine, dapsone, and a variety of other medications have been reported as being a useful alternative to steroids. Complications of the arteritis such as sudden blindness can occur 2 years or longer after initial diagnosis, even in patients who are apparently adequately treated. Thus, lifelong vigilance for reactivation of the disease is necessary.

OSTEOMYELITIS

method of
FRANK C. WILSON, M.D.
University of North Carolina
Chapel Hill, North Carolina

Skeletal infections are among the oldest medical nemeses of humankind, with unmistakable evidence of osteomyelitis found in bones antedating the birth of Christ. Pathogenic bacteria (or fungi) enter bone from the bloodstream (hematogenous osteomyelitis), directly from the external environment (exogenous osteomyelitis), or from infected contiguous soft tissues. Hematogenous infection of bone from a distant primary locus of infection is much more common in children than in adults, although the primary locus cannot always be identified. The metaphyses of growing bones are chosen because of the unique vascular anatomy imposed by the epiphyseal plates. Organisms pass through the nutrient arteries into the bone lined channels that abut the epiphyseal plates. Egress of blood flow from this point necessitates a 180-degree turn of the vessel and its exit through the same impermeable channel. The slowing of the circulation required for this turn allows the bacteria to settle, multiply, and obstruct the bone channel. Thus isolated from the normal defenses of the host, early proliferation of the organisms is unimpeded.

DIAGNOSIS

Although four clinical stages of osteomyelitis may be identified (acute, subacute, chronic, and residual), only two (acute and chronic) need be distinguished therapeutically. *In the acute stage,* the patient is systemically ill. Diagnostic laboratory indices are positive for infection, lytic lesions are observed on radiographs, and pathologic changes are characterized by dead bone, acute inflammatory cells, and pus. *In the subacute stage,* the clinical and laboratory manifestations are less pronounced, and new bone can be seen on radiographs and during pathologic examinations. *In the chronic stage,* there are no clinical signs of systemic illness, although a draining sinus may be associated with slight elevations of the white blood count and erythrocyte sedimentation rate. A sequestrum is usually present, and the exudate contains a high percentage of lymphocytes. *In the residual stage,* architectural changes appear in the bone, with or without clinical deformity.

The nature and complexity of bone infections have changed during the past 2 decades, but the critical importance of early diagnosis and of vigorous treatment has not changed. Delay in diagnosis, inappropriate antibiotic therapy, or failure to provide needed surgical drainage permits entrenchment of the infectious process, which may lead to chronicity and permanent functional or anatomic sequelae. Because of the difficulty in interpreting clinical manifestations, tardy diagnoses are more common in neonates and in patients receiving antibiotic treatment.

Since bacteremia is common in osteomyelitis, the diagnostic work-up should include blood cultures, preferably performed at the time of a fever "spike" and before antibiotics have been given. In untreated patients, these cultures will provide positive results in over 50 per cent. In post-traumatic or postoperative osteomyelitis, the offending organism can often be recovered in the drainage from overlying soft tissues. With hematogenous infection, however, identification of the pathogen usually depends upon subperiosteal or metaphyseal aspiration of pus at the point of maximal tenderness, which will yield an organism in approximately 70 per cent of cases. Roentgenographic findings, including those of bone scans, are often nonspecific in early bone infections.

As soon as bone, blood, and other foci of infection have been cultured, parenteral antibiotic therapy should be instituted using bactericidal drugs in large doses. A preliminary guide to appropriate antibiotic therapy may be obtained from Gram's stain of the aspirate. Other features also provide important clues. For example, most infections in very young children are caused by group B *Streptococcus; Pseudomonas* infections are especially prevalent in heroin addicts and in patients with puncture wounds of the foot; patients with sickle cell anemia have a propensity for *Salmonella* infections; gram-negative infections are more common in neonates and immunologically suppressed patients; and anaerobic infections are more likely in patients with diabetes or in patients with bite wounds. In the absence of such predisposing factors, *Staphylococcus aureus* is the most likely pathogen. In children over 2 years of age, *S. aureus* is responsible for approximately 80 per cent of osseous infections, most of which are penicillin-resistant.

Antibiotic Therapy

Prior to culture, initial antibiotic therapy must be sufficiently broad to cover the common and expected pathogens (Table 1). Thus, in the neonate, optimal treatment is most likely to be provided by a penicillinase-resistant penicillin coupled with an aminoglycoside. In the older child, for whom the risk of a gram-negative infection is less, a penicillinase-resistant penicillin would be sufficient. In a patient with sickle hemoglobinopathy, ampicillin or chloramphenicol should be chosen; if *Pseudomonas* and enteric bacilli are expected pathogens, a broad-spectrum penicillin, e.g., carbenicillin or piperacillin, should be combined with an aminoglycoside, such as gentamycin or tobramycin. Anaerobic infections usually respond to penicillin G or a first generation cephalosporin, such as cefazolin.

Once the invading organisms have been identified and characterized, the antibiotic regimen should be made more specific. Penicillin G is the mainstay for sensitive staphylcococci and for groups A and B streptococci; ampicillin is the drug of choice for sensitive *Haemophilus influenzae* and *Salmonella*; a penicillinase-resistant penicillin, such as nafcillin or oxacillin, is preferred for penicillinase-producing staphylococci. Gram-negative organisms, especially *Pseudomonas aeruginosa,* are particularly difficult to treat. An aminoglycoside is usually the first line of defense, although if greater activity against the organism is shown by one of the cephalosporins, that drug should be used. A new semisynthetic aminoglycoside, amikacin, has been demonstrated to be effective against some organisms resistant to gentamycin, tobramycin, and kanamycin.

When an aminoglycoside is administered, serum antibiotic levels must be monitored regularly, along with signs of nephrotoxocity and ototoxicity, which occur in 10 to 20 per cent of patients. Nephrotoxicity is more common and more dangerous; ototoxicity due to gentamycin and tobramycin is more likely to involve the auditory than the vestibular portion of the eighth nerve and is usually irreversible. Factors that predispose the patient to aminoglycoside toxicity are previous aminoglycoside treatment, impair-

TABLE 1. **Antibiotic Dosages for the Treatment of Bacterial Osteomyelitis**

Antibiotic	Recommended Daily Dosage: *Children (mg/kg)*	Recommended Daily Dosage: *Adults*	Hours Between Doses	Route of Administration
Amikacin (Amikin)	15	15 mg/kg	8–12	IV, IM
Ampicillin (Principen)	200	8–12 gm	4	IV
Cefazolin (Kefzol)	60	4–6 gm	8	IV, IM
Cefamandole (Mandol)	100	6–12 gm	4	IV, IM
Cefoperazone (Cefobid)	Not established	4–6 gm	8–12	IV, IM
Cefotaxime (Claforan)	180	8–12 gm	4	IV, IM
Chloramphenicol (Chloromycetin)	75	50 mg/kg	6	IV, PO
Clindamycin (Cleocin)	30	1.8–2.4 gm	8	IV
		1.5 gm	8	PO
Cloxacillin (Tegopen)	100	2–4 gm	6	PO
Dicloxacillin (Dynapen)	50*	2–4 gm*	6	PO
Gentamicin (Garamycin)	6	5–6 mg/kg	8	IV, IM
Kanamycin (Kantrex)	20	15 mg/kg	8	IV, IM
Nafcillin (Nafcil)	150	8–12 gm	4	IV, IM
Oxacillin (Prostaphilin)	200	8–12 gm	4	IV, IM
Tetracycline hydrochloride (Cyclopar)	50	2–4 gm	6	PO
Penicillin V potassium (V-Cillin-K)	100	12–13 million units	3–4	IV
Piperacillin (Pipracil)	Not established	18–24 gm	3–4	IV
Tobramycin (Nebcin)	8	3–5 mg/kg	6	IV, IM
Vancomycin (Vancocin)	50	2 gm	6	IV

*This dosage may exceed recommendation of manufacturer.

ment of renal function, prolonged (over 2 or 3 weeks) aminoglycoside therapy, inappropriately high dosages, and concomitant administration of other potentially ototoxic or nephrotoxic agents, particularly diuretics. Most importantly, aminoglycoside dosages must be based on lean body mass and must be reduced when renal insufficiency is present. Appropriate dosages should be confirmed by "peak and trough" serum drug level determinations.

Monitoring for ototoxicity entails testing for high tone hearing, which is usually the first measurable auditory function to diminish. Vestibular function is difficult to monitor, since electronystagmograms do not correlate well with loss of balance. Occasionally, ototoxicity is apparent only when a patient's balance is so severely impaired that crutches are required to walk.

Renal dysfunction, which is usually correctable, should be monitored several times weekly by blood urea nitrogen level, creatinine level, and urinalysis. Baseline renal and auditory measurements should be taken before aminoglycoside treatment is begun.

In general, the spectra of activity for different aminoglycosides are similar, as are their complications. Rather than administer aminoglycosides for long periods of time, one might choose to leave the patient with chronic or recurrent sinus drainage. If the infection is caused by a single pathogen, cure may be expected with aminoglycoside therapy in about two thirds of the patients; however, if the infection is caused by multiple, gram-negative organisms, complete eradication is likely in only about half of the patients.

Perhaps the major use of a third generation cephalosporin, such as cefoperazone or cefotaxime, is in the patient with a susceptible gram-negative infection that requires prolonged therapy. Although it was hoped that third generation cephalosporins would provide a less dangerous alternative to prolonged aminoglycoside therapy, this has not been realized with moxalactam therapy, in which bleeding and supercolonization with group D streptococci have occurred frequently. Cefoperazone and cefotaxime, although less active against anaerobic organisms, have been associated less often with these complications.

Penicillin-sensitive patients and methicillin-resistant staphylococci are seen with increasing frequency. In some hospitals, as many as 70 per cent of the cases of *Staphylococcus epidermidis* infections are methicillin-resistant. In such cases, vancomycin, which is also a reliable antistaphylococcal agent, should be used. Although the spectrum of vancomycin is not as broad as that of the beta-lactam antibiotics, adverse side effects, such as phlebitis and nephrotoxicity, have been minimized by improved manufacturing techniques.

Other variables being equal, the cost factor should be considered in determining whether to prescribe a generic aminoglycoside or a third generation cephalosporin, since the cost of cephalosporin therapy may be as much as thirty times that of aminoglycoside therapy.

In patients with a history of hypersensitivity to penicillin, a cephalosporin is preferred to either clindamycin or tetracycline, because recommended doses of the latter compounds are bacteriostatic rather than bactericidal. The substitution of a cephalosporin for penicillin, however, must be done very carefully, as there is a low incidence of cross allergies between penicillins and cephalosporins. Patients with a history of immediate hypersensitivity (anaphylaxis) to penicillin should not be given cephalosporin.

The following caveats should be observed in prescribing antibiotics for acute osteomyelitis: antibiotics must be tailored to the sensitivities of the offending organisms; the dosage must be adjusted for individual patients according to body weight and the presence or absence of underlying kidney or liver disease; when parenteral therapy is used, intravenous administration is usually preferable to intramuscular injection; and appropriate monitoring of serum antibiotic levels and serum chemical indicators of drug toxicity is mandatory. Consultation with experts in infectious disease is recommended when dealing with patients who have gram-negative or polymicrobial infections.

The duration of antibiotic therapy for acute osteomyelitis is controversial. Recent reports recommend that treatment be continued for 4 to 6 weeks, although there is little evidence to support treatment past 3 weeks, and complete cures have followed even more limited periods. Any generalization is dangerous, since the response to therapy depends upon many variables: the infectious agents, the duration of infection prior to treatment, specificity and dose of antibiotics, adequacy of local circulation, presence of a foreign body, and the immunologic status of the patient. Some clinicians believe that treatment should be continued until all diagnostic laboratory test indices have returned to normal; others, noting that these indices may remain abnormal even after the acute process has been arrested, rely on the clinical response. Roentgenographic features are probably the least useful parameters, since bone remodeling continues long after control of the infection.

The question of how long to continue therapy also involves practical considerations, since parenteral administration of antibiotics requires hospitalization, discomfort, considerable cost, and inconvenience. To reduce the long period of confinement, a number of investigators have, in recent years, employed oral antibiotic therapy for acute osseous infections, with cure rates comparable to those reported with parenteral therapy. This approach is based on the demonstration of comparable serum concentration and bioavailability after oral antibiotic administration. While possessing undeniable advantages, oral antibiotic therapy is hazardous if serum bactericidal activity and patient compliance cannot be carefully monitored. Since most patients with acute osteomyelitis are systemically ill, therapy is begun with parenteral antibiotics. During the next 4 or 5 days, any necessary surgical procedures can be performed and antibiotic therapy adjusted after culture and sensitivity reports are received and evaluated. The bactericidal titer of serum is tested about 1 hour after a parenteral dose of antibiotic is administered to provide a goal for oral therapy. While there is no consensus on the minimal effective serum bactericidal titer, levels of 1:8 or 1:16 are generally thought to be adequate for *Staphylococcus* and *Pseudomonas* infections; higher titers are desirable for *Streptococcus* and *H. influenzae* infections. The oral antibiotic selected depends upon bacterial susceptibilities, and the dose varies with the age of the patient. For *Staphylococcus aureus* infections, doses of penicillinase-resistant dicloxacillin usually produce greater serum bactericidal activity than comparable doses of nafcillin, oxacillin, or cephalosporins. Dicloxacillin is inactivated by gastric acid, however, and must be given 1 hour before or 2 hours after meals. For young children who require liquid suspensions, cephalosporins may be more palatable than penicillin derivatives because of their more pleasant taste. Penicillin V is the preferred agent for group A or B streptococcal and pneumococcal infections. Since oral antibiotic dosage for osteomyelitis is several times that for less severe infections, problems may be encountered in administering these antibiotics to young children. Oral therapy is not suitable for infections caused by *Pseudomonas* or coliform bacilli.

After 2 or 3 days of oral therapy, the serum bactericidal activity is determined an hour after a dose of the antibiotic is administered. If the titer is low, the dose can be increased by 50 per cent, or, if a beta-lactam antibiotic is being used, probenecid (40 mg/kg) can be added to the regimen. If the titer still remains low, another antibiotic should be selected, or parenteral therapy reinstituted.

The optimal duration for oral antibiotic therapy is unknown; however, most authorities recommend 4 to 8 weeks.

While early reports of parenteral-oral antibiotic therapy are promising, it must be cautioned that the follow-up period in most studies has been less than 2 years. Since osteomyelitis may recur many years after the original infection, it is impossible to say at this time how many cases have been permanently eradicated. Certainly this therapy should not be employed when uncertainty exists about patient compliance or about antimicrobial drug activity.

Surgery

When the local or systemic manifestations of osteomyelitis fail to respond to parenteral antibiotic administration within 48 hours, surgical drainage is indicated. After drainage of subperiosteal pus, a window is made in the subjacent metaphysis to ensure osseous decompression and drainage. The wound is packed open and may be closed secondarily after purulent drainage ceases. Closed suction drainage is not used in the treatment of acute infections.

Whether or not surgical drainage is employed, it is important to understand that the infection so weakens the bone that fracture from minor trauma is common. For this reason, traction or cast immobilization of affected long bones until remineralization occurs is desirable.

Chronic Osteomyelitis Therapy

Chronic osteomyelitis is defined by the presence of a sequestrum and represents, for whatever reason, a failure of therapy for acute osteomyelitis. Fortunately, prompt and adequate therapy has all but eliminated this devastating outcome. Small sequestra are usually resorbed through osteoclastic activity; however, large or inaccessible sequestra often cannot be dealt with by endogenous mechanisms, and their extirpation is necessary for cure.

The treatment of chronic osteomyelitis follows three lines; aggressive surgical débridement of necrotic bone and soft tissue scars, obliteration of residual defects in bone and soft tissues, and prolonged antimicrobial therapy. Even with optimal treatment, recurrence is encountered in 20 to 30 per cent of patients with this condition. The reason for the high rate is that it is frequently impossible to remove all avascular bone and soft tissue so that the remaining tissues can be perfused with antibiotics.

Since failure to control the infection often leads to amputation, a number of ingenious surgical techniques have been employed to improve perfusion and antibiotic delivery to devitalized tissues while simultaneously filling the dead space that follows aggressive surgical débridement. One approach has been to fill the defect with a muscle flap obtained locally or obtained through a free vascularized transfer—a technique that finds its greatest applicability in post-traumatic osteomyelitis of the lower limb. Local muscle flaps are preferred when available; free vascularized transfers are used when alternatives do not exist for local muscle flaps.

Another procedure involves the implantation of gentamycin-impregnated polymethyl methacrylate beads. This approach is based on the knowledge that residual monomers are released from hardened bone cement. High local concentrations of the antibiotic may be achieved, thereby avoiding the risk, expense, and inconvenience of prolonged systemic therapy. The beads do not impede drainage and can be removed for bone grafting at any time. Being inert, they do not stimulate a foreign body reaction. Comparative studies suggest that this method is as successful in eradicating infection as older suction-irrigation techniques, and it requires much less attention. Antibiotic-impregnated plaster of Paris beads have also been shown to deliver high, local concentrations of antibiotics. A further advantage of plaster of Paris beads is that they are spontaneously resorbed and replaced by normal bone in a period of weeks to months and thus do not require removal.

Bone grafting may be employed either to add bone mass to an area already weakened by débridement or to repair nonunion. In 1979, Papineau published a protocol for the management of chronic pyogenic osteomyelitis in 3 stages: *stage 1* entailed removal of necrotic tissue, *stage 2* involved cancellous bone grafting, and *stage 3* provided skin coverage. While repeated débridements are occasionally necessary to control the infection, grafting with small fragments of iliac bone restores the structural integrity of the affected bone so that weight bearing can be permitted.

Antibiotic therapy for chronic osteomyelitis should be based on a careful study of sensitivity data from evaluation of deep wound cultures, since at least a third of the cases are polymicrobial, most often with *Staphylococcus aureus* and gram-negative rods. I prefer a regimen of 3 to 4 weeks of parenteral therapy followed by 8 weeks of oral therapy. More than one antibiotic is often necessary, and changes in the flora during treatment may require changes in the drugs. Although his method is not generally accepted as adequate treatment alone, Bell has provided 10 years of follow-up information on the successful use of prolonged, high dosages of oral penicillin in a group of patients with chronic osteomyelitis. Peak serum concentrations were held above 20 micrograms per ml, and treatment was continued for 6 to 12 months in most cases, being discontinued when the patient was asymptomatic. The sedimentation rates were normal, and no sequestra were demonstrable.

COMMON SPORTS INJURIES

method of
DAVID O. HOUGH, M.D.
Michigan State University
East Lansing, Michigan

Participation in fitness, recreational, and competitive athletic activities at all ages has increased dramatically, with 54 per cent of all Americans exercising on a regular basis. Individuals who exercise regularly are more prone to overtraining or overconditioning, which may result in an overuse injury syndrome. The process of overuse relates directly to the intensity, duration, and frequency of exercise, resulting in the breakdown of body structures. Common examples of overuse injury syndrome include bursitis, tenosynovitis, tendonitis, fascitis, compartment syndrome, and stress fractures.

The goals of treatment for all sports injuries are to 1. provide proper diagnosis and early management to reduce swelling and pain, 2. institute early mobilization to restore range of motion, 3. restore strength, 4. maintain general body conditioning, 5. provide functional exercises specific to the patient's event or sport, and 6. determine when the athlete may resume participation.

Reasonable guidelines for returning to participation include the following: (1) a definite diagnosis has been made, (2) the injury will not worsen with continued activity, (3) the individual is not at greater risk of further injury, and (4) the injury will allow the individual to fairly compete and not render the individual incapable of protecting himself or herself. Finally, the physician should emphasize the importance of injury prevention through the use of proper conditioning and injury rehabilitation programs, of good equipment and facilities, of proper coaching techniques and supervision, and of adequate medical care.

Treatment of Contusions

Contusions are caused by a direct blow against the skin and are most common to the anterior thigh, arms, shoulder, and iliac crest area. The blow causes ruptured capillaries and bleeding into the subcutaneous tissues and muscle and may eventually lead to myositis ossificans traumatica. Initial treatment involves application of ice for 24 to 36 hours, compression with a thick pad (e.g., football thigh pad material), and elevation. Use of heat massage or ultrasound is contraindicated. Application of ice in the form of bags, massage, or immersion is carried out six to eight times the first day at 20 to 30 minute intervals. The extremity is initially immobilized to encourage healing and to prevent further bleeding. Resumption of muscle function is gradually encouraged within the limits of pain after several days. Early flexibility training and muscle strengthening exercises with the use of contrast baths (described later) are utilized 4 to 7 days after injury. Administration of oral, nonsteroidal anti-inflammatory agents (NSAIDs) may be helpful. Occasionally, a fluctuant seroma may need to be aspirated and drained for relief of symptoms. The athletes should continue to apply ice to the area at least twice daily once they return to participation and should wear protective padding over the injured area during competition.

Sprains and Strains

A sprain implies a damaged ligament, whereas a strain implies a damaged muscle or tendon. Sprains and strains are graded as I (mild), II (moderate), or III (severe). Their management is summarized in Table 1.

Strains commonly occur to the muscles of the back, hamstrings, quadriceps, hip adductors and flexors, and rotator cuff of the shoulder and cervical spine. These injuries can also be associated with ligamentous injuries and should be treated appropriately.

A *grade I strain* occurs with stretching of the musculotendinous unit and is associated with localized tenderness initially. Swelling may occur but is often absent. The problem often resolves within several days. The *grade II strain* implies more damage with partial tearing of involved tissues and results in soreness and minimal loss of strength. The *grade III strain* or complete rupture of the musculotendinous unit often requires surgical repair. Recognition of severe strains is often difficult due to muscle guarding, which may mask the extent of the injury.

Treatment of Strains

Initial treatment of grade I and II strains involves the use of rest, ice, compression, and elevation (RICE). Ice can be applied through ice massage, ice packs, or ice immersion four to six times daily for 20 to 30 minutes. Protection from further injury is important through the use of splinting, taping, crutches, or other immobilizing devices. After 3 to 4 days, the injured area is mobilized slowly with gentle stretching to avoid a chronic problem. Grade III sprains often require surgery and should be evaluated by an orthopedic surgeon. NSAIDs may be necessary to reduce inflammation and should be used judiciously. A discussion of NSAID therapy is provided elsewhere in this text and in many other publications. Their use is generally limited to 5 to 10 days, but in chronic problems their use may be longer. The physician should be familiar with the side effects, cost, dosage schedule, and efficacy of each NSAID. Many musculotendinous strains are prone to chronic inflammation and pain associated with loss of function. When this development occurs, the athlete will require a long period of rest (often 6 to 12 weeks) followed by a long period of rehabilitation in order to achieve pain-free, normal muscle strength and function.

Treatment of Sprains

Sprains are probably the most common injury in all sports. The joints most often affected are the ankles, knees, and shoulders. The management of all sprains is summarized next. More specific treatment of ankle and knee sprains will also be discussed.

Grade I Sprain. A Grade I sprain involves stretching of ligaments that support a joint without significant tearing. Symptoms are tenderness, swelling, often without effusion or hematoma, no pain on motion, and no instability. Treatment includes rest for the injured joint—use of crutches, soft wraps, or slings when appropriate. A compression dressing can be applied during the first 48 hours to control hemorrhage. The administration of injectable enzymes to alleviate soft tissue reactions has not proved beneficial and should be avoided. Once swelling and tenderness decrease, usually 3 to 10 days after injury, further movement of the injured joint is encouraged. Range of motion exercises are begun and often performed after the application of moist heat in a whirlpool, tub, or paraffin bath.

TABLE 1. **Management of Sprains and Strains**

Grade	Pathophysiology	Clinical Findings	Treatment*
I	Stretch without tear	No joint instability, tender with minimal effusion, normal function.	RICE initially, contrast baths.
II	Partial tear	No instability of joint, tenderness and effusion, possible hematoma, muscle function on stress testing, inability to use joint, mild loss of strength.	RICE initially, immobilization, contrast baths later, NSAIDs, surgery rare.
III	Complete tear	Severe pain, hematoma and effusion with joint instability, severe disability, and abnormal function. Muscle guarding common. Muscle strength often absent.	RICE, immobilization, contrast baths later, NSAIDs, surgery more common

*RICE = rest, ice, compression, and elevation.

In the later healing stages, contrast bath treatments are given to provide an alternating vasodilatation-vasoconstriction effect that ameliorates edema. This procedure consists of packing the injured area in ice or applying ice massage or ice immersion for 1 minute at 13 to 18 C (55 to 65 F), removing the injured joint from the ice, and applying moist heat for 4 minutes at 40 C (104 F). These treatments are done for 30 minutes each time, three to four times a day. The patient should be able to use the extremity without discomfort in 7 to 10 days. The time period varies with the joint injured and the age of the patient. Generally, joints involving more complex motions require longer recovery periods. All patients should be given written rehabilitation instructions that include flexibility and strength exercises, ice and contrast treatments, other physical therapy procedures, and other functional exercises that will help them return to participation in their activity as soon as possible.

Grade II Sprain. A grade II sprain is often difficult to recognize and treat. This injury involves partial tearing of the ligaments involved in stabilizing the joint. No joint instability, however, is demonstrable on physical examination. Further injury to a grade II sprain may result in a complete tear of the ligament if improperly treated. Symptoms generally include pain, local tenderness, swelling with effusion, and inability to use the joint.

Treatment involves rest, a compression dressing, application of ice, and external support in the form of a splint or a cast. A posterior splint is often superior to a cast in the presence of excessive joint swelling. Aspiration of the joint to remove the effusion is seldom performed unless the patient has excessive swelling resulting in neurovascular impairment. The injection of enzymes is not advised. It is often difficult to determine the severity of the injury; this determination is done through stress testing of the involved ligaments. Generally, longer periods of immobilization and rehabilitation are required for more extensive tears of the ligament. A grade II injury often requires the same treatment time as that of a fracture. Immobilization is frequently required for 2 to 3 weeks, after which time the joint is re-examined to determine whether further immobilization is needed. The amount of support is decreased as the sprain improves, employing materials that are less rigid than a cast (cast padding wrap or felt strapping). Gradually, immobilization is decreased over the next 7 to 14 days. When all external support has been removed, the joint should be mobilized using contrast bath treatments as previously described.

Problems in managing patients with grade II sprains are often encountered, usually 3 weeks post-injury when swelling is decreased and the joint feels relatively good. Return to full participation is not in the best interest of the patient; many patients with grade II sprains may require an additional 3 to 6 weeks to completely heal and to assure normal joint function. In addition to the use of contrast baths, physical therapy modalities including ultrasound, muscle stimulation, or galvanic stimulation aid earlier return to normal function. Appropriate flexibility and strengthening exercises should be initiated early in the rehabilitation period. Isometric exercises, especially for the quadriceps and hamstrings, can be done early in the treatment phase. They help reduce the rehabilitation period and minimize the atrophy of the involved muscles surrounding the injured joint.

NSAIDs are helpful in dealing with the inflammation accompanying grade II sprains and may aid in returning the athlete to earlier participation. Cortisone injections may be indicated in rare cases. Extreme caution should be exercised by the physician when injecting corticosteroids into or around tendons, as the tensile strength of the tendon may be interrupted for 4 to 6 months.

Grade III Sprain. A grade III sprain or a complete tear of one or several ligaments that maintain joint stability is associated with severe pain, blood within the joint, swelling, severe disability, abnormal motion, and joint instability. Muscle guarding is common and may make the determination of joint instability difficult. If instability cannot be demonstrated on clinical stress testing of the involved ligament, it may be necessary to anesthetize the joint and take an x-ray with the area under stress.

Initial treatment involves RICE (rest, ice, compression, and elevation). Treatment for grade III ankle sprains involving both the anterior talofibular and calcaneofibular ligament may be surgery. Most grade III knee sprains require arthroscopic surgery and possible reconstruction except for isolated grade III medial collateral ligament sprains.

Patients with grade III knee sprains are commonly treated as patients with simple injuries; they should be referred to an orthopedic surgeon for arthroscopy within 10 days of the injury. If a nonoperative approach is chosen, the knee should be immobilized in either a semirigid splint, such as a Zimmer or Universal, or a knee splint, such as a Bledsoe brace. The AirCast splint is useful in providing early immobilization for most grade II and III ankle sprains.

Application of a plaster cast is often done for rigid immobilization of the joint, providing the utmost comfort for the patient in many cases.

Immobilization time varies with the injured joint, but it is approximately the same as the time required for a fracture in the same area.

Treatment of all grade III sprains involves a complete rehabilitation program as outlined under grade I and II sprains. During the rehabilitation period, it is important for the patient to work on both muscular and cardiovascular endurance. Endurance training may be done during the intermediate phases of rehabilitation. Exercises in a pool are an excellent way to regain both strength and endurance. The athlete can begin these exercises as soon as the cast is removed or even earlier if no cast was applied. The buoyancy of water allows the performance of exercises that would otherwise be painful, especially in injuries involving weight-bearing joints. The injured athlete should strive to improve cardiovascular endurance during rehabilitation to prevent early fatigue and the possibility of reinjury upon returning to sports participation.

Agility, speed, and skills specific to the athlete's sport are regained in the final phases of rehabilitation. These activities are begun at a noncompetitive level and are gradually increased to a competitive level. Complete rehabilitation for certain injuries may require a full year. It is important that the physician be actively involved in all phases of the rehabilitation program.

Specific Therapeutic Considerations

Lateral Ankle Sprains

The most common ankle injury is the sprain of one of the lateral ligaments due to inversion stress. If the foot is plantar flexed at the time of the injury, the anterior talofibular ligament is affected, but if the foot is not flexed, the calcaneofibular ligament is affected. The degree of the sprain should be determined, as this will have impact on the treatment program. X-rays of a sprained ankle are as important in ruling out the differential diagnosis of associated fractures as they are in assessing joint instability.

The majority of ankle sprains are grade I injuries limited to the single anterior talofibular ligament. This type of injury is best treated by external support with elastic wrap or tape, which permits ankle flexion and extension but prevents inversion. Another alternative is application of the commercially available AirCast. Avoid complete immobilization of the ankle, which tends to produce heel cord tightening. Instead, encourage the patient to bear some weight with crutches and then to begin balancing and proprioceptive exercises when the pain subsides, usually within 3 to 5 days.

An acute ankle sprain rarely requires surgical repair. The exception is the case of the active young athlete with complete tears of the major lateral ligaments associated with joint instability. Other candidates for surgery are the patients with acute, complete ligamentous tears and histories of recurrent episodes of instability and the patients with unstable ankles associated with small avulsion fractures or osteochondral fractures of the talus. Long-term instability will eventually produce osteoarthritic changes in the joint, particularly evident on radiographs taken during weight-bearing positions. Reconstruction of lateral ligamentous structures is an effective way to prevent recurrent ankle instability from progressing to symptomatic osteoarthritis. A full rehabilitation program should be instituted after every ankle injury.

Medial Ankle Sprains

Deltoid ligament sprains, although rare, occur when the ankle joint is placed under stress in severe pronation. The physician should not overlook the significance of a medial ankle sprain involving the deltoid ligament, especially in the presence of joint stability. Obtain x-rays to help rule out the differential diagnosis of associated fractures of the malleous, tibia, and fibula. Tears of the tibiofibular ligament or interosseous membrane, or both, are commonly found with a deltoid ligament sprain and may lead to an unstable ankle mortice, which must be examined by x-ray. Any significant deltoid ligament sprain should be evaluated by an orthopedic surgeon to determine the necessity for immediate repair. Early care of the medial ankle sprain is similar to that of the lateral ankle sprain. The joint should be protected by rigid immobilization and use of crutches until evaluation by an orthopedic surgeon.

Criteria for Return to Activity Following an Ankle Injury

1. There should be no suggestion from the examination that a fracture is still present.
2. There should be no evidence of ligamentous instability.
3. The athlete should be able to raise up on his toes without difficulty; hop; run forward and backward; "run and cut" (the athlete runs fairly rapidly over a 20 to 30 yard distance and cuts to the right and then to the left); and run "figure 8's" at normal speed without a limp.

After these criteria are satisfied, the athlete is permitted to return to participation. Protective tape or an AirCast should be applied to support the injured ligaments. Immediately after participation, the ankle is re-evaluated and treated as indicated previously.

Management of Knee Sprains

Collateral Ligament Sprains

The isolated sprain of the medial collateral ligament is more common than that of the lateral collateral ligament. The grading system and treatment program are similar for both ligamentous sprains. Significant lateral collateral ligament sprains, however, may be associated with injuries to other secondary, restraining structures of the knee and may require thorough evaluation by an orthopedic surgeon.

Grade I knee sprains are generally managed nonsurgically. Protection with a knee immobilizer for 3 to 7 days combined with NSAID therapy and quadriceps rehabilitation (knee isometrics) will restore function of the injured ligament within 2 weeks, in most cases. The patient should not return to full activity until there is full range of motion and normal muscle strength, and effusion has subsided.

Grade II injuries require the knee to be immobilized in a splint for 10 to 14 days. The patient begins isometric quadricep exercises immediately. Immobilization in a long leg cast for 6 weeks is no longer the treatment of choice. A cast is unnecessary and often detrimental due to severe quadriceps atrophy. After several days of immobilization, the patient is able to begin gentle range of motion exercises of the knee. When the patient can move the knee through the full range of motion without swelling, a jogging program with no cutting or turning is begun. A competitive athlete generally returns to full activity within 3 to 5 weeks, while the recreational athlete may return to full activity 8 to 10 weeks following a grade II injury. When range of motion is established, start the patient on stationary bike exercises or swimming for maintenance of cardiovascular conditioning. A full-weight training program is initiated once complete range of motion is achieved.

Grade III or complete tears of the ligament have been traditionally repaired surgically. Most incidences of isolated grade III medial collateral ligament sprains will require longer periods of immobilization in a splint, often up to 4 weeks. The patient is then begun on a full rehabilitation program, as mentioned under grade II sprains, and returns to activity once normal strength and function are achieved. Grade III collateral ligament sprains associated with tears of other ligaments may require surgery. If surgery is required, the ligaments should be repaired within 10 to 14 days of injury, or the inflammatory process may significantly weaken any remaining ligament or lead to development of excessive scar tissue. An orthopedist capable of arthroscopic surgery should be consulted as early as possible, following the grade III knee sprain.

Guidelines for Return to Activity Following a Knee Injury

1. No return to activity is allowed in the presence of knee instability.
2. If the athlete has ligamentous stability and normal menisci and patella, he or she should be put through a series of functional tests: hopping on the affected leg; "running and cutting" (the athlete runs fairly rapidly over a 20 to 30 yard distance and cuts to the right and then to the left); running backwards; and running figure 8's (the athlete starts with rather large figure 8's and rapidly runs progressively smaller ones). If the athlete completes these functional tests without problems, return to play is permitted. Injection of cortisone or local anesthetics should never be attempted to allow an athlete to participate.

Anterior Cruciate Sprain

The most common mechanism of injury is external rotation of the tibia in relation to the femur. This is always associated with damage to the medial capsule and collateral structures. The anterior cruciate ligament (ACL) can also be injured when the tibia is internally rotated or hyperextended, or both. The patient often hears or feels a pop within the knee. This sign should be considered indicative of a ruptured ACL until proved otherwise. Although intense pain is initially felt, the patient is often able to continue participation for a short time. Usually a painful effusion develops within 2 to 4 hours. The most common mistake made by the examiner is to not diagnose a partial or complete ACL tear. Any questionable ACL sprain should be evaluated by an orthopedic surgeon capable of performing arthroscopy.

Treatment of isolated ACL tears or ACL tears in conjunction with medial collateral ligament sprains has been widely debated. Many orthopedic surgeons would repair an isolated tear in a young athletic patient through an augmentation or reconstruction technique. If repair of the ACL is elected, it should be done within the first 14 days following injury. Prior to an orthopedic referral, the knee should be immobilized in a Zimmer or Universal knee immobilizer. Frequent application of ice and elevation of the extremity is indicated until the patient can be evaluated by an orthopedic surgeon. The rare patient with a tense effusion may require aspiration of blood from the joint.

Dislocation

Dislocation is the loss of normal anatomic alignment of a joint caused by tearing of soft tissues around the joint. Partial dislocation or subluxation is suspected in the patient complaining of a feeling that the joint is slipping out of place in the absence of true dislocation. Recurrent injuries to a subluxated joint may result in a dislocation. All such complaints should be investigated by the physician, as it is important that the muscular structures surrounding the joint be thoroughly rehabilitated. X-rays should be obtained to determine the extent of the injury, to identify any associated fractures, and to report the position of the joint following reduction. The physician should remember that a dislocation creates a grade II or III injury to the joint, which will require appropriate initial therapy and rehabilitation. A period of immobilization should follow reduction to allow time for the soft tissue injury to heel.

The shoulder joint is a common area for partial (subluxation) or complete dislocation. The most common type is the anterior displacement of the shoulder as a result of athletic trauma. The arm is forced into abduction and extension with the head of the humerus displacing anteriorly, causing damage to the anterior structures of the shoulder and decreased stability. The anterior aspect of the shoulder is acutely tender with decreased range of motion and a positive apprehension test. Significant clicking or popping in the joint and discomfort upon reproduction of sound may indicate a glenolabrium tear. Appropriate x-rays should be obtained.

Treatment of Dislocation of the Shoulder

Treatment includes initial reduction of the dislocation following x-ray. A wide variety of reduction techniques are available. Following reduction, the shoulder is placed in a sling and swathe or a simple sling for comfort and within 1 to 3 weeks early range of motion with progressive resistance exercises are performed. The athlete is allowed to return to play when full use of the shoulder and equal strength (at least 90 per cent of the uninjured side) is obtained. The patient with recurrent subluxation and dislocation can be managed with a sling for comfort after reduction. Early range of motion exercises should be initiated. The patient may return to activity when all guidelines have been met. Surgery is indicated for recurrent subluxation and dislocation not responding satisfactorily to conservative treatment.

Many joints are subject to dislocation in athletic injuries. The principles of proper diagnosis, early management, and rehabilitation are the same for most of these injuries. Prior to competition, the athlete can be fitted with an appropriate protective sling, harness, or splint during the later rehabilitative phases of therapy.

Overuse Injuries

By far the most common category of injury seen in the office or emergency room is that of the overuse syndrome. Overuse can be a result of overtraining or overconditioning and occurs in many different sports and activities. The patient most likely to suffer an overuse injury is one who exercises on a regular basis, and the degree of injury relates directly to the amount, intensity, and frequency of the exercise performed. Repetitive stress to any body part is capable of producing tissue breakdown, resulting in an overuse syndrome or injury. The injury may cause a variety of clinical problems, such as bursitis, tendonitis, fasciitis, compartment syndrome, and stress fracture. A clinical guideline that outlines an approach to most of the musculoskeletal injuries caused by overuse is presented in Table 2.

Use of the clinical guideline is summarized as follows:

1. It is important to ascertain from the patient when pain is perceived in relation to the timing of the exercise. The more severe the problem, the more likely pain will occur before, during, and after exercise and severely affect performance.
2. Physical examination will reveal generalized tenderness in mild overuse injuries but will reveal localized tenderness, decreased range of motion, and normal function in the most severe overuse injuries.
3. The pathophysiology involved in causing the symptoms of overuse is postulated for each level of overuse injury. True overuse has occurred only in the more severe injuries—grades III to IV.
4. Diagnostic aids such as x-rays and bone scans are useful only for grade III and IV injuries.
5. Treatment of overuse syndrome varies with the severity of the injury. The range of treatment extends from reassurance and injury prevention when dealing with a grade I injury to complete rest and use of NSAIDs when dealing with a grade IV injury.

Treatment of Overuse Injuries

The following general guidelines for therapy are helpful:

Reassurance and Education of the Athlete. The physician should concentrate on the etiology of the patient's injury and evaluate intensity, duration, and frequency of training and any recent training adjustments. A review of the patient's equipment, footwear, training environment, weight-training program, as well as input from the younger patient's parents and coach may be helpful in eliciting the cause of injury. The biomechanics of the sport or exercise activity should be thoroughly discussed, and any biomechanical or training errors should be corrected as part of the treatment program. It is paramount that the physician work closely with the athlete, coach, and family when appropriate to treat and prevent overuse injuries.

Ice. Ice application is the primary mode of treatment for all overuse injuries. It is readily available, easy to use, inexpensive, and universally tolerated with few side effects. Heat in the form of contrast baths may also prove valuable in the treatment of overuse injuries.

TABLE 2. **Clinical Guide to the Treatment of Musculoskeletal Overuse Injuries**

Injury Continuum	History	Physical Examination	Patho-physiology	Diagnostic Aids	Treatment	Comments
Grade I	Transient pains, hours *after* activity "Soreness" Symptoms of less than 2 weeks' duration	Generalized tenderness	Increase in lactic acid levels Muscle breakdown Minor inflammation	None	Ice as needed	Look at training regimen "New" athlete "Getting in shape"
Grade II	Longer standing pain *late* in activity or immediately *after* activity Symptoms of 2 to 3 weeks' duration	Localized pain, but not discrete point tenderness	Mild musculotendinous (soft tissue) inflammation	None	Ice Decrease regimen by 10 to 25%	True overuse Investigate environmental factors, such as use of wrong equipment or poor technique
Grade III	Pain in *early* or *middle of* activity (closer to beginning of activity) Symptoms of 3 to 4 weeks' duration	Point tenderness Percussion tenderness Pressure elsewhere produces pain at point Other evidence of inflammation (heat, erythema, swelling, crepitation)	Major musculotendinous inflammation Periostitis Bone microtrauma	X-ray (seldom positive) Bone scan useful in about 75% of cases	Ice Decrease regimen by 25 to 75% Initial 5 to 7 day rest period with concurrent course of NSAIDs	"Pre-stress" fracture syndrome
Grade IV	Pain *before* or *early* in exercise, preventng or affecting performance Symptoms of more than 4 weeks' duration	All of the grade III signs Disturbance in function Decrease in range of motion Muscle atrophy	Breakdown in soft tissue Stress fracture Compartment syndrome (especially if swelling is major finding)	X-ray Bone scan useful in about 95% of cases	Ice Rest from exercise NSAIDs	Immobilization? (usually not)

(Reprinted from McKeag, D. B.: The concept of overuse: the primary care aspects of overuse syndromes in sports. Primary Care *11*:48, 1984.)

Rest. Rest of the extremity is important for overuse injuries. The more severe the problem, the longer the initial period of rest should be. Rest in combination with NSAIDs provides faster healing of the injured area. Many athletes are noncompliant and dissatisfied with the prescription of rest, and rest can cause muscle atrophy, deconditioning, and loss of fine motor skills, which can predispose an athlete to further injury when activity is resumed. Therefore, the athlete is usually allowed to exercise on a stationary bike or in a swimming pool with most overuse injuries to maintain cardiovascular conditioning. An active weight-training program is instituted early in the physical therapy program to maintain muscular endurance.

Anti-inflammatory Medications. Although not recommended, dimethylsulfoxide (DMSO) is used in the self-treatment of overuse injuries, although it is not an FDA approved medication. Side effects of DMSO include a scaling skin rash and a garlic or oyster-like taste. NSAIDs are common in the treatment of overuse syndromes and are prescribed for their anti-inflammatory and analgesic affects. It is best not to administer NSAIDs unless the patient is willing to completely rest the extremity. Otherwise, masking of the pain occurs and the athlete tends to return to activity too early, causing re-injury or re-aggravation of the overuse problem. Parenteral corticosteroid medication alone or in combination with an anesthetic should be reserved for selected cases of bursitis or tenosynovitis. Repeated injections may cause necrosis of the collagen at the injection site and the possibility of tendon or ligamentous rupture. For this reason, corticosteroid injections are unwarranted in most overuse injuries. Any patient with a chronic overuse injury not responding to more common modes of treatment should be referred to an orthopedic surgeon.

Surgery. Surgery may be indicated in the treatment of overuse injuries (e.g., chronic rotator cuff injuries, Achilles tendons, compartment syndromes, and certain stress fractures). Surgery should be considered only after all medical measures have been attempted.

Rehabilitation. The patient should be given complete instructions regarding return to activity that concentrate on cardiovascular conditioning and range of motion and muscle strength exercises. Patients with severe overuse problems require 6 to 10 weeks of conditioning after the injury is healed before they can return to their activity. It is common for stress fractures to take the longest time for complete rehabilitation. During this period, patients gradually increase the frequency, duration, and intensity of their training. Any evidence of pain is cause for decreasing the training program to a level that will not produce pain. Application of ice to the injured area should follow every exercise session. By maintaining a gradual program of rehabilitation, the athlete will often return to full activity with normal function and little recurrence of the overuse injury.

Section 15

Obstetrics and Gynecology

ANTEPARTUM CARE

method of
JEFFREY P. PHELAN, M.D.,
and CARL V. SMITH, M.D.
University of Southern California
Los Angeles, California

Diagnosis of Pregnancy

Early diagnosis of pregnancy allows prompt antenatal evaluation of the pregnant patient. Thus, early diagnosis allows for thorough assessment of potential medical and obstetric problems and, most importantly, aids in the establishment of an estimated date of confinement (EDC). Determination of uterine size in the first trimester and recall of the last normal menstrual period (LNMP) are important reasons to initiate early antenatal care.

Typically, early pregnancy diagnosis relies on the presence or absence of human chorionic gonadotropin (HCG) in the urine or blood. Tests to rapidly determine HCG levels are readily available today and can be divided into three major groups. First, latex agglutination tests, which depend on the presence of HCG in the urine, have a sensitivity of 1.5 to 3 Iu per ml. These tests do not, however, distinguish between luteinizing hormone (LH) and HCG. As such, false-positive test results may occur in perimenopausal women whose LH levels are frequently elevated. When prompt diagnosis of pregnancy is essential, a more sensitive assay should be considered. Secondly, radioreceptor assays, using bovine corpora lutea, are more sensitive, but, like the latex agglutination tests, do not distinguish LH and HCG. Lastly, radioimmunoassays for the B-subunit of HCG are the most sensitive and will detect levels of 1 to 5 mIu per ml of HCG in the serum. It is a specific assay for HCG and does not cross-react with LH. Because of the high sensitivity, this test can be positive within 8 days of conception.

It should be stressed that even a positive B-subunit assay is not conclusive evidence of pregnancy. Ectopic production of HCG by ovarian and other neoplasias and by gestational trophoblastic neoplasia (*e.g.*, hydatidiform mole) may occur.

A final method of pregnancy diagnosis is ultrasound. Identification of a gestational sac within the uterus is frequently possible 5 weeks after the last menses. Fetal echoes inside the gestational sac are visible by 8 to 10 weeks of gestation. Absence of such findings does not, however, absolutely rule out pregnancy. Confirmation of an intrauterine pregnancy, early in gestation, is of critical importance in patients who are at high risk for ectopic pregnancies. Factors associated with an increased risk of an ectopic pregnancy include prior adnexal surgery, history of salpingitis, and the presence of an intrauterine contraceptive device (IUD). Ultrasound diagnosis of pregnancy using the Doppler stethoscope is possible after 10 weeks of gestation.

Establishment of an Accurate EDC

Determination of an accurate EDC is the most essential ingredient in the management of normal and complicated pregnancies. All obstetric care hinges on the patient's due date. The most accurate predictor of an EDC is the woman's last menstrual period (LMP). However, before one can rely on this index, the patient's prior menstrual history should be ascertained. In a regularly menstruating and presumably ovulating patient, the LMP may be used with a reasonable degree of certainty. However, in the patient with irregular menses or a history of oral contraceptive use within the prior 3 months, alternative methods to establish the EDC should be considered.

Additional confirmation may be obtained by estimation of the uterine size in the first trimester of pregnancy. If the length of gestation by LMP corresponds with the uterine size in the first trimester of pregnancy, one can be reasonably certain of the EDC. Similarly, the height of the uterine fundus, measured from the top of the symphysis pubis to the top of the fundus, correlates well with length of gestation between 20 and 32 weeks. This distance, in centimeters, should equal the weeks of gestation.

Auscultation of the fetal heart rate with a DeLee stethoscope is another important landmark. In normal pregnancies, fetal heart tones are audible between the eighteenth and twenty-second weeks of gestation. In this same time frame, quickening or maternal perception of fetal movement is first noticed. It is important to remember that the latter is a subjective method and may vary with placental location, parity, and education of the patient.

If there is any discrepancy in these clinical landmarks, ultrasonography should be used to complement the clinical findings. Although it may be performed at any time throughout pregnancy, its accuracy diminishes with advancing gestation. In the first trimester, sonographic measurement of the fetal crown-rump length is the most accurate determination of gestational age. In many series, this measurement correlates within 1 week of the patient's due date. Measurement of the diameter of the gestational sac is also feasible but is a less reliable estimate of gestational age.

Second trimester ultrasound is also an accurate predictor of gestational age. Such a sonogram should contain measurements of biparietal diameter (BPD), occipitofrontal diameter (OFD), abdominal diameter, and femur length. From these measurements, abdominal and head circumferences can be calculated. Standard tables can then be used to determine the ultrasound estimate of gestational age. Many such tables are available and the practitioner should use one that is most appropriate for his patient population. A single ultrasound performed between 13 and 20 weeks of gestation may predict a patient's EDC within 1 to 2 weeks. Serial sonographic evaluations of the fetus, intervally consistent, should increase the accuracy.

Third trimester ultrasounds are much less accurate and may disagree with delivery date by as much as 3 weeks.

First Obstetric Visit

History. In addition to a complete menstrual history, a complete medical history should be taken. Emphasis should be placed on prior hospitalizations, surgery, drug, alcohol, and tobacco use. A thorough review of systems should also be undertaken. Special emphasis should be placed on communicable diseases such as rubella, sexually transmitted diseases (including genital herpes), and hepatitis.

Obstetric History. Prior pregnancy outcomes should be carefully documented. Important information includes the number and durations of all pregnancies, the presence or absence of medical or obstetric complications, route of delivery and any reasons for intervention, prior birth weights, and neonatal malformations or complications. If the patient has undergone a prior cesarean delivery, the indication and type of uterine incision should be documented. Additionally, a detailed family history is important. The provider should search for a history of birth defects, medical illness, known genetic disease, multiple gestation, and bleeding diathesis. The finding of any of the above merits careful assessment of risks to both mother and fetus.

Physical Examination. A complete physical examination should be performed at the initial prenatal visit. The examination should include an evaluation of the height, weight (present and prepregnant), vital signs, head, neck, breast, lungs, heart, abdomen—presence of masses (including the gravid uterus, which is palpable after 12 weeks), bruits, fetal heart tones, extremities, and pelvis. During pelvic examination, the clinician should focus on the uterine size; presence of adnexal masses; cervical examination for lacerations, lesions, dilatation, and effacement; and the adequacy of the bony pelvis.

Laboratory Tests

Routine laboratory tests, which should be obtained at the first prenatal visit, include the following: complete blood count (CBC), urinalysis with culture and sensitivity, serologic test for syphilis, rubella antibody titre, blood group and Rh type with antibody screen, and cervical cytology. Additional laboratory studies may be dictated by historic and physical findings. These laboratory investigations might include, but are not limited to, a sickle cell screen in black patients, culture for *Neisseria gonorrhoeae,* a screen for diabetes mellitus, tuberculosis skin test, and hepatitis B surface antigen.

At approximately 28 weeks of gestation, the following laboratory tests are ordered: CBC; blood type, Rh, and antibody screen; and diabetes screening for all patients.

At approximately 36 weeks, the CBC should be repeated along with blood type, Rh, and antibody screen. In patients at increased risk, serologic testing for syphilis and cervical culture for gonorrhea may be repeated.

Prenatal Education

Diet. The energy requirements during pregnancy are 15 per cent higher than in the nonpregnant state. As such, most authorities recommend an additional 300 Kcal per day throughout gestation. In addition to the increased caloric requirements, 65 gm of protein per day should be included. Following these guidelines, the average gravida will gain an additional 20 to 30 lbs. In most instances, pregnant patients may be counseled to eat three balanced meals per day, salted to taste. Sodium restriction in pregnancy has not proved to be effective in reducing the incidence of hypertension and may, in fact, be harmful. Poor weight gain may be associated with intrauterine growth retardation (IUGR). Rapid weight gain should lead the clinician to suspect pregnancy-induced hypertension.

Because most women are unable to meet the minimum nutritional requirements, use of prenatal vitamins are recommended during pregnancy. Supplementation with 30 to 60 mg per day of elemental iron is recommended due to the 6 to 7 mg per day increase in maternal requirements for iron. Folic acid requirements are also increased in pregnancy. Supplementation of folate in amounts of 400 to 800 micrograms per day is currently recommended.

Activity. In general, no activity restrictions are necessary in a normal pregnancy. Pregnant women should avoid strenuous or near-maximal physical activity. Excessive fatigue, whatever the reason, should likewise be avoided. The activity level of women whose pregnancies are complicated by IUGR, cardiac disease, hypertensive disorders, or multiple gestation should be modified accordingly. If a pregnant woman is employed, an inquiry into her work environment should be done at her initial visit. Subsequent recommendations as to continued employment or a modification of her current position should take into account the potential hazards on the job. Frequently, consultation with occupational health care providers is needed.

Medication Use. Every medication used by the gravida should be presumed to cross the placenta. In every case, the benefits of medication use should outweigh the potential risks.

Travel. Travel restrictions during pregnancy are usually not required. For reasons of comfort and fewer complications, the best time to travel is in the second trimester. Whatever the mode of transportation selected, the best means of transportation is the one by which the patient will feel most comfortable and enjoy the most. During travel, the patient should avoid excessive fatigue and should be ambulatory every 1 to 2 hours to minimize venous stasis and potential thromboembolic complications. Another factor to consider is travel to foreign countries, which may expose the patient to the risk of required immunizations in endemic areas. A more practical consideration is the potential limited access to adequate health care in the event complications arise.

Travel by automobile is the most common form of transportation by pregnant women today. Unfortunately, few pregnant women use any form of seat belt for protection. The use of a car restraint system is the best precaution anyone, including the pregnant woman, can take. In all circumstances, the seat belt should be fastened snugly. The lap belt should be positioned low on the hips and under the bulge of the abdomen.

Sexual Relations. Sexual intercourse appears to have no adverse effect on normal pregnancies before 36 weeks. After 36 weeks, some reports indicate a higher infection rate. Sexual intercourse should be avoided if there are ruptured membranes, during labor, and if there is threatened abortion or vaginal bleeding. In patients at high risk for premature labor and delivery, sexual relations should be avoided.

Genetic Counseling. Midtrimester amniocentesis should be offered to patients with the following indications: (1) maternal age 35 or greater at delivery, (2) prior delivery of a chromosomally abnormal fetus, (3) fetal sex determination in cases of X-linked recessive disorders, (4) parents with balanced translocation, (5) prior child or parent with a neural tube defect, and (6) biochemical analysis in patients at risk for an in-born error of metabolism. This list should not be considered all-inclusive, and a patient with any history of genetic disease should be referred for genetic counseling.

Immunization. As with medication use, the benefits must clearly outweigh the risks. Live virus vaccines, which include measles, mumps, and rubella, should be avoided. In the event of unavoidable travel to endemic areas, immunization with a "killed virus" vaccine may be preferable.

Vaginal Birth After Cesarean Delivery. The marked increase in the incidence of cesarean delivery in the last decade has been a recent concern. One proposed method of reducing this incidence is by permitting selected patients a trial of labor (TOL). Current recommended requirements for permitting a TOL are as follows: (1) one prior low transverse uterine incision, (2) availability of immediate cesarean delivery, (3) availability of banked blood, and (4) no obstetric indication for cesarean delivery. It would appear that the use of oxytocin and epidural anesthesia is also a reasonable consideration in this group. One can anticipate a 70 to 80 per cent success rate in the TOL group with minimal risks to mother and fetus. Investigation of patients with more than one prior cesarean delivery and the presence of a low vertical scar in the uterus is continuing. In the future, a TOL may also be a reasonable alternative in these patients.

Childbirth Education. Many organizations provide Childbirth Education to prospective parents. Practitioners should be familiar with these groups because many patients benefit from additional education. This additional information may allay their fears and be a useful adjunct to prenatal education by members of the health care team. Responding to the demands of prospective parents, many hospitals have established "birthing rooms" or alternative birth centers. These areas offer motivated prospective parents an alternative to the hazardous practice of home delivery.

Schedule of Prenatal Visits

After the initial prenatal visits, patients are seen every 4 weeks until 28 weeks of gestation, biweeky until 36 weeks, and then weekly. The following information should be checked at each prenatal visit: weight, blood pressure, fundal height, presence or absence of edema, fetal heart tones, maternal urine screen for albumin and glucose, weeks of gestation, and fetal lie and presentation in late pregnancy.

Complications of Pregnancy

Diabetes Mellitus. Because of the high frequency of latent diabetes mellitus, all pregnant patients should be screened for diabetes mellitus. Screening should include a fasting glucose level and a glucose determination one hour following oral ingestion of 50 grams carbohydrate load. Any serum value greater than 140 mg per dl warrants a 3-hour glucose tolerance test (GTT). Risk factors that indicate early screening for diabetes mellitus are glycosuria, prior delivery of an infant weighing in excess of 4000 grams, family history of diabetes, prior unexplained stillbirth with or without congenital anomalies, and history of gestational diabetes (Class A). If any two values are abnormal, a diagnosis of gestational diabetes (Class A) diabetes mellitus should be made. The upper limits of normal for plasma glucose values for the GTT are fasting: 105 mg per dl, 1 hour: 190 mg per dl, 2 hours: 165 mg per dl, and 3 hours: 145 mg per dl. Once a diagnosis of diabetes is made, the patient should undergo dietary counseling and be placed on an ADA diet consisting of 30 to 35 kcal per kg, including 1.5 grams protein per kg of actual body weight.

The prognosis of the diabetic pregnancy is related to the severity of the disease. An estimate of the perinatal risk can be obtained by categorizing according to a modification of the White Classification (Table 1).

TABLE 1. **Classification of Diabetes in Pregnancy**

A:	Gestational diabetes
B:	Maturity onset (age over 20 years), duration under 10 years, no vascular lesions
C_1A:	Age 10 to 19 years at onset
C_2:	10 to 19 years duration
D_1:	Under age 10 years at onset
D_2:	Over 20 years duration
D_3:	Benign retinopathy
D_4:	Calcified vessels of legs
D_5:	Hypertension
F:	Nephropathy
G:	Many obstetric failures
H:	Cardiopathy
R:	Proliferative retinopathy
T:	Renal transplant

The primary goal in the diabetic pregnancy is the maintenance of euglycemia, that is, fasting glucose level below 105 mg per dl and a 2-hour postprandial level below 120 mg per dl. Tight control of maternal glucose levels before conception and throughout the pregnancy is associated with a reduction in neonatal morbidity and mortality as well as congenital anomalies. Throughout the pregnancy, ketoacidosis and hypoglycemia, which have an undesirable effect on the fetus, should be avoided.

Antepartum fetal heart rate testing, traditionally the nonstress test (NST), should be initiated at 40 weeks of gestation in patients with gestational diabetes. All other patients with diabetes should be tested beginning at 34 weeks of gestation. Earlier testing should be considered in those patients whose diabetes is complicated by vascular disease, history of a prior stillbirth, or preeclampsia.

In the absence of maternal complication or an abnormal NST, delivery of gestational diabetics is generally at term. Other classes of diabetes should be delivered after assessment of fetal pulmonary maturity. The presence of phosphatidyl glycerol (PG) in amniotic fluid obtained by amniocentesis is reflective of pulmonary maturity. Generally, amniocentesis is performed at 37 to 38 weeks. In the absence of fetal macrosomatia, oxytocin induction of labor and vaginal delivery may be considered. If ultrasonographic or clinical estimates of fetal weight exceed 4000 grams, elective primary cesarean delivery should be strongly considered.

Hypertension. Approximately 9 per cent of all pregnancies are complicated by hypertension. This may be either chronic hypertension (prior to 20 weeks of gestation), pregnancy-induced hypertension (PIH) (after the 20th week), or PIH superimposed on chronic hypertension.

Chronic hypertension, newly diagnosed in pregnancy, should be treated when blood pressure is above 140/90mm Hg. The most commonly used antihypertensives in pregnancy are methyldopa and hydralazine. Both have had extensive use in obstetrics. Before initiating therapy, the following laboratory tests should be considered: 24-hour urine collection for creatinine clearance and total protein, serum BUN, creatinine, electrolytes, electrocardiogram, and chest x-ray (shielded abdomen) if appropriate. If those studies and the physical examination are normal, the patient is presumed to have essential hypertension. Medical therapy may be instituted with methyldopa in doses of 250 mg twice daily and increased to maximum of 2 grams per day to achieve a blood pressure of less than 140/90 mm Hg.

The chronic hypertensive is at risk for development of intrauterine growth retardation, intrauterine fetal death, abruptio placenta, and superimposed PIH. The latter is manifested by worsening blood pressure control, increasing proteinuria, and deteriorating renal function. NSTs should begin at 34 weeks and continue until delivery.

PIH (pre-eclampsia) can be defined as an absolute blood pressure of 140/90 mm Hg or a 30-mm Hg rise in the systolic blood pressure or a 15-mm Hg rise in the diastolic blood pressure over baseline levels. Generalized edema and protein are variably present. The treatment for pre-eclampsia at term is delivery, generally under anticonvulsant therapy with parenteral magnesium sulfate. In the preterm patient, bed rest with serial testing of renal function and the fetal heart rate may be attempted. Worsening hypertension, deteriorating renal function, or abnormal fetal heart rate testing are indications for delivery. Severe pre-eclampsia defined as blood pressure elevation to 160/110 mm Hg, 5 grams per 24 hours of proteinuria, headache, epigastric pain, oliguria, abnormal liver function tests, or fetal growth retardation are also indications for delivery.

A variant of pre-eclampsia characterized by hemolysis, elevated liver function tests, and low platelets has been described and given the eponym, the HELLP syndrome. Even though many of the patients with this disorder do not meet the blood pressure criteria for severe pre-eclampsia, these patients should be considered to have it. The subsequent management of these patients should be consistent with the management of any patient with severe pre-eclampsia.

In the gravida with severe pre-eclampsia, especially when there is oliguria, pulmonary edema or poorly controlled hypertension, central hemodynamic monitoring with a flow-directed pulmonary artery catheter may be of significant assistance in directing therapy.

Most authorities recommend continuing magnesium therapy until 24 hours postpartum or until clinical improvement occurs. This is usually heralded by a pronounced diuresis.

Urinary Tract Infection. Asymptomatic bacteriuria (ASB), defined as greater than 100,000 colonies per ml in a clean catch urine specimen may progress to acute pyelonephritis if untreated. All pregnant patients should be screened for ASB at the initial prenatal visit. Treatment should be based on the sensitivity report. Nitrofurantoin, cephalosporins, and ampicillin are appropriate antibiotics in the nonallergic patient. Once treated, periodic urine cultures should be performed. Recurrent ASB is a commonly accepted indication for prophylaxis. Nightly use of 100 mg of nitrofurantoin is an acceptable regimen.

Acute lower urinary tract infections (UTI) should be treated in a similar fashion. Acute pyelonephritis is an indication for hospitalization and parenteral antibiotic therapy. Initial treatment with cephalosporins or ampicillin is common until the sensitivity report is available. Aminoglycosides, because of their toxicity, should be reserved for serious or unresponsive infections. After completion of intravenous antibiotic therapy, prophylaxis with nitrofurantoin is initiated and continued until term. Post-treatment culture and sensitivity is essential.

Preterm Delivery. This is the most frequent cause of perinatal mortality. Antecedent risk factors for its development are premature rupture of the membranes (PROM), UTI and pyelonephritis, prior history of preterm delivery, and multiple gestation. The presence of any of these factors should prompt the clinician to educate the patient regarding the symptoms of preterm labor or PROM. The presence of either merits hospitalization for further evaluation and possible tocolysis. Agents available for tocolysis are beta-sympathomimetics (*e.g.*, ritodrine) and magnesium sulfate. Because of the enhanced risk of myocardial ischemia, combination chemotherapy with a beta-mimetic and magnesium sulfate should be avoided. Tocolytics should be used with caution when PROM and vaginal bleeding are evident. They are contraindicated in the presence of a dead fetus, an obstetric indication for delivery, maternal cardiovascular disease (beta-sympathomimetics), heavy vaginal bleeding, unexplained maternal fever, fetal distress, or advanced labor.

Maternal side effects of beta-sympathomimetics include tachycardia, hypokalemia, hyperglycemia, arrhythmia, hypotension, chest pain, and, rarely, pulmonary edema. Fetal complications include tachycardia and, rarely, metabolic effects similar to those found in the mother. Discontinuation should be considered whenever the following major side effects are encountered: maternal tachycardia (above 150), fetal tachycardia (above 200), hypotension (diastolic below 40), more than six premature ventricular contractions per minute, presence of chest pain, and signs and symptoms of pulmonary edema.

The diagnosis of PROM is confirmed by sterile speculum examination. Pooling of amnionic fluid in the posterior vaginal fornix, ferning pattern on microscopy, and an alkaline pH by nitrazene paper testing are suggestive findings of PROM. PROM in a term patient is treated by delivery. The majority of those patients will be in spontaneous labor within 12 hours.

The treatment of preterm PROM is largely

conservative in patients who are at less than 34 weeks of gestation. Vaginal pool samples for evidence of fetal pulmonary maturity (Lecithin/sphingomyelin [L/S] ratio, presence of phosphatidyl glycerol) may be performed, and, if consistent with pulmonary maturity, delivery should be considered. If conservative management is elected, the patient should be closely monitored for evidence of labor, fetal distress, or infection (chorioamnionitis). The roles of tocolysis, amniocentesis, and corticosteroids (to enhance fetal pulmonary maturity) remain controversial.

Intrauterine Growth Retardation (IUGR). As many as 40 to 50 per cent of all small for gestational age (SGA) neonates are undiagnosed prior to delivery. With the increasing use of ultrasound, more antenatal diagnoses are made. Associated risk factors for this condition include multiple gestation, reduced weight gain and low pre-pregnancy weight, maternal vascular disease, congenital anomalies, and placental or umbilical cord abnormalities. Clinical suspicion may be aroused when the uterine fundal height demonstrates poor growth or when oligohydramnios is suspected. A baseline ultrasound should be considered in high-risk pregnancy with serial ultrasound examination to determine growth. No single ultrasound parameter can be used, but serial measurements of the parameters listed earlier allow for a diagnosis of altered fetal growth. The presence of oligohydramnios should be interpreted as ominous. It should alert the clinician to the possibility of congenital anomalies or of end-stage IUGR.

Two types of IUGR have been described. Symmetric IUGR, so-called because both the head (BPD, HC) and the abdomen (AC) are affected, is more common with congenital infections and congenital or chromosomal anomalies. It is also reflective of the end-stage of asymmetric IUGR. The latter is thought to be associated with uteroplacental dysfunction and is characterized by a normal BPD for gestational age ("head-sparing") and an AC less than the 10th percentile for gestational age.

Both types of IUGR are indications for antepartum fetal heart rate testing (AFHRT). When IUGR is complicated by abnormal AFHRT, further evaluation, including assessment of fetal pulmonary maturity and evaluation for delivery, should be considered.

Abnormal Lie. In late pregnancy, determination of fetal presentation should be assessed at each clinic visit. The presence of a breech presentation or a transverse lie at 37 weeks or beyond should prompt an evaluation for its etiology. Placenta previa, uterine anomalies, and fetal anomalies are associated with an increased incidence of abnormal presentation. If none are identified, the patient should be alerted to risks of cesarean section, umbilical cord prolapse, and fetal death. If attempted vaginal delivery is accepted by the patient, she should be instructed to report to the hospital promptly after labor or membrane rupture occurs. If this and external cephalic version are unacceptable to her, strong consideration should be given for elective primary cesarean birth at 39 weeks of gestation.

Although currently controversial, an alternative approach, external cephalic version (ECV), is a reasonable consideration. If successful, it may obviate the need for cesarean delivery and lower the incidence of cord prolapse. Patients with breech presentation should be referred for evaluation between 37 and 42 weeks. Absence of congenital anomalies, a reactive NST, normal ultrasound evaluation of amniotic fluid volume, and patient acceptance are requirements for inclusion. ECV is accomplished under tocolysis with ritodrine or magnesium sulfate under continuous fetal heart rate monitoring. After attempted ECV, a second NST is performed. The patient is then discharged with a recommendation for weekly NSTs. One can anticipate a 70 to 80 per cent success rate. In addition, the procedure appears to be safe for both mother and fetus.

Patients with a transverse lie may likewise be candidates for ECV. The same inclusion criteria as for breech are used. ECV of a breech presentation occurs in our outpatient clinic area. Because of the higher theoretical risks of cord prolapse and membrane rupture, version of transverse lie patients is attempted in the labor and delivery area. Prior to attempted version, fetal pulmonary maturity is assessed sonographically. If there is evidence of maturity, ECV is attempted. If ECV is successful, induction of labor is performed. If it is unsuccessful, we proceed to cesarean delivery.

Multiple Gestation. The incidence of twin gestation is reported as 1 in 90 pregnancies. Because of the marked increase in prematurity and perinatal mortality, early diagnosis and management is essential. Routine ultrasonography would improve the rate of antenatal diagnosis but cannot be advocated currently. Patients at high risk for multiple gestation should undergo ultrasound examination. These patients are those with a family history of twins, size-date discrepancies, history of ovulation induction with the current pregnancy (clomiphene citrate or human menopausal gonadotropins), or the appearance of pregnancy-induced hypertension prior to 20 weeks of gestation. Twin pregnancies are more likely to be complicated by anemia, glucose intolerance, pregnancy-induced hypertension, IUGR, prematurity, and postpartum hemorrhage. Patients with twin gestations should be encouraged to increase their amount of bed rest, beginning in the late second or early third trimester until term. The efficacy of this approach, however, is controversial. Prophylactic cerclage placement and the routine use of oral tocolytics have not proved to be efficacious. Ultrasound monitoring of concordant fetal growth is of critical importance. Although antepartum fetal heart rate (FHR) testing is of proven value in high-risk singleton pregnancies, its role in otherwise uncomplicated twin pregnancies is as yet unproved. Certainly, with the appearance of hypertension, premature labor, and discordant growth, some form of fetal surveillance is indicated.

Similarly, the intrapartum management of term twins is controversial. Malpresentation of the first twin is a commonly used indication for cesarean delivery. At some institutions, if the first twin is in the cephalic presentation, a trial of labor is permitted with close monitoring of both twins. Immediate availability of cesarean delivery is mandatory. No apparent increase in morbidity or mortality has been found in our population, even when the second twin is breech or transverse. Familiarity with total breech extraction is necessary for the vaginal delivery of any twin pregnancy.

Isoimmunization. All gravidas should undergo blood typing and antibody screening at the initial visit. Even the Rh positive patients should undergo repeat testing in the second and third trimesters. With the widespread use of anti-D immune globulin (RhoGAM), the incidence of sensitization to the D-antigen appears to be decreasing. Antibodies to other blood group antigens (e,E,c,C, Duffy and Kell) are being seen more frequently than anti-D in many centers. Thus, even the Rh-positive patient is at risk for the development of isoimmunization. The presence of any antibody titer is an indication for evaluation by a specialist in maternal-fetal medicine. The majority of these patients will require amniocentesis to detect the presence of bilirubin pigments in the amniotic fluid (OD_{450}). Serial amniocentesis and, rarely, intrauterine fetal transfusion may be necessary.

It is currently recommended that all unsensitized Rh-negative women receive antenatal prophylaxis with 300 micrograms of RhoGAM at 28 weeks. This is designed to prevent the approximately 1 per cent of patients who will become sensitized in this period from doing so. Finally, the indications for RhoGAM administration are as follows: (1) to an Rh-negative woman after delivery of an Rh-positive infant, (2) to an Rh-negative woman after spontaneous or induced abortion or ectopic pregnancy, and (3) after second or third trimester amniocentesis. Consideration of its use should be given after external cephalic version and blunt abdominal trauma and in the conservative management of Rh-negative patients with placenta previa.

Post Dates. When the duration of pregnancy has exceeded 294 days (at least 42 weeks) from the first day of the last menstrual period, the pregnancy is considered to be post dated (PD). Approximately 10 per cent of all pregnancies continue beyond 42 weeks. Pregnancies deemed to be PD are found more frequently in women with a previous PD pregnancy and are known to be associated with certain fetal malformations such as anencephaly, hydrocephaly, and osteogenesis imperfecta. In general, the incidence of macrosomatia (4000 grams or more), postmaturity, and variable decelerations on nonstress testing is about 20 per cent of all PD pregnancies.

The current recommendations for the management of the uncomplicated PD pregnancy are controversial. Some investigators recommend fetal surveillance and selective induction of labor, whereas others prefer routine induction of labor at 42 weeks. Recent reports, however, have failed to demonstrate any advantage to this latter approach. If the former approach is elected, patients with an inducible cervix (Bishop score of 9 or greater) or with evidence of fetal macrosomatia should be considered for delivery. If the patient does not meet these criteria, fetal well-being should be assessed twice a week. The preferred approach, in our opinion, is a combination of FHR (nonstress test) and amniotic fluid volume assessment. Subsequent management of these patients will be based on the results of the fetal surveillance tests and the inducibility of the cervix. Lastly, no patient should be allowed to go beyond 44 weeks.

Antenatal Fetal Testing

Ultrasound. Currently, ultrasound cannot be recommended for all patients. It should be used for specific indications. No clinical studies on humans have indicated a risk to mother or fetus. Of prime consideration is the fact that the level of ultrasound used for diagnostic purposes is of relatively low intensity and pulsed rather than continuous. Alternatively, Doppler instruments for the detection of the FHR are of higher intensity and continuous in quality. Indications for diagnostic ultrasound imaging include, but are not limited to, the following: diagnosis of early pregnancy, size-date discrepancies, confirmation of adequate fetal growth, diagnosis of anomalies, guidance of amniocentesis, evaluation of placental location, estimation of fetal weight, documentation of fetal viability, documentation of fetal maturity, evaluation of adnexal masses, uterine tumors or anomalies, confirmation of EDC.

Ultrasound examinations are frequently classified as Level I or Level II. Level I examinations should include determination of BPD, OFD, abdominal diameter, femur length, number and position of fetuses, placental location, estimation of fetal weight, and assessment of amniotic fluid volume. This type of examination should be within the capability of all personnel who do obstetric ultrasonography. Level II examinations include all of the aforementioned information and a careful search for anomalies and is generally performed at a tertiary care facility. However, any sonographer performing a Level I examination should be alert to the presence of anomalies.

Antepartum Fetal Heart Rate Testing

In our opinion, the primary method of fetal surveillance in high-risk pregnancies is the NST. Indications for the use of the NST include post-dates, hypertensive disorders, IUGR, multiple gestation, isoimmunization, diabetes mellitus, and prior stillbirth. The NST is performed in the semi-Fowlers position, with frequent blood pressure recordings. A test is considered reactive if there are two accelerations of at least 15 beats per minute lasting at least 15 seconds in a 10-minute window. If these criteria are not met in 40 minutes of monitoring, the test is considered nonreactive. These tests are generally repeated the same day. Persistently nonreactive tests are followed by either a biophysical profile (BPP) or a contraction stress test (CST). A BPP score of 8 or greater is considered normal. A score of 6 requires retesting in 12 to 24 hours. A score of 4 or less merits evaluation of fetal pulmonary maturity and delivery. A negative CST requires 3 uterine contractions in a 10-minute window with no late decelerations. An equivocal CST is one in which nonrepetitive late decelerations occur. The presence of repetitive late deceleration, considered a positive CST, is managed the same way as a BPP score of 4 or less. The management of patients with variable deceleration is an unresolved issue. The presence of variable decelerations in term patients, particularly those with post-dates, IUGR, or decreased amniotic fluid volume should be viewed with concern. We recommend evaluation for delivery in these circumstances.

ABORTION

method of
HOOSHANG M. NIKOO, M.D.
Episcopal Hospital
Philadelphia, Pennsylvania

Incidence

The true incidence of *spontaneous abortion* is difficult to assess, but the generally accepted rate is 10 per cent. However, if fertilization and elevation of HCG hormone is considered to be true pregnancy, more than 60 per cent of fertilized ova do not reach viability and end as abortuses.

The incidence of *induced abortion* in the United States has almost tripled since the Supreme Court's 1973 decision which legalized abortion. Before 1973, almost 500,000 induced abortions were performed yearly in the United States. Over 1.5 million legal abortions were reported in 1982 and about 26 per cent of all pregnancies are terminated by abortion.

Etiology

Although there is no conclusive etiologic factor for spontaneous abortion, certain factors are known to contribute to the incidence of spontaneous abortion.

Genetic Factors. Between 40 and 60 per cent of the abortuses in the first 12 weeks of gestation have abnormal chromosomal arrangement, the most common being numeric aberration, monosomies, trisomies, or polyploidies. Parents usually have normal karyotypes, but, in 4 to 6 per cent of the parents with more than two spontaneous abortions, some balanced translocation has been reported. Maternal and paternal age has been reported to be an important factor in chromosomal abnormalities, but this has not yet been proved.

Infectious Disease. Any viral or bacterial infection that causes high fever could interfere with normal fetal development and become a factor in spontaneous abortion. Moreover, certain infectious diseases such as mycoplasmal infection of the genital tract, rubella, toxoplasmosis, and *Listeria monocytogenes* have been specifically related to an increased spontaneous abortion rate, with mycoplasma gaining more attention as a specific etiologic factor.

Endocrine Disorders. Thyroid dysfunction and Cushing's disease have been reported to cause spontaneous abortion, but not diabetes mellitus. Progesterone deficiency in early pregnancy is always considered an etiologic factor; indeed, in luteal phase defect, in which the corpus luteum has a shorter-than-normal life span, repeated early spontaneous abortion is seen. This condition is diagnosed by endometrial biopsy in the luteal phase. If a discrepancy of 48 or more hours exists between histologic and calendar dating of the cycle, a short luteal phase is suspected. In some instances, this condition is due to high levels of serum prolactin, and, in these cases, the possibility of pituitary microadenomas should be investigated.

Abnormalities of the Genital Tract. Abnormal müllerian development is a cause for midtrimester pregnancy loss. Diethylstilbestrol (DES)-exposed patients have a specific uterine abnormality, which is either a T-shaped uterine cavity or an incompetent cervix; the rate of pregnancy loss is high. Submucosal fibroids and, rarely, intramural or subserosal fibroids also cause spontaneous abortion. Incompetent cervix due to cervical trauma or congenital maldevelopment is a known factor in second trimester losses. Hysterosalpingography, a simple test, is usually sufficient for diagnosis, and corrective surgery is indicated if no other cause for repeated spontaneous abortion is found.

Environmental Factors. Exposure of pregnant women

to chemical and industrial wastes, especially to those with high levels of arsenic and lead compounds, has been shown to cause a high rate of spontaneous abortion. Chronic exposure to radiographic and anesthetic agents (occupational hazards) also correlate with an increased incidence of spontaneous abortion.

Maternal Habits. Drug, alcohol, and tobacco usage during pregnancy has been correlated with an increased incidence of spontaneous abortion. The effect of lysergic acid (LSD) usage on chromosomal breakage is well known. Cigarette smoking also has some known effect on placental development and increases the abortion rate. The effect of surgery and emotional and physical trauma in the etiology of spontaneous abortion is unclear, but laparotomies and removal of organs close to a pregnant uterus have increased the rate of abortion.

Clinical Classification

Spontaneous abortion has different clinical stages: threatened abortion, inevitable abortion, incomplete abortion, complete abortion, missed abortion, habitual abortion, and septic abortion.

Threatened abortion is the appearance of bleeding during the first half of pregnancy. Bleeding during pregnancy is abnormal, but some nonpregnancy-related bleedings are from the cervix (polyps, cervicitis, tumors), vagina, or urethra and should be differentiated by careful examination. Some small amount of bleeding in early pregnancy is due to the implantation of the zygote and is considered normal. Dark brown bleeding, usually due to necrosis of the decidua after fetal death, is abnormal. Mild abdominal cramping usually accompanies the bleeding.

Therapeutic Considerations. A thorough pelvic examination is done to rule out other causes for the bleeding.

A pelvic ultrasound examination is done not only to rule out bleeding due to ectopic pregnancy but also to confirm fetal viability. If, with the ultrasound, the fetus is seen to be alive, the prognosis for the continuation of the pregnancy is excellent, with 90 per cent of the patients able to carry the pregnancy, regardless of treatment. If no viable fetus and only an empty gestational sac are seen in the ultrasound examination, the outcome of the pregnancy is poor, regardless of treatment. Bed rest and repeat ultrasound examination in 1 week will differentiate a blighted ovum or missed abortion from a very early normal gestation.

If repeat ultrasound examination fails to reveal a viable fetus, a dilatation and evacuation (D and E) is probably necessary to terminate the pregnancy, thus preventing complications of missed abortion and septic abortion. The appearance of a living fetus will indicate a normal pregnancy with a good prognosis.

Hormones should not be used to treat threatened abortion. They are not effective and could cause prolongation and retention of a dead fetus or adverse effect on organogenesis of a living one.

Bed rest, avoiding sexual activity, and taking vaginal precautions are psychologically beneficial to the patient, but they do not have medical therapeutic value.

Inevitable abortion is the appearance of ruptured membrane, uterine contractions, vaginal bleeding, and cervical dilatation. Treatment is the same as for incomplete abortion.

Incomplete abortion involves a partially expelled fetus and placenta. Because the retained portion of the product of conception usually prevents the involution of the uterus, abdominal cramps, vaginal bleeding, cervical dilatation, and the appearance of portions of the product of conception from the cervical canal characterize this condition.

Therapeutic Considerations. After proper diagnosis, the aim should be the prompt evacuation of the uterus. This could be accomplished best by transferring the patient to the operating room (OR) or short procedure unit with OR facilities. An intravenous fluid with 1000 ml of 5 per cent glucose and 10 to 20 units of pitocin is started. An analgesic such as 50 mg of meperidine (Demerol) is given intravenously. A paracervical block is done by injecting 7 ml of 1 or 2 per cent lidocaine to the paracervical areas at 4 and 8 o'clock.

No surgical dilatation is needed, because the cervix is already dilated. A suction catheter is inserted into the canal, and, with mild negative pressure of 30 to 40 mm Hg, the suction is completed and the bleeding and pain stop. Rarely, a sharp curette is used to ascertain the completeness of the evacuation.

A whole dose of RhoGAM is given to Rh-negative patients.

A blood count is performed after the procedure to rule out anemia and excessive blood loss.

Methylergonovine (Methergine), 0.2 mg by mouth every 6 to 8 hours for 2 days, may be given.

The patient should be observed for a few hours, followed by discharge with a follow-up visit scheduled in 2 weeks. A method of contraception should be discussed at the time of discharge.

Complete abortion occurs when the entire product of conception is expelled spontaneously, the uterus contracts, and bleeding stops without interference. This usually happens at 6 to 10 weeks of gestation, after an episode of bleeding and abdominal cramps. The patient passes the sac of pregnancy and the fetus. The bleeding and abdominal cramps diminish thereafter and finally stop.

Therapeutic Considerations. The product of conception should be examined grossly and microscopically to rule out incomplete abortion or ectopic pregnancy.

An ultrasound examination should be done to rule out the possibility of retained placenta. The endometrial cavity seen as a regular line indicates the completeness of the abortion with no dilatation and curettage necessary, but a shadow that is irregular or not identifiable indicates an incomplete abortion with treatment as such.

Methylergonovine is prescribed. A whole dose of RhoGAM is given for Rh-negative patients.

A repeat serum human chorionic gonadotropin (HCG) level determined 48 to 72 hours after the abortion shows a very low level or becomes negative. This is a reassuring sign of complete abortion and rules out the possibility of ectopic pregnancy.

Missed abortion is the condition wherein the product of conception is retained in the uterus for 8 weeks or longer after the death of the fetus. Usually there is no vaginal bleeding. The early pregnancy symptoms, including morning sickness and breast enlargement and tenderness, disappear and a previously positive pregnancy test may become negative. Pelvic examination fails to reveal uterine growth, and the uterus even becomes smaller when compared with previous examinations. Ultrasound examination reveals no evidence of fetal viability, and the sac of pregnancy is usually irregularly shaped.

Carrying a dead fetus may be psychologically intolerable to some patients, even though this could facilitate the spontaneous expulsion of the fetus; but when the pregnancy is more advanced and spontaneous expulsion has not occurred within 1 month, a coagulation defect may occur. The rate of this serious complication of missed abortion could be as high as 25 per cent if missed abortion continues longer than 2 months. To prevent this complication, the uterus should be evacuated either by a suction curettage if the pregnancy is less than 14 weeks or by medical induction if the pregnancy is more advanced. The medical induction could safely be accomplished by prostaglandin instillation of $F_2\alpha$ or vaginal insertion of prostaglandin E_2, and intravenous infusion of oxytocin.

Treatment. Treatment of the coagulation defect is usually accomplished by evacuation of the uterus after stabilization of the patient. If the phenomenon is severe, serious bleeding may occur. The bleeding should be treated with an infusion of fresh-frozen plasma; a transfusion of fresh blood, if available; the administration of cryoprecipitate; a platelet transfusion; and, rarely, when the previously mentioned measures fail, a lifesaving heparin infusion.

Habitual abortion refers to three or more spontaneous, consecutive losses of pregnancy. The most common cause for early (first trimester) abortions is genetic disorders. Other etiologic factors are short luteal phase and mycoplasmal infection of the genital tract. Mid and third trimester pregnancy losses are usually due to genital tract anomalies and incompetent cervix.

Therapeutic Considerations. For early habitual abortions, therapeutic measures include a complete work-up, including endometrial biopsy, *Mycoplasma* culture, and chromosomal testing of parents. In the case of luteal phase defect, treatment includes 25 to 50 mg of progesterone given intramuscularly every other day, with 2500 units to 5000 units of HCG given intramuscularly biweekly. The treatment should start at midcycle and continue until 6 to 12 weeks of gestation if pregnancy occurs. Mycoplasmal infection is treated with erythromycin or doxycycline. Some physicians recommend a medical treatment of early habitual abortion with a 14-day course of 100 mg of doxycycline (Vibramycin) given by mouth twice daily, but the value of this method is still unclear.

TREATMENT OF INCOMPETENT CERVIX. This is defined as the spontaneous, painless opening of the cervical os and the loss of pregnancy. This typically occurs in the second trimester. The cause is either traumatic with previous mechanical dilatation of the cervix or is congenital due to abnormal cervical development.

The best-accepted treatment for incompetent cervix is a cerclage procedure. The easiest technique is the McDonald operation, which involves placing a suture at the level of the internal os. The suture is left in place until the last few weeks of pregnancy; then it is removed and a vaginal delivery is allowed. The shirodkar procedure involves placing a permanent suture at the cervix; delivery is performed by cesarean section. This procedure is more complicated and should be performed only by experienced personnel.

The success rate in correction of true incompetent cervix is more than 85 per cent with either cerclage procedure. Concomitant use of 250 mg to 500 mg of 17 medroxyprogesterone caproate in weekly injections is also recommended and may enhance the success rate.

Induced abortion is the deliberate termination of the pregnancy prior to survivability of the fetus. It is called *therapeutic abortion* when the termination is performed to safeguard the mother's health (for example, termination of a pregnancy in a cancerous uterus); it is called *elective abortion* when the termination is requested by the mother for social, economic, or other reasons.

Septic abortion is the development of infection with incomplete abortion. Typical signs of infection are present and include fever, chills, and abdominal tenderness. In more severe cases, signs of septic shock and acute renal failure may develop. Septic complication is the most common cause of death in second trimester abortion, and it is considered to be a more severe complication if the pregnancy was accompanied by an intrauterine device (IUD) in situ.

Therapeutic Considerations. Prompt evacuation of the uterus and use of proper antibiotics and adequate hydration of the patient usually prevent more serious complications.

Elective Abortions

The primary factor in choosing the particular method is gestational age. Ninety per cent of elective abortions are performed in the first trimester, and the primary means of abortion at this stage is the suction curettage. Suction curettage is, at best, to be performed under local anesthesia, and, if preceded by the insertion of a laminaria tent to the cervix, is relatively simple and very safe. The adverse effect concerning the patient's future pregnancies is minimal.

A *Laminaria* tent is a device made from the stems of a special seaweed called *Laminaria digitata*. Through its hydrophilic action, the device, if inserted properly into the cervix, will gradually dilate the cervical canal and will reduce the cervical trauma and laceration due to mechanical dilatation. The *Laminaria* is usually inserted 6 to 8 hours prior to the scheduled procedure and is removed just before starting the suction curettage.

Suction curettage is performed under aseptic conditions. If the *Laminaria* is not used, the cervix is dilated using Pratt dilators and under paracervical anesthesia. A plastic curette is inserted into the cavity. The diameter, in millimeters, of the suction curette is usually chosen to correpond to the gestation age by week; for example, a 6 mm curette is used for a pregnancy of 6 weeks, an 8 mm curette for a pregnancy of 8 weeks. The curette is then connected to the pump, and, using negative pressure created by the pump, the evacuation is started and completed. The negative pressure, at between 30 and 50 mm Hg, should not exceed 50 mm Hg. Some physicians perform a sharp curettage after the completion of suctioning, but this practice should be limited, because too vigorous a curettage could cause intrauterine synechiae and future infertility.

The intravenous use of 10 to 20 units of pitocin in 1000 ml of 5 per cent dextrose in Ringer's lactate solution is recommended to lower the blood loss. No prophylactic antibiotic is usually necessary, but if a patient has a history of pelvic inflammatory disease or with teenage patients who are at risk of developing infection, a single dose of 500 mg of doxycycline is given a few hours prior to the procedure. This significantly lowers the rate of postoperative infection.

A proper contraception should be prescribed since ovulation occurs usually 17 to 22 days after the D and E.

Midtrimester Abortion

The morbidity and mortality rates for second trimester abortion are at least four times higher than for the first trimester. The methods for midtrimester abortion are medical, surgical, or mechanical.

The medical method for midtrimester abortion includes the instillation technique with hypertonic saline. Amniocentesis is performed under aseptic conditions. Two hundred milliliters of commercially available 20 per cent saline solution is then instilled into the amniotic cavity. After the completion of the procedure, the patient is kept under observation, and, in 85 to 90 per cent of patients, spontaneous labor starts and the fetus is expelled. In more than 50 per cent of patients, the placenta is also expelled spontaneously; it should be removed surgically if not expelled spontaneously.

Injecting 40 mg of prostaglandin $F_2\alpha$ into the amniotic cavity is also a very effective way of inducing midtrimester abortion. The technique is more effective if it is combined with the intravenous infusion of pitocin after the labor is started.

Prostaglandin E_2 also has been used to induce midtrimester abortion. This product is in the form of vaginal suppositories, and the insertion of one suppository every 6 to 8 hours will start the labor in 8 to 24 hours.

Complications of the saline instillation include the development of clotting defect, water intoxication, hypernatremia, and myometrial necrosis due to extravasation of the hypertonic saline during the injection. Infection and bleeding are seen in more than 4 per cent of patients owing to placental retention. Rarely, the fetus is born alive. A very stressful condition for both patient and hospital personnel, this creates a hard medicolegal problem.

Complications related to the prostaglandin administration most commonly include diarrhea, nausea, vomiting, and hyperthermia. The most serious complication, however, is uterine rupture or expulsion of the fetus from the lower uterine segment, which may cause uterovaginal fistula formation. The complication occurs more commonly if the prostaglandins are used with an intravenous oxytocin infusion, especially if the infusion is started before the rupture of the membranes. Care should be taken to avoid this very serious complication.

Surgical methods for midtrimester abortions include the use of suction curettage to terminate pregnancies of more than 12 weeks. Currently, there is enough evidence to show this to be a safe technique when done by experienced personnel. The basic technique is similar to that of the suction curettage performed for first trimester abortion. The complication rate is less than that of the instillation techniques.

Hysterotomy is used in about 1 per cent of abortions performed in the United States. Hysterotomy, in fact, is a miniclassic cesarean section and has very high rates of mortality and morbidity compared with suction curettage. The mortality rate is almost 40 times higher, and future pregnancies should be delivered by cesarean section. Hysterotomy should be used only if other methods have failed; routine use is discouraged!

Pregnant hysterectomy could be used as a means of abortion if serious uterine pathology coexists with pregnancy and warrants a hysterectomy. It must be emphasized that such an occasion occurs rarely and should be evaluated on an individual basis.

Mechanical methods used to induce abortion include the use of bougies, bags, catheters, and other mechanical means. There is a high rate of infection with these techniques and in general they are disadvantageous.

Effect of Induced Abortion on Future Pregnancies

The effect of induced abortion on subsequent pregnancies is unclear. Studies are divided equally among no adverse effect and adverse effects, which include increased chance of pregnancy loss, premature ruptured membrane, growth retardation, increased rate of placenta previa by threefold, infertility, increased rate of ectopic pregnancy by fivefold, increased rate of first trimester vaginal bleeding, and incompetent cervix.

It is reasonable to assume that if induced abortion is performed early, if cervical trauma is minimized by using *Laminaria,* and if there is no postoperative infection, the effect of induced abortion in future pregnancies should not be significant. However, the rates of infertility and ectopic pregnancy will increase if other than the just-stated ideal conditions, especially no postoperative infection, occurs.

ECTOPIC PREGNANCY

method of
ROBERT C. KAUFMANN, M.D.
Southern Illinois University
Springfield, Illinois

The incidence of ectopic pregnancy in the United States has increased almost threefold in the last 10 years. In 1980, 52,200 ectopic pregnancies were reported. This figure is increasing at an annual rate of 11 per cent, meaning that in 1985, there will be approximately 88,000 ectopic pregnancies in the United States. Although ectopic pregnancy is still the major cause of maternal death in the first trimester of pregnancy, the death-to-case ratio has decreased from 3.5 to less than 1 death per 1000 ectopic pregnancies.

The introduction of the beta-HCG radioimmunoassays into most laboratories, the common availability of ultrasonography, and the development of laparoscopy have served to decrease the death rate from ectopic pregnancies. Beta-HCG radioimmunoassay can be used to determine whether a patient having the symptoms of ectopic pregnancy is, in fact, pregnant. If pregnancy is confirmed, ultrasonic examination can be done to determine the location. If intrauterine, the patient probably does not have an ectopic pregnancy, and one must begin to search for other causes of the patient's symptoms, because twin pregnancy with concurrent intrauterine and ectopic locations is rare. Corpus luteum cyst, threatened abortion, appendicitis, or twisted ovarian mass are the most common differential diagnoses. If no intrauterine pregnancy is found on ultrasound examination, the pregnancy is either intrauterine and of less than 5 weeks gestation or is ectopic. Laparoscopy can then be used to determine which of the aforementioned conditions is present.

The most common location of an ectopic pregnancy is within the uterine tube. Other types of extrauterine gestation, including ovarian pregnancy, cervical pregnancy, and cornual pregnancy are much less common. Once the diagnosis of ectopic pregnancy is suspected, it must be confirmed or ruled out. If confirmed, immediate treatment is required.

Treatment

Unruptured Tubal Pregnancy. When a diagnosis of unruptured tubal pregnancy is suspected, the following measures should be undertaken:

1. Hospital admission.
2. CBC, urinalysis, and type and cross-match for several units of blood.
3. Intravenous fluids and NPO for approximately 6 hours.
4. Laparoscopy.

If, at the time of laparoscopy, an unruptured ectopic pregnancy is found, a Pfannenstiel incision can be used. If, however, active bleeding is occurring, the median incision, a faster approach, should be used. If no ectopic pregnancy is found at laparoscopy, the surgery is concluded and the patient is discharged unless other conditions that require hospitalization are present.

Since more than 50 per cent of the patients will have coexisting tubal disease in the contralateral tube and another 50 per cent will have a subsequent tubal pregnancy, it is best to attempt to preserve tubal structure and function in those patients who desire future childbearing. Conservative surgery is the method of choice for unruptured tubal pregnancy in such patients. This can be accomplished by inducing a tubal abortion, by salpingotomy, or by segmental excision with or without immediate reanastomosis.

Tubal abortion is performed when the pregnancy is located at the infundibulum of the tube. The products of conception are removed by either "milking" the tube or by suction through the fimbrial opening. Areas of bleeding are controlled by cautery or fine nonreactive suture.

For unruptured pregnancies located in the ampullary portion of the tube, salpingotomy is the method of choice. In this procedure, an incision is made in the antimesenteric portion of the tube over the bulge of the pregnancy. Using gentle blunt dissection, the products of conception are "shelled out" of the tube with hemostasis being accomplished by cautery or fine nonreactive suture. The tube is closed in two layers using 5-0 or 6-0 polyglycol suture.

When the pregnancy is located proximal to the ampulla, segmental resection with or without immediate reanastomosis may be attempted. In this procedure, the portion of the tube containing the pregnancy is excised, and the cut ends of the tube are either reconnected using 8-0 nylon sutures under microscopic control or simply ligated for later repair. In situations in which the patient has no desire to maintain her fertility, salpingectomy with cornual resection is the method of choice in the treatment of unruptured tubal pregnancy. The mesosalpinx is doubly clamped, incised, and sutured with 2-0 absorbable suture in a step-wise manner until the cornu is reached. The tube is resected from the uterus by making a wedge-shaped incision into the uterus at the cornu. The defect is closed in two layers, the first being a continuous locking suture of 2-0, and the second, a continuous inverting suture of 3-0 absorbable suture.

Ruptured Tubal Pregnancy. Shock is a common complication of a ruptured tubal pregnancy that is actively bleeding. When bleeding is occurring from a ruptured tubal pregnancy and shock is present, blood pressure and pulse will usually return to normal levels once the vessels that feed the tube have been clamped. Because ruptured ectopic pregnancy has significant risks and most deaths are associated with active bleeding and shock, surgery should be undertaken as soon as the diagnosis has been made and adequate blood is available. In ruptured tubal pregnancy, conservative surgery may be possible if there has been no excessive bleeding or extensive tissue damage. In such cases, when future fertility is desired, segmental resection of the tube may be attempted. If this is not the case, salpingectomy with cornual resection should be done. In young women, conservation of the ipsilateral ovary should be attempted because of the possible need for future procedures during which ovarian conservation of the contralateral side may not be possible. In these patients, ovarian function may still be desired for hormonal reasons or possible *in vitro* fertilization procedures.

Ovarian Pregnancy. In the case of ovarian pregnancy, conservation of ovarian tissue should be attempted unless the whole ovary is involved or destroyed. Wedge resection can be carried out in most instances, and the ovarian defect can be closed with 3-0 absorbable suture. If conservative surgery is impossible, oophorectomy must be undertaken.

Abdominal Pregnancy. Abdominal pregnancy is the most serious of all ectopic pregnancies because of the risk of extensive bleeding from the placental site prior to, during, and after surgery. Laparotomy should be undertaken as soon as the diagnosis has been made and adequate blood is available. The fetus and amniotic fluid are removed with the cord being cut (but not ligated) close to the placenta. Ligation of the cord is not recommended, because it may increase the possibility of later cyst formation. The placenta is left undisturbed to prevent uncontrollable bleeding from the placental site.

Cornual or Interstitial Pregnancy. These rare varieties of ectopic pregnancy are usually not recognized until rupture and massive hemorrhage have occurred. In most cases, supportive measures and immediate operative intervention, usually hysterectomy, are required.

Cervical Pregnancy. This is a rare complication of pregnancy and is often mistaken for an incomplete abortion. When recognized, total abdominal hysterectomy is recommended, because vaginal evacuation may lead to uncontrollable hemorrhage.

Rh Prophylaxis. In all cases of ectopic pregnancy, RhoGAM should be given to unsensitized Rh-negative mothers. In cases in which greater than normal fetal to maternal transfusion is suspected, laboratory tests to determine the amount of transfusion should be done to ensure administration of adequate RhoGAM.

VAGINAL BLEEDING LATE IN PREGNANCY

method of
ROBERT A. KNUPPEL, M.D., and
JEFFREY L. ANGEL, M.D.
University of South Florida
Tampa, Florida

Obstetric hemorrhage continues to be a leading cause of maternal and fetal morbidity and mortality. Bleeding from the reproductive tract during the last half of pregnancy is associated with a higher perinatal mortality regardless of the etiology. The perinatal mortality rate is quadrupled in pregnancies that are complicated by a placenta previa or by placental abruption. There is a marked increase in the uterine blood flow associated with normal physiologic changes of pregnancy. Any vaginal bleeding during the last half of pregnancy should therefore be considered as potentially life threatening and evaluated appropriately.

Etiology. Identifiable causes of antepartum hemorrhage will be found in only 50 to 60 per cent of patients. Of these causes, placental abruption and placenta previa are the most common and potentially the most serious. Important but less common problems include pre-term labor, rupture of the uterus (scarred or unscarred), bleeding from a vasa previa, cervical abnormalities (malignancy, polyps, erosions), and coagulation defects, both acquired and congenital.

Diagnosis. Changes in the patient's pulse and blood pressure are late findings in antepartum hemorrhage and usually signify substantial blood loss. Normal vital signs, on the other hand, cannot be interpreted as precluding significant hemorrhage and impending hypovolemic shock. Gingival bleeding, petechiae, and ecchymosis may be seen if disseminated intravascular coagulation (DIC) is present. Persistent abdominal pain and tenderness may be seen with abruptio placentae or uterine rupture. Examination of the external genitalia for signs of trauma or a ruptured vulvar varicosity should be done. A gentle speculum examination of the vagina can be done in search of vaginal lacerations or cervical abnormalities. Adherent clots should not be removed. An attempt at visual estimation of the blood loss should be done, but underestimation is a common problem. A pelvic examination should not be done at this time, and one should await the "double set-up" examination.

Laboratory Data. A stat baseline hemogram is important but may give a false sense of security in the unequilibrated state. Blood obtained from the vagina can be sent for an APT test, or a Kliehauer Betke smear can be sent for identification of fetal red blood cells, which, if present, can be prognostically quite ominous. A coagulation profile including a PT, PTT, fibrinogen, fibrin degradation products, and platelets may be helpful depending on the clinical circumstances. For patients who are hypovolemic, baseline renal function tests are imperative. A Kliehauer Betke smear on the mother's blood may reveal a significant fetal maternal hemorrhage. For patients with a suspected coagulopathy, a separate red top core vac tube should be observed for clot formation. If this is not observed or if there is poor clot retraction after 8 minutes, DIC should be highly suspect.

The use of real-time ultrasound has greatly improved the diagnostic capabilities in patients with third trimester bleeding. The safest, least invasive, and most precise method of placental localization is with real-time ultrasound scanning. There are reports stating an accuracy of between 5 and 60 per cent for visualization of a retroplacental clot consistent with an abruption using sonography. The ultimate diagnostic test will be described later and is the "double set-up" examination.

General Management

Supportive measures should be established immediately. Two large-gauge intravenous catheters should be inserted in patients with significant hemorrhage. The patient should be typed and crossed for four to six units of packed red blood cells and two units of fresh frozen plasma. Hypotension should be corrected with crystalloid, colloid, packed red blood cells, and fresh frozen plasma. Platelets and vasoactive agents should be used in appropriate situations. The urinary output should be kept in the 30 to 60 ml per hour range with close observation of input and output. Invasive hemodynamic monitoring using a central intravenous catheter or Swan-Ganz catheter may be useful in patients requiring massive fluid replacement or with associated medical problems such as hypertension. The fetus should be continuously monitored, preferably with the mother in the left lateral recumbent position. Evidence of fetal distress may resolve with stabilization of the mother, and this should be considered prior to hastily delivering the fetus operatively and endangering the life of the unstable mother. At the time of delivery, O negative pedi red blood cells should be available for neonatal resuscitation.

Placental Abruption (Abruptio Placentae). Premature separation of the normally implanted placenta occurs with the frequency of approximately 1 per cent. Placental abruption severe enough to kill the fetus occurs in approximately 1 in 500 pregnancies. Pregnant patients who are at highest risk for placental abruption are those with hypertension (especially chronic hypertension with superimposed pre-eclampsia), previous abruption, and infrequently maternal trauma. The etiology of placental abruption is not known. Initially, there is bleeding into the decidua basalis and progressive placental separation as the blood tracts between the maternal surface of the placenta and the uterine decidua. Early on, the patients may be asymptomatic; however, classically patients will note the sudden onset of painful, dark red vaginal bleeding. The pain may be continuous or intermittent with regular and frequent repetitive abdominal pain. These patients may present with massive obvious external hemorrhage or with minimal bleeding and a concealed hemorrhage if the blood does not tract to the internal os and into the vagina.

The ability of the fetus to tolerate labor associated with a placental abruption will depend on the degree of separation and the amount of fetal reserve. Placental abruption, itself, is not an indication for cesarean section. If the fetus is vertex and if there is no evidence of fetal distress, vaginal delivery should be attempted. The fetus should be closely monitored with internal electronic fetal monitoring and scalp PHs if necessary. The judicious use of pitocin augmentation is recommended if necessary. The mother's blood loss should be replaced, and coagulation defects should be corrected. DIC or bleeding is not an indication for cesarean section. More frequently than not, labor is rapid and may go without incident. Cesarean section should be used when evidence of fetal distress occurs or when one is unable to adequately replace maternal blood loss or correct coagulation defects. The coagulation defects associated with placental abruption will return to normal soon after delivery. In the more severe cases of placental abruption, the incidence of DIC, renal failure, and intrauterine fetal death are increased.

Placenta Previa. There are varying degrees of placenta previa.

1. *Total placenta previa.* The placenta entirely covers the internal os.
2. *Partial placenta previa.* The placenta covers a portion of the area over the internal os.
3. *Marginal previa.* The edge of the placenta lies at the margin of the internal os.

The incidence of this varies with ultrasonography in early pregnancy revealing a 30 to 40 per cent frequency rate. The third trimester incidence is approximately 0.4 per cent. Patients with a prior cesarean section have a 4 to 6 per cent incidence of recurrent placenta previa. The bleeding associated with a placenta previa is usually secondary to progressive thinning of the lower uterine segment or progressive dilatation of the cervix. This results in tearing of placental attachments and hemorrhage from uterine vessels.

The patient notes painless bright red vaginal bleeding with or without associated contractions. The first episode of bleeding is rarely profuse enough to be fatal to the fetus or mother and can frequently be treated conservatively. Pregnancies beyond 36 weeks with a total or partial previa should be delivered by cesarean section and not treated conservatively. Pre-term pregnancies in patients who are hemodynamically stable without persistent significant bleeding or evidence of fetal distress may be treated conservatively. This includes bed rest, blood replacement to maintain a hemoglobin of greater than 10 grams per dl, tocolytics, and glucocorticoids. These patients should remain hospitalized and should deliver at between 34 and 36 weeks of gestation after documentation of pulmonary maturity. Occasionally, patients with a marginal placenta previa can be delivered vaginally with progressive descent of the head tamponading the placenta and preventing further bleeding.

The "double set-up" examination is used in cases of vaginal bleeding of unknown etiology and to determine the degree of placenta previa present. This is carried out in the operating room with the physician gowned and gloved, an anesthesiologist present, and available personnel for an emergency cesarean section. Another physician will perform a gentle but conclusive pelvic examination to determine (hopefully) the etiology of the bleeding and the potential route of delivery.

Miscellaneous Causes. Uterine rupture is an infrequent cause of third trimester bleeding but should be suspected in patients with a prior cesarean section. Vertical uterine scars versus transverse uterine scars have an incidence of uterine rupture of 2.4 and 0.6 per cent, respectively. These patients will complain of a tearing sensation followed by a marked decrease in the amount of abdominal pain and frequently cessation of fetal movement. This is a surgical emergency and should be treated as such. This frequently results in death of the fetus and potentially morbid complications in the mother.

Cervical Bleeding. The congested pregnant cervix is friable and prone to bleeding. This may occur post-coitally or after a routine pap or pelvic examination. One should always consider the possibility of malignancy and obtain a pap smear if a recent one has not been performed.

HYPERTENSIVE DISORDERS OF PREGNANCY

method of
RICHARD J. WORLEY, M.D.
University of Utah
Salt Lake City, Utah

Hypertension complicates about 6 to 8 per cent of pregnancies in healthy women and as many as one fourth or more of the pregnancies in high-risk populations. Along with infection and hemorrhage, the hypertensive disorders are important causes of both maternal and infant morbidity and mortality. In fact, in some medically advanced regions of the world, hypertension is the most prominent cause of maternal mortality. Hypertension complicating pregnancy is often relatively straightforward to manage. Major pitfalls that preclude optimal management are (1) failure to recognize the disorder, and (2) failure to act on the diagnosis when the disorder is recognized.

Classification and Diagnosis. A useful classification of hypertensive disorders in pregnancy is as follows:

1. Pregnancy-induced hypertension (PIH)
   a. Without proteinuria
   b. Pre-eclampsia (with proteinuria)
   c. Eclamspia
2. Chronic hypertension preceding pregnancy (any etiology)
3. Chronic hypertension (any etiology) with superimposed pregnancy-induced hypertension
   a. Superimposed pre-eclampsia
   b. Superimposed eclampsia

Pregnancy-induced hypertension (PIH) is defined as a blood pressure of 140/90 mm Hg during the second half of pregnancy in a previously normotensive woman. A rise in systolic blood pressure of 30 mm Hg or in diastolic pressure of 15 mm Hg over baseline values also defines the condition. The diagnosis is made when these blood pressure changes are found on at least two occasions 6 or more hours apart. The addition of proteinuria to PIH constitutes pre-eclampsia, clearly a more severe stage of the disorder. Eclampsia, the most severe state of PIH, consists of convulsions that can result from fulminating, typically untreated PIH. It is highly desirable, however, to identify PIH early in its evolution because (1) the perinatal mortality rate begins to rise with the occurrence of hypertension alone (before proteinuria appears), and (2) eclampsia can occur in women with PIH who do not have proteinuria.

Differentiating between PIH and chronic hypertension may be difficult unless the patient's blood pressure before pregnancy is known. PIH typically occurs only in the first pregnancy, but serious forms of the disorder can either recur or make their initial appearance in a subsequent pregnancy. In such cases, underlying or latent essential hypertension or other vasculorenal disease is often a contributing factor. Distinguishing between chronic hypertension and PIH is not always critical. When hypertension is severe, management is the same in both cases. When mild and unassociated with proteinuria, however, some forms of chronic hypertension in the gravida who is remote from term are less ominous than is PIH. The clinician must search carefully at each prenatal visit for any of the aforementioned signs of hypertensive disease. When found, one should manage the disorder promptly and vigorously as described in the section entitled Management.

Pathophysiology and Etiology. Vasospasm is the cardinal characteristic of PIH. Consequences for the mother are hypertension and impaired regional perfusion. When the disease is severe, function of the kidneys, liver, and brain, among other organs, may be substantially impaired. The major consequence of PIH for the fetus is reduced intervillous perfusion, typically to a value only 35 to 50 per cent of normal. Fortunately, the fetus can sustain this degree of placental compromise fairly well when it is brought about slowly. Acute reductions in placental function of this magnitude, however, can be catastrophic. So also is the further reduction in perfusion that improper treatment of PIH can produce. Although the cause of vasospasm in women with PIH is not completely understood, considerable evidence supports the view that an alteration in prostaglandin metabolism or availability is involved.

Management

See Table 1.

Hypertension at Term. Fortunately, in many instances, the fetus is mature (36 weeks or more) by the time PIH is clinically evident. By then there is no benefit in further prolonging the pregnancy, but, instead, there is a danger in doing so. Delivery is warranted, most often by inducing labor with dilute oxytocin given intravenously via an infusion pump. Women with PIH should have a hematocrit and platelet count performed, a urinalysis, and a multi-channel chemistry analysis. Because labor is the most likely time for PIH to progress to eclampsia (seizures), all such laboring women should receive the effective and safe anticonvulsant magnesium sulfate prophylactically. Infuse 4 grams of 20 per cent solution intravenously over 20 minutes, then infuse about 2 grams per hour via a continuous infusion pump. If renal output is impaired (30 ml per hour or less), a slower rate of infusion may be required to avoid magnesium toxicity, symptoms of which are loss of deep tendon reflexes, respiratory paralysis, and ultimately cardiac arrest. No less often than every 4 hours, one must thus verify that the knee jerk is present, the respiratory rate is 12 or more breaths per minute, and urinary output is adequate. It is helpful to monitor the serum magnesium concentration about every 6 hours to ensure that the value is

TABLE 1. **Management of Hypertensive Disorders During Pregnancy**

Clinical Condition	Therapy
PIH (or chronic hypertension) when the fetus is mature	Definitive Prevent convulsions Control blood pressure Deliver
Pregnancy-induced or chronic hypertension when the fetus is premature but there is either severe or superimposed pre-eclampsia, or evidence of fetal jeopardy	Definitive Prevent convulsions Control blood pressure Deliver
Eclampsia, regardless of fetal maturity	Definitive Treat convulsions Control blood pressure Stabilize mother Deliver
Mild pregnancy-induced or chronic hypertension when fetus is premature	Expectant Hospitalization Ambulatory

in the therapeutic range (4 to 8 mEq per liter) and not in the toxic range (more than 10 mEq per liter). Antihypertensive medication is warranted only when the blood pressure threatens the mother (see Severe Hypertension, which follows). Unwarranted lowering of blood pressure in women with PIH further reduces the already compromised placental blood flow. Epidural anesthesia for labor and delivery is safe in most cases of PIH when the block is induced gradually and when the anesthesiologist is experienced and knowledgable in dealing with hypertensive disorders of pregnancy. PIH typically resolves largely within 24 hours of delivery, by which time it is usually safe to discontinue magnesium sulfate prophylaxis.

Severe Hypertension. Delivery is warranted whether or not the fetus is mature. Severe hypertensive disease in pregnancy consists of any one of the following in a hypertensive gravida: blood pressure of 160/110 mm Hg or higher, proteinuria of 5 grams per 24 hours, oliguria (output less than 400 ml in 24 hours), cerebral or visual disturbances, pulmonary edema or cyanosis, deranged liver function, or thrombocytopenia. Serious fetal jeopardy is ascertained from the fetal heart rate response to nonstress (fetal movement) and stress (uterine contraction) testing, and from sonographic evaluation of fetal growth rate. Magnesium sulfate prophylaxis is mandatory. If the blood pressure is 160/110 mm Hg or higher, hydralazine should be given in a dose of 5 to 10 mg by slow intravenous infusion, then the dose increased by 5 mg every 20 minutes until the blood pressure falls to between 150/100 and 140/90 mm Hg. For the sake of the fetus it is unwise to lower the blood pressure below 140/90 mm Hg. Often labor can be induced as previously described. Limit fluid replacement to measured plus insensitive loss only. In many cases of severe PIH, central venous or Swan-Ganz monitoring is helpful. If thrombocytopenia is present, the catheter is more safely passed antecubitally, and conduction anesthesia is best avoided.

Eclampsia. The convulsions of eclampsia are a frightening and potentially lethal complication of PIH. Nevertheless, good general medical care and attention to some unique features of the problem usually lead to a favorable outcome. The patient's airway must be secured. The convulsions are treated as previously described for prophylaxis, and the blood pressure is controlled as for severe pre-eclampsia, if necessary. Before delivering the infant, however, one should allow a stabilization period of a few hours, during which both mother and fetus need time to recover from the metabolic insult of convulsions. Resist the temptation to deliver the infant by emergency cesarean section immediately after the seizure. Abnormalities in fetal heart rate are expected at this time, and they typically resolve spontaneously as the mother recovers. The highest maternal and infant morbidity and mortality rates come from inappropriate decisions to perform cesarean section in this dire situation. After stabilization, oxytocin induction of labor, rather than cesarean section, is often an appropriate and successful method of delivery.

Mild PIH or Chronic Hypertension Remote from Term. At the first sign of PIH, the physician is urged to hospitalize the patient at least long enough to ascertain that (1) the hypertension, however mild when detected, is not worsening rapidly; (2) the hypertension improves with bed rest; and (3) both the mother and fetus exhibit general signs of well-being. Biophysical evaluation of the fetus, biochemical evaluation of the mother as described for PIH at term, and blood pressure evaluation while at rest in the hospital for 12 to 36 hours may be all that is required to become convinced that the patient can be safely managed at rest at home, where a friend or relative can learn to take her blood pressure daily. The physician should see the patient weekly. In this manner, such pregnancies can often be prolonged safely for weeks. Indications for delivery are recurrence of hypertension or the presence of a mature fetus.

OBSTETRIC ANESTHESIA

method of
RICHARD B. CLARK, M.D.
University of Arkansas
Little Rock, Arkansas

The use of prepared childbirth has increased dramatically in recent times and is to be applauded. The teachings of Fernando LaMaze, if used intelligently and not carried to an extreme, are very helpful to the parturient. Breathing techniques, exercises, wife-husband interaction, and the education provided in these classes regarding the physiology of pregnancy, labor, and delivery are reassuring, reduce (and may eliminate) the need for anesthesia, and make the event more controllable, gratifying, and expeditious.

Anesthesia and Analgesia for Labor and Vaginal Delivery

Systemic Analgesia

Narcotics and some sedatives have a long history in obstetric pain relief and, if used with discretion, provide a reduction in maternal discomfort with little neonatal effect. The first narcotic, morphine, was combined with scopolamine to provide "twilight sleep." This technique, although popular for more than a century, produced many depressed infants. Morphine depresses the Apgar score more than do other narcotics. Meperidine (Demerol) became popular in the 1940s, and it, too, was combined with scopolamine, often with significant neonatal effects. Morphine is now obsolete, as is scopolamine, but meperidine, in reasonable doses (50 to 75 mg given once or twice during labor) is still quite useful and usually safe. It may be administered intravenously or intramuscularly. The latter route produces less placental transfer, therefore less effect on the infant. Meperidine should not be administered intramuscularly within 3 hours of anticipated delivery because it may affect the Apgar score. The concomitant use of tranquilizers (promethazine, Phenergan, 25 to 50 mg or hydroxyzine, Vistaril, 50 to 100 mg) reduces nausea and vomiting without increasing respiratory depression, reduces anxiety, and may potentiate the analgesic effect. Meperidine metabolites, particularly normeperidine, have been suspected of causing neonatal depression, but, if reasonable doses of meperidine are used, this effect is probably minimal. Alphaprodine (Nisentil), a potent analgesic, can cause maternal and neonatal apnea if given in excess, perhaps demonstrating less margin of safety when compared with meperidine. Two new analgesics, butorphanol (Stadol) and nalbuphine (Nubain) have been used in obstetrics and show promise. Both demonstrate a "ceiling effect" in regard to respiratory depression (and to analgesia, also) so they might be considered safer than meperidine. At the doses currently used in obstetrics, neither meperidine butorphanol, nor nalbuphine impart significant maternal or neonatal respiratory depression. Our favorite is butorphanol (1 to 2 mg). It provides good analgesia and sedation, does not cause nausea and vomiting, does not seem to produce respiratory depression, and obviates the need for tranquilizers. All narcotics have some effect on fetal heart rate variability, which is usually decreased. If narcotic depression is suspected, the narcotic antagonist naloxone (Narcan) is given to the neonate (10 micrograms per kg), preferably intravenously. This should occur infrequently if narcotic doses to the mother are kept to a minimum. Although theoretically attractive, the administration of naloxone intravenously to the mother just before delivery (with the intent of transplacental reversal of the narcotic depression of the infant) has never been approved by the Food and Drug Administration. Diazepam (Valium) should be avoided for obstetrics, because it may cause neonatal flaccidity and lower Apgar scores and may interfere with temperature regulation.

Subanesthetic concentrations of anesthetic agents may be inhaled intermittently during labor and do provide a reduction in labor pain. This has been achieved with nitrous oxide–oxygen, 50 per cent, and methoxyflurane in air, 0.1 to 0.9 per cent (the latter with a "Cyprane inhaler"). Administration of the analgesia should be discontinued if the patient seems to be losing consciousness. Nitrous oxide has never attained much popularity in the United States, but methoxyflurane was fairly widely used during the 1970s. Both techniques require a cooperative, motivated patient, and both fail in the presence of severe pain.

Regional Anesthesia for Vaginal Delivery

Nerve blocks approach the ideal in chemical obstetric pain relief. They have been shown to reduce catecholamine levels and presumably to improve uterine blood flow. Anesthesia could thus be beneficial to the fetus, as well as the mother. The mother remains awake, so there is little danger of aspiration; she can participate in the delivery; and she can relate to the infant.

Epidural Anesthesia. Lumbar epidural anesthesia is the most elegant and satisfactory of the regional blocks and is achieved by injection of a local anesthetic into the epidural space, usually at L2–3, or L3–4, when labor is well established (6 cm cervical dilatation in the prima gravida, 4 cm dilatation in the multi gravida). The epidural space is located using the loss of resistance technique. Once identified, the drug may be injected through the needle or, more commonly, a plastic catheter is advanced about 2 cm into the epidural space. The needle is removed, and the local anesthetic drugs are injected intermittently into the epidural space to provide pain relief. Because the nerve roots of T11 and T12 should be blocked during the first stage, a small volume of drug, 4 to 8 ml, is adequate. This is termed a segmental epidural (extent of anesthesia T10 to L3 or L4). A greater volume is injected before delivery (12 to 14 ml) to obtain anesthesia of the sacral roots as well.

There is considerable controversy regarding the choice of local anesthetic drug for lumbar epidural. Four drugs have recently enjoyed popularity; mepivacaine (Carbocaine), lidocaine (Xylocaine), bupivacaine (Marcaine), and chloroprocaine (Nesacaine). Mepivacaine has been shown to have some effect on the neurobehavioral score of the infant during the first few hours after birth (but not on Apgar score) and has largely fallen into disuse for obstetric anesthesia (Table 1). Lidocaine, which was the first drug that became popular for lumbar epidural, is enjoying a renaissance. All local anesthetics have some effect on fetal heart rate variability, but this is usually of minor significance (Table 1). The enthusiasm for

TABLE 1. **Fetal and Neonatal Effects of Four Local Anesthetic Drugs Used Primarily for Epidural Anesthesia.**
(Note advantages and disadvantages. Some pertinent maternal considerations are also included.)

Drug	Advantages	Disadvantages
Mepivacaine	Fairly long duration: reliable and safe for mother	Causes neurobehavioral changes; transient reduction in FHR variability
Lidocaine	No neurobehavioral effect: reliable and safe for mother	Fairly short duration; can cause minimal to moderate loss of FHR variability
Bupivacaine	Long duration; no neurobehavioral effect	Maternal cardiac toxicity? Increase in FHR variability not known to be advantage or disadvantage
Chloroprocaine	Rapidly metabolized; low or absent neonatal levels; no neurobehavioral effect; no effect on FHR variability	Short duration; rare neurologic deficit in mother

the special qualities of bupivacaine (long duration, low neonatal blood levels) and chloroprocaine (rapid metabolism, low systemic toxicity) has been tempered by reports of toxicity of these drugs. Bupivacaine has been linked with a number of maternal deaths, in which unintended intravascular injection produced convulsions and cardiac arrest, refractory to treatment in several instances. Chloroprocaine has been associated with a few cases of neurologic damage when the drug was mistakenly injected into the subarachnoid space (Table 1). This has been linked with the low pH of the drug and the presence of sodium bisulfite. If chloroprocaine is accidentally injected into the subarachnoid space, it has been suggested that the spinal fluid be drained. Since the withdrawal of 0.75 per cent bupivacaine for obstetric anesthesia, there has been a dramatic reduction of reports of maternal death associated with bupivacaine. The high concentration was used for anesthesia in obstetric surgery. Bupivacaine, 0.25 per cent, is adequate for labor and delivery and is unlikely to cause toxicity.

Both bupivacaine and chloroprocaine are safe if extensive precautions are taken to inject only into the epidural space. Regardless of which drug is used, the needle or catheter is aspirated carefully before injection to detect the presence of blood or spinal fluid. If present, no further injection should be made, and the catheter or needle should be removed. Next, a test dose of the local anesthetic is given (2 to 3 ml) to further rule out subarachnoid injection; if this is not done, a high or total spinal might ensue. If the test dose is injected into the subarachnoid space, low spinal results, and the epidural anesthetic is abandoned. Epinephrine, 10 to 15 micrograms, should be added to the local anesthetic, to detect intravascular injection (which would result in tachycardia and hypertension). Intravascular injection of the local anesthetic alone often (but not always) produces a change in sensorium, ringing in the ears, tingling about the mouth, and so on; thus, addition of epinephrine is highly desirable, especially if bupivacaine is used. The patient should be attached to an electrocardiogram (ECG) and blood pressure monitor during injection of the test dose and other doses of the local anesthetic, and blood pressure should be checked frequently. After the test dose is found to have no effect, incremental doses of the local anesthetic are given, with close observation of the patient, to further ensure the prevention of injection into an unwanted area. Chloroprocaine is unlikely to cause problems if a test dose injection is used and if the drug is given in increments. We prefer to give the test dose through the epidural catheter rather than through the needle, because the catheter might migrate into a vein or the subarachnoid space. The catheter should never be pulled back through the needle once it has passed the needle tip. We use lidocaine, 1.5 per cent, with epinephrine, 1:200,000, 2 to 3 ml, for the test dose, then give 4 to 8 ml of this solution per hour through the catheter to maintain the segmental epidural. The effect of epinephrine on uterine blood flow is controversial, but our experience is that these small amounts do not have significant effect. For delivery, we inject 12 to 14 ml chloroprocaine 3 per cent in the semi-sitting position to produce perineal anesthesia, converting the segmental epidural to a "standard" epidural (anesthesia from the tenth thoracic dermatome to the fifth sacral root).

Several of the complications of lumbar epidural have previously been mentioned. A high or total spinal can result in respiratory distress or apnea, and the patient should be ventilated with oxygen, usually through an endotracheal tube. Allergic reactions to local anesthetic can occur but are very rare. Seizures should be treated with an anticonvulsant, such as a short-acting barbiturate and oxygen. Hypotension can occur from local anesthetic systemic toxicity, but it more commonly occurs from sympathetic blockade. Hypotension is treated by displacement of the uterus to the left, off the great vessels. (Because compression of the inferior vena cava and aorta can occur even in the absence of anesthesia, pregnant patients should lie on their side, rather than in the supine position.) Fluids, such as lactated Ringer's solution are infused, and oxygen is administered. The legs may be raised to produce an autotransfusion. If these measures do not produce a systolic blood pressure above 100 mm Hg or if the systolic pressure has fallen more than 30 per cent of the pre-anesthetic level, ephedrine, 10 to 15 mg, is injected intravenously. Ephedrine is chosen because it increases blood pressure by increasing cardiac output, rather than by vasoconstriction. Neurologic damage is rare if normal patients are chosen and if the anesthetic is given properly. Cardiac arrest is treated by closed chest cardiac massage, ventilation with 100 per cent oxygen, intravenous epinephrine, appropriate therapy for arrhythmias, and so on. It may be necessary to deliver the infant to remove the aorta-caval compression produced by the gravid uterus, and to allow effective resuscitation.

Spinal Anesthesia. Spinal anesthesia is still used for obstetrics. Although it does not allay pain during labor, it is used for anesthesia for delivery, being given in the delivery room, rather than the labor room, as is epidural anesthesia. Low spinal anesthesia (T10–S5) produces rapid, satisfactory anesthesia for delivery. A low spinal anesthesia is achieved by letting the patient sit for 45 to 60 seconds, before being placed in lithotomy. A variant of spinal anesthesia, "saddle block," produces anesthesia of the perineum, but not of the abdomen. As a result, the patient can bear down more effectively and deliver spontaneously, but the patient with a "saddle block" usually continues to experience the discomfort of uterine contractions. Both types are produced by injecting tetracaine (4 mg) and dextrose 6 per cent (total volume 2 ml) in the sitting position. If the patient remains upright for 3 to 5 minutes after injection, a "saddle block" is achieved. Spinal block should not be administered during contractions, as an excessive level may ensue. Spinal anesthesia generally produces a higher anesthetic level in the pregnant than the nonpregnant patient because of the engorgement of the epidural veins, produced by occlusion of the inferior vena cava. Drug dose should be reduced by about one third. Lidocaine (5 per cent 30 to 40 mg with dextrose) can be used if a spinal block of shorter duration is desired.

CONTRAINDICATIONS. Contraindications to both spinal and epidural anesthesia include hypovolemia (particularly from hemorrhage), septicemia, spinal cord tumor, increased intracranial pressure, and many other types of active neurologic diseases, infection over the lumbar area, bleeding disorder, and patient refusal. Relative contraindications to spinal anesthesia are a history of postspinal headache, chronic backache, and chronic headache.

The most common complication occurring with spinal anesthesia is *hypotension.* It is treated with left uterine displacement, intravenous fluids, oxygen, and leg raising, but *not* Trendelenburg position. Ephedrine, 10 to 15 mg, is given intravenously if the blood pressure does not respond to the previously mentioned maneuver. The extent of the sympathetic block is the main determinant of hypotension, not the choice of the local anesthetic drug. *Postspinal headache* is caused by the loss of spinal fluid through the hole made by the spinal needle, so that the larger the needle, the greater the incidence. In our experience, using 22-gauge needles, the incidence is 11 per cent. We find 25-gauge needles too small to use easily in our practice. Postspinal headache is aggravated by the sitting position and indeed is diagnosed by this finding. Lying flat in bed for 24 hours does not prevent spinal headache, so spinal anesthesia is not a contraindication to early ambulation. Characteristically, spinal headache begins 1 to 2 days after the lumbar puncture and lasts 5 to 7 days. It is treated with bed rest, analgesics, oral or intravenous fluids (3000 ml per day), and an abdominal binder (to recompress the inferior vena cava). If these treatments are ineffective, caffeine and sodium benzoate, 500 mg, given intravenously once or twice, may help. The ultimate and definitive treatment of postspinal headache is the aseptic injection of 10 ml of the patient's own blood into the lumbar epidural space (blood patch epidural). Respiratory arrest can occur with high or total spinal anesthesia and is treated with ventilation. Convulsions from systemic local anesthetic toxicity are unknown with spinal anesthesia due to the small amount of drug used. Neurologic complications are rare and are unlikely to occur if normal patients are chosen and if the spinal block is administered correctly.

Caudal Anesthesia. Caudal epidural anesthesia was once considered the very best of obstetric anesthesia and is still used by some practitioners. Like lumbar epidural, there is no spinal headache, and the anesthesia may be initiated when labor is well established. Unlike lumbar epidural, a segmental block cannot be given, and more drug is used. It is more difficult, more painful, and more likely to fail than is the lumbar epidural. A needle is inserted into the caudal canal (a continuation of the epidural space) through the sacral hiatus (located by palpation), and the easy injection of air after placement implies proper placement. The local anesthetic drug (lidocaine, bupivacaine, or chloroprocaine) may be injected through the needle or through a catheter.

A test dose (2 to 3 ml) is always given. The initial dose is approximately 25 ml to achieve a T10 level, with repeated doses of about 15 ml every 1 to 3 hours to maintain complete pain relief. Caudal anesthesia has been almost completely superseded by lumbar epidural anesthesia because of the many advantages of the latter. The same complications can occur with caudal anesthesia as with epidural, and they are treated similarly. Because of the rapid, overwhelming complications that potentially can occur in epidural, spinal, or caudal anesthesia, the practitioner is again urged to avoid these very effective techniques unless he or she is extremely well trained in their administration, understands their theory of action, and is well versed in treating complications that may arise. It is better to achieve partial pain relief with narcotics, tranquilizers, and a pudendal block than to have a maternal and/or neonatal death!

Paracervical Block. Paracervical block is achieved by injecting 10 ml of one of the four commonly used local anesthetics on either side of the cervix, in the lateral fornices. The drug affects the pelvic plexus (Frankenhäuser's ganglion) and blocks the transmission of the pain of uterine contractions and cervical dilatation. It has no effect on perineal pain; this could be achieved by addition of a pudendal block. There is virtually no incidence of hypotension in the mother, but there is a slight chance of local anesthetic convulsion if the drug is injected intravascularly. The block is effective and rapid in onset but can cause fetal bradycardia. This bradycardia reflects true fetal distress. It is probably caused by local anesthetic intoxication of the fetus and has resulted in the virtual abandonment of paracervical block in obstetrics. Paracervical block is still useful in gynecologic practices, however, for anesthesia for dilatation and curretage.

Pudendal Block. Pudendal block is the basic regional anesthetic of the obstetrician and is simple and safe. On the other hand, it provides only anesthesia of the perineum. It is accomplished by injection of a local anesthetic (usually 10 to 15 ml of 1 per cent lidocaine per side) transvaginally below and behind the ischial spine, blocking the pudendal nerves.

General Anesthesia

For many years, general anesthesia, without endotracheal intubation, was commonly used for vaginal delivery. Over the past one or two decades, it has been fully realized that general anesthesia can lead to aspiration, a prominent cause of maternal mortality. The virtual abandonment of general anesthesia for vaginal delivery is undoubtedly a major determinant in the reduction in maternal mortality.

Pregnant patients, particularly in the third trimester, have delayed gastric emptying. The angle of the gastroesophageal junction is changed, predisposing to regurgitation. The stomach ceases to empty during labor and food ingested many hours before can be vomited and aspirated if the patient is unconscious. Gastric secretions accumulate during labor, and, even if the stomach were empty at the start of labor, these acid secretions can be a grave threat.

The most effective method for preventing this complication is to keep the mother awake—use prepared childbirth or regional block, such as epidural, spinal, or pudendal. If vomiting or regurgitation occurs, laryngeal reflexes are intact, and aspiration is less likely to occur. The use of antacids during labor and just before delivery may reduce the effect of aspiration if it occurs. Aspiration can occur in the absence of general anesthesia, for instance, with epileptic, eclamptic, or local anesthetic convulsions. Therefore, we give 15 ml particulate antacids (Maalox) every 3 hours during labor to all patients and a clear antacid (sodium citrate, Bicitra, 15 ml) before delivery if there is a significant possibility of vomiting (in cases of general anesthesia for vaginal or abdominal delivery and in every cesarean section). The aspiration of particulate antacids can be quite harmful (probably less serious than aspirating acid gastric contents), but the chronic ingestion of sodium citrate would produce a metabolic alkalosis. Therefore, we give the clear antacid only once, and that is given just before delivery. The purpose is to raise the pH above the critical level of 2.5. If general anesthesia becomes necessary, the trachea should be intubated with a cuffed endotracheal tube.

Other strategies suggested for reducing gastric contents are administration of glycopyrrolate (Robinul), cimetidine (Tagamet), and metoclopramide (Reglan). Glycopyrrolate is an anticholinergic and reduces glandular secretion. It does not pass the placenta. Administration approximately 1 hour before anesthesia is induced should reduce the amount of salivary and gastric secretion. Cimetidine is an H_2 receptor antagonist and reduces the production of hydrochloric acid. It does pass the placenta but appears to have no adverse effect on the newborn. It is widely used in anesthesia for the nonpregnant patient. Metoclopramide facilitates gastric emptying by opening the pylorus. It is used as an antiemetic, for gastroesophageal reflux, and in patients with diabetic gastroparesis. It, too, passes the placenta but appears to be without neonatal effect. Studies performed in pregnant and nonpregnant patients suggest it usually, but not always, reduces gastric volume; pH is unaffected. A combination of cimetidine and metoclopramide is especially effective. Despite the lack of neonatal effect of cimetidine and metoclopramide, neither has been approved for use in the pregnant patient. We, therefore, do not use them, and, for the time being, rely on sodium citrate and glycopyrrolate.

General anesthesia for vaginal delivery is occasionally indicated for emergencies such as forceps delivery for fetal distress, breech, and twins. An antacid and glycopyrrolate are given, the patient is pre-oxygenated, and pancuronium, 1 mg, is given intravenously to prevent fasciculations. After 2 to 3 minutes, thiopental (Pentothal), 4 mg per kg, is given intravenously, and cricoid pressure is applied (Sellick's maneuver). Succinylcholine, 100 mg, is injected intravenously. The patient is not ventilated. After 2 minutes, the trachea is intubated and the cuff is inflated. With this technique, the danger of aspiration is slight, even if the patient vomits. Nitrous oxide and oxygen (50 per cent) and a small amount of halothane (0.5 per cent) or enflurane (0.8 per cent) are administered. If uterine relaxation is needed, as for breech or second twin, 2 to 3 per cent halothane is administered until delivery, and then discontinued. Skeletal muscle relaxation, if needed, is provided by a succinylcholine infusion (0.2 per cent). A Pitocin infusion is started after delivery. After the obstetric procedure is completed, the patient is allowed to awaken. She is extubated only when she is ventilating adequately and when her laryngeal reflexes have returned. After delivery, about 8 hours are required for the stomach to empty spontaneously. General anesthesia should not be used for postpartum tubal ligation until this time has elapsed. After that, the risk of aspiration is no greater than in the nonpregnant patient.

Despite all these precautions, aspiration may occur. In this event, the patient is immediately placed in the Trendelenburg position, and the mouth and pharynx are suctioned. It may help to collect some of the vomitus in a small trap and check the pH. If the pH is below 2.5, serious problems are likely to occur. If the pH is above 2.5, there may be no pathology. It is usually desirable to expose the larynx and suction the trachea. If the amount of vomitus is small and the patient is resisting, this may be deferred. If the aspiration is massive and food particles are present, the patient is reintubated, the trachea is suctioned, and the patient is ventilated with 100 per cent oxygen. A chest x-ray is obtained. (In the supine position, aspiration usually involves the apical branch of the right lower lobe.) Arterial blood gases are measured, and the degree of intrapulmonary shunting is assessed. Signs of aspiration are cyanosis, tachypnea, and tachycardia. Mechanical ventilation of the lungs is an important part of the treatment, affecting outcome possibly more than any other maneuver. Mechanical ventilatory support is given if the Po_2 is less than 70 mm Hg or room air or if there is an alveolar-arterial oxygen difference over 140 mm Hg on 40 per cent oxygen. Positive pressure ventilation is administered with the addition of 5 to 10 cm H_2O positive end expiratory pressure (PEEP). Bronchospasm may require bronchodilator therapy. Intravenous fluids are given in appropriate amounts, and antibiotics are given if infection is present. Steroids are probably of no value.

Ketamine can be used for general anesthesia for obstetrics, at a reduced dose. For delivery, 0.5 mg per kg provides analgesia but does not induce unconsciousness, leaving the laryngeal reflexes intact.

Anesthesia for Cesarean Section

The cesarean section rate has risen from 5 per cent in the 1960s to 20 to 25 per cent in the 1980s. Anesthesia for abdominal delivery may be provided by hypnosis, acupuncture, or local, spinal, epidural, or general anesthesia; but the techniques popular in this country are the latter three. Spinal or epidural anesthetics do not usually result in neonatal sedation, but there are disadvantages; not all women wish to be awake, and there may be some discomfort. With epidural and particularly spinal anesthesia, severe hypotension may occur, which may be difficult to treat. If the mother remains awake, there is less danger of aspiration, which is more likely under general anesthesia. General anesthesia is indicated if there is extreme fetal distress, if the mother refuses regional anesthesia, or if there is a clotting abnormality, maternal hemorrhage or CNS disease, or a need for haste.

Spinal anesthesia is relatively easy to administer. Bicitra is given to every patient before spinal anesthesia is instituted in case a high spinal anesthesia ensues or if general anesthesia is required. One thousand to 1500 ml lactated Ringer's solution is given before the block to expand the blood volume and to lessen the incidence of hypotension. The loading solution should not contain more than 500 ml 5 per cent dextrose; otherwise, neonatal hypoglycemia may result. Spinal anesthesia may be given in the sitting or lateral position, and 8 to 10 mg tetracaine, with dextrose, is administered. The drug is not administered during contractions if the patient is in labor. The obese patient may develop a higher anesthetic level than expected. The dose should be reduced even more in these patients. A folded blanket is placed beneath the right hip to displace the uterus. Oxygen is administered by face mask. An anesthetic level of T6 is sought; a lower level may result in surgical discomfort, and a higher level may produce respiratory distress. If the systolic blood pressure falls below 100 mm Hg or 30 per cent of control, ephedrine, 10 to 15 mg, is given intravenously; several doses may be necessary. On a few occasions, tachyphylaxis to ephedrine resulted after multiple doses were given; we have successfully used dopamine, 5 micrograms per kg per minute, as a vasopressor. After delivery, Pitocin, 20 units, is injected into the bag of lactated Ringer's solution, and a tranquilizer (diazepam or droperidol) and a narcotic (meperidine or fentanyl) are given. Because of the possibility of a rapid onset of hypotension and/or respiratory distress, persons administering anesthesia for cesarean sections should be alert and able to rapidly recognize and treat these complications.

Epidural anesthesia is more difficult to administer than spinal anesthesia for cesarean section, but there is no postspinal headache, and the incidence of hypotension seems to be lower. The sitting or lateral position is used, the epidural space is identified by the loss of resistance technique, and the catheter is inserted 2 to 3 cm. The needle is removed, and a test dose of local anesthetic (lidocaine, 1 to 2 per cent, or bupivacaine, 0.5 per cent, 2 to 3 ml with epinephrine) is injected. If no effects occur, the anesthetizing dose is given, in increments. We prefer chloroprocaine, 3 per cent 20 to 25 ml, for the main dose. Again, a T6 level is sought. Chloroprocaine produces more rapid anesthesia (10 minutes) than does lidocaine or bupivacaine. As with spinal anesthesia, hypotension and respiratory distress may occur and must be treated. Fluid loading is performed before the epidural is administered, and hypotension is treated with ephedrine. Unlike spinal anesthesia, epidural anesthesia can result in toxic reactions to the local anesthetic, especially if the drug is given intravenously by mistake. This is treated symptomatically, with oxygen, ventilation, anticonvulsants (if there is CNS excitation), vasopressors, and even cardiopulmonary resuscitation) (CPR) if cardiac arrest occurs. Another of the many advantages of epidural anesthesia when compared with spinal anesthesia is that further doses of drug may be injected if the anesthetic level is inadequate. With spinal anesthesia, the drug is injected as a single dose; with epidural anesthesia, the drug is titrated, and subsequent doses may be given if the surgery is prolonged.

A fairly new variant of epidural anesthesia is the epidural injection of narcotics. This does not produce surgical anesthesia but gives postpartum pain relief for up to 24 hours. Morphine (Duramorph) is the only drug approved thus far, but fentanyl and butorphanol have been used experimentally. Epidural narcotics generally do not produce labor analgesia. Side effects include pruritus (treated with naloxone) and rare respiratory depression. Because respiratory depression can be insidious and can occur hours after injection, patients must be monitored for 24 hours. In obstetrics, the greatest use of epidural narcotics is for postsection pain relief.

General anesthesia continues to be popular for cesarean section. With current techniques, Apgar scores are almost as good with general as with regional anesthesia. The chance of aspiration or airway problems causes us to still prefer regional anesthesia, however. These patients are also fluid loaded before induction of anesthesia, and the uterus is displaced to the left. Currently, the patient for cesarean section under general anesthesia is given glycopyrrolate, 0.2 mg intramuscularly, and Bicitra, 15 ml, orally, an hour before surgery. No tranquilizer or narcotic is given. During preoxygenation, on the operating table, pancuronium, 1 mg, is given intravenously to prevent fasciculations, and 2 to 3 minutes later, thiopental, 4 mg per kg, is injected, followed by succinylcholine, 100 mg. The patient is not ventilated if a full stomach is suspected. In all cases, Sellick's maneuver (cricoid pressure) is performed by an assistant. The trachea is intubated, and the cuff is inflated. Surgery commences, and nitrous oxide 50 per cent, is administered with halothane 0.5 per cent, or enflurane, 0.8 per cent. A succinylcholine infusion is given as needed. Tranquilizers and narcotics are given after delivery, along with Pitocin. Despite the fact that thiopental crosses the placenta readily, fetal shunts (portal vein, ductus venosus) prevent high fetal CNS levels of the barbiturate, so there is usually little neonatal depression if no repeat doses are given. Nitrous oxide and halothane or enflurane have little effect, because they are given in low concentrations, enough to produce maternal unconsciousness. Succinylcholine does not pass the placenta unless given in very high doses. Both the induction-delivery interval and the uterine incision–delivery intervals should be kept as short as possible. Difficulties with intubation have resulted in several maternal deaths in recent years in this country, so general anesthesia for cesarean section is not approached casually. If the patient cannot be intubated and if the surgery is not elective, one approach is to administer anesthesia with a mask while the assistant continues to hold cricoid pressure. If the surgery is elective, the patient may be allowed to awaken, and a spinal or epidural may be given. If this is unacceptable, the trachea may be intubated with the aid of a fiber optic bronchoscope or by the blind nasal approach. An esophageal gastric tube airway could be used as an alternative. Ketamine, 1 mg per kg intravenously, can be used as an induction agent in patients with hemorrhagic hypotension.

Anesthesia and Medical Complications of Pregnancy

Pre-eclampsia is a common complication of pregnancy, characterized by hypertension, proteinuria, and edema. This may proceed to eclamptic convulsions. This disease has many anesthetic implications owing to the presence of hypovolemia, coagulopathies, uteroplacental insufficiency, and hypersensitivity of the vascular and central nervous systems. Intubation of these patients, even under general anesthesia, often produces severe hypertension; dramatic hypotension can result from regional anesthesia if the contracted blood volume is not treated. Some centers even avoid regional anesthesia in these patients for this reason. We have found that after liberal crystalloid infusion, hypotension is seldom a problem, so we often use epidural anesthesia and sometimes spinal anesthesia for both vaginal and abdominal deliveries. These patients are usually treated with magnesium sulfate, so smaller doses of muscle relaxants should be used, if general anesthesia is used. Central pressure monitoring, such as CVP or wedge pressure, is useful to assess volume status. Central venous pressure often ranges from 0 to 6 cm H_2O and should be raised to 6 to 8 cm before institution of regional anesthesia by the infusion of 1000 to 1500 ml crystalloid or colloid. The severe hypertension frequently occurring with intubation during general anesthesia may be blunted somewhat by the injection of lidocaine, 100 mg intravenously, just before the thiopental. Some practitioners advocate the use of nitroprusside, nitroglycerine, or trimethaphan, but we have had no experience with these drugs for pre-eclampsia.

Diabetes. Relatively common, this disease often results in large babies, frequently necessitating cesarean section. Ketoacidosis can occur in the mother during labor if the insulin requirements are not well managed. Hypoglycemia may occur if insulin administration is excessive. Insulin requirements often fall after delivery. Blood glucose determinations should be made frequently during labor, and regular insulin should be given as needed. If scheduled for elective cesarean section, half the dose of long-acting insulin is given the morning of surgery, with frequent glucose measurements. We find that the best method of managing the diabetic for vaginal or abdominal delivery is with continuous insulin infusion with frequent blood glucose determination. These determinations may be made on blood obtained from fingersticks. Epidural anesthesia is the preferred method for vaginal delivery or cesarean section.

Prematurity. Infants with a low birthweight are very sensitive to anesthetic drugs, asphyxia, and obstetric complications. Premature infants have underdeveloped renal, hepatic, and enzyme systems and have difficulty excreting anesthetic drugs. Intracranial hemorrhage is more common than in the term infant. Epidural anesthesia is considered ideal for delivery, because it avoids potentially depressing narcotic and tranquilizing drugs and permits a controlled delivery.

An added problem with prematurity is the possibility that the mother has received tocolytic drugs, such as ritodrine (Yutopar), in an attempt to inhibit labor. If this course of therapy has been unsuccessful, anesthesia for vaginal or abdominal delivery may have to be initiated, even though these drugs may produce possible metabolic derangements. Ritodrine, a beta agonist, causes many of the side effects associated with epinephrine, such as tachycardia, arrhythmias, hypopotassemia, and hyperglycemia. Pulmonary edema has been reported, which may be due to increased capillary permeability or of cardiac origin. The pulmonary edema is possibly associated with steroid therapy (given to enhance fetal lung maturation) and fluid overload.

If the tocolytic therapy has been considered unsuccessful, the drug is discontinued and the patient is made ready for delivery and anesthesia. The half-life of ritodrine is short, and the acute effects are rapidly dissipated, but the metabolic problems persist. Supplemental potassium is only given if plasma levels are as low as 2.5 mEq per liter or less. Epidural anesthesia again is considered the technique of choice.

Breech Presentation and Multiple Gestation. When these patients are delivered vaginally, a member of the anesthesia team should be present, available to provide deep general anesthesia if necessary. Management usually involves spontaneous delivery, with pudendal block and nitrous oxide analgesia. If the aftercoming head of the breech infant is trapped by the cervix, a rapid sequence induction is performed, the patient is intubated, and halothane, 2 to 3 per cent, is administered. If, in the vaginal delivery of twins, the second infant does not deliver expeditiously, the obstetrician may request uterine relaxation for an internal podalic version and breech extraction. The patient is induced, the trachea is intubated, and deep halothane anesthesia is given until delivery is complete. The patient is not extubated until she awakens.

Heart Disease. Heart disease remains a significant cause of maternal mortality. The overall incidence of heart disease in pregnancy over the past 25 years has decreased from 3.6 to 1.6 per cent. Rheumatic heart disease, despite a declining incidence, still represents the most common type of heart disease. Congenital heart disease has become more common as women with this disease, through improved medical therapy, reach the reproductive years. Pregnant women are most likely to go into failure (1) at 28 to 32 weeks of gestation, (2) during labor and delivery, or (3) immediately postpartum.

In general, most pregnant patients with heart disease benefit from epidural anesthesia during labor and delivery. Tachycardia, straining, and increased oxygen consumption are minimized. Tachycardia can lead to congestive heart failure, and the Valsalva maneuver can lead to such a reduction in cardiac output that organ blood flow is compromised. Hypotension should be avoided, and fluid administration should be adequate but not excessive. Central venous, direct arterial, and possibly pulmonary capillary wedge pressure monitoring may be indicated.

Patients in whom the use of epidural anesthesia is probably not wise are those with aortic stenosis and congenital heart disease with right-to-left shunts. Systemic hypotension can be disastrous, because cardiac output cannot rise in aortic stenosis to compensate for a fall in systemic pressure. Right-to-left shunting may be increased or allowed to occur, with a fall in peripheral resistance. Regional anesthesia is usually avoided in patients with primary pulmonary hypertension, because hypotension will increase pulmonary vascular resistance even further.

Pulmonary Disease. Pregnant patients may present with bronchitis, emphysema, cystic fibrosis, pneumonitis, bronchiectasis, sarcoidosis, and so on, but the most common pulmonary derangement in pregnancy is bronchial asthma. This obstructive lung disease usually results in hypocarbia during an acute attack as a result of hyperventilation to correct hypoxia. Hypercarbia is not seen until late, when respiratory failure has developed. Asthmatic patients often have been treated with aminophylline, steroids, and other bronchodilators, which may have affected the development of the fetus and may also complicate anesthetic management of the delivery. Regional anesthesia is preferred for both vaginal and abdominal delivery. Bronchodilator therapy may be necessary. Endotracheal intubation, necessary for general anesthesia, often precipitates bronchospasm.

POSTPARTUM CARE

method of
FRANK W. LING, M.D.
University of Tennessee
Memphis, Tennessee

The puerperium (the 6 weeks following delivery), is the time during which important physiologic changes take place to return the female reproductive tract to its nonpregnant condition. Most of the psychologic and physiologic changes may be readily anticipated such that routine postpartum orders can be of great benefit in managing the majority of normal puerperal patients while also preventing or allowing identification of complications of the postpartum period. Table 1 lists routine postpartum orders that can facilitate nursing care and alleviate time-consuming writing of individual orders for each patient. These should *not* be used for the postoperative, diabetic, hypertensive, or pre-eclamptic-eclamptic patient.

TABLE 1. **Routine Postpartum Orders**

1. Patients given caudal, spinal, or epidural anesthesia must be able to move legs before leaving recovery room.
2. BP, P fundal check, and blood loss assessment q 15 min × 4, 1 h × 2; oral temperature qid for 48 h, then 6 A.M. only (unless febrile > 100.4 F); notify physician if pulse > 110; systolic BP > 150 or <90, diastolic BP > 100; temp. > 100.4 F.
3. Continue IV at 125–150 ml q h until discontinued.
4. NPO until stable and normal observations for 1 h, then discontinue IV and place on regular diet.
5. UP ad lib, unless spinal, epidural, or saddle block; must be able to move extremities and regain sensation in legs before getting out of bed.
6. Encourage daily shower.
7. If unable to void within 4–6 h and bladder distended, catheterize with #18 Foley; if volume > 500 ml or necessary to catheterize second time, leave Foley in place 24 hours; specimen to lab for C & S when catheter removed.
8. Routine perineal and breast care daily; encourage use of supportive bra.
9. Acetaminophen #3 po q 3–4 h PRN pain; notify physician if pain relief inadequate.
10. Promethazine hydrochloride (Phenergan) 15 mg IM q 4 h PRN nausea; notify physician if second dose is required.
11. Flurazepam hydrochloride (Dalmane) 30 mg po HS PRN.
12. Dioctyl sodium sulfosuccinate 100 mg po tid.
13. Bisacodyl USP suppository PRN the P.M. of the second postpartum day if no bowel movement since delivery.
14. Hct in A.M. day after delivery. Notify physician if < 30%.
15. If mother D neg, Du neg; check ABO, Rh, and Coombs of baby and record on maternal chart.
16. Type and crossmatch for anti-D immune globulin if appropriate after laboratory evaluation.
17. Rooming in if desired.

Normal Postpartum Course

Uterus. Involution progresses throughout the 6-week puerperium, reducing the uterus in size to that of a 16- to 18-week gestation during the immediate puerperium. By 2 weeks postpartum, the uterus is usually no longer palpable abdominally. After delivery of the placenta, the uterus contracts, becomes firm, and, in this way, provides hemostasis. Uterine tone may be maintained with (1) frequent massage; (2) oxytocin, 10 units in 1000 ml D5RL, given intravenously at 100 to 200 ml per hour; or 10 units intramuscularly; or (3) methylergonovine maleate (Methergine), 0.2 mg intramuscularly or by mouth every 4 hours. Postpartum hemorrhage due to uterine atony may also be controlled with prostaglandin $F_{2\alpha}$, 0.25 mg intramuscularly.

Uterine drainage (lochia) usually does not exceed a normal menstrual flow and gradually changes from the initial discharge comprised mainly of blood to a minimal leukorrhea at 2 to 3 weeks postpartum. A perineal pad is usually adequate for hygiene. Menstruation is not expected until 6 to 8 weeks postpartum in the nonlactating woman, and it may be delayed several months in the patient who is breast-feeding.

Perineum. Routine perineal care is intended for hygienic purposes and to minimize discomfort. Gentle cleansing with water, sitz baths, and application of 50 per cent witch hazel (Tucks pad) are effective during the immediate puerperium. In addition, an ice pack will hasten resolution of labial edema.

Extension of an episiotomy or laceration into the rectal sphincter necessitates the additional routine use of a stool softener such as docusate sodium (Colace), 100 mg two to three times daily to minimize the risk of disruption of the repair. In addition, avoidance of enemas or suppositories in cases of rectal mucosa repair will minimize the risk of faulty wound healing.

Breasts. The watery colostrum is replaced by milk on the second or third day postpartum. The patient can sense the engorgement, which may become uncomfortable. If the mother is nursing, regular feedings or breast pumping is the only treatment needed. The additional use of a supportive bra is also useful to decrease the effect of gravity. Cracked nipples may be managed with topical lanolin.

For the non-nursing mother, inhibition of lactation will prevent painful engorgement. Bromocriptine mesylate (Parlodel), 2.5 mg twice daily by mouth for 14 days, is the most effective therapy. As an alternative, a patient can be given a breast binder, ice pack, and mild analgesic.

Gastrointestinal Tract. Puerperal bowel activity may be depressed by the relaxing action of progesterone on smooth muscle. Bisacodyl (Dulcolax) suppository, psyllium hydrophilic mucilloid (Metamucil), 1 tablespoon orally twice daily, or stool softeners will aid the patient who becomes uncomfortable for this reason.

Hemorrhoids may be managed using sitz baths in conjunction with hemorrhoidal preparations such as Anusol or Corticaine.

Bladder. Often, various urinary complaints follow what is otherwise a normal, uncomplicated delivery. Minimal hematuria may be attributable to capillary fragility of the bladder mucosa. Similarly, incontinence or urinary retention may be due to mucosal edema, perineal pain, or effects of conduction anesthesia. If the patient is unable to void, catheterization for 12 to 24 hours may be needed. A 2- to 3-liter diuresis should be expected in the first 24 to 36 hours postpartum.

Chills. It is not uncommon for a patient to develop transient shaking chills immediately following the third stage of labor. Contributing factors include muscle exhaustion and the usually cool temperature of the delivery room. An infectious etiology is rare. Warm blankets and reassurance are usually adequate therapy.

Hospital Care. The immediate postpartum care begins in the delivery room when special attention is given to inspection of the reproductive tract in order to prevent postpartum hemorrhage. Hemostatic suturing of lacerations and/or episiotomy in addition to complete evacuation of uterine contents is vital.

Recovery room time is minimally 1 hour, during which the patient is monitored for changes in vital signs, excessive bleeding, unusual discomfort, or inability to void. This time can also be devoted to fostering mother-infant interaction.

The average 2- to 3-day hospitalization should include rounds at least daily to inspect for potential common problems such as breast tenderness, uterine tenderness, foul-smelling lochia, leg tenderness or episiotomy complications such as hematoma, infection, or wound breakdown.

Discharge and Home Care. Possible discharge medications include analgesics, iron supplement, vitamin supplement, stool softener, hemorrhoidal preparations, contraceptives, antibiotics, and lactation suppressant. The patient should be allowed to be active as tolerated without becoming too strenuous. Mild exercises may be started immediately. Sexual intercourse need not be delayed until 6 weeks as has been commonly recommended but should be initiated when the patient is comfortable, when lochia is minimized, and when the issue of contraception has been thoroughly addressed. It is not uncommon for a nursing mother to have hypoestrogenic effects of the vaginal mucosa which produces dyspareunia. This can be managed with 1/2 applicatorful of estrogen cream applied topically to the vagina one or two times weekly. Bathing and hygiene is as usual, but douching is proscribed for at least 2 to 3 weeks.

Postpartum Examination

Although traditionally scheduled for 6 weeks postpartum, this examination is commonly performed sooner, especially for problems or if other factors such as the need to return to a job are a major concern. Several areas should be addressed.

Breast examination. Since the breast examination has usually not been performed throughout gestation, it should be performed at this time. This should be done even in nursing mothers in order to identify new lesions that may be palable despite breast engorgement.

Pelvic examination. By the time most postpartum examinations are performed, pelvic structures have usually returned to their normal nonpregnant size. Special attention should be paid to the perineum. Kegel exercises (repetitive contractions of the pubococcygeus muscles) are frequently needed to aid the return of muscle tone.

Pap smear. A routine pap smear at the postpartum examination is a part of normal health care maintenance. If performed less than 6 weeks after a delivery, normal repair of the cervix may be misinterpreted as dysplastic abnormalities. Aggressive therapy may not be warranted, because these changes will regress as healing progresses.

Contraception. The patient should have considered postpartum contraception prior to delivery so that appropriate steps could be taken upon discharge from the hospital. Oral contraceptives are not recommended for the nursing mother. IUD insertion at 6 weeks or less is associated with an incidence of uterine perforation significantly greater than insertion at 3 to 4 months postpartum.

Coital activity. Sexual activity since delivery should be reviewed in order to identify potential problems. Factors such as nursing, altered father-mother relationships, and the fatigue of child care are among the many factors that may affect a couple's ability to resume sexual activity without difficulty.

Parenting concerns. A new mother is often caught in a conflict of roles, that is, being a mother, a wife, a lover, and a wage earner. In addition, the added responsibilities of a new infant can precipitate problems with older siblings. It is not inappropriate to address these issues at the postpartum visit.

Long-term health care. The patient should be encouraged to be seen routinely for health care maintenance and should be instructed in breast self-examination. Gynecologic and obstetric health care should be placed in proper perspective with other long-term health care issues that were either identified prior to pregnancy or that became problematic during gestation.

Complications of the Puerperium

Early Postpartum Hemorrhage. Excessive blood loss is commonly due to uterine atony, lacerations, and retained placental fragments. In rare circumstances, uterine rupture is a cause of postpartum hemorrhage. The treatment to maintain uterine tone has been discussed. Oxytocin should not be given as an intravenous bolus, because it may result in severe hypotension. Similarly, methylergonovine maleate (Methergine) should not be given as an intravenous bolus. It can also exacerbate hypertension. Evidence of hypotension and tachycardia require blood transfusion and volume expanders; persistent problems may require surgery for definitive therapy.

Blood loss is expected to be greater when mediolateral episiotomies are performed. Particular attention must be paid to the presence of a laceration when forceps are used or when a difficult delivery is encountered. A vaginal pack is rarely of any benefit and may actually delay the diagnosis of postpartum hemorrhage.

Persistent uterine bleeding in the absence of lacerations or uterine atony is likely to be caused by retained placental fragments or membranes. Manual exploration of the uterine cavity can be accomplished without anesthesia but may prove difficult and uncomfortable for the patient. The rare cases of uterine rupture after a normal vaginal delivery are not necessarily associated with a great amount of pain or external blood loss. Immediate surgical management is indicated, resulting in either repair of the uterine defect or hysterectomy.

Late Postpartum Hemorrhage. The two common causes of excessive uterine bleeding at a time distant to delivery (2 to 4 weeks postpartum) are retained products of conception and subinvolution of the uterus. The former requires removal of the placental fragments, whereas the latter may be treated with Methergine, 0.2 mg orally every 4 hours for 1 to 2 days.

Fever. Febrile morbidity is usually defined as an oral temperature of 38°C (100.4 F) or higher on any two consecutive days exclusive of the first 24 hours postpartum. Therapy should not be empiric but specifically directed to abnormal findings on history or physical examination, with specific attention being paid to the respiratory tract, breasts, abdomen, genital tract, and extremities. Appropriate cultures, both anaerobic and aerobic, should be taken prior to the initiation of antibiotics. Urine should be cultured only from a catheterized specimen because of the potential contamination by normal postpartum lochia. Uterine cultures must be done from the uterine cavity and not from the cervix.

Endometritis is characteristically associated with uterine tenderness, foul-smelling lochia, and possible ileus. Infections are usually polymicrobial, and antibiotic therapy should be chosen with this in mind. Oral antibiotics are sometimes inadequate, and aggressive parenteral antibiotics may be necessary. A combination of clindamycin (Cleocin), 900 mg intravenously every 8 hours, and gentamicin sulfate, 60 to 80 mg intravenously every 8 hours, has proved to be effective. Because of the potential toxicity of both of these drugs, newer generation cephalosporins and semi-synthetic penicillins have been effectively used as first-line parenteral antibiotic therapy.

Pelvic thrombophlebitis should be suspected when a spiking temperature occurs with minimal pelvic findings. Diagnosis is made by exclusion of other sources of fever. Heparinization brings a dramatic improvement within 24 hours.

Urinary tract infection is not uncommon, with upper tract infection being the result of retrograde bacterial spread. Fever, costovertebral angle tenderness, pyuria, hematuria, and leukocytosis are characteristic findings. Intravenous medications are usually indicated, with oral agents being used after the patient has become afebrile.

Mastitis is an uncommon source of postpartum fever. Nursing need not be discontinued while antibiotics are directed to the most common organisms, that is, *Staphylococcus aureus*. A breast pump may be used to empty the breasts mechanically if the patient desires. Dicloxacillin sodium, 250 mg orally every 6 hours, is a very effective first line agent. Abscess formation is rare, and, therefore, surgical drainage is an uncommon necessity.

Infection of the episiotomy site is indicated by tenderness, erythema, and induration. Subsequent abscess may be identified. Necessary management includes heat, cleansing of the affected area, and drainage. Sitz baths two to three times daily provide all of these. Repair of the wound should *not* be attempted during the immediate postpartum period but should be delayed at least 3 months.

Postpartum Depression. Postpartum "blues" is a frequent occurrence, whereas postpartum psychosis is rare. No specific prophylactic measures except forewarning the patient can be taken, but reassurance is effective. Patients appreciate emotional support, both in the hospital and subsequently, either in the office or over the telephone.

Spinal Headache. This may occur following as many as 10 per cent of all spinal anesthesias. Typically, the headache is frontoparietal when the patient is upright. Relief is obtained when she resumes the supine position. Therapy includes bed rest in the supine or prone position and intravenous or oral fluids. Analgesics are beneficial, and the use of a blood patch (injection of fresh venous blood from the patient into the subarachnoid and epidural space at the site of puncture) is effective in more severe cases.

NEONATAL RESUSCITATION

method of
MARK C. MAMMEL, M.D.,
and MICHAEL COLEMAN, M.D.
Children's Hospital
St. Paul, Minnesota

Delivery room care should assist the neonate in making an adequate transition from intrauterine to extrauterine life. For this transition to be successful, a number of complex and interdependent physiologic changes must occur within minutes of birth. Most prominent are changes in the cardiovascular and respiratory systems.

The lung is fluid-filled in utero; the placenta performs numerous functions, including acting as the "membrane oxygenator" for the fetus. At birth, dramatic changes occur. The placenta is removed from the circulation of the neonate. The infant's lungs become the source of oxygen and the primary excretor of carbon dioxide. The neonate must establish functional residual capacity in a collapsed lung. This requires the generation of 20 to 70 cm of negative pressure in the chest—far greater than the 5 to 10 cm of negative pressure generated during normal spontaneous breathing. Fluid in the lung itself is removed partially by physical effects, such as squeezing during delivery, and by an increase in lymphatic drainage. The presence of adequate alveolar surfactant allows decreases in alveolar surface tension. This, then, prevents complete collapse of the lung with expiration and results in decreased inflation pressure requirements with each succeeding breath. Finally, by about 5 minutes of age, the newborn infant should be spontaneously breathing and pink. Failure at any step in this complex cascade can result in neonatal depression and asphyxia.

Goals of resuscitation:

(1) *Expansion of the lungs*—this step is the cornerstone of successful resuscitation. Initial lung expansion decreases pulmonary vascular resistance, establishes lung volume, and allows for termination of right-to-left intracardiac shunting.

(2) *Establishment of effective air exchange*—this step follows naturally from step 1. If assisted ventilation is necessary, 100 per cent oxygen is used. This is used even in the very premature infant to insure adequate systemic oxygenation and to maximize the effects on the pulmonary vasculature.

(3) *Support of cardiac output*—most often, the first

two steps will be sufficient to establish this goal. In an infant with a heart rate of less than 60 to 80 beats per minute or a heart rate of less than 100 beats per minute and falling, external cardiac massage is necessary to maintain adequate cardiac output. Chest compression should be continued until the heart rate is greater than 100 beats per minute without assistance.

(4) *Minimized oxygen consumption*—any increase in the metabolic demand for oxygen requires increased cardiac output and systemic oxygen delivery. The simplest way to minimize oxygen consumption is to provide adequate warmth for the infant. Babies lose heat rapidly because of immature autonomic regulation, a large surface area to volume ratio, and because their skin is wet at birth. The neonate should be adequately dried with warm towels. In addition, a warm area for resuscitation, usually by means of an overhead radiant warmer, is extremely important.

When these goals have been achieved, further attention can be directed at the underlying cause for the infant's depression. The equipment necessary for newborn resuscitation is listed in Table 1.

TABLE 1. **Resuscitation Equipment**

Bag and two face masks (sizes: premature, newborn)
Stethoscope
Suction catheter and apparatus (mechanical, DeLee trap, bulb)
Pencil-handle laryngoscope (0 and 1 size straight blades)
Source of 100% oxygen
Umbilical vessel catheterization equipment (3.5 and 5.0 French umbilical catheters, stopcocks, 3 and 10 ml syringes, sutures, #11 blade, sterile drapes)
Adequate source of radiant heat and light
Prewarmed blankets

Treatment

In resuscitating the neonate, it helps to remember an old saw: "If it works, don't fix it." It takes experience to be certain which babies are in distress and which are not. Because the newborn autonomic nervous system reacts differently from that in the older patient, seemingly harmless intervention may not be so harmless for a neonate. Excessive oropharyngeal stimulation, deep suctioning of the nasopharynx and esophagus, or inappropriate manipulation of the airway can result in unexpected and profound bradycardia, creating an emergency where none had existed.

Recognizing the severely depressed infant in need of immediate resuscitation is easy. Recognition of conditions requiring less aggressive intervention comes with experience. Infants are often classified using the Apgar score (Table 2). It is especially useful in recreating events from written records. Apgar scores are obtained at 1 and 5 minutes of age; in discussing levels of resuscitation, the range of Apgar scores will be presented. However, the infant's condition, not the Apgar score, dictates the level of resuscitation required. In addition, meconium staining will be discussed separately because of the special management necessary.

Delivery room management of the infant without meconium staining is summarized in Table 3. Whether an infant is born vaginally or by cesarean section, gentle clearing of the oropharynx with a bulb suction device or DeLee trap is done to prevent aspiration. The infant is then dried with a warm towel and placed under a radiant warmer with the head slightly dependent. Oxygen may be blown over the face if necessary, but cyanosis alone in an infant who is otherwise well is not an indication for aggressive intervention. Many normal infants are quite cyanotic until they are 5 minutes old. Apgar scores for these infants are generally 7 to 10.

Mild Depression. These infants generally have poor color and respiratory effort, slightly decreased tone, and decreased reflex response. Their heart rate is usually normal. The initial intervention for these babies after the prior steps have been carried out is to stimulate the infant gently. This can be done during the drying procedure; rubbing of the forehead and paravertebral area should be all that is necessary. During this procedure, warmed, humidified oxygen should be blown over the infant's face. If the infant does not respond rapidly to this intervention, then bag and mask ventilation should be instituted. An orogastric tube is inserted prior to beginning assisted ventilation to remove air in the stomach. Since gas follows the path of least resistance and these infants have not yet established their lung volume, significant gastric inflation can occur

TABLE 2. **Apgar Scores**

	0	1	2
Heart rate	absent	< 100/min	> 100/min
Respiratory effort	absent	weak cry	strong cry
Muscle tone	limp	slight extremity flexion	well-flexed extremities
Reflex activity	no response	some motion	crying
Color	blue, pale	baby pink, extremities blue	completely pink

TABLE 3. **Delivery Room Management of the Neonate (When Amniotic Fluid Is *Not* Meconium-Stained)**

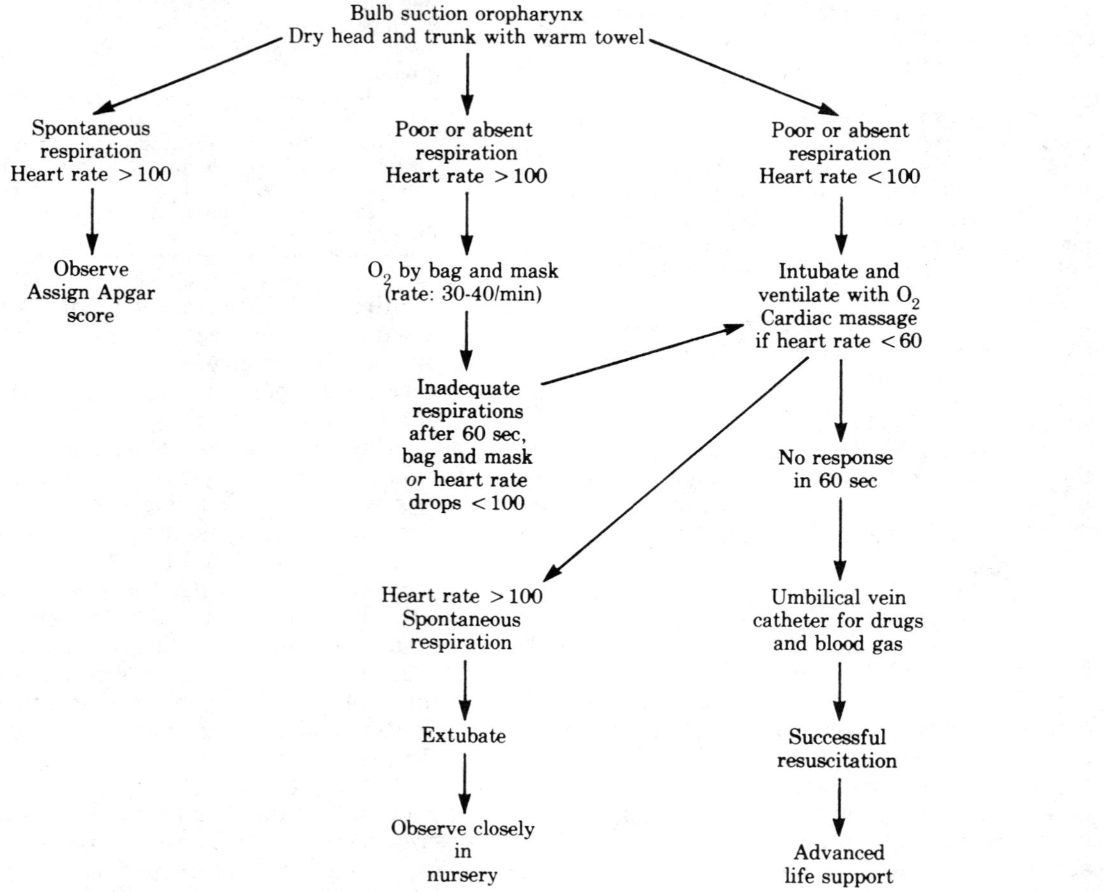

during bag and mask ventilation. Thirty to 60 breaths per minute should be provided. The neck is extended slightly; hyperextension should be avoided as this will compress the airway and compromise respiration. Auscultation is necessary to confirm that the lungs are being ventilated.

If this technique is inadequate and spontaneous respirations do not develop after 60 seconds, or if the heart rate falls to less than 100 beats per minute, the infant should be intubated with an appropriately sized endotracheal tube and given 100 per cent oxygen. Endotracheal tube lengths and diameters for different-sized babies are given in Table 4. If rapid improvement does not occur, verify the position of the endotracheal tube. If an endotracheal tube is inserted too far, it often enters the right main stem bronchus. If the vocal cords are not clearly seen during insertion, it may inadvertently be placed in the esophagus. Sound is transmitted easily throughout a neonate's body, and breath sounds may be heard over the chest when the esophagus is intubated. By far the most common reason for inadequate ventilation after endotracheal intubation is improper placement of the endotracheal tube.

If the infant's heart rate improves and respirations ensue, the endotracheal tube may be removed in the delivery room. The infant is then transferred to an observational area in the nursery. If hypotonia, poor respiratory effort, or bradycardia persists, more aggressive resuscitation is indicated (see following). These infants generally have Apgar scores of 5, 6, or 7.

TABLE 4. **Endotracheal Tubes**

Birth Weight *(gm)*	**Size** *(ID, mm)*	**Lip-to-Tip** *(cm)*
<750	2.5	7
750–2000	3.0	7–8
2000–3500	3.5	8–9
>3500	4.0	10

Moderate Depression. Infants with moderate depression have poor respiratory effort, a heart rate of approximately 100 beats per minute, and decreased tone and reflex activity and are cyanotic. Bag and mask ventilation must be instituted rapidly. These infants are unlikely to respond to stimulation alone. As noted, an orogastric tube should be inserted. Early intervention to establish respiration will usually prevent the need for intubation and pharmacologic resuscitation. Infants in this group generally have Apgar Scores of 3, 4, and 5.

Severe Depression. These infants need resuscitation immediately. They are limp, cyanotic, bradycardic, and apneic. Endotracheal intubation is mandatory. Bag and mask ventilation is indicated only during the time that the endotracheal tube is being prepared. Thirty to 60 breaths per minute of 100 per cent oxygen are delivered through the endotracheal tube. If the infant's heart rate is less than 60, external cardiac massage should be begun. Both hands should encircle the chest, with the thumbs placed over the midsternum and the finger tips over the spine. The sternum should be compressed 2 cm at approximately 100 to 150 compressions per minute.

Infants requiring intubation and cardiac massage will also require pharmacologic resuscitation. Infants requiring only intubation and ventilation generally do not require emergency medications. Only a few drugs are necessary in the delivery room. In general, inotropic agents, parasympathetic blockers, or vasopressors (other than epinephrine) should not be used. Appropriate medications and their doses are given in Table 5. Any depressed baby whose mother has received a narcotic agent within a few hours of delivery should receive naloxone (Narcan), 0.01 to 0.02 mg per kg. This can be given intravenously, intramuscularly, or into an endotracheal tube. Absorption from the alveoli is very rapid and very effective. Naloxone should not be used to avert the need for bag and mask ventilation or endotracheal intubation. The airway must always be managed prior to this step.

When intravenous medications are necessary, they are best given through a low umbilical venous catheter. Umbilical arterial catheters are more difficult to place in an emergency situation. Many emergency medications are associated with serious and permanent sequelae when given into the aorta. The umbilical venous catheter should be placed and advanced 2 to 4 cm until blood returns freely. Whereas an umbilical venous catheter may often be advanced 10 or more cm easily, without radiographic verification of position it is impossible to be certain whether the catheter is in the right atrium or within the hepatic circulation. Because the ductus venosus has low blood flow, medications given should be followed by a flush of intravenous fluid. Sodium bicarbonate is the first agent that should be given. An aliquot of 2 mEq per kg (0.5 mEq/ml) should be delivered over 1 to 2 minutes. If the infant appears to be in shock with poor capillary filling times, volume expansion can be life-saving. When anemia is suspected prior to delivery, type O negative red blood cells can be cross-matched against the mother's blood and available in the delivery room. Most of the time, this is not the case. Plasmanate, 5 per cent albumin, lactated Ringer's, or normal saline can all be used to restore the circulating volume. Ten to 20 ml per kg should be given. Blood from the placenta can also be used for this purpose; this is often not practical as it is difficult to rapidly remove enough blood from the placenta for resuscitation. If bradycardia persists following these measures, epinephrine diluted 1:10,000 should be given. One tenth ml per kg can be given intravenously or, alternatively, 1 ml can be given into the endotracheal tube. Again, the endotracheal route is very effective. At this point, before repeating these medications or adding other agents, blood gas evaluation is necessary. A second dose of bicarbonate may be given while waiting for pH results.

Intracardiac medications are a "last ditch" effort. Epinephrine can be given intracardiac if no other route is available or effective and the infant

TABLE 5. **Neonatal Resuscitation Medications for Severe Depression**

	Stock Solution	Indication	Administration
Epinephrine	1:1,000 1:10,000	Asystole Severe bradycardia	Use only 1:10,000 solution Give 0.1 ml/kg/dose IV or 0.5–1 ml per ET tube
Naloxone	0.02 mg/ml (neonatal)	Narcotic antagonism	0.01–0.02 mg/kg IV IM, or per ET tube. May repeat in 5–10 min
Sodium bicarbonate	0.5 mEq/ml (4.2%)	Acidosis with adequate ventilation	2–4 mEq/kg/dose slowly IV
Plasmanate, Ringer's lactate	——	Shock, hypotension	10–20 ml/kg IV slowly
D10W	——	Hypoglycemia	2 ml/kg/dose IV

is dying. A 23 gauge butterfly needle is inserted subxyphoid and directed toward the left shoulder. As the needle is placed, a syringe is used to aspirate. When blood returns, the needle is intracardiac and epinephrine can then be given.

Infants requiring extensive resuscitation should not be extubated in the delivery room. They should be transferred to an intensive care nursery for further evaluation and therapy, if indicated. Be certain the endotracheal tube is well secured with tape to prevent accidental extubation during transfer.

Delivery room management of very low birth weight neonates (<1250 grams) requires a more aggressive approach. Ideally, these infants should be delivered in a level III perinatal center. They frequently are unable to establish effective respirations and are more sensitive to hypoxia, hypercapnia, and acidosis than larger infants. We recommend intubation in the delivery room for all but the most vigorous of these infants.

Meconium

Meconium-staining of the amniotic fluid is a common event, occurring in approximately 10 per cent of deliveries at term. Meconium passage in infants of less than 34 weeks' gestational age is quite unusual, and its occurrence suggests the possibility of infection. Passage of meconium may result from fetal distress due to intrapartum asphyxia. It may also occur in the otherwise normal delivery. Aspiration of meconium can result in mechanical obstruction and chemical pneumonitis. Meconium aspiration syndrome is characterized by large and small airway obstruction, areas of hyperinflation and atelectasis, and respiratory failure. Mechanical ventilation of this condition is difficult. The mortality rate, though greatly improved in the last 10 years, still remains approximately 10 per cent. Because this disease is potentially preventable in most cases, an aggressive intrapartum approach has developed.

Prevention of aspiration requires a combination of obstetric and pediatric management. Though clearly shown in numerous studies that immediate endotracheal intubation after delivery is essential for some infants, the details of resuscitation still vary from place to place. We will describe our management. When the infant's head is delivered, the oropharynx and nasopharynx should be cleared with a DeLee suction trap. This has been shown to be more effective than a bulb device. If there is heavy meconium staining of the amniotic fluid, or "pea-soup meconium," all infants should be intubated and suctioned. We believe the most efficient way to clear the airway is to place a 4 by 4 inch gauze or a facemask over the endotracheal tube and apply suction with the mouth. Suction is continued as the endotracheal tube is removed. The infant is reintubated and suctioned until no meconium-stained material is returned. In addition, the stomach should be emptied via an oro- or nasogastric tube. Saline lavage of the lungs or stomach is not indicated. Remember that up to 40 per cent of infants with thick meconium may have normal Apgar scores. These infants require the same aggressive treatment their depressed counterparts receive.

The infant who is vigorous may be at greater risk for aspiration of pharyngeal or gastric contents, with resultant pneumonia. When the resuscitation team arrives after the infant has been born, the airway should still be suctioned since meconium can be removed even at 20 to 30 minutes of age.

When meconium is thin and amniotic fluid is lightly stained, management is based on the infant's condition. An infant who is depressed should receive the same treatment as the infant with thick meconium staining—that is, intubation, suctioning below the vocal cords, and removal of gastric contents. A vigorous infant, however, should be treated as a normal neonate. The vocal cords should not be visualized, and intubation need not be carried out. Visualization of the vocal cords is a common practice. Since in 20 to 50 per cent of cases staining of the vocal cords does not predict meconium in the trachea, we believe visualization without intubation is not helpful and is potentially dangerous. Ideally, positive-pressure ventilation should not be begun until the airway has been cleared, even if this requires intubation two or more times.

Ethical Considerations

Which babies do you resuscitate and when do you stop? Obviously, no single, simple answer can be given. The lower limit of viability has changed over the past few years, from 26 to 28 weeks to 24 to 26 weeks, in part because of improvement in both obstetric and neonatal care and because of more aggressive treatment of smaller babies. Nevertheless, morbidity and mortality remain extremely high in infants weighing 750 grams or less at birth. When possible, potential outcome and resuscitative options should be frankly discussed by the attending physician and the infant's parents prior to the delivery. Many times this cannot be done.

A number of steps should be followed to deal with the delivery of an extremely premature baby. First, the most experienced person available should attend these deliveries. Second, a sling scale in the delivery room allows for a rapid assessment of the neonate's weight, as well as the visual assessment of gestational age. Third, when questions arise, err on the side of the neonate. A severely depressed 24 week, 600 gram neonate with no respiration activity and a falling or absent heart rate is different from an infant of similar size and gestational age, gasping or crying and maintaining a normal heart rate. Decisions regarding the type and duration of support are best made in the intensive care unit, not in the delivery room.

At the other end of the spectrum is the larger infant with severe depression and asphyxia. These infants, even when born pulseless, require aggressive resuscitation. Studies in both the United Kingdom and the United States revealed normal outcome in the majority of infants who survived asphyxia. However, those not normal are generally seriously handicapped. Most agree that an infant who is showing little or no response after 30 minutes of resuscitation is extremely unlikely to survive, much less have a normal outcome.

Whenever an infant dies, whether in the delivery room, the intensive care unit, or outside the hospital, the parents should be encouraged to spend time with their baby. Some may wish only to see the infant; others may hold the baby for hours after death. Even when quite malformed, parents should at least see the infant; the features that are normal should be emphasized. Long-term psychologic sequelae can occur if this opportunity is denied.

CARE OF THE HIGH RISK NEONATE

method of
RALPH J. WYNN, M.D.
State University of New York
Buffalo, New York

REGIONAL PERINATAL HEALTH CARE

Although the importance of the primary care physician as a keystone in the provision of optimal neonatal health care must not be underestimated, within a regional system of perinatal health care each hospital has its own important role in permitting access of patients to the sophistication of care necessary to meet their medical needs. Hospitals with level I programs provide services for uncomplicated pregnancies and normal neonates. Level II program hospitals provide for care of selected high risk maternal and neonatal patients in addition to routine level I services. Hospitals with level III programs provide all types of perinatal care services, including consultation, transport, education, evaluation, and research.

Studies have shown that the early diagnosis of prenatal problems and the initiation of care and transfer, when indicated, are beneficial to the fetus. Maternal-fetal transport to ensure neonatal intensive care at birth further improves neonatal outcome. In addition, maternal-fetal transport has been shown to be cost effective, and it promotes early parental-infant bonding and attachment. For neonates who require intensive care, the benefits of transport by a trained team outweigh the risks when outcomes are compared with those kept at facilities unable to provide such care. I encourage you to use the consultation/transfer number of your regional center.

PERINATAL RISK ASSESSMENT

The term *high risk* defines a patient in whom the morbidity or mortality is anticipated to be greater than in the general population. Anticipatory care of the high risk neonate ideally begins in the prenatal period and permits early participation in a regionalized system of perinatal health care. Effective antepartum and intrapartum screening can alert the physician to approximately two thirds of the neonates who will require special care. Approximately 20 per cent of pregnant women can be identified in the antepartum period to be at risk, accounting for 55 per cent of the poor outcomes of pregnancy. Risk assessment must continue during the intrapartum period, as an additional 5 to 10 per cent of women will become at risk for the first time during labor. Medical and obstetric considerations, as well as the patient's lifestyle and environment, can put the neonatal-perinatal patient at risk. Table 1 is a partial list of factors that should alert the physician to the possibility that the outcome of pregnancy will be a high risk neonate. Earlier articles in this section provide a thorough discussion of obstetric management of the high risk pregnancy. Communication and cooperation between the obstetric and neonatal health care professionals provides the best care for the resultant high risk neonate.

Risk assessment must continue in the delivery room with the Apgar score (see Table 2 of the preceding article, page 835) at 1 and 5 minutes. Continued

TABLE 1. **Perinatal High Risk Factors**

Antepartum
maternal medical complication or disorders
maternal age under 16 or over 35 years
oligohydramnios or polyhydramnios
drug/substance abuse or addiction
intrauterine growth retardation
prior poor outcome of pregnancy
pregnancy-induced hypertension
lower socioeconomic status
third trimester bleeding
multiple gestation
diabetes mellitus
isoimmunization
postmaturity
Intrapartum
rupture of membranes greater than 24 hours
meconium-stained amniotic fluid
abnormal presentation or lie
prolonged second stage
chorioamnionitis
premature labor
fetal distress

assessment at 5 minute intervals while the score remains severely depressed (0 to 3) has been demonstrated in the National Collaborative Perinatal Project to relate to mortality before 1 year and chronic neurologic disability at age 7 years.

While 80 per cent of the high risk neonates can be anticipated from antepartum or intrapartum maternal risk factors, the remaining neonates first present either in the delivery room or recovery nursery. Just as the Apgar score is a means of risk assessment in the delivery room, the determination of the neonate's gestational age and its relationship to weight can be utilized in further risk identification for neonatal illness.

The assessment of neonatal maturity is quickly and easily performed, using indices of neuromuscular and physical maturity (Figure 1). While the physical maturity assessment is best performed in the first hours after birth, the neuromuscular scores may be affected by a variety of perinatal events. Anesthetic agents, narcotic analgesics, or acute asphyxia can markedly depress the neuromuscular maturity rating. Chronic, mild in utero stress such as mild toxemia or prolonged rupture of membranes frequently results in a neonate whose neuromuscular tone appears more advanced than the gestational age. If there is disparity between the physical and neuromuscular maturity ratings, the history should be reviewed closely for perinatal events, and the assessment reperformed at 24 hours of age. Continued depression of the neuromuscular rating should encourage the physician to perform a close neurologic evaluation of the neonate.

After the gestational age has been determined, based on the physical examination in conjunction with relevant obstetric data, the neonate should be plotted on a birth weight/gestational age graph (Figure 2). Although this relationship of birth weight with gestational age varies with altitude and race, these growth curves from Denver remain the most commonly used graph for this purpose. With these graphs, a neonate can be classified into one of nine possible groups based on gestation (preterm, term, post-term) and birth weight (small for gestational age [SGA], appropriate for gestational age [AGA], or large for gestational age [LGA]). Table 2 lists some of the more common causes and problems in each high risk category. Assignment of the neonate to a specific gestational age group for birth weight permits anticipation of problems and a specific care plan. Management of some of these problems is discussed later.

Risk assessment of the high risk neonate should be a continuum throughout the hospital course and a component of discharge planning. Indices of parent contact and participation in care may alert the physician to nonmedical risk factors that ultimately could affect family stability or adequacy of infant home care. Premature infants or infants requiring extended hospitalization who have single parents or infrequent visitation by the family are at increased risk for child abuse. Metabolic screening for hypothyroidism and other treatable disorders must not be forgotten. An ophthalmologist experienced in neonatal ophthalmology should dilate and examine the retinas of premature neonates exposed to oxygen when they are 6 to 8 weeks of age. Infants at risk for hearing loss should be screened by 3 months of age. A common practice is to utilize brain stem auditory evoked response (BAER) as a screening test. High risk neonatal follow-up of neurodevelopmental milestones should be regularly scheduled in those infants at greatest risk to permit early identification and intervention.

Neonatal Resuscitation

(See preceding article on Neonatal Resuscitation.

Stabilization of the High Risk Neonate

Temperature. Thermal stress to the high risk neonate can be detrimental by increasing metabolic demands on oxygen delivery and carbohydrate stores, both of which may be marginal. Keeping newborn infants warm, especially premature infants, increases their chance of survival. Temperature maintenance is the keystone of effective stabilization.

The normal skin temperature is 36.0 to 36.5 C (96.8 to 97.7 F), and the normal axillary and rectal temperature is 36.5 to 37.0 C (97.7 to 98.6 F). Rectal measurement of temperature risks rectal perforation, and unless the thermometer is inserted 5 cm (2 in), it does not measure core temperature. Measurement of axillary temperatures provides good correlation with core temperature in the neonate.

The sick neonate who will require close observation, monitoring, or procedures is best cared for under a radiant warmer. The infant's temperature should be regulated using a servocontrol skin probe securely attached. The functioning of the radiant warmer and the infant's axillary temperature should be checked frequently and recorded. A hypothermic infant should be rewarmed slowly as apnea can occur with too rapid a rise in temperature. Placing a warming pad or blanket under the very small infant will assist rewarming. Do not cover a baby under a radiant warmer as this just blocks out the heat source. It goes without saying that sick neonates should not be bathed or shampooed as these will result in evaporative heat loss!

If the infant is placed in an incubator, the concept of neutral thermal environment must be remembered: a narrow range of ambient air temperature wherein the oxygen consumption necessary to maintain normal body temperature is minimal. A normal axillary temperature does not necessarily mean that the infant is in the correct ambient temperature, as a cold-stressed infant can increase its metabolic rate to produce a normal temperature. Maintaining the environmental temperatures within this range in both incubators and oxygen hoods (Table 3) is especially

ESTIMATION OF GESTATIONAL AGE BY MATURITY RATING

Symbols: X - 1st Exam O - 2nd Exam

NEUROMUSCULAR MATURITY

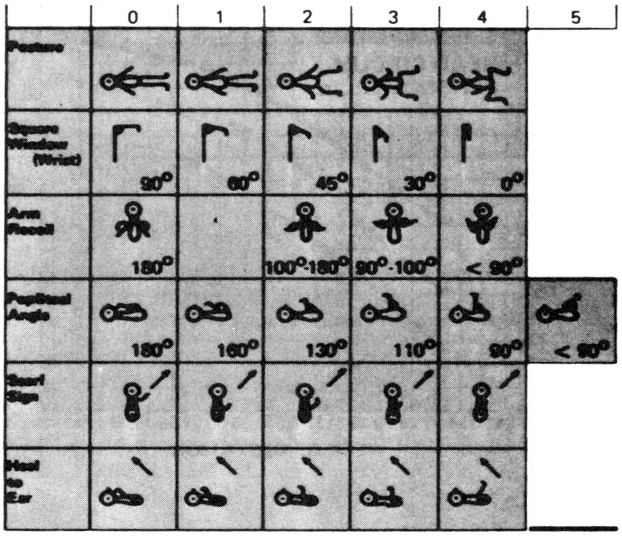

PHYSICAL MATURITY

	0	1	2	3	4	5
SKIN	gelatinous red, transparent	smooth pink, visible veins	superficial peeling &/or rash, few veins	cracking pale area, rare veins	parchment, deep cracking, no vessels	leathery, cracked, wrinkled
LANUGO	none	abundant	thinning	bald areas	mostly bald	
PLANTAR CREASES	no crease	faint red marks	anterior transverse crease only	creases ant. 2/3	creases cover entire sole	
BREAST	barely percept.	flat areola, no bud	stippled areola, 1–2 mm bud	raised areola, 3–4 mm bud	full areola, 5–10 mm bud	
EAR	pinna flat, stays folded	sl. curved pinna, soft with slow recoil	well-curv. pinna, soft but ready recoil	formed & firm with instant recoil	thick cartilage, ear stiff	
GENITALS Male	scrotum empty, no rugae		testes descending, few rugae	testes down, good rugae	testes pendulous, deep rugae	
GENITALS Female	prominent clitoris & labia minora		majora & minora equally prominent	majora large, minora small	clitoris & minora completely covered	

Gestation by Dates ____________ wks

Birth Date ____________ Hour ____________ am / pm

APGAR ____________ 1 min ____________ 5 min

MATURITY RATING

Score	Wks
5	26
10	28
15	30
20	32
25	34
30	36
35	38
40	40
45	42
50	44

SCORING SECTION

	1st Exam=X	2nd Exam=O
Estimating Gest Age by Maturity Rating	______ Weeks	______ Weeks
Time of Exam	Date ______ Hour ______ am/pm	Date ______ Hour ______ am/pm
Age at Exam	______ Hours	______ Hours
Signature of Examiner	______ M.D.	______ M.D.

Figure 1. Scoring system: Ballard JL, et al: A simplified assessment of gestational age. Pediatr Res *11*:374, 1977. Figures adapted from Sweet AY: Classification of the low-birth-weight infant, *in* Klaus MH, Fanaroff AA: Care of the High-Risk Infant. Philadelphia, WB Saunders Company, 1977, p 79. Copywright 1977, Mead Johnson & Company, Evansville IN 47721.

CLASSIFICATION OF NEWBORNS — BASED ON MATURITY AND INTRAUTERINE GROWTH

Symbols: X - 1st Exam O - 2nd Exam

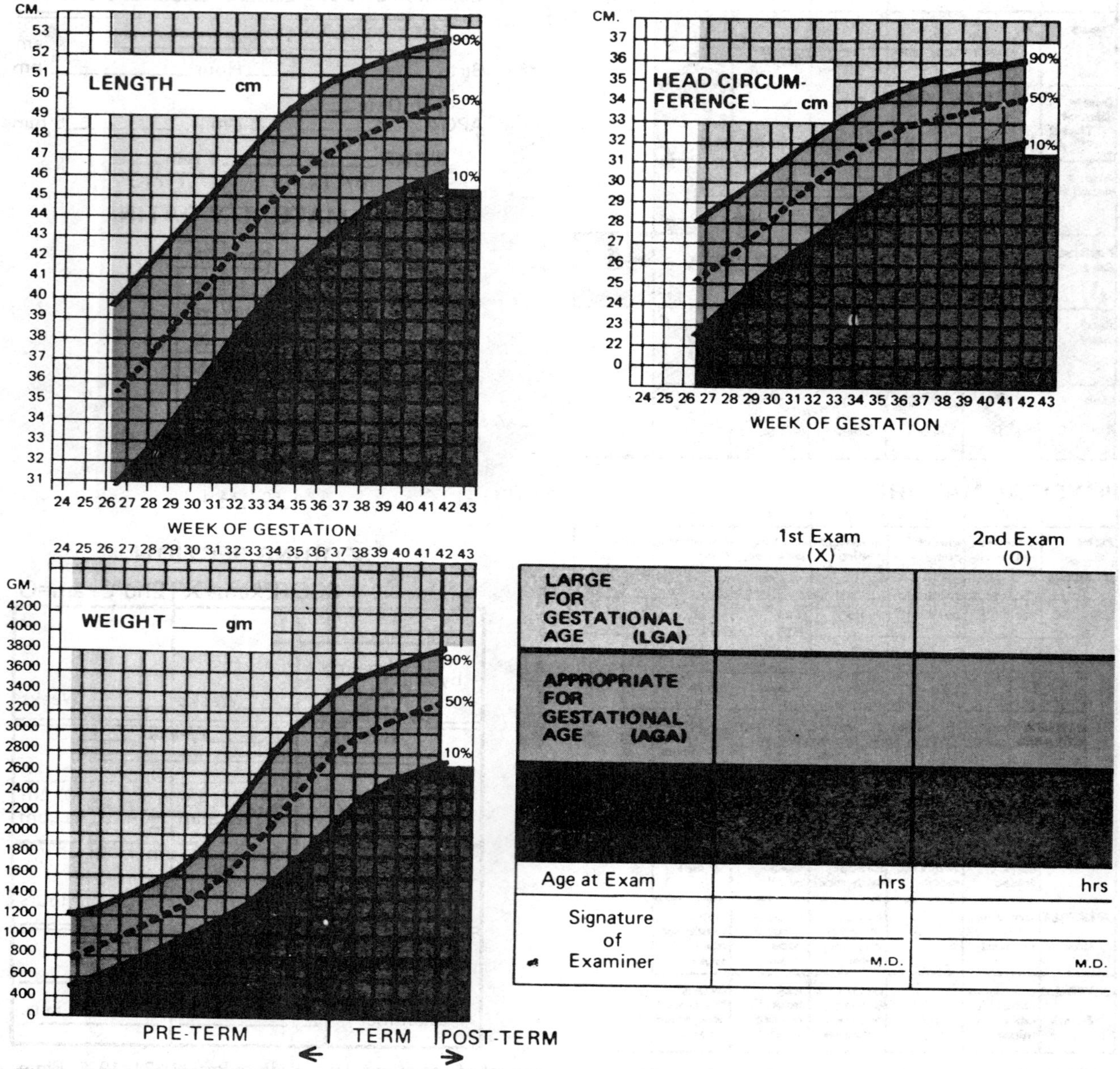

Figure 2. Adapted from Lubchenco LC, Hansman C, Boyd E: Pediatrics *37*:403, 1966; Battaglia FC, Lubehenco LC: J Pediatr *71*:159, 1967. Copyright 1977, Mead Johnson & Company, Evansville IN 47721.

TABLE 2. **Specific Problems of High Risk Infants**

Small for Gestational Age (SGA)
Causes
placental pathology/insufficiency
congenital/chromosomal anomalies
maternal disease/addiction
intrauterine infection
Problems
pulmonary hemorrhage
polycythemia
hypoglycemia
asphyxia
Large for Gestational Age (LGA)
Causes
"constitutional" (large mother)
maternal hyperglycemia
Problems
congenital anomalies
birth trauma
hypoglycemia
Preterm
Causes
prior premature labor/delivery
uterine and cervical anomalies
iatrogenic (elective delivery)
placental abnormalities
multiple gestation
Problems
hyaline membrane disease
intracranial hemorrhage
hypocalcemia
hypoglycemia
hypothermia
jaundice
sepsis
apnea
Post-Term
Causes
incorrect dates (EDC)
unknown
Problems
meconium aspiration
hypoglycemia
asphyxia

important in the premature infant. A skin servocontrol probe also can be used in most incubators. The equipment, setpoint, and incubator's and infant's temperatures should be checked and recorded on a regular basis. Keep the incubator away from cold walls, windows, and air-conditioner drafts as the infant can still lose heat by radiation in single-walled incubators. If it is necessary frequently to open incubator doors for procedures, the infant's temperature control would be better under a radiant warmer.

Oxygenation and Ventilation. Adequate oxygenation and ventilation of the high risk neonate are important to prevent tissue damage from hypoxia or acidosis. To assure that the tissues are receiving proper amounts of oxygen, arterial blood gas, hemoglobin or hematocrit, and blood pressure measurements should be obtained.

Any infant with central cyanosis should be placed in adequate amounts of environmental oxygen to alleviate cyanosis. Many incubators and infant resuscitation bags limit the oxygen concentration to 40 per cent, an outdated restriction that at one time was thought to lessen the incidence of retrolental fibroplasia. Standing orders should permit the nurse or respiratory therapist to increase the oxygen concentration to whatever percentage is necessary to alleviate cyanosis. If this does not improve the infant's condition, ventilation by bag and mask or endotracheal tube is indicated. The oxygen delivered should be both warmed and humidified. The concentration of oxygen should be monitored carefully every hour with a calibrated oxygen analyzer and recorded. Arterial oxygen tension levels should be recorded upon initiating therapy and at frequent intervals for all infants, especially those under 36 weeks' gestation. Adjustments in the inspired oxygen concentration should be made to maintain the PaO_2 at a level of 60 to 80 mm Hg. Capillary blood gases in the first day of life correlate poorly with arterial oxygen tensions. Transcutaneous monitoring of oxygen and carbon dioxide levels does not replace the arterial blood gas samples needed to assure correlation, especially in the poorly perfused neonate. Calibration and maintenance of transcutaneous monitoring equipment require patience and skill to obtain reliable results.

An infant who by auscultation is not moving air well or who by blood gas determination is found to have a respiratory acidosis with $PaCO_2$ over 60 mm Hg or pH below 7.20 is developing respiratory failure and requires ventilation. Choice of the correct endotracheal tube size and position (Table 4) remains critical. A radiograph should be obtained to assure proper tube placement and to rule out a pneumothorax which might occur in up to 25 per cent of infants in significant respiratory distress. Proper ventilation requires training and equipment that differ from those for adult care. The neonate should receive an initial respiratory rate of 40 to 60 breaths per minute with an inspiratory pressure that produces symmetric chest movement. The addition of positive end expiratory pressure (PEEP) in premature infants with hyaline membrane disease will also improve oxygenation. Contact your regional neonatal center for further specific guidelines.

To assure adequate oxygen-carrying ability of the blood, a hematocrit should be obtained, along with the arterial blood gas. In the face of pulmonary disease, an infant may not be able to completely oxygenate the blood, and thus a mild anemia could become a significant factor in decreasing the delivery of adequate oxygen to the tissues. If the venous or arterial hematocrit is less than 40 per cent, packed red blood cells may be given in a dose of 10 ml per kg slowly over 30

TABLE 3. **Neutral Thermal Environmental Temperatures**

Age and Weight	Starting Temperature (C)	Temperature Range (C)
0–6 hours		
Under 1200 grams	35.0	34.0–35.4
1200–1500 grams	34.1	33.9–34.4
1501–2500 grams	33.4	32.8–33.8
Over 2500 (and >36 weeks)	32.9	32.0–33.8
6–12 hours		
Under 1200 grams	35.0	34.0–35.4
1200–1500 grams	34.0	33.5–34.4
1501–2500 grams	33.1	32.3–33.8
Over 2500 (and >36 weeks)	32.8	31.4–33.8
12–24 hours		
Under 1200 grams	34.0	34.0–35.4
1200–1500 grams	33.8	33.3–34.3
1501–2500 grams	32.8	31.8–33.8
Over 2500 (and >36 weeks)	32.4	31.0–33.7
24–36 hours		
Under 1200 grams	34.0	34.0–35.0
1200–1500 grams	33.6	33.1–34.2
1501–2500 grams	32.6	31.6–33.6
Over 2500 (and >36 weeks)	32.1	30.7–33.5
36–48 hours		
Under 1200 grams	34.0	34.0–35.0
1200–1500 grams	33.5	33.0–34.1
1501–2500 grams	32.5	31.4–33.5
Over 2500 (and >36 weeks)	31.9	30.5–33.3
48–72 hours		
Under 1200 grams	34.0	34.0–35.0
1200–1500 grams	33.5	33.0–34.0
1500–2500 grams	32.3	31.2–33.4
Over 2500 (and >36 weeks)	31.7	30.1–33.2
72–96 hours		
Under 1200 grams	34.0	34.0–35.0
1200–1500 grams	33.5	33.0–34.0
1501–2500 grams	32.2	31.1–33.2
Over 2500 (and >36 weeks)	31.3	29.8–32.8
4–12 days		
Under 1500 grams	33.5	33.0–34.0
1501–2500 grams	32.1	31.0–33.2
Over 2500 (and >36 weeks)		
4–5 days	31.0	29.5–32.6
5–6 days	30.9	29.4–32.3
6–8 days	30.6	29.0–32.2
8–10 days	30.3	29.0–31.8
10–12 days	30.1	29.0–31.4
12–14 days		
Under 1500 grams	33.5	32.6–34.0
1501–2500 grams	32.1	31.0–33.2
2–3 weeks		
Under 1500 grams	33.1	32.2–34.0
1501–2500 grams	31.7	30.5–33.0
3–4 weeks		
Under 1500 grams	32.6	31.6–33.6
1501–2500 grams	31.4	30.0–32.7
4–5 weeks		
Under 1500 grams	22.0	31.2–33.0
1501–2500 grams	30.9	29.5–32.2
5–6 weeks		
Under 1500 grams	31.4	30.6–32.3
1501–2500 grams	30.4	29.0–31.8

Data from Scopes JW, Ahmed I: Minimal rates of oxygen consumption in sick and premature infants. Arch Dis Child *41*:407–416, 1966; Scopes JW, Ahmed I: Range of critical temperatures in sick and premature newborn babies. Arch Dis Child *41*:417–419, 1966. For his table, Scopes had the walls of the incubator 1 to 2 degrees warmer than the ambient air temperature.

(From American Academy of Pediatrics/American College of Obstetricians and Gynecologists: Guidelines for Perinatal Care. Evanston IL, 1983, pp 228–229. Copyright AAP/ACOG, 1983.)

TABLE 4. **Neonatal Endotracheal Intubation**

Neonate		Laryngoscope Blade	Endotracheal Tube		Suction Catheter
Weight (kg)	*Gestation (wk)*	*Size*	*Size (mm)*	*Distance at Lip (cm)*	**(Fr)**
0.5–1.2	24–30	0	2.5 (12 Fr)	6–7	5
1.2–2.4	30–34	0	3.0 (14 Fr)	7–8	6
2.4–3.6	34–38	1	3.5 (16 Fr)	8–9	8

to 60 minutes. Occasionally, the opposite situation exists and hyperviscosity with poor capillary flow results from polycythemia, defined as a central hematocrit greater than 65 per cent. Such infants may benefit from a partial exchange transfusion, as will be discussed later in Problems in Transition.

The third ingredient of proper tissue oxygenation relates to cardiac output and blood pressure. The severely asphyxiated or hypoglycemic neonate may have poor tissue perfusion based on cardiogenic shock, in which case volume expansion should be performed only after addition of cardiotonic drugs or correction of the hypoglycemia. The infant who is acidotic or hypothermic will appear to have poor peripheral perfusion due to vasoconstriction. Accurate measurement of systolic blood pressures can be obtained using inexpensive neonatal Doppler devices. Appropriate blood pressure cuff size must also be utilized. Systolic blood pressure below 40 to 50 mm Hg in preterm or below 50 to 60 mm Hg in term infants warrants volume expansion. A resting heart rate above 180 beats per minute in the preterm or above 150 beats per minutes in the term infant may reflect cardiac compensation for hypovolemia. In the absence of anemia, careful volume expansion with aliquots of isotonic crystalloid (normal saline) or colloid (5 per cent albumin, plasminate) in a dose of 5 to 10 ml per kg over 30 to 60 minutes should be performed. Rechecking of blood pressure, heart rate, and hematocrit is warranted.

Fluids and Glucose Homeostasis. Sick neonates are at risk for developing hypoglycemia, yet are frequently in too much respiratory distress with the risk of aspiration if fed by mouth. Establishment of a fluid line using a peripheral vein is preferable with least risk, yet can be technically difficult. An umbilical catheter situated in the umbilical vein is technically easy with only moderate risk. It can be used to draw blood for initial blood studies, cultures, and venous blood gas pH and P_{CO_2} (but not P_{O_2}) which closely approximate arterial blood gas values. The umbilical venous catheter should be used only during the initial period of stabilization or transfer. An umbilical artery catheter requires skill in placement, attention to details of location, and care and risks too great for routine use in a primary care setting.

Initial fluids for the neonate should consist of 5 per cent dextrose in water for the premature infant under 1.2 kg and 10 per cent dextrose in water for infants over 1.2 kg, at an infusion rate of 60 to 80 ml per kg per day (approximately 3 ml per kg per hour). If intravenous fluids are required beyond the first day, serum electrolytes should be checked and if normal, with adequate urine output, the dextrose solution should have approximately 25 to 30 mEq of sodium per liter and 20 to 30 mEq of potassium per liter added. The infusion rate should be gradually increased over the first week to a rate of 160 to 180 ml per kg per day by age 7 days. If the infant is under a radiant warmer or phototherapy, the fluid requirements are increased by 10 to 20 per cent. The blood glucose level should be monitored every few hours to assure glucose homeostasis with a level between 40 and 80 mg per cent. Screening with capillary whole blood reagent strips (Visidex II, Dextrostix), and with laboratory follow-up of borderline values with true glucose levels, permits appropriate adjustments of infusion rate. If the reagent strip reads zero, immediately repeat the heel stick test with a test strip from a new bottle. If it is indeed zero, or less than 20 mg per cent, do not wait for a true glucose level reading to come back from the laboratory but initiate therapy as discussed in the later section on Infants of Diabetic Mothers.

Problems of the Neonate in Transition

During the first 24 hours of life, the neonate must undergo a variety of physiologic adjustments to extrauterine life. Careful evaluation of even the normal newborn (Table 5) should be performed during the first 4 hours of life. Abnormal adjustments can be identified early and intervention initiated before deterioration occurs.

Transient Tachypnea. The neonate at birth may have a respiratory rate in excess of 60 breaths per minute with slight flaring, grunting, or retractions. As the fetal lung fluid is removed and lung compliance improves, the signs of distress should quickly dissipate and the respiratory rate

TABLE 5. **Transitional Care and Stabilization**

Risk Assessment
- Review antepartum and intrapartum history
- Classify birth weight/gestational age
- Perform physical examination

Vital Signs
- Blood pressure, upper and lower
- Respiratory rate every hour
- Temperature every hour
- Heart rate every hour

Prophylaxis
- Hemorrhagic disease (vitamin K)
- Gonococcal/chlamydial ophthalmia (1% silver nitrate or 0.5% erythromycin)

Laboratory Studies
- Cord blood if mother's blood is type O or Rh neg
- Whole blood glucose screen on admission and every hour if at risk
- Capillary hematocrit at 2–4 hrs; obtain venous sample if symptomatic or if capillary hematocrit >70%

Nutrition
- Breast, formula, or water when alert and stable
- Early feeding if at risk for hypoglycemia

decline toward 40 breaths per minute by 4 hours of age. Any infant in the transition period whose respiratory rate or distress is increasing should be thoroughly and quickly evaluated for sepsis, surfactant deficiency disease (hyaline membrane disease, shock lung), spontaneous pneumothorax, or congenital anomaly (tracheoesophageal fistula, diaphragmatic hernia). The diagnosis of exclusion is transient tachypnea of the newborn (TTN), a condition resulting from delayed resorption of fetal lung fluid. Arterial blood gas should be measured and supplemental warm, humidified oxygen supplied as indicated. An orogastric tube should be placed to vent so that gaseous abdominal distention from aerophagia does not worsen the respiratory distress. Fluids and glucose must be provided either by gavage, if the baby is only tachypneic, or by the intravenous route if it is in distress. Nipple feeds can result in aspiration, while delay in feeding can result in hypoglycemia. If there is any concern regarding sepsis, appropriate therapy should be initiated without delay.

Persistence of the Fetal Circulation. Near-term, term, or post-term infants who have been exposed to a variety of nonspecific perinatal events can develop right to left shunting through the foramen ovale or ductus arteriosus as a result of high pulmonary artery resistance. Perinatal asphyxia, neonatal hypoxia, hypothermia, hypoglycemia, metabolic acidosis, or aspiration syndromes are common precipitating factors. Infants in respiratory distress or requiring oxygen should have all these parameters evaluated. Mild transient tachypnea or aspiration syndromes inappropriately cared for in the early stages can suddenly decompensate. Administration of high concentrations of oxygen to obtain a stable PaO_2 of 80 to 100 mm Hg is an initial priority. Do not remove the infant from oxygen for even a brief period. Efforts should be made to correct immediately any acidosis, hypothermia, hypotension, or hypoglycemia. Do not stress the infant with loud noise or unnecessary handling. Contact your regional neonatal center early as this potentially fatal entity requires the most sophisticated level of care available.

Polycythemia. While anemia reduces the oxygen-carrying capacity of the blood, polycythemia with its resultant hyperviscosity impedes the microcirculatory delivery of oxygen to the tissues. The tissue hypoxia can result in a variety of systems disorders, including respiratory distress, congestive heart failure, necrotizing enterocolitis, diffuse thrombotic disease, and seizures. While virtually all the symptoms are related to the increase in whole blood viscosity, its measurement is not readily available. The venous hematocrit, however, is a readily available measurement with some correlation to viscosity. A hematocrit of 60 per cent is associated with a viscosity three to five times greater than that of a 40 per cent hematocrit level.

Although controversy exists in the literature about long-term benefits of correction of hyperviscosity, it has been well shown that such correction can alleviate the short-term symptoms and morbidity. At the Children's Hospital of Buffalo, hematocrit screening by warmed heel stick is routinely performed on all neonates by 4 hours of age. In those infants with warmed capillary hematocrit counts of greater than 70 per cent, a venous hematocrit is determined. A hematocrit count is performed at 1 hour and again at 4 hours of age in infants who are at increased risk for polycythemia. A partial exchange transfusion is expeditiously performed on all infants with a venous hematocrit count greater than 70 per cent and in those infants with hematocrit values greater than 60 per cent who have symptoms of insufficient microcirculation. The partial exchange is performed via an umbilical venous catheter using aliquots of crystalloid or colloid solution to lower the hematocrit to a level of 50 per cent. To calculate the partial exchange volume, the following formula is used:

Volume of exchange (ml) =

$$\text{blood volume} \times \frac{\text{observed} - \text{desired}}{\text{observed}} \text{ hematocrit}$$

The blood value of a fullterm neonate is 80 ml per kg. Simple phlebotomy or volume transfusions are ill advised as they may risk hypo- or hypervolemia. A common error in the management of polycythemia is permitting a hematocrit value to remain elevated over the next several days. The red cell mass and plasma volume normally equilibrate to a hematocrit level that rises over the first 4 to 6 hours after birth and remains constant for the first weeks of life. Delays in decreasing blood viscosity may be the reason for the lack of improvement in long-term outcomes of these infants.

Infants of Diabetic Mothers. Approximately 1 per cent of neonates are the product of a diabetic pregnancy. With proper care of the mother, the fetus, and the neonate, most of these infants will be normal. Perhaps no other single group of neonates presents the plethora of transitional problems as does the infant of a diabetic mother (IDM). The problems include respiratory distress, hypoglycemia, hypocalcemia, polycythemia, hyperbilirubinemia, and congenital anomalies. For a variety of maternal and fetal reasons, many of these infants are delivered preterm. It is most important that such infants have a birth weight and gestational age plotted to properly assign risks. While often large for gestational age, physiologically and developmentally these infants must be managed based on the gestational age.

Respiratory distress occurs commonly in this group of infants. Preterm delivery, with delayed surfactant maturation in the IDM, can result in hyaline membrane disease. A high incidence of delivery by cesarean section without labor can result in delayed resorption of fetal lung fluid. An increased risk of neonatal sepsis, presenting as respiratory distress, is a result of a higher frequency of urinary tract infections in diabetic pregnancy. All such infants must be appropriately evaluated and managed as discussed in other sections.

If appropriate preventive management is not taken, approximately 50 per cent of IDMs will become hypoglycemic (blood glucose below 40 mg per cent); of these, one half will be symptomatic. Good control of maternal blood glucose during pregnancy and labor is a critical determinant of neonatal glucose homeostasis. If the maternal control has been very good and the neonatal blood sugar as measured in the delivery room is less than 100 mg per dl, these infants often can be managed by hourly screening of capillary whole blood glucose and initiation of early feedings. For infants who manifest evidence of poor maternal glucose homeostasis by being large for gestational age or showing retarded intrauterine growth or who have elevated blood glucose levels in the delivery room, an infusion of glucose water by peripheral vein should be initiated early.

A 10 per cent dextrose in water solution at 90 to 120 ml per kg per day will provide the 6 to 8 mg per kg per minute continuous infusion necessary for glucose homeostasis. Frequent monitoring of glucose levels to maintain them at 40 to 80 mg per cent, with initiation of frequent feedings while slowly decreasing the intravenous infusion, will lessen the labile swings in glucose and insulin levels. If the infant becomes hypoglycemic, minibolus infusions of 200 mg of glucose per kg are preferred over the use of glucagon or large bolus glucose infusions that result in hyperglycemia, thus potentiating the vicious cycle of hyperinsulinemia followed by hypoglycemia.

Impaired responsiveness of the parathyroid glands results in hypocalcemia (serum calcium less than 7.5 or 8 mg per cent) in up to 25 per cent of IDMs. If the serum calcium drops below 6 mg per cent or the infant becomes symptomatic, supplemental calcium should be provided and the serum calcium level monitored. Calcium gluconate, 200 to 400 mg per kg per day well diluted in the intravenous or enteral fluids, is one approach to calcium supplementation. All calcium preparations are extremely irritating to veins and intestinal tissues and should be used with caution and close monitoring.

The IDM has an increased incidence of polycythemia and hyperviscosity. Early screening and management are indicated, as the large red cell mass and decreased tissue perfusion can worsen the hypoglycemia. Because of alterations in the deformability of the red blood cell membrane, hyperviscosity in the microcirculation can occur at hematocrit levels in the 60 to 65 per cent range. Partial exchange transfusion, as discussed earlier, should be considered in the management of these infants.

Serum bilirubin levels tend to rise more quickly in the IDM. The pathogenesis is unclear but might relate to a combination of factors including birth trauma, increased red cell mass, and delayed passage of meconium resulting from a functional small left colon. Monitoring of stooling, hydration, and serum bilirubin will lessen the finding of a dangerously high serum bilirubin level at the time of discharge.

Congenital anomalies are two to four times more frequent among IDMs than in normal controls. They commonly affect multiple organ systems, especially cardiovascular, genitourinary, central nervous, respiratory, and musculoskeletal. Close evaluation of the newborn IDM will identify them and permit early initiation of appropriate therapy.

Major Causes of Neonatal Morbidity and Mortality

With increasing awareness of prematurity and medical advances in the pharmacologic inhibition of premature labor and induction or replacement of lung surfactant and effective ventilator support, other disorders have become more prevalent as causes of significant neonatal morbidity and mortality.

Perinatal Asphyxia. Following successful resuscitation, stabilization requires prompt and meticulous attention to the basic aspects of transitional care. These include, but are not limited to, neutral thermal environment, adequate tissue oxygenation, effective ventilation, and glucose homeostasis. The need for transfer should be individualized and discussed with your regional neonatal center.

Management of fluid and electrolyte balance in the postasphyxiated neonate requires close monitoring of weight, urinary output, and serum chemistries. Oliguria (urine output less than 2 ml per kg per hour) is a common sign of asphyxial insult to the kidneys, with resultant acute tubular necrosis, or to the brain, with inappropriate antidiuretic hormone secretion. Initial fluid restriction of 40 to 60 ml per kg per day of a 10 or 12.5 per cent dextrose in water solution lessens dilutional hyponatremia and cerebral edema. Since these infants are at risk for hypocalcemia, 200 to 400 mg per kg per day of calcium gluconate can be added. Weight, urine output, and serum chemistries should be evaluated two or three times a day. As urine output increases, sodium (3 to 4 mEq per kg per day) and potassium (1 to 2 mEq per kg per day) should be added to the intravenous infusion.

Neonatal seizures classically occur 12 to 24 hours after the asphyxial insult. These seizures are rarely the familiar massive tonic-clonic movements of children or adults. They can be myoclonic jerks, clonic or tonic movements of one extremity, or, most commonly, subtle types presenting as apnea, vasomotor changes, facial twitching, posturing, or chewing or sucking motions. A high index of suspicion is necessary to provide the close observation necessary to identify and initiate appropriate therapy. Metabolic disturbances such as hypoglycemia or hypocalcemia should be evaluated and treated. Sepsis should be considered if clinical or historical risk factors exist. Initiation of anticonvulsant therapy should not be delayed while arranging transfer or further neurologic testing with electroencephalogram or computed brain imaging. Phenobarbital, with a volume of distribution of 1 liter per kg, will give a serum level of 10 μg per ml for each 10 mg per kg loading dose. Thus, to reach a therapeutic level of 20 to 30 μg per ml, the neonate must receive a total phenobarbital load of 20 to 30 mg per kg. Intramuscular administration of loading doses of 10, 10, 5, and 5 mg per kg at hourly intervals lessens the risk of respiratory depression and achieves a therapeutic phenobarbital level. In many infants, seizures will cease after a total dose of 20 mg per kg and no further loading is necessary. Asphyxiated neonates eliminate phenobarbital slowly, and routine initiation of maintenance dosing can result in drug accumulation. Phenobarbital levels should be monitored and maintenance dosing initiated as indicated.

Referral of infants with postasphyxial seizures for pediatric neurologic evaluation and long-term developmental followup is optimal. No extemporaneous prognosis nor incriminations should be made as these cases are rich grounds for litigation. The multidisciplinary evaluation, support, and follow-up team appoach offered at a regional neonatal center benefits both the patient and the family.

Sepsis. The clinical presentation of sepsis in the neonate is so varied and nonspecific that its diagnosis is often delayed, with disastrous results. A perinatal history of prolonged rupture of membranes or chorioamnionitis will increase the index of suspicion in some but not all cases. The white blood cell count with a leukopenia (less than 5000 per mm^3) or an absolute band to total neutrophils ratio of greater than 0.2 supports a diagnosis of sepsis. Antigen detection of serum or urine specimens by latex agglutination (Wellogen) is a highly sensitive indicator of neonatal group B streptococcal (GBS) sepsis. Radiographic findings in neonatal pneumonia are too similar to those of either hyaline membrane disease or transient tachypnea to be of value. For this reason, it is prudent to treat all infants with respiratory distress as potentially having sepsis. Early onset GBS infection is the most common cause of neonatal sepsis, with an attack rate varying from 1.3 to 4.0 per 1000 live births and a mean case fatality rate of 55 per cent. Although presenting as a generalized septicemia with pneumonia, approximately 30 per cent of infants have concomitant meningitis. This must be taken into consideration for antibiotic dosing until results of a spinal tap can be obtained.

Before beginning antibiotic therapy, a blood culture and complete blood count should be obtained. Ideally, a suprapubic urine culture and spinal tap should be performed unless the patient's condition would be compromised or they would delay initiation of antibiotic therapy. Gastric aspirates and endotracheal secretions for Gram stain and culture are used by some centers with mixed results. Simple surface cultures of the skin, umbilicus, or ear produce confusing information and correlate poorly with true bacterial sepsis. Only 1 to 2 per cent of neonates with GBS colonization develop GBS sepsis.

Initiation of antibiotic therapy in the septic

neonate is a true emergency. It is ideally given intravenously after appropriate cultures and studies are obtained. However, administration of the antibiotics should not be delayed because of inability to obtain a blood culture or intravenous line. The septic infant can transform from moderately ill to moribund within a matter of hours. Initial antibiotic therapy for presumed sepsis is with ampicillin and an aminoglycoside (Table 6). Gentamicin is the aminoglycoside most commonly used in our nursery, given by slow intravenous infusion over 20 to 30 minutes. The frequency of administration is adjusted based on maturity and urine output, with monitoring of levels in those patients at risk. This adjustment in dosing is the result of the published experience of our institution and others regarding gentamicin serum levels. If GBS is the confirmed bacterial agent, penicillin G alone in the doses indicated can be utilized. Therapy should continue for 10 days in sepsis or pneumonia and for 2 to 3 weeks in meningitis. Vigorous supportive therapy is required as most of these infants will have difficulty with temperature and glucose homeostasis. Ventilatory assistance and aggressive treatment of shock may be necessary.

Congenital Anomalies. Life-threatening congenital anomalies require prompt recognition, stabilization, and transfer of the patient to a regional center where further evaluation and corrective surgical repairs can be undertaken. The role of the primary care physician and hospital staff in the initiation of appropriate stabilization techniques and support of the family is most important. Four relatively common congenital anomalies in which early intervention is beneficial will be discussed briefly. Basic stabilization, as noted, is always the first important task.

Heart defects are among the most common abnormalities. The group of anomalies in which perfusion of the pulmonary or systemic circulation depends on patency of the ductus arteriosus presents problems early in the neonatal period. As the ductus begins to close in response to extrauterine oxygenation, the infant develops either increasing cyanosis with hypoxemia or decreasing peripheral perfusion with resultant tissue hypoxia, metabolic acidosis, and congestive heart failure. The cyanotic lesions that present in the first hours of life include transposition of the great arteries, tetralogy of Fallot, and hypoplastic right heart lesions (pulmonary stenosis/atresia, tricuspid atresia). Obstruction to systemic blood flow from coarctation of the aorta and hypoplastic left heart complex (mitral atresia, aortic atresia, hypoplastic aortic arch) usually present with increasing respiratory distress from pulmonary vascular congestion, followed by a picture of cardiogenic shock before 6 days of age. Determination of the specific lesion is facilitated by echocardiography performed by a skilled pediatric cardiologist. After basic stabilization and glucose homeostasis have been accomplished, sepsis as a differential diagnosis should be considered and antibiotic agents provided.

The major advance in providing medical care for these duct-dependent congenital heart lesions has been the availability of prostaglandin E_1 (PGE_1, Prostin VR), which produces a relaxation

TABLE 6. **Initial Antibiotic Therapy for the Neonate**

	Sepsis	*Meningitis*
Ampicillin[1]		
preterm	25 mg/kg q 12 hr	50 mg/kg q 12 hr
term 0–7 days	25 mg/kg q 8 hr	50 mg/kg q 8 hr
term > 7 days	25 mg/kg q 6 hr	50 mg/kg q 6 hr
Gentamicin[2]		
preterm:		
<28 wk gestational age	2.5 mg/kg q 24 hr	2.5 mg/kg q 24 hr
28–34 wk gestational age	2.5 mg/kg q 18 hr	2.5 mg/kg q 18 hr
>34 wk gestational age	2.5 mg/kg q 12 hr	2.5 mg/kg q 12 hr
term 0–7 days	2.5 mg/kg q 12 hr	2.5 mg/kg q 12 hr
term > 7 days	2.5 mg/kg q 8 hr	2.5 mg/kg q 8 hr
Penicillin G*[3]		
preterm	100,000 units/kg q 12 hr	200,000 units/kg q 12 hr
term 0–7 days	75,000 units/kg q 8 hr	50–125,000 units/kg q 8 hr
term >7 days	50,000 units/kg q 6 hr	50–100,000 units/kg q 6 hr

*Note that the doses of aqueous penicillin G are approximately four times higher than the usual dose per kg. This is related to the higher MIC of GBS. See text.

[1]From McCracken GH Jr, Nelson JD (eds): Antimicrobial Therapy for Newborns. 2nd ed. New York, Grune & Stratton, 1983.

[2]From Szefler S, et al: Relationship of gentamicin serum concentrations to gestational age in preterm and term neonates. J Pediatr *97*:312–315, 1980.

[3]From Baker CJ: Group B streptococcal infections in neonates. Pediatr Rev *1*:5–15, 1979.

of the constricting ductus arteriosus, thereby permitting better perfusion of either the pulmonary or systemic circulation across a patent ductus arteriosus. The medication is given most commonly by peripheral vein in a starting dose of 0.05 μg per kg per minute. Consultation should be sought from your regional neonatal center prior to initiation, and facilities must be available to manage the side effects, which include apnea, bradycardia, and seizures.

The neonate with a diaphragmatic hernia presents a great challenge for the team at a regional center. Small defects are often picked up incidentally on a chest radiograph obtained for mild respiratory distress. Large defects usually present in the delivery room with the infant who cries at birth, then quickly becomes cyanotic. The abdomen is classically scaphoid but facemask bagging will quickly cause distention and worsen the distress as gas-filled bowel further displaces the already hypoplastic lungs. Management is aided by delivery room recognition with immediate endotracheal tube intubation and ventilation, with a rapid rate, low peak inspiratory pressures, and minimal end expiratory pressure. The hypoplastic lungs are very prone to iatrogenic pneumothoraces. A gastric tube should be placed and connected to low intermittent suction to maintain decompression of the bowel. Maintenance of temperature and glucose homeostasis will lessen the development of metabolic acidosis, which will worsen the pulmonary hypertension and right-to-left shunting, resulting in the cycle of persistent fetal circulation. Although mortality remains high despite aggressive management, proper stabilization and expedient transfer improve the chances for survival.

Defects of the anterior abdominal wall are readily apparent at delivery. Herniation of the intra-abdominal contents through a defect of the umbilical ring is an omphalocele, and it is usually covered by a sac composed of amnion and peritoneum. The sac is sometimes ruptured during delivery. The size of the defect varies considerably, from a small defect at the base of the umbilical cord to a sac that includes not only the gastrointestinal tract but also the liver. More than 50 per cent of cases have other serious congenital anomalies.

Gastroschisis is a defect of the anterior abdominal wall just lateral to the umbilicus. Unlike the case in omphalocele, there is no peritoneal sac, and the exposed bowel wall is often thick and edematous from the irritating effects of the amniotic fluid. Once delivered, infants with exposed abdominal wall defects rapidly lose heat and fluid. If the sac is intact, it should be covered with a dry sterile dressing. Exposed bowel should be covered with a sterile saline dressing. Place the entire lower half of the infant, including the eviscerated bowel, in a sterile intestine bag, which decreases evaporative heat and fluid loss. A nasogastric tube should be inserted to decompress the stomach and prevent bowel distention. A blood culture should be obtained and antibiotics (ampicillin and gentamicin) administered. A good peripheral intravenous line should be started early, with an initial volume expansion of 10 to 20 ml per kg using an isotonic colloid or crystalloid solution. A glucose infusion should then be maintained and blood pressure, heart rate, and temperature closely monitored to permit early identification and correction of hypovolemia or hypothermia. Good stabilization permits low risk surgical repair and good outcome in the absence of other congenital anomalies.

Obstruction of the alimentary tract can occur anywhere along its length and will produce one or more of four cardinal signs: polyhydramnios, bilious vomiting, abdominal distention, and failure to pass meconium, depending upon its location. The earliest-noted of these is esophageal atresia, which usually has an accompanying tracheoesophageal fistula. Associated anomalies of the cardiovascular, genitourinary, gastrointestinal, and musculoskeletal systems are very common. Choking, coughing, and cyanosis at first feeding, with excessive salivation, respiratory distress, or increasing gastric distention, are frequent presenting symptoms. These infants are in double jeopardy from aspiration of oral secretions or feedings and the reflux of gastric acid into the lungs. Emergency care consists of placing a double lumen suction catheter in the blind upper esophageal pouch for continuous suction and positioning the infant in a prone, head-elevated position. After insuring adequate stabilization, the infant should then be transferred for further evaluation and treatment.

Appropriate basic stabilization and attention to some of the details specific to the congenital anomaly can improve morbidity and mortality rates in these birth defects. The outcome is complicated by the high incidence of other congenital anomalies. The ethical dilemma of providing only supportive care or palliative surgery is difficult and requires a full team evaluation. In view of the increasing attempts at governmental and legal challenges to such decisions, it is best to provide effective initial stabilization and obtain consultation from your regional neonatal center. Support of the parents is a continuing and necessary challenge.

Continuing Care of the High Risk Infant

An important component of regional perinatal health care is the return of neonates to a hospital with facilities, equipment, and personnel capable of providing continuing care. While physiologic systems maturation of the premature infant continues under the supervision of the primary health care physician and staff, the parents have the opportunity to reidentify the high risk neonate as part of their family unit.

Nutrition. The goal of nutrition in the premature infant is to provide for optimal growth with a weight gain of 20 to 30 grams per day. The weight, length and head circumference should be plotted weekly on a standard extrauterine growth curve. Serum electrolytes, especially sodium, total protein, calcium, phosphorus, and hematocrit, should be followed one to two times per week. Provision of 120 calories per kg per day is usually required after the first week of life. Small for gestational age (SGA) infants frequently require close to 150 calories per kg per day for growth. If the infant is not in a neutral thermal environment or is losing unrecognized heat by radiation, calories are burned for heat instead of stored as growth. Remember, a normal infant temperature does not mean that ideal ambient thermal conditions have been achieved. The most common cause of growth failure in the stable premature infant receiving adequate calories is unrecognized thermal stresses.

Premature infants less than 34 weeks' gestational age should receive feedings by intermittent gavage equally divided every 2 or 3 hours. Placement of the tube and the volume and nature of the gastric aspirate should also be checked prior to each feeding. If the aspirate volume is increasing or bilious, radiographic evaluation for bowel pathology should be considered. Plain films will usually detect signs of obstruction, ileus, or necrotizing enterocolitis. Maturation of an intact suck-swallow gag reflex is usually developed by 33 to 34 weeks' gestational age, and nipple feeding can then be slowly started if it does not cause thermal or respiratory stress.

Most neonatologists believe that colostrum and breast milk from the infant's own mother provide both immunologic and nutritional advantages. Problems in storage and processing of banked breast milk markedly lessen the number of macrophages and concentration of immunoglobulins. The use of freshly expressed colostrum or breast milk lessens bacterial contamination and maximizes the availability of host resistance factors. Nutritionally, breast milk is usually better tolerated in the sick preterm neonate.

A significant problem of breast milk in the rapidly growing infant is the low levels of protein, sodium, calcium, and phosphorus found in the breast milk of mothers of full-term infants and after approximately 4 to 6 weeks in the milk of mothers of preterm infants. At this stage it often becomes necessary to modify the breast milk either by adding human milk fortifier (Similac Natural Care, Enfamil Human Milk Fortifier), mixing part breast milk and part premature formula, or temporarily using one of the formulas for premature infants. It is very important to encourage the mother and assure her that there is nothing wrong with her milk but that her infant is growing very rapidly. This stage of rapid growth with increased needs extends until the infant weighs approximately 1800 grams or until 34 weeks' gestational age when nipple feeds usually can be offered.

The alternative to breast milk is the use of a cow's milk protein-based formula. Soy bean–based formulas are not recommended as a routine protein source for premature infants. One of the special premature formulas available from Mead-Johnson, Ross, or Wyeth nutritional laboratories should be used. These low solute load preparations provide higher levels of protein, sodium, calcium and phosphorus, resulting in approximate in utero accretion rates and consistent growth. The carbohydrate source is approximately 50 per cent glucose polymers and the fats are partially medium chain triglycerides. These two modifications result in better gastrointestinal tolerance. When the infant attains 1800 grams or 34 weeks' gestational age, the usual full-term formulas will sustain continued growth and provide adequate levels of electrolytes and minerals.

Vitamin supplementation is an integral component of nutritional management of the growing premature infant. Infants on breast milk should receive 20 to 50 mg of vitamin C, 400 units of vitamin D, 5 to 10 IU of vitamin E, and 50 to 100 μg of folic acid daily. A multivitamin preparation such as Poly-Vi-Sol or Vi-Daylin, at a dose of 0.5 ml twice daily, will provide these minimums except for folic acid, which must be added. The vitamin drops increase the osmolality when added to the feeding and can cause feeding intolerances. Much conflicting information is appearing in the literature regarding the role of large doses of vitamin E in mitigating retrolental fibroplasia or bronchopulmonary dysplasia. The commercially available preparation of oral vitamin E has an extremely high osmolality and has been incriminated in producing necrotizing enterocolitis.

At discharge, the breast-feeding premature infant should be switched to a multivitamin preparation that contains 0.25 mg of fluoride and iron. For the infant receiving one of the premature infant formulas, the necessity and type of supplementation vary with the formula. While all the formulas contain insufficient amounts of vitamin D for infants below 1500 grams, the use of a routine multivitamin preparation can result in very high amounts of the fat-soluble vitamin A with one brand of premature formula. The health care provider should select a premature formula and calculate and supplement additional vitamins as indicated, with the caution of hyperosmolality from the vitamin preparation. Upon discharge, formula-fed premature infants may benefit from continued supplementation of a multivitamin preparation. The supplementation of fluoride should be based on the fluoride content of the local water supply. Iron supplementation will be discussed in the next section.

Anemia of Prematurity. A physiologic decline in the serum hemoglobin concentration develops in the stable growing premature infant, reaching a nadir at 4 to 8 weeks of age of 8.0 to 8.5 grams per cent or even down to 7.0 to 7.5 grams per cent in infants with birth weights of less than 1000 grams. The pathogenesis of this decline is the result of several factors, including a decrease in red blood cell mass, decrease in hematopoietic activity, and a rapidly expanding plasma volume. Like transient tachypnea of the neonate, physiologic anemia in the premature infant is a diagnosis of exclusion. One must be sure that the particular infant's anemia is not the result of the increased hemolysis from vitamin E deficiency nor blood loss from excessive or unreplaced phlebotomy sampling. The use of premature formula or breast milk with appropriate vitamin supplementation diminishes the incidence of vitamin E deficiency anemia. It has been our practice to keep a cumulative record of the blood drawn from each infant and if it exceeds 10 per cent in under 10 days the infant is transfused with packed red blood cells. Infants with an ongoing requirement for supplemental oxygen are also transfused to maintain a hemoglobin concentration of 12 to 13 grams per dl or a hematocrit of 35 to 40 per cent.

Management of the stable premature infant with physiologic anemia should be individualized. Hemoglobin concentrations or hematocrit and reticulocyte counts are followed one to two times a week. Iron supplementation of 2 to 4 mg per kg is added to the folic acid and vitamin E supplements when the reticulocyte count is first noted to rise. Infants who develop symptoms of poor oxygen delivery during the anemia of prematurity may benefit from transfusion of packed red blood cells. These symptoms or signs include poor weight gain, tachypnea, tachycardia, and apnea. A transfusion of 10 ml of red blood cells per kg given over 30 to 60 minutes usually raises the hemoglobin concentration by 1 to 2 grams per dl. Frequent replacement transfusions can result in a rebound in fetal hemoglobin production and will result in a delay or even further hinder adaptation.

Apnea and Bradycardia. Apnea during the first 24 hours of life is never a normal phenomenon, and sepsis should be aggressively treated until another cause is proved. Approximately 25 per cent of all low birth weight infants and over 80 per cent of infants weighing less than 1000 grams experience episodes of apnea during their neonatal course. Utilization of monitoring techniques will result in an even higher incidence in the premature infant. While monitoring of all prematures is recommended, the detection of significant apnea or bradycardia is at times more an art than science. Proper placement of chest leads, correct sensitivity adjustment, choice of alarm settings, and charting of observations are all critical factors in separating true apnea or bradycardia from monitor malfunctions or periodic breathing.

Management of apnea or bradycardia is first aimed at investigating and treating the causes. Further measures are then taken to avoid triggering reflexes from suction catheters, cold stimulus to the face, or hyperinflation during ambu bagging. Maintain the infant in an ambient temperature in the low zone of thermoneutrality. Place the infant in the prone position with head slightly elevated, to lessen gastroesophageal reflux. Avoid baby seats where the infant's poor tone can result in positional obstruction to the airway. If the spells are infrequent they usually can be managed by monitoring and tactile stimulation. Oscillating mattresses can reduce apnea by increasing vestibular input to the brain stem. Methylxanthines are effective in the treatment of apnea of prematurity. The dosing of either caffeine or theophylline must take into consideration the decreased protein-binding of the drug and the serum half-life, which has a wide range in the neonate. Regional preferences exist as to which methylxanthine to utilize. Theophylline is readily available commercially in both intravenous and numerous oral formulations. Caffeine, felt to have a wider therapeutic index, is usually prepared extemporaneously. They are both safe when used under well-monitored conditions with a suggested therapeutic level of 8 to 12 mg per liter. For theophylline, a loading dose of 7 mg per kg followed by a maintenance dose of 1.5 mg per kg per dose every 8 hours should be given. For caffeine, a loading dose of 10 mg per kg followed by a maintenance dose of 2.5 mg per kg is given once daily. The major complications of methylxanthines are dose related, including tachycardia, emesis, abdominal distention, jitteriness, and seizures. Diuresis also occurs, and serum electrolytes, especially sodium, should be monitored in the infant of less than 34 weeks' gestational age. More severe apnea or bradycardia may respond to the administration of continuous positive airway pressure, using nasal prongs or an endotracheal tube. Ventilator support may become necessary in the most severe cases.

If the apnea or bradycardia is simply a function of immaturity of control mechanisms, it usually resolves by about 34 to 36 weeks' gestational age. Discontinuation of methylxanthine therapy with continued observation and monitoring for another 10 to 14 days is indicated. If apnea or bradycardia persists, a detailed work-up of the nervous and cardiopulmonary systems should be performed. If uncertainty exists as to whether the episodes are true apneic or bradycardiac spells or monitoring equipment alarms, obtaining a 12 hour sleep study can be helpful. These cardiorespiratory impedance pneumograms are easily obtained but require judgment and skill in their interpretation.

The most difficult aspect of management of this group of infants is making the decision regarding home monitoring. Often this decision is predetermined by parental interpretation of information in the lay literature. Parents must be aware that home monitoring is expensive and has not yet been well established as preventive treatment of sudden infant death syndrome. If home monitoring is to be used, a well-organized system for providing 24 hour technical, psychosocial, and medical support for the patient and family must be available. Such decisions should be made in consultation with your regional neonatal or apnea evaluation unit.

Bronchopulmonary Dysplasia. Mechanical ventilation in the premature infant has improved survival but has resulted in a 10 to 30 per cent incidence of a chronic respiratory insufficiency termed bronchopulmonary dysplasia (BPD). These infants have a prolonged need for an oxygen-enriched environment with close attention to the details of supportive care in maintenance of nutrition, cardiopulmonary function, and hemoglobin concentration.

Fluid restriction utilizing 24 calories per ounce formulas to limit intake to 150 ml per kg per day is a common practice. Infants with BPD often require gavage feeding because nipple feeding is limited with their increased work of breathing. Furosemide has been shown to improve pulmonary function on a short-term basis. If diuretics are used, serum electrolytes must be monitored and replacement of potassium, sodium and chloride provided. Severe fluid restriction and use of furosemide have been known to produce nephrolithiasis.

Oxygen needs are difficult to monitor in infants with BPD because the stress of arterial blood gas sampling makes them hypoxic. Noninvasive transcutaneous oxygen monitoring or ear lobe oximetry of oxygen saturation are useful tools in these infants. Many develop systemic hypertension on an unexplained basis, with left ventricular hypertrophy. Other infants develop cor pulmonale with right-sided congestive heart failure resistant to management. Delivery of oxygen to the tissues should be supported by maintenance of a hemoglobin concentration of 12 to 13 grams per dl. Transfusions of packed red blood cells should be given cautiously to avoid fluid overload.

After discharge, this group of infants remains at high risk, with poor growth, developmental delay, and reactive airway disease. For unknown reasons, respiratory syncytial virus (RSV) produces severe respiratory compromise. They rapidly progress from an upper respiratory illness to pulmonary insufficiency and cardiopulmonary arrest. Viral illness in infants who required prolonged ventilation or oxygen-enriched environments should be taken seriously and managed aggressively.

Caring for Families of High Risk Neonates

The birth of a high risk neonate is a devastating blow to the parents and often to everyone else involved, including the medical staff. A newborn infant is the culmination of a community's best efforts and embodies their hopes for the future. The "Gerber Baby" image promoted by our culture gives parents very little preparation for dealing with all the realities of parenthood. During the period following birth the parents undergo a high degree of anxiety regarding the neonate's survival. This stress is further complicated by feelings of guilt in looking at possible personal reasons for the poor outcome of pregnancy.

Consumer pressure for family-centered birthing and bonding can at times place the high risk neonate in jeopardy. While this approach is perhaps beneficial for the majority of labors and deliveries, the presence of high risk assessment factors mandates appropriate monitoring of the fetus and effective resuscitation and stabilization of the neonate. The touching scene of the parents "bonding" with the neonate on the delivery bed will become soured if the infant develops meconium aspiration or hypoxia during the process. Bonding is a complex process better delineated perhaps in animals than in humans. A study performed in England revealed that this feeling of attachment developed over a prolonged period, with only 24 per cent of parents noting its onset at the time of birth. The medical needs of the high risk neonate must be a first priority, with appropriate support provided to the parents.

The parents of high risk neonates need help adapting their previously conceived image of the baby to reality, relieving the associated guilt, developing a mutual interaction with the baby, and learning how to care for their infant. A supportive health care team and parent groups will provide the parents with opportunities to communicate and share their stress. Return transport, parent involvement in the nursery, and rooming-in prior to discharge all assist parents in taking over the responsibility of meeting the needs of their special baby. The siblings of high risk neonates should be an integral part of these discussions, visitation, and involvement.

When an infant dies, it is especially important to recognize that the parents will express shock, denial, guilt, anger, and depression. It is an often difficult, but extremely important, task to help the family in their grieving. Opportunities to discuss their reactions should be readily available to the family around the time of death and over the next 3 to 6 months. Discomfort in dealing with the death of a neonate often makes difficult appropriate interaction between health care providers and the family. Occasional meetings of the medical and nursing staffs on the topic of grieving and meeting the needs of the family can be beneficial to the staff in caring for the family of the next infant who dies.

Discharge of the High Risk Neonate

Discharge planning, like risk assessment, must be a continuum throughout the hospital stay of the high risk infant. The anticipated medical needs of the neonate and the psychosocial support requirements of the family must be regularly reviewed. A periodic meeting of the health care team, both from hospital and community, should be utilized to develop a comprehensive plan for each patient and family. This information must be made available to the primary health care providers upon discharge.

NORMAL INFANT FEEDING

method of
HERBERT H. POMERANCE, M.D.
University of South Florida
Tampa, Florida

Human milk is intended as the food for human infants. Historically, the inability of some mothers to provide milk for their infants was an overriding problem, solved in varying ways. At times, this was by employment of a wet-nurse, a practice well documented in ancient writings. Sometimes it was by obtaining milk from other mammals, mainly the cow, but also the goat and, in some areas, the ass. The scientific era of the mid-nineteenth century ushered in attempts to formalize the nutritional values of milk and thus there was created a greater interest in nonhuman milks.

Increasing knowledge of the components of cow's milk led to greater use of cow's milk as the substitute. In turn, this led to the establishment of "milk stations" designed to provide clean and more standardized feedings for infants. Such milk stations were in operation from the late 1890s on. Early use of whole milk (often raw) quickly revealed that it could not be tolerated by young infants. After a number of trials, diluted milk with added carbohydrate, adjusted to the caloric value of whole milk, became commonplace. Some simplification occurred with the use of evaporated milk, and a major improvement followed the more recent advent of prepared formulas. These newer formulas contain protein, which is reduced in quantity and heat-treated; carbohydrate readjusted to original levels; replaced fat content; and the same caloric content (0.66 cal per ml or 20 cal per oz) as cow's milk and human milk.

It was inevitable that, after a whole generation of experience and increasing dependence upon prepared formulas, a resurgence of interest in breast-feeding would next occur. This has coincided with the greater knowledge that, although cow's milk formulas represent a highly acceptable substitute for a mother who is unable, or perhaps unwilling, to breast-feed, they do have drawbacks. Although the protein concentration has been adjusted downward, the lactoproteins are still bovine proteins. Although the butterfat has been replaced with combinations of unsaturated and saturated fats, these still differ from the combination present in human milk. Although dilution has reduced the sodium content, it is still, in most instances, substantially higher than that of human milk. In other words, despite the *relative* acceptability of cow's milk formulas, it must be acknowledged that "cow's milk was meant for calves."

Preparation for Breast-feeding

Breast-feeding is *the* feeding of choice for the new infant. However, even with the present "favorable climate" toward the idea of breast-feeding, most mothers need some preparation for this pleasant and important task. Although this preparation should really begin in school education programs, most often the pediatrician is the one who must provide the basic information and support. Here he or she is helped measurably if an introductory counseling session with the prospective parents is part of a prenatal interview. Such interviews are more and more common today and are highly recommended in the new "Guidelines for Health Supervision" of the American Academy of Pediatrics. Feelings can be explored, as can conceptions and misconceptions. Paternal roles often so important to maternal success can be developed. Early details of techniques can be discussed.

In addition, the pediatrician needs to talk over a preference for breast-feeding with the obstetricians from whom the newborn referrals come. This will avoid emotional confusion in the prospective parents, an event that might result from differing physician philosophies.

During the first postpartum visit, the pediatrician must once more reinforce support of breast-feeding and in addition must now ensure that the mother learns how to breast-feed properly. In contrast to past practice, considerable support and actual teaching now come from nursing personnel.

Techniques of Breast-Feeding

It has been said that there are two prerequisites to breast-feeding: being postpartum and wanting to. Essentially this is true, with prolactin production a major factor. The "wanting to" translates into a need for proper instruction in the technique, so that the mother not only begins but also enjoys and continues breast-feeding. To this end, the pediatrician and nurses need to combine their efforts effectively to address the following issues:

1. The mother must be seated comfortably when feeding her baby. The same system that prescribes early ambulation for the postpartum mother often prescribes the almost impossible task of feeding the baby in a reclining position. A straight chair, allowing feet to be flat on the floor, perhaps with a pillow on the lap, is the preferable position.

2. The mother must hold her infant properly. The baby should not be supine on the lap pillow, although the infant may rest there intermittently. Cradled on the mother's arm, the baby is in a semiupright position.

3. The mother must be shown the proper way to support the breast with the opposite hand, usually with thumb and index finger above and the remaining fingers below the nipple, allowing necessary manipulation.

4. The mother must understand how the rooting reflex works, and that contact between the cleansed nipple and the baby's face is not bad but instead activates rooting. She will then understand that pressure against the infant's outer (exposed) cheek will be counterproductive, since the infant will then turn away from the nipple.

5. The mother must know that stimulation to production of milk comes from regular emptying of the breasts, both of them at first, perhaps progressing to, or almost to, one per feeding. Most often, the mother who uses both breasts initially is able to gradually increase the time on one while decreasing the time on the other, alternating breasts with each feeding.

6. The mother should feed her infant using a flexible schedule. Her nipples will not tolerate too frequent feedings. The infant also will do better with a semblance of timing, since refilling of the breasts requires a number of hours.

7. The mother must be educated about proper nutrition, understanding that if she produces roughly a liter of milk per day, she needs about 660 extra calories (1000×0.66 cal per ml). An excessive diet, however, will result only in weight gain in the mother. Although most physicians suggest that milk be included in the mother's diet, it is not essential and should be used in moderation.

In addition, the teachers must themselves be aware that it is unwise to give preliminary formula feedings to infants before placing them to breast; that the first feeding at breast should be quite early, as soon as the mother is stable; that it is inadvisable to offer cow's milk formula as a "supplement"; that very early jaundice is not caused by breast-feeding; and that jaundice at about a week of age, said to be due to estrogenic hormone secretion into the milk, is not cause for more than a temporary interruption of breast-feeding.

Armed in this fashion, the mother can progress rapidly from "novice" to "expert." In addition, a close relationship will develop between mother and infant, ideally with the father sharing deeply in this closeness.

Later Management

Once lactation is established, other considerations become important. One is the need for *vitamins*. A difference of opinion exists. Some physicians prescribe a multivitamin for the mother during lactation, to increase the vitamin content of the milk. "Prenatal" vitamins may be continued, but a standard "low potency" product is preferable. Others prefer to provide a standard product to the infant, either a complete multivitamin or an "A-C-D" preparation.

Questionable also is the need for *iron* supplementation. Here too there is differing opinion. Most feel that iron supplementation is not necessary. Although the amount of iron in breast milk is small, absorption is very efficient, and thus iron need not be added for 6 to 9 months.

The mother may, when the infant is 1 month of age, be ready to *modify the feeding schedule* to allow a more relaxed family life. One of the adjustments may be to allow substitution with a middle-of-the-night formula feeding. Some mothers like this as a relief, to allow an 8 hour sleep period. Thus it is valuable only if another (preferably the father) does the feeding; if the mother must get up to give the feeding, breast-feeding is easier.

An increasingly important element of some new mothers' lives is the need to *return to gainful employment*. The need to work is not a contraindication to breast-feeding. Often, work schedules and feeding schedules can be suitably modified to avoid conflict. Sometimes arrangements can be made for a short "time out" during work hours so that the infant may be brought to the mother for feeding.

Finally the question must be approached as to when *weaning* from the breast should occur. A great variability exists in maternal desires, and these desires should be honored. Probably 6 months is an average time for most mothers, with some continuing longer and some stopping sooner. If breast-feeding is stopped before 1 year of age, a prepared formula should be continued until that time.

Feeding with Cow's Milk

A few mothers are unable to breast-feed. Others do not wish to do so. For these mothers, a variety of formulas, for example of altered cow's milk, are available. Much evidence now exists to suggest that, although human milk is best both nutritionally and emotionally, the modern prepared formula is an acceptable substitute. The available formulas can be purchased in powdered, concentrated, or ready-to-feed forms. If the mother is going to bottle-feed her infant from the beginning, or if she must switch early, she must know several important things.

1. The infant should never be fed in bed in the supine position. For both psychologic reasons and physical safety, the baby should be held in the mother's arms. A semi-upright position will minimize air-swallowing and the possibility of aspiration. Despite this, bottle-fed infants swallow more air than do breast-fed infants and need more attention to "burping."

2. Flexible schedules should be maintained. It appears reasonable that just as the old rigid feeding times were illogical, so also are untempered demand feedings. A so-called "modified demand" schedule, based on the knowledge that the emptying time of the stomach is approximately 4 hours, rests on an understanding of gastrointestinal physiology.

3. Vitamin supplements are not necessary during the first year, because of fortification of the commercial formulas. Premature infants, because of their rapid rate of growth, are an exception and need extra vitamin D. On the other hand, the need for iron may be a problem. Many infants have a significant enteric blood loss (overt or covert) because of bovine lactoprotein sensitivity and need iron supplementation if a cow's milk formula is used. Opinions differ with regard to whether this iron should be in the formula or extrinsic, routine or only on indication.

Again, it should be remembered that unaltered cow's milk should never be used until the infant is 1 year of age.

It must also be pointed out, and mothers should be made aware, that while the additional food she must eat while breast-feeding may cost her 50 cents per day, a can of concentrated formula (a day's supply) is now roughly $1.25, and the 1 quart ready-mix formulas are about $1.80. The occasional family that demands the use of ready-mixed 8 ounce bottles or cans may spend over $4.00 per day.

Solid Foods

The history of introducing solid foods to infants goes back to the very early practice of having the mother chew the food and transfer it to the infant's mouth. Unsanitary as this may seem, it provided both suitable consistency and some predigestion. The advent of the prepared commercial baby foods signaled an era of contest between mother and mother, mother and doctor, and even doctor and doctor, to see who could begin more varieties of foods earlier. It became a status symbol to be the mother who held the record for early food starts, with cereals and other foods begun as early as 2 weeks of age or less. Little attention was paid to physiologic need, or to the safety of giving these foods at such an early age. No attention was given to the fact that many of the commercial products had little nutritive value, and since they were "seasoned to taste" (mothers' taste, not babies' taste), they contained considerable added sugar and salt, the latter adding to the already excessive salt content of cow's milk.

Although all the commercial foods have now been changed to contain no added sugar or salt, it remains true that most foods for small infants can be produced at home, using the normal family foods. Blenders, grinders, mills, and even shredding with forks can be used to create desired consistency. The food can be mixed with a little water, poured into ice cube trays, frozen, then stored in plastic bags. Such foods provide better nutrition and certainly are less expensive. Spinach, carrots, and beets, however, should not be frozen at home, as they contain nitrates (removed in commercial processing) that may convert to nitrites during storage and produce hemolytic anemia.

Considerable study has been given recently to the timing of the need for additional foods. Theoretically, no solids are needed until 6 months of age, and then only in small amounts, increasing gradually to 1 year of age. In actual practice, most infants need some small supplementation, because of appetite and growth rate, by about 4 months of age, with gradual increase thereafter.

The Bottom Line

The aim of every mother and physician should be to equip the child for eventual existence—for better or worse—in our adult world. This is an on-going job, but it should begin in infancy. The breast-fed baby may be able to progress directly to a cup. The bottle-fed baby should never be left with a bottle to act as a pacifier; the "pacified" infant is often seen at play at 3 or 4 years of age with a bottle still dangling from the mouth. The mother who puts "solids" into a bottle with an enlarged-hole nipple will find difficulty in reversing this practice, perhaps even at age 4 years. A little forethought by the mother and a little anticipatory guidance by the physician will go a long way.

DISEASES OF THE BREAST

method of
R. ROBINSON BAKER, M.D.
Johns Hopkins University
Baltimore, Maryland

BENIGN DISEASE

With the onset of regular menstrual periods the breast begins to undergo monthly cyclic changes secondary to the relative concentration of estrogen and progesterone produced by the ovary. Prior to the onset of menses there may be significant fluid accumulation in the breasts resulting in swelling and, in some cases, pain and tenderness. These symptoms are extremely variable. Some women have practically no symptoms, whereas others complain of rather severe swelling, pain, and tenderness. The symptoms are usually most severe 2 to 3 days prior to the menstrual period and subside with the onset of menses. In some cases they are noted with ovulation and continue until the onset of menses. The physical findings associated with these symptoms are also variable, particularly in relation to the menstrual cycle. If the patient is examined just prior to her menstrual period, the breast tissue can be remarkably tender, indurated, and nodular. In contrast, following the onset of menses there can be a remarkable resolution of these findings.

These symptoms and physical findings have for many years been attributed to "fibrocystic disease." These clinical findings in fact should not be called a disease, since they are present in most women at some phase of their menstrual career. No treatment is usually necessary, and the patient can be reassured that these symptoms do not increase the risk of breast cancer. A small percentage of patients have rather severe pain and tenderness, which may or may not be associated with nodularity and induration on physical examination. These symptoms are probably related to a relative excess of estrogen compared with progesterone. They are almost surely not due to the ingestion of excessive amounts of xanthines, as suggested by Minton.

Treatment

Women with severe persistent pain and tenderness can be treated with two different drugs. Danazol (Danocrine), an inhibitor of pituitary gonadatropins, decreases the estrogenic stimulation of the breasts. Tamoxifen (Nolvadex), an antiestrogen, combines with the estrogen receptors in the cytoplasm of the ductal cells and thus prevents estrogen stimulation. In the past women with severe symptoms have been treated by bilateral subcutaneous mastectomies and the restoration of breast contour with a silastic implant. Since all of the breast tissue cannot be excised through a limited incision, these procedures are associated with numerous complications and seldom relieve all the symptoms. Subcutaneous mastectomies should, therefore, never be performed for symptomatic fibrocystic disease.

Although periodic swelling, pain, and tenderness are the most common complaints referrable to the breasts, significant numbers of women seek medical attention because of a discrete, usually solitary, mass. The etiology of the mass varies with age. Fibroadenomas are most commonly encountered in women under age 30. They are usually asymptomatic and freely mobile. A specific diagnosis can and should be established by excision under local anesthesia. Cysts are most commonly seen in women between 30 and 45 years of age. In contrast to a fibroadenoma, cysts are frequently tender, particularly prior to the menstrual period. They fluctuate in size and are most prominent prior to the onset of menses. A diagnosis can be established by needle aspiration. Cytologic examination of fluid is advisable if the fluid is bloody. Any other fluid can be discarded.

Another common complaint is a nipple discharge. The discharge can vary from colorless fluid to frank blood. The vast majority of nonbloody discharges are of no consequence and no further work-up is necessary. If milky and profuse, a serum prolactin level should be obtained to rule out the possibility of a pituitary tumor. Bloody discharges are of more concern. They are most frequently due to an intraductal papilloma in premenopausal women and to an intraductal carcinoma in postmenopausal women. A mass is usually not palpable. Localization can at times be accomplished by radial palpation and excision of the area that produces the bloody discharge. Mammograms or ductograms are occasionally necessary for localization prior to excision.

Infections of the breast are usually encountered in lactating women. They can present as an area of erythema and tenderness or as an abscess. They are almost invariably secondary to a staphylococcal infection. In the absence of a definite abscess, treatment consists of warm compresses and appropriate antibiotics. An abscess is incised and drained. The wall of the abscess should be excised for histologic study to rule out an inflammatory breast carcinoma. Periareolar infections can be seen in nonlactating women. These lesions are notoriously indolent infections and are due to a staphylococcal infection in the sebaceous glands beneath the areolar skin. Excision and drainage are occasionally necessary. The incision should be left open and allowed to granulate in. Recurrence is not unusual.

Cosmetic problems vary with the mores of the society. Relatively small breasts can be increased in size by the placement of a silicone prosthesis between the chest wall and the breast. This is a relatively simple operation and is associated with excellent cosmetic results. Large pendulous breasts can be reduced in size by a reduction mammoplasty, a considerably more extensive procedure compared with an augmentation mammoplasty.

PRIMARY BREAST CANCER

Breast cancer is the commonest cause of death from cancer in females in the United States. An estimated 9 per cent of women in the United States will die of breast cancer in 1985. Women at increased risk include those with a positive family history and nulliparous women or women whose first pregnancy occurs after age 30. Other risk factors include a history of radiation exposures, a history of early menarche or late menopause, obesity, and hypothyroidism. Of these risk factors, a positive family history is of greatest significance, particularly if the patient's mother, sister, or maternal aunts have had breast cancer prior to age 45. A history of bilateral breast cancer in the family further increases these risks, and women whose mother or sisters have had bilateral breast cancer prior to age 45 probably have a 40 per cent chance of developing breast cancer. All of these risk factors are unusual, however, and the majority of women with breast cancer have none of these risk factors in their past history.

Diagnostic Considerations

Screening for breast cancer should be an integral part of any medical evaluation. Physical examination and mammography are the only procedures of proven value. Thermography, sonography, and transillumination of the breast are of no value as screening procedures. The frequency of the physical examination varies with the patient's history. A woman with a positive family history, particularly if the relative has had cancer prior to age 45, should be seen three times per year. Other patients are seen at yearly intervals, but every patient should be taught to examine her breasts at monthly intervals and report any significant findings.

A baseline screening mammogram should be obtained when the patient is in the late 30s and probably at 3 to 4 year intervals until the patient is 50 years of age. After 50 years of age the patient should have yearly screening mammograms in addition to the physical examination. Those women at increased risk of breast cancer, particularly those with a positive family history, should have screening mammograms at an earlier age and probably at more frequent intervals prior to age 50.

Breast cancer is most commonly encountered in women 55 to 60 years of age. It is not uncommon in women in their 70's or 80's. Approximately 20 per cent of breast cancers are seen in women under 50 years of age. Only 2 per cent of breast cancers occur in women under 35, and less than 1 per cent are encountered in women under 30.

The histologic type of cancer has some influence on the prognosis and clinical management. Seventy five per cent of breast cancers arise in the ductal system and are called ductal cancers or, because they frequently elicit a fibrous response around them, scirrhous duct cancers. Approximately 30 per cent of these tumors are multifocal in origin in the ipsilateral breast. Carcinomas arising in the lobules, lobular carcinoma, are the second commonest histologic type of tumor, comprising approximately 5 per cent of all breast cancers. In general lobular carcinomas have the same prognosis as scirrhous duct carcinomas. These tumors have a slightly higher incidence of multicentric origin, particularly in the opposite breast, compared with scirrhous duct cancers. Medullary carcinomas, papillary carcinomas, and tubular carcinomas constitute approximately 20 per cent of breast cancers and are associated with a slightly better prognosis and have a lesser incidence of multifocal origin.

Two types of noninvasive cancers are encountered, particularly since the introduction of mammography. Intraductal carcinomas are confined to the ducts; similar carcinomas in situ can be encountered in the lobules. The prognosis of these two lesions is considerably different. At least 50 per cent of intraductal cancers will become invasive and capable of metastasis within 5 years of diagnosis. Remarkably, these tumors are seldom bilateral. In contrast, the incidence of bilaterality is considerably greater in lobular carcinoma in situ, but these tumors have a considerably better prognosis. Patients with lobular carcinoma in situ have an approximate 25 per cent chance of developing an invasive tumor in either breast within 25 years of the diagnosis.

The prognosis in invasive breast cancer varies with the size of the primary tumor and the presence or absence of lymph node metastasis. Women with primary tumors less than 2 cm in size and no evidence of lymph node metastasis have an approximate 90 per cent chance of 10 year survival. The prognosis worsens as the size of the primary tumor increases, but the presence or absence of lymph node metastasis is the most accurate means of predicting prognosis at the present time. Patients with primary tumors less than 5 cm in size and no evidence of lymph node metastasis have an approximate 80 per cent chance of 10 year survival. Those patients with one to three nodes containing metastatic tumor have an approximate 40 per cent chance of survival, and those patients with four or more lymph nodes containing metastatic tumor have a 10 per cent chance of survival.

In addition to the histologic examination of primary breast cancers and axillary lymph nodes, these tumors should also be analyzed for the presence of estrogen and progesterone receptor proteins. These determinations have both prognostic and therapeutic potential. Tumors that contain both estrogen and progesterone receptor proteins are more indolent tumors and may also be associated with a better prognosis. Although long-term follow-up studies have not been completed, the patient with estrogen and progesterone receptor proteins in the tumor and one to two axillary lymph nodes containing metastatic tumor probably has the same prognosis as the patient with no evidence of estrogen and progesterone receptor proteins and no evidence of axillary lymph node metastasis. The estrogen and progesterone receptor protein studies are also of importance in adjuvant therapy as well as in the treatment of metastatic breast cancer.

Breast cancers can present as a nonpalpable x-ray abnormality detected by mammography or as a palpable mass. The clinical management varies with the mode of presentation and the age of the patient.

Treatment

Small nonpalpable cancers can be detected by mammography. The most characteristic lesion is a focal area of microcalcifications. Following localization of the lesion in reference to the nipple, the area is excised. X-ray views of the specimen are obtained to be sure the appropriate area has been removed. The specimen is then submitted for histologic study. I prefer not to perform a frozen section because the histologic findings are often subtle and the pathologist would rather evaluate them with permanent histologic sections. Further management is discussed with the patient after review of the permanent histologic sections.

The clinical management of the patient with a palpable mass varies with the patient's age and clinical findings. A discrete, palpable mass in any woman, regardless of age, should be excised for histologic study if it is not a cyst that disappears on needle aspiration. This general principle is true even if a mammogram reveals no evidence of malignant change. Approximately 15 to 20 per cent of malignant lesions are not detected by mammography in premenopausal women, and, to a lesser extent, postmenopausal women.

In the absence of overt signs of malignancy on mammography or physical examination, a discrete mass is usually excised under local anesthesia, particularly in premenopausal women. The majority of premenopausal women do not wish to undergo general anesthesia, breast biopsy, frozen section, and possible mastectomy. They would prefer to discuss various therapeutic options after a precise histologic diagnosis has been established by permanent histologic sections. If there are overt signs of malignant disease on mammography or physical examination, however, a biopsy under general anesthesia, frozen section, and possible definitive therapy should be discussed with the patient, since a biopsy under local anesthesia is usually unnecessary.

Once a diagnosis of breast cancer is established or suspected, all patients should have chest x-ray films made and serum alkaline phosphatase levels assessed. If the chest x-ray view reveals no evidence of metastasis and the serum alkaline phosphatase level is within normal limits, further diagnostic studies, such as a bone scan and CAT scan of the liver, are not indicated if the primary tumor is 5 cm or less in size. Occult metastasis will only be detected in approximately 1 per cent of such patients. Those women with an abnormal serum alkaline phosphatase level or women with tumors larger than 5 cm should have a bone scan and CAT scan of the liver performed since the presence of detectable occult metastasis in these patients is in the range of 20 per cent.

The treatment of breast cancers 5 cm or less in size is controversial. Certain facts are well established. Scirrhous duct cancers and lobular carcinomas are multicentric in origin in at least 30 per cent of the cases. Local excision of a primary tumor is thus associated with an approximate 25 per cent incidence of subsequent recurrence in the ipsilateral breast. Radiation of the breast probably offers the same chance of local control of the cancer in the breast as a mastectomy if the primary tumor is grossly excised by the biopsy procedure. Satisfactory reconstruction of the breast following mastectomy can be obtained in most cases, particularly in women with moderate sized well supported breasts. The cosmetic results of reconstruction are not as satisfactory, however, as those obtained following radiation. Excision of the axillary lymph nodes for histologic study is the most accurate means of determining prognosis and, therefore, the indications for adjuvant therapy.

The standard form of therapy for breast cancer remains a mastectomy and axillary lymph node dissection (modified radical mastectomy). Reconstruction is discussed with all patients preoperatively. Those women with small or moderate sized well supported breasts are offered simultaneous reconstruction. Patients with large pendulous breasts are not good candidates for simultaneous reconstruction since symmetry can only be obtained by an extensive reduction mammoplasty on the contralateral breast.

Radiation of the breast and axillary lymph node dissection is an alternative in women who cannot tolerate a mastectomy. Women under age 40 with a tumor less than 3 cm in size are faced with a difficult decision. Those patients without axillary lymph node metastasis have an excellent chance of cure. Should such patients trade cosmesis for 5,000 to 6,000 rads to the chest wall? Long-term follow-up studies of patients under age 40 are not available at the present time but heavy doses of radiation are bound to have an adverse long-term effect on some of these patients.

Adjuvant therapy for breast cancer has been under intensive study for a number of years. A number of prospective randomized studies are in progress and additional information should be available within the next several years. On the basis of currently available information the following statements can be made. Postoperative radiation following a mastectomy and axillary lymph node dissection decreases the incidence of local recurrence on the chest wall and in the axilla and supraclavicular fossa but has no effect on survival. Adjuvant chemotherapy in the form of cytoxin, methotrexate, and 5-fluorouracil is of benefit in premenopausal women with one to three nodes containing metastatic tumor. If the tumor contains both estrogen receptors and progesterone receptors, the addition of an antiestrogen, tamoxifen, further increases the benefit of the adjuvant therapy. The value of any other forms of adjuvant chemotherapy and/or hormonal therapy has not been established by completed randomized prospective trials. There is suggestive evidence that adjuvant chemotherapy in the form of cytoxin, methotrexate, 5-fluorouracil, vincristine, and prednisone or adriamycin combined with various other chemotherapeutic agents may be of benefit in both pre- and postmenopausal women with multiple axillary lymph node metastasis but the appropriate studies have not been completed at this time. Similarly there is suggestive evidence that tamoxifen alone for indefinite periods of time is of benefit in postmenopausal women with axillary lymph node metastases.

The routine follow-up of patients who have been treated for primary breast cancer is also controversial. I see these patients at 3 to 4 month intervals. Mammograms of the contralateral breast and chest x-ray films are obtained yearly. In the absence of symptoms or physical findings suggestive of metastasis, I do not perform routine bone scans or CAT scans of the liver nor is the serum screened for tumor markers such as CEA antigens. To my knowledge there is no evidence that the treatment of asymptomatic metastasis is of any value to the patient, and screening procedures that are suggestive of metastasis but not diagnostic can produce severe anxiety in patients.

METASTATIC BREAST CANCER

Treatment

Metastatic breast cancer is generally treated with systemic chemotherapy and/or additive or ablative hormonal therapy. Treatment varies according to the menopausal status of the patient and the presence or absence of estrogen and progesterone receptors in the tumor cells.

Premenopausal women with positive estrogen/progesterone receptors have an excellent chance of response to procedures that eliminate or neutralize the effect of systemic estrogen. Ovarian excision eliminates a major source of estrogen, or the systemic effect of estrogen on the breast cancer cells can be blocked by tamoxifen. The chances of response vary with the concentrations of estrogen and progesterone receptor protein in the tumor cells. If both estrogen and progesterone receptors are present the chance of response for significant periods of time is 80 per cent; the chance of response decreases as the relative concentration of estrogen and progesterone receptors decreases. Those patients who have a recurrence of symptoms after either oophorectomy or tamoxifen therapy are candidates for chemotherapy.

Premenopausal women with metastatic breast cancer and negative estrogen and progesterone receptors are candidates for some type of chemotherapy. First line drugs are combinations of cytoxin, methotrexate, and 5-fluorouracil. If the patient has received these drugs as surgical adjuvant chemotherapy, subsequent chemotherapy would then most likely consist of adriamycin, vincristine, and possibly prednisone. The chance of significant response is in the range of 20 per cent.

The treatment of postmenopausal women with metastatic breast cancer is also dependent on the presence or absence of estrogen and progesterone receptor proteins in the tumor cells. If these proteins are present, postmenopausal women have an excellent chance of responding to tamoxifen for significant periods of time. If the estrogen/progesterone receptors are absent or present in low concentration, chemotherapy again is the treatment of choice. The drugs employed are similar to those discussed in premenopausal women.

The common sites of metastatic breast cancer include bone, particularly the spine and pelvis, the liver, lungs, brain, and retroperitoneal tissues. Although treatment is generally systemic, unique problems can arise in certain organ systems.

If x-ray films reveal evidence of extensive metastatic disease in the spine and/or if the patient develops symptoms of spinal cord compression, these metastatic areas should be radiated in an effort to prevent further compression of the spinal cord and paraplegia. X-ray films of the femur should be obtained in any patient with significant pain on weight bearing. Extensive metastatic lesions in the femur can be treated by insertion of a metal prosthesis and radiation, thus preventing the morbidity of a pathologic fracture. Brain metastases, which are usually heralded by a severe headache, can be documented by a CAT scan. The headaches will subside with high doses of corticosteroids. The metastatic lesions in the brain usually respond to radiation. A pleural effusion secondary to implants of metastatic tumor on the visceral and parietal pleural surfaces can be eliminated by insertion of a chest tube. If the visceral and parietal pleura can be approximated by suction, a sclerosing agent can be injected into the pleural space and a symphysis obtained between the visceral and parietal pleura, thus preventing subsequent effusions. Pain from isolated bone metastasis can be relieved by radiation, which is frequently employed in patients who are also on some type of systemic chemotherapy and/or hormonal therapy.

ENDOMETRIOSIS

method of
CARL J. LEVINSON, M.D.
Children's Hospital of San Francisco
San Francisco, California

Endometriosis is a difficult disease, complex to understand and awkward to treat. The etiology is unknown. The incidence appears to be increasing. There is an association with infertility, and with few therapeutic modalities. It is characterized by the presence of functional endometrial glands, most often with endometrial stroma, in sites outside the uterine cavity. It most frequently affects the ovary, the posterior uterine wall, the uterosacral ligaments, and the pelvic peritoneum over the rectum, small bowel, and ureter. The overt pathology is manifested by bleeding into the ectopic endometrial tissue (responding to cyclic hormonal changes) interspersed with attempts of the body to "heal itself" by fibrosis. In turn, these adhesions result in obstruction (e.g., tubal, sigmoid) or distortion of normal anatomic relationships. Ovarian endometriomas interfere with the normal ovulatory process.

Prevention

Since it is generally agreed that retrograde menstruation occurs commonly, it is unlikely that a pelvic examination during menstruation will be of any importance in forcing cells through the tubes. Therapy to the cervix should be limited to absolutely necessary procedures, since certain operations (cryosurgery, conization) may predispose to subsequent stenosis of the cervix. If the patient has a uterine anomaly predisposing to retrograde menstruation, it should be corrected as soon as possible; this includes cervical stenosis, rudimentary horns that are obliterated, and partial vaginal atresia. There is a clinical impression that endometriosis seems to occur less in patients who have used oral contraceptives over an extended period of time. This seems logical in view of the fact that the quantity of menstrual flow is reduced. A career woman planning to delay child-bearing should consider the use of oral contraceptives as a means of birth control, especially if there appears to be a familial incidence of the disease. Early child-bearing is effective but remains a social, not a medical, decision.

Infertility Associated with Endometriosis

The mechanism of infertility in patients who have endometriosis is not clear, particularly in those with mild disease and without distorted pelvic structures. It is much easier to explain if there are ovarian endometriomas, peritubal adhesions, fixation of the tube away from the ovary, tubal obstruction, a fixed retroverted uterus, or severe dysmenorrhea/dyspareunia resulting in decreased coitus. The finding of increased concentrations of prostaglandins in the peritoneal fluid of patients with endometriosis has raised consideration regarding disruption of tubal motility, altered release of the ovum, and interference with steroid production. The luteinized unruptured follicle syndrome appears to be more frequent in association with endometriosis. Although new theories develop on a regular basis, the answer is still not evident regarding the mechanism of infertility in patients who have minimal endometriosis.

Therapy

Categories to be considered for a special therapeutic approach include (1) women not wishing for pregnancy (with mild, moderate, or severe disease), either young and delaying pregnancy or older with no wish for future pregnancy, and (2) women wishing for pregnancy, who have mild, moderate, or severe disease.

As indicated earlier, not many modalities are available for the treatment of endometriosis. Nevertheless, therapy remains confusing to physicians and patients since a wide variety of factors must be considered. How old is the patient? Does she wish for pregnancy now or later? Is the disease process extensive or minimal? Has there been previous hormonal or surgical therapy? Is there residual disease after hormonal or surgical therapy? Will hormonal therapy facilitate conservative surgery? Should radical surgery (total abdominal hysterectomy and bilateral salpingo-oophorectomy) be considered? If radical surgery is considered in a relatively young individual, should any ovarian tissue be preserved? What are the relative benefits between pseudopregnancy and pseudomenopause? What is the proper dosage and length of time for danazol (Danocrine) therapy (pseudomenopause)? What is the role of uterine suspension and/or presacral neurectomy in the course of conservative surgical treatment? Is microsurgery a factor in the prognosis? Is it necessary to attempt to remove every visible particle of endometriosis during conservative surgery? Is there any benefit to cauterizing a lesion of minimal endometriosis at the time of laparoscopy if there is no interference with the pelvic structures? What is the role of laser therapy for endometriosis, either by the laparoscope or intra-abdominally?

All therapy for endometriosis can be categorized into (1) observation, (2) conservative or radical surgery, (3) hormonal therapy, or (4) a combination of these. The therapy should be individualized based on the woman's age, the severity of the symptoms, the extent of the disease, and the desire for pregnancy.

No Desire for Pregnancy—Young Patient

If a woman does not wish for pregnancy, if the endometriosis is discovered coincidentally (laparoscopy performed for some other reason), and if the disease is mild and without symptoms, no therapy should be instituted. If the symptoms are mild, they can usually be controlled by mild analgesics. Such a patient may be started on oral contraceptive therapy for birth control (if there are no contraindications).

With moderate disease, either pseudopregnancy or pseudomenopause, suppressive therapy is indicated, rather than surgery. For pseudopregnancy she should be placed on a continuous regimen of oral contraceptives of low estrogen, high potency progestin for 6 to 9 months. Following this, cyclic oral contraceptives of the same type should be continued. If oral therapy cannot be used, intramuscular medroxyprogesterone acetate (Depo-Provera) is used at a dose of 200 mg intramuscularly, with 150 mg every 3 to 4 weeks for 6 to 9 months. The side effects of medroxyprogesterone acetate include delay in return to ovulation after therapy, breakthrough bleeding, and occasionally amenorrhea and weight gain. Danazol (Danocrine) may also be used for such a patient, starting with 400 mg daily for 6 to 9 months. The side effects of danazol are primarily edema with weight gain and acne; occasionally one may see hirsutism and a reduction in breast size. Danazol is a testosterone derivative without estrogenic or progestational activity that acts as a weak androgen. It is known to induce atrophy within the endometrium and the ovarian follicle as well. Although this dose of danazol will suppress ovulation, there is occasional breakthrough bleeding. Fortunately, ovulation returns within 4 to 6 weeks after cessation of the drug.

The patient not wishing pregnancy at this time who has severe disease may have to undergo conservative (or even radical) surgery if symptoms such as rupture of an endometrioma warrant. Preoperative danazol therapy may be necessary. If endometriotic tissue is left in the pelvis at the end of the operative procedure, postoperative danazol therapy can be used.

Desire for Pregnancy

The woman with endometriosis, often over 30 years of age, who presents with infertility represents a complex problem for physician and patient alike. If the diagnosis is made, as often happens, in the course of a routine laparoscopy done at the end of an infertility evaluation, the extent of the disease is usually minimal. If minimal, most operators will cauterize the lesions when seen, although there is recent evidence that this may not be beneficial. After laparoscopy, therapy may be simple observation for 6 months or low dose (400 mg daily) danazol therapy for 4 to 6 months. I prefer to observe these patients.

If the same patient just described has moderate endometriosis with distortion of the pelvic organs, she is best treated by conservative surgery. Although some have recommended preoperative therapy with danazol, this does not facilitate the surgery nor does it appear to improve the statistics. Such conservative surgery would consist of excision, cautery, or laser of endometriotic tissue; careful lysis of adhesions (utilizing microsurgical techniques if necessary); uterine suspension (if the uterus is retroverted or the cul-de-sac is raw), and presacral neurectomy. The presacral neurectomy is my choice and is especially indicated when dysmenorrhea or dyspareunia are prominent symptoms. The value of presacral neurectomy in improving fertility statistics has not yet been shown.

The same infertile patient with severe endometriosis should receive preoperative therapy with danazol, 400 to 800 mg daily, for 6 months; this serves to reduce the size of many of the lesions and diminish pelvic vascularity. The size of ovarian endometriomas is not affected; rupture has occasionally been reported. Conservative surgery (as described previously) is then performed. Surgery for endometriosis is among the most difficult of gynecologic procedures. The tissue is often dense, and planes of cleavage are absent. Nevertheless, it is well to be aware of the principles involved in microsurgery, such as meticulous hemostasis, careful handling of tissue, lavage rather than sponging, careful approximation of peritoneal edges, reperitonealization wherever possible, use of magnification where needed, and careful restructuring of the normal anatomy. The recurrence of adhesions following surgery is a frequent problem. It is not yet clear what, in addition to the techniques already discussed, can be done to prevent this recurrence. Some operators utilize high doses of parenteral dexamethasone (Decadron) and promethazine (Phenergan), whereas others prefer to instill high molecular weight dextran 70 (Hyskon) into the pelvis at the end of the procedure. Neither clinical nor experimental evidence has proved the benefit of one over the other.

No Desire for Pregnancy—Family Completed

For the patient at the end of her reproductive era and not wishing further pregnancies, definitive surgical therapy is often indicated. This includes total abdominal hysterectomy, removal of both adnexa, and removal of any other obvious endometriosis. Postoperatively, lesions elsewhere (bowel, urinary tract) will usually dissolve. Such radical therapy is easily accepted by the patient over age 40 or with severe symptoms.

If such a patient is near menopause, danazol may be used for 9 to 12 months to provide relief of symptoms. There is a small risk of recurrence following this pseudomenopause. The risk will increase each year until natural menopause occurs. Medroxyprogesterone (Depo-Provera) may be utilized in the same fashion with less risk than in the younger patient, since recurrence of ovulation is not significant.

If menopausal symptoms occur following castration, these can usually be relieved by low dose estrogen without the risk of recurring symptoms. Symptoms may indeed recur following radical surgery. It is often difficult to determine the etiology for these in the absence of positive pelvic findings. Psychologic elements are often important.

DYSFUNCTIONAL UTERINE BLEEDING

method of
G. WILLIAM BATES, M.D.
University of Mississippi
Jackson, Mississippi

Dysfunctional uterine bleeding results when a woman becomes anovulatory for any reason and has irregular, unpredictable uterine bleeding. In the normal ovulatory menstrual cycle, estradiol-17β (E_2) stimulates endometrial proliferation; progesterone (P) is secreted after ovulation. Progesterone arrests endometrial proliferation and converts the proliferative endometrium into a secretory endometrium. When a woman continues to secrete estrogen but fails to ovulate, endometrial growth and proliferation continue unchecked by progesterone, and irregular uterine bleeding of varying severity results.

Dysfunctional uterine bleeding occurs most commonly at the extremes of a woman's reproductive life span—in the early postmenarchal years or in the late perimenopausal years—when ovulatory cycles have not become fully established or when they are waning. Furthermore, dysfunctional uterine bleeding occurs in association with polycystic ovarian disease (PCOD), exogenous obesity, weight loss disorders, and mild congenital adrenal hyperplasia. Thus, when dysfunctional bleeding is not the result of anovulation at the extremes of the reproductive years, a specific underlying cause for anovulation should be diagnosed and treated. If obesity is suspected as the cause of dysfunctional uterine bleeding, I advocate a weight reduction diet and an exercise program in conjunction with hormonal therapy.

Treatment

The therapeutic objective in treating dysfunctional uterine bleeding is to convert a proliferative endometrium into a secretory endometrium and establish cyclic withdrawal bleeding. This objective can be accomplished in several ways, depending on the desires of the patient. If the woman is not interested in pregnancy and wants long-term control of her bleeding problem, the simple approach is to initiate hypothalamic-pituitary-ovarian suppression with a combination oral contraceptive regimen. My choice of agents is mestranol, 50 micrograms, and norethindrone, 1 mg (Norinyl 1/50 or Ortho-Novum 1/50). This combination is well-tolerated and has minimal side effects.

If a woman refuses to take the oral contraceptive tablets or if there is a contraindication to the use of oral contraceptives, medroxyprogesterone acetate (Provera) is the second drug of choice. Provera, 10 mg per day for the first 10 days of each calendar month, converts the proliferative endometrium into a secretory endometrium. With the withdrawal of Provera, controlled, predictable uterine bleeding occurs. In some women, the use of Provera may induce ovulation by its action on pituitary gonadotropin secretion. When this mode of therapy is chosen in a sexually active woman, she should be advised that she needs some form of contraception if pregnancy is not desired.

Many women with dysfunctional uterine bleeding desire pregnancy. This poses a dual therapeutic challenge for the physician—to control the bleeding *and* induce ovulation. In this situation, begin with administration of Provera to produce a secretory endometrium, induce withdrawal uterine bleeding, and suppress pituitary gonadotropin secretion. After one cycle of Provera, follow with clomiphene citrate (Clomid, Serophene), 50 mg per day for 5 days. Begin on the fifth day of the cycle after Provera withdrawal bleeding begins. If ovulation induction is successful, the dysfunctional uterine bleeding will be corrected.

Most women with dysfunctional uterine bleeding can be controlled with the administration of oral contraceptives or progestins. However, some situations cannot be managed by the administration of these agents alone. The most difficult cases to manage are adolescent women and perimenopausal women with severe menorrhagia. In these patients the physician is tempted to perform a dilatation and curettage (D & C), but a surgical approach does not correct the underlying problem of altered hormonal stimulation of the endometrium.

In these seemingly intractable cases, I administer medroxyprogesterone acetate, 20 mg orally every 4 to 6 hours. If the rate of uterine bleeding does not begin to slow within 1 to 2 hours, I add large doses of conjugated equine estrogens (Premarin), 25 mg intravenously. If the bleeding does not stop within a short time of estrogen administration, I will repeat this dose of Premarin twice at 4 hour intervals. The administration of conjugated estrogens to a woman with dysfunctional uterine bleeding serves to stabilize the endometrium. After the rate of uterine bleeding slows, begin medroxyprogesterone acetate or oral contraceptives. When the progestin therapy is discontinued, withdrawal bleeding will occur since the endometrium has changed from a proliferative endometrium to a secretory endometrium. Warn the patient (or if the patient is an adolescent, warn her parents) of this bleeding! Otherwise, she will be alarmed that her dysfunctional uterine bleeding has recurred. Once the first withdrawal bleeding occurs, begin cyclic administration of oral contraceptives or medroxyprogesterone acetate as described previously to establish regular, predictable withdrawal bleeding.

Remember—dysfunctional uterine bleeding is a symptom of anovulation. The therapeutic regimens recommended herein do not correct the problem. They are designed only to convert the proliferative endometrium to a secretory endometrium. The underlying problem remains to be identified and solved.

AMENORRHEA

method of
M. YUSOFF DAWOOD, M.D.
University of Illinois
Chicago, Illinois

There is no uniform agreement about the duration of menstruation absence that constitutes amenorrhea. Amenorrhea may be clinically diagnosed and meaningful evaluation begun if menstruation is absent for more than 3 months or three cycle lengths in individuals who previously had menstruation at regular intervals or if menarche is not established by 16 years of age regardless of development of secondary sexual characteristics.

CLASSIFICATION OF AMENORRHEA

Some form of classification is necessary to aid therapy. It is essential to differentiate between physiologic and pathologic causes.

Physiologic Causes

Physiologic conditions such as pregnancy, postpartum breast-feeding, some forms of delayed menarche, and menopause produce amenorrhea. Pregnancy is the commonest cause of amenorrhea and must be ruled out before undertaking costly investigations and starting unwarranted therapy. Indeed, physiologic amenorrhea usually warrants no specific therapy. With menopause, however, therapy with estrogen replacement and calcium supplements is helpful (see hereafter). With constitutional or idiopathic delayed puberty or menarche, specific therapy is often not needed.

Pathologic Causes

There are five major categories of amenorrhea (Table 1). An overview of the pathophysiologic mechanisms of amenorrhea is helpful in developing a rational basis of therapy despite apparently similar therapies for different causes of amenorrhea.

Hypothalamic Causes. With hypothalamic dysfunction, there is inadequate gonadotropin-releasing hormone (GnRH) release due to a disturbance of either the frequency or amplitude of GnRH "pulses," resulting in nonpulsatile luteinizing hormone (LH) and follicle-stimulating hormone (FSH) secretion. Clinically a normoestrogenic or hypogonadal state ensues. In hypothalamic amenorrhea, there is exaggerated negative feedback or absent positive feedback of estradiol on LH secretion, quite unlike polycystic ovarian syndrome (PCO), in which there is an intact but excess ovarian or adrenal androgen steroid feedback effect on the hypothalamus. In hypothalamic hypogonadotropic amenorrhea, the endogenous opioid-dopaminergic system may inhibit GnRH release or pulsatility. This mechanism is responsible for some forms of psychogenic or psychologic-induced amenorrhea and exercise-induced amenorrhea. Neuropharmacologic agents may interfere with neurotransmission through dopamine or serotonin to elevate prolactin (PRL) levels and through disruption of noradrenergic effects to inhibit GnRH secretion. Tumors and granulomatous disease of the hypothalamus disrupt the hypothalamic neural pathways responsible for modulating pituitary gonadotropin release.

Pituitary Causes. Pituitary lesions cause amenorrhea through hyperprolactinemia and/or partial or complete hypopituitarism. Thus there is either deficient FSH and LH secretion or the hyperprolactinemia antagonizes the actions of FSH and LH on the ovaries. In prolactinomas and pituitary stalk damage, PRL secretion is increased with or without FSH and LH changes. In the empty sella syndrome, hyperprolactinemia is common. Postpartum pituitary necrosis results in reduced or absent FSH and LH secretion. Some pituitary tumors may increase secretion of all pituitary hormones including FSH and LH. With pituitary causes of amenorrhea, there is hypoestrogenism, which is an important consideration in therapy.

Ovarian Causes. In primary ovarian failure there is absence or loss of viable ovarian follicles with resultant failure of estradiol production. With premature ovarian failure (premature menopause), it is unclear whether it is an extreme variation of the normal menopause or a pathologic loss of viable follicles, possibly due to ovarian autoimmunity. In "resistant ovary syndrome" the ovarian follicles are insensitive to FSH secondary

TABLE 1. **Classification of Pathologic Causes of Amenorrhea**

Causative Level	Main Groups of Causes	Specific Clinical Cause
Hypothalamic	Neuropharmacologic agents	Psychotropic drugs
		Antihypertensive drugs
	Weight (fat) loss	Simple loss
		Anorexia nervosa
		Exercise (jogging, running, aerobic dancing)
	Psychologic stress	Employment or school
		Personal relationships
		Emotional disturbance
		Moving
	Tumors	Craniopharyngioma
		Teratomas, gliomas
	Granulomatous disease	Tuberculosis
		Hand-Schüller-Christian disease
		Sarcoidosis
Pituitary	Neoplasm	Prolactinomas
		Other pituitary adenomas
	Traumatic	Radiation or surgery of pituitary
		Head trauma (traffic accidents)
		Postpartum pituitary ischemic necrosis
		Gonadal dysgenesis (Turner's syndrome)
Ovarian	Genetic	Premature menopause
		Resistant ovary syndrome
	Trauma	Inflammatory destruction
		Radiation of ovary
		Cytotoxic drugs
		Vascular or surgical insult
	Ovarian hyperandrogenism	Polycystic ovarian disease
Uterine-Vaginal	Traumatic	Uterine synechiae
	Congenital	Imperforate hymen
		Vaginal septum
		Vaginal atresia
	Hormonal	Contraceptive steroids (progestogens)
Adrenal-Thyroid	Adrenal hyperandrogenism	Polycystic ovarian syndrome
		Adrenal adenomas
		Cushing's syndrome
	Adrenal insufficiency	Polyendocrine autoimmune syndrome
		Tuberculosis
		Granulomatous disease
		Hemorrhage
	Thyroid dysfunction	Hypothyroidism
		Hyperthyroidism

to ovarian gonadotropin receptor abnormality. With ovarian failures, there is hypoestrogenism.

In contrast, in PCO and other ovarian hyperandrogenic states, excess extra ovarian estrogens accumulate through peripheral aromatization of androgens. This either enhances or suppresses LH secretion. The positive feedback on LH is accompanied by a negative feedback on FSH, giving rise to an increased LH-FSH ratio. Dopaminergic sensitivity may be altered in PCO, thus affecting gonadotropin secretion and also causing hyperprolactinemia. With more severe hyperandrogenism, gonadotropins may be suppressed and hypoestrogenism may ensue. In the adult type of adrenal hyperplasia due to an attenuated steroid enzyme deficiency, gonadotropin and steroid hormone levels may be similar to those seen in PCO.

Uterine or Anatomic Causes. Anatomic derangement interfering with the menstrual outflow tract produces amenorrhea. In most instances, surgical correction is necessary for restoration of menstruation. With other congenital causes, such as an imperforate hymen, vaginal septum, and partial vaginal atresia with uterus, cryptic menstruation occurs.

Thyroid-Adrenal Causes. With adrenal hyperandrogenism, the mechanism causing amenorrhea is similar to that of ovarian hyperandrogenism. In contrast, adrenal insufficiency may cause amenorrhea through a polyendocrine autoimmunity, including ovarian autoimmunity causing ovarian failure, or through hypothalamic effects secondary to the systemic illness causing the adrenal insufficiency.

Thyroid dysfunction produces amenorrhea through a hypothalamic mechanism such as hyperprolactinemia as in hypothyroidism with elevated thyroid-stimulating hormone (TSH) and thyrotropin-releasing factor (TRF) levels. With hypothyroidism, testosterone estradiol binding globulin (TeBG) is reduced and the metabolic clearance rate (MCR) of testosterone is increased, causing a shift to testosterone and estradiol. Hyperthyroidism increases TeBG and reduces the MCR of testosterone with a resultant shift to androstenedione and estrone, which is hormonally similar to the situation in PCO.

TREATMENT

There are four specific goals in the therapy of amenorrhea. (1) To restore a normoestrogenic state if hypoestrogenism exists so that its preventable long-term sequelae can be avoided or minimized. (2) To prevent any prolonged unopposed estrogen or hyperestrogen stimulatory effects on target tissues such as the endometrium and consequent endometrial hyperplasia or carcinoma. (3) To restore fertility in those desiring conception. (4) To reassure the patient psychologically that she is capable of menstruating and that there is no life-threatening basis for her amenorrhea if no such cause exists. Therapy of amenorrhea is either medical or surgical or, in some instances, a combination of both.

Surgical Therapy

Surgical correction of anatomic defects of the uterus and vagina is necessary for restoration of menstruation except when the uterus is absent. Hymenotomy is necessary for imperforate hymen; resection is done for vaginal septum. Uterine synechiae requires dilatation and curettage or hysteroscopic lysis followed by intrauterine device insertion and estrogen therapy for 4 to 6 months (see hereafter).

With hormone-producing ovarian tumors (granulosa cell tumor, thecomas, arrhenoblastoma, hilar cell tumor, lipoid cell tumor), resection or oophorectomy is necessary. With severe forms of PCO or hyperthecosis, when the hirsutism is not responding to medical therapy, bilateral ovarian wedge resection using microsurgical techniques to prevent adhesions can be employed, albeit infrequently. It should not be done for amenorrhea or infertility.

Surgery is employed with pituitary or hypothalamic tumors. Transsphenoidal resection of pituitary adenomas gives good results. The choice of surgery versus medical therapy of prolactinomas, including both micro- and macroadenomas, can be debated. Experience with both methods of therapy suggests that initially medical therapy (see hereafter) is preferable to surgery, since the latter can be resorted to should the former fail. With surgery, menstruation takes longer to return and it may never return in those with very high PRL levels, which decrease to a lower but still abnormally high level. Medical therapy should therefore be chosen, especially for microprolactinomas (less than 10 mm). For macroadenomas, tumor resection should be done prior to allowing pregnancy.

Medical Therapy

Judicious choice and skillful use of hormones invariably form the basis of successful medical therapy of amenorrhea.

Sex Steroids

Estrogen, progestogens, or both in the form of oral contraceptives (OC) are used. Pregnancy *must* be excluded before giving any sex steroid hormone. Progestogens (either progesterone, 100 to 150 mg intramuscularly, or medroxyprogesterone acetate [Provera], 10 mg orally once daily for 5 days) can be given to evaluate the endogenous estrogen status and integrity of the menstrual outflow tract or for therapy. Withdrawal bleeding reflects adequate estrogenization and an intact uterus and vagina. Sometimes the patient may start to cycle with this therapy and only follow-up is necessary.

Secondary Amenorrhea with Adequate Estrogen. If pregnancy is not desired, treatment is directed toward the prevention of unopposed estrogen effects on the endometrium. An oral contraceptive can be given. Withdrawal bleeding is induced with either intramuscular progesterone or oral Provera (as previously described). On the fifth day of menstrual flow, an oral contraceptive is given for 3 weeks and stopped for 1 week; this cycle is repeated. If the patient is unable to tolerate the OC, she can be treated cyclically with Provera, 10 mg daily from days 16 through 25 with the first day of menstrual flow being day 1. The initial menstrual flow can be established with either intramuscular progesterone or Provera as previously described for diagnostic evaluation. For this category of patients, the treatment should continue for 6 months, then stopped and the patient re-evaluated. For some, menstrual cyclicity resumes and no further specific therapy other than follow-up is necessary. If menstrual cycling does not resume within 3 to 6 months after stopping therapy, the same hormone therapy is restarted.

For PCO patients, an OC is given if pregnancy is not desired and hirsutism is significant. The OC suppresses pituitary gonadotropin secretion and endometrial growth, prevents unopposed estrogen effect, and induces cyclical withdrawal bleeding. The resultant ovarian suppression secondary to pituitary suppression reduces ovarian androgen output, whereas the OC induces sex hormone binding globulin, thereby reducing circulating free testosterone, and inhibits the enzyme 5a-reductase, which converts testosterone to the tissue-active 5a-dihydrotestosterone. In this setting, an OC is given for a year or more.

Secondary Amenorrhea with Inadequate Estrogen. Therapy should be directed toward the cause of the amenorrhea responsible for the hypoestrogenic state. Hypothyroidism and hyperprolactinemia require specific therapies. With hypopituitarism, ovarian hyperandrogenism, or ovarian destruction, cyclic estrogen and progestogen therapy or an oral contraceptive is given to prime sex steroid target tissues, prevent potential adverse effects of hypoestrogenism, and restore cyclic bleeding if pregnancy is not wanted. The cyclic estrogen and progestogen regimen is similar to that described for primary amenorrhea and absent secondary sexual characteristics.

Menopause. Currently, menopause should be treated to alleviate the short-term symptoms of hot flashes and sleep and psychoemotional disturbances and to prevent the long-term development of osteoporosis. Thus the aim of therapy is not restoration of menstruation. In the absence of contraindications, such as breast carcinoma or deep vein thrombosis, replacement therapy with estrogen is indicated. Certainly patients with a reduced weight for height ratio or who are extremely thin require estrogens for prevention of osteoporosis. Encourage the patient to stop smoking, as it increases the risk for developing osteoporosis. Unopposed estrogen use increases the risk of developing endometrial carcinoma 3 to 11 times, which is directly related to the duration and dose of estrogen used but can be significantly reduced by the cyclic administration of a progestogen for 10 days each month. Recent studies suggest that even in the absence of the uterus, the addition of progestogens could be helpful to the breast in terms of reducing the risk of breast cancer.

Currently, estrogen replacement therapy can be given by one of two regimens. In those patients with a uterus, an estrogen such as conjugated equine estrogens (Premarin), 0.625 to 1.25 mg daily, is given orally for 25 days with a progestogen such as Provera, 10 mg daily from days 16 through 25 followed by 5 days of no medication. This cycle is repeated. In patients without a uterus, the alternate regimen of conjugated equine estrogens (Premarin), 0.625 to 1.25 mg, is given daily for 30 days with Provera, 10 mg daily, from days 21 through 30. To simplify this regimen, the patient can take both Premarin and Provera from the first of the calendar month until she runs out of the 10 Provera tablets and continue with the estrogen tablets until the end of the month. The cycle is repeated at the beginning of each calendar month.

Other estrogens that could be used include ethinyl estradiol, 5 to 10 micrograms daily, micronized estradiol (Ogen), or estriol-17B-hemisuccinate. Norethindrone (Norlutin), 10 mg, or norethindrone acetate (Norlutate, Aygesting), 10 mg, could be substituted for medroxyprogesterone acetate. However, the 19-norgestogens such as norethindrone and norgestrol increase the plasma triglyceride and low density lipoprotein levels but decrease high density lipoprotein levels, a profile more closely associated with the development of arteriosclerosis. Provera induces little or no change in the lipid profile.

The minimum effective dose for prevention of osteoporosis, 0.625 mg Premarin daily, should be given first and increased to 0.9 and 1.25 mg daily when necessary. The side effects of OC do not need to be considered in postmenopausal estrogen replacement therapy, since the dose of estrogen used in patients in menopause is much smaller than even the low dose OC. Premarin 0.625 mg is equivalent to 5 micrograms ethinyl estradiol.

If the patient is intolerant of 10 mg Provera, 5 mg daily for 10 days can be tried. Patients who have no problems with estrogen replacement therapy should be maintained on it until near death to prevent osteoporosis. Additional calcium supplements (1,200 mg/day) should be given and weight bearing exercises encouraged.

Primary Amenorrhea. Good secondary sex characteristics suggest adequate endogenous estrogens, and menarche may be initiated with intramuscular progesterone or oral Provera (as previously described). If cyclic menstruation is established, no further specific treatment is necessary. If further menstruation does not occur, OC may be given as previously described for up to 3 months, then stopped to see if menstruation occurs. If not, there could be other causes for the amenorrhea.

If there are inadequate estrogens and poor development of secondary sexual characteristics, estrogen therapy is necessary to stimulate and develop them. Conjugated estrogens such as Premarin, 2.5 to 3.75 mg daily, or ethinyl estradiol, 50 micrograms daily, can be given orally and cyclically for 25 days with Provera, 10 mg daily on days 16 through 25 followed by 5 days of no medication. This should induce menstruation and stimulate secondary sexual characteristics. Therapy should be continued for 3 to 6 months and stopped once secondary sexual characteristics develop and there is no gonadal failure. If there is ovarian failure, switch to OC given in the usual way until age 40, when it is replaced with postmenopausal estrogen replacement therapy (see hereafter).

Induction of Ovulation

Bromocriptine. Bromocriptine (Parlodel), a dopamine agonist, is currently the drug of choice for the treatment of hyperprolactinemic amenorrhea. It also induces ovulation in these patients. After ruling out pregnancy and hypothyroidism, bromocriptine, 2.5 mg orally, is given daily and increased to 5 mg daily after a week. With galactorrhea, 80 per cent of patients notice total cessation or marked reduction of lactation within 2 months of therapy. Ovulatory cycles and menstruation are established by 3 to 6 months of therapy in 80 per cent of patients. PRL levels are rapidly brought down (within hours) and are often normalized within 1 or 2 weeks. If 5 mg of bromocriptine daily is inadequate, increase the dosage to 7.5 mg.

The commonest side effect of bromocriptine is nausea and sometimes vomiting. These can be avoided by adjusting the intake of bromocriptine with food, taking it before going to bed, and keeping the daily dose to 5 mg whenever possible. Therapy is continued for up to 6 months, stopped and the patient reassessed. Not infrequently there is a slight rebound in PRL levels after stopping therapy. Other dopamine agonists such as lergotrile mesylate (Pergolide) are also effective but are not currently approved.

The choice between surgery and bromocriptine for microprolactinomas has been discussed previously. Currently, medical therapy with bromocriptine is preferred. Recent studies show that it is often not necessary to increase the dose beyond 7.5 to 10 mg daily to induce regression.

For induction of ovulation in hyperprolactinemic amenorrhea, bromocriptine, 2.5 mg twice daily, is given for 4 weeks after inducing a withdrawal bleeding with intramuscular progesterone. Alternatively, bromocriptine, 2.5 mg twice daily, is given until the basal body temperature indicates that ovulation has occurred. Subsequently, if no menstruation occurs, pregnancy must be excluded, menses induced with intramuscular progesterone, and bromocriptine therapy restarted. Pregnancy rates of 70 to 90 per cent have been obtained with no increased incidence of spontaneous abortion or congenital malformations. Because of the higher rate of symptoms of tumor enlargement with macroadenomas (17 per cent) as opposed to microadenomas, it is currently prudent to have the macroadenomas removed surgically before inducing pregnancy.

Clomiphene Citrate (Clomid, Serophene). Clomiphene citrate, a racemic mixture of a nonsteroidal substance with estrogenic and antiestrogenic properties, has been widely used for inducing ovulation in amenorrheics with an intact functional pituitary gland. It competitively binds with hypothalamic estrogen receptors and prevents their replenishment. FSH and LH secretion is increased, whereas ovarian estradiol continues to build up without prematurely recruiting the estradiol negative and positive feedbacks on LH and FSH. The side effects of clomiphene are minimal and tolerable. They include nausea, vomiting, headache, hot flashes, visual disturbances, rash, ovarian hyperstimulation, and multiple pregnancy to (five- to sevenfold; twins 8 per cent). Ovarian hyperstimulation is infrequent and usually mild. Clomiphene is usually the agent of choice for inducing ovulation except if the pituitary is destroyed, in which case human menopausal gonadotropins (hMG) or bromocriptine (if hyperprolactinemia is present) should be used. Thus clomiphene is used in hypothalamic amenorrhea, chronic anovulation, and PCO when fertility is desired. In PCO with hyperprolactinemia, bromocriptine is preferred. Before starting clomiphene, if there is a hypoplastic uterus or hypoestrogenism, estrogen therapy as described previously is given to prime the tissues.

Although clomiphene can be given in an amenorrheic patient after excluding pregnancy, it is preferable to induce menstruation with intramuscular progesterone. Clomiphene citrate, 50 mg daily, is taken on days 5 through 9 of the cycle. Ovulation can be expected on days 12 through 18, during which time coitus should occur frequently. If ovulation occurs, this dose is continued for three cycles. If there is no menses, pregnancy is excluded, menstruation induced with intramuscular progesterone, and clomiphene started again. With three ovulatory cycles and no pregnancy, the same clomiphene dose regimen is repeated and human chorionic gonadotropin (hCG), 5,000 IU intramuscularly, is given on days 14 and 16. If there is no pregnancy, the clomiphene dose is increased to 100 mg per day, 150 mg, 200 mg, and finally 250 mg per day for 5 days as before. If ovulation occurs at each dose level, the same dose regimen should be tried for three cycles. hCG may again be added on days 14 and 16 or 15 and 17. If ovulation does not occur with one dose level, the clomiphene dose should be increased stepwise at each successive cycle. It is sensible to stop for one cycle after every six cycles of clomiphene therapy, as pregnancy not infrequently occurs in the postclomiphene cycle. If no pregnancy occurs with the maximum dose of clomiphene, it is a clomiphene failure and hMG (Pergonal) should be employed. Pregnancy rates with clomiphene are about 40 per cent, although ovulation may be as high as 75 to 80 per cent.

Menopausal Gonadotropins. The prescribing of hMG (Pergonal) should be limited to physicians with special training or experience. Although in Sweden and Australia it is possible to obtain and use human pituitary extracts that contain FSH and LH to induce ovulation, in most parts of the world, including the U.S., menotropin (Pergonal), which is urinary FSH and LH, is used instead. Each ampule of menotropin contains 75 IU FSH and 75 IU LH. Ovarian hyperstimulation syndrome and multiple pregnancies occur more frequently with menotropin than with clomiphene. The high cost and potential side effects of menotropin limit its wide use.

Menotropins are indicated in amenorrheics desiring pregnancy but who have a destroyed pituitary or have failed to respond to clomiphene. For menotropins to be effective, the ovaries must be functional and have recruitable follicles. Usually 2 ampules of Pergonal are given intramuscularly daily, starting from day 5 or as early as day 3, and the dose is adjusted from day to day. No remarkable response is likely to occur in the first 4 to 5 days of injection. Response is monitored with serum estradiol (E_2), cervical mucus examination, and ultrasound of the ovaries for number and size of follicles developed. Serum E_2 should increase stepwise with a logarithmic increase of 50 per cent each day over the last 5 to 6 days to reach E_2 levels of 600 to 800 pg/ml but not more than 1,500 pg/ml. To avoid ovarian hyperstimulation, hCG should not be given if serum E_2 is 1,500 pg/ml or more. Optimal follicle diameter should be 18 to 25 mm.

Usually after the last dose of Pergonal, one day should elapse with no medication, and hCG, 5,000 IU, is given the following day and 48 hours later. Daily coitus for 4 to 5 days is recommended at this time. The usual length of Pergonal treatment is 8 to 12 days, with 15 to 28 ampules and as many as 60 ampules required per induction cycle. Treatment may be reinitiated with the next cycle. It is impossible to teach Pergonal induction of ovulation by the book or by laboratory tests. Personal experience and skill in Pergonal therapy have to be clinically developed. Minimal overstimulation appears necessary for successful outcome of Pergonal therapy. Pregnancy rates of up to 70 to 80 per cent can be achieved if no other infertility factors exist.

Clomiphene has been used in combination with Pergonal to reduce the quantity of Pergonal and, therefore, the cost. Clomiphene, 150 mg daily, is given from days 5 through 9 followed by pergonal and hCG when the follicles are mature enough (by serum E_2 and ultrasonography of the ovaries) to trigger ovulation.

Gonadotropin-Releasing Hormone. Recently, GnRH has been employed in many clinical trials to induce ovulation. GnRH is now available in the U.S. (Factorel). It appears useful in hypothalamic amenorrhea and is cheaper than Pergonal. It is given subcutaneously in pulsatile doses every 90 minutes with an automatic programmable pump. The optimal doses are yet to be worked out, but currently the dose used is 2.5 to 20 micrograms. An alternate route of administration is intravenous but also in a pulsatile fashion. Ensuing pregnancies have so far reported no higher incidence of anomalies. The advantage appears to be less risk of ovarian hyperstimulation and cheaper cost than Pergonal. Future promise resides in the potential use of GnRH agonists with longer half-lives that can be given as an intermittent nasal snuff.

Adrenal Steroids. Glucocorticoids are used for amenorrhea due to congenital adrenogenital syndrome, hirsutism/amenorrhea due to adrenal hyperandrogenism, and adrenal insufficiency. Dexamethasone, 0.5 mg, is given orally once each night and may be increased to twice daily. Alternatively, prednisolone, 5 mg twice daily, methylprednisolone, 4 mg twice daily, and triamcinolone, 4 mg twice daily, can be given. In mild adrenogenital syndrome with amenorrhea, glucocorticoid therapy should be continued for at least 4 months or up to three menstrual cycles if menses are established after the first 3 months. If there is associated primary amenorrhea and poor development of secondary sexual characteristics, adrenal steroid replacement therapy should be continued until puberty and menarche are established. If the amenorrhea is due to adrenal insufficiency, both glucocorticoid and aldosterone therapies need to be given for life.

Thyroid. If the amenorrhea is due to hypothyroidism, sodium levothyroxine (Synthyroid, Levothyroid), starting with 0.05 mg daily and increasing up to 0.15 mg, or desiccated thyroid extract, starting with 16 mg daily, is given and the dose titrated by clinical evidence of euthyroidism (sleeping pulse rate, hand tremors, and so on). If there is hypothyroidism due to panhypopituitarism, adrenal steroids (glucocorticords and aldosterone) are also given as for primary adrenal insufficiency. Thyroid extracts or thyroxine should never be given for amenorrhea without any documented laboratory evidence of hypothyroidism. Patients with hypothyroidism associated with elevated TSH and PRL levels should be given thyroid hormone but not bromocriptine. Hyperthyroidism requires medical treatment with antithyroid medications; methimazole (Tapazole), 5 mg three times daily, or carbimazole can be given. Alternatively, partial thyroidectomy can be done or radioactive iodine therapy given.

DYSMENORRHEA

method of
ANDREW J. FRIEDMAN, M.D.,
and ISAAC SCHIFF, M.D.
Harvard Medical School
Boston, Massachusetts

Dysmenorrhea, or painful menses, occurs in the majority of women in their reproductive years. Two types exist, primary and secondary, and a proper diagnosis is essential for successful therapy. Primary dysmenorrhea is defined as painful menses with no identifiable pelvic pathology. In secondary dysmenorrhea pelvic pathology must be demonstrated. Common etiologies of secondary dysmenorrhea include endometriosis, pelvic inflammatory disease, congenital malformations of the müllerian system, uterine myomas or polyps, ovarian cysts, adenomyosis, and pain secondary to the presence of an intrauterine device.

The symptom complex of primary dysmenorrhea includes colicky lower abdominal pain, which may radiate to the lower back and upper thighs. Many women also experience concurrent headache, nausea, fatigue, diarrhea, and, rarely, syncope. These symptoms usually begin within 24 hours of the onset of menstrual flow and rarely last beyond the first 2 to 3 days of menses. Primary dysmenorrhea occurs only in ovulatory cycles. It usually begins within a few years after menarche and reaches its peak incidence in the mid 20's.

In secondary dysmenorrhea, pain is not always limited to the time of menses and is less often related to the first day of flow. Infertility, abnormal bleeding, and dyspareunia may accompany this disorder but are uncommon in primary dysmenorrhea. Patients with secondary dysmenorrhea are usually older than those with primary dysmenorrhea, but this is not always the case.

Management

Primary Dysmenorrhea

It is important to approach the patient with primary dysmenorrhea with sensitivity and an understanding attitude. In the adolescent age group, dysmenorrhea is the most common cause of absenteeism from school. Often the patient is young, self-conscious, and has never had a pelvic examination. A gentle approach will reassure a patient who may be under the impression that her discomfort is purely psychologic in origin. A complete history and physical examination is essential to rule out the presence of organic disease suggestive of secondary dysmenorrhea.

Once the diagnosis of primary dysmenorrhea is suspected, prostaglandin synthetase inhibitors may be tried. These can be administered for the first 2 or 3 days of each cycle beginning with the first evidence of menstrual flow to ensure that the patient is not pregnant. Different types of prostaglandin synthetase inhibitors exist, and each is effective in 80 to 90 per cent of cases. These inhibitors appear to suppress menstrual fluid prostaglandins directly by inhibiting the endometrial prostaglandin biosynthesis and release that occur during the first 48 hours of menstruation. Commonly used prostaglandin synthetase inhibitors include naproxen (Naprosyn), 250 mg three to four times daily; naproxen sodium (Anaprox), 275 mg three to four times daily; ibuprofen (Motrin), 400 to 600 mg four times daily; and mefenamic acid (Ponstel), 250 to 500 mg three to four times daily. All of these are usually well tolerated but may have upper gastrointestinal side effects (i.e., dyspepsia). If one inhibitor does not work another may be tried, but a 6 month trial is considered adequate. Contraindications to prostaglandin synthetase inhibitor use include allergy or bronchospasm in response to aspirin or aspirin-like comounds and peptic ulcer disease. After 6 months without pain relief, diagnostic laparoscopy with or without hysteroscopy should be considered to rule out previously unsuspected organic disease.

If no medical contraindications exist, low dose oral contraceptive agents may not only provide protection against unwanted pregnancy but will provide relief from dysmenorrhea in over 90 per cent of patients. By suppressing endometrial tissue growth, oral contraceptives probably work by decreasing total prostaglandin production. If no success is obtained after a 3 to 4 month trial, this regimen should be re-evaluated.

Secondary Dysmenorrhea

Successful treatment of secondary dysmenorrhea depends on an accurate diagnosis of the process responsible for menstrual discomfort. Endometriosis may often be treated successfully by medical therapy with pseudomenopause induction (Danazol, 200 mg two to four times daily) or pseudopregnancy (continuous oral contraceptives). Conservative surgery may also be used in women desirous of maintaining their reproductive potential. Total abdominal hysterectomy with bilateral salpingo-oophorectomy is often successful in alleviating symptoms in women with endometriosis who have completed childbearing. In patients with dysmenorrhea from intrauterine devices who wish to keep them, prostaglandin synthetase inhibitors may relieve discomfort if pelvic inflammatory disease can be ruled out. If this is not successful or if there is a suspicion of pelvic inflammatory disease, removal of the device with or without initiation of broad spectrum antibiotic therapy may be necessary. Dysmenorrhea secondary to congenital müllerian duct anomalies, uterine myomas, and adenomyosis are often best treated surgically. Pelvic inflammatory disease is best treated with broad spectrum antibiotics. If antibiotic therapy is unsuccessful surgical intervention may be necessary. Ovarian cysts often respond to gonadotropin suppression with oral contraceptives but may require surgical intervention if they persist or enlarge.

THE MENOPAUSE

method of
ROBERT B. GREENBLATT, M.D.
Medical College of Georgia
Augusta, Georgia

What should be the attitude of the physician in the management of the protean complaints associated with the menopausal period? There are clinicians who believe that only vasomotor disturbances (hot flushes, sweats) and atrophic vaginitis are directly due to the estrogen deficiency and that these manifestations may be treated with oral estrogens, in cyclic fashion, in the smallest dose for the shortest period of time. They dismiss all other symptoms (e.g., depression, migrainoid headaches, nervousness, sexual dysfunction) as spurious or incidental. Many will not admit that metabolic changes that occur subsequent to the relative lack of gonadal steroids have any relevance to the promotion of osteopenia, alterations in lipoprotein ratios that contribute to an increased risk of heart attacks, or the inexorable march of catabolism that hastens the aging process.

We take a different view and believe that the menopause is a hormonal deficiency state and, like all endocrinopathies, should be managed as vigorously as need be without a time limitation. We believe that alterations in the hormonal milieu result in autonomic nervous system imbalance, metabolic disorders, and psychogenic disturbances and that hormone replacement therapy should be offered the woman who needs or seeks relief from the psychophysical aberrations directly or indirectly related to the estrogen deprivation.

Some women require hormonal therapy for years rather than months, continuously instead of cyclically, and in much larger doses than the minimal doses often recommended. When oral medication proves unsatisfactory for one reason or another, intramuscular injections or pellet implantation may often be rewarding. The incidence of cancer of the endometrium or breasts need not increase as a result of long-term therapy if cyclic progestogens in adequate doses are added to the estrogen regimen. Furthermore, it is our belief (as biased, perhaps, as that of the opponents of hormone replacement therapy) that the physician should render effective physiologic support throughout the increasing length of human life.

HORMONE-DEPENDENT NEUROVEGETATIVE SYMPTOMS

New information challenges the restrictive assessment of what constitutes the menopausal syndrome. Hitherto, mood changes and psychogenic manifestations, so frequently associated with "the change of life," were regarded as purely coincidental and not hormone related. Recent reports of investigators from the United States and abroad, employing estrogens and a placebo in double blind studies, have shown that such manifestations as depression, anxiety, and headaches are hormone responsive, the implications being that estrogens are psychotonic agents. The neurovegetative symptoms of the menopause were hormone responsive even if hormone dependency had not been proven.

Depression. The monoamino oxidase content of the brain matches the prodigious production of gonadotropins by the pituitary in estrogen deficiency states. To argue that nonpsychotic depression and other mood changes are not hormone dependent in the menopausal woman is to ignore the role of cerebral hormones (dopamine, norepinephrine, serotonin) in hypothalamic-pituitary physiology. Several studies have shown that free tryptophan was restored toward normalcy in the depressed menopausal woman by the administration of estrogens in large dosage.

Menopausal Headaches. Menstrual headache, held in abeyance during pregnancy, is often experienced by many women. The very fact that the high levels of estrogen and progesterone of pregnancy hold headaches in abeyance in women who suffer from menstrual migraine indicates that certain migrainoid headaches have some kind of hormonal basis. Menopausal women with frequent migrainoid headaches may obtain relief if estrogen concentration can be sustained at high levels for prolonged periods. Thus, administration of estradiol pellets to hysterectomized women (with and without testosterone pellets) maintains high estrogen levels for 5 to 6 months and has proven most efficacious in a high percentage of cases. The headaches often return as the estrogen levels fall after the fifth month.

Sexual Dysfunction. Sexual libido is a complex phenomenon that can be studied only in the human. State of health and psychogenic, anatomic, neurologic, and hormonal factors play important roles. Many sex therapists believe that most problems of sexual dysfunction are psychogenic and should be treated as such. Sexual dysfunction in the postmenopausal woman may be attributable to dryness of the vagina, causing dyspareunia. Estrogens usually are helpful. In women in whom estrogens are not helpful, the addition of androgens to the regimen yields surprisingly good results.

In a double blind randomized study we noted that women under treatment for severe hot flushes preferred a preparation that proved to be a mixture of an estrogen and androgen because not only were the hot flushes eliminated but the frequency and intensity of the sexual climax were increased. Placebos resulted in a 16 per cent amelioration of hot flushes but did little to enhance sexual gratification.

Nongynecologic Conditions: Osteoporosis and Cardiovascular Disease. The prevention of osteoporosis by estrogens (along with exercise and adequate calcium intake) is now well established if hormonal therapy is started within 3 years of the onset of the menopause. Even after marked osteopenia has occurred, bone mass accrual can be enhanced by the addition of progesto-

TABLE 1. **Hormonal Replacement Preparations**

Generic Name	Trade Name	Manufacturer	Dose
Oral Estrogens			
conjugated estrogens (USP)	Premarin	Ayerst	0.3–2.5 mg
micronized estradiol-17β	Estrace	Mead Johnson	1–2 mg
estrone sulfate	Estratab	Reid-Provident	0.625–1.25 mg
	Evex	Syntex	
piperazine estrone sulfate	Ogen	Abbott	0.75–3 mg
ethinyl estradiol	Estinyl	Schering	0.02–0.05 mg
diethylstilbestrol	Diethylstilbestrol Enseals	Lilly	0.1–5 mg
Injectable Estrogens			
estradiol cypionate	Depo-Estradiol	Upjohn	5 mg
Vaginal Preparations	Premarin Cream	Ayerst	
	Dienestrol Cream	Ortho	
	Estrace Cream	Mead Johnson	
Pellets for Implantation			
estradiol 17β	Progynon*	Progynon Associates	25 mg
	Estropel*	Bartor Pharmacal Co.	25 mg
testosterone, 75 mg	Oreton	Progynon Associates	75 mg
	Testopel	Bartor Pharmacal Co.	75 mg
Oral Androgens			
methyltestosterone	Android	Brown	2.5–5 mg
fluoxymesterone	Halotestin	Upjohn	5–10 mg
Injectable Androgens			
testosterone cypionate	Depo-Testosterone	Upjohn	100 mg per ml
testosterone enanthate	Delatestryl	Squibb	200 mg per ml
Oral Progestogens			
medroxyprogesterone acetate	Provera	Upjohn	5–10 mg
	Amen	Carnrick	10 mg
	Curretabs	Reid-Provident	10 mg
norethindrone acetate	Norlutate	Parke Davis	5 mg
	Aygestin	Ayerst	5 mg
norgestrel	Ovrette	Wyeth	0.075 mg
norethindrone	Nor Q.D.	Syntex	0.35 mg
	Norlutin	Parke Davis	5 mg
Injectable Progestogens			
hydroxyprogesterone caproate	Delalutin	Squibb	125–250 mg per ml
medroxyprogesterone acetate	Depo-Provera	Upjohn	100 mg per ml
Progesterone Suppositories	25–50 mg suppositories can be compounded by the pharmacy		
Estrogen-Androgen Combinations			
estrone sulfate/methyltestosterone	Estratest†	Reid Provident	1.25 mg/2.5 mg
conjugated estrogens/methyltestosterone	Premarin MT†	Ayerst	1.25 mg/10 mg

*Presently available by obtaining an IND from the FDA.
†Available at half strength.

gens to the estrogen regimen. Coronary heart disease occurs with increasing frequency in postmenopausal women, and this is believed to be due to the reversal of the ratio of high density lipoprotein cholesterol to low density lipoprotein cholesterol. Estrogens help restore the balance and reduce myocardial infarction by almost 60 per cent.

Treatment

Hormonal replacement therapy is the primary treatment mode for the symptoms of menopause (Table 1).

Contraindications

Estrogens should not be used or should be used only after careful evaluation in women with a history of endometrial or breast malignancy, deep vein thrombophlebitis or thromboembolic phenomena, or active liver or gallbladder disease and in those in whom severe headaches are "induced" by hormonal therapy. Androgens may increase hairiness already present or may induce the growth of unwanted hair. Occasionally, a mild voice change, slight enlargement of the clitoris, and acne may result from the androgen therapy. In such instances, androgen therapy should be discontinued.

The appropriate use of gonadal steroids can help to maintain physical and mental health. There are, however, some hazards associated with hormone replacement therapy, but the benefits far outweigh the risks. An appreciation of the concept of an extended view of the menopause will permit the physician to offer comfort to many women who have been denied the benefits of hormonal therapy.

When hormonal replacement therapy should be used, what agents should be used, and how long therapy should continue are decisions each physician has to make as he evaluates each patient. For some estrogens alone, and for others combinations of estrogens and androgens and/or progestogens, are the hormones of choice.

VULVOVAGINITIS

method of
RAYMOND H. KAUFMAN, M.D.,
and DALE BROWN, JR., M.D.
Baylor College of Medicine
Houston, Texas

Pruritus and abnormal discharge are the predominant symptoms of vulvovaginitis. The discharge may be excessive in amount, may vary in color and consistency, and may be frothy, malodorous, or cheesy. Pruritus may range from mild to severe, and at times the patient may also complain of associated vulvar burning. Not uncommonly, the patient will have been seen by many physicians and treated with numerous medications. Frequently, treatment is prescribed without complete examination of the patient or sufficient confirmation of diagnosis.

It is important that an accurate diagnosis be established before therapy is initiated. Although clinical examination alone can often be misleading, the practitioner should recognize the primary symptoms and signs of the various disorders. In the overwhelming majority of cases, use of saline and KOH wet mounts and measurement of vaginal pH can provide reliable diagnosis of common vulvovaginal infections.

CANDIDIASIS

Candidiasis comprises approximately one half of all the vaginitides. No one questions the prominent role played by individual susceptibility in the development of candidiasis. It is seen most often in women in the childbearing years and may appear in 15 to 20 per cent of patients in late pregnancy as opposed to an estimated 4 to 6 per cent of nonpregnant patients. Pregnancy is the most common predisposing factor to candidal infection. The majority of premenarcheal or postmenopausal patients developing vaginal candidiasis either are diabetic or have recently taken antibiotics or estrogens. Use of oral contraceptives is reported to increase susceptibility to candidiasis, but this relationship has never been substantiated. Since the introduction of antibiotics the incidence of candidiasis has increased severalfold. The degree of irritant reaction observed may be related to susceptibility of mucocutaneous tissues to allergenic or endotoxic substances derived from the cells of the *Candida* organisms.

Pruritus, the primary symptom, is reported in approximately 90 per cent of patients with infection. Erythema of the vulva is the sign most often observed.

Treatment

The most effective and safe medications available are vaginal candidacidal agents. Clotrimazole (Gyne-Lotrimin or Mycelex-G) suppositories and miconazole (Monistat) suppositories or cream should be used intravaginally nightly for 1 week. These two drugs appear equally effective in establishing microbiologic control and relief of associated clinical symptoms. A 3 day course of treatment with either clotrimazole or miconazole has recently been advocated. The preliminary data appear to be quite promising. A steroid cream (1 per cent hydrocortisone) applied topically is justified for reduction of the inflammatory reaction and relief of itching until the candidacide has taken effect. Gentian violet (1 to 2 per cent), the oldest and most reliable treatment, may cause severe chemical irritation and may be esthetically displeasing; but there is no question that it may produce immediate relief for the patient.

Reinfection, which is usually endogenous in origin, is a problem. Occasionally it may be explained by the practice of oral genital sex. Continuous vaginal candidacidal therapy for 3 or 4 weeks, even during the menstrual period, is used in patients with chronic or recurrent infection. In addition, the use of intravaginal candidacides at bedtime for 7 to 10 days before subsequent menstrual periods for 2 or 3 months is recommended. When these measures are unsuccessful, the use of an antifungal agent every 3 to 4 days on a regular basis may keep the patient symptom free. Whenever a patient with a history of recurrent candidal infections receives a course of antibiotic therapy, intravaginal candidacides should be considered. If the previously mentioned measures fail to prevent recurrence of infection, a 2 week course of oral ketoconazole (Nizoral), 200 mg once daily for both patient and sexual partner, may be beneficial. However, the use of this drug for vulvovaginal candidiasis has not as yet been approved by the FDA.

Balanoposthitis in the uncircumcised partner may also be a source of infection. Cleansing of the preputial folds and topical application of a candidacidal agent will reduce the infection rate.

PRIMARY CUTANEOUS CANDIDIASIS OF THE VULVA

This is a disease favored by warm, humid climates in which maceration and changes in the skin provide a good environment for the growth of fungi. Lesions tend to be moist and weeping and are found primarily on the labia majora, genital crural folds, perianal region, and inner thighs.

Treatment

Treatment consists of topical application of amphotericin B or nystatin in lotion form. Application of Castellani's paint or 1 to 2 per cent gentian violet affords rapid relief, although the prolonged use of these agents may cause untoward side effects. Lotrimin Cream 1 per cent is also effective. To ensure effectiveness, preparations must be used daily for at least 14 days.

DIABETIC VULVITIS

Although diabetes is a predisposing factor, it is of little overall significance in the general problem of vulvovaginal candidiasis. What is referred to as diabetic vulvitis is usually a chronic neurodermatitis secondary to recurrent or persistent candidiasis.

Treatment

In addition to treatment for diabetes and associated candidiasis, pruritus is controlled by the topical use of corticosteroid preparations, such as 0.025 per cent fluocinolone acetonide cream (Synalar), 0.05 per cent flurandrenolide cream (Cordran), or 1 per cent hydrocortisone cream (Cortef).

TRICHOMONIASIS

Currently, trichomoniasis accounts for 10 per cent of all vaginal infections with the cardinal symptom being discharge. The majority of patients acquire the disease through sexual intercourse; however, vulvar contact between homosexuals is sometimes a mode of transfer. *Trichomonas vaginalis* causes infection not only in the vagina but also in the Skene's ducts and the lower urinary tract of women as well as the lower urinary tract in men.

Treatment

Systemic oral therapy with metronidazole (Flagyl, Protostat) should be given to both men and women simultaneously in a single dose of 2 grams or 500 mg twice daily for 5 days. The drug may be contraindicated in patients with some types of blood dyscrasia or disease of the central nervous system. Treatment should be withheld during the first trimester of pregnancy. Topical agents are ineffective. Douching with medicated preparations such as Betadine or Vagisec may afford some protection but is not curative. Condoms may be safeguards against reinfection.

Occasionally, patients will not respond to the standard therapy for trichomoniasis. Possibilities to be considered are that the patient has been reinfected by another sexual partner or that her consort has in turn been reinfected and then infected her. Exclusion of these explanations suggests that the infection is resistant to therapy with Flagyl or that the medication has been inadequately absorbed. If the latter is the case, the use of Flagyl, 500 mg three times daily for 10 days, may be of benefit in eradicating the infection.

Gardnerella vaginalis VAGINITIS

The bacteria *Gardnerella vaginalis* is never indigenous in the vagina, never commensal, and consistently induces a recognizable vaginal disease. An abnormal state is produced in the vagina that alters the consistency and biochemical reaction of vaginal secretions. It is seen in approximately 10 to 15 per cent of married women in private office practice and up to 50 per cent of sexually active unmarried females. Many patients are unaware of the symptoms and signs until they have been treated and the organism eliminated from the vagina. It is considered a sexually transmitted disease and is frequently associated with other venereal diseases.

The diagnosis is made by the finding of the "clue cell" on saline wet mount. Because of the interaction of the *Gardnerella vaginalis* bacterium with that of the anaerobic bacteria present in the vagina, a malodor is produced that is described as fishy, musty, and amine-like.

Treatment

All patients should be treated once the diagnosis is established. Oral metronidazole, 500 mg twice daily for 6 days, is given simultaneously to both sexual partners. Cephradine, 500 mg four times daily for 6 days, eliminates *Gardnerella vaginalis* from the vagina and relieves the clinical symptoms of the disease but has little effect on the anaerobic flora within the vagina. Topical applications of antibiotic creams containing various sulfa products are ineffective in treating this infection. Douching will temporarily remove malodorous secretions but will not eradicate the infection.

In the patient with frequently recurrent or "persistent" infection, consideration must be given to the fact that the patient is being reinfected by her sexual partner. This possibility should be explored before one assumes that the patient's infection is resistant to the medication used.

DESQUAMATIVE INFLAMMATORY VAGINITIS

This is a rarely seen condition in which the patient complains of persistent, irritating vaginal discharge that is not responsive to the usual forms of local medication. Examination reveals acute inflammation of all or part of the upper half of the vagina, especially the exposed surfaces of the posterior fornix and ectocervix. The gross and histopathologic appearance of the vaginal tissues is that of an atrophic vaginal mucosa; however, the patient almost invariably is one who is in the reproductive years and is having regular menstrual cycles.

Treatment

The use of intravaginal cortisone suppositories (Cort-Dome Vaginal Suppositories, one half inserted twice daily) has been found to be the only successful agent in treating this problem. The suppositories must be used for a prolonged period of time—3 to 6 months—if symptomatic relief is to be obtained. Even then, symptoms may recur after treatment is discontinued.

Torulopsis glabrata (Candida Glabrata)

Candida Glabrata is a marginal or weak pathogen that produces mild vulvovaginitis in approximately 8 per cent of patients found to have candidiasis. Diagnosis by wet mount potassium hydroxide preparation will reveal the presence of spores similar to those of *Candida* but with conspicuous absence of hype.

Treatment

The use of gentian violet or commercial compounds containing this chemical (Genapax) is preferable to use of the new fungicidal agents. (To ensure prevention of toxic shock syndrome, it is important that medicated tampons be changed every 4 to 6 hours.) The recurrence rate of this infection is high, and some patients seem to be resistant to treatment.

ATROPHIC VAGINITIS

Thinning of the vaginal mucosa secondary to estrogen deficiency is responsible for atrophic vaginitis. In most instances, the patients are asymptomatic; the most common symptoms when they do occur are persistent vaginal discharge and occasional bloody vaginal spotting. The vagina has a pale pink tan appearance, and there is loss of the vaginal folds and rugae. Occasionally, the denuded surfaces of the upper vagina adhere to each other. Wet mount preparation will reveal a predominance of parabasal cells and polymorphonucleocytes in the smear.

Treatment

Treatment is best accomplished with an intravaginal estrogen cream (Premarin Vaginal Cream, Dienestrol Vaginal Cream). One half applicatorful should be inserted into the vagina nightly for 2 to 3 consecutive nights and once weekly thereafter.

HERPES GENITALIS

This is a sexually transmitted disease seen in all age groups with a mean age for primary disease of 26 years and for recurrent disease of 36 years. Vulvar burning, itching, dysuria, pain, and dyspareunia may be exquisite. The virus may be recovered from acute lesions by culturing a ruptured vesicle.

Treatment

Acyclovir (Zovirax) as a 5 per cent ointment is useful in reducing pain and decreasing duration of viral shedding in the primary infection. It is applied to lesions every 3 hours at least six times each day for 5 to 7 days. The drug is not curative and does not prevent recurrence in either primary or secondary infections. In severe initial infections, intravenous acyclovir in a dose of 5 mg per kg every 8 hours for 5 days has been found effective in shortening the duration of clinical symptoms and decreasing duration of viral shedding.

The use of topical and intravenous acyclovir is of benefit primarily in immunosuppressed patients and nonimmunosuppressed patients with initial disease. Their use is of little or no value in the treatment of recurrent genital herpes infections.

Oral acyclovir has been demonstrated to be effective in decreasing the duration of viral shedding and the duration of the frequency of new lesion formation and in shortening the healing time in individuals with primary genital herpes infections. A dose of 200 mg five times daily for 5 to 7 days is recommended. The time of viral shedding is significantly shorter in individuals with recurrent infection who take acyclovir than in a control population. The effectiveness in shortening the duration of viral shedding and preventing new lesion formation is increased if the patients self-initiate therapy when they note signs or symptoms of recurrence. The recommended dose of acyclovir is 200 mg three to five times daily for 5 days. Acyclovir has also proven effective in preventing recurrences when the medication is used chronically in doses varying from 200 mg twice daily to 200 mg five times daily. It is anticipated, however, that approximately 25 to 35 per cent of individuals taking oral acyclovir on a daily basis will still have "breakthrough" recurrences. In individuals who have used the medication for 3 to 6 months on a daily basis, recurrences have developed after medication is discontinued in a pattern similar to that seen prior to institution of treatment.

Symptomatic relief produced by tranquilizers and narcotics is often needed. Additional measures such as hot baths or use of compresses of boric acid solution diluted 1:10 parts of water may afford some relief.

CONTACT VULVOVAGINITIS

Contact vulvovaginitis is usually induced by agents initially applied for therapeutic or hygienic purposes. For example, nitrofurazone (Furacin) is associated with reactions in approximately 1 per cent of all patients using this medication. A cumulative primary irritation may develop after primary exposure to some varieties of intravaginal medications.

Treatment

Removal of the causative agent in addition to use of wet compresses, such as 1:20 Burow's solution or a concentrated boric acid solution, may afford immediate relief. Steroid ointments, fluocinolone acetonide (Synalar 0.025), hydrocortisone acetate (Cortef Ointment), or triamcinolone acetonide (Aristocort) may significantly reduce the symptoms.

CONDYLOMA ACUMINATA

Condyloma acuminata is caused by one of several strains of papilloma virus and is acquired by sexual contact. Because the incubation period may be 3 to 6 months, identification of the specific sexual contact from whom infection was obtained is sometimes difficult. Condyloma acuminata may involve the vulva, vagina, and cervix as focal, isolated lesions or as multiple, diffuse, confluent papillary structures.

Many patients with condyloma acuminata also acquire other sexually transmitted infections such as trichomoniasis, *Gardnerella vaginalis* vaginitis, and gonorrhea; these should be treated prior to attempting to eradicate the condylomata.

Treatment

Isolated, small lesions can be treated effectively with 20 per cent podophyllin in a tincture of benzoin solution. The podophyllin is applied directly to the lesions, and contact with the adjacent normal skin is avoided. Patients are instructed to wash the medication off the vulva in approximately 4 to 6 hours. The use of podophyllin within the vagina is not advisable, since the substance can be absorbed and occasionally can result in toxic reactions. Podophyllin should not be utilized during pregnancy. Tri- or bichloracetic acid may also be applied to individual lesions. This will usually result in immediate blanching with ultimate sloughing of the condylomata within several days. When any caustic agent, such as podophyllin or tri- or bichloracetic acid, is used the patient should be re-examined in 7 to 10 days and given additional treatment for any lesions that have not responded to therapy.

Treatment with 5-fluorouracil (5 per cent Efudex) has been found to be effective in eradicating persistent or recurrent lesions. The ointment is applied directly to the lesions on a daily basis for approximately 1 week or can be inserted into the vagina, using one half applicatorful daily for 1 week. Side effects such as blistering and ulceration of the tissues are often noted.

Large condylomata or those that persist despite relatively conservative treatment can be removed with the carbon dioxide laser. It is important, however, that the entire lesion down to the skin level be removed. Cryocautery has also been used effectively in treating condyloma acuminata of the vulva, vagina, and cervix; it is important that the ice ball extend down to the adjacent skin or mucosa. Large lesions with a sessile base can be removed with the electric cutting knife. Such lesions may be separated from the adjacent skin with the cutting loop. Occasionally, small lesions can be electrodesiccated and curetted off the underlying tissues. Extensive lesions found during pregnancy can be treated with the carbon dioxide laser, cryocautery, or a combination of electric cutting loop and electrodesiccation with curettage. If large lesions are present on the vulva and the vagina at the time the patient goes into labor, cesarean section may be indicated. Infants delivered vaginally of mothers who have condylomata have an increased incidence of laryngeal papillomas. These papillomas may not develop until many months after delivery.

MOLLUSCUM CONTAGIOSUM

This is a sexually transmitted viral infection caused by the pox virus. Lesions produced are distinctive and consist of nodules that are umbilicated and contain a white core of curdylike material.

Treatment

Use of a small dermal curette will aid in the removal of the entire papule. Bleeding is controlled by local application of Monsel's solution.

VESTIBULAR ADENITIS

Vestibular adenitis is a recently described clinical entity associated with extreme discomfort during coitus as well as irritation and burning in the region of the vulvar vestibule. Careful examination of the vestibule will reveal evident areas of punctation and hyperemia. These findings are frequently prominent around the opening of the Bartholin ducts onto the vestibule. Palpation of the vestibular tissues with a cotton-tipped applicator frequently reproduces the patient's symptoms.

Treatment

Vestibular adenitis is best treated by excision of the vestibular mucosa along with the underlying paravestibular glands followed by undermining the vaginal mucosa, which is then pulled down to cover the defect.

TOXIC SHOCK SYNDROME

method of
P. JOAN CHESNEY, M.D.
University of Wisconsin
Madison, Wisconsin

Toxic shock syndrome (TSS) is fatal in 3 to 5 per cent of cases, usually as a result of irreversible respiratory failure, refractory cardiac arrhythmias, or severe bleeding. Such deaths could potentially be prevented by early recognition, rapid intensive monitoring, and treatment of each of the well-described multisystem components of this disease. As outlined in Table 1, most of the sequelae are probably toxin-mediated, but some appear to be related to the degree and duration of hypotension and are also potentially preventable.

Pathogenesis

TSS appears to be mediated by a toxin produced by certain strains of *Staphylococcus aureus*. As with other bacterial toxin-mediated diseases, the bacteria themselves are usually present in only a single focus and often only in relatively small numbers. With few exceptions, blood, urine, and cerebrospinal fluid (CSF) cultures are negative. Typically there is often no inflammatory reaction around the wounds or infection site that would suggest the presence of a staphylococcal infection. Thus, numerous case reports suggest that in a patient with TSS all recent surgical wounds and any suspected sites should be opened, irrigated, and cultured even when no clinical evidence of inflammation is apparent.

TABLE 1. **Sequelae of Toxic Shock Syndrome**

Probably Mediated by Toxin
Desquamation of skin of fingers, toes, soles, palms at 7 to 14 days: DIAGNOSTIC
Desquamation of mucous membranes of mouth and GI tract at 4 to 10 days: UNCOMMON
Pruritic maculopapular rash at 10 to 14 days: COMMON
Prolonged myalgias and muscle weakness: UNCOMMON
Neuropathies/carpal tunnel syndrome: RARE
CNS dysfunction—impaired memory and poorly sustained concentration: RARE
Prolonged myocardial dysfunction: RARE
Recurrences in menses-associated cases: COMMON
Probably Related to Hypotension
Gangrene: RARE
Chronic renal failure: RARE
Hair and nail loss (2 to 3 months): COMMON
Pulmonary emboli: RARE
Possibly Related to Prolonged Anemia or Myocardial Dysfunction
Prolonged fatigue: COMMON

The toxins that mediate this syndrome and their mechanism of action are not yet defined with certainty. Toxic shock syndrome toxin (TSST-1), a protein of 24,000 molecular weight, is a valuable marker for the *S. aureus* strains isolated from menstrually associated cases of TSS. Whereas 95 per cent of such isolates make TSST-1, in one study as few as 63 per cent of *S. aureus* isolates from nonmenstrually related cases produce TSST-1, suggesting the likely involvement of other unidentified toxins.

A number of studies using animal models provide evidence for TSST-1 being of etiologic importance in TSS in that, when injected into different animal species in relatively high doses, TSST-1 reproduces many of the manifestations of TSS. Based on animal studies and the similarity of some aspects of the human disease to gram negative septic shock, several investigators have suggested the possibility that endotoxins may be important in the pathogenesis of TSS. Pretreatment of rabbits with TSST-1 reduces the 50 per cent lethal dose (LD50) of endotoxin by several thousandfold. In other words, the rabbits become exquisitely sensitive to endotoxin after receiving TSST-1, suggesting that both TSST-1 and endotoxin may be important in the pathogenesis of TSS. There is as yet no evidence from the human disease to support this theory.

The most important pathophysiologic effect of the toxin mediating this syndrome is extensive capillary leakage of intravascular fluid resulting in a rapidly progressive hypovolemia. In addition to the ensuing poor tissue perfusion, the toxin appears to have direct toxic effects on the myocardium, kidneys, lungs, liver, muscles, lymphoid tissue, and, possibly, the central and peripheral nervous systems. Hence, the two most important principles of management are rapid restoration of the intravascular volume and inactivation and/or elimination of the toxin.

Treatment

As noted in Table 2, immediate and appropriate monitoring for the early recognition of the well-described acute complications should be established in all hospitalized patients.

Although antimicrobials have not been proved to modify the outcome of the acute illness, their use is clearly indicated to eradicate organisms from the infected site, to treat the rare patient with positive blood or urine cultures, and to prevent recurrences in menstrually associated cases.

In vitro, concentrations of clindamycin (Cleocin) below the minimal inhibitory concentration of *S. aureus* have been shown to "turn off" the production of TSST-1 despite continued growth

TABLE 2. **Monitoring of Toxic Shock Syndrome Patients**

Initial	
Clinical	*Laboratory*
Blood pressure	Electrolyte–acid base status
Urine output	Serum calcium/phosphorus
Respiratory rate	Chest x-ray
Heart rate	Electrocardiogram
Heart sounds	Coagulation status
Pulmonary sounds	BUN/creatinine
Temperature	Liver function tests
Weight	Stool guaiac
Level of consciousness	Cultures of infected focus, blood, and urine
Prolonged Hypotension (> **2 hr**)	
Central venous pressure	
Pulmonary artery wedge pressure	
Mean arterial pressure	
Cardiac index	
Arterial blood gases	
M-mode and two-dimensional echocardiograms	

of the organism. This phenomenon is not seen with other antibiotics such as ampicillin. The significance of this phenomenon has yet to be studied in humans. TSS-associated strains of *S. aureus* are usually resistant to penicillin and ampicillin but uniformly sensitive to the beta-lactamase–resistant (BLR) penicillins, all cephalosporins, clindamycin (Cleocin), and vancomycin (Vancocin).

The antimicrobial of first choice in the treatment of *S. aureus* infection is a BLR penicillin. For patients allergic to penicillin, vancomycin hydrochloride (Vancocin) or clindamycin hydrochloride (Cleocin) is the drug of first choice. BLR penicillin is administered at a maximal intravenous dose appropriate for the patient's age until the patient is afebrile and has not required pressor agents for 2 to 3 days. Then an oral BLR penicillin is administered, 100 mg per kg per day every 6 hours not to exceed 4 grams. Clindamycin hydrochloride may be used at 25 mg per kg per day. Combined intravenous and oral therapy should continue for 10 to 14 days. In bacteremic patients, the possibility of additional therapy for endocarditis should be considered.

Of greater importance than antimicrobial selection is the identification of the infected focus, removal of all foreign bodies (tampons, gauze packing, prosthesis, and so on), and drainage and irrigation of any purulent material. The correct techniques for removing and/or eradicating any toxins are not known, as the tissue distribution, sites, and mechanisms for inactivation of TSST-1 (if this is the most important toxin) and other unidentified toxins are not yet known.

One patient with TSS due to a *S. aureus* infection of a herniorrhapy incision did not recover for 5 days despite aggressive resuscitation and intravenous nafcillin (Nafcil) administration until povidone-iodine (Betadine) irrigation and soaks of a well-drained, normal appearing but still infected wound were instituted. Saline irrigations and povidone-iodine (Betadine) irrigations and soaks of infected foci including the vagina should be considered as additional means of eradicating the source of toxin. Povidone-iodine (Betadine) is readily absorbed from the vagina after only a 2 minute application, leading to five- to fifteenfold increases in serum total iodine and inorganic iodide concentrations within 15 minutes. This finding should be noted when this form of therapy is considered.

Aggressive management of hypovolemic TSS patients as outlined in Table 3 is crucial. Numerous reports document the initial hemodynamic changes as a markedly decreased systemic vascular resistance (SVR), decreased mean arterial pressure (MAP), and increased cardiac output (CO). In some patients, however, after an initial phase of increased CO, myocardial contractility decreases, presumably owing to a toxin-mediated cardiomyopathy. This results in a decreased CO, increased pulmonary artery wedge pressure (PAWP), and increased CVP. This stage of myocardial dysfunction may not be readily apparent from the nonspecific ECG findings but will be quickly recognized from increased CVP and pulmonary artery wedge pressure readings, a decreased cardiac index, and an abnormal echocardiogram. Early recognition of myocardial failure should lead to changes in management such as decreasing the amount of fluid volume administered and considering afterload reduction, a subject beyond the scope of this discussion. Whereas dopamine may be effective in the early stages before myocardial dysfunction develops, dobutamine or a combination of both is preferable when myocardial damage has been demonstrated.

The use of methylprednisolone sodium succinate (Solu-Medrol) within the first 2 to 3 days of onset of TSS has been shown to significantly reduce the severity of illness and duration of fever in one retrospective study of 25 patients who received steroid and 20 who did not. All 45 patients were in shock or had postural hypotension and all fulfilled the CDC criteria for TSS. A number of in vitro and animal model studies provide reasons why steroids might be efficacious for TSS. Although most medical centers will use steroids, their use should still be considered investigational.

If an unstable blood pressure persists despite aggressive management and if an unsuspected site of infection with continued toxin production cannot be found, anecdotal case reports suggest that naloxone hydrochloride (Narcan) or techniques that might remove toxins from the blood such as plasmapharesis or hemodialysis might be

TABLE 3. **Supportive and Symptomatic Therapy**

Hypovolemia and Hypotension
Initial therapy:
1. Large bore intravascular catheter
2. Rapid administration of 20 to 40 ml per kg of crystalloid over 1 hr to stabilize blood pressure (BP) and achieve urine output of ≥ 2 ml per kg per hr
3. Oxygen
4. Methylprednisolone sodium succinate (Solu-Medrol), 30 mg per kg bolus and continue at 15 mg per kg q6h for two doses

If no response after 1 hour
1. Transfer to ICU
2. Continue crystalloid at 20 ml per kg per hr; may require many times maintenance to restore BP
3. Establish central venous pressure (CVP) line
4. Correct electrolyte/calcium/acid base status

If no response after 2 to 4 hours
1. Place pulmonary artery Swan-Ganz and arterial catheters
2. Establish status of myocardium and lungs
3. Consider use of dopamine hydrochloride (Dopamine HCl) or dobutamine hydrochloride (Dobutrex) for myocardial dysfunction
4. Appropriate therapy of myocardial dysfunction if needed
5. Look for sources of bleeding

If BP remains unstable after 12 to 24 hours
1. Look for continued source of toxin production
2. Consider naloxone hydrochloride (Narcan)
3. Consider other techniques for toxin removal (see text)

Adult Respiratory Distress Syndrome (ARDS)
Anticipate ARDS: oxygen, intubation, PEEP

Electrolyte and Acid-Base Status
Correct initial hyponatremia and acidosis

Hypocalcemia
Anticipate hypocalcemia and tetany
Maintain physiologic levels

Acute Renal Failure
Avoid nephrotoxic drugs
Monitor and dialyze if necessary

Thrombocytopenia and DIC
Fresh frozen plasma and platelets if needed

Edema: Pericardial and Pleural Effusions
Maintain adequate intravascular volume before using diuretic to mobilize extravascular fluid

Hypoferrinemia and Anemia
No treatment unless blood loss

Hepatic Dysfunction
Avoid drugs conjugated in the liver

Central Nervous System Dysfunction
Anticipate irrational behavior, seizures

useful. These forms of therapy have not been studied and should be considered investigational.

Other multisystem manifestations commonly present in hospitalized patients with TSS are listed in Table 3. Each complication should be managed using standard guidelines, and anticipation and early recognition of these complications are of great importance. Although hypocalcemic tetany is uncommon, hypocalcemia that appears to be mediated by a toxin-induced calcitonin-like molecule is common. Close attention to maintaining physiologic calcium concentrations may be important.

Peripheral edema, pleural effusions, and pericardial effusions can sequester massive volumes of fluid so that unexpectedly large volumes of fluid are often required to restore the intravascular volume. Once the patient's blood pressure is stable, the judicious use of diuretics will help to mobilize fluid.

The hypoferrinemia, most often incidentally detected on routine chemistry panels, is a physiologic response to acute inflammation and need not be treated.

Prevention

Adequate therapy of the initial episode of TSS is the cornerstone of prevention of recurrence in menstrually associated TSS. Without therapy, up to 65 per cent of women who develop their initial episode of TSS during menses will experience at least one more episode during subsequent menses. Subsequent episodes may be mild or severe. Recurrence is rare in patients who have had nonmenstrually associated TSS. Women who develop TSS with menses take many months to develop an antibody titer to TSST-1. Patients with nonmenstrual TSS develop a significant antibody titer soon after their illness.

Administering a BLR penicillin during the acute illness and discontinuing tampon use will decrease the recurrence rate to less than 5 per cent. Such women may remain susceptible to TSS until they have developed a significant anti–TSST-1 antibody titer. Serum antibody levels to TSST-1 could be monitored; tampon use can be cautiously resumed once "significant" levels are achieved. Such individuals may also continue to be at risk as long as they are colonized with TSST-1–producing strains of *S. aureus*. Thus, repeat vaginal cultures several months after the initial episode may be of help in identifying persistent carriers. Aside from continuing to avoid tampon use, optimal management of such carriers is not known.

The patterns of tampon use that will minimize the risk of TSS are unclear. Although superabsorbent tampons clearly increase the risk of TSS in epidemiologic studies, such tampons *cannot* be identified by the consumer based on manufacturers' labels. Using pads at night and removing tampons and seeking medical help when any symptoms suggestive of TSS develop are two recommendations with which most investigators would concur. The optimal frequency for changing tampons to minimize risk is not clear.

Certain precautions may prevent the initial episode of TSS. Physicians should instruct their patients to use tampons judiciously. In the future individuals at risk of developing TSS may be identified, i.e., those patients with no antibody to toxins and colonization by toxin-producing *S. aureus*. Treatment of these women may include administration of toxoid and/or eradication of carriage. In menstruating women who have had TSS, tampon use should be discontinued until antibody to TSST-1 is present.

PELVIC INFLAMMATORY DISEASE

method of
CHARLES R. B. BECKMANN, M.D., MHPE
University of Illinois
Chicago, Illinois

An estimated 1 per cent of all sexually active women will suffer pelvic inflammatory disease (PID) during their lifetime. Effective treatment is imperative considering that (1) women in their early reproductive years are the most commonly infected, including an estimated 1 in 8 teenagers; (2) the high associated incidence of infertility, ectopic pregnancy, chronic pelvic pain, and recurrent infection; and (3) the multibillion dollar cost of these infections each year. Treatment involves three steps: thoughtful diagnosis and laboratory/surgical evaluation, considered therapy, and timely follow-up and re-evaluation of the diagnosis and/or therapy.

Treatment

Diagnosis

Accurate diagnosis of PID is difficult. Clinical criteria include abdominopelvic pain with or without peritonitis; cervical and adnexal tenderness (with or without adnexal fullness); plus one or more of the following: temperature greater than 38 C (100.4 F), leukocytosis greater than 10,000 per microliter, and elevated ESR. Yet, about one in three patients with the diagnosis of PID actually has other problems, the most common being ectopic pregnancy, appendicitis, endometriosis, threatened or incomplete abortion, or a functional ovarian cyst.

Several steps may be taken to help arrive at an accurate diagnosis.

1. Serum B-hCG levels should be obtained in all fertile patients regardless of sexual or contraceptive history.
2. A gram stain of cervical secretions should be obtained. As upper genital tract infection is rare in the absence of lower tract disease, a normal pattern of few white cells and abundant lactobacilli is not usual in a patient with PID. Endocervical cultures for *Neisseria gonorrheae* and *Chlamydia trachomatis* may be useful, but aerobic/anaerobic cultures from this area are of little value.
3. Culdocentesis should be performed. Turbid fluid or pus supports the diagnosis. Gram stain and culture and sensitivity of the aspirate may be useful. Care must be taken, however, not to rupture an abscess.
4. Diagnostic laparoscopy is the "gold standard," as it allows a firm diagnosis in virtually all cases as well as facilitates sampling for culture and sensitivity from the fallopian tubes themselves, perhaps the most useful culture is the treatment of PID.
5. An RPR and urinanalysis/culture and sensitivity should be obtained, with further evaluation if indicated.

Therapy

There are two decisions to be made regarding therapy: outpatient or inpatient therapy, and choice of antibiotic regimen. The latter is based on the understanding that PID is a polymicrobial infection, usually involving both anaerobic and aerobic organisms during its natural course. *Neisseria gonorrheae* and *Chlamydia trachomatis* are commonly found, singly or together, in many patients with PID as well as many other organisms including *Streptococcus, Staphylococcus,* and *Bacteroides* species. Broad spectrum antibiotic coverage is thus essential.

Outpatient Therapy. Outpatient therapy may be considered in patients with mild disease and a high degree of certainty of correct diagnosis. Given the difficulties encountered in both judgments, however, many argue that all patients should be treated as inpatients with intravenous antibiotics. Suggested outpatient regimens include probenecid, 1 gram orally, plus either cefoxitin (Mefoxitin), 2 grams intramuscularly, aqueous procaine penicillin G, 4.8 million units intramuscularly, or ampicillin, 3.5 grams orally, followed by tetracycline, 500 mg orally four times daily, or doxycycline (Vibramycin), 100 mg orally twice daily, either for 14 days.

Inpatient Therapy. Suggested indications for inpatient therapy include a patient who is unable to take medications and/or fluids, a noncompliant patient, a temperature greater than 38 C (100.4 F), peritonitis, suspected or confirmed abscess, pregnancy, IUD, a medical problem that may be exacerbated by infection, status as an "infertility" or low parity patient, and an uncertain diagnosis. Suggested regimens include clindamycin (Cleocin), 600 mg intravenously every 6 hours, plus gentamicin (Garamycin)/tobramycin (Nebcin), 2 mg per kg intravenously as an initial dose followed by 1.5 mg per kg intravenously, every 8 hours, to be continued for at least 4 days and at least 48 hours after the patient defervesces. Then give clindamycin (Cleocin), 450 mg orally 4 times daily, to complete 14 days of therapy. Alternatively, give cefoxitin (Mefoxitin), 2 grams intravenously every 8 hours, plus doxycycline (Vibramycin), 100 mg intravenously every 12 hours, to be continued for at least 4 days and at least 48 hours after the patient defervesces. Then give doxycycline, 100 mg orally twice daily, to complete 14 days of therapy.

With either outpatient or inpatient regimen, an IUD should be removed after an appropriate interval for adequate serum antibiotic levels to be reached. Patients should have adequate fluid intake, antipyretic and analgesic administration as needed, and should abstain from sexual activity during the treatment interval.

Follow-up at 24, 48, and 72 hours is essential. If the patient does not improve, either the diagnosis is incorrect or the therapy is inadequate. Re-evaluation is mandatory, most probably including diagnostic laparoscopy if not previously done. If the patient is being treated as an outpatient, inpatient evaluation and treatment are almost always indicated.

LEIOMYOMAS OF THE UTERUS

method of
DEBORAH J. DOTTERS, M.D.,
and WILLIAM DROEGEMUELLER, M.D.
University of North Carolina
Chapel Hill, North Carolina

Uterine leiomyomas, or "fibroids," are one of the most common benign tumors found in women. It is estimated that 20 per cent of women over the age of 30 have leiomyomas. The peak incidence is between the ages of 35 and 50. However, myomas may occur in teenagers and postmenopausal women. For unknown reasons, they occur five times more frequently in blacks than in whites.

Leiomyomas are spherical masses formed by whorls of smooth muscle. They are usually surrounded by a pseudocapsule of compressed myometrium. Leiomyomas are often multiple, producing an irregular uterine contour. Within the uterus they may occur in a subserous, intramural, or submucous location. Outside the uterus they may occur in the cervix, the broad ligament, the omentum, or free in the peritoneal cavity. Their growth appears to be dependent upon estrogen, as they often enlarge during pregnancy and regress after menopause.

Diagnosis

The symptoms of leiomyomas are related to their size and location. Small fibroids are usually asymptomatic. As they enlarge, they may produce symptoms of pelvic pressure, pain, backache, and urinary frequency. Submucous myomas may cause menorrhagia or intermenstrual bleeding. The etiology of bleeding cannot be assumed to originate from the myomas, and endometrial sampling should be performed to rule out carcinoma.

The diagnosis of leiomyomas is most often made by pelvic examination. The myomatous uterus is characteristically knobby and irregularly enlarged. Radiographically, fibroids may appear as pelvic calcifications. An intravenous pyelogram may show lateral displacement or obstruction of the ureters. Ultrasound is occasionally helpful in differentiating uterine myomas from an adnexal mass.

Degeneration of myomas occurs when they outgrow their blood supply. This usually leads to hyalinization or calcification. Carneous, or "red," degeneration presents with severe pain, leukocytosis, low grade fever, and occasionally, an acute abdomen. During pregnancy, management is expectant, with intravenous narcotics and hydration; surgery should be avoided. Sarcomatous degeneration is rare but should be suspected if a myoma rapidly enlarges, particularly in a postmenopausal woman.

Myomas are often associated with poor reproductive function, including infertility and repetitive first trimester abortion. Implantation over a myoma can result in marked impairment in blood supply to the placenta, leading to intrauterine growth retardation. Rapid growth of myomas during pregnancy may distort the endometrial cavity, causing fetal malpresentation and/or dystocia in labor.

Treatment

The surgical management of myoma depends on several factors, including the patient's age, her reproductive desires, the severity of her symptoms, and the size of the myoma. An asymptomatic woman with a uterus less than 12 weeks' size is best managed expectantly, with pelvic examination every 6 months to assess the size and shape of the uterus. Conservative surgery, e.g., abdominal myomectomy, is indicated for women who wish to retain their childbearing potential. Common indications for myomectomy include infertility, a pelvic mass larger than 12 weeks' size, persistent bleeding not responsive to medical management, chronic pelvic pain and pressure, and a poor reproductive history related to the presence of the myoma. The success rate for term pregnancy following myomectomy is 40 to 50 per cent. However, one quarter of women who have undergone myomectomy subsequently require hysterectomy for symptoms related to recurrent myomas.

Submucous fibroids may occasionally prolapse through the cervical os, causing cramps, bleeding, and discharge. Vaginal myomectomy is indicated in this situation. Small submucous myomas may be resected under direct visualization using a hysteroscope and electrocautery. Hysterectomy is reserved for women with myomas greater than 12 weeks' size who have completed their childbearing and whose symptoms are severe.

There are small series in the literature describing successful medical management of myomas using high dose medroxyprogesterone or LH-RH agonists. The therapeutic rationale of these medications is to decrease the level of circulating estrogens. These reports, although preliminary, look promising as a future alternative to surgical management.

The use of oral contraceptives or estrogens in women with myomas demands careful follow-up with pelvic examination to determine uterine size. These medications should be discontinued if significant growth occurs.

CANCER OF THE UTERINE CORPUS

method of
FRANCISCO AMPUERO, M.D.
University of New Mexico
Albuquerque, New Mexico

Cancer of the uterine corpus is the most frequent malignancy of the female genital tract; the incidence of these tumors has increased over the last two decades, and today uterine cancer is more frequent than squamous cell cancer of the cervix. The greater availability of medical care, an increase in the number of women who reach the critical age for development of endometrial cancer, and environmental and unknown factors have all been implicated in the increased incidence. Endometrial cancer is predominantly a disease of post menopause; the mean age for cancer of the uterine corpus is 60 years, the range extends from 16 to 88 years, and the average is 57 to 59 years of age. Approximately 5 per cent will have adenocarcinoma before the age of 40, and 20 to 25 per cent will be diagnosed before the menopause; 80 per cent of patients with the disease are at least 50 years old or older.

Some of the risk factors associated with endometrial cancer are obesity, nulliparity, late menopause, diabetes mellitus, hypertension, anovulatory menstrual cycle, and the use of exogenous estrogens.

Although only about 20 per cent of patients with postmenopausal bleeding have a malignant disease of the genital tract, bleeding is nevertheless the first symptom of endometrial cancer in 90 per cent of cases. In 10 per cent, a serous discharge may be the presenting symptom, demanding attention before actual bleeding occurs. In the young or premenopausal patient, irregular or intermittent bleeding may be the presenting symptom, and, as for the patient with postmenopausal bleeding, further investigation is required. Other symptoms, including foul-smelling discharge, pain, leg edema, and adenopathy, are unimportant from the point of view of early diagnosis and are usually a sign of advanced disease.

Cytologic detection by routine cervical Pap smear is not nearly as successful in detecting endometrial cancer as it is in detecting early cervical cancer. Only about 30 per cent of patients with adenocarcinoma of the endometrium will have an abnormal Pap smear on routine screening. Fractional dilatation and curettage or endometrial biopsies are the cornerstones in the diagnosis of endometrial cancer.

Endometrial biopsy or aspiration curettage as an outpatient procedure may facilitate the diagnosis of endometrial cancer but does not always provide an adequate and complete sample. Diagnostic dilatation and curettage under general or spinal anesthesia by the fractional technique is the final diagnostic method for this malignancy. Fractional dilatation and curettage provides accurate information with regard to the histologic grade of the tumor as well as the size of the uterine cavity and the important parameter of cervical stromal involvement. The procedure should include biopsies of any suspicious lesions in the portio followed by careful clockwise sampling of the endocervical mucosa; the curettings so obtained should be labeled endocervical curettage.

The next step is to sound the uterine cavity to determine its depth from the external os to the uterine fundus. This is followed by dilatation of the endocervical canal and a meticulous curettage of the endometrial cavity including the anterior and posterior walls as well as the fundus.

After the histologic diagnosis of endometrial cancer has been established, a pretreatment evaluation should be performed to determine the presence of regional or distant metastasis. We routinely examine the patient under anesthesia and include cystoscopy, proctosigmoidoscopy, chest radiography, IVP, barium enema, and blood chemistries. If indicated by the physical findings or in the patient with more advanced disease, an abdominal pelvic CAT scan is performed, as this may provide important information with respect to the extent of the disease in the pelvis, retroperitoneal lymph nodes, and liver. Accurate determination of the extent of the disease is important in planning therapy. The currently used FIGO staging of endometrial cancer is shown in Table 1.

In decreasing order of frequency, the histologic subtypes of endometrial cancer are adenocarcinoma, adenoacanthoma, adenosquamous clear cell carcinoma, papillary adenocarcinoma, and secretory carcinoma. Although relatively rare, papillary and clear cell carcinomas are important because of their aggressive nature. Uterine sarcomas represent about 3 per cent of all uterine cancers.

The histologic differentiation of endometrial cancer

TABLE 1. **Staging Classification of Endometrial Carcinoma (FIGO)**

Stage I
The carcinoma is confined to the corpus
Stage IA: The length of the uterine cavity is 8 cm or less
Stage IB: The length of the uterine cavity is more than 8 cm
Stage I cases should be subgrouped with regard to the histologic type of the adenocarcinoma as follows:
G1: Highly differentiated adenomatous carcinoma
G2: Moderately differentiated adenomatous carcinoma with partly solid areas
G3: Predominantly solid or entirely undifferentiated carcinoma

Stage II
The carcinoma has involved the corpus and the cervix but has not extended outside the uterus

Stage III
The carcinoma has extended outside the uterus but not outside the true pelvis

Stage IV
The carcinoma has extended outside the true pelvis or has obviously involved the mucosa of the bladder or rectum; a bullous edema as such does not permit allotment of a case to stage IV

Stage IVA
Spread of growth to adjacent organs

Stage IVB
Spread of growth to distant organs

is important not only as a prognostic indicator but in determining therapy.

There are seven different prognostic factors in endometrial cancer: histologic type, histologic grade, depth of invasion, lymph node metastasis, extent of disease (stage), peritoneal cytology, and uterine size. These factors need to be carefully considered before determining the therapeutic modality for each patient with carcinoma of the uterine corpus.

Treatment

The prescription of a treatment plan depends upon several factors. (1) An accurate pathologic diagnosis that includes careful histologic grading of the tumor. (2) The determination of the stage of the disease, i.e., its local, regional, or distant metastatic spread. (3) Careful pretreatment evaluation of the patient's general medical condition to determine her ability to tolerate surgery. (4) Selection of the mode of treatment best suited for each individual patient.

The treatment of endometrial cancer originally developed along two separate lines (radiation therapy and surgery), but in the last decades the trend has been toward combined therapy.

Stage I Endometrial Cancer

Of all patients diagnosed as having endometrial cancer, 75 per cent will have the disease confined to the uterine corpus. It is clear today that the mainstay of therapy in endometrial cancer is total abdominal hysterectomy and bilateral salpingo-oophorectomy combined with radiation therapy when indicated by the prognostic factors. Radiotherapy alone should be reserved for the patient who is a poor surgical candidate, i.e., one with severe cardiac or pulmonary disease, uncontrolled diabetes mellitus, or other medical problems that absolutely contraindicate surgery.

In those patients who are good surgical candidates, the histologic grade of the tumor is important in determining the treatment modality. We treat patients with stage I, grade I tumors with a total abdominal hysterectomy and bilateral salpingo-oophorectomy. The uterus is carefully examined by the pathologist in the operating room, and if there is evidence of deep myometrial invasion, pelvic and para-aortic lymph node sampling is performed. Patients with deep myometrial invasion and positive pelvic or para-aortic nodes receive additional radiation therapy and/or chemotherapy as indicated by the extent of the disease.

We treat patients with grades 2 and 3 tumors with preoperative intracavitary radiation therapy using tandem and colpostats by the afterloading technique with cesium 137. Five thousand mg hours are prescribed, providing approximately 7,000 rads to the vaginal surface, 3,000 rads to point A, and about 16,000 to 18,000 rads to the endometrial surface. The purposes of preoperative intracavitary radiation are to destroy the vitality of the endometrial surface of the tumor, to diminish implantation metastasis and dissemination by operative manipulation, to seal lymphatics and vascular channels in the tumor bed, and to enhance operative clearance, thereby preventing operative dissemination.

We prefer preoperative intracavitary radiation to postoperative intravaginal application because, although statistically unproven, preoperative application permits administration of radiation therapy to the entire, intact intercommunicating system of uterine, cervical, and vaginal lymphatics and is likely to be more effective than postoperative radiation therapy to the vaginal cuff. The day following removal of the intracavitary sources, we perform a total abdominal hysterectomy, bilateral salpingo-oophorectomy, and pelvic and para-aortic node sampling. We prefer to perform the hysterectomy immediately after the intracavitary radiation therapy in order to preserve important information regarding the depth of myometrial invasion that can be otherwise altered if surgery is performed 4 to 6 weeks later.

At the time of exploratory laparotomy, a thorough visual and palpatory examination of the abdominal cavity is carried out. Pelvic peritoneal washings are obtained using 100 ml of normal saline and sent for cytologic analysis. If ascites is present, an adequate sample should be sent for cytologic evaluation.

Next, an extrafascial total abdominal hysterectomy is performed. The retroperitoneal spaces along the pelvic vessels are opened, and any suspicious lymph nodes are removed and sent for histologic evaluation. If no suspicious nodes are present, the lymph-bearing tissues along the common, external, and internal iliac vessels are removed from the bifurcation of the aorta to the obturator fossa above the obturator nerve. Next the peritoneum over the aorta and vena cava is incised from the bifurcation to the duodenum, and the lymph-bearing tissue overlying the vena cava and the aorta is removed. We also routinely perform an omental biopsy.

Following careful histologic examination of the uterus, ovaries, and lymph nodes, additional postoperative external radiation therapy is given to the pelvis when there is invasion of the myometrium to more than one third of its thickness, extension into the cervix with stromal invasion, or metastases to the pelvic nodes. A total dose of 4,500 to 5,000 rads is given over a 4 to 5 week period.

About 10 per cent of patients with stage I disease will have positive peritoneal cytologies, and the treatment of patients in this group still remains controversial. The use of radioactive P32 chemotherapy or hormonal therapy has been suggested in addition to external radiation therapy. We treat patients with positive cytologies with oral cyclophosphamide (Cytoxan), 200 mg per square meter for 5 days a month for a total of 12 courses.

Those patients with myometrial invasion to less than one third, no cervical extension, and negative pelvic nodes and peritoneal cytology do not receive further therapy.

If there is evidence of extrapelvic disease to the para-aortic nodes, extended field radiation therapy to the para-aortic area is given to a dose of 4,500 rads followed by systemic chemotherapy. Metastatic disease to other areas within the abdomen is treated with chemotherapy using a combination of adriamycin (Doxorubicin), 40 mg per square meter intravenously; cyclophosphamide (Cytoxan), 600 mg per square meter intravenously; and cis-platinum (Cisplatin), 50 mg per square meter intravenously. This dosage is repeated every 3 weeks for the first 3 courses and then every 4 weeks for a total of 12 courses. Patients with well-differentiated tumors may benefit from progestational agents.

Patients with papillary serous tumors deserve special attention, as these tumors, although relatively well-differentiated histologically, are very aggressive. Deep myometrial invasion is significantly more common than in other types of uterine adenocarcinomas, ovarian metastasis is present in 19 per cent of patients with these tumors, and a marked propensity for endolymphatic spread as well as a tendency to spread over the peritoneal surface in an ovarian cancer–like fashion is frequently observed. We treat these tumors with total abdominal hysterectomy, bilateral salpingo-oophorectomy, and total omentectomy followed by radiation therapy to the pelvis if disease is confined to the uterus. If the disease is present outside the pelvis or if cytologies are positive, we recommend aggressive chemotherapy with a combination of adriamycin, cis-platinum, and cyclophosphamide, although the sensitivity of these tumors to these agents has not been established. Because of the high incidence of intraperitoneal recurrence, others have recommended the use of whole abdominal radiation therapy.

Papillary serous adenocarcinoma tends to overlap with clear cell carcinomas of the endometrium tumors that also tend to have a poor prognosis. In both situations these prognostically unfavorable tumors may be judged to be well-differentiated and hence prognostically favorable because of the relatively benign histologic appearance.

Stage II Endometrial Cancer

Of all patients with endometrial cancer, 14.7 per cent will be stage II at the time of diagnosis. The basis of diagnosis of stage II endometrial cancer is tumor invasion of the cervical stroma. The presence of "floaters" or cells detached from the endometrial cavity and retrieved from the endocervical canal during the fractional dilatation and curettage does not denote stage II disease. It is well recognized that tumor extension into the cervical stroma increases the propensity for extrauterine spread, especially to the pelvic lymph nodes. The incidence of metastasis to the pelvic lymph nodes for stage II is 35 per cent.

Because of the increased risk of extrauterine extension, we treat stage II patients with a combination of radiation therapy and surgery. Tandem and colpostats are used to deliver 5,000 mg hours for a total dose of 3,000 rads to point A and 7,000 rads to the vaginal surface. This is followed by external whole pelvis radiation therapy delivering 4,500 to 5,000 rads in 4 to 5 weeks. Two to 4 weeks after completing radiation therapy, extrafascial total abdominal hysterectomy and bilateral salpingo-oophorectomy are performed. At the time, thorough exploration of the abdomen, peritoneal cytologies, para-aortic node sampling, and omental biopsy are performed. If negative, no further treatment is given. Patients with extrapelvic disease receive external radiation therapy or systemic chemotherapy.

In the past, radical hysterectomy and pelvic lymphadenectomy had been advocated to treat patients with stage II endometrial cancer. However, very often patients with endometrial cancer are not suitable candidates for radical surgery. Diabetes, hypertension, and arteriosclerotic disease are some of the common medical problems seen in this group of patients. Pelvic lymphadenectomy is usually not only technically difficult but often suboptimal in the frequently obese patient with endometrial cancer. In addition, 35 per cent of patients with stage II endometrial cancer have metastases to the pelvic nodes and require additional external radiation therapy. It is well known that adding radiation therapy to a radical surgical procedure increases the chances for radiation therapy complications in the form of vesicovaginal or rectovaginal fistulas. In our opinion, these factors make the use of radical hysterectomy of very limited value in the treatment of stage II disease.

With adequate therapy, the expected 5 year survival in patients with stage II endometrial cancer is 57.4 per cent.

Stages III and IV Adenocarcinoma of the Endometrium

Only 7.2 per cent of patients with endometrial cancer will have stage III disease at the time of diagnosis. We initially treat these patients with external radiation therapy to the whole pelvis; 5,000 rads in 4 to 5 weeks are delivered. Upon completion of radiation therapy, patients are reevaluated and, providing the extrauterine tumor response has been optimal, a total abdominal hysterectomy and bilateral salpingo-oophorectomy are considered. Those patients with residual tumor are considered for additional boost with a limited smaller field and/or chemotherapy.

Patients with stage IV disease represent only 3 per cent of patients with endometrial cancer. The treatment includes a combination of radiation therapy, surgery, and/or systemic chemotherapy depending on the extent of the disease and site of the metastasis.

Recurrent endometrial cancer may occur within the radiation field in the pelvis or distant sites, i.e., lung, liver, or intraperitoneal dissemination. These patients are treated with systemic multiple agent chemotherapy (adriamycin, cisplatinum, and cyclophosphamide) or hormonal therapy if the tumors are histologically well-differentiated. Metastatic disease outside of the field of radiation therapy tends to have a better response to chemotherapy or hormonal therapy than pelvic recurrence following radiation therapy. Patients with solitary lung metastasis may benefit from segmental lung resection followed by systemic chemotherapy or hormonal therapy providing that the local tumor has been controlled and that there is no evidence of other metastatic disease outside of the lung.

The response to hormonal therapy depends on the histologic grade of the tumor. Well-differentiated tumors have a better and more prolonged response. Overall response in endometrial cancer, including partial and complete responses to hormonal therapy, is about 25 per cent.

CANCER OF THE UTERINE CERVIX

method of
ROBERT L. GIUNTOLI, M.D.
University of Pennsylvania
Philadelphia, Pennsylvania

During the last three decades there has been a dramatic decline in deaths from cervical cancer in the United States. This decline has largely been due to the wide use of cytology, colposcopy, and early treatment. The tools to totally eliminate cervical cancer as a cause of death are available. The reduction in the death rate from cervical cancer has been followed by an increase in the number of cases of premalignant diseases of the cervix, as witnessed by an increase in the number of women who are found to have abnormal cytology.

DETECTION

Cytology is the leading diagnostic tool for early detection. The Pap smear is associated with a 10 to 40 per cent false negative rate. This is why any gross lesion must be biopsied. The Pap smear should include endocervical and cervical specimens. A vaginal smear by itself is not accurate.

The old classification system is no longer considered adequate and is replaced by the cervical intraepithelial neoplasia (CIN), or dysplasia, systems.

Class I	Normal
Class II	Mild dysplasia or CIN I
Class III	Moderate dysplasia or CIN II
Class IV	Severe dysplasia, carcinoma in situ or CIN III
Class V	Invasive cancer

This classification cannot convey an accurate diagnosis. Regardless of the terminology adopted, communication between the clinician and pathologist is needed.

COLPOSCOPY AND BIOPSY

Cytology is used for screening and determining which patients have an abnormal condition. Colposcopy is used to determine the location of the abnormal area. Biopsy is used to determine what abnormality is present. Colposcopy and cytology cannot determine the degree of abnormality; only the biopsy can determine if the area is abnormal and the type of abnormality. Any patient with an abnormal Pap smear or a gross lesion should undergo colposcopic examination (Figure 1).

For the majority of patients with CIN disease, colposcopy with excisional biopsy is adequate for diagnosis and complete therapy as long as there is close follow-up care. Excisional biopsy provides tissue for thorough evaluation and is less likely to decrease fertility or effect visualization of the squamocolumnar junction for future colposcopic evaluation.

CONE BIOPSY

Cone biopsy is performed when colposcopy is inadequate or when excisional biopsy does not provide an adequate sample. A cone biopsy is not only diagnostic but therapeutic. The indications for a cone biopsy include the following:

1. The entire lesion is not seen colposcopically.
2. The entire squamocolumnar junction is not seen colposcopically.
3. The lesion extends into the endocervical canal.
4. The endocervical curettage contains CIN III disease.
5. There is progression of the disease.
6. Microinvasion is present on colposcopically directed biopsy.

A review of the colposcopic records at the University of Pennsylvania of women referred for evaluation of their abnormal Pap smear revealed that 2 per cent of CIN I, 9 per cent of CIN II, and 30 percent of CIN III underwent conization. If a hysterectomy was performed within 24 to 48 hours of the conization, residual disease was found in two thirds of the hysterectomy specimens.

Long-term follow-up subsequent to conization revealed that recurrence is associated with the depth of glandular involvement and not with involvement of

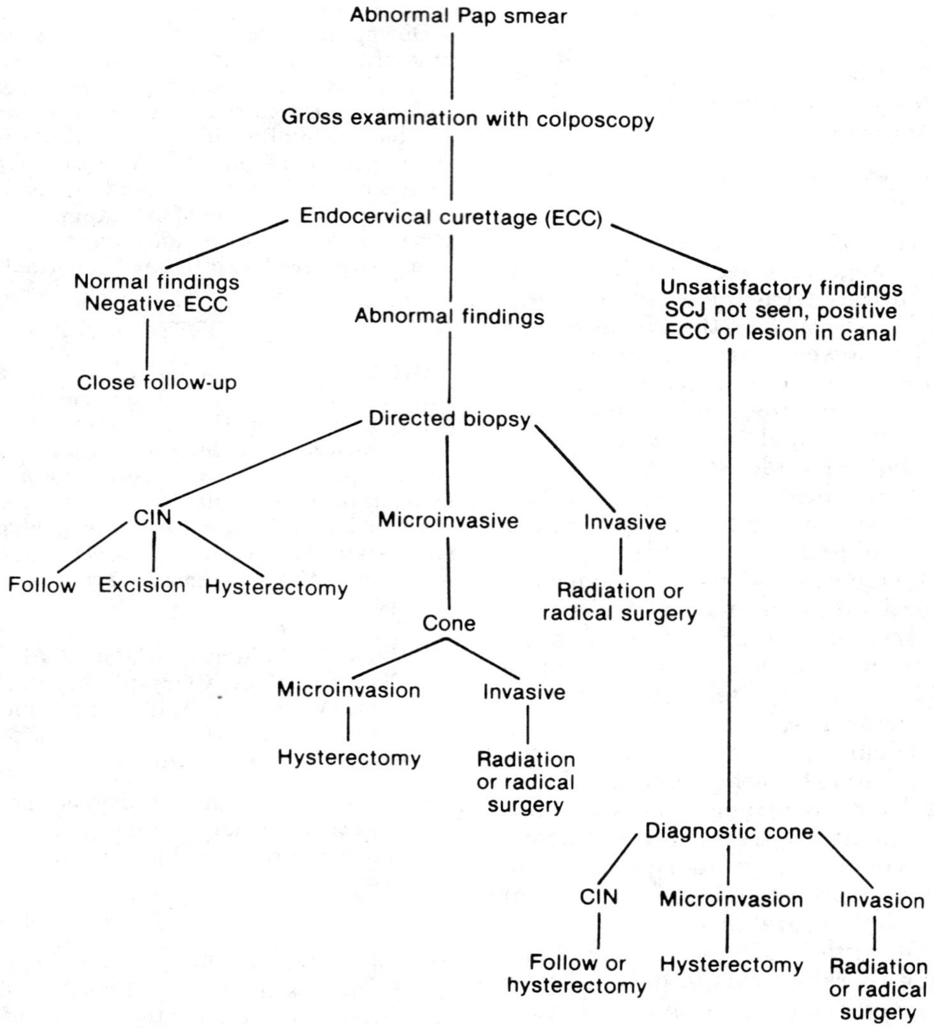

Figure 1. Treatment plan for cervical intraepithelial neoplasia.

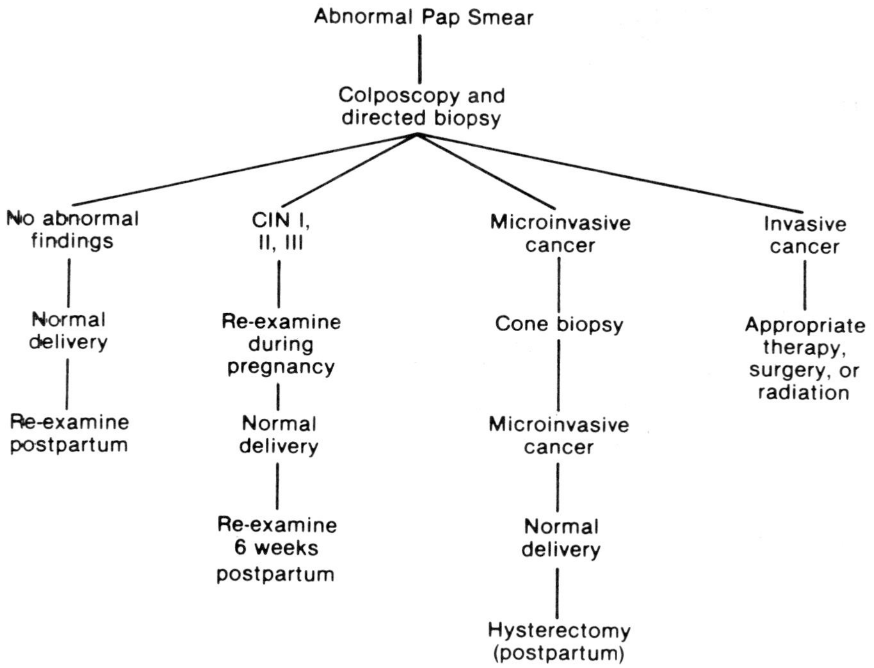

Figure 2. Therapy for the pregnant patient.

the margins. The recurrence rate is much greater when the involved glands are 3 mm or greater below the basement membrane.

CRYOSURGERY AND LASER THERAPY

Cryosurgery and laser therapy are useful in treating many gynecological problems but are not the techniques of choice in treating CIN. These techniques result in destruction of tissues needed for diagnosis and may interfere with fertility and obscure the squamocolumnar junction, rendering future colposcopic evaluation inadequate.

A study of patients treated at the University of Pennsylvania without cryosurgery and laser evaporation revealed that 45 per cent had normal findings following colposcopy, 35 per cent had normal findings following colposcopy with biopsies, and 10 per cent had conization, less than 1 per cent had invasive cancer, and 14 per cent had stable disease. Most of the women with stable disease had infertility problems and requested conservative management.

PREGNANCY

Colposcopic evaluation of the cervix during pregnancy is technically difficult. There is thick tenacious mucus, the squamocolumnar junction is difficult to visualize, and the increased vascularity limits the size and number of biopsies. The majority of pregnant women with abnormal cytology can be managed conservatively with colposcopy and limited biopsies. If there is no evidence of invasion, a vaginal delivery is permitted, and the patient is recolposcoped 6 weeks post partum.

A cone biopsy during pregnancy is rarely indicated and should only be performed when suspected invasion or colposcopic biopsy–proven microinvasion is found. Conization during pregnancy is ideally performed during the second trimester. If microinvasion is found on cone biopsy, the pregnancy is allowed to continue and a vaginal delivery permitted, with hysterectomy recommended at the time of delivery or 6 weeks post partum.

The treatment of invasive cancer during pregnancy varies with trimester and the patient's desires and medical status. If the cancer is found early in the pregnancy, a radical hysterectomy with pelvic and para-aortic node dissection or radiation therapy is recommended. The 5 year survival and loss of fetus rates are the same. If the cancer is found during the third trimester, the pregnancy is allowed to continue to viability, at which time a cesarean section, radical hysterectomy, and node dissection might be performed. A cesarean section followed by radiation therapy is an alternative to surgery; both have the same 5 year survival rates (Figure 2).

STAGING SYSTEM

The FIGO classification of cervical cancer is a clinical system (Table 1). Biopsy, physical examination, and intravenous pylography are the only methods allowed in determining the stage of cervical cancer.

The most important aspect in evaluating the patient with cervical cancer is the clinical stage, since this will determine the type of treatment and the prognosis. The evaluation should include the following: x-ray films: chest, IVP, barium enema; blood work: CBC, platelets, chemistry; scans: liver, spleen, CT; biopsies

TABLE 1. **FIGO Classification in Carcinoma of the Cervix Uteri**

PREINVASIVE CARCINOMA	
Stage 0	Carcinoma in situ.
Stage I	Carcinoma strictly confined to cervix.
	Stage IA Microinvasive carcinoma (early stromal invasion).
	Stage IB All other cases of stage I. Occult cancer should be marked "occ."
Stage II	The carcinoma extends beyond the cervix but has not extended to the pelvic wall. The carcinoma involves the vagina but not the lower third.
	Stage IIA No obvious parametrial involvement.
	Stage IIB Obvious parametrial involvement.
Stage III	The carcinoma has extended to the pelvic wall. On rectal examination there is no cancer-free space between the tumor and the pelvic wall. The tumor involves the lower third of the vagina. All cases with a nonfunctioning kidney should be included, unless they are known to be due to other causes.
	Stage IIIA No extension to the pelvic wall.
	Stage IIIB Extension to the pelvic wall and/or hydronephrosis or nonfunctioning kidney.
Stage IV	The carcinoma has extended beyond the true pelvis or clinically involves the mucosa of the bladder or rectum. A bullous edema as such does not permit a case to be allotted to stage IV.
	Stage IVA Spread of the growth to adjacent organs.
	Stage IVB Spread to distant organs.

of any glands or suspected metastases; EKG; evaluation of all findings; cystoscopy and sigmoidoscopy. All of these studies ensure proper therapy and the best results.

Treatment

The treatment of cervical intraepithelial neoplasia is controversial. Therapy is determined by the stage, class, and evaluation of the disease and the desires of the patient.

Stage 0

CIN III is not included in any statistics of invasive cancer but is considered a premalignant condition. If left untreated, over 70 per cent progress to invasive carcinoma. Treatment includes conization or simple hysterectomy and is determined by the patient's desire to have children. Conservative therapy is chosen for those who wish to have more children, whereas hysterectomy is considered the treatment of choice in those who are not interested in further childbearing.

Stage IA

Stage IA is treated by simple hysterectomy without node dissection. This may be either vaginal or abdominal. The ovaries are usually not removed, since this is not a hormonal-dependent tumor.

Stage IB or IIA

Stage IB or early IIA can be treated by either a radical hysterectomy with pelvic and para-aortic node dissection or radiation therapy. The advantages of surgery include preservation of ovarian function and avoiding exposing the young patient to the long-term effects of radiation changes.

Stages II, III, and IV

Stages IIB, III, and IV are best treated with radiation therapy. The standard radiation therapy for cervical carcinoma includes external and internal irradiation. The external therapy consists of 4,500 to 5,000 rads, delivered over 5 weeks, using 15 × 15 cm anterior and posterior portals. Internal radiation is given by a Fletcher-Suit applicator and tandem with cesium sources to deliver 3,000 rads to point A, which is 2 cm into the external os and 2 cm lateral from the endocervical canal; 1,000 rads is delivered to point B, which is 5 cm lateral to the center. This is given in one or two applications.

Recurrent Cancer

If there is recurrence after surgery, radiation therapy is used. If there is recurrence after radiation and the carcinoma is limited to the pelvis, a pelvic exenteration is performed removing the bladder, vagina, cervix, uterus, and rectum. The cure rate over 5 years is 35 to 65 per cent. Approximately 50 per cent of patients with recurrent disease have resectable disease limited to the pelvis.

Chemotherapy has been used, but the results are poor. The agents being used are only in the early stages of development. Much more research and newer drugs are needed.

CARCINOMA OF THE VULVA

method of
HOWARD D. HOMESLEY, M.D.
Bowman Gray School of Medicine of Wake Forest University
Winston-Salem, North Carolina

Vulvar carcinoma accounts for less than 1 to 2 per cent of genital tract malignancies. Carcinoma of the vulva is the fourth least common gynecologic malignancy, being exceeded in descending order by cancer of the endometrium, ovary, and cervix. Carcinoma of the vulva usually presents in elderly women, with the highest incidence in the seventh decade. Approximately 95 per cent of vulvar carcinomas are squamous cell carcinoma. Radical vulvectomy and bilateral inguinal node dissection is the usual method of surgical therapy in the United States.

In the past decade, there has been either an increased awareness or an actual increased incidence of vulvar intraepithelial neoplasia (VIN) or preinvasive lesions of the vulva, which can usually be treated with conservative local wide resection. Concurrently, there has been an attempt to define a subset of patients with small, superficially invasive vulvar lesions suitable for less radical surgical procedures. Thus, treatment of vulvar lesions can be individualized, based on careful assessment of significant clinical and histopathologic findings.

Preinvasive Lesions of the Vulva

Vulvar Intraepithelial Neoplasia (VIN)

Vulvar intraepithelial neoplasia (VIN) is a histologic continuum from mild, moderate, and severe dysplasia to carcinoma in situ, including the Bowen's disease variant of carcinoma in situ. VIN is analogous to cervical intraepithelial neoplasia (CIN). VIN is now frequently diagnosed in premenopausal patients, not uncommonly in patients in their 20s. The most common complaints are irritative symptoms related to the vulva, such as pruritus, discharge, or local discomfort. Every patient with a complaint of vulvar irritation, either acute or chronic, must undergo careful examination of the vulva. Any presumed inflammatory lesion of the vulva that does not respond rapidly to topical therapy requires biopsy. Any lesion that presents as ulcerated, indurated, or nodular should be biopsied immediately. Condylomatous-like lesions, especially extensive, coalescent, or flat areas, should be biopsied, as the most experienced examiner may be unable to distinguish clinically among carcinoma in situ, early invasive carcinoma, and extensive condylomatous vulvar lesions.

The best technique to determine the site for biopsy includes visual and colposcopic inspection of the vulva. For the latter, 1 per cent acetic acid is first applied to the vulva. Discrete white, slightly raised areas of carcinoma in situ can be appreciated colposcopically.

To enhance areas of VIN lesions, 1 per cent toluidine blue dye can be applied to the vulva, allowed to dry, and rinsed away with 1 per cent acetic acid. Areas that retain this nuclear stain have increased nuclear density and are considered suspicious for VIN. As an office procedure, the vulva can be biopsied using local anesthesia, either with a dermal punch or a knife incision. Discrete lesions 2 to 3 cm in size can be completely excised in the office under local anesthesia.

Patients with VIN may have multiple sites of intraepithelial neoplasia involving the vulva (VIN), vagina (VAIN), and cervix (CIN). These patients require full evaluation for concurrent or subsequent development of genital intraepithelial neoplasia (GIN) in any of these sites.

Wide local excision of single or multiple VIN lesions with primary closure can be accomplished. Recently, effective and better cosmetic results have been obtained with CO_2 laser excision or vaporization of VIN lesions. Laser vaporization is very useful in the young, sexually active patient in whom full preservation of vulvar anatomy and sexual function is important. Often these patients may have extensive lesions and may require multiple treatments for recurrent or new VIN lesions. Multiple biopsies of suspected VIN lesions are mandatory to confirm the diagnosis prior to performance of laser vaporization. Laser excision for histologic verification can be combined with extensive laser vaporization.

Topical chemotherapy with 5-fluorouracil cream (Efudex) applied twice daily to treat VIN has been advocated as a conservative approach, especially in younger women. However, local excision or CO_2 laser vaporization usually is more satisfactory for almost all patients than is topical chemotherapy, which is not as effective and often must be continued for at least 6 to 8 weeks.

Paget's Disease

Paget's disease of the vulva is usually an intraepithelial lesion but can be associated with an invasive adenocarcinoma in underlying apocrine glands. The usual presentation is as a pruritic, bright red, scaling, raised area with some white patches. For Paget's disease a vulvectomy is performed. If invasive carcinoma is discovered, bilateral inguinal node dissection is recommended. Frozen sections and multiple permanent sections are required to determine the free margins of surgical resection in patients with Paget's disease as lesion extent is often greater than is clinically appreciated.

Vulvar Dystrophy

Vulvar dystrophies, which have been classified into either atrophic, hypertrophic, or mixed, with or without atypia, usually present postmenopausally and can be confused with VIN and invasive lesions of the vulva. The malignant potential for vulvar dystrophies is less than 5 per cent. However, in a recent study of the Gynecologic Oncology Group (GOG), a National Cancer Institute–sponsored collaborative group of nearly 40 institutions in the United States, 35 per cent of patients with invasive squamous cell carcinoma of the vulva had the associated finding of vulvar dystrophy. Use of 1 per cent toluidine blue and 1 per cent acetic acid can determine the best site for biopsy of the patient with suspected vulvar dystrophy. Because of the malignant potential, these patients must have scrupulous follow-up.

The usual therapy for patients with hypertrophic dystrophy consists of application of topical steroid medication. Atrophic dystrophy or lichen sclerosus et atrophicus often can be controlled with topical 2 per cent testosterone proprionate in petrolatum applied two to three times daily. Vulvectomy had been used in the past as last resort therapy; however, this is of limited benefit as this chronic condition often recurs. CO_2 laser vaporization for vulvar dystrophy appears to be of similar limited benefit, although large numbers of patients have not been treated by this method. CO_2 laser vaporization has been attempted only after all other management has failed to control symptoms.

Invasive Carcinoma of the Vulva

FIGO Staging. Previously nearly all patients with invasive squamous cell carcinoma of the vulva were treated primarily with radical vulvectomy and bilateral inguinal node dissection regardless of FIGO staging (Table 1). This approach has been based upon the characteristic initial regional inguinal node spread pattern of invasive carcinoma of the vulva. FIGO staging is determined by lesion size, clinical assessment of inguinal node status for presence or absence of node metastasis, and lesion location. Stage I lesions confined to the vulva are not associated with any clinical evidence of palpably suspicious groin nodes. However, lesions larger than 2 cm in diameter can be either stage II (no clinically suspicious nodes) or stage III (clinically suspicious inguinal nodes). Regardless of lesion diameter size, if clinically suspicious inguinal nodes are present the patient is classified as stage III.

Actual inguinal node status is of paramount significance in planning individualized treatment. Five year survival in patients with negative groin nodes is about 90 per cent. When inguinal node metastasis is present, 5 year survival is 40 to 45 per cent. Therefore, the presence or absence of inguinal node metastasis is a primary prognostic determinant of success of treatment by radical vulvectomy and bilateral inguinal node dissection.

Lymph Node Spread Pattern. Most commonly, lymphatic spread of a unilateral lesion is to the ipsilateral regional lymphatics, with first involvement of superficial and deep inguinal lymph nodes. Subsequent metastasis is then to the pelvic nodes through the femoral canal involving Cloquet's node, which is medial to the femoral vein beneath the inguinal ligament. The external iliac nodes, obturator nodes, and subsequently the common iliac nodes are involved. Direct extension to the pelvic nodes such as the external iliac, obturator, internal iliac, and common iliac nodes without involvement of the groin nodes is rare. However, a lesion involving the clitoris or midline of the vulva can spread unilaterally or bilaterally to inguinal lymph nodes.

TABLE 1. **FIGO Classification for Staging of Carcinoma of the Vulva**

STAGE I	All lesions confined to the vulva with a maximum diameter of 2 cm or less and no suspicious groin nodes
STAGE II	All lesions confined to the vulva with a diameter greater than 2 cm and no suspicious groin nodes
STAGE III	Lesions extending beyond the vulva without grossly positive groin nodes or lesions confined to the vulva with suspicious or grossly positive groin nodes
STAGE IV	Lesions extending beyond the vulva with grossly positive nodes or involvement of mucosa of rectum, bladder, urethra, or bone. Patients with distant or palpable deep pelvic masses are included with stage IV

Prognostic Factors. The Gynecologic Oncology Group (GOG) has performed a study to determine the significance of various prognostic factors related to the FIGO staging factors of lesion size, clinical status of inguinal lymph nodes, and lesion location. Lesion size can be readily assessed and is an important prognostic factor upon which therapy can be based. However, clinical examination of inguinal nodes by experienced examiners is fraught with a 25 to 30 per cent error in assessing histologic incidence of inguinal lymph node metastasis. Lesion location, except for midline lesions of the clitoris or perineum that might be associated with bilateral inguinal node metastasis, is more often a reflection of lesion extent whereby extensive lesions can involve the urethra, vagina, or anus. Other factors that have been considered to be of possible prognostic importance are depth of tumor invasion and histologic grade.

From an assessment of over 500 patients by the GOG, it is apparent, as noted in Table 2, that there is a relationship between FIGO stage and incidence of groin node metastasis. The 2 cm or less stage I lesion is noted to have a 10 per cent incidence of positive groin node metastasis. When the lesion is greater than 2 cm in diameter, the incidence of positive nodal metastasis is markedly increased to 31 per cent. There is a much higher inguinal node involvement in stages III (55 per cent) and IV (40 per cent) patients.

The importance of lesion size is more apparent, as noted in Table 3, where there is no major difference in lymph node metastasis in patients with lesions less

TABLE 2. **Relationship of FIGO Stage to Positive Groin Nodes***

FIGO Stage	Per Cent of Positive Groin Nodes (No. of Patients)
I	10 (142)
II	31 (191)
III	55 (195)
IV	40 (5)
TOTAL	35 (533)

*Gynecologic Oncology Group—Protocol 36.

TABLE 3. **Relationship of Tumor Diameter to Positive Groin Nodes***

Tumor Diameter (cm)	Per Cent of Positive Groin Nodes (No. of Patients)
≤1	16 (55)
1.1–2	18 (120)
2.1–3	34 (161)
3.1–4	56 (73)
4.1–5	43 (44)
>5.1	51 (71)

*Gynecologic Oncology Group—Protocol 36.

than 1 cm or 1 to 2 cm in diameter. The lower incidence of 10 per cent for lesions 2 cm or less in size, as noted in Table 2 for stage I, can be accounted for because stage I patients cannot have suspicious clinical groin node metastasis. If the lesion is less than 2 cm in size but clinicallly suspicious inguinal nodes are present, then 16 to 18 per cent of the patients may have inguinal node metastasis (Table 3). However, there is a dramatic increase in inguinal node metastasis in patients with lesions larger than 2 cm (34 to 56 per cent).

There does appear to be a relationship between depth of penetration of the tumor and inguinal node metastasis (Table 4). This appears to become greatly increased beyond 2 mm of tumor penetration. However, the probability of lymph node metastasis is primarily based on the combined assessment of depth of penetration of tumor and lesion size. There is a close correlation in that the greater the lesion size the deeper the tumor penetration. Thus, a lesion of less than 2 cm and less than 2 mm of invasion would have a low incidence of inguinal node metastasis; however, a small lesion with deep invasion may still be at high risk of having inguinal node spread even if there were no palpably suspicious inguinal nodes present.

There are conflicting reports because of lack of standardization of histologic grading of vulvar carcinoma as to the value of grading the tumors in order to predict inguinal node involvement. The GOG criteria for histologic grading is defined as the per cent of tumor area with an undifferentiated pattern: grade 1, less than 30 per cent; grade 2, 30 to 49 per cent; and grade 3, greater than 50 per cent. GOG histologic grading does correlate with inguinal node status (Table 5).

The most important prognostic factors in the GOG analysis related to positive inguinal nodes were identified in order of descending significance as clinically palpable nodes, undifferentiated histologic grade, depth of tumor penetration, and tumor diameter. However, one must combine all characteristics of the lesion to most accurately predict inguinal node status. When the nodes were not clinically palpable, the risk of positive nodes was 5 per cent in grade 1 tumors of 2 cm or less in diameter. This increased to 34 per cent in grade 3 tumors of more than 2 cm in diameter. The tumor location, conventional histologic grading, and vascular involvement did not correlate with positive inguinal nodes.

TABLE 4. **Relationship of Depth of Tumor Invasion to Positive Groin Nodes***

Depth of Tumor Invasion (mm)	Per Cent of Positive Groin Nodes (No. of Patients)
≤1	4 (28)
2	9 (54)
3	19 (54)
4	31 (64)
5	37 (52)
6–10	46 (175)
>11	51 (80)

*Gynecologic Oncology Group—Protocol 36.

Low Risk Disease. From analysis of over 500 patients by the GOG and review of reports of others, the risk of groin node metastasis can now be classified into low risk and high risk based on assessment of the combination of lesion size, depth of penetration of the tumor, and possibly histologic grading along with groin node clinical examination. The reproducibility of histologic grading results awaits confirmation by other pathologists as there has been no prior standardization of histologic grading of vulvar lesions.

Five year survival for stage I carcinoma of the vulvar patients treated with radical vulvectomy and bilateral groin dissection exceeds 90 per cent when the patient has no evidence of inguinal lymph node metastasis at operation. When the lesion is not in the midline, it is rare for there to be contralateral lymph node involvement without ipsilateral metastasis. Therefore, currently a GOG study is attempting to define which patients may be suitable for less extensive therapy than radical vulvectomy and bilateral groin dissection. This is a cautious approach to define low risk disease. The patient with a unilateral lesion first undergoes a wide local excision with greater than 2 cm skin margins and deep resection of subcutaneous fat of vulvar lesions 2 cm or less in diameter. The excised lesion is then evaluated for depth of penetration. If less than a 5 mm invasion from the lesion surface is noted, an ipsilateral groin node dissection is performed. If there is no evidence of inguinal node metastasis, then it is anticipated that the patient is at low risk for having recurrent disease. If positive inguinal nodes are present, the standard operation of radical vulvectomy and bilateral inguinal dissection is performed.

High Risk Disease. In patients with clinically positive or confirmed inguinal node metastasis, CT scan–directed fine needle aspiration of para-aortic nodes or extraperitoneal or transperitoneal exploration of the abdomen can confirm extensive distant metastasis to para-aortic lymph nodes, which would militate against vulvar resection. When exenterative procedures or radical resection are unacceptable, extensive radiation therapy, often combining external beam and implant therapy, may offer control for locally advanced vulvar

TABLE 5. **Relationship of GOG Histologic Grade to Positive Groin Nodes***

GOG Histologic Grade	Per Cent Positive Groin Nodes (No. of Patients)
I	16 (179)
II	44 (141)
III	57 (141)

*Gynecologic Oncology Group—Protocol 36.

carcinoma and even possible cure if the tumor is confined to the treatment field.

Radiation Therapy

If the inguinal nodes are positive for metastasis, then pelvic lymphadenectomy has been recommended. Because of the poor prognosis in patients with pelvic node metastasis, recently the GOG has explored the role of radiation therapy in control of regional metastasis to groin and pelvic nodes. A randomized study was performed to determine the benefit and morbidity of adding adjunctive radiation to the pelvic and groin for patients with positive groin nodes, compared with surgery alone consisting of radical vulvectomy, bilateral groin dissection, and pelvic dissection on the positive groin node side(s). Radiation therapy to the bilateral groin, obturator foramen, and external and internal iliac nodes was given. Patients received 4500 to 5000 rads to the plane of the pelvis, halfway between the superior border of the obturator foramen and the L5-S1 interspace, at the rate of 180 to 200 rads per day. A second dose calculation was made to the center of the inguinal and femoral nodal area at a depth of 2 to 3 cm from the anterior surface. In 5 to 6.5 weeks, a 4500 to 5000 rad tumor dose was given. Electron beams were used for anterior boosts.

Radiation therapy added to radical vulvectomy and bilateral groin dissection was superior to pelvic node dissection alone. Survivals were significantly higher for the radiation group, and there were fewer groin recurrences.

Chemotherapy

Chemotherapy has not proved useful in therapy of advanced or recurrent squamous cell carcinoma of the vulva. In the GOG cisplatin study in vulvar carcinoma, no substantial activity was detected.

Malignant Melanoma

Although rare, malignant melanoma is the second most common vulvar malignancy. Traditionally radical vulvectomy and bilateral inguinofemoral lymphadenectomy has been the recommended therapy for all patients with malignant melanoma. However, the histopathologic features of assessment of levels of invasion and tumor volume measurement of maximum diameter of the primary lesion may be as predictive as for nonvulvar melanomas. Currently, the GOG is collecting histopathologic data on all FIGO stages of malignant melanoma in order to clarify the proper role of less radical surgery, such as hemivulvectomy and ipsilateral inguinal node dissection in patients with favorable small, superficial lesions.

Surgical Technique

Radical Vulvectomy. Radical vulvectomy can be performed before or after the bilateral groin node dissection. The groin node dissection can be done first to allow for lymph node analysis by frozen section in case pelvic node dissection is planned if inguinal nodes are positive. To perform the radical vulvectomy a circumferential incision is made to permit removal of the entire vulva and most of the mons pubis. The incision is begun on the mons pubis and carried laterally along the labiocrural folds bilaterally to join at the perineum. The inner margin of resection is along the vaginal mucosa, whereby the labia majora and the labia minora with clitoris are completely resected. The lateral incisions are carried deeply to expose the tendons of the underlying muscles of the urogenital diaphragm. Upon removal of the specimen, the perineum is reconstructed with approximation of the levator muscles anterior to the rectum. Primary closure usually can be accomplished by reapproximation of mobilized skin and vaginal mucosa.

Inguinal Node Dissection. Either bilateral vertical or transverse inguinal incisions or one incision can be made extending medially from the anterior superior iliac spine above the inguinal ligament, curving to the midline above the mons pubis and extending in a similar fashion to the opposite anterior superior iliac spine. After completing the skin incision, skin flaps are developed with exposure of the external oblique fascia superior to the inguinal ligament, the fascia lata lateral to the femoral vessels, and the fascia of the adductor longus muscle medially. Distally the femoral artery and vein are exposed beyond the entrance of the saphenous vein into the femoral vein. The group of inguinal lymph nodes superficial to the cribriform fascia can be dissected as a separate superficial group of nodes at this time. Ligatures are placed distally across lymphatics and ligated separately to reduce lymphatic drainage and minimize later lymphocyst development. The fascia lata is divided longitudinally and retracted medially. The superficial external pudendal artery is ligated. The saphenous vein at its entrance into the femoral vein is ligated. All deep inguinal node tissue is resected distally from the femoral canal at the inguinal ligament for 8 to 10 cm. Nodal tissue medial to the femoral vein is designated Cloquet's node and submitted as a separate specimen. The resection of the superficial and deep groin nodes is accomplished in a similar fashion bilaterally.

Pelvic Node Dissection. The pelvic node dissection is carried out only on the side containing positive inguinal nodes. If bilateral positive inguinal nodes are detected, a bilateral pelvic node dissection is performed. An incision is made through the aponeurosis of the external oblique muscle paralleling the inguinal ligament. The incision is extended along the inguinal ligament upward to the anterior superior iliac spine. The internal oblique muscle bundle is divided. The round ligament and the inferior epigastric vessels are divided and ligated. The peritoneum is retracted upward and medially. The pelvic lymph nodes, including the external iliac, obturator, and internal iliac, are dissected to the bifurcation of the iliac vessels and submitted as separate specimens. The common iliac nodes are also removed. The wound is closed by reapproximation of internal and external oblique fascia. If the incision is extended, retroperitoneal node dissection can include sampling of the para-aortic nodes. If noninvasive means have not detected para-aortic spread in patients with very extensive inguinal nodal metastasis, retroperitoneal exposure of the para-aortic nodes can be performed first to determine the most distant spread of disease.

Operative Technique. One must attempt to avoid trauma to the margins of the skin flaps to improve healing. After the tissue has been undermined and before closure, vascular compromise can be recognized, especially at the edge of the lower groin skin flap. This can be prophylactically resected for a 4 to 5 cm width prior to closure to reduce the need for later debridement. The electrocautery can be used to make the incision and coagulate bleeders during the procedure. The vulvar incision can be modified, depending upon lesion location.

Retroperitoneal and/or groin dissection lymphatic drainage postoperatively is best achieved with Hemovac or a Jackson-Pratt type of suction drainage. The sartorius muscles can be transposed over the femoral vessels by division proximally of the sartorius muscle near its insertion at the anterior iliac spine. The transposed sartorius muscles will cover the femoral vessels if extensive necrosis of inguinal skin occurs.

Perioperative Management. Commonly, broad-spectrum prophylactic antibiotics are given perioperatively. Patients can be ambulated within 24 to 48 hours. Intermittent venous calf compression can be used to prevent deep venous thrombosis. The most common complication is wound infection. Usually this is controlled with local debridement. Most patients remain in the hospital postoperatively for 14 to 21 days. Long-term disability secondary to moderate and severe lymphedema of the lower extremities occurred in 3 and 10 per cent of the GOG patients. Surgical mortality is 1 to 2 per cent.

THROMBOPHLEBITIS IN OBSTETRICS AND GYNECOLOGY

method of
CHI V. DANG, M.D., PhD,
and WILLIAM R. BELL, M.D.
The Johns Hopkins Hospital Medical Institutions
Baltimore, Maryland

Thrombophlebitis is the occurrence of a thrombus within the lumen of a vein associated with inflammation of the vessel wall or perivascular tissue. Symptoms and signs of thrombophlebitis are caused by the obstruction of venous outflow or the associated inflammation. Venous thrombi are formed usually in association with stasis of blood flow with or without damage of the vessel wall. The venous thrombus, consisting of cellular elements and plasma proteins held together by fibrin, adheres to the vessel wall at its point of initiation and has a free-floating portion that may grow or fracture to form an embolus or emboli.

Venous thromboembolism, the second commonest cause of maternal mortality during pregnancy, may result in serious sequelae, primarily because of the risk of fatal pulmonary embolism. Thrombi from the lower extremities embolize to the pulmonary circulation with a frequency of approximately 20 per cent. Major emboli often arise from veins above the knee, which result from proximal propagation of calf venous thrombosis. The overall mortality from symptomatic pulmonary embolism is about 30 per cent.

Thrombophlebitis may occur in the superficial veins or in the deep veins of the extremities or body cavities. Superficial thrombophlebitis is more common than deep vein phlebitis. In the hospitalized patient superficial phlebitis usually results from intravenous therapy. Deep vein phlebitis occurs most commonly in the midgastrocnemius area in postoperative patients. Gynecologic patients are managed in the same manner as other surgical patients. Thrombophlebitis must be considered and managed differently in the pregnant patient. During normal pregnancy a hypercoagulable state may occur as the result of increases in factors VII, VIII, IX, and fibrinogen and a decline in fibrinolytic activity. This probably accounts for the fivefold increased risk for thrombosis in pregnant women as compared with nonpregnant women in the same age group.

SUPERFICIAL THROMBOPHLEBITIS

Superficial thrombophlebitis commonly results from intravenous therapy and occurs in about 1 per cent or less of pregnancies. In the pregnant patient, superficial thrombophlebitis is about six times more common in the postpartum than during the antepartum period. Spontaneous superficial thrombophlebitis may occur in the lower extremities and is usually more common in the calf veins than in those of the thigh. Superficial thrombophlebitis involving either the upper or lower extremities is usually benign and self-limiting and extremely rarely results in emboli. The diagnosis is certain with the presence of a warm, erythematous, tender, and palpable firm knot or cord in the course of a superficial vein. Lymphangitis is the other entity in the differential diagnosis and is not associated with a knot or cord. Hospitalization is necessary when the phlebitis extends into the inguinal area within the long saphenous trunk. Extension of phlebitis into the deep veins may terminate in fatal pulmonary embolism.

Superficial thrombophlebitis of either lower or upper extemities is managed by elevation of the involved area 10 cm above the right atrium, avoidance of dependency, application of warm wet compresses or heating pads, and bed rest to avoid weight bearing on the involved extremity. When the acute discomfort has disappeared (usually 3 to 4 days), the patient should gradually return to normal daily activities. The residual cord will slowly disappear within several months. If systemic symptoms such as fever, diaphoresis, anorexia, and generalized malaise are associated with superficial thrombophlebitis, the patient should be treated as previously mentioned and in addition be fully anticoagulated with heparin. When these abnormal features disappear (4 to 7 days), the heparin anticoagulation should be discontinued and normal activities progressively resumed. Subsequent warfarin therapy is usually not necessary. Prophylactic anticoagulation therapy appears unjustified, and the use of elastic hose has not been proven efficacious. Anti-inflammatory agents such as salicylates should be avoided in the antepartum period because of possible premature closure of the fetal ductus arteriosus.

DEEP VENOUS THROMBOSIS

Deep venous thrombisis (DVT) is infrequent (less than 0.5 per cent of pregnancies) in the gravid state, but it may occur in 20 per cent of the postoperative gynecologic patients as determined by the ^{125}I-fibrinogen test. An increased risk for DVT is associated with surgery for gynecologic malignancies. The clinical diagnosis of DVT is difficult and may be mimicked by other disease processes. Induration of the muscle, unilateral edema, calf tenderness, and unilateral ankle swelling occur in order of decreasing frequency with DVT. A sudden swelling of an entire leg showing increased superficial venous pattern and tenderness over the femoral triangle suggest deep ileofemoral thrombophlebitis. Ascending venography is the most accurately reliable technique to identify venous thrombosis in the upper and lower extremities. Disadvantages are discomfort, expense, and a 1 per cent or less frequency of postvenography phlebitis. Venography is not recommended for the pregnant patient because of radiation-related risks. Similarly, ^{125}I-fibrinogen cannot be used. Noninvasive testing should be used extensively. Impedance phlethysmography is most accurate for identifying thrombosis in the venous system proximal to the knee and is suitable for the pregnant patient.

When the deep venous system is occluded by thrombi, prompt fibrinolysis or anticoagulation is indicated. If thrombus formation is present in the thigh and extends into the inferior vena cava or is present in the upper extremity, thrombolytic therapy is indicated. If DVT is limited distal to the popliteal area, heparin therrapy is probably the treatment of choice. Thrombolytic therapy may be considered if heparin therapy fails. The patient should be at bed rest with elevation of the involved extremity 10 cm above the level of the right atrium to decrease edema and the associated discomfort.

SEPTIC THROMBOPHLEBITIS

Septic thrombophlebitis is present in virtually 100 per cent of patients with septicemia and DVT. In addition to the treatment for DVT (as previously discussed), aggressive treatment with generous doses of the indicated antibiotics is necessary. A third generation cephalosporin, moxalactam (Moxam), should be avoided because of associated hemorrhagic complications due to hypoprothrombinemia and platelet dysfunction. If medical therapy fails, surgical extirpation of the involved vessel may be necessary.

The syndrome of puerperal ovarian vein thrombophlebitis is characterized by the cardinal feature of lower abdominal pain, usually associated with fever, occurring 2 to 3 days after delivery. The right ovarian vein is affected more often than the left ovarian vein, and in about 40 per cent of cases a deep tender abdominal mass is palpable. Pelvic thrombophlebitis is thought to be a serious sequela to puerperal metritis. Sonography and computed axial tomography may be helpful in identifying this disorder. Full dose heparinization (as hereafter) and generous doses of antibiotics (covering gram-negative and anaerobic organisms) should be immediately instituted. If adequate anticoagulation and antibiotic treatment fail in 3 to 5 days, operative intervention appears justified.

Treatment

Thromboprophylaxis

Prophylactic treatment with low dose heparin, 5,000 USP units subcutaneously every 12 hours, should be considered in high risk pregnant patients in the third trimester until the onset of labor. Low dose heparin with or without dihydroergotamine may be used in the gynecologic patient. Ambulation, when not contraindicated, should be encouraged.

Heparin Therapy

Heparin is the drug of choice for treatment of DVT in the pregnant patient because it does not cross the placental barrier. Baseline studies including prothrombin time (PT), activated partial thromboplastin time (APTT), Lee-White clotting time, and a complete blood count (red cells, white cells, and platelets) are obtained before starting therapy. Continous intravenous infusion therapy is initiated by a loading dose of heparin, 5,000 USP units of heparin intravenously over 10 minutes (10,000 units of heparin for weight greater than 95 kg), followed by a constant infusion,

24,000 to 30,000 units of heparin in 1 liter of 5 per cent dextrose, to be infused over 24 hours.

Theraputic anticoagulation is achieved when the Lee-White clotting time (normal 8 to 15 minutes) is greater than 20 minutes and less than 40 minutes. If APTT is used, it should be two to three times baseline normal APTT. The Lee-White clotting time or APTT should be determined at 6, 12, and 24 hours after the initiation of therapy, every 12 hours for 2 to 3 days, and then once daily for the duration of intravenous heparin therapy. The patient should remain at bed rest until weight can be supported by the affected extremity without discomfort. Warfarin therapy (see later section) should be started 48 hours before the discontinuation of heparin in gynecologic patients. Following full dose heparin therapy, subsequent therapy in the pregnant patient may be achieved by adjusted dose subcutaneous heparin therapy, since warfarin should be avoided. Subcutaneous heparin, 10,000 units, is administered every 12 hours. The dose is set by adjusting the dose given over the first 3 days of therapy to maintain the APTT, measured 6 hours after injection, at 1.5 times the control normal APTT. After the dose is adjusted no further monitoring is necessary for the long-term (12 weeks) therapy. Therapy should be stopped in the peripartum period and may be resumed post partum.

Thrombolytic Therapy

Two thrombolytic agents, streptokinase (SK) and urokinase (UK), are approved for use. Streptokinase is derived from cultured streptococci, and urokinase is collected from human urine and fetal kidney cell cultures. UK is much more expensive than SK and is reserved for patients with potential adverse allergic reactions to SK.

Thrombolytic therapy is indicated in proximal thrombophlebitis above the knee and especially when pulmonary embolism is suspected or documented in addition to DVT. It should not be used in the peripartum period and is not recommended for use in the pregnant patient. However, if a refractory situation is encountered and by default thrombolytic therapy is selected, SK is probably the agent of choice since it does not cross the placental barrier. Theoretically, thrombolytic therapy may induce premature separation, and therefore caution is suggested. Thrombolytic therapy has the advantage over heparin therapy of faster dissolution of thrombi and results in less postphlebitic changes and venous insufficiency because of venous valve function preservation. Significant thrombolysis is achieved when thrombolytic therapy is initiated within 7 days of the onset of symptoms. Patients with obstructing pelvic or abdominal neoplasms responded as well as patients without obstructing tumors. Disadvantages are febrile and allergic reactions with SK. Thrombolytic therapy is absolutely contraindicated in patients with active bleeding, recent cerebrovascular accident, intracranial neoplasms, or head trauma. Relative contraindications are recent (less than 10 days) major surgery, obstetric delivery, organ biopsy, puncture of noncompressible organ, serious GI bleeding, serious trauma, and severe arterial hypertension. Minor relative contraindications include pregnancy, minor trauma, left-sided intracardiac thrombus, bacterial endocarditis, diabetic hemorrhagic retinopathy, hemostatic defects, and age of 75 years or greater.

Baseline laboratory studies (hematocrit valve, platelet count, PT, APTT, and thrombin time [TT]) are performed before therapy. If heparin has been started, it should be discontinued 2 to 3 hours before beginning thrombolytic therapy. A loading dose of SK, 250,000 units, or UK, 4,000 units per kg body weight, is given intravenously over 30 minutes followed by a continous infusion of SK, 100,000 units per hour, or UK, 2,000 units per kg body weight per hour. The thrombin time is determined at 4 hours after starting the continous infusion and every 12 hours for the duration of thrombolytic therapy. It should be between 1.5 to 5 times the preinfusion normal TT.

Thrombolytic therapy is continued for 48 to 72 hours, as the mean lysis time for DVT is 36 hours. Full dose intravenous heparinization is started without a loading dose 3 hours after terminating thrombolytic therapy. Warfarin may be started 2 days before the end of the 7 to 10 day course of heparin.

Warfarin Therapy

Warfarin therapy should be avoided during pregnancy, especially in the first trimester, since warfarin crosses the placenta and has been reported to cause congenital malformations. In addition, significant fetal losses result from fetal hemorrhage owing to the trauma of delivery. During the second and third trimesters of pregnancy or in the gynecologic patient warfarin may be instituted with the awareness of possible drug/warfarin interactions. Although warfarin may appear in breast milk, it is not associated with hemorrhage or prolonged PT in breast-fed infants and thus may be used in the postpartum period.

Warfarin therapy is started by giving 20 to 25 mg warfarin on day 1 and 5 mg on day 2; PT is checked on the morning of day 3. The maintenance dose is that amount of warfarin required to prolong the PT to between 18 and 25 seconds (normal control 11 to 12 seconds). The duration of warfarin therapy is 3 weeks for a young active patient with known traumatic etiology for DVT, 6 weeks for a patient without risk factors, and 6 months for patients with risk factors such as immobilization, obesity, congestive heart failure, past history of DVT, or diabetes mellitus.

Surgical Therapy

Surgical therapy for DVT includes ligation or removal of the affected vessels and partial interruption of venous flow to prevent embolic events. None of these modalities reverses the thrombotic process. In general venous interruption for the management of DVT is not necessary. Surgical therapy may be employed in rare situations where patients cannot be treated medically or when therapy fails, as in some cases of septic thrombophlebitis.

CONTRACEPTION

method of
KRISTEN L. ENGDAHL HOFFMAN, M.D.
University of Nebraska
Omaha, Nebraska

Unlike 30 years ago, physicians have many options to present to their patients regarding birth control. Neither birth control pills, intrauterine devices, nor barrier methods are perfect methods of preventing pregnancy nor are they without risk. Some methods have systemic risks that may be unacceptable in certain patients. Physicians are placed in the position of advising "situational contraception" for patients.

One of the first questions that is asked is "how effective is the method?" As the patient gets older, gets married, raises her socioeconomic status, and uses the method for a period of time, her failure rate decreases. Theoretical and actual use effectiveness of a method are not the same. In a study of currently married women who became pregnant within the first year of contraceptive use in the mid 1970's, pregnancy rates were 2 per cent for oral contraceptive users, 5 per cent for IUD users, 10 per cent for condom users, 18 per cent for spermicide users, and 19 per cent for diaphragm users. Even if 10 million women use the pill perfectly, the failure rate of 1 per cent will cause 100,000 unintended pregnancies per year.

There are risks involved in using any form of contraception. Oral contraceptive–related deaths per year are 5 per 100,000 users. In contrast, maternal mortality associated with pregnancy is twice that rate. Carrying a pregnancy to term is simply more risky than contraceptive use.

Management

Barrier Methods

Vaginal Spermicide. The active ingredients in vaginal spermicides are either nonozynol-9 or octoxinol-9, both of which kill and immobilize sperm. An inert base—either a foam, jelly, cream, suppositories, or sponge—holds the spermicide near the cervix. Each differs in the time of insertion prior to ejaculation. Foam is effective for only 30 minutes prior to ejaculation. Jellies and creams should be used with a diaphragm. Suppositories may take 10 to 30 minutes to dissolve before effectiveness begins. Vaginal sponges are effective in the vagina for up to 24 hours after insertion.

There are few risks with spermicides. Failures are due to improper use and nonuse. Some people experience a burning and some an allergic reaction. Changing either the spermicide or the inert base may eliminate this problem. Toxic shock syndrome may be associated with contraceptive sponge use. Although several studies have suggested that the use of spermicides at the time of conception or during pregnancy may cause birth defects, this has not been proven. Some studies show an additional protection against venereal disease. The vaginal sponge has the added benefit of 24 hour effectiveness with each insertion.

Condom. Condoms are rubber or processed collagenous tissue sheaths that are placed over the erect penis to act as a barrier between the semen and the vagina. There are essentially no differences among condoms made in the U.S. except their shape and the presence or absence of lubrication or spermicide. The failure rate when consistently used with foam approaches that of birth control pills.

The risks of condoms are minor. Those allergic to the rubber should use natural skin condoms. Males who complain of decreased sensitivity or inability to maintain an erection may benefit by changing to natural skin condoms or those with lubrication. Some couples dislike the interruption of foreplay associated with condom use.

The benefits of condoms include low cost, ready availability (i.e., no prescription is needed), and safety. They also offer protection against venereal disease.

Diaphragm. The diaphragm is a dome-shaped rubber cup with a flexible outside rimspring that is either arcing, coiled, or flat. It is fitted by a physician over the cervix, resting between the posterior fornix and the pubic bone. Spermicide is placed in the diaphragm so that it is next to the cervical opening. The effectiveness of this device depends on its function as both a barrier between the semen and the cervix and a spermicide holder.

The risks of this method are minimal. Several cases of toxic shock have been noted with the diaphragm. Users may also experience recurrent cystitis or allergy to rubber or spermicide. Some patients complain of increased vaginal discharge.

Pelvic discomfort from the diaphragm resting on the bladder or rectum may be due to poor fit.

The benefit of this method is that, like the condom, it provides some protection against sexually transmitted disease.

Barrier methods can be offered to women who cannot or will not use systemic hormonal contraception. They are also useful for those who wish not to expose themselves to the higher risk of pelvic inflammatory disease with an intrauterine device (IUD), back-up for birth control pills in the first month of use or when pills may have been missed, and breast-feeding mothers. Some physicians also recommend barrier methods during the first several months of IUD use.

Intrauterine Devices

There are four types of intrauterine devices available for use in the United States. The nonmedicated devices are loops that do not have to be replaced intermittently. The medicated devices contain either copper or progesterone and must be replaced at 3 to 4 or 1 year intervals, respectively. The IUD has several mechanisms of action. The local foreign body inflammatory response may lead to lysis of the blastocyst or sperm and/or prevention of implantation. The IUD effects ovum transport through the fallopian tubes and increases production of prostaglandins locally, which may inhibit implantation. Copper-imbedded IUDs compete with zinc, which inhibits carbonic anhydrase and possibly alkaline phosphatase activity. Progesterone IUDs disrupt the proliferative secretory maturation process by impairing implantation.

The risks of this method may be significant. Pregnancy complications can occur with an IUD in place. If an intrauterine pregnancy occurs the spontaneous abortion rate increases to about 55 per cent. If an intrauterine pregnancy occurs the IUD should be removed, since the rate of spontaneous abortion decreases and the chance of maternal morbidity and/or mortality declines following removal. There is approximately a 5 per cent chance of ectopic pregnancy with an IUD in place. Therefore, IUD wearers complaining of amenorrhea and abdominal pain must be evaluated carefully.

Uterine perforation is associated with IUD use. Most perforations are fundal, and more occur in postpartum breast-feeding women. Perforation is associated with pain at insertion, gradual disappearance of IUD string, bleeding post insertion, and pregnancy. Women should be taught to check for their IUD string after each menses and before each episode of coitus. If the string is not felt, it is best to rule out pregnancy and then attempt to locate the IUD in the uterus with a sound, curette, uterine packing forceps, or IUD retriever. However, if this is unsuccessful, localization may be done by ultrasound. Laparoscopy, culpotomy, or laparotomy may be necessary to remove the IUD from an extratuterine position if it is not retrieved by hysteroscopy or probing under anesthesia.

Pelvic inflammatory disease (PID) and possible resultant infertility account for the most serious complications of IUD use. However, only one half of 1 per cent of women using this method are hospitalized each year for PID. PID with significant salpingitis should not be treated with the IUD in place. However, in cases of mild endometritis, the patient may be given the option of leaving the IUD in place during treatment. Many clinicians culture the IUD upon removal for actinomyces, a branching anaerobic gram positive bacterium that may cause PID. PID in the presence of an IUD may be unilateral and may be confused with ectopic pregnancy, which must be ruled out.

IUD users may discontinue use for several less serious reasons. Bleeding may occur intermenstrually for 2 to 3 months or patients may experience menorrhagia. If bleeding is associated with partial expulsion of the IUD or a fall in hematocrit, it should be removed. Antiprostaglandin agents taken at the time of menses may decrease the flow if no other problems are found with the IUD. Cramping and bleeding may be improved with use of the progesterone-bearing IUD.

Intrauterine contraception has as its major benefit the fact that it is a one time effective contraceptive method that does not have to be ingested daily or used at each intercourse.

The best candidates for IUD use are women who have finished their childbearing but are not ready for sterilization, are spacing children, or are breast-feeding. Other candidates are women who cannot use hormonal contraception or who prefer the convenience of an IUD.

Contraindications to the use of the IUD include active or past PID, possible pregnancy, abnormal bleeding, multiple sexual partners, uterine pathology including abnormal cytology, impaired response to infection or coagulation, dysmenorrhea, cervical stenosis, small uterine cavity, valvular heart disease, allergy to copper, and history of ectopic pregnancy. Most clinicians prefer not to place IUDs in nulligravid young women for fear of future infertility. Proper written informed consent on the dangers of infection and infertility should be obtained.

IUD patients should be seen 1 month after insertion to check placement and string length. Some clinicians recommend a barrier method mid cycle for the first 1 to 3 months.

Oral Contraceptives

Oral contraceptives are the most effective reversible method of contraception. Their mechanism of action is multiple. Their main mechanism is suppression of ovulation by inhibition of the hypothalamic releasing factors, thereby blocking pituitary gonadotropin activity and secondarily blocking ovarian activity. They also impair tubal transport of the egg, sperm penetration of the cervical mucus, and endometrial implantation of the fertilized ovum.

The risks of oral contraceptives may be divided between those caused by the estrogen and those caused by the progesterone. Estrogen may cause nausea, breast tenderness, fluid retention, early cycle breakthrough bleeding, and amenorrhea. The progesterone component causes the cardiovascular effects of atherosclerosis, heart attack, and hypertension along with anxiety, weight gain, depression, acne, and late cycle breakthrough bleeding. Patients who have minor problems related to one component or the other may need a change in the composition of the oral contraceptive.

Early cycle breakthrough bleeding may be treated by adding 20 mg ethinyl estradiol or 1.25 mg of conjugated estrogens for 7 days. Switching to a pill containing high dose estrogen may be necessary; however, most clinicians would prefer to stay at 50 micrograms or below. Late cycle breakthrough bleeding can be corrected by increasing the progestin content. Amenorrhea for 1 month should not cause alarm, especially if the patient has been using pills for a prolonged time and her early morning basal body temperature is less than 98 F. However, a patient who has missed two periods should have a pregnancy test and pelvic exam.

Some myths about oral contraceptive use should be dispelled. They do not cause genetic abnormalities in the fetus if the mother has discontinued pill use prior to conception. In addition, they do not cause such endocrine problems as infertility, delayed pituitary maturation, or growth inhibition.

Absolute contraindications for oral contraceptives are pregnancy, undiagnosed bleeding, history of thromboembolic event, personal history of breast or reproductive organ cancer, and abnormal liver function studies. The relative contraindications are more often debated. These are age greater than 40 for nonsmokers or 35 for smokers, diabetes, hypertension, gallbladder disease, gestational cholestasis, impaired renal function, hyperlipidemia, and breast-feeding. Several entities that are not contraindications to pill use are myomas, recurrent monilia, migraines, and varicose veins. Only about 2 to 3 per cent of women have true contraindications to pill use.

The oral contraceptive has the most noncontraceptive benefits of any method. Among these are protection against ovarian and endometrial cancer, even after discontinuation. Iron deficiency anemia and curettages are decreased owing to decreased menstrual flow and regulation of cycles. Hospitalization for function cysts and PID are reduced significantly in users. Office visits and absenteeism due to dysmenorrhea drop with pill use.

The initial evaluation of a woman for oral contraceptive use entails a history and physical examination, looking for contraindications, weight, blood pressure, and lab work to include hematocrit, cytology, gonorrhea culture, serology, and urinalysis. Some women may need glucose tolerance testing and a liver and/or lipid profile. Many people check blood pressure 3 months after starting the pill. Subsequent yearly follow-up exams should follow these guidelines. For a woman starting on the pill, a 30 to 35 microgram estrogen pill is recommended. Currently there are no known advantages to biphasic or triphasic estrogen pills. Most doctors suggest starting the pill the Sunday after the menses starts, 3 weeks post partum if not lactating, or 1 week postabortally. It should be stopped 30 days before major surgery, one to two cycles before conception (to be able to know last menstrual period for dating), and when triglycerides are greater than 170, cholesterol is greater than 270, glucose tolerance testing is greater than 140, blood pressure diastolic is greater than 110 once or 90 three times, and blood pressure systolic is greater than 150 once.

Section 16

Psychiatric Disorders

ALCOHOLISM

method of
BARRY I. LISKOW, M.D.
Veterans Administration Medical Center
Kansas City, Missouri

As with many diseases, early diagnosis of alcoholism aids in its successful treatment. In contrast to other diseases, however, the physician is often faced with the problem of not only diagnosing the illness but also convincing a resistant patient that the diagnosis is correct and that treatment is available, necessary, and efficacious. This type of denial on the patient's part, coupled with the physician's frequent uncertainty regarding the diagnosis and treatment of alcoholism, has led to the tendency by physicians to ignore all but the most obvious of drinking problems. This attitude, though understandable, is no longer tenable given the growing evidence that early diagnosis and vigorous intervention benefit many alcoholics.

Identification/Diagnosis

The diagnosis of alcohol dependence is made on the basis of a pattern of pathologic alcohol use, impairment in social or occupational functioning due to alcohol use, and either evidence of tolerance to alcohol or of withdrawal upon cessation or reduction in drinking. Patients, however, especially early in the course of the disease, frequently deny specific problems related to alcohol. Hence, the physician must be alert to data from the patient's history, physical examination, and laboratory results that indicate a possible problem with alcohol. For example, patients with alcohol problems often have gastrointestinal complaints, including epigastric pain, nausea, vomiting, and diarrhea, which may occur more often early in the week and in the morning. They may relate a history of job difficulties due to frequent absences from work (often on Monday mornings and Friday afternoons), marital difficulties, and moving traffic violations. Inquiry regarding alcohol's relation to any problems uncovered should be made. Any unusual reactions to such inquiries should be observed—for example, hostility, evasiveness, or excessive jocularity. Alcohol on the patient's breath, multiple bruises, or cigarette burns between the fingers may be observed on physical examination. The pattern of any abnormal laboratory results should be noted. Elevated mean corpuscular volume and levels of uric acid and liver enzymes (especially ALT and AST) are frequently found in active alcoholics. A blood alcohol level of greater than 150 mg per cent in an apparently sober patient is strong evidence of tolerance to alcohol and a likely alcohol problem. The presence of any or all of these signs and symptoms does not prove the presence of an alcohol problem in the face of a patient's denial, but the more that are present, the more confident the physician can be that the patient is alcohol dependent. The ability to recognize what are often subtle signs and symptoms, however, requires that the physician maintain a high index of suspicion regarding the possible presence of alcohol dependence in all patients.

Confrontation

The next step, and the beginning of treatment for the alcohol-dependent individual, is to confront the patient with the diagnosis. Such confrontation needs to be done in a straightforward, nonaccusatory, and nonjudgmental manner. The evidence for the diagnosis as gathered from the patient's history, from additional history from significant others if available, and from physical and laboratory examinations is presented to the patient.

Some patients accept the diagnosis of a drinking problem but insist that they can stop anytime. These patients can be asked to go without alcohol for 3 to 4 weeks. Most alcohol-dependent patients have periods of sobriety lasting up to several months or longer, and many patients, though not all, will be able to successfully comply with this period of sobriety. When such patients return for their follow-up appointment, if they have been successful, the request is lengthened to 6 months and later to 1 year. Few alcohol-dependent patients can maintain sobriety on their own for this length of time (and if they can, they may be spontaneous remitters or not alcoholics) and will frequently be willing to accept treatment when failure occurs.

Another type of patient may agree that he or she has a drinking problem but makes it clear that he is only seeking treatment because he is being forced to do so by a spouse, an employer, or the courts. Although such an attitude is discouraging to the physician, it might be less so if it is realized that such a patient often does as well with treatment as more compliant patients.

Detoxification

Once the need for treatment is accepted, the physician must decide on the need for detoxification and, if needed, whether it should be accomplished in an inpatient or outpatient setting. The need for detoxification is based on an assessment of the length of the current episode of drinking, the amount drunk during this episode, the severity of withdrawal symptoms (tremulousness, autonomic hyperactivity, impaired orientation, presence of hallucinations, and so on), and the patient's medical condition. A pint of liquor a day or its equivalent in beer or wine drunk for 2 weeks will result in withdrawal symptoms in most individuals with a cessation or sudden decrease in drinking. In general, patients drinking heavily for longer than 10 days and who have a previous history of alcohol withdrawal seizures or delirium tremens should be hospitalized, as should all patients with intercurrent medical problems such as pneumonia, head injuries, malnutrition, and so forth. Patients without medical problems and without a prior history of severe withdrawal symptoms often can be managed as outpatients or in nonmedical detoxification centers unless their withdrawal symptoms are severe (seizures, disorientation, hallucinations).

It has been clearly demonstrated that benzodiazepines reduce the incidence of alcohol withdrawal seizures and delirium tremens in the detoxifying, alcohol-dependent patient and make such patients subjectively more comfortable. Although various studies have indicated that 80 to 95 per cent of patients can be successfully detoxified without medication, there is no reliable method of determining which 5 to 20 per cent of patients need benzodiazepines (although those with intercurrent infections and with a prior history of delirium tremens or seizures are probably at greatest risk). Hence, it is best to use these medications in most patients who are withdrawing from alcohol. If the benzodiazepines are used for treating withdrawal in an outpatient setting, it is important that a significant other be with the patient and dispense the medication as prescribed. The patient should visit the physician every day during detoxification, or if that is not possible, telephone contact with the patient or the significant other should be maintained daily.

The long-acting benzodiazepines—for example, chlordiazepoxide (Librium) and diazepam (Valium)—are preferable to short-acting ones because more stable blood levels can be achieved and the dosing intervals are not as critical. Chlordiazepoxide and diazepam should be given orally and are more effective by this route than intramuscularly. It is important, because these are long-acting agents, that they begin to be tapered on the second day of withdrawal and that they continue to be tapered daily thereafter. Rarely are more than 4 to 5 days needed to complete the withdrawal period. Seldom is more than 300 mg of chlordiazepoxide or 100 mg of diazepam necessary the first day and often considerably less may be needed. The dose is then decreased after the first day by 20 to 30 per cent per day, depending on the patient's clinical status. If the patient is excessively drowsy or ataxic, the dose is decreased faster or held; if the patient is showing excessive or severe withdrawal symptoms, such as tremor, tachycardia, or diaphoresis, the dose is increased or the percentage of decrease reduced.

It is usually not necessary to give anticonvulsant medication, except of course to those patients with a chronic seizure disorder. Patients who have a history of alcohol withdrawal seizures may be given phenytoin for 5 days, although the necessity of doing so has not been clearly established. Patients who sustain an apparent alcohol withdrawal seizure should have its cause investigated. If the seizure is determined to be due to alcohol withdrawal, continuous therapy with anticonvulsants beyond 5 days is neither necessary nor indicated. Finally, because alcohol-dependent patients are frequently malnourished to various degrees, all patients should be given multivitamins and minerals during the detoxification phase of treatment, and for those with obvious nutritional deficits such therapy should be continued for several months.

Patients who are in delirium tremens (profound disorientation, psychomotor agitation, hallucinations, and delusions) must, of course, be hospitalized. A vigorous search for intercurrent medical problems and for other possible causes for the delirium needs to be done. Treatment consists of intravenous diazepam (Valium), 5 to 10 mg intravenously every 5 minutes, until the patient is lightly sedated, followed by 100 mg of diazepam or 300 mg of chlordiazepoxide (Librium) orally in divided doses the first day, followed by declining oral doses as indicated earlier. The benzodiazepines will not change the course of the delirium, which will last 1 to 5 days, but will reduce the patient's psychomotor agitation and hence make restraints less necessary and thus prevent the patient from becoming exhausted. Finally, thiamine, 100 mg intramuscularly, should be given to patients with delirium tremens as well as to all inpatient alcohol-dependent patients, to prevent or treat Wernicke's encephalopathy. Fluid and electrolyte balance must also be carefully monitored, as patients may be either overhydrated or dehydrated during withdrawal.

Rehabilitation

A successfully detoxified patient is ready to enter the rehabilitation phase of treatment. The primary care physician should become knowledgeable regarding the availability of specialized inpatient and outpatient alcohol treatment facilities and of Alcoholics Anonymous (AA) and Al-Anon groups in the community. A knowledge of the use of disulfiram (Antabuse) is also helpful, whether used by the physician in a treatment program or simply prescribed by the physician who is providing medical services to patients receiving rehabilitation in community alcohol programs.

1. Specialized inpatient and outpatient units generally have a full array of treatment modalities, including individual, couple, and family counseling, as well as a variety of groups including educational, assertiveness, and relaxation training, and leisure planning. The decision to hospitalize a patient is based on a number of factors, including such nonmedical issues as insurance coverage and availability of inpatient versus outpatient resources. Inpatient care is justified for patients in crisis (for example, following recent loss of job, marriage, or financial resources), those who have repeatedly failed outpatient treatment, and those with psychiatric illnesses in addition to alcoholism. The last group might do best in an inpatient unit in a psychiatric hospital or in a general hospital with an active psychiatric consultation service. Recent research has found little benefit of long-term (4 to 12 weeks) over short-term (2 to 4 weeks) inpatient programs and has found little benefit of inpatient over outpatient alcohol rehabilitation for most patients. However, presently most resources for alcohol rehabilitation continue to be located on inpatient services.

The philosophy of virtually all alcohol rehabilitation programs is abstinence. Undoubtedly some patients can return to controlled drinking, but they are a minority and it is not possible currently to determine which patients can do so.

2. Alcoholics Anonymous (AA) provides the alcohol-dependent patient with a support group of individuals with the same illness and is available 24 hours a day, 7 days a week. Some patients object to the spiritual (religious) orientation of Alcoholics Anonymous whereas others apparently appreciate and benefit from such an orientation. Many AA groups do not emphasize this aspect, and most large communities have several AA groups. Patients, therefore, should be encouraged to attend at least four to five meetings and, if necessary, several different AA groups, thus increasing their chances of finding a group with which they are comfortable. The physician can benefit by visiting AA groups in the community (they all have open meetings to which the public is invited and most are very willing to cooperate with physicians) and referring patients to preferred groups.

3. Al-Anon is a support group for the spouses of alcohol-dependent patients. The groups usually emphasize the need for spouses to recognize their own needs, to quit their futile attempts to force their spouses to stop drinking, and to realize that only when their spouses admit their drinking problem and decide to deal with it will their alcoholism be on the way to cure. Some spouses have difficulty with this philosophy, but many find it helpful in alleviating their own sense of impotence and guilt. A companion group, Alateen, is available in many communities for teenage children of alcohol-dependent patients. The groups are oriented toward helping teenagers understand alcoholism and deal with their feelings toward their alcoholic parents. Recent emphasis has been given in these groups to informing teenagers of research findings indicating that the children of alcoholics are at much increased risk for developing alcoholism. Such teenagers are strongly counselled to avoid all alcohol, given their increased susceptibility to developing alcohol dependence. The primary care physician should also emphasize these findings to parents and children.

4. Disulfiram (Antabuse), if regularly ingested, inhibits the metabolism of acetaldehyde (the first metabolic breakdown product of alcohol) to carbon dioxide and water and hence results in a toxic reaction when alcohol is drunk. The reaction can occur 12 hours after the first disulfiram dose and up to 2 weeks after the last dose and begins approximately 20 minutes after alcohol is ingested. The reaction consists of hypotension, flushing, nausea, vomiting, pounding headache, diaphoresis, and weakness and lasts 1 to 4 hours; rarely there is a fatal outcome. Only patients who have been fully informed of disulfiram's effects and dangers, who are free of severe cardiac, renal, and hepatic disease, who have no organic mental disorder, and who have given informed consent should be considered for disulfiram therapy. The standard dose is 250 mg daily, usually given at night to take advantage of its soporific effects. At this dose, side effects are few and include drowsiness, metallic taste, and dermatitic reactions.

Disulfiram does not decrease the desire to drink but concentrates the decision whether to drink to one point in time per day. Once the disulfiram is taken, the alcohol-dependent patient knows he or she cannot drink safely for 2 weeks. There is now evidence that the value of disulfiram is enhanced if the drug is given under the supervision of a significant other, for example, a spouse or employer. If the physician, patient, and significant other agree to such administration, it is important that the physician make clear that the significant other is the physician's agent acting under the physician's instructions and that the doctor must be called if the patient refuses to take the medication. In this manner, any anger the patient develops toward supervised therapy will be deflected to the treating physician where it can be appropriately handled by reviewing with the patient the evidence of the alcohol problem and the continued need for disulfiram.

There are no specific data regarding the length of time disulfiram should be taken, but 6 months to 1 year is reasonable for most patients. Patients who wish to stop after this period of time and who appear confident and comfortable in their sober life-style should be allowed to do so, with close followup for several months.

5. Group therapy and individual counseling focus on educating alcoholics about alcoholism, including its medical, psychologic, and social effects and teaching such patients how to begin a sober life-style. This may involve changing friends, social activities, and occasionally jobs. The difficult transition to this new life-style is emphasized; it requires a major commitment and can be discouraging. Methods of coping with current and anticipated problems are taught through such modalities as relaxation training, assertiveness training, and psychotherapy groups to deal with psychologic problems; couples and family groups to address marital and family difficulties; leisure counseling to manage new amounts of free time effectively; and vocational rehabilitation to help with employment problems. The full range of these services, while not needed by every patient, is available in most comprehensive inpatient and outpatient treatment centers.

6. Specialized treatment units are offered by several alcohol centers and generally involve a program of aversion therapy. Patients drink alcohol, shortly after which vomiting is induced by either injectable or oral emetics. Such pairing of drinking and vomiting theoretically leads to a conditioned avoidance of drinking alcohol. The treatment is generally applied in private alcohol inpatient settings for middle to upper class patients, with little attention given to other treatment modalities. Cure rates reported by these treatment centers are high, in the range of 50 to 80 per cent abstinence on 2 year followup. However, cure rates tend to be high, regardless of treatment, in this socioeconomic group. If such a treatment center is available, the primary care physician should become familiar with the treatment and the type of patients who appear to benefit from this modality.

Role of the Primary Care Physician

The major role of the primary care physician in addressing the issue of alcoholism in patients is the identification of and, if necessary, confrontation with the alcohol-dependent patient regarding the diagnosis and need for treatment. Some patients, depending on the severity of their alcohol problem and the physician's time, interest, and expertise, may be treated by their primary care physician. Such treatment entails detoxification, use of disulfiram if the patient is a willing and appropriate candidate, and referral of the patient to Alcoholics Anonymous and the family to Al-Anon and Alateen. Initially, after detoxification, weekly 20 to 30 minute office visits should be offered to discuss the patient's progress, to provide education about alcohol, and to offer support regarding a sober life-style. It is essential that the focus of these weekly sessions be kept on the alcohol problem and that the patient not be allowed to dwell on other problems, although they can and should be noted and discussed as they relate to alcohol. Abstinence should be the goal of therapy and psychoactive drugs avoided. If psychiatric problems become apparent, they should be evaluated. The most common psychiatric symptoms will be those related to depressive and anxiety disorders. If the primary care physician is confident in the treatment of these disorders, appropriate psychotropic medication can be initiated. However, because such symptoms are very common in the first several weeks after detoxification, such treatment should not be initiated unless the patient has persistent anxiety or depressive symptoms for 3 weeks or longer beyond detoxification.

After a month of weekly visits, contact can be reduced to twice monthly and then to monthly. There is no rule regarding the length of therapy but a minimum of 1 year is reasonable, with the understanding after that time that the patient can return whenever necessary.

Relapses should be handled as would relapses with any chronic illness. Patients should be reassured that a relapse does not mean that they will never overcome their problem, that methods that have been taught can and will be reapplied and are often successful on reapplication, and that new procedures, if needed, will be initiated (for example, initiation of disulfiram therapy in a patient who previously refused the medication, or hospitalization for a patient who has been previously treated as an outpatient).

NARCOTIC POISONING

method of
GEORGE R. GAY, M.D.
Haight-Ashbury Free Medical Clinics
San Francisco, California

The colorful history of opium and its derivatives has been voluminously documented throughout recorded time, dating from the ideographs of the Sumerians some 4,000 years B.C. Morphine, opium's principal alkaloid (approximately 10 per cent by weight), was first isolated by Friedrick Sertürner in 1803 and was named for Morphius, the Greek god of dreams. The Greek word "narkōtikos," meaning "to benumb or deaden," lent the descriptive term "narcotic" to morphine (the prototype) and to its subsequently discovered natural, synthetic, and semisynthetic congeners as well as to agents of similar pharmacologic actions (Table 1). "Narcotic-analgesic" and "opioid" are other terms commonly applied to this class of drug, which pharmacologically combines the actions of an analgesic (to relieve pain), a hypnotic (to produce sleep), and a euphoriant (to bring about a feeling of well-being or a loss of care). (Diacetylmorphine [heroin], with a greater capacity to cross the blood brain barrier than morphine, appears to have the highest euphoriant property of the opioids.)

Narcotics exert a twofold analgesic action on the central nervous system: the pain threshold is elevated and the psychologic stress response to pain is alleviated. Clinically, the picture is one of a sedated, drowsy, mentally obtunded individual with impaired physical performance. Psychologic dependence as well as a true tissue—physical—dependence rapidly develops. Tolerance also rapidly evolves. Nausea and vomiting may be seen owing to action on the chemoreceptor trigger zone of the medulla, and a dose-related respiratory depression arises through a direct action on brain stem respiratory centers (which no longer respond to increasing carbon dioxide and decreasing oxygen tensions). Thus is produced an emergent critical life-threatening situation.

One is tempted to associate narcotic poisoning (or "overdose") with the classically dramatic illicit drug diacetylmorphine (heroin). But in reality, in such an overdose one must suspect *multiple concurrent drug abuse*. In particular, suspect alcohol and any of a multitude of available sedative-hypnotic agents and major and minor tranquilizers (e.g., short-acting barbiturates, chloral hydrate, methaqualone, glutethimide, all benzodiazepines, "muscle relaxants," monoamine oxidase inhibitors, tricyclic antidepressants, and phenothiazines). In these cases, pharmacologically additive and often synergistic effects may lead to a most profound central nervous system depression.

Treatment of Narcotic Poisoning

Immediate attention to airway and adequate oxygenation is a sine qua non. Of vital (but secondary) importance in establishing diagnosis is *any* available history, a thorough physical examination, and a collection of blood, urine, and gastric contents for a subsequent toxicologic analysis.

The classic narcotic poisoning victim presents with pinpoint pupils (anoxia or concurrent other drug use may muddy this sign), areflexia, marked respiratory depression with slow periodic (Biot) or Cheyne-Stokes respiration, and a cyanotic, clammy pallor. Needle marks may or may not be present or apparent.

Assure Adequate Oxygenation

Treatment must be precise and immediate, with all attention given to establishing and protecting the airway. If spontaneous respiratory effort and oropharyngeal (gag) reflexes are present and evidence of aspiration of vomitus is not present (lungs are clear and breath sounds good), then endotracheal intubation may not be immediately necessary.

1. Promptly place the patient in a head down left lateral position (protect the more vulnerable right mainstem bronchus from aspiration).
2. Clear the contents of the mouth and oropharynx. Mucus, blood, vomitus, gum, or tobacco may be present. (Ideally an adequate suction machine would be at hand; practically, manual cleaning with fingers and a handkerchief or shirttail may have to suffice.)
3. Tip the head slightly back, grasping the jaw at the angles of the mandible and at the point of the chin (being careful not to overextend the neck, creating a "sniffing-like" position). Pull the tongue forward, making sure it is not occluding the posterior oropharynx. Insert an oropharyngeal or nasopharyngeal airway (if indicated and if tolerated). (A nasal airway is better tolerated, but may occasionally cause nosebleed.) It may be necessary to hold the tongue forward with your fingers during initial airway establishment.
4. Breathe for (or assist) the patient if he is apneic or in obvious respiratory distress. Use mouth-to-mouth or mouth-to-nose respiration or an Ambu bag if one is handy. An esophageal obturator airway (EOA) may be employed at this point. Make sure that air is entering the lungs, i.e., that the chest (not stomach) is expanding. Listen for vesicular breath sounds with a stethoscope. Do not initially stop to look for or call for endotracheal equipment. This is an emergency of the most acute nature, and hesitation can spell disaster. Endotracheal intubation should be carried out after the patient has been properly oxygenated and stabilized. In any event, never exceed 2 minutes in any intubation attempt (try holding your breath against a timed 2 minutes—then desist if unsuccessful—reoxygenate, and try again).

TABLE 1. **Narcotic Agonist Agents**

Generic Name	Trade Name	Street Name	Dose (mg)*	Plasma Half-Life (hr)	Withdrawal Symptoms	Special Features
opium		OP, O, Black, Stuff	0.3–0.6 PO or PR only		Like morphine	Can be smoked; taken orally; administered rectally. Op. tincture: laudanum. Op. camphorated tincture: paregoric.
morphine		M, Miss Emma, Dreamer	10	2–3	Prototype	Oral, IM, SC, IV.
diacetylmorphine (heroin)†		Junk, Boy, H, Horse, China White, Persian Heroin	3–8	2.5–3	Like morphine	Speedball (with cocaine). Snorted, smoked, SC, IM, or IV.
dihydromorphinone (hydromorphone)	Dilaudid	Dillys, Little D	1.5	2–4	Like morphine	Oral, rectal, SC, IM, or IV.
dihydrohydroxymorphinone (Oxymorphone)	Numorphan	Number, N	1.0–1.5	2–4	Like morphine	SC, IM, IV, or rectal.
methylmorphine (codeine)	Codeine	Cough syrup, Turps, Schoolboys	120	2.5–3	Less severe than morphine, extended	Oral, SC, or IM.
dihydrocodeinone (hydrocodone)	Hycodan	Hyke	5–10 (oral only)	2–4	Between morphine and codeine	Oral; a preferred cough syrup narcotic.
dihydrohydroxycodeinone (oxycodone)	Percodan	Perks	10–15 (oral only)	3–4	Like morphine	Oral. The preferred diverted drug. Percodan or Percodan-demi with ASA; Percocet or Tylox with acetaminophen.
methadone	Dolophine	Dolls, Tang, Meth	7.5–10	24–48	Extended, severe, like morphine	Oral, IM, SC.
meperidine	Demerol	Big D, Dem, Pethidine	80–150	3	Like morphine	SC, IM, IV, or oral.
alphaprodine	Nisentil	Nice	30–60	1.5	Like meperidine	SC, IM, or IV.
propoxyphene	Darvon	Dummies	260 (PO only)	10–12	Like methadone	Oral (HCl 65 mg, Napsylate 100 mg).
fentanyl	Sublimaze	Sub, China White	0.1	0.5	Like morphine	IV or powder. Sold as heroin or China White.
levo-alpha-acetyl methadol	LAAM	LAAM	10	48–72+	Like methadone	Ultra long-acting methadone congener.

*Dosage based on equivalent amount of agent injected subcutaneously to the standard of 10 mg morphine.
†Since 1978, particularly on the West Coast, smoking and snorting heroin has become acceptable at social gatherings. This is often associated with the smoking of cocaine ("basing") and (since 1984) the smoking of methamphetamine.

Assess Cardiovascular System

1. Check the pulse for rate and rhythm. Check precordial, femoral, radial, or temporal pulses. (A palpable temporal artery pulse roughly assures a systolic blood pressure of 80 or above and hence adequate circulation to the brain.) Do not be lulled into complacency by the strong, full pulse of hypoxia, which may be premonitory to aberrant and then terminal arrhythmia and cardiac cessation.

2. Begin external cardiac massage if the heartbeat is absent. Determine ECG status as soon as possible; then institute appropriate action.

3. In severe cases of narcotic poisoning, the patient's cardiovascular system may be so depressed that pulmonary edema develops. (This is also not unusual in cases of meperidine [Demerol] or propoxyphene [Darvon] overdose or as a hypersensitive or "allergic" reaction to illicit drug "filler" or admixture.) Also, vomiting and pulmonary aspiration may have occurred, giving the signs of pulmonary edema. Intubation or tracheostomy plus continuous positive pressure res-

piration may be literally life-saving in this situation.

4. Dehydration may be evident, but maintain a conservative fluid replacement regimen until effective cardiac output (as reflected clinically by monitored end-diastolic pressure) is assured. If the patient's color is good, chest is clear of rales and rhonchi, and the jugular veins are flat—yet blood pressure is below 100 mm systolic—try the rapid infusion of 250 cc of dextrose/electrolyte solution, aiming for a systolic response of 100 or above. A Swann-Ganz catheter would be most helpful; a simple central venous pressure monitor line is of advantage. Pressor agents (e.g., dopamine) should be immediately available but used judiciously if at all.

Narcotic Antagonist Therapy (Table 2)

Naloxone. Give naloxone (Narcan), 0.4 mg intravenously. (A reasonable variation is to dilute 1 ml of naloxone [0.4 mg] to 10 cc in normal saline, then titrate with less than 0.4 mg per dose.) Naloxone dosages (usually in increments of 0.4 mg per dose) may be repeated at 2 to 3 minute intervals, monitoring continuously for any sign of narcotic reversal (e.g., increase in rate and depth of respiration, increase in heart rate and blood pressure, signs of central nervous system arousal). This dosage of naloxone may be repeated up to 15 times (which may be necessary for the methadone-configured molecule of propoxyphene [Darvon] overdose, whereupon a truly dramatic arousal may be seen). Recent individual case reports as well as the author's own repeated clinical experience indicate that such high dose naloxone reversal therapy may serve to produce central nervous system arousal in patients comatose from alcohol overdose alone.

One must also be cautious not to precipitate an "instant cold turkey" syndrome, with abrupt full reversal of all narcotic effects in an addicted individual. In this case, a comatose (but calm) patient is suddenly transformed into a violent, retching, completely unhappy and unmanageable one. It is possible, however, to reverse titrate this patient "downward" with morphine given by 2 mg bolus intravenously at 3 to 5 minute intervals until a state of light "renarcotization" is achieved.

Start 5 per cent dextrose in one half molar lactated Ringer's solution using a large bore intravenous cannula. Naloxone reversal may be seen within 20 to 30 seconds of intravenous

TABLE 2. **Mixed Narcotic Agonist-Antagonists and Pure Narcotic Antagonists**

Generic Name	Trade Name	Street Name	Dose (mg)*	Plasma Half-Life (hr)	Agonist Activity	Special Features
Mixed Agonists-Antagonists						
pentazocine	Talwin	T's, T's & Blues, Blue Velvets†	30–50 (agonist action)	2–3	Mild morphine-like agonist activity, 2+	PO, IM, IV, SC
levallorphan	Lorfan		1–1.5 (agonist action)	0.5	Morphine-like agonist activity, 1+	Formerly used as antagonists; now obsolete (pentazocine, levallorphan, nalorphine)
nalorphine	Nalline		10–15 (agonist action)	0.5	Morphine-like agonist activity, 1+	
butorphanol	Stadol		1	2.5–3.5	Mild morphine-like agonist activity, 3+	IM, IV, SC; not classified under Controlled Substances Act
nalbuphine	Nubain		10	3–4	Mild morphine-like agonist activity, 3+	IM, IV, SC; not classified under Controlled Substances Act
Pure Antagonists						
naloxone	Narcan		0.4–1.2	1–3	None	Injectable, extremely safe
naltrexone	Trexan		50–100 (oral)	24–48	None	Dose-related hepatic toxicity, recommended *not* to be given until 7 to 10 days after last narcotic dose‡

*Dosage based on equivalent amount of agent injected subcutaneously to the standard of 10 mg morphine.

†T's & Blues, aka Blue Velvets, is Talwin combined with tripelennamine (pyribenzamine), known as the "Poor Man's Heroin." Seen predominantly in the midwestern (namely, Chicago) region.

‡Acute withdrawal symptoms will occur if given any earlier. Hospitalization recommended for administration of this agent, with Narcan test (0.8 mg IV or subcutaneous). May take massive dose of narcotic to overcome naltrexone; self-attempt may cause overdose. The naltrexone patient requiring narcotic-analgesia (e.g., surgery) warrants special monitoring.

administration (one circulation time) in the case of "pure" narcotic poisoning, which is extremely rare. Given intramuscularly, the drug may take 20 minutes or longer to act. If the patient has sclerosed or "collapsed" veins, as many addicts do, try the external jugular or femoral veins, or, if all else fails, inject into the vascular-rich muscle of the base of the tongue.

Naloxone is a "pure" narcotic antagonist in its action, with *no* potential for dangerous additive "agonist" effect (as was seen with the older agents nallorphine [Nalline] and levallorphan [Lorfan]). One may consider the use of from 4 to 8 mg total of naloxone to be in no way contraindicated in a narcotic poisoning resuscitative effort.

The respiratory depressant effects of narcotic poisoning contribute significantly to increased intracranial cerebrospinal fluid pressure, and this may be augmented by any pre-existing head injury or one sustained concomitant to the overdose. In such a case, naloxone is not only safe but may serve to unmask any underlying head injury and its signs.

If coma still supervenes after the administration of naloxone, one may consider administering 50 per cent glucose as a bolus of 50 ml intravenously. This effectively treats hypoglycemic states such as those seen in insulin overdose. (An early blood sugar determination will help to dictate such therapy.)

Acidosis should be corrected by the administration of sodium bicarbonate, 50 ml (3.75 grams), repeated as necessary. Serial arterial blood gas sampling should be employed as clinically indicated.

The intubated comatose patient should have a large bore orogastric tube placed, and (after aspiration of available contents for toxicologic analysis) gastric lavage should be carried out with 500 ml of isotonic saline. Activated charcoal, 100 grams, should then be instilled in 250 ml of isotonic saline and left in place to adsorb any residual orally ingested toxic agents.

Hospitalization. By now all available history (from relatives, friends, or an arousing patient) should be complete, as should the clinical search and evaluation to rule out all other possible etiologic factors in the patient presenting in an obtunded or comatose state other than acute narcotic poisoning (e.g., head trauma with possible intracranial bleeding or subdural or epidural hematoma, disorders of blood sugar or electrolytes, hepatic or uremic coma, or evidence of severe systemic sepsis).

Continue in-hospital monitoring for possible narcotic relapse ("renarcotization") with naloxone infusion of 0.4 mg at 2 to 3 hour intervals as necessary for a full 72 hours. The half-life of naloxone is less than that of most available narcotics, and naloxone is clinically effective for only 2 to 3 hours. Many narcotics will sustain respiratory depressant effects for longer than this (e.g., 24 to 48 hours for methadone, or up to 72 hours for L-alpha-acetyl methadol [LAAM]).

Aftercare. The diagnosis of narcotic poisoning in and of itself indicates some degree of psychologic dysfunction, and appropriate personalized referral and care should be arranged (e.g., psychiatric counseling in the case of attempted suicide).

Likewise, in this age of universal availability of a myriad of prescribed as well as illicit drugs, combined with an often open peer acceptance of drug use, the individual who unintentionally overdoses will almost without exception be found to be a multiple drug abuser. As pharmacologic complexity increases, so do the problems of sustained abstinence and social rehabilitation. Proper individualized counseling and peer support systems must be devised and actualized.

Treatment of Withdrawal

Withdrawal from narcotics may be discomfiting in the extreme, with signs of "super flu" (hypersalivation, runny eyes and nose, fever, chills, and diaphoresis). Nausea, vomiting, abdominal cramps, and diarrhea may be present as may photophobia (due to dilation of the pupils), musculoskeletal pains and cramps, and "jitteriness" and insomnia to a marked degree. These symptoms will largely subside within 5 days, with some residual insomnia and a vague generalized

TABLE 3. **Non-Narcotic Treatment of Withdrawal Symptom Complexes**

Symptom Complex	Treatment
Pain (generalized aches, "deep bone pain")	Aspirin or acetaminophen (in normal clinical dosages); ibuprofen (Motrin, Advil, etc.), 600 mg; propoxyphene napsylate (Darvon-N), 200 mg; propoxyphene hydrochloride (Darvon), 130 mg, or clonidine, 0.1 mg every 6 hrs.
Sleeplessness	Chloral hydrate, up to 1.0 to 1.5 grams at bedtime.
Nervousness	Phenobarbital, 30 to 60 mg every 6 to 8 hrs.
Gastrointestinal distress	Belladonna leaf extract, phenobarbital (Belphen No. 1), oxyphenonium bromide and phenobarbital (Antrenyl-phenobarbital), or dicyclomine hydrochloride (Bentyl), 2 capsules every 4 to 6 hrs. Note: For pronounced nausea and vomiting, 5 to 15 mg prochlorperazine (Compazine) orally or 10 mg by rectal suppository every 4 to 6 hours.

irritability and muscular aches and pains, which gradually lessen and disappear after several weeks. During this time decreased rapid eye movements (REM) and absence of dreaming are also noted. (The report of resumed normal dream patterns is an optimistic clinical sign.)

Four withdrawal symptom complexes are commonly treated: (1) pain (muscle, joint, and "bone aches"); (2) sleeplessness; (3) nervousness; and (4) gastrointestinal complaints (Table 3).

The "poly drug abuser" exhibits all of these symptoms, plus a time variable (usually after 3 to 7 days of abstinence) *crisis state* that may entail generalized tonic and clonic seizure, hypertensive and hyperpyrexic crisis, and occasional cardiovascular collapse and exitus. This life-threatening complex of events is seen particularly when narcotic abuse is coupled with chronic alcoholism and/or sedative-hypnotic and/or "tranquilizer" abuse. This patient requires hospitalization and close and expectant observation for at least 7 days. Likewise, as might be expected, aftercare is increased in complexity. A monitored, extended aftercare program is mandatory.

Narcotic Poisoning in Infants

This potential tragedy is almost without exception an accidental happening, often occurring in the household of a methadone-maintained adult who keeps available a methadone citrus drink preparation. Occasionally implicated in infant narcotic poisoning as well are the common antidiarrheal agents diphenoxylate plus atropine (Lomotil) and loperamide (Imodium).

Unfortunately, an increasing number of narcotics are routinely kept around the home, often within reach of a toddler. These may include flavored antitussive syrups containing codeine or hydrocodone; tablets or capsules of propoxyphene (Darvon), pentazocine (Talwin), meperidine (Demerol), and others; and aspirin or acetaminophen mixtures with codeine or oxycodone.

The onset of respiratory depression, coma, and cardiovascular collapse is extremely rapid in cases of infant narcotic poisoning (within 30 minutes to one hour). Treatment must be prompt, and whatever heroic measures deemed necessary must be instituted in these cases. Antagonist treatment is naloxone, 0.01 mg per kg, by intravenous bolus administration, to be repeated at 3 to 4 minute intervals until adequate spontaneous respiration is restored and protective oropharyngeal reflexes are again present. The same dosage is then repeated as necessary (during constant intensive care monitoring) over a 72 hour hospital stay. Explicit instructions and counseling are given to the adults of the household to prevent this from recurring.

PSYCHONEUROSIS

method of
THOMAS H. HOLMES, M.D.
University of Washington
Seattle, Washington

Psychoneuroses

The psychoneuroses are among the commonest disorders in middle class America. The classification includes a wide variety of names, such as anxiety neuroses, phobias, childhood fears, obsessive compulsive thinking, and angry, acting out behavior. The content of problems encountered is typical of middle class America and includes money, children, and sex. The mental status is usually normal. These patients have intact retention and recall and they are oriented as to time and place. They have good intellectual capacity and the ability to free associate. The one feature common throughout is the motive. The characteristic of the motive in these disorders is that it lacks relevance and pertinence to the situation. The application of this "wrong" motive leads to strong emotion, disrupting behavior, and compelling, driving thoughts. The degree of discomfort and impaired productivity can range from slight to incapacitating. It is this state that drives patients to see the doctor in search of the restoration of some degree of comfort and productivity.

In common with most other diseases, the psychoneuroses have their onset in a setting of life change or critical life situation. The bodily reaction to this critical stimulus produces the signs and symptoms of the neurosis. This stimulus-response is a part of the stress reaction. Stress can be defined as the subset of pathology having to do with the new etiology. Pathology can be defined as the result of an interaction between a host and the stimulus or etiologic situation. The parameters of a stimulus situation are contained in Table 1. The reactions contain the emotional state of the individual and the bodily reaction of the organ system or systems affected.

Anxiety is the psychologic and physiologic response to a life situation or onset of events often culminating in a crisis. The emotion is one of an overwhelming feeling composed of two states—apprehension and tension. The individual is aware of danger or threat to his security and prepares his body to cope with the danger once it is defined. The onset of anxiety commonly occurs in childhood and undergoes exacerbations and remissions throughout life. The physiologic accompaniments of this state are breathlessness, pounding heart, tachycardia, cold sweaty palms, reduction in blood flow to the gastrointestinal tract, increase in muscle blood flow, and increase in free fatty acids. The variety of names attached to this reaction range from the hyperventilation syndrome to acute and chronic anxiety. In its various forms it is one of the most common disorders encountered by a physician.

TABLE 1. **The Social Readjustment Rating Scale**

Life Event	Mean Value	Life Event	Mean Value
1. Death of spouse	100	25. Outstanding personal achievement	28
2. Divorce	73	26. Wife beginning or ceasing work outside the home	26
3. Marital separation from mate	65	27. Beginning or ceasing formal schooling	26
4. Detention in jail or other institution	63	28. Major change in living conditions (e.g., building a new home, remodeling, deterioration of home or neighborhood)	25
5. Death of a close family member	63	29. Revision of personal habits (dress, manners, association, etc.)	24
6. Major personal injury or illness	53	30. Troubles with the boss	23
7. Marriage	50	31. Major change in working hours or conditions	20
8. Being fired at work	47	32. Change in residence	20
9. Marital reconciliation with mate	45	33. Changing to a new school	20
10. Retirement from work	45	34. Major change in usual type and/or amount of recreation	19
11. Major change in the health or behavior of a family member	44	35. Major change in church activities (e.g., a lot more or a lot less than usual)	19
12. Pregnancy	40	36. Major change in social activities (e.g., clubs, dancing, movies, visiting, etc.)	18
13. Sexual difficulties	39	37. Taking out a mortgage or loan for a lesser purchase (e.g., for a car, TV, freezer, etc.)	17
14. Gaining a new family member (e.g., through birth, adoption, oldster moving in, etc.)	39	38. Major change in sleeping habits (a lot more or a lot less sleep, or change in part of day when asleep)	16
15. Major business readjustment (e.g., merger, reorganization, bankruptcy, etc.)	39	39. Major change in number of family get-togethers (e.g., a lot more or a lot less than usual)	15
16. Major change in financial state (e.g., a lot worse off or a lot better off than usual)	38	40. Major change in eating habits (a lot more or a lot less food intake, or very different meal hours or surroundings)	15
17. Death of a close friend	37	41. Vacation	13
18. Changing to a different line of work	36	42. Christmas	12
19. Major change in the number of arguments with spouse (e.g., either a lot more or a lot less than usual regarding child-bearing, personal habits, etc.)	35	43. Minor violations of the law (e.g., traffic tickets, jaywalking, disturbing the peace, etc.)	11
20. Taking out a mortgage or loan for a major purchase (e.g., for a home, business, etc.)	31		
21. Foreclosure on a mortgage or loan	30		
22. Major change in responsibilities at work (e.g., promotion, demotion, lateral transfer)	29		
23. Son or daughter leaving home (e.g., marriage, attending college, etc.)	29		
24. Trouble with in-laws	29		

The more change an individual experiences, the more likely illness will follow. Of people with 300 or more Life Change Units for the past year, almost 80% get sick in the near future; with 150 to 299 Life Change Units, about 50% get sick in the near future; and with fewer than 150 Life Change Units, only about 30% get sick in the near future.

(From Holmes TH, Rahe RH: The Social Readjustment Rating Scale. J Psychosom Res *11*:213, 1967.)

Depression is the feeling of hopelessness commingled with feelings of self-importance, anger, guilt, and deprivation. Hopelessness implies that the outlook is gloomy and dull, without the expectation of anything favorable happening. Anger implies intent to attack, injure, or destroy. Self-importance implies a sense of exalted superiority. Guilt implies that the individual has done those things that he should not have done or has left undone those things that he should have done. Deprivation implies a sense of loss. Depression is a fairly common dimension of the neurosis and is a syndrome that is often difficult to cope with.

Techniques of Psychotherapy

Psychotherapy is a technique for understanding, guiding, and reeducating the patient. With the varying degrees of dramatic change that occur in the patient's psychological state and bodily function, symptoms are alleviated, signs of disease subside, and productivity and comfort are partially or fully restored. Psychotherapy is executed within a doctor-patient relationship in which communication is the essence. Communication can be defined as the exchange of information in which that which is conveyed and that which is perceived are consonant. The technique of psychotherapy can be divided into how to listen and how to ask questions.

How to Listen

There are certain generalizations about listening that apply to the therapeutic relationship. The speech pattern of most psychoneurotics has a time component. Most patients speak 80 per cent of the time ± 10 per cent. The doctor speaks 10 per cent of the time ± 5 per cent. There is a certain amount of time for silence. In an hour's interview, the patient speaks about 48 minutes and the doctor about 6 minutes. Aside from a rare yes or no response, most patients talk between 15 seconds and 2 minutes. The physician speaks with 4 second cues, often accompanied by a head nod and the statement of "uh-huh." Occasionally the physician may speak as long as 7 seconds and close out the interview with a 12 second comment.

During this transaction, the physician is seated comfortably with a certain amount of tension being present, looking at the patient's eyes or where the eyes would be if he or she has not shielded them. The physician's communication is one of understanding and tolerance. No moral judgment is made. Translated into other terms, the physican's purpose in using short questions is to keep the patient talking about personal preoccupations and concerns. As long as new material is produced, the interview is profitable. The physician selects for reinforcement from among the many topics introduced by the patient those considered to have the greatest salience. The reinforcement will convey to the patient the physician's conviction about what is wrong, how things might be changed, and what the patient's assets are. The implication is that the patient should take these critical variables home for further reflection and consideration.

How to Ask Questions

The interview or art of interrogation usually begins with a general question having to do with the reason the patient has consulted the physician. Such a question would be, "What is your problem?" "What brings you to see me?" or "How can I help?" In response to the question, the patient will usually give a definition of the problem as she or he sees it. This usually is included in a time frame that lasts from 30 seconds to 1 minute 20 seconds. Out of the information given, the doctor will select one portion for reinforcement. The fragment chosen by the physician for reinforcement includes what the physician considers the most salient or relevant lead to pursue. As the patient discusses the present illness, usually included are what the patient considers relevant portions of the history, which encompasses family finances, occupational situation, childhood, and education. These segments of the history will usually flow in a meaningful sequence that includes the setting or crisis in which the occurrence takes place and will make a cohesive package of the apparently diverse information. Again, from this information the physician selects one bit for reinforcement, repeating the last phrase uttered by the patient. "Tell me more about . . ." or "Give me an example of . . ." would be adequate to keep the interview moving. About 30 minutes is sufficient to get the problem defined, and the physician is then free to fill in the gaps in the history left by the patient's free association.

What kinds of questions are the most economical in terms of the yield for the cue? If the question provokes a yes or no answer, the physician would respond with an open-ended question. The question "Tell me about your story" provides a series of facts evolving from free association. The interview proceeds in a manner not unlike the use of the microscope in examining a piece of tissue. Gross inspection is similar to the question "Tell me about . . ." A piece of information is selected on which to focus attention. This is the equivalent of low power observation. Out of that universe of discourse another bit is selected to pursue at higher magnification. Out of this set of information, the final bit is selected for "oil immersion" scrutiny. This provides the irreducible verbal communication, which amounts to the patient's attitude. The doctor proceeds through this phase of the interview by moving from the statement "Tell me about . . ." to the question "It's as though you feel like doing what, if anything?"

An example of this type of interviewing is a patient whose main problem is backache. In response to the statement "Tell me about . . ." the patient will give the doctor some information about the backache and go on to define the setting in which the backache occurred. This will include bits of family history, occupational history, and so on. The backache complaint is then selected for further elucidation. This is low power. As the patient discusses pain in greater detail he or she will tell where it occurs and define its quality and quantity. This is the equivalent of high, dry power observation. The next questions reflect oil immersion observation and pursue the way the patient feels and what action, if any, he feels like taking. This is the attitude dominating the patient's behavior and is in part responsible for the muscle tension, which is responsible for the backache itself. This definition of the attitude identifies that part of the patient's life style that the physician's attempts at therapy are designed to modify.

In the technique of question asking, the word "Why" should never be used; it carries the connotation that the physician is passing a negative judgment on the patient and that punishment should follow. The physician's answer to the question under discussion should not be used to formulate a new question. This will coerce the patient into using the doctor's answer rather than the patient's unique response.

Subsequent interviews usually start with the patient responding to an open-ended question, "What's gone on during the interval?" The same sequence follows each visit, and attention is focused on what has happened during the interval. Once this has been defined, an attempt is made to establish its source: "Can you remember the first time this happened or the first time you felt this way?" The physician then proceeds to reinforce the new data by establishing their parameters and details.

The sequence of events usually provides the format for subsequent meetings.

The occasional 7 second speech by the physician formulates briefly what has been said and establishes the basis for asking a new question. For example, "You said your mother-in-law came to visit and that parts of the visit were traumatic. Can you give me an example of the difficulty?"

In terminating the interview, the physician gives a succinct summary of the salient features that provide a basis for the diagnosis. The patient is then asked if there are questions about the process, and another appointment is set up.

With some exceptions, appointments at weekly intervals usually serve best. This allows enough time for reflection on what has been discussed and for the occurrence of new problems that provide the basis for the next visit, but not so much time that the material becomes stale.

Most acute psychiatric problems can be managed within about eight visits. This allows the doctor an opportunity to understand the problem and provide reassurance and an enhanced sense of personal worth, as well as a new direction in the format of the patient's life. By this time the physician should have a feel for continuing the interviews or for their termination. One always holds out to the patient the continuing availability of the doctor. Patients are never discharged; a prolongation of the time between interviews is preferred. It is suggested that the patient return at most once a year, preferably just before Christmas.

Special Observations

During the course of the interview the physician utilizes all of his senses to gather relevant information. Attention is paid to the rate of speech, changes in timbre or quality of voice, pitch of voice, and volume. Smiles and laughs are important to note. It should be remembered that there are many forms of the smile and the laugh. Increase in cardiac output can be noted by observing the rise and fall of the chest or movement of the crossed leg. The skin of the face will show pallor or redness and at times frank sweating. The handshake may be cool or warm, firm or limp, sweaty or dry.

Special note should be taken of the occurrence of blushing during the interview. Blushing is a physiologic state of vasodilatation of exposed skin blood vessels accompanied by a feeling of resentment. It is wise to question the patient since such feelings are likely to involve the physician. Such questions as "Was that a sensitive question?" or "Did that question involve sensitive topics for you?" often provide entree to the patient's attitudes and feelings about the physician. Getting them out in the open is a good way to defuse them.

Weeping among patients, especially female patients, is common. It connotes a sense of helplessness, loneliness, being left out in the cold, and a wish that the problem would go away. The doctor accepts the appearance of tears with no change in emotional set. A period of quiet ensues, after which the patient may continue to talk. If not, inquiry can be made about the feeling that accompanies the tears, the meaning of the situation present at the beginning of tears, or the patient's interpretation of the meaning of the tears. This statement provides the orientation or direction for the ensuing conversation.

The occurrence of anger is most often identified by perceiving controlled quietness in the patient. Words may become terse and directed at the physician. The doctor does not immediately label the feeling but instead asks questions to identify the feeling and encourages the patient to verbalize. If the doctor is the object of the anger, it becomes even more important to allow ventilation to occur. Inquiry is directed toward previous occurrences of the feeling, the people involved, and the setting in which it occurred.

Not uncommonly, one encounters patients who are on the periphery of the neurosis. The silent, monosyllabic patient who talks less than 10 seconds is likely exhibiting varying degrees of depression. The polysyllabic or dramatic monologist is likely in a manic state. The suspicious patient who goes into great detail in presenting the sequence of facts uses this technique to provide the data base for the existence of a paranoid state. The patient who continually gives the same story and is difficult to divert likely has some form of psychosis.

Patients Who Ask Questions

The physician responds to questions from the patient as though they are another bit of historical information. It is necessary to understand what the question means and the reason for asking the question at that particular point in the interview. Rather than giving a direct answer it is preferable to turn the question and afford the patient the opportunity to give his own answer or assess his own reason for the question. This technique usually ensures the continuation of the interview, provides more insight for the therapist about the patient, and avoids having the physician commit himself to an answer that lacks relevance and pertinence.

Outcome of Interview

Talking freely to an understanding doctor provides a great deal of reassurance. Pursuing what seems to be the patient's own problem, reinforced by the occasional "uh-huh" or short sentence, provides much needed emotional support and reassurance. This allows the patient to look at himself in a somewhat more objective manner, to recognize and acknowledge his own deviances and indiscretions, and to devise his own techniques for rearranging and redirecting his life.

As the interview progresses the physician has the opportunity to explain the psychophysiologic aspects of the problem or the psychodynamics involved. The judicious use of drugs on a temporary basis is sometimes indicated. The occasional use of the physical examination can be very reassuring. The doctor can test the patient's hand temperature, take the pulse, listen to the heartbeat, check the reflexes, or examine the joints. A statement of the findings, whether positive or negative, is often reassuring to the patient.

Occasional meetings with the family group are indicated. By moderating the exchange between involved people, new perspectives about the patient's problem can be achieved, and a more balanced understanding of the communication between the family members can be constructed.

Insight, defined as awareness of the relationship of relevant and pertinent variables, can sometimes be achieved by the patient, but it is not necessary for a favorable outcome. Providing the patient with an awareness of the complexity of the problem and identifying his present coping techniques may be accomplishing the most that is possible under the circumstances. Although advice should seldom be given, there are times, after the patient achieves some understanding of the dynamics involved, when a gentle constructive statement can be given.

Prognosis

The outcome of the attempted therapy is variable, but for the most part, effective and helpful. One does not aim for a state free from signs and symptoms; rather, one seeks to achieve fewer signs and symptoms of less intensity. As the time progresses, new situations will be encountered that bring about an exacerbation of the state and require further work, as though the illness is new. The illness is most likely to resolve with less effort, and the interval between this exacerbation and the next will be greater.

As the patients are followed over time, one is impressed with the subtleties of the changes that occur. Symptoms, when they do occur, are less acute but seldom disappear completely. The real achievement is in the quality of life-style. The emphasis is on the relative comfort of the patient and the fullness and satisfaction of the patient's life itself.

Attributes that predict a favorable treatment outcome are:

1. Recognition of failure of present patterns of adjustment and a desire for help.
2. Confidence in and ability to cooperate with the physician.
3. Flexibility of personality structure.
4. Disorder of recent origin.
5. Capacity and willingness to assume responsibility in treatment.
6. Past record of constructive interpersonal relationships.
7. Past record of ability to derive satisfaction from occupation, religion, sports, lodges, and other activities.
8. Willingness of family to cooperate.

DELIRIUM

method of
JEFFREY L. HOUPT, M.D.
Emory University
Atlanta, Georgia

Delirium is a psychiatric disorder of organic etiology. Diagnosis is based on a symptom complex that includes clouding of consciousness, cognitive impairment, and behavioral change. Treatment is directed at correcting the underlying organic abnormality, although environmental manipulation and appropriate psychotropic drugs are useful aids in management.

The symptoms of delirium are multiple. They range from quiet torpor to agitation and hallucinations. Some patients experience moderate amounts of anxiety, whereas others are agitated. Some show a schizophrenic-like thought disorder, whereas others do not. All patients, however, show an alteration in level of awareness and cognitive impairment if tested.

The most significant feature of delirium is the pattern of symptom emergence. Behavioral symptoms as well as the alteration in consciousness and cognitive impairment vary during the course of the day. This change in mental status follows a "sine wave" pattern. Those patients who show predominant disturbance at night with lucidity during the day are frequently referred to as "sundowners." It is not uncommon for these patients to have a normal or nearly normal mental status during the day, only to be abnormal a few hours later.

Diagnostic Considerations

Keeping in mind this fluctuating clinical course, the following four criteria should be met in order to make the diagnosis. Patient should show evidence of (1) clouding of consciousness, (2) disorientation and/or memory impairment, (3) at least two of the following behavioral symptoms: (a) perceptual disturbances such as misinterpretations, illusions, or hallucinations; (b) incoherent speech; (c) changes in sleep/wakefulness cycle; and (d) increased or decreased psychomotor activity, and (4) a reasonable association between a specific organic factor and the change in behavior (from the history, physical examination, or laboratory tests).

Clouding of consciousness (a reduced clarity of awareness of the environment) is inferred when the patient demonstrates a reduced capacity to shift, focus, or sustain attention to environmental stimuli. Disorientation generally occurs with respect to time, sometimes to place, and almost never to person. Memory impairment can most easily be tested by asking the patient to recall three objects after 5 minutes or by naming the last six presidents in reverse order. A more formal brief bedside examination would include calculations (serially subtracting 3 from 50 or 7 from 100), digit span (repeating six digits both forward and in reverse order), and naming address, phone number, family names, birthdate, and birthplace.

Because physicians spend limited amounts of time on the ward, obsevations from the nursing staff are most useful. In most instances, a presumptive diagnosis can be made from a description of the behavioral change and a review of the nursing notes. In addition, a number of factors are known to predispose to delirium, and thus the patient's previous history alerts the clinician to the possibility. Progressive age, alcoholism, history of head trauma, sensory impairment (blindness, deafness), major organ system failure (hepatic, renal, pulmonary, cardiovascular, endocrine), multiple medications (particularly those with central nervous system effects), placement in the intensive care unit, and surgical operations are all predisposing factors to delirium. Any change in behavior associated with any of these predisposing factors should immediately alert the clinician to the possibility of a delirious state.

Etiologic Evaluation

The fundamental principle of assessment of delirium is to determine the underlying physiologic malady causing the altered behavioral state. Although the list of causes is potentially extensive, evaluation takes a reasonably brief period of time.

First, the clinician should review the history of the predisposing factors and determine which, if any, are present and the nature of their severity. Second, the physician should review electrolytes, glucose, liver, and renal function tests, CBC, arterial blood gases, chest x-ray films, and ECG as well as the medications being taken by the patient, particularly their cumulative doses. Finally, if a cause still escapes detection, further metabolic and neurologic evaluation is indicated.

Two principles should be kept in mind. First, the acuteness of metabolic insult is important in the development of delirium. Thus a rapid change in electrolyte or hematocrit may cause delirium, whereas a slower progressive change of the same magnitude may not. Second, multiple minor metabolic abnormalities may be cumulative and together may account for delirium, whereas each of them taken independently would not be significant.

Treatment

Treatment should be directed at finding the underlying abnormality. Although many deliria are transient and resolve without determination of the causative agent, an extensive search for underlying causes is important, since, in some cases, untreated delirium will lead to a dementia. It is also important to recognize that even though a delirium can be modified and managed through the use of psychotropic agents and environmental manipulation, the clinical improvement can occur in the face of ongoing organic insult. Thus the clinician should pursue the work-up for physiologic abnormality until such time as the clinician is reasonably sure that ongoing acute processes have been discovered and corrected.

Both environmental manipulation and psychotropic drugs can be of use in managing the delirious state, however. Because psychotropic drugs carry their own potential side effects, environmental manipulation should be used as a primary resource. These include utilizing family members, familiar items from the home to help orient the patient, special efforts to introduce the patient to procedures that are taking place and to assist in his orientation to time and place by the nursing staff, and the use of a light on in the room at night (often invaluable for patients who sundown). Family members can often be of significant help by remaining at the patient's bedside and assisting in orienting the patient and quelling his fears. Every effort should be made to liberalize hospital rules if the family proves to be an adjunct in the patient's treatment. In addition, calendars on the wall or familiar photographs or a radio are often of major assistance.

Patients whose delirium is a threat to their welfare or to that of others on the ward because of the behavioral abnormalities and who do not respond to simpler environmental manipulations should be managed with psychotropic medications. Benzodiazepines are indicated in those cases where the delirium is due to sedative hypnotic withdrawal, as in alcohol withdrawal states; anticholinesterase agents such as physostigmine are indicated in those cases where the delirium is determined to be caused by cholinergic agents.

Most cases of delirium, however, are of a nonspecific cause and are characterized by agitation. In these cases, haloperidol (Haldol) is of use. In most cases, 1 to 2 mg two to three times daily orally or intramuscularly are useful. In some cases, up to 5 mg intramuscularly are necessary if the initial smaller dose is unsuccessful in controlling behavior. General rules of thumb are as follows: the intramuscular route of Haldol achieves two to three times the plasma level as the oral route; peak action of the intramuscular route is achieved in 30 minutes, whereas the oral route requires 4 to 6 hours; more than 20 mg intramuscularly of haloperidol is rarely needed within the first 24 hours; and if the patient has not responded, further evaluation and consultation are required.

Many antipsychotic drugs have significant interactions with other drugs. The effects of narcotics, sedative hypnotics, and anticholinergic drugs are all enhanced when combined with antipsychotics. In addition, antipsychotics can induce hypotension if combined with sympathomimetics, inhalation anesthetics, or conduction anesthetics because of the alpha-blocking properties of the antipsychotics. This is particularly true in patients who are hypovolemic.

The prevention of severe behavioral disturbance from delirium is best accomplished by early recognition of the syndrome. Thus the clinician should be aware of the predisposing factors of delirium and the early changes in orientation and cognitive impairment that accompany the behavioral abnormalities. Early detection and appropriate treatment can prevent many of the severe secondary disturbances associated with this disorder.

AFFECTIVE DISORDERS

method of
DAVID S. JANOWSKY, M.D.
University of California, San Diego
San Diego, California

Disorders of mood, including mania and depression, are very common emotional disturbances, with estimates of incidence over a lifetime ranging between 6 and 25 per cent of people, depending on the definitions used. Depression, at the extreme, includes (1) a mood component (feeling sad, blue, unhappy, down in the dumps); (2) a motoric component (being slowed down, having sagging features, having prolonged latency to speak, or being agitated); (3) cognitive manifestations (feeling worthless, hopeless, useless, pessimistic, and a failure; (4) physiologic features (middle and late insomnia, decreased REM sleep, constipation, diurnal mood variation, fatigue, impotence, decreased libido); and (5) a motivational disturbance (lack of interest in usual pleasurable and necessary activities, inability to experience pleasure, lack of motivation).

Depression

Interpersonal Approaches

Once an accurate diagnosis is made, the cornerstone of psychotherapy for the depressive patient is the effective instillation of hope and an attempt to deal positively with feelings of hopelessness, helplessness, and worthlessness in an empathetic, warm, and caring way. Since depression is often associated with a poor evaluation of one's abilities, significant decisions should be deferred during depressive episodes. The clinician knows that depression is a disorder that ultimately will remit or will be responsive to treatment. However, the depressive does not know this and thinks just the opposite is true.

Little is known about the specific comparative efficacies of different psychotherapies, and indeed clinician personality variables seem very important. Therapists who are empathetic, genuine, warm, and accepting consistently have the best psychotherapeutic results compared with those who lack such skills.

With respect to specific psychotherapies for depression, there is fairly good evidence that interpersonal therapy, a technique aimed primarily at supporting the patient in his or her life and identifying and working through issues causing conflict and negative emotion, leads to improved social functioning, compared with a lack of therapy. Cognitive therapy, aimed at defining and extinguishing faulty negative thinking, using primarily behavioral techniques, also has proved efficacious.

The Suicidal Patient. It is important to note that all depressed patients are suicide risks to a greater or lesser extent. Suicide potential is the limiting factor in treating depressed patients on an ambulatory basis, and this risk should be directly, repeatedly, and explicitly assessed by asking the patient about his or her suicidal ideas. There must be sensitivity to the behavioral clues for suicide, such as statements about wishing to be dead, a sudden unexpected alleviation of depressive symptoms, or a "wrapping up" of the obligations of one's life.

Hospitalization is appropriate at many points in the treatment of moderate-to-severe depression, especially when psychologic and psychopharmacologic approaches fail or suicide seems a concrete risk. The clinician should attempt to prevent patients from using the "suicide option," and should display no ambivalence regarding this.

Psychopharmacologic Treatment

The most popular psychopharmacologic approaches to the treatment of depression are the use of conventional or first generation tricyclic antidepressants and new generation antidepressants. Major indications for these drugs include the treatment of biologic depressions (major depressive disorder, bipolar disorder) and selected cases of minor or reactive depression. These drugs may also be helpful in the treatment of dysthymic disorder, mixed anxiety-depression syndromes in the alleviation of panic attacks, and as treatments for insomnia and enuresis.

The conventional and newer antidepressants are 60 to 75 per cent effective, compared with placebo or no treatment in which approximately 30 per cent of the patients respond. Overall, any of the conventional antidepressants (imipramine [Tofranil], amitriptyline [Elavil], desipramine [Norpramin], nortriptyline [Aventyl], protriptyline [Vivactil], doxepin [Sinequan, Adapin], and trimipramine [Surmontil]); the newer antidepressants (trazodone [Desyrel], amoxapine [Asendin], maprotiline [Ludiomil], nomifesin [Merital]); or the soon to be released antidepressant bupropion [Wellbutrin]) has a similar efficacy in large groups of depressed patients.

General Principles of Use. Most antidepressants require between 1 and 2 or more weeks to exert therapeutic effects. Therefore, the patient must be advised not to expect immediate relief. Antidepressant drugs are often given in inadequate doses. Although optimal doses vary among drugs, most antidepressants require final doses of 150 to 300 mg orally each day. Protriptyline (Vivactil) requires about half this amount and trazodone (Desyrel) and amoxapine (Asendin) require one third to one half more. Dosages generally should be started at 25 mg per day and can be increased to peak amounts over 10 to 20 days. Obtaining serum antidepressant levels may be useful in determining compliance or toxicity, but such levels are probably not very useful in determining efficacy, at least in the outpatient setting.

Doses of antidepressants in the elderly should be increased relatively slowly, and lower starting doses and peak amounts (beginning at 10 mg per day and increasing the dose to 75 to 100 mg per day) are often safe and effective, although full doses may be necessary in a given patient.

In general, antidepressant drugs can be given as a single dose at bedtime, except when problems such as A-V conduction defects or benign prostatic hypertrophy contraindicate such a schedule.

Maintenance of antidepressant drug treatment over a period of months to years will decrease the relapse rate in patients with recurrent unipolar depression. It is probably best to keep patients on full antidepressant doses during maintenance therapy.

Specificity. In the past decade, much has been written about specific types of neurochemical depressions. However, overall, antidepressant efficacies appear unrelated to their specific neurotransmitter-altering properties, such as being primarily serotonergic or noradrenergic.

Antidepressant Side Effects. In choosing an antidepressant drug, the side effect profile is the most important guide. Central nervous system effects frequently include drowsiness and sedation, as well as difficulties in concentration and fine tremor. Furthermore, with increasing age, progressively more patients develop a confusional syndrome due to the central anticholinergic effects of antidepressants. Less common are seizure induction and incoordination, as well as the activation of pre-existing psychotic symptoms and the induction of mania or hypomania in bipolar patients.

Of the conventional antidepressants, doxepin (Sinequan), amitriptyline (Elavil), and trimipramine (Surmontil) are the most sedating. These drugs may be useful in the treatment of depressed and anxious insomniac patients, although there is no real relationship between sedation and the ultimate alleviation of actual core depressive symptoms. Conversely, sedation and "foggyheadedness" are major reasons for noncompliance. Of the newer antidepressants, trazodone (Desyrel) and maprotiline (Ludiomil) are especially sedating, as is alprazolam (Xanax), an antianxiety agent showing antidepressant efficacy. Somewhat less sedating antidepressants are desipramine (Norpramin), imipramine (Tofranil), and amoxapine (Asendin). The recently approved drug nomifesin (Merital) and the investigational drug bupropion (Wellbutrin) appear to have few if any sedating properties and indeed may be activating and capable of causing insomnia.

Although all antidepressants can cause seizures, it currently appears that maprotiline (Ludiomil) is especially dangerous in this regard. Furthermore, early studies suggest that bupropion (Wellbutrin) has the potential to cause frequent seizures. Nomifesin (Merital) and possibly trazodone (Desyrel) to date appear to have relatively little seizure-producing potential. Upon withdrawal, alprazolam (Xanax), when given chronically in 4 to 6 mg per day antidepressant doses, can cause seizures and other barbiturate-like withdrawal effects.

In addition, there is evidence that nomifesin (Merital) and bupropion (Wellbutrin), due to their dopaminergic properties, may be especially prone to cause behavioral activation, insomnia, excitement, and, in the case of nomifesin, activation of psychotic symptoms and manic episodes.

Generally, antidepressants do not cause extrapyramidal effects. Amoxapine (Asendin), due to its dopamine-blocking properties, can cause parkinsonian symptoms, akathesia (motor restlessness), and galactorrhea, associated with increases in serum prolactin, as well as in rare instances the semipermanent or permanent neuromotor dysfunction tardive dyskinesia. Therefore, use of amoxapine for more than 3 to 4 months is not recommended.

Anticholinergic effects are a very common cause of distress in patients receiving antidepressants and most commonly include blurred vision, tachycardia, dry mouth, and constipation. In predisposed patients with benign prostatic hypertrophy, urinary obstruction may occur, as may increases in intraocular pressure in patients with closed-angle glaucoma.

Amitriptyline (Elavil), doxepin (Sinequan, Adapin), protriptyline (Vivactil), and trimipramine (Surmontil) have the most anticholinergic effects of the conventional antidepressants. Imipramine and desipramine, although having fewer anticholinergic properties than the former drugs, still have these effects. Similarly, amoxapine (Asendin) and maprotiline (Ludiomil), while less anticholinergic than amitriptyline (Elavil) and trimipramine (Surmontil), still are moderately anticholinergic. Trazodone (Desyrel), in contrast, appears to have virtually no anticholinergic properties, a characteristic indicating its special use in the elderly. Nomifesin (Merital) and bupropion (Wellbutrin) appears to have some, although minimal, anticholinergic effects, as does alprazolam (Xanax).

The speed of onset of an antidepressant may be important in certain patients. There is evidence that amoxapine (Asendin) and possibly maprotiline (Ludiomil), trazodone (Desyrel), and alprazolam (Xanax) have faster onsets of action (5 to 7 days) than do other antidepressants. Bupropion (Wellbutrin) appears to have a slow onset of action.

The cardiovascular effects of the antidepressant drugs represent a major drawback to their use. Hypotension is probably the most common cardiovascular effect and may lead to fainting episodes with trauma, especially in the elderly, as well as rare cases of myocardial infarction and cerebral ischemia. Also common is anticholinergic-induced tachycardia. In addition, antidepressants have been reported to have cardiac depressant effects and to worsen congestive heart failure. Many of the conventional and newer antidepressants have quinidine-like effects which exaggerate atrial-ventricular conduction defects, including first degree A-V block and right and left bundle branch block in predisposed patients. Generally, the cardiotoxic and hypotensive effects of the antidepressant drugs are correlated with patient age and cardiac status.

With respect to conventional antidepressant hypotensive effects, nortriptyline (Aventyl) appears to be the least hypotension-inducing. Imipramine (Tofranil), amitriptyline (Elavil), and trimipramine (Surmontil) appear prone to cause hypotension, although most conventional antidepressants can also cause lowered blood pressure, as can maprotiline (Ludiomil), amoxapine (Asendin), and trazodone (Desyrel). Preliminary findings suggest that nomifesin (Merital) and bupropion (Wellbutrin) are relatively less hypotension-inducing.

With respect to quinidine-like effects, all conventional antidepressants can cause conduction abnormalities, especially in people with pre-existing defects. In addition, similar cardiac problems have been reported with maprotiline (Ludiomil) and amoxapine (Asendin). Trazodone (Desyrel) appears not to cause conduction defects but may increase premature ventricular contractions and intensify bradycardia. Bupropion (Wellbutrin), nomifesin (Merital), and alprazolam (Xanax) appear to cause minimal cardiotoxicity. With respect to the induction of allergic reactions, skin rashes have been reported relatively frequently with bupropion.

Rapid withdrawal of antidepressants may lead to motor restlessness, headaches, anxiety, dysphoria, insomnia, muscle aches, and nausea, all probably due to the unmasking of cholinergic receptors. This syndrome can be prevented by slowly withdrawing the antidepressant drug over a 1.5 to 2 week period.

Treatment of Side Effects. Generally, treatment of the side effects of a given antidepressant is based on proper initial selection and judicious switching of antidepressants to one with less of a given troublesome side effect, if problems occur. However, bethanechol (Urecholine), 10 to 50 mg every 4 to 6 hours, may be helpful in the treatment of peripheral anticholinergic effects (use not listed by maker). The centrally acting cholinomimetic physostigmine (Antilirium) may be useful in the treatment of the central anticholinergic syndrome (confusional state) induced by antidepressant drugs. Giving an antidepressant at night may eliminate conscious perception of side effects, since these tend to occur in conjunction with peak blood levels, when the patient is asleep. Propranolol, 30 to 60 mg per day, may be useful for tremor (use not listed by maker).

Overdoses in Depressed Patients. A major problem for the depressed patient is the tendency to attempt suicide. Potentially suicidal patients should be given only small amounts of drugs (7 to 10 day quantities), and drugs should be kept under lock and key and dispensed by a family member. Of the antidepressants, trazodone (Desyrel), nomifesin (Merital), and bupropion (Wellbutrin) appear relatively safe in an overdose, at least when taken without other drugs such as alcohol or barbiturates. Maprotiline (Ludiomil) and possibly amoxapine (Asendin) appear especially dangerous in an overdose.

Combination Therapies

There is some evidence that giving an antidepressant drug in combination with other drugs may be useful. Levothyroxine (Synthroid), in doses of 25 micrograms per day, appears to salvage imipramine nonresponders and to increase imipramine's speed of onset. Doses of L-tryptophan of 2 to 4 grams per day added to an antidepressant regimen sometimes have been shown useful in refractory depression, as has the addition of relatively low (300 to 900 mg per day) doses of lithium carbonate. There is also some evidence that methylphenidate (5 to 15 mg three times daily) added to an antidepressant regimen may be effective. Finally, it may be useful in patients with psychotic depression (those with delusions and hallucinations) to add conventional doses of an antipsychotic drug, such as haloperidol (Haldol), up to 15 mg per day, along with an antidepressant regimen.

Monoamine Oxidase Inhibitors

Generally, the monoamine oxidase inhibitors (MAOIs), like phenelzine (Nardil) or tranylcypromine (Parnate), should be considered a second line of therapy in the treatment of depression. These drugs generally have been underused, owing to their reputation for causing dangerous sympathetic reactions. Nevertheless, they are probably useful in "biologic" depressions as well as in the more neurotic or "atypical" depressions. There is some evidence that MAOIs may be especially useful in depressed geriatric patients, as well as in patients with panic attacks and in the treatment of post-traumatic neurosis. Their most feared side effect is the induction of hypertensive crises. This occurs following the ingestion of tyramine-containing foods or legally prescribed, over-the-counter, or illicit psychostimulants or meperidine (Demerol). Examples of such agents or foods include diet pills; amphetamines; cocaine; cold capsules containing such psychostimulants as phenylpropranolamine, ephedrine, or phenylephrine; bronchodilators; fava beans; aged cheeses; lager beers; pickled herring; canned figs; soybean products; chicken livers; yeast extract products; excessive caffeine; and excessive alcohol.

Hypertensive crises often present as a severe throbbing occipital headache, diaphoresis and prostration, neck stiffness, nausea, convulsions, hyperpyrexia, vomiting, and hypertension. These effects can be very serious, even fatal. An alpha-adrenergic blocking agent such as phentolamine or chlorpromazine is the primary treatment of choice. Furthermore, the tricyclic antidepressants have infrequently been reported to induce hypertensive crises in MAO-treated patients. This occurs most often when a tricyclic antidepressant is added to a MAOI regimen, rather than the opposite. At least a 10 day wash-out should occur between beginning a tricyclic antidepressant after MAOI treatment or vice versa. MAOI effects and vulnerability to side effects can persist for about 2 weeks after drug discontinuation.

More common than the hypertensive crisis is the induction of hypotension by MAOIs, as well as the impairment of ejaculation, overstimulation and insomnia, activation of mania in bipolar patients, and psychosis activation in schizophrenics. Induction of confusion, nausea, vomiting, diarrhea, and lethargy can also occur. A very rare but sometimes lethal hepatic neurosis can occur. Anticholinergic, quinidine-like, and sedating effects tend to occur less frequently than with the conventional and newer antidepressants. Therefore, the MAOIs may be especially indicated in patients with cardiac disease or when anticholinergic effects are dangerous. However, MAOI efficacy is confounded by the fact that the elderly often receive multiple drugs that can interact with MAOIs, and that this population may have difficulty being compliant.

Doses of phenelzine (Nardil), the most widely used MAOI in the USA, range from 30 to 90 or more mg per day (approximately 1 mg per kg body weight), given in 15 or 30 mg divided doses to avoid the drug's insomniac effects. MAOIs tend to show therapeutic effects somewhat more slowly than do the tricyclic and newer antidepressants, and therapeutic effects may require several weeks of full dosages.

Psychostimulants

Although generally discouraged by governmental agencies because of their abuse potential, psychotogenic effects, and tolerance development, the psychostimulants may have some usefulness in the treatment of affective disorders. There is evidence that certain elderly patients may benefit from long-term treatment with methylphenidate (Ritalin), and that the short-term euphoria-antidepressant effects of these drugs may be useful as an adjunct to treatment with conventional antidepressants.

Electroconvulsive Treatment (ECT)

Mostly because of political and esthetic reasons, ECT is used as a second or third line treatment and, in many centers is used rarely if at all. ECT is a remarkably effective (80 to 90 per cent) and safe treatment for major depressive disorder and bipolar depression. The major side effect of ECT is temporary confusion and memory loss, which ultimately usually extends only around the period of treatment.

Contemporary electroconvulsive therapy is given in conjunction with administration of atropine, a short-acting muscle relaxant such as succinylcholine, concurrent artificial respiration, and airway maintenance. Pretreatment with a short-acting barbiturate renders the patient unconscious before succinylcholine administration. Few contraindications to ECT exist. Any increase in intracranial pressure, existence of a brain tumor, or cerebral or arterial aneurysm is a contraindication. Of course, contraindications to the use of a barbiturate anesthesia or to succinylcholine may preclude the use of ECT or dictate use of ECT without pretreatment.

Generally, patients receive a series of 8 to 12 or more treatments over 2 to 4 weeks. Unilateral application of ECT electrodes over the nondominant hemisphere, rather than bilateral administration, decreases memory loss but retains efficacy.

Mania

Psychologic Treatment

Along with a generally supportive approach, the psychologic treatment of mania involves the formation of a relationship with the patient that undercuts the exaggerated tendency to deny illness and to stop treatment, so as to regain "high" feelings. Many manic patients, while seeming plausible, are self-destructive in their grandiosity, overspend, are overimposing, and show extremely poor judgment. When the manic patient is going out of control, it is important for the physician to exert as much therapeutic control as possible, no matter how persuasive the manic's logic seems, and to seriously consider hospitalization. Hospitalization is indicated if the mania is progressing, especially if drug noncompliance is occurring.

Manic patients often do not appear sick. This, combined with their ability to attack therapists', coworkers' and family's soft spots, to "con," to push limits, to project responsibility onto others, and to alternately treat those close to them as esteemed and despised, makes them difficult to handle psychologically. A physician dealing with a manic patient should be aware of these characteristics and be on guard against forgetting that mania is an illness and regarding the patient as hateful. Finally, working out a "hypomanic alert" with the patient, coworkers, and family—a system for reporting early key symptoms of mania specific for the patient—may allow prompt institution of treatment.

Drug Treatment

A major advance in the treatment of mania is the use of lithium carbonate. Lithium is effective in treating about 85 per cent of manic attacks. It probably has a prophylactic value in preventing bipolar manic and depressive swings and recurrent depressions, decreasing both the frequency and amplitude of these. As with the tricyclic antidepressants, lithium usually has a 7 to 14 day lag phase before it begins to work. Therefore, coadministration of an antipsychotic drug (perphenazine [Trilafon], 8 to 64 mg per day), especially in highly manic patients, may be indicated. This part of the treatment can be stopped after several weeks, when manic symptoms decrease and lithium becomes effective.

Lithium is a relatively toxic drug. Therefore, it is necessary to monitor serum lithium levels as often as twice weekly during the first several weeks of treatment, and subsequently twice a month and ultimately monthly or every other month. Serum levels needed to treat an acute manic episode generally range between 1.0 and 1.5 mEq per liter, with levels taken 12 hours after oral dosing. Sometimes even higher serum levels are required, whereas low levels may be adequate in the elderly and in selected other patients. Levels of 0.6 to 1.0 mEq per liter are generally needed to maintain prophylaxis. The actual dose of $LiCO_3$ given may vary widely; doses as low as 900 mg per day to 3 to 4 grams per day may be needed. Acutely manic patients seem to require more lithium to attain a given blood level.

Since bipolar disorders are often recurrent and a high chance of suicide exists, the chronic administration of lithium over a period of years is indicated in patients who tend to relapse.

Noncompliance is a major problem in the treatment of mania. Reasons given for noncompliance include the missing of the "high" of mania. Furthermore, side effects often occur, including memory problems, muscle weakness, tremor, poor coordination, feeling mentally dull, polyurea, thirst, nocturia, weight gain, edema, and feeling depressed. In addition, lithium-treated patients often feel nauseated, have muscle weakness, and may have diarrhea, aggravation of acne, maculopapular rashes, and alopecia. Cardiac and other defects in the fetus during the first trimester of pregnancy may also occur. At more toxic doses, lithium can cause extreme lethargy, severe tremor, disorientation, confusion, delirium, ataxia, myoclonic jerks, and central nervous system depression. Toxic blood levels of lithium are only two to three times therapeutic levels. Fortunately, the severe effects of lithium tend to develop slowly and insidiously, so that toxic blood levels in an overdose are less dangerous than those that increase slowly over time.

Sodium depletion due to diet, excessive sweating, or diuretics can rapidly cause serum lithium levels to rise to dangerous levels, and close monitoring of lithium levels is indicated in these above conditions.

Furthermore, chronic use of lithium tends to cause a reversible suppression of the thyroid in up to 25 per cent of cases. Finally, although some evidence exists that renal fibrosis may occur in addition to a reversible diabetes insipidus–like syndrome, there is actually little evidence that irreversible renal changes occur.

Treatment of lithium side effects involves giving the drug in small, frequent doses, lowering the dose when possible, and giving lithium along with meals. The beta-adrenergic blocking agents propranolol (Inderal), 30 to 60 mg per day, and metoprolol (Lopressor) have been reported useful in the treatment of lithium-induced tremor. Supplemental thyroid is the treatment of choice in lithium-induced hypothyroidism.

Because of its numerous side effects, it is advised that baseline renal function studies (creatinine, BUN, urinalysis), a complete blood count, thyroid function studies, and serum electrolyte levels be obtained prior to lithium therapy. Although lithium's cardiovascular effects are generally minimal, T wave flattening is common and sinoatrial conduction defects have occurred, especially in the elderly; a baseline electrocardiogram is suggested. Electrolytes, renal function, and thyroid tests should be repeated every 6 months.

Recently, the antiseizure medication carbamazepine (Tegretol) has been shown to be effective in the treatment of approximately 60 per cent of manic patients, as well as to be useful in the prophylaxis of bipolar swings (this use is not listed in the manufacturer's directive). Furthermore, carbamazepine may be useful in the treatment of lithium-resistant manic patients, and a synergistic effect with both drugs used together has been reported in several cases. Generally, it is best to use carbamazepine as a back-up drug for lithium and to give these drugs separately rather than together.

The most dramatic side effects of carbamazepine are hematologic. Severe agranulocytosis, as well as suppression of white blood cells and platelets, has been reported rarely. Other significant side effects include nausea, vomiting, dizziness, ataxia, incoordination, and tremor.

Efficacious doses of carbamazepine vary from patient to patient. However, dosages of 600 to 1200 mg per day are common in the treatment of mania, and prophylaxis may occur at doses of 200 to 600 mg per day. Blood levels usually lie between 6 and 12 micrograms per ml, but no solid blood level–efficacy relationship has been discovered, although blood levels may be helpful in determining compliance and documenting toxicity.

SCHIZOPHRENIA

method of
JOHN M. DAVIS, M.D.
University of Illinois
Chicago, Illinois

Although the cause of schizophrenia remains unknown, treatment with antipsychotic drugs has radically altered its natural course. Prior to the discovery of antipsychotic drugs, approximately two out of three patients who developed schizophrenic symptoms spent most of their lives in a psychotic condition in a state hospital. With drug treatment, some patients make an almost complete recovery, whereas others function at a reasonable or borderline level except during brief hospitalizations for relapses. Today it is relatively uncommon for patients to spend their lives in continuous hospitalization. There are two variants of schizophrenic spectrum disease: classic DSM III schizophrenia and schizophreniform disease (a psychotic episode without a chronic course of over 6 months). The acute episodes of both variants of this disorder are treated similarly, namely, with antipsychotic drugs. Maintenance medication to prevent relapse is used for classic schizophrenia. The efficacy of antipsychotic drugs is well substantiated by a large number (over 100) of double blind controlled studies. With only placebo treatment, about 25 per cent of patients who presented with an acute episode were much improved at 6 weeks. However, 45 per cent further deteriorated at 6 weeks. The remaining placebo-treated patients were equally divided between those showing no change and those manifesting minimal improvement. With drug treatment, 70 per cent of those patients were much improved at 6 weeks and over 90 per cent showed some degree of improvement at 6 weeks, with only a small minority either showing no change or worsening at this time point.

MECHANISM OF ACTION

The antipsychotic drugs lessen or eliminate virtually all of the symptoms of schizophrenia, such as hallucinations and delusions, and are the only agents that do so. They speed up retarded schizophrenics but slow down excited schizophrenics, so on this psychomotor dimension they normalize. The appropriate term for these drugs is "antipsychotics." The term "antischizophrenics" would be too specific because the antipsychotic drugs also normalize the psychosis in psychotic depression or paranoid disorders, have an antimanic effect in mania, and have an antipsychotic effect in organic psychosis.

Working with psychologists Holzman and Hurt, I quantified the degree of improvement in thought disorder and was able to show that the time course of the average antipsychotic drug in producing improvement in symptoms exactly parallels that of the improvement in thought disorder. The biochemical mechanism of action of the antipsychotic drugs is now known; their therapeutic effect occurs through blocking dopamine receptors. The antipsychotic action lies in the stereo specific isomer blocking dopamine rather than in the dopaminergically inactive isomers. There is an almost perfect correlation between dose to achieve dopamine blockade and dose used clinically. If one reduces brain dopamine levels by synthesis inhibition, a lower dose of neuroleptic would be needed for effective treatment of schizophrenia.

Since the cause of schizophrenia is unknown, we cannot specify exactly how an antidopaminergic mechanism of action has a beneficial effect. "Tranquilizer" is an inappropriate term. Normal persons often find these drugs slightly unpleasant, and in no sense do they produce a happy sedation. Antipsychotics with marked sedative properties are no more effective than antipsychotics with minimal or no sedative properties. Their antidopaminergic mechanism of action is qualitatively different from the mechanism of sedation. For example, they do not block benzodiazepine receptors.

Just after their discovery, when chlorpromazine and meprobamate were first prescribed, the term "major and minor tranquilizers" was used. At that time, it was incorrectly thought that the majority of mental illnesses were defenses against anxiety. Mental illness was said to vary with the depth of regression from schizophrenia (severe regression), to depression (moderate regression), to the neuroses (mild regression). This type of thinking has led to the idea that chlorpromazine is to be used for severe anxiety and meprobamate for mild cases. This is false. Antipsychotics are not indicated in nonpsychotic depression, severe generalized anxiety, or panic attacks. Unipolar depression should be treated by antidepressants (or electroconvulsive therapy [ECT]) (Table 1) and acute episodes of bipolar depression by lithium or antidepressants or both (or ECT) with lithium for maintenance. Generalized anxiety is treated by buspirone (Buspar) or a benzodiazepine and panic attack by tricyclics, MAO inhibitors, or alprazolam. Panic attack disease should not be treated acutely or chronically with antipsychotics or with chronic benzodiazepines (other than alprazolam), except possibly in a single panic attack in which 1 tab can be used for a transitory effect. We need to dispel the old notion of major and minor tranquilizers.

TABLE 1. **Treatment of Drug-Responsive Psychiatric Disorders**

Disorder	Treatment: *Acute Episode*	*Maintenance*
Schizophreniform	antipsychotic	none
Schizophrenia	antipsychotic	antipsychotic
Manic phase bipolar	lithium	lithium
"Severe mania"	lithium plus antipsychotic	lithium
Bipolar depressed phase	lithium with antidepressant	lithium
Bipolar psychotic depression	lithium or antidepressant plus antipsychotic	lithium
Unipolar depression	antidepressant	antidepressant (? lithium)
Unipolar depression with psychosis	antidepressant plus antipsychotic	not studied
Generalized anxiety	benzodiazepine or buspirone	not well studied
Panic attack disease	reassurance	alprazolam MAO inhibitor (phenelzine) tricyclics

There is a qualitative difference between classes of psychotropic drugs. There are five basic drug responsive entities in psychiatry (schizophreniform disease, mania, depression, generalized anxiety, and panic attack disease), and each has a different constellation of symptoms, course, and drug response. A recent study found that psychotic depression responds poorly to antidepressants alone and should be treated with a combined antipsychotic-antidepressant drug or with ECT. Antipsychotics are sometimes needed in acute mania. With lithium, there is a lag period of about 5 to 20 days between initiation of treatment and antimanic response. Although antipsychotics combined with lithium can produce a more rapid response, if possible I prefer lithium alone in mild to moderate mania because a response to lithium alone indicates that lithium would be the drug of choice for maintenance. A low dose of antipsychotic is sometimes helpful in severe agitation in the elderly, but long-term use should be avoided.

Treatment of Acute Episode

Since there is a loss of reality testing in psychosis, patients can be dangerous to others or themselves (suicide, self-destructive behavior, inability to care for self). The physician must determine the potential for such serious harm and arrange hospitalization if necessary. Sometimes the essential support to protect the patient can be provided without hospitalization by involving the family or resorting to hospital alternatives. In administering medication, the clinician should first determine the degree of urgency. An intramuscular injection has a more rapid action: a reasonable plasma level of antipsychotic drug occurs approximately 30 minutes after intramuscular injection versus approximately 1½ hours after oral administration. The bioavailability of oral preparations is such that plasma level after oral medication is one third to one half of the plasma level after intramuscular injection. However, it is possible to switch to oral tablets after the first injection in the patient who will take oral medication.

The dose of antipsychotic drugs is administered at periodic intervals as determined by urgency, e.g., 4 tablets a day for the typical patient versus hourly injections or tablets for a violent patient. The dose is titrated based on the patient's therapeutic response and side effects after each dose. If some lessening of the psychosis is not apparent, the dose needs to be increased. Patients do manifest reduction of psychotic symptoms even 1 hour after intramuscular injection. The time course of improvement is such that one third to one half of the improvement that would ultimately occur takes place within the first week, and most of the remaining improvement is seen by 6 weeks. Although there is improvement within hours, the time course of improvement is measured in days and weeks. The half-life of improvement is about 1 week.

There are five classes of antipsychotic compounds: the phenothiazines, the thioxanthenes (thiothixene), the butyrophenones (haloperidol), the dibenzoxazepines (loxapine), and the indoles (molindone). We believe that all exert their therapeutic action in the same manner by blocking dopamine receptors and hence are identical in their therapeutic action. The only exception to this is promazine, which, although possessing antipsychotic properties, is clearly less effective than the other neuroleptics. The drugs do, however, differ in side effects, and the clinician may choose a given drug according to the side effect he wishes to avoid at the expense of a different side effect that he thinks is tolerable. There is a trade-off between side effects. Thioridazine has the fewest extrapyramidal side effects but is more sedating and anticholinergic. The so-called high potency neuroleptics, e.g., thiothixene, haloperidol, trifluoperazine, and fluphenazine, cause fewer sedative-anticholinergic but more extrapyramidal side effects.

At one time, it was suggested that there might be different antipsychotics for different subtypes of schizophrenia, e.g., one for the excited schizophrenic, and another for the retarded schizophrenic. This has proven to be false. All psychotics respond equally well to all psychotic drugs. If a patient does not respond to a given neuroleptic, the physician should alter the dose. If dose adjustment fails, some clinicians favor switching to a different antipsychotic. Some patients respond favorably to the second antipsychotic. This may be because that particular patient is a slow responder and may have responded to the initial drug with a longer duration of treatment. Controlled studies are needed.

In Table 2 are listed the antipsychotic drugs and a rough estimate of their antipsychotic doses. I recommend starting out with a modest dose (roughly 600 to 900 mg chlorpromazine equivalence) for the first few days or cut back slightly for the next week (400 to 800 mg) or two and then again switch to maintenance medication (200 to 500 mg). It is important to titrate the dose according to the patient's clinical response and side effects. In patients who appear oversedated, the clinician may consider trying a lower dose or switching to a less sedative neuroleptic. In patients who experience no side effects and no clinical response, the dose should be increased. I recommend gradually increasing the dose in nonresponding patients until a clinical response occurs.

There have been approximately 25 dose response studies in psychiatry. These studies reveal that massive doses, on average, produce no better therapeutic effect than standard doses (below 900 mg chlorpromazine equivalence). There are also studies that find that doses in the realm 300 mg chlorpromazine equivalence or less produce a poorer response than somewhat higher doses. There is, however, substantial individual variability, so one schizophrenic may do well on 300 mg chlorpromazine equivalence, whereas another may require 500 mg, and a third may need 800 mg.

There are wide individual differences in plasma drug levels in patients given comparable doses of different antipsychotic drugs. There have been approximately 10 controlled studies correlating plasma level to therapeutic efficacy using a reliable experimental design. Most of these studies find nonresponders to have either unusually low or unusually high plasma or RBC levels. However, there is a good deal of scatter in the data. The use of plasma levels is restricted to research at this point in time, as more information is needed before we can use them on a routine clinical basis. Variability in rate of metabolism is one of the reasons that clinicians must adjust the individual dose clinically.

Does treating an acute episode with antipsychotic drugs alter the natural course of schizophrenia? If we inspect the outcome of patients at the present time in comparison with the outcome before antipsychotic drugs were discovered (e.g., outcome in the 1920's or 1930's), we find a much more favorable outcome at present. Further data are provided from a random assignment study where patients were assigned for 6 months to 1 year to one of the following: (1) a controlled group of milieu therapy only, (2) a no drug psychotherapy group, (3) a drugs alone group, or (4) a drugs and psychotherapy group. The patients in the no drug group had a relatively poor outcome in the first 6 months to 1 year, and eventually this aspect of the study was terminated and these patients received drugs. During the next 3 to 5 years, patients were allowed to receive any indicated treatment. Based on a 3 to 5 year follow-up study, the initial treatment with drugs did improve the long range outcome. When we take as the index of outcome the number of days in the hospital during the follow-up period after first release, patients in the drug groups were

TABLE 2. **Antipsychotic Drugs**

Generic Name	Trade Name	Equivalence	Dose (mg)	Side Effects *EPS*	*Sedative*	*Anticholinergic*
thioridazine	Mellaril	100	400–800	+	+ + +	+ + +
chlorpromazine	Thorazine	100	400–800	+ +	+ + +	+ + +
perphenazine	Trilafon	9	18–60	+ +	+ +	+ +
mesoridazine	Serentil	55	100–400	+ +	+ +	+ +
trifluoperazine	Stelazine	2.8	6–40	+ + +	+	+
fluphenazine*	Prolixin, Permitil	1.2	3–40	+ + +	+	+
haloperidol	Haldol	1.6	3–40	+ + +	+	+
molindone	Moban	6	10–60	+ + +	+	+
loxapine	Loxitane	9	20–100	+ + +	+	+
thiothixene	Navane	5	10–50	+ + +	+	+

*Depot form fluphenazine decanoate 0.67 mg per day = 1.2 mg per dose orally or 25 mg injection every 2 weeks equals slightly less than 300 micrograms chlorpromazine orally each day.

found to spend one third to one half the number of days in hospital as those who initially did not receive drugs.

Maintenance Medication

The schizophreniform variant of pyschosis is one in which a patient has a single psychotic episode without relapse. Generally speaking, the physician should treat an initial psychotic episode with antipsychotic drugs and continue treatment for an average of 6 months (3 to 12 months). However, if the patient makes an excellent recovery after only one controlled episode, long-term maintenance treatment is generally not indicated.

What is the natural course of "process" schizophrenia? I observed that a graph of the percentage of patients relapsing over time resembled the curve seen in studies of drug half-lives in the body. I inspected the existing data for various controlled studies of patients switched to placebo and found that patients relapse with a constant rate over time of about 10 per cent per month. For example, if we start with 100 chronic schizophrenics who relapse at 10 per cent per month, we find in the first month 10 per cent or 10 relapsed, leaving 90; the next month 10 per cent of 90, or 9, relapsed, leaving 81; the following month, 10 per cent of 81, or 8, relapsed, leaving 73; then 10 per cent of 73, or 7, relapsed, leaving 66; and so on. We averaged the data from 30 double blind placebo studies lasting usually 4 to 6 months. Over 50 per cent of the placebo group relapsed as compared with only approximately 20 per cent of the drug group.

Maintenance treatment is certainly indicated if the patient has continuing symptomatology. If the patient has had several relapses in the past and we predict that he will relapse in the future because it occurred previously, then maintenance medication is recommended. The criteria for maintenance treatment are (1) presence of continuing symptoms, (2) frequency of past relapses, and (3) severity of past relapses. One of the reasons antipsychotic drugs do not completely eliminate relapses is that many patients fail to take their medication as prescribed. For patients who are not dependable about taking their oral medication, one of several forms of intramuscular depot preparations, such as fluphenazine decanoate (Prolixin), can be injected once every 2 weeks. A haloperidol decanoate formulation is being developed for monthly injection. It has been suggested that patients off drug can be closely monitored for early signs of relapse (anxiety, sleeplessness, depression, and dysphoria), which would then be treated with antipsychotic drug to abort a relapse. But some researchers think that once a schizophrenic relapse occurs, it cannot be easily aborted. Yet if interrupted treatment proves feasible, it might be a viable alternative to continous maintenance treatment. Empirical studies are in progress, but until these data are available we would recommend maintenance treatment. If a patient is showing nonspecific signs of relapse, the clinician should quickly increase the dose of antipsychotic in an effort to abort a relapse.

In an attempt to treat negative symptoms, such as withdrawal or apathy, antipsychotics with either tricyclic antidepressants or MAO inhibitors have also been tried but without success. In a controlled study the psychomotor stimulant amphetamine was added to an antipsychotic, but the results were inferior to antipsychotic alone. Empirically from time to time we do encounter someone incorrectly diagnosed as schizophrenic who, in fact, has an affective disorder or who has two disorders and may respond to tricyclic drugs. There also is a role for ECT in patients with severe depression, acute suicidal tendencies, and mania; catatonic excitement; or a very severe psychosis and treatment-resistant depression. The role of psychotherapy, particularly family therapy, is equally important to drug treatment, but space considerations do not allow a full discussion.

Side Effects

The autonomic side effects from the anticholinergic and antiadrenergic properties of antipsychotics are dry mouth, blurred vision, cutaneous flushing, constipation, urinary retention, paralytic ileus, mental confusion, miosis, mydriasis, and postural hypotension. Patients may develop some tolerance to the autonomic side effects such that they tend to be troublesome only during the early stages of treatment. For dry mouth, the patient should rinse out the mouth frequently with water but not chew sugar-containing gum because this is a good culture medium for *Monilia* species and may increase dental cavities. Pilocarpine may provide transitory relief.

Orthostatic (postural) hypotension frequently develops, particularly in the first few days of treatment, and patients do faint. When using high doses of intramuscular medication, it would be prudent to measure the patient's blood pressure (lying and standing) during the first days of treatment. Support hosiery may help. The patient should be instructed to rise gradually from bed, sit at first with legs dangling, wait a minute before standing, and sit or lie down if feeling faint. When orthostatic hypotension occurs, the patient should lie down with his feet higher than his head.

Although thioridazine produces EKG abnormalities consisting of broadened, flattened, or clove T-waves and increased Q-R intervals, these abnormalities are not associated with any significant clinical problem. Although sudden death rarely occurs in patients on antipsychotics, we cannot as yet accurately determine whether the drugs are causally or coincidentally associated with its occurrence. The introduction of antipsychotics has not altered the incidence of sudden death in mental patients. Sudden death might be caused by the stresses of the psychosis rather than by the drugs used. Until research establishes that there is a causal, not coincidental, relationship, the physician should be aware of erroneously attributing sudden death to antipsychotic medication.

Patients may also develop sedative side effects in the first few weeks, particularly to the sedative neuroleptics. A fair degree of tolerance exists for the side effects. If a seizure occurs, treat with either a lower dose or the addition of an anticonvulsant. When antipsychotic drugs are abruptly discontinued, a syndrome of withdrawal, nausea, and vomiting can occur. This is an anticholinergic withdrawal symptom produced by the concomitant discontinuance of the anticholinergic antiparkinsonian drugs, so both the antipsychotic and the anticholinergic should be gradually discontinued over the course of a few days or weeks. Antipsychotic drugs do not produce withdrawal symptoms of the barbiturate or narcotic type. Following administration of chlorpromazine rarely agranulocytosis can occur (in approximately 1 case in 500,000), usually within 6 weeks after initiation of treatment. A contact dermatitis can also develop in patients who handle chlorpromazine. A photosensitivity resembling severe sunburn can occur with chlorpromazine use, and patients should avoid sunlight and apply sunscreens. Long-term high dose use of chlorpromazine can produce a blue gray, metallic skin discoloration as well as lens opacity, which does not impair vision. Chlorpromazine can produce an obstructive jaundice. Thioridazine in very high doses (in excess of 1600 mg) (this exceeds maker's recommended dose of 800 mg/day) can produce a retinitis pigmentosa, which inteferes with vision and which may not be reversible. The antipsychotic drugs interact with dopamine receptors in the pituitary to produce an elevation of prolactin, with consequent breast engorgement and lactation in females and, to a lesser extent, in males. Delayed ejaculation has been reported to occur with thioridazine use.

Extrapyramidal Effects

We classify extrapyramidal side effects (EPS) as follows: (1) the parkinsonian syndrome (mask-like facies, tremor at rest, rigidity, shuffling gait), (2) a broad range of bizarre movements of the tongue, face, neck, arms, legs, and so on with salivation (torticollis, oculogyric crisis, and opisthotonos), (3) akathisia (a motor restlessness in which the patient has a great urge to move about), and (4) tardive dyskinesia. Diagnosis is occasionally difficult because dystonia can be confused with bizarre mannerisms, akathisia with agitation, and parkinsonian motor retardation with schizophrenic apathy. The acute dystonias occur in the first few days or weeks of treatment. They appear in patients receiving even small single doses of antipsychotics, e.g., a single dose of prochlorperazine (Compazine) for nausea. A therapeutic intramuscular trial of an antiparkinsonian drug—benztropine (Cogentin) or diphenhydramine (Benadryl), in which there is a response in minutes—is helpful in diagnosis. If this is unsatisfactory, diazepam, methylphenidate (Ritalin), or caffeine may be effective.

Parkinsonian syndrome and akathisia occur in the first few weeks of treatment and if not treated can persist in a fairly constant state. Although the classic tremor, mask-like facies, shuffling gait, and rigidity are obvious, patients can additionally manifest a more subtle form, with emotional blunting or a zombie-like appearance (apathy, lack of spontaneity, relative inability to participate in social activities, lifelessness).

Treatment involves either decreasing the dose of the antipsychotic medication or adding an antiparkinsonian drug, e.g., benztropine (Cogentin), procyclidine (Kemadren), and so on, and amantadine (Symmetrel). In akathisia, the patient is driven by motor restlessness and is not preoccupied with the psychologic content of whatever he is agitated about. There is a new body of evidence that propranolol is the treatment of choice; however, more studies are needed for confirmation. Akathisia is also treated with anticholinergic antiparkinsonian drugs, including amantadine or diazepam, and/or switching to a different antipsychotic.

Although prophylactic antiparkinsonian drugs will prevent some 60 per cent of the side effects that would otherwise occur, I do not advocate routine prophylactic use of antiparkinsonian drugs, preferring to add these medications if the side effects develop. Prophylaxis should only be attempted when there is a specific clinical reason for that particular patient, such as a history of severe EPS in the past. As patients may, to some degree, develop tolerance to the parkinsonian side effects, we would recommend the gradual discontinuance of antiparkinsonian medication after several months of treatment and continuous treatment only when there is clinical evidence that the patient still needs the antiparkinsonian medication (e.g., recurrence of symptoms).

Tardive dyskinesia (TD) is an important extrapyramidal side effect that presents relatively late in the course of antipsychotic drug treatment, generally after several years of treatment; rarely is it manifested sooner than 6 months of treatment. TD is characterized by (1) buccofacial mandibular or buccolingual movements (sucking, smacking, lateral fly-catching movements of the tongue, lateral jaw movements), (2) choreiform and/or athetoid movements of the arms and legs, and (3) neck and trunkal dystonias. The abnormal movements of TD are similar, indeed almost identical, to those seen in Huntington's chorea. They are absent during sleep. Since continued antipsychotic drug treatment suppresses the symptoms of TD, it is not unusual to find their appearance when the dose of neuroleptic is decreased or withdrawn entirely. This variant is sometimes referred to as emergent or withdrawal tardive dyskinesia, whereas the term "transient tardive dyskinesia" refers to TD symptoms that remit within some arbitrary time period. Persistent tardive dyskinesia refers to cases that do not remit in this arbitrary time period. Many of these remit after an even longer time period. The great majority of these cases are mild, but some are moderate, and a few (1 to 2 percent) are severe. Many patients with severe TD improve a year or two following discontinuance of neuroleptics. Indeed, some patients show spontaneous improvement despite continued neuroleptic therapy. Other cases seem irreversible.

Prevalence surveys of TD find that roughly 20 per cent of patients who receive or have received antipsychotic medication exhibit TD-like symptoms and about 5 per cent of drug-free controls who have never received antipsychotic medication have such movements. This is called spontaneous dyskinesia and, in general, is found in elderly controls. The true prevalence rate of TD is 15 per cent (20 per cent in drug-treated patients minus the 5 per cent in controls). In longitudinal studies, where patients were assessed at baseline and over time, the approximate incidence was about 3 per cent per year. That is, about 3 per cent of the patients would develop TD the first year, 6 per cent the second year, 9 per cent the third year, 12 per cent the fourth year, 15 per cent the fifth year, 18 per cent the sixth year, 21 per cent the seventh year. At some point, we would anticipate that this rate of development would level off. From available evidence, TD does not seem to be an inevitable progressive disease. Many cases level off after the development of only mild symptoms and do not seem to progress. If possible, neuroleptic drugs should be discontinued when a patient develops TD. When discontinuance is impossible because of the severity of psychosis or high frequency of relapse, treatment should consist of the lowest possible dose. Our current theory is that TD is caused by an increased number of dopamine receptor sites consequent to pharmacologic denervation through dopamine blockade. Certain drugs might dampen or worsen the expression of tardive dyskinesia in brief (few weeks) studies, but there is no (known) drug that, in a permanent sense, can cause the true remission of TD symptoms.

Malpractice suits for TD may emanate from the failure to obtain documented informed consent, the inappropriate prescription of antipsychotics to patients when there is no specific indication, or the failure to quickly diagnose TD. After the patient has recovered from an acute episode (or at least recovered as much as that particular patient is capable of recovering), the clinician should explain to him the benefits and the side effects, including TD. The physician will be maximally protected if such an explanation is (1) made in the presence of the family as well as of a social worker or nurse or other witness and (2) recorded in the chart, including responses from patient and family indicating an understanding of what was explained. All physicians need to have a prepared mind to diagnose tardive dyskinesia. For example, it is quite possible for patients to take antipsychotics needlessly for years without medical approval, so physicians must also have a prepared mind to stop the patients from taking unnecessary medication. We emphasize that long-term neuroleptics should not be used chronically unless there are very clear indications. Since there clearly are patients who require long-term treatment with neuroleptics, TD may be viewed as an inevitable consequence of good medical practice. What we wish to avoid is unnecessary cases of TD where neuroleptics are used for simple anxiety or simple depression when another drug would have been more specific.

PANIC DISORDER AND AGORAPHOBIA

method of
ROBERT S. BROWN, JR., M.D.
University of Virginia
Charlottesville, Virginia
and JAMES C. BALLENGER, M.D.
Medical University of South Carolina
Charleston, South Carolina

While anxiety is normally part of all our lives, pathologic anxiety states that lead to occupational and social dysfunction require medical treatment. Anxious patients who suffer discrete episodes of severe and sudden panic anxiety (panic attacks) in the presence of generalized anxiety, especially if accompanied by phobic avoidance, are now considered fundamentally different from those anxious patients without panic anxiety. The presence of panic attacks is highly predictive of response to tricyclic antidepressants, monoamine oxidase inhibitors, and alprazolam. These medications have dramatically improved our ability to treat these disorders, within 60 to 95 per cent of patients reporting marked alleviation (or resolution) of symptoms. Correct recognition of the disorder, adequate doses of medication, proper length of treatment, and attention to the secondary phobic avoidance are keys to successful treatment.

The incidence of panic disorders is believed to be between 2 and 6 per cent of the general population, and 75 per cent have not been correctly diagnosed. Eighty per cent of patients are female, with an average of 12 years from the onset of symptoms until effective therapy is begun. There is an increased frequency of alcohol and sedative abuse in this population as patients attempt to medicate themselves to reduce their severe anxiety. The suicide rate approaches and may surpass that for major depression. Studies examining the family incidence of panic disorder point to a multifactorial mode of inheritance and predict that males need more predisposing genetic and environmental factors to be affected clinically.

Panic Disorder

When patients with panic anxiety are examined as a group, certain symptoms are characteristic. The syndrome generally begins in young adults with a sudden, intense, overwhelming episode of anxiety (a panic attack) in which the patient experiences horrible panic, usually accompanied by the fear of impending death. Panic attacks are manifested by marked physical symptoms of anxiety, including tachycardia, palpitations, chest pain, shortness of breath, hyperventilation, choking sensations, faintness, trembling, hot and cold flashes, gastrointestinal distress, ataxia, and sweating, although no traditional medical explanation is found on examination. The panic attack as experienced by these patients can be reproduced in the laboratory by the infusion of sodium lactate, strongly suggesting a biologic etiology.

As the individual suffers additional panic attacks, the fear of dying is replaced with the fear of losing control of behavior, sanity, or bodily functions. Early in the course of the disorder, patients often go to a hospital emergency room, convinced they are having a heart attack. Panic attacks occur spontaneously and often awaken the patient from sleep. These attacks comtinue to occur at home, in automobiles, stores, malls, and restaurants, and on bridges. Although the panic anxiety generally lasts only a few minutes (sometimes hours), afterwards the patient is left fatigued, frightened, and shaken. Panic attacks tend to become, at least in part, situational and occur in public places where the circumstances are difficult or embarrassing. Patients almost always seek out the security of home or the hospital when panic attacks occur. Anticipatory anxiety develops as patients fear the occurrence of the next attack, and this is soon accompanied by avoidance behavior. Patients may develop an avoidance of traveling alone away from the home into public places, a behavioral pattern called agoraphobia.

Agoraphobia

The word agoraphobia, literally translated, means fear of people in the market place, but this is a misnomer. What actually develops is avoidance or dread of situations in which a panic attack would be difficult to handle or where a "dignified exit" would be impossible. This is especially true of crowded public places and often includes an automobile that someone else is driving. In our studies, avoidance behavior begins an average of 3 months after the first panic attack (range: 1 day to 7 years). While for most the illness waxes and wanes, two thirds of patients gradually worsen, with approximately 5 per cent actually becoming housebound. The agoraphobic patient's reclusiveness complicates adequate diagnosis and treatment and may require a house call.

Treatment

Effective pharmacotherapy of this evolved from studies that demonstrated that both monoamine oxidase inhibitors (MAOIs) and tricyclic antidepressants (TCAs) were effective in a high percentage of cases (80 to 100 per cent). The bulk of clinical experience has been with imipramine (Tofranil), a TCA, and phenelzine (Nardil), a MAOI. The effects of the antidepressants have been described as "patholytic," for not only are the panic attacks blocked and the secondary avoidance behavior reduced, but improvement in depression and in the extensive physical symptoms is also seen. Recent evidence suggests that the triazolobenzodiazepine alprazolam (Xanax) is also effective in this condition. Caffeine reduction is strongly recommended in these patients, many of whom are sensitive to its effects.

The only aspect of pharmacotherapy of this disorder that is not straightforward is management of patient fears that the medication may harm or even kill them. This initial *phobic* response is heightened in the one third who seem to be initially "hypersensitive" to medications. They develop stimulatory side effects with the TCAs or MAOIs and experience increases in tachycardia, palpitations, insomnia, sweating, anxiety, faintness, and "full feelings in the head." What needs to be emphasized repeatedly to patients is that these side effects are expected, transient, and safe. Although as many as 25 per cent discontinue medications because of these symptoms, in our experience almost all can reach the maximum dose gradually if they are properly prepared and given much encouragement. These side effects nearly always disappear within the first 2 or 3 weeks of treatment.

We frequently begin treatment with imipramine, reserving phenelzine for difficult treatment cases or for patients who respond inadequately to imipramine. Although phenelzine is probably the most effective medication in this disorder, the medication and dietary restrictions required during therapy are significant. Sympathomimetic drugs, including methyldopa, L-dopa, dopamine, and tryptamine-containing substances, as well as epinephrine- and norepinephrine-containing medications (Novocain, "cold pills"), are to be avoided when phenelzine is used. In addition, tyramine-rich foods such as pods of broad beans, aged cheeses, beer, wines, pickled herring, yogurt, liver, and yeast extract should be avoided because of the risk of hypertensive crisis. Some include restriction of excessive amounts of caffeine and chocolate. The necessity for these restrictions is usually quite frightening to the patients.

Treatment with imipramine can begin with 10 mg per day, often with the first pill in the physician's office for the reassurance that gesture offers the patient. The dosage can be increased by 10 mg daily to 50 mg, and then by 25 mg increments every 2 to 3 days to a total daily dose of 150 to 200 mg. Doses of imipramine in this range can be taken at bedtime, avoiding the need for divided doses. Dosage recommendations are primarily based on the clinical experience that most patients seem to tolerate and need about 150 mg of imipramine daily to block the panic attacks. An occasional patient will require more imipramine with doses in the 200 to 300 mg range daily. We have observed only a few patients such as described by Klein and Zitrin who cannot tolerate more than 5 to 25 mg of imipramine daily and who recover at these low doses. When phenelzine is used, the initial dose is 15 mg per day, with increases of 15 mg every 2 to 4 days, to a total dose of 60 mg per day (divided doses). Most clinicians give half at 8 A.M. and the remainder at noon to avoid insomnia. As with TCAs, response generally occurs after 6 to 12 weeks. Some patients require higher doses of phenelzine (to 90 mg daily) for a complete response.

Preliminary evidence with alprazolam in this condition is encouraging, with some patients reporting reduced or blocked panic attacks in less than a week. The initial dose is 0.5 mg three times daily, and the majority appear to need between 4 and 7 mg of alprazolam daily (7 mg exceeds maximum dose recommended by maker). It generally takes 3 to 6 weeks to reach these higher levels. Side effects encountered include primarily sedation and less commonly irritability, depressed libido, and decreased concentration and recall. Side effects are generally easily managed by reducing the dose by 1 mg or by slowing the rate of increases. Seizures have been reported with abrupt discontinuation of alprazolam, and patients must be tapered no more rapidly than with a 1 mg per day decrease every 4 days. Clinical experience favors an even slower taper (1 mg per day decrease every 1 to 3 weeks) to minimize withdrawal symptoms and the anxiogenic effect of these symptoms. A number of clinicians have combined imipramine and alprazolam in the initial treatment of the patient with severe panic anxiety in the hopes that the alprazolam will serve to diminish the patient's immediate discomfort while the imipramine dose is being increased into the therapeutic range. Most patients are treated for a total of 3 to 12 months before taper of medications is attempted.

The patients with a great deal of secondary avoidance behavior benefit from exposure treatments, of which various types are available. We offer a program that educates the patient about the illness and the central importance of panic attacks in the development of secondary anticipatory anxiety and avoidance behavior. After adequate levels of medication are achieved, patients are then encouraged to systematically and repeatedly re-expose themselves to their feared or phobic situations. Although perhaps initially accompanied by a therapist, spouse, or friend, later they need to confront these situations alone and repeatedly. These treatments result in considerable improvement or recovery for as many as 95 per cent of patients with panic attacks and agoraphobia.

Section 17

Physical and Chemical Injuries

BURNS

method of
ALBERT E. CRAM, M.D.
University of Iowa
Iowa City, Iowa

Skin is the largest and one of the most complex organs in the body. Significant thermal injury to the integument produces drastic multisystem derangements. Immediate effects of burn injury include the loss of an effective barrier to microbial invasion and the loss of the selective barrier to fluid evaporation. Toxins released from the burn site into the general circulation have wide ranging deleterious effects, the earliest of which include a generalized "capillary leak" and depression of myocardial function. This two pronged attack on peripheral perfusion demands aggressive fluid replacement, or shock, renal failure, and death will ensue.

The effect of burn injury on antimicrobial defense mechanisms is overwhelming. Normal neutrophil functions of chemotaxis, phagocytosis, and bactericidal activity are all depressed. Both normal and alternate pathways of complement activation are adversely affected. The lymphocyte system and macrophage activities are significantly impaired, and all of these factors render the burn victim susceptible to invasive infection and sepsis. Infection remains the leading cause of death in burn injury, and the risk of sepsis remains high until the wounds have healed or closure is obtained by skin grafting.

There are more subtle dysfunctions of the hematopoietic, coagulation, gastrointestinal, renal, and endocrine systems. The intense catabolic effect of thermal injury further compounds the multisystemic dysfunction and demands intense therapeutic efforts. The psychologic impact of the injury is often severe and may require intensive acute and chronic therapy.

The development of specialized burn care facilities with a multidisciplinary approach to the comprehensive needs of the patient has resulted in steady improvement in burn injury survival figures. Survival from burns covering 60 to 70 per cent of the body surface area is now commonplace, and recovery from larger injury is no longer rare.

TREATMENT

Initial Assessment

Initial assessment and treatment should proceed simultaneously in the burn patient. All clothing and jewelry should be removed at once. Assessment of the airway and respiration should receive top priority. The provision of humidified oxygen is recommended throughout the initial assessment phase. Cardiovascular assessment and treatment are aimed at ensuring adequate peripheral perfusion. Since burn injuries may involve explosions, falls, or motor vehicle trauma, the secondary survey should consist of a thorough search for traumatic injuries other than the obvious burn. Shock in the first hour after burn injury should lead to a presumption of occult hemorrhage, and indicated diagnostic procedures such as peritoneal lavage should not be delayed.

The history will alert the examiner to preexisting illness and may raise the index of suspicion for occult injury, which is often masked owing to the pain associated with the burn wound. A tetanus immunization history should be elicited and a booster given if indicated. Patients not previously immunized should receive human antitoxin in addition to initiation of the toxoid series.

Evaluation of the cutaneous injury should include an estimate of burn size and depth. A rough guide to burn size can be obtained using the "Rule of Nines," in which the head and neck represent 9 per cent of the body surface area, the anterior and posterior trunk 18 per cent each, the arms 9 per cent each, and the legs 18 per cent each. When using the Rule of Nines method allowances should be made for the larger head and smaller legs in infants and children. It is useful to remember that the patient's palmar surface is equal to 1 per cent of the body surface area when attempting to assess scattered burns. A more accurate guide can be obtained using a Lund-Browder chart. The wound is drawn while observing the patient and burn size is calculated using age specific guidelines.

Estimation of burn depth is often difficult immediately after injury and fortunately is less critical than accurate burn size estimation in the initial evaluation. First degree burns are erythematous, dry, and very painful lesions that involve only the epidermal layer. These injuries usually heal in a matter of several days. Second degree burns may be divided into superficial and deep injuries depending on the depth of dermal injury. Superficial second degree burns are frequently erythematous, moist wounds with evidence of blister formation. Deep second degree burns are frequently pale to chalky white, painful, and moist in appearance. These burns involve the deeper layer of the dermis and on occasion are hypesthetic and very difficult to differentiate from full thickness injury. Full thickness burns (third degree) result from thermal destruction of the full dermal layer. These injuries may appear white or charred. Blisters have already burst and the wound is anesthetic and dry. Any hair remaining in the area of full thickness injury is easily and painlessly removed.

At the completion of the physical examination, an estimate of burn severity should be made utilizing the guidelines in Table 1. The patient's age and burn size have the most obvious direct correlation with burn severity. Infants and patients older than 60 are at extremely high risk. The presence of an inhalation injury exerts a marked deleterious effect on survival and is said to double the mortality for any given burn size. Burns of the face, hands, feet, and perineum result in increased morbidity. Significant burns of these areas should be treated in centers with burn expertise. Pre-existing chronic illness and the presence of other injuries place the patient at great risk. Injuries categorized as moderate should always be treated on an inpatient basis, and major injuries are best managed in a facility with special burn expertise.

TABLE 1. **Classification of Burns**

Minor
- Less than 2 per cent third degree
- Less than 15 per cent second degree

Moderate
- 15 to 30 per cent second degree
- 2 to 10 per cent third degree

Severe
- Greater than 30 per cent body surface area second degree
- Greater than 10 per cent third degree
- Involvement of hands, face, feet, or perineum
- Burns in the presence of:
  - Associated injuries
  - Significant pre-existing disease
  - Extremes of age
  - Inhalation injury
  - Electrical injury

Respiratory Injury

The earliest threat to respiratory function is loss of a patent airway. Early swelling in the hypopharyngeal area with edema of the false vocal cords may result in partial or complete airway occlusion. This complication is usually associated with burns of the face and neck, but major airway and parenchymal injury need not be present. Physical signs of impending airway obstruction include increasing hoarseness, tachypnea, stridor, restlessness, and an inability to swallow oral secretions. This problem develops during the period of increased vascular permeability and may lead to airway obstruction within hours of the injury. Early endotracheal intubation is the treatment of choice since tracheostomy should be avoided if possible.

When this complication is suspected, an early inspection of the upper airway is indicated. A cocaine spray will reduce nasal swelling and anesthetize the nasopharynx to facilitate the examination. A flexible fiberoptic laryngoscope or bronchoscope is threaded through the largest endotracheal tube the nasal passage will accommodate. The scope is advanced into the hypopharyngeal region and, after observing the laryngeal structures, is advanced into the trachea. The endotracheal tube is then advanced using the fiberoptic scope as a stent. Early intubation is advocated since intubation may be difficult or impossible in the late stage of upper airway edema.

Major airway damage occurs owing to the inhalation of the toxic products of combustion. The chemical injury to the trachea and major bronchi produces progressive inflammation, edema, and loss of ciliary function. These changes set the stage for later microbial invasion and subsequent infection. A history of burns suffered in a closed space or loss of consciousness at the scene suggests inhalation injury.

Physical findings suggestive of major airway injury include facial burns, singed nasal vibrissae, soot in the oropharynx, soot-stained sputum, and the wheezing breath sounds associated with bronchospasm. The diagnosis can be confirmed by bronchoscopic examination. Treatment includes the administration of humidified oxygen and good tracheobronchial toilet. If bronchospasm is present it should be treated with bronchodilators. Major airway injury is usually progressive over a 3 to 5 day period. Mortality from this injury is usually due to the development of microbial invasion with pulmonary and systemic sepsis.

Parenchymal injury occurs when toxic products of combustion reach sufficient concentration at the alveolar level. In addition to the inflammatory response and edema also seen in major airway injury, there is a loss of surfactant. Progressive hypoxemia and hypercarbia develop over a period of hours to several days. Severity depends on the relative toxicity of the combustion products inhaled as well as the concentration and length of exposure. Death may occur early owing to hypoxemia or late owing to bacterial or mycotic infection.

The history and physical signs of parenchymal injury are identical to those seen with major airway injury. Chest x-ray films are usually normal for 48 to 72 hours unless there was preexisting pulmonary disease. Injection of radioactive xenon with immediate lung scan will disclose areas of delayed clearance. Bronchoscopic findings will usually be identical to those seen in major airway injury. Serial blood gases provide the best guide to the need for ventilatory support. Progressive hypoxemia or hypercapnia indicates the need for volume ventilation with increased oxygen concentration and positive end expiratory pressure. Aggressive tracheobronchial toilet must occasionally be supplemented by bronchoscopic removal of mucous plugs. Sputum cultures should be used to guide antibiotic therapy if pulmonary infection supervenes. Steroids should not be administered to patients with concomitant inhalation and cutaneous injury.

Carbon monoxide inhalation results in production of carboxyhemoglobin. Levels of carboxyhemoglobin greater than 10 per cent are abnormal and patients should be given 100 per cent oxygen. The half-life of carboxyhemoglobin is approximately 45 minutes under these circumstances. Levels above 60 per cent are associated with permanent neurologic deficit.

Respiratory embarrassment may occur when full thickness circumferential burns of the chest are present. The leathery eschar restricts expansion of the rib cage as edema develops. The patient experiences increasing difficulty in air exchange and may asphyxiate unless escharotomy is performed. Incisions through the full thickness burn in the anterior axillary line usually relieve the problem. Incisions should be carried through the dermis to allow separation of the wound edges. Occasionally it is necessary to connect the two vertical incisions with one or more horizontal incisions across the lower chest or upper abdomen.

Fluid Resuscitation

Evaporative fluid loss from the burn wound and the increased capillary permeability lead to a rapid depletion of intravascular volume. The quantity of fluid loss is proportional to the size of the burn, and a number of resuscitation formulae have been proposed to prevent the ensuing hypovolemic shock. We prefer the "Parkland formula" because of its simplicity and efficacy. The formula, outlined in Table 2, requires an accurate assessment of burn size and an accurate determination of body weight.

One half of the calculated fluid needs is given in the first 8 hours, with the remainder being given in the next 16 hours. Fluid requirements during the second 24 hours are usually about one half the requirements in the first 24 hours. Although this formula accurately predicts the fluid needs of most patients, it should be used only as a guideline and starting point. The goal of resuscitation is to maintain peripheral perfusion without producing fluid overload. The level of consciousness, vital signs, and especially the urine output provide adequate parameters for altering the fluid administration rate in most patients. Urine output in adults should be maintained at 40 to 50 ml per hour. In infants 1 ml per pound and in children 1 ml per kg serve as indications of the adequacy of resuscitation. Extremely deep burns and inhalation injury usually lead to fluid requirements in excess of the Parkland formula prediction.

Occasionally patients, especially those with pre-existing renal or cardiac disease, may require more invasive monitoring. Central venous pressure monitoring seldom provides more reliable information than the hourly urine output and vital signs. On the rare occasions when more invasive monitoring seems indicated, we recommend insertion of a Swan-Ganz line with measurement of pulmonary artery wedge pressures and cardiac output. This technique increases the risk of endocarditis and should be used only if the resuscitation is not proceeding smoothly.

Due to the large quantity of fluid required in

TABLE 2. **Resuscitation Formula**

4 ml lactated Ringer's × body surface area burned × weight in kg

One half given in the first 8 hours post burn, the remainder in the ensuing 16 hours

Example: 50 per cent burn in an 80-kg patient
4 ml × 50 × 80 = 16,000 ml lactated Ringer's solution

8,000 ml in first 8 hours
4,000 ml in each of next two 8 hour periods
Adjust to maintain urine output at 50 ml per hour

large burns, two large bore (16 gauge or larger) intravenous catheters should be inserted. It may be necessary to perform a cutdown if percutaneous needle access cannot be obtained. Although we try to locate venous access in unburned areas, we do not hesitate to place needles through the burn wounds when no other access is available. Normal capillary permeability is usually restored some time between 8 and 30 hours post injury. Fluid requirements can then usually be met by the enteral route, and intravenous lines should be removed as soon as they are no longer needed.

Wound Management

Wound closure, whether obtained by spontaneous healing in superficial wounds or by surgical means in deeper wounds, is the goal of all wound care. Ideal wound care should eliminate or minimize bacterial colonization of the wound and provide an optimal environment for wound healing. Wound management should also minimize the development of hypertrophic scar.

Small superficial burns involving only the epidermal layers will usually heal in 5 to 7 days. When there is only erythema and the epidermis remains intact, gentle wound cleansing and prevention of further trauma will produce good wound healing. When deeper burns produce small blisters these may be left intact. If the blisters have broken spontaneously or through inadvertent trauma, the necrotic outer layer should be removed and an antimicrobial cream such as silver sulfadiazine (Silvadene) applied.

Partial thickness burns that involve the entire epidermis and portions of the dermis will heal by epithelial migration from surviving hair follicles, sebaceous glands, and sweat glands unless these epidermal appendages are destroyed by infection. Prevention of wound infection is the key to healing in the medium thickness second degree burn. Those wounds that epithelialize within 14 days almost never produce hypertrophic scar. The incidence of hypertrophic scar begins to rise slowly between 14 and 21 days, and wounds that require more than 21 days to heal almost always produce some residual hypertrophic scar. Bacterial invasion of the wound can result in conversion of the partial thickness wound to a full thickness injury.

Full thickness burns can only heal by epithelial migration and contracture. This mechanism can successfully close only small full thickness injuries. Full thickness injuries greater than 4 cm in diameter are best treated by skin grafting.

We prefer to debride blisters in wounds larger than 5 cm in diameter. The wound is then cleansed with a mild agent such as Hibiclens and dressed in a synthetic dressing if it appears to be relatively superficial. We use Biobrane as the synthetic dressing of choice. This dressing is held in place with a gauze wrap. The Biobrane is inspected at intervals for fluid accumulation, which should be removed by needle aspiration. The dressing may be left in place and allowed to separate spontaneously as the wound heals. If infection occurs beneath the dressing the Biobrane should be removed and after debridement an antimicrobial agent should be applied.

Deeper partial thickness injury is treated by debridement and application of an antimicrobial cream such as silver sulfadiazine (Silvadene). The agent is applied as a thin layer covered by a single layer of gauze held in place by commercially available elastic net. This dressing is changed daily, and it is often necessary to provide narcotic pain relief prior to the dressing change. Silvadene may cause a neutropenia in some patients, and either this reaction or an allergic reaction may necessitate a change in topical antimicrobial medication.

Mafenide acetate (Sulfamylon) is a popular burn antimicrobial agent that is applied in a thin layer over the burn wound. This agent has the advantage of penetrating the eschar better than any other agent, and it therefore achieves good antimicrobial levels at the interface between the eschar and the viable deep tissue. Sulfamylon has the disadvantage of causing pain when applied to a partial thickness wound, probably owing to its acid pH. In addition, Sulfamylon is a carbonic anhydrase inhibitor and, used on large body surface area burns, may result in significant acidosis.

Surgical Intervention

Surgical intervention may be indicated within hours of the burn injury if extremities exhibit full thickness circumferential involvement. Third space fluid loss into a space that can no longer expand results in compression of the venous and arterial systems. Symptoms include pain and then numbness. Signs include distal venous dilatation in the face of decreased or absent pulses in severe cases. Escharotomy should be carried out by incising through the dermis on the medial and lateral sides of the involved extremity, avoiding incision across flexor and extensor surfaces.

Whenever the wound appears unlikely to heal within 14 to 21 days, consideration should be given to early excision and graft. In the case of obvious full thickness burns, we prefer to begin excision and grafting as soon as the fluid resuscitation phase of treatment is complete. Burn wound excision is a formidable procedure and should be attempted only by those with training and experience in the technique.

Excision of the burn wound may be accomplished by either tangential technique or complete excision to fascia. Tangential excision is preferred when the wound depth is indeterminate. Sequential thin slices of eschar are removed until punctate capillary bleeding indicates a viable wound bed. Tangential excision of extremities utilizing tourniquets will decrease blood loss, but this technique requires significant expertise to recognize an adequate depth of excision. Complete excision to fascia is often less bloody but does produce a greater cosmetic defect. Excision of greater than 15 per cent of the body surface area at one operation is extremely hazardous, so frequent sequential excisions are necessary with large burns. Excellent anesthesia and blood bank support are essential to success in excisional therapy.

Once excised, the resulting wound must be covered. Failure to provide adequate coverage of the surgically created wound will result in formation of new eschar and the need for further debridement. The obvious cover of choice is split thickness autograft. With large body surface area burns it is frequently impossible to obtain enough autograft for wound closure. Temporary closure with viable cadaver homograft is the current second choice when autograft donor sites are inadequate to provide coverage. In the massively burned patient in whom immunosuppression secondary to the burn injury is significant, we have seen survival of cadaver homograft for up to several months.

Other choices for temporary closure include porcine xenograft, placental membranes, and synthetic materials such as Biobrane. The "artificial skin" described by Burke is not yet commercially available, and the epidermal culture techniques appearing in the literature remain experimental. All but the epidermal culture techniques ultimately require autograft for permanent closure.

In large burns it is usually necessary to increase autograft coverage by utilizing a meshing device to "expand" the skin. Mesh ratios from 1.5:1 up to 9:1 are available, but the quality of skin coverage drops drastically with expansion ratios greater than 3:1. With expansions greater than 1:1.5 it is necessary to cover the autograft with xenograft or Biobrane. The wound is then dressed as described hereafter.

Following application of the graft, our dressing technique involves placement of a sterile nylon mesh sutured to surrounding normal skin, followed by a multilayer dressing soaked in 0.5 per cent silver nitrate solution. Dressings are kept moist by an outer layer of treated stockinette and frequent addition of silver nitrate. Dressings are changed daily down to the nylon net. The net is removed after the graft shows evidence of good vascularization, usually on the fifth postoperative day.

Antibiotics

Systemic antibiotic coverage should be reserved for patients with suspected or proven sepsis. We do provide coverage against streptococcal infection by the administration of penicillin during the first 5 days post burn. Systemic gram negative antibiotic administration should be reserved for patients with suspected or proven sepsis. Early recognition of sepsis is critical but may be difficult in the patient with major thermal injury. Subtle changes in the level of consciousness, ileus, marked leukocytosis or sudden neutropenia, azotemia, fluid retention, and fever above 39 C should raise the suspicion of sepsis. Blood cultures should be drawn and systemic antibiotics, usually an aminoglycoside, should be given pending culture results. Prophylactic use of broad spectrum antibiotics is contraindicated, since it increases the risk of infection with resistant bacteria and fungi.

Nutrition

Major thermal injury results in a marked catabolic response. The detrimental effect of this deficit on wound healing and immune mechanisms cannot be overstated. Recovery from thermal injury requires aggressive nutritional support.

The ileus seen with burns usually resolves within 48 hours. During the period of ileus the stomach should be decompressed by a nasogastric tube, and antacid therapy should be administered via the tube to prevent stress ulceration. Antacid therapy is sufficient when it maintains gastric pH above 5.

Immediately upon resumption of bowel activity enteral feedings should begin using a high calorie, high protein formula. Caloric needs are calculated using the formula in Table 3.

In most cases combined tube feedings and oral intake will be sufficient to meet caloric and protein needs. Occasionally patients will require

TABLE 3. **Caloric Requirements**

Calories	
Adult	(20 Kcal × kg body weight) + (70 Kcal × per cent burn)
Child	(60 Kcal × kg body weight) + (35 Kcal × per cent burn)
Protein	
Adult	(1 gram × kg body weight) + (3 grams × per cent burn)
Child	(3 grams × kg body weight) + (1 gram × per cent burn)

central venous nutrition despite the increased risk of sepsis from long-term intravenous catheter insertion. Strict aseptic insertion technique and frequent line changes will decrease but not eliminate the risk.

Pain Management

During the initial capillary leak phase, pain relief must be given intravenously. We prefer intravenous morphine sulfate since it is both effective and inexpensive; 2 mg increments are administered until the patient is comfortable. Narcotic antagonists should be available, but careful titration to the point of pain relief seldom results in significant respiratory depression. Later in the course of therapy narcotics can be given by the intramuscular or oral route. Pain relief requirements should decrease as wound closure is obtained. Addiction is extremely rare unless the patient was a drug abuser prior to injury.

Physical Therapy

Physical and/or occupational therapists should be involved in the care plan from the onset. Extremities should be positioned in extension to prevent contracture, and splinting across burned joints is usually necessary to maintain extension. Early aggressive passive and active range of motion is critical to obtain maximal functional recovery. Early physical therapy is especially important to recovery of hand function. The need for pressure garments and rigid pressure devices to control hypertrophic scar should be assessed prior to discharge.

Electrical Injury

Electrical injury can occur through direct current contact or via arc injury. Direct current injury may produce severe deep muscle or visceral organ injury depending on the amount and duration of current and its pathway through the body. Entrance and exit sites are usually obvious, but fluid resuscitation needs cannot be calculated from the visible surface wounds. Injury to muscle may often be obvious from functional deficits apparent on physical examination. Neurologic injury may be central or peripheral depending on current pathway, and often the patient will have unusual permanent neurologic deficits. More occult sequelae such as cataract formation require vigilant follow-up examination.

Resuscitation for large electrical injury involves insertion of large bore intravenous lines and administration of lactated Ringer's solution at rates rapid enough to establish 100 ml per hour urine output. With significant vascular or muscle injury the urine will contain myoglobin and/or hemoglobin pigment. If peripheral perfusion is adequate the urine will be alkaline and the pigment will clear without damage to the kidneys. If the urine is acid an increase in fluid administration rate and the addition of 1 ampule of sodium bicarbonate to each liter of fluid is indicated. When the initiation of fluid resuscitation has been delayed it may be necessary to give mannitol, 25 grams immediately following insertion of the intravenous lines.

Patients should have an EKG, and any patients with evidence of myocardial injury or arrhythmia should receive continuous EKG monitoring. Patients who arrest at the scene of the injury may do so because of either cardiac arrhythmia or centrally induced apnea. If such patients can be resuscitated at the scene without anoxic brain injury they usually do well.

Stable cardiovascular and renal function can usually be achieved within 12 to 24 hours of injury. The patient who has obvious or suspected muscle injury can then be explored surgically. Obvious necrotic muscle should be removed, but we prefer to preserve any muscle that appears questionably viable. This technique often requires several sequential exploratory procedures, but it leads to preservation of more muscle and results in improved functional recovery.

Occult vascular injury often leads to progressive ischemia as patent but injured vessels thrombose. Our experience with attempts to modify coagulation in these cases has been uniformly discouraging. Repeated examination of peripheral perfusion is necessary in all injured extremities. Fasciotomy is carried out during exploration of muscle compartments. Arc injuries, which often involve only skin and subcutaneous tissue, are treated as full thickness flame burns.

Chemical Injury

Agents that damage skin by chemical reaction are far too numerous and diverse in mode of action to discuss individually. Initial treatment consists of copious water lavage. It is virtually impossible to use too much lavage, and errors in treatment usually involve inadequate removal of the offending chemical. During lavage, if the offending chemical agent can be identified, inquiry for specific measures can be directed to the regional poison control facility. Depth of injury is especially difficult to judge in chemical injury. Tangential excision earlier than 5 to 7 days post injury frequently results in inadequate excision and graft loss. In all other respects chemical burns are treated by the techniques used in flame and scald burns.

DISTURBANCES DUE TO COLD

method of
WILLIAM H. DOOLITTLE, M.D.
Fairbanks Memorial Hospital
Fairbanks, Alaska

FROSTBITE

General Considerations and Pathophysiology

Frostbite is a not uncommon injury incurred during exposure to freezing temperatures and involves the actual freezing of tissue. In the usually encountered clinical cases developing over time in freezing environmental temperatures, ice crystals develop in the extracellular space, creating a shift of cellular water, denaturation of intracellular proteins, and alteration of cellular function on a hierarchic basis related to the temperature constants of the cellular enzyme systems. The damage under these circumstances, within certain limitations, is considered to be largely reversible with appropriate rewarming. Less frequently, a more rapid cooling of tissue occurs—supercooling—which results in the intracellular development of ice crystals.

With rewarming by recommended methods there is immediate return of circulation, at least in resuscitatable tissues, and then, depending on the extent of injury, microcirculatory flow stops and intravascular thrombus develops. The exact mechanism of this phenomenon is not well defined, but one need not seek a special new mechanism to explain microcirculatory failure once one accepts the fact that the vascular endothelium is disrupted by the freezing/thawing event. Most even modestly successful experimental inroads and any but the most basic clinical interventions depend on the fact that microvascular injury and failure underlie tissue loss in frostbite.

Epidemiology

Exposure at a given temperature, wind chill, and duration might be expected to result in a freezing injury. Should the patient be concurrently exposed to specific illness or a medication or drug that accelerates heat loss from the extremities, the extent of the injury might be predicted to be greater. Frostbite is more likely to occur in blacks, smokers, those with antecedent cold injuries (not necessarily the same part of the body), and those whose home of origin is in warmer latitudes. Although these conditions increase the statistical likelihood of sustaining freezing injury on exposure, it should be remembered that cold injury is a completely preventable disease. Individuals with specific susceptibility must increase their protective vigil, and they should further be aware that the lower the temperature the greater the expression of their susceptibility. For example, cigarette smoking is not a significant risk at −17 C. Below −28 C the impact of smoking becomes a significant variable.

Clinical Manifestations

The first sign that cold injury is an imminent risk is development of painful cold, usually associated with a decrease in sensation (and a decrease in dexterity if the involved part is the hand). From this point there is progressive loss of sensation and function, and when freezing actually occurs there is no awareness of change because of the cold-induced anesthesia. For this reason frostbite has been called a painless injury.

Occasionally the ears or parts of the face are involved in an even more superficial injury called frostnip. In this injury a very distinct "ping" is described at the time of crystallization of tissue water. In frostnip the tissue has an actual frosted appearance and is by inspection clearly superficial, very localized, and readidly reversed with the heat of the warmed hand. On the other hand, frostbitten tissue has a pale, white appearance and is firm to touch, cold, without sensation, and without the usual tissue turgor. Involved joints are frequently impossible to move with reasonable force, and at this point, along with an appropriate history of exposure, a diagnosis of frostbite can be made with assurance.

The depth and prognosis of the injury are much more difficult to define. Except for the most superficial injuries where pliability is usually maintained, it is difficult to have a prognostic accuracy of much greater than 50 per cent before thawing and 65 per cent immediately after thawing. Sophisticated study of microvascular blood flow improves the post-thaw prognostication but is frequently beyond the capability of even moderate-sized hospitals and, more importantly, never achieves a level of reliance that significantly modifies treatment.

Treatment

First Aid

The major effort in the field management of frostbite is to prevent further injury. Frostnip represents little problem. Rewarming with the warm hand of the patient or a comrade with subsequent protection of the part from further cold exposure is all that is required. Clearly defined frostbite or appearance of tissue that makes it impossible to exclude frostbite requires further judgment based on the circumstances of the injury. If definitive care is readily accessible, either field rewarming and transport to a definitive care facility, or, if the distances are short and transportation reliable, removal to the next echelon of care without attempted field rewarming is appropriate. If, on the other hand, there is risk that, following rewarming, reinjury may occur, or if, as in the case of foot injury, weight bearing is essential for extrication, then the part should be left frozen until arrival at the definitive care facility. Freeze-thaw-refreeze injuries inevitably result in extensive tissue loss. Spontaneous rewarming should probably be discouraged, again depending on the situation, and rapid rewarming instituted as described hereafter.

Definitive Treatment

Rapid rewarming is universally accepted as the method of choice for thawing frozen tissue. The part is immersed in a water or, preferably, a circulating bath at a temperature of 38 to 43 C. Temperatures much above this risk tissue injury. If careful control of the bath temperature is not possible, then the error should be toward the lower temperature, using a temperature that is comfortable to a euthermic hand or other equally sensitive part. Ideally, the bath should contain an antiseptic solution, e.g., povidone-iodine (Betadine) and the treatment continued until the tissue is again pliable and, usually, a brisk reactive hyperemia develops. Return of sensation is not a reliable end point, since sensory nerve integrity relates to the extent of the injury and previous exposure. The time required to accomplish thawing is approximately 45 minutes. During the bath as much of the frozen part as possible should be cleansed to avoid future contamination.

After rewarming, and after each subsequent daily whirlpool, the injured part should be carefully dried and aseptically debrided of any loose superficial tissue of decompressed blebs that may have ruptured. Digits should be separated with sterile gauze or cotton pledgets and dressings limited to those required for protection from injury and contamination. The usual surgical principles of wound management apply. Aseptic techniques are essential, protection from physical injury paramount, and any definitive surgical procedures should be deferred until clear demarcation occurs as discussed hereafter.

Frequently, after rewarming and before separation of the bleb, superficial sensation returns to the injured part and is a favorable sign. Usually blebs develop over the injured areas from 6 to 48 hours following rapid rewarming. Full, tense, clear blebs involving the full area of freezing are generally correlated with a favorable outcome with very limited tissue loss (skin and some atrophy of the volar fat pad of involved digits). Scattered, small, irregular or hemorrhagic blebs usually denote more severe injury and a higher risk of tissue loss. Blebs should be left intact and allowed to spontaneously resolve. This should not be interpreted as a strict interdiction of debridement of an intact bleb, but the loss of integrity of the bleb increases the risk of infection and the resultant increase in tissue loss. Ruptured blebs should be debrided to avoid "closed space" infection.

Physiotherapy

The injured part should be whirlpooled in an antiseptic solution twice daily and in the interim maintained slightly elevated to avoid dependent edema. The patient should be encouraged to engage in active movement of the part from the first day and analgesia provided as required. The amount of analgesia required is usually small and frequently is accomplished with salicylates or acetaminophen with or without codeine. Although the rate of functional loss in frostbitten hands is considerably less than that of a comparably deep burn, the risk of contractures still exists and mandates early and active efforts at range of motion.

Drug Therapy

We have spoken of the need for sufficient analgesia to allow for early range of motion. Antibiotics have no advantage when used in a prophylactic role and should be reserved for specifically and culturally identified infections. The use of topical antibiotics or antiseptic agents has had advocates but generally offers little significant advantage, even in open wounds, over frequent dressing changes, fine mesh gauze, and good aseptic technique. Tetanus toxoid should probably be given according to standard recommendations and based on the clinical perception of the risk. The same judgmental considerations relate to the use of tetanus antitoxin in those not previously immunized.

Interventions designed specifically to enhance microvascular flow by preventing intravascular coagulation or increasing fibrinolysis in occluded vessels have been generally disappointing. The disappointment has been in part related to the difficulty in developing a reliable prognostication without treatment. Anticoagulation, thrombolysis, carrier substances used with either of the foregoing, and "desludging" agents have had and continue to have advocates. Experimental studies plagued by the same vagaries of predictability have shown some encouraging results. The most significant changes have occurred in experimental studies where these agents were used prior to injury.

Probably the most defensible current position is the use of inhibitors of platelet aggregation as early as possible in the course, even before thawing. Aspirin, 300 mg twice daily, along with dipyridamole, 50 mg twice daily, have at least some theoretic advantage and, in the absence of any specific contraindications, very little risk. (This use of dipyridamole and aspirin is not listed in the manufacturer's official directive.) The disruption in the microvasculature occurs within at least 30 minutes of rewarming, and, therefore, any preventive measures must be instituted very soon after recognition of the problem. Unfortunately, many cases of frostbite present only after spontaneous rewarming, the average in one study being 2 hours post spontaneous rewarming. Vasodilators probably have no place in the current management of frostbite.

Surgery

Only the most conservative surgical approach is defensible in frostbite. Early in the course, debridement of disrupted blebs is the rational limit. Subsequent release of constricting eschar over hands or feet is imperative. Occasionally, and equally imperative, is the performance of a fasciotomy to preserve existing circulation. Amputation should be deferred until clear demarcation is evident. It is uncommon, especially in hands, for amputation to be appropriate prior to 3 weeks and then, of course, at the most distal level possible. In denuded areas, especially overlying superficial tendons or joints, split thickness autologous skin grafts may help preserve length and function in selected cases. In earlier years some held enthusiasm for sympathectomy to increase survival and diminish late complications of frostbite, but little clinical evidence remains to support this position at the present time.

IMMERSION FOOT (TRENCHFOOT, LIFEBOAT LEG)

General Considerations and Pathophysiology

Immersion foot is an ischemic injury resulting from nonfreezing exposure to wet cold, usually associated with stasis. It occurs more commonly in military populations where operational constraints prevent careful foot hygiene and foot protection and require longer periods of unbroken field duty. The initial pathology appears to be vascular reactivity, where cold exposure leads initially to vasoconstriction and to a reactive hyperemia and tissue edema. The vascular integrity is progressively compromised, and ischemia results in progressive swelling, infarction necrosis, and cutaneous bullae or vesicles.

Clinical Manifestations

The foot is frequently pale but gives way to an intense hyperemia, with swelling, bullae, and variable sensory and motor deficits. Cellulitis is often present and a wet gangrene may quickly follow. As vasodilatation occurs, pulses return and pain may become intense. Vasomotor instability is a common late sequela with recurrent dependent edema and lividity. As with frostbite, a dyshidrosis occurs and is lasting and occasionally incapacitating.

Treatment

Unlike frostbite, trenchfoot should be rewarmed at much lower temperatures. Room temperature suffices (approximately 22 C), and the foot should be kept elevated to avoid further vascular compromise by extravascular fluid sequestration. Blebs should be left intact if possible but debrided when appropriate according to the same principles described for frostbite.

Physiotherapy

Early active exercise should be encouraged to restore muscle and vascular tone and promote resumption of normal function as soon as possible.

Drug Therapy

Analgesics represent the major pharmacologic intervention. Vasoactive drugs have little or no place in trenchfoot. In contrast to frostbite, antibiotics are probably warranted early in the course of trenchfoot, since clinical evidence of infection is frequently present. Careful cultural control is still in order. Because of the risk of venous stasis and subsequent thrombosis, close observation for indication for anticoagulation is essential. Where available, Doppler venous examination early and serially may provide such indication.

Surgery

Surgical intervention here, as in frostbite, is reserved for relief of constricting compartmental swelling and superficial debridement. Only late in the course is there sufficiently clear indication to warrant amputation.

HYPOTHERMIA

General Considerations and Pathophysiology

Accidental hypothermia is a medical emergency with a mortality that hovers near 50 per cent. It is defined as a core temperature of 34.4 C or below and can occur in relatively temperate climates and in diverse clinical settings. It must be considered in all cases of blunted sensorium or unconsciousness with a history or likelihood of cold exposure and *should* be considered in any case of an unconscious patient until the core temperature has been reliably established. Awareness that profoundly hypothermic patients may present as clinically dead with no observable respirations, recordable blood pressure, or discernible pulse is the first step to successful resuscitation. In such cases only the finding of electric activity on an electrocardiograph may signal reversible disease. Although the dramatic presentation just described may be unusual, it is not unusual to have less serious levels of hypothermia go undetected even on medical floors, with the result that patients slip into irreversibility.

Clinical Manifestations

There is no hard and fast clinicopathologic correlation between a given core temperature and a particular clinical deficit. Some patients seem remarkably resistant to the depressant effects of low body temperatures and others even more remarkably sensitive. The most common explanation of such a variation is concomitant disease or injury. Along with the establishment of body temperature, a search must be made (through both history and physical findings) for associated problems that sometimes take precedence over the hypothermia or at the least modify the therapeutic approach. Table 1 describes the clinical events usually recognizable at the temperatures noted. This focuses on the level of consciousness as the variable most influencing management.

Although much has been made of the rate of heat loss in hypothermia, the issues of greatest prognostic significance are probably the core temperature on arrival, the level of consciousness, and the presence of coexisting disease. The first two relate to the risk of developing uncontrollable cardiac arrhythmias, which is the usual terminal event in hypothermia, and the last has most to do with survival in the post-rewarming period.

Treatment

Clearly, the hypothermic emergency requires specific treatment and the sine qua non of that treatment is ADD HEAT. The method by which the heat is added can be with warmed blankets; with chemical heating pads applied to the trunk and axillae and groins under blankets; with heated, humidified oxygen if available; or with heated intravenous infusions. The only unacceptable technique is to specifically prevent rewarming by deliberately continuing cold exposure.

Definitive Treatment

Although each case must be individualized, the point of departure between aggressive and less aggressive rewarming is the level of consciousness when that is presumed primarily related to the hypothermia. The clinical perception of the contribution of concomitant illness or injury to the unconsciousness will of course modify the approach. Table 2 outlines the approach for the conscious patient and Table 3 for the unconscious patient. For both, the investigative studies in Table 4 apply. There is probably no justification for purely passive rewarming in clinical hypothermia, so Table 5 outlines active rewarming techniques for both shell first and core first programs. Notable by its absence is warm water immersion rewarming. Although physiologically reasonable, it has sufficient technical and logistic disadvantages that it should be discouraged, at least for the seriously ill or profoundly hypothermic patient. It should be reconsidered when there is concomitant freezing injury that cannot be rapidly rewarmed at the usual temperatures using bedside whirlpool.

As in the cases of heated inhaled air or oxygen and heated intravenous infusions, there is some crossover between core techniques and purely external methods. The major effort is to restore normal physiologic function as soon as possible to prevent the immediate complications of hypothermia, which are primarily cardiovascular, and to bring the patient to the point where his own defenses can fend off coexisting problems. Special recognition is necessary for the possibility of late depression from previously administered or ingested drugs. If ingested substances are suspected, then early nasogastric intubation and lavage are important. Needless to say the lavaging fluids should be warmed to at least 40 C.

In the event of cardiopulmonary collapse, which in hypothermia relates primarily to car-

TABLE 1. **Clinical Corollaries of Levels of Hypothermia**

Responsive (34.5 to 32 C)
- Shivering
- Blood pressure elevated
- Pulse elevated
- Respirations elevated
- Peripheral vasoconstriction
- Cold-induced diuresis
- Confusion or disorganized thought processes

Poorly Responsive (31.5 to 26.5 C)
- Shivering stops
- Blood pressure decreased
- Pulse decreased
- Respirations decreased
- Peripheral vasoconstriction
- May be unconscious; usually rousable

Unresponsive (under 26.5 C)
- Poikilothermic
- Blood pressure unrecordable?
- Pulse unobtainable?
- Respiration undetectable?
- Cardiac arrhythmias by ECG
- Atrial then ventricular
- Unresponsive

TABLE 2. **Conscious Patient**

1. Lab work as in Table 4
2. Inspect for concomitant injury
3. Continuous cardiac monitoring
4. Establish central venous line; avoid entering heart
5. Administer fluids at 40 C
6. Monitor vital signs every 5 to 10 minutes until warmed
7. Monitor I & O (Input and Output)
8. Begin external active rewarming
9. Reassess frequently

TABLE 3. **Unconscious Patient**

1. Gentle handling
2. Indwelling urinary bladder catheter
3. Begin core rewarming (see Table 5)
4. Partially correct metabolic abnormalities until rewarming complete
5. Cautious nasogastric intubation and lavage
   Aspirates to lab for toxicology screens
   Lavage with warm fluids at 40 C
6. CPR as required (see text)

Note: Prior to initiating these steps, follow guidelines in Table 2.

TABLE 4. **Laboratory Investigations**

Baseline Laboratory Studies	
	Hemogram with platelets
	Urinalysis (measure temperature)
	Electrolytes, blood urea nitrogen, creatinine, glucose, amylase, liver profile, prothrombin time, partial thromboplastin time
	Blood gases with temperature correction
Other Baseline Data	
	ECG
	Chest x-ray films
Special Circumstance Studies	
	Blood, urine, sputum cultures
	Toxicology—urine, blood, gastric aspirates, blood alcohol
	Lumbar puncture
	Triiodothyronine, thyroxine
	Magnesium
	Stool guaiac
	EEG
	Computed axial tomography of the head

diac arrest or ventricular fibrillation, full CPR must be commenced, despite concerns over induction of ventricular fibrillation by physical stimuli, and rewarming instituted concurrently. Tracheal intubation in a deeply hypothermic patient may be unexpectedly difficult. Although the cold heart is predictably less responsive to resuscitative medications or delivered direct current energy, at least initial attempts must be made along conventional lines while rewarming is taking place. No major investment in time to the exclusion of rewarming should be made in these efforts. Aside from the judgmental procedures outlined, three important rules must constantly be kept uppermost in the operator's mind: (1) keep constant vigilance for coexisting disease or injury; (2) avoid irrevocable therapeutic commitment—things will change momentarily; (3) THINK HEAT.

Laboratory Studies

The electrocardiogram will frequently show a characteristic intraventricular conduction delay referred to as Osborne waves or "J waves." Although these have been advertised as unique to hypothermia, such is not the case and they can be seen in other conditions including CNS disease and some electrolyte disturbances.

TABLE 5. **Methods of Rewarming in Accidental Hypothermia**

Active External (Shell First) Rewarming	
	Electric blankets
	Circulating blankets
	Heated objects
Active Core Rewarming	
	Vaporized, heated oxygen/air
	Heated intravenous solutions
	Peritoneal dialysis
	Hemodialysis—especially in association with dialyzable intoxications
	Arteriovenous shunt with heat exchanger

Drug Therapy

Several major problems must be addressed in hypothermia in addition to the provision of heat.

Fluid Volume and Electrolyte Disorders. Unless there is specific information to the contrary or unless the duration of exposure was extremely brief, as in cold water immersion, one can usually assume a depletion of total body fluid volumes. A warmed solution of physiologic fluids is appropriate, beginning at relatively high flows of 150 ml per hour or slightly more until new observations dictate different flow rates. Observed deficits should be only partially corrected to avoid serious overshoot when rewarming has occurred. Fluids initially should contain no potassium until laboratory values are received. These values should be frequently checked.

Cardiovascular Drugs. Since arrhythmias are a major concern during rewarming, some advanced planning is appropriate. Cardiac monitoring is essential. Vigilance to avoid overload and identify the emerging signs of some pre-existing heart disease after cardiac work increases during rewarming is essential. These problems can be treated according to usual convention once rewarming has occurred. A trial of lidocaine (Xylocaine) should be attempted in efforts to control ventricular ectopy, although the likelihood of success is small until rewarming is under way. Other type 1 antiarrhythmic drugs should probably be avoided. Whatever agents are used, the physician should be aware that conjugation of drugs in the liver is delayed during hypothermia and toxicity may occur at lower levels because of decreased clearance. Bretylium tosylate (Bretylol) has been used experimentally in hypothermia-induced ventricular fibrillation, but clinical experience with this agent is lacking. The role of the beta-blockers and the calcium channel blockers in this very difficult setting still remains to be seen, and very little clinical data have been reported.

Blood Sugar. Hyperglycemia, euglycemia, and hypoglycemia all occur with hypothermia. While awaiting specific results, it is usually reasonable to administer at least 50 ml of 50 per cent dextrose in the unconscious patient.

Antibiotics. Pulmonary complications on an aspiration or infectious basis are common in accidental hypothermia. Following cultural control, antibiotics should be instituted according to the dictates of the specific setting.

Corticosteroids. There is no regular indication for steroid supplementation in hypothermia unless, following initial rewarming, the patient develops some new systemic collapse for which pharmacologic doses of corticosteroids are appropriate.

Complications

The major common complications of hypothermia are pancreatitis, pneumonia, renal shutdown (probably due to acute tubular necrosis in most instances), and disseminated intravascular coagulopathy. Management of these problems is by usual convention, and once core temperature has returned to normal no special allowances need be made. Other complications are related more to coexisting disease or injury than to the specific effects of hypothermia.

DISTURBANCES DUE TO HEAT

method of
JOHN B. De HOFF, M.D., MPH
University of Maryland
Baltimore, Maryland

Preparation for Heat Casualties

Expect heat casualties as seasonal hot weather approaches, where workplace environments subject employees to high ambient temperatures, or during sports activities such as late summer football practice or long distance running events.

Review detailed procedures with all staffs well in advance of anticipated difficulties, and assure that adequate solutions, drugs, and equipment are on hand and in working order.

Select a treatment area, post clearly written instructions, and assemble equipment; provide for safekeeping of emergency material throughout the time period of expected heat difficulties. If ice is to be used, assure its ready availability. Obtain a tub or small boat if immersion of heat victims in ice water is planned. Make sure that other emergency equipment is safely on hand and that all staff know what they will do. Include night and holiday shifts in orientation and training sessions because heat casualties occur at any hour.

Instruct foremen or training directors in how to prevent heat-related emergencies. Describe early symptoms. Conduct drills in first aid and early management of victims.

General Considerations

An environment hotter than 35 C (95 F), exposure to high radiant heat, increased metabolic heat production from work or sports, or disease-induced fever usually causes perspiration, which aids body cooling by evaporation. Interference with normal loss of heat by radiation, convection, conduction, or sweat evaporation may lead to serious changes in organ function and temperature regulation. High humidity or temperature, low air flow, poor acclimatization, poor preconditioning for sports, obesity, belladonna-like drugs, or electrolyte disturbances from reduced fluid or salt intake may rapidly cause critical body disturbances and possibly lead to a fatal outcome. Conditions that lead to moderate or severe heat injuries include elevated environmental temperatures, high humidity, excessive radiant heat loads on workers, or training demands on unacclimated or novice runners.

Heat stroke and hyperpyrexia usually develop slowly, with increasing restlessness and irritability, decreased interest in work, and tachycardia. A critical state appears abruptly when the flushed face becomes ashen, the skin is hot and dry, and breathing becomes labored. If cooling is not promptly instituted, collapse and coma ensue, frequently with convulsions.

Malignant hyperthermia, not related to anesthesia or drugs, is increasingly reported. It can occur in moderate environmental temperatures. It is defined as an autosomal dominant metabolic disease with high mortality. The target organ is skeletal muscle, with rapid swelling and rhabdomyolysis.

Heat exhaustion (anhidrotic, with or without salt or water depletion) appears insidiously or quickly with severe fatigue or even collapse, profuse perspiration, pale or flushed skin, rapid pulse, and central nervous system symptoms. All athletes, especially runners and heavily muscled football interior linemen, and elderly people require close observation for detection of anhidrosis or circulatory collapse, the first stages of heat stroke.

Skin conditions that predispose to heat injury include miliaria rubra with continued heat intolerance, intertrigo, tropical anhidrotic asthenia, and hereditary anhidrotic ectodermal dysplasia. Prevention is the best treatment.

Heat cramps—painful tonic spasms of skeletal muscles—occur abruptly with or without evidence of heat exhaustion.

HEAT STROKE

Treatment

Treatment must be individualized for each patient and special combinations of disturbed physiology or organ damage.

First Aid

Begin treatment immediately when heat stroke is suspected, recognized, or diagnosed. Remove the patient from exposure to sun or heat, preferably to an air-conditioned room or first aid facility. While awaiting transportation, remove all clothing from the patient, permitting the briefest of covering for modesty. Wet the patient and litter-stretcher with cool or room temperature water, and direct air flow from high velocity fans from head to foot. Apply packs of crushed ice to the head and the back of the neck. Continue cooling efforts en route to the hospital or other emergency facility.

Cooling Techniques

Two methods are available for rapid cooling of heat stroke victims. Immersion in an ice water bath is the one more commonly used in North America and other geographic areas with elevated summer humidity. A large tub or child's rubber boat is used, with adequate surrounding space for the therapy team to work freely. Although ice water baths for persons with rectal temperatures over 41 C (105 F) are uncomfortable, they do not cause shock or significantly decrease skin blood flow.

The second method, rapid cooling by evaporation, can be accomplished in environments with low humidity and is effective when the rectal temperature of a patient is 41 C (105 F) or lower. Nylon net or mesh supported on a pipe frame or a loosely woven rattan litter permits air flow from strong fans to circulate freely around the victim. Tepid water sprays are used to encourage evaporation and resultant heat loss.

Remove the patient from the ice water bath or discontinue electric fan air flow when rectal temperature reaches 38.3 C (101 F), and continue to monitor the body temperature. A rapidly falling core temperature will cause a continued drop in the rectal temperature, or there may be a subsequent temperature increase, which requires that active cooling techniques be reinstituted.

Supportive Therapy

Have ready or prepare flow charts on which data and certain observations can be entered serially, thus providing necessary information for gauging resuscitation efforts. Measure at regular and frequent intervals rectal or other core temperatures determined by electronic thermometers, pulse rate, blood pressure, accurate respiratory rate, urinary output by indwelling catheter, and central venous pressure. Request emergency laboratory examinations to assess serum electrolytes, including glucose, tissue enzymes, and coagulation times.

Establish an intravenous line, using a large bore needle or cannula, and administer Ringer's lactate solution to correct dehydration and maintain an adequate circulatory volume. Administer replacement fluids with care, because hypovolemia may not be extreme in younger adults, and elderly persons may easily suffer circulatory overload. Closely monitor the central venous pressures and the pulse and respiratory rates, and observe the patient carefully for early signs of pulmonary congestion.

Digitalis may help combat high output failure. Beta adrenergic drugs may be useful in hypotensive patients; do not use alpha adrenergic drugs. Oxygen may be needed by nasal catheter; intubation or tracheostomy may be needed for ventilatory assistance. Be alert for respiratory alkalosis due to tachypnea or metabolic acidosis secondary to renal failure. Early use of mannitol, 12.5 grams per liter of intravenous fluid, may promote renal blood flow and diuresis; renal dialysis may be needed should renal failure occur.

Supplementary Medications

Chlorpromazine (Thorazine), 50 to 100 mg intravenously, may be used to control shivering and to limit any consequent heat production. Diazepam (Valium), 10 mg intravenously, helps control seizures when they develop. Heparin, 5,000 to 7,500 units every 4 hours, is helpful in managing a bleeding tendency due to consumption coagulopathy. Fibrinogen may be needed to combat hypofibrinogenemia; fresh whole blood or platelet transfusions may be needed if platelets fall below 50,000 per ml. Avoid atropine and other anticholinergic drugs that inhibit sweating. Corticosteroids are of little or no value. Antibiotics should be used only when indicated for the treatment of recognized infections; fatal candidiasis has followed prophylactic antibiotic use. Reduce or adjust with care any medication being used to treat emotionally ill persons; psychotropic or neuroleptic drugs may have contributed to heat stroke. Do not use dextrans because they prolong bleeding time.

Malignant hyperthermia requires prompt action and continued monitoring. Use no beta-blockers. Hyperventilate with oxygen. Administer bicarbonate and mannitol solutions intravenously. Consider 50 per cent dextrose IV with insulin to prevent hypokalemia. Dantrolene sodium IV, 1 mg per kg, will help control tachycardia and muscle rigidity.

The Elderly and the Very Young

Heat stroke carries a high mortality in persons over 50 years of age (from three to eight times that in younger people) and is often mistaken for cardiorespiratory disease. Elderly patients are unable to compensate hemodynamically, cannot respond with tachycardia, do not adequately perfuse the skin for needed heat loss, and suffer hypovolemia. Care must be taken not to overcorrect any abnormality, yet treatment must be prompt and thorough owing to the high risk of this group. Thirst is a poor guide to hydration in these persons, and oliguria, dysphagia, and dry mucous membranes result.

Children with febrile infections are exposed to the risk of hyperpyrexia when bundled in blankets by anxious parents. Children have also suffered fatal heat injury when left unattended in closed cars parked in the summer sun. Principles of treatment are unchanged, but close monitoring of clinical signs and laboratory measurements is required.

HEAT EXHAUSTION

Symptoms of heat exhaustion include gastrointestinal upset, dizziness, weakness, faintness, and thirst. Signs include hypotension, hyperventilation, tachycardia, and syncope. In acclimated athletes, heat exhaustion is usually due to fluid loss and hypovolemia, but in unacclimated persons it may be due to sodium loss or a combination of fluid loss and hyponatremia. Heat exhaustion may spiral rapidly into heat stroke, or early stages of heat stroke in obtunded individuals may be misdiagnosed as heat exhaustion. Constant consideration of heat stroke as a possible diagnosis will save persons with severe heat exhaustion symptoms and signs.

Treatment

Treatment starts by cooling the patient. Remove outer or heavy clothing. Sponge the patient's body with cool water and help evaporation with air currents or a fan. Place the patient in a cool or air-conditioned environment. Encourage the patient to relax to diminish heat production. If nausea exists, start intravenous isotonic saline and 5 per cent dextrose solution. When nausea is relieved, urge room temperature water by mouth to assure adequate rehydration.

HEAT CRAMPS

Treatment

Place the patient in a cool or air-conditioned environment. Insist on oral rehydration with cool water. Consider starting intravenous isotonic saline or Ringer's lactate solution. Carefully observe all athletes and elderly persons for several hours, until it is certain that they are out of danger from heat.

PREVENTION

Direct special preventive efforts to young athletes and all long distance runners, active elderly persons employed in heavy industry or outdoor occupations, senescent city dwellers, and nursing home proprietors and attendants.

Athletes and Runners

Conduct orientation sessions with coaches, trainers, and athletes prior to starting practice. Describe the signs and symptoms of heat-related illnesses, and obtain agreement on prevention and first aid processes. Provide facilities for emergency medical treatment, and arrange for evacuation if necessary. Develop schedules of work and rest to provide for acclimation in 4 to 12 days. Commence practice in lightweight and light-colored clothing. Establish a WBGT (wet-bulb globe temperature) index system, and enforce hourly determination in critical periods, with prompt limitation of sports practices as indicated. (Consult sports medicine techniques for detailed guidance.)

Do not provide salt tablets; gastric pooling of oral fluids occurs, and severe hypokalemia has been reported. Avoid highly promoted packaged beverages, because hypertonicity delays hydration.

Long distance runners, especially novices, and joggers or other recreational runners may suffer severe heat exhaustion or even heat stroke. Careful race organization (time of year, route preparation), mandatory competitor education (acclimatization, awareness of premonitory symptoms), and careful medical preparation (first aid, available oral and intravenous fluids, rapid cooling equipment) will minimize heat casualties.

Lightweight clothing with a light-colored head covering is recommended to reduce absorption of solar heat. Runners should overhydrate by drinking plain water 1 or 2 hours before racing and attempt to maintain hydration by drinking 150 ml of water frequently during the run. Have on hand ample quantities of water to wet down runners quickly by "splashing" during races. Novice runners should be especially cautioned to be alert for early signs of decompensation and not to overexert in high ambient temperatures or humidity.

Workers

Outdoor workers or those in heavy industry, military commanders, and especially persons over 50 years of age should be cautioned about the dangers of high temperatures, either by physicians-in-charge or through general information releases from local health departments through the press, radio stations, and local television channels. Heavy protective clothing increases pyrexia risks. Clear heat-related cases before return to duty.

The Elderly

Elderly persons, with or without known chronic conditions, who live alone in small apartments are at high risk and should be counseled before heat waves occur. General physical activity should be reduced in times of high environmental heat stress; room air conditioners are recommended, or other air-conditioned facilities should be sought for temporary relief.

Nursing home proprietors and physician advisers should prepare for heat waves and for breakdown of air-conditioning systems should they be present. Nurses and aides should be responsible for hydration of specific patients, and fluid intake should be recorded during hot spells. Rectal temperatures must be taken at least twice daily. Clinical staffs on all shifts should know the signs of heat exhaustion and heat stroke, and emergency procedures should be at hand. Bedridden and other patients should be monitored for hyperpyrexia and signs of dehydration. Other causes for elevated temperatures, such as pneumonia or urinary tract infections, should not be overlooked. Mortality is high in nursing home patients during heat waves, but deaths can be reduced with careful preparation and attention to details.

The Emotionally Ill

Emotionally ill persons for whom psychotropic drugs have been prescribed must be closely monitored in hot weather. Family members and other care givers need specific instructions about possible severe pyrexia. Deinstitutionalized patients who care for themselves are at high risk. Chronic schizophrenics have a diminished perception of unusually hot weather.

SPIDER BITES AND SCORPION STINGS

method of
CLAUDE A. FRAZIER, M.D.
Asheville, North Carolina

Black Widow Spider *(Latrodectus mactans)*

The black widow spider (female) is, as her name implies, black: shiny black with bright, distinctive markings, usually hourglass in shape, on the underside of her abdomen. Some species have substituted brilliant red or orange dots or a simple splotch for the more decorative hourglass. About a half inch in length, the black widow is found everywhere in the United States with the exception of Alaska. She builds her untidy web in dark corners, in rock and lumber piles, and under stones and loose tree bark. Most bites occur through accidental contact, since the spider is shy and tries to avoid such encounters.

Symptoms of Envenomization

The venom of the black widow is neurotoxic, causing an ascending motor paralysis and destruction of peripheral nerve endings. Pain caused by the bite is not great at first, with most patients reporting a pinprick sensation. Within 1 to 3 hours, however, the pain increases greatly, becoming a dull numbing ache that may persist from 12 to 48 hours. The characteristic abdominal rigidity, sometimes mistaken for appendicitis, develops in 15 to 30 minutes. The bite itself is visible as two small punctures surrounded by erythema and perhaps some edema.

Systemic symptoms include weakness, tremor, severe muscular pain and muscle spasms, excessive salivation and sweating, weak pulse, bradycardia, and tightness in the chest and pain upon inspiration, with the patient often grunting upon expiration. Severe abdominal pain is characteristic along with abdominal rigidity. The skin may become extremely sensitive, with rigidity and spasms of large muscle groups occurring. Paralysis, stupor, and convulsions, especially convulsions in the case of young children, are possible.

Treatment

The only local treatment advisable is to cleanse the wound area and apply ice packs to slow absorption of the venom. Application of a tourniquet, incision of the wound, and suction to remove venom are all contraindicated; such steps may only increase the discomfort of the patient and increase the necrosis of the wound.

It is vital that the patient be transported to a physician or hospital as quickly as possible to receive antivenin which, if administered early, minimizes the severity of symptoms. Since antivenin is of equine origin, it is essential that the patient be tested for serum hypersensitivity before use. For this purpose, the packaged antivenin includes a 1 ml vial of normal horse serum, diluted in a ratio of 1:10, for testing and desensitization. The kit also includes a 2.5 ml vial of sterile water for restoring the serum, which is administered intramuscularly; the packaged instructions should be followed carefully. Usually, the 2.5 ml dose is sufficient, but in severe cases, in children under 12 years and in patients who are also in shock, the antivenin may be given intravenously in a 10 to 50 ml saline solution over a 15 minute period. Some patients may also require a second 2.5 ml intramuscular dose, which can be administered 1 to 2 hours following the initial dose.

A 10 per cent solution of calcium gluconate, 10 ml, should be given intravenously immediately to relieve muscle pain and can be repeated as needed. Muscle relaxants also may be given over an 8 to 16 hour period to relieve muscle spasms and pains. In severe cases, the corticosteroids may be of value; if pain is unbearable, morphine and phenobarbital may be given simultaneously, but as they are respiratory depressants and as black widow venom can cause respiratory paralysis, care must be taken if these drugs are employed. Prolonged warm baths may offer relief from the pain and discomfort. Hospitalization is desirable.

Brown Recluse Spider *(Loxosceles reclusa)*

Once thought of as a hazard only in the South Central United States, the brown recluse spider now probably ranges throughout the country. Including leg span, the brown recluse is about 1 to 1.5 inches in length. Its color ranges from tan to dark brown, with its most distinctive feature being a dark, violin-shaped marking from eyes to waist. Due to its penchant for seeking shelter in warm, dry areas, the spider's encounters with humans are probably more frequent than physicians realize. It has been suggested that many people are bitten by the spider, but few suffer severely. Some reactions to the spider's venom have been dubbed "clinically benign," with lesions that are mildly necrotic in comparison with other cases in which necrosis can be severe enough to require skin grafting. It is possible for one reason or another (e.g., because the spider used its venom in obtaining its last meal, or because the spider is very young) that the amount of venom injected is so minute as to cause only a mild toxic reaction. In any case, the venom of the brown recluse is necrotoxic and can be hemolytic.

Symptoms of Envenomization

The bite initially causes little or no pain. There is a transient erythema at the puncture site, followed within 2 to 8 hours by a bleb or blister and by pain in the area that can range from mild to severe. The vesiculation becomes surrounded by an irregular area of ischemia. Within 3 to 4 days, this area becomes somewhat star-shaped, hard, and dark purple in color. Within a week or two the central area becomes depressed and ulcerated and heals slowly with scarring and keloid formation.

Systemic symptoms can include fever, chills, nausea, vomiting, joint pain, weakness, and scarlatiniform rash. Potentially fatal hemolysis—thrombocytopenia and hemolytic anemia—presents serious complications, which are signaled by reddish urine. Fatalities, due mainly to hemolysis or renal failure, more often occur among children bitten by the brown recluse than among adult victims.

Treatment

No local treatment other than cleansing and the application of ice packs is necessary. Supportive treatment and the use of systemic corticosteroids and parenteral antihistamines constitute the treatment of choice and should be administered within 24 hours of the bite—the sooner the better for the prognosis and the less the damage of the necrotoxins at the bite area. A dose of 80 mg of methylprednisolone given intramuscularly should be followed by 60 mg of prednisone orally daily for 3 days, then tapered off over a 10 to 14 day period.

A 10 per cent solution of calcium gluconate in 10 ml injections, repeated as needed, helps relieve numbness and muscle weakness, while meperidine, 50 to 100 mg administered intramuscularly, can be administered to relieve pain.

To combat hemolysis, a dose of 5 per cent dextrose with bicarbonate and whole blood may be administered intravenously. Measures to combat shock and measures to combat renal failure such as dialysis and blood transfusions may be necessary, as well as heparin therapy if diffuse intravascular coagulation occurs.

Antibiotics are indicated for the development of secondary infection, and tetanus prophylaxis may be wise, considering the size and depth of the lesion.

It is possible that an antivenom for the brown recluse will be available in the near future. Researchers have developed an antivenom that has been successfully tested with laboratory animals; if side effects for humans appear minimal, approval for human use may be sought from the Food and Drug Administration.

Scorpions *(Centruroides sculpturatus and Centruroides gertschii)*

While there are some 30 species of scorpions in the United States, only two are dangerously venomous; and while scorpion stings can be painful and allergic reactions to the venoms are a possibility, it is the venom of *C. sculpturatus* and *C. gertschii*, found mainly in Arizona, that is potentially fatal. Their venom includes neurotoxins, cardiac toxins, and agglutinins.

Scorpions range from less than an inch to 4 inches in size and are somewhat like miniature lobsters in appearance with long, segmented tails at the end of which is the noticeable stinger. They are nocturnal, hiding during the day beneath stones, logs, and debris. The two most venomous species are yellow-greenish or lemon-yellow in color.

Symptoms

The sting causes severe pain, followed by a sensation of pins and needles, but, unlike the sting of less harmful scorpions, there is neither edema nor discoloration. Systemic symptoms develop within 1 to 3 hours, beginning usually with numbness in the limb (the usual site of the sting). The patient becomes drowsy, and complains of itching of the nose, throat, and mouth. Jaw muscles tighten and speech becomes impaired. Lymphangitis and lymphadenitis may occur in the area of the sting. Other symptoms can include restlessness and muscle spasms (the latter beginning with involuntary twitching), nausea, vomiting, incontinence, and convulsions. Respiratory and/or circulatory distress are possible. Fatalities usually occur within the first 3 hours of being stung and are generally the result of respiratory failure or pulmonary edema. Children under 3 years of age are the most likely to succumb.

Treatment

Local treatment consists of immediate application of ice on and above the sting site. If the sting is on a limb the limb should, if possible, be immersed in ice water reaching well above the sting. A tourniquet should be placed as close above the sting as possible and removed within 5 minutes, the venomized area remaining in the ice water. Keep the patient warm.

Specific antivenin does exist for the two dangerous species and should be administered as quickly as possible. Calcium gluconate, 10 ml of a 10 per cent solution, should be administered intravenously to relieve pain and may be repeated as needed, while atropine may be used to relieve excessive salivation. Slowly administer intravenously 60 to 100 mg of sodium phenobarbital to combat convulsions. Morphine and other opiates are contraindicated, however, since they increase toxic effects.

On occasion, less harmful species of scorpions can cause anaphylactic shock reactions as well as generalized allergic symptoms. It is the aforementioned species, however, that occasionally cause fatalities among adults and that are especially dangerous to small children.

SNAKEBITE

method of
WILLIAM E. LOCKHART, JR.
Alpine, Texas

When walking through an area where snakes may be a danger, it is important to take a companion along and to wear kneehigh boots and cuffed gloves. Hands and feet should never be put where they cannot be seen, as under brush or logs. The hiker should always carry a hickory hoe handle for defense. The more remote the area, the stricter the precautionary measures should be.

Management

In cases of snakebite, it is important to remember three important precautions in giving first aid in the field: no skin incision, no tourniquet, and no antivenin or other drugs. Rapid, safe transport to a hospital is the first priority. The second priority is to pack the bite area with ice made from fresh (not salt) water, which does not cause frostbite; no other refrigerant is recommended. The third priority is to capture and kill the snake for identification at the hospital. Identification is important because in patients bitten by the Mojave rattlesnake *(Crotalus scutulatus)*, whose bite is extremely toxic, specific antivenin is available. Also, the bite of the immature diamondback snake *(Crotalus atrox)* may cause afibrinogenemia.

Respiratory failure following a snakebite is rare but requires aggressive management. Oxygen must be kept flowing into the lungs, even if a tracheostomy and a mechanical respirator are required. Shock is best managed by giving lactated Ringer's solution intravenously with 1.0 gram of hydrocortisone sodium succinate (Solu-Cortef, Upjohn), repeated as needed.

In the emergency room a vertical incision is made under local anesthesia in the area of the fang wounds. The incision, about 3 inches long, should extend down through the subcutaneous tissue and the deep fascia, care being taken to avoid injury to nerves and arteries. The subcutaneous and subfascial tissues are then explored by blunt dissection. If envenomation has occurred, as indicated by darkening of the tissues as a result of capillary hemorrhage and evidence of the action of enzymes on tissues, all envenomated tissue should be removed with a sharp, small uterine curet and suction. Only by the use of such incisions is it possible to determine immediately whether there has been subfascial envenomation.

Since most patients sustaining snakebites arrive at a hospital emergency room within 1 hour after being bitten, one usually can remove as much as 90 per cent of the venom from the tissues; this is especially important if the patient cannot tolerate horse serum antivenin. One also must realize that subfascial envenomation can occur without subcutaneous envenomation, an extremely serious situation. In some cases of deep envenomation, as in bites involving the hand, debridement cannot be carried out because of the value of the anatomic structures.

The patient who has sustained a snakebite should be admitted to the hospital for observation, relief of pain, tetanus prophylaxis, and perhaps antivenin and antibiotic administration. Fibrinogen and hemoglobin levels should be determined immediately and then every 4 hours during the first day.

Antivenin is indicated if afibrinogenemia occurs or if significant venom remains in the tissues after debridement and in patients bitten by the Mojave rattlesnake, in which case species specific antivenin can be used. If antivenin is to be given, 0.1 ml of 1:10 horse serum is administered intradermally first to test for sensitivity. If a positive reaction occurs, no antivenin should be given. There is no safe method of rapidly desensitizing a patient who is allergic to horse serum.

In giving antivenin, at least 5 units of the antivenin should be mixed in 1 liter of 0.9 per cent saline solution and administered intravenously at a rate of 125 drops per minute. A "piggyback" container of 500 ml of lactated Ringer's solution should be ready to be mixed with 1.0 gram of hydrocortisone sodium succinate if urticaria or asthma develops. Both 1 per cent Neo-Synephrine (1 ml) and 1:1000 epinephrine (1 ml) should also be at hand. The former is preferred because it is less cardiotoxic and, in my experience, has always resolved anaphylaxis. Epinephrine is dangerous to use in cases of envenomation because of the hazard of ventricular fibrillation and sudden death. However, if Neo-Synephrine treatment is not successful, epinephrine should be used; a maximum of 0.1 ml is injected into the "piggyback" tubing.

ACUTE POISONINGS

method of
HOWARD C. MOFENSON, M.D., FAAP, FAACT,
THOMAS R. CARACCIO, Pharm.D.,
and JOSEPH GREENSHER, M.D., FAAP, FAACT
Long Island Regional Poison Control Center
East Meadow, New York

BASIC MANAGEMENT OF POISONINGS

The severity of the manifestations of acute poisoning exposures varies greatly with the age and intent of the victims. Accidental poisoning exposures make up 80 to 85 per cent of all poisoning episodes and are most frequent in children under 5 years of age. Many of these episodes are actually ingestions of relatively nontoxic substances that require minimal medical care. Intentional poisonings comprise 10 to 15 per cent of poisonings and often require the highest standards of medical and nursing care and the occasional use of sophisticated equipment for recovery. Suicide deaths are a significant number, and the use of toxic substances is often involved. The majority of the drug-related suicide attempts involve a central nervous system depressant, and "coma management" is vital to the treatment.

Sixty per cent of patients who take a drug overdose do so with their own prescribed medication and 15 per cent with drugs prescribed for relatives. The top poisoning categories for all ages are over the counter analgesics, sedative-hypnotics, benzodiazepines, cleaning agents and petroleum products, alcohol and abuse substances, pesticides, tricyclic antidepressants, plants, carbon monoxide, and opioids.

The assistance of Lauren Leader and Helene Jacobs in the preparation of this manuscript is gratefully acknowledged.

Assessment and Maintenance of Vital Functions

Upper airway obstruction is the most common cause of death in intoxicated patients outside the hospital. Any patient who is comatose and has absent protective airway reflexes is able to tolerate an endotracheal tube (cuffed for those over ages 7 to 9 years) and should have it inserted as soon as possible.

Ventilation is required if the respiratory rate and depth are inadequate.

The circulatory status is best assessed by the blood pressure and heart rate and rhythm. The circulatory clinical status and tissue perfusion may be inferred from the skin temperature, the return of color after pressure blanching (capillary filling), and the urine output. Intra-arterial blood pressure measurements are essential for adequate monitoring.

If the circulation fails to improve after adequate ventilation and oxygenation, then a 15 to 20 cm elevation of the foot of the bed may aid by increasing the venous return to the heart. A fluid challenge also may improve the circulatory status if hypovolemia is the cause. If these measures fail, plasma expanders and similar products may be required. As a last resort vasopressors may be needed. If these measures fail to produce a response, a central venous pressure (CVP) or a pulmonary artery wedge pressure (PAWP) line should be inserted to monitor for heart failure and fluid overload.

The level of consciousness of all intoxicated patients should be assessed and the time of assessment recorded. The Glasgow Coma Score used in head trauma is not useful in intoxications, as alcohol, depressant drugs, and hypotension may give falsely lowered scores. The Reed Coma Scale is preferred (Table 1).

Prevention of Absorption and Reduction of Local Damage

Ocular exposure should be immediately treated with water or saline irrigation for 20 minutes with eyelids fully retracted. Do not use neutralizing chemicals. All caustic and corrosive injuries should be evaluated by an ophthalmologist.

Dermal exposure is treated immediately with rinsing, not a forceful flushing in a shower, which might result in deeper penetration of the toxic substance. The skin should be rinsed with copious amounts of water for at least 30 minutes. Hair shampoo, cleansing of fingernails and navel, and irrigation of the eyes is necessary in an extensive exposure. The clothes may have to be discarded. Leather goods are often irreversibly contaminated and must be abandoned. Caustics (alkali) often require hours of irrigation until the "soapy"

TABLE 1. **Level of Consciousness (Reed's Coma Scale)**

Stage	Conscious Level	Pain Response	Reflexes	Respiration	Circulation
0	asleep	normal	normal	normal	normal
1	coma	decreased	normal	normal	normal
2	coma	none	normal	normal	normal
3	coma	none	none	normal	normal
4	coma	none	none	abnormal	abnormal

Stages 3 and 4 require intubation and placement in intensive care unit.
Stage 4 needs intervention to sustain life.

feeling of the burn is gone. Dermal absorption may cccur with pesticides, hydrocarbons, and cyanide.

Injected exposures to drugs and toxins or those introduced by envenomation may require a proximal tourniquet and early incision and suction. (See Antidotes 4 and 5 in Table 4.)

Inhalation exposures to toxic substances are treated by immediately removing the victim from the contaminated environment.

Gastrointestinal exposure is the most common route of poisoning and requires an estimate of what, when, and how much of the toxic substance was ingested. If there is a possibility of potential intoxication, gastrointestinal decontamination is performed rather than waiting for symptoms to develop.

Gastrointestinal Decontamination

To decrease the gastrointestinal absorption, emesis should be induced or gastric aspiration and lavage performed. Neither of these methods is completely effective; each removes only 30 to 50 per cent of the ingested substance. They are recommended up to 3 to 4 hours postingestion; however, to elect *not* to remove a potential toxin after 4 hours requires reliance on an often unreliable history of the substance and the time of ingestion. Therefore, it is safer to evacuate the stomach up to 12 hours after an ingestion in most significant intoxications.

Emesis

Relative contraindications to the induction of emesis are (1) in petroleum distillate ingestion of high viscosity agents, (2) with agents that are likely to rapidly produce coma (short-acting barbiturates) or convulsions (propoxyphene, camphor, isoniazid, strychnine) in less than 30 minutes and therefore may predispose to aspiration during emesis; and (3) in prior significant vomiting.

Absolute contraindications to the induction of emesis are (1) in caustic (alkali) or corrosive (acid) ingestions; (2) in convulsions because of the danger of aspiration and possible induction of laryngospasm; (3) in coma because of the possibility of aspiration with the loss of protective airway reflexes; (4) in absence of a cough reflex. Absence of the gag reflex is not a reliable indication of lack of airway protection since a number of healthy people lack gag reflexes; (5) in hematemesis in which vomiting may produce additional damage; (6) in an infant under 6 months of age, because of immature protective airway reflexes; and (7) with foreign bodies—emesis is ineffective and risks ostruction or aspiration.

Inducing Emesis. *Syrup of ipecac* is the preferred method; but never fluid extract of ipecac, which is too potent, or salt water, which has produced fatal hypernatremia. Emesis is not recommended to be induced at home in children under 1 year of age but can be performed in a medical facility under supervision when indicated. The dose of syrup of ipecac in the 6 to 9 month old infant is 5 ml; in the 9 to 12 month old, 10 ml; and in the 1 to 5 year old, 15 ml. In children over 5 years and in adults, the dose is 30 ml. The dose may be repeated *once* if the child does not vomit in 15 to 20 minutes. The vomitus should be inspected for remnants of pills or toxic substances and the appearance and odor noted.

Apomorphine is a parenteral emetic that must be freshly prepared. Its use is fraught with complications although it produces more rapid onset of emesis than syrup of ipecac. We do not recommend its use in the cooperative patient.

Gastric aspiration and lavage may be preferable to the induction of emesis in cooperative adolescents or adults because a large tube can be introduced through the oral cavity. *Contraindications* to gastric aspiration and lavage in intoxicated patients are (1) caustic (alkali) and corrosive (acid) ingestions because of esophageal perforation risk, (2) uncontrolled convulsions because of the danger of aspiration and injury during the procedure, (3) petroleum distillate products, (4) coma or absent protective airway reflexes, which require the insertion of an endotracheal tube to protect against aspiration, (5) significant cardiac dysrhythmias, which should be controlled first, and (6) hematemesis, which may be a relative contraindication.

The best results with gastric aspiration and lavage are obtained with the largest possible orogastric tube that can be reasonably passed (nasogastric tubes are not large enough for this purpose). In adults, use large bore orogastric Lavacuator hose or a #36 Fr Ewald tube; in children, use a #22–28 Fr orogastric-type tube.

The amount of fluid used will vary with age and size but in general an adult is lavaged with 300 ml per lavage and a child, 100 ml.

Continuous gastric "dialysis" has been used for substances that have an enterohepatic recirculation or are actively secreted into the gastrointestinal tract, such as tricyclic antidepressants (Tofranil) and local anesthetics such as mepivacaine (Carbocaine) (Table 2).

Activated charcoal is produced by combustion of organic material in the absence of air until the carbon particle is formed. There are few *relative contraindications* to activated charcoal: (1) it should not be administered prior to, concomitantly with, or shortly after syrup of ipecac since it may adsorb the ipecac and interfere with its emetic properties, (2) it should not be given prior to, concomitantly with, or shortly after oral antidotes such as *N*-acetylcysteine since it may adsorb these drugs and interfere with their therapeutic action, and (3) it does not effectively adsorb caustics and corrosives and may produce vomiting or cling to the esophageal or gastric mucosa and falsely appear as a burn on endoscopy. Activated charcoal has no *absolute contraindications,* but it does not effectively absorb alcohols, boric acid, caustics, corrosives, cyanide, metals, and drugs insoluble in aqueous acid solution (Table 3). Activated charcoal is a stool marker indicating that the toxin has passed through the gastrointestinal tract and that no further significant absorption from the original ingestion will occur.

The dose of activated charcoal is 1 gram per kg per dose orally with a minimum of 30 grams. The usual adolescent and adult dose is 60 to 100 grams. It is administered as a slurry mixed with water or by orogastric tube. It is too thick to get down by nasogastric tube. It should not be mixed with milk, marmalade, or starch because these interfere with charcoal's adsorptive action. Charcoal may be mixed with sorbitol which acts as a cathartic and does not interfere with charcoal's adsorptive capacity.

TABLE 2. **Substances with Enterohepatic Recirculation**

Chloral hydrate
Colchicine
Digitalis preparations (digoxin, digitoxin)
Glutethimide
Halogenated hydrocarbons (DDT derivatives)
Isoniazid
Methaqualone
Phenothiazines
Phenytoin
Salicylates
Tricyclic antidepressants

TABLE 3. **Toxic Substances Not Effectively Adsorbed by Activated Charcoal**

Alcohols
Antimalarial agents
Boric acid
Caustic alkali
Corrosive acids
Cyanide
2-4-Dichlorophenylacetic acid
Glutethimide
Insecticides (malathion, DDT)
Iron
Meprobamate
Methyl salicylate
Mineral acids
Phenylbutazone (Butazolidin)
Quinidine
Tolbutamide (Orinase)

Activated charcoal may be administered orally every 4 hours and may be especially beneficial in intoxications that have an enterohepatic recirculation (Table 3). Repeated dosing with oral activated charcoal has been shown to increase the clearance of intravenous barbiturates even in the absence of enterohepatic recirculation.

Catharsis is used to hasten the elimination of any remaining toxin in the gastrointestinal tract. Cathartics are *relatively contraindicated* (1) when ileus is indicated by absence of bowel sounds, (2) in intestinal obstruction or evidence of intestinal perforation, and (3) in cases with a pre-existing electrolyte disturbance. Magnesium sulfate is contraindicated in renal failure; sodium sulfate, in heart failure or diseases requiring sodium restriction. Magnesium sulfate (Epsom salts) or sodium sulfate (Glauber's salts) is administered in doses of 250 mg per kg per dose as 20 per cent solutions. The adolescent and adult doses are 30 grams. Cathartics may be repeated every 4 hours as long as bowel sounds are present or until the black stools of activated charcoal are passed.

Dilutional treatment is indicated for the immediate management of caustic and corrosive poisonings but is otherwise not useful. *Contraindications* to dilution are (1) inability of the patient to swallow, resulting in aspiration of the diluting fluid, and (2) signs of upper airway obstruction, esophageal perforation, and shock. The administration of large quantities of diluting fluid—above 30 ml in children and 250 ml in adults—may produce vomiting, re-exposing the vital tissues to the effects of local damage and possible aspiration.

Neutralization has not been proved to be scientifically effective.

The Use of Antidotes (Table 4)

Antidotes are available for only a relatively small number of poisons. An available antidote should be administered only after the vital functions are established. Table 4 summarizes the commonly used antidotes and their indications and methods of administration. Most informational, so-called first aid measures and antidotes on commercial product labels are notorious for their inaccuracy; it is preferable to contact the regional poison control center than to follow recommendations on these labels.

Enhancement of Elimination

The medical methods for elimination of the absorbed toxic substances are diuresis, dialysis, hemoperfusion, exchange transfusion, plasmapheresis, enzyme induction, and inhibition. The methods to increase urinary excretion of toxic chemicals and drugs are being studied extensively, but the other modalities have not been well evaluated.

In general, these methods are needed in only a minority of instances and should be reserved for life-threatening circumstances or when a definite benefit is anticipated.

Diuresis increases the renal clearance of compounds that are partially reabsorbed in the renal tubules. *Forced-fluid diuresis* is based on the principle that it will shorten exposure for reabsorption at the *distal* renal tubules. The risks of diuresis are fluid overload, with cerebral and pulmonary edema, and disturbances in acid-base and electrolyte balance. Failure to produce a diuresis may imply prerenal or renal failure. If renal failure is present, dialysis should be considered.

Osmotic diuresis is meant to increase the osmotic gradient and prevent reabsorption from the *proximal* loop and *distal* tubules. Mannitol is used to initiate this type of diuresis, and then fluids are added in sufficient amounts to produce a diuresis similar to forced-fluid diuresis.

Acid and alkaline diuresis is based on the principle that to inhibit reabsorption of certain toxic agents the urinary pH can be adjusted so the substance is maintained in its ionized form, which interferes with its passage back into the blood. Electrolyte and acid-base monitoring is necessary. Hypokalemia and hypocalcemia are frequent complications. *Acid diuresis* is accomplished by using ammonium chloride (see Antidote 2, Table 4). Ascorbic acid may be used as an adjunct. It enhances the elimination of weak bases such as amphetamines, fenfluramine (Pondimin), and quinine and has been extensively studied in phencyclidine intoxication. *Alkaline diuresis* with sodium bicarbonate can be utilized in the therapy of weak acids, such as salicylates, and long-acting barbiturates, such as phenobarbital (see Antidote 31, Table 4).

Dialysis is the extrarenal means of removing certain toxins from the body or as a substitute for the kidney when renal failure occurs. Dialysis is never the first measure instituted; however, it may be life-saving later in the course of the severe intoxication. It is needed only in a small minority of intoxications (Table 5). *Peritoneal dialysis* is only one twentieth as effective as hemodialysis. It is easier to use and less hazardous to the patient but also less reliable in removing the toxin. *Hemodialysis* is the most effective means of dialysis but requires experience with sophisticated equipment. *The patient-related criteria for dialysis* are anticipated prolonged coma and the likelihood of complications, renal impairment, and deterioration despite careful medical management.

Hemoperfusion is the extracorporeal exposure of the patient's blood to an adsorbing surface (charcoal or resin). This procedure has extended extracorporeal removal to a large range of substances that were either poorly dialyzable or nondialyzable. *Hemoperfusion may be used for agents that have* high protein-binding, low aqueous solubility, and poor distribution in the plasma water. In these cases hemodialysis was relatively ineffective. Hemoperfusion has proved useful in glutethimide (Doriden) intoxication, barbiturate overdose even with short-acting barbiturates, theophylline, tricyclic antidepressants, and chlorophenothane (DDT). The commonly used types are activated charcoal and resin cartridges. In general, supportive care is all that is required. Analysis of studies with hemodialysis and hemoperfusion does not indicate that they reduced morbidity or mortality substantially except in certain cases (Table 6).

Supportive Care, Observation, and Therapy of Complications

The comatose patient is on the threshold of death and must be stabilized initially by establishing an airway. Intubation should be attempted in any comatose patient. This is the best means to check for the presence of the protective airway reflexes.

An intravenous line should be inserted in all comatose patients and blood collected for appropriate tests, including toxicologic analysis (10 ml of clotted blood, initial gastric aspirate, 100 ml of urine). The initial management of the comatose patient should include the administration of 100 per cent oxygen, 100 mg of thiamine intramuscularly, 50 per cent glucose as an intravenous

Text continued on page 954

TABLE 4. **Antidotes**

Drug	Indications	Comments
1. ***N*-Acetylcysteine** (NAC, Mucomyst), Mead Johnson. **Dose:** *Adult,* 140 mg/kg PO of 5% solution as loading dose, then 70 mg/kg PO every 4 hr for 17 doses as maintenance dose. *Child,* same as adult. Packaged: 10 and 20% solution in 4, 10, and 30 ml vials.	Acetaminophen toxicity. Most effective within first 16 hours (to make more palatable, administer through a straw inserted into closed container of soda or juice) **AR:** Stomatitis, nausea, vomiting	See Acetaminophen. Contact regional poison control center for details of its use The full course of therapy is required in any patient whose level falls in the toxic range IV preparation experimental
2. **Ammonium chloride** USP, usually given via nasogastric tube. **Dose:** *Adult,* 2 gm every 6 hr in 60 ml dose to maximum of 12 gm/day or 1.5 gm as 1–2% IV q 6 hr up to 6 gm/day. *Child,* 75 mg/kg (2.75 mEq/kg) 4 times/day to maximum of 2–6 gm/day IV or PO. Packaged: 325, 500, and 1000 mg tablets; 2.14% in 500 ml, 21.4% in 30 ml, 26.75% in 20 ml.	For acidification of urine to enhance excretion of compounds such as amphetamine, strychnine, phencyclidine (weak bases with low volume of distribution, low protein binding, and excreted in the urine unchanged) Absorption may be erratic, depending upon the toxic substances ingested **AR:** Adequate doses frequently cause gastric irritation, nausea, vomiting	Goal in acid diuresis is to keep urine pH 4.5–5.5 and output 3–6 ml/kg/hr. Monitor blood pH, keep at 7.2–7.3 A diuretic may be used to enhance acid diuresis Contraindications: weak acid drugs, rhabdomyolysis and myoglobinuria, liver dysfunction, renal dysfunction, closed head injury
3. **Amyl nitrite.**	See 13, Cyanide kit	
4. **Antivenin Polyvalent** for *Crotalidae* (Pit Vipers), Wyeth. IV only. **Dose:** 3–5 × 10 ml vials in 500 ml over 1 hour; 3–20 vials may be used in first 6 hr. Packaged: 1 vial (10 ml) lyophilized serum, 1 vial (10 ml) bacteriostatic water for injection, 1 vial (1 ml) normal horse serum.	Venoms of crotalids (pit vipers) of North and South America **AR:** (Shock anaphylaxis) Reaction occurs within 30 min. Serum sickness usually occurs 5–44 days after admin. The postimmunization period may be less than 5 days, especially in those who have received horse serum products in the past. Symptoms include fever, edema, arthralgia, nausea, and vomiting, as well as pain and muscle weakness	Consider consulting with regional poison control center and herpetologist Administer IV Preliminary sensitivity test Never inject in fingers, toes, or bite site
5. **Antivenin,** North American coral snake, Wyeth. IV only. **Dose:** 3–5 vials (30–50 ml) by slow IV injection. First 1–2 ml should be injected over 3–5 min. Packaged: 1 vial antivenin, 10 ml, 1 vial bacteriostatic water 10 ml, for injection	*Micrurus fulvis* (Eastern coral snake); *Micrurus tenere* (Texas coral snake) **AR:** Anaphylaxis (sensitivity reaction). Usually 30 min after administration. Signs/Symptoms: Flushing, itching, edema of face, cough, dyspnea, cyanosis. Neurologic manifestations—usually involve the shoulder and arms. Pain and muscle weakness are frequently present and permanent atrophy may develop	Same as for Antivenin polyvalent for Crotalidae. Will not neutralize the venom of *Micrurus euryxanthus* (Arizona or sonoran coral snake)
6. **Atropine** (various manufacturers). **Dose:** *Adult,* initial dose of 2–4 mg IV. Dose every 2–5 min as necessary until cessation of secretions. Severe poisoning may require doses up to 2000 mg. *Child:* Initial dose of 0.05 mg/kg to a max of 2 mg, dose every 2–5 min as necessary until cessation of secretions. Packaged: 0.3 mg/ml in 30 ml; 0.4 mg/ml in 0.5, 1, 20, and 30 ml vials; 1 mg/ml in 1 and 10 ml vials.	Diagnostic aid; therapy in carbamate and organophosphate insecticide poisonings. Rarely needed in cholinergic mushroom intoxication (*Muscaria, Clitocybe, Inocybe* spp) **AR:** flushing and dryness of skin, blurred vision, rapid and irregular pulse, fever, and loss of neuromuscular coordination	If cyanosis—establish respiration first If severe signs of atropinization, may correct with physostigmine
7. **BAL**	See 16, Dimercaprol	
8. **Bicarbonate**	See 31, Sodium Bicarbonate	

Table continued on opposite page

TABLE 4. **Antidotes** *(Continued)*

Drug	Indications	Comments
9. **Botulism antitoxin,** Connaught Med. Research Labs. **Dose:** *Adult,* 1 vial IV stat then 1 vial IM, repeat in 2–4 hours if symptoms appear in 12–24 hr. *Child,* Check with State Health Dept.	Prevention or treatment of botulism	Contact state health department for full management guidelines
10. **Calcium Disodium Edetate** (EDTA), versenate, Riker. **Dose:** *Adult,* Max 4 gm. *Child,* 1 gm. *Moderate Toxicity,* IM or IV, 50 mg/kg/day for 3–5 days. *Severe Toxicity,* IV or IM, 75 mg/kg/day for 4–5 days. Doses divided into 3–6 doses daily. **Max dose:** 4 gm/day IV. Dilute 1 gm in 250–500 ml saline or D5W, infuse over 4 hr twice daily for 5 days. *Child,* Max 1 gm. For lead levels over 69 μg/dl or encephalopathy: Add BAL alone initially, 4 mg/kg, then combination BAL and EDTA at different sites. Doses for combination: 12.5 mg/kg IM. (See text for latest recommendations.) Packaged: 200 mg/ml. 5 ml amps.	Lead poisoning **AR:** 1. Thrombophlebitis 2. Nausea, vomiting 3. Hypotension 4. Transient bone morrow suppression 5. Nephrotoxicity, reversible tubular necrosis (particularly in acid urine) 6. Fever 4–8 hr after infusion 7. Increased prothrombin time	Hydrate first and establish renal flow. Avoid plain sodium EDTA since hypocalcemia may result Procaine 0.25–1 ml. of 0.5% for each ml of IM EDTA to reduce pain Do not use EDTA orally Limit use to 5 days (otherwise loss of other ions and cardiac dysrhythmias may occur) **MP:** Calcium levels, urinalysis, renal profile, erythrocyte protoporphyrin, blood lead, and liver profile
11. (A) **Calcium gluconate,** various manufacturers. **Dose:** *Adult,* 10 gm in 250 ml of water PO or by NG tube. 30 gm max daily dose. Packaged: 500, 650 mg, 1 gm tabs.	To precipitate fluorides, magnesium salts, and oxalates after oral ingestion.	
(B) **Calcium gluconate 10%.** **Dose:** IV 0.2 to 0.5 ml/kg/dose up to 10 ml/dose or 7.2–18 mg/kg of elemental calcium up to 360 mg over 5–10 min with continuous ECG monitoring. Titrate to adequate response. Packaged: 10% in 10 ml vial.	Calcium antogonists poisoning, e.g., nifedipine (Procardia), Verapamil (Calan), Diltiazem (Cardiazem). Hypocalcemia as result of poisonings. Black widow spider envenomation	Repeat dose as needed Monitor plasma calcium levels and ECG during IV administration
(C) **Infiltration of calcium gluconate.** **Dose:** Infiltrate each square cm of the affected dermis and subcutaneous tissue with about 0.5 ml of 10% calcium gluconate using a 30 gauge needle. Repeat as needed to control pain. Packaged: 10% in 10 ml vial.	Hydrofluoric acid (HF) (if irrigation with cool water fails to control the pain) **AR:** IV bradycardia, asystole, necrosis with extravasation	Infiltration with calcium gluconate should be considered if HF exposure results in immediate tissue damage, and erythema and pain persist following adequate irrigation
12. **Chlorpromazine,** various manufacturers. **Dose:** *Adult,* 1 mg/kg/dose IV/IM or 0.5 mg/kg/dose if taken with barbiturate or if exhausted. Packaged: 25 mg/ml in 1, 2, and 10 ml vials.	Give only in *pure* amphetamine OD, with life-threatening manifestations. (Diazepam [Valium] is preferred.) *Toxicity:* CNS depression, coma, hypotension, extrapyramidal syndrome, agitation, fever, convulsions, dry mouth, cardiac arrhythmias, ECG changes	Do not use if any signs of atropinization are present or "street drug" amphetamine. Watch for hypotension. In general it is safer to use diazepam (Valium) or haloperidol (Haldol)

*Consult regional poison control center before administration of antidotes. AR = Adverse reactions of antidotes; MP = Monitor parameters.

Table continued on following page

TABLE 4. **Antidotes** *(Continued)*

Drug	Indications	Comments
13. **Cyanide antidote kit,** Lilly. **Dose:** *Adult,* amyl nitrite. Inhale for 30 sec of every min. Use a new ampule every 3 min. Reapply until sodium nitrite can be given. Then inject IV 300 mg (10 ml of 3% solution) of Na nitrite at a rate of 2.5 to 5 ml/min. Then inject 12.5 gm (50 ml of 25% sol) of Na thiosulfate. *Child,* use the following chart for children's dosage. Packaged: 2–10 ml ampules sodium nitrite injection; 2–50 ml ampules Na thiosulfate injection; 0.3 amyl nitrite inhalant.	Cyanide poisoning **AR:** Hypotension, methemoglobinemia	*Note:* If a child is given the adult dose of Na nitrite a fatal methemoglobinemia may result. *Do not use methylene blue* for excess methemoglobinemia. Observe for hypotension and have epinephrine available Cyanide kits should have amyl nitrite changed annually Administer oxygen 100% between inhalations of amyl nitrite. Monitor hemoglobin, arterial blood gases, methemoglobin concentration (nitrite given to obtain a methemoglobin of 25%)
Hemoglobin of Child	*Initial Child Dose of Sodium Nitrite 3% (do not exceed 10 ml)*	*Initial Child Dose of Sodium Thiosulfate (do not exceed 12.5 gm)*
8 gm	0.22 ml/kg (6.6 mg/kg)	1.10 ml/kg
10 gm	0.27 ml/kg (8.7 mg/kg)	1.35 ml/kg
12 gm	0.33 ml/kg (10 mg/kg)	1.65 ml/kg
14 gm	0.39 ml/kg (11.6 mg/kg)	1.95 ml/kg
If hemoglobin level not known, use 12 gm dosage.		
14. **Deferoxamine mesylate** (DFOM, Desferal), Ciba. **Therapeutic Dose:** *Adult,* 90 mg/kg IM or IV every 8 hr to a max of 1 gm/injec. May repeat every 4–12 hr, but do not exceed 6 gm in 24 hr. *Child,* same as adult, IM or IV. IV administration can be given by slow infusion at rate not exceeding 15 mg/kg/hr. May be repeated as described for IM route. Packaged: 500 mg/amp (powder).	Iron intoxication. Therapeutic—see dose in left column. *Diagnostic* trial. Give deferoxamine, 20 mg/kg IM (up to 1 gm). If serum iron exceeds TIBC, unbound iron is excreted in urine, producing a "vin rose" color (pink orange) **AR:** Flushing of the skin, generalized erythema, urticaria, hypotension, and shock may occur. Blindness has occurred rarely in patients receiving long-term, high dose, DFOM therapy Contraindicated in patients with renal disease or anuria	Therapy is usually continued until urine color and/or iron levels are normal. Therapy is rarely required over 24 hours Oral route of administration to prevent absorption is controversial Establish a good renal flow To be effective, DFOM should be administered in first 12–16 hr In mild to moderate iron intoxication, IM or IV route. In severe intoxication or shock, IV route only Monitor serum iron levels, urine output, and urine color
15. **Diazepam** (Valium), Roche. **Dose:** *Adult,* 5–10 mg IV (max 20 mg) at a rate of 5 mg/min until seizure is controlled. May be repeated 2 or 3 times. *Child,* 0.1–0.3 mg/kg up to 10 mg IV slowly over 2 min. Packaged: 5 mg/ml, 2 ml, 10 ml vials.	Any intoxication that provokes seizures when specific therapy is *not* available, e.g., amphetamines, PCP, barbiturate and alcohol withdrawal **AR:** Confusion, somnolence, coma, hypotension	Intramuscular absorption is erratic Establish airway and administer 100% oxygen and glucose

Table continued on opposite page

TABLE 4. **Antidotes** *(Continued)*

Drug	Indications	Comments
16. **Dimercaprol** (BAL) in oil, Hynson, Westcott, and Dunning. **Dose:** Recommendations vary, contact regional poison control center. Given deep IM only. For severe lead poisoning. See 10, EDTA. For *mild arsenic or gold*—2.5 mg/kg 4 times daily for 2 days, then 2 times on the third day, and once daily thereafter for 10 days. For *severe arsenic or gold*—3–5 mg/kg 4 times daily for 3 days, then twice daily thereafter for 10 days. For *mercury*—5 mg/kg initially, followed by 2.5 mg/kg one or two times daily for 10 days. *Lead*—See text for latest recommendations. Packaged: 100 mg/ml in 3 ml amp.	For lead, arsenic, gold, mercury, copper, nickel, and antimony poisoning **AR:** 50% of patients have reactions: fever (30% of children), hypertension, tachycardia, may give hemolysis in G-6-PD deficiency patients. Doses greater than recommended may cause various adverse effects: nausea, vomiting, headache, chest pain, tachycardia, and hypertension	Contraindicated in instances of hepatic insufficiency, with the exception of postarsenic jaundice Should be discontinued or used only with extreme caution if acute renal insufficiency is present Monitor blood pressure and heart rate (both may increase), urinalysis, qualitative urine excretion of heavy metal Contraindicated in iron, silver, uranium, selenium, and cadmium poisoning
17. **Diphenhydramine** (Benadryl), Parke Davis. **Dose:** *Adult,* 10–50 mg IV over 2 min. *Child,* 1–2 mg/kg IV, 50 mg over 2 min. Packaged: 10 mg/ml, in 10 and 30 ml vials, 50 mg/ml in 1, 5, 10, and 30 ml vials.	Dystonia induced by phenothiazines and related drugs **AR:** Fatal dose, 20–40 mg/kg	Continue with oral diphenhydramine, 5 mg/kg/day to 25 mg 3 times a day for 72 hours to avoid recurrence
18. **EDTA**	See 10, Calcium disodium edetate	
19. **Ethanol** (ETOH) **Dose:** *Loading*—Administer 7.6–10.0 ml/kg of 10% ETOH in D5W over 30 min IV or 0.8–1.0 ml/kg 95% ETOH PO in 6 oz of orange juice over 30 min. **Maintenance Dose:** Volume of 10% ETOH needed IV (not on dialysis). *Average Patient,* 1.4 ml/kg/hr IV or (0.15 ml/kg/hr PO 95%). *Chronic drinker,* 1.96 ml/kg/hr IV or (0.2 ml/kg/hr PO 95%). *Nondrinker,* 0.83 ml/kg/hr IV or (0.09 ml/kg/hr PO 95%). If patient is on dialysis, add 91 ml/hr in addition to regular maintenance dose. Packaged: 10% ethanol in D5W 1000 ml; 95% ethanol.	Methanol, ethylene glycol **AR:** DNS depression, hypoglycemia	Monitor blood glucose, electrolytes, arterial blood gases, and ethanol levels. The ethanol levels should be kept at approximately 100 mg/dl Ethanol-induced hypoglycemia may occur. Dialysis, preferably hemodialysis, should be considered in severe intoxication not controlled by ethanol alone
20. **Fab** (antibody fragment). **Dose:** Dose may vary, effective but still experimental. (Investigational status.) Dosage details will be specified by investigator on procuring drug.	Digoxin and digitoxin intoxication with life-threatening intoxication, refractory dysrhythmias, hyperkalemia	Contact regional poison control center Preliminary sensitivity test Administer through a 22 micron filter
21. **Glucagon.** **Dose:** 50–150 μg/kg over 1 min IV followed by a continuous infusion of 1–5 mg/hr in dextrose and then taper over 5–12 hr. Packaged: 1 mg (1 unit) vial, with 1 ml diluent with glycerine and phenol; also, both come in 10 ml size.	Propranolol and other beta blockers intoxication **AR:** Generally well tolerated—most frequent are nausea, vomiting. However, these effects may be caused by hypoglycemia rather than the drug	Do not dissolve the lyophilized glucagon in the solvent packaged with it when administering IV infusion because of possible phenol toxicity Effects of single dose observed in 5–10 min and last for 15–30 min A constant infusion may be necessary to sustain desired effects
22. **Methylene blue,** American Quinine and others. **Dose:** *Adult,* 0.1–0.2 ml/kg of 1% solution (1–2 mg/kg) over 5 min IV. *Child,* Same as adult. Packaged: 1% 10 ml ampules. May repeat in 1 hr if necessary.	Methemoglobinemia **AR:** GI (nausea, vomiting), headache, hypertension, dizziness, mental confusion, restlessness, dyspnea when IV dose exceeds 7 mg/kg Treatment is unnecessary unless methemoglobin is over 30% or respiratory distress	Saliva, urine, and other body fluids may turn blue *Contraindications:* Renal insufficiency, cyanide poisonings when sodium nitrite is used to induce methemoglobinemia Monitor hemolysis, methemoglobin level, and arterial blood gases

*Consult regional poison control center before administration of antidotes. AR = Adverse reactions of antidotes; MP = Monitor parameters.

Table continued on following page

TABLE 4. **Antidotes** *(Continued)*

Drug	Indications	Comments
23. **Naloxone** (Narcan). **Dose:** *Adult,* 0.4–2.0 mg IV and repeat as needed to reverse signs or symptoms of toxicity. If no response is observed after 10 mg, diagnosis of narcotic-induced toxicity should be questioned. Continuous infusion may be beneficial in long-acting narcotics: 4–8 mg to each liter of D5W and infuse at 100 ml/hr to deliver 0.4–0.8 mg/hr to improve ventilation, but not to produce withdrawal; may need to repeat bolus after 0.5 hour. *Child,* Initial dose is 0.01 mg/kg IV. If no response, a subsequent dose of 0.1 mg/kg may be administered. Packaged: 0.02 mg/ml, 0.4 mg/ml ampule, and 10 ml multidose vial.	Narcotic, opiate, CNS depression. This drug is relatively free of adverse reactions Should be administered with caution in pregnancy. It is used only to reverse depression and hypoxia	Does not cause CNS depression Routes: IV or endotracheal are preferred Other routes that may be used include intramuscular, rectal, and subcutaneous Pentazocine (Talwin), propoxyphene (Darvon), and codeine may require larger doses
24. **Nicotinamide,** various manufacturers. **Dose:** *Adult,* 500 mg IM or IV slowly, then 200–400 mg q 4 hr. If symptoms develop, the frequency of injections should be increased to every 2 hr (max 3 gm/day). *Child,* one half suggested adult dose. Packaged: 100 mg/ml; 2, 5, 10, 30 ml vials; 25 and 50 mg tablets.	Vacor poisoning; phenylurea pesticide intoxication. *Note:* Vacor 2% is available only to professional exterminators. 0.5% Vacor is available to the general public and can be toxic to children if swallowed **AR:** Large doses—flushing, pruritus, sensation of burning, nausea, vomiting, anaphylactic shock	Nicotinamide is most effective when given within 1 hr of ingestion Do not use niacin or nicotinic acid in place of nicotinamide Monitor liver profile
25. **Oxygen 100%.** **Dose:** *Adult,* 100% oxygen by inhalation or 100% oxygen in hyperbaric chamber at 2–3 atm. *Child,* same as adult.	Carbon monoxide poisoning	Half-life of carboxyhemoglobin is 240 min in room air 21% oxygen. But, if a patient is hyperventilated with 100% oxygen, the half-life of carboxyhemoglobin is 90 min. If in chamber at 3 atm, half-life is 25–30 min
26. **Penicillamine** (Cuprimine, Merck; Depen, Wallace). **Dose:** 250 mg 4 times daily PO for up to 5 days for long-term (20–40 days) therapy; do not exceed 40 mg/kg/day. Packaged: 125 and 250 mg capsules.	Heavy metals, lead, mercury, copper, arsenic **MP:** Routine urinalysis, white differential blood count, hemoglobin determination, direct platelet count, renal and hepatic profiles, collect 24 hr urine, quantify for heavy metal **AR:** Leukopenia (2%); thrombocytopenia (4%); GI nausea, vomiting, anaphylactic shock, diarrhea (17%); fever, rash, renal and hepatic injury	This is not considered standard therapy for lead poisoning after chelation therapy May produce ampicillin-like rash, allergic reactions, neutropenia, and nephropathy Contraindication: Hypersensitivity to penicillin
27. **Physostigmine salicylate** (Antilirium), O'Neil. **Dose:** *Adult,* 1–2 mg IV over 2 min; may repeat every 5 min to max dose of 6 mg. IM, 1–2 mg; may repeat every 20 min to a max dose of 6 mg. *Child,* IV, 0.5 mg over 2 min to a max dose of 2 mg. Packaged: 1 mg/ml, 2 ml/amp.	Used if conventional therapy fails for coma, convulsions, severe cardiac dysrhythmias, severe hypertension, hallucinations secondary to anticholinergics, antihistamines, and anticholinergic plants **AR:** Death—respiratory paralysis, hypertension/hypotension, bradycardia/tachycardia, hypersalivation, respiratory difficulties/convulsions (cholinergic crisis)	IV administration should be at a slow controlled rate, no more than 1 mg/min Rapid administration can cause bradycardia, hypersalivation, leading to respiratory difficulties and possible convulsions Can be reversed by atropine Lasts only 30 min Contraindicated in asthma, cardiovascular disease, intestinal obstruction

Table continued on opposite page

TABLE 4. **Antidotes** *(Continued)*

Drug	Indications	Comments
28. **Pralidoxime chloride** (2-PAM, Protopam), Ayerst. **Dose:** *Adult,* 1 gram IV at 0.5 gm/min or infused in 150 ml saline over 30 min. Repeat every 8–12 hr when needed; if severe, 0.5 gm/hr infusion. *Child,* 25–50 mg/kg IV over 2 min or IM. Repeat every 8–12 hr when needed; run an infusion at a lower rate than in adults. Packaged: 1 gm/20 ml vials.	Organophosphate insecticide poisoning. Not usually needed in carbamate insecticide poisoning. Most effective if started in first 24 hours **AR:** Rapid IV injection has produced tachycardia, muscle rigidity, transient neuromuscular blockade. IM: conjunctival hyperemia, subconjunctival hemorrhage, especially if concentrations exceed 5%. *Oral:* Nausea, vomiting, diarrhea, malaise	Should be used only after initial treatment with atropine. Draw blood for RBC cholinesterase level prior to giving 2-PAM. The use of 2-PAM may require a reduction in the dose of atropine **MP:** Monitor renal profile and reduce dose accordingly
29. **Propranolol** (Inderal). **Dose:** *Adult,* 0.1–0.15 mg/kg IV, administered in increments of 0.5 to 0.75 mg every 1–2 min with continuous ECG and blood pressure monitoring up to 10 mg. *Child,* 0.01–0.015 mg/kg/dose slow IV push with repeat dose every 6–8 hr as needed. *Oral* dose when stable, 40 mg every 8 hr. Packaged: 1 mg/ml; tab: 10, 20, 40, 60, 80, 90 mg; cap: 20, 80, 160 mg.	Cocaine intoxication Has not been scientifically proved to be safe and effective. Anecdotal reports only **AR:** Bradycardia, hypotension, pallor; neurologic effects include hallucinations, coma, and seizures	Not a specific antidote; used for catecholamine storm and dysrythmias
30. **Pyridoxine—Vitamin B_6.** **Dose:** *Unknown amount ingested:* 5 gm over 5 min IV. *Known amount:* Add 1 gm/gm of INH ingested IV over 5 min. Packaged: 50 and 100 mg/ml; 10, 30 ml.	Isoniazid (INH), hydrazine **AR:** Unlikely due to the fact that B_6 is water soluble. However, nausea, vomiting, somnolence, and paresthesia have been reported from chronic high doses	Pyridoxine is given as 5–10% solution IV mixed with water. It may be repeated every 5–20 min until seizures cease. Some administer pyridoxine over 30–60 min **MP:** Correct acidosis, monitor liver profile, acid-base parameters
31. **Sodium bicarbonate.** **Dose:** Lavage 1–5% solution IV 1–3 mEq/kg as needed. To keep pH 7.5 where alkalinization is desired to correct acidosis to a pH greater than 7.2 Two mEq/kg raises pH 0.1 unit. *Child,* Same as adult. Packaged: 50 ml, 44.6 mEq/ampule.	To promote urinary alkalinization for agents such as salicylates, phenobarbital (weak acids with low volume of distribution excreted in urine unchanged) To correct severe acidosis May use in lavage solution for IRON poisonings To promote protein-binding in cyclic antidepressant intoxication **AR:** Large doses in patients with renal insufficiency may cause metabolic alkalosis. In patients with ketoacidosis, rapid alkalinization with sodium bicarbonate may reportedly result in clouding of consciousness, cerebral dysfunction, seizures, hypoxia and lactic acidosis	Alkaline diuresis. The assessment of the need for bicarbonate should be based on both the blood and urine pH. Maintain the blood pH at 7.5. Keep the urinary output at 3–6 ml/kg/hr May use a diuretic to enhance diuresis Potassium is necessary to produce alkaline diuresis Monitor electrolytes, calcium, pH of both urine and blood, arterial blood gases
32. **Sodium nitrite.**	See 13, Cyanide kit	
33. **Sodium thiosulfate.**	See 13, Cyanide kit	
34. **Vitamin K** (Aquamephyton) Merck. **Dose:** *Adult,* 2.5–10 mg IM, depending on potential for hemorrhage. Severe bleeding, 5–25 mg slow IV push. Rate 1 mg/min. Repeat every 4–8 hr depending on prothrombin time. *Child,* 1–5 mg IM. Packaged: 2 mg/ml in 0.5 ml ampules, 2.5 or 5 ml vials.	Warfarin (coumarin), salicylate intoxication	Fatalities from anaphylactic reaction have been reported following IV route. It takes 24 hr for vitamin K to be effective. Doses over 25 mg may be hepatotoxic. The need for further vitamin K is determined by the prothrombin time test. If severe bleeding, fresh blood or plasma transfusion

*Consult regional poison control center before administration of antidotes. AR = Adverse reactions of antidotes; MP = Monitor parameters.

TABLE 5. **Indications and Contraindications for Dialysis**

Immediate Consideration of Dialysis
- Ethylene glycol with refractory acidosis
- Methanol with refractory acidosis and levels consistently over 50 mg/dl
- Lithium levels consistently elevated over 4 mEq/liter
- *Amanita phalloides*

Indications on Basis of Patient's Condition (Coma greater than Stage 3 of Reed Classification)

Alcohol*	Iodides
Ammonia	Isoniazid*
Amphetamines	Meprobamate
Anilines	Paraldehyde
Antibiotics	Potassium*
Barbiturates* (long-acting)	Quinidine
Boric acid	Quinine
Bromides*	Salicylate*
Calcium	Strychnine
Chloral hydrate*	Thiocyanates
Fluorides	(Certain other drugs also dialyzable)

*Most useful

Indicated for General Supportive Therapy
- Uncontrollable metabolic acidosis or alkalosis
- Uncontrollable electrolyte disturbance, particularly sodium or potassium
- Overhydration
- Renal failure
- Hyperosmolality not responding to conservative therapy
- Marked hypothermia
- Nonresponsive Stage 3 or greater coma (Reed Classification)

Contraindicated on Pharmacologic Basis Except for Supportive Care
- Antidepressants (tricyclic and MAO inhibitors)
- Antihistamines
- Barbiturates (short-acting)
- Belladonna alkaloids
- Benzodiazepines (Valium, Librium)
- Digitalis and derivatives
- Hallucinogens
- Meprobamate (Equanil, Miltown)
- Methyprylon (Noludar)
- Opioids (heroin, Lomotil)
- Phenothiazines (Thorazine, Compazine)
- Phenytoin (Dilantin)

TABLE 6. **Plasma Concentrations Above Which Removal by Extracorporeal Means May Be Indicated**

Drug	Plasma Concentration *(mg/dl)*	Method of Choice
Phenobarbital	10	HP > HD
Other barbiturates	5	HP
Glutethimide	4	HP
Methaqualone	4	HP
Salicylates	80	HD > HP
Ethchlorvynol	15	HP
Meprobamate	10	HP
Trichloroethanol	5	HP
Paraquat	0.1	HP > HD
Theophylline	6 (chronic), 10 (acute)	HP
Methanol	50	HD
Ethylene glycol	unknown	HD
Lithium	4 mEq/liter	HD
Ethanol	500	HD

(Modified from Haddad L, Winchester JF (eds): Clinical Management of Poisoning and Drug Overdose. Philadelphia, WB Saunders Company, 1983, p 162.)

bolus, and 2 to 10 mg of naloxone (Narcan) intravenously. Other causes associated with coma and mimicking intoxications should be eliminated by examination and laboratory tests (trauma, infection, cerebrovascular accident, hypoxia, and endocrine-metabolic causes).

Pulmonary edema complicating poisoning may be cardiac or noncardiac. Fluid overload during forced diuresis may cause the cardiac variety, particularly if the drugs have an antidiuretic effect (opioids, barbiturates, and salicylates). Some toxic agents produce increased pulmonary capillary permeability and other agents may cause a massive sympathetic discharge resulting in neurogenic pulmonary edema (opioids and salicylates). Management consists of minimizing the fluid administration, diuretics, and oxygen. If renal failure is present, dialysis may be necessary. The noncardiac type of pulmonary edema occurs with inhaled toxins such as ammonia, chlorine, and oxides of nitrogen or with drugs such as salicylates, opioids, paraquat, and intravenous ethchlorvynol (Placidyl). This type does not respond to cardiac measures, and oxygen with intensive respiratory management using mechanical ventilation with positive end-expiratory pressure (PEEP) is necessary.

Hypotension and circulatory shock may be caused by heart failure owing to myocardial depression, hypovolemia (fluid loss or venous pooling), decrease in peripheral vasculature resistance (adrenergic blockage), or loss of vasomotor tone caused by central nervous system depression.

Renal failure may be due to tubular necrosis as a result of hypotension, hypoxia, or a direct effect of the poison on the tubular cells (salicylate, paraquat, acetaminophen, carbon tetrachloride). Hemoglobinuria or myoglobinuria may precipitate in the renal tubules and produce renal failure.

Cerebral edema in intoxications is produced by hypoxia, hypercapnia, hypotension, hypoglycemia, and drug-impaired capillary integrity. Computed axial tomography may aid in diagnosis. Therapy consists of correction of the arterial blood gases, the metabolic abnormalities, and the hypotension. Reduction of the increased intracranial pressure may be accomplished by 20 per cent mannitol, 0.5 gram per kg, run in over a 30 minute period, and hyperventilation to reduce the Pa_{CO_2} to 25 mm Hg. The head should be elevated, and intracranial pressure monitoring should be considered. Fluid administration should be minimized.

Seizures are caused by many substances, such as amphetamines, camphor, chlorinated hydrocarbon insecticides, cocaine, isoniazid, lithium, phencyclidine, phenothiazines, propoxyphene, strychnine, tricyclic antidepressants, and drug withdrawal from ethanol and sedative-hypnotics. Isolated brief convulsions require no therapy, but recurring or protracted seizures require intravenous diazepam (Valium) and phenytoin.

Cardiac dysrhythmias occur with poisoning. A wide QT occurs with phenothiazines and a wide QRS occurs with tricyclic antidepressants, quinine, or quinidine overdose. Digitalis, cocaine, cyanide, propranolol, theophylline, and amphetamines are among the more frequent toxic causes of dysrhythmias. Correction of metabolic disturbances and adequate oxygenation will correct some of the dysrhythmias; others may need antidysrhythmic drugs or a cardiac pacemaker.

Metabolic acidosis with an increased anion gap is seen with many agents in overdose. Assessment of the arterial blood gases, electrolytes, and osmolality may be a clue to the etiologic agent. Intravenous sodium bicarbonate may be needed when the pH is below 7.1.

Hematemesis can be produced by caustics and corrosives, iron, lithium, mercury, phosphorus, arsenic, mushrooms, plant poisons, fluoride, and organophosphates. Therapy consists of fluid and blood replacement and iced saline lavage if there is no esophageal damage.

Toxicokinetics for the Practicing Physician

Toxicokinetics is clinical pharmacokinetics from the viewpoint of the toxicologist. Pharmacokinetics is a mathematical description of what the body does to a drug. Knowledge of the toxicokinetics of a specific toxic agent will allow the physician to plan a rational approach to the definitive management of the intoxicated patient after the vital functions have been stabilized.

The LD_{50} (the lethal dose for 50 per cent of experimental animals) and the *MLD* (the minimum lethal dose) are seldom relevant in human intoxications but indicate potential toxicity of the substance. *Protein-binding* of toxic agents influences the volume distribution, elimination, and action of the drug. Diuresis and dialysis are usually reserved for drugs with less than 50 per cent protein-binding. The *therapeutic blood range* is the concentration of any drug at which the majority of the treated population can be expected to receive therapeutic benefit. The *toxic blood range* is the concentration at which this majority would be expected to have toxic manifestations. The range is not an absolute value. *Blood concentrations* are a quantitative aid in determining whether more specific measures need to be instituted in correlation with the clinical manifestations. The *apparent volume distribution (Vd)* is the percentage of body mass in which the drug is distributed. It is determined by dividing the amount absorbed by the blood concentration. When a substance has a large volume distribution, as in most lipid-soluble chemicals (above 1 liter per kg), and is concentrated in the body fat it will not be available for diuresis, dialysis, or exchange transfusion. *Elimination routes* of detoxification will allow the physician to make therapeutic decisions, such as using ethanol to interfere with the metabolism of methanol and ethylene glycol into more toxic metabolites. *Urine identification* is qualitative and only allows the identification of an agent.

Never manage a poisoned patient solely by laboratory tests and always treat manifestations, not the laboratory test. The laboratory toxicology analyst should be given whatever historical information is available so the agent can be sought and identified as rapidly as possible. Toxicologic analysis is like a miniresearch project, unlike most other laboratory tests. *Specimens* for toxicologic analysis require the patient's name, date, time of ingestion, time specimen was drawn, therapeutic drugs administered, patient's manifestations, and other relevant data. The toxicologic specimens that should be obtained for analysis are (1) vomitus, or initial gastric aspiration, (2) blood, 10 ml (ask the analyst about the type of container and anticoagulant), and (3) urine, 100 ml.

COMMON POISONS AND THERAPY

Abbreviations Used in Following List of Common Poisons

t½	=	half-life (time required for blood level to drop by 50 per cent of the original value)
Vd	=	volume of distribution (liter per kg)
TLV	=	threshold limit value in air
TWA	=	time-weighted average
PPM	=	parts per million in air and water

Conversion Factors

1 gram	=	1000 milligrams (mg)
1 milligram (mg)	=	1000 micrograms (μg)
1 microgram (μg)	=	1000 nanograms (ng)

Blood levels:

1 microgram per ml	=	100 micrograms per dl
	=	1 milligram per liter
	=	1000 nanograms per ml
100 mg per dl	=	0.1 gram per dl = 100 mg per dl
	=	1000 mg (1 gram) per liter
	=	1.0 mg per ml

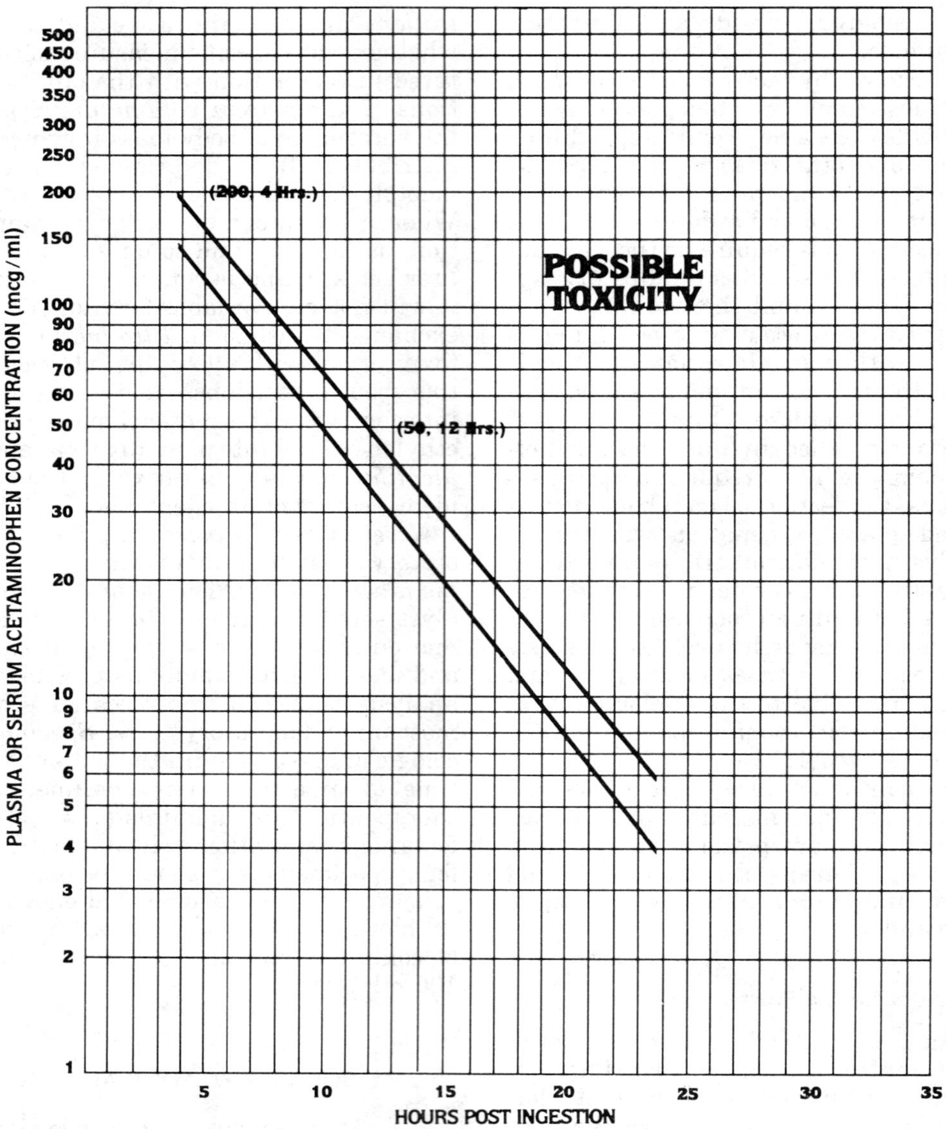

Figure 1. Nomogram for acetaminophen intoxication. Start *N*-acetylcysteine therapy if levels and time coordinates are above the lower line on the nomogram. Continue and complete therapy even if subsequent values fall below the toxic zone. The nomogram is useful only in acute, single ingestions. Serum levels drawn before 4 hours may not represent peak levels. (From Rumack BH, Matthew H: Acetaminophen poisoning and toxicity. Pediatrics *55*:871, 1975. © American Academy of Pediatrics, 1975.)

Acetaminophen, APAP (Tylenol). *Toxic dose:* Child, 3 or more grams; adult, 7.5 or more grams. Liver toxicity, 140 mg per kg. *Toxicokinetics:* Absorption time, 0.5 to 1 hour. Vd, 0.9 liter per kg. Route of elimination by liver. Draw peak blood level after 4 hours in overdose. *Manifestations:* First 24 hours: malaise, nausea, vomiting, and drowsiness, followed by a latent period of 24 hours to 5 days; then hepatic symptoms, disturbances in clotting mechanism, and renal damage. *Management:* (1) Activated charcoal has been contraindicated when *N*-acetylcysteine is contemplated; use gastric lavage. However, recently activated charcoal may be given in the first few hours or alternated 2 hours after the *N*-acetylcysteine. It should be removed prior to instilling the *N*-acetylcysteine. (2) *N*-Acetylcysteine for toxic overdose (see Antidote 1, Table 4). Start and give a full course if a toxic dose has been ingested or if blood concentrations are above the toxic line on the nomogram shown in Figure 1. (3) Dialysis (peritoneal/hemodialysis) in severe cases when antidote is not administered in time. *Laboratory aids:* APAP level, optimally at 4 to 6 hours. Plot levels on nomogram in Figure 1 as a guide for treatment. Monitor liver and renal profiles daily.

Acids. See Caustics and Corrosives.

Alcohols

1. **Ethanol** (grain alcohol). *Manifestations:* Blood

ethanol levels over 30 mg per dl produce euphoria; over 50, incoordination and intoxication; over 100, ataxia (the person is legally drunk in most states); over 300, stupor; and over 500, coma. Levels of 500 to 700 mg per dl may be fatal. Chronic alcoholic patients tolerate higher levels and the correlation may not be valid. *Management:* (1) Gastrointestinal decontamination up to 1 hour postingestion. Activated charcoal and saline cathartics are not indicated. (2) 50 per cent glucose intravenously if the blood glucose level is less than 60 mg per dl. (3) Thiamine, 100 mg intramuscularly, if chronic alcoholism is suspected, to prevent Wernicke-Korsakoff syndrome. (4) Hemodialysis is indicated in severe cases when conventional therapy is ineffective (rarely needed). (5) Treat seizures with diazepam (Valium) followed by phenytoin (Dilantin) if unresponsive. (6) Treat withdrawal with hydration and chlordiazepoxide (Librium) or diazepam. Large doses of sedatives may be required for delirium tremens. *Laboratory aids:* Arterial blood gases, electrolytes, blood ethanol levels, glucose, determine anion and osmolar gap, and check for ketosis. Chest radiograph to determine whether aspiration pneumonia is present. Liver function tests and bilirubin levels.

2. **Isopropanol** (rubbing alcohol). Normal propyl alcohol is related to isopropanol but is more toxic. *Manifestations:* Ethanol-like intoxication with acetone odor to breath, acetonuria, acetonemia without systemic acidosis, gastritis. *Management:* (1) Gastrointestinal decontamination. Activated charcoal and cathartics not indicated. (2) Hemodialysis in life-threatening overdose (rarely needed). *Laboratory aids:* Isopropyl alcohol levels, acetone, glucose, arterial blood gases.

3. **Methanol** (wood alcohol). *Toxic dose:* One teaspoonful is potentially lethal for a 2 year old and can cause blindness in an adult. The toxic blood level of methanol is above 20 mg per dl, the potentially fatal level over 50 mg per dl. *Manifestations:* Hyperemia of optic disk, violent abdominal colic, blindness, and shock. *Management:* (1) Gastrointestinal decontamination. Activated charcoal and saline cathartics are not indicated. (2) Treat acidosis vigorously with sodium bicarbonate intravenously. (3) Initiate ethanol therapy (Antidote 19, Table 4). (4) Folinic acid and folic acid have been used successfully in animal investigations. (5) Consider hemodialysis if the blood methanol level is greater than 50 mg per dl or if significant metabolic acidosis or visual or mental symptoms are present. *Note:* The ethanol dose has to be increased during dialysis therapy. (6) Ophthalmology consultation. *Laboratory aids:* Methanol and ethanol levels, electrolytes, glucose, and arterial blood gases.

Alkali. See Caustics and Corrosives.

Amitriptyline (Elavil). See Tricyclic Antidepressants.

Amphetamines (diet pills, various trade names). *Toxicity:* Child, 5 mg per kg; adult, 12 mg has been reported as lethal. *Toxicokinetics:* Peak time of action is 2 to 4 hours. t½, 8 to 10 hours in acid urine (pH less than 6.0) and 16 to 31 hours in alkaline urine (pH, 7.5). *Route of elimination:* Liver, 60 per cent; kidney, 30 to 40 per cent at alkaline urine pH; at acid urine pH, 50 to 70 per cent. *Manifestations:* Dysrhythmias, hyperpyrexia, convulsions, hypertension, paranoia, violence. *Management:* (1) Gastrointestinal decontamination up to 4 hours. (2) Control extreme agitation or convulsions with diazepam. Thorazine may be dangerous if ingestion is not pure amphetamine. (3) Treat hypertensive crisis with diazoxide. (4) Acidification diuresis with ammonium chloride (Antidote 2, Table 4) in life-threatening intoxications when conservative measures have failed. (5) Treat hyperpyrexia symptomatically. (6) If unusual neurologic symptoms, consider cerebrovascular accident. (7) Observe for suicidal depression that may follow intoxication. (8) In life-threatening agitation use haloperidol (Haldol). (9) Significant life-threatening tachydysrhythmia may respond to beta blockers (propranolol) (Antidote 29, Table 4). *Laboratory aids:* Monitor for rhabdomyolysis (creatine phosphokinase), myoglobinuria, hyperkalemia, and disseminated intravascular coagulation. Toxic blood level, 10 μg per dl.

Aniline. See Nitrites and Nitrates.

Anticholinergic Agents. Examples are antihistamines—hydroxyline (Atarax), diphenhydramine (Benadryl); antipsychotics (neuroleptics)—phenothiazines (Thorazine); antidepressant drugs (tricyclic antidepressants)—imipramine (Tofranil); antiparkinson drugs—trihexyphenidyl (Artane), benzotropine (Cogentin); over the counter sleep, cold, and hayfever medicine (methapyrilene); ophthalmic products (atropine); plants—jimsonweed *(Datura stramonium),* deadly nightshade *(Atropa belladonna),* henbane *(Hyoscyamus niger);* and antispasmodic agents for the bowel (atropine). *Toxicokinetics:* See Table 7, next page. *Manifestations:* Anticholinergic signs—hyperpyrexia, dilated pupils, flushing of skin, dry mucosa, tachycardia, delirium, hallucinations, coma, and convulsions. *Management:* (1) Gastrointestinal decontamination up to 12 hours postingestion. (2) Control seizures with diazepam. (3) Control ventricular dysrhythmias with lidocaine. (4) Physostigmine (Antidote 27, Table 4) for life-threatening anticholinergic effects refractory to conventional treatments. (5) Treat urinary retention. (6) Treat cardiac dysrhythmias only if patient is not perfusing tissues adequately or is hypotensive.

Anticonvulsants. See Table 8, next page. *Toxic dose:* Specific anticonvulsant blood levels and the clinical manifestations will indicate toxicity. In general, the ingestion of five times the therapeutic dose is expected to have the potential for toxicity. *Management:* (1) Gastrointestinal decontamination up to 12 hours postingestion. (2) Monitor specific anticonvulsant blood levels. (3) The effectiveness of hemoperfusion and dialysis has not been established.

Antidepressants. See Tricyclic Antidepressants.

Antifreeze. See Alcohols (Methanol) and Ethylene Glycol.

Antihistamines. See Anticholinergic Agents.

Arsenic and Arsine Gas. *Toxic dose:* In humans, the inorganic arsenic trioxide toxic dose is 5 to 50 mg; the potential fatal dose is 120 mg. Organic arsenic is less toxic. The maximum allowable concentration for prolonged exposure is 0.05 ppm. See Table 9, page 959. Humans are more sensitive than rodents to arsenic. Acute poisoning results from accidental ingestion of arsenic-containing pesticides. (Ant traps sold in some States contain arsenic.) *Toxicokinetics:* Rapidly absorbed by inhalation and ingestion. Crosses placenta

TABLE 7. **Toxicokinetics of Anticholinergic Agents**

Drug	*Potential Total Dose*	*Peak Effect*	*Vd*	*t½*	*Excretion Route*
Atropine	Child: 10–20 mg; adult: 100 mg	1–2 hours, may be prolonged in overdose	2–4 liters/kg	13–38 hr	Renal 50–70%, hepatic 30–50%
Diphenhydramine	100–500 mg; 2 oz has been fatal in 2 year old	3–4 hours but may be prolonged in overdose	3–4 liters/kg	5–8 hr	Renal (some hepatic)

and can cause fetal damage. Distributes into spleen, liver, kidneys. *Excretion:* In urine, 90 per cent. Following acute ingestion, it takes 10 days to clear a single dose; chronic ingestion takes up to 70 days. *Arsine gas:* Forms when active hydrogen comes in contact with arsenic. This may occur when zinc, antimony, lead, or iron is contaminated with arsenic and comes in contact with acid. This causes arsine inhalation intoxication characterized by a latent period of 2 to 48 hours and a triad of abdominal pain, jaundice (due to hemolysis), and hematuria. *Manifestations:* Gastroenteritis, neurologic and cardiac abnormalities, subsequent renal involvement. A garlic odor to the breath may be a clue. Smaller doses and prolonged low level exposure produce subacute (stomatitis) and chronic (peripheral neuropathy) symptoms.

Management: (1) Gastrointestinal decontamination. Follow with abdominal radiographs, as arsenic is radiopaque. (2) Intravenous fluids to correct dehydration and electrolyte deficiencies. (3) Treat shock with oxygen, blood, and fluids as needed. (4) In severe cases, administer BAL (dimercaprol) (Antidote 16, Table 4). (5) In chronic poisoning, D-penicillamine (Antidote 26, Table 4) may be used to chelate arsenic. Therapy should be continued until the urine arsenic is less than 50 μg per liter. (6) Hemodialysis is effective in acute poisoning and can be used concurrently with chelation therapy in severe cases, especially if renal failure develops. (7) Arsine intoxication is treated by exchange transfusion and hemodialysis if renal failure occurs. BAL is ineffective. *Laboratory aids:* Blood arsenic and 24 hour urine arsenic levels. 50 μg per liter of arsenic in urine indicates excessive exposure, but diets rich in seafood may excrete 200 μg per day. View values over 100 with suspicion. Monitor electrocardiogram and renal function. Normal blood arsenic level is less than 7 μg per dl (false values occur in inexperienced laboratories).

Aspirin. See Salicylates.

Atropine. See Anticholinergic Agents.

Barbiturates. See Table 10, next page. *Management:* (1) Gastrointestinal decontamination up to 8 to 12 hours. Activated charcoal in repeated doses of 60 to 100 grams has been shown to reduce the serum half-life and increase the nonrenal clearance over 50 per cent. Give every 4 hours while in coma. (2) Supportive and symptomatic care is all that is necessary in the majority of cases. (3) Forced alkaline diuresis (if not in shock), for phenobarbital intoxication. Sodium bicarbonate, 44 to 88 mEq/liter, and potassium chloride,

TABLE 8. **Anticonvulsants**

Drug	**Peak Time of Action/Hrs** *(steady state)*	**Vd** *(liters/kg)*	**t½** *(hr)*	**Route of Elimination** *(per cent)*	**Protein-Binding** *(per cent)*	**Blood Level** *(μg/ml)*	**Comment***
Carbamazepine (Tegretol)	6–12 (2–4 days)	0.8–1.4	30–60	Liver (98)	70	Therapeutic, 5–12	Related to tricyclic antidepressants, can cause dysrhythmias
Ethosuximide (Zarontin)	24–48 (5–8 days)	0.6–0.8	24–56	Liver (80–90) Renal (10–20)	0	Therapeutic, 40–100	
Phenytoin (Dilantin)	Oral, 6–12 IV, 1 (5–10 days)	0.6–1.0	20–30; varies in toxic doses: zero order kinetics	Liver (95)	87–93	Therapeutic, 10–20; toxic, 20–30: nystagmus only, 30–40: ataxia, 40+: coma, convulsions	Dysrhythmias with parenteral use only
Primidone (Mysoline)	3–4? (4–7 days)	0.6	Parent, 3–12; metabolites, 30–36	Liver	70–80	Therapeutic, 8–12 primidone and 10–25 phenobarbital (PB); toxic, over 50 primidone and over 40 PB (see Barbiturates)	Metabolized to active metabolites phenylethylmalonamide and PB; overdose gives white crystals in urine†
Valproic acid (Depakene)	? (1–4 days)	0.3–0.5	8–15	Liver (80–100)	20	Therapeutic, 60–100	Produces nausea and vomiting, changes in liver function
Clonazepam (Clonipin)	? (4–12 days)		20–60	Liver (98)	90	Therapeutic, 20–70 ng/ml	

*Manifestations: The major manifestations of these agents are depression of consciousness and respiratory depression. Other significant manifestations are mentioned in this column.

†Primidone produces whorls of shimmering white crystals in the urine from precipitation of intact primidone in massive overdose.

TABLE 9. **Comparative Acute Toxicities of Some Common Arsenicals**

Arsenical	Oral LD_{50} in Rats *(mg/kg)*	Estimated Mortality in Human Poisoning (%)
Arsenic trioxide	385	12
Sodium arsenite	42	65
Calcium arsenite	ca. 275	?
Lead arsenite	1500+	5
Ortho crabgrass killer*	3719	none known

*Product containing 8 per cent each of only mildly toxic octyl NH_4 and dodecyl NH_4 methanearsonate. (From Done AK: . . . And old lace. Emergency Med 5:246, 1973.)

20 mEq/liter, should be given at a rate to produce a urine flow of 3 to 6 ml/kg/hr and a urine pH of 7 to 8. Additional sodium bicarbonate (1 to 2 mEq/liter) and potassium chloride (20 to 40 mEq/liter) may be needed to achieve an optimal urine pH. Assure adequate hydration and renal function prior to alkalinization. Not useful for other barbiturates (Antidote 31, Table 4). (4) In severe cases not responding to conservative measures, consider hemodialysis and hemoperfusion. (5) Treat any bullae as a local second degree skin burn. (6) Give intensive care monitoring to comatose patient. *Treatment of withdrawal: In an emergency,* use pentothal or diazepam intravenously. If the patient is stable, a pentobarbital tolerance test may be given. 200 mg of pentobarbital is given orally and the patient examined after 1 hour for signs of intoxication (nystagmus, slurred speech, and ataxia). If none are present, the dose is repeated every 3 hours until these signs develop. This is the stabilizing dose; the patient is maintained on this dose for 72 hours and then changed to phenobarbital, 30 mg substituted for each 100 mg of pentobarbital. The phenobarbital is tapered, decreasing by 10 per cent or 30 mg every 3 to 5 days. *Laboratory aids:* Emergency plasma barbiturate concentrations rarely alter management.

Benzene. See Hydrocarbons.

Benzodiazepines (BZP). See Table 11. *Toxicity:* Low toxic potential. More than 500 mg has been ingested without respiratory depression. Benzodiazepines have an additive effect with sedatives such as alcohol and barbiturates. Most patients intoxicated with BZP alone recover within 24 hours. Many of these agents have active metabolites with a long plasma t½, so performance in skilled tasks such as driving may be impaired. Withdrawal occurs infrequently and is delayed. *Manifestations:* Central nervous system depression. Deep coma leading to respiratory depression suggests presence of other drugs. *Management:* (1) Gastrointestinal decontamination. (2) Supportive and symptomatic care. (3) Withdrawal, if it occurs, is treated like barbiturate withdrawal. *Laboratory aids:* Document benzodiazepines in urine. Quantitative blood levels are not useful.

Bleach. Household bleaches are 4 to 6 per cent sodium hypochlorite. Commerical types are 10 to 20 per cent. *Manifestations:* Difficulty in swallowing; pain in mouth, throat, chest, or abdomen. General household strength bleach does not produce burns; commercial strength bleach may. Inhalation of gases produced by mixing chlorine bleach with acids (toilet bowl cleaner and rust removers—chlorine gas) or with household ammonia (chloramine gas) is irritating to mucous membranes, eyes, and upper respiratory tract. *Management:* (1) Ingestion—Do not induce emesis. Dilute with water or milk. Avoid acids. (2) Esophagoscopy

TABLE 10. **Barbiturates; Examples and Elimination***

	Long-Acting		Intermediate	Short-Acting	
Generic name	Barbital	Phenobarbital	Amobarbital	Pentobarbital	Secobarbital
Trade name	Veronal	Luminal	Amytal	Nembutal	Seconal
Slang name	—	Purple hearts	Blue heaven	Yellow jackets	Red devils
pK_a	7.74	7.24	7.25	7.96	7.9
Detoxification	renal	renal 30%/ hepatic 70%	hepatic 98%	hepatic 90–100%	hepatic 90–100%
Onset: IV	22 min	12 min	—	0.1 min	0.1 min
PO	over 6 hr	3–6 hr (peak 12–18 hr)	less than 3 hr (peak 3–4 hr)	10–15 min (peak 2–4 hr)	10–15 min (peak 2–4 hr)
Protein-binding (%)	5	29	—	35	44
Hypnotic dose (mg)	300–500	100–200	50–200	50–100	50–100
Fatal dose (grams)	10	8	5	3	3
Toxic dose (mg/kg)	8	8	3–5	3–5	3–5
Therapeutic level (μg/ml)	5–8	15–35	5–8	1–4	3–5
Toxic level (μg/ml)	over 30	over 40	10–30	over 10	over 5
Lethal level† (μg/ml)	over 100	over 100	over 50	over 35	over 15
Duration of action	over 6	over 6	less than 3	less than 3	less than 3
Half-life (hr)	58–96	24–96	16–24	36–50	25–50
Rate of metabolism (hr)	—	0.7	2.5	—	—
Volume distribution, liter/kg	—	0.75	0.5–1.1	0.65–1.5	0.65–1.5

Manifestations

Low dose: Euphoria, ataxia, incoordination, nystagmus on lateral gaze

High dose: Flaccid coma, hypotension, respiratory depression, pulmonary edema (particularly with the short-acting barbiturates), subcutaneous bullae (6%), dermatographia

*Classification into long-acting, intermediate, and short-acting has no relationship to the duration of coma.

†These levels are not absolute, and tolerance occurs.

TABLE 11. **Benzodiazepines (BZP)**

Drug	Oral Dosage Range	Peak Oral Plasma Levels *(Hr)*	Half-Life *(Hr)*	Major Active Metabolites *(Half-Life in Hr)*	Elimination Rate
ANXIOLYTICS					
Diazepam (Valium)	6–40 mg/day	1–2	20–50	desmethyldiazepman (30–60)	slow
Chlordiazepoxide (Librium, Libritabs, various other)	15–100 mg/day	2–4	5–30	Desmethylchlordiazepoxide, demoxepam, desmethyldiazepam	slow
Clorazepate (Tranxene)	15–60 mg/day	—	30–60	desmethyldiazepam	slow
Prazepam (Centrax)	20–60 mg/day	6	78	3-hydroxyprazepam, desmethyldiazepam	slow
Halazepam (Paxipam)	60–160 mg/day	1–3	7	*n*-3-hydroxyhalazepam, desmethyldiazepam	slow
Oxazepam (Serax)	30–120 mg/day	1–2	5–10	None	rapid to intermediate
Lorazepam (Ativan)	2–6 mg/day	2	10–20	None	intermediate
Alprazolam (Xanax)	0.75–4 mg/day	0.7–1.6	12–19	α-hydroxyalprazolam	intermediate
HYPNOTICS					
Flurazepam (Dalmane)	15–60 mg	—	50–100	desalkylflurazepam (50–100)	slow
Flunitrazepam (Rohypnol—investigational, Roche)	1–2 mg	< 1	—	7-aminoflunitrazepam (23) *N*-desmethylflunitrazepam (31)	—
Temazepam (Restoril)	15–30 mg	2–3	9–12	None	intermediate
Triazolam (Halcion)	0.125–0.5 mg	0.5–1.5	2.3	α-hydroxytriazolam	rapid

only if unusually large amounts have been ingested, the patient is symptomatic, or the product was stronger than the average household bleach. (3) Inhalation—Remove from contaminated area. Observe for pulmonary edema.

Botulism. See article on Foodborne Illnesses in Section 1.

Brake Fluid. See Ethylene Glycol.

Calcium Channel Blockers. Used in treatment of effort angina and supraventricular tachycardia. See Table 12, this page. *Manifestations:* Hypotension, bradycardia within 1 to 5 hours, central nervous system depression, and gastric distress. *Management:* (1) Gastrointestinal decontamination. (2) Treat hypotension and bradycardia with calcium gluconate or chloride. See Antidote 11, Table 4. Dopamine may be used if necessary. (3) Heart block—may respond to IV calcium, atropine sulfate, 0.5 to 1 mg, or isoproterenol. (4) Ventricular pacing may be required in the severely intoxicated patient. (5) Patients receiving digitalis run the risk of toxicity and should be carefully monitored. *Laboratory aids:* Specific drug levels, blood sugar and calcium, electrocardiogram.

TABLE 12. **Calcium Channel Blockers**

	Nifedipine	Verapamil	Diltiazem
Trade name	Procardia	Calan, Isoptin	Cardizem
Onset of action	Oral: < 20 min	Oral: < 1 hr	Oral: < 15 min
	sublingual: < 3 min	—	—
	IV: < 1 min	IV: < 2 min	—
Peak effect	Oral: 1–2 hr	5 hr	30 min
Half-life (hr)	2.5–5	2–7	2–6
Route of elimination	Liver/kidney	Liver/kidney	Liver/kidney
Toxic level (ng/ml)	> 100	> 300	> 200

Camphor (External analgesic rubs, Vicks Vaporub 4.8 per cent, Campho-Phenique 11 per cent). Many camphorated oil products were removed from the marketplace in September, 1982. Five milliliters of camphorated oil (20 per cent camphor) equals 1 gram of camphor. *Toxicity:* Adult, 5 grams; child, 1 gram has been fatal. *Toxicokinetics:* Onset of manifestations, 5 to 90 minutes. Readily and rapidly absorbed through the skin, mucous membranes, and gastrointestinal tract and crosses the placenta. Route of elimination: Rapidly metabolized in liver to the glucuronide form which is excreted in urine. Pulmonary excretion causes a distinctive odor on the breath. *Manifestations:* Nausea, vomiting, and burning epigastric pain. Seizures may occur suddenly and without warning within 5 minutes of ingestion. Apnea and vision disturbances may occur. *Management:* (1) Induction of emesis is contraindicated because of early seizures. (2) Remove residual drug by gastric lavage. (3) Administer activated charcoal and a saline cathartic. Avoid giving oils or alcohol. (4) Treat seizures with IV diazepam. (5) Treat apnea with respiratory support. (6) Hemoperfusion with Amberlite XAD-4 or lipid dialysis may be needed in cases unresponsive to conventional therapy.

Carbon Monoxide (CO). This is an odorless gas produced from incomplete combustion; it is found also as an in vivo metabolic breakdown product of methylene chloride (paint removers). See Table 13, this page. Admit patients with carboxyhemoglobin levels of 25 per cent, or 15 per cent if the patient has cardiac or liver disease, is pregnant, or is a child. Observe for the symptoms described in Table 13. Contrary to popular belief, the skin rarely shows a cherry-red color in the live patient. *Toxicokinetics:* CO is rapidly absorbed through the lungs. The rate of absorption is directly related to alveolar ventilation. Elimination occurs through the lungs. The $t\frac{1}{2}$ in room air equals 5 to 6 hours; in 100 per cent oxygen, 90 minutes; in hyperbaric oxygen, 20 minutes. The nomogram pictured in Figure 2 can be used to decide quickly whether serious CO intoxication is likely to have occurred and to select patients at high risk or early management in the intensive care unit.

Management: (1) Remove from contaminated area and expose to fresh air. Establish vital functions. (2) 100 per cent oxygen to all patients until the carboxyhemoglobin level falls to 5 to 10 per cent. Assisted ventilation may be necessary. (3) Monitor arterial blood gases and carboxyhemoglobin levels. Determine carboxyhemoglobin level at time of exposure by using nomogram. *Note:* A near normal carboxyhemoglobin level does not rule out significant CO poisoning. (4) If pH is below 7.1 after correction of hypoxia and adequate ventilation, give sodium bicarbonate to correct acidosis. (5) Consider hyperbaric oxygen for severe cases with disturbance in mentation. (6) Treat seizures with intravenous diazepam. (7) Monitor electrocardiogram, chest radiograph, serum creatinine phosphokinase (CPK), and lactate dehydrogenase (LDH). (8) Treat cerebral edema with elevation of the patient's head, minimizing intravenous fluid, hyperventilation, and, if needed, mannitol and intracranial pressure monitor. (9) Re-evaluate after recovery for neuropsychiatric sequelae. *Laboratory aids:* Arterial blood gases show metabolic acidosis and normal oxygen tension but reduced oxygen saturation.

Carbon Tetrachloride. See Hydrocarbons.

Caustics and Corrosives. Common acid substances are hydrochloric acid, sulfuric acid (battery acid), carbolic acid (phenol), nitric acid, oxalic acid, hydrofluoric acid, and aqua regia (mixture of hydrochloric and nitric acids). These are used as cleaning agents. Common alkali substances are sodium or potassium hydroxide (lye), sodium hypochlorite (Clorox) (bleach), sodium carbonate (nonphosphate detergents), potassium permanganate, ammonia, electric dishwashing agents, cement, and flat disk batteries. *Toxicity:* Acids produce mucosal coagulation necrosis. They usually do not penetrate deeply (exception: hydrofluoric acid). The gastric mucosa is the primary site of injury. Alkalis produce liquefaction necrosis and saponification and penetrate deeply. Oropharyngeal and esophageal damage by solids is more frequent than by liquids. Liquids are more likely to produce gastric damage as well. *Toxic dose:* Adult potential fatal dose of concentrated acid/alkali is 5 ml. The absence of oral burns does not exclude the possibility of esophageal burns (10 to 15 per cent).

Management: (1) Dilute with milk or water immediately up to 30 ml in children or 250 ml in adults. Neutralization with acidic or alkalinic agents is contraindicated. Dilute only if patient can swallow. (2) Gastrointestinal decontamination is contraindicated. However, in acid ingestions some authorities advocate nasogastric intubation and aspiration in the early postingestion phase. Patient should receive only intravenous fluids following dilution until surgical consultation. Dermal and ocular decontamination should be carried out when appropriate. (3) Esophagoscopy may be indicated postingestion to assess severity of burn. (4) Steroids are controversial. Some recommend steroids administered if burns are found or esophagoscopy is not performed. (5) Antibiotics are not useful prophylactically. (6) Barium swallow may be necessary at 10 days to 3 weeks to assess severity of damage. (7) Dilation may need to be performed at 2 to 4 week intervals if evidence of stricture. (8) Intraposition of the colon may be necessary if dilation fails to provide an adequate-sized esophagus. (9) Inhalation manage-

TABLE 13. **Carbon Monoxide (CO)**

CO in Atmosphere	Duration of Exposure	Saturation of Blood (%)	Symptoms
up to 0.01	indefinite	1–10	None
0.01–0.02	indefinite	10–20	Tightness across forehead, slight headache, dilation of cutaneous vessels
0.02–0.03	5–6 hr	20–30	Headache, throbbing temples
0.04–0.06	4–5 hr	30–40	Severe headache, weakness and dizziness, nausea and vomiting, collapse. Leukocytosis
0.07–0.10	3–4 hr	40–50	Above, plus increased tendency to collapse and syncope, increased pulse and respiratory rate
0.11–0.15	1.5–3 hr	50–60	Increased pulse and respiratory rate, syncope, Cheyne-Stokes respiration, coma with intermittent convulsions
0.16–0.30	1–1.5 hr	60–70	Coma with intermittent convulsions, depressed heart action and respirations, death possible
0.50–1.00	1–2 min	70–80	Weak pulse, depressed respirations, respiratory failure and death

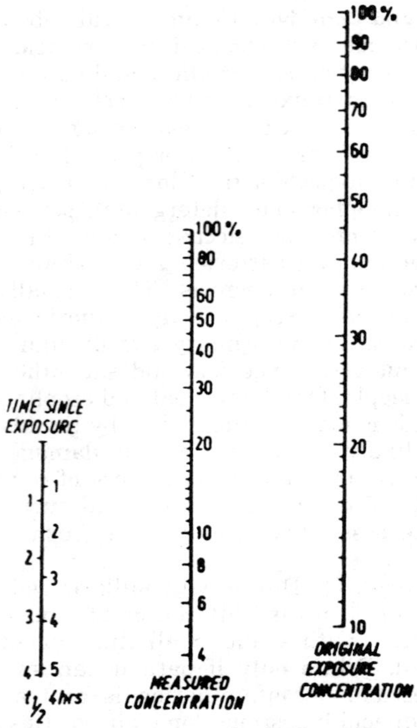

Figure 2. Nomogram for calculating carboxyhemoglobin concentration at time of exposure. The time since exposure is given on two scales to allow for the effects of previous oxygen administration on the half-life of carboxyhemoglobin (left-hand scale assumes a half-life of 3 hours). *Note:* The nomogram assumes a half-life of carboxyhemoglobin of 4 hours in a subject breathing room air. Most patients will not have received supplementary oxygen before admission, and at best this will have been administered via a face mask, giving a maximum fractional inspired oxygen concentration of 50 to 60 per cent with little effect on carboxyhemoglobin elimination. The scale on the left side of the time column makes allowances for prior oxygen supplements by assuming a short half-life of 3 hours. The nomogram may help decide quickly whether serious carbon monoxide intoxication is likely to have occurred and may help select patients at high risk for early management in the intensive care unit. The nomogram may be an oversimplification because patients usually are not resuscitated with constant concentrations of oxygen, and many patients may hyperventilate, thus changing elimination characteristics. (From Clerk et al: Blood carboxyhemoglobin and cyanide levels in fire. Lancet, *1*:1332, 1981.)

ment requires immediate removal from the environment, and clinical, x-ray, and arterial blood gas evaluation when appropriate. Oxygen and respiratory support may be required.

Chloral Hydrate. See Sedative Hypnotics.

Chlordane. See Organochlorine Insecticides.

Chlordiazepoxide (Librium). See Benzodiazepines.

Chlorine Gas. Chlorine gas is a yellow-greenish gas with an irritating odor used in bleach, manufacture of plastics, and for water purification. Exposure usually results from transportation mishaps, industrial accidents, chemistry experiments, the mixing of household cleaners with bleach containing hypochlorite, and accidental release around swimming pools. Its density is greater than that of air, and an odor is detected at concentrations of less than 0.5 ppm. Chlorine acts as an oxidizing agent and also acts with tissue water to form hypochlorite and hydrochloric acid and generate free oxygen radicals. *Toxic dose and management:* The threshold limit value is less than 1 ppm; 4 ppm is tolerated for 0.5 hour; 15 ppm immediately irritates mucous membranes of eyes, ears, nose, and throat; 30 ppm produces choking and chest pain; 60 ppm produces pulmonary edema; 400 ppm for 30 minutes is lethal; and 1000 ppm is fatal in a few minutes.

Management: (1) Remove from contaminated environment and stabilize vital functions. Decontamination procedures for dermal and ocular contamination as indicated. Protect rescue personnel with breathing apparatus. Classification—If symptomless or with a cough that clears up in less than 1 hour, rest for 12 hours and report if symptoms occur; no vigorous exercise for 24 hours. If symptoms persist beyond period of exposure, admit to hospital and treat with bronchodilators (use theophylline, not epinephrine) and humidified oxygen. Noncardiac pulmonary edema is treated with positive end expiratory pressure; corticosteroids are controversial; furosemide (Lasix) may be used. For conjunctival irritation, copious water irrigation and fluorescein stain for corneal damage. For dermal burns, copious water irrigation and treat burns conventionally. *Laboratory aids:* Chest radiograph (may not reflect damage for 24 hours), arterial blood gases, cardiac monitor for dysrhythmias.

Chlorpromazine (Thorazine). See Phenothiazines.

Clinitest Tablets. See Caustics and Corrosives.

Cocaine (Benzoylmethylecgonine). *Toxic dose*: The potential fatal dose is 1200 mg, but death has occurred with 20 mg parenterally. *Toxicokinetics*: Peak effect (intranasal), 30 to 60 minutes; intravenous, 2 minutes. Duration, $<$ 3 hours. Route of elimination: 80 per cent liver; 20 per cent kidney. *Manifestations*: Hypertension, convulsions, hyperthermia, and cardiac dysrhythmias. *Management*: (1) Supportive care. Cardiac and thermal monitoring. Lidocaine may be ineffective for cardiac dysrhythmias. Control anxiety and convulsions with diazepam. Propranolol intravenously (Antidote 29, Table 4) can be used to control life-threatening hypertension and tachycardia (controversial). A nonthreatening environment to reduce all sensory stimuli and protect patient from injury is required.

Codeine. See Opioids.

Corrosives. See Caustics and Corrosives.

Cyanide. See Table 14, next page. Hydrocyanic acid and sodium and potassium salts act rapidly and are extremely poisonous. The acid is extremely volatile, producing cyanide, which has a distinctive odor of bitter almonds and can produce death within minutes after inhalation. Cyanide interferes with the cytochrome oxidase system. *Classes of cyanides and derivatives*: (1) Hydrogen cyanide and simple salts in large doses act to produce death in 15 minutes. (2) Halogenated cyanides such as cyanogen chloride—irritant and vesicant gases that may produce pulmonary edema. (3) Nitriles such as acrylonitrile and acetonitrile. Cyanides are used as fumigants (hydrogen cyanide), in synthetic rubber (acrylonitrile), in fertilizers (cyanamide), in metal refining (salts), and in the home in some silver and furniture polishes. Cyanide in the seeds of fruit stones is harmful only if the capsule is

TABLE 14. **Forms of Cyanide and Their Toxicity**

Common Forms	Toxicity
Hydrocyanic acid	PFD* = 50 mg (0.5 mg/kg)
Potassium/sodium cyanide	PFD = 150–300 mg (2 mg/kg)
Calcium and ferric or ferrocyanides	Low order of toxicity; PFD = 50 grams
Sodium nitroprusside	5 mg/kg causes acute toxicity; PFD = 3–4 grams (195–260 mg)
Bitter almonds	
oil	2 oz kills immediately
almonds	50–60 bitter almonds; each contain 0.001 gram of hydrogen cyanide
pulp	240 grams
Peach seed	100 grams of moist seeds = 88 mg of cyanide
Apricot	
wild	100 grams of moist seed = 217 mg of cyanide
cultivated	100 grams = 8.7 mg of cyanide
Laetrile (amygdalin); cyanogenic glycoside in kernels of apricots	
Hydrogen cyanide inhalation; acrylonitrile, cyanamide, cyanogen chloride, cyanides, nitroprussides (produced in fire involving polyurethane foams)	Maximum allowable concentration, 10 ppm TLV* = 5 mg/m^3 in air for cyanide salts 0.2–0.3 mg/liter is immediately fatal 0.13 mg/liter (130 ppm) is fatal in 1 hour
Hydrogen cyanide liquid	Rapidly absorbed through skin

*PFD, Potential fatal dose; TLV, Threshold limit values

broken. *Manifestations*: Seizures, stupor, cardiac dysrhythmias, pulmonary edema, lactic acidemia, decreased arterial venous oxygen difference. Bright red venous blood.

Management: (1) Immediately, 100 per cent oxygen. If inhaled, remove patient from contaminated atmosphere. (2) Cyanide antidote kit, Poisoning Antidote 13, Table 4. Use antidote only if certain of diagnosis and significant toxicity (impairment of consciousness). (3) Gastrointestinal decontamination by gastric lavage. *No* syrup of ipecac. Activated charcoal not very effective (1 gram binds only 35 mg of cyanide). (4) Treat seizures with intravenous diazepam. (5) Correct acidosis. (6) Other antidotes: In Europe, dicobalt edetate, 600 mg, is used intravenously, followed by 300 mg if the response is not satisfactory. Hydroxycobalamin (vitamin B_{12}) may be a useful antidote but must be given before or slightly after exposure in very large doses. Dose: 1800 mg of B_{12} per dl of KCN is usually required (forms cyanocobalamin).

DDT and Derivatives. See Organochlorine Insecticides.

Desipramine (Norpramin, Pertofrane). See Tricyclic Antidepressants.

Diazepam (Valium). See Benzodiazepines.

Digitalis Preparations. See Table 15, this page. *Manifestations*: Abdominal pain, nausea, vomiting, diarrhea, dysrhythmias, heart block, central nervous system depression, colored-halo vision. *Management*: (1) Gastrointestinal decontamination up to 12 hours. Repeated doses of activated charcoal may interrupt enterohepatic recirculation. (2) Treat with phenytoin ventricular premature contractions, including bigeminy, trigeminy, quadrigeminy, ventricular tachycardia, and atrial tachycardia with block. Lidocaine also may be administered for ventricular dysrhythmias. (3) Treat bradycardia and second and third degree AV block with atropine. External pacing may be needed. (4) Treat hyperkalemia (above 6 mEq/liter with intravenous glucose 5 to 10 per cent, intravenous sodium bicarbonate, intravenous insulin (insulin is not used in children), and Kayexalate retention enema (25 per cent in sorbitol 25 per cent) in severe cases. If hyperkalemia is present (ominous sign), insertion of a pacemaker should be considered seriously. Hemodialysis is treatment of choice for severe or refractory hyperkalemia. (5) Direct current countershock should be a last resort in life-threatening dysrhythmias. (6) Specific Fab antibody fragments (Antidote 20, Table 4) have been used for life-threatening cardiac dysrhythmias, hyperkalemia, and cases refractory to conventional measures. *Laboratory aids*: Monitor electrocardiogram and potassium and digitalis levels. Draw digoxin levels 6 to 8 hours postingestion.

Diphenhydramine (Benadryl). See Anticholinergic Agents.

Doxepin (Sinequan, Adapin). See Tricyclic Antidepressants.

Ethchlorvynol (Placidyl). See Sedative Hypnotics.

Ethyl Alcohol. See Alcohols.

Ethylene Glycol (solvent, antifreeze). *Toxic dose*: Death has occurred after a 60 ml ingestion; fatal dose = 1.4 ml per kg of 100 per cent solution. The threshold limit value (TLV) is 50 ppm. *Toxicokinetics*: Time of onset, 30 minutes to 12 hours for central nervous system and metabolic abnormalities to occur (Phase I). Twelve to 36 hours postingestion, cardiopulmonary depression (Phase II). In Phase III (2 to 3 days postingestion), renal failure occurs. The $t_{1/2}$ is 3 hours (during ethanol therapy this is prolonged to 17 hours). *Management*: (1) Gastrointestinal decontamination up to 2 to 4 hours postingestion. Activated charcoal and cathartics are not indicated. (2) Treat seizures with

TABLE 15. **Digitalis Preparations**

	Digoxin	Digitoxin
Trade name	Lanoxin	Crystodigin
Onset time PO	1.5–6 hr	3–6 hr
Peak	4–6	6–12
Half-life	31–40 hr	4–6 days
Protein-bound (%)	25	90
Vd	7–8 liters/kg	0.6 liter/kg
Route of elimination	Renal, 75 per cent	Liver, 80 per cent
Toxic blood levels	2.4 ng/ml	> 30 ng/ml
Enterohepatic route	Small	Large

intravenous diazepam followed by phenytoin if unresponsive. (3) Correct acidosis with intravenous sodium bicarbonate. (4) Initiate ethanol therapy to block metabolism. (Antidote 19, Table 4). (5) Early hemodialysis is indicated if the ingestion was large; if the blood ethylene glycol level is greater than 100 mg per dl; if severe acid-base or electrolyte abnormalities occur despite conventional therapy; or if renal failure occurs. (6) Thiamine and pyridoxine have been recommended but not extensively studied. *Laboratory aids*: Complete blood count, electrolytes, urinalysis (look for oxalate crystals), and arterial blood gases. Obtain ethylene glycol and ethanol levels, plasma osmolarity (use freezing point depression method). Calcium, creatinine, and BUN studies. An ethylene glycol level of 100 mg per dl is usually toxic (levels are very difficult to obtain).

Flurazepam (Dalmane). See Benzodiazepines.

Glutethimide (Doriden). See Sedative Hypnotics.

Hallucinogens

1. **LSD** (lysergic acid diethylamide). *Toxic dose*: ≥ 35 μg. Street doses are typically 50 to 300 μg. *Toxicokinetics*: Peak effect, 1 to 2 hours. Duration, 12 to 24 hours. $t\frac{1}{2}$, 3 hours. Route of elimination, bile.

2. **Morning-Glory Seeds** *(Rivea corymbosa* or *Ipomoea)*. These have one tenth the potency of LSD.

3. **Mescaline/Peyote** (trimethoxyphenylethylamine or *Lophophora williamsii*). *Toxic dose*: ≥ 5 mg per kg. Each button of mescaline contains 45 mg (4 to 12 produce symptoms). *Toxicokinetics*: Peak effect, 4 to 6 hours. Duration, 14 hours.

4. **Psilocybin**: Similar in effect to LSD but short-acting. Peak effect, 90 minutes. Duration, 5 to 6 hours.

5. **Nutmeg** *(Myristica)*. *Toxic dose*: 5 to 15 grams (1 to 3 nutmegs). Peak effect, 3 to 6 hours. Duration, up to 60 hours.

6. **Marijuana** *(Cannabis sativa)* (δ-9-tetrahydrocannabinol, THC). One joint equals 500 mg of marijuana; when smoked, 50 per cent is destroyed. *Toxicokinetics*: Time of onset, 2 to 3 minutes (smoked). Duration, 2 to 3 hours. $t\frac{1}{2}$, 28 to 47 hours (shorter for chronic user). *Note*: 1 per cent of the metabolite can be detected in urine up to 2 weeks after use. *Manifestations*: Visual illusions, sensory perceptual distortions, depersonalization, and derealization. *Management*: "Talk-down" technique.

7. **Inhalants**: Nitrites (amyl and isobutyl nitrite)—act immediately; aromatic hydrocarbon in airplane model glues, plastic cements (benzene, toluene, xylene)—see hydrocarbons; *nitrous oxide* and *halogenated hydrocarbons*.

8. **Tryptamine Derivatives** (DMT, dimethyltryptamine; DET, diethyltryptamine; DPT, dipropyltryptamine). Rapid onset of action, but duration is only 1 to 2 hours.

9. **STP** or **DOM** (2,5-dimethoxy-4-methyl-amphetamine) acts like LSD but lasts 72 hours or longer.

10. **MDA** (3-methoxy-4,5-ethylenedioxy amphetamine), related to amphetamine, produces a mild LSD-like reaction lasting 6 to 10 hours (love pill).

See also Alcohols, Amphetamines, Anticholinergic Agents, Barbiturates, Cocaine, Opioids, Phencyclidine, Phenothiazines, and Tricyclic Antidepressants.

Haloperidol (Haldol). See Phenothiazines.

Heroin. See Opioids.

Hydrocarbons

1. **Petroleum Distillates**: gasoline (petroleum spirit), 2 to 5 per cent benzene; kerosene (coal oil, kerosene, jet aviation fuel No. 1, charcoal lighter fluid); petroleum naphtha (cigarette lighter fluid, ligroin, racing fuel); petroleum ether (benzine); turpentine (pine oil, oil of turpentine); and mineral spirits (Stoddard solvent, white spirits, varasol, mineral turpentine, petroleum spirit). *Manifestations*: Materials aspirated during the process of ingestion may produce pneumonitis. Hypoxia associated with aspiration is the cause of central nervous system depression, not absorption. It is *unlikely* that a child accidentally or an adult during siphoning would ingest sufficient quantity to warrant the induction of emesis.

2. **Aromatic Hydrocarbons.** *Benzene*, a solvent used in manufacturing dyes, phenol, and nitrobenzene, has a threshold limit value (TLV) of 10 ppm by inhalation according to the Occupational Safety and Health Administration (OSHA). The National Institute for Occupational Safety and Health (NIOSH) value is 1 PPM. The adult ingested toxic dose is 15 ml. Chronic exposure may cause leukemia. Two hundred ppm is fatal in 5 minutes. *Toluene,* used in manufacturing TNT, has an OSHA TLV of 200 ppm by inhalation; the NIOSH figure is 100. The adult ingested toxic dose is 50 ml. *Styrene* has an OSHA TLV of 100 ppm by inhalation. *Xylene,* used in the manufacture of perfumes, has an OSHA TLV of 100 ppm by inhalation. The adult ingested toxic dose is 50 ml. *Manifestations*: Asphyxiation, central nervous system depression, defatting dermatitis, and aspiration pneumonitis. A bite into a tube of household plastic cement by a young child does not warrant the induction of emesis. Ingestion of hydrocarbon with a benzene fraction over 5 per cent may warrant induction of emesis.

3. **Aliphatic Halogenated Hydrocarbons.** See Table 16, next page, for common examples. *Manifestations*: Myocardial sensitization and irritability, hepatorenal toxicity, and central nervous system depression. Dichloromethane may be converted into carbon monoxide in the body. Trichloroethylene concentrates in the fetus (pregnant women should not be exposed) and causes a disulfiram (Antabuse) reaction ("degreasers flush") when associated with ingestion of ethanol. The decision to induce emesis must be based on the toxicity of the agent.

4. **Dangerous Additives.** Dangerous additives to the hydrocarbons, such as heavy metals, nitrobenzene, aniline dyes, insecticides and demothing agents, may warrant the induction of emesis.

5. **Heavy Hydrocarbons.** These have high viscosity, low volatility, and minimal absorption, so emesis is unwarranted. Examples are asphalt (tar), machine oil, motor oil (lubricating oil, engine oil), diesel oil (engine fuel, home heating oil), petrolatum liquid (mineral oil, suntan oils), petrolatum jelly (Vaseline), paraffin wax, transmission oil, cutting oil, and greases and glues.

6. **Products Treated as Petroleum Distillates.** Essential oils (e.g., turpentine, pine oil) are treated as petroleum distillates. Mineral seal oil (signal oil), found in some furniture polishes, is a heavy, viscous oil that *never* warrants emesis; it can produce severe pneumonia if aspirated. It has minimal absorption.

TABLE 16. **Common Examples of Aliphatic Halogenated Hydrocarbons**

	Estimated Fatal Dose (Ingested)	TLV-TWA (PPM)	Synonyms
Trichloroethane 1, 1, 1	5.7 grams/kg	350	Methyl chloroform, Triethane, chlorethane, Glamorene spot remover, Scotchgard
Trichloroethane 1, 1, 2	580 mg/kg	10	Vinyl trichloride
Trichloroethylene	Controversial, 3–5 ml/kg	50	—
Tetrachloroethanene	Not known	5	Acetylene tetrachloride
Dichloromethane	25 ml	100	Methylene chloride
Tetrachloroethylene	5 ml	50	Tetrachloroethene Perchloroethylene
Dichloroethane	0.5 ml/kg	200	—
Carbon tetrachloride	3–5 ml	5	—

Management: Dermal decontamination. Removal from the enviroment in inhalation.

First Aid Treatment. See Table 17, this page. *The use of activated charcoal, oils, and cathartics is not advised in petroleum distillate ingestions. General management*: (1) In the asymptomatic patient: observe several hours for development of respiratory distress. (2) In the symptomatic patient: supportive respiratory care for respiratory distress. Bronchospasm may be treated with intravenous aminophylline. Avoid epinephrine. Monitor ECG; arterial blood gases; liver, pulmonary, and renal function; serum electrolytes; serial radiographs. Observe for intravascular hemolysis and disseminated intravascular coagulation. If cyanosis is present that does not respond to oxygen or the arterial PaO_2 is normal, suspect methemoglobinemia that may require therapy with methylene blue. Steroids have not been shown to be beneficial. Antimicrobials are not useful in prophylaxis. (Fever or leukocytosis may be produced by the chemical pneumonitis itself.) It is not necessary to treat pneumatoceles. Most infiltrations resolve spontaneously in 1 week except for lipoid pneumonia, which may last up to 6 weeks.

Imipramine (Tofranil). See Tricyclic Antidepressants.

Iron. The iron content of some preparations appears in Table 18, next page. *Toxic dose*: Range, 20 to 60 mg per kg or greater of elemental iron. Dose to induce emesis, ⩾ 20 mg per kg. The potential fatal dose is 180 mg per kg (600 mg of elemental iron). *Toxicokinetics*: Absorption occurs chiefly in the small intestine. For excretion there is no normal route except blood loss or gastrointestinal desquamation. *Manifestations*: Phase I—Mucosal injury possibly with hematemesis (1 to 6 hours postingestion). Phase II—patient appears improved (6 to 48 hours). Phase III—cardiovascular collapse and severe metabolic acidosis. Phase IV—sequelae of intestinal stricture and obstruction or anemia (weeks to months). Patients asymptomatic for 6 hours rarely develop serious intoxication manifestations.

Management: (1) Gastrointestinal decontamination. Emesis should be induced in ingestions of elemental iron of over 20 mg per kg. Emesis should be followed by gastric lavage if large amounts have been ingested (over 60 mg per kg). The solution to be used for lavage is 1 to 1.5 per cent sodium bicarbonate to form ferrous carbonate salts which are poorly absorbed. One hundred milliliters of this solution should be left in

TABLE 17. **First Aid Treatment for Hydrocarbon Ingestion**

Symptoms	Contents	Amount	First Aid
None	Petroleum distillate only	Less than 2 ml/kg	None
None	Heavy hydrocarbon	More than 2 ml/kg	None*
	Mineral seal oil		None
	Petroleum distillate	Minimum, 30 ml	Consider emesis induction†
None	Petroleum distillate with dangerous additive	Depends on toxicity of additive	Consider emesis induction†
	Aromatic and halogenated hydrocarbons	Depends on toxicity of hydrocarbon	Consider emesis induction†
Loss of protective airway reflex; convulsions	Petroleum distillate with dangerous additive	Depends on toxicity of additive	Consider endotracheal intubation prior to gastric aspiration and lavage
Breathing difficulty	Aromatic and halogenated hydrocarbons	Depends on toxicity of individual hydrocarbon	Consider endotracheal intubation prior to gastric aspiration and lavage

*Emesis may be necessary if machine oil contains triorthocresyl phosphate (TOCP) which causes weakness, sensory impairment and "partially reversible damage to the spinal cord."

†Emesis induction is rarely indicated if the patient has already vomited. Emesis usually should be induced with proper positioning.

TABLE 18. **Iron Content of Some Preparations**

Salt	Elemental Iron Content (%)	Average Tablet Strength (mg)	Iron Content Per Tablet (mg)
Ferrous sulfate	20	300	60
Ferrous sulfate (dried)	29.7	200	65
Ferrous gluconate	11.6	320	36
Ferrous fumarate	33	200	67

the stomach (prepared by dilution of a sodium bicarbonate ampule with saline). The use of deferoxamine (Desferal) in the gastrointestinal tract is controversial. The use of diluted Fleet's enema solution risks severe hypertonic phosphate poisoning. (2) Postlavage abdominal radiograph—if significant amounts of residual radiopaque material are present, consider removal by endoscopy or surgery since coalesced tablets have produced hemorrhagic infarction and perforation peritonitis. (3) Protect the mucosal surfaces with demulcents if damage is evident. (4) Diagnostic chelation test—deferoxamine (Antidote 14, Table 4). (5) Indications for chelation therapy with deferoxamine are serum iron greater than total iron binding capacity, or positive diagnostic chelation test; serum iron over 500 mg per dl; and systemic signs of intoxication independent of serum iron level. Chelation should be performed within 12 to 18 hours to be effective.

Laboratory aids: Serum iron levels correlate with the clinical course. Iron levels drawn at 2 to 6 hours that are below 350 mg per dl predict an asymptomatic course; levels of 350 to 500 are associated with mild gastrointestinal symptoms (rarely serious); and levels greater than 500 suggest the possibility of serious Phase III manifestations. White blood cell counts greater than 15,000, blood glucose levels over 150 mg per dl, radiopaque material present on abdominal radiograph, vomiting, and diarrhea predict iron levels greater than 300 mg per dl. Monitor complete blood counts, blood glucose, serum iron, stools, and vomitus for occult blood; electrolytes; acid-base balance; urinalysis and urinary output; liver function tests; BUN; and creatinine. Obtain type and match of blood in severe cases. Abdominal radiographs. Follow-up is necessary for sequelae in significant intoxications—GI series for intestinal strictures and anemia secondary to blood loss.

Isoniazid (INH, Nydrazid). This is an antituberculosis drug frequently used in suicides by American Indians and Eskimos. *Mechanism of toxicity:* It produces pyridoxine deficiency (doubles excretion of pyridoxine). *Toxic dose:* 1.5 grams, 35 to 40 mg per kg, produces convulsions; severe toxicity is seen at 6 to 10 grams; 200 mg per kg is an obligatory convulsant. *Toxicokinetics:* Absorption is rapid, with a peak in 1 to 2 hours (clinical symptoms may start in 30 minutes). Volume distribution is 0.6 liter per kg. It passes the placenta and into breast milk at 50 per cent of the maternal serum level. Not protein-bound. Elimination is by the liver, which produces a hepatotoxic metabolite, acetylisoniazid. The t½—Slow acetylators (2 to 4 hours) may develop peripheral neuropathy (50 per cent of blacks and caucasians). Fast acetylators (0.7 to 2 hours) may develop hepatitis (90 per cent of orientals and a majority of patients with diabetes). Excreted unchanged, 10 to 40 per cent. *Major toxic manifestations:* Visual disturbances, convulsions (90 per cent or more with one or more seizures), coma, resistant severe acidosis (due to lactate secondary to hypoxia, convulsions, and metabolic blocks).

Management: (1) Control seizures with large doses of pyridoxine, 1 gram for each gram of isoniazid ingested (Antidote 30, Table 4). If the dose ingested is unknown, give at least 5 grams of pyridoxine intravenously. (2) Correct acidosis with fluids and sodium bicarbonate (pyridoxine may spontaneously correct the acidosis). (3) Diazepam may be used as a supplement to control the seizures if pyridoxine is ineffective (20 per cent of cases). (4) After patient is stabilized or if asymptomatic, gastrointestinal decontamination procedures may be carried out, keeping in mind the rapid onset of convulsions. Asymptomatic patients should be observed for 4 hours. (5) Hemodialysis is rarely needed but may be used as an adjunct for uncontrollable acidosis and seizures. Hemoperfusion has not been adequately evaluated. Diuresis is ineffective. *Laboratory aids:* Isoniazid toxic levels are above 8 μg per ml. Monitor the blood glucose (often hyperglycemia), electrolytes (often hyperkalemia), bicarbonate, and arterial blood gases. Monitor the temperature closely (often hyperpyrexia).

Isopropyl Alcohol. See Alcohols.

Kerosene. See Hydrocarbons.

Lead. Acute lead poisoning is rare. *Acute toxic dose:* 0.5 gram. *Management:* (1) Gastrointestinal decontamination. (2) Supportive care, including measures to deal with the hepatic and renal failure and intravascular hemolysis. (3) EDTA in all severe cases if lead levels confirm absorption. **Chronic** lead poisoning occurs most often in children 1 to 6 years of age who are exposed in their environment and in adults in certain occupations or from illicit whiskey. *Chronic toxic dose:* Determined by blood lead level and clinical findings. Over 30 μg per dl indicates excess body burden. A chronic dose of 0.6 mg a day will increase the body burden, 2.5 mg a day will result in toxicity in 4 years, and 3.5 mg a day will cause toxicity in a few months. *Toxicokinetics:* Absorption—10 to 15 per cent of the ingested dose is absorbed in adults; in children up to 40 per cent is absorbed with iron deficiency anemia. Inhalation absorption is rapid and complete. Vd—95 per cent present in bone. In blood, 95 per cent is in red blood cells. t½, 35 days; in bone, 10 years. The major elimination route for inorganic lead is renal. Organic lead is metabolized in the liver to inorganic lead; 9 per cent is excreted in the urine per day. *Manifestations of acute symptoms of chronic lead poisoning* (ABCDE): Anorexia, apathy, anemia; behavior disturbances; clumsiness; developmental deterioration; and emesis. Manifestations of encephalopathy are "PAINT:" *P*, persistent forceful vomiting, *A*, ataxia, *I*, intermittent stupor and lucidity, *N*, neurologic coma and convulsions, *T*, tired and lethargic. In adults one may see peripheral neuropathies and "lead gum lines."

Management: (1) Gastrointestinal decontamination

TABLE 19. **Choice of Chelation Therapy Based on Symptoms and Blood Lead Concentration**

Clinical Presentation	*Treatment*	*Comments*
Symptomatic children		
Acute encephalopathy	BAL, 450 mg/M²/day $CaNa_2$-EDTA, 1500 mg/M²/day (EDTA not used alone if blood Pb >72 μg/dl or symptoms)	Start with BAL, 75 mg/M² IM every 4 hours After 4 hours start continuous infusion of $CaNa_2$-EDTA, 1500 mg/M²/day Therapy with BAL and $CaNa_2$-EDTA should be continued for 5 days Interrupt therapy for 2 days Treat for 5 additional days, including BAL if blood Pb remains high Other cycles may be needed depending on blood Pb rebound.
Other symptoms	BAL, 300 mg/M²/day $CaNa_2$-EDTA, 1000 mg/M²/day Monitor BUN, creatinine, AST, ALT, urine	Start with BAL, 90 mg/M² IM every 4 hours After 4 hours start $CaNa_2$-EDTA, 1000 mg/M²/day, preferably by continuous infusion, or in divided doses IV (through a heparin lock) Therapy with $CaNa_2$-EDTA should be continued for 5 days BAL may be discontinued after 3 days if blood Pb <50 μg/dl Interrupt therapy for 2 days Treat for 5 additional days, including BAL if blood Pb remains high (>50 μg/dl) Other cycles may be needed depending on blood Pb rebound
Asymptomatic children		
Before treatment, measure venous blood lead		
Blood Pb >70 μg/dl	BAL, 300 mg/M²/day $CaNa_2$-EDTA 1000 mg/M²/day	Start with BAL, 50 mg/M² IM every 4 hours After 4 hours start $CaNa_2$-EDTA, 1000 mg/M²/day, preferably by continuous infusion, or in divided doses IV (through a heparin lock) Treatment with $CaNa_2$-EDTA should be continued for 5 days BAL may be discontinued after 3 days if blood Pb <50 μg/dl Other cycles may be needed depending on blood Pb rebound
Blood Pb 56 to 69 μg/dl	$CaNa_2$-EDTA, 1000 mg/M²/day	$CaNa_2$-EDTA for 5 days, preferably by continuous infusion, or in divided doses (through a heparin lock) Alternatively, if lead exposure is controlled, $CaNa_2$-EDTA may be given as a single daily outpatient dose IM or IV Other cycles may be needed depending on blood Pb rebound
Blood Pb 25 to 55 μg/dl		
Perform $CaNa_2$-EDTA provocation test to assess lead excretion ratio		
If ratio >0.70	$CaNa_2$-EDTA, 1000 mg/M²/day	Treat for 5 days IV or IM, as above
If ratio 0.60 to 0.69		
Age <3 years	$CaNa_2$-EDTA, 1000 mg/M²/day	Treat for 3 days IV or IM, as above
Age >3 years	No treatment	Repeat blood Pb and $CaNa_2$-EDTA provocation test periodically
If ratio <0.60	No treatment	Repeat blood Pb and $CaNa_2$-EDTA provocation test periodically

(From Piomelli S: Am J Pediatr *105*:527, 1984, with permission.)

with enemas if radiopaque foreign bodies are noted. Do not delay therapy until clear. (2) Remove from exposure. For children, see Table 19. *Laboratory aids:* (1) Provocation mobilization test—50 mg per kg of EDTA intramuscularly for 1 dose and collect the urine for 6 to 8 hours. A ratio of micrograms excreted in the urine to milligrams of Ca-EDTA administered greater than 0.6 represents an increased lead body burden and chelation should be administered. (2) CBC, serum iron, or ferritin; repeat blood lead levels and EP. (3) Flat plate of the abdomen and long bone radiographs (knees usually). (4) Renal function tests. (5) Electrolytes, serum calcium, phosphorus, blood glucose.

Lindane. See Organochlorine Insecticides.

Lithium (Eskalith, Lithane). Most cases of intoxication have occurred as therapeutic overdoses. The toxic dose is determined by serum levels although intoxication has occurred with levels in the therapeutic range.

Toxicokinetics: Absorption is rapid, with complete peaking in 1 to 4 hours. Vd is 0.5 to 0.9 liter per kg. It is not protein bound. The t½ therapeutically is 18 to 24 hours. Eighty-nine to 98 per cent is excreted by the kidney unchanged, one third to two thirds in 6 to 12 hours. Excretion is decreased in the presence of hyponatremia and dehydration. The cerebrospinal fluid concentration is one half the plasma concentration. The breast milk level is 50 per cent of the maternal serum level—toxic to the nursling. *Manifestations:* The first sign of toxicity may be diarrhea. Fine tremor of hands, lethargy, weakness, polyuria and polydipsia, goiter and hypothyroidism, and fasciculations are side effects. Severe toxicity is manifest by ataxia, impaired mental state, coma, seizures (limbs held in hyperextension with eyes open in "coma vigil"). Cardiovascular manifestations are dysrhythmias, hypotension, flat T waves, and increased QT interval.

Management: (1) Gastrointestinal decontamination may not be useful after 2 hours because of rapid absorption. In slow release preparations, decontamination may be useful up to 24 hours postingestion. Activated charcoal is not indicated. (2) Hospitalize if intoxication is suspected because seizures may occur unexpectedly. (3) Restore normothermia and fluid and electrolyte balance, particularly sodium. If diabetes insipidus is present, an infusion of sodium may give hypernatremia. Current evidence supports saline infusion as enhancing excretion of lithium. (4) Forced diuresis has no role, unless the glomerular filtration rate is low. Consider only when the lithium level is not above 2.5 mEq per liter and fails to fall below 1 mEq per liter within 30 hours. (5) Hemodialysis is the treatment of choice for severe intoxication. Lithium is the most dialyzable toxin known. Long runs of 12 hours or longer should be used until the lithium level is less than 1 mEq per liter because of extensive reequilibration rebound. Follow levels every 4 hours after dialysis. Dialysis may have to be repeated. Expect a time lag in neurologic recovery. If hemodialysis is not available or delayed, peritoneal dialysis can be used but is less effective. (6) Monitor ECG. Refractory dysrhythmias may be treated with magnesium sulfate and sodium bicarbonate. (7) Aminophylline may increase lithium excretion and decrease lithium reabsorption but has not been extensively studied. (8) Avoid thiazides and spironolactone diuretics, which increase lithium levels.

Laboratory aids: Lithium level determinations should be performed every 4 hours. Although they do not always correlate with the manifestations at low levels, they are predictive in severe intoxications. Levels of 0.6 to 1.2 mEq per liter are usually therapeutic. Levels over 4.0 mEq per liter are severely toxic. Other tests to be monitored are CBC (lithium causes leukocytosis), renal function, thyroid, ECG, and electrolytes. Factors that predispose to lithium toxicity are febrile illness, sodium depletion, concomitant drugs (thiazide and spironolactone diuretics), impaired renal function, advanced age, and fluid loss in vomiting and diarrheal illness.

Lomotil (Diphenoxylate and Atropine). See Opioids and Anticholinergic Agents.

LSD (Lysergic Acid Diethylamide). See Hallucinogens.

Marijuana. See Hallucinogens.

Meperidine (Demerol). See Opioids.

Meprobamate (Equanil, Miltown). See Sedative Hypnotics.

Mercury. Management: (1) Inhalation of elemental mercury—remove from exposure. (2) Ingestion of mercuric salt—gastrointestinal decontamination. A protein solution such as egg white or 5 per cent salt-poor albumin can be given to reduce to mercurous ion (less toxic). Give activated charcoal and cathartic. (3) Chelating agents (do not use Ca-EDTA because of nephrotoxicity): Dimercaprol (BAL) enhances mercury excretion through the bile as well as the urine and would be the choice if there were renal impairment from the mercury (Antidote 16, Table 4). Penicillamine (Antidote 26, Table 4) or *N*-acetyl DL-penicillamine (investigational use). BAL in methyl mercury intoxication increases the brain mercury and appears to be contraindicated; penicillamine and its analogue should be used (decreases mercury in brain). A new chelator, 2,3-dimercaptosuccinic acid, holds promise of less toxicity and more specific therapy but is not yet available. (4) Monitor fluid and electrolytes, renal function, hemoglobin levels. Obtain blood and urine mercury levels (consult the laboratory for proper collection technique and containers). (5) Hemodialysis early in the symptomatic patient is useful. (6) New but not established approaches are Polythiol resin to bind the methyl mercury excreted in the bile; heat and sauna treatment to increase mercury excretion through perspiration; and a regional dialyzer system using L-cysteine. (7) Surgical excision of *local injection sites. Laboratory aids:* (1) Blood levels are below 2 to 4 μg per dl and urine levels below 10 to 20 μg per liter in 90 per cent of adult population. Levels above 4 μg per dl in blood and 20 μg per liter in urine probably should be considered abnormal. Blood levels are not always reliable. Exposed industrial workers' urine levels are 150 to 200 μg. (2) In asymptomatic patients with urine levels under 300 μg per liter, a chelating challenge with BAL or penicillamine may bring a significant increase that may aid in establishing the diagnosis. (3) Approximately 150 μg per liter in urine is equivalent to 3.5 μg per dl in blood. (4) Methyl mercury is excreted mainly through the feces, so urine mercury would not be a reliable measurement. (5) Mercury is also excreted in the sweat and saliva. The parotid fluid level is approximately two thirds that of the blood. Since the hair is porous, it may absorb mercury from the atmosphere; however, hair concentrations of 400 to 500 μg are likely to be associated with neurologic symptoms.

Methadone. See Opioids.

Methanol. See Alcohols.

Methaqualone. See Sedative Hypnotics.

Methyprylon (Noludar). See Sedative Hypnotics.

Narcotic Analgesics. See Opioids.

Nitrites (NO_2) and Nitrates (NO_3). These are readily available in both inorganic and organic forms. Organic nitrates used for angina pectoris are listed in Table 20. Inorganic nitrates have more toxicologic importance in natural foods and contaminated well water. *Potential fatal doses:* Nitrite, 1 gram; nitrate, 10 grams; nitrobenzene, 2 ml; nitroglycerine, 0.2 gram; and aniline dye (pure), 5 to 30 grams. *Toxicokinetics:* Onset of action of nitroglycerin sublingually is 1 to 3 minutes, with a peak action of 3 to 15 minutes and a duration of 20 to 30 minutes. Other routes have a slower onset (2 to 5 minutes) and longer duration of action (1.5 to 6 hours). Nitrites are potent oxidizing agents converting ferrous to ferric iron, which cannot carry oxygen. Normally, humans have 0.7 per cent of methemoglobin which is converted by methemoglobin reductase into oxygen-carrying hemoglobin. Liver detoxification by dinitration is the route of elimination. *Toxic manifes-*

TABLE 20. **Organic Nitrates for Angina Pectoris**

Drug and Route	Trade Name	Onset (*Min*)	Duration (*Hr*)
Nitroglycerine			
oral	many	varies	4–6
sublingual	many	1–3	¼–½
2% ointment	Nitrobid Nitrol	varies	3–6
Isosorbide dinitrate	Isordil		
sublingual		1–3	1.3–3
oral		2–5	4–6
chewable		2–5	2–3
timed release		varies	—
Pentaerythritol tetranitrate, oral	Peritrate	2–5	3–5
Erythril tetranitrate, oral	Cardilate	2–5	4–6

tations depend on the level of methemoglobinemia. At 10 per cent, "chocolate cyanosis" occurs; at 10 to 20 per cent, headache, dizziness, and tachypnea occur; and at 50 per cent mental alterations are present and coma and convulsions may occur. Headache, flush, and sweating are due to the vasodilatory effect; hypotension, tachycardia, and syncope may also occur. Severe hypoxia may produce pulmonary edema and encephalopathy. Levels above 50 per cent produce metabolic acidosis and ECG changes; cardiovascular collapse occurs at levels of 70 per cent.

Management: (1) Dermal decontamination, if indicated. Aniline dyes may be removed with 5 per cent acetic acid (vinegar). (2) Gastrointestinal decontamination if ingested. (3) Hypotension can be treated by the Trendelenburg position and fluid challenge. Vasoconstrictors (dopamine or norepinephrine) are rarely needed. (4) Methylene blue (Antidote 22, Table 4) is indicated for methemoglobin levels above 40 per cent, dyspnea, metabolic acidosis (lactic acidosis), or an altered mental state. (5) Oxygen, 100 per cent, or a hyperbaric chamber should be used in symptomatic cases if methylene blue fails or is not effective, e.g., chlorate intoxication or G-6-PD deficiency. *Laboratory aids:* Methemoglobin levels, arterial blood gases. Blood has a chocolate-brown appearance and fails to turn red on exposure to oxygen.

Nortriptyline (Aventyl, Pamelor). See Tricyclic Antidepressants.

Opioids (Narcotic Opiates). See Table 21. The major metabolic pathway differs for each opioid but they are 90 per cent metabolized in the liver. Patients should be observed for central nervous system and respiratory depression and hypotension. Pulmonary edema is a potentially lethal complication of mainlining (intravenous use). *Manifestations:* All opiate agonists produce miotic pupils (except meperidine and Lomotil early), respiratory and central nervous system depression, physical dependence, and withdrawal. *Management:* (1) Supportive care particularly an endotracheal tube and assisted ventilation. (2) Gastrointestinal decontamination up to 12 hours postingestion as opiates delay gastric emptying time, but this is of no benefit if overdose is by injection. Convulsions occur rapidly with propoxyphene (Darvon) and codeine overdose, and this may be an indication not to use an emetic for gastrointestinal decontamination in this drug overdose. (3) Naloxone (Narcan) (Antidote 23, Table 4) may be given in bolus intravenous doses and by continuous drip, starting with 4 to 8 mg in 1 liter of fluid. Naloxone must be titrated against the clinical response and precipitation of withdrawal in narcotic addicts. It should be repeated as often as necessary since many opioids in overdose can last 24 hours to 48 hours whereas the action of naloxone lasts only 2 to 3 hours. *Larger doses are needed for codeine, pentazocine, and propoxyphene.* (4) Pulmonary edema does not respond to naloxone and needs respiratory supportive care. Fluids should be given cautiously in opioid overdose, because these agents stimulate antidiuretic hormone effect and pulmonary edema is frequent. (5) *If the patient is comatose, give 50 per cent glucose* (3 to 4 per cent of comatose narcotic overdose patients have hypoglycemia). (6) *If the patient is agitated,* consider hypoxia rather than withdrawal and treat as such. (7) *Observe for withdrawal* (nausea, vomiting, cramps, diarrhea, dilated pupils, rhinorrhea, piloerection). If these occur, stop naloxone.

OPIOID ADDICT WITHDRAWAL SCORE. Symptoms of withdrawal are diarrhea, dilated pupils, gooseflesh, hyperactive bowel sounds, hypertension, insomnia, lacrimation, muscle cramps, restlessness, tachycardia, and yawning. Each sign or symptom is given 0, 1, or 2 points, depending on the severity. A score of 1 to 5 is mild; 6 to 10, moderate; and 11 to 15, severe. Seizures are very unusual with withdrawal. They indicate severity regardless of the rest of the score. *Management:* Mild withdrawal is treated with diazepam orally, 10 mg every 6 hours; moderate withdrawal with intramuscular diazepam; and severe withdrawal with diazepam and diphenoxylate (Lomotil) for the diarrhea. Methadone orally may be used, 20 to 40 mg every 12 hours, decreased by 5 mg every 12 hours. When 10 mg is reached, add Lomotil. Clonidine (Catapres), 6 mg per kg every 6 hours, can be used with informed consent. (This is an unlisted use of clonidine; the maker states that relief from withdrawal symptoms has been reported with 0.8 mg/day.)

PROPOXYPHENE (DARVON). *Manifestations:* Onset may be as early as 30 minutes after ingestion. Convulsions occur early. Patients may develop diabetes insipidus, pulmonary edema, and hypoglycemia. *Elimination:* Metabolism is 90 per cent by demethylation in the liver. Peak plasma level of 1 to 2 hours after oral dose. Half-life is 1 to 5 hours. As little as 10 mg per kg has caused symptoms, and 35 mg per kg has caused cardiopulmonary arrest. Therapeutic blood level is less than 200 μg per ml. *Treatment* (in addition to the general management): (1) Emesis can be dangerous because of the rapid onset of seizures. (2) Indications for naloxone are respiratory depression, seizure activity, coma, and miotic pupils. Signs of naloxone effect are dilation of pupils, increased rate and depth of respirations, reversal of hypotension, and improvement of obtunded or comatose state. (3) Naloxone and intravenous glucose should be tried first to control seizures. If these fail, diazepam may be tried.

Organochlorine Insecticides (DDT Derivatives). See Table 22 for a listing of these agents. The *toxic dose* varies

TABLE 21. **Opioids (Narcotic Opiates)**

Drugs *Generic*	*Trade*	Equivalent IM Dose* *(Mg)*	Oral* *(Mg)*	Peak Action *(Hr)*	Half-Life *(Hr)*	Duration *(Hr)*	Potential Toxic Dose *(Mg)*
Alphaprodine	Nisentil	45	—	0.5	—	1–2	—
Butorphanol	Stadol	2	12	—	3	3–4	—
Camphorated tincture of opium	Paregoric	25	—	—	—	4–5	—
Codeine	various	120	200	—	3	3–6	800
Diacetylmorphine	Heroin	3.0	60	—	0.5	3–4	100
Dihydrocodeine	Hycodan	5–10	—	—	—		100
Diphenoxylate	Lomotil	40–60	—	delayed by atropine	—	—	—
Fentanyl	Sublimaze	0.2	—	0.5	—	1–2	—
Hydromorphine	Dilaudid	1.5	6.5	0.5–0.75	2–3	4–5	100
Meperidine	Demerol	75–100	300	0.5–1	3	4–6	1000
Methadone	Dolophine	10.0	20	4	—	4–6	120
Morphine	various	10.0	60	0.75–1	2–3	4–6	200
Nalbuphine	Nubain	10.0	60	—	5	3–6	—
Oxycodone	Percodan	15	30	—	—	3–4	—
Oxymorphone	Numorphan	1.0	6.5	1	2–3	4–5	—
Pentazocine	Talwin	60	180	0.75	2	4–7	—
Propoxyphene	Darvon	240	—	2–4	12–36	2–4	500

"Ts and blues" are a combination of pentazocine (Talwin) and tripelennamine (Pyribenzamine) used intravenously. Pentazocine now has naloxone added to it to counter this abuse. Innovar is fentanyl plus droperidol, used as an IV anesthetic.

*Dose equivalent to 10 mg of morphine.

greatly. Chlorophenothane (DDT), 200 to 250 mg per kg, is fatal; 16 mg per kg causes seizures. Methoxychlor, 500 to 6000 mg per kg, is fatal. Chlordane, 200 mg per kg is fatal (chlordane house air guidelines are below 5 μg per M^3; the occupational threshold limit value (TLV) is 500 μg per M^3). These insecticides interfere with axon transmission of nerve impulses. Metabolism varies; they resist degradation in human tissue and the environment. They accumulate in adipose tissue; the elimination route is via the liver. *Manifestations:* CNS stimulation, convulsions, late respiratory depression, increased myocardial irritability. Endrin produces liver toxicity with guarded prognosis. Chronic exposure causes liver and kidney damage. *Management:* (1) Dermal decontamination, discard contaminated leather goods. Protect personnel. Gastrointestinal decontamination, no oils. Many are dissolved in petroleum distillates, presenting an aspiration hazard. (2) No adrenergic stimulants (epinephrine) should be used because of myocardial irritability. (3) Cholestyramine, 4 grams every 8 hours, has been reported to increase the fecal excretion. (4) Anticonvulsants, if needed.

Organophosphate Insecticides (OPI). These may cause (a) irreversible inhibition of cholinesterase, either direct (TEPP) or delayed (parathion or malathion), or (b) reversible inhibition of cholinesterase (carbamates). Examples of OPI are listed in Table 23. Absorption is

TABLE 22. **Organochlorine Pesticides (DDT Derivatives)**

Chemical Name	Trade Name	Toxicity Rating	Elimination Time	Comment
Endrin	Hexadrin	Highest	hrs–days	Banned
Lindane	1% in Kwell; Benesan; Isotox; Gamene	Moderate to high	hrs–days	Scabicide; general garden insecticide
Endosulfan	Thiodan	Moderate	hrs–days	
Benzene hexachloride	BHC, HCH	Moderate	wks–mos	Banned, produces porphyria (cutanea tarda)
Dieldrin	Dieldrite	High	wks–mos	
Aldrin	Aldrite	High	wks–mos	
Chlordane (10% is heptachlor)	Chlordan	High	wks–mos	Restricted; termiticide
Toxophene	Toxakil Strobane-T	High	hrs–days	
Heptachlor	—	Moderate	wks–mos	Malignancy in rats
Chlorophenothane	DDT	Moderate	mos–yrs	Banned in 1972
Mirex	—	Moderate	mos–yrs	Banned; red anticide
Chlordecone	Kepone	Moderate	mos–yrs	Tidewater, Virginia, contamination
Methoxychlor	Marlate	Low	hrs–days	
Perthane	—	Low	hrs–days	
Dicofol	Kelthane	Low	hrs–days	
Chlorobenzilate	Acaraben	Low	hrs–days	Banned

TABLE 23. **Examples of Organophosphate Insecticides (OPI)**

Common Name	*Synonym*	*EFD**
Agricultural Products (highly toxic; LD_{50} is 1–50 mg/kg)		
Tetraethyl pyrophosphate	TEPP, Tetron	0.05
Phorate	Thimet	
Disulfoton†	Di-Syston	0.2
Demeton†	Systox	
Terbufos	Counter	
Chlortriphos	Calathion	
Mevinphos	Phosdrin	0.15
Parathion	Thiophos	0.10
Methamidophos	Monitor	delayed neuropathy
Monocrotophos	Azodrin	
Octamethyl-diphosphoramide	OMPA, Schradan	
Azinphosmethyl	Guthion	0.2
Ethyl–nitrophenyl thiobenzene PO_4	EPN	
Animal Insecticides (moderately toxic; LD_{50} is 30–500 mg/kg)		
DEF	DeGreen	
Dichlorvos	DDVP, Vapona	
Coumaphos	Co-ral	
Trichlorfon	Dylox	
Ronnel	Korlan	10.0
Dimethoate	Cygon, De-Fend	
Fenthion	Baytex	long-acting
Leptophos	Phosvel	
Chlorfenvinophos (tick dip)	Supona, Dermaton	
Household and Garden Pest Control (low toxicity; LD_{50} is 60–1300 mg/kg)		
Malathion	Cythion	60.0
Diazinon‡	Spectracide, Dimpylate	25.0
Chlorpyrifos‡	Lorsban, Dursban	
Temephos	Abate	

*EFD, Estimated fatal dose (grams/70 kg).
†Most OPI degrade in the environment in a few days to nontoxic radicals. These are taken up by the plants and fruits.
‡Some classify these as moderately toxic.

by all routes. The onset of acute toxicity is usually before 12 hours and always before 24 hours. *Toxic manifestations:* Early, cholinergic crisis—cramps, diarrhea, excess secretion, bronchospasms, bradycardia. Later, sympathetic and nicotine effects occur—twitching, fasciculations, weakness, tachycardia and hypertension, and convulsions. Central nervous system effects are anxiety, confusion, emotional lability, and coma.

Management: (1) Basic life support and decontamination with careful protection of personnel. (2) Atropine (Antidote 6, Table 4), if symptomatic, every 10 to 30 minutes until drying of secretions and clear lungs occur. Maintain for 12 to 24 hours, then taper the dose and observe for relapse. (3) Intravenous pralidoxime (2-PAM) may be required after atropinization (Antidote 28, Table 4). It should be given in the first 24 hours. It is used in the presence of weakness, respiratory depression, or muscle twitching. Its use may require reduction in the dose of atropine. (4) Careful dermal and gastrointestinal decontamination when stable. (5) Suction secretions until atropinization drying is achieved. Intubation and assisted ventilation may be needed. (6) *Do not* use morphine, aminophylline, phenothiazine, or reserpine-like drugs or succinylcholine. *Laboratory aids:* Draw blood for red blood cell cholinesterase before giving pralidoxime. Levels are usually more than 50 per cent depressed for severe symptoms. Monitor chest radiograph, blood glucose, arterial blood gases, ECG, blood coagulation status, liver function, and the urine for the metabolite alkyl phosphate *p*-nitrophenol. *Note:* If the diagnosis is probable, do not delay therapy until it is confirmed by laboratory tests. Atropine is both a diagnostic and therapeutic agent. A test dose of 2 mg in adults and 0.05 mg per kg in children may be administered parenterally. In the presence of severe cholinesterase inhibition, the patient fails to develop signs of atropinization.

It is not medically advisable to administer atropine or pralidoxime prophylactically to workers exposed to organophosphate pesticides.

Carbamates (esters of carbonic acid). Carbamates cause reversible carbamylation of acetylcholinesterase. Pralidoxime is usually not indicated in the management but atropine may be required. The major differences from OPI are (1) toxicity is less and of shorter duration; (2) they rarely produce overt central nervous system effects because of poor penetration; and (3) cholinesterase returns to normal rapidly so that blood values are not useful in confirming diagnosis. Some common examples of carbamates are Ziram, Temik (alkicarb) (taken up by plants and fruit), Matacil (aminocarb, carazol), Vydate (oxamyl), Isolan, furadan (Carbofuran), Lannate (methomyl, Nudrin), Zectran (mexacarbate), and Mesural (methiocarb). These agents are all highly toxic. Moderately toxic are Baygon (propoxur) and Sevin (carbaryl). Some of these agents may be formulated in wood alcohol and have the added toxicity of methyl alcohol.

Paradichlorbenzene. See Hydrocarbons.

Paraquat and Diquat. Paraquat is a quaternary ammonia herbicide rapidly inactivated in the soil by clay particles. Nonindustrial preparations of 0.2 per cent are unlikely to cause serious intoxications. *Toxic dose:* Commercial preparations such as Gramoxone 20 per cent are very toxic; one mouthful has produced death. Systemic absorption in the course of occupational use is apparently minimal. Paraquat on marijuana leaves is pyrolyzed to nontoxic dipyridyl. *Toxicokinetics:* "Hit and run" toxin. Less than 20 per cent is absorbed. The peak is 1 hour postingestion. The route of elimination is the kidney. Most of the dose is eliminated in the first 40 hours; it is detected in urine for 15 days. Volume distribution is over 500 liters per kg. *Manifestations:* Local corrosive effect on skin and mucous membranes. Acute renal failure in 48 hours (often reversible). Pulmonary effects in 72 hours are progressive, and oxygen aggravates the pulmonary fibrosis. Diquat does not produce effects on the lungs but produces convulsions and gastrointestinal distention. Long-term exposure may give cataracts. Chlormequat's target organ is the kidney.

Management: (1) Gastrointestinal decontamination despite corrosive effects should be done cautiously with a nasogastric tube; administer local adsorbent. Polystyrene sulfonate (Kayexalate) may be the best agent to prevent absorption—orally, 15 grams in water with 10 to 20 ml of 70 per cent sorbitol every 2 to 3 hours. This may be better than bentonite, fuller's earth, and activated charcoal. Dermal and ocular decontamination as needed. (2) Hemodialysis and hemoperfusion may be carried out in tandem. Hemoperfusion with charcoal alone is the present choice; however, the results are still poor. Continue hemoperfusion until blood paraquat levels cannot be detected. (3) Diuresis may be of value but consider the risk of fluid overload. (4) Niacin, 500 mg per kg every 4 hours to convert to nicotinamide adenine dinucleotide. (5) Avoid oxygen unless absolutely necessary (Pa_{O_2} below 60 mm Hg) because this aggravates fibrosis. Some use hypoxic air, Fi_{O_2} 10 to 20 per cent, and propranolol (Antidote 29, Table 4). (6) Corticosteroids may help prevent adrenal cortical necrosis. *Laboratory aids:* Blood levels above 2 μg per ml at 4 hours or above 0.10 at 16 hours are usually fatal. Blood levels and advice may be obtained from the Chevron Environmental Health Center, (415) 233–3737. Monitor renal, liver, and pulmonary functions and chest radiographs. Urine test for paraquat exposure: alkalinization and sodium dithionite give an intense blue-green color in exposure.

Parathion. See Organophosphate Insecticides.

Pentazocine (Talwin). See Opioids.

Perphenazine. See Phenothiazines.

Petroleum Products. See Hydrocarbons.

Phencyclidine (Angel Dust, PCP, Peace Pill, Hog). This is the "drug of deceit" because it is substituted for many other drugs, such as THC and mescaline. There are now at least 38 analogues. Smoking may give cyanide poisoning. Improper mixing has caused explosions. *Toxic dose:* Two to five mg smoked or "snorted" produces drunken behavior, agitation and excitement. Five to ten mg produce stupor, coma, and myoclonus convulsions. Ten to 25 mg smoked, snorted, or orally results in prolonged coma and respiratory failure. It is usually fatal over 25 mg (250 mg per ml blood concentration). *Toxicokinetics:* Weak base. Rapidly absorbed when smoked, snorted, or ingested and secreted into stomach gastric juice. Absorbed in alkaline intestine, but ion-trapping takes place in acid gastric media. Half-life is 30 to 60 minutes. Lipophilic drug with extensive Vd. The onset of action if smoked is 2 to 5 minutes (peak in 15 to 30 minutes); orally, 30 to 60 minutes. The duration at low doses is 4 to 6 hours and normality returns in 24 hours. At large overdoses coma may last 6 to 10 days (waxes and wanes). An adverse reaction in overdose occurs in 1 to 2 hours. *Route of elimination:* By liver metabolism (50 per cent). Urinary excretion of conjugates and free PCP. *Manifestations:* Sympathomimetic, cholinergic, cerebellar. Observe for violent behavior, paranoid schizophrenia, self-destructive behavior. Clues to diagnosis are bursts of horizontal, vertical, and rotary nystagmus, coma with eyes open.

Management (avoid overtreatment of mild intoxications): (1) gastrointestinal decontamination up to 4 hours postingestion, but this may not be effective because it is rapidly absorbed. Insert nasogastric tube into stomach for administration of activated charcoal, a cathartic, and ammonium chloride every 6 hours, because PCP is secreted into the stomach even if it is smoked or snorted. (2) Protect patient and others from harm. "Talk down" is usually ineffective. Low sensory environment. Diazepam (Valium) may be used orally or intramuscularly in the uncooperative patient. (3) For behavioral disorders and toxic psychosis—haloperidol (Haldol), 2 to 5 mg, or diazepam or both. (4) Seizures and muscle spasm—control with diazepam, 2.5 mg, up to 10 mg (Antidote 15, Table 4). (5) Dystonia reaction—diphenhydramine (Benadryl) intravenously (Antidote 17, Table 4). (6) Hyperthermia—external cooling. (7) Hypertensive crisis (dopaminergic)—diazoxide, 3 to 5 mg per kg intravenously up to 300 mg bolus, or propranolol, 1 mg intravenously up to 10 mg (Antidote 29, Table 4), or nitroprusside. (8) Acid diuresis ion-trapping (controversial). Ammonium chloride through nasogastric tube (Antidote 2, Table 4): Clamp tube for a half hour after instillation. Repeat every 6 hours to keep urine pH less than 5.5 (blood pH varies from 7.2 to 7.4). Administer sufficient fluid and a diuretic, if necessary, to produce a diuresis of 3 to 6 ml per kg per hour. Blood pH is often reduced to 7.2 intermittently with this therapy. Ascorbic acid may be administered intravenously (2 grams in 500 ml every 6 hours) as an adjunct. Ammonium chloride may be given intravenously if excess gastric bleeding occurs. Continue ammonium chloride therapy while the patient is in coma. Cranberry juice may be given orally every 6 hours for 10 days to 2 weeks as an adjunct to keep the urine acidified (cranberry juice is metabolized to hippuric acid). (9) No phenothiazines in the acute phase of intoxication because they lower the convulsive threshold. May be needed later for psychosis.

Laboratory aids: (1) CPK level will be clue to the amount of rhabdomyolysis occurring and the chance of myoglobinuria developing. Values up to 20,000 have been reported. (2) Test urine for myoglobin and pigmented casts. Test urine with ortho-toluidine; a positive test without red blood cells on microscopic examination suggests myoglobinuria. (3) Monitor urine and blood pH and urinary output if acidifying patient. (4) Phencyclidine level. (5) BUN, ammonia, electrolytes, blood glucose (20 per cent have hypoglycemia). (6) Test for PCP in gastric juice; levels are 40 to 50 times higher than in blood. *Complications:* Rhabdomyolysis, myoglobinuria, and renal failure. Dopaminogenic—hypertensive crisis, CVA, encephalopathy, and malignant hyperthermia. Schizophrenic paranoid psychosis (induced in chronic users or precipitated in acute users). Loss of memory for months. Teratogenic cases have been reported. Children have been intoxicated from inhalation in a room where adults were smoking PCP. PCP-induced depression and suicide.

Phenobarbital. See Barbiturates.

Phenothiazines and Other Major Neuroleptics. Phenothiazines are represented by aliphatic compounds: chlorpromazine (Thorazine), promethazine (Phenergan), promazine (Sparine), triflupromazine (Vesprin), methoxypromazine (Tentone); piperazine compounds (dimethylamine series); acetophenazine (Tindal), fluphenazine (Prolixin), prochlorperazine (Compazine), perphenazine (Trilifan), trifluoperazine (Stelazine); and piperidine compounds: mepazine (Pacatal), mesoridazine (Serentil), thioridazine (Mellaril), pipamazine (Mornidine). Non-phenothiazines are the thioxanthines: clorprothixene (Taractan), thiothixene (Navane); butyrophenones: haloperidol (Haldol), droperidol (Inapsine); dibenzoxazepines: loxapine (Loxitane, Daxolin); and dihydroindolones: molindone (Moban, Lidone). These have pharmacologic properties similar to those of the phenothiazines. *Manifestations:* Clues to phenothiazine overdose are miosis, tremor, hypotension, hypothermia, respiratory depression, radiopaque pills on radiograph of abdomen, and increased QT waves in the electrocardiogram. Anticholinergic actions are also present. Major problems are respiratory depression, myocardial toxicity (quinidine-like), neurogenic hypotension (antidopaminogenic), and idiosyncratic reaction, which may occur at therapeutic levels. Idiosyncratic reaction consists of opisthotonos, torticollis, orolingual dyskinesis, and oculogyric crisis (painful upward gaze) and can be mistaken for a psychotic episode. Extrapyramidal crisis is frequent in children and women. Death is usually due to cardiac effects. Phenothiazines are metabolized by the liver into many metabolites. Some remain in the body longer than 6 months.

Management: (1) Gastrointestinal decontamination. Emesis induction may be useful if symptoms have not occurred. If symptoms are already present, many of these agents have antiemetic action so lavage may be required. Always provide gastric lavage to comatose patients after the airway is protected regardless of the time of ingestion because of inhibition of gastric motility. (2) Extrapyramidal signs (idiosyncratic reaction) can be treated with diphenhydramine (Benadryl) (Antidote 17, Table 4), or benztropine (Cogentin), 1 to 2 mg intravenously slowly. Symptoms recur, and these drugs should be continued orally for 2 to 3 days. *This is not the treatment of overdose,* only of the idiosyncratic reaction. (3) Monitor ECG for dysrhythmias and treat with antidysrhythmic agents. (4) Hypotension is treated with the Trendelenburg position or fluid challenge or both. Vasopressors are used only if these fail. Dopamine (Intropin) should not be used to treat the hypotension because these drugs are antidopaminogenic. If a pressor agent is needed, use norepinephrine (Levarterenol, Levophed). (5) Physostigmine may be used for life-threatening anticholinergic symptoms. (6) A radiograph of the abdomen is useful to detect undissolved tablets, which may be radiopaque. (7) Treat hypo- or hyperthermia with external physical measures (not drugs).

Laboratory aids: A ferric chloride test of urine can confirm exposure to phenothiazines if there is a sufficient blood level. Blood levels are *not* useful in management.

Phenylpropanolamine (PPA). See Amphetamines.

Primidone. See Anticonvulsants.

Propoxyphene. See Opioids.

Propranolol and Beta Blockers. Some of these agents available in the USA at this time are listed in Table 24. *Toxic dose:* Varies considerably. *Toxicokinetics*: Peak action is 1 to 2 hours orally and lasts 24 to 48 hours. In drugs with long half-lives, e.g., nadolol, it may take many days to recover from overdose toxicity (see Table 23). *Manifestations*: Observe for bradycardia and hypotension. Fat-soluble drugs have more CNS effects. Partial agonists may produce tachycardia and hypertension (oxprenolol, pindolol).

Management: (1) Gastrointestinal decontamination up to 2 hours postingestion. (2) Treat hypoglycemia (frequent in children) and hyperkalemia. (3) Control convulsions. (4) Cardiovascular manifestations: Bradycardia—if hemodynamically stable and asymptomatic, no therapy. If unstable (hypotension or atriovenous block), use atropine, isoproterenol, glucagon, and pacemaker. Ventricular tachycardia or premature beats—use lidocaine, phenytoin, or overdrive pacing. Myocardial depression and hypotension—correct dysrhythmias, Trendelenburg positioning, and fluids. Monitor with pulmonary arterial wedge pressure (PAWP) catheter. If low cardiac output with low PAWP, give more fluids. If low cardiac output with normal PAWP, use glucagon (Antidote 21, Table 4). Avoid quinidine, procainamide, and disopyramide (Norpace). Glucagon is probably the choice drug since it works through adenylcyclase mechanism not affected by the beta blockers. It is given as a bolus and may be continued as an infusion (Antidote 21, Table 4). If bronchospasm—give aminophylline. Hemodialysis or hemoperfusion for low volume distribution drugs with low protein binding and water-soluble (nadolol and atenolol), particularly if evidence of renal failure. If hypoglycemia—give intravenous glucose. *Laboratory aids*: Monitor blood glucose, potassium, ECG, PAWP. Fatal blood level of propranolol is 0.8 to 1.2 mg per dl (8 to 12 μg per ml).

Quinidine and Quinine (Antidysrhythmic and Antimalarial Agents). *Toxic dose* in child is 1 gram; in adult is 2 to 8 grams. There is 95 to 100 per cent absorption, peak action in 2 to 4 hours. Half-life is 3 to 4 hours (quinidine gluconate, 8 to 12 hours). Large Vd. Metabolized predominantly by the liver. *Manifestations*: Cinchonism (headache, nausea, vomiting, tinnitus, deafness, diplopia, dilated pupils). Myocardial depression, dysrhythmias, ECG changes—prolongation of PR, QRS, and QT intervals. Skin rashes and flushing. Hemolysis in G-6-PD deficiency. Dementia reported. *Management*: (1) Gastrointestinal decontamination. (2) Monitor ECG and liver functions. (3) May need antidysrhythmic drugs and pacemaker and alkalinization.

Salicylate Intoxication. *Toxic dose:* See Table 25. Methyl salicylate (oil of wintergreen): 1 ml equals 1.4 grams of salicylate. One teaspoonful equals 21 adult aspirins. *Toxicokinetics*: Plasma concentration is significant in 30 minutes and peaks in 1 to 2 hours. Half-life is 3 to 6 hours (therapeutic) to 12 to 36 hours (toxic). Urine pH influences urine salicylate elimination. *Manifestations of acute ingestion* (see Table 25): The metabolic disturbance in adults and older children is usually respiratory alkalosis; in children under 5 years of age the initial respiratory alkalosis will usually change to metabolic or mixed metabolic acidosis and respiratory alkalosis with acidosis predominating within a few hours.

Management: (1) Gastrointestinal decontamination is useful up to 12 hours postingestion as some factors delay absorption (food, enteric-coated tablets, other drugs); pylorospasm may delay emptying; and concre-

TABLE 24. **Propranolol and Beta Blockers**

	Solubility and Absorption (%)	Membrane Stabilizer	Relative Potency (Propranolol = 1)	Plasma Half-life	Elimination	Protein Bound	VD (Liter/Kg)
Atenolol (Tenormin) Dose: 50–100 mg MDD = 100 mg	water (46–62)	no	1.0	6–9	95% renal	3–10	0.7
Metoprolol (Lopressor) Dose: 50–400 mg MDD = 450 mg	fat (over 95)	no	1.0	3–4	hepatic	10	5.6
Nadolol (Corgard) Dose: 40–320 mg MDD = 320 mg	water (15–25)	+/−	1.0	17–23	70% renal	25	2.1
Pindolol* (Visken) Dose: 20–60 mg MDD = 60 mg	fat (over 90)	no	6.0	3–4	hepatic (40% renal)	57	2.0
Propranolol† (Inderal) Dose: 40–160 mg MDD = 480 mg	fat (100)	+ +	1.0	2–3	hepatic (less than 1% renal)	90–95	3.6
Timolol‡ (Blocadren) Dose: 20 mg MDD = 60 mg Ophthalmologic (Timoptic, 0.25–0.5%) Dose: 1 drop twice daily	fat (over 90)	no	6.0	3	hepatic (20% renal)	less than 10	1.5

*Partial agonists
†Substantial first pass
‡Mitochondrial calcium protection during ischemia
MDD, maximum daily dose

tions may form. A cathartic and activated charcoal should be administered every 4 hours until stools are black. Concretions may be removed by lavage, endoscopy, or gastrostomy. (2) Intravenous fluid should be given as recommended in Table 26. Alkalinization enhances salicylate excretion. Potassium is essential to produce adequate alkalinization. Monitor *both* the urine and blood pH. Do not use the urine pH alone to assess the need for alkalinization (Antidote 31, Table 4). (3) Fluid retention can be treated with mannitol (20 per cent), 0.5 gram per kg over 30 minutes, or furosemide, 1 mg per kg intravenously. (4) Hyperpyrexia should be treated with external cooling. (5) Abnormal bleeding or hypoprothrombinemia will need vitamin K, 10 mg intramuscularly and, if bleeding continues, fresh blood or platelet transfusion (Antidote 34, Table 4). (6) Dialysis (hemodialysis) or hemoperfusion is indicated if there is persistent acidosis (pH<7.1) and lack of response to fluid and/or alkali in 6 hours; if serum salicylate levels are initially greater than 160 mg per dl or greater than 130 mg per dl at 6 hours postingestion (do *not* use the salicylate level as the sole criterion for dialysis); if there are coma and uncontrollable seizures; congestive heart failure, acute

TABLE 25. **Salicylate Intoxication from Acute Single Ingestion of Salicylate Categories**

Category	Approx. Dose to Consider GI Decontamination*	Approx. Toxic Dose	Manifestations
Ill or dehydrated child or on ASA	40 mg/kg (½ baby aspirin/lb)	—	—
Well child	80 mg/kg (1 baby aspirin/lb)	—	—
Mild toxicity	yes	150–200 mg/kg	vomiting, hyperventilation, tinnitus
Moderate toxicity	yes	200–300 mg/kg	hyperventilation, fever, vertigo, agitation, hallucination, stupor
Severe toxicity	yes	300–400 mg/kg	hyperventilation, coma, convulsions, shock
Potential fatal dose	yes	500 mg/kg	—

*The usual contraindications to GI decontamination should be followed.

TABLE 26. **Recommendations for Fluid Management in Salicylate Intoxication**

	Rate of Administration (*ml/kg/hr*)	Duration	Composite of Fluid *Na*	*K*	*Cl*	HCO_3	*Glucose (%)*
Initial hydration	15–20	1–2 hr	75	0	50	25	5–10
Subsequent hydration	4–8	until ASA level is therapeutic	40 (55)*	35	50	20 (35)*	5–10
Maintenance	2–3	prn	25	20	25	20	5

*For severe acidosis. *Note:* For severe acidosis (pH < 7.15), give 1–2 mEq/kg of $NaHCO_3$ additionally every 1–2 hours. Monitor carefully for cerebral edema, pulmonary edema, and inappropriate secretion of antidiuretic hormone.

renal failure, and progressive deterioration despite good management. (7) Chronic toxicity is usually a more severe intoxication because of the cumulative pharmocokinetics of salicylates. Management needs are outlined in Table 27.

Laboratory aids: The metabolic acidosis of salicylism has a moderately elevated anion gap. Hyper- or hypoglycemia may exist. Serum salicylate levels used in conjunction with the Done nomogram (Figure 3, next page) are useful predictors of expected severity following *acute single ingestions*. The Done nomogram is *not* useful in chronic intoxications, methyl salicylate, phenyl salicylate, or homomethyl salicylate ingestions. The salicylate level for use in the Done nomogram should be obtained 6 hours postingestion. Before 6 hours, levels in the toxic range should be treated and levels below the toxic range should be repeated if a potentially toxic dose is ingested. Monitor urine output, urine pH, electrolytes, arterial blood gases, blood glucose, prothrombin time, renal function, serum salicylate level, and urine salicylate with the ferric chloride test. Arterial blood pH should be kept at 7.5. *Prognosis*: Persistent vigorous treatment of salicylate ingestions is essential as recovery has occurred despite decerebrate rigidity.

Sedative Hypnotics, Nonbarbiturate. See Table 28. *Management* is primarily supportive (especially intubation and ventilator therapy with continuous positive airway pressure (CPAP) for adult respiratory distress syndrome) and with the use of hemoperfusion or hemodialysis in patients who are severely intoxicated and fail to respond to good supportive care and whose intoxication is life-threatening. (1) *Chloral hydrate* management includes cautious gastrointestinal decontamination. Avoid the use of epinephrine and catecholamines that may produce dysrhythmias. Propranolol, 0.1 mg per kg in 1 mg increments, appears to be more effective than lidocaine for ventricular dysrhythmias. (2) *Ethchlorvynol* management includes GI decontamination up to 12 hours postingestion. Resin hemoperfusion (Amberlite XAD-4) is the best method of extracorporeal removal when other measures fail in a life-threatening situation (ingestion of over 10 grams or 100 mg per kg, with serum levels of over 100 μg per ml in the first 12 hours or 70 μg per ml after 12 hours in patients with prolonged life-threatening coma). External rewarming if temperature is below 32 C. (3) *Glutethimide* management includes GI decontamination up to 24 hours postingestion. Concretions may form. Resin hemoperfusion appears to be the best method of extracorporeal removal in life-threatening protracted coma when the patient has ingested over 10 grams and has a serum level of over 30 μg per ml. Treat hyperthermia with external cooling. (4) *Meprobamate* management includes GI decontamination up to 12 hours postingestion, with charcoal hemoperfusion in prolonged coma with life-threatening complications. Concretions may form in the stomach and may require breaking up or surgical removal. (5) *Methaqualone* management includes GI decontamination. Forced diuresis, dialysis, and hemoperfusion are not indicated. Fatalities are rare. (6) *Methyprylon* management includes GI decontamination and may require treatment of the hypotension with vasopressors of the alpha adrenergic variety—levarterenol (Levophed). The hypotension usually does not respond to position or fluids alone. This is a dialyzable drug but usually this is not necessary. Fatalities are rare.

Strychnine. Primarily available as a rodenticide and component of cathartics and "tonics." Adulterant of "street drugs," particularly marijuana and cocaine. *Toxic dose*: 5 to 10 mg; fatal in doses of 15 to 30 mg. *Toxicokinetics*: Rapid absorption. Manifestations may occur within 15 to 30 minutes. Low protein-binding.

TABLE 27. **Management of Chronic Salicylate Intoxication**

Classification	Urine pH	Blood pH	Hydration	Add Sodium Bicarb (*mEq/L*)	Add Potassium (*mEq/L*)
Mild	alkaline	alkaline	+	+	0
Moderate	acid	alkaline	diuresis	40	40
Severe	acid	acid	diuresis	80 80	40* 80†

*Normal serum potassium and/or ECG.
†Normal serum potassium and/or abnormal ECG showing sign of potassium deficiency.

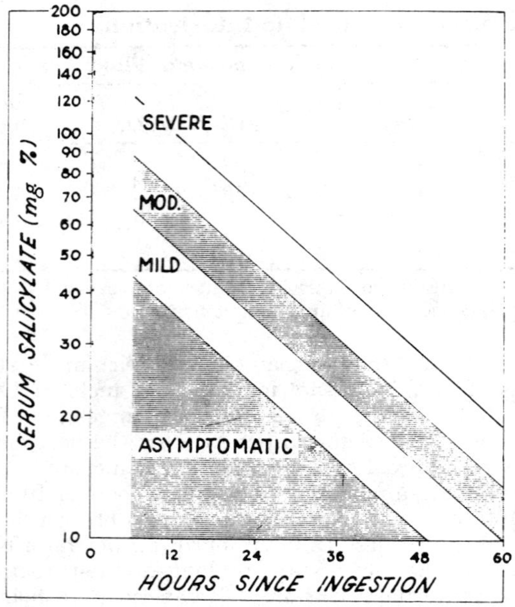

Figure 3. The Done nomogram for salicylate intoxication. For limitations of use, see *Laboratory aids*. (From Done A: Salicylate intoxication: Significance of measurements of salicylate in blood in cases of acute ingestion. Pediatrics *26*:800, 1960. © American Academy of Pediatrics, 1960.)

Hepatic metabolism, which appears to be saturable. Twenty per cent is excreted in urine. Has been found in the urine up to 48 hours after a 700 mg dose. *Manifestations*: Interferes with postsynaptic neurotransmitter inhibition by glycine. Hyperacusis is often the first sign. Mild cases—face stiffness (trismus and risus sardonicus). Moderate cases—extensor muscle thrusts. Severe cases—tetanic convulsions with opisthotonos. Death occurs within 1 to 3 hours after ingestion. The prognosis for survival improves if the patient survives beyond 5 hours. The complications of intoxication are lactic acidosis, hyperthermia, rhabdomyolysis and renal damage from precipitation of myoglobin in the renal tubules, and death from hypoxia. *Management*: (1) Emesis appears contraindicated because of rapid absorption and the early onset of seizures. Gastric aspiration and lavage may be used after the seizures are controlled. Activated charcoal should be given and repeated. (2) Control convulsions with diazepam or phenobarbital. (3) Supportive care for respiratory depression. (4) Acid diuresis and dialysis do not appear to be justified on the basis of available studies. (5) Paralysis with assisted ventilation is useful.

Tear Gas (Lacrimators). CS (chlorobenzylidine), "riot control"; CN powder (chloroacetophenone, 1 per cent); Mace (chloroacetophenone). *Management.* Dermal and ocular decontamination. Protect attendants from contamination. Ophthalmologic evaluation. Oxygen therapy may be needed for dyspnea and respiratory distress.

Theophylline. *Toxic dose*: Acute, single dose greater than 10 mg per kg yields mild toxicity. Greater than 20 mg per kg, moderate manifestations. *Toxicokinetics*: Absorption is complete. Peak levels occur within 60 to 90 minutes after ingestion of liquid preparations; 1 to 3 hours after regular tablets; and 3 to 10 hours after slow release preparations. Vd, 0.3 to 0.7 liter per kg. Protein-binding, 15 to 40 per cent. t½ varies: 3.5 hours average in a child and 4.5 hours in an adult (range from 3 to 9 hours). In neonates and young infants the drug's half-life is much longer. Overdose increases the half-life. *Elimination*: Hepatic metabolism, 90 per cent (demethylation and oxidation); 8 to 10 per cent is excreted unchanged in the urine. *Manifestations*: Acute toxicity generally correlates with blood levels; chronic toxicity does not. Ten to 20 μg per ml is the therapeutic range, but some mild gastrointestinal toxicity may occur. Twenty to 40 μg per ml is moderate toxicity, with gastrointestinal and CNS stimulation. Over 50 μg per ml—seizures and dysrhythmias may occur but they may also occur at lower levels and without gastrointestinal symptoms. Children tolerate higher serum levels. Chronic intoxication is more serious and difficult to treat. Many factors increase theophylline concentration.

Management: (1) Gastrointestinal decontamination in acute overdose, up to 4 hours with regular preparations and up to 8 to 12 hours with slow release preparations. Test aspirate or vomitus for blood. Give activated charcoal every 4 hours and a cathartic. Do not induce emesis if hematemesis exists. (2) Monitor ECG, obtain theophylline levels every 4 hours until in the therapeutic range of 10 to 20 μg per ml. (3) Control seizures with diazepam. If coma, convulsions, and vomiting exist, intubate immediately. (4) Hypotension is treated with fluid challenge and if this fails, vasopressors. (5) Hematemesis is managed with iced saline lavage and blood replacement if needed. (6) Charcoal hemoperfusion is the management of choice in life-threatening convulsions, dysrhythmias, hematemesis, or intractable vomiting refractory to conventional measures. Differences in slow release preparations from regular preparations: little or no gastrointestinal symptoms with high levels; peak concentration times may be 10 to 24 hours postingestion; and onset of seizures may occur 10 to 12 hours postingestion. *Laboratory aids*: Monitor theophylline levels, check for occult blood in vomitus and stools, monitor vital signs and hemoglobin and hematocrit (for hemorrhage). Monitor cardiac, renal, and hepatic function, electrolytes, blood glucose, arterial blood gases, and acid-base balance.

Toluene. See Hydrocarbons.

Tranquilizers. See Sedative Hypnotics.

Tricyclic Antidepressants (TCAD). These agents are generally rapidly absorbed from the gastrointestinal tract, but absorption may be prolonged in overdose owing to anticholinergic action. Their bioavailability has considerable variation among patients, and they are highly bound to plasma and tissue proteins. Protein-binding decreases with decreasing pH. The Vd is large, usually 10 to 20 liters per kg. The TCAD are metabolized primarily in the liver. *N*-Demethylation of the tertiary amines yields the active secondary amine metabolites; hydroxylation gives rise to inactive metabolites. Forty per cent is excreted in the feces and only 3 per cent in the urine unchanged. The t½ varies

TABLE 28. **Nonbarbiturate Sedative Hypnotic Drugs**

	Absorption and Toxic Dose	Peak Hours	VD L/kg	Protein-Bound (%)	Elimination Route	Serum Half-life (hrs)	Toxic Level (μg/ml)	Manifestations and Comment*
Chloral hydrate (Noctec)	Rapid TD, 2 grams FD, 4–10 grams	1–2	0.6	40	Hepatic 90% to active metabolite trichloroethanol (TCE)	4–8	100 (80 TCE—very toxic)	Pearlike odor. Dysrhythmias (especially ventricular), hepatotoxic irritant to mucosa of GI tract; ARDS; radiopaque capsules
Ethchlorvynol (Placidyl)	Rapid TD, 2.5 grams	2–4	3–4	35–50	Hepatic 90%	(1–6) 21–105 in toxic dose	20–80	Prolonged coma up to 200 hr, apnea, hypothermia, pulmonary edema, pink gastric aspirate, pungent odor
Glutethimide (Doriden) (highest mortality of all sedative hypnotics, 14%)	Slow, erratic TD, 5 grams FD, 10 grams	6	large, 10–20	50	Hepatic 98% to toxic metabolite 4-hydroxyglutarimide (4HG)	10	20–80	Prolonged, cyclic coma up to 120 hr, anticholinergic signs, convulsions, apnea recurrent, hyperthermia
Meprobamate (Equanil, Miltown)	Rapid TD, 10 grams	4–8	1.0	20	Hepatic 90%	6–16	30–100, 200	Coma, convulsions, pulmonary edema, apnea, concretions in stomach
Methaqualone (Quaaludes, "Love Drugs")	Rapid TD, 800 mg FD, 125 mg/kg	1–3	2–6	80	Hepatic 90%	10–40	8–10	Hypertonia, hyperreflexia, convulsions, apnea, act "drunk," bleeding tendencies
Methyprylon (Noludar)	Rapid TD, 3 grams	2–4	1–2		Hepatic 97%	3–6; over 8 in toxic dose	30	Hyperactive coma lasts 30 hr, miosis, persistent hypotension, pulmonary edema. Mortality rare

*Comment includes other features besides the typical manifestations of all these agents—coma, respiratory depression, psychologic and physiologic withdrawal, hypotension, hypothermia (except glutethimide hyperthermia).
TD, Toxic dose; FD, Fatal dose.

from 9 to 198 hours. In an overdose, the half-life may be much longer. Tricyclic tertiary amines (metabolized to active metabolites) are amitriptyline (Elavil), imipramine (Tofranil), and doxepin (Sinequan). Tricyclic secondary amines (metabolized to nonactive metabolites) are desipramine (Norpramin, Pertofrane), protriptyline (Vivactil), and nortriptyline (Aventyl). Tricyclic dibenzoxazepine (metabolized to a major metabolite) is amoxapine (Asendin).

Manifestations: The onset of action varies from less than 1 hour to 12 hours after ingestion. The phases of intoxication are (1) consciousness with dry mouth, mydriasis, ataxia, increased deep tendon reflexes, and changes in the ST segment; (2) Stages I and II coma with hypertension, tachycardia above 160, mydriasis, and supraventricular tachycardia; and (3) Stages III and IV coma with hypotension, heart rate under 120, respiratory depression, tonic clonic seizures, and ventricular dysrhythmias. The central nervous system effects occur early, and seizures are common. *Cardiovascular toxicity* is frequent in the serious poisonings and results from anticholinergic effects, sympathomimetic activity (by blocking reuptake of catecholamines), quinidine activity, catecholamine depletion, and alpha adrenergic blockage. Cardiotoxic effects include cardiac dysrhythmias, hypertension, hypotension, and pulmonary edema.

Toxic dose: The TCAD have a narrow margin of safety. In a child, a 375 mg dose and in adults, as little as 500 to 750 mg has been fatal. The following dosages may serve as a guide to the degree of toxicity: Less than 10 mg per kg produces light coma, mydriasis, and tachycardia and has a good prognosis. At 20 mg per kg, Stage III manifestations are produced. At 30 mg per kg, fatalities may result. At 50 mg per kg, the mortality rate is increased. Over 70 mg per kg is rarely survived. Therapeutic blood levels are in the range of 50 to 170 ng per ml. A blood level of 1000 ng per ml or greater is generally associated with a QRS interval greater than 100 msec and indicates severe overdose. This is not an absolute correlation because QRS duration varies from minute to minute and also with acid-base changes.

CYCLIC ANTIDEPRESSANTS: Amoxapine (Asendin) allegedly has less cardiotoxicity. Patients with amoxapine overdose may develop the syndrome of seizures, rhabdomyolysis, and acute renal tubular necrosis. Recent reports indicate more fatalities with amoxapine than with TCAD. Maprotiline (Ludiomil) is a tetracyclic compound with pharmacologic effects similar to the existing tricyclic antidepressant drugs. Trazodone HCl (Desyrel) is an antidepressant chemically unrelated to the other antidepressants. It is claimed that this agent does not cause electrocardiographic changes.

Management: (1) Maintenance of vital functions. ICU care until there are no abnormalities in the ECG for 24 to 48 hours. (2) Gastrointestinal decontamination if the patient is alert. Intact pills have been recovered by lavage up to 18 hours after ingestion. Suspected cases should have ECG monitoring. (3) Activated charcoal every 4 to 6 hours and continuous nasogastric suction for the first 48 hours may interrupt enterohepatic recycling of tricyclic antidepressants. (4) Control seizures with intravenous diazepam. Intravenous phenytoin (Dilantin) may be added for seizures not responding to diazepam alone. For refractory seizures, physostigmine may be used (Antidote 27, Table 4). (5) Life-threatening delirium and hallucinations can be treated with physostigmine. Physostigmine was the drug of choice, but recently its use has been advocated only when conventional therapy has failed. (6) All cardiovascular complications of TCAD should *first* be treated by alkalinization of blood with sodium bicarbonate to a pH of 7.5 to 7.55 (Antidote 31, Table 4). Serum potassium levels should be followed, as a sudden increase in blood pH can aggravate or precipitate hypokalemia. Specific cardiovascular complications should be treated as follows: *Hypotension*—norepinephrine (Levophed), a predominantly alpha adrenergic drug, is preferred over dopamine. (Hypertension that occurs early rarely requires treatment.) *Serious conduction defects* are best managed with phenytoin and may need temporary transvenous pacemaker. *Sinus tachycardia* usually does not require treatment. If the tachycardia persists despite alkalinization and the patient is unstable, physostigmine may be used. *Supraventricular tachycardia* that does not respond to alkalinization alone may be treated with phenytoin, physostigmine, or synchronized cardioversion. *Ventricular tachycardia*—after alkalinization and phenytoin, intravenous lidocaine (for one dose only) may be required for persistent ventricular tachycardia. Synchronized cardioversion may be needed if lidocaine fails. *Ventricular fibrillation* should be treated with DC countershock. *Laboratory aids*: Arterial blood gases with blood pH, ECG, serum electrolytes, BUN and creatinine, serum phenytoin level, urine output, and, in severe cases, central venous pressure and/or pulmonary wedge pressure.

Trichloroethylene. See Hydrocarbons.

Turpentine. See Hydrocarbons.

Xylene. See Hydrocarbons.

Section 18

Appendices and Index

LABORATORY VALUES OF CLINICAL IMPORTANCE

method of
REX B. CONN, M.D.
Emory University
Atlanta, Georgia

INTRODUCTION

The quantitative procedures carried out in a clinical laboratory represent measurements of substances normally present within rather narrow ranges of concentration. In order to use such data, we must know the values to be expected in a normal individual and what is considered a significant deviation from normal. Actually, there can be no sharp dividing line between abnormal and normal values, since there is a gradual transition during any pathological process from what is clearly normal to what is clearly a pathological condition.

In medicine, it is a logical impossibility to define normality, and the term "reference values" has replaced the earlier term "normal values." Reference values are derived from statistical studies on subjects believed to have no condition that might affect the measurements under consideration. The traditional and most widely used statistical approach is to carry out the measurement on a large group of subjects and to set the reference limits at the mean value plus or minus two standard deviations. Since values obtained for many measurements are not Gaussian in distribution, additional steps are frequently used in calculation of the reference ranges. The important consideration is that the reference ranges derived by these statistical methods contain only 95 per cent of the reference population. Thus, a value slightly outside the reference range might be due either to chance distribution or to an underlying pathological process.

A single reference range for all individuals may be inadequate for some clinical measurements. Values obtained on presumably normal persons may vary because of age, sex, body build, race, environment, and state of gastrointestinal absorption. The use of reference values is that for many procedures the reference range will vary with the method used. This is particularly true for enzyme measurements and measurements based upon immunochemical principles.

THE INTERNATIONAL SYSTEM OF UNITS FOR LABORATORY MEASUREMENTS (LE SYSTÈME INTERNATIONAL D'UNITÉS)

An extensive modification of the metric system has been adopted by clinical laboratories in many countries. This adaptation is the International System of Units (Le Système International d'Unités), usually abbreviated S.I. Units. Whereas the metric system utilizes the centimeter, the gram, and the second as basic units, the International System uses the meter, the kilogram, and the second as well as four other basic units.

The International System is a coherent approach to all types of measurement that utilizes seven dimensionally independent basic quantities: mass, length, time, thermodynamic temperature, electric current, luminous intensity, and amount of substance. Each of these quantities is expressed in a clearly defined *basic unit* (Table 1).

Two or more basic units may be combined to provide *derived units* (Table 2) for expressing other measure-

Table 1. BASIC UNITS

Property	Basic Unit	Symbol
Length	metre	m
Mass	kilogram	kg
Amount of substance	mole	mol
Time	second	s
Thermodynamic temperature	kelvin	K
Electric current	ampere	A
Luminous intensity	candela	cd

Table 2. DERIVED UNITS

Derived Property	Derived Unit	Symbol
Area	square metre	m^2
Volume	cubic metre	m^3
	litre	l
Mass concentration	kilogram/cubic metre	kg/m^3
	gram/litre	g/l
Substance concentration	mole/cubic metre	mol/m^3
	mole/litre	mol/l
Temperature	degree Celsius	C = K − 273.15

ments such as mass concentration (kilograms per cubic meter) and velocity (meters per second). Standardized prefixes (Table 3) for basic and derived units are used to express fractions or multiples of the basic units so that any measurement can be expressed in a value between 0.001 and 1000.

Medical Applications

The most profound change in laboratory reports will result from expressing concentration as amount per volume (moles per liter) rather than mass per volume (milligrams per 100 milliliters). The advantages of the former expression can be seen in the following:

Conventional Units

1.0 gram of hemoglobin
Combines with 1.37 ml. of oxygen
Contains 3.4 mg. of iron
Forms 34.9 mg. of bilirubin

S.I. Units

1.0 mmol of hemoglobin
Combines with 4.0 mmol of oxygen
Contains 4.0 mmol of iron
Forms 4.0 mmol of bilirubin

Chemical relationships between lactic acid and pyruvic acid and the glucose from which both are derived, as well as the relationship between bilirubin and the binding capacity of albumin, are other examples of chemical relationships that will be clarified by using the new system.

There are a number of laboratory and other medical measurements for which the S.I. Units appear to offer little advantage, and some that are disadvantageous because the change would require replacement or revision of instruments such as the sphygmomanometer. The cubic meter is the derived unit for volume; however, it is inappropriately large for medical measurements, and the liter has been retained. Thermodynamic temperature expressed in kelvins is not more informative for medical measurements. Since the Celsius degree is the same as the Kelvin degree, the Celsius scale is used. Celsius rather than centigrade is the preferred term.

Table 3. STANDARD PREFIXES

Prefix	Multiplication Factor	Symbol
atto	10^{-18}	a
femto	10^{-15}	f
pico	10^{-12}	p
nano	10^{-9}	n
micro	10^{-6}	μ
milli	10^{-3}	m
centi	10^{-2}	c
deci	10^{-1}	d
deca	10^{1}	da
hecto	10^{2}	h
kilo	10^{3}	k
mega	10^{6}	M
giga	10^{9}	G
tera	10^{12}	T

Selection of units for expressing enzyme activity presents certain difficulties. Literally dozens of different units have been used in expressing enzyme activity, and interlaboratory comparison of enzyme results is impossible unless the assay system is precisely defined. In 1964, the International Union of Biochemistry attempted to remedy the situation by proposing the International Unit for enzymes. This unit was defined as the amount of enzyme that will catalyze the conversion of 1 micromole of substrate per minute under standard conditions. Difficulties remain, however, as enzyme activity is affected by the temperature, pH, the type and amount of substrate, the presence of inhibitors, and other factors. Enzyme activity can be expressed in S.I. Units, and the katal has been proposed to express activities of all catalysts, including enzymes. The katal is that amount of enzyme that catalyzes a reaction rate of 1 mole per second. Thus, adoption of the katal as the unit of enzyme activity would provide no more information than is obtained when results are expressed in International Units.

Hydrogen ion concentration in blood is customarily expressed as pH, but in S.I. Units it would be expressed in nanomoles per liter. It appears unlikely that the very useful pH scale will be discarded.

Pressure measures, such as blood pressure and partial pressures of blood gases, would be expressed in S.I. Units using the Pascal, a unit that can be derived from the basic units for mass, length, and time. This change probably will not be adopted in the early phases of the conversion to S.I. Units. Similarly, a proposed change in expressing osmolality in terms of the depression of freezing point is inappropriate, because osmolality may be calculated from vapor pressure as well as freezing point measurement.

Conventions

A number of conventions have been adopted to standardize usage of S.I. Units:

1. No periods are used after the symbol for a unit (kg not kg.), and it remains unchanged when used in the plural (70 kg not 70 kgs).
2. A half space rather than a comma is used to divide large numbers into groups of three (5 400 000 not 5,400,000).
3. Compound prefixes should be avoided (nanometer not millimicrometer).
4. Multiples and submultiples are used in steps of 10^3 or 10^{-3}.
5. The degree sign for the temperature scales is omitted (38 C not 38°C).
6. The preferred spelling is metre not meter, litre not liter.
7. Report of a measurement should include infor-

mation on the system, the component, the kind of quantity, the numerical value, and the unit. For example: *System,* serum. *Component,* glucose. *Kind of quantity,* substance concentration. *Value,* 5.10. *Unit,* mmol/l.

8. The name of the component should be unambiguous; for example, "serum bilirubin" might refer to unconjugated bilirubin or to total bilirubin. For acids and bases, the maximally ionized form is used in naming the component; for example, lactate or urate rather than lactic acid or uric acid.

Tables of Reference Values

Tables accompanying this article indicate "normal values" for most of the commonly performed laboratory tests. The title of the tables has been changed from the "normal values" of previous years to "reference values" to conform to current usage. The reference value is given in conventional units, and the **value in S.I. Units is calculated from these figures. Notes (page 1322) provide additional information.**

REFERENCE VALUES IN HEMATOLOGY

	Conventional Units		S.I. Units		Notes
Acid hemolysis test (Ham)	No hemolysis		No hemolysis		
Alkaline phosphatase, leukocyte	Total score 14–100		Total score 14–100		
Carboxyhemoglobin	Up to 5% of total		0.05 of total		a
Cell counts					
Erythrocytes					
Males	4.6–6.2 million/cu. mm.		$4.6–6.2 \times 10^{12}/l$		
Females	4.2–5.4 million/cu. mm.		$4.2–5.4 \times 10^{12}/l$		
Children (varies with age)	4.5–5.1 million/cu. mm.		$4.5–5.1 \times 10^{12}/l$		
Leukocytes					
Total	4500–11,000/cu. mm.		$4.5–11.0 \times 10^{9}/l$		
Differential	*Percentage*	*Absolute*			
Myelocytes	0	0/cu. mm.	0/1		b
Band neutrophils	3–5	150–400/cu. mm.	$150–400 \times 10^{6}/l$		
Segmented neutrophils	54–62	3000–5800/cu. mm.	$3000–5800 \times 10^{6}/l$		
Lymphocytes	25–33	1500–3000/cu. mm.	$1500–3000 \times 10^{6}/l$		
Monocytes	3–7	300–500/cu. mm.	$300–500 \times 10^{6}/l$		
Eosinophils	1–3	50–250/cu. mm.	$50–250 \times 10^{6}/l$		
Basophils	0–0.75	15–50/cu. mm.	$15–50 \times 10^{6}/l$		
Platelets	150,000–350,000/cu. mm.		$150–350 \times 10^{9}/l$		
Reticulocytes	25,000–75,000/cu. mm. 0.5–1.5% of erythrocytes		$25–75 \times 10^{9}/l$		b
Bone marrow, differential cell count					
	Range	*Average*	*Range*	*Average*	
Myeloblasts	0.3–5.0%	2.0%	0.003–0.05	0.02	a
Promyelocytes	1.0–8.0%	5.0%	0.01–0.08	0.05	
Myelocytes: Neutrophilic	5.0–19.0%	12.0%	0.05–0.19	0.12	
Eosinophilic	0.5–3.0%	1.5%	0.005–0.03	0.015	
Basophilic	0.0–0.5%	0.3%	0.00–0.005	0.003	
Metamyelocytes	13.0–32.0%	22.0%	0.13–0.32	0.22	
Polymorphonuclear neutrophils	7.0–30.0%	20.0%	0.07–0.30	0.20	
Polymorphonuclear eosinophils	0.5–4.0%	2.0%	0.005–0.04	0.02	
Polymorphonuclear basophilis	0.0–0.7%	0.2%	0.00–0.007	0.002	
Lymphocytes	3.0–17.0%	10.0%	0.03–0.17	0.10	
Plasma cells	0.0–2.0%	0.4%	0.00–0.02	0.004	
Monocytes	0.5–5.0%	2.0%	0.005–0.05	0.02	
Reticulum cells	0.1–2.0%	0.2%	0.001–0.02	0.002	
Megakaryocytes	0.3–3.0%	0.4%	0.003–0.03	0.004	
Pronormoblasts	1.0–8.0%	4.0%	0.01–0.08	0.04	
Normoblasts	7.0–32.0%	18.0%	0.07–0.32	0.18	
Coagulation tests					
Antithrombin III (synthetic substrate)	80–120% of normal		0.8–1.2 of normal		
Bleeding time (Duke)	1–5 min.		1–5 min		
Bleeding time (Ivy)	Less than 5 min.		Less than 5 min		
Bleeding time (Template)	2.5–9.5 min.		2.5–9.5 min		
Clot retraction, qualitative	Begins in 30–60 min. Complete in 24 hrs.		Begins in 30–60 min Complete in 24 h		

Coagulation time (Lee-White)	5–15 min. (glass tubes) 19–60 min. (siliconized tubes)	5–15 min (glass tubes) 19–60 min (siliconized tubes)	
Euglobulin lysis time	2–6 hr. at 37°	2–6 h at 37 C	
Factor VIII and other coagulation factors	50–150% of normal	0.50–1.5 of normal	a
Fibrin split products (Thrombo-Wellco test)	Less than 10 mcg./ml.	Less than 10 mg/l	
Fibrinogen	200–400 mg./dl.	5.9–11.7 μmol/l	c
Fibrinolysins	0	0	
Partial thromboplastin time, activated (APTT)	20–35 sec.	20–35 sec.	
Prothrombin consumption	Over 80% consumed in 1 hr.	Over 0.80 consumed in 1 h	a
Prothrombin content	100% (calculated from prothrombin time)	1.0 (calculated from prothrombin time)	a
Prothrombin time (one stage)	12.0–14.0 sec.	12.0–14.0 s	
Tourniquet test	Ten or fewer petechiae in a 2.5 cm. circle after 5 min.	Ten or fewer petechiae in a 2.5 cm circle after 5 min	
Cold hemolysin test (Donath-Landsteiner)	No hemolysis	No hemolysis	
Coombs' test			
Direct	Negative	Negative	
Indirect	Negative	Negative	
Corpuscular values of erythrocytes (values are for adults; in children, values vary with age)			
M.C.H. (mean corpuscular hemoglobin)	27–31 picogm.	0.42–0.48 fmol	d
M.C.V. (mean corpuscular volume)	80–96 cu. micra	80–96 fl	
M.C.H.C. (mean corpuscular hemoglobin concentration)	32–36%	0.32–0.36	a
Haptoglobin (as hemoglobin binding capacity)	100–200 mg./dl.	16–31 μmol/l	d
Hematocrit			
Males	40–54 ml./dl.	0.40–0.54	a
Females	37–47 ml./dl.	0.37–0.47	
Newborn	49–54 ml.dl.	0.49–0.54	
Children (varies with age)	35–49 ml./dl.	0.35–0.49	
Hemoglobin			
Males	14.0–18.0 grams/dl.	2.17–2.79 mmol/l	d
Females	12.0–16.0 grams/dl.	1.86–2.48 mmol/l	
Newborn	16.5–19.5 grams/dl.	2.56–3.02 mmol/l	
Children (varies with age)	11.2–16.5 grams/dl.	1.74–2.56 mmol/l	
Hemoglobin, fetal	Less than 1% of total	Less than 0.01 of total	a
Hemoglobin A_{1c}	3–5% of total	0.03–0.05 of total	a
Hemoglobin A_2	1.5–3.0% of total	0.015–0.03 of total	a
Hemoglobin, plasma	0–5.0 mg./dl.	0–0.8 μmol/l	d
Methemoglobin	0–130 mg./dl.	4.7–20 μmol/l	e
Osmotic fragility of erythrocytes	Begins in 0.45–0.39% NaCl Complete in 0.33–0.30% NaCl	Begins in 77–67 mmol/l NaCl Complete in 56–51 mmol/l NaCl	
Sedimentation rate			
Wintrobe: Males	0–5 mm. in 1 hr.	0–5 mm/h	
Females	0–15 mm. in 1 hr.	0–15 mm/h	
Westergren: Male	0–15 mm. in 1 hr.	0–15 mm/h	
Females	0–20 mm. in 1 hr.	0–20 mm/h	
(May be slightly higher in children and during pregnancy)			

Table continued on following page

REFERENCE VALUES FOR BLOOD, PLASMA AND SERUM

(For some procedures the reference values may vary depending upon the method used)

	Conventional Units	S.I. Units	Notes
Acetoacetate plus acetone, serum			
Qualitative	Negative	Negative	
Quantitative	0.3–2.0 mg./dl.	3–20 mg/l	
Adrenocorticotropin (ACTH), plasma			
6 A.M.	10–80 picogm./ml.	10–80 ng/l	
6 P.M.	Less than 50 picogm./ml.	Less than 50 ng/l	
Alanine aminotransferase *see* Transaminase			
Aldolase, serum	0–11 milliunits/ml. (30°)	0–11 units/l (30 C)	f
Aldosterone			
Adult, supine	3–10 ng./dl.	0.08–0.3 nmol/l	
standing			
male	6–22 ng./dl.	0.17–0.61 nmol/l	
female	5–30 ng./dl.	0.14–0.8 nmol/l	
Alpha amino nitrogen, serum	3.0–5.5 mg./dl.	2.1–3.9 mmol/l	
Ammonia (nitrogen), plasma	15–49 mcg./dl.	11–35 μmol/l	
Amylase, serum	25–125 milliunits/ml.	25–125 units/l	
Anion gap	8–16 mEq./l.	8–16 mmol/l	
Ascorbic acid, blood	0.4–1.5 mg./dl.	23–85 μmol/l	
Aspartate aminotransferase *see* Transaminase			
Base excess, blood	0 ± 2 mEq./liter	0 ± 2 mmol/l	
Bicarbonate, serum	23–29 mEq./liter	23–29 mmol/l	
Bile acids, serum	0.3–3.0 mg./dl.	3.0–30.0 mg/l	
Bilirubin, serum			
Direct	0.1–0.4 mg./dl.	1.7–6.8 μmol/l	
Indirect	0.2–0.7 mg./dl. (Total minus direct)	3.4–12 μmol/l (Total minus direct)	
Total	0.3–1.1 mg./dl.	5.1–19 μmol/l	
Calcium, serum	4.5–5.5 mEq./liter 9.0–11.0 mg./dl. (Slightly higher in children) (Varies with protein concentration)	2.25–2.75 mmol/l (Slightly higher in children) (Varies with protein concentration)	a
Calcium, ionized, serum	2.1–2.6 mEq./liter 4.25–5.25 mg./dl.	1.05–1.30 mmol/l	
Carbon dioxide content, serum			
Adults	24–30 mEq./liter	24–30 mmol/l	
Infants	20–28 mEq./liter	20–28 mmol/l	
Carbon dioxide tension (P_{CO_2}), blood	35–45 mm. Hg	35–45 mm Hg	g
Carotene, serum	40–200 mcg./dl.	0.74–3.72 μmol/l	
Ceruloplasmin, serum	23–44 mg./dl.	230–440 mg./l	h
Chloride, serum	96–106 mEq./liter	96–106 mmol/l	
Cholesterol, serum			
Total	150–250 mg./dl.	3.9–6.5 mmol/l	
Esters	68–76% of total cholesterol	0.68–0.76 of total cholesterol	a

Cholinesterase			
Serum	0.5–1.3 pH units	0.5–1.3 pH units	f
Erythrocytes	0.5–1.0 pH unit	0.5–1.0 pH unit	f
Copper, serum			
Males	70–140 mcg./dl.	11–22 μmol/l	
Females	85–155 mcg./dl.	13–24 μmol/l	
Cortisol, plasma			
(8 A.M.)	6–23 mcg./dl.	170–635 nmol/l	
(4 P.M.)	3–15 mcg./dl.	82–413 nmol/l	
(10 P.M.)	Less than 50% of 8 A.M. value	Less than 0.5 of 8 A.M. value	
Creatine, serum	0.2–0.8 mg./dl.	15–61 μmol/l	
Creatine kinase, serum (CK, CPK)			
Males	12–80 milliunits/ml. (30°)	12–80 units/l (30 C)	f
	55–170 milliunits/ml. (37°)	55–170 units/l (37 C)	f
Females	10–55 milliunits/ml. (30°)	10–55 units/l (30 C)	f
	30–135 milliunits/ml. (37°)	30–135 units/l (37 C)	f
Creatine kinase isoenzymes, serum			
CK-MM	Present	Present	
CK-MB	Absent	Absent	
CK-BB	Absent	Absent	
Creatinine, serum	0.6–1.2 mg./dl.	53–106 μmol/l	
Cryoglobulins, serum	0	0	
Fatty acids, total, serum	190–420 mg./dl.	7–15 mmol/l	i
nonesterified, serum	8–25 mg./dl.	0.30–0.90 mmol/l	
Ferritin, serum	20–200 nanogm./ml.	20–200 μg/l	
Fibrinogen, plasma	200–400 mg./100 ml.	5.9–11.7 μmol/l	c
Folate, serum	1.8–9.0 nanogm./ml.	4.1–20.4 nmol/l	
Erythrocytes	150–450 nanogm./ml.	340–1020 nmol/l	
Follicle-stimulating hormone (FSH), plasma			
Males	4–25 milliunits/ml. (I.U.)	4–25 IU/l	
Females	4–30 milliunits/ml. (I.U.)	4–30 IU/l	
Postmenopausal	40–250 milliunits/ml. (I.U.)	40–250 IU/l	
Gamma glutamyltransferase			
Males	6–32 milliunits/ml. (30°)	6–32 units/l (30 C)	f
Females	4–18 milliunits/ml. (30°)	4–18 units/l (30 C)	f
Gastrin, serum	0–200 picogm./ml.	0–200 ng/l	
Glucose (fasting)			
Blood	60–100 mg./dl.	3.33–5.55 mmol/l	
Plasma or serum	70–115 mg./dl.	3.89–6.38 mmol/l	
Growth hormone, serum	0–10 nanogm./ml.	0–10 μg/l	
Haptoglobin, serum	100–200 mg./dl.	16–31 μmol/l	d
	(As hemoglobin binding capacity)	(As hemoglobin binding capacity)	
Hydroxybutyric dehydrogenase, serum (HBD)	0–180 milliunits/ml. (30°)	0–180 units/l (30 C)	f
17-Hydroxycorticosteroids, plasma	8–18 mcg./dl.	0.22–0.50 μmol/l	j
Immunoglobins, serum			
IgG	550–1900 mg./dl.	5.5–19.0 g/l	
IgA	60–333 mg./dl.	0.60–3.3 g/l	
IgM	45–145 mg./dl.	0.45–1.5 g/l	
IgD	0.5–3.0 mg./dl.	5–30 mg/l	
IgE	<500 nanogm./ml.	<500 μg/l	
	(Varies with age in children)	(Varies with age in children)	

Table continued on following page.

REFERENCE VALUES FOR BLOOD, PLASMA AND SERUM (*continued*)

(For some procedures the reference values may vary depending upon the method used)

	Conventional Units	S.I. Units	Notes
Insulin, plasma (fasting)	5–25 microunits/ml.	5–25 milliunits/l	
Iodine, protein bound, serum	3.5–8.0 mcg./dl.	0.28–0.63 μmol/l	k
Iron, serum	75–175 mcg./dl.	13–31 μmol/l	
Iron binding capacity, serum			
Total	250–410 mcg./dl.	45–73 μmol/l	
Saturation	20–55%	0.20–0.55	a
Lactate, blood, venous	4.5–19.8 mg./dl.	0.5–2.2 mmol/l	
arterial	4.5–14.4 mg./dl.	0.5–1.6 mmol/l	
Lactate dehydrogenase, serum (LD, LDH)	45–90 milliunits/ml. (I.U.) (30°) 100–190 milliunits/ml. (37°)	45–90 units/l (30 C) 100–190 milliunits/ml (37 C)	f
LDH_1	22–37% of total	0.22–0.37 of total	a
LDH_2	30–46% of total	0.30–0.46 of total	
LDH_3	14–29% of total	0.14–0.29 of total	
LDH_4	5–11% of total	0.05–0.11 of total	
LDH_5	2–11% of total	0.02–0.11 of total	
Leucine aminopeptidase, serum	14–40 milliunits/ml. (30°)	14–40 units/l (30 C)	f
Lipase, serum	0–1.5 units (Cherry-Crandall)	0–1.5 units (Cherry-Crandall)	f
Lipids, total, serum	450–850 mg./dl.	4.5–8.5 g/l	m
Lipoprotein cholesterol, serum			
LDL cholesterol	60–180 mg./dl.	600–1800 mg/l	
HDL cholesterol	30–80 mg./dl.	300–800 mg/l	
Luteinizing hormone (LH), serum			
Males	6–18 milliunits/ml. (I.U.)	6–18 IU/l	
Females, premenopausal	5–22 milliunits/ml. (I.U.)	5–22 IU/l	
midcycle	3 times baseline	3 times baseline	
postmenopausal	Greater than 30 milliunits/ml. (I.U.)	Greater than 30 IU/l	
Magnesium, serum	1.5–2.5 mEq./liter 1.8–3.0 mg./dl.	0.75–1.25 mmol/l	
5′-Nucleotidase, serum	3.5–12.7 milliunits/ml. (37°)	3.5–12.5 units/l (37 C)	f
Nitrogen, nonprotein, serum	15–35 mg./dl.	10.7–25.0 mmol/l	
Osmolality, serum	285–295 mOsm./kg. serum water	285–295 mmol/kg serum water	n
Oxygen, blood			
Capacity	16–24 vol. % (varies with hemoglobin)	7.14–10.7 mmol/l (varies with hemoglobin)	o
Content Arterial	15–23 vol. %	6.69–10.3 mmol/l	o
Venous	10–16 vol. %	4.46–7.14 mmol/l	o
Saturation Arterial	94–100% of capacity	0.94–1.00 of capacity	a
Venous	60–85% of capacity	0.60–0.85 of capacity	a
Tension, pO_2 Arterial	75–100 mm. Hg	75–100 mm Hg	g
P_{50}, blood	26–27 mm. Hg	26–27 mm. Hg	g
pH, arterial, blood	7.35–7.45	7.35–7.45	p
Phenylalanine, serum	Less than 3 mg./dl.	Less than 0.18 mmol/l	
Phosphatase, acid, serum	0.11–0.60 milliunits/ml. (37°) (Roy, Brower, Hayden)	0.11–0.60 units/l	f
Phosphatase, alkaline, serum (ALP)	20–90 milliunits/ml. (30°) (Values are higher in children)	20–90 units/l (30 C) (Values are higher in children)	f
Phosphate, inorganic, serum			
Adults	3.0–4.5 mg./dl.	1.0–1.5 mmol/l	
Children	4.0–7.0 mg./dl.	1.3–2.3 mmol/l	

Phospholipids, serum	6–12 mg./dl.	1.9–3.9 mmol/l	
	(As lipid phosphorus)	(As lipid phosphorus)	
Potassium, serum	3.5–5.0 mEq./liter	3.5–5.0 mmol/l	
Prolactin, serum			
Males	1–20 nanogm./ml.	1–20 μg/l	
Females	1–25 nanogm./ml.	1–25 μg/l	
Protein, serum			
Total	6.0–8.0 grams/dl.	60–80 g/l	m
Albumin	3.5–5.5 grams/dl.	35–55 g/l	q
	52–68% of total	0.52–0.68 of total	a
Globulin			
Alpha$_1$	0.2–0.4 gram/dl.	2–4 g/l	m
	2–5% of total	0.02–0.05 of total	a
Alpha$_2$	0.5–0.9 gram/dl.	5–9 g/l	m
	7–14% of total	0.07–0.14 of total	a
Beta	0.6–1.1 grams/dl.	6–11 g/l	m
	9–15% of total	0.09–0.15 of total	a
Gamma	0.7–1.7 grams/dl.	7–17 g/l	m
	11–21% of total	0.11–0.21 of total	a
Protoporphyrin, erythrocyte	27–61 mcg./dl. packed RBC	0.48–1.09 μmol/l packed RBC	
Pyruvate, blood	0.3–0.9 mg./dl.	0.03–0.10 mmol/l	
Sodium, serum	136–145 mEq./liter	136–145 mmol/l	
Sulfates, inorganic, serum	0.8–1.2 mg./dl.	83–125 μmol/l	
Testosterone, plasma			
Males	275–875 nanogm./dl.	9.5–30 nmol/l	
Females	23–75 nanogm./dl.	0.8–2.6 nmol/l	
Pregnant	38–190 nanogm./dl.	1.3–6.6 nmol/l	
Thyroid-stimulating hormone (TSH), serum	0–7 microunits/ml.	0–7 milliunits/l	
Thyroxine, free, serum	1.0–2.1 nanogm./dl.	13–27 pmol/l	
Thyroxine (T_4), serum	4.4–9.9 mcg./dl.	57–128 nmol/l	
Thyroxine binding globulin (TBG), serum (as thyroxine)	10–26 mcg./dl.	129–335 nmol/l	
Thyroxine iodine, serum	2.9–6.4 mcg./dl.	229–504 nmol/l	k
Tri-iodothyronine (T_3), serum	150–250 nanogm./dl.	2.3–3.9 nmol/l	
Tri-iodothyronine (T_3) uptake, resin (T_3RU)	25–38%	0.25–0.38 uptake	a
Transaminase, serum			
SGOT (aspartate aminotransferase, AST)	8–20 milliunits/ml. (30°)	8–20 units/l (30 C)	
	7–40 milliunits/ml. (37°)	7–40 units/l (37 C)	
SGPT (alanine aminotransferase, ALT)	8–20 milliunits/ml. (30°)	8–20 units/l (30 C)	f
	5–35 milliunits/ml. (37°)	5–35 units/l (37 C)	f
Triglycerides, serum	40–150 mg./dl.	0.4–1.5 g/l	r
		0.45–1.71 mmol/l	
Urate, serum			
Males	2.5–8.0 mg/dl.	0.15–0.48 mmol/l	
Females	1.5–7.0 mg./dl.	0.09–0.42 mmol/l	
Urea			
Blood	21–43 mg./dl.	3.5–7.2 mmol/l	
Plasma or serum	24–49 mg./dl.	4.0–8.2 mmol/l	
Urea nitrogen			
Blood	10–20 mg./dl.	7.1–14.3 mmol/l	k
Plasma or serum	11–23 mg./dl.	7.9–16.4 mmol/l	
Viscosity, serum	1.4–1.8 times water	1.4–1.8 times water	
Vitamin A, serum	20–80 mcg./dl.	0.70–2.8 μmol/l	
Vitamin B_{12}, serum	180–900 picogm./ml.	133–664 pmol/l	

REFERENCE VALUES FOR URINE

(For some procedures the reference values may vary depending upon the method used)

	Conventional Units	S.I. Units	Notes
Acetone and acetoacetate, qualitative	Negative	Negative	
Albumin			
Qualitative	Negative	Negative	
Quantitative	10–100 mg./24 hrs.	10–100 mg/24 h 0.15–1.5 µmol/24 h	q
Aldosterone	3–20 mcg./24 hrs.	8.3–55 nmol/24 h	
Alpha amino nitrogen	50–200 mg./24 hrs.	3.6–14.3 mmol/24 h	
Ammonia nitrogen	20–70 mEq./24 hrs.	20–70 mmol/24 h	
Amylase	1–17 units/hr.	1–17 units/h	
Amylase/creatinine clearance ratio	1–4%	0.01–0.04	f
Bilirubin, qualitative	Negative	Negative	
Calcium			
Low Ca diet	Less than 150 mg./24 hrs.	Less than 3.8 mmol/24 h	
Usual diet	Less than 250 mg./24 hrs.	Less than 6.3 mmol/24 h	
Catecholamines			
Epinephrine	Less than 10 mcg./24 hrs.	Less than 55 nmol/24 h	
Norepinephrine	Less than 100 mcg./24 hrs.	Less than 590 nmol/24 h	
Total free catecholamines	4–126 mcg./24 hrs.	24–745 nmol/24 h	s
Total metanephrines	0.1–1.6 mg./24 hrs.	0.5–8.1 µmol/24 h	t
Chloride	110–250 mEq./24 hrs. (Varies with intake)	110–250 mmol/24 h (Varies with intake)	
Chorionic gonadotropin	0	0	
Copper	0–50 mcg./24 hrs.	0–0.80 µmol/24 h	
Cortisol, free	10–100 mcg./24 hrs.	27.6–276 mmol/24 h	
Creatine			
Males	0–40 mg./24 hrs.	0–0.30 mmol/24 h	
Females	0–100 mg./24 hrs. (Higher in children and during pregnancy)	0–0.76 mmol/24 h (Higher in children and during pregnancy)	
Creatinine	15–25 mg./kg. body weight/24 hrs.	0.13–0.22 mmol · kg^{-1} body weight/24 h	
Creatinine clearance			
Males	110–150 ml./min.	110–150 ml/min	
Females	105–132 ml./min. (1.73 sq. meter surface area)	105–132 ml/min (1.73 m^2 surface area)	
Cystine or cysteine, qualitative	Negative	Negative	
Dehydroepiandrosterone	Less than 15% of total 17-ketosteroids	Less than 0.15 of total 17-ketosteroids	a
Males	0.2–2.0 mg./24 hr.	0.7–6.9 µm/24 h	
Females	0.2–1.8 mg./24 hr.	0.7–6.2 µm/24 h	
Delta aminolevulinic acid	1.3–7.0 mg./24 hrs.	10–53 µmol/24 h	
Estrogens			
Males			
Estrone	3–8 µg./24 hrs.	11–30 nmol/24 h	
Estradiol	0–6 µg./24 hrs.	0–22 nmol/24 h	
Estriol	1–11 µg./24 hrs.	3–38 nmol/24 h	
Total	4–25 µg./24 hrs.	14–90 nmol/24 h	u
Females			
Estrone	4–31 µg./24 hrs.	15–115 nmol/24 h	
Estradiol	0–14 µg./24 hrs.	0–51 nmol/24 h	
Estriol	0–72 µg./24 hrs.	0–250 nmol/24 h	
Total	5–100 µg./24 hrs. (Markedly increased during pregnancy)	18–360 nmol/24 h (Markedly increased during pregnancy)	u

Glucose (as reducing substance)	Less than 250 mg./24 hrs.	Less than 250 mg/24 h	
Hemoglobin and myoglobin, qualitative	Negative	Negative	
Homogentisic acid, qualitative	Negative	Negative	
17-Hydroxycorticosteroids			
Males	3–9 mg./24 hrs.	8.3–25 μmol/24 h	j
Females	2–8 mg./24 hrs.	5.5–22 μmol/24 h	
5-Hydroxyindoleacetic acid			
Qualitative	Negative	Negative	
Quantitative	Less than 9 mg./24 hrs.	Less than 47 μmol/24 h	
17-Ketosteroids			
Males	6–18 mg./24 hrs.	21–62 μmol/24 h	l
Females	4–13 mg./24 hrs.	14–45 μmol/24 h	
	(Varies with age)	(Varies with age)	
Magnesium	6.0–8.5 mEq./24 hrs.	3.0–4.3 mmol/24 h	
Metanephrines (see Catecholamines)			
Osmolality	38–1400 mOsm./kg. water	38–1400 mmol/kg water	n
pH	4.6–8.0, average 6.0	4.6–8.0, average 6.0	p
	(Depends on diet)	(Depends on diet)	
Phenolsulfonphthalein excretion (PSP)	25% or more in 15 min.	0.25 or more in 15 min	a
	40% or more in 30 min.	0.40 or more in 30 min	
	55% or more in 2 hrs.	0.55 or more in 2 h	
	(After injection of 1 ml PSP intravenously)	(After injection of 1 ml PSP intravenously)	
Phenylpyruvic acid, qualitative	Negative	Negative	
Phosphorus	0.9–1.3 gm./24 hrs.	29–42 mmol/24 h	
Porphobilinogen			
Qualitative	Negative	Negative	
Quantitative	0–0.2 mg./dl.	0–0.9 μmol/l	
	Less than 2.0 mg./24 hrs.	Less than 9 μmol/24 h	
Porphyrins			
Coproporphyrin	50–250 mcg./24 hrs.	77–380 nmol/24 h	
Uroporphyrin	10–30 mcg./24 hrs.	12–36 nmol/24 h	
Potassium	25–100 mEq./24 hrs.	25–100 mmol/24 h	
	(Varies with intake)	(Varies with intake)	
Pregnanediol			
Males	0.4–1.4 mg./24 hrs.	1.2–4.4 μmol/24 h	
Females			
Proliferative phase	0.5–1.5 mg./24 hrs.	1.6–4.7 μmol/24 h	
Luteal phase	2.0–7.0 mg./24 hrs.	6.2–22 μmol/24 h	
Postmenopausal phase	0.2–1.0 mg./24 hrs.	0.6–3.1 μmol/24 h	
Pregnanetriol	Less than 2.5 mg./24 hrs. in adults	Less than 7.4 μmol/24 h in adults	
Protein			
Qualitative	Negative	Negative	
Quantitative	10–150 mg./24 hrs.	10–150 mg/24 h	m
Sodium	130–260 mEq./24 hrs.	130–260 mmol/24 h	
	(Varies with intake)	(Varies with intake)	
Specific gravity	1.003–1.030	1.003–1.030	
Titratable acidity	20–40 mEq./24 hrs.	20–40 mmol/24 h	
Urate	200–500 mg./24 hrs.	1.2–3.0 mmol/24 h	
	(With normal diet)	(With normal diet)	
Urobilinogen	Up to 1.0 Ehrlich unit/2 hrs.	Up to 1.0 Ehrlich unit/2 h	
	(1–3 P.M.)	(1–3 P.M.)	
	0–4.0 mg./24 hrs.	0–4.0 mg/24 h	
Vanillylmandelic acid (VMA) (4-hydroxy-3-methoxymandelic acid)	1–8 mg./24 hrs.	5–40 μmol/24 h	

REFERENCE VALUES FOR THERAPEUTIC DRUG MONITORING

Drug	Therapeutic Range	Toxic Levels	Proprietary Names
Antibiotics			
Amikacin, serum	15–25 mcg./ml.	Peak: >35 mcg./ml. Trough: > 5–8 mcg./ml.	Amikin
Chloramphenicol, serum	10–20 mcg./ml.	>25 mcg./ml.	Chloromycetin
Gentamicin, serum	5–10 mcg./ml.	Peak: >12 mcg./ml. Trough: >2 mcg./ml.	Garamycin
Tobramycin, serum	5–10 mcg./ml.	Peak: >12 mcg./ml. Trough: >2 mcg./ml.	Nebcin
Anticonvulsants			
Carbamazepine, serum	5–12 mcg./ml.	> 12 mcg./ml.	Tegretol
Ethosuximide, serum	40–100 mcg./ml.	> 100 mcg./ml.	Zarontin
Phenobarbital, serum	10–30 mcg./ml.	Vary widely because of developed tolerance	
Phenytoin, serum (diphenylhydantoin)	10–20 mcg./ml.	>20 mcg./ml.	Dilantin
Primidone, serum	5–12 mcg./ml.	>15 mcg./ml.	Mysoline
Valproic acid, serum	50–100 mcg./ml.	> 100 mcg./ml.	Depakene
Analgesics			
Acetaminophen, serum	10–20 mcg./mlds.	>250 mcg./ml.	Tylenol Datril
Salicylate, serum	100–250 mcg./ml.	>300 mcg./ml.	
Bronchodilator			
Theophylline (aminophylline)	10–20 mcg./ml.	>20 mcg./ml.	
Cardiovascular drugs			
Digitoxin, serum	15–25 nanogm./ml. (Specimen obtained 12–24 hrs. after last dose)	>25 nanogm./ml.	Crystodigin
Digoxin, serum	0.8–2 nanogm./ml. (Specimen obtained 12–24 hrs. after last dose)	>2.4 nanogm./ml.	Lanoxin

Disopyramide, serum	2–5 mcg./ml.	>5 mcg./ml.	Norpace
Lidocaine, serum	1.5–5 mcg./ml.	>5 nanogm./ml.	Anestacon Xylocaine
Procainamide, serum	4–10 mcg./ml. *10–30 mcg./ml. (*Procainamide + N-Acetyl Procainamide)	>16 mcg./ml. *>30 mcg./ml.	Pronestyl
Propranolol, serum	50–100 nanogm./ml.	Variable	Inderal
Quinidine, serum	2–5 mcg./ml.	>10 mcg./ml.	Cardioquin Quinaglute Quinidex Quinora
Psychopharmacologic drugs			
Amitriptyline, serum	*120–150 nanogm./ml. (*Amitriptyline + Nortriptyline)	*>500 nanogm./ml.	Amitril Elavil Endep Etralon Limbitrol Triavil
Desipramine, serum	*150–300 nanogm./ml. (*Desipramine + Imipramine)	*>500 nanogm./ml.	Norpramin Pertofrane
Imipramine, serum	*150–300 nanogm./ml. (*Imipramine + Desipramine)	*>500 nanogm./ml.	Antipress Imavate Janimine Presamine Trofranil
Lithium, serum	0.8–1.2 mEq./liter (Specimen obtained 12 hrs. after last dose)	>2.0 mEq./liter	Lithobid Lithotabs
Nortriptyline, serum	50–150 nanogm./ml.	>500 nanogm./ml.	Aventyl Pamelor

REFERENCE VALUES IN TOXICOLOGY

	Conventional Units	S.I. Units	Notes
Arsenic, blood	3.5–7.2 mcg./dl.	0.47–0.96 μmol/l	
Arsenic, urine	Less than 100 mcg./24 hrs.	Less than 1.3 μmol/24 h	
Bromides, serum	0	0	
	Toxic levels: Above 17 mmol/l	Toxic levels: Above 17 mmol/l	
Carbon monoxide, blood	Up to 5% saturation	Up to 0.05 saturation	
	Symptoms occur with 20% saturation	Symptoms occur with 0.20 saturation	a
Ethanol, blood	Less than 0.005%	Less than 1 mmol/l	
Marked intoxication	0.3–0.4%	65–87 mmol/l	
Alcoholic stupor	0.4–0.5% mcg./dl.	87–109 mmol/l	
Coma	Above 0.5%	Above 109 mmol/l	
Lead, blood	0–40 mcg./dl.	0–2 μmol/l	
Lead, urine	Less than 100 mcg./24 hrs.	Less than 0.48 μmol/24 h	
Mercury, urine	Less than 10 mcg./24 hrs.	Less than 50 nmol/24 h	

REFERENCE VALUES FOR CEREBROSPINAL FLUID

	Conventional Units	S.I. Units	Notes
Cells	Fewer than 5/cu. mm.; all mononuclear	Fewer than 5/μl; all mononuclear	
Chloride	120–130 mEq./liter	120–130 mmol/l	
	(20 mEq./liter higher than serum)	(20 mmol/l higher than serum)	
Electrophoresis	Predominantly albumin	Predominantly albumin	
Glucose	50–75 mg./dl.	2.8–4.2 mmol/l	
	(20 mg./dl. less than serum)	(1.1 mmol/l less than serum)	
IgG			
Children under 14	Less than 8% of total protein	Less than 0.08 of total protein	a,m
Adults	Less than 14% of total protein	Less than 0.14 of total protein	
Pressure	70–180 mm. water	70–180 mm water	g
Protein, total	15–45 mg./dl.	0.150–0.450 g/l	m
	(Higher, up to 70 mg./dl., in elderly adults and children)	(Higher, up to 0.70 g/l, in elderly adults and children)	

REFERENCE VALUES FOR GASTRIC ANALYSIS

	Conventional Units	S.I. Units	Notes
Basal gastric secretion (1 hour)			
Concentration	(Mean ± 1 S.D.)	(Mean ± 1 S.D.)	
Males	25.8 ± 1.8 mEq./liter	25.8 ± 1.8 mmol/l	
Females	20.3 ± 3.0 mEq./liter	20.3 ± 3.0 mmol/l	
Output	(Mean ± 1 S.D.)	(Mean ± 1 S.D.)	
Males	2.57 ± 0.16 mEq./hr.	2.57 ± 0.16 mmol/h	
Females	1.61 ± 0.18 mEq./hr.	1.61 ± 0.18 mmol/h	
After histamine stimulation			
Normal	Mean output 11.8 mEq./hr.	Mean output 11.8 mmol/h	
Duodenal ulcer	Mean output 15.2 mEq./hr.	Mean output 15.2 mmol/h	
After maximal histamine stimulation			
Normal	Mean output 22.6 mEq./hr.	Mean output 22.6 mmol/h	
Duodenal ulcer	Mean output 44.6 mEq./hr.	Mean output 44.6 mmol/h	
Diagnex blue (Squibb): Anacidity	0–0.3 mg. in 2 hrs.	0–0.03 mg in 2 h	
Doubtful	0.3–0.6 mg. in 2 hrs.	0.3–0.6 mg in 2 h	
Normal	Greater than 0.6 mg. in 2 hrs.	Greater than 0.6 mg in 2 h	
Volume, fasting stomach content	50–100 ml.	0.05–0.11	
Emptying time	3–6 hrs.	3–6 h	
Color	Opalescent or colorless	Opalescent or colorless	
Specific gravity	1.006–1.009	1.006–1.009	
pH (adults)	0.9–1.5	0.9–1.5	p

GASTROINTESTINAL ABSORPTION TESTS

	Conventional Units	S.I. Units	Notes
d/Xylose absorption test	After an 8 hour fast, 10 ml./kg. body weight of a 0.05 solution of d-xylose is given by mouth. Nothing further by mouth is given until the test has been completed. All urine voided during the following 5 hours is pooled, and blood samples are taken at 0, 60, and 120 minutes. Normally 0.26 (range 0.16–0.33) of ingested xylose is excreted within 5 hours, and the serum xylose reaches a level between 25 and 40 mg./100 ml. after 1 hour and is maintained at this level for another 60 minutes.	No change	
Vitamin A absorption	A fasting blood specimen is obtained and 200,000 units of vitamin A in oil is given by mouth. Serum vitamin A level should rise to twice fasting level in 3 to 5 hours.	No change	

REFERENCE VALUES FOR FECES

	Conventional Units	S.I. Units	Notes
Bulk	100–200 grams/24 hrs.	100–200 g/24 h	
Dry matter	23–32 grams/24 hrs.	23–32 g/24 h	
Fat, total	Less than 6.0 grams/24 hrs.	Less than 6.0 g/24 h	
Nitrogen, total	Less than 2.0 grams/24 hrs.	Less than 2.0 g/24 h	
Urobilinogen	40–280 mg./24 hrs.	40–280 mg/24 h	
Water	Approximately 65%	Approximately 0.65	a

REFERENCE VALUES FOR IMMUNOLOGIC PROCEDURES

	Conventional Units
Lymphocyte Subsets	
T cells	60–85%
B cells	1–20%
Helper cells	35–60%
Suppressor cells	15–30%
H/S ratio	1.5–2.5
Complement	
C3	85–175 mg./dl.
C4	15–45 mg./dl.
CH_{50}	25–55 H_{50} units/ml.
Tumor Markers	
Carcinoembryonic Antigen (CEA)	
(Roche)	Less than 5 nanog./ml.
(Abbott)	Less than 4.1 nanog./ml.
Alpha-fetoprotein (AFP)	Less than 10–30 nanog./ml. (depends on method)

REFERENCE VALUES FOR SEMEN ANALYSIS

	Conventional Units	S.I. Units	Notes
Volume	2–5 ml.; usually 3–4 ml.	2–5 ml; usually 3–4 ml	
Liquefaction	Complete in 15 min.	Complete in 15 min	
pH	7.2–8.0; average 7.8	7.2–8.0; average 7.8	p
Leukocytes	Occasional or absent	Occasional or absent	
Count	60–150 million/ml.	60–150 million/ml	
	Below 60 million/ml. is abnormal	Below 60 million/ml is abnormal	
Motility	80% or more motile	0.80 or more motile	a
Morphology	80–90% normal forms	0.80–0.90 normal forms	a

ORAL GLUCOSE TOLERANCE TEST

The oral glucose tolerance test (OGTT) may be unnecessary if the fasting plasma glucose concentration is elevated (venous plasma ≥140 mg/dl or 7.8 mmol/l) on two occasions. The OGTT should be carried out only on patients who are ambulatory and otherwise healthy and who are known not to be taking agents that elevate the plasma glucose (see reference 10). The test should be conducted in the morning after at least 3 days of unrestricted diet (≥150 grams of carbohydrate) and physical activity. The subject should have fasted for at least 10 hours but no more than 16 hours. Water is permitted during the test period; however, the subject should remain seated and should not smoke throughout the test.

The dose of glucose administered should be 75 grams (1.75 grams per kg of ideal body weight, up to a maximum of 75 grams for children). Commercial preparations containing a suitable carbohydrate load are acceptable. If criteria for gestational diabetes are used, a dose of 100 grams of glucose is required.

A fasting blood sample should be collected, after which the glucose dose is taken within 5 minutes. Blood samples should be collected at 30 minute intervals for 2 hours (for gestational diabetes fasting 1, 2 and 3 hours). The following diagnostic criteria have been recommended by the National Diabetes Data Group:

Normal OGTT in Nonpregnant Adults	Fasting venous plasma glucose <115 mg/dl (6.4 mmol/l) ½ h, 1 h, or 1½ h OGTT venous plasma glucose <200 mg/dl (11.1 mmol/l) 2 h OGTT venous plasma glucose <140 mg/dl (7.8 mmol/l)
Diabetes Mellitus in Nonpregnant Adults	Both the 2 hour sample *and* some other sample taken between administration of the 75 gram glucose dose and 2 hours later must show a venous plasma glucose ≥200 mg/dl (11.1 mmol/l)
Impaired Glucose Tolerance in Nonpregnant Adults	Three criteria must be met: Fasting venous plasma glucose <140 mg/dl (7.8 mmol/l) ½ h, 1 h, or 1½ h OGTT value ≥200 mg/dl (11.1 mmol/l) 2 h OGTT venous plasma glucose between 140 and 200 mg/dl (7.8 and 11.1 mmol/l)
Gestational Diabetes	Two or more of the following values after a 100 gram oral glucose challenge must be met or exceeded: (values are for venous plasma glucose) Fasting 105 mg/dl 5.8 mmol/l 1 h 190 mg/dl 10.6 mmol/l 2 h 165 mg/dl 9.2 mmol/l 3 h 145 mg/dl 8.1 mmol/l

NOTES

a. Percentage is expressed as a decimal fraction.
b. Percentage may be expressed as a decimal fraction; however, when the result expressed is itself a variable fraction of another variable, the absolute value is more meaningful. There is no reason, other than custom, for expressing reticulocyte counts and differential leukocyte counts in percentages or decimal fractions rather than in absolute numbers.
c. Molecular weight of fibrinogen = 341,000 daltons.
d. Molecular weight of hemoglobin = 64,500 daltons. Because of disagreement as to whether the monomer or tetramer of hemoglobin should be used in the conversion, it has been recommended that the conventional grams per deciliter be retained. The tetramer is used in the table; values given should be multiplied by 4 to obtain concentration of the monomer.
e. Molecular weight of methemoglobin = 64,500 daltons. See note d above.
f. Enzyme units have not been changed in these tables because the proposed enzyme unit, the katal, has not been universally adopted (1 International Unit = 16.7 nkat).
g. It has been proposed that pressure be expressed in the Pascal (1 mm Hg = 0.133 kPa); however, this convention has not been universally accepted.
h. Molecular weight of ceruloplasmin = 151,000.
i. "Fatty acids" includes a mixture of different aliphatic acids of varying molecular weight. A mean molecular weight of 284 has been assumed in calculating the conversion factor.
j. Based upon molecular weight of cortisol 362.47.
k. The practice of expressing concentration of an organic molecule in terms of one of its constituent elements originated when measurements included a heterogeneous class of compounds (nonprotein nitrogenous compounds, iodine-containing compounds bound to serum proteins). It was carried over to expressing measurements of specific substances (urea, thyroxine), but the practice should be discarded. For iodine and nitrogen 1 mole is taken as the monoatomic form, although they occur as diatomic molecules.
l. Based upon molecular weight of dehydroepiandrosterone 288.41.
m. Weight per volume is retained as the unit because of the heterogeneous nature of the material measured.
n. The proposal that osmolality be reported as freezing point depression using the millikelvin as the unit has not been received with universal enthusiasm. The milliosmole is not an S.I. unit, and the unit used here is the millimole.
o. Volumes per cent might be converted to a decimal fraction; however, this would not permit direct correlation with hemoglobin content, which is possible when oxygen content and capacity are expressed in molar quantities. One millimole of hemoglobin combines with 4 millimoles of oxygen.
p. Hydrogen ion concentration in S.I. units would be expressed in nanomoles per liter; however, this change has not received general approval. Conversion can be calculated as antilog (−pH).
q. Albumin is expressed in grams per liter to be consistent with units used for other proteins. Concentration of albumin may be expressed in mmol/l also, an expression that permits assessment of binding capacity of albumin for substances such as bilirubin. Molecular weight of albumin is 65,000.
r. Most techniques for quantitating triglycerides measure the glycerol moiety, and the total mass is calculated using an average molecular weight. The factor given assumes a mean molecular weight of 875 for triglycerides.
s. Calculated as norepinephrine, molecular weight 169.18.
t. Calculated as metanephrine, molecular weight 197.23.
u. Conversion factor calculated from molecular weights of estrone, estradiol, and estriol in proportions of 2:1:2.

REFERENCES

1. AMA Drug Evaluations, 4th ed. Chicago, American Medical Association, 1980.
2. Baron, D. N., Broughton, P. M. G., Cohen, M., Lansley, T. S., Lewis, S. M., and Shinton, N. K.: J. Clin. Path. *27*:590, 1974.
3. Dybkaer, R.: Am. J. Clin. Path. *52*:637, 1969.
4. Gilman, A. G., Goodman, L. S., and Gilman, A.: Pharmacologic Basis of Therapeutics, 6th ed. New York, Macmillan, 1980.
5. Henry, J. B.: Clinical Diagnosis and Management by Laboratory Methods, 17th ed. Philadelphia, W. B. Saunders Company, 1984.
6. Henry, R. J., Cannon, D. C., and Winkleman, J. W.: Clinical Chemistry—Principles and Techniques, 2nd ed. New York, Harper & Row, 1974.
7. International Committee for Standardization in Hematology, International Federation of Clinical Chemistry and World Association of Pathology Societies: Clin. Chem. *19*:135, 1973.
8. Lehmann, H. P.: Am. J. Clin. Path. *65*:2, 1976.
9. Miale, J. B.: Laboratory Medicine—Hematology, 6th ed. St. Louis, C. V. Mosby, 1982.
10. National Diabetes Data Group: Diabetes *28*:1039, 1979.
11. Page, C. H., and Vigourex, P.: The International System of Units (S.I.). U.S. Department of Commerce, National Bureau of Standards, Special Publication 330, 1974.
12. Physicians' Desk Reference. 38th ed. Oradell, N.J., Medical Economics Company, 1984.
13. Scully, R. E., McNeely, B. U., and Galdabini, J. J.: N. Engl. J. Med. *302*:37, 1980.
14. Tietz, N. W.: Clinical Guide to Laboratory Tests. Philadelphia, W. B. Saunders Company, 1983.
15. Tietz, N. W.: Reference ranges and laboratory values of clinical importance. *In* Wyngaarden, J. B., and Smith, L. H. Jr.: Cecil Textbook of Medicine, 16th ed. Philadelphia, W. B. Saunders Company, 1982.
16. Williams, W. J., Beutler, E., Erslev, A. J., and Lichtman, M. A., Hematology, 3rd ed. New York, McGraw-Hill Book Company, 1983.
17. Young, D. S.: N. Engl. J. Med. *292*:795, 1975.

Some of the values have been established by the Clinical Pathology Laboratories, Emory University Hospital, Atlanta, Georgia, and have not been published elsewhere.

Index

Note: Page numbers followed by (t) refer to tables; page numbers in *italics* refer to illustrations.

NO POSTAGE
NECESSARY
IF MAILED
IN THE
UNITED STATES

BUSINESS REPLY MAIL

FIRST CLASS PERMIT NO. 5152 NEW YORK, NEW YORK

POSTAGE WILL BE PAID BY ADDRESSEE

CBS Educational & Professional Publishing
W.B. Saunders Company
Order Fulfillment Department
383 Madison Avenue
New York, NY 10017

NO POSTAGE
NECESSARY
IF MAILED
IN THE
UNITED STATES

BUSINESS REPLY MAIL

FIRST CLASS PERMIT NO. 5152 NEW YORK, NEW YORK

POSTAGE WILL BE PAID BY ADDRESSEE

CBS Educational & Professional Publishing
W.B. Saunders Company
Order Fulfillment Department
383 Madison Avenue
New York, NY 10017